*Coté and Lerman's*

# A Practice of Anesthesia for Infants and Children

*Coté and Lerman's*

# A Practice of Anesthesia for Infants and Children

## FIFTH EDITION

**Charles J. Coté, MD, FAAP, MA(Hon)**

Professor of Anaesthesia
Harvard Medical School
Division of Pediatric Anesthesia
MassGeneral Hospital for Children
Department of Anesthesia, Critical Care, and Pain Medicine
Massachusetts General Hospital
Boston, Massachusetts

**Jerrold Lerman, MD, FRCPC, FANZCA**

Clinical Professor of Anesthesiology
State University of New York at Buffalo
Staff Anesthesiologist, Department of Anesthesia
Women and Children's Hospital of Buffalo
Buffalo, New York
Clinical Professor of Anesthesiology
University of Rochester
Staff Anesthesiologist, Department of Anesthesia
Strong Memorial Hospital
Rochester, New York

**Brian J. Anderson, MB, ChB, PhD, FANZCA, FCICM**

Adjunct Professor
Department of Anaesthesiology
University of Aukland School of Medicine
Attending, Paediatric Anaesthesia and Intensive Care Unit
Starship Children's Hospital
Auckland, New Zealand

ELSEVIER
SAUNDERS

# ELSEVIER
## SAUNDERS

1600 John F. Kennedy Blvd.
Ste 1800
Philadelphia, PA 19103-2899

A PRACTICE OF ANESTHESIA FOR INFANTS AND CHILDREN:
FIFTH EDITION
ISBN: 978-1-4377-2792-0

**Library of Congress Cataloging-in-Publication Data**
Coté and Lerman's a practice of anesthesia for infants and children / [edited by] Charles J. Coté,
Jerrold Lerman, Brian J. Anderson.—5th ed.
    p. ; cm.
  Practice of anesthesia for infants and children
  Rev. ed. of: A practice of anesthesia for infants and children / [edited by] Charles J. Coté,
Jerrold Lerman, I. David Todres. 4th ed. c2009.
  Includes bibliographical references and index.
  ISBN 978-1-4377-2792-0 (hardcover : alk. paper)
  I. Coté, Charles J.   II. Lerman, Jerrold.   III. Anderson, Brian J.   IV. Practice of anesthesia for infants
and children.   V. Title: Practice of anesthesia for infants and children.
  [DNLM: 1. Anesthesia.   2. Child.   3. Infant. WO 440]
  617.9′6083–dc23
                                                                          2012036940

*Executive Content Strategist:* William R. Schmitt
*Content Development Specialist:* Taylor Ball
*Publishing Services Manager:* Anne Altepeter
*Project Manager:* Louise King
*Design Manager:* Amy Buxton
*Cover Photography:* J. Stefaniak, Medical Photographer, Women and Children's Hospital of Buffalo,
                Buffalo, New York

Printed in China

Last digit is the print number:   9   8   7   6   5   4   3   2   1

*We dedicate this edition of* A Practice of Anesthesia for Infants and Children *to all physicians around the world who have the pleasure of caring for children in the operating room, ICU, or other venues where anesthesia services are vital. In particular, we especially thank all who take care of children and deliver the best possible care with the resources available. Our specialty has grown exponentially in the past 20 years. As a result of new licensing laws, medications are now more thoroughly investigated before they are released for use in children. Ultrasound technology has made regional anesthesia and invasive line insertion far safer than in the past. The quality of airway devices continues to improve. Noninvasive continuous cardiac output devices may provide the next generation of monitors to safeguard the care of our children. Depth-of-anesthesia monitors also continue to evolve, but currently are unreliable in young infants and children younger than 5 years. We hope that in the near future advances will ensure that these devices are reliable in the infant and young child to both assess the depth of anesthesia as well as differentiate moderate from deep sedation and deep sedation from general anesthesia.*

*We also dedicate this book to the children we work for every day. We would like to assure the families we work with that their children are safe from harm. Consequently, it is imperative that we investigate the possible harmful effects of anesthetics on the developing brain in infants and children and determine if this is a laboratory phenomenon or an issue that is potentially harmful to humans. If it is the latter, then we must develop methods or new medications to block these adverse effects so that children can continue to undergo anesthesia safely. Our challenge in this next decade is to determine if the laboratory studies concerning anesthetic agent toxicity are a tempest in a teacup or a real threat to our children.*

*This edition of* A Practice of Anesthesia for Infants and Children *highlights key advances and questions in our specialty that we hope will continue to inspire anesthesiologists worldwide.*

**Charles J. Coté**
**Jerrold Lerman**
**Brian J. Anderson**

# CONTRIBUTORS

Brian J. Anderson, MB, ChB, PhD, FANZCA, FCICM
Adjunct Professor
Department of Anaesthesiology
University of Auckland School of Medicine
Attending, Paediatric Anaesthesia and Intensive Care Unit
Starship Children's Hospital
Auckland, New Zealand
*The Practice of Pediatric Anesthesia; Pharmacokinetics and Pharmacology of Drugs Used in Children; Orthopedic and Spinal Surgery*

Dean B. Andropoulos, MD, MHCM
Professor
Departments of Anesthesiology and Pediatrics
Baylor College of Medicine
Chief of Anesthesiology
Texas Children's Hospital
Houston, Texas
*Cardiopulmonary Bypass and Management*

Miriam Anixter, MD
Assistant Professor of Anesthesia
University of Pittsburgh School of Medicine
Attending Anesthesiologist
Children's Hospital of Pittsburgh of University of Pittsburgh
    Medical Center
Pittsburgh, Pennsylvania
*Organ Transplantation*

Philip Arnold, BM, FRCA
Consultant in Paediatric Anaesthesia, Jackson Rees Department
    of Paediatric Anaesthesia
Alder Hey Children's Hospital
Honorary Lecturer
University of Liverpool
Liverpool, United Kingdom
*Medications for Hemostasis*

Patricia R. Bachiller, MD
Instructor in Anaesthesia
Harvard Medical School
Division of Pediatric Anesthesia
MassGeneral Hospital for Children
Department of Anesthesia, Critical Care, and Pain Medicine
Massachusetts General Hospital
Boston, Massachusetts
*Neonatal Emergencies*

Richard Banchs, MD
Fellow, Pediatric Anesthesia
Department of Anesthesiology
Women and Children's Hospital of Buffalo
State University of New York at Buffalo
Buffalo, New York
*General Abdominal and Urologic Surgery*

M.A. Bender, MD, PhD
Associate Professor
Department of Pediatrics
Division of Hematology/Oncology
University of Washington School of Medicine
Director, Odessa Brown Sickle Cell Program
Odessa Brown Children's Clinic
Seattle, Washington

Charles B. Berde, MD, PhD
Professor of Anaesthesia (Pediatrics)
Harvard Medical School
Sara Page Mayo Chair and Chief, Division of Pain Medicine
Department of Anesthesia, Perioperative,
    and Pain Medicine
Boston Children's Hospital
Boston, Massachusetts
*Acute Pain*

Frederic A. Berry, MD
Emeritus Professor of Anesthesiology and Pediatrics
Department of Anesthesiology
University of Virginia Health Sciences Center
Charlottesville, Virginia
*Medicolegal Issues*

Richard H. Blum, MD, MSE, FAAP
Assistant Professor of Anaesthesia
Harvard Medical School
Senior Associate in Anesthesia and Medical Director Post
    Anesthesia Care Unit
Department of Anesthesia, Perioperative, and Pain Medicine
Boston Children's Hospital
Boston, Massachusetts
*Pediatric Equipment*

Adrian T. Bösenberg, MB, ChB, FFA (SA)
Professor
University of Washington
Pediatric Anesthesiologist and Director, Regional Anesthesia
Department of Anesthesiology and Pain Management
Seattle Children's Hospital
Seattle, Washington
*Pediatric Anesthesia in Developing Countries*

Karen A. Brown, MD, FRCPC
Professor, Department of Anesthesia
Queen Elizabeth Hospital of Montreal Foundation Chair in
    Pediatric Anesthesia
McGill University Faculty of Medicine
Staff Anesthesiologist
The Montreal Children's Hospital
Montreal, Quebec, Canada
*Otorhinolaryngologic Procedures*

Roland Brusseau, MD
Instructor in Anaesthesia
Harvard Medical School
Assistant in Perioperative Anesthesia
Department of Anesthesia, Perioperative, and Pain Medicine
Boston Children's Hospital
Boston, Massachusetts
*Fetal Intervention and the EXIT Procedure*

James Cain, MD
Associate Professor
Department of Anesthesiology
University of Pittsburgh School of Medicine
Director of Trauma Anesthesiology
Children's Hospital of Pittsburgh of University of Pittsburgh
    Medical Center
Pittsburgh, Pennsylvania
*Organ Transplantation*

Joseph H. Chou, MD, PhD
Instructor in Pediatrics
Harvard Medical School
Medical Director, Neonatal Intensive Care Unit
MassGeneral Hospital for Children
Boston, Massachusetts
*Neonatal Emergencies*

Franklyn Cladis, MD
Associate Professor
Department of Anesthesiology
University of Pittsburgh School of Medicine
Attending Anesthesiologist
Children's Hospital of Pittsburgh of University of Pittsburgh
    Medical Center
Pittsburgh, Pennsylvania
*Organ Transplantation*

Jeffrey B. Cooper, PhD
Professor of Anaesthesia
Harvard Medical School
Department of Anesthesia, Critical Care, and Pain Medicine
Massachusetts General Hospital
Boston, Massachusetts
Executive Director, Center for Medical Simulation
Cambridge, Massachusetts
*Simulation in Pediatric Anesthesia*

Charles J. Coté, MD, FAAP, MA(Hon)
Professor of Anaesthesia
Harvard Medical School
Division of Pediatric Anesthesia
MassGeneral Hospital for Children
Department of Anesthesia, Critical Care, and Pain Medicine
Massachusetts General Hospital
Boston, Massachusetts
*The Practice of Pediatric Anesthesia; Preoperative Evaluation,*
    *Premedication, and Induction of Anesthesia; Pharmacokinetics and*
    *Pharmacology of Drugs Used in Children; Strategies for Blood*
    *Product Management and Reducing Transfusions; The Pediatric*
    *Airway; Burn Injuries; Regional Anesthesia; Sedation for*
    *Diagnostic and Therapeutic Procedures Outside the Operating*
    *Room; Procedures for Vascular Access; Pediatric Equipment*

Joseph P. Cravero, MD
Lecturer in Anaesthesiology
Harvard Medical School
Senior Associate
Department of Anesthesia, Perioperative, and Pain Medicine
Boston Children's Hospital
Boston, Massachusetts
*Anesthesia Outside the Operating Room; Sedation for Diagnostic and*
    *Therapeutic Procedures Outside the Operating Room*

Mark W. Crawford, MBBS, FRCPC
Associate Professor of Anesthesiology
Faculty of Medicine
University of Toronto
Anesthesiologist-in-Chief and Director of Research
The Hospital for Sick Children
Toronto, Ontario, Canada
*Plastic and Reconstructive Surgery*

Peter Crean, MBBCh, FRCA, FFARCS
Consultant Paediatric Anaesthetist
Royal Belfast Hospital for Sick Children
Belfast, United Kingdom
*Essentials of Neurology and Neuromuscular Disorders*

Andrew J. Davidson, MBBS, MD, FANZCA
Associate Professor, Department of Paediatrics
University of Melbourne
Staff Anaesthetist, Anaesthesia and Pain Management
Director of Clinical Research
Royal Children's Hospital
Melbourne, Victoria, Australia
*Surgery, Anesthesia, and the Immature Brain*

Peter J. Davis, MD, FAAP
Professor of Anesthesiology and Pediatrics
University of Pittsburgh School of Medicine
Anesthesiologist-in-Chief
Department of Anesthesiology
Children's Hospital of Pittsburgh of University of Pittsburgh
    Medical Center
Pittsburgh, Pennsylvania
*Essentials of Hepatology; Organ Transplantation*

**Laura K. Diaz, MD**
Assistant Professor of Anesthesiology and Critical Care
    Medicine
University of Pennsylvania School of Medicine
Staff Anesthesiologist, Division of Cardiothoracic Anesthesia
The Cardiac Center at the Children's Hospital of Philadelphia
Philadelphia, Pennsylvania
*Mechanical Circulatory Support*

**James A. DiNardo, MD**
Professor of Anaesthesia
Harvard Medical School
Chief, Division of Cardiac Anesthesia
Francis X. McGowan, Jr., MD, Chair in Cardiac Anesthesia
Department of Anesthesia, Perioperative, and Pain Medicine
Boston Children's Hospital
Boston, Massachusetts
*Cardiac Physiology and Pharmacology*

**Michael J. Eisses, MD**
Associate Professor
Department of Anesthesiology
University of Washington School of Medicine
Attending Anesthesiologist
Seattle Children's Hospital
Seattle, Washington
*Essentials of Hematology*

**Frank Engbers, MD, FRCA**
Staff Anesthesiologist
Department of Anesthesia
Leiden University Medical Center
Leiden, The Netherlands
*Total Intravenous Anesthesia and Target-Controlled Infusion*

**Thomas Engelhardt, MD, PhD, FRCA**
Honorary Senior Lecturer
University of Aberdeen Faculty of Medicine
Consultant Paediatric Anaesthetist
Department of Anaesthesia
Royal Aberdeen Children's Hospital
Aberdeen, United Kingdom
*Plastic and Reconstructive Surgery*

**John E. Fiadjoe, MD**
Assistant Professor
Department of Anesthesiology and Critical Care Medicine
The Children's Hospital of Philadelphia
Perelman School of Medicine at the University of Pennsylvania
Philadelphia, Pennsylvania
*The Pediatric Airway*

**Paul G. Firth, MBChB, BA**
Assistant Professor of Anaesthesia
Harvard Medical School
Division of Pediatric Anesthesia
MassGeneral Hospital for Children
Attending Anesthesiologist
Department of Anesthesia, Critical Care, and Pain Medicine
Massachusetts General Hospital
Boston, Massachusetts
*Essentials of Pulmonology*

**John W. Foreman, MD**
Professor of Pediatrics
Duke University School of Medicine
Chief, Division of Pediatric Nephrology
Duke University Medical Center
Durham, North Carolina
*Essentials of Nephrology*

**Michelle A. Fortier, PhD**
Assistant Professor-in-Residence
Anesthesiology and Perioperative Care
University of California, Irvine School of Medicine
UCI Center on Stress and Health
Orange, California
*Perioperative Behavioral Stress in Children*

**Mark E. Gerber, MD**
Clinical Assistant Professor of Otolaryngology
NorthShore Medical Group
Ann & Robert H. Lurie Children's Hospital of Chicago
Chicago, Illinois
*The Pediatric Airway: Laryngeal Web; Laryngeal Edema (videos)*

**Ralph Gertler, MD**
Consultant Pediatric Cardiac Anesthesiologist
Institute of Anesthesiology
German Heart Centre of the State of Bavaria
Technical University Munich
Munich, Germany
*Essentials of Cardiology; Cardiopulmonary Bypass and Management*

**Elizabeth A. Ghazal, MD**
Assistant Professor of Anesthesiology
Department of Anesthesiology
Loma Linda University School of Medicine
Loma Linda, California
*Preoperative Evaluation, Premedication, and Induction of Anesthesia*

**Kenneth Goldschneider, MD**
Associate Professor, Clinical Anesthesia and Pediatrics
University of Cincinnati College of Medicine
Department of Anesthesiology
Director, Pain Management Center
Cincinnati Children's Hospital Medical Center
Cincinnati, Ohio
*Chronic Pain*

**Eric F. Grabowski, MD, Dr Sci**
Associate Professor of Pediatrics
Harvard Medical School
Director, MassGeneral Comprehensive Hemophilia Treatment
    Center
Director, Cardiovascular Thrombosis Laboratory
Co-Director, Pediatric Stroke Service
MassGeneral Hospital for Children
Massachusetts General Hospital
Boston, Massachusetts
*Strategies for Blood Product Management and Reducing Transfusions*

**Charles M. Haberkern, MD, MPH**
Professor
Department of Anesthesiology and Pain Medicine
Adjunct Professor
Department of Pediatrics
University of Washington School of Medicine
Staff Anesthesiologist
Seattle Children's Hospital
Seattle, Washington
*Essentials of Hematology*

**Gregory B. Hammer, MD**
Professor of Anesthesia and Pediatrics
Stanford University School of Medicine
Stanford, California
Director of Research, Anesthesia
Lucile Packard Children's Hospital at Stanford
Palo Alto, California
*Anesthesia for Thoracic Surgery*

**Raafat S. Hannallah, MD**
Professor of Anesthesiology and Pediatrics
The George Washington University Medical Center
School of Medicine and Health Sciences
Faculty, Anesthesiology and Pain Medicine
Principal Investigator, Children's Research Institute
Center for Clinical and Community Research
Children's National Medical Center
Washington, DC
*Otorhinolaryngologic Procedures*

**Jeana E. Havidich, MD**
Associate Professor of Anesthesiology
Department of Anesthesiology
Dartmouth Medical School
Hanover, New Hampshire
Dartmouth-Hitchcock Medical Center
Lebanon, New Hampshire
*The Postanesthesia Care Unit and Beyond*

**Reiko Hayashi, MD**
Staff Anesthesiologist
Department of Anesthesia and Intensive Care
National Center for Child Health and Development
Tokyo, Japan
*General Abdominal and Urologic Surgery*

**Andre L. Jaichenco, MD**
Head Chief of the Service of Anesthesiology
The National Pediatric Hospital S.A.M.I.C.
Prof. Dr. Juan P. Garrahan
Buenos Aires, Argentina
*Infectious Disease Considerations for the Operating Room*

**Zeev N. Kain, MD, MBA**
Professor of Anesthesiology, Pediatrics, and Psychiatry
Chair, Department of Anesthesiology
Associate Dean of Clinical Research
University of California, Irvine School of Medicine
UCI Center on Stress and Health
Orange, California
*Perioperative Behavioral Stress in Children*

**Richard F. Kaplan, MD**
Professor of Anesthesiology and Pediatrics
School of Medicine and Health Sciences
The George Washington University Medical Center
Chief, Division of Anesthesiology and Pain Medicine
Children's National Medical Center
Washington, DC
*Sedation for Diagnostic and Therapeutic Procedures Outside the
    Operating Room*

**Manoj K. Karmakar, MD, FRCA, DA(UK), FHKCA, FHKAM**
Associate Professor and Director of Pediatric Anesthesia
Department of Anesthesia and Intensive Care
The Chinese University of Hong Kong/Prince of Wales
    Hospital
Hong Kong, China
*Ultrasound-Guided Regional Anesthesia*

**T. Bernard Kinane, MD**
Associate Professor of Pediatrics
Harvard Medical School
Chief, Pediatric Pulmonary Unit
Department of Pediatrics
MassGeneral Hospital for Children
Massachusetts General Hospital
Boston, Massachusetts
*Essentials of Pulmonology*

**Yoichi Kondo, MD**
Chief of Pain Services
Department of Anesthesia and Intensive Care
National Center for Child Health and Development
Tokyo, Japan
*General Abdominal and Urologic Surgery*

**Elliot J. Krane, MD**
Professor of Anesthesia and Pediatrics
Stanford University School of Medicine
Stanford, California
Director, Pediatric Pain Management Service
Lucile Packard Children's Hospital at Stanford
Palo Alto, California
*Essentials of Endocrinology*

**Pooja Kulkarni, MD**
Assistant Professor of Clinical Pediatrics
Department of Pediatrics
Columbia University Medical Center
New York, New York
*Cardiopulmonary Resuscitation*

**C. Dean Kurth, MD**
Professor of Anesthesia and Pediatrics
University of Cincinnati College of Medicine
Anesthesiologist-in-Chief
Department of Anesthesiology
Cincinnati Children's Hospital Medical Center
Cincinnati, Ohio
*The Extremely Premature Infant (Micropremie)*

**Wing H. Kwok, MBChB, FANZCA, FHKCA, FHKAM**
Clinical Associate Professor (Honorary), Consultant in
  Anesthesia
Department of Anesthesia and Intensive Care
The Chinese University of Hong Kong/Prince of Wales
  Hospital
Hong Kong, China
*Ultrasound-Guided Regional Anesthesia*

**Geoffrey K. Lane, BPharm, MBBS, FRACP, FCSANZ, FACC**
Lead Clinician
Cardiac Catheterization and Interventional Cardiology Service
The Royal Children's Hospital
Melbourne, Australia
*Interventional Cardiology*

**Gregory J. Latham, MD**
Assistant Professor
Department of Anesthesiology
University of Washington School of Medicine
Staff Anesthesiologist
Seattle Children's Hospital
Seattle, Washington
*Essentials of Hematology*

**Jerrold Lerman, MD, FRCPC, FANZCA**
Clinical Professor of Anesthesiology
State University of New York at Buffalo
Staff Anesthesiologist, Department of Anesthesia
Women and Children's Hospital of Buffalo
Buffalo, New York
Clinical Professor of Anesthesiology
University of Rochester
Staff Anesthesiologist, Department of Anesthesia
Strong Memorial Hospital
Rochester, New York
*The Practice of Pediatric Anesthesia; Pharmacokinetics and Pharma-
  cology of Drugs Used in Children; General Abdominal and
  Urologic Surgery; Plastic and Reconstructive Surgery; Malignant
  Hyperthermia*

**Steven Lichtenstein, MD**
Clinical Associate Professor of Anesthesiology
University of Pittsburgh School of Medicine
Attending Anesthesiologist
Children's Hospital of Pittsburgh of University of Pittsburgh
  Medical Center
Pittsburgh, Pennsylvania
*Organ Transplantation*

**James Limb, FRCA**
Honorary Lecturer, Department of Sedation
University of Newcastle School of Dental Sciences
Newcastle, United Kingdom
Consultant Paediatric Anaesthetist
Department of Anaesthesia
Darlington Memorial Hospital
Darlington, United Kingdom
*Total Intravenous Anesthesia and Target-Controlled Infusion*

**Ronald S. Litman, DO**
Professor of Anesthesiology and Pediatrics
Perelman School of Medicine at the University of Pennsylvania
Department of Anesthesiology and Critical Care
The Children's Hospital of Philadelphia
Philadelphia, Pennsylvania
*The Pediatric Airway*

**Andreas W. Loepke, MD, PhD, FAAP**
Associate Professor of Clinical Anesthesia and Pediatrics
University of Cincinnati College of Medicine
Staff Anesthesiologist Division of Pediatric Cardiac Anesthesia
Department of Anesthesiology
Cincinnati Children's Hospital Medical Center
Cincinnati, Ohio
*Surgery, Anesthesia, and the Immature Brain*

**Christine L. Mai, MD**
Instructor in Anaesthesia
Harvard Medical School
Attending Anesthesiologist
Division of Pediatric Anesthesia
MassGeneral Hospital for Children
Department of Anesthesia, Critical Care, and Pain Medicine
Massachusetts General Hospital
Boston, Massachusetts
*Simulation in Pediatric Anesthesia*

**Shobha Malviya, MD**
Professor of Anesthesiology
University of Michigan
Associate Director
Division of Pediatric Anesthesiology
C.S. Mott Children's Hospital
Ann Arbor, Michigan
*Acute Pain*

**Bruno Marciniak, MD**
Pediatric Anesthesiologist
Department of Anesthesiology and Critical Care Medicine
Centre Hospitalier Universitaire de Lille
Lille, France
*Growth and Development*

**J.A. Jeevendra Martyn, MD, FRCA, FCCM**
Professor of Anaesthesia
Harvard Medical School
Anesthetist-in-Chief
Shriners Hospitals for Children
Director, Clinical and Biochemical Pharmacology Laboratory
Massachusetts General Hospital
Boston, Massachusetts
*Burn Injuries*

**Linda J. Mason, MD**
Professor of Anesthesiology and Pediatrics
Director of Pediatric Anesthesia
Department of Anesthesiology
Loma Linda University School of Medicine
Loma Linda, California
*Preoperative Evaluation, Premedication, and Induction of Anesthesia*

**Linda C. Mayes, MD**
Arnold Gesell Professor of Child Psychiatry
Pediatrics and Psychology
Yale University School of Medicine
Staff Physician
Child Study Center
New Haven, Connecticut
*Perioperative Behavioral Stress in Children*

**Craig D. McClain, MD, MPH**
Assistant Professor of Anaesthesia
Harvard Medical School
Associate in Anesthesia
Department of Anesthesia, Perioperative, and Pain Medicine
Boston Children's Hospital
Boston, Massachusetts
*Fluid Management; Pediatric Neurosurgical Anesthesia*

**Angus McEwan, MBChB, FRCA**
Consultant Paediatric Anaesthetist
Great Ormond Street Hospital for Children
London, United Kingdom
*Anesthesia for Children Undergoing Heart Surgery*

**Michael L. McManus, MD, MPH**
Associate Professor of Anaesthesia (Pediatrics)
Harvard Medical School
Senior Associate
Department of Anesthesia, Perioperative, and Pain Medicine
Boston Children's Hospital
Boston, Massachusetts
*Fluid Management*

**Wanda C. Miller-Hance, MD**
Professor of Pediatrics and Anesthesiology
Baylor College of Medicine
Associate Director of Pediatric Cardiovascular Anesthesiology
Director of Intraoperative Echocardiography
Texas Children's Hospital
Houston, Texas
*Essentials of Cardiology; Anesthesia for Noncardiac Surgery in Children with Congenital Heart Disease*

**Katsuyuki Miyasaka, MD, PhD, FAAP, FCCP**
Director, Perioperative and Acute Care Center
St. Luke's International Hospital
Tokyo, Japan
*General Abdominal and Urologic Surgery*

**Neil S. Morton, MD, FRCA**
Reader in Paediatric Anaesthesia and Pain Management
University of Glasgow
Consultant in Paediatric Anaesthesia and Pain Management
Royal Hospital for Sick Children
Glasgow, United Kingdom
*Total Intravenous Anesthesia and Target-Controlled Infusion*

**Marilyn C. Morris, MD, MPH**
Associate Professor of Clinical Pediatrics
Department of Pediatrics
Columbia University Medical Center
New York, New York
*Cardiopulmonary Resuscitation*

**Jerome Parness, MD, PhD**
Visiting Professor
Departments of Anesthesiology/Pharmacology and Chemical Biology
University of Pittsburgh School of Medicine
Staff Anesthesiologist
Children's Hospital of Pittsburgh of University of Pittsburgh Medical Center
Pittsburgh, Pennsylvania
*Malignant Hyperthermia*

**Deirdre Peake, MB Bch, BAO, MRCPI**
Consultant Paediatric Neurologist
Royal Belfast Hospital for Sick Children
Belfast, United Kingdom
*Essentials of Neurology and Neuromuscular Disorders*

**David M. Polaner, MD, FAAP**
Professor of Anesthesiology and Pediatrics
University of Colorado School of Medicine
Attending Pediatric Anesthesiologist, Acute Pain Service
Director, Transplant Anesthesia
Children's Hospital Colorado
Aurora, Colorado
*Regional Anesthesia; Acute Pain*

**Erinn T. Rhodes, MD, MPH**
Assistant Professor of Pediatrics
Harvard Medical School
Director, Type 2 Diabetes Program
Director, Inpatient Diabetes Program
Division of Endocrinology
Boston Children's Hospital
Boston, Massachusetts
*Essentials of Endocrinology*

**Marcus Rivera, MD**
Assistant Professor of Pediatrics
Director, Intestinal Care Program
Division of Gastroenterology, Hepatology, and Nutrition
Golisano Children's Hospital at Upstate Medical University
Syracuse, New York
*Essentials of Hepatology*

Jesse D. Roberts, Jr., MD, MS, FAAP
Associate Professor of Anaesthesia
Harvard Medical School
Associate Anesthetist, Pediatrician, and Associate Scientist
Departments of Anesthesia, Critical Care, and Pain Medicine,
    Pediatrics, and Medicine
Massachusetts General Hospital
Director of Newborn Research
MassGeneral Hospital for Children
Boston, Massachusetts
*Neonatal Emergencies*

Mark A. Rockoff, MD, FAAP
Professor of Anaesthesia
Harvard Medical School
Associate Anesthesiologist-in-Chief
Department of Anesthesia, Perioperative, and Pain Medicine
Boston Children's Hospital
Boston, Massachusetts
*Pediatric Neurosurgical Anesthesia*

Thomas M. Romanelli, MD, FAAP
Assistant Professor
Division of Pediatric Anesthesiology
Monroe Carell Jr. Children's Hopsital at Vanderbilt
Nashville, Tennessee
*Neonatal Emergencies*

Allison Kinder Ross, MD
Professor of Anesthesiology and Pediatrics
Duke University School of Medicine
Chief, Division of Pediatric Anesthesia
Duke University Medical Center
Durham, North Carolina
*Essentials of Nephrology*

Charles L. Schleien, MD, MBA
Chairman of Pediatrics
Hofstra/North Shore–Long Island Jewish School of Medicine
Pediatrician-in-Chief
North Shore–Long Island Jewish Health System
New Hyde Park, New York
*Cardiopulmonary Resuscitation*

Annette Y. Schure, MD, DEAA
Senior Associate in Cardiac Anesthesia
Department of Anesthesia, Perioperative, and Pain Medicine
Boston Children's Hospital
Instructor in Anaesthesia
Harvard Medical School
Boston, Massachusetts
*Cardiac Physiology and Pharmacology*

Erik S. Shank, MD
Assistant Professor of Anaesthesia
Harvard Medical School
Associate Chief
Division of Pediatric Anesthesia
MassGeneral Hospital for Children
Department of Anesthesia, Critical Care, and Pain Medicine
Massachusetts General Hospital
Associate Chief
Department of Anesthesia
Shriners Hospital for Children
Boston, Massachusetts
*Burn Injuries*

Adam Skinner, BSC, MBChB, MRCP, FRCA
Consultant Paediatric Anaesthetist
Department of Anaesthesia
Royal Children's Hospital
Melbourne, Victoria, Australia
*Medications for Hemostasis; Interventional Cardiology*

Sulpicio G. Soriano, MD, FAAP
Professor of Anaesthesia
Harvard Medical School
BCH Endowed Chair in Pediatric Neuroanesthesia
Senior Associate in Anesthesia
Department of Anesthesia, Perioperative, and Pain Medicine
Boston Children's Hospital
Boston, Massachusetts
*Pediatric Neurosurgical Anesthesia*

James P. Spaeth, MD
Associate Professor of Anesthesia and Pediatrics
University of Cincinnati College of Medicine
Director of Cardiac Anesthesia
Associate Chief, Anesthesia Division
Department of Anesthesiology
Cincinnati Children's Hospital Medical Center
Cincinnati, Ohio
*The Extremely Premature Infant (Micropremie)*

Robert H. Squires, MD
Professor of Pediatrics
University of Pittsburgh School of Medicine
Clinical Director
Pediatric Gastroenterology, Hepatology, and Nutrition
Children's Hospital of Pittsburgh of University of Pittsburgh
    Medical Center
Pittsburgh, Pennsylvania
*Essentials of Hepatology*

Christopher P. Stowell, MD, PhD
Associate Professor of Pathology
Harvard Medical School
Director, Blood Transfusion Service
Massachusetts General Hospital
Boston, Massachusetts
*Strategies for Blood Product Management and Reducing Transfusions*

**Paul A. Stricker, MD**
Assistant Professor
Perelman School of Medicine at the University of Pennsylvania
Attending Anesthesiologist
Department of Anesthesiology and Critical Care Medicine
The Children's Hospital of Philadelphia
Philadelphia, Pennsylvania
*The Pediatric Airway*

**Rajeev Subramanyam, MB BS, MD, DNB, MNAMS**
Pediatric Anesthesiologist
Department of Anesthesiology
University of Toronto Faculty of Medicine
Chief Fellow
The Hospital for Sick Children
Toronto, Ontario, Canada
*Plastic and Reconstructive Surgery*

**Santhanam Suresh, MD, FAAP**
Anesthesiologist-in-Chief
Ann & Robert H. Lurie Children's Hospital of Chicago
Professor of Anesthesiology and Pediatrics
Northwestern University Feinberg School of Medicine
Chicago, Illinois
*Regional Anesthesia*

**Yasuyuki Suzuki, MD**
Director
Department of Anesthesia and Intensive Care
National Center for Child Health and Development
Tokyo, Japan
*General Abdominal and Urologic Surgery*

**Alexandra Szabova, MD**
Assistant Professor
University of Cincinnati College of Medicine
Anesthesia
Cincinnati Children's Hospital Medical Center
Cincinnati, Ohio
*Chronic Pain*

**Demian Szyld, MD, EdM**
Assistant Professor, Emergency Medicine
New York University School of Medicine
Associate Medical Director
New York Simulation Center for the Health Sciences
The City University of New York
New York University Langone Medical Center
New York, New York
*Simulation in Pediatric Anesthesia*

**Andreas H. Taenzer, MD, MS, FAAP**
Associate Professor of Anesthesiology and Pediatrics
Geisel School of Medicine at Dartmouth
Hanover, New Hampshire
Co-Director, Pediatric Anesthesiology
Director, Pediatric Pain Service
Dartmouth-Hitchcock Medical Center/Children's Hospital at Dartmouth
Lebanon, New Hampshire
*The Postanesthesia Care Unit and Beyond*

**Takako Tamura, MD**
Clinical Director
Department of Anesthesia and Intensive Care
National Center for Child Health and Development
Tokyo, Japan
*General Abdominal and Urologic Surgery*

**Joseph R. Tobin, MD**
Professor and Chairman
Department of Anesthesiology
Wake Forest University Health Sciences
Winston-Salem, North Carolina
*Ophthalmology*

**†I. David Todres, MD**
Professor of Pediatrics
Harvard Medical Unit
Chief, Ethics Unit
Division of Pediatric Anesthesia
MassGeneral Hospital for Children
Department of Anesthesia, Critical Care, and Pain Medicine
Massachusetts General Hospital
Boston, Massachusetts
*The Pediatric Airway (video)*

**Susan T. Verghese, MD**
Professor of Anesthesiology and Pediatrics
The George Washington University Medical Center
Faculty, Anesthesiology
Principal Investigator, Children's Research Institute Center for Clinical and Community Research
Department of Anesthesiology
Children's National Medical Center
Washington, DC
*Otorhinolaryngologic Procedures*

**Samuel H. Wald, MD**
Professor of Clinical Anesthesiology
Department of Anesthesiology
David Geffen School of Medicine at UCLA
Los Angeles, California
*Procedures for Vascular Access*

**David B. Waisel, MD**
Associate Professor of Anaesthesia
Harvard Medical School
Senior Associate in Anesthesia
Department of Anesthesia, Perioperative, and Pain Medicine
Boston Children's Hospital
Boston, Massachusetts
*Ethical Issues in Pediatric Anesthesiology*

**R. Grey Weaver, Jr., MD**
Associate Professor
Department of Ophthalmology
Wake Forest University School of Medicine
Winston-Salem, North Carolina
*Ophthalmology*

†Deceased.

David E. Wesson, MD
Professor of Surgery
Baylor College of Medicine
Associate Surgeon-in-Chief
Texas Children's Hospital
Houston, Texas
*Trauma*

Rebecca W. West, JD
Assistant Professor of General Medicine
University of Virginia School of Medicine
Chief Executive Officer, Piedmont Liability Trust
Charlottesville, Virginia
*Medicolegal Issues*

Melissa Wheeler, MD
Chief of Anesthesiology
Shriners Hospitals for Children
Chicago, Illinois
*The Pediatric Airway: Stretching of the Trachea (video)*

Delbert R. Wigfall, MD
Associate Dean of Medical Education
Professor of Pediatrics
Division of Pediatric Nephrology
Duke University School of Medicine
Durham, North Carolina
*Essentials of Nephrology*

Niall C. Wilton, MRCP, FRCA
Clinical Director
Paediatric Anaesthesia and Operating Rooms
Department of Paediatric Anaesthesia
Starship Children's Hospital
Auckland, New Zealand
*Orthopedic and Spinal Surgery*

Joseph I. Wolfsdorf, MB, BCh
Professor of Pediatrics
Harvard Medical School
Clinical Director and Associate Chief
Director, Diabetes Program
Chair in Endocrinology
Division of Endocrinology
Boston Children's Hospital
Boston, Massachusetts
*Essentials of Endocrinology*

Grace Lai-Sze Wong, MBBS, FANZCA, FHKCA, FHKAM
Associate Consultant, Specialist in Pediatric Anesthesia
Department of Anesthesiology
Queen Mary Hospital
Clinical Assistant Professor, Department of Anesthesia
The University of Hong Kong
Hong Kong SAR, The People's Republic of China
Consultant Paediatric Anaesthetist, Department of Anaesthesia
Royal Hospital for Sick Children, Yorkhill
Glasgow, United Kingdom
*Total Intravenous Anesthesia and Target-Controlled Infusion*

Masao Yamashita, MD
Post-Doctorate Fellow
Electron Microscopy Lab
University of Sheffield
Sheffield, United Kingdom
*Regional Anesthesia: Hanging Drop Technique (video)*

Myron Yaster, MD
Richard J. Traystman Professor
Departments of Anesthesiology, Critical Care Medicine, and
     Pediatrics
Johns Hopkins University School of Medicine
Attending, Johns Hopkins Hospital
Baltimore, Maryland
*Sedation for Diagnostic and Therapeutic Procedures Outside
     the Operating Room*

David A. Young, MD, MEd, MBA
Associate Professor
Departments of Anesthesiology and Pediatrics
Baylor College of Medicine
Texas Children's Hospital
Houston, Texas
*Trauma*

# PREFACE

*A Practice of Anesthesia for Infants and Children, Fifth Edition,* has evolved from its predecessors. Jerrold Lerman joined as co-editor in the previous edition, and we have greatly strengthened our editorial team with the addition of Brian J. Anderson in this edition. Dr. Anderson brings not only a further international perspective to the editorship that reflects the mission of our text, but also a specific expertise in pharmacology.

This book has blossomed from its humble beginnings as a synopsis of local practice to an international authoritative and evidence-based tome. In addition to pediatric anesthesiologists, the list of contributors includes pediatric subspecialists, internists, two surgeons, and a lawyer. More than 20 of the pediatric anesthesiologists are also board-certified pediatricians, and several have subspecialty board certification in cardiology and neonatology. The inclusion of 110 authors from 10 countries and six continents speaks to the global nature of this edition.

In the fifth edition, we have exploited the advances in state-of-the-art publishing, including Internet access. The book has the same feel and style as the previous edition, divided into 10 color-coded sections: Introduction, Drug and Fluid Therapy, The Chest, The Heart, The Brain and Glands, The Abdomen, Other Surgeries, Emergencies, Pain, and Special Topics. This format enables the reader to find chapters and topics of interest easily and quickly. To maintain a size similar to that of the previous edition, we have again shifted all but a few select references from each chapter to the accompanying Expert Consult website, with hypertext links to the original publications. We also have combined a few chapters. Color illustrations, photographs, and graphics maximize clarity and enhance visual appeal; many new video clips, figures, tables, and appendices also are available online.

In keeping with our mission to create a comprehensive text, we have again sought contributions from a number of pediatric subspecialists, who have shared their perspectives on and insights into basic pediatric physiology and the pathophysiologic implications of diseases in children. In each case, these specialists have been paired with a pediatric anesthesiologist to ensure the basic science is intertwined with a practical clinical perspective.

The largest chapter of the book covers pharmacology and includes more than 1900 references. As in previous editions, the chapter has benefited from very significant contributions from Dr. Anderson, who now has assumed the role of first author. Written by all three editors, the chapter's usefulness is enhanced by including three different perspectives in pediatric pharmacology. It includes older and less frequently used medications to address the wide range of practices used around the world. Given the rapidly increasing interest in total intravenous anesthesia (TIVA) in children, the TIVA chapter also now provides online computer simulations.

The pediatric airway chapter includes a more extensive discussion of the numerous supraglottic devices as well as emergency airway management strategies and equipment currently available for use in infants and children. This chapter has been enhanced with online video clips. The transfusion chapter has been updated with contributions from a pediatric hematologist specializing in hemophilia and the director of the Blood Transfusion Service at the Massachusetts General Hospital.

All of the chapters on specialized topics—including thoracic anesthesia, orthopedics, plastic surgery, general and urologic surgeries; the cardiac chapters, including cardiopulmonary bypass, medications used for hemostasis, cardiac assist devices, and the cardiac catheterization laboratory; as well as the practice of anesthesia in medically disadvantaged countries—have been extensively updated. In the section on the abdomen, the chapter on organ transplantation remains the centerpiece.

Perhaps the most important addition is a chapter on anesthesia and the developing brain. This topic remains a major concern for pediatric anesthesiologists at the time of printing. The chapters that address the extremely premature infant, the ex-utero intrapartum treatment procedure and trauma, medical-legal issues, and infectious diseases have been extensively revised.

The increasing importance of training residents to diagnose and treat pain in children is highlighted in several chapters that include an extensive discussion on pain scoring systems for both "normal" and cognitively impaired children. Likewise, these topics are covered at length in chapters devoted to landmark- and ultrasound-guided regional anesthesia, also supplemented with online video clips. A wholly new chapter addresses medical simulation in children, with several demonstrative video clips on the website. Further sophistication of medical simulation may ultimately improve the safety of anesthesia.

Finally, the accompanying website has been greatly expanded in audio-visual content to include myriad illustrations, figures, video clips, and sample order forms. The addition of videos, in particular, affords users the opportunity to view a hands-on approach to procedures such as ultrasound- and landmark-guided nerve blocks, catheter insertions, radiologic investigations, ultrasound procedures, and echocardiograms, as well as various levels of sedation and analgesia. A pocket reference card also provides general recommendations for dosages of commonly used medications by weight and other useful guides such as LMA sizes, ETT sizes, and other quick references.

Undertaking this revision has been quite a journey, often appearing to be a microcosm of the world and life in general. Once again many of our contributors have experienced various challenges, such as the loss of loved ones, personal crises, and illnesses, during the writing of their chapters. Despite these obstacles, the authors have succeeded in crafting masterful chapters to create what we think is a state-of-the-art text on pediatric anesthesia. Furthermore, the entire text and e-only content is also available for purchase as an eBook.

In assembling this edition, we have spent many days and nights debating controversial issues. We think we have arrived at a middle ground that addresses the diversity of pediatric anesthesia practice. It is our hope that these discussions, combined with the global perspective offered by our contributing authors, strengthen the quality of our text while showcasing the diversity of our specialty.

We believe *A Practice of Anesthesia for Infants and Children, Fifth Edition*, will continue to provide the basis for residency and fellowship training in pediatric anesthesia, and be a valuable resource to practicing pediatric anesthesiologists and other pediatric care providers around the world.

**Charles J. Coté, MD, FAAP, MA(Hon)**
**Jerrold Lerman, MD, FRCPC, FANZCA**
**Brian J. Anderson, MB, ChB, PhD, FANZCA, FCICM**

# ACKNOWLEDGMENTS

We wish to thank the chairpersons of the departments of anesthesiology, pediatrics, surgery, and internal medicine around the world who supported the academic endeavors of their staff and thus made it possible for them to contribute to *A Practice of Anesthesia for Infants and Children, Fifth Edition.* In particular, we thank all of the wives, husbands, significant others, children, friends, secretaries, and staff members who lent their support to this wonderful international family of experts that has come together to produce this edition.

**Charles J. Coté, MD, FAAP, MA(Hon)**
**Jerrold Lerman, MD, FRCPC, FANZCA**
**Brian J. Anderson, MB, ChB, PhD, FANZCA, FCICM**

# CONTENTS

# VIDEO CONTENTS

# INTRODUCTION

# The Practice of Pediatric Anesthesia

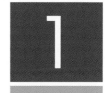

## CHARLES J. COTÉ, JERROLD LERMAN, AND BRIAN J. ANDERSON

| | |
|---|---|
| **Preoperative Evaluation and Management** | Hearing |
| Parents and Child | Touch |
| The Anesthesiologist | **Airway and Ventilation** |
| **Informed Consent** | **Fluids and Perfusion** |
| **Operating Room and Monitoring** | **Conduct of the Anesthesia Team** |
| **Induction and Maintenance of Anesthesia** | **The Postanesthesia Care Unit** |
| **Clinical Monitors** | **Postoperative Visit** |
| Sight | **Summary** |

IN THIS CHAPTER WE outline the basis of our collective practice of pediatric anesthesia. These basic principles of practice can be applied regardless of the circumstances; they provide the foundation for safe anesthesia.

## Preoperative Evaluation and Management

### PARENTS AND CHILD

Anesthesiologists must assume an active role in the preoperative assessment of children. Ideally, the anesthesiologist performing the preoperative evaluation will also anesthetize the child. A complete medical and surgical history; family history; medical record review; evaluation and review of laboratory, radiologic, and other investigations; and physical examination are performed on every child who is to be anesthetized (see Chapter 4). When appropriate, the child should receive preoperative medical therapy to optimize his or her medical condition or conditions (e.g., children with seizure disorders or reactive airway disease) before receiving anesthesia. In addition, the emotional state of the child and family must be considered and appropriate psychological and, if necessary, pharmacologic support provided. The anesthesia team, working in concert with surgical colleagues, nursing, and child-life specialists, should find appropriate and creative techniques (e.g., use of videotapes, booklets, hospital tours, and trained paramedical personnel) to prepare the child and family. The marked increase in the number of outpatient surgical procedures has reduced the time available for interaction among the anesthesiologist, the family, and the child. Despite this reduced contact time, these support techniques should not be neglected.

Familiarity with a child's clinical and psychological status as well as the parental concerns is essential to delivering quality anesthesia care. To achieve the very best outcome for each child, it is essential to meet with the child and the parents (or caregiver or legal guardian) together and establish rapport preoperatively. There are many developmental issues that surround the hospital experience: for example, teenagers fear loss of control, awareness, and pain; younger children fear mutilation from their surgery; and toddlers fear separation from their parents (see Chapter 3). However, for children who are old enough to understand (usually age 5 years and older), it is reasonable to explain in simple terms what anesthesia involves and what will transpire on entering the operating room. It is vital to speak directly to the child because he or she is the person having the surgery. Children at the age of reason have the same fears as adults, but have greater difficulty articulating them. It is important to explain the differences between "sleep" from anesthesia medicine and the sleep they get at home. Even if they undergo anesthesia for hours, they will feel as if they were unconscious for only the time it takes to blink the eyelids once. Many children are also fearful of awakening during the surgery and others are fearful of not awakening at the end of surgery. Children require reassurance that *they will not feel anything during surgery, that they will not wake up during the procedure, and that they will awaken at the conclusion of the surgery.*

The possibility of postoperative pain and the relief the child will receive in the form of nerve blocks and analgesics must be clearly presented to the child and the parents. It is also important to explain to the child and the family what they can anticipate on entering the operating room and to explain the special monitoring you, as the anesthesiologist, will provide for the child. A simple explanation of the monitors can be very reassuring to parents and interesting for many children. For example, the pulse oximeter can be described as a *"Band-Aid–like device"* that lights up red and measures the oxygen in the bloodstream during anesthesia and recovery; the blood pressure cuff can be characterized as an *"arm hugger"* or *"muscle tester";* and the electrocardiogram leads can be called *"little sticky things that don't hurt so we can watch the heart beat."* Simple descriptions of the measurements may also be soothing. For example, you can say: *"We measure the oxygen you (your child) are (is) breathing, we measure the amount of the anesthesia medicines you (your child) are (is) breathing, and we measure the carbon dioxide you (your child) are (is) breathing so as to ensure that your (your child's) breathing is just right throughout the anesthesia."* Sometimes asking teenagers if they have studied carbon dioxide in school science class helps them to better understand the monitors and provides reassurance, as well as making it more interesting. The detail with which this is presented will vary from family to family and child to child as well as with the anesthesiologist's understanding of the needs of the child and family. By the end of the interview, however, the child and the parents should understand that you will be providing the quality of care that ensures the child's safety during anesthesia, thus reducing the child's and parents' anxiety. Explanation is also needed to describe how anesthesia will be induced, although the degree of detail used will again depend on the developmental level of the child. For young children, one can describe a plan to breathe "laughing gas" through a flavored mask, with a flavor that he or she chooses. Older children can be given the option of an intravenous (IV) induction, with nitrous oxide by mask to establish IV access painlessly; or if they are afraid of needles, they might be given the option of an inhalational induction.

If parents are to be present during induction, it is essential to describe to them how they can assist in comforting the child and prepare them for what they might observe and experience to avoid any misconceptions. Parents should not be pressured into feeling that they must be present for induction. It must be clear that, if at any time during the induction there is a new or additional risk to the child, they may be asked to leave the operating room and will be escorted to the parent waiting room. Remind them that their presence at induction is for their child's benefit and is a privilege, not a right. Thus, if there are issues with a difficult airway, if a rapid induction of anesthesia is needed, or if the child is very young, it would be inappropriate for the parents to be present and not in the child's best interest for physicians and nurses to be distracted at a time when everyone's attention needs to be focused on the child.

It is helpful and essential to explain to the parents specific changes in the child that might be observed at the time of anesthetic induction:

1. As your child is anesthetized, the eyes may roll up: *"You might see your child's eyes roll up and this is completely normal and happens to all of us when we fall asleep; it is just that we are not looking for it."*

2. *"As people fall asleep they often make snoring noises and other noises from their throat; if your child does this it is completely normal."*

3. *"As the anesthetic reaches the brain, the brain sometimes gets excited and causes movement of the arms and legs that are without purpose, or it may cause them to turn their head from side to side. This means the anesthetic is having its effect and even though your child appears to be partly awake, he (or she) has received enough anesthesia to ensure that he (or she) does not remember this."*

4. *"If your child becomes frightened, we will increase the amount of the anesthesia medicine rapidly and calm your child as quickly as possible."*

5. If the child is to have an IV induction, then informing the parents that the child might suddenly look pale and that the start of anesthesia will be very rapid is also helpful so as to avoid confusion about what the parents will observe.

These preemptive explanations are important to undermine the parents' anxiety at a time when you need to focus on the child. It is common for parents to decline to be present during induction once they hear these explanations. Finally, it is prudent to reassure the parents that for surgeries that are emetogenic and in children who have been or are prone to emesis, that appropriate prophylactic therapy will be administered before the child recovers. Similarly, explain to them that if pain is anticipated, it will be managed aggressively in the operating room and in the recovery room. Anesthesiologists can provide valuable assistance in this respect because of their knowledge of the pharmacology of sedative and opioid medications (see Chapter 6), as well as their ability to perform neuraxial and peripheral nerve blocks (see Chapters 41 to 43). The possible need for postoperative intensive care, including assisted ventilation, should be anticipated and fully discussed with the parents and child (if the child is of an appropriate age). If special monitoring is required in the operating room or postoperatively, this should be explained and the child assured that the IV catheters, airway devices, and all invasive monitoring devices will be placed after induction of anesthesia to avoid causing discomfort and will be removed as soon as the child's postoperative condition permits.

The anesthesiologist who sits down, who speaks slowly and clearly while answering questions, and who is neither distracted nor in a rush to leave, presents a very different image to the child and parents from the anesthesiologist who stands tapping his or her toes, speaks quickly, and has one foot pointed toward the door. Details regarding the anesthetic should not be recited in a cold and technical manner, but rather with communication that addresses the parents' and the child's questions and concerns. This dialogue is frequently afforded too little time, leaving the parents and child insecure and apprehensive, their questions unanswered. Body language is especially important during this preoperative interview. If the family speaks a different language than the anesthesiologist, then a medical interpreter should be sought.

## THE ANESTHESIOLOGIST

Anesthesiologists must fully understand the proposed surgical or investigative procedure to facilitate the planning of an appropriate level of monitoring and selection of anesthetic drugs and technique. The anesthesiologist must anticipate the needs of the surgeon or proceduralist in terms of positioning the child, the need for or avoidance of muscle relaxants, considerations regarding specific procedures (e.g., the surgeon's need for motor and sensory evoked potentials may influence choices of anesthetic technique), IV fluid and blood product management (see Chapters 8 and 10), as well as the need for strategies to alleviate perioperative pain and anxiety. For complex cases, the anesthesiologist and surgeon should formulate a plan preoperatively and explain the plan to the parents and child. All important medical issues that require clarification should be investigated during the preoperative evaluation and planning process. It is useful to discuss your concerns with the appropriate medical consultants (e.g., the neurologist for the management of seizure medications in the perioperative period, the hematologist for the child with hemophilia, and others as indicated). To maximize the benefit from these consultations, it is important to focus on the specific anesthetic or medical issue of concern. Consultant recommendations must be carefully reviewed and should reflect the consultant's understanding of the anesthesia process and what it is that you require regarding the child's medical condition that will assist you in the delivery of anesthesia (see Chapters 11, 14, 22, 25, 26, and 28).

All children should be fasted preoperatively. Infants must receive special consideration; prolonged abstinence may lead to dehydration or hypoglycemia (see Chapters 4 and 8). Children may surreptitiously circumvent the preoperative fasting orders, especially if the period of fasting is prolonged or other children in the vicinity are in possession of food. One must always be prepared for the possibility of a full stomach and its sequelae. For example, the risk of pulmonary aspiration of gastric contents is increased in some children (e.g., who are obese and who had previous esophageal surgery, difficult intubation, or hiatal hernia). In these children, the anesthetic management should be modified to minimize the risk of regurgitation and aspiration. Preoperative consideration must be given to proper psychological support, appropriate premedication, and the timing of the premedication (see Chapters 3 and 4). Psychological support of the child and parents must never be neglected, no matter how calm they might appear. Premedication may be administered on the ward or in the waiting area; however, once any medication is administered, the child must be observed for compromise in cardiopulmonary function. If the child is premedicated on the ward, transport to the operating room must be undertaken with caution and with appropriate monitoring. A critically ill child must be accompanied by skilled staff who will ensure continued infusion of vasoactive medications and who are skilled in the management of any emergencies that could arise during transport (see Chapter 38). In some, premedication may be omitted because of the critical nature of a child's illness or because a child is especially cooperative.

## Informed Consent

The benefits and risks of the anesthetic procedure must be presented in clear, easily understood terms. At the same time, it is important not to present this in a manner that unduly frightens the child or parents. The details of such a presentation will depend, in part, on the severity of the underlying medical and surgical conditions and how these affect anesthetic management and the planned procedure. Thus, risk can be presented in general terms, such as:

■ *"The risks of anesthesia are generally proportional to the health of the child. For example, if a child has a heart, lung, or kidney disorder, etc., then the risk from anesthesia is increased. In your child's case these are our concerns"* (and then elaborate the particular patient's issues, such as reactive airway disease, apnea of prematurity, etc.). *"Knowing these problems ahead of time may reduce the anesthetic risk for your child because we can modify our anesthetic prescription according to your child's specific needs. However, there is always the possibility of allergic or unusual responses to anesthetic medications that we cannot predict, and that is why I shall carefully observe and monitor your child as I have described."*

We are designing the "anesthetic prescription" specifically for the particular needs of their child, and this notion should be described exactly this way to the parents. We are physicians and

not technicians, and just as the pediatrician writes a prescription for antibiotics, anesthesiologists write the treatment prescription for anesthesia and administer it.

If a child is critically ill or has a disease process that is an immediate threat to his or her life, then this must be explained to the family. If a parent asks about the mortality risk, then all one can say is that the mortality related to anesthesia in most advanced countries is very small, less risky than crossing a busy thoroughfare on foot. Statistically, the incidence varies from one in several hundred thousand for healthy children undergoing routine procedures to a much greater rate for those who are critically ill. Nonetheless, the mortality for any specific child cannot be predicted with certainty. Recent concerns regarding possible anesthetic agent–induced neurotoxicity (see Chapter 23) has become a common question from parents of neonates or toddlers. Again, reassurance regarding the lack of substantive human data, the importance of our monitors, and our experience will help allay their concerns.

## Operating Room and Monitoring

For the anesthesiologist to successfully carry out a proposed anesthetic plan, the child's medical record must be examined for pertinent information before induction of anesthesia. For children who have already been assessed preoperatively, the record should be reviewed again for new information that may have been added since the initial evaluation. It is most important that the child's identification bracelet is checked, especially if the anesthetizing team is different from the preoperative evaluation team. A "time-out" and checklist for nurses, surgeon, and anesthesiologist to confirm the child's name, the planned surgical procedure, and the site of the surgical procedure (right or left side or bilateral); airway concerns; the need for prophylactic antibiotics; allergies and anaphylaxis; and availability of special equipment and large IV access are also reviewed. This review constitutes a vital safety net that we provide in the operating room (Fig. 1-1). All equipment for induction and maintenance of anesthesia, including suction and all necessary monitoring devices, must be functioning and reliable (see Chapter 51). *Equipment must be checked by the anesthesia team before induction of anesthesia.*

The monitoring should be appropriate for the child's clinical condition and surgical procedure. In every situation, basic monitoring is essential; to this are added special monitoring devices as they become necessary. The basic monitors are the anesthesiologist's eyes, ears, and hands, which confer the ability to observe a child's color and chest movements, to listen for heart tones and breath sounds, and to palpate the arterial pulse and temperature of the skin. A precordial or esophageal stethoscope is a very useful and simple device that allows constant assessment of heart tones and the quality of breath sounds even when our attention is focused away from physiologic monitors. All children, except those undergoing the briefest noninvasive procedures, should have IV access to allow for fluid administration and to provide a route for rapid and predictable drug administration. If IV access is already in place, it is essential to ensure its functionality and size before anesthesia is induced. Fluid replacement with balanced salt solution is particularly important in children who have undergone prolonged fasting or who have ongoing third-space losses, although glucose-containing solutions may be preferable under specific circumstances (see Chapter 8). Continuous monitoring of the electrocardiogram,

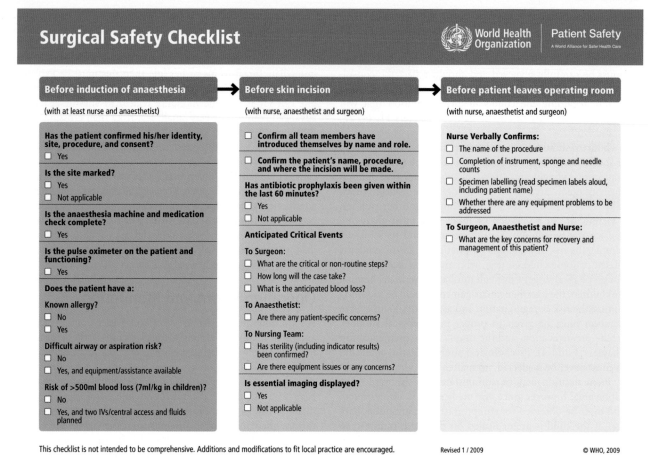

**FIGURE 1-1** WHO Surgical Safety Checklist. (From World Health Organization, Geneva, 2009. Available from: http://www.who.int/patientsafety/safesurgery/en/)

temperature, inspired oxygen concentration, oxygen saturation, expired carbon dioxide, and intermittent blood pressure determination are considered routine. Expired carbon dioxide monitors (especially those that display the waveform) and pulse oximetry are extremely important in the early detection of potential anesthetic-related events that, if undetected, could result in serious morbidity or mortality. Identifying the anesthetic agent and monitoring its concentration breath by breath is also helpful but not mandatory. The role of wakefulness-monitoring devices in children remains unestablished, especially in children who are younger than 2 years of age (see Chapters 6 and 51). Near infrared spectroscopy is being used increasingly during cardiac surgery; it provides a useful monitor of cerebral (i.e., organ) oxygenation.

Invasive hemodynamic monitoring (e.g., direct arterial blood pressure, central venous pressure) may be required for major surgery if extensive blood loss or major fluid shifts are anticipated, or if a child is medically unstable. Urine output provides indirect data of the intravascular volume and organ perfusion in the presence of normal renal function. Monitoring urinary output is particularly useful for prolonged operations, for procedures involving major blood loss, when there is the potential for rapid or massive blood loss, when wide variations in blood pressure and fluid balance can be anticipated, or during induced hypotensive anesthesia. *In general, if a particular variable would be monitored in an adult, then the same approach should be adopted for a child.*

Invasive monitoring procedures are sometimes forsaken in a child because inexperience with pediatric techniques causes the anesthesiologist to dismiss these procedures as being "excessive." These monitors, however, allow the accurate measurement of blood pressure, cardiac output, filling pressures, and cardiac and pulmonary function. In turn, they provide a safe mechanism for assessing the response to pharmacologic interventions, as well as the responses to administration of blood products, fluids, and vasoactive medications (see Chapter 48).

*A cautionary note:* With increased sophistication in monitoring, anesthesiologists have become more distanced than ever from their patients. Relying totally on mechanical monitoring devices to detect clinical abnormalities is dangerous. *The focus must always be on the child and the surgical field. Monitors may fail, and if the anesthesiologist focuses attention on the monitor in an effort to interpret it, rather than attending directly to the child, the child may suffer.* This is the reason that a precordial stethoscope is so useful; strong heart sounds in the face of failed monitors provides some degree of assurance that the child is not in severe trouble. *Disabling monitor alarms for an extended period of time is a serious breach of safety and practice standards.* One of the editors knows of a child for whom all monitor alarms and sounds were disabled during anesthesia, who was discovered dead at the conclusion of the procedure after an unrecognized, unintended tracheal extubation. Most importantly, the tone of the pulse oximeter should be audible by everyone in the operating room to detect decreasing oxygen saturation.

# Induction and Maintenance of Anesthesia

Significant differences in the physiology and behavior of a child, especially a neonate, in comparison with an adult, mandate that the anesthesiologist not consider a child merely a small adult. In an infant, the rate of uptake of inhalation anesthetic agents is more rapid than in an adult. An infant's response to most oral and IV medications is also different; therefore, if changes need to be made, the inspired concentration of an inhalation agent should be adjusted more gradually and the doses of medication diluted and titrated more carefully than in older children and adults (see Chapter 6).

In principle, the approach to an anesthetic procedure in a child is similar to that in an adult. In practice, however, it is often advisable to modify the sequence of application of monitoring devices. In a relatively stable child, induction of anesthesia may proceed with only a pulse oximeter and possibly a precordial stethoscope, while the remaining monitors are applied after induction. This sequence often avoids a prolonged preparation phase during which a child may have more time to become anxious and distressed. In critically ill children, however, omitting some monitors in order to avoid upsetting them is imprudent, especially if it compromises the child's well-being during anesthesia. In a struggling, upset child, some monitors may display accurate measurements before induction of anesthesia, whereas others do not. The pulse oximeter may not provide reliable measurements in a struggling child until the finger or toe is relaxed.

# Clinical Monitors

In children as in adults, monitoring begins with the basic observations of a child's general condition: the heart rate, blood pressure, respirations, and temperature. The most important aspect of basic monitoring consists of using the senses of sight, hearing, and touch to integrate all the data provided by patient observations and the monitors.

### SIGHT
Constantly observing a child's chest excursions (depth and symmetry), the color of the nail beds, oral mucosa, and capillary refill provides vital information about the adequacy of ventilation and perfusion. Observation of the surgical field provides an immediate indication of the extent of fluid shifts and blood loss, the color of the blood in the surgical field, evidence of muscle relaxation, depth of anesthesia, and various physiologic problems that may occur during the surgery (e.g., surgical retraction causing venous obstruction).

### HEARING
Constantly listening to the pitch of the pulse oximeter as well as the heart tones and breath sounds through a precordial or esophageal stethoscope provides instant and continuous feedback about oxygenation (pulse oximeter), heart rate and rhythm, an impression of the cardiac output (changes in intensity of heart sounds), and the adequacy of ventilation (wheezing, stridor, laryngeal spasm, no air exchange). This information is particularly helpful in diagnosing arrhythmias, hypovolemia, anesthetic overdose, and airway obstruction. It may also be helpful to listen to the sounds of surgery, such as the sudden change in the noise of the suction device with rapid blood loss or the surgeon's comments regarding technical difficulties with the procedure.

### TOUCH
Intermittently examining a child—especially palpating peripheral pulses and the skin—provides information that may confirm the auditory input about heart rate, cardiac output, blood pressure, perfusion, and temperature.

# Airway and Ventilation

The most important consideration in the safe practice of pediatric anesthesia is attention to the adequacy of the airway. Airway obstruction occurs readily because of the unique characteristics of the infant and child airway (see Chapter 12). Thus the anesthesiologist must maintain constant vigilance of the airway to ensure that it remains clear at all times. Airway obstruction may lead to hypoventilation, although the causes of hypoventilation may be central (opioids or inhalation agents) or peripheral (muscle relaxants) in origin. Thus anesthesiologists must always place emphasis and attention on constantly monitoring the adequacy of ventilation, particularly when administering anesthesia via a facemask. This is necessary because the expired carbon dioxide tension may underestimate the true carbon dioxide tension as a result of a poor mask fit with air leaks, in combination with an obstructed airway. The capnogram is usually very accurate during mask anesthesia with a circle breathing circuit. Failure to detect an appropriate end-tidal carbon dioxide tension suggests inadequate ventilation, a mask leak, or reduced pulmonary blood flow, with the result that the child's condition may deteriorate from lack of an adequate airway or dilution of the anesthetic gas concentrations.

Although it is desirable to optimize ventilation by maintaining an arterial carbon dioxide pressure within the normal range (35 to 45 mm Hg), most healthy infants and children are not harmed by mild to moderate overventilation; however, severe underventilation has more serious implications.

Constantly monitoring the inspired concentration of oxygen, the expired concentration of carbon dioxide, and the oxygen saturation is a valuable adjunct to the senses of sight, hearing, and touch. *Failure to ventilate adequately is probably the most important factor in the morbidity and mortality of children undergoing anesthesia.*

# Fluids and Perfusion

Appropriate intraoperative fluid management is especially important in infants and children. Because of the relatively small blood volumes of infants and children, hypovolemia may develop rapidly after what may appear to be a trivial amount of blood loss. Fluid shifts may occur in infants because they were fasted for a prolonged period preoperatively. Replacement of lost blood and basic fluid administration must be carefully titrated (using rate-limiting devices), because overhydration readily occurs. The anesthesiologist should have a clear plan for the type and volume of fluid for perioperative administration. Preoperative calculation of maintenance, deficit, and potential third-space losses helps in formulating this fluid management plan, although for children beyond 1 year of age, the fluid replacement strategy has been greatly simplified. A well-planned outline results in a rational and safe approach both to fluid maintenance and to correction of fluid deficit and losses (see Chapters 8 and 10). The anesthesiologist should have immediate access to indwelling IV cannulae; obstructions in the line, loose connections, disconnections, or interstitial cannulae result in children not receiving intended fluid therapy or medications, sometimes with disastrous consequences.

## Conduct of the Anesthesia Team

The anesthesiologist must concentrate exclusively on the child and the monitors throughout the procedure. The child's safety is in his or her hands, and any inattention may place the child's life in jeopardy. Should members of the anesthesia team need to replace each other during the anesthetic procedure, it is essential that the "baton of responsibility" be passed in a smooth and coordinated manner. A clear dialogue between team members must be established about the nature of the surgery, the child's underlying conditions, anesthetic agents and other medications, fluid and blood product management, and any problems that have developed during the anesthetic procedure. Drugs on the anesthesia machine must be clearly labeled by name and dosage. For infants, dilution of drugs or the use of tuberculin syringes may improve the safety of drug administration by limiting the amount of drug in each syringe and allowing more accurate dose administration, although a disproportionate amount of the small volumes of a drug—as in the case of undiluted drugs administered from a tuberculin syringe—may be trapped in the dead space of claves and/or stopcocks, resulting in an underdosing of the drug.

Ongoing communication between the anesthesiologist and surgeon is important if the anesthesiologist is to anticipate potential changes in a child's physiologic status due to surgical manipulations, and deal with them immediately, appropriately, and effectively.

The conclusion of an anesthetic procedure is fraught with potential problems. The anesthesiologist should not be left alone in the operating room without a nurse or other physician, nor should he or she relax vigilance while a child is awakening and being transferred to the recovery room or intensive care unit. It is during this stage that airway obstruction, desaturation, vomiting and aspiration, and excitement are likely to occur.

Records of an anesthetic procedure must be accurate and complete; however, anesthesiologists must avoid the compulsion to complete these during the procedure if a child's condition warrants special attention.

## The Postanesthesia Care Unit

The anesthesiologist's responsibility to a child continues into the postanesthesia care unit (PACU). Transport to the PACU must be carried out with appropriate monitoring, attention to a clear airway, and adequate ventilation, oxygenation, and perfusion. If necessary, battery-powered infusion pumps should be used to maintain accurate infusions of vasoactive drugs. If needed, oxygen should be administered by facemask. Alternately, oxygen saturation may be monitored during transport; administering oxygen and monitoring pulse oximetry may give misleading information regarding the adequacy of ventilation. Oxygen should be available during transport. For children who are not yet fully awake, transport in the "tonsil position" or "recovery position" (lateral decubitus position) rather than the common practice of transport in the supine position is recommended so that, should vomiting occur, it will flow away from the larynx and will be seen immediately. In general, oxygen should be administered to children who have not yet awakened. The mask should be observed for condensation with each breath to assess the respiratory rate as well as gas movement with respiration.

On arrival in the PACU, a clear summary of the medical and surgical problems of the child; important intraoperative events; timing of antibiotics, analgesics, local anesthetics, or nerve blocks; and details of the anesthetic procedure are given to the PACU personnel. The PACU must be equipped with age- and size-appropriate resuscitation equipment. Vital signs (oxygen saturation, heart rate, blood pressure, respirations, temperature, and pain score) should be recorded on admission to the PACU and at appropriate intervals during the child's stay (see Chapter 46). If appropriate, specific instructions should be given relating to fluid management; the administration of oxygen, analgesics, antiemetics, and other medications; blood tests (e.g., hematocrit, blood gases, electrolytes, and coagulation profile); and radiographs. Once the anesthesiologist is certain that the child is stable from a cardiopulmonary standpoint and that all vital information has been provided to the PACU staff, the anesthesiologist should inform the parents that the child has arrived safely in the PACU, provide them with a summary of the anesthetic procedure, and then proceed to the next case. If the child requires special attention (airway issues, hypotension, possible ongoing blood loss, etc.) in the PACU, then the anesthesiologist should reassess the child personally before the child is discharged.

## Postoperative Visit

If the child has been admitted to the hospital for more than an overnight observation, it is good practice to visit the child and family postoperatively to assess the postanesthetic clinical course and discuss the child's reaction to the anesthetic. A note documenting the visit should also be inserted into the child's record. All too often the anesthesiologist appears only preoperatively and is never seen again by the family, especially if there was a poor outcome. If the public is to understand and respect the profession of anesthesiology as a vital medical specialty, close interaction and trust among parents, child, and anesthesiologist are essential. A follow-up telephone call from the nursing staff is also useful in identifying and managing anesthesia-related postoperative issues.

## Summary

This introductory chapter has outlined the fundamentals of safe pediatric anesthesia practice. The chapters that follow elaborate on these principles; our collective experience has been used to guide practicing anesthesiologists. We reiterate specific points throughout to emphasize their importance and to present several different perspectives on those issues.

# Growth and Development

BRUNO MARCINIAK

AS AN INFANT GROWS and matures, vital changes occur that affect the child's response to disease, drugs, and the environment. Growth is an increase in physical size, and development is an increase in complexity and function. An overview of the subject is presented so that anesthesiologists can appreciate the uniqueness of developing children from both physical and psychological perspectives.

The physician should understand the main developmental changes that occur over time, as well as how these changes affect both responses to diseases and to drug pharmacokinetics and pharmacodynamics.

## Normal and Abnormal Growth and Maturation

Growth is the quantitative development of the body and maturation is the acquisition of new functionalities; both phenomena occur during pregnancy and after birth. Prenatal growth is the most important phase in development, comprising organogenesis in the first 8 weeks (embryonic growth), followed by the functional development of organ systems and maturation of the fetus to full term (fetal growth). Rapid growth occurs particularly in the second trimester; a major increase in weight from subcutaneous tissue and muscle mass occurs in the third trimester. Environmental agents may affect the human embryo in a negative way. The duration of gestation and the weight of an infant have an important relationship (Table 2-1).

The term *prematurity* has conventionally been applied to infants weighing less than 2500 g at birth, but the designation *preterm infant* is more appropriate and is defined as one born before 37 completed weeks of gestation. A *term or full-term infant* is one born between 37 and 42 completed weeks of gestation. *A postterm infant* is one born after 42 completed weeks of gestation.

Preterm infants are further classified according to their actual birth weight. A low–birth-weight (LBW) infant is one weighing less than 2500 g regardless of the duration of the pregnancy. A very low–birth-weight (VLBW) infant weighs less than 1500 g, and an extremely low–birth-weight infant weighs less than 1000 g. In addition, infants weighing less than 750 g are now being called "*micropremies*"; there is very little published information regarding the anesthetic management of this vulnerable subpopulation of neonates (see Chapter 35). Common neonatal problems as they relate to age and birth weight are presented in Table 2-2.

After birth, physical growth continues at a rapid pace during the first 6 months of extrauterine life but slows by about 2 years of age. Physical growth accelerates a second time during the pubertal period. A simple way to remember how rapidly the infant grows is that birth weight doubles by 6 months of age and triples by 1 year. Length doubles by 4 years of age. This scale, however, does not affect all organs or functions in the same way. It is important to be able to assess correctly and precisely the stage of development of the child, because any abnormal slowdown requires investigation to find the cause.

**TABLE 2-1** The Relationship of Gestational Age to Weight

| Gestation (weeks) | Mean Weight (grams) |
| --- | --- |
| 28 | 1165 ± 109 |
| 32 | 1760 ± 128 |
| 36 | 2621 ± 274 |
| 40 (full term) | 3351 ± 448 |

Data from Naeye RL, Dixon JB. Distortions in fetal growth. Pediatr Res 1978;12: 987-91.

## GESTATIONAL AGE ASSESSMENT

The gestational age of an infant may be assessed in one of three ways. The most accurate means of assessing gestational age is by measuring the crown-rump length of the fetus during a first-trimester ultrasonographic examination. Another method involves calculating gestational age from the first day of the mother's last menstrual period, but this is commonly inaccurate, leading to errors in estimation. Finally, the Dubowitz scoring system is a well-accepted method combining neurologic and physical criteria of the infant to provide an accurate assessment of gestational age.[1,2] A summary of the more significant neurologic and physical signs of maturity is presented in Table 2-3.

## WEIGHT AND LENGTH

Assessment of growth is measured by changes in weight, length, and head circumference. Percentile charts are valuable for monitoring the child's growth and development. Deviation from growth within the same percentile for a child of any age is of greater significance than any single measurement (Figs. 2-1 and 2-2). Weight is a more sensitive index of well-being, illness, or poor nutrition than length or head circumference and is the most commonly used measurement of growth. Change in weight reflects changes in muscle mass, adipose tissue, skeleton, and body water and thus is a nonspecific measure of growth. Measurement of length provides the best indicator of skeletal growth because it is not affected by changes in adipose tissue or water content.

Term infants may lose 5% to 10% of their body weight during the first 24 to 72 hours of life from loss of body water. Birth weight is usually regained in 7 to 10 days. A daily increase of 30 g (210 g/week) is satisfactory for the first 3 months. Thereafter, weight gain slows so that at 10 to 12 months of age it is 70 g each week (Table 2-4).

*When plotting the weight of a preterm infant on a growth chart, it is common to use the infant's corrected gestational age (postmenstrual age; postconceptual age is taken from conception and is approximately 2 weeks shorter) instead of his or her chronologic age (postnatal age, i.e., from birth) during the first 2 years of the infant's life in order to correct for prematurity.*

Weight and length are important but changes affect the composition of the body itself, especially total body water, which decreases at the expense of the extracellular compartment, with adult levels attained at 1 year of age.[3,4] This finding has implications for drug dosing and distribution in the infant. Males have a greater percentage of water, whereas females have a slightly greater percentage of fat. The percentage decrease in extracellular water is greater than the decrease in total body water because of the simultaneous increase in intracellular water (Table 2-5).[5]

Another, more precise way to assess development is to calculate the body surface area (BSA).[6]

**TABLE 2-2** Common Neonatal Problems with Respect to Weight and Gestation

| Gestation | Relative Weight | Neonatal Problems at Increased Incidence |
| --- | --- | --- |
| Preterm (<37 weeks) | SGA | Respiratory distress syndrome |
| | | Apnea |
| | | Perinatal depression |
| | | Hypoglycemia |
| | | Polycythemia |
| | | Hypocalcemia |
| | | Hypomagnesemia |
| | | Hyperbilirubinemia |
| | | Viral infection |
| | | Thrombocytopenia |
| | | Congenital anomalies |
| | | Maternal drug addiction |
| | | Fetal alcohol syndrome |
| | AGA | Respiratory distress syndrome |
| | | Apnea |
| | | Hypoglycemia |
| | | Hypocalcemia |
| | | Hypomagnesemia |
| | | Hyperbilirubinemia |
| | LGA | Respiratory distress syndrome |
| | | Hypoglycemia: infant of a diabetic mother |
| | | Apnea |
| | | Hypocalcemia |
| | | Hypomagnesemia |
| | | Hyperbilirubinemia |
| Normal (37-42 weeks) | SGA | Congenital anomalies |
| | | Viral infection |
| | | Thrombocytopenia |
| | | Maternal drug addiction |
| | | Perinatal depression |
| | | Hypoglycemia |
| | AGA | — |
| | LGA | Birth trauma |
| | | Hyperbilirubinemia |
| | | Hypoglycemia: infant of a diabetic mother |
| Postmature (>42 weeks) | SGA | Meconium aspiration syndrome |
| | | Congenital anomalies |
| | | Viral infection |
| | | Thrombocytopenia |
| | | Maternal drug addiction |
| | | Perinatal depression |
| | | Aspiration pneumonia |
| | | Hypoglycemia |
| | AGA | — |
| | LGA | Birth trauma |
| | | Hyperbilirubinemia |
| | | Hypoglycemia: infant of a diabetic mother |

*AGA*, Appropriate for gestational age; *LGA*, large for gestational age; *SGA*, small for gestational age.

**TABLE 2-3** Neurologic and External Physical Criteria to Assess Gestational Age

| Physical Examination | Preterm (<37 weeks) | Term (≥37 weeks) |
|---|---|---|
| Ear | Shapeless, pliable | Firm, well formed |
| Skin | Edematous, thin skin | Thick skin |
| Sole of foot | Creases on anterior third | Whole foot creased |
| Breast tissue | Less than 1 mm diameter | More than 5 mm diameter |
| Genitalia | | |
| Male | Scrotum poorly developed Testes undescended | Scrotum rugated Testes descended |
| Female | Large clitoris, gaping labia majora | Labia majora developed |
| Limbs | Hypotonic | Tonic (flexed) |
| Grasp reflex | Weak grasp | Can be lifted by reflex grasp |
| Moro reflex | Complete but exhaustible (>32 weeks) | Complete |
| Sucking reflex | Weak | Strong, synchronous with swallowing |

**TABLE 2-4** Approximate Relationship of Age to Weight

| Age (years) | Weight (kg) |
|---|---|
| 1 | 10 |
| 3 | 15 |
| 5 | 19 |
| 7 | 23 |

**TABLE 2-5** Relationship of Age to Body Water

| Age | Body Water (percent) | Extracellular | Intracellular |
|---|---|---|---|
| Fetus | 90 | 60 | 25 |
| Preterm | 80 | 55 | 30 |
| Full-term | 70 | 50 | 35 |
| 6-12 months | 60 | 30 | 40 |

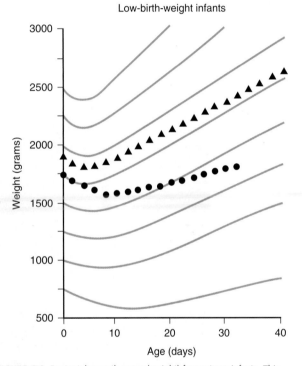

**FIGURE 2-2** Postnatal growth curve (weight) for preterm infants. This figure represents normal growth curves for preterm infants. *Triangles* indicate a normal preterm infant. *Circles* demonstrate failure to thrive in an infant with bronchopulmonary dysplasia.

$$BSA\,(m^2) = \sqrt{Body\ length\ (cm) \times Body\ weight\ (kg)/3600}$$

BSA can also be described using an allometric equation with an exponent of ⅔ (see Chapter 6):

$$BSA \propto weight^{2/3}$$

## HEAD CIRCUMFERENCE

Head size reflects growth of the brain and correlates with intracranial volume and brain weight. Changing head circumference reflects head growth and is a part of the total body growth process; it may or may not indicate underlying involvement of

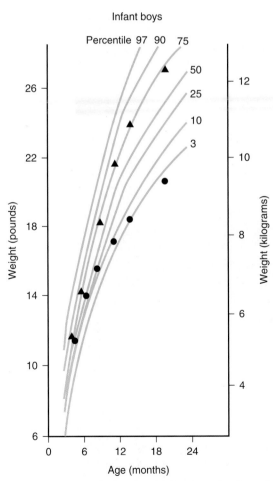

**FIGURE 2-1** Postnatal growth curve (weight) for term male infants. This figure represents normal growth curves. *Triangles* indicate a normal child. *Circles* demonstrate failure to thrive in a child with severe renal failure.

the brain. An abnormally large or small head may indicate abnormal brain development, which must alert the anesthesiologist to possible underlying neurologic problems. A large head may indicate a normal variation, familial feature, or pathologic condition (e.g., hydrocephalus or increased intracranial pressure), whereas a small head may indicate a normal variant, familial feature, or pathologic condition such as craniosynostosis or abnormal brain development.

During the first year of life, head circumference normally increases 10 cm, and it increases 2.5 cm in the second year. By 9 months of age, head circumference reaches 50% of adult size, and by 2 years it is 75%. Head circumference is closely followed on standard percentile growth curves. As with weight, deviations of growth of the head within the same percentile are more significant than a single measurement.

The anterior fontanel should be palpated to assess whether it is sunken (dehydration) or bulging abnormally (suggesting increased intracranial pressure as in hydrocephalus, infection, hemorrhage, or increased partial pressure of carbon dioxide in the arterial blood [$PaCO_2$]). If it is bulging, the sutures should be palpated for abnormal separation as a result of increased intracranial pressure. The anterior fontanel closes between 9 and 18 months of age; the posterior fontanel closes by 2 to 4 months of age (Fig. 2-3). Cranial molding occurs particularly in LBW infants and is usually of no clinical importance.

## FACE

Although the cranial vault increases rapidly in size, the face and base of the skull develop at a slower rate. At birth, the mandible is small; but as a child develops, forward growth occurs, reducing the obliquity of the mandibular angle. Failure of prenatal development of the mandible may be associated with severe congenital defects (e.g., Pierre Robin, Treacher Collins, or Goldenhar syndromes). These syndromes often have other associated anomalies. After 2 years of age, the cranial vault increases only marginally in size, whereas the facial configuration undergoes substantive changes. The upper jaw grows rapidly to accommodate the developing teeth. In addition, the frontal sinuses develop by 2 to 6 years of age, and the maxillary, ethmoidal, and sphenoidal sinuses appear after 6 years of age.

## TEETH

The first tooth, usually a lower incisor, erupts at approximately 6 months after birth (deciduous dentition). Eruption of all deciduous teeth is usually complete by 28 months of age. Permanent teeth appear at 6 years, with the shedding of the deciduous teeth; this process takes place during the next 6 to 8 years. Abnormally developed teeth occur with hereditary disorders, Down syndrome, cerebral palsy, medications (eg., tetracycline) and nutritional defects. Preterm infants may show severe enamel hypoplasia in their primary dentition.[7,8]

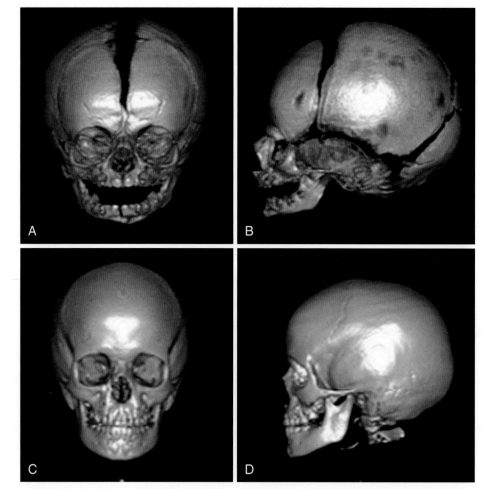

**FIGURE 2-3** Cranial development. **A** and **B** depict the skull of a neonate with wide-open suture. **C** and **D** depict the skull of a 7-year-old boy with fused sutures.

## COMPORTMENT AND BEHAVIOR

The neurologic status and social acquisition of the child are part of the development assessment and will be described later in this chapter.

## Airway and Respiratory System

Airway development includes a large number of structures including cranial vault and base, cranioverterbal development, face, branchial apparatus, larynx and oral cavity.

These structures are involved in the respiratory function (to provide enough oxygen and to remove carbon dioxide) but also to separate the circulation of air from the circulation of liquid and food. A variety of processes, including ventilation, perfusion, and diffusion, are involved in fulfilling these functions. Specifically, the anesthesiologist has to consider these developmental changes because of their implication in airway management and ventilation.

### UPPER AIRWAY DEVELOPMENT

During the course of development, the infant upper airways undergo deep anatomic modifications that include changes in size, shape, and interrelationship; this is particularly prominent during the first few years of life.

The face and the nasal chamber, the oropharynx with the tongue, and the laryngotracheal lumen are the three main parts of the upper airway involved. The development of the neurocranium will lead to the maturation of the cranial vault and skull base, and the development of the viscerocranium to the skeletal part of the face. The primordial areas involved in forming the covering of the tongue appear early in the second month of development.

The larynx is developed embryologically from ectodermal, endodermal, and mesodermal tissues that are derived from the third, fourth, and sixth branchial arch and pouch apparatus. The development of the larynx and airway in the neonate is outlined in detail in Chapter 12. The laryngeal opening (epiglottis and vocal cords) in a neonate and 2-year-old boy are shown in Figure 2-4. Note the omega-shaped long epiglottis and the pearly white vocal cords in the neonate.

The skull base grows rapidly until age 6 years, with relatively slower growth thereafter. The cranial base flexes postnatally in a rapid growth trajectory that is complete by 2 years of age.

The depth of the nasopharynx increases due to remodeling of the palate as well as changes in the angulation of the skull base. During childhood, the soft tissues of the pharyngeal structures surrounding the upper airway grow proportionally to the skeletal structures. After birth, the dimensions of the nasal cavity increase very rapidly. During the first year of life, the total minimal cross-sectional area is increased by 67%, and the volume of the anterior 4 cm of the nasal airways by 36%.[9]

The volume of the oral cavity in the neonate is proportionally less than that in the adult, owing to a significantly shorter mandibular ramus. The volume of the oral cavity significantly increases during the first 12 months because of rapid growth in the height of the mandibular ramus.

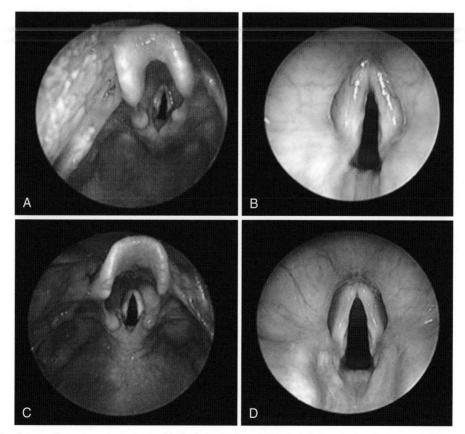

**FIGURE 2-4** Larynx development from neonate to 2 years old. The larynx in the neonate (**A** and **B**), with the long epiglottis (**A**) and the vocal cords (**B,** close-up). The larynx in a 2-year-old (**C** and **D**), with a shorter epiglottis (**C**) and the vocal cords (**D,** close up).

Compared with the adult, the tongue in the neonate contains considerably less fat and soft tissue, but overall is large in size relative to the dimensions of the mouth, with relatively larger extrinsic musculature and a less developed superior longitudinal muscle resulting in a flat dorsal surface with poor lateral mobility (see also Chapter 12).

## RESPIRATORY SYSTEM DEVELOPMENT

The development of the respiratory system begins during week 4 of gestation. Three "laws" that describe the temporal development of the conducting airways, alveoli, and pulmonary vessels govern normal lung growth.

*Airways:* The bronchial tree down to and including the terminal bronchioles forms by week 16 of gestation. The acinus, consisting of all the airway structures distal to the terminal bronchiole and the entire gas-exchanging apparatus, develops throughout the remainder of gestation.

*Alveoli:* Alveoli develop mainly after birth, increasing in number until approximately 8 years of life and in size until growth of the chest wall ceases.

*Pulmonary vessels:* Arteries and veins accompanying the bronchial tree form by week 16 of gestation. Those vessels lying within the acinus follow the development of the alveoli. The appearance and growth of arterial smooth muscle lags behind the sprouting of new vessels and is not completed until late adolescence.

## TRANSITION TO AIR BREATHING

Fetal breathing movements have been detected as early as 11 weeks of gestational age; they are interspersed with long periods of apnea and produce little tidal movement of lung fluid.[10,11] The critical event in the change from placental to pulmonary gas exchange is the first inspiration, which initiates pulmonary ventilation, promotes the clearance of lung fluid, and triggers the change from the fetal to the neonatal pattern of circulation.

The first breath is a gasp that generates a transpulmonary distending pressure of 40 to 80 cm $H_2O$.[12] This moves the tracheal fluid (100 times more viscous than air), overcomes surface forces that develop as the air–fluid interface reaches the small airways, and overcomes tissue resistance. In some children, the removal of lung fluid may be delayed, producing the syndrome called *transient tachypnea of the newborn*.[13] Tachypnea lasts for 24 to 72 hours and is associated with a characteristic chest radiographic appearance consisting of increased perihilar markings, fluid in the interlobar fissures, and streaky linear opacities in the parenchyma.

With the onset of pulmonary ventilation, pulmonary blood flow sharply increases. Decreased pulmonary vascular resistance (PVR) and increased peripheral systemic vascular resistance (loss of the umbilical circulation) are the two crucial events involved in the immediate transition from the fetal circulation to the normal postnatal pattern. The increase in systemic afterload causes an immediate closure of the flap valve mechanism of the foramen ovale and reverses the direction of shunt through the ductus arteriosus. Until these fetal shunt pathways close anatomically, the pattern of circulation is unstable. Increased pulmonary vascular reactivity in response to hypoxia and acidosis may precipitate a reversal to right-to-left shunting ("flip-flop" circulation).

In the first few minutes of life, a state of "normal" asphyxia exists as a result of impairment of placental blood flow during labor. The partial pressure of oxygen in arterial blood ($PaO_2$) and pH are low, whereas the $PaCO_2$ is increased immediately after birth, but these parameters change rapidly in the first hour of life. Extrapulmonary shunting through fetal channels and intrapulmonary shunting, probably through unexpanded regions of the lung, persist for some time after birth, so that in neonates the physiologic right-to-left shunt is about three times that in adults.[14]

## MECHANICS OF BREATHING
### Chest Wall and Respiratory Muscles

The accessory muscles of inspiration are relatively ineffective in infants because of an unfavorable anatomic rib configuration. In infancy, the ribs extend horizontally from the vertebral column, moving little with inspiration.[15] These factors increase the workload on the diaphragm. Consequently, and in contrast to an adult, thoracic cross-sectional area is fairly constant throughout the breathing cycle, and inspiration occurs almost entirely as a result of diaphragmatic descent.

The chest wall of a neonate is floppy because it comprises noncalcified cartilage, its musculature is poorly developed, and the ribs are incompletely calcified.[16,17] As the work of breathing increases, diaphragmatic displacement must also increase to maintain the tidal volume. The increased workload may lead to diaphragmatic fatigue and respiratory failure or apnea, especially in preterm infants.[18,19]

The tendency to respiratory muscle fatigue is the result of the metabolic characteristics of the diaphragm, which has very little type I (slow twitch, high oxidative capacity) muscle fibers (see Fig. 12-11).

### Elastic Properties of the Lung

Changes in the static pressure–volume relationship of the lungs during growth are caused by increases in volume and changes in the elastic properties of lung tissue. Volume is the principal factor that determines lung compliance, which increases throughout childhood. Specific lung compliance remains relatively constant throughout childhood.[20] In contrast, specific compliance of the chest wall declines throughout childhood and adolescence, reflecting the progressive calcification of the ribs and the increasing bulk of the thoracic muscles.

### Static Lung Volumes

Detailed information expressing static lung volumes on the basis of body weight are detailed in Table 2-6.

### Total Lung Capacity

Adults have a markedly greater total lung capacity (TLC) than infants (Fig. 2-5). This difference reflects the fact that TLC is an effort-dependent parameter, depending on the strength and efficiency of the inspiratory muscles, which can be estimated by the maximum inspiratory pressure at functional residual capacity (FRC). An adult can generate negative pressures in excess of 100 cm $H_2O$; negative inspiratory pressures as high as 70 cm $H_2O$ have been recorded for neonates, a surprisingly high value in view of their underdeveloped musculature and highly compliant chest wall. This may be a consequence of the small radius of curvature of an infant's rib cage, which by the Laplace relationship converts a small tension into a large pressure difference.[21]

### Functional Residual Capacity

FRC is similar on a per-kilogram basis at all ages, but the mechanical factors on which it is based are different in infants and adults.[22] In adults, FRC is the same as the volume at which the elastic forces generated by the passive recoil of the chest wall are

**TABLE 2-6** Age-Dependent Respiratory Variables

|  | Newborn | 6 months | 12 months | 3 years | 5 years | 12 years | Adult | Units |
|---|---|---|---|---|---|---|---|---|
| F | 50 ± 1 | 30 ± 5 | 24 ± 6 | 24 ± 6 | 23 ± 5 | 18 ± 5 | 12 ± 3 | Breaths per min |
| TV | 21 | 45 | 78 | 112 | 270 | 480 | 575 | mL |
|  | 6-8 |  |  |  |  |  | 6-7 | mL/kg |
| VE | 1050 | 1350 | 1780 | 2460 | 5500 | 6200 | 6400 | mL/min |
|  | 200-260 |  |  |  |  |  | 90 | mL/kg/min |
| VA | 665 |  | 1245 | 1760 | 1800 | 3000 | 3100 | mL/min |
|  | 100-150 |  |  |  |  |  | 60 | mL/kg/min |
| VD/VT | 0.3 |  |  |  |  |  | 0.3 |  |
| VO2 | 6-8 |  |  |  |  |  | 3-4 | mL/kg/min |
| VC | 120 |  |  | 870 | 1160 | 3100 | 4000 | mL |
| FRC | 80 |  |  | 490 | 680 | 1970 | 3000 | mL |
|  | 30 |  |  |  |  |  | 30 | mL/kg |
| TLC | 160 |  |  | 1100 | 1500 | 4000 | 6000 | mL |
|  | 63 |  |  |  |  |  | 82 | mL/kg |
| pH | 7.3-7.4 |  | 7.35-7.45 |  |  |  | 7.35-7.45 |  |
| PaO2 | 60-90 |  | 80-100 |  |  |  | 80-100 | mm Hg |
| PaCO2 | 30-35 |  | 30-40 |  |  |  | 37-42 | mm Hg |

Modified from O'Rourke PP, Crone RK. The respiratory system. In: Gregory GA, editor. Pediatric anesthesia. 2nd ed. New York: Churchill Livingstone; 1989.

*F,* Frequency; *FRC,* functional residual capacity; *PaCO₂,* arterial carbon dioxide tension; *PaO₂,* arterial oxygen tension; *TLC,* total lung capacity; *TV,* tidal volume; *VA,* alveolar ventilation; *VC,* vital capacity; *VD/VT,* dead space/tidal volume; *VE,* minute ventilation; *VO₂,* oxygen consumption.

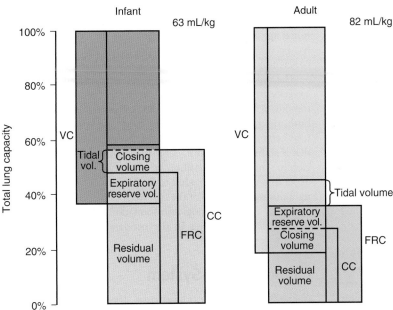

**FIGURE 2-5** Lung volumes in infants and adults. Note that, in infants, tidal volume breathing occurs at the same volume as closing volume. *CC,* Closing capacity; *FRC,* functional residual capacity; *VC,* vital capacity. (Modified from Nelson NM. Respiration and circulation after birth. In: Smith CA, Nelson NM editors. The physiology of the newborn infant. Springfield, Ill.: Charles C Thomas; 1976. p. 207.)

balanced by the recoil of the lung (Fig. 2-6); this is the volume attained at end-expiration with an open glottis.

An important clinical implication of the dynamic control of FRC is that an apneic infant has a disproportionately smaller reserve of intrapulmonary oxygen on which to draw than a similarly affected adult. This, combined with their increased metabolic rate, contributes to the rapid development of hypoxemia if the airway is lost in the anesthetized infant.

## Closing Capacity

As exhalation proceeds to completion, small airways in dependent regions of the lung close, leading to air trapping in the affected areas. Closing capacity is closely related to age, declining throughout childhood and adolescence and increasing thereafter throughout adult life (see Fig. 2-5). This pattern of change has been related to the development and deterioration of lung elastic tissue and its effect on recoil pressure. The latter is the principal determinant of transmural pressure and therefore patency of the smallest airways, which lack intrinsic stability because they contain no cartilage.

Closing volume is within the range of tidal breathing in some adults older than 40 years and some children younger than 10 years (see Fig. 2-5). It is not possible to measure closing volume in children younger than 5 years, but because elastic recoil pressure decreases to very low levels in infancy (see Fig. 2-6); it is likely that some airways remain closed throughout tidal

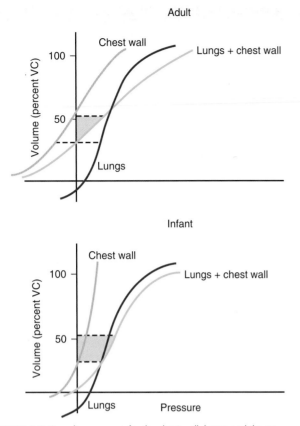

**FIGURE 2-6** Compliance curves for the chest wall, lungs, and thorax (combination of chest wall and lungs) in infants and adults. (Modified and reproduced with permission from Pérez Fontán JJ, Haddad GG. Respiratory physiology. In: Behrman RE, Kliegman RM, Jenson HB, editors. Nelson textbook of pediatrics. 17th ed. Philadelphia: WB Saunders; 2003. p. 1363.)

breathing. This conclusion is supported by the finding that infants have a large "trapped gas volume" that is not in free communication with the conducting airways. Age-related changes in $PaO_2$, which parallel the changes in the difference between FRC and closing volume, may also be related to airway closure.[21]

## AIRWAY DYNAMICS

### Resistance and Conductance

Airway resistance declines markedly with growth from 19 to 28 cm $H_2O$/L/sec in neonates to less than 2 cm $H_2O$/L/sec in adults.[22,23] Airway resistance is greater in preterm than in full-term infants. On the other hand, specific airway conductance (reciprocal of resistance) is greater in preterm infants, and it continues to decline throughout the first 5 years of life.[24,25]

### Distribution of Resistance

The distribution of airway resistance changes markedly around the age of 5 years. Airway resistance per gram of lung tissue is constant at all ages in the "central airways" (trachea to the twelfth to fifteenth bronchial generation), whereas it decreases markedly around the age of 5 years in the "peripheral airways" (twelvth to fifteenth generation to the alveoli).

### Inspiratory and Expiratory Flow Limitation

Tracheal compliance in neonates is twice that of adults; it is even greater in preterm infants and appears to be a consequence of

cartilaginous immaturity. The functional importance of this finding is that dynamic collapse of the trachea may occur with inspiration and expiration (see Fig. 12-10).

### Regulation of Breathing

In neonates as in adults, $PaO_2$, $PaCO_2$, and pH control pulmonary ventilation, with $PaO_2$ acting mainly through peripheral chemoreceptors in the carotid and aortic bodies and $PaCO_2$ and pH acting on central chemoreceptors in the medulla. Unlike an adult, an infant's response to hypercapnia is not potentiated by hypoxia. In fact, hypoxia may depress the hypercapnic ventilatory response in term and preterm infants.[26]

High concentrations of oxygen depress the neonate's respirations, whereas low concentrations stimulate it. The hypoxic response is not sustained. However, sustained hypoxia leads first to a return to baseline ventilation and then to ventilatory depression. This pattern of response persists in normal term infants for the first week of life, after which the response to sustained hypoxia is replaced by a sustained increase in ventilation.[27] This pattern persists longer in preterm infants.

Periodic breathing commonly occurs in neonates and should be distinguished from clinical apnea, which occurs in as many as 25% of all preterm infants but especially in the most premature. Apnea of prematurity may be a life-threatening condition. Ventilatory pauses are prolonged and are associated with desaturation of arterial oxygen, bradycardia, and loss of muscle tone.

Prematurity is an important risk factor for life-threatening apnea in infants undergoing general anesthesia.[28] The risk of postanesthetic respiratory depression is inversely related to gestational age and postconceptual age at the time of anesthesia.[29] It has been stated that infants may be at risk up to 60 weeks after conception.[29-31]

The reduced $PaO_2$ of neonates is compensated by a greater oxygen-carrying capacity due to increased hemoglobin concentrations, which decline during the first several weeks of life. At birth, the hemoglobin content of the blood is made up of 50% fetal hemoglobin, which has an in vivo oxygen-dissociation curve that is shifted to the left in comparison with normal adult hemoglobin. The shift in position of the oxygen-dissociation curve depends on the ratio of adult to fetal hemoglobin. It shifts to the right during the course of the first week of life, reflecting a switch from fetal to adult hemoglobin formation.[20] Normal $PaCO_2$ and pH are somewhat lower in the neonatal period than in later infancy (see Table 2-6).

## Cardiovascular System

An understanding of cardiovascular development is important for anesthesiologists. This section briefly considers developmental changes in heart rate, blood pressure, cardiac output, and the electrocardiogram; more detailed descriptions are found in Chapters 14 and 16.

### HEART RATE

Autonomic control of the heart in utero is mediated predominantly through the parasympathetic nervous system. It is only shortly after birth that sympathetic control appears. In neonates, the heart rate may have a wide variation that is within normal limits.

In older children, a significant number of arrhythmias and conduction abnormalities are also encountered, with marked fluctuations in heart rate due to variations in autonomic tone.

The mean heart rate in neonates in the first 24 hours of life is 120 beats per minute. It increases to a mean of 160 beats per minute at 1 month, after which it gradually decreases to 75 beats per minute at adolescence (Table 2-7).[32]

## BLOOD PRESSURE

Mean systolic blood pressure in neonates and infants increases from 65 mm Hg in the first 12 hours of life to 75 mm Hg at 4 days and 95 mm Hg at 6 weeks. There is little change in mean systolic pressure between 6 weeks and 1 year of age; between 1 year and 6 years, there is only a slight change, followed by a gradual increase.[33,34] These measurements apply to infants and children who are awake and quiet. The blood pressure in preterm infants in the first 12 hours is less than that in full-term infants; a gradual increase in blood pressure occurs after birth–68/43 mm Hg on day 1 of life compared with 90/55 mm Hg on day 90 of life (Table 2-8).[35,36] It has also been noted that infants with birth asphyxia and those who require mechanical ventilation have reduced blood pressures.[37] Blood pressure measured in the lower leg is less than in the upper arm.[38]

Blood pressure in adolescents and adults who were born preterm is greater than in those who were born full-term. However, the slower fetal growth in preterm, LBW infants was not identified as an independent predictor of this greater blood pressure later in life.[39]

**TABLE 2-7** The Relationship of Age to Heart Rate*

| Age | Mean Heart Rate in Beats per Minute (range) |
| --- | --- |
| Premature | 120-170 |
| 0-3 months | 100-150 |
| 3-6 months | 90-120 |
| 6-12 months | 80-120 |
| 1-3 years | 70-110 |
| 3-6 years | 65-110 |
| 6-12 years | 60-95 |
| >12 years | 55-85 |

Data from Hartman ME, Cheifetz IM. Pediatric Emergencies and Resuscitation. In: Kliegman RM, Stanton ST BF, Geme III JW, Schor NF, Behrman RE, editors. Nelson Textbook of Pediatrics. 19th ed. Philadelphia: Elsevier; 2011. p. 280.
*Note that the heart rate will be lower during sleep.

**TABLE 2-8** The Relationship of Age to Blood Pressure*

| Age | Normal Blood Pressure (mm Hg) | |
| --- | --- | --- |
| | Mean Systolic | Mean Diastolic |
| Premature | 55-75 | 35-45 |
| 0-3 months | 65-85 | 45-55 |
| 3-6 months | 70-90 | 50-65 |
| 6-12 months | 80-100 | 55-65 |
| 1-3 years | 90-105 | 55-70 |
| 3-6 years | 95-110 | 60-75 |
| 6-12 years | 100-120 | 60-75 |
| >12 years | 110-135 | 65-85 |

Data from Hartman ME, Cheifetz IM. Pediatric Emergencies and Resuscitation. In: Kliegman RM, Stanton ST BF, Geme III JW, Schor NF, Behrman RE, editors. Nelson Textbook of Pediatrics. 19th ed. Philadelphia: Elsevier; 2011. p. 280.
*Note that the blood pressure will be lower during sleep or during anesthesia.

## CARDIAC OUTPUT

Determination of cardiac output and blood pressure allows calculation of systemic vascular resistance. It provides important information relating to the left ventricular afterload and allows rational application of vasoactive (e.g., vasoconstrictor, vasodilator) and inotropic drugs. Measurement of cardiac output may be carried out by the Fick method (using oxygen extraction) or thermodilution using a pulmonary artery flow-directed catheter. In neonates, the latter technique is rarely used because shunts at the atrial and ductal level introduce errors when interpreting the results.

Pulsed Doppler determinations of cardiac output provide reasonable noninvasive estimates of cardiac output for clinical application in neonates. Cardiac output, normalized for body weight, in neonates between 780 and 4740 g at birth, remains fairly constant, changing approximately 10% over the weight range.[40] The range of cardiac output in both full-term and preterm neonates is 220 to 350 mL/kg/min, two- to threefold greater than in adults.[40,41] Between birth and the end of the first year, mean cardiac output normalized for body weight (or surface area), remains fairly constant at $204 \pm 45$ mL/kg/min.[42] The relatively large cardiac output (mL/min/kg) in neonates reflects their greater metabolic rate (expressed per kilogram) and oxygen consumption compared with adults. Basal metabolic rate has been shown to increase as size decreases in all species[43] (see Chapter 6).

Pulsed Doppler estimation of cardiac output has also been found useful in assessing left ventricular myocardial dysfunction in neonates after perinatal asphyxia and acidosis, as well as its response to therapy.[35,44,45] In older children, measurements of cardiac output are necessary in circulatory shock.[46] New noninvasive techniques using changes in impedance may be useful in the future (see Chapter 51).

## NORMAL ELECTROCARDIOGRAPHIC FINDINGS FROM INFANCY TO ADOLESCENCE

The P wave reflects atrial depolarization and varies little with age. The PR interval increases with age (mean value for the first year is 0.10 second, increasing to 0.14 second at 12 to 16 years).[47] The duration of the QRS complex increases with age, but prolongation greater than 0.10 second is abnormal at any age.

At birth, the QRS axis is right sided, reflecting the predominant right ventricular intrauterine development. It moves leftward in the first month as left ventricular muscle hypertrophies. Thereafter, the QRS follows a gradual change away from the initial marked right-sided axis.

In addition, T waves are upright in all chest leads. Within hours, they become isoelectric or inverted over the left chest; by the seventh day, the T waves are inverted in $V_{4R}$ ($V_4$ position under the right clavicle), $V_1$, and across to $V_4$; from then on, the T waves remain inverted over the right chest until adolescence, when they become upright over the right side of the chest again. Failure of T waves to become inverted in $V_{4R}$ and $V_1$ to $V_4$ by 7 days may be the earliest electrocardiographic evidence of right ventricular hypertrophy.[48,49]

# Renal System

The complex development of the human kidney begins in week 4 of gestation and continues into adulthood. Serious renal malfunctioning is usually associated with growth retardation.

Urine production begins in utero at 10 to 12 weeks of gestation and is excreted into the amniotic cavity, helping to maintain amniotic fluid volume. The fetus maintains its metabolic homeostasis through the placenta. It is only after birth that the kidney assumes this responsibility. More than 90% of neonates will have voided urine within the first 24 hours after birth. All normal infants should have voided by 48 hours after birth.[50]

Tubular function begins to develop after 34 weeks of gestation and increases during the first two years of life.[51] The number and function of the $Na^+/K^+$-ATPase transporters, are reduced at birth (activity increases 5- to 10-fold during the postnatal period). All transporters reliant on the $Na^+$ gradient are also reduced in function. The renal tubular threshold is decreased for sodium (identifying the risk for hyponatremia), for glucose (increased risk for osmotic polyuria), and for bicarbonates (increased risk for metabolic acidosis).

Nephrogenesis is complete by 36 weeks of gestation. Renal blood flow and glomerular filtration rate (GFR) are reduced and correlate with gestational age. GFR is 20% to 25% of adult levels at term. They increase rapidly in the postnatal period due to an increase in cardiac output and a decrease in renal vascular resistance.[52] Adult rates are achieved by approximately two years of age[53] (see Fig. 6-11). A reduced GFR significantly affects the neonate's ability to excrete saline and water loads, as well as drugs. At birth, the serum creatinine concentration reflects the maternal concentration, but decreases during the first days of life. Over the course of early childhood, creatinine clearance slowly increases, reaching adult values between 2 and 3 years of age. Due to the rapid growth and increase in muscular mass, normal serum creatinine values increase with age and are greater in males.

In utero, the fetus maintains a mild respiratory acidosis, with a similar plasma bicarbonate concentration, but a greater $PaCO_2$ than its mother. After birth, infants have a reduced plasma bicarbonate concentration and $PaCO_2$ than older children and adults. They have a comparatively greater basal acid production and are less able to respond to an acid load. Endogenous acid production in small children is between 50% and 100% greater per kilogram when compared with adults. This is primarily due to the deposition of $Ca^{2+}$ in bone, a process that produces 0.5 to 1 mEq per liter of acid per day. Bicarbonate absorption from the gastrointestinal tract is an important source of base to neutralize this nonvolatile acid, and in part, explains the tendency of infants to become profoundly acidotic when suffering from gastroenteritis. The infant or small child is living near its limit of acid compensation and is therefore prone to develop acidosis during the course of an acute illness or starvation.

Neonates and preterm infants are obligate salt losers; they cannot excrete a large salt load or concentrate urine effectively. Immaturity of distal tubular function and relative hypoaldosteronism explain the risk of hyperkalemia in preterm infants.

# Digestive and Endocrine System

## HEPATIC SYSTEM

Development of the liver and bile ducts begins as an outgrowth of the foregut; by 10 weeks of gestation, the biliary tract has completed its development. The vitelline veins give rise to the portal and hepatic veins. Hepatic sinusoids form the ductus venosus, the bridge between the hepatic vein and the inferior vena cava. Most umbilical venous blood from the placenta passes through the ductus venosus to the inferior vena cava. The remainder passes via the portal vein through the liver to the hepatic veins. The portal venous drainage to the left lobe is less than to the right lobe, leading to a relative underdevelopment of the left lobe. The ductus venosus closes soon after birth.

At 12 weeks of gestation there is evidence of gluconeogenesis and protein synthesis; at 14 weeks, glycogen is found in liver cells. Although by late gestation liver cell morphology is similar to that of adults, the functional development of the liver is immature in neonates and more so in preterm infants. The liver has a major role in metabolism, controlling carbohydrate, protein, and lipid delivery to the tissues. Toward the end of pregnancy, large amounts of glycogen appear in the liver, and, as a result, preterm and small-for-gestational-age (SGA) infants with smaller stores of glycogen may develop hypoglycemia. Bile acid secretion in neonates is reduced, and malabsorption of fat occurs.

The liver is the site for the synthesis of proteins; this process is active in fetal and neonatal life. In fetal life, the main serum protein is alpha-fetoprotein. This protein first appears at 6 weeks of gestation and reaches a peak at 13 weeks. Albumin synthesis starts at 3 to 4 months of gestation and approaches adult values at birth; in preterm infants, the level is reduced. Proteins involved in clotting are also formed in the liver but their concentrations in preterm and full-term neonates are less than normal for the first few days after birth. Hematopoiesis occurs in the fetal liver, with peak activity at 7 months of gestation. After 6 weeks of age, hematopoiesis is confined to the bone marrow except under pathologic conditions, such as hemolytic anemia (see Chapter 28).

The capacity to enzymatically break down proteins is reduced at birth. This is particularly important in preterm infants, when the intake of a large protein load can result in dangerous levels of serum amino acid concentrations. In the first weeks of life, drug metabolism is less efficient than in later life. In addition to less effective hepatic metabolism, altered drug binding by serum proteins and immature renal function contribute to the problem (see Chapter 6).

### Physiologic Jaundice

Hyperbilirubinemia (defined as a total serum bilirubin level >5 mg/dL) is an especially important problem in neonates. About 60% of term and 80% of preterm neonates develop jaundice in the first week of life, with a total bilirubin concentration greater than 5 mg/dL.[54] The mechanisms for producing jaundice are outlined in Table 2-9.[55,56] In term neonates, the normal total bilirubin concentration is usually less than 5 mg/dL (86 μmol/L), rarely >12 mg/dL without a risk factor and peaks at 3 to 4 days. In preterm infants, the bilirubin concentration peaks at 10 to 12 mg/dL on the fifth to seventh postnatal day. After this period, the concentration gradually decreases reaching adult values (less than 2 mg/dL) by 1 to 2 months in both term and preterm infants. The concentration of indirect bilirubin is also increased in the first few days after birth. The cause of nonhemolytic physiologic hyperbilirubinemia is excessive bilirubin production from breakdown of red blood cells and increased enterohepatic circulation of bilirubin with deficient hepatic conjugation due to depressed glucuronyl transferase activity. The relationship between breast feeding and hyperbilirubinemia has been well documented. It is usually delayed in onset (after the third day of life), its cause remains unclear, and it occurs in about 1% of

| TABLE 2-9 Causes of Jaundice in Neonates |
| --- |
| Excess bilirubin production |
| Impaired uptake of bilirubin |
| Impaired conjugation of bilirubin |
| Defective bilirubin excretion |
| Increased enterohepatic circulation of bilirubin |

**TABLE 2-10** Pathologic Causes of Jaundice in Neonates

| |
|---|
| Antibody-induced hemolysis (Rh and ABO) |
| Hereditary red blood cell disorders (e.g., glucose-6-phosphate dehydrogenase deficiency, which gives rise to hemolysis from drugs or infection) |
| Infections (e.g., neonatal hepatitis, sepsis, severe urinary tract infections) |
| Hemorrhage into the body (e.g., intracerebral) |
| Biliary atresia |
| Metabolic (e.g., hypothyroidism, galactosemia) |

breastfeeding infants. An earlier hypothesis ascribing it to inhibition of glucuronyl transferase by $3\alpha$, $20\beta$-pregnanediol activity has not been substantiated.

Important pathologic causes of jaundice in neonates are presented in Table 2-10. The relative rarity of cholestasis is in sharp contrast with the very common finding of jaundice during the first weeks of life, and therefore, a false diagnosis of physiologic or breast milk jaundice is easily made. Symptoms indicative of cholestasis such as dark urine and pale stools are often unrecognized.[57]

Once the distinction between physiologic and hemolytic hyperbilirubinemia has been made, the underlying cause can then be treated and efforts can be directed at preventing bilirubin encephalopathy (kernicterus) by the use of phototherapy and, in selected cases, exchange transfusions. Phototherapy reduces serum bilirubin concentrations by converting bilirubin through structural photoisomerization and photooxidation into excretable products.[58] A possible relationship between neonatal blue-light phototherapy and the development of benign or malignant melanocyte lesions has been suggested[59]; further studies are required to clarify this concern.

Sick preterm infants are especially at risk for kernicterus and are more aggressively treated at reduced bilirubin concentrations than full-term infants. Increasingly common is a form of cholestatic jaundice in LBW infants receiving prolonged hyperalimentation. Its mechanism is unclear, but it may be due to inhibition of bile flow by amino acids.[60-63] Future therapy for hyperbilirubinemia in LBW infants may include the use of tin-mesoporphyrin, which inhibits the production of bilirubin.[64,65]

## GASTROINTESTINAL TRACT

In an embryo, the digestive tract consists of the developing foregut and hindgut. These rapidly elongate so that a loop of gut is forced into the yolk sac. At 5 to 7 weeks, this loop twists around the axis of the superior mesenteric artery and returns to the abdominal cavity. Maturation occurs gradually from the proximal to the distal end. Blood vessels and nerves (Auerbach and Meissner plexuses) are developed by 13 weeks of gestation, and peristalsis begins. The pancreas arises from two outgrowths of the foregut; a diverticulum of the foregut gives rise to the liver.

Enzyme levels of enterokinase and lipase increase with gestational age but are lower at birth compared with older children. Full-term neonates and preterm infants handle protein loads reasonably well, although preterm infants may have difficulty with large loads. Fat digestion is limited, particularly in preterm infants, who absorb only 65% of adult levels. Neonatal duodenal motility undergoes marked maturational changes between 29 and 32 weeks of gestation. This is one factor limiting tolerance of enteral feeding before 29 to 30 weeks of gestation. Central nervous system abnormalities will delay these maturational changes.[66]

Swallowing is a complex process that is under central and peripheral control. The reflex is initiated in the medulla, through cranial nerves to the muscles that control the passage of food through the pharyngoesophageal sphincter. In the process, the tongue, soft palate, pharynx, and larynx all are smoothly coordinated. Any pathologic condition of these structures can interfere with normal swallowing. Neuromuscular incoordination, however, is more likely to be responsible for any dysfunction. This is particularly evident when the central nervous system has sustained damage either before or during delivery.

Lower esophageal pressures are reduced at birth but increase steadily reaching adult values 3 to 6 weeks postnatally. Daily vomiting or "spitting up" may be seen in half of all infants between 0 and 3 months of age and up to two-thirds of 4- to 6-month-old infants.[67] Most of these infants suffer no ill effect ("happy spitters") and grow well.[68] This condition usually begins in the first weeks of life and resolves spontaneously by 9 to 24 months of age as solid food is introduced and the child assumes the upright position. Between 1:300 and 1:1000 infants have reflux that is significant enough to warrant treatment to prevent complications.[69]

Meconium is the material contained in the intestinal tract before birth. It consists of desquamated epithelial cells from the intestinal tract, bile, pancreatic and intestinal secretions, and water (70%). Meconium is usually passed in the first few hours after birth; virtually all term neonates pass their first stool by 48 hours. However, passage of the first stool is usually delayed in LBW neonates, probably because of immaturity of bowel motility and lack of gut hormones due to delayed enteral feeding. Meconium ileus occurs in cystic fibrosis or Hirschsprung disease.[58]

The gastrointestinal transit time in the infant is less than that of an adult and increases with age. The normal physiologic range of stool frequency varies greatly (from 10 times a day to 1-2 times a week[70] and more often in breastfed infants. The frequency of bowel movements gradually declines over the first years of life, reaching adult habits at about 4 years of age.

Necrotizing enterocolitis is an acquired gastrointestinal disease associated with significant morbidity and mortality in prematurely born neonates. The disease affects about 10% of preterm neonates weighing less than 1500 g or 1% to 5% of all neonatal intensive care unit admissions (see also Chapters 35 and 36). Combined with enteral feeds and bacterial colonization, inflammatory mediators are released, leading to a propagated inflammatory response with both pro- and antiinflammatory influences.[71]

## PANCREAS

The placenta is impermeable to both insulin and glucagon. The islets of Langerhans in the fetal pancreas, however, secrete insulin from week 11 of fetal life; the amount of insulin secretion increases with age. After birth, insulin response is related to gestational and postnatal age and is more mature in term infants.

Maternal hyperglycemia, particularly when uncontrolled, results in hypertrophy and hyperplasia of the fetal islets of Langerhans. This leads to increased levels of insulin in the fetus, affecting lipid metabolism and giving rise to a large, overweight infant characteristic of a mother with poorly controlled diabetes (infant of a diabetic mother, IDM). Hyperglycemia alone is not instrumental in this effect; IDM may also be the result of an increase in serum amino acids found in diabetic mothers. Hyperinsulinemia of the fetus persists after birth and may lead to rapid development of serious hypoglycemia. In addition to severe hypoglycemia, these infants have an increased incidence of congenital anomalies.

Infants who are SGA are frequently hypoglycemic, and this may be the result of malnutrition in utero. In addition, hepatic glycogen stores are inadequate, and deficient gluconeogenesis exists. Preterm infants may be hypoglycemic without demonstrable symptoms, necessitating close monitoring of blood glucose levels.

Full-term neonates undergo a metabolic adjustment postnatally with regard to glucose. Studies have defined values for glucose levels that should be cause for concern: plasma glucose levels less than 35 mg/dL in the first 3 hours of life; less than 40 mg/dL between 3 and 24 hours; and less than 45 mg/dL after 24 hours.[72] Others have defined hypoglycemia in full-term infants as a plasma glucose concentration of less than 30 mg/dL in the first day of life or less than 40 mg/dL in the second day of life.[73] It is important to recognize that infants may develop serious hypoglycemia that could lead to irreversible central nervous system damage, even though they demonstrate no symptoms. Other infants may present with convulsions, but signs may also be subtle (e.g., lethargy, somnolence, and jitteriness).

Hyperglycemia (plasma glucose 150 mg/dL or greater) occurs in stressed neonates, particularly LBW infants infused with glucose-containing solutions. Hyperglycemia commonly occurs in infants undergoing elective surgery under general anesthesia; infusion of glucose-containing solutions may increase the risk of hyperglycemia. Thus it is advisable that intraoperative glucose levels be monitored. A study in infants undergoing surgery under general anesthesia showed that postsurgical plasma glucose values were significantly greater than postinduction values; insulin changes were minimal.[74] The risk of hyperglycemia is considerably greater in infants weighing less than 1000 g compared with infants of 2000 g or more.[73] Hyperglycemia may also lead to osmotic diuresis and dehydration and has been associated with an increased incidence of intraventricular hemorrhage and a neurologic handicap.

## Hematopoietic and Immunologic System

The blood volume of a full-term neonate depends on the time of cord clamping, which modifies the volume of placental transfusion. The blood volume is 93 mL/kg when cord clamping is delayed after delivery, compared with 82 mL/kg with immediate cord clamping.[75,76] Within the first 4 hours after delivery, however, fluid is lost from the blood and the plasma volume contracts by as much as 25%. The larger the placental transfusion, the larger this loss of fluid in the first few hours after birth, with resultant hemoconcentration. The blood volume in preterm infants is greater (90 to 105 mL/kg) than it is in full-term infants because of increased plasma volume.

### HEMOGLOBIN

The normal hemoglobin range in the neonate is between 14 and 20 g/dL. The site of sampling must be considered when interpreting these values for the diagnosis of neonatal anemia or hyperviscosity syndrome. Capillary sampling (e.g., heel stick) generally overestimates the true hemoglobin concentration because of stasis in peripheral vessels that results in a loss of plasma and produces hemoconcentration. The net effect may be an increase in hemoglobin by as much as 6 g/dL As a result, venipuncture is preferred over capillary sampling. In 1% of infants,

fetal-maternal transfusion before the umbilical cord is cut may explain many of the "lower normal" hemoglobin values reported.

Erythropoietic activity from the bone marrow decreases immediately after birth in both full-term and preterm infants. The cord blood reticulocyte count of 5% persists for a few days and declines below 1% by 1 week. This is followed by a slight increase to 1% to 2% by the 12th week, where it remains throughout childhood. Preterm infants have greater reticulocyte counts (up to 10%) at birth. Abnormal reticulocyte values reflect hemorrhage or hemolysis.

In term infants, the hemoglobin concentration decreases during the 9th to 12th week to reach a nadir of 10 to 11 g/dL (hematocrit 30% to 33%) and then increases. This decrease in hemoglobin concentration is due to a decrease in erythropoiesis and to some extent due to a shortened life span of the red blood cells. In preterm infants, the decrease in the hemoglobin level is greater and is directly related to the degree of prematurity; also, the nadir is reached earlier (4 to 8 weeks).[77] In infants weighing 800 to 1000 g, the decrement may reach a very small concentration, 8 g/dL. This "anemia" (physiologic anemia of the newborn) is a normal physiologic adjustment to extrauterine life. Despite the reduction in hemoglobin, the oxygen delivery to the tissues may not be compromised because of a shift of the oxygen-hemoglobin dissociation curve (to the right), secondary to an increase of 2,3-diphosphoglycerate.[78] In addition, fetal hemoglobin is replaced by adult-type hemoglobin, which also results in a shift in the same direction. In neonates, especially preterm infants, reduced hemoglobin concentrations may be associated with apnea and tachycardia.[79] Vitamin E administration does not prevent anemia of prematurity; no significant difference was noted between vitamin E–supplemented and unsupplemented groups in terms of hemoglobin concentration, reticulocyte and platelet counts, or erythrocyte morphology in infants at 6 weeks of age.[80] Infants with anemia of prematurity have been found to have an inadequate production of erythropoietin (the primary regulator in erythropoiesis). Some centers are now using recombinant human erythropoietin in VLBW infants to stimulate erythropoiesis and decrease the need for transfusions.[81,82]

After the third month, the hemoglobin concentration stabilizes at 11.5 to 12 g/dL, until about 2 years of age. The hemoglobin values of full-term and preterm infants are comparable after the first year. Thereafter, there is a gradual increase in the hemoglobin concentration to mean values at puberty of 14 g/dL for females and 15.5 g/dL for males.

### LEUKOCYTE AND IMMUNOLOGY

The white blood cell count may normally reach 21,000/mm$^3$ in the first 24 hours of life and 12,000/mm$^3$ at the end of the first week, with the number of neutrophils equaling the number of lymphocytes. It then decreases gradually, reaching adult values at puberty. At birth, neutrophil granulocytes predominate but rapidly decrease in number so that during the first week of life and through 4 years of age the lymphocyte is the predominant cell. After the fourth year, the values approximate an adult's. Neonates have an increased susceptibility to bacterial infection, which is related in part to immaturity of leukocyte function. Sepsis may be associated with a minimal leukocyte response or even with leukopenia. Spurious increases in the white blood cell content may be due to drugs (e.g., epinephrine). The incidence of neonatal sepsis correlates inversely with gestational age and may be as great as 58% in VLBW infants.[83]

## PLATELETS

Thrombocytopenia is a common hematologic finding in neonates, occurring in 1% to 2% of healthy term neonates.[84] Mechanical ventilation has been associated with a significant decrease in the platelet count in neonates.[85] There appears to be an inverse correlation between gestational age or birth weight and the severity of platelet reduction. A study of neonatal thrombocytopenia and its impact on hemostatic integrity showed that thrombocytopenic infants are at greater risk for bleeding than equally sick nonthrombocytopenic infants (see Chapter 18).

## COAGULATION

At birth, vitamin K–dependent factors (i.e., II, VII, IX, and X) are 20% to 60% of adult values; in preterm infants, the values are even less. The result is prolonged prothrombin times, normally encountered in full-term and preterm infants. Synthesis of vitamin K–dependent factors occurs in the liver, which, being immature, leads to relatively lower levels of the coagulation factors, even with the administration of vitamin K. It takes several weeks for the levels of coagulation factors to reach adult values; the deficit is even more pronounced in preterm infants. Vitamin K prophylaxis has been evaluated,[86] and the findings show that the majority of cases of neonatal vitamin K deficiency occur in normal neonates. Thus, all neonates should receive prophylactic vitamin K soon after birth to prevent hemorrhagic disease of the neonate. Its omission could lead to serious and life-threatening consequences, especially if surgery is undertaken. However, in theory, the increasing risk of bleeding is balanced by the protective effects of physiologic deficiencies of coagulation inhibitors, as well as by the decreased fibrinolytic capacity. Developmental hemostasis should be considered, as well as laboratory variations of coagulation tests that may render any diagnosis of bleeding disorder in infants difficult to establish.[87]

Infants of mothers who have received anticonvulsant drugs during pregnancy may develop a serious coagulopathy similar to that encountered with vitamin K deficiency.[88] Vitamin $K_1$ administered to neonates usually reverses this bleeding tendency, but deaths have occurred despite therapy. Other risk factors include maternal use of drugs such as warfarin, rifampin, and isoniazid. Breastfeeding may also be associated with severe vitamin K deficiency.

## POLYCYTHEMIA

Neonatal polycythemia (central hematocrit greater than 65%) occurs in 3% to 5% of full-term neonates.[89] Using M-mode echocardiography, a study of neonates demonstrated an increase in PVR with hyperviscosity.[90] Partial exchange transfusion to reduce the hematocrit and decrease the blood viscosity improves systemic and pulmonary blood flow and oxygen transport, although one review questioned the efficacy when the exchange transfusion was conducted after 6 hours of life in asymptomatic infants.[91] The increased organ blood flow should prevent the cardiovascular and neurologic symptoms associated with the hyperviscosity syndrome.

# Neurologic Development and Cognitive Development Issues

## NEUROLOGIC DEVELOPMENT

Reduction of perinatal mortality during the past decade has not resulted in the expected reduction in the prevalence of cerebral palsy (1 : 500 live births). The most common etiologies of cerebral palsy are perinatal ischemic stroke, white matter disorder, and intrauterine inflammation.[92] Less than 5% of cerebral palsy results from perinatal asphyxia. The strongest predictors of cerebral palsy appear to be congenital anomaly, low birth weight, low placental weight, multiple fetuses, or abnormal fetal position before labor and delivery.[93]

The nervous system is anatomically complete at birth; functionally it remains immature with the continuation of myelination and synaptogenesis. Myelination is usually complete by 7 years of age. An infant's normal mental development depends on the maturation of the central nervous system. This development may be affected by physical illness, inadequate psychosocial support, or bad nutrition conditions in preterm babies. In a randomized trial of diet in preterm babies, a suboptimal diet resulted in reduced intelligence quotients 7 to 8 years later.[94]

Recent controversies concerning the potential adverse effects of anesthesia on the developing brain show how delicate this organ is and how its development may be affected by environmental agents[95,96] (see Chapter 23).

The rate of brain growth is different from the growth rate of other body systems. The brain has two growth spurts, neuronal cell multiplication between 15 and 20 weeks of gestation, and glial cell multiplication commencing at 25 weeks and extending into the second year of life. Myelination continues into the third year. Malnutrition during this phase of neural development may have profound handicapping effects.

Plasma membrane transport selectively promotes the passage of essential substrates such as glucose, organic acids, and amino acids across the blood-brain barrier. Hypoxemia and ischemia may lead to a breakdown in this barrier, with resulting edema and increased intracranial pressure. Injury to the blood-brain barrier may result from abnormal entry of calcium or formation of free radicals. Further studies of the mechanism of this breakdown will lead to rational approaches to therapy. In preterm infants stressed by hypoxia, the blood-brain barrier may become particularly permeable to the water-soluble unbound bilirubin, with possible damage to the brain.[97]

Normal neonates show various primitive reflexes, which include the Moro response and grasp reflex. Milestones of development are useful indicators of mental development and possible deviations from normal. It should be appreciated, however, that these milestones represent the *average,* and infants can vary in their rates of maturation of different body functions and still be within the normal range.[98] The Denver Developmental Screening Test is useful for assessing these milestones. The test focuses on four areas: (1) gross motor function, (2) fine motor and adaptive skills, (3) language, and (4) personal and social skills. Developing infants rapidly acquire motor skills. For effective movement, an infant needs postural control, which develops in a cephalocaudal direction. It starts with head control and progresses to sitting, standing, walking, and finally running (Table 2-11).

**TABLE 2-11** Relationship of Motor Milestones to Age

| Motor Milestone | Age |
| --- | --- |
| Supports head | 3 months |
| Sits alone | 6 months |
| Stands alone | 12 months |
| Balances on one foot | 3 years |

**TABLE 2-12** Relationship of Fine Motor/Adaptive Milestones to Age

| Fine Motor/Adaptive Milestones | Age |
| --- | --- |
| Grasps rattle | 3 months |
| Passes cube hand to hand | 6 months |
| Pincer grip | 1 year |
| Imitates vertical line | 2 years |
| Copies circle | 3 years |

**TABLE 2-13** Relationship of Language Milestones to Age

| Language Milestones | Age |
| --- | --- |
| Squeals | 1.5-3 months |
| Turns to voice | 6 months |
| Combines two words | 1.5 years |
| Composes short sentences | 2 years |
| Gives entire name | 3 years |

**TABLE 2-14** Relationship of Personal-Social Milestones to Age

| Personal-Social Milestones | Age |
| --- | --- |
| Smiles spontaneously | 3 months |
| Feeds self crackers | 6 months |
| Drinks from cup | 1 year |
| Plays interactive games | 2 years |

Adaptive skills are performed through well-coordinated fine motor movements (Table 2-12). Abnormal development may be reflected in a delay in appearance of a particular milestone or in its pathologic persistence with maturation in a child. For example, at 20 weeks, a child reaches and retrieves objects, frequently placing them in his or her mouth. As an infant matures, however, this behavior pattern usually ceases at 12 to 13 months of age; in infants with a developmental delay, this practice may continue much longer.

Language development correlates closely with cognitive skills (Table 2-13). Personal and social skills are modified by environmental factors and cultural patterns (Table 2-14). Development of walking, speech, and sphincter control are most important. For appropriate evaluation consider familial patterns, level of intelligence, and physical illness. Deafness may cause delayed speech.

## DEVELOPMENTAL ISSUES

Children with developmental issues are delayed in *many* aspects of both cognitive and motor development. Smiling, vocalization, sitting, walking, speech, and sphincter control are delayed. When there is a delay in the eye following an object and the head turning in response to sound, blindness and deafness may erroneously be diagnosed. Drooling, common in young infants, is frequently prolonged for years in neurologically delayed children. Initially, a mentally handicapped infant appears to be inactive and may be seen as a "good child." The child later demonstrates constant and sometimes uncontrollable overactivity. In diagnosing a developmental abnormality, anesthesiologists must be aware of possible pitfalls: Infants born prematurely will be delayed and should be assessed in terms of their conceptional age. Infants with cerebral palsy or sensory deficits (auditory and visual) may have normal mental development, but the handicap may interfere with assessment of mental status. The effects of drugs should be considered (e.g., barbiturates for epilepsy).

## ACKNOWLEDGMENT

The author wishes to acknowledge the prior contributions of Robert M. Insoft and I. David Todres to this chapter.

## REFERENCES

Please see www.expertconsult.com

# Perioperative Behavioral Stress in Children

ZEEV N. KAIN, MICHELLE A. FORTIER, AND LINDA C. MAYES

INTEREST IN CHILDREN'S PERIOPERATIVE behavior has increased dramatically over the past 20 years. Specifically, the recognition of the importance of developmental factors in perioperative research has created a dramatic growth of investigation in this area. In this chapter, we discuss developmental considerations that are relevant to the child's perioperative experience (cognitive development, attachment and separation, temperament). We then offer a review and synthesis of recent data on preoperative anxiety and maladaptive behavioral and cognitive outcomes associated with surgery and anesthesia.

## Developmental Issues

### COGNITIVE DEVELOPMENT AND UNDERSTANDING OF ILLNESS

The perioperative period is stressful for many individuals undergoing surgery, and this is especially true for children. Children's stress during the perioperative period results from multiple sources, one of which is a limited understanding of illness and the need for surgery. Early developmental theorists (e.g., Piaget,[1,2] Werner[3]) suggested that a child's understanding of illness changes qualitatively as cognitive maturation occurs. The most widely cited model for understanding a child's perspective on illness posits that the child's understanding of illness evolves from prelogical explanations, such as phenomenism (e.g., magical thinking), to concrete-logical explanations, such as contamination (e.g., eating bad food), to formal-logical explanations (e.g., physiologic causes), and differences in understanding occur according to the child's differentiation between the self and others.[4]

Children's understanding of the treatments for illnesses is thought to follow a similar developmental pattern. In terms of surgery, a child's concepts are particularly underdeveloped. Young children have difficulty defining "an operation," suggesting that it is the same as being sick, going for a doctor's checkup, or taking a nap.[5] Given these developmental considerations, it is not surprising that young children are more likely to have misconceptions about hospitalization and surgery than are older children and adults,[6] and therefore are at unique and disparate risk for perioperative stress.

### ATTACHMENT

Attachment style is another developmental consideration unique to children in the perioperative setting. Although adults also undergo separation from family, the separation of children from their parents is particularly stressful and affected by the parent-child relationship.

Coping with separation is a lifelong challenge that is inevitable and necessary for a child's normal, healthy development.[7] Separation experiences, such as saying good-bye at school or sleeping overnight at a friend's house, facilitate normal childhood psychological growth and personality organization by mobilizing opportunities for learning and adaptation. Other separation experiences, especially those occurring in the context of loss, illness, or other stressors, can precipitate states of confusion, anger, and anxiety. Brief separations, such as those associated with surgery, are most stressful for infants, toddlers, and preschool-aged children. Indeed, for school-aged children, responses to separation may reflect, in part, response patterns established early in the preschool years.[7] For children with biologically based vulnerabilities, such as a sensitivity to novelty and changes in routines, even expected separations may impose a greater degree of stress than for less sensitive children.[7] Similarly, for children with developmental delay, separation may be experienced with a degree of anxiety and developmental stress more like that experienced by a younger child.

Attachment affects a child's response to separation and is shaped through early experiences with the primary caregiver. Through these interactions, an infant has the opportunity to develop a sense of trust and security in the reliability and predictability of his or her relationship and the world.[8] The style of attachment exhibited by infants is evident in their responses to brief separations from the primary caregiver and is conceptualized as *secure*, *insecure*, or *anxious*.

Children who are more "securely attached" to their parents deal more adaptively with the stress of brief separation and with the novelty of the hospital experience. Such children are more willing to explore their world and respond positively to their caregivers' return, using the caregivers as a secure, stable base from which to approach strangers and new situations.[9,10] In contrast, children classified as "anxiously attached" to their parents tend to be distressed in unfamiliar situations, like the perioperative environment, even in the presence of their caregivers. When their parents return after brief separations, these infants exhibit anger and distress and avoid physical contact. Another form of "insecure attachment" is avoidance. Avoidant children do not explore their surroundings as much as securely attached infants, rarely show distress at separation, and tend to ignore their parents on reuniting. Conversely, "insecurely attached" infants are more easily distressed by even brief separations and spend more time trying to stay close to their parents. They are less likely to explore and adapt positively to new situations.

## TEMPERAMENT

Responses of young children to the stress of the perioperative period also reflect the child's temperament. Temperament refers to stable emotional and behavioral responses (e.g., emotionality, activity, attention, reactivity, sociability, etc.) that appear in infancy and are thought to be primarily genetic in nature.[11] Three main dimensions have been proposed to classify infant temperament: emotionality, activity, and sociability.[12] *Emotionality* refers to the ease with which an infant becomes aroused or anxious, especially in situations that might lead to fear, such as perioperative settings. *Activity* refers to the infant's customary level of energy and intensity of behavior. *Sociability* reflects the infant's tendency to approach or avoid others. These behavioral dimensions of temperament are also reflected in physiologic responses related to anxiety.[13,14] In long-term studies, infants who are inhibited in the face of novelty continue to be so through early school age.[15] Thus, temperament as a behavioral descriptor appears to characterize an enduring cluster of traits reflecting reactivity and anxiety regulation in the face of novelty.

In light of these issues, the child's developmental level is an important consideration in the perioperative period, especially as it relates to the child's perioperative behavior. The remainder of this chapter addresses specific behavioral issues related to surgery in children, including anxiety in the preoperative period as well as postoperative behavioral outcomes, such as emergence delirium, sleep, and other maladaptive behavioral changes.

# Preoperative Anxiety

Anxiety in children undergoing anesthesia and surgery is characterized by feelings of tension, apprehension, and nervousness.[16] This response is attributed to separating from parents, loss of control, uncertainty about anesthesia, and uncertainty about the surgery and its outcome.[16] It is estimated that 40% to 60% of children develop significant fear and anxiety before their surgery.[17] Furthermore, separation from parents and induction of anesthesia have been found to be the most stressful times during the surgical and anesthesia experience. Some children verbalize their fears explicitly, whereas others express their anxiety only by behavioral changes. Children may appear scared or agitated, breathe deeply, tremble, stop talking or playing, and start to cry. Some may wet or soil themselves, display increased motor tone, and actively attempt to escape from medical personnel.[18] These behaviors may give children some sense of control in the situation and thereby diminish the damaging effects of a sense of helplessness.[16,18] In addition to the behavioral manifestations detailed here, several studies have documented that anxiety before surgery is associated with neuroendocrine changes, such as increased serum cortisol, epinephrine, growth hormone, and adrenocorticotropic hormone levels, as well as increased natural killer cell activity.[19,20] Significant correlations between heart rate, blood pressure, and behavioral ratings of anxiety have also been reported.[21,22]

## RISK FACTORS

Preoperative anxiety is a clinically important phenomenon that should be treated as any other clinical phenomenon or disease. In epidemiologic terms, *all* diseases are characterized operationally by risk factors, interventions, and outcomes; preoperative anxiety is no exception. We review the phenomenon of preoperative anxiety using the classic epidemiologic model of a disease (Fig. 3-1).

Identifying the risk factors for preoperative anxiety is important because the routine use of pharmacologic and behavioral interventions is associated with both advantages and disadvantages. Routine administration of sedative premedication may increase indirect pharmacy costs, the need for nursing staff, and appropriately monitored bed space in the preoperative holding area. Children undergoing extremely short outpatient procedures may also experience delayed discharge. Similarly, behavioral preparation programs administered preoperatively are associated with increased hospital operational costs. Likewise, anxious children can use hospital resources that would be reduced with appropriate pharmacologic preparation. Thus, identifying children who are at a particularly high risk for developing extreme anxiety and distress before surgery would help guide the most effective use of limited resources.

Variation in children's behavioral responses to the perioperative experience has its origin in at least four domains:

- Age and developmental maturity
- Previous experience with medical procedures and illness
- Individual capacity for affect regulation and trait (baseline) anxiety
- Parental state (situational) and trait anxiety

Previous studies that examined the behavioral responses to induction of anesthesia in children did so in terms of these four domains.[23-27] Children between the ages of 1 and 5 years are at greatest risk for developing extreme anxiety and distress. This is not surprising because separation anxiety often does not peak until 1 year of age and children older than the age of 5 years can more easily cope with new and unpredictable situations. A history of previous stressful medical encounters, such as with previous hospitalization, affects how a child reacts to new medical encounters; these are important risk factors for preoperative anxiety. Children who are shy and inhibited, as identified by temperament tests, and those who lack good social adaptive abilities, are also at increased risk for developing anxiety and distress before surgery.[27]

Parental characteristics also have a strong influence on a child's behavior during the perioperative experience. Children of parents who are more anxious, children of parents who use avoidance coping mechanisms, and children of separated or divorced parents all appear to be at high risk for developing preoperative anxiety.[28] Because children of anxious parents are more likely to experience high levels of preoperative anxiety, it is important to identify the predictors of increased *parental* preoperative anxiety. Parent gender (mothers are more anxious than fathers[29]), the child's age (under 1 year), children with repeated hospital admissions, and the child's temperament are all predictors of increased parental preoperative anxiety.[28,30,31,32] Identification of children and parents who are at the greatest risk for preoperative anxiety

Behavioral perioperative stress

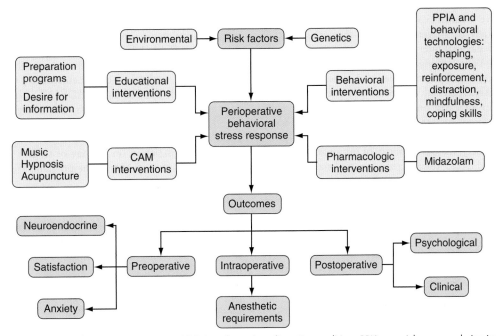

**FIGURE 3-1** Operational overview of perioperative anxiety. *CAM,* Complementary alternative medicine; *PPIA,* parental presence during induction of anesthesia.

and distress allows for appropriate intervention for this "at risk" population.

## BEHAVIORAL INTERVENTIONS

Pharmacologic (e.g., administration of premedications) and behavioral (e.g., psychological preparation programs) interventions are used to treat preoperative anxiety and distress in children and their parents.[17,33]

### Preoperative Preparation Programs

Psychological preparation for children undergoing anesthesia and surgery has been widely advocated. These preparation programs may provide narrative information, an orientation tour of the operative facility, role rehearsal using dolls, modeling using videotapes or a puppet show, child life preparation, or coping education and relaxation skills.[34,35,36]

Although there is general agreement in the medical community about the benefit of preparation programs, recommendations regarding the content of behavioral preoperative preparation differ widely. Early programs were information oriented and often incorporated modeling techniques using videos or a puppet show.[37,38] These techniques were augmented in the late 1980s with child life preparation and coping skills education.[35] Child life specialists are trained individuals who facilitate development of coping skills and the adjustment of children and parents to the perioperative environment by providing play experiences, presenting information about events and procedures, and establishing supportive relationships with children and parents.[36] Currently, the development of coping skills is considered the most effective preoperative intervention, followed by modeling, play therapy, operating room (OR) tour, and printed material.[39] Interestingly, coping skills preparation with child life specialists was associated with less anxiety on the day of surgery when compared to lesser rated techniques; however, no differences were found

immediately or up to 2 weeks after surgery.[40] Thus, from a cost-effectiveness point of view, one must decide whether the additional cost associated with child life specialists is justified by reduction of anxiety *only* during the preoperative period.

It is important that preparation programs are tailored to the individual, age-appropriate needs of each child. Several variables have been identified as influencing the response of children to preparation programs.[28] For example, children who are 6 years of age or older benefit most if they participate in a preparation program more than 5 days before the scheduled surgery and benefit least if the program is given only 1 day before surgery. In fact, older children prepared a week in advance showed an *increase* in anxiety level during and immediately after the preparation program, but demonstrated a gradual decrease in anxiety during the 5 days before the time of surgery.[41] To avoid increasing excessive anticipatory anxiety, older children should be given enough time to process the new information and to rehearse newly acquired coping skills. It is also important to realize that there may be a *negative* effect of a preparation program on children younger than 3 years of age. This may be a result of their inability to distinguish fantasy from reality.[1] A reality-based preparation program may do little to calm young children and may even exacerbate anxiety or sensitize the young child to the surgery. From age 3 to 6 years, children demonstrate an increasing ability to distinguish fantasy from reality and by the age of 6 this distinction is usually accomplished.[1] Therefore, to provide the most benefit, both the age of the child and timing must be factored into delivery of the program.

In addition to age and timing, previous experience in a hospital setting also influences the effectiveness of a preparation program. A child who was previously hospitalized is more likely to develop an exaggerated emotional response to a behavioral preoperative preparation program and the perioperative experience.[28,41-43] Information about what will occur, as demonstrated by sensory expectation and doll play, does *not* provide new information for these children. Furthermore, if the child has had a previous negative medical experience, the routine preparation may increase anxiety by triggering negative memories. In this case, alternative behavioral interventions, such as extensive individualized coping-skills training combined with desensitization and actual practice, may be better suited and indicated.[42]

Because increased parental preoperative anxiety has been shown to result in increased preoperative anxiety in their children, preparation programs for surgery should also be directed at parents.[23] Although various interventions are routinely used to reduce a child's anxiety, there is a paucity of information regarding interventions directed toward reducing parental anxiety.[44] One study demonstrated that parental preoperative anxiety decreased after viewing an educational videotape.[45] Most studies to date suggest that preoperative preparation programs for children reduce preoperative anxiety and enhance coping.[35,41,46]

Children whose parents have been taught to be active in distracting their child during stressful medical events may evidence lower anxiety compared to parents who receive no intervention.[47] Indeed, this was the case in a randomized controlled trial evaluating a family-centered behavioral preparation program (ADVANCE) (Table 3-1). Parents and children who received

ADVANCE were less anxious before and during induction of anesthesia than parents and children who did not receive this program. In fact, ADVANCE was as successful as midazolam in managing children's compliance with and anxiety at induction of anesthesia (Table 3-2).[48] It is important to note that ADVANCE also decreased the time spent in the postanesthesia care unit and decreased the analgesic requirements during the postoperative period. A major disadvantage of ADVANCE, however, is its high cost and personnel requirements. Accordingly, efforts to dismantle this multimodal intervention indicate that behavioral shaping through exposing children to the anesthesia mask before surgery and distraction on the day of surgery proved to be the most effective components of the program.[49]

### Parental Presence during Induction of Anesthesia

It is well established that most parents and children prefer to remain together during procedures such as immunization, bone marrow aspiration, and dental treatment.[50,51] Several survey studies have also indicated that most parents prefer to be present during induction of anesthesia regardless of the child's age or previous surgical experience.[52,53] This is even the case for those parents who have had previous experience with pharmacologic interventions. Indeed, parents of children undergoing repeated surgery were likely to request parental presence regardless of their experience with prior parental presence or premedication with midazolam.[54] That is, even if children were calm after midazolam during their first surgery, parents still preferred to be present during induction of anesthesia during subsequent surgeries.

It is important to note, however, that parental presence during induction of anesthesia (PPIA) does not necessarily equate with appropriate choice of interventions. For example, mothers who were most highly motivated to be present at induction of anesthesia also reported high levels of anxiety and their children were more distressed at induction.[55] Indeed, more than 90% of parents report some degree of anxiety during the anesthesia induction process.[56] The most upsetting factors include seeing their child become flaccid during induction and separation from their child.[56] This observation was confirmed by a study that examined heart rate, blood pressure, and skin conductance levels in mothers as they observed their child's induction of anesthesia.[57] Mothers

---

**TABLE 3-1** The ADVANCE Preoperative Preparation Program

**A**nxiety reduction

**D**istraction on the day of surgery

**V**ideo modeling and education before surgery

**A**dding parents to the child's surgical experience and promoting family-centered care

**N**o excessive reassurance—a suggestion made to parents for communication with children about surgery

**C**oaching of parents by researchers to help them succeed

**E**xposure/shaping of the child via induction mask practice (the mask placed over the child's nose and mouth to deliver anesthetic drugs)

Reproduced with permission from Kain ZN, Caldwell-Andrews AA, Mayes LC, et al. Family-centered preparation for surgery improves perioperative outcomes in children: a randomized controlled trial. Anesthesiology 2007;106:65-74.

---

**TABLE 3-2** Perioperative Outcomes of the ADVANCE Program

| | Study Group | | | | | |
| --- | --- | --- | --- | --- | --- | --- |
| | Control (n = 99) | Parental Presence (n = 94) | ADVANCE (n = 96) | Midazolam (n = 98) | P Value[‖] | Effect Size (95% CI)[¶] |
| **Children's Anxiety (mYPAS)** | | | | | | |
| Holding area | 36 ± 16 | 35 ± 16 | 31 ± 12* | 37 ± 17 | 0.001 | 0.54 (0.78-0.30) |
| Introduction of mask at induction | 52 ± 26 | 50 ± 26 | 43 ± 23[†] | 40 ± 24 | 0.018 | 0.33 (0.58-0.08) |
| **Postanesthesia Care Unit** | | | | | | |
| Fentanyl consumption (μg/kg) | 1.37 ± 2.00 | 0.81 ± 1.00 | 0.41 ± 1.00[‡] | 1.23 ± 2 | 0.016 | 0.54 (0.75-0.24) |
| Time until discharge (min) | 120 ± 48 | 122 ± 44 | 108 ± 46[§] | 129 ± 44 | 0.040 | 0.34 (0.60-0.09) |

Reproduced with permission from Kain ZN, Caldwell-Andrews AA, Mayes LC, et al. Family-centered preparation for surgery improves perioperative outcomes in children: a randomized controlled trial. Anesthesiology 2007;106:65-74.
CI, Confidence interval; mYPAS, modified Yale Preoperative Anxiety Scale.
ADVANCE group anxiety scores:
*Significantly less than those in all other groups, P < 0.01.
[†]Significantly less than those in the control and parental presence groups, P < 0.05.
[‡]Significantly less than those in the control and midazolam groups, P < 0.01.
[§]Significantly less than those in the midazolam group, P < 0.01.
[‖]P values for parental presence and control groups = 0.07.
[¶]Cohen's d effect sizes were calculated for the intervention group vs. other groups combined.

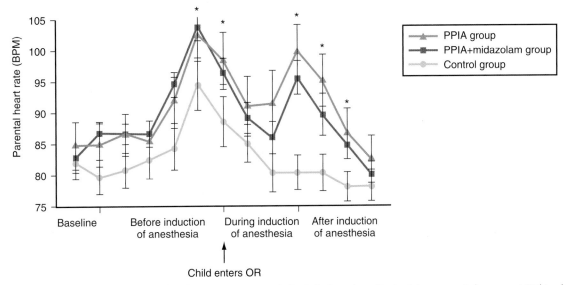

**FIGURE 3-2** Changes in parental heart rate from baseline measurement until after induction of anesthesia. Data are reported as mean ± SE (standard error). *Asterisks* indicate time points at which differences between groups are statistically significant ($P < 0.05$). *BPM,* Beats per minute; *OR,* operating room; *PPIA,* parental presence during induction of anesthesia. (From Kain ZN, Caldwell-Andrews AA, Mayes LC, et al. Parental presence during induction of anesthesia: physiological effects on parents. Anesthesiology 2003;98:58-64.)

who were present during induction of anesthesia showed a moderate increase in heart rate and blood pressure (Fig. 3-2). However, no cardiac arrhythmias or ischemic episodes were noted. Another study examined whether parental auricular acupuncture would reduce parental preoperative anxiety and thus allow children to benefit from parental presence during induction of anesthesia.[58] A multivariate model demonstrated that children whose mothers had received the acupuncture intervention were significantly less anxious on entrance to the OR and during placement of the anesthesia mask on their child's face.

Potential benefits from PPIA include minimizing the need for premedication and avoiding the screaming and struggling of the child that may result on separation from the parents. Whether PPIA decreases child anxiety during induction and affects the long-term behavior effects of surgery and anesthesia remain controversial. Common objections to PPIA include concern about disruption of the OR routine, compromising operative sterility, crowded ORs, and a possible adverse reaction of the parent. For some children, their behavioral response to stress may be more negative when a parent is present than when the parent is absent.[59] In several reports, PPIA resulted in disruptive behavior, parents refusing to leave the room when requested, and even removal of a child from the OR by a grandmother during the second stage of anesthesia.[60,61] However, one report has described a 4-year experience with 3086 children in a freestanding ambulatory surgery center in which no parent needed to be escorted from the OR because of undue anxiety and only two parents developed syncope, with prompt recovery.[62] Despite objections, the prevalence of PPIA is becoming more common in the United States. In fact, there has been an increase in the overall prevalence in PPIA from 1995 to 2002, and geographic differences in PPIA use decreased during the 7-year period (Fig. 3-3).[63,64]

The experimental evidence to date does not clearly support the routine use of PPIA.[65-67] Although early studies suggested reduced anxiety and increased cooperation if parents were present during induction,[68,69] more recent investigations indicate that routine PPIA may *not* always be beneficial.[65-67] Characteristics of

the parent and child have an impact on the effectiveness of parental presence. For example, older children (over 4 years), children with a "calm" and less active baseline temperament, parents with less situational anxiety, and parents with lower external locus of control benefit most from PPIA.[30,65] The match between parent and child anxiety level also appears to be important. Calm children with anxious parents do more poorly during induction when compared with calm children with calm parents or anxious children with either calm or anxious parents.[30] When interpreting the results of these studies, however, several factors should be considered. First, the design of a randomized controlled study, while considered a gold standard in research, may *not* reflect the practice of *all* anesthesiologists. That is, although a randomized controlled study is applicable to centers that offer PPIA for *all* parents, it may not be applicable to centers in which each request for PPIA is considered individually based on personality characteristics of each child and parent. Such centers may have different results with PPIA than were demonstrated in experimental studies. Second, allowing PPIA without adequate preparation of the parent may be counterproductive. Some parent behaviors, such as criticism, excessive reassurance, and commands, are associated with greater distress.[70]

Given these drawbacks, interest in this area has begun to shift toward an emphasis on what parents actually do during induction of anesthesia. The development of a new tool for assessing child and adult behavior in the perioperative setting (Perioperative Child-Adult Medical Procedure Interaction Scale [P-CAMPIS]) has been developed to facilitate such research (Fig. 3-4).[71] Preliminary validation of this measure indicates that parental behavior affects the child's anxiety during induction much as it affects a child's distress during immunizations.

## The Preoperative Interview

Although not obvious, the preoperative interview is a behavioral intervention that is routinely administered to *all* children undergoing anesthesia and surgery.[72] It is clear that anesthesiologists have an ethical and legal responsibility to disclose to children

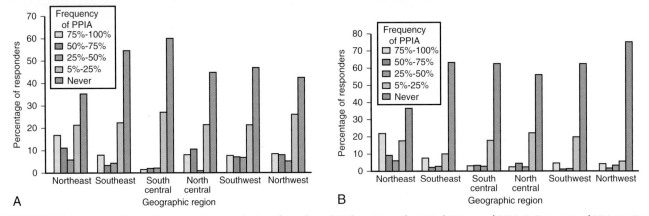

**FIGURE 3-3 A,** Frequency of parental presence during induction of anesthesia (*PPIA*) practice in the United States as of 2002. **B,** Frequency of PPIA practice in the United States as of 1995/1996. Data reported are medians (range, 0%-100%). (From Kain ZN, Caldwell-Andrews AA, Krivutza DM, et al. Trends in the practice of parental presence during induction of anesthesia and the use of preoperative sedative premedication in the United States, 1995-2002: Results of a follow-up national survey. Anesth Analg 2004;98:1252-9.)

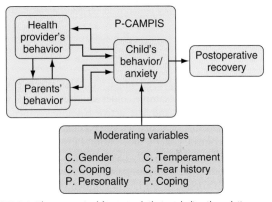

**FIGURE 3-4** The conceptual framework that underlies the relation between a child's preoperative anxiety, parental behaviors, health care provider's behaviors, moderating variables, and postoperative recovery. *C,* Child; *P,* parent; *P-CAMPIS,* Perioperative Child-Adult Medical Procedure Interaction Scale. (From Caldwell-Andrews AA, Blount RL, Mayes LC, Kain ZN. Behavioral interactions in the perioperative environment: a new conceptual framework and the development of the perioperative child-adult medical procedure interaction scale. Anesthesiology 2005;103:1130-5.)

and parents detailed anesthetic risk information when obtaining informed consent, but how far this disclosure must extend remains controversial. A common reason given for not providing detailed anesthetic risk information is that it may increase the child's or parents' anxiety. Comparative studies investigating anxiety levels in adult patients given a limited amount of information, versus more detailed information concerning procedural and anesthetic risks, report conflicting results. Although early studies provided mixed data regarding whether detailed information delivered preoperatively increased anxiety,[73-75] several studies in the United States and Australia have demonstrated that patients and parents who received detailed information, including numerical estimates of anesthesia-related complications, were no more anxious than those given minimal information regarding risks.[76-78] Furthermore, parents have expressed their desire to have as much perioperative information about their child's

surgery as possible,[77] and even children have expressed a desire for detailed perioperative information, including information about pain, anesthesia, and potential complications.[79] Thus, the presentation of very detailed anesthetic information of what might go wrong should not increase parental or patient anxiety and has the advantage of allowing for fully informed choices. It should be emphasized, however, that anesthesiologists should note the particular coping style of the parents. Parents use different strategies to cope with or handle difficult, unclear, or unpleasant life experiences, such as a child undergoing surgery. Whereas some parents try to avoid information about unpleasant or unclear situations ("avoidance behavior"), others may seek any available information ("monitoring behavior").[80] Although a "monitoring" parent will benefit from a large amount of perioperative information, an "avoiding" parent may react to the information with increased anxiety and distress. Thus, the amount of information provided should be tailored to the needs of the individual parent.

## HEALTH CARE PROVIDER INTERVENTIONS

In addition to behavioral interventions targeting children and their parents, a promising new line of research supports the use of behavioral interventions targeting health care providers—both anesthesiologists and nurses. Specifically, an empirically derived intervention titled Provider-Tailored Intervention for Perioperative Stress (P-TIPS) was shown to be successful in changing anesthesiologist and nurse behaviors in the perioperative setting and represents a new clinical avenue for decreasing perioperative anxiety in children.[81] The development of P-TIPS was based on research documenting that adult behaviors (parents and health care providers) affect children's distress during invasive medical procedures, including surgery. Specifically, the use of distraction, nonprocedural talk, and humor are conceptualized as "coping promoting" behaviors and have been shown to decrease children's distress.[82-88] Conversely, adults' use of reassurance, apology, empathy, criticism, or allowing the child too much control over the medical procedure are conceptualized as "distress promoting" behaviors and lead to increased distress in children.[82,87-90] With P-TIPS, a new behavior that affected child distress also emerged: medical reinterpretation (i.e., reconceptualizing medical experiences and equipment as nonthreatening) and was found to increase a child's coping when used with medical experiences that were in the child's immediate environment, but increase distress when used in reference to objects outside of the immediate environment.[87]

Preliminary investigation revealed that P-TIPS was successful at both increasing desired behaviors (coping promoting) and decreasing undesired (distress promoting) behaviors among health care providers.[81] Both resident and attending anesthesiologists were included in this study and evidenced behavior change, as did OR nurses, who were charged with not only changing their own behaviors, but with changing parent behaviors in the perioperative setting as well. In fact, nurses demonstrated appropriate behavior change and, in turn, parents demonstrated increases in desired and decreases in undesired behaviors. One important benefit to the type of approach offered by P-TIPS is that it is not necessary to conduct individual training with parents of children undergoing surgery, rather health care providers who interact with multiple children and parents are targeted, which reduces both logistical and financial constraints of behavioral interventions.

### PHARMACOLOGIC INTERVENTIONS

The primary goals of administering a premedication to children are to facilitate an anxiety-free separation from their parents and a smooth, stress-free induction of anesthesia. Other effects that may be achieved by pharmacologic preparation of the child include amnesia, anxiolysis, prevention of physiologic stress (e.g., avoiding tachycardia in patients with cyanotic congenital heart disease), and analgesia (see Chapter 4).

The pattern of use of sedative premedications in the United States has changed over the past decade. Premedication use varied widely among age groups and geographic locations in 1996.[63] Premedicant sedative drugs were least often prescribed for children younger than 3 years of age and most often prescribed for adults younger than 65 years of age (25% vs. 75%). When analyzed by geographic location, sedative premedications were used least often in the southwest and northeast regions and most often in the southeast region. A follow-up study revealed several interesting changes (Fig. 3-5).[64] Most notably, the overall number of children undergoing surgery with premedication increased from 30% to 50%. There was also significantly less geographic variability in premedication use in 2002 than there was in 1996. In both years, the most commonly used sedative premedicant in the

preoperative holding area was midazolam, followed by ketamine, transmucosal fentanyl, and meperidine. When data from several survey studies were reviewed, it was noted that anesthesiologists from the United States who allowed PPIA *least* used sedative premedication most frequently.[63,91] Thus, most anesthesiologists in the United States use either parental presence or sedative premedication to treat preoperative anxiety in children.

### PHARMACOLOGIC INTERVENTIONS VERSUS BEHAVIORAL INTERVENTIONS

When pharmacologic interventions are directly compared with behavioral interventions, children receiving a sedative are less anxious and more compliant than those who are accompanied to the OR by a parent.[67] Interestingly, parental anxiety is also decreased when the child receives a premedication. Examining both sedative premedication and PPIA revealed that a combination of PPIA and sedative premedication was more effective than medication alone for reducing parent anxiety and improving parent satisfaction.[92] However, PPIA offered no additional anxiolysis for children who received a sedative preoperatively. Nonetheless, parents who accompanied their sedated children into the operating rooms were themselves significantly less anxious and more satisfied both with the separation process and with the overall anesthetic, nursing, and surgical care provided. It is important to note that these parents had no preparation for their presence at anesthesia induction. Premedication combined with an advanced behavioral preparation resulted in similar outcomes on child and parent anxiety at induction and child compliance with induction.[48] Furthermore, children who received behavioral preparation evidenced significantly less emergence delirium and required less analgesia in the recovery room compared with children who received only premedication.

In conclusion, although sedative premedications are effective for treatment of preoperative anxiety, they should *not* be used routinely in all children undergoing surgery. Their use should be directed to children who are at a significant risk for the development of preoperative anxiety. Variables, such as age, duration of surgery, and potential recovery delays, should also be considered. However, it is important to not withhold premedication if that premedication would likely be of benefit to a selected child. For example, a child undergoing a very brief procedure who is very anxious would likely benefit from a premedication regardless of the negative effects on recovery and discharge.

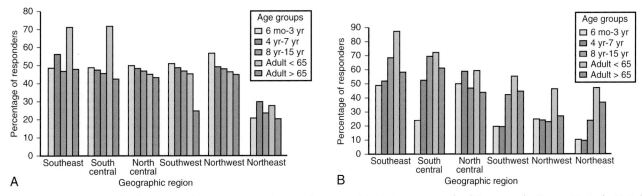

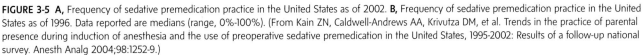

**FIGURE 3-5 A,** Frequency of sedative premedication practice in the United States as of 2002. **B,** Frequency of sedative premedication practice in the United States as of 1996. Data reported are medians (range, 0%-100%). (From Kain ZN, Caldwell-Andrews AA, Krivutza DM, et al. Trends in the practice of parental presence during induction of anesthesia and the use of preoperative sedative premedication in the United States, 1995-2002: Results of a follow-up national survey. Anesth Analg 2004;98:1252-9.)

# Postoperative Outcomes

Four decades ago, it was proposed that moderate levels of preoperative anxiety in adult patients were associated with good postoperative behavioral recovery, whereas low and high levels of preoperative anxiety were associated with poor behavioral recovery.[93] Although this theory is intriguing, these studies were based on descriptive data from nonrandom, limited samples and retrospective reports of questionable validity. Subsequent studies have reported a linear rather than a curvilinear relationship between anxiety level and postoperative behavioral recovery.[94,95,96,97] In addition, increased preoperative anxiety in adult patients correlates with increased postoperative pain, increased postoperative analgesic requirements, prolonged recovery and hospital stay, and behavioral changes after surgery.[23,98-101] Anxious children have been shown to experience significantly more pain both during the hospital stay and over the first 3 days at home[102] (Fig. 3-6). During home recovery, anxious children also consumed significantly more codeine and acetaminophen compared with nonanxious children. Anxious children also had a greater incidence of emergence delirium (9.7% vs. 1.5%), postoperative anxiety, and sleep problems compared with nonanxious children. The investigators concluded that preoperative anxiety in young children undergoing surgery is associated with a more painful postoperative recovery and a greater incidence of disrupted sleep and other problems.[102] Moreover, a recent study suggests that perioperative anxiety—not just preoperative anxiety—is associated with poorer surgical outcomes.[103] That is, children have traditionally been conceptualized as anxious or nonanxious via assessment of anxiety in children before surgery, such as in the presurgical holding area or at the point of induction in the OR. By contrast, this study examined anxiety in children throughout the perioperative continuum (pre- and postoperatively) and replicated findings of associations between perioperative anxiety and both postoperative pain and new-onset behavioral changes.[103]

The assumption that minimal preoperative anxiety predicts good postoperative outcomes underlies many interventions in which the aim is to reduce preoperative anxiety. To date, preoperative preparation studies in adult patients have used diverse postoperative outcome measures, including intensity of pain, analgesic requirements, postsurgical complications, length of hospital stay, patient satisfaction, blood cortisol levels, changes in blood pressure and heart rate, and behavioral indices of recovery.[96,104-111] Reviews of this research, while critical of the methodology, concluded that psychologically prepared adult patients

may have improved postoperative recovery.[99,104,112,113] As noted previously, children who received the ADVANCE preoperative program were less anxious preoperatively and experienced a reduced incidence of emergence delirium, had a briefer stay in the recovery area, reported less postoperative pain, and required fewer analgesics as compared with a control group.[48]

## EMERGENCE DELIRIUM

The first maladaptive behavioral change in children that may be evident after surgery is emergence delirium. This phenomenon is characterized by nonpurposeful restlessness and agitation, thrashing, crying or moaning, and disorientation. Published studies have reported up to 18% of all children undergoing surgery and anesthesia develop emergence delirium.[114] Factors such as young age, previous surgery, type of procedure, and type of anesthetic all affect the incidence of emergence delirium.[114,115] Preoperative anxiety has also been shown to be related to emergence delirium.[115,116] Furthermore, preoperative anxiety, emergence delirium, and postoperative maladaptive behavior changes have been shown to be closely related phenomena. One study found that the odds of children experiencing marked symptoms of emergence delirium increased in proportion with their preoperative anxiety scores, and that the odds of the onset of new maladaptive behavioral changes also increased with the presence of emergence delirium.[102] This finding is highly significant to practicing clinicians, who can now predict the development of adverse postoperative phenomena, such as emergence delirium and postoperative behavioral changes, based on levels of preoperative anxiety.

## SLEEP CHANGES

Changes in sleep patterns in the postoperative period have been well documented in adults and children. One study reported that 47% of children experienced sleep disturbances after anesthesia[117] and approximately 14% of children showed significant decreases in percentage of time spent asleep (in both REM and non-REM sleep) after surgery. The most common predictor of sleep difficulties after surgery has been postoperative pain,[118] but psychological variables have also been shown to be important. Specifically, parental personality measures of anxiety and child measures of externalizing behavior have both been found to predict sleep efficiency in children after surgery.

## OTHER BEHAVIORAL CHANGES

In addition to sleep, changes in daytime behavior in children after surgery and anesthesia have also been documented. A number of studies have indicated that up to 60% of children undergoing outpatient surgery may develop negative *postoperative* behavioral changes within 2 weeks after surgery.[119-121] These negative postoperative behaviors include sleep and eating disturbances, separation anxiety, apathy, withdrawal, and new-onset enuresis.[23,103,121] In fact, some children may develop long-lasting psychological effects that could have an impact on their responses to subsequent medical care. Interference with normal development has also been described.[122] A significant number of children demonstrate new negative behaviors postoperatively, such as new onset of general anxiety, nighttime crying, enuresis, separation anxiety, temper tantrums, and sleep or eating disturbances. These behaviors may occur in up to 44% of children 2 weeks after surgery; about 20% of these children continue to demonstrate negative behaviors up to 6 months postoperatively.[23] The postoperative negative behavioral changes are likely the result of an interaction between the distress the child experiences during the

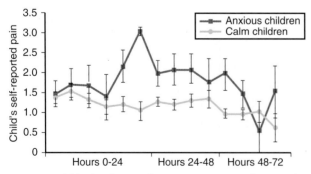

**FIGURE 3-6** Children's self-reported postoperative pain as a function of preoperative anxiety. (From Kain ZN, Mayes LC, Caldwell-Andrews AA, et al. Preoperative anxiety, postoperative pain, and behavioral recovery in young children undergoing surgery. Pediatrics 2006;118:651-8.)

perioperative period and the individual personality characteristics of the child. Previously, variables such as the age and temperament of the child and the state and trait anxiety of the parent have been identified as predictors for the occurrence of negative postoperative behavioral changes.[23] There is a paucity of data, however, regarding a possible association between the distress the child experiences during induction of anesthesia and the occurrence of these negative postoperative behavioral changes. One investigation concluded that extreme anxiety, such as that which occurs with a "stormy induction" of anesthesia, was associated with an increased incidence of postoperative negative behavioral changes.[123] The investigators recommend that anesthesiologists advise parents of children who are anxious during induction of anesthesia of the increased likelihood that their children will develop postoperative negative behavioral changes, such as nightmares, separation anxiety, and aggression toward authority.[123]

Because the anxiety level of the child and mother in the preoperative holding area predicts the occurrence of negative postoperative behavioral problems,[23] it can be hypothesized that if sedative premedications reduce anxiety of the child and the parents in the preoperative holding area, they may also have an effect on negative postoperative behavioral outcomes.[70] One investigation of premedicated children found a significantly reduced incidence of negative behavioral changes during week 1 after surgery.[124] This study suggests that reducing anxiety in the holding area has a beneficial effect on the behavior of the child preoperatively, as well as in the immediate postoperative period.[124]

## Intraoperative Clinical Outcomes

It is commonly believed that increased anxiety before surgery is associated with increased intraoperative anesthetic requirements.[95,125] This belief, however, is based on early studies of questionable scientific validity,[126,127] many of which did not use validated scales to measure anxiety or control for potential confounding variables, such as sedative premedication and the surgical procedure.[22] One investigation indicated that an increased baseline (i.e., trait) anxiety is associated with increased intraoperative anesthetic requirements in adults. The investigators in that study controlled for the surgical procedure, used bispectral electroencephalographic analysis (bispectral index) monitoring to ensure the same anesthetic depth in all patients, and used a total intravenous anesthetic technique to ease the calculation of the anesthetics used.[128] As such, it does seem clear that an increased baseline, or trait, anxiety is associated with increased intraoperative anesthetic requirements.

Although several review articles suggest that increased anxiety before surgery and anesthesia is associated with postoperative nausea and vomiting,[129] experimental data suggest that a child's anxiety in the preoperative holding area is not predictive of postoperative nausea and vomiting either in the postanesthesia care unit or at home.[130]

## Summary

Approximately 3 million children undergo anesthesia and surgery in the United States every year. It is reported that 40% to 60% of these children develop behavioral stress before their surgery. Multiple interventions have been proposed to treat the preoperative behavioral stress response in children. Currently, however, there is a trend toward a *reduction* in both behavioral and pharmacologic preoperative interventions aimed at children. One possible reason for this trend may be that some physicians believe that reducing parental anxiety during the preoperative period is a surrogate outcome. Rather than evaluating the effects of various preoperative interventions on the transient preoperative behavior, some believe that we should concentrate on research directed at demonstrating that a reduction in preoperative anxiety can dramatically change postoperative outcomes. It is well established that low levels of preoperative anxiety are associated with good postoperative behavioral recovery, whereas moderate and high levels of preoperative anxiety are associated with poor postoperative behavioral recovery. A far more intriguing question is the possible association between preoperative anxiety and postoperative clinical recovery; quality research needs to be developed regarding the relationship between preoperative anxiety and postoperative recovery. Further, shifting research focus toward development of economically and clinically feasible interventions that can be delivered to the large numbers of children undergoing surgery each year is vital. Accordingly, incorporating web-based technologies and changes in institutional practice (i.e., changing health care provider behaviors) represent two promising new avenues of intervention.

## ANNOTATED REFERENCES

Kain ZN, Caldwell-Andrews AA, Mayes LC. Parental intervention choices for children undergoing repeated surgeries. Anesth Analg 2003;96:970-5.

*Children were assigned to parental presence at induction (PPIA), premedication with midazolam, PPIA + premedication, or no intervention at initial surgery. Children were then followed up at subsequent surgery and parental preference for intervention was assessed. Of parents whose children were assigned to PPIA, 70% would choose PPIA as intervention again. Of those assigned to premedication, only 23% would choose premedication again. Regardless of prior intervention, parents at subsequent surgery favored PPIA. Children's and parents' anxiety also affected parental preference for intervention.*

Kain ZN, Caldwell-Andrews AA, Mayes LC, et al. Family-centered preparation for surgery improves perioperative outcomes in children: a randomized controlled trial. Anesthesiology 2007;106:65-74.

*This study evaluated the efficacy of a family-centered behavioral preparation program (ADVANCE) for children undergoing outpatient surgery (n = 408). Children were randomly assigned to no intervention, ADVANCE + PPIA, PPIA without advance, and midazolam premedication. Children in ADVANCE + PPIA displayed significantly less anxiety at induction than no intervention or PPIA alone. Anxiety and compliance in the ADVANCE + PPIA group were comparable to premedication. ADVANCE + PPIA was superior to all other groups on postoperative recovery variables.*

Kain ZN, Hofstadter MB, Mayes LC, et al. Midazolam: Effects on amnesia and anxiety in children. Anesthesiology 2000;93:676-84.

*These researchers assessed children's memory at baseline and in four randomly assigned groups (5, 10, and 20 minutes post midazolam administration, and no midazolam [control]) of children (n = 118). Compared with controls, recall memory was impaired for children in the 10- and 20-minute post-midazolam groups. All midazolam groups demonstrated recognition deficits when compared with controls. In terms of perioperative anxiety, significant effects of midazolam were evidenced at approximately 15 minutes.*

Kain ZN, Mayes LC, Caldwell-Andrews AA, et al. Preoperative anxiety and postoperative pain and behavioral recovery in young children undergoing surgery. Pediatrics 2006;118:651-8.

*This study assessed preoperative anxiety and postoperative pain and behavioral outcomes after surgery in 241 children. Children who displayed more preoperative anxiety were rated as having higher pain after surgery by their parents. Anxious children also consumed more analgesics at home after surgery and were more likely to experience emergence delirium and postoperative sleep disturbances.*

Kain ZN, Mayes LC, Wang SM, et al. Parental presence during induction of anesthesia vs. sedative premedication: which intervention is more effective? Anesthesiology 1998;89:1147-56.

*Eighty-eight children undergoing outpatient surgery were randomly assigned to parental presence at anesthesia induction, midazolam premedication, or no intervention. Children in the midazolam group exhibited significantly less perioperative anxiety than children in the parental presence or no intervention groups.*

## REFERENCES

Please see www.expertconsult.com

# Preoperative Evaluation, Premedication, and Induction of Anesthesia

## ELIZABETH A. GHAZAL, LINDA J. MASON, AND CHARLES J. COTÉ

4

## Preparation of Children for Anesthesia

### FASTING

Infants and children are fasted before sedation and anesthesia to minimize the risk of pulmonary aspiration of gastric contents. In a fasted child, only the basal secretions of gastric juice should be present in the stomach. In 1948, Digby Leigh recommended a 1-hour preoperative fast after clear fluids. Subsequently, Mendelson reported a number of maternal deaths that were attributed to aspiration at induction of anesthesia.[1] During the intervening 20 years, the fasting interval before elective surgery increased to 8 hours after all solids and fluids. In the late 1980s and early 1990s, an evidence-based approach to the effects of fasting intervals on gastric fluid pH and volume concluded that fasting more than 2 hours after clear fluids neither increased nor decreased the risk of pneumonitis should aspiration occur.[2-10] In the past, the risk for pneumonitis was reported to be based on two parameters: gastric fluid volume greater than 0.4 mL/kg and pH less than 2.5; however, these data were never published in a peer-reviewed journal.[1,11] In a monkey, 0.4 mL/kg of acid instilled endobronchially, equivalent to 0.8 mL/kg aspirated tracheally, resulted in pneumonitis.[12] Using these corrected criteria for acute pneumonitis (gastric residual fluid volume greater than 0.8 mL/kg and pH less than 2.5), studies in children demonstrated no additional risk for pneumonitis when children were fasted for only 2 hours after clear fluids.[2-9]

The incidence of pulmonary aspiration in modern routine elective pediatric or adult cases without known risk factors is small.[13-16] This small risk is the result of a number of factors including the preoperative fasting schedule. The half-life to empty clear fluids from the stomach is approximately 15 minutes (Fig. 4-1); as a result, 98% of clear fluids exit the stomach in children by 1 hour. Clear liquids include water, fruit juices without pulp, carbonated beverages, clear tea, and black coffee. Although fasting for 2 hours after clear fluids ensures nearly complete emptying of the residual volume, extending the fasting interval to 3 hours introduces flexibility in the operative schedule. The potential benefits of a 2-hour fasting interval after clear fluids include a reduced risk of hypoglycemia, which is a real possibility in children who are debilitated, have chronic disease, are poorly nourished, have metabolic dysfunction, or are preterm or formerly preterm infants.[17-20] Additional benefits include decreased thirst, decreased hunger (and thus reduced temptation that the fasting child will "steal" another child's food), decreased risk for hypotension during induction, and improved child cooperation.[2,11,21]

A scheduled operation on a preterm infant or neonate may occasionally be delayed, thus extending the period of fasting to a point that could be potentially dangerous (i.e., from hypoglycemia or hypovolemia). In this circumstance, the infants should be given glucose-containing intravenous maintenance fluids before induction of anesthesia. Alternatively, if the period may be protracted, the infant should be offered clear fluids orally until 2 hours before induction.

Breast milk, which can cause significant pulmonary injury if aspirated,[22] has a very high and variable fat content (determined by maternal diet), which will delay gastric emptying.[21] *Breast milk*

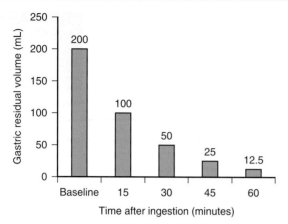

**FIGURE 4-1** Clear liquids are rapidly absorbed from the stomach with a half-life of approximately 15 minutes. In this figure, for example, 200 mL of apple juice would be reduced to 12.5 mL after 60 minutes. (Data abstracted from Hunt JN, MacDonald M. The influence of volume on gastric emptying. J Physiol 1954;126:459-74.)

| TABLE 4-1 Preoperative Fasting Recommendations in Infants and Children | |
|---|---|
| Clear liquids* | 2 hours |
| Breast milk | 4 hours |
| Infant formula | 6 hours† |
| Solids (fatty or fried foods) | 8 hours |

From Warner MA, Caplan RA, Epstein B. Practice guidelines for preoperative fasting and the use of pharmacologic agents to reduce the risk of pulmonary aspiration: application to healthy patients undergoing elective procedures. A report by the American Society of Anesthesiologists Task Force on Preoperative Fasting. Anesthesiology 1999;90:896-905.
*Include only fluids without pulp, clear tea, or coffee without milk products.
†Some centers allow plain toast (no dairy products) up to 6 hours prior to induction.

*should not be considered a clear liquid.*[23] Two studies estimated the gastric emptying times after clear fluids, breast milk, or formula in full-term and preterm neonates.[24,25] The emptying times for breast milk in both age groups were substantively greater than for clear fluids, and the gastric emptying times for formula were even greater than those for breast milk. With half-life emptying times for breast milk of 50 minutes and for formula of 75 minutes, fasting intervals of at least 3.3 hours for breast milk and 5 hours for formula are required. More importantly, perhaps, was the large (15%) variability in gastric emptying times for breast milk and formula in full-term infants (E-Fig. 4-1). Based in part on these data, the Task Force on Fasting of the American Society of Anesthesiologists (ASA) issued the following guidelines: for breast milk, 4 hours; and for formula, 6 hours (Table 4-1).[10]

Children who have been chewing gum must dispose of the gum by expectorating it, not swallowing it. Chewing gum increases both gastric fluid volume and gastric pH in children, leaving no clear evidence that it affects the risk of pneumonitis should aspiration occur.[26] Consequently, we recommend that if the gum is discarded, then elective anesthesia can proceed without additional delay. If, however, the child swallows the gum, then surgery should be cancelled, because aspirated gum at body temperature may be very difficult to extract from a bronchus or trachea.

Children can never be trusted to fast. Therefore, anesthesiologists must always be suspicious and question children just before induction as to whether they have eaten or drunk anything (although the veracity of the answer may always be questioned as well). It is not unusual to find bubble gum, candy, or other food in a child's mouth. This is another reason to ask children to open their mouth fully and stick out their tongue during the preoperative examination of the airway.

When the anesthesiologist suspects that the child has a full stomach, induction of anesthesia should be adjusted appropriately. The incidence of pulmonary aspiration of gastric contents during elective surgery in children ranges from 1:1163 to 1:10,000, depending on the study.[13-15,27] In contrast, the frequency of pulmonary aspiration in children undergoing emergency procedures is several times greater, 1:373 to 1:4544.[27] Risk factors for perianesthetic aspiration included neurologic or esophagogastric abnormality, emergency surgery (especially at

night), ASA physical status 3 to 5, intestinal obstruction, increased intracranial pressure, increased abdominal pressure, obesity, and the skill and experience of the anesthesiologist.[14]

The majority of aspirations in children occur during induction of anesthesia, with only 13% occurring during emergence and extubation. In contrast, 30% of the aspirations in adults occur during emergence. Bowel obstruction or ileus was present in the majority of infants and children who aspirated during the perioperative period in one study, with the risk increasing in children younger than 3 years of age.[27] A combination of factors predispose the infant and young child to regurgitation and aspiration, including decreased competence of the lower esophageal sphincter, excessive air swallowing while crying during the preinduction period, strenuous diaphragmatic breathing, and a shorter esophagus. In one study, almost all cases of pulmonary aspiration occurred either when the child gagged or coughed during airway manipulation or during induction of anesthesia when neuromuscular blocking drugs were not provided or before the child was completely paralyzed.[27]

When children do aspirate, the morbidity and mortality are exceedingly small for elective surgical procedures and generally reflect their ASA physical status. In general, most ASA 1 or 2 patients who aspirate clear gastric contents have minimal to no sequelae.[13,27] If clinical signs of sequelae from an aspiration in a child are going to occur, they will be apparent within 2 hours after the regurgitation.[27] The mortality rate from aspiration in children is exceedingly low, between zero and 1:50,000.[13,14,27]

### PIERCINGS

Body piercing is common practice in adolescents and young adults. Single or multiple piercings may appear anywhere on the body. To minimize the liability and risk of complications from metal piercings, they must be removed before surgery. Complications that may occur if they are left in situ during anesthesia are listed in E-Table 4-1.[28-30]

### PRIMARY AND SECONDARY SMOKING
#### Primary Smoking

Unfortunately, cigarette smoking is not only limited to adults. Each day, about 6000 American adolescents smoke their first cigarette. Of these, 50% will become regular smokers. Even though two thirds of these adolescents will regret taking up the habit and will want to quit, three quarters of them will not succeed because they are addicted to the nicotine. Sadly, about one third of those who cannot quit will die prematurely due to smoking.[31] Even though the rate of new smokers in North America has waned in the past 2 decades, this has been offset by the increasing rate of new smokers in other continents. Media, peer influence, and secondhand smoke exposure play a significant role in influencing initiation of smokers in this age group.[32]

Smoking is known to increase blood carboxyhemoglobin concentrations, decrease ciliary function, decrease functional vital capacity (FVC) and the forced expiratory flow in midphase ($FEF_{25\%-75\%}$), and increase sputum production. There is extensive evidence that smokers undergoing surgery are more likely to develop wound infections and postoperative respiratory complications.[33] Although stopping smoking for 2 days decreases carboxyhemoglobin levels and shifts the oxyhemoglobin dissociation curve to the right, stopping for at least 6 to 8 weeks is necessary to reduce the rate of postoperative pulmonary complications.[34,35]

We seldom interview our patients 8 weeks before surgery, but because the perioperative period is the ideal time to abandon the smoking habit permanently, anesthesiologists can perhaps play a more active role in facilitating this process. Physician communication with adolescents regarding smoking cessation has been shown to positively impact their attitudes, knowledge, intentions to smoke, and quitting behaviors.[36] In summary, during the preoperative visit with adolescents, anesthesiologists should inquire about cigarette smoking and emphasize the need to stop the habit by offering measures to ameliorate the withdrawal (e.g., nictoine patch).

### Secondary Smoking

The World Health Organization has estimated that approximately 700 million children, or almost half of the children in the world, are exposed to environmental tobacco smoke (ETS).[37] Children exposed to ETS are more likely to have asthma, otitis media,[38] atopic eczema, hay fever,[39] and dental caries.[40] There is also an increased rate of lower respiratory tract illness in infants with ETS exposure.[41,42]

Several authors have demonstrated that ETS results in increased perioperative airway complications in children. In one study[43] of children receiving general anesthesia, urinary cotinine, the major metabolite of nicotine, was used as a surrogate of ETS. A strong association was found between passive inhalation of tobacco smoke and airway complications on induction and emergence from anesthesia. Other investigators confirmed that ETS exposure was associated with an increased frequency of respiratory complications during emergence and recovery from anesthesia.[44]

The evidence against ETS is clearly overwhelming. During the preoperative visit, the anesthesiologist must question the child's exposure to ETS by asking parents or guardians about smoking within the household. This is an opportune time to educate parents and guardians about the dangers of ETS for their children.

## PSYCHOLOGICAL PREPARATION OF CHILDREN FOR SURGERY

The perioperative period is stressful and anxiety-provoking for the child and family; many parents express more concern about the risks of anesthesia than those of the surgery. The factors that influence the ability of the child and family to cope with the stress of surgery include family dynamics, the child's developmental and behavioral status and cultural biases, and our ability to explain away misperceptions and misinformation.

Because of logistics and today's practice constraints, there is limited time to evaluate family dynamics and establish rapport. It is therefore vital for the anesthesiologist to interact directly with the child in a manner that is consistent with the child's level of development. A specific child-oriented approach by the anesthesiologist, surgeon, nurses, and hospital staff is required. Preoperative evaluation is usually simplified once the basic concepts of how to evaluate a child are understood.

Although the preoperative evaluation and preparation of children are similar to those of adults from a physiologic standpoint, the psychological preparation of infants and children is very different (see also Chapter 3). Many hospitals have an open house or a brochure to describe the preoperative programs available to parents before the day of admission.[45] However, printed material should not replace verbal communication with nursing and medical staff.[46] Anesthesiologists are encouraged to participate in the design of these programs so that they accurately reflect the anesthetic practice of the institution. The preoperative anesthetic experience begins at the time parents are first informed that the child is to have surgery or a procedure that requires general anesthesia. Parental satisfaction correlates with the comfort of the environment and the trust established between the anesthesiologist, the child, and the parents.[47] If parental presence during induction is deemed to be in the child's best interest, a parental educational program that describes what the parent can expect to happen if he or she accompanies the child to the operating room can significantly decrease parents' anxiety and increase their satisfaction.[48] The greater the understanding and amount of information the parents have, the less anxious they will be, and this attitude, in turn, will be reflected in the child.[49,50]

Informed consent should include a detailed description of what the family can anticipate and our role to protect the welfare of the child. Before surgery, the anesthetic risks should be discussed in clear terms but in a reassuring manner by describing the measures that will be taken to carefully and closely monitor the safety of the child. Mentioning specific details and the purpose of the various monitoring devices may help diminish the parents' anxiety by demonstrating to them that the child will be anesthetized with the utmost safety and care. A blood pressure cuff will *"check the blood pressure,"* an electrocardiographic monitor will *"watch the heartbeat,"* a stethoscope will help us *"to continuously listen to the heart sounds,"* a pulse oximeter will *"measure the oxygen in the bloodstream,"* a carbon dioxide analyzer will *"monitor the breathing,"* an anesthetic agent monitor will *"accurately measure the level of anesthesia,"* and an intravenous catheter will be placed *"to administer fluid and medications as needed."* Children who are capable and their parents should be given ample opportunity to ask questions preoperatively. Finally, they should be assured that our "anesthetic prescription" will be designed specifically for their child's needs, taking into account the child's underlying medical conditions and the needs of surgery to ensure optimal conditions for surgery, the safety of the child, and analgesia.

It has been shown that parents desire comprehensive perioperative information, and that discussion of highly detailed anesthetic risk information does not increase parent's anxiety level.[51] Inadequate preparation of children and their families may lead to a traumatic anesthetic induction and difficulty for both the child and the anesthesiologist, with the possibility of postoperative psychological disturbances.[52] Numerous preoperative educational programs for children and adults have evolved to alleviate some of these fears and anxiety. They include preoperative tours of the operating rooms, educational videos, play therapy, magical distractions, puppet shows, anesthesia consultations, and child life preparation.[53] The timing of the preoperative preparation has been found to be an important determinant of whether the intervention will be effective. For example, children older than 6 years of age who participated in a preparation program more than 5 to 7 days before surgery were least anxious during separation from their parents, those who participated in no preoperative preparation were moderately anxious, and those who received the information 1 day before surgery were the most anxious. The predictors of anxiety correlated also with the child's baseline temperament and history of previous hospitalizations.[54] Children of different ages vary in their response to the anesthetic experience (see also Chapter 3).[55] Even more important may be the child's trait anxiety when confronted with a stressful medical procedure.[56]

### Child Development and Behavior

Understanding age-appropriate behavior in response to external situations is essential (E-Table 4-2). Infants younger than 10 months of age tolerate short periods of separation from their parents. Many do not object to an inhalation induction and frequently respond to the smell of the inhalation agents by sucking or licking the mask. These infants usually do not need a sedative premedication.

Children between 11 months and 6 years of age frequently cling to their parents. In an unfamiliar environment such as a hospital, preschool children tend to become very anxious, especially if the situation appears threatening. Their anxiety may be exacerbated if they sense that their parents are anxious. Efforts to educate the parents to allay their anxiety can also reduce the child's anxiety.[45,57,58] A heightened anxiety response may lead to immediate postoperative maladaptive behavior, such as nightmares, eating disturbances, and new-onset enuresis. Compared with other patients, children 2 to 6 years of age are more likely to exhibit problematic behavior when separated from their parents (see also Chapter 3).[55] Children who display one or more of the predictive risk factors would probably benefit from a sedative premedication.[59-62] They are generally more content if their parents accompany them during induction or if they are sedated in the presence of their parents in a nonthreatening environment before entering the operating room (see later discussion).

Children older than 6 years of age and those who attend preschool or kindergarten are more willing to accept brief periods of separation from their parents. They tend to be more independent because of their school experience. They are better able to communicate and have a greater understanding of their environment. Their sense of curiosity and interest in new things and their trust of adults can be used to elicit their cooperation for a mask induction of anesthesia without the need for premedication.

Children ages 4 to 10 years may exhibit psychological factors that are predictive of postoperative behavior (e.g., abnormal sleep patterns, parental anxiety, aggressive behavior).[63,64] In addition, children who have pain on the day of the operation have behavioral problems that continue well after the pain has been relieved.[65] Therefore, preventing postoperative pain decreases and limits the duration of postoperative behavioral problems.

Special aspects of a child's perception of anesthesia should be anticipated; children often have the same fears as adults but are unable to articulate them. The reason and need for a surgical procedure should also be carefully explained to the child. It is important to reassure children that anesthesia is not the same as the usual nightly sleep but rather a special sleep caused by the medicines we give during which they cannot be awakened and no matter what the surgeon does, they cannot feel pain. Many children fear the possibility that they will wake up in the middle of the anesthetic and during surgery. They should be reassured that they will awaken only after the surgery is completed.

The words the anesthesiologist uses to describe to the child what can be anticipated must be carefully chosen, because children think concretely and tend to interpret the facts literally. Examples of this are presented by the following anecdotes:

*Example 1:* A 4-year-old child was informed that in the morning she would receive a "shot" that would "put her to sleep." That night, a frantic call was received from the mother, describing a very upset child; the child thought she was going to be "put to sleep" like the veterinarian had permanently "put to sleep" her sick pet.

*Example 2:* A 5-year-old child admitted for elective inguinal herniorrhaphy received a heavy premedication and was deeply sedated on arrival in the operating room. After discharge, the parents frequently discovered him wandering about the house at night. On questioning, the child stated that he was "protecting" his family. He stated: "I don't want anyone sneaking up on you and operating while you are sleeping."

In the first example, the child's concrete thought processes misunderstood the anesthesiologist's choice of words. The second case represents a problem of communication: the child was never told he would have an operation.

The importance of proper psychological preparation for surgery should not be underestimated. Often, little has been explained to both patient and parents before the day of surgery. Anesthesiologists have a key role in defusing fear of the unknown if they understand a child's age-related perception of anesthesia and surgery (see Chapter 3). They can convey their understanding by presenting a calm and friendly face (smiling, looking at the child and making eye contact), offering a warm introduction, touching the patient in a reassuring manner (holding a child's or parent's hand), and being completely honest. Children respond positively to an honest description of exactly what they can anticipate. This includes informing them of the slight discomfort of starting an intravenous line or giving an intramuscular premedication, the possible bitter taste of an oral premedication, or breathing our magic laughing gas through the flavored mask.

The postoperative process, from the operating room to the recovery room, and the onset of postoperative pain should be described. Encourage the child and family to ask questions. Strategies to maintain analgesia should be discussed, including the use of long-acting local anesthetics; nerve blocks; neuraxial blocks; patient-controlled, nurse-controlled, or parent-controlled analgesia or epidural analgesia; or intermittent opioids (see also Chapters 41, 42, and 43).

As children age, they become more aware of their bodies and may develop a fear of mutilation. Adolescents frequently appear quite independent and self-confident, but as a group, they have unique problems. In a moment their mood can change from an intelligent, mature adult to a very immature child who needs support and reassurance. Coping with a disability or illness is often very difficult for adolescents. Because they are often comparing their physical appearance with that of their peers, they may become especially anxious when they have a physical problem. In general, they want to know exactly what will transpire during the course of anesthesia. Adolescents are usually cooperative, preferring to be in control and unpremedicated preoperatively. The occasional overly anxious or rambunctious adolescent, however, may benefit from preanesthetic medication.

Monitoring the attitude and behavior of a child is very useful. A child who clings to the parents, avoids eye contact, and will not speak is very anxious. A self-assured, cocky child who "knows it all" may also be apprehensive or frightened. This know-it-all behavior may mask the child's true emotions, and he or she may decompensate just when cooperation is most needed. In some cases, nonpharmacologic supportive measures may be effective. In the extremely anxious child, supportive measures alone may be insufficient to reduce anxiety, and premedication is indicated.

Identifying a difficult parent or child preoperatively is not always easy, especially if the anesthesiologist first meets the child or family on the day of surgery and has limited time to assess the situation. Occasionally, we receive a warning regarding a difficult parent or child from the surgeon or nursing staff, based on their encounters with the family. With experience, some anesthesiologists are able to identify difficult parents and children during the short preoperative assessment and make appropriate adjustments to the anesthetic management plan.

The "veterans" or "frequent flyers" of anesthesia can also be difficult in the perioperative period. They have played the anesthesia and surgical game before and are not interested in participating again, especially if their previous experiences were negative. These children may benefit the most from a relatively heavy premedication; reviewing previous responses to premedication will aid in the adjustment of the current planned premedication (e.g., adding ketamine and atropine to oral midazolam so as to achieve a greater depth of sedation).

It is important to observe the family dynamics to better understand the child and determine who is in control, the parent or the child. Families many times are in a state of stress, particularly if the child has a chronic illness; these parents are often angry, guilt ridden, or simply exhausted. Ultimately, the manner in which a family copes with an illness largely determines how the child will cope.[66] The well-organized, open, and communicative family tends to be supportive and resourceful, whereas the disorganized, noncommunicative, and dysfunctional family tends to be angry and frustrated. Dealing with a family and child from the latter category can be challenging. There is the occasional parent who is overbearing and demands total control of the situation. It is important to be empathetic and understanding but to set limits and clearly define the parent's role. He or she must be told that the anesthesiologist determines when the parent must leave the operating room; this is particularly true if an unexpected development occurs during the induction.

## Parental Presence during Induction

One controversial area in pediatric anesthesia is parental presence during induction. Some anesthesiologists encourage parents to be present at induction, whereas others are uncomfortable with the process and do not allow parents to be present. Inviting a parent to accompany the child to the operating room has been interpreted by some courts as an implicit contract on the part of the caregiver who invited the parent to participate in the child's care; in one case, the institution was found to have assumed responsibility for a mother who suffered an injury when she fainted.[67] Each child and family must be evaluated individually; what is good for one child and family may not be good for the next.[68-71] (See Chapter 3 for a full discussion of this and other anxiolytic strategies in children.)

If the practice of having parents present at induction is to work well, then the anesthesiologist must be comfortable with such an arrangement. No parent should ever be forced to be present for the induction of anesthesia, nor should any anesthesiologist be forced into a situation that compromises the quality of care he or she affords a child in need.

Parents must be informed about what to anticipate in terms of the operating room itself (e.g., equipment, surgical devices), in terms of what they may observe during induction (e.g., eyes rolling back, laryngeal noises, anesthetic monitor alarms, excitation), and when they will be asked to leave. They must also be instructed regarding their ability to assist during the induction process, such as by comforting the child, encouraging the child to trust the anesthesiologist, distracting the child, and consoling the child (Video 4-1). Personnel should be immediately available to escort parents back to the waiting area at the appropriate time. Someone should also be available to care for a parent who wishes to leave the induction area or who becomes lightheaded or faints. An anesthesiologist's anxiety about parents' presence during induction decreases significantly with experience.[72]

Explaining what parents might see or hear is essential. We generally tell parents the following:

*As you see your child fall asleep today, there are several things you might observe that you are not used to seeing. First, when anyone falls asleep, the eyes roll up, but since we are sleeping we do not generally see it. You may see your child do that today, and I do not want you to be frightened by that—it is expected and normal. The second thing is that as children go to sleep from the anesthesia medications, the tone of the structures in the neck decreases, so that some children will begin to snore or make vibrating noises. Again, I do not want you to be frightened or think that something is wrong. We expect this, and it is normal. The third thing you might see is what we call "excitement." As the brain begins to go to sleep, it can actually get excited first. About 30 to 60 seconds after breathing the anesthesia medications, your child might suddenly look around or suddenly move his or her arms and legs. To you it appears that he is awakening from anesthesia or that he or she is upset. In reality, this is a good sign, because it indicates to us that your child is falling asleep and that 15 to 30 seconds later he or she will be completely anesthetized. Also you should know that even though your child appears to be awake to you, in reality he or she will not remember any of that. As soon as your child loses consciousness, we will ask you to give your child a kiss and step out of the operating room.*

This kind of careful preparation provides to the parents the confidence that the anesthesiologist really knows what he or she is talking about, and it avoids frightening the parents. In general, the more information provided, the lower the parental anxiety levels.

Occasionally, the best efforts to relieve a child's anxiety by parental presence or administration of a sedative premedication (or both) are not successful, and an anticipated smooth induction may not go as planned. There are three options that may be used depending on the age of the child: (1) renegotiate (which is seldom successful), (2) hold the mask farther away from the child's face, or (3) suggest an intravenous or intramuscular induction. Sedation can be considered if it was not already used and may be intramuscular, oral, inhalational (nitrous oxide), or given by another route). If an intramuscular shot or intravenous induction is proposed, the child will usually choose the mask. If the

**TABLE 4-2** Review of Systems: Anesthetic Implications

| System | Factors to Assess | Possible Anesthetic Implications |
|---|---|---|
| Respiratory | Cough, asthma, recent cold | Irritable airway, bronchospasm, medication history, atelectasis, infiltrate |
| | Croup | Subglottic narrowing |
| | Apnea/bradycardia | Postoperative apnea/bradycardia |
| Cardiovascular | Murmur | Septal defect, avoid air bubbles in intravenous line |
| | Cyanosis | Right-to-left shunt |
| | History of squatting | Tetralogy of Fallot |
| | Hypertension | Coarctation, renal disease |
| | Rheumatic fever | Valvular heart disease |
| | Exercise intolerance | Congestive heart failure, cyanosis |
| Neurologic | Seizures | Medications, metabolic derangement |
| | Head trauma | Intracranial hypertension |
| | Swallowing incoordination | Aspiration, esophageal reflux, hiatus hernia |
| | Neuromuscular disease | Neuromuscular relaxant drug sensitivity, malignant hyperpyrexia |
| Gastrointestinal/hepatic | Vomiting, diarrhea | Electrolyte imbalance, dehydration, full stomach |
| | Malabsorption | Anemia |
| | Black stools | Anemia, hypovolemia |
| | Reflux | Possible need for full-stomach precautions |
| | Jaundice | Drug metabolism/hypoglycemia |
| Genitourinary | Frequency | Urinary tract infection, diabetes, hypercalcemia |
| | Time of last urination | State of hydration |
| | Frequent urinary tract infections | Evaluate renal function |
| Endocrine/metabolic | Abnormal development | Endocrinopathy, hypothyroid, diabetes |
| | Hypoglycemia, steroid therapy | Hypoglycemia, adrenal insufficiency |
| Hematologic | Anemia | Need for transfusion |
| | Bruising, excessive bleeding | Coagulopathy, thrombocytopenia, thrombocytopathy |
| | Sickle cell disease | Hydration, possible transfusion |
| Allergies | Medications | Possible drug interaction |
| Dental | Loose or carious teeth | Aspiration of loose teeth, bacterial endocarditis prophylaxis |

situation is totally out of control, either elective surgery can be rescheduled or intramuscular ketamine can be used if the parents choose to proceed. These situations are particularly difficult for the parents and the caregivers but must be handled on an individual basis.

## HISTORY OF PRESENT ILLNESS

The medical history of a child obtained during the preanesthetic visit allows the anesthesiologist to determine whether the child is optimized for the planned surgery, to anticipate potential problems due to coexisting disease, to determine whether appropriate laboratory or other tests are available or needed, to select optimal premedication, to formulate the appropriate anesthetic plan including perioperative monitoring, and to anticipate postoperative concerns including pain management and postoperative ventilatory needs. The history of the present illness is described to the physicians by the parents and verified by the referring or consultant surgeon's notes. If the child is old enough, it is helpful to obtain the child's input. The history should focus on the following aspects:

- A review of all organ systems (Table 4-2) with special emphasis on the organ system involved in the surgery
- Medications (over-the-counter and prescribed) related to and taken before the present illness, including herbals and vitamins, and when the last dose was taken
- Medication allergies with specific details of the nature of the allergy and whether immunologic testing was performed
- Previous surgical and hospital experiences, including those related to the current problem

- Timing of the last oral intake, last urination (wet diaper), and vomiting and diarrhea. It is essential to recognize that decreased gastrointestinal motility often occurs with an illness or injury.

In the case of a neonate, problems that may have been present during gestation and birth may still be relevant in the neonatal period and beyond (E-Table 4-3). The maternal medical and pharmacologic history (both therapeutic and drug abuse) may also provide valuable information for the management of a neonate requiring surgery.

## PAST/OTHER MEDICAL HISTORY

The past medical history should include a history of all past medical illnesses with a review of organ systems, previous hospitalizations (medical or surgical), childhood syndromes with associated anomalies, medication list, herbal remedies, and any allergies, especially to antibiotics and latex. Whether the child was full-term or preterm at birth should be discerned; if preterm, any associated problems should be noted, including admission to a neonatal intensive care unit, duration of tracheal intubation, history of apnea or bradycardia (including oxygen treatment, home apnea monitor, intraventricular hemorrhage), and congenital defects.

Examination of previous surgical and anesthesia records greatly assists in planning the anesthesia. Particular attention should be paid to any difficulties encountered with airway management, venous access, or emergence. The response to or need for premedication and the route of administration utilized should be noted.

## Herbal Remedies

Increasing numbers of children are ingesting herbal medicine products. During the preoperative interview, anesthesiologists should include specific inquiries regarding the use of these medications because of their potential adverse effects and drug interactions. Hospital surveys suggest that the use of herbal remedies ranges from 17% to 32%[73-75] of presurgical patients, and 70% of these patients do not inform their anesthesiologist of such use.

In Hong Kong, 80% of patients undergoing major elective surgery use prepacked over-the-counter traditional Chinese herbal medicines, and 8% use medicines prescribed by traditional Chinese medicine practitioners.[76] The prescription users of traditional Chinese medicines experienced a greater incidence of adverse perioperative events. In particular, this group was twice as likely to have hypokalemia or impaired hemostasis (i.e., prolonged international normalized prothrombin ratio [INR] and activated partial thromboplastin time [aPTT]) than nonusers, although there was no significant difference in the incidence of perioperative events between self-prescribed users and nonusers. To further complicate this subject, there is an important difference between Chinese and Western herbs. Traditional Chinese herbal medicines consist of multiple herbs that are combined for their effects, whereas Western herbs are usually ingested as a single substance.[77]

Herbal medicines are associated with cardiovascular instability, coagulation disturbances, prolongation of anesthesia, and immunosuppression.[78] The most commonly used herbal medications reported are garlic, ginseng, *Ginkgo biloba*, St. John's wort, and echinacea.[79] The three "g" herbals, together with feverfew *(Tanacetum parthenium)*, potentially increase the risk of bleeding during surgery. The amount of active ingredient in each preparation may vary, the dose taken by a child may also vary, and detection of a change in platelet function and other subtle coagulation disturbances may be difficult. St. John's wort is the herb that most commonly interacts with anesthetics and other medications, usually via a change in drug metabolism, because it is a potent induction of the cytochrome P-450 enzymes (e.g., CYP3A4) and P-glycoprotein. A potentially fatal interaction between cyclosporine and St. John's wort has been well documented.[80-83] Heart, kidney, or liver transplant recipients who were stabilized on a dose of cyclosporine experienced decreased plasma concentrations of cyclosporine and, in some cases, acute rejection episodes after taking St. John's wort. A summary of the most commonly used herbal remedies and their potential perioperative complications is shown in E-Table 4-4.

To avoid potential perioperative complications, the ASA has encouraged the discontinuation of all herbal medicines 2 weeks before surgery,[84] although this recommendation is not evidence based. Indeed, some herbs such as valerian, a treatment for insomnia *(Valeriana officinalis)*, should *not* be discontinued abruptly but tapered; otherwise, abrupt discontinuation may result in a paradoxical and severe reaction.[85] Each herb should be carefully evaluated using standard resource texts, and a decision should be made regarding the timing of or need for discontinuation as determined on a case-by-case basis.[86]

## Anesthesia and Vaccination

Children may present for surgery after having been recently immunized. The anesthesiologist and surgeon must then consider (1) whether the immunomodulatory effects of anesthesia and surgery might affect the efficacy and safety of the vaccine and (2) whether the inflammatory responses to the vaccine will alter the perioperative course.

What do anesthesiologists think about anesthesia and vaccination? An international survey[87] revealed that only one third of responding anesthesiologists had the benefit of a hospital policy, ranging from a formal decision to delay surgery to an independent choice by the anesthesiologist. Sixty percent of respondents would anesthetize a child for elective surgery within 1 week of receiving a live attenuated vaccine (such as oral polio vaccine or measles, mumps, and rubella [MMR] vaccine), whereas 40% would not. The survey also revealed that 28% of anesthesiologists would delay immunization for 2 to 30 days after surgery.

Is there a consensus statement on anesthesia and vaccination? A scientific review of the literature associating anesthesia and vaccination in children resulted in recommendations for the care of children under these circumstances.[88] The review demonstrated a brief and reversible influence of vaccination on lymphoproliferative responses that generally returned to preoperative values within 2 days. Vaccine-driven adverse events (e.g., fever, pain, irritability) might occur but should not be confused with perioperative complications. Adverse events to inactivated vaccines such as diphtheria-tetanus-pertussis (DPT) become apparent from 2 days and to live attenuated vaccines such as MMR from 7 to 21 days after immunization.[88] Therefore, appropriate delays between immunization and anesthesia are recommended by type of vaccine to avoid misinterpretation of vaccine-associated adverse events as perioperative complications. Because children remain at risk of contracting vaccine-preventable diseases, the minimum delay seems prudent, especially in the first year of life. Likewise, it seems reasonable to delay vaccination *after* surgery until the child is fully recovered. Other immunocompromised patients, such as human immunodeficiency virus (HIV)-positive children, cancer patients, and transplant recipients, have distinct underlying immune impairments, and the influence of anesthesia on vaccine responses has not been comprehensively investigated.

## Allergies to Medications and Latex

The details pertaining to all allergies to medications and materials should be described in the child's record. These include the age of onset, frequency, severity, investigations, and treatments. The vast majority of reported allergies on children's charts are either nonimmunologic reactions or known (or unknown) drug adverse effects. The most common medication- and hospital-related allergies in children are penicillin and latex allergy.

Most cases of reported penicillin allergy consist of a maculopapular rash after oral penicillin. This occurs in 1% to 4% of children receiving penicillin or in 3% to 7% of those taking ampicillin, usually during treatment.[89] Rarely are signs or symptoms that suggest an acute (immunoglobulin E–mediated) allergic reaction present (i.e., angioedema), and even less frequently is skin testing conducted to establish penicillin allergy. Given the frequency of penicillin allergy, most of these unverified allergies in fact are not allergies to penicillin but rather minor allergies to the dye in the liquid vehicle or a consequence of the (viral) infection. If the child has not received penicillin for at least 5 years since the initial exposure and has not been diagnosed with a penicillin allergy by an immunologist or allergist, then a reexposure is warranted. If the child has been tested immunologically for penicillin allergy, then it is best to avoid this class of antibiotics. Although there is a 5% to 10% cross-reactivity between first-generation cephalosporins and penicillin, there is no similar cross-reactivity with second- and third-generation cephalosporins. To date, there have been no fatal anaphylactic reactions in penicillin allergic children from a cephalosporin.[89]

Latex allergy is an acquired immunologic sensitivity resulting from repeated exposure to latex, usually on mucous membranes (e.g., children with spina bifida or congenital urologic abnormalities who have undergone repeated bladder catheterizations with latex catheters, those with more than four surgeries, those requiring home ventilation). It occurs more frequently in atopic individuals and in those with certain fruit and vegetable allergies (e.g., banana, chestnut, avocado, kiwi, pineapple).[90-96] For a diagnosis of latex anaphylaxis, the child should have personally experienced an anaphylactic reaction to latex, skin-tested positive for anaphylaxis to latex, or experienced swelling of the lips after touching a toy balloon to the lips or a swollen tongue after a dentist inserted a rubber dam into the mouth.[96] The avoidance of latex within the hospital will prevent acute anaphylactic reactions to latex in children who are at risk.[97] Latex gloves and other latex-containing products should be removed from the immediate vicinity of the child. Prophylactic therapy with histamine $H_1$ and $H_2$ antagonists and steroids do not prevent latex anaphylaxis.[90,98] Latex anaphylaxis should be treated by removal of the source of latex, administration of 100% oxygen, acute volume loading with balanced salt solution (10 to 20 mL/kg repeated until the systolic blood pressure stabilizes), and administration of intravenous epinephrine (1 to 10 μg/kg according to the severity of the anaphylaxis). In some severe reactions, a continuous infusion of epinephrine alone (0.01 to 0.2 μg/kg/min) or combined with other vasoactive medications may be required for several hours.

### Family History

It is important to inquire about a family history, particularly focusing on a number of conditions, including malignant hyperthermia, muscular dystrophy, prolonged paralysis associated with anesthesia (pseudocholinesterase deficiency), sickle cell disease, bleeding (and bruising) tendencies, and drug addiction (drug withdrawal, HIV infection). The precise relationship to the proband must be documented.

### LABORATORY DATA

The laboratory data obtained preoperatively should be appropriate to the history, illness, and surgical procedure. Routine hemoglobin testing or urinalysis is not indicated for most elective procedures; the value of these tests is questionable when the surgical procedure will not involve clinically significant blood loss.[99] There are insufficient data in the literature to make strict hemoglobin testing recommendations in healthy children. A preoperative hemoglobin value is usually determined only for those who will undergo procedures with the potential for blood loss, those with specific risk factors for a hemoglobinopathy, formerly preterm infants, and those younger than 6 months of age. Coagulation studies (platelet count, INR, and PTT) may be indicated if major reconstructive surgery is contemplated, especially if warranted by the medical history, and in some centers before tonsillectomy. In addition, collection of a preoperative type-and-screen or type-and-crossmatch sample is indicated in preparation for potential blood transfusions depending on the nature of the planned surgery and the anticipated blood loss.

In general, routine chest radiography is not necessary; studies have confirmed that routine chest radiographs are not cost-effective in children.[100,101] The oxygen saturation of children who are breathing room air is very helpful. Baseline saturations of 95% or less suggest clinically important pulmonary or cardiac compromise and warrant further investigation.

Special laboratory tests, such as electrolyte and blood glucose determinations, renal function tests, blood gas analysis, blood concentrations of seizure medication and digoxin, electrocardiography, echocardiography, liver function tests, computed tomography (CT), magnetic resonance imaging (MRI), or pulmonary function tests, should be performed when appropriate.

### PREGNANCY TESTING

Although pregnancy rates among teenagers in the United States are declining,[102] a small percentage of young women may still present for elective surgery with an unsuspected pregnancy. In 2003, the birth rate in girls aged 15 to 19 years was 41.6 births per 1000, and for girls aged 10 to 14 years it was 0.6 per 1000. However, routine preoperative pregnancy testing in adolescent girls may present ethical and legal dilemmas, including social and confidentiality concerns. This places the anesthesiologist in a predicament when faced with a question of whether to perform routine preoperative pregnancy screening.[102] Each hospital should adopt a policy regarding pregnancy testing to provide a consistent and comprehensive policy for all females who have reached menarche.

A survey of members of the Society for Pediatric Anesthesia practicing in North America revealed that pregnancy testing was routinely required by approximately 45% of the respondents regardless of the practice setting (teaching versus nonteaching facilities).[99] A retrospective review of a 2-year study of mandatory pregnancy testing in 412 adolescent surgical patients[103] revealed that the overall incidence of positive tests was 1.2%. Five of 207 patients aged 15 years and older tested positive, for an incidence of 2.4% in that group. None of the 205 patients younger than the age of 15 years had a positive pregnancy test.

The most recent ASA Task Force on Preanesthesia Evaluation[104] recognized that a history and physical examination may not adequately identify early pregnancy and issued the following statement: *"The literature is insufficient to inform patients or physicians on whether anesthesia causes harmful effects on early pregnancy. Pregnancy testing may be offered to female patients of childbearing age and for whom the result would alter the patient's management."*[105] Because of the risk of exposing the fetus to potential teratogens and radiation from anesthesia and surgery, the risk of spontaneous abortion, and the risk of apoptosis reported in the rapidly developing fetal animal brain, elective surgery with general anesthesia is not advised during early pregnancy. Therefore, if the situation is unclear, and when indicated by medical history, it is best to perform a preoperative pregnancy test. If the surgery is required in a patient who might be pregnant, then using an opioid-based anesthetic such as remifentanil and the lowest concentration of inhalational agent or propofol that provides adequate anesthesia is preferred.

## Premedication and Induction Principles

### GENERAL PRINCIPLES

The major objectives of preanesthetic medication are to (1) allay anxiety, (2) block autonomic (vagal) reflexes, (3) reduce airway secretions, (4) produce amnesia, (5) provide prophylaxis against pulmonary aspiration of gastric contents, (6) facilitate the induction of anesthesia, and (7) if necessary, provide analgesia. Premedication may also decrease the stress response to anesthesia and prevent cardiac arrhythmias.[106] The goal of premedication for each child must be individualized. Light sedation, even though it may not eliminate anxiety, may adequately calm a child so that the induction of anesthesia will be smooth and a pleasant experience. In contrast, heavy sedation may be needed for the very anxious child who is unwilling to separate from his or her parents.

Factors to consider when selecting a drug or a combination of drugs for premedication include the child's age, ideal body weight, drug history, and allergic status; underlying medical or surgical conditions and how they might affect the response to premedication or how the premedication might alter anesthetic induction; parent and child expectations; and the child's emotional maturity, personality, anxiety level, cooperation, and physiologic and psychological status. The anesthesiologist should also consider the proposed surgical procedure and the attitudes and wishes of the child and the parents.

The route of administration of premedicant drugs is very important. Premedications have been administered by many routes including the oral, nasal, rectal, buccal, intravenous, and intramuscular routes. Although a drug may be more effective and have a more reliable onset when given intranasally or intramuscularly, most pediatric anesthesiologists refrain from administering parenteral medication to children without intravenous access. Many children who are able to verbalize report that receiving a needle puncture was their worst experience in the hospital.[107,108] In most cases, medication administered without a needle will be more pleasant for children, their parents, and the medical staff. Oral premedications do not increase the risk of aspiration pneumonia unless large volumes of fluids are ingested.[109] In general, the route of delivery of the premedication should depend on the drug, the desired drug effect, and the psychological impact of the route of administration. For example, a small dose of oral medication may be sufficient for a relatively calm child, whereas an intramuscular injection (e.g., ketamine) may be best for an uncooperative, combative, extremely anxious child. Intramuscular administration may be less traumatic for this type of child than forcing him or her to swallow a drug, giving a drug rectally, or forcefully holding an anesthesia mask on the face.[110]

Since Water's classic work in 1938 on premedication of children, numerous reports have addressed this subject.[111] Despite the wealth of studies, no single drug or combination of drugs has been found to be ideal for all children. Many drugs used for premedication have similar effects, and a specific drug may have various effects in different children or in the same child under different conditions.

## MEDICATIONS

Several categories of drugs are available for premedicating children before anesthesia (Table 4-3). Selection of drugs for premedication depends on the goal desired. Drug effects should be weighed against potential side effects, and drug interactions should be considered. Premedicant drugs include tranquilizers, sedatives, hypnotics, opioids, antihistamines, anticholinergics, $H_2$-receptor antagonists, antacids, and drugs that increase gastric motility.

### Tranquilizers

The major effect of tranquilizers is to allay anxiety, but they also have the potential to produce sedation. This group of drugs includes the benzodiazepines, phenothiazines, and butyrophenones. Benzodiazepines are widely used in children, whereas phenothiazines and butyrophenones are infrequently used.

**TABLE 4-3** Doses of Drugs Commonly Administered for Premedication

| Drug | Route | Dose (mg/kg) |
|---|---|---|
| **Barbiturates** | | |
| Methohexital | Rectal | (10% solution) 20-40 |
| | Intramuscular | (5% solution) 10 |
| Thiopental | Rectal | (10% solution) 20-40 |
| **Benzodiazepines** | | |
| Diazepam | Oral | 0.1-0.5 |
| | Rectal | 1 mg/kg |
| Midazolam | Oral | 0.25-0.75 |
| | Nasal | 0.2 |
| | Rectal | 0.5-1 |
| | Intramuscular | 0.1-0.15 |
| Lorazepam | Oral | 0.025-0.05 |
| **Phencyclidine** | | |
| Ketamine* | Oral | 3-6 |
| | Nasal | 3 |
| | Rectal | 6-10 |
| | Intramuscular | 2-10 |
| **$\alpha_2$-Adrenergic Agonist** | | |
| Clonidine | Oral | 0.004 |
| **Opioids** | | |
| Morphine | Intramuscular | 0.1-0.2 |
| Meperidine† | Intramuscular | 1-2 |
| Fentanyl | Oral | 0.010-0.015 (10-15 µg/kg) |
| | Nasal | 0.001-0.002 (1-2 µg/kg) |
| Sufentanil | Nasal | 0.001-0.003 (1-3 µg/kg) |

*With atropine 0.02 mg/kg.
†Only a single dose is recommended due to metabolites that may cause seizures.

### Benzodiazepines

Benzodiazepines calm children, allay anxiety, and diminish recall of perianesthetic events. At low doses, minimal drowsiness and cardiovascular or respiratory depression are produced.

*Midazolam*, a short-acting, water-soluble benzodiazepine with an elimination half-life of approximately 2 hours, is the most widely used premedication for children.[112,113] The major advantage of midazolam over other drugs in its class is its rapid uptake and elimination.[114] It can be administered intravenously, intramuscularly, nasally, orally, and rectally with minimal irritation, although it leaves a bitter taste in the mouth or nasopharynx after oral or nasal administration, respectively.[115-121] Peak plasma concentrations occur approximately 10 minutes after intranasal midazolam administration, 16 minutes after rectal administration, and 53 minutes after oral administration.[114,121,122] The relative bioavailability of midazolam is approximately 90% after intramuscular injection, 60% after intranasal administration, 40% to 50% after rectal administration, and 30% after oral administration, compared with intravenous administration (see Chapter 6).[122,123] After oral or rectal administration, there is incomplete absorption and extensive hepatic extraction of the drug during the first pass through the liver—hence, the need for large doses through these routes. Most children are adequately sedated after receiving a midazolam dose of 0.025 to 0.1 mg/kg intravenously, 0.1 to 0.2 mg/kg intramuscularly, 0.25 to 0.75 mg/kg orally, 0.2 mg/kg nasally, or 1 mg/kg rectally.

Orally administered midazolam is effective in calming most children and does not increase gastric pH or residual volume.[124,125] The current formulation of oral midazolam (2 mg/mL) is a commercially prepared, strawberry-flavored liquid. Two multicenter studies yielded slightly different responses to this preparation of oral midazolam in children.[126,127] In one study, 0.25, 0.5, and 1.0 mg/kg all produced satisfactory sedation and anxiolysis within 10 to 20 minutes,[127] whereas in the other study, 1.0 mg/kg provided greater anxiolysis and sedation than 0.25 mg/kg.[126] These differing results may be attributed to the older ages of children in the former study.[126]

Recent evidence suggests that the required dose of midazolam increases as age decreases in children, similar to that for inhaled agents and intravenous agents.[128] An increased clearance in younger children contributes to their increased dose requirement.[129] Thus, greater doses may be required in younger children to achieve a similar degree of sedation and anxiolysis. However, the formulation of the oral solution may also attenuate its effectiveness.[130,131] A number of medications that affect the cytochrome oxidase system, significantly affect the first-pass metabolism of midazolam, including grapefruit juice, erythromycin, protease inhibitors, and calcium-channel blockers that decrease CYP3A4 activity, which in turn increases the blood concentration of midazolam and prolongs sedation.[132-138] Conversely, anticonvulsants (phenytoin and carbamazepine), rifampin, St. John's wort, glucocorticoids, and barbiturates induce the CYP3A4 isoenzyme, thereby reducing the blood concentration of midazolam and its duration of action.* The dose of oral midazolam should be adjusted in children who are taking these medications.

Concerns have been raised about possible delayed discharge after premedication with oral midazolam. Oral midazolam, 0.5 mg/kg, administered to children 1 to 10 years of age did not affect awakening times, time to extubation, postanesthesia care unit, or hospital discharge times, after sevoflurane anesthesia.[139] Similar results have been reported in children and adolescents after 20 mg of oral midazolam, however, detectable preoperative sedation in this group of children was predictive of delayed emergence.[140] In children aged 1 to 3 years undergoing adenoidectomy as outpatients, premedication with oral midazolam, 0.5 mg/kg, slightly delayed spontaneous eye opening by 4 minutes and discharge by 10 minutes compared with placebo; children who had been premedicated, however, exhibited a more peaceful sleep at home on the night after surgery.[141]

Likely the greatest effect of oral midazolam on recovery occurs with its use in children undergoing myringotomy and tube insertion, a procedure that normally takes 5 to 7 minutes. In this surgery, the use of this premedication must be carefully considered. Oral midazolam decreased the infusion requirements of propofol by 33% during a propofol-based anesthesia, although the time to discharge readiness was delayed.[142] After oral midazolam premedication (0.5 mg/kg), induction of anesthesia with propofol, and maintenance with sevoflurane, emergence and early recovery were delayed by 6 and 14 minutes, respectively, in children 1 to 3 years of age compared with unpremedicated children, although discharge times did not differ.[143] Increased postoperative sedation may be attributed to synergism between propofol and midazolam on γ-aminobutyric acid (GABA) receptors.[144]

One notable benefit of midazolam is anterograde amnesia; children who were amnestic about their initial dental extractions tolerated further dental treatments better than those who were not amnestic.[145] It appears that memory becomes impaired within 10 minutes and anxiolytic effects are apparent as early as 15 minutes after oral midazolam.[146]

Although anxiolysis and a mild degree of sedation occur in most children after midazolam, a few develop undesirable adverse effects. Some children become agitated after oral midazolam.[147] If this occurs after intravenous midazolam (0.1 mg/kg), intravenous ketamine (0.5 mg/kg) may reverse the agitation.[148] Adverse behavioral changes have been reported in the postoperative period after midazolam premedication. One study found that oral midazolam suppresses crying during induction of anesthesia but may cause adverse behavioral changes (nightmares, night terrors, food rejection, anxiety, and negativism) for up to 4 weeks postoperatively compared with placebo[149]; this finding has not been substantiated.[59] One undesirable effect associated with midazolam, independent of the mode of administration (rectal, nasal, or oral), is hiccups (approximately 1%); the etiology is unknown.

Anxiolysis and sedation usually occur within 10 minutes after intranasal midazolam,[150] although it may be less effective in children with an upper respiratory tract infection (URI) and excessive nasal discharge.[121] Intranasal midazolam does not affect the time to recovery or discharge after surgical procedures at least 10 minutes in duration.[151,152] Although midazolam reduces negative behavior in children during parental separation, nasal administration is not well accepted because it produces irritation, discomfort, and a burning aftertaste that may overshadow its positive sedative effects.[153-155] Another theoretical concern for the nasal route of administration of midazolam is its potential to cause neurotoxicity via the cribriform plate.[121] There are direct connections between the nasal mucosa and the central nervous system (CNS) (E-Fig. 4-2). Medications administered nasally reach high concentrations in the cerebrospinal fluid very quickly.[156-158] To date, no such sequelae have been reported. Because midazolam with preservative has been shown to cause neurotoxicity in animals, we recommend only preservative-free midazolam for nasal administration.[159,160]

Sublingual midazolam (0.2 mg/kg) has been reported to be as effective as, and better accepted than, intranasal midazolam.[161] Oral transmucosal midazolam given in three to five small allotments (0.2 mg/kg total dose) placed on a child's tongue (8 months to 6 years of age) was found to provide satisfactory acceptance and separation from parents in 95% of children.[162]

There is another pharmacodynamic difference among benzodiazepines that is important to consider when these drugs are administered intravenously. Entry into the CNS is directly related to fat solubility.[163,164] The greater the fat solubility, the more rapid the transit into the CNS. The time to peak CNS electroencephalographic effect in adults is 4.8 minutes for midazolam but only 1.6 minutes for diazepam (see Fig. 47-7). Therefore, when administering intravenous midazolam, one must wait an adequate interval between doses to avoid excessive medication and oversedation.

*Diazepam* is only used for premedication of older children. In infants and especially preterm neonates, the elimination half-life of diazepam is markedly prolonged because of immature hepatic function (see Chapter 6). In addition, the active metabolite (desmethyldiazepam) has pharmacologic activity equal to that of the parent compound and a half-life of up to 9 days in adults.[165] The most effective route of administration of diazepam is intravenous, followed by oral and rectal. The intramuscular route is not recommended because it is painful and absorption is erratic.[166-170] The combination of oral midazolam 0.25 mg/kg and diazepam

---

*See http://www.medicine.iupui.edu/clinpharm/ddis/p450_Table_Oct_11_2009.pdf (accessed July 1, 2012).

0.25 mg/kg has been shown to provide better sedation at induction of anesthesia and less agitation during emergence than oral midazolam 0.5 mg/kg in children undergoing adenotonsillectomy.[171] The average oral dose for premedicating healthy children with diazepam ranges from 0.1 to 0.3 mg/kg; however, doses as large as 0.5 mg/kg have been used.[172] A rectal solution of diazepam is more effective and reliable than rectally administered tablets or suppositories.[170,173] The recommended dose of rectal diazepam is 1 mg/kg, and the peak serum concentration is reached after approximately at 20 minutes.[173] When compared with rectal midazolam, rectal diazepam is less effective.[174]

*Lorazepam* (0.05 mg/kg) is reserved primarily for older children. Lorazepam causes less tissue irritation and more reliable amnesia than diazepam. It can be administered orally, intravenously, or intramuscularly and is metabolized in the liver to inactive metabolites. Compared with diazepam, the onset of action of lorazepam is slower and its duration of action is prolonged. Whereas these characteristics make it a suitable premedication for inpatients, there are disadvantages for outpatients. When given the night before surgery to children undergoing reconstructive burn surgery, oral lorazepam, 0.025 mg/kg, significantly decreased preoperative anxiety.[175] The intravenous formulation of lorazepam is avoided in neonates because it may be neurotoxic.[176,177]

## Barbiturates

Barbiturates are among the oldest medications used for premedication in children, but they are infrequently used for this purpose any longer. The advantages of barbiturates include minimal respiratory or cardiovascular depression, anticonvulsant effects, and a very low incidence of nausea and vomiting. The major disadvantage of barbiturates is hyperanalgesia. In some cases, a small dose administered to children with pain may intensify the pain and cause them to become uncooperative.

The relatively short-acting barbiturates *thiopental* and *methohexital* may be given rectally to premedicate young children who refuse other modes of sedation. These drugs are usually administered in the presence of the parents who may hold the toddler until he or she is sedated.[178] The usual dose of rectal thiopental is 30 mg/kg. This dose produces sleep in about two thirds of the children within 15 minutes.[179,180] The elimination half-life of intravenous thiopental (9 ± 1.6 hours) is almost threefold greater than that of methohexital (3.9 ± 2.1 hours) owing to a slower rate of hepatic metabolism.[181] There are few data comparing the elimination kinetics of rectally administered barbiturates.

As in the case of thiopental, rectal methohexital is rarely used for premedication any longer. For rectal premedication, a 10% solution of 25 mg/kg or a 1% solution of 15 mg/kg administered via a shortened suction catheter provides effective sedation within 10 to 15 minutes.[182-184] In some cases, the sedation may be profound, resulting in airway obstruction and laryngospasm. Hence, all children should be closely monitored with a source of oxygen, suction, and a means for providing ventilatory support; rectally administered methohexital has been reported to cause apnea in children with meningomyelocele.[185,186] Children chronically treated with phenobarbital or phenytoin are more resistant to the effects of rectally administered methohexital, probably because of enzyme induction.[183,187]

Recovery after methohexital is relatively rapid, but the time required to return to full consciousness after a 30-minute or shorter surgical procedure is slightly prolonged compared with the time needed after 5 mg/kg of intravenous thiopental for the induction of anesthesia.[188]

Additional disadvantages of rectal methohexital include unpredictable systemic absorption, defecation after administration, and hiccups. Contraindications to methohexital include hypersensitivity, temporal lobe epilepsy, and latent or overt porphyria.[189-191] Rectal methohexital is also contraindicated in children with rectal mucosal tears or hemorrhoids because large quantities of the drug can be absorbed, resulting in respiratory or cardiac arrest.

## Nonbarbiturate Sedatives

*Chloral hydrate* and *triclofos* are orally administered nonbarbiturate drugs that are used to sedate children; both have slow onset times and are relatively long acting. They are converted to trichloroethanol, which has an elimination half-life of 9 hours in toddlers (see Fig. 47-3).[192] Chloral hydrate is frequently used by nonanesthesiologists to sedate children.[193-195] It is rarely used by anesthesiologists because it is unreliable, has a prolonged duration of action, is unpleasant to taste, and is irritating to the skin, mucous membranes, and gastrointestinal tract. An oral dose (50 to 100 mg/kg with a total maximum dose of 2 g) is most effective when administered 1.5 to 2 hours before anesthesia (see Chapters 6 and 47). Its use in neonates is not recommended because of impaired metabolism,[196,197] nor is chronic administration recommended because of the theoretical possibility of carcinogenesis.[198] Children with hepatic failure may have prolonged action of chloral hydrate, and greater doses can produce significant respiratory depression in children with liver disease. Commercially prepared chloral hydrate is no longer available in the USA but a powdered form can be reconstituted by the hospital pharmacy for oral administration.

## Opioids

Opioids may be useful to provide analgesia and sedation in children who have pain preoperatively, but they also confer side effects including nausea, vomiting, respiratory depression, sedation, and dysphoria. Therefore, all children who receive an opioid premedication should be continuously observed and monitored with pulse oximetry.

*Morphine sulfate*, 0.05 to 0.1 mg/kg intravenously, may be given to children with preoperative pain. It is also effective when given orally; rectal administration is not recommended owing to erratic absorption. Neonates are more sensitive to the respiratory depressant effects of morphine, and it is rarely used to premedicate that age group.[199]

*Fentanyl* was introduced in a "lollipop" delivery system known as oral transmucosal fentanyl citrate (OTFC) for premedication in children in the United States but is no longer available for that indication. Its current use is to treat breakthrough cancer pain. It is nonthreatening and more readily accepted by children than other routes as a premedicant and facilitates separation from parents.[200] Fentanyl is strongly lipophilic, and OTFC is readily absorbed from the buccal mucosa, with an overall bioavailability of approximately 50%.[201,202] The optimal dose for premedication is 10 to 15 μg/kg with minimal desaturation and preoperative nausea.[203,204] The onset of sedation is within 10 minutes, although the blood concentrations of fentanyl continue to increase for up to 20 minutes after completion. Recovery from anesthesia after a premedication of 10 to 15 μg/kg of oral fentanyl is similar to that after 2 μg/kg intravenously.[203] Doses greater than 15 μg/kg are not recommended because of opioid adverse effects, particularly respiratory depression. The incidence of the opioid-associated adverse effects is increased when the interval between completion of "lollipop" and induction of anesthesia is prolonged.[204-207]

Ondansetron given after the induction of anesthesia does not affect the frequency of opioid-related nausea and vomiting.[208] Fentanyl has also been administered nasally (1 to 2 µg/kg) but primarily after induction of anesthesia as a means of providing analgesia in children without intravenous access.[209]

*Sufentanil* is 10 times more potent than fentanyl and is administered nasally in a dose of 1.5 to 3 µg/kg. Children are usually calm and cooperative, and most separate with minimal distress from their parents.[150] In a study that compared the adverse effects of nasally administered midazolam and sufentanil, midazolam caused more nasal irritation, whereas sufentanil caused more postoperative nausea and vomiting and reduced chest wall compliance. In addition, children in the sufentanil group were discharged approximately 40 minutes later than those in the midazolam group.[154] The potential adverse effects and prolonged hospital stay after nasal sufentanil makes it an unpopular choice for premedication.

*Tramadol* is a weak µ-opioid receptor agonist whose analgesic effect is mediated via inhibition of norepinephrine reuptake and stimulation of serotonin release. Tramadol is devoid of action on platelets and does not depress respirations in the clinical dose range.[210] Serum concentrations peak by 2 hours after oral dosing with clinical analgesia maintained for 6 to 9 hours. Tramadol is metabolized by CYP2D6 and is subject to variable responses based on polymorphisms of this enzyme.[211] When oral tramadol (1.5 mg/kg) was given to children who had been premedicated with oral midazolam (0.5 mg/kg), it provided good analgesia after multiple dental extractions with no adverse respiratory or cardiovascular effects.[212] Intravenous tramadol (1.5 mg/kg) given before induction of general anesthesia has been compared with local infiltration of 0.5% bupivacaine (0.25 mL/kg) for ilioinguinal and iliohypogastric nerve blocks. Tramadol was as effective as the regional blocks in terms of pain control, although the incidence of nausea and vomiting was greater in the tramadol group. Time to discharge was similar in both groups.[213]

*Butorphanol* is a synthetic opioid agonist-antagonist with properties similar to those of morphine that can be administered nasally.[214] It is as effective as equipotent doses of intramuscular meperidine and morphine, with an onset of analgesic action in about 15 minutes and peak activity within 1 to 2 hours in adults. The most frequent adverse effect is sedation that resolves approximately 1 hour after administration. A dose of 0.025 mg/kg administered nasally immediately after the induction of anesthesia was shown to provide good analgesia after myringotomy and tube placement at the expense of an increased incidence of emesis at home compared with nonopioid analgesics such as acetaminophen.[215]

When fentanyl or other opioids are combined with midazolam, they produce more respiratory depression than opioids or midazolam alone.[216] If opioids are used in combination with other sedatives such as benzodiazepines, the dose of each drug should be appropriately reduced to avoid serious respiratory depression. For example, if fentanyl is indicated to control pain in a child who has already received midazolam, the fentanyl dose should be titrated in small increments (0.25 to 0.5 µg/kg) to prevent hypoxemia and hypopnea or apnea.

*Codeine* is a commonly prescribed oral opioid that must undergo *O*-demethylation in the liver to produce morphine to provide effective analgesia. Between 5% and 10% of children lack the cytochrome isoenzyme (CYP2D6) required for this conversion and therefore do not derive analgesic benefit. On the other hand, a very small percentage of children are ultrarapid metabolizers who rapidly convert this prodrug to morphine (see Chapter 6 for further discussion). As a result, they may experience the more severe adverse effects and complications associated with morphine (the codeine metabolite) in addition to analgesia, particularly if excessive or frequent doses of codeine are prescribed. If these same children have been sensitized to opioids because of intermittent or chronic hypoxia, the adverse events may result in respiratory and cardiac arrest.[217]

Codeine can be administered orally or intramuscularly but should not be administered intravenously because of the risk of seizures.[217a] The usual oral dose of oral codeine is 0.5 to 1.5 mg/kg with an onset of action within 20 minutes and a peak effect between 1 and 2 hours. The elimination half-life of codeine is 2.5 to 3 hours. The combination of codeine with acetaminophen is effective in relieving mild to moderate pain. This combination was found to provide superior analgesia compared with acetaminophen alone after myringotomy and placement of pressure-equalizing tubes.[218,219] Codeine, like all opioids, may result in nausea and vomiting (see Chapter 6).

## Ketamine

*Ketamine* is a phencyclidine derivative that produces dissociation of the cortex from the limbic system, producing reliable sedation and analgesia while preserving upper airway muscular tone and respiratory drive.[218] Ketamine may be administered by intravenous, intramuscular, oral, nasal transmucosal, and rectal routes. The disadvantages of ketamine include sialorrhea, nystagmus, an increased incidence of postoperative emesis, and possible undesirable psychological reactions such as hallucinations, nightmares, and delirium, although to date no psychological reactions have been reported after oral ketamine. Concomitant administration of midazolam may eliminate or attenuate these emergence reactions.[220,221] The addition of atropine or glycopyrrolate is recommended to decrease the sialorrhea caused by ketamine.[222]

Intramuscular ketamine is an effective means of sedating combative, apprehensive, or developmentally delayed children who are otherwise uncooperative and refuse oral medication. A low dose of 2 mg/kg is sufficient to adequately calm most uncooperative children in 3 to 5 minutes so that they will accept a mask for inhalation induction of anesthesia and does not prolong hospital discharge times even after brief procedures.[110] However, the combination of intramuscular ketamine (2 mg/kg) and midazolam (0.1 to 0.2 mg/kg) significantly prolongs recovery and discharge times, making the ketamine-midazolam combination inappropriate for brief ambulatory procedures.[223]

Larger doses of intramuscular ketamine are particularly useful for the induction of anesthesia in children in whom there is a desire to maintain a stable blood pressure and in whom there is no venous access, such as those with congenital heart disease. Larger doses (4 to 5 mg/kg) sedate children within 2 to 4 minutes, and very large doses (10 mg/kg) induce deep sedation that may last from 12 to 25 minutes. Larger doses and repeated doses may be associated with hallucinations, nightmares, vomiting, and unpleasant, as well as prolonged, recovery from anesthesia.[110,224] Concentrations of ketamine of 100 mg/mL are available in the United States and several other countries for intramuscular injection. It is imperative to label these syringes to avoid a syringe swap with syringes containing more dilute concentrations of ketamine. Oral ketamine alone and in combination with oral midazolam is an effective premedication and has been used to alleviate the distress of invasive procedures (e.g., bone marrow aspiration) in pediatric oncology patients.[225,226] In a dose of 5 to 6 mg/kg, oral ketamine alone sedates most children within 12 minutes and provides sufficient sedation in more than half of the children to permit establishing intravenous access.[223,227] A larger dose of 8 mg/kg prolongs recovery from anesthesia, although by 2 hours the recovery was no different from that after 4 mg/kg.[228] Doses of up to 10 mg/kg have been described as a premedicant for children having procedures for burns; the relative bioavailability was 45%, and absorption was slow with an absorption half-life of 1 hour in this cohort.[229]

The combination of oral midazolam and ketamine provides more effective preoperative sedation than either drug alone. This oral lytic cocktail is a good alternative for children who were not adequately sedated with oral midazolam alone. The combination of oral ketamine (3 mg/kg) and midazolam (0.5 mg/kg) did not prolong recovery after surgical procedures that lasted more than 30 minutes.[230]

Nasal transmucosal ketamine in a dose of 6 mg/kg is also an effective premedication for children, with sedation developing by 20 to 40 minutes.[231] In theory, nasally administered ketamine could cause neural tissue damage if it reaches the cribriform plate (see E-Fig. 4-2). Because the preservative in ketamine is neurotoxic, preservative-free ketamine may be safer to administer by the nasal route, although this has not been established.[232] If ketamine is given by this route, we recommend the 100 mg/mL concentration to minimize the volume that must be instilled.

Rectal ketamine (5 mg/kg) produces good anxiolysis and sedation within 30 minutes of administration.[233] However, the rectal route does not provide reliable absorption.

### α₂-Agonists

*Clonidine*, an α₂-agonist, causes dose-related sedation by its effect in the locus ceruleus.[234] After oral administration, the plasma concentration peaks at approximately 60 minutes,[235] similar to rectal administration, which peaks at about 50 minutes.[236] An oral dose of 3 μg/kg given 45 to 120 minutes before surgery produces comparable sedation to that of diazepam or midazolam.[237] Oral clonidine combined with 0.15 mL/kg of apple juice 100 minutes before the induction of anesthesia does not affect the gastric fluid pH and volume in children.[238] Clonidine acts both centrally and peripherally to reduce blood pressure, and therefore it attenuates the hemodynamic response to intubation.[239] It appears to be devoid of respiratory depressant properties, even when administered in an overdose.[234] The sedative and CNS properties of clonidine reduce the dose of intravenous barbiturate required for induction of anesthesia[239] as well as the minimum alveolar concentration (MAC) of sevoflurane for tracheal intubation[240] and the concentration of inhaled anesthetic required for the maintenance of anesthesia, as evidenced by the hemodynamic stability.[241-243] Oral clonidine (2 or 4 μg/kg) reduces MAC for tracheal extubation (MAC-ex) for sevoflurane by 36% and 60%, respectively. These doses neither prolonged emergence from anesthesia nor led to airway-related complications.[244]

During the first 12 hours after surgery, oral clonidine (4 μg/kg) reduced the postoperative pain scores and the requirement for supplementary analgesics.[245,246] In children scheduled for tonsillectomy, those who received oral clonidine (4 μg/kg) exhibited more intense anxiety on separation and during induction than those who received oral midazolam (0.5 mg/kg). However, those who received clonidine had reduced mean intraoperative blood pressures; reduced duration of surgery, anesthesia, and

emergence; and decreased need for supplemental oxygen during recovery but greater postoperative opioid requirements, greater pain scores, and greater excitement. Parenthetically, these observations are not consistent with previously reported analgesic and anesthetic properties of clonidine. Even though discharge readiness, postoperative emesis, and 24-hour analgesic requirements were similar in both groups, midazolam was judged to be the better premedicant for children undergoing tonsillectomy.[247] Oral clonidine (4 μg/kg) reduces the incidence of vomiting after strabismus surgery compared with a placebo, clonidine (2 μg/kg), and oral diazepam (0.4 mg/kg).[248]

Although oral clonidine offers several desirable qualities as a premedication, particularly sedation and analgesia, the need to administer it 60 minutes before induction of anesthesia makes its use impractical in many busy outpatient settings.[247] One study found that an oral dose of 4 μg/kg attenuated the hyperglycemic response to a glucose infusion and the surgical stress in children undergoing minor surgery, possibly by inhibiting the surgical stress release of catecholamines and cortisol. Children who were involved in surgeries that lasted 1.7 hours did not develop hypoglycemia, but in the absence of intraoperative glucose infusions, there is a risk of hypoglycemia during operations of prolonged duration.[249]

*Dexmedetomidine* is a sedative with properties that are similar to those of clonidine except that it has an eightfold greater affinity for the α₂-adenoreceptors than clonidine. Based on bioavailability studies in adults,[250] it is well absorbed through the oral mucosa. In a study of 13 children aged 4 to 14 years, of whom 9 had neurobehavioral disorders, an oral dose of 2 μg/kg of dexmedetomidine provided adequate sedation for a mask induction within 20 to 30 minutes of administration. It was postulated that a larger dose of 3 to 4 μg/kg might be more effective.[251]

Intranasal administration of 1 and 1.5 μg/kg dexmedetomidine produced significant sedation after 45 minutes with a peak effect at 90 to 150 minutes as compared with placebo. In addition, decreases in systolic blood pressure and heart rate were reported.[252]

In children with burns, both 2 μg/kg intranasal dexmedetomidine and 0.5 mg/kg oral midazolam administered 30 to 45 minutes before induction of anesthesia provided adequate conditions for induction of anesthesia and emergence, although dexmedetomidine produced more sleep preoperatively.[253] Oral midazolam (0.5 μg/kg given 30 minutes before surgery), oral clonidine (4 μg/kg given 90 minutes before surgery), and transmucosal dexmedetomidine (1 μg/kg given 45 minutes before surgery) all produced similar preanesthetic sedation and response to separation from parents in a comparative trial, although children who received dexmedetomidine and clonidine experienced attenuated mean arterial pressure and heart rate preoperatively and reduced pain scores postoperatively compared with midazolam.[254]

### Antihistamines

Antihistamines are rarely used for premedication in children, in part because their sedative effects are quite variable. They are very rarely given to infants but may occasionally be indicated for older children, especially those who are hyperkinetic.

*Hydroxyzine* is mainly administered for its tranquilizing properties[255,256]; it also has antiemetic, antihistaminic, and antispasmodic properties, with minimal respiratory and circulatory effects. It is commonly administered with other classes of drugs as an intramuscular "cocktail" in a dose of 0.5 to 1.0 mg/kg.

*Diphenhydramine* is an $H_1$ blocker with mild sedative and antimuscarinic effects. The dose in children is 2.5 to 5 mg/kg/day (maximum 300 mg/day) in four divided doses orally, intravenously, or intramuscularly. Although the duration of action is 4 to 6 hours, it does not appear to interfere with recovery from anesthesia.[257] The combination of oral diphenhydramine (1.25 mg/kg) and oral midazolam (0.5 mg/kg) has been used to provide sedation for healthy children undergoing MRI.[258] The combination was more effective than midazolam alone without a delay in discharge and recovery times.

### Anticholinergic Drugs

In the past, anticholinergic agents were used (1) to prevent the undesirable bradycardia associated with some anesthetic agents (halothane and succinylcholine), (2) to minimize the autonomic vagal reflexes manifested during surgical manipulations (e.g., laryngoscopy, strabismus repair), and (3) to reduce secretions. The most commonly used anticholinergic drugs are atropine, scopolamine, and glycopyrrolate. Anticholinergics also provide undesirable effects including tachycardia, dry mouth, skin erythema, and hyperthermia due to inhibition of sweating. Atropine and scopolamine cross the blood-brain barrier and may cause CNS excitation manifested as agitation, confusion, restlessness, ataxia, hallucinations, slurred speech, and memory loss if given in excessive doses.

Because most modern inhalational anesthetics are not associated with bradycardia and succinylcholine is infrequently used in children, the routine use of an anticholinergic drug is not generally warranted. Most anesthesiologists administer these agents only when indicated, such as before intravenous succinylcholine, combined with ketamine, before laryngoscopy and intubation in neonates, and when surgery stimulates vagal reflexes, such as during strabismus repair. In the majority of cases, anticholinergics need not be given preoperatively but rather should be given after intravenous access is established.

The recommended doses of anticholinergics are *atropine*, 0.01 to 0.02 mg/kg, and *scopolamine*, 0.005 to 0.010 mg/kg. Atropine is more commonly used and blocks the vagus nerve more effectively than scopolamine, whereas scopolamine is a better sedative, antisialagogue, and amnestic. Infants who are at risk for or show early evidence of a slowing of the heart rate should receive the atropine before the heart rate actually decreases to ensure a prompt onset of effect to maintain cardiac output.[259] *Glycopyrrolate* is a synthetic quaternary ammonium compound that does not cross the blood-brain barrier. It is twice as potent as atropine in decreasing the volume of oral secretions, and its duration of effect is three times greater. The recommended dose of glycopyrrolate (0.01 mg/kg) is half that of atropine. The routine use of an anticholinergic drug for the sole purpose of drying secretions is probably unwarranted, because a dry mouth can be a source of extreme discomfort for a child. Therefore, it is best to reserve the use of glycopyrrolate for specific indications such as to limit sialorrhea associated with ketamine.

### Topical Anesthetics

The child's exaggerated fear of the needle makes topical anesthetic creams an attractive alternative to intradermal infiltration and intramuscular injections. There are several needleless methods to minimize procedural pain, each with its own limitations.

*EMLA* cream (eutectic mixture of local anesthetic, Astra Zeneca, Wilmington, Del.) is a mixture of two local anesthetics (2.5% lidocaine and 2.5% prilocaine). One-hour application of EMLA cream to intact skin with an occlusive dressing provides adequate topical anesthesia[260] for a variety of superficial procedures, including intravenous catheter insertion, lumbar puncture, vaccination, laser treatment of port-wine stains, and neonatal circumcision.[261-266] However, EMLA causes venoconstriction and skin blanching, both of which obscure superficial veins, making intravenous cannulation more difficult.[267] The prilocaine in EMLA may cause methemoglobinemia,[268] although, a 1-hour application at a maximum dose of 1 gram did not induce methemoglobinemia when applied to intact skin in full-term neonates and infants younger than 3 months of age.[269] Lidocaine toxicity has been reported when EMLA was applied to mucosal membranes for extended periods.[270]

*Ametop* is a topical local anesthetic (4% tetracaine) that is available in the United Kingdom, Europe, and Canada (Smith and Nephew, Lachine, Quebec) but not in the United States. Its indications are identical to those of EMLA, but its properties are different. When applied to intact skin under an occlusive dressing, it anesthetizes the skin within 30 to 40 minutes, and it produces no venoconstriction or skin blanching and zero risk of methemoglobinemia.

*ELA-Max* (4% lidocaine) is another topical anesthetic cream that decreases the pain associated with dermatologic procedures[271] and intravenous catheter insertion after only a 30-minute application.[272] ELA-Max causes some blanching of the skin, like EMLA cream but to a lesser extent, and dilates the veins better than EMLA cream.[273]

The *S-Caine Patch* (ZARS, Inc., Salt Lake City) is a eutectic mixture of lidocaine and tetracaine (70 mg of each per patch) that uses a controlled heating system to accelerate delivery and effectiveness of the local anesthetic. After 20 minutes of application, the pain associated with venipuncture is reduced. This patch causes mild and transient local erythema and edema and no blanching of the skin.[274] Other noninvasive topical anesthetic delivery systems are available, such as lidocaine iontophoresis using an impregnated electrode, a current generator, and a return pad to carry ionized lidocaine through the stratum corneum.[275] This technique provides similar pain relief for insertion of intravenous catheters in children as EMLA cream but requires extra equipment and training for proper application.[276] Lidocaine iontophoresis also causes a stinging pain that some children experience during current application, and potential skin burns from the electrodes.[277] Needle-free injection systems for lidocaine are also available for pain free insertion of intravenous cannulae or other needle-based procedures.[277a,277b]

### Nonopioid Analgesics

*Acetaminophen* is the most common nonopioid analgesic used for treatment of postoperative pain in children. It can be administered orally preoperatively, rectally immediately after induction of anesthesia but before the start of surgery, or intravenously (where available) once intravenous access has been established.

The oral doses of acetaminophen for antipyresis, 10 to 15 mg/kg, are as effective as ketorolac, 1 mg/kg,[278] given 10 or more minutes postoperatively for myringotomies and tube placement.[279] Oral acetaminophen is very rapidly absorbed with a bioavailability of 0.9-1.[279] Neonates may have a lower incidence of hepatotoxicity because the immature hepatic enzyme systems in neonates produce less toxic metabolites than in older children.[280-282] When given preemptively, acetaminophen has opioid-sparing properties that enhance analgesia in children after tonsillectomy.[283,284] Preoperative oral acetaminophen and codeine provided superior analgesia to acetaminophen alone after myringotomy and tube placement.[219] However, in children undergoing tonsillectomy, there was no difference in the level of pain control provided by acetaminophen and acetaminophen with codeine. Postoperative oral intake was significantly higher in children treated with acetaminophen alone.[285] A relationship between concentration and analgesic effect for pain relief after tonsillectomy has been observed in children. An effect compartment concentration of 10 mg/L was associated with a reduction of pain by 2.6 units (using a visual analogue scale ranging from 0 to 10).[286]

The time to the peak blood concentration of acetaminophen after rectal administration of 10, 20, and 30 mg/kg ranges between 60 and 180 minutes after administration. In addition, the equilibration half-time between plasma and effect compartment is approximately 1 hour.[286] This slow absorption and delayed effect site concentrations require acetaminophen administration immediately after induction of anesthesia to provide sufficient time to achieve therapeutic blood concentrations by the end of surgery (primarily for operations that will take 1 hour or longer).[287] Furthermore, doses of 10 to 30 mg/kg rectal acetaminophen may not achieve peak or sustained blood concentrations that ensure effect (Fig. 4-2). Thus, an initial dose of rectal acetaminophen of 40 mg/kg has been recommended, followed by 20 mg/kg rectally every 6 hours. This dosing regimen was subsequently confirmed.[288] After 45 mg/kg rectal acetaminophen, the mean maximum blood concentration was 13 μg/mL (range 7 to 19), and the mean time to that maximum concentration was approximately 200 minutes.[289] Several other single-dose rectal administration studies reported similar results.[289,290]

For children undergoing tonsillectomy, a preoperative oral dose of 40 mg/kg plus 20 mg/kg rectally 2 hours later was associated with satisfactory pain scores for about 8 hours after administration.[279] With doses of 40 to 60 mg/kg rectally administered after induction of anesthesia but before surgery, children required less rescue morphine postoperatively and less analgesia at home than children who received either a placebo or 20 mg/kg of acetaminophen rectally.[284] In addition, the children who received larger doses of acetaminophen experienced less postoperative nausea and vomiting. However, until further safety data are developed, the initial dose of acetaminophen should not exceed 40 to 45 mg/kg with a total 24-hour dose of not more than 100 mg/kg in order to avoid hepatic toxicity. Acetaminophen administered rectally in a loading dose of 40 mg/kg and then 20 mg/kg either orally or rectally every 6 hours after elective craniofacial surgery yielded greater plasma concentrations and lower pain scores than those who received oral acetaminophen; this was in part related to some children vomiting the oral acetaminophen.[291] Note that these are excessive oral doses which cannot be recommended.

Excessive fasting, a very large loading dose of acetaminophen, and sevoflurane anesthesia may deplete glutathione stores and thus contribute to the development of hepatic failure.[292] The coadministration of antiepileptic drugs has also been implicated in hepatotoxicity from acetaminophen.[293] *Because hepatic toxicity is a real and potentially fatal complication of an acetaminophen overdose, a complete medication history of acetaminophen consumption and concomitant drugs should be completed preoperatively, and the recommended maximum daily dose should not be exceeded.*

There are two different intravenous formulations of acetaminophen available in some countries.[294] One is a prodrug of acetaminophen (*propacetamol*) with a bioavailability of 50%. It may

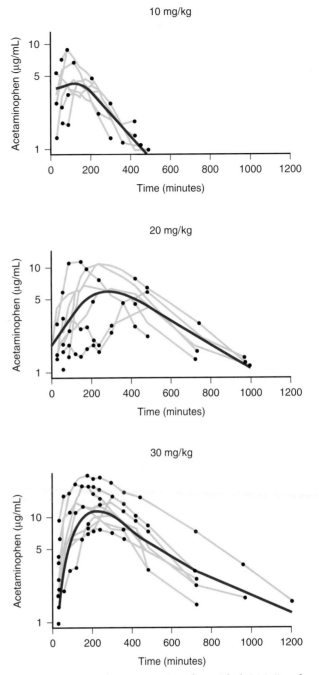

**FIGURE 4-2** Acetaminophen concentrations after rectal administration of 10, 20, or 30 mg/kg were recorded. Values for serum concentration of acetaminophen (*solid circles, teal lines*) are plotted against time for each child. Thick (*magenta*) lines indicate "average" values. Note that only children who received 30 mg/kg achieved the antipyretic threshold of 10 to 20 μg/mL, but that even at this dose that range was not sustained. These data suggest the need to use a larger loading dose (approximately 40 mg/kg) followed by subsequent doses of 20 mg/kg every 6 hours; see text for details. (From Birmingham PK, Tobin MJ, Henthorn TK, et al. Twenty-four-hour pharmacokinetics of rectal acetaminophen: an old drug with new recommendations. Anesthesiology 1997;87:244-52.)

be administered in a dose of 30 mg/kg (15 mg/kg acetaminophen) every 6 hours to children 2 to 15 years of age. In a placebo-controlled trial in febrile children, this dose of propacetamol was superior to placebo.[295] Pharmacokinetic studies indicate that such a dose of propacetamol maintains mean steady-state blood concentrations of acetaminophen of 10 μg/mL.[296] Therapeutic blood concentrations are achieved in neonates 10 days of age or younger with 15 mg/kg of propacetamol four times daily, but neonates older than 10 days require twice the dose, or 30 mg/kg at the same frequency.[297] Hemostatic effects of large (60 mg/kg) doses of propacetamol in adult volunteers showed transient but reversible inhibition of platelet aggregation as well as decreased thromboxane activity. Although these effects were less than those after ketorolac (0.4 mg/kg), the combination of acetaminophen and ketorolac may prolong these effects.[298]

A new intravenous formulation of paracetamol (15 mg/kg) was introduced and compared with propacetamol, 30 mg/kg, for postoperative pain relief after inguinal hernia repair. The outcomes were similar, but intravenous paracetamol was better tolerated at the injection site.[299]

In a study of 50 children, ages 2 to 5 years, undergoing elective adenoidectomy or adenotonsillectomy, intravenous acetaminophen 15 mg/kg or rectal acetaminophen 40 mg/kg resulted in equivalent pain scores. The time to the first rescue analgesic in the rectal acetaminophen group (median 10 hours, attributed to its slow absorption) was greater than in the intravenous acetaminophen group (median 7 hours), although few children in either group required any rescue analgesics during the first 6 hours.[300] Intravenous acetaminophen (15 mg/kg) has been compared with intramuscular meperidine 1 mg/kg in children undergoing tonsillectomy. When compared with meperidine, intravenous acetaminophen resulted in comparable analgesia but less sedation and earlier readiness for discharge.[301] In children undergoing dental restoration with the same medications and doses, children in the acetaminophen group had greater pain scores but earlier readiness for recovery room discharge.[302]

Current dosing recommendations for intravenous paracetamol in children and adolescents 2 to 12 years old weighing less than 50 kg is 15 mg/kg every 6 hours with a maximum of 75 mg/kg/day. In infants 1 month to 2 years of age, dosing from the pharmacokinetic data suggests a dose reduction of 33%, 10 mg/kg every 4 hours or 12.5 mg/kg every 6 hours with a maximum dose of 50 to 60 mg/kg/day. In full-term neonates up to 28 days of age, the dose of intravenous acetaminophen should be reduced by 50% to 7.5 mg/kg every 6 to 8 hours with a maximum daily dose of 30 mg/kg. This dosing regimen produces a similar pharmacokinetic profile as in children older than 2 years of age.[303,304] The major concern in this age group is accidental overdose of acetaminophen and hepatic toxicity. Three near-fatal cases of infants who received 10- and 20-fold overdoses of intravenous acetaminophen have been reported.[305,306] Careful documentation of the dose of intravenous acetaminophen is warranted in infants.[307]

Combinations of nonsteroidal antiinflammatory drugs (NSAIDs) can be more effective in pain management than single-agent therapy.[308] Children undergoing suboccipital craniotomy who received a combination of oral acetaminophen (10 mg/kg) and ibuprofen (10 mg/kg) alternating every 2 hours had better pain scores and decreased opioid and antiemetic interventions compared with those who received analgesic medications only when requested.[309]

*Ibuprofen* is a commonly used NSAID. In children undergoing a variety of surgical procedures, rectal ibuprofen (40 mg/kg/day in divided doses) was given for up to 3 days supplemented with intravenous or intramuscular morphine as clinically indicated. The need for supplemental morphine during the 3-day study period was less for those who received the rectal ibuprofen than for those without ibuprofen.[310] Children undergoing bilateral myringotomy who were given either oral ibuprofen (10 mg/kg) or acetaminophen (15 mg/kg) demonstrated similar pain scores.[311] Rectal ibuprofen alone provided insufficient analgesia for children undergoing ambulatory adenoidectomy.[312]

A combination of acetaminophen and codeine provides superior analgesia to ibuprofen after tonsillectomy. Furthermore, the children who received ibuprofen had a significant increase in bleeding time.[313] In an unblinded study, ibuprofen provided similar postoperative analgesia as acetaminophen with codeine after tonsillectomy with less nausea and vomiting and no increase in bleeding.[314] The combination of acetaminophen with ibuprofen, but not with rofecoxib, reduced the need for early analgesia by 50% in children undergoing tonsillectomy compared with acetaminophen alone.[315] Ibuprofen provides analgesia superior to placebo and equal to acetaminophen in children undergoing dental procedures.[316] Ibuprofen should not be used in children with impaired renal function or in those who are hypovolemic because of the increased risk of renal toxicity.[317,318]

*Ketorolac* is an NSAID that can be administered parenterally or orally, intraoperatively, or postoperatively. Ketorolac has an opioid-sparing effect, reducing the incidence of adverse effects of opioids such as respiratory depression, nausea, and vomiting. Features that may limit the usefulness of this drug include gastrointestinal irritation, antiplatelet effects, and limited safety data. In children, small cohort pharmacokinetic studies failed to demonstrate any age-related differences in pharmacokinetics.[319] However, stereospecific pharmacokinetics of ketorolac in infants and toddlers aged 6 to 18 months showed differences in pharmacokinetics between the R(+) and S(−) isomers with more rapid elimination of the analgesic S(−) isomer. Thus, smaller dose intervals of 4 hours rather than 6 hours may be needed in infants older than 6 months to achieve serum concentrations comparable to the adult effective concentration ($EC_{50}$).[320]

Ketorolac diminishes emergence agitation and pain when given intravenously after induction for myringotomy and tube insertion.[321] However, ketorolac (1 mg/kg) provided no better pain relief than rectal acetaminophen (35 mg/kg) in children undergoing tonsillectomy with or without adenoidectomy.[322] Ketorolac (1 mg/kg) intramuscularly or intravenously before tonsillectomy increased intraoperative and postoperative blood loss compared with codeine (1.5 mg/kg) intramuscularly[323] or morphine (0.1 mg/kg) intravenously.[324,325] In the same study, there was no difference in awakening time or readiness for discharge among the treatment groups. In contrast, when ketorolac was given as a single dose at the end of tonsillectomy there was no increase in posttonsillectomy hemorrhage, although duration of hospitalization and the likelihood of overnight admission decreased.[326] Ketorolac is a useful adjunct when given intravenously to supplement the local anesthesia infiltrated by the surgeon during inguinal herniorrhaphies.[327] Ketorolac (0.9 mg/kg) is an effective alternative to morphine (0.1 mg/kg), with less nausea and vomiting[328] and less postoperative morphine requirement if continued at a dose of 0.5 mg/kg intravenously every 6 hours in infants and children.[329] This has also been confirmed in orthopedic surgery with the added benefit of decreased length of stay.[330] Single doses of ketorolac (0.8 mg/kg) are opioid sparing and decrease the frequency of urinary retention in orthopedic surgery when combined with patient-controlled analgesia with morphine.[331] In children undergoing strabismus surgery, ketorolac provides equivalent analgesia to fentanyl (1 μg/kg) and morphine (0.1 mg/kg), with less postoperative nausea and vomiting.[332,333] In children undergoing ureteral reimplantation, ketorolac decreases the incidence and severity of postoperative bladder spasms with no decrease in hematocrit or increase in serum creatinine.[334,335]

Because ketorolac can increase bleeding time, we recommend discussing its use with the surgeon and administering the drug only after achieving hemostasis and completion of surgery. The safe use of this drug in infants younger than 6 months of age has been questioned, although a review of 53 infants who received ketorolac 48 hours after cardiac surgery that was continued for 3 days showed a minimal increase in serum creatinine and blood urea nitrogen at 48 hours after institution of the therapy but no increase in bleeding episodes.[336,337] This is too small a sample to forecast the safety of ketorolac in the entire population of surgical children. Furthermore, creatinine and blood urea nitrogen are too insensitive as indices of renal function. Despite the varied doses described earlier, the recommended dose should be limited to 0.5 mg/kg, with a maximal dose of 15 mg for children who weigh less than 50 kg and 0.5 mg/kg up to 30 mg every 6 hours for those who weigh more than 50 kg. A new metered nasal formulation may simplify administration.

*Rofecoxib*, an NSAID cyclooxygenase-2 (COX-2) inhibitor, offers the advantages of minimal effects on renal, gastrointestinal, and platelet functions.[338-341] However, the use of COX-2 inhibitors is currently under reevaluation owing to the increased risk of myocardial and neurologic sequelae after their long-term use in adults[342]; risks in the pediatric population have not been described.

### Antiemetics

Antiemetic administration should be considered in children undergoing high-risk procedures such as tonsillectomy and strabismus repair as well as those who have a history of motion sickness or prior history of postanesthesia nausea and vomiting. The uses of these medications are presented elsewhere in the text (see Chapters 6, 31, and 32).

### Corticosteroids

Children who have been taking chronic corticosteroid therapy (e.g., for asthma, Crohn disease, lupus, acute lymphocytic leukemia) and those who have discontinued chronic corticosteroid therapy in the last 6 months may suffer from suppression of the hypothalamic-pituitary-adrenal axis.[343] There is a paucity of evidence to support the need for supplemental corticosteroids in children in the perioperative period who have been taking chronic corticosteroid therapy. In the past, hypotension was reported in those who were taking chronic corticosteroid therapy and underwent general anesthesia or another stress. This may be attributed to hypovolemia. Nonetheless, many endocrinologists continue to recommend a dose of supplemental corticosteroids before or shortly after induction of anesthesia for "stress" corticosteroid coverage. The usual recommended dose is 1 to 2 mg/kg of hydrocortisone intramuscularly or intravenously or an equivalent dose of dexamethasone (0.05 to 0.1 mg/kg) approximately 1 hour before the induction of anesthesia or as soon as intravenous access is established. For more complicated operations, the corticosteroid dose may be repeated every 6 hours for up to 72 hours (see Chapter 25).

### Insulin

Optimal management of diabetic children undergoing surgery entails maintaining glucose homeostasis, avoiding hyperglycemia with resultant osmotic diuresis, impaired wound healing, and increased infection rate, and avoiding hypoglycemia. Anesthesiologists should work together with the endocrinologist or primary care physician to design a plan for each child's specific diabetes treatment regimen, glycemic control, intended surgery, and anticipated postoperative care. Diabetes mellitus is the most common endocrine problem encountered in children. The preoperative fasting time should be the same as that recommended for nondiabetic children. Every attempt should be made to schedule these children as the first case of the day to minimize the fasting period. Preoperative laboratory tests generally include hematocrit, serum electrolytes, and glucose levels; blood glucose concentrations should be measured at frequent intervals during the perianesthetic period. Several protocols have been crafted to control the blood sugar in children who are diabetic[344]; these are described in more detail in Chapter 25 (see also Figs. 25-1 to 25-9, which describe a variety of management strategies).

### Antibiotics

Antibiotics are frequently administered to prevent or reduce infection in surgical patients. The appropriate timing of antibiotics is now a source of performance benchmarking for some insurance carriers, making communication with surgeons essential for the success of this anesthesiology-directed quality assessment measure. For prophylaxis against endocarditis in children with structural heart disease, antibiotics should ideally be administered either intravenously 30 to 60 minutes or orally 1 hour before the induction of anesthesia and surgery. In reality, in children these antibiotics are usually administered after induction of anesthesia and establishment of intravenous access (see also Tables 14-2 and 14-3).[345]

### Antacids, H₂ Antagonists, and Gastrointestinal Motility Drugs

The risk of aspiration during induction of or emergence from anesthesia is increased in children who are developmentally delayed, have gastroesophageal reflux, experienced previous esophageal surgery, had a difficult airway, were obese, or had undergone a traumatic injury. Preanesthetic administration of drugs that reduce gastric fluid volume and acidity may decrease the risk of pulmonary acid aspiration syndrome (Table 4-4).[1,346] Gastric fluid pH may be increased by drinking a nonparticulate antacid such as sodium citrate; particulate antacids should be avoided because they can cause severe pneumonitis if aspirated.

*Cimetidine* and *ranitidine* are H₂-receptor antagonists that decrease gastric acid secretion, increase gastric fluid pH, and

**TABLE 4-4** Doses of Antacids, H₂ Antagonists, and Gastrointestinal Motility Drugs

| Drug | Dose |
|---|---|
| **Antacids** | |
| Bicitra | 30 mL (0.5-1 mL/kg up to 30 mL) |
| **Prokinetic** | |
| Metoclopramide | 0.1-0.15 mg/kg |
| **H₂ Antagonists** | |
| Cimetidine | 5-10 mg/kg |
| Ranitidine | 2-2.5 mg/kg |
| Famotidine | 0.3-0.4 mg/kg |

reduce gastric residual volume.[347,348] These drugs can be given orally, intravenously, or intramuscularly.

*Metoclopramide* is often administered with an $H_2$-receptor antagonist to increase lower esophageal sphincter tone, relax the pyloric sphincter and the duodenal bulb, and promote gastric emptying by increasing peristalsis of the duodenum and jejunum. The drug effect is apparent 30 to 60 minutes after oral administration and 1 to 2 minutes after intravenous administration.[349] Adverse effects such as extrapyramidal signs relate to the effect of metoclopramide on the CNS through blockade of dopaminergic receptors.

# Induction of Anesthesia

## PREPARATION FOR INDUCTION

Adequate preparation includes warming the operating room and ensuring that warming devices are functioning properly (e.g., heat lamps, warming blanket, forced air warmer) before the child's arrival, especially for young infants. The preinduction checklist should include a variety of sizes of masks, oral airways, laryngoscope blades, tracheal tubes (one-half size larger and one-half size smaller than the anticipated size), an appropriate size laryngeal mask airway (LMA), and functioning wall suction. The anesthesia machine and monitoring equipment should be prepared before the child's arrival in the operating room to ensure that all appropriate equipment is on hand and to minimize any last-minute commotion. One of the most essential monitors used during the induction of anesthesia is the precordial stethoscope. The bell from the stethoscope should have a double-stick adhesive attached and ready for application before induction. A chair or stool for the child's parent to sit on helps avoid fainting episodes should the parent be present at induction of anesthesia. Ensuring a quiet, calm operating room environment, free of clanging instruments and loud conversations among the staff, allows for a smoother and less upsetting induction.

There are a variety of techniques for inducing general anesthesia. The technique used depends on a number of factors, including the child's developmental age, understanding and ability to cooperate, and previous experiences; the presence of a parent; and the interaction of these factors with the child's underlying medical or surgical conditions.

## INHALATION INDUCTION

The most common method of inducing anesthesia in children is inhalation by mask of the nonpungent inhalational anesthetic agent sevoflurane or halothane. The anesthesiologist should be flexible and adapt an approach that suits the child, depending on age, degree of sedation, and cooperation.

If the child is already asleep on arrival in the operating room, it is possible to utilize the "steal induction" technique. The child is not touched or disturbed. After priming of the breathing circuit with $N_2O$ in $O_2$, the mask is gently placed near the child's face and gradually brought closer and closer until it is tightly applied to the face. After the child has been breathing $N_2O$ for 1 to 2 minutes, sevoflurane is administered in a single stepwise increase in concentration to 8% (halothane may be delivered in increasing concentrations as tolerated). Adequate monitoring must be instituted as soon as possible, and the child is then transferred to the operating table. This technique is atraumatic and avoids exposing the child to the strange operating room surroundings while awake. However, it is possible that the child

may suffer psychological harm when he or she awakens to pain without realizing what has transpired.

The optimal induction sequence in toddlers is to avoid making them feel vulnerable by having the children pick a flavor of lip balm to flavor the mask and having them seated (not lying supine) on the operating room bed with the back supported by the anesthesiologist's chest or on the anesthesiologist's or the parent's lap (E-Fig. 4-3A, Video 4-2). They may be distracted by asking them to try to "blow up the balloon" by taking deeper and deeper breaths, where the balloon refers to the reservoir bag. If the child is seated on the parent's or anesthesiologist's lap, it is strongly advised that this be undertaken only with children who are wearing diapers or are sitting on a thick blanket to limit the spread of urine should the bladder empty during induction. The anesthesia machine should be within easy reach during such an induction, to allow control of the bag, pop-off valve, and vaporizer without interruption. An assistant should be at hand to help position and hold the child when needed. Other distraction techniques may be used, including allowing them to bring their favorite toy or security blanket into the operating room (see E-Fig. 4-3B). Older children may be distracted by allowing them to play electronic hand-held games or to watch a movie on a portable electronic device.

If a parent wishes to accompany a young child to the operating room, we may allow the child to remain in the parent's lap for the induction. We request that the child be sitting facing forward in the parent's lap so that there is free access to the child's face. It is vital to instruct the parent that he or she must hold the child in a "bear hug"—that is, have the arms tightly wrapped around the child and holding the child's arms in such a way that the child cannot reach up to the face mask—and to warn the parents that as the child loses consciousness the child will become limp. This approach can be difficult with either an inexperienced anesthesiologist or a very strong child who vigorously rotates his or her neck from left to right, preventing the tight application of a face mask. It is also important to have an experienced individual in front of the child and parent to hold onto the child as induction proceeds and help place the child on the operating room table after successful induction. At this point we invite the parent to kiss their child and then the parent is escorted to the waiting room (E-Fig. 4-4, *A* and *B*).

Some children refuse to have the face mask placed anywhere near their face. They may have an unknown fear of masks or may have been traumatized previously with high concentrations of sevoflurane or halothane administered at the outset through the face mask, without premedication or pretreatment with nitrous oxide. One solution to this problem is to remove the mask, place the elbow of the breathing circuit between one's fingers, and then cup your hands below the child's chin. Because nitrous oxide is heavier than air, cupped hands act like a reservoir. The hands are gradually brought closer and closer to the face, while the child is distracted, until they gently cover the mouth. Once the child is becoming sedated, 8% sevoflurane can be introduced and the mask placed on the face. Younger infants who refuse a mask may be soothed by placing one's small finger ("pinky") in the child's mouth to suck on as the face mask is gently advanced to the nose and mouth for an inhalation induction (Fig. 4-3, *A* and *B*).

### Inhalation with Sevoflurane

The traditional mask induction of anesthesia is accomplished by placing the mask lightly on the child's face and administering a mixture of $N_2O$ in $O_2$ (2:1) for 1 or 2 minutes until the full effect

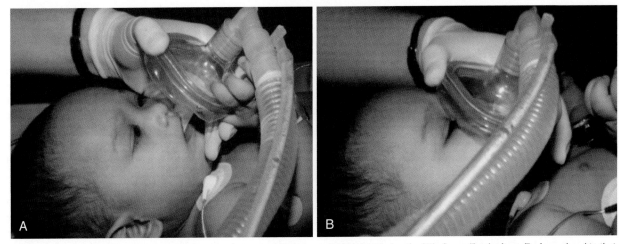

**FIGURE 4-3 A,** Infants 6 months of age or younger are often consoled during induction by placing the little finger ("pinky finger") of your hand in their mouth while you hold the face mask near their face with the rest of the hand. In general, they are so hungry that they will stop crying and eagerly suckle on your pinky finger. **B,** As the infant loses consciousness, the intensity of the suckling diminishes, the pinky finger is gently removed, and the face mask is fully applied.

of $N_2O$ is achieved. Offering children the choice of a scented mask or "sleepy air," such as bubble gum or strawberry flavor, applied to the inside of the face mask may disguise the odor of the plastic. Sevoflurane is then introduced and can be rapidly increased to 8% in a single stepwise increase, without significant bradycardia or hypotension in otherwise healthy children. After anesthesia is induced, the sevoflurane concentration should be maintained at the maximum tolerable concentration until intravenous access is established, but this concentration should be reduced if controlled ventilation is initiated so as to avoid overdose. The reason for maintaining delivery of a high concentration of sevoflurane is to minimize the risk of awareness during the early period of the induction sequence. Data from unmedicated children (aged ≥3 years) indicate that sevoflurane is associated with small increases in heart rate, although heart rate does decrease to 80 to 100 beats per minute in some children after breathing sevoflurane for a period of time.[350] In contrast to halothane,[351] sevoflurane does not increase the myocardial sensitivity to epinephrine.[352] In a study of three techniques for delivering sevoflurane for induction of anesthesia, minimal differences were detected among the three: incremental increases in sevoflurane (2%, 4%, 6%, and 7%) in oxygen, a high concentration of sevoflurane (7%) in oxygen, and a high concentration of sevoflurane in a 1:1 mixture of $N_2O$ and $O_2$.[353] When $N_2O$ was added, there was a decreased time to loss of the eyelash reflex and a decreased incidence of excitement during the induction. Agitation or excitement in early induction (shortly after loss of eyelash reflex) with sevoflurane has been observed; this is discussed in detail in Chapter 6.

### Inhalation Induction with Halothane

Halothane has largely been replaced by sevoflurane for inhalation induction of anesthesia because of halothane's slower wash-in and emergence and greater incidence of bradycardia, hypotension, and arrhythmias. When anesthesia is induced with halothane, the inspired concentration is gradually increased by 0.5% every two to three breaths up to 5%. Alternatively, a single-breath induction of anesthesia with 5% halothane can yield a rapid induction of anesthesia without triggering airway reflex responses.[354]

The inspired concentration of halothane should be decreased as soon as anesthesia is established to avoid heart rate slowing and myocardial depression. The child will autoregulate the depth of anesthesia as long as he or she is allowed to breath spontaneously; however, if respirations are controlled, then anesthetic overdose may easily occur (see Chapter 6).[355,356] Halothane sensitizes the heart to catecholamines, and ventricular arrhythmias may commonly be seen, especially during periods of hypercapnia or light anesthesia.[357]

If vital signs become abnormal during induction, the concentration of halothane should be reduced or discontinued and the circuit flushed with 100% oxygen. If bigeminy or short bursts of ventricular tachycardia occur, then the following strategies should be considered: (1) hyperventilation (to reduce the arterial carbon dioxide tension [$PaCO_2$]) (2) deepening of the halothane anesthesia, or (3) changing to an alternate potent inhalation agent.[357] There is no role for intravenous lidocaine to treat these arrhythmias.

During inhalation induction with either sevoflurane or halothane, if the oxygen saturation decreases (and there is no mechanical cause for the desaturation such as partial dislodgement of the oximeter probe, patient clenching of fingers or toes, or blood pressure cuff inflating), 100% oxygen should be administered until the oxygen saturation returns to normal while the cause of the desaturation is addressed. If the cause of the desaturation is not related to upper airway obstruction, the most common cause in a healthy child is a ventilation-perfusion mismatch due to segmental atelectasis. Recruitment of alveoli may be achieved by applying a sustained inflation of the lungs to 30 cm $H_2O$ for 30 seconds or as tolerated.[358] This may be difficult to complete before tracheal intubation, because the stomach may inflate. In such a case, recruitment should be abandoned. Alternatively, mild to moderate upper airway obstruction from collapse of the hypopharyngeal structures or the development of mild laryngospasm causes hypoventilation and desaturation. In general, this upper airway obstruction is readily relieved by gently applying a tight mask fit, closing the pop-off valve sufficiently to generate 5 to 10 cm of positive end-expiratory pressure, and allowing the distending pressure of the bag to stent open the airway until the child is adequately anesthetized to tolerate the placement of an oral airway (see Fig. 12-10 and Fig. 31-6). Cephalad pressure should be applied to the superior pole of the condyle of the mandible to sublux the temporomandibular joint. because this maneuver opens the mouth and pulls the tongue off the posterior and nasopharyngeal walls, opening the laryngeal inlet (Video 4-3, *A* and *B*).[359] This maneuver may supplant the need for an oral airway. It is very important to avoid applying digital pressure to the soft tissues of the submental triangle, because this pushes the tongue and soft tissues into the hypopharynx, occluding the oropharynx and nasopharynx. If the child develops symptomatic bradycardia, then oxygenation and ventilation must first be established, followed by intravenous atropine (0.02 mg/kg) and, if necessary, chest compressions and intravenous epinephrine (see Chapter 39).

### Inhalation Induction with Desflurane

Desflurane is very pungent, as evidenced by severe laryngospasm (49%), coughing, increased secretions, and hypoxemia during induction.[360] Therefore, *desflurane is not recommended for inhalation induction in children* but may be used safely for maintenance of general anesthesia after the trachea has been intubated.

### Hypnotic Induction

Hypnosis can reduce anxiety and pain in children with chronic medical problems and those undergoing painful procedures[361,362] as well as reduce preoperative anxiety. Hypnosis is an altered state of consciousness with highly focused attention, based on the principle of dissociation.[363] Hypnosis results in a state of inner absorption that leads to a reduction in awareness of immediate physical surroundings and experiences. Children are more likely to be absorbed in fantasy, and their natural power of play making them more hypnotizable than adults.[364] Although an anesthesiologist may not have training in hypnosis, he or she can use hypnotic suggestions to help children even though an actual trance state is not induced. It may be helpful to engage children in age-appropriate scenarios, such as going to the zoo, a fancy tea party, a baseball game, or flying a jet. Words should be spoken slowly and rhythmically with descriptions of sights and sounds that are familiar to the child as well as repeated suggestions of "feeling good." The hypnotic suggestions distract the child so that the smell of anesthetic agent becomes the scent of the zoo animals, the tea brewing, the aviation fuel, and so on. Any number of stories can be told with the same result as long as one remembers to repeatedly say things that can be identified by the child and that fit with what the child is experiencing at the time of induction.

When hypnosis was administered 30 minutes before surgery, it significantly reduced preoperative anxiety at the time of face mask application and the frequency of behavior disorders postoperatively when compared with oral midazolam, 0.5 mg/kg.[365] Hypnosis provided a relaxed state of well-being and enabled children to actively participate in anesthesia, thus leaving them with a pleasant memory. Unlike the anterograde amnesia associated with midazolam, hypnosis offers the benefit of maintaining a pleasant memory to prevent fear during future anesthetics.

### Modified Single-Breath Induction

The single-breath induction is especially appealing to children who desire to fall asleep "really fast" with a face mask, because loss of consciousness is achieved much more rapidly than with a traditional escalating dose technique. It works best with older children, although some as young as 3 years of age can be anesthetized with this technique if they are cooperative. Before beginning, the child should be coached through a mock induction by instructing him or her to "breathe in the biggest breath, possible" through the mouth (not the nose) and then "breathe all the way out until there is no more air in the lungs." If the child is used to swimming and holding the breath underwater, this makes the exercise much easier. Once this has been practiced a few times, then a practice run is repeated with only the mask (no circuit) on the face.

Before induction, the circuit and reservoir bag are primed with 70% $N_2O$ in $O_2$ and the maximum concentration of concentration of halothane or sevoflurane the vaporizer can deliver. This is achieved by running modest fresh gas flows through the circuit and intermittently emptying the reservoir bag manually into the scavenger system (i.e., with the circuit Y-connector occluded). Once the circuit is primed with the maximum concentration of inhalation agent, the mask is placed on the Y-connector, then the distal end of the circuit is occluded (to avoid contaminating the operating room), and the child is instructed to take a deep breath of room air and to exhale all the air and hold expiration. The face mask is then placed securely over the child's mouth and nose while he or she is instructed to take in the "deepest breath ever through their mouth" and "hold it, now just breathe normally." Loss of consciousness, as noted by loss of the eyelash reflex, occurs within 15 to 30 seconds after this vital capacity breath (Fig. 4-4, *A*, *B* and *C*, and Video 4-4).[354,366]

## INTRAVENOUS INDUCTION

Intravenous induction is usually reserved for older children, those who request an intravenous induction, those with a previously established intravenous catheter, those with potential cardiovascular instability, and those who need a rapid-sequence induction (RSI) because of a full stomach. There are many different options as far as medications that can be used for an intravenous induction in a child (Table 4-5). Ideally, all children should breathe 100% oxygen before intravenous induction; if the face mask is met with objections, oxygen may be insufflated without a mask by simply holding the Y-connector of the circuit between your fingers over or near the child's face.

### Thiopental

Thiopental (sodium pentothal) has been replaced by propofol as the most commonly used intravenous induction agent. The recommended induction dose of thiopental in healthy, unpremedicated children is 5 to 6 mg/kg[367]; neonates require a smaller dose (3 to 4 mg/kg).[368] Debilitated or severely ill patients, those who are hypovolemic, and those who have been premedicated may also require a smaller dose for induction of anesthesia. The beta-elimination half-life of thiopental in neonates is twice that in

| TABLE 4-5 Doses of Commonly Used Intravenous Induction Agents | |
| --- | --- |
| Drug | Dose (mg/kg) |
| Thiopental or thiamylal* | 5-8 |
| Methohexital | 1-2.5 |
| Propofol | 2.5-3.5 |
| Etomidate | 0.2-0.3 |
| Ketamine | 1-2 |

*No longer available in the United States.

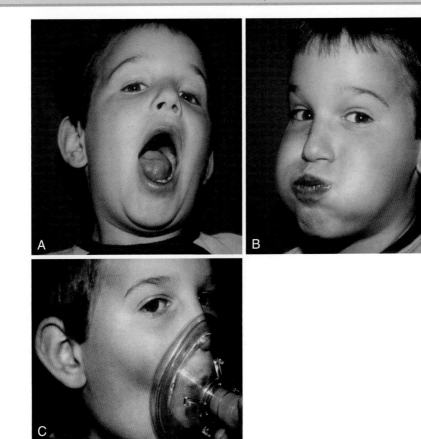

FIGURE 4-4 A single-breath induction is another useful method that is most appropriate for children 5 to 10 years of age. It is important to practice several times without the mask attached to the circuit before the actual induction (see text for details of preparing the circuit). This allows the child to become familiar with the feel of the mask as it is applied to the face and to properly time the sequence of events. **A** and **B,** Typically, we ask the child to take "the biggest breath possible and hold it." Then we ask the child to "breathe all the way out until you have no more air in your lungs and hold it" and place the face mask on the child's face. **C,** We then ask the child to take in "the biggest breath you have ever taken, hold it, then breathe normally." If a full vital capacity breath is taken with a good mask seal around the mouth and nose, most children will lose their lid reflex within 15 to 30 seconds, which is similar to intravenous induction agents.

their mothers (15 versus 7 hours), so a single dose may produce excessively prolonged effect in neonates.[369] This drug is no longer available in the United States.

### Methohexital

Methohexital is an ultra-short-acting oxybarbiturate that is infrequently used for induction. The induction dose for unpremedicated children ranges from 1.0 to 2.5 mg/kg[370]; premedicated children require a smaller dose. Recovery after intravenous administration is more rapid than after thiopental.[371] Larger doses cause skeletal muscle hyperactivity, myoclonic movements, and hiccups.[370] Pain at the injection site is common, necessitating pretreatment with intravenous lidocaine.

### Propofol

Propofol is the most commonly used nonbarbiturate intravenous induction agent in children. The induction dose of propofol varies with age: the median effective dose ($ED_{50}$) for a satisfactory induction in healthy infants 1 to 6 months old is 3.0 ± 0.2 mg/kg, and in healthy children 10 to 16 years old it is 2.4 ± 0.1 mg/kg.[372] The 95% effective dose ($ED_{95}$) in healthy unpremedicated children 3 to 12 years of age is 2.5 to 3.0 mg/kg.[373] The early distribution half-life is about 2 minutes, and the terminal elimination half-life is about 30 minutes.[374] Clearance is very large (2.3

± 0.6 L/min) and exceeds liver blood flow.[374] Advantages to propofol for induction of anesthesia include a reduced incidence of airway-related problems (e.g., laryngospasm, bronchospasm), more rapid emergence,[375,376] and a reduced incidence of nausea and vomiting.[377,378] The major disadvantage of propofol is pain at the site of injection, especially when administered in small veins (e.g., the back of the hand).[372] The administration of lidocaine (0.5 to 1.0 mg/kg) while applying tourniquet pressure proximal to the injection site (mini-Bier block) for 30 to 60 seconds before injecting the propofol effectively eliminates the pain in more than 90% of patients. However, younger children may not tolerate even the discomfort from the Bier block, which is the reason to consider using nitrous oxide to as an alternative and equally effective strategy (see Chapter 6). Other techniques reported to attenuate the pain include mixing lidocaine (0.5 to 1 mg/kg) with the propofol (but this should be done within 60 seconds of administration of the propofol), mixing thiopental with the propofol, refrigerating the propofol, pretreating with an opioid or ketamine, and diluting propofol to a 0.5% solution.[379-388]

In addition to its use as an induction agent, propofol can be administered by infusion for total intravenous anesthesia (see Chapter 7) because of its relatively low context-sensitive half-life. It is especially useful for pediatric patients undergoing non–operating room procedures such as CT, MRI, radiotherapy, bone marrow biopsy, upper and lower gastrointestinal endoscopy, and lumbar puncture.

### Etomidate

Etomidate is a hypnotic induction agent that provides marked cardiovascular stability. Etomidate is available for use in the United States and several other countries, but it is not available in many others due to concern for adrenal suppression. It is indicated for the induction of anesthesia in children with sepsis, cardiac instability, cardiomyopathy, or hypovolemic shock. The recommended induction dose is 0.2 to 0.3 mg/kg depending on the cardiovascular status of the child. Etomidate causes pain and myoclonic movements when injected intravenously[389] and may suppress adrenal steroid synthesis (see also Chapter 6).[390]

### Ketamine

Ketamine is a very useful induction agent for children with cardiovascular instability, especially in hypovolemic states, or for those who cannot tolerate a reduction in systemic vascular resistance, such as those with aortic stenosis or congenital heart disease in whom the balance between pulmonary and systemic blood flow is vital for maintaining cardiovascular homeostasis. In children whose circulation is already maximally compensated by endogenous catecholamines, ketamine is a myocardial depressant that can result in systemic hypotension.[391] The induction dose of ketamine in healthy children is 1 to 2 mg/kg. The dose should be reduced in the presence of severe hypovolemia. Smaller doses of intravenous ketamine (0.25 to 0.5 mg/kg) have also been used successfully for procedural sedation.

Ketamine causes sialorrhea, psychomimetic side effects (hallucinations, nightmares), and postoperative nausea and vomiting. The administration of an antisialagogue and midazolam is recommended to attenuate these side effects.

### INTRAMUSCULAR INDUCTION

Although it is preferable to avoid intramuscular injections in children, there are occasions when this route may be indicated, such as for the uncooperative child or adolescent who refuses all other routes of sedation (oral, intranasal, intravenous), those susceptible to malignant hyperthermia, those with congenital heart disease, and those who have poor venous access. In infants, but especially in older children, intramuscular ketamine is a very useful medication because it is available in a concentrated solution (100 mg/mL) (see earlier discussion).[110] In infants and very small children, intramuscular methohexital (10 mg/kg of a 5% solution) produces a state of anesthesia within several minutes.

### RECTAL INDUCTION

Rectal drug administration is ideally suited for an extremely frightened young child who rejects other forms of premedication and for those who are developmentally delayed. It is usually limited to children younger than 5 or 6 years of age or smaller than 20 kg, owing to volume limitations on the fluid injected and concern over emotional consequences. Methohexital, thiopental, ketamine, and midazolam have all been investigated as agents for rectal induction. For unpremedicated children, the induction doses are 30 to 40 mg/kg thiopental, 20 to 25 mg/kg methohexital,[392] 1.0 mg/kg midazolam,[393] and approximately 5 mg/kg ketamine.

Disadvantages of rectal drug administration include failure to induce anesthesia because of poor drug bioavailability or defecation and delayed recovery from anesthesia after brief

procedures due to the variability of rectal drug absorption. Conversely, there can be a very rapid drug uptake leading to respiratory compromise.

### FULL STOMACH AND RAPID-SEQUENCE INDUCTION

A full stomach is one of the most common problems that pediatric anesthesiologists face. The preferred method to secure the airway in the presence of a full stomach is intravenous RSI. Before this is undertaken, the anesthesiologist must ensure that the proper equipment is at hand: two functioning laryngoscope blades and handles (should a bulb or contact fail, a spare is available), two suctions (should the suction be blocked by vomitus or blood, a second is available), anesthetic medications, a checked anesthesia workstation with a checked breathing circuit, tracheal tubes of appropriate sizes, and stylet. All monitors should be properly functioning, and, at a minimum, the pulse oximeter, blood pressure cuff, and precordial stethoscope should be applied (in a crying, struggling child the pulse oximeter may not function properly until after anesthetic induction).

After intravenous access is established, the child should breathe 100% oxygen (preoxygenated) if possible. Studies of adult patients demonstrated that oxygen saturation remains greater than 95% for 6 minutes after only four vital capacity breaths of 100% oxygen.[394] Similar studies have not been performed in either cooperative or uncooperative children; however, without preoxygenation, younger infants and children desaturate very rapidly after induction of anesthesia, and much more rapidly than older children and adults.[395,396] One study demonstrated a more rapid increase in the inspired oxygen concentration in infants compared with older patients and that preoxygenation to a fractional concentration of $O_2$ in expired gas ($FEO_2$) of 0.9 can be achieved in 100 seconds.[397] Even with a crying child, it is possible to increase the arterial oxygen tension ($PaO_2$) by enriching the immediate environment with high gas flows of oxygen.

Preoxygenation should not be carried out in such a way that it upsets a child. Premedication (e.g., intravenous midazolam, 0.05 to 0.1 mg/kg) in divided doses may alleviate fear and anxiety before induction. It is important to preoxygenate children to avoid positive-pressure ventilation before tracheal intubation because positive-pressure ventilation might distend the already full stomach, leading to regurgitation and aspiration. After preoxygenation (and atropine 0.02 mg/kg), anesthesia is induced with intravenous thiopental (5 to 6 mg/kg),[367] propofol (3 to 4 mg/kg),[398,399] ketamine (1 to 2 mg/kg), or etomidate (0.2 to 0.3 mg/kg), followed immediately by 2 mg/kg of succinylcholine. Succinylcholine is still the paralytic agent of choice for rapid onset and short duration. However, high-dose rocuronium may be used as an alternative muscle relaxant for RSI if succinylcholine is contraindicated. Intubating conditions 30 seconds after 1.2 mg/kg rocuronium were similar to those after 1.5 mg/kg succinylcholine.[400] The mean time to return 25% of the twitch response was 46 ± 23 minutes (range, 30 to 72 minutes) for rocuronium compared with 5.8 ± 3.3 minutes (range, 1.5 to 8.2 minutes) for succinylcholine. However, if thiopental is used for induction of anesthesia and followed by rocuronium, the thiopental must be cleared from the tubing before the rocuronium is administered to prevent thiopental from precipitating.[401] The availability of a new reversal agent (sugammadex) for rocuronium (and potentially vecuronium) may reduce concern about the risks associated with a prolonged duration of action of rocuronium, particularly in the presence of a difficult airway, and eliminate the need for intravenous succinylcholine (see Chapter 6).

**TABLE 4-6** Contraindications to Cricoid Pressure

| Contraindication | Potential Complication |
|---|---|
| Active vomiting | • Possible rupture of esophagus |
| Airway issues | • Fractured cricoid cartilage may be made worse.<br>• Sharp foreign body in larynx may result in further laryngeal injury. |
| Esophageal issues | • Zenker diverticulum<br>• Sharp foreign body in upper esophagus may result in further esophageal injury. |
| Vertebral/neurologic issues | • Unstable cervical spine may result in spinal cord injury.<br>• Sharp foreign body in the neck may result in injury to other structures in the neck. |

From Thiagarajah S, Lear E, Keh M. Anesthetic implications of Zenker's diverticulum. Anesth Analg 1990;70:109-11.

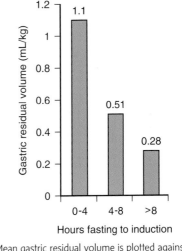

**FIGURE 4-5** Mean gastric residual volume is plotted against hours of fasting before anesthetic induction in emergency pediatric cases. These data suggest that a 4-hour fast, if it does not compromise patient safety, may reduce gastric residual volume and therefore reduce (but not eliminate) risk for aspiration. (Data abstracted from Schurizek BA, Rybro L, Boggild-Madsen NB, Juhl B. Gastric volume and pH in children for emergency surgery. Acta Anaesthesiol Scand 1986;30:404-8.)

Cricoid pressure (Sellick maneuver) should be applied as anesthesia is induced, and the pressure should be maintained until the tracheal tube has been successfully placed between the vocal cords.[402,403] Unfortunately, few apply cricoid pressure as originally described by Sellick. The neck is not hyperextended, and a hard neck rest is not placed beneath the cervical curve. By obliterating the esophageal lumen, cricoid pressure is intended to prevent regurgitated material from passing from the stomach to the pharynx. Before induction of anesthesia, the cricoid ring is palpated between the thumb and the middle finger, and as soon as the child loses consciousness, pressure is steadily increased using the index finger. To prevent passive gastroesophageal reflux, a force of 30 to 40 Newtons (3 to 4 kg of force) must be applied to the upper esophagus (in adults), which creates an intraluminal pressure of approximately 50 cm $H_2O$ in the upper esophagus.[404] However, active vomiting may create esophageal pressures in excess of 60 cm $H_2O$ that could overcome cricoid pressure and result in regurgitation and pulmonary aspiration. Alternatively, if cricoid pressure is not relieved immediately, spontaneous rupture of the esophagus (Boerhaave syndrome) may occur. Hence, the contraindications to cricoid pressure should be carefully reviewed to avoid complications from this maneuver (Table 4-6). Gastric insufflation is prevented in children by cricoid pressure during mask ventilation with peak inspiratory pressures up to 40 cm $H_2O$.[405] The Sellick maneuver should seal the esophagus in the presence of a nasogastric tube,[406] but removal of the nasogastric tube before intubation provides a better mask fit on the face and exposure for laryngoscopy and intubation. If the nasogastric tube is left in place, leaving it open to atmospheric pressure will vent liquid and gas present in the stomach.

The results of surveys from the United Kingdom showed that cricoid pressure was used in only 40% to 50% of children in whom it was indicated.[407,408] Reluctance to apply cricoid pressure may be attributed to a number of reasons, including the indications for its use and how often it is applied with the correct position and pressure.[409-411] In adults evaluated with MRI, the esophagus was situated lateral to the cricoid cartilage in more than 50% of patients without cricoid pressure and was laterally displaced more than 90% of the time when cricoid pressure was applied.[412] In addition, cricoid pressure may distort the anatomy of the upper airway, making laryngoscopy more

difficult, and it must sometimes be released to facilitate a clear view of the larynx and tracheal intubation, particularly in infants.[413] Cricoid pressure also decreases the tone of the upper and lower esophageal sphincters.[404,414] However, properly applied cricoid pressure can facilitate intubation with RSI and mask ventilation.

Evidence suggests that the gastric residual volume in children undergoing emergency surgery is greater if a child is anesthetized within 4 hours after hospital admission (1.1 mL/kg).[415] If, on the other hand, surgery can be delayed for at least 4 hours, then the mean gastric residual volume is on average much less (0.51 mL/kg)[415]; this gastric residual volume is in fact similar to that observed in children who have fasted for routine surgical procedures (Fig. 4-5).[1] This does not imply that these children should not be regarded as having a full stomach; rather, the risk may be somewhat reduced if surgery can be delayed several hours. In addition, evidence suggests that in emergency cases, the gastric residual volume depends in part, on the time interval between the last food ingestion and the time of the injury as well as the severity of the injury.[415] Children who last ate more than 4 hours before the injury have a gastric residual volume similar to those who fasted as if it were elective surgery (Fig. 4-6). *There is some comfort in these numbers, but one should never consider such children as not having a full stomach but rather as having a less full stomach.* Additionally, the possible value of $H_2$-blocking agents, metoclopramide, and clear antacids may be considered, but their use in this regard is not evidence based.

A modified RSI may be preferred in small infants who will likely desaturate during brief periods of apnea and will therefore require assisted ventilation before the trachea is secured. Neonates may be intubated awake if indicated; this may provide a greater margin of safety because it preserves spontaneous ventilation as well as laryngeal reflexes. Skillfully performed awake intubation in neonates is not associated with either significant adverse cardiovascular responses or neurologic sequelae[416] and may be preferred in infants with hemodynamic instability.[417]

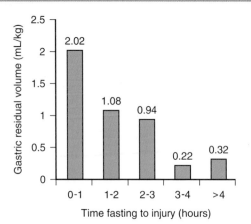

**FIGURE 4-6** Mean gastric residual volume is plotted against time from last food ingestion to time of injury. These data suggest that the longer the time from ingestion to injury, the lower the risk for pulmonary aspiration of gastric contents. Also, if more than 4 hours has elapsed between the time of last food ingestion and time of injury, the risk is similar to that for patients with routine fasting. However, even with a 4-hour fasting time period, these patients must still be treated as though they have a full stomach. It should be noted that these volumes also relate to the severity of injury (increased volumes with increased injury severity). (Data abstracted from Bricker SRW, McLuckie A, Nightingale DA. Gastric aspirates after trauma in children. Anesthesia 1989;44:721-4.)

## Special Problems

### THE FEARFUL CHILD

This is a difficult problem without a satisfactory solution. The child's fear is generally based on the child's developmental status, the hospital environment, and the impending surgery. This is why it is so vital that as much information as possible be presented and queries as to why the child is afraid are so important. Frequently, a few well-directed questions and honest answers will resolve most of the child's concerns. Often, allowing a parent to hold the child during induction of anesthesia or allowing the child to hold the anesthetic mask himself or herself, will stop the flow of tears and settle the child's emotional upheaval. In other situations, one commonly practiced solution is to use intramuscular ketamine.

### AUTISM

Autism is characterized by a delay in the development of socialization and communication skills and is the best-studied form of pervasive developmental disorders. Other types include Asperger syndrome, Rett syndrome, and childhood disintegrative disorder. Autism is a clinical diagnosis, with an onset before the age of 3 years. The diagnostic criteria as listed in the *Diagnostic and Statistical Manual of Mental Disorders* (DSM-IV) are (1) qualitative impairment in social interaction, (2) qualitative impairment in verbal and nonverbal communication, and (3) restricted repetitive and stereotypical patterns of behavior, interests, and activities.

The overall estimated prevalence of autism spectrum disorders (ASD) is 1 in 88 (11.3 per 1000), which is an increase over previous estimates of 1 in 150 (6.4 per 1000) owing to better ascertainment and a broadening of the diagnostic concept.[418,418a] Autism affects boys more commonly than girls in a ratio of 4:1 to 5:1 with equal distribution in all socioeconomic groups.[419] Behavior

and cognitive training is the most effective therapy, but it must be initiated at as early an age as possible to achieve the best possible neurologic improvement. Serotonin reuptake inhibitors may suppress aggression and repetitive behavior.[420-422] Naltrexone may be used to decrease the effects of the hypersecretion of endorphins.[422,423] Seizures are present in about 25% of autistic children and usually manifest in adolescence.[420,421,424]

The perioperative period can be a stressful time for the child with autism and his or her family. These children do not respond well to any change in their routine and may challenge the ingenuity of the anesthesiologist. They are very sensitive to stimuli such as light, sound, touch, and pain. The hospital setting is anxiety provoking and usually upsets most autistic children until they become totally disruptive and uncooperative.

The anesthesiologist's approach to the autistic child depends on the severity of the disorder. Information regarding the child's previous anesthetic experience, assessment of the child's behavior and idiosyncrasies, and bonding with parents or caregivers should be accomplished during the preanesthetic visit. Sedative premedication can work very well in these children. The decision to administer premedication needs to be made on an individual basis (see "Premedication and Induction Principles"). Oral midazolam (0.5 to 1 mg/kg)[126] is the most commonly used preoperative anxiolytic for children, although other choices include oral ketamine (6 mg/kg)[227] and a combination of oral midazolam (0.5 mg/kg) and ketamine (3 mg/kg).[230] The overly anxious child may be uncooperative with oral medication and may require intramuscular ketamine. Parents can also offer insight into which strategies would make their child's life easier during this difficult time. It is important to take the time to address parental concerns and establish a trust relationship with the family.

There is great variation in the severity of autism and hospital needs of these children.[425] The focus for optimal management of these children in one institution was on early communication to provide a flexible and individualized admission process and anesthetic plan.[425] A quiet room may offer advantage preoperatively for more severe cases. Where premedication was indicated, oral midazolam (0.5 mg/kg) was effective for mild cases and oral ketamine (7 mg/kg) was most reliable for moderate and severe cases. The oral medication was mixed in the child's favorite clear liquid.

Although parental presence during induction combined with oral midazolam is no more beneficial in reducing a child's anxiety than oral midazolam alone,[125] for this population parental presence is most often beneficial (since the child knows and trusts their parent or parents) in helping the child reach the operating room. Finally, the appropriate use of parents in the postanesthesia care unit can facilitate the transition from surgery to recovery. Studies have shown that children who are reunited with their parents sooner require less pain medication and are discharged earlier in an ambulatory setting.[426]

### ANEMIA

The minimum hematocrit necessary to ensure adequate oxygen transport in children has not been well established. Preoperative hemoglobin testing, however, is of limited value in healthy children undergoing elective surgery when minimal blood loss is expected.[427] Children with chronic anemia, such as those with renal failure, do not require preoperative transfusion because of compensatory mechanisms, such as increased 2,3-diphosphoglycerate, increased oxygen extraction, and increased cardiac output. Elective surgery for children who are anemic should take into consideration their medical history, underlying diseases (e.g., hemoglobinopathies, von Willebrand, sickle cell, other factor deficiency), the nature of the surgery, and its urgency. Most pediatric anesthesiologists would recommend a hematocrit greater than 25% before elective surgery in the absence of chronic disease. If significant blood loss is anticipated and the surgery is elective, then the cause of anemia should be investigated and treated and the surgery postponed until the hematocrit is restored to the normal range. *Healthy children scheduled for elective surgery that is not expected to cause substantive bleeding should not routinely receive a blood transfusion just to bring their hematocrit to an arbitrary limit such as 30%.*

Physiologic anemia of infancy occurs between 2 and 4 months of postnatal age. At this time, there is an increased production of hemoglobin A and an increase in red cell 2,3-diphosphoglycerate, which contribute to a right shift of the oxygen-hemoglobin dissociation curve (see Chapter 9). Therefore, in infants 2 to 4 months of age, a reduced hemoglobin value is acceptable. Anemia, with a hematocrit of less than 30%, in formerly preterm infants represents a special category of patients who may have an increased incidence of postoperative apnea (see later discussion), but transfusion is still not recommended.[428]

## UPPER RESPIRATORY TRACT INFECTION

Most anesthesiologists agree that the presence of an acute purulent upper respiratory tract infection (URI), fever, change in mental state or behavior, or signs pertaining to a lower respiratory tract infection (i.e., wheezing and rales) are sufficient grounds to postpone elective surgery for approximately 4 weeks.[429] However, the child with a nonpurulent active or recent URI (within 4 weeks) often presents a conundrum, even for the most experienced anesthesiologist.

Between 20% and 30% of all children have a runny nose during a significant part of the year. In the preanesthetic evaluation, we must rely on history, physical examination, and, rarely, laboratory data to decide whether to proceed with the anesthesia. A differential diagnosis of a child with a runny nose is presented in Table 4-7.

The perioperative and postoperative risks of anesthetizing children with URIs are poorly understood. In part, this stems from study bias in that procedures for many children with symptomatic URIs are cancelled before the day of surgery, thus precluding them from inclusion in the studies. Another difficulty is the variable definition of a URI, which limits the external validity of these studies. Finally, study design flaws or inadequacies including retrospective, nonrandomized, and nonblinded studies have created inconsistencies among the published results.

A number of perioperative risks have been studied.[429] The risk of postintubation croup was similar in children who had an active URI and those who did not. However, some children in that study had "tight-fitting" tracheal tubes, which may have confounded the results.[430] Intraoperative complications including atelectasis and cyanosis were described in a series of children with a history of a recent URI. Very severe complications have been associated with the administration of anesthesia in children with recently infected airways, although the study was retrospective and lacked a case-matched control population.[431] In another retrospective study, the incidence of intraoperative complications in children with URIs was similar to that in children without URIs.[432] This study included children with an active URI at the time of anesthesia and some whose tracheas were intubated. However, the authors did report a greater incidence of respiratory complications in those who had recently had a URI. In a prospective cohort study in which children who were scheduled for myringotomy and tube placement for chronic ear infection were matched with controls who did not have a URI, the morbidity from face mask general anesthesia was no different from that in the children who did not have a URI.[433] However, it is difficult to evaluate this study because bronchospasm would not be expected without tracheal intubation.[434,435] Bronchospasm occurs more frequently in children whose tracheas are intubated and who have active URIs.[435] The incidence of bronchospasm in children with a URI (41:1000) is 10-fold greater than it is in those without a URI. Mechanical stimulation of the airway appears to be an important trigger for bronchospasm.[434] The incidence of laryngospasm in children with a URI (96:1000) is fivefold greater than it is in children without a URI (17:1000).[436] The incidence of minor but not major intraoperative hemoglobin desaturation events in children with a URI is greater than in those without a URI.[435] Lastly, the incidence of all respiratory-related adverse events combined in children with a URI was 9-fold greater than in those without a URI and 11-fold greater in children who had a URI and required tracheal intubation.[437]

When the a tracheal tube and LMA were compared in children with a URI, the incidence of mild bronchospasm, major desaturation events, and overall respiratory events was reduced in the presence of a LMA, although the incidence of laryngospasm was similar with the two airway devices.[438,439]

Prognostic factors of adverse anesthetic events in children with URIs who were scheduled for elective surgery include the type of airway management (tracheal intubation > LMA), that the parent states that the child has a "cold," the presence of nasal congestion, snoring, passive smoking, the induction agent (thiopental > halothane > sevoflurane ~ propofol), sputum production, and whether the neuromuscular agent was antagonized.[440] Propofol depresses laryngeal reflexes and may decrease airway responsiveness by relaxation of bronchial smooth muscle.[441,442] Several variables, including wheezing, fever, malaise, and age, could not be excluded as predictors of adverse events because procedures in some children were deferred or cancelled after their preoperative visit.

| **TABLE 4-7** Differential Diagnosis of a Child with a Runny Nose |
| --- |
| **Noninfectious Causes** |
| Allergic rhinitis: seasonal, perennial, clear nasal discharge; no fever |
| Vasomotor rhinitis: emotional (crying); temperature changes |
| **Infectious Causes** |
| *Viral infections* |
| Nasopharyngitis (common cold) |
| Flu syndrome (upper and lower respiratory tract) |
| Laryngotracheal bronchitis (infectious croup) |
| *Viral exanthems* |
| Measles |
| Chickenpox |
| *Acute bacterial infections* |
| Acute epiglottitis |
| Meningitis |
| Streptococcal tonsillitis |

In a similar study, three children with a recent or active URI required unanticipated admission to hospital.[443] Logistic regression determined that the risk factors associated with adverse outcomes in children with URIs included the presence of copious secretions ($P = 0.0001$), nasal congestion ($P = 0.014$), passive (parental) smoking ($P = 0.018$), and reactive airway disease ($P = 0.028$), as well as whether the child had been a premature infant ($P = 0.007$). ASA status did not correlate with adverse outcomes. Age has not been an independent predictor of adverse events in children with URIs in most studies, although this study suggested that the incidence of bronchospasm in infants younger than 6 months old with active URIs was greater (20.8% versus 4.7%, $P = 0.08$) than in older children.[443] This same study also demonstrated that the incidence of oxygen desaturation in children younger than 2 years of age was greater than it was in older children (21.5% versus 12.5%, $P = 0.023$). Tracheal intubation in children younger than 5 years of age was an independent risk factor for postoperative respiratory adverse events ($P = 0.0002$).[443] Neither the duration of anesthesia nor the depth of anesthesia at the time of extubation (awake versus deep) was a risk factor. Children with active URIs who were anesthetized and maintained with sevoflurane had the smallest incidence of adverse events. The greatest incidence of adverse respiratory events occurred in children undergoing airway surgery (e.g., tonsillectomy and adenoidectomy, direct laryngoscopy, bronchoscopy). This study concluded that children with active and recent URIs (within 4 weeks) are at greater risk for adverse respiratory events, particularly if there is a history of reactive airway disease, of surgery involving the airway, or of prematurity, passive smoke inhalation, nasal congestion or copious secretions, or requirement for a tracheal tube.

In another study that examined the risk factors for adverse anesthetic events in children with URIs, adverse respiratory events were greater in children who were premedicated with midazolam, in those who were extubated while deeply anesthetized, and in those who had peak URI symptoms that occurred within the preceding 4 weeks. However, specific preoperative symptoms were not useful in predicting respiratory adverse events during emergence from anesthesia.[444]

Cancellation of cardiac surgery carries special import because of the risk that the child's heart will deteriorate or the disease process will progress (e.g., pulmonary hypertension) as well as the extensive time, materials, and personnel committed to a planned case. In a prospective study of children scheduled for cardiac surgery, the incidences of respiratory adverse events (29.2% versus 17.3%, $P < 0.01$), multiple postoperative complications (25% versus 10.3%, $P < 0.01$), and bacterial infection (5.2% versus 1.0%, $P = 0.01$) were greater in those with a URI than in those without.[445] Logistic regression identified the presence of a URI as an independent risk factor for both postoperative infections and multiple postoperative complications. Although the duration of the intensive care unit stay was greater for children with URIs (80 ± 90 versus 60 ± 60 hours, $P < 0.01$), the duration of hospital stay was not (8.4 versus 7.8 days, $P > 0.05$).

A national survey suggested that more experienced anesthesiologists are less likely to cancel surgery because of the presence of a URI.[446] Cancellation may also impose emotional and economic burdens on the parents.[447,448] Factors that should be considered when deciding whether to proceed with elective surgery in a child with a URI are summarized in Table 4-8.

On the basis of the best evidence available at the present time, a child with a mild URI that is not of acute onset may be safely

**TABLE 4-8** Factors Affecting Decision for Elective Surgery in a Child with Upper Respiratory Tract Infection

| Proceed with Caution | Consider Cancellation |
|---|---|
| • Child has "just a runny nose," no other symptoms, "much better" | • Parents confirm symptoms: fever, malaise, cough, poor appetite, just developed symptoms last night |
| • Active and happy child | • Lethargic, ill-appearing |
| • Clear rhinorrhea | • Purulent nasal discharge |
| • Clear lungs and symptoms have leveled off or have improved | • Wheezing, rales that do not clear |
| • Older child | • Child <1 year, ex-premie |
| • Social issues: hardship for parents to be away from work, insurance will run out | • Other factors: history of reactive airway disease, major operation, endotracheal tube required |
| • No fever | • Fever >38.5° C |
| • Outpatient procedure that will not expose immunocompromised children to possible infectious agent | • Inpatient procedure that may result in exposure of immunocompromised children to viral/bacterial infection |

From Tait AR, Malviya S. Anesthesia for the child with an upper respiratory tract infection: still a dilemma? Anesth Analg 2005;100:59-65.

anesthetized for minor surgical procedures; if a tracheal tube is required, then the risk of bronchospasm, laryngospasm, and desaturation events increases.[430,432-437,440,443] It is reassuring to note that most such adverse perioperative events are not associated with significant morbidity; that is, the severity of oxygen-hemoglobin desaturation is similar in children with and without a URI.[435] Such children may also be more susceptible to mild episodes of oxygen desaturation in the recovery room. Once again, these episodes are readily treated with supplemental oxygen administration.[449]

Insofar as which techniques will help to prevent complications from a URI, pretreating healthy children who either had a URI within the preceding 6 weeks or had an active URI with bronchodilators, either inhaled ipratropium or albuterol, before anesthesia provided no benefit. In addition, there was no association between either a recent URI or an active URI and the incidence of desaturation, wheezing, coughing, stridor, or laryngospasm causing desaturation.[450] However, in another study, children with a recent URI (≤2 weeks in duration) who received preoperative salbutamol experienced a significantly reduced incidence of laryngospasm, bronchospasm, oxygen desaturation (<95%) and severe coughing with an LMA or tracheal tube.[451] Humidification, intravenous hydration, and anticholinergics may also decrease perioperative complications,[446] although the results of at least one study suggested that glycopyrrolate did not reduce the incidence of perioperative adverse respiratory events when it was given after induction of anesthesia to children with URIs.[452]

If a child is recovering from a URI, the child's physical examination should be near normal. If this is true, anesthesia can generally proceed without increasing the risks substantively. However, if the child with a URI requires prolonged tracheal intubation, the clinician must use his or her judgment and experience together with consultation with the parents and surgeon to determine whether to proceed with or postpone anesthesia.[434-436,446,453]

If the decision is to postpone anesthesia, then how long should one wait before undertaking general anesthesia? Bronchial hyperreactivity, which is associated with URIs in children, shows spirometric changes in the lungs for as long as 7 weeks after a URI.[453,454] Although studies suggest that surgery should be postponed for at least 7 weeks after resolution of a URI, this plan is impractical because most children will be infected with a new URI by that time. Postponing surgery until 2 weeks after resolution of the URI is a common but as yet unproven strategy. In fact, some data suggest that the incidence of adverse respiratory events is just as great in this population as it is in those who were anesthetized during the acute phase of the URI.[433,455] This 2-week waiting period may be acceptable in a child with uncomplicated nasopharyngitis.[456] Unfortunately, there is no consensus on the optimal time interval before surgery is rescheduled. In a survey of anesthesiologists, most wait 3 to 4 weeks before proceeding with surgery.[446] The rationale for this time period is that the risk of respiratory complications is unchanged for 4 to 6 weeks.[443]

In conclusion, there are always risks associated with anesthesia, even in children without URIs. In children with URIs, we must wait 4 to 6 weeks or longer for these risks to return to baseline. Therefore, in children who have had a URI, we can tailor our anesthetic management to further decrease these risks (by using propofol, an LMA, or a face mask instead of a tracheal tube), but the risk cannot be reduced to zero. Good judgment, common sense, clinical experience, and informed consent from the parents or guardians must be used when deciding whether to proceed or postpone the surgery. All of these deliberations and discussions including the risks and benefits should be documented in the chart (see Chapter 11 for additional discussion and perspectives).

## OBSTRUCTIVE SLEEP APNEA SYNDROME

Sleep apnea is a sleep-related breathing disorder in children characterized by a periodic cessation of air exchange, with apnea episodes lasting longer than 10 seconds and an apnea-hypopnea index (AHI) indicating that the total number of obstructive episodes per hour of sleep is greater than 1 (AHI 1-5 = mild OSA, 6-10 = moderate OSA, >10 = severe OSA).[457] Sleep apnea may be defined as central (absent gas flow, lack of respiratory effort), obstructive (absent gas flow, upper airway obstruction and paradoxical movement of rib cage and abdominal muscles) or mixed (due to both CNS defect and obstructive problems). Diagnosis is made by clinical assessment (see later discussion), nocturnal pulse oximetry, or polysomnography studies.

Obstructive sleep apnea syndrome (OSAS) is manifested by episodes that disturb sleep and ventilation. These episodes occur more frequently during rapid-eye-movement (REM) sleep and increase in frequency as more time is spent in REM sleep periods as the night progresses. OSAS occurs in children of all ages (about 2% of all children) but more commonly in children 3 to 7 years of age. It occurs equally in boys and girls, although the prevalence is greater in African American children.[458]

Signs of OSAS are sleep disturbances (including daytime sleepiness), irritability, night terrors, nocturnal enuresis, snoring loud enough to hear through a closed door, pauses and/or gasps during the night, failure to thrive resulting from poor intake due to tonsillar hypertrophy, speech disorders, and decreased size (decreased growth hormone release during disturbed REM sleep). With the worldwide increase in childhood obesity, the presence of obesity in children with OSAS

exacerbates the signs and symptoms of OSAS. Parents of obese children should be specifically asked about such signs and symptoms. This syndrome can cause significant cardiac, pulmonary, and CNS impairment due to chronic oxygen desaturation. Indeed, both OSAS and obesity are systemic inflammatory responses.[459] When they occur together in a child, the severity of the signs and symptoms are greater than if only one had occurred, and resolution of the OSAS after tonsillectomy is less likely. In children with OSAS and morbid obesity, the incidences of hypertension and diabetes are greater than in the absence of these disorders. Therefore it is important to evaluate the cardiovascular status; although right ventricular dysfunction with pulmonary hypertension is classic, biventricular hypertrophy can develop. It is more likely to occur in children with severe OSAS but has been reported in children with only mild OSAS.[460] Cardiac evaluation is recommended for any child with signs of right ventricular dysfunction, systemic or pulmonary hypertension, or multiple episodes of desaturation below 70%. Electrocardiography and chest radiography are insensitive diagnostic tests; rather, echocardiography is recommended.[461] Relief of the tonsillar/adenoidal obstruction can reverse many of these disorders and prevent progression of others (pulmonary hypertension and cor pulmonale) within 6 months after tonsillectomy, although approximately 30% of children with severe OSAS will not have resolution of the OSAS after tonsillectomy.

Children with OSAS may be premedicated with caution with oral midazolam. Despite an incidence of self-limited preoperative desaturation of less than 1.5%, post-premedication monitoring of hemoglobin saturation in these children would seem reasonable.[462] Avoidance of premedication may, however, be more advantageous postoperatively.

Children who are at increased risk for postoperative upper airway obstruction after tonsillectomy and/or adenoidectomy for OSAS include age younger than 2 years, craniofacial anomalies, failure to thrive, hypotonia, morbid obesity, previous upper airway trauma, cor pulmonale, a polysomnogram with a respiratory distress index (RDI) greater than 40 or $O_2$ saturation nadir less than 85%, and a child undergoing an additional uvulopalatopharyngoplasty (UPPP).[463] *Nocturnal desaturation to less than 85% upregulates the genes responsible for control of opioid receptors, resulting in an increased sensitivity to opioids; opioid requirement is reduced by approximately 50%, making standard doses of opioids a relative overdose in children with severe OSA.* This has been demonstrated in both animals and humans.[464,465] To attenuate the risk of perioperative respiratory complications, opioids should be carefully titrated to the respiratory responses during surgery, and if an increased sensitivity to opioids is detected, all perioperative opioids should be reduced accordingly (see Chapter 31 for further details).[466] If nocturnal upper airway obstruction continues after tonsillectomy, ancillary strategies that have been met with variable success have been used: nasal continuous positive airway pressure (CPAP) or bi-level positive airway pressure (BiPAP), nasal steroids, oxygen therapy, and weight loss, although nasal CPAP/BiPAP is rarely tolerated in children.[463]

The American Academy of Pediatrics (AAP) Clinical Practice Guidelines[458] provide recommendations for inpatient monitoring of children at high risk for postoperative complications who have OSAS and are undergoing adenotonsillectomy (Table 4-9). It should be noted that there is an ongoing concern regarding where these children should undergo surgery (in an ambulatory center or in a hospital) and the monitoring these children should have postoperatively (extended observation followed by

**TABLE 4-9** The American Academy of Pediatrics Clinical Practice Guidelines: Risk Factors for Postoperative Respiratory Complications in Children with OSAS Undergoing Adenotonsillectomy

Age younger than 3 years

Severe OSAS on polysomnography

Cardiac complications of OSAS (e.g., right ventricular hypertrophy)

Recent respiratory infection

Craniofacial disorders

Neuromuscular disorders

Cerebral palsy

Down syndrome

Failure to thrive

Obesity

Prematurity

Sickle cell disease

Central hypoventilation syndromes

Genetic, metabolic, or storage disease

Chronic lung disease

Modified from Clinical practice guideline: diagnosis and management of childhood obstructive sleep apnea syndrome. Pediatrics 2002;109:704-12.
OSAS, Obstructive sleep apnea syndrome.

**TABLE 4-10** Candidate Criteria for Identification and Assessment of OSA*

**A: Clinical Signs and Symptoms Suggesting Obstructive Sleep Apnea (OSA)**

*1. Predisposing physical characteristics*

a. ≥95th percentile for age and gender
b. Craniofacial abnormalities affecting the airway (e.g., Down syndrome)
c. Anatomic nasal obstruction
d. Tonsils nearly touching or touching in the midline (kissing tonsils)

*2. History of apparent airway obstruction during sleep (two or more of the following are present; if patient sleep is not observed by another person, then only one of the following needs to be present)*

a. Snoring (loud enough to be heard through a closed door)
b. Frequent snoring
c. Observed pauses in breathing during sleep
d. Awakened from sleep with choking sensation
e. Frequent arousal from sleep
f. Intermittent vocalizations during sleep
g. Parental report of restless sleep, difficulty breathing, or struggling respiratory efforts during sleep
h. Parental report of enuresis

*3. Somnolence (one of the following is present)*

a. Frequent somnolence or fatigue despite adequate "sleep"
b. Falls asleep easily in a nonstimulating environment (e.g., watching television) despite adequate "sleep"
c. Parent or teacher comments that the child appears sleepy during the day, is easily distracted, is overly aggressive, or has difficulty concentrating
d. Child is often difficult to arouse at usual awakening time

**B: Determination of Severity**

a. If a child has signs or symptoms in two or more of the above categories, there is a significant probability that he or she has OSA. The severity of OSA may be determined by sleep study. If a sleep study is not available, such patients should be treated as though they have moderate sleep apnea unless one or more of the signs of symptoms above is severely abnormal (e.g., ≥95th percentile for age and gender, respiratory pauses that are frightening to the observer, child snores loudly enough to be heard through a closed door, child regularly falls asleep within minutes after being left unstimulated), in which cases patients should be treated as though they have severe sleep apnea.
b. If a sleep study has been done, the result should be used to determine the perioperative anesthetic management of a child. (Review the polysomnogram for evidence of nocturnal desaturations <85%, which increases sensitivity to opioids.) However, because sleep laboratories differ in their criteria for detecting episodes of apnea and hypoxemia, the Task Force recommends that the sleep laboratory's assessment (none, mild, moderate, or severe) take precedence over the actual apnea-hypopnea index (AHI, the number of episodes of sleep-disordered breathing per hour). If the overall severity is not indicated, it may be determined by using the following table:

| Severity of OSA | Adult AHI | Pediatric AHI |
| --- | --- | --- |
| None | 0-5 | 0 |
| Mild OSA | 6-20 | 1-5 |
| Moderate OSA | 21-40 | 6-10 |
| Severe OSA | >40 | >10 |

Modified from Gross JB, Bachenberg KL, Benumof JL, et al. Practice guidelines for the perioperative management of patients with obstructive sleep apnea: a report by the American Society of Anesthesiologists Task Force on Perioperative Management of Patients with Obstructive Sleep Apnea. Anesthesiology 2006;104: 1081-93.
*Note: This table has been modified for children; the scoring system is intended only as a guide and has not been validated.

discharge home or overnight observation). In addition to the AAP guidelines, the ASA considers this such a growing problem for both adults and children that they also have formulated a Practice Guideline. Tables 4-10 and 4-11 (modified for children) help to clarify the identification and assessment of children potentially at risk for OSA and offer a proposed (although as yet unvalidated) risk assessment scoring system.[467] This system attempts to characterize those patients who are at significantly increased risk for perioperative complications.

Among children 1 to 18 years of age with OSAS, those without complicating medical conditions such as neuromuscular disease, obesity, or craniofacial abnormalities but with mild sleep apnea may have either no or some improvement in their airway obstruction on the night of surgery. Based on current literature, one may consider discharging children 3 to 12 years of age home on the day of surgery after an extended period of observation (4 to 6 hours), if they meet these criteria. However, those with moderate to severe OSA (particularly obese children) may actually experience worse OSA on the night of their surgery.[468,469] These children should receive reduced doses of opioids and be admitted for overnight monitoring with pulse oximetry and an apnea monitor.[470]

## ASYMPTOMATIC CARDIAC MURMURS

The presence of a cardiac murmur is a common finding in children[471] and may have significant anesthetic implications. Never underestimate the potential implications of a newly diagnosed heart murmur. A history should be obtained to delineate the nature of the murmur. In most cases, the parents will report that the murmur was detected previously by the child's pediatrician and determined to be an "innocent flow murmur" without any anatomic or physiologic abnormalities. When a pediatric cardiologist confirms the classic clinical features of an innocent murmur, an echocardiogram seldom reveals heart disease, especially if the child is older at presentation.[472] *However, even an experienced cardiologist can occasionally make a misdiagnosis; the only certain means to exclude a structural defect within the heart is with*

## TABLE 4-11 OSA Risk Scoring System: Example*

### A. Severity of Sleep Apnea Based on Sleep Study (or Clinical Indicators if Sleep Study Is Not Available: Point Score 0-3†‡)

*Severity of OSA*

| | |
|---|---|
| None | 0 |
| Mild | 1 |
| Moderate | 2 |
| Severe | 3 |

### B. Invasiveness of Surgery and Anesthesia: Point Score 0-3

*Type of surgery and anesthesia*

| | |
|---|---|
| Superficial surgery under local or peripheral nerve block anesthesia without sedation | 0 |
| Superficial surgery with moderate sedation or general anesthesia | 1 |
| Peripheral surgery with spinal or epidural anesthesia (with no more than moderate sedation) | 1 |
| Peripheral surgery with general anesthesia | 2 |
| Airway surgery with moderate sedation | 2 |
| Major surgery with general anesthesia | 3 |
| Airway surgery with general anesthesia (e.g., tonsillectomy) | 3 |

### C. Requirement for Postoperative Opioids: Point Score 0-3

*Opioid requirement*

| | |
|---|---|
| None | 0 |
| Low-dose oral opioids (tonsillectomy) | 1 |
| High-dose oral opioids, parenteral or neuraxial opioids | 3 |

### D. Estimation of Perioperative Risk—Overall Score Equals the Score for "A" Plus the Greater of the Score for "B" or "C": Possible Score 0-6§

Modified from Gross JB, Bachenberg KL, Benumof JL, et al. Practice guidelines for the perioperative management of patients with obstructive sleep apnea: a report by the American Society of Anesthesiologists Task Force on Perioperative Management of Patients with Obstructive Sleep Apnea. Anesthesiology 2006;104: 1081-93.

*Note: This table has been modified for children. A scoring system similar to this table may be used to estimate whether a child is at increased perioperative risk of complications from OSA. This example has not been clinically validated, and such a scoring system is simply meant to provide guidance.

†One point may be subtracted if a patient has been on continuous positive airway pressure (CPAP) for noninvasive positive-pressure ventilation before surgery and will be using his or her appliance consistently during the postoperative period.

‡One point should be added if a child with mild or moderate OSA also has a resting arterial carbon dioxide tension greater than 50 mm Hg.

§Children with a score of 4 may be at increased perioperative risk from OSA; children with a score of 5 or 6 maybe at significantly increased perioperative risk from OSA.

## TABLE 4-12 Grading of Heart Murmurs

| | |
|---|---|
| Grade I | Heard only with intense concentration |
| Grade II | Faint, but heard immediately |
| Grade III | Easily heard, of intermediate intensity |
| Grade IV | Easily heard, palpable thrill/vibration on chest wall |
| Grade V | Very loud, thrill present, audible with only edge of stethoscope on chest wall |
| Grade VI | Audible with stethoscope off the chest wall |

Modified from Emmanouilides GC, Allen HD, Riemenschneider TA, Gutgesell HP. Moss and Adams heart disease in infants, children, and adolescents including the fetus and young adult. 5th ed. Baltimore: Williams & Wilkins; 1995.

## TABLE 4-13 Symptoms and Signs of Heart Disease

- Feeding difficulties: disinterest, fatigue, diaphoresis, tachypnea, dyspnea
- Poor exercise tolerance
- Tachypnea, dyspnea, grunting, nasal flaring, and intercostal, suprasternal, or subcostal retractions
- Frequent respiratory tract infections (a result of compression of airways by plethoric vessels leading to stasis of secretions and atelectasis)
- Central cyanosis (involving warm mucous membranes: tongue and buccal mucosa) or poor capillary refill
- Absent or abnormal peripheral pulses

Modified from Pelech AN. Evaluation of the pediatric patient with a cardiac murmur. Pediatr Clin North Am 1999;46:167-88.

*an echocardiogram.*[473] In general, nonpathologic murmurs occur during systole and are soft and nonradiating with normal feel to peripheral pulses; there are normal blood pressures in both upper and lower extremities. However, if the murmur is harsh and difficult to localize, if there are bounding pulses, if the murmur is louder than grade II/VI, or if it is accompanied by other findings (Tables 4-12 and 4-13), then further evaluation is warranted.[474] If the murmur has not been detected previously, referral to a pediatric cardiologist is indicated or an echocardiogram by an experienced pediatric echocardiographer should be obtained before induction of anesthesia.[475]

## FEVER

The presence of a low-grade fever before elective surgery poses a dilemma whether to proceed with anesthesia or to delay. In general, if a child has only 0.5° C to 1.0° C of fever and no other symptoms, this degree of fever is not a contraindication to general anesthesia. However, if the fever is associated with a recent onset of rhinitis, pharyngitis, otitis media, dehydration, or any other sign of impending illness, it is prudent to postpone the procedure. If the planned surgery is of an urgent nature, every effort should be made to reduce the fever before induction of anesthesia, primarily to reduce oxygen demands. Reduction of the fever should not include aspirin, because aspirin may interfere with platelet function and is associated with Reye syndrome. Ibuprofen may be associated with an increase in bleeding time[313] and should be avoided before surgery. On the other hand, acetaminophen has no effect on platelet function and is an excellent antipyretic. It is rapidly absorbed when administered orally, producing adequate blood concentrations within several minutes. In contrast, rectal administration requires at least 60 minutes to achieve a significant blood concentration.[287,476] There is no evidence that an existing fever predisposes to a malignant hyperthermic reaction.[477]

## POSTANESTHESIA APNEA IN FORMERLY PRETERM INFANTS

The formerly preterm infant may have a multitude of residual problems owing to intensive care therapy, prolonged intubation, and still-maturing organogenesis. The incidence of subglottic stenosis is increased in this population. These infants are also prone to developing perioperative respiratory complications.[478] At the time surgery is scheduled, these infants may or may not have intermittent apnea spells, although they often appear normal for their age. Since the original descriptions of this subgroup of infants, a number of prospective studies have defined

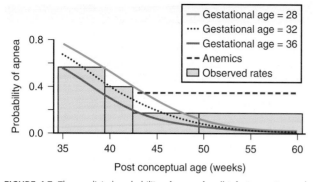

**FIGURE 4-7** The predicted probability of apnea for all infants was inversely related to gestational age at the time of birth and postconceptional age at the time of surgery. The probability of apnea was the same regardless of postconceptional age or gestational age for infants with anemia. *(dashed magenta line)* (From Coté CJ, Zaslavsky A, Downes JJ, et al. Postoperative apnea in former preterm infants after inguinal herniorrhaphy: a combined analysis. Anesthesiology 1995;82:807-8.)

the population at greatest risk for postoperative apnea.[428,478-487] Formerly premature infants of less than 44 weeks postconceptional age (PCA) are at a greater risk for apnea after general anesthesia than are those older than 44 weeks PCA, although the risk of postanesthetic apnea in preterm infants who are older than 44 weeks PCA remains substantial (approximately 5%).[488] In an analysis of eight published prospective papers from four institutions conducted over 6 years, the incidence of apnea varied inversely with the both gestational age and PCA (E-Fig. 4-5).[488] For example, consider two infants who are now 45 weeks PCA: one was born at 28 weeks and the other at 32 weeks of gestation. The risk of apnea in the 28-week gestational age infant is twice that in the 32-week gestational age infant (Fig. 4-7).[488] Similarly, consider two infants of the same gestational age: one anesthetized at 45 weeks PCA and the other at 50 weeks PCA. The younger-PCA infant would be at greater risk for postoperative apnea.

The diagnosis of apnea in the postoperative period depends on the type of apnea device used to monitor the infants (E-Fig. 4-5). For example, simple observation and impedance pneumography are more likely to miss an apneic episode than are continuous recording devices.[488-490] Preterm infants with anemia (hematocrit <30%) are more prone to apnea, and the incidence is unrelated to PCA or gestational age (see Fig. 4-7).[428,488] It appears that the risk for apnea exceeds 1% with statistical certainty until approximately 56 weeks PCA in infants with a gestational age of 32 weeks or 54 weeks PCA in those with a gestational age of 35 weeks, if one excludes anemic infants and those with obvious apnea in the recovery room. This analysis determined that (1) apnea was strongly and inversely related to both gestational age and PCA; (2) ongoing apnea at home is a risk factor; (3) small-for-gestational-age infants are protected from apnea compared with appropriate- and large-for-gestational-age infants; (4) anemia is a significant risk factor, particularly for infants of more than 44 weeks PCA; and (5) a history of necrotizing enterocolitis, neonatal apnea, respiratory distress syndrome, bronchopulmonary dysplasia, or operative use of opioids or muscle relaxants did not correlate with postoperative apnea.[488] Each clinician must decide how to balance the risk of an unrecognized apnea with the benefit of proceeding with the surgery in terms

of cost savings and not hospitalizing the infant for overnight monitoring.[491] The most practical and appropriate plan is to admit and monitor all formerly preterm infants who are less than 60 weeks PCA until they are free of apnea for a minimum of 12 hours.

In a subsequent study of preterm infants, four anesthetic techniques were compared: sevoflurane induction and maintenance, halothane induction and maintenance, halothane induction/desflurane maintenance, and thiopental induction/desflurane maintenance.[492] No major episodes of apnea occurred in any of the 40 formerly preterm infants who were less than 60 weeks PCA and undergoing hernia repair, although there was at least one episode of breath-holding or self-limited apnea in each group. In view of the small sample size in this study, the upper 95% confidence interval that no apnea episodes will occur in all formerly preterm infants is only 92%. *Although the majority of formerly preterm infants in a microanalysis of eight studies were anesthetized with halothane,[488] apnea has been reported with all anesthetics, including sevoflurane, desflurane, and regional anesthesia (spinal or caudal epidural, discussed later).[493,494]*

The preoperative evaluation of these infants requires discussion with the pharmacy regarding the availability of intravenous caffeine, discussion with the intensive care unit regarding availability of a monitored bed postoperatively, and discussion with the family regarding the perioperative risks of anesthesia and apnea. If the child is receiving theophylline or caffeine preoperatively, this therapy should be continued postoperatively.[495] If the child is not receiving theophylline or caffeine preoperatively, there is no evidence to support the administration of aminophylline postoperatively, but there is weak evidence that caffeine (10 mg/kg) may prevent postoperative apnea spells in high-risk infants.[486,487] The pharmacokinetics of caffeine in preterm and full-term neonates suggest that a single intravenous dose of caffeine will have a clinical effect that may last for several days. However, the pharmacokinetics of caffeine change dramatically with age: in older infants (e.g., those who are 60 weeks PCA), the half-life of caffeine is reduced to approximately 5 hours (E-Fig. 4-6).[496] Larger, well-controlled studies are indicated before caffeine can be advocated for all infants at risk for postoperative apnea. A Cochrane review of prophylactic caffeine to prevent postoperative apnea after general anesthesia in formerly preterm infants concluded that although caffeine can be used to prevent postoperative apnea, bradycardia, and episodes of oxygen desaturation in growing preterm infants, there was insufficient evidence to adopt this as routine anesthetic practice.[497] *If caffeine is administered to a formerly preterm infant, postoperative admission and overnight respiratory monitoring are still required, because caffeine is not 100% effective in preventing postoperative apnea.*

Apnea may be related to many causes besides prematurity (Fig. 4-8). The most common causes after surgery, however, relate to metabolic derangements, pharmacologic effects, or CNS immaturity. Metabolic causes of apnea such as hypothermia, hypoglycemia, hypocalcemia, acidosis, and hypoxemia should also be considered and avoided (see Chapters 35 and 36). Pharmacologic effects cannot be avoided, because administering anesthesia requires the use of drugs, and most drugs used in anesthesia depress the respiratory system either directly or indirectly. Most inhalation agents, opioids, and sedatives depress the central response to carbon dioxide in adults in a dose-related fashion.[498] Respiratory depression is probably even more likely to occur in neonates who have an immature respiratory center. Studies of adults have demonstrated both ablation of the

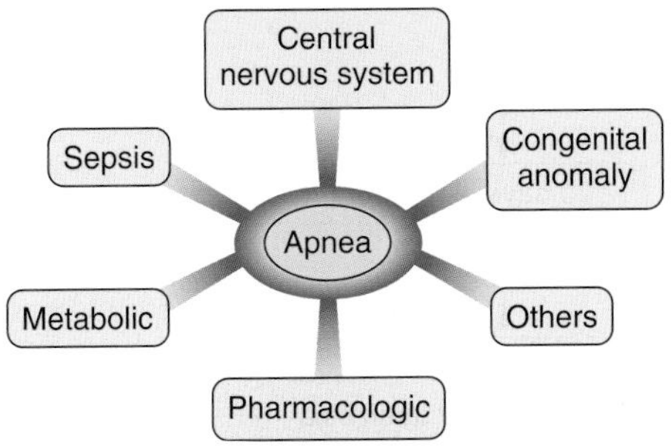

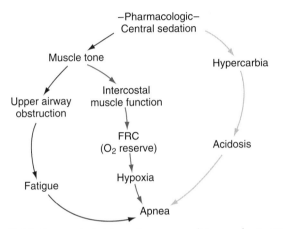

**FIGURE 4-8** Apnea, defined as the absence of movement of air at the mouth or nose, may have many causes. Those that anesthesiologists are most often involved with are of metabolic, pharmacologic, or respiratory origins.

**FIGURE 4-9** Pharmacologic interventions may result in several sequences of events leading to apnea. *FRC,* Functional residual capacity.

response to hypoxia and potentiation of that response by hypercarbia in the presence of halothane in concentrations as low as 0.1%; therefore, residual anesthetic action may contribute to the development of apnea in infants.[499] In addition, most pharmacologic agents used in anesthesia decrease muscle tone of the upper airway, thus contributing to the development of upper airway obstruction, more labored breathing, fatigue, and apnea in the perioperative period.[485] Potent inhalation anesthetic agents also decrease intercostal muscle tone, reducing functional residual capacity and thereby increasing the propensity to develop hypoxemia (Fig. 4-9).[500]

Regional anesthesia has been used to reduce the risk of postoperative apnea associated with general anesthesia. Regional techniques may offer advantages over general anesthesia, but apnea has been associated with regional anesthesia techniques.[480,501-503] In a study that compared spinal with general anesthesia, the incidence of desaturation and bradycardia but not apnea was reduced in the spinal group.[493] In a review of four studies that utilized regional (spinal, epidural, caudal) versus general anesthesia in formerly preterm infants undergoing inguinal herniorrhaphy in early infancy, there was no convincing evidence to support the use of spinal anesthesia as part of the standard practice in inguinal herniorrhaphy, although there was some evidence that spinal anesthesia reduced the incidence of postoperative apnea in an infant population who were not given additional sedation.[504] Additive drugs used to prolong the duration of a spinal or caudal block, such as clonidine, have been associated with

apnea.[505-508] Spinal anesthesia is also associated with a significant failure rate and the need for multiple attempts to achieve accurate placement of the needle,[509,510] although in experienced hands, the success rate for placing a spinal block was 97.4% and an adequate level of spinal anesthesia was achieved in 95.4% of infants. *In summary, formerly preterm infants should not be anesthetized as outpatients even when a regional technique has been used; they require admission for postoperative monitoring overnight for apnea.*

With respect to full-term neonates, three reports have described infants who developed apnea after apparently uneventful general anesthesias.[511-513] Therefore, if a full-term infant who is younger than 44 weeks PCA demonstrates any abnormality of respiration after anesthesia, we recommend that they be admitted overnight for monitoring for apnea. The algorithms in Figure 4-10 can be used as a decision tree for outpatient surgery in the term and formerly preterm infant.

## HYPERALIMENTATION

Intravenous alimentation is frequently used as a means of life support and to prepare children for surgery. It is important for anesthesiologists to identify the composition and rate of administration of these fluids so that potential intraoperative complications can be avoided. Most of these solutions are hypertonic, have high glucose content, and must be administered through a centrally placed intravenous route.

The basic principles of care are as follows:

1. Avoid contaminating the line. It is best not to puncture the line for administering medications or changing fluid.
2. Do not discontinue the glucose-containing solution, because the relative hyperinsulinemic state could induce hypoglycemia, the signs of which might be masked by general anesthesia. In contrast, intralipid infusions should be discontinued before surgery, because it is a culture medium if contaminated.
3. An infusion device should be used at all times so that the rate of infusion is constant. Accidental rapid infusion of large amounts of hyperalimentation fluid can cause a hypertonic nonketotic coma.[514] There is no consensus on the intraoperative management of hyperalimentation solutions. Some clinicians reduce the infusion rate by 33% to 50% to avoid hyperglycemia resulting from a reduced metabolic rate due to the effects of anesthetic agents and a reduced body temperature, whereas others leave the infusion rate unchanged to avoid intraoperative hypoglycemia.
4. Perioperative and intraoperative monitoring of glucose, potassium, sodium, and calcium, as well as acid-base status, is important for long procedures.
5. Preoperative confirmation of correct intravascular line placement (radiography or aspiration of blood) is important to avoid intraoperative complications such as hydrothorax or hemothorax.

## DIABETES

Diabetes mellitus is the most common endocrine problem encountered in children. Preoperative assessment should include a thorough knowledge of the child's insulin schedule. The preoperative fasting time should be the same as that recommended for nondiabetics. Every attempt should be made to schedule a diabetic child as the first case of the day to minimize the fasting period. Several protocols have been advocated for glycemic control in diabetics. An intravenous infusion that contains 5% glucose and electrolytes at a maintenance infusion rate should

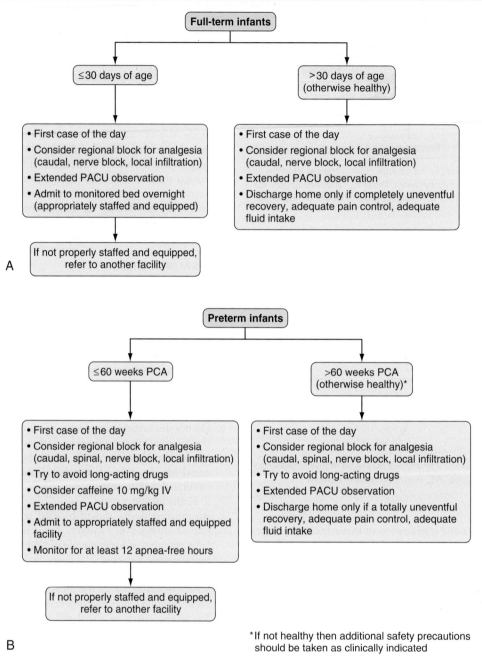

**FIGURE 4-10** Algorithms used as a decision tree for outpatient surgery in term infants (**A**) and in former preterm infants (**B**). *PACU,* Postanesthesia care unit; *PCA,* postconceptional age.

be started to avoid hypoglycemia. Blood glucose concentrations should be monitored just prior to induction, intraoperatively, and postoperatively until the child is back on a routine schedule. A more detailed discussion of the perioperative management of the child with diabetes is presented in Chapter 25.

### BRONCHOPULMONARY DYSPLASIA

Bronchopulmonary dysplasia is a form of chronic lung disease associated with prolonged mechanical ventilation and oxygen toxicity in preterm neonates. Antenatal glucocorticosteroids, early surfactant therapy, and gentler ventilation modalities currently utilized have reduced the severity of lung injury. The clinical manifestations of bronchopulmonary dysplasia include

tachypnea, dyspnea, and airway hyperactivity, as well as oxygen dependence. These infants suffer from hypoxemia, hypercarbia, abnormal functional airway growth, tracheomalacia, bronchomalacia, subglottic stenosis, increased pulmonary vascular resistance, and congestive heart failure. Pulmonary function abnormalities, including a reduced functional residual capacity, reduced diffusion capacity, airway obstruction, and reduced exercise tolerance, may persist into the school-age years. Many also suffer neurodevelopmental problems and seizures. Some also have a cardiomyopathy due to corticosteroid therapy in the neonatal period or the combination of corticosteroid therapy and viral infections; others have systemic hypertension. These children are often cared for at home on oxygen therapy with diuretics, digoxin, and β₂-agonists. Preoperative preparation should focus on optimizing oxygenation, reducing airway hyperactivity, and correcting electrode abnormalities caused by chronic diuretic therapy. Particular attention should be paid to fluid balance and avoiding excessive hydration. Chronic hearing problems may be an additional concern and may necessitate avoiding nitrous oxide. Adequate expiratory time to avoid excessive positive-pressure ventilation is important, and the potential for subglottic stenosis may necessitate using a smaller than expected tracheal tube. Use of an LMA may offer some advantage in select situations by reducing the incidence of coughing, wheezing, and hoarseness.

## SEIZURE DISORDER

Management of children with seizure disorders requires a knowledge of the antiseizure medications, medication schedule, and possible interactions between these medications and anesthetic drugs. The stress of surgery and anesthesia may lower the seizure threshold and cause a seizure. Seizure medications should be continued until the time of elective surgery. Characterization of the clinical manifestations of the seizure is useful so as to be able to diagnose potential seizures postoperatively. If the child is expected to have a significant problem with oral intake postoperatively, then a game plan with the child's neurologist should be developed so as to build a transition to intravenous antiseizure medications. Preoperative and postoperative management of anticonvulsant blood concentrations may also ensure proper therapeutic effect (see also Chapter 22).

## SICKLE CELL DISEASE

Whenever a child presents with either sickle cell disease or sickle cell trait, the anesthetic and postanesthetic management must be modified (see also Chapters 9 and 11). It is important to obtain a detailed family history, and if the child has not been previously tested, a sickle preparation should be obtained. If a sickle test is positive and the surgery is elective, then surgery should be postponed pending a hemoglobin electrophoresis to more carefully delineate the nature of the hemoglobinopathy. It must be emphasized that the status of hydration and oxygenation is critical for all children with sickle cell disease or trait. A secure intravenous route with hydration of at least 1.5 times maintenance is recommended well into the postoperative period, especially after procedures in which ileus may result. Meticulous attention to detail to ensure stable cardiovascular and ventilatory status establishes adequate oxygenation to prevent sickling. Pulse oximetry is of particular value in managing these children by providing an early warning of desaturation. Children with hemoglobin SC are especially at risk because they have a relatively normal hemoglobin level yet are extremely vulnerable to sickling. Further recommendations regarding management of these children, including indications for preoperative transfusion to bring the hemoglobin concentration to 10 g/dL, are discussed in Chapter 9.

## ACKNOWLEDGMENT

We wish to thank John F. Ryan, MD, Letty M. P. Liu, I. D. Todres, MD, Nishan G. Goudsouzian, MD, and Leila Mei Pang, MD, for their prior contributions to these topics.

## ANNOTATED REFERENCES

Craven PD, Badawi N, Henderson-Smart DJ, O'Brien M. Regional (spinal, epidural, caudal) versus general anaesthesia in preterm infants undergoing inguinal herniorrhaphy in early infancy [review]. Cochrane Database Syst Rev 2003;CD003669.

*The review found that there is not enough evidence from trials to show whether spinal block improves outcome for a preterm infant having surgery for inguinal hernia.*

Henderson-Smart DJ, Steer P. Prophylactic caffeine to prevent postoperative apnea following general anesthesia in preterm infants [review]. Cochrane Database Syst Rev 2001;CD000048.

*Caffeine can be used to prevent postoperative apnea/bradycardia and episodes of oxygen desaturation in growing preterm infants if clinically necessary. There is a need to determine with further studies which infants might benefit most by this treatment.*

Holzman RS. Clinical management of latex-allergic children. Anesth Analg 1997;85:529-33.

*Latex-allergic children can be safely anesthetized if exposure to latex in the medical environment is avoided, and administration of prophylactic medication to decrease the response is unnecessary.*

Kain ZN, Mayes LC, Wang SM, Hofstadter MB. Postoperative behavioral outcomes in children: effects of sedative premedication. Anesthesiology 1999;90:758-65.

*Premedication of children with midazolam is not only beneficial in reducing preoperative anxiety but also results in fewer negative behavioral changes during the first postoperative week.*

Schwengel DA, Sterni LM, Tunkel DE, Heitmiller ES. Perioperative management of children with obstructive sleep apnea. Anesth Analg 2009;109:60-75.

*An excellent review article on the diagnosis, treatment, and anesthetic management of children with obstructive sleep apnea syndrome.*

Skinner CM, Rangasami J. Preoperative use of herbal medicines: a patient survey. Br J Anaesth 2002;89:792-5.

*Self-administration of herbal medicine is common in patients presenting for anesthesia. Because of the potential for side effects and drug interactions, it is important for anesthesiologists to be aware of their use. This is a good overview of herbal medicines and potential perioperative complications with their use.*

Tait AR, Malviya S, Voepel-Lewis T, et al. Risk factors for perioperative adverse respiratory events in children with upper respiratory tract infections. Anesthesiology 2001;95:299-306.

*Several risk factors for perioperative adverse respiratory events in children were identified: use of an endotracheal tube (<5 years of age), history of prematurity, history of reactive airway disease, paternal smoking, surgery involving the airway, presence of copious secretions, and nasal congestion.*

Warner MA, Warner ME, Warner DO, Warner LO, Warner EJ. Perioperative pulmonary aspiration in infants and children. Anesthesiology 1999;90:66-71.

*The frequency of perioperative pulmonary aspiration in children is quite low. Serious respiratory morbidity is rare, and there were no associated deaths in this review. Infants and children with clinically apparent pulmonary aspiration in whom symptoms did not develop within 2 hours did not have respiratory sequelae.*

## REFERENCES

Please see www.expertconsult.com.

# Ethical Issues in Pediatric Anesthesiology

**5**

DAVID B. WAISEL

THERE ARE TWO OVERARCHING THEMES of this chapter: (1) Anesthesiologists must take seriously "the experience, perspective, and power of children,"[1] and (2) anesthesiologists should treat every child and family with the grace and consideration with which they would want their own child and family treated.

Taking seriously the experience of children means involving interested children in developmentally appropriate decision making. Anesthesiologists should not solicit a child's views without intending to seriously consider them. *Pro forma* solicitations are harmful.

Treating every child like your own means taking time to allow premedication to work, even if it leads to criticism for a delayed anesthesia start time start. It means rigorously following sterile practice protocols for central lines. It means patiently explaining anesthetic options to the parents as many times as needed.

Bioethics helps motivated physicians to identify and resolve ethical dilemmas. Solving ethical dilemmas is not solely a matter of being moral. Consider a child with an upper airway respiratory infection. Usually, the surgery would be postponed, but suppose the child has missed two previous surgical dates because of an unstable home situation. While the anesthesiologist is explaining the risks of proceeding, the mother distractedly says to proceed because "we're already here." The anesthesiologist has to determine what is in the child's best interest by weighing the risks of proceeding or not proceeding, the duty to ensure that the child receives necessary health care, the weight to be given the mother's consent to proceed, and the duty to "do no harm." Mindful anesthesiologists will seek to identify lurking conflicts of interest in considering whether to proceed.

## Informed Consent

The American Academy of Pediatrics (AAP) bases pediatric informed consent on assent, informed permission, and the best interests standard.[1]

### THE INFORMED CONSENT PROCESS
#### Assent: The Role of the Patient
Although most children cannot legally consent to medical care, children should share in decision making to the extent that their development permits (Table 5-1). As children grow older, participation in decision making should increase, depending on both their maturity and the consequences involved in the decision.[2]

School-age children are developing decision-making capacity, so anesthesiologists should seek both informed permission from the parent and assent and participatory decision making from the child. School-age children are capable of using logic and reason and are able to define and relate multiple aspects of a situation. Such situations may include whether to sedate a 6-year-old before an inhalation induction, whether to use an inhalation or intravenous induction of anesthesia in an 8-year-old, and whether to place an epidural for postoperative analgesia in a 12-year-old.

Many adolescents older than 14 years of age have the ability to use abstract thought, apply complex reasoning, foresee outcomes, simultaneously evaluate multiple options, and understand concepts such as probability. Anesthesiologists should try to fulfill the ethical requirements of consent while obtaining assent. Although some adolescents have cognitive abilities similar to those of adults, adolescents may be hindered by insufficient emotional development. Situations involving these aspects may include obtaining consent from a 14-year-old for anesthesia for scoliosis surgery or from a 16-year-old for an awake thoracic epidural placement for a pectus repair.

### Informed Permission and the Best Interests Standard
Parents have traditionally acted as the surrogate decision makers for their children, and legally they give consent. But surrogate consent does not fulfill the spirit of consent, which is based on obtaining an individualized autonomous decision from the patient receiving the treatment. The AAP has suggested that the proper role for the surrogate decision maker is to provide *informed permission*.[1] Informed permission has the same requirements as informed consent, but it recognizes that the doctrine of informed consent cannot apply.

The *best interests standard* requires decision makers to select the objectively best care. It acknowledges that the cornerstone of informed consent, the right to self-determination, is inapplicable when it is impossible to know or surmise from previous interactions a child's likely preference. Using this standard requires determining (1) who will make the decision and (2) what is the

**TABLE 5-1** Graduated Involvement of Minors in Medical Decision Making*

| Age | Decision-Making Capacity | Techniques |
|---|---|---|
| <6 year | None | Best interests standard |
| 6-12 year | Developing | Informed permission Informed assent |
| 13-18 year | Mostly developed | Informed assent Informed permission |
| Mature minor | Developed, as legally determined by a judge, for a specific decision. Although particulars vary by state, the mature minor doctrine in general requires adolescents to be at least 14 years old and tends to permit decisions of lesser risk. | Informed consent |
| Emancipated minor | Developed as determined by statutes defining eligible situations (e.g., being married, in the military, economically independent). | Informed consent |

*This broad outline should be viewed as a guide. Specific circumstances should be taken into consideration.

best care. The difficulties arise in assuming that there is always one best choice, because if there is, it should not matter who makes the decision. In our society, acceptable decision making is broadly defined. Parents capable of participating in the decision-making process are the appropriate primary decision makers. This is in part due to society's respect for the concept of the family and the assumption that parents care greatly for their children. Although a child's preferences cannot be known, it is reasonable to assume that because children will incorporate some of the parents' values as they mature, parental values are a good first approximation for the child's future values.[3] A few have argued that the presumption that parents are the best decision makers needs to be more closely examined.[4] These objections center on the legitimacy of the parents' knowledge of the preferences of the child's future self. Although these concerns are theoretically interesting and help physicians understand the complexities of the best interests standard, the standard is that parents have extensive leeway in determining what is in a child's best interests.

One way to decide what is in the best interests of the child is to define what choices fall outside the range of acceptable decision making. Criteria to make this determination include the extent of harm to the child deriving from the intervention or its absence, the likelihood of success, and the overall risk-to-benefit ratio. In the classic Baby Doe case, a child was born with Down syndrome and duodenal atresia and was permitted to die without intervention. Public discussion ensued, and it was thought that not repairing a correctable lesion was outside the bounds of acceptable undertreatment. The case spurred passage of so-called Baby Doe regulations, which define what care must be given to certain infants. In this effort to avoid unacceptable undertreatment, some believe that such regulations cause unacceptable overtreatment of patients, primarily because regulations are crude instruments for dissecting complex clinical situations.

Parents can make bad decisions. Although anesthesiologists must respect the diversity values and the parent–child relationship, decision making that imperils the health of a child needs to be challenged. If parents are choosing unacceptable treatments, anesthesiologists should determine the basis of their judgment, address those specific concerns, and involve other clinicians both to offer an assessment of the appropriateness of care and to engage the parents in discussion. Charging parents with not acting in the child's best interests is serious and can have significant social, fiscal, and familial ramifications. If the parents remain steadfast, however, anesthesiologists should report the situation to proper child welfare authorities for possible legal action.

### Disclosure

The "reasonable person" standard, the legal standard for most of the United States, requires that the information disclosed be sufficient to satisfy a hypothetical reasonable person. However, this standard does not define exactly what information should be given, and it does not take into account the patient's desires and needs. The "subjective person" standard suggests that informed consent should be matched to the wants and needs of the decision makers. Although the subjective person standard better fulfills the spirit of informed consent, its greater ambiguity makes it difficult to use as a legal standard.

Rather than rely on a rote informed consent process, anesthesiologists should seek to satisfy the needs of the decision makers by meeting their information and decision-making needs. Patients and surrogates differ in the extent to which they prefer to receive information and to participate in decision making.[5-8] In general, 10% to 15% of patients may prefer less information than their peers. Overall, a quarter of patients want to be the primary decision maker, a quarter want the physician to be the primary decision maker, and half want some form of shared decision making.[6,9,10]

Anesthesiologists should inform families about matters that the anesthesiologist feels must be communicated and about options that affect the perioperative experience (e.g., regional versus general anesthesia). Following this baseline, anesthesiologists can then ask whether the decision makers wish to know more. By being attentive to the words and actions of the decision makers, anesthesiologists can tailor the process. The likelihood of being sued based on informed consent malpractice issues is very rare. Patient-driven interactions likely reduce malpractice lawsuits.[11]

Performing patient-centered informed consent often requires communication of the anesthesiologist's opinion along with an explanation of the supporting reasons. With this information, the patient is better able to determine which anesthetic approach provides the most desired benefits.

### Informed Refusal

The requirements to achieve an informed refusal of a procedure are similar to the requirements for informed consent in that decision makers should be substantially well versed about the risks, benefits, and alternatives before declining. When parents refuse what clinicians believe is necessary care for a child who cannot participate in the decision-making process, clinicians may invoke the best interests standard. This situation is more complicated when the child expresses significant decision-making capacity and refuses nonemergent procedures. Anesthesiologists should respect the right of children (typically those over the age of 10 years) not to assent to a procedure, and they should not coerce the child to proceed. In children, particularly adolescents, the distinction between persuasion and coercion is critical. *Persuasion,* the act of using argument and reason to influence a patient's decision, is appropriate. *Coercion,* the outright use of a credible threat, manipulation, or misleading information, is not. Achieving the child's assent may necessitate further discussions with the child, parents, and other providers, and such discussions may best take place away from the operating room.

Consider a 15-year-old who is scheduled for an elective knee arthroscopy. The day before the procedure, she gave assent and her parents gave informed permission for anesthesia and surgery. She is now crying in the preoperative area and refusing to cooperate. Rather than forcibly or surreptitiously sedating her, the anesthesiologist should discuss her concerns. If she is unable to discuss the issues, the anesthesiologist should consider removing her from the area and giving her time to regain composure before readdressing the situation. Simple actions often allow the situation to be resolved. If the withdrawal of assent was in part related to anxiety, the child may assent to receiving ample premedication before returning to the holding area. Anesthesiologists must obtain her assent before administering the sedation, however, and not simply assume that forceful or surreptitious administration is justified.

### Doctor, If This Were Your Child, What Would You Do?

Physicians should respond to requests for advice by using medical facts to explain how different paths support specific values, so that decision makers can choose the most concordant path. However, the question, "If this were your child, what would you do?" can be asked for a number of different reasons, forcing physicians to put the question into a broader context.[12,13]

For example, parents may be declaring that they are having difficulty comprehending the overwhelming information and need help making a reasonable decision. Perhaps they are actually asking what would give their child the best chance of getting better. In this situation, physicians should explain the reasons and values underlying their personal choice.

Parents may be looking for support that they are making the right choice in an untenable situation. Physicians should answer with their best judgment if they agree with the family. If they disagree, physicians should lend support through comments such as, "Other parents in the same situation have made the same choice," or by acknowledging that it is normal to feel uncertain.[12] If the family persists in asking what they should do, physicians may wish to acknowledge that their choice might have been different. Physicians should emphasize, however, that parental values are more valid than physician values when referring to their own child.

Parents may be asking for help in making a life-altering decision. One way of approaching this question is to offer a process for answering the question (e.g., "I would talk with the chaplain"). Physicians should feel comfortable admitting that are unable to determine what they would do if in the same situation. Honesty reinforces the difficulty of the decision for the parents.

### Disclosure and Apology of Medical Errors

Hiding medical errors is indecent and breaches informed consent.[14] Fear, inadequate support, and lack of education prevent physicians from disclosing and apologizing appropriately.[14-18] Forthrightly disclosing medical errors, although upsetting, often strengthens the patient–physician relationship. Learning about a hidden medical error destroys trust and rapidly (and often appropriately) triggers legal action.

Physician apologies or sympathetic comments often are prohibited as legal evidence of wrongdoing.[19] Nonetheless, disclosing and apologizing may influence whether patients pursue legal action and whether such action is successful.[20,21] Sincere (not *pro forma*!) apologies and subsequent redress to prevent future occurrences improves the patient–physician relationship, minimizing the likelihood of legal action.[11]

Physicians without expertise in disclosure and apology often botch the process. Disclosure is a process over time. Initial disclosure should take place as soon as possible after an event and should center on the medical implications.[22-24] Do not speculate about cause or fault. When disclosing, it is wise to bring along an appropriate colleague who can help with the disclosure by providing psychological support for the patient and family. Soon thereafter, a specific, permanent liaison to the family should be identified. The liaison should be available to arrange meetings, explain the results of the investigation into the cause of the event, and describe plans to prevent future events. The liaison should be trained and experienced in apology and disclosure (e.g., a colleague in risk management).

*An apology expresses regret or sorrow. Sincere apologies followed by consistent actions are priceless; insincere apologies are costly.* It is always appropriate to apologize for the adverse effects of an event. And although the standard teaching is that physicians should not assume responsibility for an event before an investigation is performed, it seems bizarre to dissemble about clear errors. As an example, after reassuring the parents that their child is unharmed, I would readily admit that because I had inadvertently given a muscle relaxant instead of an anticholinesterase, their child will require a brief stay in the intensive care unit until ready for tracheal extubation. To evade responsibility (e.g., "Somehow one drug was given when another was intended") for a clear error mocks the apology.

Anesthesiologists should also acknowledge, apologize, and recommend remedies for future difficult situations such as multiple intravenous catheter insertions or a very stressful anesthetic induction.

## SPECIAL SITUATIONS IN PEDIATRIC INFORMED CONSENT
### Confidentially for Adolescents

The obligation to maintain confidentiality requires physicians to protect patient information from unauthorized and unnecessary disclosure. Confidentiality is necessary for an open flow of information.[25] The anesthesiologist enhances trust by interviewing the adolescent in private, acknowledging the adolescent's concerns about confidentiality, and following through on promises. Emancipated and mature minors have a right to complete confidentiality. For other adolescents, if maintaining confidentiality entails minimal harm, physicians should encourage adolescents to be forthright with parents but respect their decision not to be. If maintaining confidentiality may result in serious harm to the adolescent, physicians may be ethically justified in notifying the parents.[25]

### The Pregnant Adolescent

Anesthesiologists face confidentially issues when an adolescent has a positive pregnancy test before anesthesia. Given the principles of confidentiality, it is ethically appropriate to inform only the adolescent of the positive pregnancy test.[26] Because many locales statutorily prohibit sharing pregnancy information with anyone other than the adolescent, anesthesiologists must share this information with the adolescent without letting the parents know. Anesthesiologists should involve pediatricians, gynecologists, and social workers with expertise in adolescent issues in this discussion.

Matters may become more complex if the surgeon, anesthesiologist, adolescent, and other advisors believe the case should be postponed and the adolescent chooses not to inform her parents about the pregnancy test. Anesthesiologists must be careful not to inadvertently inform the parents of the pregnancy test while postponing anesthesia and surgery. Nor should anesthesiologists betray the adolescent by saying, "The case is postponed. If you want to know why, ask your daughter." Although such a statement is factually true and within the letter of the law of confidentially, terse obliqueness scorns the spirit of confidentially.

As a parent of an impregnable adolescent, I understand the desire of anesthesiologists to tell the parents. But I would suggest that anesthesiologists who feel that way are too narrowly applying their own experiences and expectations. Not all parents are wise and gentle, and not all homes are safe and healthy. Confidentially statutes specifically address concerns about child abuse in pregnant adolescents.

To what extent anesthesiologists should protect the adolescent's confidentiality is debatable. Nonetheless, because the parents have no legal right to that information, I believe that more active deception, although less desirable, is appropriate if necessary. Successful deception avoids initiating diagnostic evaluations or treatment and does not unduly worry parents. For example, attributing the delay to "hearing a new murmur" or an abnormal laboratory value "just found" are poor reasons to give to parents. Vague, unremarkable reasons such as "an oncoming cold" are best.

It is rare to condone deception. Deception should not be undertaken without serious reservations. But under certain circumstances, the obligation to the patient may supersede prohibitions on deception. At times, the harms of not deceiving outweigh the harms of deceiving.

### The Adolescent and Abortion

Even though pediatric patients who are pregnant may be considered emancipated, many states require some form of parental involvement, such as parental consent or notification, before an elective abortion.[27,28] If a state requires parental involvement, the ability of the minor to circumvent this regulation by seeking relief from a judge, known as *judicial bypass,* must be available. Requirements and enforcement of statutes vary from state to state.[29] The need for parental involvement in a minor's planned abortion is not always legally straightforward, and it may be best to consult with hospital counsel in determining these issues. Although this is clearly an area in which honorable people disagree, it is worth noting that both the AAP and the American Medical Association (AMA) have affirmed these rights.[25,29,30]

### Children of Jehovah's Witnesses

Jehovah's Witnesses interpret biblical scripture as prohibiting transfusion therapy because blood holds the "life force" and anyone who takes blood will be "cut off from his people" and not earn eternal salvation.[27,28] Adults may refuse transfusion therapy because it is assumed they are making an informed decision about the risks and benefits of transfusion. However, based on the obligations of the state to protect the interests of

incompetent patients, courts have uniformly intervened when parents desire to refuse transfusion therapy on behalf of their children.

Obtaining informed permission and assent for the care of a ward of a Jehovah's Witness should address transfusion therapy. Anesthesiologists should clarify which therapy is acceptable. Synthetic colloid solutions, dextran, erythropoietin, desmopressin, and preoperative iron are usually acceptable. Note that erythropoietin is available in two forms: lyophilized, and dissolved in saline with trace concentrations of albumin. Jehovah's Witnesses who accept albumin will accept either formulation, whereas those who refuse albumin should be offered the lyophilized formulation. Some Jehovah's Witnesses will accept the removal and return of blood in a continuous loop (e.g., cell saver blood). The family should understand, however, that in a life-threatening situation, the anesthesiologist will seek a court order authorizing the administration of life-sustaining blood. In instances in which the likelihood of requiring blood is high or the local judiciary is not that familiar with case law for Jehovah's Witnesses, the anesthesiologist may choose to obtain a court order in advance of the operation.

A common concern is the sudden need for an emergent transfusion in a healthy child undergoing a low-risk procedure. In emergencies, based on the obligation to protect children, anesthesiologists should take the legally correct and ethically appropriate action to protect the child by transfusing blood without a court order. A court order may then be sought if desired.

For procedures that may be safely delayed, decision makers may consider postponing the procedure until the child is of sufficient age and maturity to decide about transfusion therapy. The complexity is whether the delay may increase the risk or decrease the likelihood of a good outcome. This decision requires the same balancing act as for determining the best interests for a child. Relevant factors include the quantitative change in risk or benefit and the significance of the type of risk or benefit. For example, it may be easier to wait on a procedure that is purely cosmetic than on a procedure for which waiting entails a small chance of causing a permanent injury. If individual clinicians choose to honor the wishes of a mature minor, they must ensure the fidelity of the agreement by making certain that postoperative and on-call clinicians will honor the mature minor's wishes.

### Emergency Care

Anesthesiologists should provide necessary emergent care for minors who do not have a parent available to give legal consent.[31] Emergencies include problems that could cause death, disability, and the increased risk of future complications.

The right of an adolescent to refuse emergency care treatment turns on the adolescent's decision-making capacity and the resulting harm from refusal of care.[1] If the harm is significant and the adolescent's rationale is decidedly short-term or filled with misunderstanding, it becomes necessary to consider whether the adolescent has sufficient decision-making capacity for this decision. In this situation, it may be appropriate to consider what is in the best interests of the adolescent. For example, a 15-year-old football player with a cervical fracture might refuse emergency stabilization, stating that he does not want to live life without football. Most would hold that his conclusion overly values short-term implications, especially in light of the suddenness of the injury, and that he should receive emergency treatment.

**THE IMPAIRED PARENT**

Parents may be unable to fulfill surrogate responsibilities because of acutely impaired judgment, such as being intoxicated.[32] Anesthesiologists will then have to weigh the benefits of waiting for appropriate legal consent against what is in the best interests of the child. It may be in the child's best interests to proceed with a routine procedure in the situation of an impaired parent who is unable to give legal consent. Anesthesiologists may wish to consult legal and risk management colleagues for guidance.

# End-of-Life Issues

## FORGOING POTENTIALLY LIFE-SUSTAINING TREATMENT

### Perioperative Limitations on Life-Sustaining Medical Therapy

The concept of limiting potentially life-sustaining medical therapy (LSMT) is the same for children as is for adults. Decision makers choose to limit LSMT because they do not consider the potential burdens worth the potential benefits.[33] The AAP, the American Society of Anesthesiologists (ASA), and the American College of Surgery mandate reevaluation of any limitations on LSMT before proceeding to the operating room.[34-36]

Readers will note a shift from the term "Do Not Resuscitate" to terms similar to "Life-Sustaining Medical Therapy." One purpose of this shift is to emphasize that desired limitations on medical treatment are continuous rather than dichotomous. The term "potentially" is often used to modify LSMT to emphasize the uncertainty about whether a therapy will be life sustaining.

Reevaluation of LSMT preferences for the perioperative period starts with clarifying the patient's goals for the proposed surgery and end-of-life care (Table 5-2). Anesthesiologists should involve the patient, family, and other clinicians such as surgeons, intensivists, and pediatricians in determining what is in the best interests of the child.

---

**TABLE 5-2** Components of a Pediatric Perioperative LSMT Discussion

- Planned procedure and anticipated benefit to child
- Advantages and opportunities of having specific, identified clinicians providing therapy for a defined period
- Likelihood of requiring resuscitation
- Reversibility of likely causes for resuscitation
- Description of potential interventions and their consequences
- Chances of successful resuscitation including improved outcomes of witnessed arrests compared to unwitnessed arrests
- Ranges of outcomes with and without resuscitation
- Responses to iatrogenic events
- Intended and possible venues and types of postoperative care
- Postoperative timing and mechanisms for reevaluation of the limitations on LSMT
- Establishment of an agreement (which may include a full resuscitation status) through a goal-directed approach
- Documentation

Adapted from Truog RD, Waisel DB, Burns JP. DNR in the OR: a goal-directed approach. Anesthesiology 1999;90:289-95; and Fallat ME, Deshpande JK. Do-not-resuscitate orders for pediatric patients who require anesthesia and surgery. Pediatrics 2004;114:1686-92.
*LSMT*, Life-sustaining medical therapy.

---

Benefits of potentially LSMT include an improved quality of life and prolongation of life under certain circumstances. Burdens include intractable pain and suffering, disability, and events that cause a decrement in the quality of life, as viewed by the patient.[37] These guidelines help in considering short- and long-term goals and putting into appropriate context specific fears such as long-term ventilatory dependency, pain, and suffering.

Legitimate procedures for a child with limitations on LSMT include procedures that decrease pain, provide vascular access, enable the child to be at home, treat an urgent problem unrelated to the primary problem (e.g., appendicitis), or treat a problem that may be related but is not considered a terminal event (e.g., bowel obstruction). But seeking these interventions does not obviate the desire to avoid potential postresuscitation burdens such as need for extensive ventilator support, cognitive deficits, or physical limitations.

The goal-directed approach for perioperative limitations on LSMT permits decision makers to guide therapy by prioritizing outcomes rather than procedures.[33] After defining desirable outcomes, decision makers have anesthesiologists use their clinical judgment to determine how specific interventions will affect achieving the specific goals. Predictions about the success of interventions made at the time of the resuscitation are more accurate than predictions made preoperatively, when the quality and nature of the problems are unknown. Therapy may be guided by goals rather than specific procedures (as is done on the ward), because during the perioperative period children are cared for by dedicated anesthesiologists for brief, defined periods. It is helpful to define a goal-directed approach by discussing the acceptable burdens, the desirable benefits, and the likelihood of distinct outcomes. Most decision makers choose a goal-directed approach indicating that they would desire therapy if the interventions and burdens were temporary and reversible (i.e., if they could return to the present state without suffering too much).

Prior determination of acceptable postoperative LSMT is less critical in pediatrics, because usually parents are available in the postoperative period to make decisions regarding therapy. Nonetheless, when a sufficiently mature child participates in discussions about LSMT, anesthesiologists should ensure that the discussion incorporates the child's preferences for postoperative trials of therapy. The willingness to undergo a trial of therapy indicates a belief that the burdens of the trial (e.g., a few days of ventilator support) may be worth the benefits (e.g., extubation of the trachea) initially, but at some point the increasing burdens may not be worth the decreasing likelihood of the benefits.

### Barriers to Honoring Preferences for Resuscitation

Barriers to honoring limitations center on clinician attitudes, time pressures, and inadequate knowledge about policy, law, and ethics.[38-43] In short, whereas patients prioritize functional status in choosing to limit LSMT, clinicians tend to base their opinions on diagnosis and life expectancy.

Anesthesiologists may falsely believe that law or hospital policy requires full resuscitation during the perioperative period. Physicians who act in accordance with statutory requirements are often explicitly protected from liability when they honor a child's or family's refusal of resuscitation.[44] Given the well-established right of children and parents to refuse medical treatment and the paucity of cases finding physicians liable for honoring limitations on LSMT, the risk of liability for honoring an appropriately documented perioperative limitation on LSMT is not high and is likely to be lower than the risk of not honoring the limitations.[44]

Iatrogenic problems such as cardiac arrest do not obviate decisions to limit LSMT.[45] To decision makers, the cause of the arrest is irrelevant. Decision makers care about the factors they considered in requesting limited resuscitation, including likelihood of successful resuscitation and physical and mental status after the arrest. The benefits of continued therapy after certain types of iatrogenic arrests should be addressed as part of the perioperative discussion.[45]

### Inadvisable Care

Treatments with low likelihoods of success may be considered inadvisable because of the burden to the child, cost, or uncertain benefit. Discussions about inadvisable treatment should bear in mind the goals of the treatment and the likelihood of achieving a defined result. When offering the likelihood of a result, physicians should be clear whether the information used to form the estimation is based on intuition, clinical experience, or rigorous scientific studies. Scoring systems that are useful for population predictions in determining potentially inadvisable care should be considered as contributory but not determinative for decision making for individuals.

Decision making for a child near the end of life should be based on the best interests of the child. A useful approach to resolving conflicts has been proposed by the Commission for the Study of Ethical Problems in Medicine and Biomedical and Behavioral Research (Table 5-3).[3] In short, physicians may override parental preferences only if a therapy is clearly beneficial (e.g., blood transfusion for anemia). When physicians override parental preferences, the appropriateness of the treatment and the process of decision making should undergo an external review, which will often be medical, ethical, or legal in nature.

The improvement in long-term outcomes for the most preterm babies makes it very hard to predict the likelihood of successful treatment in very young children. The best information suggests that for those infants at the threshold of viability (22 to 25 weeks), survival increases with each week of gestation but the rate of moderate or worse disability does not improve and remains at 30% to 50%.[46,47]

Policies to help resolve differences of opinion about applying treatments with low likelihoods of success are important. Good policies are procedure based, are public, reflect the moral values

of the community, and include processes for identifying stakeholders, initiating and conducting the policy, commencing appellate mechanisms, and determining relevant information.[48]

### IMPROVING COMMUNICATION IN PEDIATRIC INTENSIVE CARE UNITS

Pediatric intensivists should emphasize interdisciplinary communication, tailor the communication style to the parents, and maximize meaningful parental participation in the child's care.[49] The goal is to be an empathic professional who establishes compassionate relationships with the child and family by managing emotional, informational, and care needs.[50] In almost all conversations, clinicians should explain the meaning of the conversation in terms of overall care.[51] Table 5-4 lists characteristics of good communication in the intensive care unit.

### PALLIATIVE CARE

Anesthesiologists, in their role as pain management specialists, as intensive care unit doctors, or in the operating room, may participate in pediatric palliative care.[52,53] Palliative care emphasizes relationship-centered care and should be available to children with a wide variety of diseases (Table 5-5).[54] Although pediatric palliative care has struggled for recognition, in 2011 there are signs of improvement.[55,56]

### EUTHANASIA

Although euthanasia has been permitted in the Netherlands for some time, only recently have there been reports of euthanasia for children. Sixteen-year-olds may now request euthanasia, and 12- to 15-year-olds may request euthanasia with their parent's approval. On reflection, it is reasonable for teenagers to want to minimize suffering and pain at the end of life. Similar to euthanasia in the adult patient, the adolescent must have decision-making capacity; must clearly, voluntarily, and repeatedly request to die; must have an incurable condition associated with severe, unrelenting, and intolerable suffering; and should not be making the request due to inadequate comfort care.[56,57] In the Netherlands, the deliberate ending of a neonate's life is permitted under certain circumstances depending on the neonate's life expectancy and intensive care dependency.[57,58]

### DONATION AFTER CARDIAC DEATH

In organ procurement after a declaration of death through neurologic criteria (i.e., brain death), the child is declared dead before being brought to the operating room. The organs are then retrieved while body homeostasis is maintained through mechanical ventilation, pharmacologic therapy, and other standard resuscitative techniques.[59]

Concern about limited availability of organs for transplantation has resulted in the now widely accepted concept of donation after cardiac death (DCD).[60,61] In DCD, the child is not declared dead before being brought to the operating room for organ retrieval. Instead, after it is determined that therapy should be withdrawn based on a standard benefits and burdens assessment, the child is brought to the operating room and therapy is withdrawn. If the child dies after life-sustaining therapy is withdrawn, he or she is declared dead by cardiac criteria and the organs are retrieved. Ethical issues regarding DCD protocols center on whether the protocols seriously alter the dying process by shifting decision making away from the best interests of the dying child and by interfering with the family's ability to be with their dying child (Table 5-6).

| TABLE 5-3 | Suggested Grid for Resolving Disputes about Appropriate Care | |
|---|---|---|
| | **Parents Prefer to** *Accept* **Treatment** | **Parents Prefer to** *Forgo* **Treatment** |
| Physicians consider treatment *clearly beneficial* | Treat | Provide treatment during review process |
| Physicians consider treatment to be of *ambiguous or uncertain benefit* | Treat | Forgo |
| Physicians consider treatment to be *inadvisable* | Provide treatment during review process | Forgo |

From President's Commission for the Study of Ethical Problems in Medicine and Biomedical and Behavioral Research. Deciding to forgo life-sustaining treatment: ethical, medical and legal issues in treatment decisions. Washington, D.C.: U.S. Government Printing Office; 1983.

**TABLE 5-4** Parents' Desires for Communication in the Intensive Care Units

1. **Honest and complete information** should be tailored to the parents' needs and information-receiving preferences. Comprehension of the child's potential trajectories permits better participation in care and a greater chance of appropriate end-of-life care.

2. **Ready access to staff** should include periodic scheduled informal visits to the bedside and the availability of e-mail interactions. The goal is to provide the parents with easy and frequent opportunities to have their questions answered, with sufficient repetition and clarification of the "big picture."

3. To maximize successful **communication**, clinicians should actively assess the parents' preferences for communication and decision making. This includes considering how to relate information to parents when clinicians have different management opinions. Parents frequently recognize that there are differences between options, and some prefer to hear the range of options whereas others prefer to hear only the recommended option.

4. **Emotional expression and support by staff** are critical to parents. To do this successfully, clinicians should adapt their style to parents' preferences. Most clinicians should adopt practices that give parents more room to control the conversation, including talking less, listening more, and tolerating silence as parents gather themselves to continue communicating.

5. Parents respond and benefit from the **relational aspects of compassion, mercy, authenticity, and integrity**.[52] More colloquially, the relational aspect is referred to as "being there," interacting with the parents as a caring person with feelings and emotions.[53] For example, although some clinicians may believe it is inappropriate to show emotion, parents appreciate compassion and some level of distress at the sharing of bad news, rather than cold hard professionalism.[51]

6. **Preservation of the integrity of the parent–child relationship** means enabling parents to continue in their self-identified and prominent role as decision maker and protector. Loss of this role harms parents and may impair their ability to participate in decision making for the child.

7. **Faith and spiritual matters** are highly personal, and parents may feel uncomfortable expressing their faith in an institutional setting. Spiritual matters should be accepted and integrated into the intensive care unit practice to assist those who benefit from spiritual support.

8. **Parents' lifelong views of these events** are profoundly colored by vivid memories and strong feelings about seminal discussions. How difficult discussions are handled and the quality of the communication among clinicians and families often become the bases for the family's lifelong narrative of these events.

Modified from Meyer EC, Ritholz MD, Burns JP, Truog RD. Improving the quality of end-of-life care in the pediatric intensive care unit: parents' priorities and recommendations. Pediatrics 2006;117:649-57.

**TABLE 5-5** Palliative Care

| | |
|---|---|
| WHO | All children suffering from chronic, life-threatening, and terminal illnesses are eligible; this includes<br>• Diseases for which curative therapy may fail (e.g., malignancies with poor prognoses)<br>• Diseases that require long periods of hospitalization to prolong life (e.g., severe epidermolysis bullosa, immunodeficiencies)<br>• Progressive diseases for which treatment is palliative (e.g., severe osteogenesis imperfecta)<br>• Severe nonprogressive disabilities that place the child at risk for coexisting diseases<br>Do-not-resuscitate orders should not be required<br>Prognosis for short-term survival is not required |
| WHAT | Child-focused, family-oriented, and relationship-centered care that focuses on relief of suffering and enhancing quality of life<br>Prioritization of participation of the child and family in decision making<br>Caring for the child as a unique individual<br>Caring for the family as a functional unit<br>Care is not directed at shortening life |
| HOW | An interdisciplinary team is always available to families to provide continuity<br>Facilitation and documentation of communication are critical tasks of the team<br>Highly skilled, expert care is provided |
| WHY | Respite care and support are essential for families |
| WHERE & WHEN | Care is coordinated across all sites of care delivery<br>Care is incorporated into mainstream medical care<br>Bereavement care should be provided as long as it is needed |

From U.S. Department of Human Services: 45 CFR 46 Subpart D. Additional protection for children involved as subjects in research. 2009.

## Clinical and Academic Practice Issues

### PEDIATRIC RESEARCH

The anesthesiologist Henry K. Beecher was one of the first to propose different requirements for pediatric research as compared to adult research.[62] Pediatric research is closely examined because children are incapable of consenting to experiments, and because the developing child is at greater risk for long-term harm.[62] Federal guidelines give four categories of pediatric research, with each ascending category requiring greater scrutiny of the risk-to-benefit ratio, especially in research without

therapeutic benefit for the subject (Table 5-7).[63] Whereas obtaining the assent of the child whenever possible is important for therapeutic medical procedures, it is absolutely essential in the context of research, along with the informed permission of the parents.

### Minimal Risk

Minimal risks are defined as those risks that are not greater in and of themselves than those ordinarily encountered in daily life or during the performance of routine physical or psychological examinations. Most interpret this to mean the risks encountered

**TABLE 5-6** Ethical Issues Surrounding Donation after Cardiac Death (DCD)

| | |
|---|---|
| Should interventions be permitted prior to withdrawal of care? | The burdens from the interventions are not in the best interests of the child. On the other hand, the burdens of the interventions are mostly theoretical and may improve the quality of the transplanted organs. |
| Should withdrawal of therapy occur in the intensive care unit (ICU) or in the operating room? | Withdrawing therapy in the operating room may increase the quality of the organs transplanted. Withdrawing therapy in the ICU is likely to be less jarring to the family and more consistent with the premise of withdrawing therapy for the child's benefit. In addition, it may remove some of the awkwardness that may occur if the child does not die within the defined interval. |
| Who should withdraw therapy? | To be consistent with the premises of withdrawal of therapy, it should be the same person who would normally withdraw therapy from the child. Even if the decision is made to withdraw therapy in the operating room, an anesthesiologist who has not been caring for the child should not be asked to withdraw therapy because of the physical location of the event. |
| How long should cessation of cardiac function exist for a child to be declared dead? | Proposed times may be based on the premises of how long it would take to autoresuscitate compared with how long it would take to be resuscitated through medical intervention. |
| What are the contents of a good DCD policy? | • Acceptable interventions before withdrawing therapy<br>• Acceptable locations of withdrawing therapy<br>• Amount of time to wait until death before forgoing procurement<br>• Which individual should withdraw therapy<br>• What to do if the family will not leave after death is declared |

**TABLE 5-7** Federal Classification of Pediatric Research

1. Research not involving greater than minimal risk
   a. IRB determines minimal risk
   b. IRB finds and documents that adequate provisions are made for soliciting assent from children and permission from their parents or guardians
2. Research involving greater than minimal risk but presenting the prospect of direct benefit to the individual subject
   a. IRB justifies the risk by the anticipated benefit to the subjects
   b. The relationship of the anticipated benefit to the risk is at least as favorable as that presented by available alternative approaches
   c. Adequate provisions are made for assent and permission
3. Research that involves greater than minimal risk and no prospect of direct benefit to the individual subject but is likely to yield generalizable knowledge about the subject's disorder or condition
   a. IRB determines that the risk represents a minor increase over minimal risk
   b. The intervention or procedure presents experiences to subjects that are reasonably commensurate with those inherent in their actual or expected medical, dental, psychological, social, or educational situations
   c. The intervention or procedure is likely to yield generalizable knowledge ... which is of vital importance for the understanding or amelioration of the subject's disorder or condition
   d. Adequate provisions are made for assent and permission
4. Research not otherwise approvable, which presents an opportunity to understand, prevent, or alleviate a serious problem affecting the health or welfare of children

From U.S. Department of Human Services: 45 CFR 46 Subpart D. Additional protection for children involved as subjects in research. 2009.
*IRB,* Institutional review board.

**TABLE 5-8** Strategies Used by Drug Companies to Influence Physicians

1. Teach sales people subtle verbal and nonverbal techniques to influence physicians.
2. Instruct sales people to misdirect and to dissemble when questioned about possible complications.
3. Cherry-pick which data are distributed to physicians.
4. Prohibit distribution of studies that may criticize the product. (One strategy is to classify concerning studies as background studies and then prohibit distribution of background studies.)
5. Seek "opinion leaders" to speak in favor of the product.
6. Continue the well-established gift-giving strategy to subconsciously curry favor with the physician and to develop a positive association about the product and the company.

Individuals are poor at estimating the risk levels of activities and often correlate risk to familiarity, control of the activity, and reversibility of the potential harms.[65] Institutional review boards (IRB) may reject low-risk studies because they involve unfamiliar matters while approving studies that have excessive risks.

### Minor Increase over Minimal Risk

The pediatric research category that involves "greater than minimal risk and no prospect of direct benefit to the individual subject but is likely to yield generalizable knowledge about the subject's disorder or condition ... which is of vital importance" (see Table 5-8) is based on the idea that it is acceptable to expose a child to a "minor increase over minimal risk" under certain conditions.[66] Parsing the regulation may help clarify this somewhat unhelpful definition. One suggestion has been that *minor increase* means that the pain, discomfort, or stress must be transient, reversible, and not severe.[64] *Condition* of the subject should be used to mean a set of characteristics "that an established body of scientific or clinical evidence has shown to negatively affect children's health and well-being or to increase the risk of developing a health problem in the future."[64] Interpreting condition to include "having the potential to have the condition" permits

in daily life by healthy children, such as running in the backyard, playing sports, or riding in a car.[64,65] A less favored relative interpretation uses as a benchmark those risks encountered in the daily lives of children who will be enrolled in the research. In other words, if a child were living in a manner that exposed the child to risk (e.g., undergoing repeated general anesthesia), then it would be acceptable to expose the child up to that level of risk in a study.

otherwise healthy children to participate in research for diseases that they may develop (e.g., cellulitis). The term *vital importance* implies that the evidence supporting the relevance of the study should require a higher order of proof.

### Socioeconomic Concerns and Distribution of Risk

Socioeconomically disadvantaged children living in urban areas may be overrepresented in research studies because urban academic centers in disadvantaged areas perform the majority of clinical research.[67] Children living in socioeconomically disadvantaged areas are often more affected by diseases associated with their environment, such as asthma or nutritional disorders complicated by limited access to stocked grocery stores. One could argue that this unequal burden of risk, primarily manifested by greater participation of socioeconomically disadvantaged children in research studies, is reasonable because these children are more likely to develop these diseases and therefore are more likely to benefit from the research.[68] Most reject that view and believe that in some sense, socioeconomically advantaged patients gratuitously gain the benefits of the research without sharing the risks. The disproportionate risk borne by one segment of society compared with another likely breeches the most accepted interpretation of the core ethical value of justice.

Socioeconomically disadvantaged families may be more likely to be influenced by the small gifts offered to research participants. Aside from compensating for costs (e.g., parking vouchers), gifts should not of themselves encourage participation. The problem is that gifts that represent a small expression of gratitude for some families may provide an incentive for participation for socioeconomically disadvantaged families.[69]

### IMPERATIVE FOR PHARMACOLOGIC RESEARCH

Through the mid-1990s, more than 70% of new molecular entities were without pediatric drug labeling. Inadequate information exposed children to age-specific adverse reactions, ineffective treatment due to inappropriate dosing, and lack of access to new drugs because physicians tended to prescribe less effective, known medications. Inadequate research into pediatric drugs forced physicians to prescribe drugs in nonstandard ways, such as sprinkled or crushed tablets. Even when there is some pediatric labeling, there is scant labeling for children younger than 2 years of age. In 2009, a survey of a Canadian pediatric tertiary hospitals found that even when comparing off-label use to contemporary pediatric references (an unofficial and very liberal interpretation), 16% of drug administrations during the perioperative period were considered off-label. Based on a more traditional standard of the *Canadian Compendium of Pharmaceutical Specialties*, 55% of drugs administered were used off-label.[70]

The following selective history highlights the overall intent to ensure (1) that children get the same benefits of pharmacologic advances as adults and (2) that research is performed in the youngest children. Readers should also learn from this history that persistent advocacy is often required before regulatory change can be successfully obtained. In 1962, the Kefauver-Harris Amendments (passed after the thalidomide disaster) required that drug companies demonstrate safety and efficacy before marketing a drug. Because the vast majority of drugs did not undergo pediatric-specific investigation, this requirement actually led to less pediatric labeling, with the package insert (drug label) often reading, "Safety and efficacy have not been demonstrated for children <12 years," because of the expense of getting this information (see also Chapter 6). In 1994, the U.S. Food and Drug Administration (FDA) began requiring sponsors to explain why pediatric labeling cannot occur but did not require sponsors to perform pediatric studies.

The 1997 FDA Modernization Act and the 1998 Final Rule were legislative initiatives designed to gain more data from drug companies through pediatric studies in exchange for the benefit of an additional 6 months of patent exclusivity. This effort was further codified with the passage of the Best Pharmaceutical Act for Children in 2002. With these requirements, the FDA mandated pediatric studies if a new drug might be used in a substantial number of children, if it might provide a meaningful therapeutic benefit, or if inadequate labeling could pose significant risks. The pharmaceutical industry responded with an explosion of pediatric studies. However, the exclusivity provision did not encourage study of generic drugs or drugs with insufficient sales. Further, once exclusivity was credited for older pediatric age groups, there was no incentive to conduct studies in younger groups.

In December 2003, the Pediatric Research Equity Act required pediatric studies for all drugs and biologic products that have a new indication, new dosage form, new route, new dosing regimen, or new active ingredient. Studies could be waived if they were impracticable, if the therapy would be ineffective or unsafe in pediatric patients, or if there would be no meaningful therapeutic benefit over existing therapies and the moiety would not used in a substantial number of children.

Other nations have adopted similar regulatory requirements and incentives to encourage drug research. The European Union offers scientific help for performance of studies and requires that drug applications contain pediatric information that covers "all paediatric age groups and all necessary age-appropriate formulations," unless an exception is granted.[71] Performing pediatric testing earns patent extensions even if the drug is not approved for pediatric use.

### MANAGING POTENTIAL CONFLICTS OF INTEREST

A *conflict of interest* is "a set of conditions in which professional judgment concerning a primary interest (such as a patient's welfare or the validity of research) tends to be unduly influenced by a secondary interest."[72] Because these conditions in an individual are internal, they are best characterized by describing situations that may create the potential for conflicts of interest. Focusing on potential conflicts of interest moves the concept away from attacking an individual's morals and toward more uniform definitions. Conflicts of interest may be induced by financial, personal, and professional benefits such as prestige, promotion, and personal gratification.[73] Anesthesiologists should be mindful of these potential conflicts, and attempt to identify them to better understand the likelihood of compromised judgment.

### Conducting Research

Perhaps the most powerful conflict in conducting research is the loss of equipoise that can come from originating and developing an idea. Other sources of conflict related to research center on academic promotion and reputation. Physician disclosures do not help identify conflicts of interest. In one study, only 80% of physicians disclosed payments related to the research, and only 50% disclosed payments from the same company but unrelated to the product being discussed. Indirect payments were just as likely to influence behavior as direct payment.[74]

In 2009, an anesthesiologist was accused of falsifying data that had encouraged multimodal pain therapy. A routine audit had found the irregularities that initiated the subsequent evaluation (supporting the benefits of oversight). Major journals retracted articles. Steven Shafer, editor of *Anesthesia and Analgesia*, was quoted as saying, "We are left with a large hole in our understanding of this [multimodal pain therapy]."[75] Shafer called the scandal "a tragedy" for the profession, for patients, and for the anesthesiologist involved personally. Given that the anesthesiologist's studies were "robust" and influential, "the big chunk of what people have based their [multimodal] protocol on is gone."[75,76] It is important to emphasize that the anesthesiologist's coauthors were deceived by him and were not complicit. If fact, they assisted in assessing the legitimacy of articles that were not retracted.[77]

Conflicts of interest also come from industry support of research. To be clear, the academic–anesthesia-industry research complex is necessary to continue the rapid advancement of science. Rigorous oversight minimizes these abuses. Researchers need to be involved in trial development, must have access to raw data, and must be able to publish without the company's authorization. Cozy relationships between powerful members of the local academic community and industry should be examined and brought to light to minimize influence and potential conflicts of interest.

### Interaction with Industry

Anesthesiologists need to be suspicious of industry attempts to "selflessly" educate clinicians.[78] Physicians should independently evaluate information supplied by industry. Industry representatives and materials routinely overrepresent the benefits and underrepresent the risks of drugs (Table 5-8)."[79] Wisely, there has been a strong movement in academic centers to stiffen rules about physician exposure to industry representatives.[80]

Risks associated with industry misrepresentation will increase as increasing physician workload decreases time for study. For these reasons, it is instructive to look more closely at this problem. Evidence published in the 2000 VIGOR study indicated that the popular antiinflammatory drug rofecoxib (Vioxx) dramatically increased the rate of myocardial infarction in patients. In 2001, the FDA determined that physicians should be made aware of the cardiovascular effects of rofecoxib, and in 2004 it was withdrawn from the market. Congressman Henry Waxman later wrote the following[81]:

> Merck, the manufacturer of Vioxx, … has an excellent reputation within the drug industry and supports many products, such as vaccines, that are medically essential but not very profitable…. Yet as we learned, even a company like Merck can direct its sales force to provide clinicians with a distorted picture of the relevant scientific evidence….

On February 7, 2001, the Arthritis Drugs Advisory Committee of the Food and Drug Administration (FDA) … voted unanimously that physicians should be made aware of VIGOR's cardiovascular results.

The next day, Merck sent a bulletin to its rofecoxib sales force [which] ordered, "DO NOT INITIATE DISCUSSIONS ON THE FDA ARTHRITIS ADVISORY COMMITTEE … OR THE RESULTS OF THE … VIGOR STUDY." It advised that if a physician inquired about VIGOR, the sales representative should indicate that the study showed a gastrointestinal benefit and then say, "I cannot discuss the study with you."

Merck further instructed representatives to show those doctors who asked whether rofecoxib caused myocardial infarction a pamphlet called "The Cardiovascular Card." This pamphlet, prepared by Merck's marketing department, indicated that rofecoxib was associated with 1/8 the mortality from cardiovascular causes of that found with other antiinflammatory drugs.

> The Cardiovascular Card … did not include any data from the VIGOR study. Instead, it presented a pooled analysis of preapproval studies, in most of which low doses of rofecoxib were used for a short period of time. None of these studies were designed to assess cardiovascular safety…. In fact, FDA experts had publicly expressed "serious concerns" … about using preapproval studies as evidence of the drug's cardiovascular safety….
>
> [B]ut it would be a mistake to restrict the lessons learned to a single company. The testimony we heard indicated that Merck's marketing practices may be less aggressive and more ethical than many of its competitors. It should be noted that Merck eventually paid $950 million USD to settle criminal charges and civil claims related to unlawful marketing of Vioxx and misleading statements about its safety.

### Production Pressure

Anesthesiologists are prone to production pressure, which has been defined as "the internal or external pressure on the anesthetist to keep the operating room schedule moving along speedily."[82,83] Almost half of surveyed anesthesiologists reported seeing what they considered unsafe anesthetic practices in response to this production pressure.[84] As a consequence, anesthesiologists may not want to take the time to allow a child to ask questions about the anesthetic, to adequately premedicate an anxious child, or to engage the parents in a lengthy discussion about postponing the surgery because the child has a mild upper respiratory infection. Anesthesiologists should also be cognizant of their level of skill in providing anesthesia. For example, the "routine" tonsillectomy may be beyond some anesthesiologists' ability in a child with multiple congenital deficits. Anesthesiologists have an obligation to the patient and themselves to only provide care that is within their skills and to recognize when economic and administrative pressures may induce them to do otherwise.

### THE FETUS

The positions of the AAP and the American College of Obstetricians and Gynecologists (ACOG) are helpful in considering care of the fetus (Table 5-9).[85-87] The statements indicate subtle differences when the interests of the mother and fetus diverge, such as when the mother wishes to refuse a treatment that would likely be beneficial for the fetus. Broadly, the AAP advocates more for the fetus, particularly when the intervention poses a small risk to the mother and can effectively treat a problem for the fetus that would otherwise cause irreversible harm. ACOG is more concerned about complex issues of overriding maternal autonomy, such as the criminalization of not complying with medical recommendations.

### PHYSICIAN OBLIGATIONS, ADVOCACY, AND GOOD CITIZENSHIP

An implicit social contract obligates physicians to serve society beyond directly caring for patients. Society supports medical students, physicians in training, and physicians through providing opportunities to train, to perform research, and, perhaps most importantly, to learn from and with patients.[88] In return, society expects pediatric anesthesiologists to "manage all things pediatric anesthesia" (Table 5-10).[89-91] Individual anesthesiologists are not expected to fulfill every obligation. "Units" of anesthesiologists,

**TABLE 5-9** Positions of the AAP and the ACOG Regarding Ethical Considerations and Maternal Choices in Fetal Therapy

| American Academy of Pediatrics (AAP) | American College of Obstetricians and Gynecologists (ACOG) |
|---|---|
| **Priority** | |
| Respect for principle of maternal autonomy | Respect for principle of maternal autonomy |
| Fetal concerns may trump maternal autonomy | Fetal concerns may not trump maternal autonomy |
| **Type of Medical Treatment Worthy of Judicial or Physical Intervention** | |
| If the intervention has been demonstrated to be effective | If there is a high probability of serious harm to the fetus without intervention |
| If nonintervention will lead to significant and irreversible harm | If there is a high probability of significant benefit to the fetus from the intervention |
| If there is minimal maternal risk from the intervention | If there is a relatively small risk to the pregnant woman from the intervention |
| | If no comparably effective, less invasive options are available |
| | Intervention only under extraordinary circumstances of conflict |
| **Use of Physical Intervention** | |
| Physical intervention may be acceptable if judicial authorization has been obtained | Physical intervention is never acceptable |
| **Psychosocial Aspects** | |
| Psychosocial aspects of overriding a woman's autonomy are not addressed | Significant concern about overriding maternal autonomy, including<br>• criminalization of noncompliance with medical recommendations<br>• loss of trust in the health care system<br>• social costs of compromising liberty |
| **Conflict Resolution** | |
| Does not ask physicians to consider subordinating their view | Physicians should make reasonable attempts to explain recommended treatments and to persuade the woman to comply |
| Does not suggest it is reasonable to transfer the patient's care | Physicians should subordinate their values if necessary, because it is the woman's decision |
| | Suggests it may be reasonable to transfer care |

Data from Brown SD, Truog RD, Johnson JA, Ecker JL. Do differences in the American Academy of Pediatrics and the American College of Obstetricians and Gynecologists positions on the ethics of maternal-fetal interventions reflect subtly divergent professional sensitivities to pregnant women and fetuses? Pediatrics 2006;117:1382-7; American Academy of Pediatrics, Committee on Bioethics. Fetal therapy: ethical considerations. Pediatrics 1999;103:1061-3; American College of Obstetricians and Gynecologists. Committee Opinion 321: Maternal decision making, ethics, and the law. Obstet Gynecol 2005;106:1127-37.

such as private practice groups, academic departments, and state societies, should fulfill these obligations collectively.

### Participating in Patient Safety Efforts

Medical errors come from human mistakes and system flaws.[92] Anesthesiologists have an obligation to work to reduce system flaws, including participating in quality improvement activities and data collection, following policies meant to improve care in high-risk situations (e.g., nosocomial infections), and actively engaging in policies designed to reduce medical errors, such as universal standards of patient identification.[93]

Although physicians may not see the big picture and therefore resent doing "extra" steps, it is vital for physicians to accept on faith that participation is good patient care.[94] Surreptitiously circumventing policies may harm patients, does not permit remediation of the policy, and weakens the fidelity of the entire system, encouraging others to "make their own rules."[95] When anesthesiologists believe that policies are harmful or unnecessary, they are obligated to raise these questions through appropriate channels.

### Treating Suffering

Cassel described suffering as an intensely personal feeling that can be defined as "the state of severe distress associated with events that threaten the intactness of the person."[96] Suffering should be considered when managing pain, and adequate steps should be taken to find and alleviate sources of suffering. Factors that contribute to a child's suffering include not knowing the origin or meaning of the pain, believing that pain is a punishment, and fearing that the pain will never be relieved.[96]

Anesthesiologists minimize suffering by clearly communicating about these issues with parents and children and affording children as much control of their care as possible.

### Suspicion of Child Abuse

Child abuse includes acts of physical abuse, sexual abuse, emotional abuse, and neglect. Anesthesiologists should be particularly sensitive to bruises or burns in the shape of objects, injuries to soft tissue areas such as the upper arms, unexplained mouth and dental injuries, fractures in infants, height and weight less than the 5th percentile, and injures that are not explained by the history (see also Chapter 38).[97,98] Children who have physical or mental handicaps are particularly prone to abuse.[99] Anesthesiologists, like all physicians, are legally required to report the suspicion of child abuse or neglect to appropriate authorities. Indeed, in most jurisdictions, a physician can be criminally prosecuted if found liable for failing to report suspected child abuse.

### THE ETHICS CONSULTATION SERVICE

The ethical dilemmas that occur in the practice of anesthesiology may be difficult for the practitioner to resolve alone. Ethics committees and their consulting services act in an advisory role to help clinicians, patients, and families amicably resolve ethical dilemmas. Anesthesiologists may find ethics consultation helpful with questions about informed consent, decision-making capacity, and resuscitation decisions and in resolving disagreements among patients, families, and clinicians.

Although most ethics consultation services use a small group (typically three people) to perform consultations, some use the

| TABLE 5-10 | Examples of Obligations of Anesthesiologists to Participate and Advocate |
|---|---|

**Obligations of Pediatric Anesthesiologists**

Treat every child with the grace and consideration you would want for your child and family

Tailor the perioperative experience to the individual

Respond to problems that may harm children (e.g., impaired colleagues)

Practice mindfulness and critical self-reflection

Actively engage in continuing medical education

Support advancement of the science

Participate in quality improvement initiatives such as Wake Up Safe

Participate in professional organizations such as the Society for Pediatric Anesthesia and the American Academy of Pediatrics Section on Anesthesiology and Pain Medicine

Prepare future generations through teaching, mentoring, creating opportunities, and developing systems to enable anesthesiologists to fulfill these obligations

**Community Advocacy and Participation**

Raise public awareness about a health or social issue

Participating in public advocacy and lobbying

Encourage a medical society to act on an issue that concerns the public health

Serve in a local organization, political interest group, or political organization

Topics of particular relevance to pediatric anesthesiologists:
- Pediatric obesity
- Pediatric sedation in hospitals
- Child abuse
- Health care access
- Role of subspecialty training in improving care for children

entire committee and some use a single individual.[100] Physicians, nurses, social workers, chaplains, administrators, and lay people serve on ethics committees and perform consultations. Common characteristics of ethics consultation services are that they permit anyone to request an ethics consultation; that they require notification (not permission) of the patient, parents, and attending physician prior to the consultation; and that choosing to follow the recommendations is wholly voluntary.

Following consultations, clinicians feel greater satisfaction in managing cases with ethical conflicts, not only because of their heightened awareness of the expert consulting services available but also because of their increased knowledge and comfort in dealing with these issues. Ethics committees are also available to consult on policy development and to organize continuing educational programs.

## ANNOTATED REFERENCES

Cassel EJ. The nature of suffering and the goals of medicine. N Engl J Med 1982;306:639-46.
*Physicians relieve suffering. Cassel's 30-year-old treatise is the unparralled explanation of suffering.*

Committee on Bioethics, American Academy of Pediatrics. Informed consent, parental permission, and assent in pediatric practice. Pediatrics 1995;95:314-17.
*This article is the basis of informed consent for children. Pay particular attention to the introduction, in which Dr. William Bartholome (in abstentia) exhorts clinicians to respect "the experience, perspective and power of children."*

Consensus statement of the Society of Critical Care Medicine's Ethics Committee regarding futile and other possibly inadvisable treatments. Crit Care Med 1997;25:887-91.
*This article explicates the importance of recognizing the ethical and clinical differences between advisable and inadvisable treatments.*

Fallat ME, Deshpande JK. Do-not-resuscitate orders for pediatric patients who require anesthesia and surgery. Pediatrics 2004;114:1686-92.
*This article is a complete explanation of perioperative do-not-resuscitate orders for children.*

Gruen RL, Pearson SD, Brennan TA. Physician-citizens: public roles and professional obligations. JAMA 2004;291:94-8.
*Gruen et al. provide a thoughtful perspective on the public and professional obligations of physicians. They provide a path on how to fulfill these obligations.*

Kon AA. Answering the question: "Doctor, if this were your child, what would you do?" Pediatrics 2006;118:393-7.
*Kon helps anesthesiologists understand this deceptively simple question.*

Shafer SL. Tattered threads. Anesth Analg 2009;108:1361-3.
*Shafer elegantly articulates the harms of false data.*

Waxman HA. The lessons of Vioxx: drug safety and sales. N Engl J Med 2005;352:2576-8.
*Waxman's recounting of public testimony eviscerates the reassuring murmerings of industry.*

## REFERENCES

Please see www.expertconsult.com

# DRUG AND FLUID THERAPY

# Pharmacokinetics and Pharmacology of Drugs Used in Children

BRIAN J. ANDERSON, JERROLD LERMAN, AND CHARLES J. COTÉ

THE PHARMACOKINETICS AND PHARMACODYNAMICS of most medications, when used in children, especially neonates, differ from those in adults.[1-11] Children exhibit different pharmacokinetics (PK) and pharmacodynamics (PD) from adults because of their immature renal and hepatic function, different body composition, altered protein binding, distinct disease spectrum, diverse behavior, and dissimilar receptor patterns.[1,3,12-19] PK differences necessitate modification of the dose and the interval between doses to achieve the desired clinical response and to avoid toxicity.[7,20-22] In addition, some medications may displace bilirubin from its protein binding sites and possibly predispose an infant to kernicterus.[23-28] The capacity of the end organ, such as the heart or bronchial smooth muscle, to respond to medications may also differ in children compared with adults (PD effects). In this chapter we discuss basic pharmacologic principles as they relate to drugs commonly used by anesthesiologists.

# Pharmacokinetic Principles and Calculations

Changes in drug concentrations within the body over time are referred to as *pharmacokinetics*. The principles and equations that describe these changes can be used to adjust drug doses rationally to achieve more effective drug concentrations at the site of action.[29-33] The equations in this section are intended for general and practical use, whereas the more rigorous mathematical intricacies of PK are covered elsewhere.[34-37]

Within the body, a drug may diffuse between several body fluids and tissues at different rates, yet the consistent change in its circulating concentration may be used to characterize its kinetics and to guide dosages. The rate of removal of drug from the circulation is usually described using either first-order or zero-order exponential equations. The difference between these two types of rates has important implications for drug treatment.

## FIRST-ORDER KINETICS

Most drugs are cleared from the body with first-order exponential rates in which a constant fraction or constant proportion of drug is removed per unit of time. Because the proportion of drug cleared remains constant, the higher the concentration, the greater the amount of drug removed from the body. Such rates can be described by exponential equations that fit the following form:

$$C = C_0 e^{-kt} \qquad \text{(Eq. 1)}$$

where C is the concentration at time t, $C_0$ is the starting concentration (a constant determined by the dose and distribution volume), and $k$ is the elimination rate constant with units of time$^{-1}$. First-order indicates that the exponent is raised to the first power ($-kt$ in Equation 1). Second-order equations are those that are raised to the second power, such as $e^{(z)^2}$. First-order exponential equations, such as Equation 1, may be converted to the form of the equation of a straight line (y = mx + b) by taking the natural logarithm of both sides, after which they may be solved by linear regression.

$$\ln C = \ln C_0 + (-kt) \qquad \text{(Eq. 2)}$$

If ln C (i.e., natural logarithm of C) is graphed versus time, the slope is $-k$, and the intercept is ln $C_0$. If log C (i.e., common logarithm of C) is graphed versus time, the slope is $-k/2.303$, because ln x equals 2.303 log x. When graphed on linear–linear axes, exponential rates are curvilinear and on semilogarithmic axes, they produce a straight line.

## HALF-LIFE

Half-life, the time for a drug concentration to decrease by one half, is a familiar exponential term used to describe the kinetics of many drugs. *Half-life is a first-order kinetic process, because the same proportion or fraction of the drug is removed during equal periods of time.* As described earlier, the greater the starting concentration, the greater the amount of drug removed during each half-life.

Half-life can be determined by several methods. If concentration is converted to the natural logarithm of concentration and graphed versus time, as described in Equation 2, the slope of this graph is the elimination rate constant, *k*. For both accuracy and precision, at least three concentration-time points should be used to determine the slope, and they should be obtained over an interval during which the concentration decreases at least in half. In clinical practice, for infants and small children, however, *k* is often estimated from just two concentrations obtained during the terminal elimination phase. With multiple data points, the slope of ln C versus time may be calculated easily by least squares linear regression analysis. Half-life ($T_{1/2}$) may be calculated from the elimination rate constant, *k* (time$^{-1}$), as follows:

$$T_{1/2} = \frac{Natural\ Logarithm\ (2)}{k} = \frac{0.693}{k} \qquad \text{(Eq. 3)}$$

Graphic techniques may be used to determine half-life from a series of timed measurements of drug concentration. The concentration-time points should be graphed on semilogarithmic axes and used to determine the best fitting line either visually or by linear regression analysis. This approach is illustrated in Figure 6-1, in which the best-fitting line has been drawn to the concentration-points and crosses a concentration of 20 µg/mL at 100 minutes and a concentration of 10 µg/mL at 200 minutes. The concentration has decreased by one half in 100 minutes, so the half-life is 100 minutes. The elimination rate constant is (0.693/100) min$^{-1}$ or 0.00693 min$^{-1}$.

Elimination half-life is of no value in characterizing disposition of many intravenous (IV) anesthetic drugs during dosing periods relevant to anesthesia. A more useful concept is that of the context-sensitive half-time (CSHT) where "context" refers to the duration of the infusion. This is the time required for the plasma drug concentration to decrease by 50% after terminating the infusion.[38] The CSHT is the same as the elimination half-life for a one-compartment model and does not change with the duration of the infusion. However, most drugs in anesthesia conform to multiple compartment models and the CSHTs are markedly different from their respective elimination half-lives.

CSHT may be independent of the duration of the infusion (e.g., remifentanil, 2.5 minutes); moderately affected (propofol, 12 minutes at 1 hour, 38 minutes at 8 hours); or display marked prolongation (e.g., fentanyl, 1 hour at 24 minutes, 8 hours at 280 minutes). This is a result of return of drug to plasma from peripheral compartments after stopping the infusion. Peripheral compartment sizes and clearances differ in children from adults and at termination of the infusion such that more or less drug remains in the body in children for any given plasma concentration compared with adults. The CSHT for propofol in children, for example, is greater than that in adults.[39] The CSHT gives insight into the PK of a drug, but the parameter may not be clinically relevant; the percentage decrease in concentration required for recovery from the drug effect is not necessarily 50%.

### FIRST-ORDER SINGLE-COMPARTMENT KINETICS

The number of exponential equations required to describe the change in concentration determines the number of compartments. Although a drug may diffuse among several tissues and body fluids, its clearance often fits first-order, single-compartment kinetics if it quickly distributes homogeneously within the circulation and is removed rapidly from the circulation through metabolism or excretion. This may be judged visually, if a semilogarithmic graph of the change in drug concentration fits a single straight line. Kinetics may appear to be single-compartment, when they are really multiple compartments, if drug concentrations are not measured soon enough after IV administration to detect the initial distribution phase (α phase).

### FIRST-ORDER MULTIPLE-COMPARTMENT KINETICS

If drug concentrations are measured several times within the first 15 to 30 minutes after IV administration as well as during a more prolonged period, more than one rate of clearance is often present. This can be observed as a marked change in slope of a semilogarithmic graph of concentration versus time (Fig. 6-2). The number and nature of the compartments required to describe the clearance of a drug do not necessarily represent specific body fluids or tissues. When two first-order exponential equations are required to describe the clearance of drug from the circulation, the kinetics are described as first-order, two-compartment (e.g., central and peripheral compartments) that fit the following equation (Fig. 6-2)[31]:

$$C = Ae^{-\alpha t} + Be^{-\beta t} \qquad \text{(Eq. 4)}$$

where concentration is C, t is time after the dose, A is the concentration at time 0 for the distribution rate represented by the purple line graph with the steepest slope, α is the rate constant for distribution, B is the concentration at time 0 for the terminal elimination rate, and β is the rate constant for terminal elimination. Rate constants indicate the rates of change in concentration and each corresponds to the slope of the respective line divided by 2.303 for logarithm concentration versus time.

Such two-compartment or biphasic kinetics are frequently observed after IV administration of drugs that rapidly distribute out of the central compartment of the circulation to a peripheral compartment.[31] In such situations, the initial rapid decrease in concentration is referred to as the α or distribution phase and

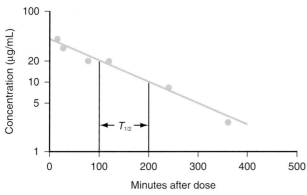

**FIGURE 6-1** Graphic determination of half-life. Half-life can be determined from a series of concentration time-points on a semilogarithmic graph, if the kinetics are first-order exponential. The concentrations are plotted on semilogarithmic axes; the best-fit line is drawn to the points; convenient concentrations are chosen that decrease in half, such as 20 µg/mL and 10 µg/mL, as illustrated; and the interval between those concentrations is the half-life, which is 100 minutes in the illustration.

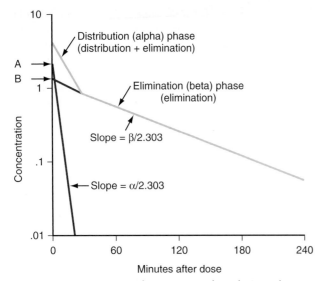

**FIGURE 6-2** Two compartment kinetics in a semilogarithmic graph. The initial rapid decrease in serum concentration reflects distribution and elimination followed by a slower decrease because of elimination. *A* is the concentration at time 0 for the distribution rate. Subtraction of the initial decrease in concentration resulting from elimination, using the concentrations from the elimination line extrapolated back to time 0 at *B*, produces the lower line with a steep slope = $\alpha$(distribution rate constant)/2.303. The terminal elimination phase has a slope = $\beta$(elimination rate constant)/2.303.

represents distribution to the peripheral (tissue) compartments in addition to drug elimination. The terminal ($\beta$) phase begins after the inflection point in the line when elimination starts to account for most of the change in drug concentration. To determine the initial change in concentration as a result of distribution (Fig. 6-2), the change in concentration that results from elimination must be subtracted from the total change in concentration. The slope of the line representing the difference between these two rates is the rate constant for distribution.

These parameters (A, B, $\alpha$, $\beta$) have little connection with underlying physiology and an alternative parameterization is to use a central volume and three rate constants ($k_{10}$, $k_{12}$, $k_{21}$) that describe drug distribution between compartments. Another common method is to use two volumes (central, V1; peripheral, V2) and two clearances (CL, Q). Q is the intercompartment clearance and the volume of distribution at steady state (Vdss) is the sum of V1 and V2. A more detailed mathematical discussion may be found elsewhere.[31,40]

Although many drugs demonstrate multiple-compartment kinetics, traditional studies of kinetics in neonates did not include enough samples immediately after dosing to determine more than one compartment. For clinical estimates of dose and dosing intervals, it is often not necessary to use multiple-compartment kinetics. To minimize cost, limit blood loss, and simplify PK calculations, dose adjustments are often based on only two plasma concentrations (peak and trough), and linear, single-compartment kinetics (such as that of gentamicin and vancomycin) is assumed. Because the elimination rate constant should be determined from the terminal elimination phase, it is important that peak concentrations of multiple-compartment drugs not be drawn prematurely, that is, during the initial distribution phase. If drawn too early, the concentrations will be greater than those during the terminal elimination phase (Fig. 6-2), which will

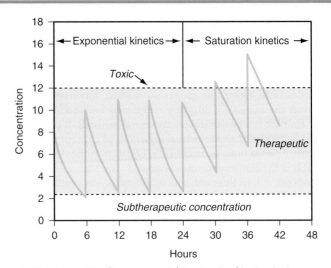

**FIGURE 6-3** Transition from exponential to saturation kinetics. During every-6-hour dosing, concentrations during the first 24 hours reflect exponential kinetics with a half-life of 3 hours ($k = 0.231$/hr) followed by a change to saturation kinetics at 24 hours with elimination of 1 mg/hr, leading to drug accumulation to toxic concentrations.

overestimate the slope and the terminal elimination rate constant. Population modeling has improved analysis and interpretation of such data.[41,42]

## ZERO-ORDER KINETICS

The elimination of some drugs occurs with loss of a *constant amount per time, rather than a constant fraction per time*. Such rates are termed zero-order, and because $e^0 = 1$, the change in the amount of drug in the body fits the following equation[40]:

$$-dA/dt = k_0 \qquad \text{(Eq. 5)}$$

where dA is the change in the amount of drug in the body (in milligrams), dt is the change in time, and $k_0$ is the elimination rate constant with units of amount per unit time. After solving this equation, it has the following form:

$$A = A_0 - k_0 t \qquad \text{(Eq. 6)}$$

where $A_0$ is the initial amount of drug in the body and A is the amount of drug in the body (in milligrams) at time t.

Zero-order (also known as Michaelis-Menten) kinetics may be designated saturation kinetics, because such processes occur when excess amounts of drug saturate the capacity of metabolic enzymes or transport systems. In this situation, only a constant amount of drug is metabolized or transported per unit of time. If kinetics are zero order, a graph of serum concentration versus time is linear on linear-linear axes and is curved when graphed on linear-logarithmic (i.e., semilogarithmic) axes. Clinically, first-order elimination may become zero order after administration of excessive doses or prolonged infusions or during dysfunction of the organ of elimination. Certain drugs administered to neonates exhibit zero-order kinetics at therapeutic doses and may accumulate to excessive concentrations, including thiopental, theophylline, caffeine, diazepam, furosemide, and phenytoin.[43] Some drugs (e.g., phenytoin, ethyl alcohol) may exhibit mixed-order kinetics (i.e., first order at low concentrations and zero order after enzymes are saturated at higher concentrations). For these drugs, a small increment in dose may cause disproportionately large increments in serum concentrations (Fig. 6-3).

## APPARENT VOLUME OF DISTRIBUTION

The apparent volume of distribution (Vd) is a mathematical term that relates the dose to the circulating concentration observed immediately after administration. It might be viewed as the volume of dilution that can be used to predict the change in concentration after a dose is diluted within the body (i.e., a scaling factor). Vd does not necessarily correspond to a physiologic body fluid or tissue volume, hence the designation "apparent." For drugs that distribute out of the circulation or bind to tissues, such as digoxin, Vd may reach 10 L/kg, a physical impossibility for a fluid compartment in the body. This illustrates the mathematical nature of Vd. The units used to express concentration are amount per unit volume, and it may help to remind the reader of the following equation that expresses the relation between dose in amount per kilogram and the Vd in volume per kilogram that dilutes the dose to produce the concentration:

$$\text{Concentration (mg/L)} = \frac{\text{Dose (mg/kg)}}{\text{Vd (L/kg)}} \quad \text{(Eq. 7)}$$

If concentration is expressed with the unconventional units of milligrams per liter rather than micrograms per milliliter (which is equivalent), it is easier to balance the equation. This equation serves as the basis for most of the PK calculations because it is easily rearranged to solve for Vd and dose. It is also important to note that this equation represents the change in concentration after a rapidly administered IV dose of a drug whose elimination is great compared with its time for distribution. After a mini-infusion (e.g., of vancomycin or gentamicin), a more complex exponential equation may be required to account for drug elimination during the time of infusion.[40] For neonates in whom drug elimination is relatively slow, only a small fraction of drug is eliminated during the time of infusion, and such adjustments can be omitted, whereas more complex equations may be needed in older children.

Knowledge of the apparent Vd is essential for dosage adjustments. Vd may be calculated by rearranging Equation 7.

$$\text{Vd (L/kg)} = \frac{\text{Dose (mg/kg)}}{\text{C (postdose)} - \text{C (predose) (mg/L)}} \quad \text{(Eq. 8)}$$

The concentration after a drug infusion, C (postdose), must be measured after the distribution phase to avoid overestimating the peak concentration that would, in turn, lead to an erroneously low Vd. For the first dose, the predose concentration is 0.

### Pharmacokinetic Example

The following example illustrates the application of these PK principles using a four-step approach: (1) calculate Vd; (2) calculate half-life; (3) calculate a new dose and dosing interval based on a desired peak and trough; and (4) check the peak and trough of the new dosage regimen.

For example, vancomycin was administered in a dose of 15 mg/kg IV over 60 minutes every 12 hours. The following plasma concentrations were measured on the third day of treatment (presumed steady-state). The predose or trough concentration was 12 mg/L; the peak concentration, measured 60 minutes after the *end* of the infusion, was 32 mg/L.

$$\begin{aligned}
\text{Vd (L/kg)} &= \frac{15 \text{ mg/kg}}{32 \text{ mg/L} - 12 \text{ mg/L}} \\
&= \frac{15 \text{ mg/kg}}{20 \text{ mg/L}} \\
&= 0.75 \text{ L/kg}
\end{aligned}$$

*Step 1:* Substituting the data into Equation 8, we calculate Vd.

*Step 2:* At steady-state, peak and trough concentrations reach the same levels after each dose. The time between the peak and trough concentrations is 10 hours, that is, 12 hours minus 1 hour infusion minus 1 hour to peak concentration. Half-life may be solved by rearranging Equation 2 to solve for $k$ (elimination rate constant) and substituting the calculated $k$ into Equation 3. In this case, the calculated elimination rate constant is $0.098$ hour$^{-1}$ and the corresponding half-life is 7.1 hours. However, a practical and clinically applicable "bedside" approach may be used without need for logarithmic calculations. For example, the plasma concentration decreased from 32 to 16 mg/L in one half-life and then from 16 to 12 mg/L in a fraction of the second half-life. At the end of the second half-life, the concentration would have decreased to 8 mg/L. Because 12 mg/L is the midpoint between the first and second half-lives, 1.5 half-lives have elapsed during the 10 hours between the peak and trough. Thus, if one assumes a linear decline, the half-life may be estimated as 6.67 hours (10 hours ÷ 1.5 half-lives). Note that the error between the actual half-life of 7.1 hours and the estimated half-life (6.67 hours) is a result of the linear assumptions of this calculation between half-lives. In fact, first-order elimination is a nonlinear process and concentration will actually decline from 32 mg/L to 22.6 mg/L during the first 50% of the first half-life rather than from 32 mg/L to 24 mg/L using this linear approach. The same occurs during subsequent half-lives. However, the small error associated with this method is often acceptable for rapid bedside estimates of PK parameters.

*Step 3:* A new dosage regimen must be calculated if the concentrations are unsatisfactory. Accordingly, one must decide on a desired peak and trough concentration. If, for example, the desired vancomycin peak and trough concentrations were 32 mg/L (20 to 40 mg/L) and 8 mg/L (5 to 10 mg/L), respectively, then Equation 8 may be rearranged to solve for the new dose.

$$\begin{aligned}
\text{Dose (mg/kg)} &= \text{Vd (L/kg)} \times [\text{C (peak desired)} - \\
&\quad\quad \text{C (trough desired) (mg/L)}] \\
\text{Dose (mg/kg)} &= 0.75 \text{ L/kg} \times (32 \text{ mg/L} - 8 \text{ mg/L}) \\
\text{Dose (mg/kg)} &= 18 \text{ mg/kg}
\end{aligned} \quad \text{(Eq. 9)}$$

The current dose produces a peak of 32 mg/L that is in the recommended therapeutic range, and lengthening the dosing interval to 2 half-lives ($13\frac{1}{3}$ hours) after the peak is reached (2 hours after beginning the dose infusion) will produce a trough concentration of 8 mg/L. The dose interval should be increased to 16 hours and the dose increased to 18 mg/kg.

*Step 4:* Estimating peak and trough concentrations with the new regimen provides a good double check against a mathematical error. Sixteen hours after the 15 mg/kg dose is administered (or approximately 2 half-lives after the measured peak), the trough should be approximately 8 mg/L. At this time, administration of 18 mg/kg will raise the concentration by 24 mg/L (assuming a Vd of 0.75 L/kg) to a peak concentration of 32 mg/L.

## REPETITIVE DOSING AND DRUG ACCUMULATION

When multiple doses are administered, the dose is usually repeated before complete elimination of the previous one. In this situation, peak and trough concentrations increase until a steady-state concentration ($C_{ss}$) is reached (Fig. 6-3). The average $C_{ss}$ (Avg$C_{ss}$) can be calculated as follows[32]:

$$\text{AvgC}_{ss} = \frac{1}{\text{Clearance}} \times \frac{f \times D}{\tau}$$

$$= \frac{1}{k \times \text{Vd}} \times \frac{f \times D}{\tau} \qquad \text{(Eq. 10)}$$

$$= \frac{1.44 \times T_{1/2}}{\text{Vd}} \times \frac{f \times D}{\tau} \qquad \text{(Eq. 11)}$$

In Equations 10 and 11, f is the fraction of the dose that is absorbed, D is the dose, $\tau$ is the dosing interval in the same units of time as the elimination half-life, $k$ is the elimination rate constant, and 1.44 equals the reciprocal of 0.693 (see Equation 3). The magnitude of the average $C_{ss}$ is directly proportional to the ratio of $T_{1/2}/\tau$ and D.[32]

### STEADY STATE

Steady state occurs when the amount of drug removed from the body between doses equals the amount of the dose.[33,37] Five half-lives are usually required for drug elimination and distribution among tissue and fluid compartments to reach equilibrium. When all tissues are at equilibrium (i.e., steady state), the peak and trough concentrations are the same after each dose. However, before this time, constant peak and trough concentrations after intermittent doses, or constant concentrations during drug infusions, do not prove that a steady state has been achieved because drug may still be entering and leaving deep tissue compartments. During continuous infusion, the fraction of steady-state concentration that has been reached can be calculated in terms of multiples of the drug's half-life.[32] After three half-lives, the concentration is 88% of that at steady state. When changing doses during chronic drug therapy, the concentration should usually not be rechecked until several half-lives have elapsed, unless elimination is impaired or signs of toxicity occur. Drug concentrations may not need to be checked if symptoms improve.

### LOADING DOSE

If the time to reach a constant concentration by continuous or intermittent dosing is excessive, a loading dose may be used to reach plateau in the concentration more rapidly. This frequently is applied to initial treatment with digoxin, which has a 35- to 69-hour half-life in term neonates and an even longer half-life in preterm infants.[44] Use of a loading dose increases the circulating concentration of drug earlier in the therapeutic course, but for the equilibration to reach a true steady-state still requires treatment for five or more half-lives. Loading doses must be used cautiously, because they increase the likelihood of drug toxicity, as has been observed with loading doses of digoxin.[3,16,17,44]

Dose calculations using a 1-compartment model (Eq. 9) may not be applicable to many anesthetic drugs that are characterized using multi-compartment models. The use of V1 results in a loading dose too high, while the use of Vdss results in a loading dose too low. Too high a dose may cause transient toxicity, although slowing the rate of administration may prevent excessive concentrations during the distributive phase.

The time to peak effect (Tpeak) is dependent on clearance and effect-site equilibration half-time ($T_{1/2}$keo). At a submaximal dose, Tpeak is independent of dose. At supramaximal doses, maximal effect will occur earlier than Tpeak and persist for longer duration because of the shape of the response curve (see later discussion). The Tpeak concept has been used to calculate optimal initial bolus doses,[45] because V1 and Vdss poorly reflect the required scaling factor. A new parameter, the volume of distribution at the time of peak effect-site concentration (Vpe) is used and is calculated.

$$Vpe = \frac{V1}{\left(\dfrac{Cpeak}{C_0}\right)} \qquad \text{(Eq. 12)}$$

where $C_0$ is the theoretical plasma concentration at $t = 0$ after the bolus dose, and Cpeak is the predicted effect-site concentration at the time of peak effect-site concentration. Loading dose (LD) can then be calculated as

$$LD = Cpeak \cdot Vpe \qquad \text{(Eq. 13)}$$

## Population Modeling

Pediatric anesthesiologists have embraced the population approach for investigating PK and PD. This approach, achieved through nonlinear mixed effects models, provides a means to study variability in drug responses among individuals representative of those in whom the drug will be used clinically. Traditional approaches to interpretation of time-concentration profiles relied on "rich" data from a small group of subjects. In contrast, mixed effects models can be used to analyze "sparse" (2 to 3 samples) data from a large number of subjects. Sampling times are not crucial for population methods and can be fit around clinical procedures or outpatient appointments. Sampling time-bands rather than exact times is equally effective and allows flexibility in children.[45,46] Interpretation of truncated individual sets of data or missing data is also possible with this type of analysis, rendering it particularly useful for pediatric studies. Population modeling also allows pooling of data across studies to provide a single robust PK analysis rather than comparing separate smaller studies that are complicated by different methods and analyses.

Mixed effects models are "mixed" because they describe the data using a mixture of fixed and random effects. Fixed effects predict the average influence of a covariate, such as weight, as an explanation of some of the variability between subjects in a parameter like clearance. Random effects describe the remaining variability between subjects that are not predictable from the fixed effect average. Explanatory covariates (e.g., age, size, renal function, sex, temperature) can be introduced that explain the predictable part of the between-individual variability. Nonlinear regression is performed by an iterative process to find the curve of best fit.[47,48]

## Pediatric Pharmacokinetic Considerations

Growth and development are two major aspects of children not readily apparent in adults. How these factors interact is not necessarily easy to determine from observations because they are quite highly correlated. Drug clearance, for example, may increase with weight, height, age, body surface area, and creatinine clearance. One approach is to standardize for size before incorporating a factor for maturation.[49]

### SIZE

Clearance in children 1 to 2 years of age, expressed as L/hr/kg, is commonly greater than that observed in older children and adolescents. This is a size effect and is not because of bigger livers or increased hepatic blood flow in that subpopulation. This "artifact of size" disappears when allometric scaling is used.

*Allometry* is a term used to describe the nonlinear relationship between size and function. This nonlinear relationship is expressed as

$$y = a \cdot BodyMass^{PWR} \qquad \text{(Eq. 14)}$$

where $y$ is the variable of interest (e.g., basal metabolic rate [BMR]), $a$ is a scaling parameter and $PWR$ is the allometric exponent. The value of $PWR$ has been the subject of much debate. BMR is the commonest variable investigated and camps advocating for a $PWR$ value of $\frac{2}{3}$ (i.e., body surface area) are at odds with those advocating a value of $\frac{3}{4}$.

Support for a value of $\frac{3}{4}$ comes from investigations that show the log of BMR plotted against the log of body weight produces a straight line with a slope of $\frac{3}{4}$ in all species studied, including humans. Fractal geometry mathematically explains this phenomenon. The $\frac{3}{4}$-power law for metabolic rates was derived from a general model that describes how essential materials are transported through space-filled fractal networks of branching tubes.[50] A great many physiologic, structural, and time related variables scale predictably within and between species with weight ($W$) exponents ($PWR$) of $\frac{3}{4}$, 1, and $\frac{1}{4}$, respectively.[51] These exponents have applicability to PK parameters, such as clearance (CL exponent of $\frac{3}{4}$), volume (V exponent of 1) and half-time (T$_{1/2}$ exponent of $\frac{1}{4}$).[51] The factor for size ($Fsize$) for total drug clearance may be expressed:

$$Fsize = \left(\frac{W}{70}\right)^{3/4} \qquad \text{(Eq. 15)}$$

Remifentanil clearance in children aged 1 month to 9 years is similar to adult rates when scaled using an allometric exponent of $\frac{3}{4}$.[52] Nonspecific blood esterases that metabolize remifentanil are mature at birth.[53]

## MATURATION

Allometry alone is insufficient to predict clearance in neonates and infants from adult estimates for most drugs.[54,55] The addition of a model describing maturation is required. The sigmoid hyperbolic or Hill model[56] has been found useful for describing this maturation process ($MF$).

$$MF = \frac{PMA^{Hill}}{TM_{50}^{Hill} + PMA^{Hill}} \qquad \text{(Eq. 16)}$$

The $TM_{50}$ describes the maturation half-time, while the Hill coefficient relates to the slope of this maturation profile. Maturation of clearance begins before birth, suggesting that postmenstrual age ($PMA$) would be a better predictor of drug elimination than postnatal age.[51] Figure 6-4 shows the maturation profile for dexmedetomidine, expressed as both the standard per-kilogram model and by using allometry. Clearance is immature in infancy. Clearance, expressed as per kilogram, is greatest at 2 years of age, decreasing subsequently with age. This "artifact of size" disappears with use of the allometric model.

## ORGAN FUNCTION

Changes associated with normal growth and development can be distinguished from pathologic changes describing organ function.[49] Morphine clearance is reduced in neonates because of immature glucuronide conjugation, but clearance was lower in critically ill neonates than healthier cohorts,[57-59] possibly attributable to reduced hepatic function. The impact of organ function alteration may be concealed by another covariate. For example, positive pressure ventilation may be associated with reduced clearance. This effect may be attributable to a consequent reduced

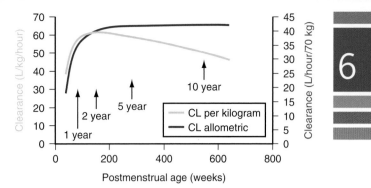

**FIGURE 6-4** The clearance (*CL*) maturation profile of dexmedetomidine, expressed using the per-kilogram model and the allometric $\frac{3}{4}$-power model. This maturation pattern is typical of many drugs cleared by the liver or kidneys. (Data extracted from Potts AL, Anderson BJ, Warman GR, et al. Dexmedetomidine pharmacokinetics in pediatric intensive care—a pooled analysis. Pediatr Anesth 2009;19:1119-29.)

hepatic blood flow with a drug that has perfusion limited clearance (e.g., propofol, morphine).

Pharmacokinetic parameters ($P$) can be described in an individual as the product of size ($Fsize$), maturation ($MF$) and organ function ($OF$) influences, where $Pstd$ is the parameter value in a standard size adult without pathologic changes in organ function[49]:

$$P = Pstd \cdot Fsize \cdot MF \cdot OF \qquad \text{(Eq. 17)}$$

## Pharmacodynamic Models

Pharmacokinetics is what the body does to the drug, while *pharmacodynamics* is what the drug does to the body. The precise boundary between these two processes is ill defined and often requires a link describing movement of drug from the plasma to the effect-site and its target. Drugs may exert effects at nonspecific membrane sites, by interference with transport mechanisms, by enzyme inhibition or induction, or by activation or inhibition of receptors.

### SIGMOID Emax MODEL

The relation between drug concentration and effect may be described by the Hill equation or Emax model (see maturation model above)[56]:

$$Effect = E0 + \frac{(Emax \cdot Ce^{N})}{(EC_{50}^{N} + Ce^{N})} \qquad \text{(Eq. 18)}$$

where $E0$ is the baseline response, $Emax$ is the maximum effect change, $Ce$ is the concentration in the effect compartment, $EC_{50}$ is the concentration producing 50% $Emax$, and $N$ is the Hill coefficient defining the steepness of the concentration-response curve (Fig. 6-5). Efficacy is the maximum response on a dose or concentration-response curve. $EC_{50}$ can be considered a measure of potency relative to another drug, provided N and Emax for the two drugs are the same. A concentration-response relationship for acetaminophen has been described using this model. An $EC_{50}$ of 9.8 mg/L, N = 1, and an Emax of 5.3 pain units (on a visual analog scale [VAS] of 0 to 10) was reported.[60] Midazolam PD in adults have been similarly defined using electroencephalographic (EEG) responses.[61,62]

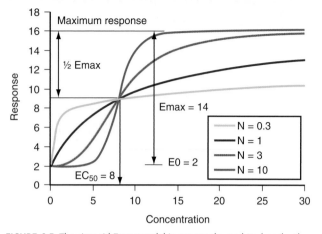

**FIGURE 6-5** The sigmoid Emax model is commonly used to describe the relationship between drug response and concentration. Changing the Hill coefficient (*N*) dramatically alters the shape of the curve.

### QUANTAL EFFECT MODEL

The potency of anesthetic vapors may be expressed by minimum alveolar concentration (MAC), and this is the concentration at which 50% of subjects move in response to a standard surgical stimulus. MAC appears, at first sight, to be similar to $EC_{50}$, but is an expression of quantal response rather than magnitude of effect. There are two methods of estimating MAC. Responses can be recorded over the clinical dose range in a large number of subjects and logistic regression applied to estimate the relationship between dose and quantal effect; the MAC can then be interpolated. Large numbers of subjects may not be available, so an alternative is often used. The "up and down" method described by Dixon[63,64] estimates only the MAC rather than the entire sigmoid curve. It usually involves a study of only one concentration in each subject and, in a sequence of subjects, each receives a concentration depending on the response of the previous subject; the concentration is either decreased if the previous subject did not respond or increased if they did. The MAC is calculated either as the mean concentration of equal numbers of responses and no-responses or is the mean concentration of pairs of "response–no response."

### LOGISTIC REGRESSION MODEL

When the pharmacologic effect is difficult to grade, then it may be useful to estimate the probability of achieving the effect as a function of plasma concentration. Effect measures, such as movement/no movement or rousable/nonrousable, are dichotomous. Logistic regression is commonly used to analyze such data and the interpolated $EC_{50}$ value refers to the probability of response. For example, an $EC_{50}$ of 0.52 mg/L for arousal after ketamine sedation in children has been estimated using this technique.[65]

## Linking Pharmacokinetics with Pharmacodynamics

A simple situation in which drug effect is directly related to concentration does not mean that drug effects parallel the time course of concentration. This occurs only when the concentration is low in relation to $EC_{50}$. In this situation the half-life of the drug may correlate closely with the half-life of drug effect.

Observed effects may not be directly related to serum concentration. Many drugs have a short half-life but a long duration of effect. This may be attributable to induced physiologic changes (e.g., aspirin and platelet function) or may be a result of the shape of the Emax model. If the initial concentration is very high in relation to the $EC_{50}$, then drug concentrations five half-lives later, when we might expect a minimal concentration, may still exert considerable effect.

There may also be a delay as a result of transfer of the drug to the effect site (e.g., neuromuscular blockers), a lag time (e.g., diuretics), physiologic response (e.g., antipyresis), active metabolite (e.g., propacetamol), or synthesis of physiologic substances (e.g., warfarin). A plasma concentration-effect plot can form a hysteresis loop because of this delay in effect. Hull and Sheiner introduced the effect compartment concept for neuromuscular blockers.[66,67] A single first-order parameter ($T_{1/2}keo$) describes the equilibration half-time. This mathematical trick assumes that the concentration in the central compartment is the same as that in the effect compartment at equilibrium, but that a time delay exists before drug reaches the effect compartment. The concentration in the effect compartment is used to describe the concentration-effect relationship.[68]

Adult $T_{1/2}keo$ values are well described (e.g., morphine, 16 minutes; fentanyl, 5 minutes; alfentanil, 1 minute; propofol, 3 minutes). This $T_{1/2}keo$ parameter is commonly incorporated into target controlled infusion pumps in order to achieve a rapid effect-site concentration. The adult midazolam $T_{1/2}keo$ of 5 minutes may be prolonged in the elderly, resulting in overdose if this is not recognized during dose titration.[66]

The $T_{1/2}keo$ for propofol in children has been described. As expected, a shorter $T_{1/2}keo$ with decreasing age based on size models has been described.[67,69] Similar results have been demonstrated for sevoflurane and changes in the EEG.[70] If the effect-site is targeted and peak effect (Tpeak) is anticipated to be later than it actually is because it was determined in a teenager or adult, this will result in excessive dose in a young child.

## Drug Distribution

### PROTEIN BINDING

Acidic drugs (e.g., diazepam, barbiturates) tend to bind mainly to albumin while basic drugs (e.g., amide local anesthetic agents) bind to globulins, lipoproteins and glycoproteins. In general, plasma protein binding of many drugs is decreased in the neonate relative to the adult in part because of reduced total protein and albumin concentrations (Fig. 6-6).[71] Many drugs that are highly protein bound in adults have less of an affinity for protein in neonates (E-Fig. 6-1).[71-75] Reduced protein binding increases the free fraction of medications, thus providing more free medication and greater pharmacologic effect.[1,3,12,14,17] This effect is particularly important for medications that are highly protein bound, because the reduced protein binding increases the free fraction of the medication to a greater extent than for low protein bound drugs. For example, phenytoin is 85% protein bound in healthy infants but only 80% in those who are jaundiced. This equates to a 33% increase in the free fraction of phenytoin when jaundice occurs (E-Fig. 6-2). Differences in protein binding may have considerable influence on the response to medications that are acidic and are, therefore, highly protein bound (e.g., phenytoin, salicylate, bupivacaine, barbiturates, antibiotics, theophylline, and diazepam).[17] In addition, some medications, such as phenytoin, salicylate, sulfisoxazole, caffeine, ceftriaxone, diatrizoate

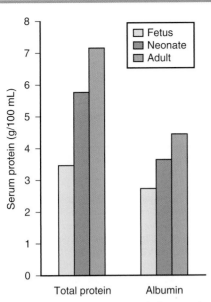

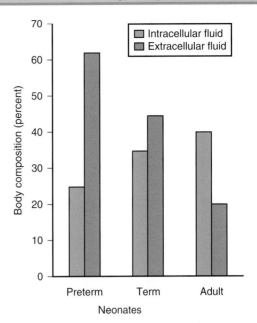

**FIGURE 6-6** Changes in total serum protein and albumin values that occur with maturation. Note that total protein and albumin are less in fetuses than in neonates and less in neonates than in adults. The result may be altered pharmacokinetics and pharmacodynamics for drugs with a high degree of protein binding, because less drug is protein bound and more is available for clinical effect. (Data from Ehrnebo M, Agurell S, Jalling B, et al. Age differences in drug binding by plasma proteins: studies on human foetuses, neonates and adults. Eur J Clin Pharmacol 1971;3:189-93.)

**FIGURE 6-7** Changes in the intracellular and extracellular compartments that occur with maturation. Note the large proportion of extracellular water in preterm and term infants. This large water compartment creates an increased volume of distribution for highly water-soluble medications (e.g., succinylcholine, gentamicin) and may account for the large (by weight) loading dose required for some medications to achieve a satisfactory clinical response. (Data from Friis-Hansen B. Body composition during growth: in-vivo measurements and biochemical data correlated to differential anatomical growth. Pediatrics 1971;47:264-74.)

(Hypaque), and sodium benzoate, compete with bilirubin for binding to albumin (see E-Fig. 6-2). If large amounts of bilirubin are displaced, particularly in the presence of hypoxemia and acidosis, which open the blood-brain barrier, kernicterus may result.[24,25,72,75-77] Because these metabolic derangements often occur in sick neonates coming to surgery, special care must be taken when selecting medications for the anesthetic.[77] Medications that are basic (e.g., lidocaine or alfentanil) are generally bound to plasma $\alpha$1-acid glycoprotein; $\alpha$1-acid glycoprotein concentrations in preterm and term infants are less than in older children and adults. Therefore, for a given dose, the free fraction of a drug is greater in preterm and term infants.[78-80] Protein binding changes are important for the relatively unusual case of a drug that is more than 95% protein bound, with a high extraction ratio and a narrow therapeutic index, that is given parenterally (e.g., lidocaine administered IV), or a drug with a narrow therapeutic index that is given orally and has a very rapid $T_{1/2}$keo (e.g., antiarrhythmic drugs; propafenone, verapamil).[81]

Maturational changes in tissue binding also affect drug distribution. Myocardial digoxin concentrations in infants are 6-fold greater than those in adults, despite similar serum concentrations. Erythrocyte/plasma concentration ratios of digoxin in infants are one-third smaller during loading digitalization than during maintenance digoxin therapy. These findings are consistent with a greater Vd of digoxin in infants and may explain, in part, the unusually large therapeutic doses needed in infants.[82]

## BODY COMPOSITION

Preterm and term infants have a much greater proportion of body weight in the form of water than do older children and adults (Fig. 6-7).[19] The net effect on water-soluble medications is a greater Vd in infants, which in turn increases the initial (loading) dose, based on weight, to achieve the desired target serum

concentration and clinical response.[1,3,14,83,84] Term neonates often require a greater loading dose (milligrams per kilogram) for some medications (e.g., digoxin, succinylcholine, and aminoglycoside antibiotics) than older children.[83-87] However, neonates also tend to be sensitive to the respiratory, neurologic, and circulatory effects of many medications and therefore tend to be more responsive to these effects at reduced blood concentrations than are children and adults. Preterm infants are usually more sensitive than term neonates and in general require even smaller blood concentrations.[1] On the other hand, dopamine may increase blood pressure and urine output in term neonates only at doses as large as 50 μg/kg/min. This dose, which would induce intense vasoconstriction in adults, suggests that neonates are less sensitive in their cardiovascular responsiveness.[3,85,88-91] *It is important to carefully titrate the doses of all medications that are administered to preterm and term infants to the desired response.*

Compared with children and adolescents, preterm and term neonates have a smaller proportion of body weight in the form of fat and muscle mass; with growth, the proportion of body weight composed of these tissues increases (Fig. 6-8).* Therefore, medications that depend on their redistribution into muscle and fat for termination of their clinical effects likely have a larger initial peak blood concentration. These medications may also have a more sustained blood concentration because neonates have less tissue for redistribution of these medications. An incorrect dose may result in prolonged undesirable clinical effects (e.g., barbiturates and opioids may cause prolonged sedation and

*References 1, 3, 4, 19, 89, 92, 93.

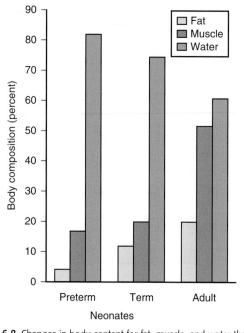

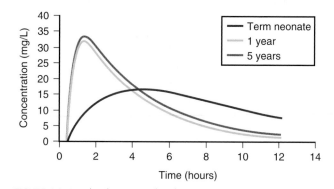

FIGURE 6-9 Simulated mean predicted time-concentration profiles for a term neonate, a 1-year-old infant, and a 5-year-old child given paracetamol elixir. The time to peak concentration is delayed in neonates because of slow gastric emptying and reduced clearance. (Reproduced with permission from Anderson BJ, van Lingen RA, Hansen TG, Lin YC, Holford NH. Acetaminophen developmental pharmacokinetics in premature neonates and infants: a pooled population analysis. Anesthesiology 2002;96:1336-45.)

FIGURE 6-8 Changes in body content for fat, muscle, and water that occur with maturation. Note the small percentage of fat and muscle mass in preterm and term infants. These factors may greatly influence the pharmacokinetics and pharmacodynamics of medications that redistribute into fat (e.g., barbiturates) and muscle (e.g., fentanyl) because there is less tissue mass into which the drug may redistribute. (Data from Friis-Hansen B. Body composition during growth: in-vivo measurements and biochemical data correlated to differential anatomical growth. Pediatrics 1971;47:264-74.)

respiratory depression). The possible influence of small muscle mass on the response to muscle relaxants is exemplified by achieving neuromuscular blockade at smaller serum concentrations in infants.[85]

## Absorption

Anesthetic drugs are mainly administered through the IV and inhalational routes, although premedication and postoperative pain relief is commonly administered enterally. Drug absorption after oral administration is slower in neonates than in children because of delayed gastric emptying (Fig. 6-9).

Adult enteral absorption rates may not be reached until 6 to 8 months after birth.[94,95] Congenital malformations (e.g., duodenal atresia), co-administration of drugs (e.g., opioids), or disease characteristics (e.g., necrotizing enterocolitis) may further affect the variability in absorption. Delayed gastric emptying and reduced clearance may dictate reduced doses and frequency of repeated drug administration. For example, a mean steady state target paracetamol concentration greater than 10 mg/L at trough can be achieved by an oral dose of 25 mg/kg/day in preterm neonates at 30 weeks, 45 mg/kg/day at 34 weeks, and 60 mg/kg/day at 40 weeks PMA.[96] Because gastric emptying is slow in preterm neonates, dosing may only be required twice a day.[96] In contrast, the rectal administration of some drugs (e.g., thiopental, methohexital) is more rapid in neonates than adults. However, the interindividual absorption and relative bioavailability variability after rectal administration may be more extensive compared to oral administration, making rectal administration less suitable for repeated administration.[97]

The larger relative skin surface area, increased cutaneous perfusion, and thinner stratum corneum in neonates increase systemic exposure of topical drugs (e.g., corticosteroids, local anesthetic creams, antiseptics). Neonates have a greater tendency to form methemoglobin because of reduced methemoglobin reductase activity compared with older children. Furthermore, fetal hemoglobin is more readily oxidized compared with adult hemoglobin. Combined with an increased transcutaneous absorption, these have resulted in reluctance to apply repeat topical local anesthetics, such as EMLA (lidocaine-prilocaine) cream, in this age group.[98] Similarly, cutaneous application of iodine antiseptics in neonates may result in transient hypothyroidism.

## Metabolism and Excretion

### HEPATIC METABOLISM

The liver is one of the most important organs involved in drug metabolism. Hepatic enzymatic drug metabolism usually converts the medication from a less polar state (lipid soluble) to a more polar, water-soluble compound (see later discussion). Although no categorical statement applies to all drugs and enzymes, the activities of most of these enzymes are reduced in neonates.[3,4,16,20,22,87,99-104] Another important factor that influences hepatic degradation is hepatic blood flow. As the infant matures, a greater proportion of the cardiac output is delivered to the liver, therefore increasing drug delivery and potentially increasing drug metabolism. Some medications are extensively metabolized by the liver or other organs (e.g., the intestines or lungs) and are referred to as having high extraction ratios. This extensive metabolism produces a "first pass" effect in which a large proportion of an enteral dose is inactivated as it passes through the organ before reaching the systemic circulation. Metabolism via cytochrome P-450 in the intestinal wall may occur during drug absorption.[105-107] Certain foods may induce or inhibit intestinal cytochromes, resulting in food–drug interactions.[108] The concentrations of these enzymes in neonates are less than in older children. These enzymes may also be affected by diseases such as cystic fibrosis or celiac disease.[109,110] Further metabolism may occur as the portal venous circulation from the small intestine passes through the liver before returning to the heart.[105,107] In contrast, IV administration circulates drug to the liver or intestine for metabolism in proportion to the organ blood flow. Some of the drugs that exhibit extensive first-pass metabolism include propranolol, morphine, and midazolam.[111-118]

The opening or closing of a patent ductus may have profound effects on drug delivery to metabolizing organs in preterm infants.[119,120] The ability to metabolize and conjugate medications improves considerably with age as a result of both increased enzyme activity and increased delivery of drug to the liver. Other factors influence the rate of hepatic maturation and metabolism (e.g., sepsis and malnutrition may slow maturation, whereas previous exposure to anticonvulsants, such as phenytoin or phenobarbital, may hasten maturation).[3,89,99,100,104,121-125] The elimination half-lives of diazepam, thiopental, and phenobarbital are markedly increased in neonates compared with adults (i.e., the elimination half-life for thiopental in the neonate (17.9 hours) is almost three times that in children (6.1 hours) and 50% greater than that in adults (12 hours) (E-Fig. 6-3).[12,74,126,127] In general, the half-lives of medications that are eliminated by the liver are prolonged in neonates, decreased in children 4 to 10 years of age, and reach adult values in adolescents, mirroring clearance changes with age (see Fig. 6-4).

Metabolism through biotransformation to more polar forms is required for many drugs before they can be eliminated. Two types of drug biotransformation can occur: Phase I and Phase II reactions. Phase I reactions transform the drug via oxidation, reduction, or hydrolysis. Phase II reactions transform the drug via conjugation reactions, such as glucuronidation, sulfation, and acetylation, into more polar forms.[29,30] Although the liver is the primary site for biotransformation, other organs are also involved, including the lungs and kidneys. Hepatic drug metabolism activity appears as early as 9 to 22 weeks gestation, when fetal liver enzyme activity may vary from 2% to 36% of adult activity.[128] It is inaccurate to generalize that the preterm neonate cannot metabolize drugs. Rather, the specific pathway(s) of drug metabolism must be considered.

Metabolism of many drugs involves the cytochrome P-450 (CYP) enzyme system. Multiple isoforms of the CYP enzyme system exist with different substrate specificities for different drugs.[129-131] Induction and inhibition of these enzymes by different drugs and chemicals requires a thorough understanding of both the nomenclature of the CYP system, as well as the specific isoforms responsible for metabolism of the drugs used in pediatric anesthesia. There are both genetic and ethnic polymorphisms leading to clinically important differences in the capacity to metabolize drugs; these differences can make individual drug responses in some cases unpredictable.[132-136] In the future it may be possible to tailor drug doses to the individual's requirements by determining the child's unique metabolic capacity.[137,138]

### CYTOCHROMES P-450: PHASE I REACTIONS

CYPs are heme-containing proteins that provide most of the phase I drug metabolism for lipophilic compounds in the body.[129] The generally accepted nomenclature of the cytochrome P-450 isozymes begins with CYP, and groups enzymes with more than 36% DNA homology into families designated with an Arabic number, followed by letters for the subfamily of closely related proteins (greater than 77% homology), followed by a number for the specific enzyme gene, such as CYP3A4.[139,140] Isozymes that are important in human drug metabolism are found in the *CYP1, CYP2,* and *CYP3* gene families. Table 6-1 outlines the CYP isozymes and their common substrates.

For many drugs, the reduced metabolism in neonates relates to reduced total quantities of CYP enzymes in the hepatic microsomes.[141] Although the concentrations of CYP enzymes increase with gestational age, they may reach only 50% of adult values at term.[141] In neonates, reduced CYP decreases clearance for many drugs, including theophylline, caffeine, diazepam, phenytoin, and phenobarbital.[87,127,130,131,142-144] Although many isozymes are immature in the neonate, some CYP isozymes exhibit near-adult activity whereas others produce unique metabolic pathways in the neonatal period that invalidate broad generalizations about neonatal drug metabolism (see Table 6-1).

### DEVELOPMENTAL CHANGES OF SPECIFIC CYTOCHROMES

Cytochrome P-450 1A2 (CYP1A2) accounts for much of the metabolism of caffeine (1, 3, 7-trimethylxanthine)[145,146] and theophylline (1,3-dimethylxanthine),[147,148] which are methylxanthines frequently used to treat neonatal apnea and bradycardia. CYP1A2 activity is nearly absent in the fetal liver and remains minimal in the neonate.[149] This limits *N*-3- and *N*-7-demethylation of caffeine in the neonatal period that prolongs elimination in preterm and term neonates.[146,150] Elimination is through the immature renal system and consequent clearance is reduced. Adult levels of activity are reached between 4 and 6 months postnatally.[151,152] A similar PK pattern of reduced metabolism at birth occurs with theophylline, in which CYP1A2 catalyzes 3-demethylation and 8-hydroxylation.[147,148] Theophylline clearance reaches adult levels by 4 to 5 months, coincident with changes in CYP1A2 reflected in urine metabolite patterns.[153]

Other CYP enzymes that are reduced or absent in the fetus include CYP2D6 and CYP2C9.[121,122,154] CYP2D6, which is involved in the metabolism of β-blockers, antiarrhythmics, antidepressants, antipsychotics, and codeine, is absent in the fetal liver and is eventually expressed postnatally (see Table 6-1).[122,123] In contrast to the slow maturation of CYP1A2 and CYP2D6, CYP2C9, which are responsible for the metabolism of nonsteroidal antiinflammatory drugs (NSAIDs), warfarin, and phenytoin, have minimal activity antenatally[121] and then develop rapidly postnatally.[119,144]

CYP3A is the most important cytochrome involved in drug metabolism, because of the broad range of drugs that it metabolizes and because it comprises the majority of adult human liver CYP (see Table 6-1).[155] CYP3A is detectable during embryogenesis as early as 17 weeks, primarily in the form of CYP3A7,[149] and reaches 75% of adult activity by 30 weeks gestation.[122] In vivo, CYP3A activity appears to be mature at birth[124]; however, there is a poorly understood postnatal transition from the fetal CYP3A7 to the predominant adult isoform CYP3A4.[156,157]

### PHASE II REACTIONS

The other major route of drug metabolism, designated phase II reactions, involves synthetic or conjugation reactions that increase the hydrophilicity of molecules to facilitate renal elimination.[29,30] The phase II enzymes include glucuronosyltransferase, sulfotransferase, *N*-acetyltransferase, glutathione *S*-transferase, and methyltransferase. The phase II enzymes also show developmental changes during infancy that influence drug clearance (Table 6-2).[131,158-160]

Most conjugation reactions have limited activity during fetal development.[161] One of the most familiar synthetic reactions in young infants involves conjugation by uridine diphosphoglucuronosyltransferases (UGT). This enzyme system includes

**TABLE 6-1** Developmental Patterns and Activities for Important Cytochrome P-450 Enzymes (Phase I Reactions) in the Neonate

| Enzymes | Selected Substrates | Inducers | Inhibitors | Developmental Changes |
|---|---|---|---|---|
| CYP1A2 | Acetaminophen, caffeine, theophylline, warfarin | Cigarette smoke, charcoal-broiled meat, omeprazole, cruciferous vegetables | α-Naphthoflavone | Not present to an appreciable extent in human fetal liver. Adult levels reached by 4 months of age and may be exceeded in children 1-2 years of age. Inhibited by phenobarbital and phenytoin. |
| CYP2A6 | Warfarin, nicotine | Barbiturates | Tranylcypromine | |
| CYP2C9 | Diclofenac, phenytoin, torsemide, S-warfarin tolbutamide | Rifampin | Sulfaphenazole, sulfinpyrazone | Not apparent in fetal liver. Inferential data using phenytoin disposition as a nonspecific pharmacologic probe suggests low activity during the first week of life, with adult activity reached by 6 months of age and peak activity reached by 3-4 years of age. Metabolism induced by rifampin and phenobarbital and inhibited by cimetidine. |
| CYP2C19 | Phenytoin, diazepam, omeprazole, propranolol | Rifampin | Tranylcypromine | |
| CYP2D6 | Amitriptyline, captopril, codeine, dextromethorphan, fluoxetine, hydrocodone, ondansetron, propafenone, propranolol, timolol | None known | Fluoxetine, quinidine | Low to absent in fetal liver but uniformly present at 1 week of postnatal age. Poor activity (approximately 20% of adult values) at 1 month of postnatal age. Adult competence reached by 3-5 years of age. Metabolism inhibited by cimetidine. |
| CYP3A4 | Acetaminophen, alfentanil, amiodarone, budesonide, carbamazepine, diazepam, erythromycin, lidocaine, midazolam, nifedipine, omeprazole, cisapride, theophylline, verapamil, R-warfarin | Carbamazepine, dexamethasone, phenobarbital, phenytoin, rifampin | Azole antifungals, ethinyl estradiol, naringenin, troleandomycin, erythromycin | CYP3A4 has low activity in the first month of life, with approach toward adult levels by 6-12 months postnatally. |
| CYP3A7 | Dehydroepiandrosterone, ethinyl estradiol, various dihydropyrimidines | Carbamazepine, rifampin | Azole antifungals | CYP3A7 is functionally active in the fetus; approximately 30% to 75% of adult levels of CYP3A4. Induced by carbamazepine, dexamethasone, phenobarbital, phenytoin, and rifampin. Enzyme inhibitors include azole antifungals, erythromycin, and cimetidine. |

Adapted from Leeder JS, Kearns GL. Pharmacogenetics in pediatrics: implications for practice. Pediatr Clin North Am 1997;44:55-77.

**TABLE 6-2** Developmental Patterns for Important Conjugation (Phase II) Reactions in the Neonate

| Enzymes | Selected Substrates | Developmental Patterns |
|---|---|---|
| Uridine diphosphoglucuronyltransferase (UDP-GT) | Chloramphenicol, morphine, acetaminophen, valproic acid, lorazepam | Ontogeny is isoform specific. In general, adult activity is achieved by 6-18 months of age. May be induced by cigarette smoke and phenobarbital. |
| Sulfotransferase | Bile acids, acetaminophen, cholesterol, polyethylene, glycols, dopamine, chloramphenicol | Ontogeny seems to be more rapid than UDP-GT; however, it is substrate specific. Activity for some isoforms may exceed adult values during infancy and childhood, e.g., that responsible for acetaminophen metabolism. |
| N-Acetyltransferase 2 | Hydralazine, procainamide, clonazepam, caffeine, sulfamethoxazole | Some fetal activity present by 16 weeks. Virtually 100% of infants between birth and 2 months of age exhibit the slow metabolizer phenotype. Adult activity present by 1-3 years of age. |

Adapted from Leeder JS, Kearns GL. Pharmacogenetics in pediatrics: implications for practice. Pediatr Clin North Am 1997;44:55-77.

numerous isoforms and is also responsible for glucuronidation of endogenous compounds, such as bilirubin (by UGT1A1).[161] As with the maturation of bilirubin conjugation, UGT activity is limited immediately postnatally and the different isoforms mature at different rates postnatally.[162] Dosage adjustments are often needed to avoid toxicity in neonates from drugs that require conjugation by UGT for clearance. Experience with chloramphenicol in the 1960s illustrated this lesson when neonates received standard pediatric doses of chloramphenicol without understanding the immaturity of UGT and its role in the elimination of chloramphenicol. Infants accumulated high concentrations of chloramphenicol and developed fatal circulatory collapse, a condition known as the gray baby syndrome.[163-165] Although the clearance of chloramphenicol is low during the neonatal period, appropriate dosage adjustments and monitoring allow safe treatment of preterm and term infants with chloramphenicol.[166]

Morphine, acetaminophen, dexmedetomidine and lorazepam also undergo glucuronidation. The major steps in the metabolic disposition of morphine in children and adults is glucuronidation in the 3- and 6-position.[111,167] The limited ability of neonates to metabolize morphine by glucuronidation necessitates

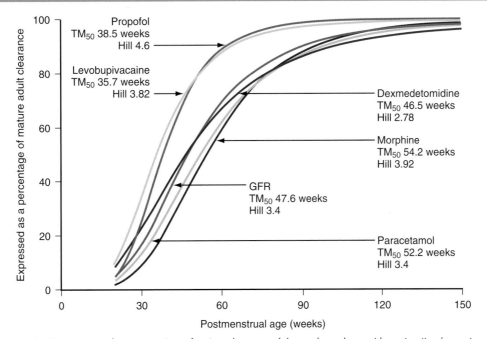

**FIGURE 6-10** Clearance maturation, expressed as a percentage of mature clearance, of drugs where glucuronide conjugation (paracetamol, morphine, dexmedetomidine) plays a major role. These profiles are closely aligned with glomerular filtration rate (*GFR*). In contrast, cytochrome P-450 isoenzymes also contribute to propofol and levobupivacaine metabolism and cause a faster maturation profile than expected from glucuronide conjugation alone. *Hill*, Hill coefficient; *TM*$_{50}$, maturation half-time. (Maturation parameter estimates from Anderson BJ, Holford NH. Mechanistic basis of using body size and maturation to predict clearance in humans. Drug Metab Pharmacokinet 2009;24:25-36; Anand KJ, Anderson BJ, Holford NH, et al. Morphine pharmacokinetics and pharmacodynamics in preterm and term neonates: secondary results from the NEOPAIN trial. Br J Anaesth 2008;101:680-9; Potts AL, Warman GR, Anderson BJ. Dexmedetomidine disposition in children: a population analysis. Pediatr Anesth 2008;18:722-30; Allegaert K, Hoon JD, Verbesselt R, Naulaers G, Murat I. Maturational pharmacokinetics of single intravenous bolus of propofol. Pediatr Anesth 2007;17:1028-34; Chalkiadis GA, Anderson BJ. Age and size are the major covariates for prediction of levobupivacaine clearance in children. Pediatr Anesth 2006;16:275-82; Rhodin MM, Anderson BJ, Peters AM, et al. Human renal function maturation: a quantitative description using weight and postmenstrual age. Pediatr Nephrol 2009;24:67-76; Anderson BJ, Holford NH. Tips and traps analyzing pediatric PK data. Pediatr Anesth 2011;21: 222-37.)

dosage adjustment.[58,168,169] Detailed studies have shown that morphine clearance,[168,170] in particular 3- and 6-glucuronide formation, is limited at birth and increases with birth weight,[169] gestational age,[129] and postnatal age.[58,167] In some studies, morphine clearance, expressed as per kilogram, approaches adult values by 1 month,[58,171] although others reported that the clearance does not reach adult values until at least 5 to 6 months.[168,172] Overall, the maturation of glucuronosyltransferase enzymes varies among isoforms, but, in general, adult activity is reached by 6 to 18 months of age.[140] Some of the confusion relating to maturation rates is attributable to the use of the per kilogram size model. The use of allometry with a maturation model has assisted understanding. The time courses of maturation of drug metabolism for morphine,[57] acetaminophen,[173] dexmedetomidine,[174] and glomerular filtration rate[175] (GFR) are strikingly similar (Fig. 6-10) with 50% of size-adjusted adult values being reached between 8 and 12 weeks (TM$_{50}$) after full-term delivery. All three drugs are cleared predominantly by UGT that converts the parent compound into a water soluble metabolite that is excreted by the kidneys and the clearance maturation profiles of these drugs matches that of GFR maturation. Glucuronidation is also the major metabolic pathway of propofol metabolism, although multiple CYP isoenzymes, including CYP2B6, CYP2C9, or CYP2A6, contribute to its metabolism and cause a faster maturation profile than expected from glucuronide conjugation alone.[176] A phase I reaction (CYP3A4) is the major enzyme system for oxidation of levobupivacaine and clearance through this pathway is faster than those associated with UGT maturation.[57,173,175,177-180]

In contrast to glucuronosyltransferase, the sulfotransferase enzyme system is well developed in the neonate, and for some compounds it may compensate for limited glucuronidation. In adults, the primary pathway for acetaminophen metabolism is glucuronidation, yet its half-life is only moderately prolonged in neonates compared with older infants and adults.[181-183] This occurs partly because of the increased Vd in neonates (T$_{1/2}$ α Vd/ CL) and partly because the neonate forms more sulfate than glucuronide conjugate, leading to a greater percent of the dose excreted as the acetaminophen-sulfate conjugate.[96,182-185] Unfortunately, this does not confer safety from hepatotoxicity. The toxic metabolite is created through the oxidative pathway mediated by CYP2E1.

## ALTERATIONS IN BIOTRANSFORMATION
Transition from the intrauterine to the extrauterine environment is associated with major changes in blood flow. There may also be an environmental trigger for the expression of some metabolic enzyme activities resulting in a slight increase in maturation rate above that predicted by postmenstrual age.[176,179] Many biotransformation reactions, especially those involving certain forms of CYP, are inducible before birth through maternal exposure to drugs, cigarette smoke, or other inducing agents. Postnatally, biotransformation reactions may be induced through drug exposure (see Tables 6-1 and 6-2) and may be slowed by hypoxia,

asphyxia, organ damage, and/or illness. The reduced thiopental clearance estimated from data when the drug was given to control neonatal seizures that resulted from hypoxic-ischemic insults, may not be applicable to healthy neonates undergoing anesthesia.[186]

## GENOTYPIC VARIATIONS IN DRUG METABOLISM
Genetic variations can have impact on both PK and PD[187] Single nucleotide changes or polymorphisms (SNPs) in the DNA sequence in CYP enzymes usually decrease but may also increase metabolic activity for a specific drug or drug substrate.[188] Some of the explanation for variations in drug responses within large populations that are described as "biologic variation" likely relate to genetic differences in drug metabolism, receptor binding, and intracellular coupling to effector mechanisms. Following the recognition that certain individuals had exaggerated hypotensive responses to debrisoquine, the enzyme responsible for its metabolism, CYP2D6 became one of the first drug-metabolizing enzyme deficiencies identified.[189-191] Earlier studies had shown that individuals might possess normal or reduced metabolic activity (poor metabolizers) for debrisoquine and sparteine.[190,192] The frequency of poor metabolizers varied among ethnic groups, occurring in approximately 7% of Caucasians[132] and in 0% to 1% of Chinese and Japanese.[193]

Codeine, is primarily a prodrug that undergoes metabolic activation by CYP2D6 O-demethylation to morphine.[194] Without O-demethylation, codeine confers a small fraction of the analgesic molar potency of morphine, and much of its analgesic effect is likely contributed by a metabolite, codeine 6-glucuronide,[195] although evidence suggests that up to 11% of codeine is also metabolized to hydrocodone.[196] For the 2% to 10% of the population who are CYP2D6 poor metabolizers, codeine causes limited opioid effects.[197,198] Gastrointestinal motility is affected only in extensive metabolizers, suggestive of a morphine-dependent mechanism of action.[199] Individuals with duplicated active CYP2D6 genes are classified as ultra-extensive metabolizers.[199a] A 29-month-old previously healthy child experienced apnea resulting in brain injury, following a dose of codeine 2 days after an uneventful anesthetic for tonsillectomy. A genetic polymorphism leading to ultra-rapid metabolism of codeine into morphine, resulting in narcosis and apnea, was proposed.[200]

For other drugs, ranging from propranolol to warfarin to methotrexate, reduced metabolism through genetic polymorphisms of other enzymes lead to exaggerated effects when administered in conventional doses.[127] Similar variations in activity have been reported for many of the CYPs involved in drug metabolism in humans.[201] The potential importance of genotyping is demonstrated for patients scheduled to receive treatment with methotrexate; genotyping has become a routine part of the evaluation before treatment, for detection of reduced activity of thiopurine methyltransferase that may be lethal with conventional dosages.[202,203] Genotyping has been proposed before drug treatment and as a guide to drug selection when specific SNPs have been correlated with adverse drug reactions or clinically significant alterations in metabolism.[138] Although hundreds of possible SNPs have been identified that account for much of the variation in drug effects among individuals, specific SNPs of CYP2C9, CYP2C19, CYP2D6, CYP3A, and uridine diphosphate-glucuronosyltransferase 1A1 (UGT1A1) account for a sufficient number of adverse pharmacologic outcomes to warrant clinical testing when it becomes feasible.[138] Until genotyping for many more abnormalities in drug metabolizing enzymes, receptors,

and channels becomes a routine part of drug treatment, careful attention to a history of adverse drug reactions in the child and first-degree relatives, and careful attention to recording current reactions, are the best guides to detect clinically important variations in drug metabolism.

## EXTRAHEPATIC ROUTES OF METABOLIC CLEARANCE
Many drugs undergo metabolic clearance at extrahepatic sites. Remifentanil and atracurium are degraded by nonspecific esterases in tissues and erythrocytes. Clearance, expressed per kilogram, is increased in younger children,[52,204-207] likely attributable to size, because clearance is similar when scaled to a 70-kg person using allometry.[52] Nonspecific blood esterases that metabolize remifentanil are mature at birth.[53]

Ester local anesthetics are metabolized by plasma butyrylcholinesterase, which is thought to be reduced in neonates. The *in vitro* plasma half-life of 2-chloroprocaine in umbilical cord blood is twice that in maternal blood,[208] but there are no *in vivo* studies of the effects of age on its metabolism. Succinylcholine clearance is increased in neonates when expressed as per kilogram, suggesting butyrylcholinesterase activity is mature at birth.[209,210]

## RENAL EXCRETION
Renal function in preterm and term infants is less efficient than in adults, even after adjusting for the differences in body weight. This reduced efficiency is related to the combination of incomplete glomerular development, low perfusion pressure, and inadequate osmotic load to produce full countercurrent effects.[211-216] However, glomerular filtration and tubular function both develop rapidly during the first few months of life,[175] and are nearly mature by 20 weeks of age, and fully mature by 2 years of age (Figs. 6-10 and 6-11).[212-216] For these reasons, *drugs that are excreted primarily through glomerular filtration or tubular secretion, such as aminoglycoside and cephalosporin antibiotics, have a prolonged elimination half-life in neonates* (E-Fig. 6-4).[217-219]

In the presence of renal failure, one or two doses of drugs that are excreted via the kidneys often achieve and maintain

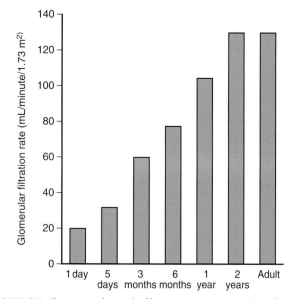

**FIGURE 6-11** Changes in glomerular filtration rate versus age. Note the rapid development of glomerular function during the first year of life. Abnormal or immature renal function may delay drug excretion. (Data from Chantler C. Clinical Pediatric Nephrology. Philadelphia: JB Lippincott; 1976.)

prolonged therapeutic drug concentrations if there is no alternate pathway of excretion. Whenever administering a medication to a preterm or term infant, one must consider the contribution of renal function in the termination of the drug's action.

The PK and PD of the old muscle relaxant, curare, exemplify the complex interaction of increased Vd, smaller muscle mass, and decreased rate of excretion as a result of immaturity of glomerular filtration. The initial dose (per kilogram) of curare needed to achieve neuromuscular blockade is similar in infants and adults.[85] In infants, however, this blockade is achieved at reduced serum concentrations compared with older children or adults, corresponding to differences in muscle mass and receptor immaturity. A larger Vd (total body water) accounts for the equivalent dose for each kilogram of body weight, and the reduced glomerular function in infants compared with older children or adults accounts in part for the longer duration of action.[85] As in the case of drugs excreted by the liver, there is a triphasic developmental response to drugs excreted by the kidneys when expressed as per kilogram (see Fig. 6-4): a prolonged half-life in neonates (immature renal function), a shortened half-life in young children, and a greater elimination half-life in adolescents and adults (size related).

Reduced protein binding in neonates and preterm infants increases the free fraction of drugs delivered to the kidneys and liver for metabolism; however, reduced clearance results in a greater potential for toxicity.[1,3,16,17] An important example is the immature clearance of bupivacaine, which resulted in high plasma concentrations that caused seizures in neonates given epidural infusions at rates greater than that at which it was metabolized.[220]

## Central Nervous System Effects

Laboratory data have demonstrated the lethal dose in 50% of animals ($LD_{50}$) for many medications to be significantly less in neonates than in adult animals.[221,222] The sensitivity of human neonates to most of the sedatives, hypnotics, and opioids is clinically well known and may in part be related to increased brain permeability (immature blood-brain barrier or damage to the blood-brain barrier) for some medications.[223-229] Laboratory studies have demonstrated greater brain concentrations of morphine and amobarbital in infant than in adult animals.[230]

However, respiratory depression, measured by carbon dioxide response curves or by arterial oxygen tension are similar from 2 to 570 days of age at the same morphine blood concentration.[231] Altered PK may contribute to apparent morphine sensitivity in neonates. A reduced clearance and a reduced Vd in neonates will result in greater plasma concentrations in this age group compared with children given similar weight-scaled doses,[232,233] and this greater concentration contributes more to respiratory depression, than does increased brain permeability.

Small molecules are thought to access fetal and neonatal brains more readily than in adults.[234] Blood-brain barrier function improves gradually, possibly reaching maturity by full-term.[234] Kernicterus, for example, is more common in preterm than in full-term neonates. In contrast to drugs bound to plasma proteins, unbound lipophilic drugs passively diffuse across the blood-brain barrier equilibrating very quickly. This may contribute to bupivacaine's propensity for producing seizures in neonates. Decreased protein binding, as in the neonate, results in a greater proportion of unbound drug that is available for passive diffusion.

In addition to passive diffusion, there are specific transport systems that mediate active transport. Pathologic CNS conditions can cause blood-brain barrier breakdown and alter these transport systems. Fentanyl is actively transported across the blood-brain barrier by a saturable ATP-dependent process; ATP-binding cassette proteins, such as P-glycoprotein, actively pump out opioids, such as fentanyl and morphine.[235] P-glycoprotein modulation significantly influences opioid brain distribution and onset time, as well as the magnitude and duration of analgesic response.[236] Modulation may occur during disease processes, fever, or in the presence of other drugs (e.g., verapamil, magnesium).[235] Genetic polymorphisms that affect P-glycoprotein–related genes may explain differences in the sensitivity to CNS-active drugs.[237]

Incomplete myelination in infants may make it easier for drugs that are not particularly lipid soluble to enter the brain at a greater rate than if the blood-brain barrier were intact.[223,224,230,238] When considering the use of any centrally acting medication in children younger than 1 year of age, and particularly those younger than 48 weeks postmenstrual age, one must balance the potential risks and benefits. Dosage must be carefully calculated and titrated to allow the lowest dose that provides the required patient response. Careful monitoring of vital signs is important, because prolonged effects or adverse clinical responses may occur in children of any age, but particularly in infants in whom CNS maturation may be incomplete.

## Pharmacodynamics in Children

Children's responses to drugs have much in common with the responses in adults.[239] The perception that drug effects differ in children arises because the drugs have not been adequately studied in pediatric populations who have size and maturation related effects, as well as different diseases. Neonates and infants, however, often have altered PD. A series of examples are presented below.

The MAC for almost all anesthetic vapors is less in neonates than in infants, which is in turn greater than that observed in children and adults.[240] MAC of isoflurane in preterm neonates less than 32 weeks gestation was 1.28%, and MAC in neonates 32-37 weeks gestation was 1.41%.[241] This value rose to 1.87% by 6 months before decreasing again over childhood.[241] The cause of these differences is uncertain and may relate to maturation changes in cerebral blood flow, γ-aminobutyric acid (GABA) class A receptor numbers, or developmental shifts in the regulation of chloride transporters.

Neonates have an increased sensitivity to the effects of neuromuscular blocking drugs (NMBDs).[85] The reason for this is unknown but it is consistent with the observation that there is a threefold reduction in the release of acetylcholine from the infant rat phrenic nerve as well as a relatively reduced muscle mass.[242-245] The increased Vd, however, means that a single NMBD dose (calculated as mg/kg) in the neonate results in blockade at a reduced plasma concentration while reduced clearance prolongs the duration of effect.

Cardiac calcium stores in the endoplasmic reticulum are reduced in the neonatal heart because of immaturity. Exogenous calcium has greater impact on contractility in this age group than in older children or adults. There are some data to suggest greater sensitivity to warfarin in children, but the mechanism is not determined.[246] Amide local anesthetic agents induce shorter block duration and require a larger weight-scaled dose to achieve similar dermatomal levels, when given by subarachnoid block to infants. This may be due, in part, to myelination, spacing of nodes of Ranvier and length of nerve exposed, increased relative volume of CSF, as well as other size factors. There is an age-dependent expression of intestinal motilin receptors and the modulation of gastric antral contractions in neonates. Prokinetic agents may not be useful in very preterm infants, partially useful in older preterm infants, and useful in full-term infants. Similarly, bronchodilators in infants are less effective because of the paucity of bronchial smooth muscle that can cause bronchospasm.

## MEASUREMENT OF PHARMACODYNAMIC ENDPOINTS

Outcome measures are more difficult to assess in neonates and infants than in children or adults. Measurement techniques, disease and pathology differences, inhomogeneous groups, recruitment issues, ethical considerations, and endpoint definitions for establishing efficacy and safety often confuse data interpretation.[247]

Common effects measured include anesthesia depth, pain responses, depth of sedation, and intensity of neuromuscular blockade. A common effect-measure used to assess depth of anesthesia is the EEG or a modification of detected EEG signals (spectral edge frequency, bispectral index [BIS], entropy). Physiologic studies in adults and children indicate that EEG-derived anesthesia depth monitors can provide an imprecise and drug-dependent measure of arousal. Although the outputs from these monitors do not closely represent any true physiologic entity, they can be used as guides for anesthesia, and in so doing, may improve outcomes in adults. In older children the physiology, anatomy, and clinical observations indicate the performance of the monitors may be similar to that in adults. In infants, however, their use cannot yet be supported in theory or in practice.[248,249] During anesthesia, the EEG in infants is fundamentally different from the EEG in older children; there remains a need for specific neonate-derived algorithms if EEG-derived anesthesia depth monitors are to be used in neonates.[250,251] Examples of problems with BIS monitoring in infants and young children include the observations that BIS numbers paradoxically increase when sevoflurane concentrations exceed 3%, there is often a difference between the right and left side of the brain, equivalent MAC concentrations produce different BIS values with each agent, and values in children tend to be greater than values in adults at equivalent MAC concentrations.[252-256]

The Children's Hospital of Wisconsin Sedation Scale has been used to investigate ketamine in the emergency department.[65,257] However, despite the use of such scales in procedural pain or sedation studies, few behavioral scales have been adequately validated in this setting and inter-observer variability can be substantial.[258-260] Most scores are validated for the acute, procedural setting and perform less well for subacute or chronic pain or stress.

## THE TARGET CONCENTRATION APPROACH

The goal of treatment is the target effect. A PD model is used to predict the target concentration given a target effect. Population estimates for the PD model parameters and covariate information are used to predict typical PD values in a specific patient. Population estimates of PK model parameter estimates and covariate information are then used to predict typical PK values in a typical patient. For example, a dexmedetomidine steady-state target concentration of 0.6 µg/L may be achieved with an infusion of 0.33 µg/kg/hr in a neonate, 0.51 µg/kg/hr in a 1-year-old, and 0.47 µg/kg/hr in an 8-year-old.[180] This target concentration strategy is a powerful tool for determining clinical dose.[261] Monitoring of serum drug concentrations and Bayesian forecasting may be used to improve dosing in individual patients.

This target effect approach is intrinsic to pediatric anesthesiologists using target-controlled infusion systems. These devices target a specific plasma or effect-site concentration in a typical individual and this concentration is assumed to have a typical target effect. The target concentration is one that achieves a target therapeutic effect (e.g., anesthesia) without excessive adverse effects (e.g., hypotension). Unfortunately, these devices have still not been approved by the FDA for use in the United States.

## DEFINING TARGET CONCENTRATION

An effect-site target concentration has been estimated for many drugs used in anesthesia, analgesia and sedation. For example, a propofol target concentration of 3 mg/L (0.003 mg/mL) in a typical patient can be achieved using preprogrammed target-controlled infusion devices. For older children a BIS monitor can then be used to manually adjust the infusion rate to achieve a desired target effect in the specific individual. The luxury of such a feedback system is not available for most drugs and unfortunately may be of little value in neonates and infants.

A target concentration of 10 µg/L may be used for morphine analgesia. Observations in children after cardiac surgery found that steady state serum concentrations greater than 20 µg/L resulted in hypercarbia ($PaCO_2$ greater than 55 mm Hg) and depressed $CO_2$ response curve slopes. During washout, morphine concentrations more than 15 µg/L resulted in hypercarbia in 46% of children, whereas concentrations less than 15 µg/L were associated with hypercarbia in 13% of children. No age-related differences in respiratory effect were seen in these studies at the same serum morphine concentration.[231] Observation or self-reporting pain scales are used as part of the feedback loop for dose incremental changes.

The target concentration may vary, depending on the desired target effect. The target concentration for ketamine analgesia (0.25 mg/L) is quite different from that of anesthesia (2 mg/L), and BIS monitoring would be totally useless because ketamine causes central excitation thereby increasing bispectral monitoring numbers.[262-265]

# Drug Interactions

There are many common examples of drug interactions that increase or decrease responses mediated through either PK or PD routes. Phenobarbitone induces CYP3A4 metabolism, increasing ketamine requirements for radiologic sedation.[266] An increase in the $T_{1/2}keo$ of *d*-tubocurarine with increasing inspired halothane concentrations has been demonstrated.[267] Halothane is a negative inotrope[268] and reduces skeletal muscle blood flow,[269] so it seems reasonable to interpret changes in $T_{1/2}keo$ as a result of changes in organ blood flow. Inhalation anesthetic agents can also prolong the duration of block and this affect is agent specific. When compared with halothane, sevoflurane potentiates the effects of vecuronium to a greater extent. When compared with balanced anesthesia, sevoflurane and halothane decrease the dose requirements of vecuronium by 60% and 40%, respectively.[270]

Anesthetic drug interactions traditionally have been characterized using isobolographic analysis or multiple logistic regression. Minto proposed a model based on response-surface methodology.[271] Computer simulations based on interactions at the

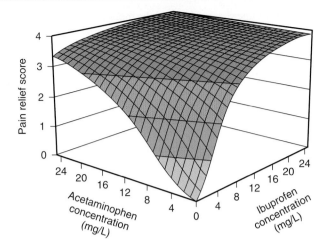

**FIGURE 6-12** The response surface of analgesic effect for acetaminophen and ibuprofen. Concentrations are those in the effect compartment. The concentration response for acetaminophen is plotted on the x-y axis, while that for ibuprofen is on the z-y axis. The "surface" is that plotted between these axes. Each point on the surface is a measure of the pain relief provided by acetaminophen and ibuprofen combination. (From Hannam J, Anderson BJ. Explaining the acetaminophen-ibuprofen analgesic interaction using a response surface model. *Pediatr Anesth* 2011;21:1234-40, with permission.)

effect-site predicted that the maximally synergistic three-drug combination (midazolam, propofol, and alfentanil) tripled the duration of effect compared with propofol alone. The response surface for ibuprofen and acetaminophen is shown in Figure 6-12. The addition of acetaminophen to ibuprofen improved analgesia when the dose of ibuprofen was less that 100 mg (5 mg/kg) in a 5-year-old child.[272] Response surfaces can describe anesthetic interactions, even those between agonists, partial agonists, competitive antagonists, and inverse agonists.[271]

Synergism between propofol and alfentanil,[273] as well as propofol and remifentanil,[274] has also been demonstrated using response-surface methodology. Remifentanil alone had no appreciable effect on response to shaking and shouting or response to laryngoscopy while propofol could ablate both responses. Modest remifentanil concentrations dramatically reduced the concentrations of propofol required to ablate both responses.[275] When comparing the different combinations of midazolam, propofol, and alfentanil, the responses varied markedly at each endpoint assessed and could not be predicted from the responses observed with each individual agent.[276] Similar response-surface methodology has been used to investigate the combined administration of sevoflurane and alfentanil,[273] and remifentanil and propofol,[274] on ventilation. These combinations have a strikingly synergistic effect on respiration, resulting in severe respiratory depression in adults. These synergistic associations can be extended to pediatric sedation techniques. It is little wonder that the use of three or more sedating medications compared with one or two medications is strongly associated with adverse outcomes.[274]

## The Drug Approval Process, the Package Insert, and Drug Labeling

One area of concern has been the general lack of approval of many medications for populations of pediatric patients. This is particularly ironic because most of the changes in legislation

pertaining to pharmaceuticals have been a result of adverse events in infants and children. The 1938 Federal Food, Drug, and Cosmetic Act[277] replaced the original Federal Food and Drugs Act of 1906 (Wiley Act)[278] because nearly 100 individuals, mostly children, were poisoned by diethylene glycol (an antifreeze analogue for vehicles) that had been added to an elixir of sulfanilamide. This new legislation prohibited the addition of poisonous substances (unless they were demonstrated to be safe in low concentrations) and instituted other measures to protect the consumer. The next major piece of legislation was the Kefauver-Harris Amendments, which were passed in 1962 as a result of the thalidomide catastrophe.[279] This legislation strengthened the safety standards by requiring the drug company to demonstrate effectiveness before marketing. The U.S. Food and Drug Administration (FDA) then allowed drugs to be marketed to adults as "safe and effective," but now the drug label was required to indicate that "safety and effectiveness had not been established in children" because no trials in children had been carried out. This had an enormous negative impact on drug development for children and led Shirkey to coin the now common expression "therapeutic orphans" when referring to drug development for children.[280]

Until the late 1990s, nearly 80% of approved medications contained language within the drug label (package insert) that excluded children of varying ages. The majority of the drugs used in the operating room (OR) and the intensive care unit (ICU) today have similar language.[281] Common examples of disclaimers for drugs used in our daily practice include those for bupivacaine ("Until further experience is gained in children younger than 12 years, administration of Sensorcaine [bupivacaine HCl] injection is not recommended")[282] and for fentanyl ("It should not be administered to children 2 years of age or younger because safety in this age group has not yet been established").[283] Such disclaimers are placed in the package insert because the contents of the package insert must, by law, be based on "adequate, well controlled studies involving children."[279,284-286] Any use of a drug that is not specifically described in the package insert is considered "unapproved" or "off label." The reason for the lack of labeling for children is that the appropriate controlled clinical trials were never supported by industry and the FDA did not have the legislative power to force the pharmaceutical companies to perform pediatric studies.[287] In 1994, the FDA passed a new interpretation of the original Food, Drug, and Cosmetic Act[277,285] that allowed manufacturers to review the published medical literature and submit these data to the FDA to support revised pediatric labeling.[286] This did result in additional changes in the drug label for approximately 100 medications. Unfortunately, for drugs that are no longer under patent protection, there was no financial incentive to force the issue, so many drugs remain unlabeled for children despite the many papers published describing their safe use in children of all ages.

During the early stages of the AIDS epidemic, there was great pressure placed on the FDA to reduce the time for the drug approval process. New legislation was passed to raise funds to pay for additional consultants and experts to help the FDA with this process (The Prescription Drug User Fee Act [PDUFA]).[288] This legislation was renewed in 1997, 2002, 2007, and was reaffirmed for the fourth time in July 2012 (PDUFA V). The monies from these fees (~ $1,170,000 per full application) greatly reduced the time from a New Drug Application until a drug reaches market, and the most recent iteration has expanded funding to support marketing safety and pharmacoepidemiology activities, as well as increased inspection of non-USA based pharmaceutical manufacturing facilities. Approximately 55 feasibility and in-depth studies were launched under PDUFA IV.[289]

Additional changes at the FDA occurred in the late 1990s when The Food and Drug Administration Modernization Act[290] and The Final Rule were passed.[291] Tacked onto this legislation was the Better Pharmaceutical Act for Children, which granted 6 months' patent extension in exchange for pediatric studies of drugs that were still patent protected. This was later replaced with the Best Pharmaceutical Act for Children (BPCA) in 2002, which earmarked money for the National Institutes of Health (NIH) to support study of drugs no longer patent protected.[292] This was subsequently challenged as giving excessive legal power to the FDA, but further legislation reinstituted the legal power to the FDA to now require drug companies to conduct research in children if the drug would have use in children (The Pediatric Research Equity Act).[293] Legislation passed in 2007 that renewed PDUFA IV was a much larger bill entitled the Food and Drug Administration Amendments Act of 2007. This bill renewed PDUFA IV, the Medical Device User Fee and Modernization Act, and BPCA.[294] Of importance to researchers was the new requirement for registration of all clinical trials with an archive of thousands of trials that is easily searchable for clinicians as well as the public.[295] Many journals now will not publish clinical pharmaceutical trials that have not been registered. Since the first legislation for children passed in 1998, there has been an explosion of pediatric drug trials (more than 600 requested or carried out from 1997 until 2011) and new drug labels have been created for nearly 400 drugs. Unfortunately, the definition of a pediatric

study is still somewhat unclear and the money that was supposed to be earmarked to the NIH for generic drug trials has not been fully provided, so deficiencies in labeling for older drugs still persist.

It is important for clinicians to understand that, despite language on the label regarding use in children, they are perfectly within their medical and legal rights to use these drugs in children. "Unapproved use does not imply an improper use and certainly does not imply an illegal use."[296,297] The use of a drug in a child is the decision of the individual physician and may be based on the available literature, despite the fact that formal FDA approval and labeling have not been achieved.[284,285] The Committee on Drugs of the American Academy of Pediatrics is very clear on this issue: "Lack of approval for a specific use should not prevent physicians from prescribing an available drug in the best interest of their patients."[296,297]

# Inhalation Anesthetic Agents

## PHYSICOCHEMICAL PROPERTIES

The potent synthesized inhaled anesthetics are ether anesthetics based on either a methyl ethyl (enflurane, isoflurane, and desflurane) or a methyl isopropyl (sevoflurane) polyhalogenated ether skeleton (Table 6-3). The single exception in chemical structure is halothane, which is a polyhalogenated alkane. Of the methyl ethyl ether anesthetics, isoflurane and enflurane are identical in chemical structure but are stereoisomers. Desflurane differs from isoflurane in the single atomic substitution of a fluoride for a chlorine atom on the α-carbon of isoflurane. Sevoflurane differs

**TABLE 6-3** Pharmacology of Inhaled Anesthetics

| | Halothane | Enflurane | Isoflurane | Sevoflurane | Desflurane | Xenon |
|---|---|---|---|---|---|---|
| **Pharmacology** | | | | | | |
| Chemical structure | (structure) | (structure) | (structure) | (structure) | (structure) | |
| Molecular weight | 197.4 | 184.5 | 184.5 | 200.1 | 168 | 131 |
| Boiling point (° C) | 50.2 | 56.5 | 48.5 | 58.6 | 23.5 | −108 |
| Vapor pressure (mm Hg) | 244 | 172 | 240 | 185 | 664 | |
| Saturation concentration (%) | 34 | 24 | 34 | 26 | 93 | |
| Odor | Mild, pleasant | Etheric | Etheric | Pleasant | Etheric | None |
| **Solubility** | | | | | | |
| $\lambda_{b/g}$ adults | 2.4 | 1.9 | 1.4 | 0.66 | 0.42 | 0.14[§] |
| $\lambda_{b/g}$ neonates* | 2.14 | 1.78 | 1.19 | 0.66 | — | — |
| $\lambda_{brain/b}$ adults[†] | 1.9 | 1.3 | 1.6 | 1.7 | 1.2 | |
| $\lambda_{brain/b}$ neonates[‡] | 1.5 | 0.9 | 1.3 | — | — | |
| $\lambda_{fat/b}$ adults | 51.1 | — | 45 | 48 | 27 | |
| **MAC** | | | | | | |
| $MAC_{adults}$ | 0.75 | 1.7 | 1.2 | 2.05 | 7.0 | 71[¶] |
| $MAC_{neonates}$ | 0.87 | — | 1.60 | 3.2 | 9.2 | |

$\lambda$, Partition coefficient; *b/g*, blood/gas; *brain/b*, brain/blood; *fat/b*, fat/blood; *MAC*, minimum alveolar concentration (%).
*Data from Lerman J, Gregory GA, Willis MM, Eger EI 2nd. Age and solubility of volatile anesthetics in blood. Anesthesiology 1984;61:139-43; Malviya S, Lerman J. The blood/gas solubilities of sevoflurane, isoflurane, halothane, and serum constituent concentrations in neonates and adults. Anesthesiology 1990;72:793-6.
[†]Data from Yasuda N, Targ AG, Eger EI II. Solubility of I-653, sevoflurane, isoflurane, and halothane in human tissues. Anesth Analg 1989;69:370-3.
[‡]Data from Lerman J, Schmitt-Bantel BI, Gregory GA, et al. Effect of age on the solubility of volatile anesthetics in human tissues. Anesthesiology 1986;65:307-11.
[§]Data from Steward A, Allott PR, Cowles AL, Maplseon WW. Solubility coefficients for inhaled anaesthetics for water, oil and biological media. Br J Anaesth 1973;45;282-93.
[¶]de Jong RH, Eger EI II. MAC expanded: AD$_{50}$ and AD$_{95}$ values of common inhalation anesthetics in man. Anesthesiology 1975;42;384-9.

from isoflurane in the substitution of a trifluoromethyl group for the chlorine atom. Although the general chemical structures of the four ether inhalational agents are similar, the single atomic substitutions confer substantially different physicochemical and pharmacologic properties that are described below and contrasted to the properties of halothane (see Table 6-3). All of these agents are liquids at room temperature and pressure.

In contrast to the potent inhaled anesthetics, nitrous oxide and xenon exist in gaseous form under atmospheric conditions. Nitrous oxide is a byproduct of chemical processes, whereas xenon is a naturally occurring element (0.05 ppm in the atmosphere), the latter being produced for clinical use by fractional distillation of atmospheric gas. Environmentally, nitrous oxide depletes the ozone layer, whereas xenon is environmentally inert. There is a wealth of data on the pharmacology of nitrous oxide in humans but far less on xenon in adults and none, to date, in children.

## PHARMACOKINETICS OF INHALED ANESTHETICS

The rate of increase or equilibration of the partial pressures of alveolar to inspired anesthetic (also known as the wash-in) is a function of the rate of delivery of anesthetic to, and uptake from, the lungs. Six factors determine the wash-in of inhalational anesthetics (Table 6-4)[298]: the first three determine the delivery of anesthetics to the lungs, and the second three determine their rate of removal (uptake) from the lungs. The wash-in, defined as the ratio of the alveolar to inspired anesthetic partial pressures ($F_A/F_I$, or fractional alveolar to fractional inspired partial pressures), increases from zero to a value of unity (1), when the inspired and alveolar partial pressures have equilibrated (Fig. 6-13).[299] Although not shown in the figure, the wash-in of xenon is exceedingly rapid based on its physicochemical properties (see Table 6-3).[300] For the $F_A/F_I$ to increase toward equilibration, the rate of delivery of anesthetic to the lungs must substantially exceed its uptake from the lungs.

Salanitre and Rackow first demonstrated that the rate of increase of $F_A/F_I$ of halothane in infants and children was more rapid than in adults (Fig. 6-14).[301] Subsequent studies substantiated similar relationships for isoflurane, enflurane, and nitrous oxide.[302,303] The more rapid rate of increase of $F_A/F_I$ in neonates compared with adults has been attributed to four factors (Table 6-5); the order in the table reflects their relative contributions to

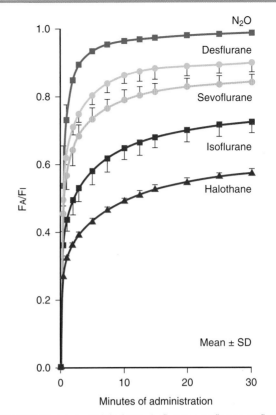

**FIGURE 6-13** Wash-in (or $F_A/F_I$) of $N_2O$, desflurane, sevoflurane, isoflurane, and halothane in adults. The order of wash-in ($N_2O$ > desflurane > sevoflurane > isoflurane > halothane) is inversely related to their solubilities in blood. *FA*, Fractional alveolar partial pressure of anesthetic; *FI*, fractional inspired partial pressure of anesthetic; *SD*, standard deviation. (Redrawn from Yasuda N, Lockhart SH, Eger EI 2nd, et al. Comparison of kinetics of sevoflurane and isoflurane in humans. Anesth Analg 1991;72:316-24.)

**TABLE 6-4** Determinants of the Wash-In of Inhalational Agents

- Inspired concentration
- Alveolar ventilation
- Functional residual capacity
- Cardiac output
- Solubility
- Alveolar to venous partial pressure gradient

**TABLE 6-5** Determinants of the Rapid Wash-In of Inhalational Agents in Infants Compared to Adults

- Greater ratio of alveolar ventilation to functional residual capacity
- Greater fraction of the cardiac output distributed to the vessel-rich group
- Reduced tissue/blood solubility
- Reduced blood/gas solubility

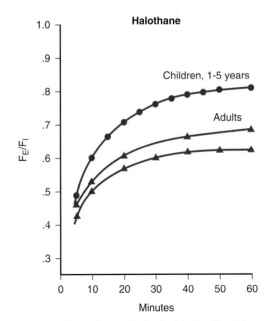

**FIGURE 6-14** Rate of rise of expired to inspired fractional partial pressures (*FE/FI*) of halothane in children and adults. (Redrawn from Salanitre E, Rackow H. The pulmonary exchange of nitrous oxide and halothane in infants and children. Anesthesiology 1969;30:388-94.)

the rapid wash-in. Based on these factors and the solubilities of sevoflurane and desflurane, we speculate that the wash-in curves of sevoflurane and desflurane in neonates and infants will be comparable to those in adults. This amounts to a safety factor for these anesthetics that was not previously afforded with halothane.

### Factors Affecting Delivery of Anesthetics to the Lungs
#### Inspired Concentration
The effect of the inspired concentration on the FA/FI of anesthetics relates only to those that are administered in high concentrations (i.e., nitrous oxide). The greater the FI of nitrous oxide, the more rapid the increase of FA/FI.[304] This effect, known as the concentration effect (second gas effect), depends on both a concentrating effect and an increase in alveolar ventilation that results from an increased uptake of nitrous oxide.[298] Hence, agents that depend on alveolar ventilation for their wash-in (i.e., the more soluble anesthetics) will have a more rapid wash-in when administered with nitrous oxide. This effect diminishes as the solubility of the anesthetic decreases and as time passes.[305-307] Although the rate of increase of FA/FI of nitrous oxide in adults is rapid, it is even more rapid in neonates and infants.[301,303]

#### Alveolar Ventilation and Functional Residual Capacity
The ratio of alveolar ventilation to functional residual capacity (Va/FRC) is the primary determinant of the rate of the delivery of anesthetic to the lungs. The greater the Va/FRC ratio, the more rapid the FA/FI (E-Fig. 6-5). However, the ratio does not affect all anesthetics similarly: more soluble anesthetics (i.e., halothane) are affected to a greater extent than are less soluble anesthetics (i.e., sevoflurane and desflurane). The reason for this differential effect of Va/FRC relates to the relative delivery of anesthetic to and uptake from the lungs: in the case of soluble anesthetics (halothane), uptake from the lungs is substantial, thereby limiting the increase in FA/FI to the delivery of anesthetic to the lungs. Hence, changes in the alveolar ventilation will directly affect the FA/FI of anesthetics in proportion to their blood solubilities. In terms of age-related effects of FA/FI, the Va/FRC ratio accounts for most of the differences between the FA/FI of anesthetics in neonates and adults (see Table 6-5). The Va/FRC ratio is approximately 5:1 in neonates compared with only 1.5:1 in adults. The greater Va/FRC ratio in neonates may be attributed to the threefold greater metabolic rate and, therefore, threefold greater alveolar ventilation in neonates compared with adults. This is true for both spontaneous and controlled ventilation, depending on the settings used during controlled ventilation.

### Factors Affecting the Uptake (Removal) of Anesthetics from the Lungs
#### Cardiac Output
The rate of increase in FA/FI is inversely related to changes in cardiac output: that is, the smaller the cardiac output, the more rapid the increase in FA/FI and vice versa (E-Fig. 6-6). As cardiac output diminishes, removal of anesthetic from the lungs diminishes and the rate of equilibration of FA/FI increases. Thus, a child in heart failure who receives an inhalational induction may achieve greater anesthetic concentrations in the lungs more rapidly than expected compared with a child with a normal cardiac output. This very serious problem may be exacerbated if the "overpressure" technique has been used, because it may cause an acute anesthetic-induced myocardial depression and decompensation of cardiac output. Conversely, in a high cardiac output

state (as in the case of anxiety), the greater blood flow through the lungs removes anesthetic from the alveoli, thus reducing the alveolar partial pressure of anesthetic, which slows the rate of equilibration of FA/FI. The impact of changes in cardiac output on FA/FI depends, in part, on the solubility of the anesthetic: the more soluble the anesthetic (e.g., halothane), the greater the effect of changes in cardiac output on FA/FI and the less soluble the anesthetic (sevoflurane and desflurane), the less the effect.[298] This is another safety feature of the less soluble anesthetics.

Paradoxically, the greater cardiac index in neonates actually speeds the increase in FA/FI. This has been attributed to the preferential distribution of the cardiac output to the vessel-rich group (VRG) of tissues (brain, heart, kidney, splanchnic organs, and endocrine glands) in neonates. The VRG receives a greater proportion of the cardiac output in neonates compared with adults because it comprises 18% of the body weight in the former compared with only 8% in the latter. As a result of the increased blood flow to the VRG, the partial pressures of anesthetics in the VRG equilibrate with those in the alveoli more rapidly in neonates than in adults. Because the uptake of anesthetic by tissues other than those in the VRG in neonates is small, the rapid increase in FA/FI in the VRG and blood suggests that the partial pressure of anesthetic in venous blood returning to the lungs rapidly approaches the partial pressure in the alveoli. Uptake of anesthetic from the lungs then diminishes, as discussed later. The net effect of the greater cardiac output in neonates is paradoxical in that it speeds the equilibration of anesthetic partial pressures in the VRG and thus speeds the equilibration of FA/FI. This also accounts for part of the "downward spiral" that occurs when an excessive concentration of inhaled agent (particularly the soluble anesthetic halothane) is administered to a neonate or infant during controlled ventilation, as discussed later.

#### Solubility
Inhalational agents partition into two compartments in body fluids and tissues: (1) an aqueous phase and (2) a protein/lipid phase. This partitioning is analogous to the distribution of gases such as oxygen in blood between the aqueous phase (dissolved fraction) and hemoglobin (bound fraction). Because inhaled anesthetics move along partial pressure gradients and not concentration gradients within and between fluids and tissues, the rate of increase of FA/FI and, therefore, the anesthetic partial pressure in blood determines how rapidly anesthetics move into and out of tissues and affect organ function (e.g., central nervous and cardiac systems).

The rate of increase of FA/FI of inhalational anesthetics, which varies inversely with the solubility of the anesthetic in blood, follows the order: nitrous oxide > desflurane > sevoflurane > isoflurane > enflurane > halothane > methoxyflurane (see Table 6-3 and Fig. 6-13).[298,299] Although the solubilities of nitrous oxide and desflurane are similar, the rate of increase in FA/FI of nitrous oxide is more rapid than that after desflurane because of the concentration effect from administering 70% nitrous oxide. After a stepwise change in the inspired partial pressure of less soluble anesthetics, the alveolar partial pressure equilibrates rapidly with the new inspired partial pressure. Because the washout of these anesthetics is equally rapid (see later discussion), the alveolar partial pressure can be adjusted to previous values rapidly by decreasing the inspired partial pressure. Thus, anesthetic depth can be controlled more rapidly with a less soluble (i.e., desflurane or sevoflurane) than with a more soluble inhalational anesthetic (i.e., halothane).

The blood solubility of xenon is one-third that of nitrous oxide and desflurane (see Table 6-3). Although the tissue solubility of xenon has not been determined, its low blood solubility would suggest that its wash-in is the most rapid of the inhalational anesthetics.

Age is an important determinant of the solubility of inhalational anesthetics in blood. The blood solubilities of halothane, isoflurane, enflurane, and methoxyflurane are 18% less in neonates than they are in adults (E-Fig. 6-7; see also Table 6-3).[308] Serum cholesterol and proteins (including albumin) account for these age-related differences in blood solubilities.[308,309] In contrast, the blood solubility of the less soluble anesthetic sevoflurane is similar in neonates and adults.[309] Factors that do not appear to significantly affect the blood solubility of most anesthetics include age-related differences in hemoglobin, serum concentration of $\alpha$1-acid glycoprotein, and prematurity.[308,309]

The tissue/gas solubilities of the inhalational anesthetics in the VRG in neonates are approximately one-half those in adults (E-Fig. 6-8).[310] The reduced tissue solubilities of halothane, isoflurane, enflurane, and methoxyflurane in neonates are attributable to two differences in the composition of tissues: (1) greater water content and (2) decreased protein and lipid concentrations. In terms of the uptake and distribution of anesthetics in tissues, the tissue/blood solubilities determine the speed of equilibration of anesthetics in tissues. The reduced tissue solubilities of inhalational anesthetics decrease the time for partial pressure equilibration of anesthetics (see time constant discussion, later). Although the partial pressures of inhalational agents in tissues cannot easily be measured in vivo, they may be estimated by their concentrations in the exhaled or alveolar gases. The solubilities of the inhalational anesthetics in the brain of adults vary approximately 50% from desflurane to halothane (see Table 6-3). In the case of neonates, the reduced tissue solubilities of inhalational anesthetics speed the rate of increase in FA/FI compared with the rates in adults. In the cases of sevoflurane and desflurane, their respectively low but similar blood solubilities and likely similar tissues solubilities in neonates and adults offer a safety factor in neonates compared with adults, because tissue equilibration of these relatively insoluble inhalational anesthetics should be similar in both age groups. In contrast, the reduced tissue solubility of halothane in neonates likely results in a more rapid and unexpected anesthetic effect compared with the time course in adults.

We can estimate the time to equilibration of anesthetic partial pressures in tissues by calculating the time constant for equilibration in the tissue. For example, the time constant (tau $\tau$) for equilibration of anesthetic partial pressure in the brain is based on the expression:

$$\tau_{brain} = \frac{\text{Volume of the brain (mL)} \times \text{Brain/blood solubility}}{\text{Brain blood flow (mL/min)}}$$

where one time constant is the time for 63% equilibration of brain to blood anesthetic partial pressures. If the blood flow to the brain is approximately 50 mL/min/100 g of brain tissue and the brain/blood solubility ratio for an inhalational anesthetic is 2.0 (assuming the density of brain tissue is 1 g/mL), then the time constant is:

$$\tau_{brain} = \frac{100 \text{ mL} \times 2}{50 \text{ mL/min}}$$

Knowing that three time constants achieve 95% equilibration, and four time constants achieve 98%, then the time to 95% equilibration is 12 minutes, and to 98% equilibration is 16 minutes. If the brain/blood solubility ratio were halved to 1.0, as it might be in the case of the neonate, then the time to 95% equilibration would decrease by 50% to 8 minutes. *Thus, the time to equilibration of anesthetic partial pressure within the brain of the neonate would be approximately one half that of the adult but still requires 8 minutes!* This holds true for the more soluble anesthetics, such as halothane, whose tissue solubility in neonates is diminished compared with adults[310] but not for the less soluble anesthetics, such as desflurane and sevoflurane, whose tissue solubilities may be similar in neonates and adults.

Whereas the PK of inhalational anesthetics during the first 15 to 20 minutes depends primarily on the characteristics of the VRG, the PK during the subsequent 20 to 200 minutes depends primarily on those of the muscle group.[298] The solubility of inhalational anesthetics in skeletal muscle varies directly with age in a logarithmic relationship.[310] Thus, the lower solubility of inhalational anesthetics in the muscle of neonates and the smaller muscle mass speed the increase in FA/FI during this period compared with that in adults. This effect of age on the solubility of anesthetics in muscle has been attributed to age-dependent increases in protein concentration (i.e., muscle bulk) during the first 5 decades of life and in fat content during the subsequent 3 decades of life.[310] Overall, the reduced solubility combined with the reduced muscle mass in neonates (and infants) decreases uptake by the muscle group, leaving the FA/FI to equilibrate more rapidly in neonates compared with adults.

The net effect of these differences between neonates and adults is to speed the equilibration of anesthetic partial pressures in alveoli and tissues, and thereby speed the rate of increase in FA/FI in neonates compared with adults.[301,302] This is particularly true for the more soluble anesthetics, such as halothane. However, the difference in the rate of wash-in of less soluble anesthetics, such as sevoflurane and desflurane, between neonates and adults may be diminished.

### *Alveolar to Venous Partial Pressure Gradient*

The difference in the anesthetic partial pressures between the alveolus and venous blood returning to the heart is a measure of the driving force of inhalational anesthetics from the alveoli into the bloodstream. As the anesthetic partial pressures in the VRG, muscle group, and others approach equilibration and less anesthetic is taken up by those tissues, the anesthetic partial pressure in the blood returning to the heart is similar to that when it left the alveoli. Thus, the driving force for anesthetics to move along a partial pressure gradient from the alveoli to the blood is diminished. This reduces the partial pressure gradient and diminishes the uptake of anesthetic from the alveoli.

### Second Gas Effect

When two anesthetics are administered simultaneously, the wash-in of the anesthetic administered in a small concentration may be increased if the uptake of the second anesthetic is relatively large.[298] Nitrous oxide is the only anesthetic for which the uptake may be relatively large compared with that of the potent inhalational anesthetics, as described earlier. There is evidence, however, that casts doubt on the clinical relevance of the second gas effect.[311,312] These data suggest that the concentrating effect, if it exists in humans at all, is a small and weak effect. This may be of minor importance in any regard, as induction of anesthesia may be hastened by using the overpressure technique, which refers to administering much greater inspired concentrations of inhalational anesthetic than the target goal.

## Induction

The more rapid increase in FA/FI of insoluble anesthetics compared with soluble anesthetics is generally thought to result in a more rapid induction of anesthesia. However, this is not necessarily true. Whereas the wash-in of inhalational anesthetics is determined by the PK of the agents, the speed of induction of anesthesia depends not only on the wash-in but also on (1) the potency or MAC of the agent, (2) the rate of increase of the inspired concentration, (3) the maximal inspired concentration, and (4) respirations (including airway irritability and the mode of ventilation [spontaneous or controlled]). It is the combination of these four factors that determines the relative rate of induction of anesthesia.

The rate of wash-in of inhalational anesthetics into the lungs varies inversely with their solubilities in blood. Although anesthetics that are less soluble (e.g., sevoflurane and desflurane) wash into the lungs more rapidly than more soluble anesthetics (e.g., halothane), the more rapid increase in FA/FI of less soluble anesthetics is offset by their greater MAC (see Table 6-3). To ensure that induction of anesthesia is as rapid with less soluble anesthetics as it is with more soluble anesthetics, two criteria must be satisfied. First, the inspired concentration of the less soluble anesthetic must be increased in greater increments (based on the relative MAC values and wash-in profile, where MAC is defined as the minimum alveolar [or end-tidal or end-expiratory] anesthetic concentration at which 50% of subjects do not move in response to a noxious stimulus) than the more soluble anesthetic and, second, the maximum inspired concentration of the less soluble anesthetic must provide an alveolar concentration that is equipotent with that of the more soluble anesthetic. Theoretically, the overpressure technique should provide rapid and similar rates of induction of anesthesia with anesthetics of differing solubilities. However, if the maximum inspired anesthetic concentrations from the vaporizers preclude the delivery of equipotent concentrations or if airway irritability (as in the case of coughing and breath holding) interrupts the smooth delivery of anesthetic, induction of anesthesia will not be comparable.

To illustrate this, contrast the rate of equilibration of FA/FI for sevoflurane and halothane during the first few minutes of induction of anesthesia (see Fig. 6-13). Data on the wash-in of inhalational anesthetics in adults is used because comparable data for children are not available. In adults, FA/FI for halothane reaches 0.35 in the first few minutes of anesthesia. Given the previous data from Salanitre and Rackow,[301] FA/FI in children should increase more rapidly than that in adults, reaching perhaps 0.45 in the same time frame. For the maximum inspired concentration of halothane of 5%, the alveolar or end-tidal concentration achieved in the first few minutes in a child is $0.45 \times 5\% = 2.25\%$. With a MAC for halothane in children of ~1.0%, this is equivalent to 2.25%/1% or 2.25 MAC multiples. Contrast this to the wash-in of sevoflurane during the same time frame. The FA/FI for sevoflurane reaches 0.5. Because of its low blood solubility, the FA/FI for sevoflurane in children is likely to be similar to that in adults. With a vaporizer that delivers a maximum sevoflurane inspired concentration of 8%, the alveolar or end-tidal concentration in children achieved in the first few minutes is $0.5 \times 8\% = 4\%$. Given that the MAC for sevoflurane in children is 2.5%, 4% sevoflurane is equivalent to 4%/2.5% or 1.6 MAC multiples. This number of MAC multiples for sevoflurane is approximately 25% less than that achieved with halothane. This model will result in even greater differences between halothane and sevoflurane if the sevoflurane vaporizer is limited to 5% or 7%, as it is in some countries.

A similar but more clinically important case can be made for neonates (with a MAC for halothane of ~0.87%) in whom the FA/FI for halothane reaches 0.5 in the first few minutes of anesthesia, resulting in an alveolar concentration of $5\% \times 0.5/0.87\%$ or 2.9 MAC multiples. Although the FA/FI for sevoflurane in neonates (with a MAC for sevoflurane of 3.3%) also reaches 0.5 in the first few minutes of anesthesia, the alveolar concentration reaches $8\% \times 0.5/3.3\%$ or only 1.2 MAC multiples. In this case, the MAC multiples of sevoflurane are 60% less than those of halothane. Thus it is difficult to rapidly induce a deep level of anesthesia with sevoflurane in neonates and infants, as it was with halothane in the past. Conversely, an anesthetic overdose during induction with sevoflurane in a neonate is far less likely to occur than with halothane.

These two examples illustrate several extremely important features of the pharmacology of sevoflurane that distinguish it from halothane. First, it may be difficult to rapidly achieve a deep level of anesthesia with sevoflurane in children (as was previously achieved with halothane) when sevoflurane is the sole anesthetic. Hence, inserting an IV catheter or performing laryngoscopy or bronchoscopy immediately after induction of anesthesia with sevoflurane may result in a physiologic or motor (withdrawal) response, even if the inspired concentration remains at 8%. We caution against decreasing the inspired concentration of sevoflurane (and nitrous oxide) as soon as the eyelash reflex is lost or the child appears to have lost consciousness, because a deep level of anesthesia has not been achieved (despite theoretical fears of seizure-like activity, see below). In such cases, supplemental IV anesthetics may be required to rapidly deepen the level of anesthesia. Second, these examples illustrate an important safety feature of sevoflurane. With the current vaporizer design, excessive concentrations of sevoflurane cannot be administered to neonates and infants because their large MAC values more than offset their reduced solubilities. These insights contribute to the cardiovascular safety profile of sevoflurane and may help to explain why the morbidity and mortality associated with sevoflurane in children appear to be less than are associated with halothane.[313]

### Control of Anesthetic Depth

Two feedback responses modulate the depth of anesthesia during inhalational anesthesia: (1) a negative-feedback respiratory response and (2) a positive-feedback cardiovascular response. The feedback responses refer to the relationships between the inspired concentration of anesthetic and depth of anesthesia. After an increase in the inspired concentration, a negative feedback response refers to a decrease in the depth of anesthesia, whereas a positive-feedback system refers to an increase in the depth of anesthesia. Two examples that follow are used to illustrate the importance of these responses in clinical pediatric anesthesia practice.

During spontaneous respirations, as the partial pressure of inhaled anesthetics increases, alveolar ventilation decreases, thereby limiting both the wash-in of anesthetics and the depth of anesthesia achieved (E-Fig. 6-9, *A*).[314] This negative-feedback response is a protective mechanism that permits the safe use of inspired concentrations of inhalational anesthetics that are severalfold greater than MAC (overpressure technique) during spontaneous respirations. Excessive depth of anesthesia cannot normally be achieved during spontaneous respirations (irrespective of the inspired concentrations of anesthetics, even if multiple anesthetics are administered simultaneously), because of the negative-feedback effect such anesthetic concentrations have to depress minute ventilation. As alveolar ventilation decreases and the wash-in of anesthetics slows, the uptake of anesthetic by blood slows and the delivery of anesthetics to the VRG slows. When the partial pressure of anesthetics in the VRG exceeds that in blood, anesthetics move along their partial pressure gradients from the VRG into blood and other tissues, thus decreasing the depth of anesthesia. As the depth of anesthesia decreases, alveolar ventilation again increases and uptake of anesthetic from the alveoli resumes. *Thus, spontaneous ventilation protects against an anesthetic overdose by virtue of its negative feedback effect on respirations.*

In contrast to the negative-feedback loop of spontaneous ventilation, the positive-feedback effect of controlled ventilation relentlessly delivers inhaled anesthetic to the alveoli, increasing FA/FI, but at the same time diminishing cardiac output (E-Fig. 6-9, *B*).[314] The decrease in cardiac output limits the uptake of anesthetic from the alveoli, further increasing FA/FI. Hence, as cardiac output decreases, FA/FI increases and the depth of anesthesia increases, thereby further decreasing cardiac output. For a specific minute ventilation in a neonate, the speed at which cardiovascular collapse occurs is reflected in part by the maximum number of MAC-multiples the vaporizer can deliver (Table 6-6). This is a positive-feedback loop. This response creates a downward spiral that may result in death, if it is not interrupted.

In a model of uptake and distribution, dogs who breathed spontaneously received up to 4% inspired concentrations of halothane[314]; the anesthetic was tolerated without cardiovascular collapse because the negative feedback response of respiratory depression prevented excessive concentrations of anesthetic from depressing the VRG. In contrast, when ventilation was controlled, cardiovascular collapse occurred at inspired concentrations 4% or more, and some dogs succumbed. High concentrations of halothane (i.e., as those used in the overpressure technique) are commonly administered during inhalational inductions, either as stepwise increases in inspired concentrations or as a single-breath large concentration. *These large concentrations are tolerated provided that spontaneous respiration is maintained. If, however, ventilation is controlled, then the negative respiratory feedback loop is bypassed and cardiovascular collapse becomes possible.* This is of particular concern in neonates and small infants who are more susceptible to the cardiodepressant effects of inhaled agents.[298]

**TABLE 6-6** Minimum Alveolar Concentration (MAC) Multiples for a Neonate Allowed by Current Vaporizers

| Agent | Maximum Vaporizer Output (%) | MAC (%) | Maximum Possible MAC Multiples |
|---|---|---|---|
| Halothane | 5 | 0.87 | 5.75 |
| Isoflurane | 5 | 1.20 | 4.2 |
| Sevoflurane | 8 | 3.3 | 2.42 |
| Desflurane | 18 | 9.16 | 1.96 |

See text for further discussion.
*MAC,* Minimum alveolar concentration.

## Shunts

Two types of shunts exist in the lungs and heart: left-to-right or right-to-left. Left-to-right shunts refer to conditions in which blood recirculates through the lungs (usually via an intracardiac defect, such as a ventricular septal defect). In contrast, right-to-left shunts refer to conditions in which venous blood returning to the heart bypasses the lungs as in an intracardiac shunt (cyanotic heart disease) or intrapulmonary shunt (pneumonia or an endobronchial intubation). The effects of shunts on the rate of increase in FA/FI are poorly understood. In general, left-to-right shunts do not significantly affect the PK of inhalational anesthetics (they may affect IV medications), provided cardiac output remains unchanged. In contrast, right-to-left shunts can significantly delay the equilibration of FA/FI of inhalational anesthetics. The magnitude of the delay with a right-to-left shunt depends on the solubility of the anesthetic: the wash-in of less soluble anesthetics is delayed to a greater extent than that of the more soluble anesthetics.[298] These effects are independent of the location of the shunt: intracardiac or intrapulmonary.

To understand the effects of right-to-left shunts on the PK of inhalational anesthetics, it is useful to consider a simplified model of a right-to-left shunt using the lung to mimic the shunt. In this model, each lung is represented by one alveolus and each is perfused by one pulmonary artery (Fig. 6-15). When a tracheal tube is positioned with its tip at the mid-trachea level (Fig. 6-15, *A*), ventilation is divided equally between both alveoli, thereby yielding equivalent anesthetic partial pressures in both pulmonary veins ($P\bar{v} = 1$). However, if the tip of the tracheal tube is advanced into the right main-stem bronchus (equivalent to a right-to-left shunt) (Fig. 6-15, *B*), all of the ventilation is delivered to one alveoli, that is, the ventilation to that alveoli is doubled, whereas ventilation to the nonventilated lung is zero. Under these conditions, total ventilation remains unchanged. For the remainder of this discussion, it is important to recognize that with a right-to-left shunt, the end-tidal and blood anesthetic partial pressures will differ, the magnitude of which will depend on the solubility of the anesthetic.

When a more soluble anesthetic (e.g., halothane) is administered through a tracheal tube that is positioned in the right main-stem bronchus (to model a right-to-left shunt), doubling the ventilation to that lung speeds the increase in FA/FI (effect of changes in ventilation on the wash-in of soluble anesthetics) (E-Fig. 6-5) such that it compensates, for the most part, for the absence of ventilation to the contralateral lung (Fig. 6-15, *B*).[298] The more soluble the anesthetic, the closer the partial pressure of anesthetic in the combined pulmonary vein that drains both the ventilated and nonventilated lungs approximates the partial pressure from delivering the anesthetic to lungs without a right-to-left shunt. The net effect of a right-to-left shunt on the FA/FI of a more soluble inhalational anesthetic is thus negligible.

In contrast, when a less soluble anesthetic (e.g., sevoflurane or desflurane) is administered in the presence of such a right-to-left shunt, doubling the ventilation to the lung minimally increases the FA/FI, because ventilation has a limited effect on the speed of increase of FA/FI of less soluble anesthetics (see E-Fig. 6-5 and Fig. 6-15, *C* ).[298] Consequently, the increase in FA/FI in the ventilated lung is insufficient to offset the absence of anesthetic in the blood draining the nonventilated lung. The *net effect is to almost halve* the anesthetic partial pressure in the combined pulmonary vein. The less soluble the anesthetic, the greater the discrepancy between the anesthetic partial pressure in the pulmonary vein that drains the ventilated and nonventilated

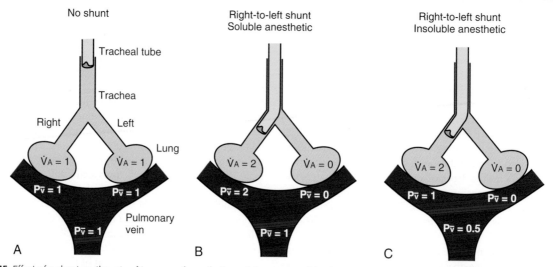

**FIGURE 6-15** Effect of a shunt on the rate of increase of anesthetic partial pressure in blood using a model. **A,** Normal situation with no shunt, equal alveolar ventilation ($\dot{V}_A$) to both lungs, and normocapnia. **B,** The effect of a right-to-left shunt (via an endobronchial intubation) with a more soluble anesthetic (e.g., halothane). Ventilation and therefore normocapnia are maintained, and hypoxic pulmonary vasoconstriction is negligible. In this case, the increased ventilation to the ventilated lung speeds the increase in FA/FI (wash-in) and offsets the effect of the shunt. Results in terms of the mixed pulmonary venous partial pressure of the anesthetic ($P\bar{v} = 1$) are similar to those in **A. C,** The effect of a shunt with a less soluble anesthetic (e.g., desflurane or sevoflurane). Because the increase in alveolar ventilation does not increase FA/FI in the ventilated lung, there is a dramatic reduction in the anesthetic partial pressure in the blood ($P\bar{v} = 0.5$). (Redrawn from Lerman J. Pharmacology of inhalational anaesthetics in infants and children. Paediatr Anaesth 1992;2:191-203.)

lungs and the partial pressure when the tube is in the trachea. The overall effect of a right-to-left shunt is to slow induction of anesthesia or even limit the depth of anesthesia that can be achieved with less soluble anesthetics.[315,316]

Few studies have documented the clinical importance of such a shunt.[315,316] Clinical situations that have posed challenges with these shunts include children with right-to-left cardiac shunts and infants with chronic lung disease. In the past, very soluble anesthetics, such as methoxyflurane (blood/gas solubility of 12), would have been unaffected by a right-to-left shunt. In the case of halothane, the most soluble anesthetic currently available, anesthesia remained quite effective in children with right-to-left shunts even though the ratio of arterial to inspired partial pressures lagged behind the ratio when the shunt was closed.[316] The most likely explanation was that the 5% inspired concentration of halothane from the vaporizer permitted a 5 × MAC overpressure effect. Although the ratios of the arterial to inspired partial pressures of sevoflurane and desflurane have not been measured in children with right-to-left shunts, we expect they will pose even greater difficulties than halothane, particularly with their limited overpressure effect (i.e., the maximal inspired concentrations of the vaporizers are limited to 3 × MAC or less [see Table 6-6]). Our experience suggests that when we use these less soluble anesthetics in such circumstances (e.g., bronchoscopy for a bronchial foreign body), IV anesthetics are needed to achieve an adequate depth of anesthesia in infants and younger children.

### Washout and Emergence

The washout of inhalational anesthetics follows an exponential decay (the inverse of the wash-in curves, see Fig. 6-13) and during emergence, this is achieved by setting the inspired concentration to zero.[299] The order of the washout (and speed of emergence) of the inhalational anesthetics parallels their blood solubilities: desflurane > sevoflurane > isoflurane > halothane > methoxyflurane (see Table 6-3).[299,317] For most inhalational anesthetics, metabolism does not contribute substantively to the washout. Halothane

is the one exception; its washout is as rapid as that of isoflurane, likely because its metabolism is 15- to 20-fold greater than that of isoflurane (see later discussion). The order of the washout of anesthetics in children should be similar to that in adults whereas the washout in neonates and infants is likely to be more rapid than that in adults for the same reasons the rate of wash-in is more rapid (see Table 6-5). Further studies are required to substantiate this notion.

Although some advocate switching inhalational anesthetics to a less soluble agent toward the end of surgery for economy and to facilitate a rapid emergence, there is a dearth of data to support such a practice in children. In fact, it has been suggested that switching from isoflurane to desflurane 30 minutes before the end of anesthesia in adults does not speed emergence.[318]

A number of other strategies have been used to speed emergence and recovery from anesthesia. In adults, discontinuing nitrous oxide accelerates the washout of and emergence from inhalational anesthesia.[319] Most recently, charcoal filters added to anesthesia breathing circuits adsorb anesthetics and have been shown to speed emergence.[320] Hypercapnic hyperventilation with a charcoal filter to adsorb the inhaled anesthetic has been shown to speed emergence from isoflurane, sevoflurane, and desflurane anesthesia in adults by about 60%.[321,322]

When comparing the speed of recovery after anesthesia, the results are heavily influenced by the study design. Studies in which the anesthetic concentration is maintained at a fixed MAC multiple until the end of surgery usually demonstrate a pattern of recovery that parallels the solubilities of the anesthetics in blood, at least during the early recovery period: halothane > isoflurane > sevoflurane > desflurane (see earlier).[323-328]

However, in the clinical setting, the inspired concentrations of inhalational anesthetics are usually tapered toward the end of surgery and this attenuates these differences. Second, differences in the speed of recovery among anesthetics parallels the duration of anesthesia; for example, differences will be less for brief surgery and greater for surgery of greater duration.[324,329-331] Third, failure to prevent or treat pain before emergence will trigger a much more rapid and stormy emergence after less soluble than after more soluble anesthetics.[324,327] A more sophisticated approach to the washout of inhalational anesthetics is to use the CSHT, which is a measure of the time to decrease the anesthetic partial pressure by 50%. Using a computer model and PK data from adults, the CSHTs of the potent inhalational anesthetics enflurane, isoflurane, sevoflurane, and desflurane were similar (less than 5 minutes) and were unaffected by the duration of the anesthetic.[332] The 80% decrement times were similar for desflurane and sevoflurane (less than 8 minutes) whereas those for isoflurane and enflurane were greater (30 and 35 minutes, respectively). However, after 6 hours of simulated anesthesia, the 90% decrement times differed substantially: 14 minutes for desflurane, 65 minutes for sevoflurane, 86 minutes for isoflurane, and 100 minutes for enflurane. These data suggest that the early recovery (up to 80% decrement in partial pressure) after inhalational anesthesia is similar among these four anesthetics (although sevoflurane and desflurane are more rapid), but after 6 hours (i.e., prolonged anesthesia) 90% decrement is achieved much more rapidly with desflurane than with the remainder.

In animal models, recovery of motor function (an indicator of more complete recovery than simple measurement of expired anesthetic concentrations) parallels the wash-out of inhalational anesthetics from fastest to slowest: desflurane < sevoflurane < isoflurane < halothane.[333] Notably, the time to recover increases in parallel with the duration of anesthesia.[333] In pediatric studies in which the recovery times after two or more anesthetics were compared, the end-tidal concentrations of the anesthetics were maintained at approximately 1 MAC until the conclusion of surgery, after which the anesthetics were abruptly discontinued.[323,324,334] In this paradigm, the rates of recovery paralleled the rates of wash-out, which in turn paralleled the solubilities of the inhalational anesthetics, including xenon and desflurane.[335] In clinical practice, however, anesthetic concentrations are gradually tapered as the end of surgery approaches. This practice may attenuate the differences in the rates of recovery among inhalational anesthetics.

## PHARMACODYNAMICS OF INHALED ANESTHETICS
### Minimum Alveolar Concentration

MAC is defined as the minimum alveolar (or end-tidal or end-expiratory) anesthetic concentration at which 50% of patients do not move in response to a noxious stimulus. The classic stimulus for MAC in humans is skin incision; throughout the remainder of this chapter, MAC will refer to this stimulus. MAC has also been determined in response to other stimuli, including tracheal intubation, insertion of a laryngeal mask airway, tracheal extubation, and awake responsiveness. The difference in the potency (or MAC) of inhalational anesthetics varies inversely with the lipid solubility of these anesthetics; that is, as the lipid solubility decreases, the potency decreases in parallel (i.e., MAC increases) (see Table 6-3).

In children, MAC varies significantly with age. For example, the MAC of halothane increases as age decreases, reaching a maximum value in infants 1 to 6 months of age (1.20 ± 0.06%) and then decreases by about 30% to (0.87 ± 0.03%) in full-term neonates.[336,337] Similar relationships hold true for isoflurane and desflurane (Figs. 6-16 and E-Fig. 6-10).[338,339] However, the relationship for sevoflurane differs from that of the other inhalational anesthetics in that the MAC of sevoflurane does not increase steadily as age decreases (Fig. 6-17).[340] In fact, the MAC

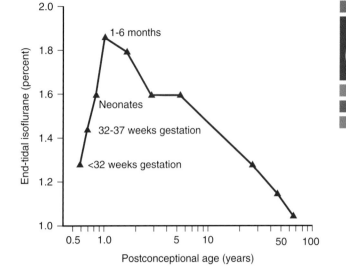

FIGURE 6-16  MAC (minimum alveolar concentration) of isoflurane in preterm and full-term neonates, infants, and children. MAC increased with gestational age in infants younger than 32 weeks gestation (1.3%), reaching a zenith in infants 1 to 6 months of age of 1.87% and decreased thereafter with increasing age to adulthood. Postconceptional age is the sum of the gestational age and postnatal age in years. (Data from Cameron CB, Robinson S, Gregory GA. The minimum anesthetic concentration of isoflurane in children. Anesth Analg 1984;63:418-20 and LeDez KM, Lerman J. The minimum alveolar concentration (MAC) of isoflurane in preterm neonates. Anesthesiology 1987;67:301-7.)

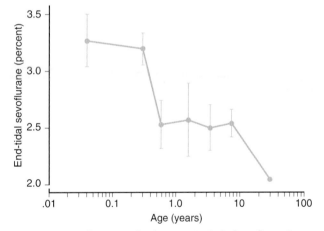

FIGURE 6-17  MAC (minimum alveolar concentration) of sevoflurane in neonates, infants, and children. MAC is greatest in full-term neonates (3.3%), less in infants 1-6 months of age (3.2%), and then decreases 25%, to 2.5%, for all infants and children 6 months to 10 years of age. Age is postnatal age in years. MAC of sevoflurane in adults, 30 years of age, shown for completeness. All MAC measurements were performed with sevoflurane in 100% oxygen using a single skin incision. (Data from Lerman J, Sikich N, Kleinman S, Yentis S. The pharmacology of sevoflurane in infants and children. Anesthesiology 1994;80:814-24.)

of sevoflurane in neonates and infants younger than 6 months of age is 3.3%, whereas in older infants and children, it is 2.5%.[340-342] The explanation for this different relationship for sevoflurane remains unclear.

The MAC of inhalational anesthetics in preterm neonates has been determined only for isoflurane (see Fig. 6-16). The (mean ± SD) MAC of isoflurane in preterm neonates younger than

32 weeks gestation ($1.28 \pm 0.17\%$) is 10% less than it is in neonates of 32 to 37 weeks gestational age ($1.41 \pm 0.18\%$), which in turn is 12% less than it is in full-term neonates ($1.60 \pm 0.03\%$).[241] The etiology of these age-dependent changes in MAC remains elusive. Several possible causes have been proposed, including maturational changes in the CNS and neurohumoral factors, but none of them have been confirmed.

Other factors are known to affect MAC. The melanocortin-1 receptor gene has been shown to affect the MAC of desflurane. That is, 90% of adults who were either homozygous or heterozygous for mutations of this gene (i.e., redheads) required 20% more anesthesia than those who had no mutations (brunettes).[343] A similar relationship should hold true for children with these mutations. Hypothermia decreases MAC. In children 4 to 10 years, the MAC of isoflurane decreases 5% per degree Celsius.[344]

Cerebral palsy and severe cognitive impairment reduce the MAC of halothane approximately 25% compared with healthy children.[345] Although tetanic stimulation was used to elicit a pain response, this stimulus underestimates the MAC compared with skin incision.[346] Nonetheless, the MAC of halothane in healthy children was similar to published data with skin incision.[337] Chronic anticonvulsant therapy decreased the MAC of halothane in handicapped children by 15%, compared with those without anticonvulsants, from $0.71\% \pm 0.10\%$ to $0.62\% \pm 0.03\%$.[345] Several factors may account for the decrease in MAC in children with cognitive impairment, including central sensory impairment, increased pain threshold or insensitivity, and a disequilibrium of inhibitory and excitatory regulatory neurons within the spinal cord in these children.[347,348] Although the acute administration of barbiturates and benzodiazepines decreases MAC,[349,350] chronic administration of similar medications does not.[351] The effects of specific anticonvulsants, such as valproic acid and phenytoin, on the MAC of inhalational anesthetics in children remain unclear.

The MAC for nitrous oxide has been estimated to be 104% in adults[352]; comparable data do not exist in children. The additivity of MAC fractions of inhalational anesthetics (as well as nitrous oxide) is well established. For example, the total anesthetic delivered when 0.5 MAC of one agent and 0.5 MAC of a second agent are administered is 1 MAC. In adults, the concept of additivity has been confirmed for all inhalational anesthetics, including sevoflurane and desflurane, in combination with nitrous oxide.[353,354] In children, the concept of MAC additivity holds true when nitrous oxide is combined with halothane or isoflurane[355,356] but not when nitrous oxide is combined with sevoflurane or desflurane.[219,220,238] Nitrous oxide 60% decreases the MAC of sevoflurane only 20% and that of desflurane 26% (Table 6-7).[339,340,357] The MAC response to tracheal intubation during sevoflurane anesthesia in children is also attenuated with nitrous oxide.[358] The explanation for the differential additivity effect of nitrous oxide in children remains unclear.

The MAC for xenon in middle-aged adults is about 70%.[359,360] The MAC of xenon in children has not been determined.

The MAC responses to stimuli other than skin incision have also been determined in children (Table 6-8). The MAC for tracheal intubation is 10% to 50% greater than the MAC for skin incision for halothane,[361,362] enflurane,[363] and sevoflurane,[358,364,365] whereas the MAC for tracheal extubation is 10% to 25% less than the MAC for skin incision for isoflurane,[366] desflurane,[367] and sevoflurane.[368,369] The MAC values for laryngeal mask airway insertion and removal during sevoflurane differ by 15%.[362,370] The MAC response to tracheal intubation during sevoflurane

**TABLE 6-7** Percent MAC Reduced in 2-Year-Olds with 60% Nitrous Oxide

| Agent | MAC with Oxygen (%) | MAC with 60% Nitrous Oxide | Percent MAC Reduced |
|---|---|---|---|
| Halothane | 0.91 | 0.37 | 65 |
| Desflurane | 8.67 | 6.4 | 26 |
| Sevoflurane | 2.5 | 2.0 | 20 |

From Gregory GA, Eger EI 2nd, Munson ES. The relationship between age and halothane requirements in man. Anesthesiology 1969;30:488-91; Taylor RH, Lerman J. Minimum alveolar concentration of desflurane and hemodynamic responses in neonates, infants, and children. Anesthesiology 1991;75:975-9; Lerman J, Sikich N, Kleinman S, Yentis S. The pharmacology of sevoflurane in infants and children. Anesthesiology 1994;80:814-24; Murray DJ, Mehta MP, Forbes RB, Dull DL. Additive contribution of nitrous oxide to halothane MAC in infants and children. Anesthesia Analgesia 1990;71:120-4; Fisher DM, Zwass MS. MAC of desflurane in 60% nitrous oxide in infants and children. Anesthesiology 1992;76:354-6.
*MAC*, Minimum alveolar concentration.

**TABLE 6-8** MAC Values in Children

| | MAC (%) | References |
|---|---|---|
| Tracheal intubation | Halothane: 1.33 | 361 |
| | Enflurane: 2.93 | 363 |
| | Sevoflurane: 2.69, 2.66, 2.83 | 342, 358, 364 |
| Tracheal extubation | Isoflurane: 1.4 | 366 |
| | Sevoflurane: 1.70, 2.3 | 368, 369 |
| | Desflurane: 7.7 | 367 |
| LMA insertion | Sevoflurane: 2.0 | 364 |
| LMA extubation | Sevoflurane 1.84 | 370 |
| | Desflurane (with 1-1.3 μg/kg Fentanyl) 3.56% | 1909 |
| Tracheal intubation/ skin incision ratio* | Halothane, enflurane, sevoflurane: 1.33 | Calculated from MAC data |
| MAC awake | Sevoflurane: 0.66 (2-5 years) and 0.43 (5-12 years) | 1910 |

*LMA*, Laryngeal mask airway; *MAC*, minimum alveolar concentration.
*Calculated using the above MAC data.

anesthesia in children is attenuated in the presence of adjuvants, such as clonidine (E-Table 6-1).[365] Conflicting evidence exists regarding the relative potencies of stereoisomers or enantiomers of chiral inhalational anesthetics.[371-373] Studies in animals suggest that the $(+)S$ optical enantiomer may be more potent than the $(-)R$ enantiomer, as evidenced by its ability to enhance potassium conductance in neurons.[371,372] In adults, the $(-)R$ enantiomer of isoflurane was nominally (17%) more potent than the $(+)S$ enantiomer.[373]

## Central Nervous System

All potent inhalational anesthetics depress the central nervous system (CNS), as evidenced by dose-dependent decreases in the cerebral vascular resistance and the cerebral metabolic rate for oxygen ($CMRO_2$). The decrease in vascular resistance causes a reciprocal increase in cerebral blood flow (CBF) that begins at approximately 0.6 MAC.[374] The extent of the increase in CBF, however, depends on the inhalational anesthetics: halothane > enflurane ~ desflurane > isoflurane > sevoflurane.[374-377] In adults, the cerebral vasculature remains responsive to $CO_2$ under general anesthesia but decreases with increasing MAC, disappearing at 1.5 MAC in the case of desflurane.[378] The net effect of inhalational anesthetics is a dose-dependent increase in the ratio of the CBF to $CMRO_2$.

The effects of inhalational anesthetics on the CNS in children have not been fully elucidated. Autoregulation of CBF does not appear to vary with age in children up to 1.5 MAC sevoflurane.[379,380] CBF velocity in children varies directly with the end-tidal $CO_2$ during halothane and isoflurane anesthesia.[381] CBF velocity increases as the concentrations of halothane[382] and desflurane[383] increase. Compared with halothane, however, sevoflurane does not increase CBF velocity, suggesting it may be the preferred anesthetic.[384] Based on current evidence, sevoflurane and isoflurane remain the preferred inhalational anesthetics for neuroanesthesia in children at low MAC values (less than 1 MAC) and in the presence of mild hyperventilation (see Chapter 24).

In children, the EEG activity during halothane anesthesia differs substantially from that of sevoflurane. In the case of halothane, the EEG is characterized by slow waves superimposed on fast rhythms (α and β waves), whereas in the case of sevoflurane, the EEG is characterized by mainly sharp slow waves.[385] Furthermore, the shift of power of the EEG from low (1 to 4 Hz) to medium frequencies (8 to 30 Hz) is greater for halothane than it is for sevoflurane. The clinical relevance of these EEG differences remains unclear at this time, but may explain in part the inconsistencies reported with processed EEG monitoring in children anesthetized with various inhalation anesthetics (see later discussion).

Enflurane was the first inhalational anesthetic to be associated with seizure activity both clinically and electroencephalographically in humans.[386,387] High concentrations of enflurane and a respiratory alkalosis were associated with seizure activity.

Both myoclonic movement of the extremities and transient spike and wave complexes on EEG have been reported during sevoflurane anesthesia in children.[385,388-391] Diffuse spike and wave complexes were noted on EEG at 5% and 7% inspired concentrations in two children with histories of epilepsy.[389] In a third child without a history of seizures, a 30-second burst of spike and wave complexes was recorded during sevoflurane anesthesia, but identified only after the event resolved.[392] The EEG data were analyzed in children who were premedicated with midazolam and then anesthetized with halothane or sevoflurane. There was no evidence of seizure activity.[385] Cortical epileptiform EEG activity has been reported during 1 to 2 MAC sevoflurane in adults with one episode of seizures that occurred with a $pCO_2$ of 34 mm Hg.[393] This prompted some to recommend limiting the depth of anesthesia with sevoflurane to minimize epileptiform EEG activity or even clinically evident seizure activity.[394] However, the co-administration of other anesthetic medications, such as midazolam, nitrous oxide, and opioids, may attenuate epileptiform EEG activity.[393] Furthermore, the notion of limiting the depth of sevoflurane anesthesia by reducing the concentration of sevoflurane as soon as the eyelash reflex is lost has not been shown to benefit children, and may actually increase the risk of awareness (see later discussion).

The association between myoclonic movement and seizures during induction of sevoflurane anesthesia remains tenuous. To prevent involuntary movements during induction, we recommend that the inspired concentration of sevoflurane be increased in a single stepwise manner from 0% to 8% (see Induction, earlier). If apnea occurs, ventilation should be assisted gently, while avoiding hyperventilation.

Awareness during inhalational anesthesia has been reported to occur with an incidence of 0.2% to 1.2% during sevoflurane anesthesia in children,[395-397] which exceeds that in adults. The reason(s) for this discrepancy remains unclear. These studies do suggest that children who experience awareness do not develop long-term sequelae.[398] Concerns over awareness during anesthesia has increased interest in the use of processed EEG monitoring in children.[399] Processed EEG monitoring during anesthesia has been evaluated using a number of EEG signals and techniques, processing signals in a "black box" and displaying a single numerical result. The most widely studied monitor to date is the BIS monitor, which displays the value on a scale between 0 and 100 (see Chapter 51). In adults, BIS readings below 60 are thought to be associated with a small risk of awareness and recall, whereas readings greater than 70 are associated with a large risk for awareness. The BIS value has been studied in children to a limited degree to date, but its validity and role in the anesthetic management of infants and children under 5 years of age remain in question. One concern is that the EEG algorithm in current BIS software is derived from adult EEG data, not from children. Despite use of an algorithm derived from adults, BIS measurements in children appear, for the most part, to track the depth of anesthesia, and these values correlate with the end-tidal concentration of the anesthetic. However, several unexplained curiosities have been reported. The BIS readings for halothane in children exceed those for isoflurane, desflurane, and sevoflurane at equipotent anesthetic concentrations.[255,256,400] This has been attributed to the differential effects of anesthetics on the EEG. The BIS readings for a specific sevoflurane concentration decreases with increasing ages.[252,255,401] The validity of processed EEG monitoring in children younger than 5 years has not been established. In children, the BIS values actually increased between 3% and 4% with sevoflurane, a paradoxical response to date unexplained.[401] A further concern is the enormous interindividual variability in processed EEG monitoring, making it difficult to define thresholds for awareness or lack thereof.[401] Interestingly, spontaneous ventilation increases the variability in the BIS readings.[402] The issue is further complicated by the fact that ketamine, nitrous oxide, and opioids do not depress the EEG in a dose-dependent manner. Discrepant BIS readings have been reported from the right and left sides of the brain[403] as well as in the prone position.[404] The BIS readings in children with cognitive impairment are reported to be 28 points less than those in unimpaired children at the same anesthetic concentration, although the authors failed to account for the reduced MAC in the impaired group.[405] Had they done so, the BIS readings may have been identical. The aggregate of this evidence undermines the validity of processed EEG monitoring in children.

### Cardiovascular System

Inhalational anesthetics (with the exception of xenon) affect the cardiovascular system either directly (by depressing myocardial contractility, altering the conduction system, or by dilating the peripheral vasculature) or indirectly (by affecting the balance of parasympathetic and sympathetic nervous systems and neurohumoral, renal, or reflex responses). The cardiovascular responses to inhalational anesthetics in children are further complicated by maturational changes in the cardiovascular system and its responsiveness to these anesthetics. When all of these developmental changes are taken into consideration there is a reduced margin of safety between adequate anesthesia and severe cardiopulmonary depression in infants and children compared with adults.

The salient features of the immature cardiovascular system in infants and children at both the macroscopic and microscopic levels have been reviewed.[406]

Assessment of cardiovascular variables in infants and children presents a challenge for clinicians. Although blood pressure (BP) and electrocardiography are standard monitors of hemodynamics in infants and children of all ages, measures of cardiac output and myocardial contractility are much more difficult to quantitate accurately. Two-dimensional echocardiography and impedance cardiometry have been used to estimate cardiac output and myocardial contractility in infants and children,[407-410] although the echocardiographic measurements are subject to variability depending on the preload and afterload. Load-independent derived echocardiographic variables (stress-velocity and stress-shortening indices) have improved the accuracy of echocardiographic estimates of myocardial function and are used with increasing frequency.[411] Transesophageal echocardiography is used much more frequently in children, although its use is limited to children with congenital heart disease undergoing cardiac surgery.

In children, several factors determine the BP responses to inhalational anesthetics, including the particular anesthetic studied, the dose, the presence of a premedication, the level of preoperative anxiety, and the systemic pressure measured: systolic, diastolic, or mean. Most studies demonstrate modest, dose-dependent decreases in BP with all of the inhalational anesthetics, although the magnitudes of the changes vary. In a direct comparison of sevoflurane and halothane, systolic BP decreased 7.5% at 1 MAC sevoflurane and 12.5% at 1 MAC halothane, but returned to awake values at 1.5 MAC with both anesthetics.[411] In children older than 1 year of age, systolic BP decreased 0% to 11% at 1 MAC sevoflurane, and 22% to 28% at 1 MAC desflurane, compared with awake values.[339,340] At 1 MAC, mean BP in children decreased 15% to 25% with isoflurane and sevoflurane.[408,410] All of the inhalational anesthetics (in concentrations up to 1.5 MAC) modestly depress the systemic BP in children.

Myocardial contractility decreases to a greater extent during halothane (up to 1.5 MAC) than during isoflurane or sevoflurane anesthesia, as evidenced by decreases in cardiac output and ejection fraction in healthy children.[409,410,412] Cardiac index decreased to similar extents with halothane and sevoflurane at 1 and 2 MAC: 10% at 1 MAC and 20% to 35% at 2 MAC.[410] Ejection fraction decreased 30% at 0.5 and 1.5 MAC halothane compared with awake values, but is unchanged at equipotent concentrations of isoflurane.[408] The addition of nitrous oxide to halothane or isoflurane in infants and small children depresses myocardial function to a similar extent as equipotent anesthetic concentrations of halothane or isoflurane in oxygen.[412] In children, halothane decreases myocardial contractility in a dose-dependent manner and to a greater extent than the ether anesthetics. Isoflurane and sevoflurane decrease myocardial contractility to a lesser extent than halothane and are preferred for children with limited cardiovascular reserves. IV atropine restores the decrease in myocardial function, in part, associated with halothane anesthesia,[412-415] whereas IV balanced salt solution restores the decrease in myocardial function associated with isoflurane anesthesia.[409]

The mechanism by which inhalational anesthetics depress myocardial function remains controversial. Studies in both animal and human myocardial cells suggest that halothane, isoflurane, and sevoflurane directly depress myocardial contractility by decreasing intracellular $Ca^{2+}$ flux. Inhalational anesthetics decrease the $Ca^{2+}$ flux by their action on the calcium channels themselves, ion exchange pumps, and the sarcoplasmic reticulum.[406] Evidence suggests that inhalational anesthetics attenuate contractility of ventricular myocytes via voltage-dependent L-type calcium channels (which are responsible for release of large amounts of calcium from the sarcoplasmic reticulum).[416,417]

That neonates and infants are more sensitive to the depressant actions of inhalational anesthetics than are older children is supported by experimental evidence of maturational differences between neonatal and adult rat, rabbit, and feline myocardium.[417-420] Structural differences that may account, in part, for the changes in myocardial sensitivity to inhalational anesthetics with age, include a reduction in contractile elements, immature sarcoplasmic reticulum, and functional differences in calcium sensitivity of the contractile elements, calcium channels, and the sodium-calcium pump in the neonatal myocardium.[406,416-418,420-423] The determinants of $Ca^{2+}$ homeostasis in neonatal ventricular myocardial cells depend on transsarcolemmic $Ca^{2+}$ flux to a far greater extent than on the sarcoplasmic reticulum.[406] This is based on a growing body of experimental evidence that includes the finding that the concentration of the $Na^+$-$Ca^{2+}$ exchange protein in the neonatal myocardium, a protein that regulates transsarcolemmic flux of $Ca^{2+}$, exceeds that in adult cells by 2.5-fold and that its concentration decreases with age as the concentration of L-type voltage-dependent calcium channels increases.[418] Furthermore, halothane reversibly inhibits the $Na^+$-$Ca^{2+}$ exchange protein in immature myocardial cells.[418] The sarcoplasmic reticulum is poorly developed in neonatal myocardial cells, and this finding weighs heavily against the sarcoplasmic reticulum being the major source of $Ca^{2+}$ required for myocardial contractility. Further research is required before the contribution of each aspect of $Ca^{2+}$ homeostasis to myocardial contractility in the neonate can be confirmed.

Ever since the introduction of halothane into clinical practice, clinicians have been aware of a greater incidence of hypotension and bradycardia in neonates who were anesthetized with halothane than in adults. However, this was not the case when *equipotent* concentrations (approximately 1 MAC) of halothane[337,414] were administered to neonates and older infants 1 to 6 months of age. Subsequent studies demonstrated that isoflurane,[424] sevoflurane,[340] and desflurane[339] all decreased systolic pressure in neonates to similar extents as in older infants 1 to 6 months of age. Interestingly, systolic BP decreased 30% in response to 1 MAC sevoflurane in neonates and infants 1 to 6 months of age, which was substantially greater than the 5% decrease in older infants and children up to 12 years of age.[340] In the case of desflurane, systolic BP decreased 30% in response to 1 MAC desflurane across all age groups.[339] These data suggest that systolic BP decreases up to 30% in response to 1 MAC of all inhalational anesthetics in infants and children, and that caution should be exercised when administering these anesthetics to infants and children who are at risk for hemodynamic instability, or in whom greater concentrations of inhaled anesthetics are required. On the basis of echocardiographic determinations, cardiac output and ejection fraction decrease in a dose-dependent fashion from awake to 1.5 MAC halothane and isoflurane in neonates and infants.[407] In a comparison of sevoflurane and halothane up to 1.5 MAC in infants, sevoflurane maintained cardiac index but decreased BP and systemic vascular resistance.[425] Myocardial contractility decreased in a dose-dependent manner with halothane as well as with sevoflurane, although the decrease with the former exceeded that with the latter.

The baroreceptor reflex response is also depressed in infants with either halothane[426] or isoflurane,[427] albeit to a greater extent with halothane. In view of the greater incidence of hypotension in neonates and infants than older children, an intact baroreceptor reflex could offset in part, the cardiovascular consequences. However, inhalational anesthetics blunt this response, leaving the infant vulnerable to the direct cardiodepressant actions of the anesthetics. Prophylactic anticholinergics augment the cardiac output by increasing the heart rate.

Two studies evaluated the effects of inhalational anesthesia on the hemodynamics of children with congenital heart disease undergoing cardiac surgery.[428,429] Sevoflurane maintained cardiac index and heart rate with less hypotension and negative inotropic effect than halothane. Isoflurane maintained cardiac index and ejection fraction, increased heart rate, and caused less depression of mean arterial pressure than halothane.[428] Sevoflurane was also associated with fewer episodes of severe hypotension and reduced need for vasopressors and chronotropes during emergence than halothane.[429]

Inhalational anesthetics also vary in their effect on cardiac rhythm. Halothane slows the heart rate, in some cases leading to junctional rhythms, bradycardia, and asystole. This response is dose dependent. Three mechanisms have been proposed to explain the genesis of halothane-associated dysrhythmias: a direct effect on the sinoatrial node, a vagal effect, or an imbalance in the parasympathetic and sympathetic tone. It has also been suggested that the etiology of the bradycardia during halothane anesthesia may be a withdrawal of sympathetic tone. Bradycardia is particularly marked in the neonate, presumably because parasympathetic influences predominate over the sparse sympathetic innervation of the myocardium in this age group. Junctional rhythms are also common during halothane anesthesia. Atrial or ventricular ectopic beats are rare, except in the presence of hypercapnia.[430] In infants and children anesthetized with halothane, 10 µg/kg atropine increases heart rate by 50% or more and promotes sinus rhythm.[431] This dose of atropine also increases BP in infants and children 2 years of age and older.

Halothane also sensitizes the myocardium to catecholamines, particularly in the presence of hypercapnia and "light anesthesia."[430] Halothane decreases the threshold for ventricular extrasystoles during epinephrine administration threefold.[432-434] In contrast, isoflurane, desflurane, and sevoflurane maintain or increase heart rate during the early induction period of anesthesia,* although a slowing of the heart rate has been reported during sevoflurane anesthesia. When bradycardia occurs in an anesthetized child, hypoxia must be considered first before other causes, such as a direct drug effect (i.e., high concentration of halothane). Isoflurane, desflurane, and sevoflurane do not sensitize the myocardium to catecholamines to the same extent as does halothane, and ventricular arrhythmias are rare.[432,433,438] The mechanism by which the sinus node controls automaticity is incompletely understood but may include K[+] currents, hyperpolarization-activated current, and T and L forms of Ca[2+] currents.[406] Moreover, developmental changes in these channels likely account, in part, for the differential effects of inhalational anesthetics on heart rate with age.[421]

Recent concerns of a relationship between inhalational anesthetics and prolonged QT interval that progressed to induce cardiac arrest or torsades de pointes have emerged. Although the

ether inhalational anesthetics prolong the QTc interval (with greater than 500 milliseconds being abnormal),[439,440] this alone appears to be insufficient to induce torsades de pointes. Torsades de pointes also requires the transmural dispersion of repolarization. This is defined as the variability in the rate of repolarization across the myocardium, from epi- to endocardium. The rate of repolarization may be estimated by the interval in the peak to end of the T wave on a 12-lead electrocardiogram. Evidence has demonstrated that the risk of torsades de pointes during sevoflurane anesthesia is minimal because the transmural dispersion of repolarization is limited.[441]

Paroxysmal increases in BP (both systolic and diastolic pressures) and heart rate have been reported in adults after a rapid increase in the inspired concentration of isoflurane or desflurane.[442] This occurs as a result of a massive sympathetic response, mediated by norepinephrine and/or epinephrine, that culminates in tachycardia and hypertension.[443,444] Further increases in the inspired concentration of the inciting anesthetic while attempting to attenuate the tachycardia and hypertension are ineffective and may perpetuate or augment the response. In order to restore vital signs to normal, the inciting anesthetic should be discontinued and replaced with another anesthetic. Repetitive small increases (1%) in the inspired concentration of the putative anesthetic produces transient but attenuated catecholamine bursts and cardiovascular responses compared with larger increases in concentration.[445,446] Fentanyl (2 µg/kg), esmolol, and clonidine have all been shown to be effective in preventing, attenuating, or eliminating these responses.[447-449] The origin of these responses is unknown, although the rapidity of the response points to the lung.[450] Others, however, dispute this notion, contending that two sites must be responsible for triggering the sympathetic discharge; the lung and the VRG,[451] with the latter mediating the greater response.[451,452] Neuroexcitatory responses have not been reported in children with isoflurane, desflurane, or sevoflurane.[453]

Xenon offers an immense advantage over the ether-based inhalational anesthetics in that it maintains circulatory stability. This anesthetic may have a niche role when anesthetizing infants and children with congenital and acquired heart disease. However, the effects of xenon on the hearts in children have not been studied. Although the MAC of xenon in adults is very large (see Table 6-3), MAC for xenon in children may be even greater. If the MAC exceeds the adult values, this may limit not only the dose that may be administered to children (e.g., much less than 1 MAC) but it may limit the inspired concentration of oxygen as well. Notwithstanding the MAC of xenon in children, this anesthetic will certainly be much less effective in children with cyanotic congenital heart disease, as it is the least soluble anesthetic and its large MAC restricts the MAC multiple that may be administered.

### Respiratory System

During spontaneous ventilation, both tidal volume and respiratory rate vary with the specific anesthetic, depth of anesthesia, and nociception. The increased respiratory rate during inhalational anesthesia in children has been attributed to sensitization of the stretch receptors within the lung as well as possible central effects. Inhalational anesthetics significantly affect respiration in infants and children in a dose-dependent fashion via effects on the respiratory center, chest wall muscles, and reflex responses. Halothane depresses minute ventilation by decreasing tidal volume and attenuating the response to carbon dioxide.[454-457]

---

*References 324, 339, 340, 408, 410, 424, 425, 435-437.

This depression is offset, in part, by an increase in the respiratory rate.[454,457] These ventilatory responses to halothane are age dependent; minute ventilation in infants decreases to a greater extent than in children.[456] In infants and young children anesthetized with halothane, intercostal muscle activity is attenuated before the diaphragm.[454,458] This effect is most pronounced in preterm and full-term neonates and infants, and when a tracheal tube is used in place of a laryngeal mask airway.[459] The movement of the chest and abdomen during the respiratory cycle is one of synchronized protrusion of the abdomen and collapse of the chest wall during inspiration (with some intercostal indrawing) and indrawing of the abdomen and flattening of the chest wall during expiration. This is commonly referred to as the "rocking horse" movement of the chest (similar to the phenomenon that occurs during upper airway obstruction in infants and children). This results in loss of FRC and is of particular concern in infants younger than 2 years of age who have decreased type I muscle fibers in both the diaphragm and intercostal muscles (see Fig. 12-11). This explains why infants fatigue easily and why positive end-expiratory pressure is useful in this age group. Isoflurane, enflurane, sevoflurane, and desflurane also depress ventilatory drive, decrease tidal volume, and attenuate the response to carbon dioxide.[455,457,460-466] The increase in respiratory frequency that follows respiratory depression (decreased tidal volume) may not restore minute ventilation to preanesthetic levels.

Sevoflurane depresses respiration to a similar extent as halothane up to 1.4 MAC but depresses respiration to a greater extent at concentrations greater than 1.4 MAC.[460] This results from a direct effect of sevoflurane on respiratory frequency.[463] Although respiratory effort may decrease rapidly during sevoflurane or desflurane anesthesia, their low blood solubilities and rapid washout profiles in part ensure that this is a self-limiting phenomenon during spontaneous respirations. Sevoflurane decreases the tone of the intercostal muscles to a lesser extent than halothane.[458,462] The compensatory changes in respiratory rate differ among the anesthetics; respiratory rate increases at 1.4 MAC or more with halothane, is unchanged with isoflurane, but decreases at 1.4 MAC or less with sevoflurane and enflurane.[455,457] This inadequate compensatory response to respiratory depression with sevoflurane and enflurane suggests that when children are anesthetized with those anesthetics, spontaneous ventilation must be monitored carefully to avoid hypopnea or apnea. Sevoflurane maintains or decreases airway resistance in children with normal airways, and those with asthma or a recent upper respiratory tract infection. Insertion of a tracheal tube during sevoflurane anesthesia increases airway resistance without sequelae.[467,468]

Desflurane depresses respiration in children during spontaneous respiration at greater than 1 MAC by decreasing tidal volume.[466] However, desflurane does increase airway resistance in children with asthma and respiratory tract infections to a greater extent than sevoflurane.[468] Desflurane is probably best avoided in these children.

Studies of the upper airway in children anesthetized with inhalational anesthesia have sought to explain the pathophysiology of airway obstruction. Sevoflurane at 1 MAC causes more upper airway obstruction than halothane.[469] In escalating doses between 0.5 and 1.5 MAC, sevoflurane decreased the cross-sectional area of the airway by one third, predominantly in the anteroposterior dimension.[470] This effect primarily results from pharyngeal wall collapse, which can be easily offset with positive end-expiratory pressure (see Chapter 12).

**TABLE 6-9** In Vivo Metabolism of Inhalational Anesthetics

| Inhalational Agent | Percent Metabolized | Reference |
|---|---|---|
| Methoxyflurane | 50 | 1911 |
| Halothane | 20 | 1912 |
| Sevoflurane | 5 | 486 |
| Enflurane | 2.4 | 1913 |
| Isoflurane | 0.2 | 1914 |
| Desflurane | 0.02 | 1915 |

## Renal System

Potent inhalational anesthetics may affect renal function via four possible mechanisms: cardiovascular, autonomic, neuroendocrine, and metabolic. Although the first three mechanisms pose no direct threat to renal function, the fourth mechanism, metabolic, is a serious clinical concern that has resulted in renal dysfunction after inhalational anesthesia.

Inhalational anesthetics are metabolized in vivo by the CYP isozyme system to varying extents (Table 6-9). Metabolism of inhalational anesthetics may release both inorganic and organic fluoride moieties.[471] It is the inorganic fluoride that is released from these ether anesthetics that has stimulated interest in renal dysfunction after inhalational anesthesia.

Isoflurane and desflurane undergo limited metabolism in vivo, resulting in very small plasma concentrations of inorganic fluoride, even after 131 MAC hours of isoflurane.[472] In contrast, halothane is metabolized to a substantially greater extent but releases most of the fluoride in an organic form, trifluoroacetate. Trifluoroacetate has, however, been linked to halothane hepatitis (see later discussion). The metabolism of enflurane, sevoflurane, and methoxyflurane yields greater plasma concentrations of inorganic fluoride than isoflurane. The metabolism of sevoflurane yields both inorganic and organic fluoride moieties.[473] The organic form, hexafluoroisopropanol, is rapidly conjugated and excreted by the kidneys[473] and poses no threat to humans. Peak plasma concentrations of inorganic fluoride after exposure to inhalational anesthetics follow a similar order to that in Table 6-9: methoxyflurane > sevoflurane > enflurane > isoflurane > halothane ~ = desflurane.[474-478] In the case of methoxyflurane, two metabolites are produced: inorganic fluoride and oxalic acid. Both were implicated in the pathogenesis of renal dysfunction, although, clinically, the renal injury was more consistently associated with inorganic fluoride.[479] Subsequent studies demonstrated that subclinical nephrotoxicity occurred after more than 2.5 MAC hours of methoxyflurane, provided the plasma concentration of inorganic fluoride exceeded 50 μmol/L; nephrotoxicity occurred after more than 5 MAC hours if the concentration of inorganic fluoride exceeded 90 μmol/L.[480] These clinical concerns led to the voluntary withdrawal of methoxyflurane from clinical practice.

In contrast to adults, renal dysfunction was not a feature after methoxyflurane anesthesia in children. The peak plasma concentrations of inorganic fluoride in children anesthetized with methoxyflurane were significantly less than in adults after an equivalent anesthetic exposure.[481] The reduced plasma concentrations of fluoride in children were attributed to several causes, including a decreased metabolism of methoxyflurane, greater uptake of fluoride by bone, increased excretion of fluoride ions, or a reduced renal sensitivity to fluoride.[481]

That the plasma concentrations of inorganic fluoride in children who were anesthetized with sevoflurane were similar to or greater than those after enflurane[482-484] raised concerns about possible renal dysfunction after prolonged exposure. However, inorganic fluoride concentrations after relatively brief anesthetics in children are similar to those in adults: less than 20 µmol/L after about 1 MAC hour, which decreases to less than 10 µmol/L by 4 hours after discontinuation of anesthesia.[465] Nonetheless, the peak plasma concentrations of inorganic fluoride paralleled the MAC hour exposure to sevoflurane in both children and adults.[484] Concerns regarding the risk of renal dysfunction after sevoflurane were heightened after reports that the peak plasma concentration of inorganic fluoride in some adults exceeded the purported threshold for nephrotoxicity (50 µmol/L).[485] Despite the high plasma concentrations of inorganic fluoride after sevoflurane anesthesia, there was no evidence of renal dysfunction. These reports, together with a dearth of evidence in the toxicology literature, suggested that fluoride-mediated nephrotoxicity may be independent of the plasma concentration of inorganic fluoride.

Kharasch and colleagues postulated that inhalational anesthetic-induced nephrotoxicity might be anesthetic specific. They determined that the primary isozyme responsible for the degradation of enflurane, isoflurane, sevoflurane, and methoxyflurane anesthetics was CYP450 2E1,[471,486-488] with secondary isozymes including CYP450 2A6 and 3A.[489] Subsequently, they reported large quantities of CYP450 2E1 not only within the liver, but also within the kidneys.[486] They also noted that the affinity of renal CYP450 2E1 for methoxyflurane was fivefold greater than it was for sevoflurane.[489] This provided further evidence that the renal dysfunction after ether inhalational anesthetics resulted from the local production of inorganic fluoride within the renal medulla rather than extrarenal production, and that certain anesthetics were more prone to release of inorganic fluoride than others (e.g., methoxyflurane much more so than sevoflurane). Because CYP450 2E1 has a greater affinity for methoxyflurane than sevoflurane, we now understand why renal dysfunction occurs after methoxyflurane and not after sevoflurane.[489] The lack of an association between sevoflurane, plasma inorganic fluoride concentration, and renal dysfunction in children and adults supports this new understanding of the mechanism of renal dysfunction after inhalational anesthesia. Consequently, the risk of renal dysfunction after sevoflurane is independent of the duration of exposure to sevoflurane. Sevoflurane does not pose any greater risk for perioperative renal disease than other maintenance anesthetics.[490] A second theoretical cause of sevoflurane-associated renal dysfunction is compound A, a product of alkaline hydrolysis of sevoflurane in the presence of carbon dioxide absorbents (see later discussion).

### Hepatic System
In vivo metabolism of inhalational anesthetics varies with age, increasing to adult values within the first 2 years of life. The developmental changes in metabolism may be attributed to several factors, including reduced activity of the hepatic microsomal enzymes, reduced fat stores, and more rapid elimination of inhalational anesthetics in infants and children compared with adults. Halothane, isoflurane, enflurane, sevoflurane, and desflurane have all been associated with postoperative liver dysfunction and/or liver failure in adults, although the relationship between sevoflurane and desflurane and liver dysfunction remains tenuous.[491-494] In children, halothane and sevoflurane have been associated with transient hepatic dysfunction.[495-498] Indeed, several pediatric cases of transient postoperative liver failure and one case of fulminant hepatic failure and death have

been attributed to "halothane hepatitis" that was confirmed serologically with antibodies to halothane-altered hepatic cell membrane antigens.[495] The exact mechanism of the hepatic dysfunction after halothane exposure remains unclear, although some clinicians have speculated that it is caused by an immunologic response to a metabolite of halothane. This putative toxic metabolite, a trifluoroacetyl halide compound, is produced during oxidative metabolism of halothane. It is thought that this compound induces an immunologic response in the liver by binding covalently to hepatic microsomal proteins, thereby forming an immunologically active hapten. A subsequent exposure to halothane then incites an immunologic response in the liver.[499] Hepatic enzymes may also be induced by previous administration of drugs, such as barbiturates, phenytoin, and rifampin. Although some have admonished clinicians for administering repeat anesthetics with halothane in children, it is our opinion that, in view of the millions of uneventful repeat halothane anesthetics in infants and children worldwide, insufficient evidence exists to support such an admonition.

## CLINICAL EFFECTS
### Induction Techniques
Although the physicochemical characteristics of the ether series of anesthetics would predict that anesthesia could be induced smoothly and more rapidly with these agents than with halothane,[308,310] this has not proved to be the case. All of the ether anesthetics (except sevoflurane) irritate the upper airway in children, resulting in a high incidence of breath holding, coughing, salivation, excitement, laryngospasm, and hemoglobin–oxygen desaturation.[435,500-509] Clinical studies with desflurane in children demonstrated a high incidence of breath holding, laryngospasm, and desaturation during inhalational induction (approximately 50%).[435,509] As a result, a "black box" warning was issued against the use of desflurane for induction of anesthesia in infants and children. Before the introduction of desflurane, some advocated inducing anesthesia in children with isoflurane.[502-506] For example, it has been suggested that the quality and speed of induction of anesthesia with isoflurane in oxygen in infants and children is similar to that with halothane.[503] However, airway reflexes were commonly triggered with isoflurane despite the use of a number of strategies to attenuate them,[507,509,510] including slowly increasing the inspired concentration, and scented masks. Given the smooth induction characteristics, economy, and availability of sevoflurane, there are no reasons to consider other anesthetics for induction of anesthesia in infants and children.

In contrast to the noxious effects of the methyl ethyl ether series of anesthetics on the airway, sevoflurane does not irritate the upper airway and is well tolerated when administered by mask to infants and children at any concentration.* The introduction of sevoflurane has challenged and displaced halothane as the induction agent of choice in children in most countries. The incidences of coughing, breath holding, laryngospasm, and hemoglobin–oxygen desaturation during induction with sevoflurane, whether by slow incremental increases in concentration or a single breath, are similar to those that occur during halothane (Table 6-10). The observation that the airway reflex responses are infrequent after a single-breath induction with 8% sevoflurane or 5% halothane casts doubt on the adage that high concentrations of inhalational anesthetics trigger airway reflex responses.[515-517] In fact, the induction is so smooth with sevoflurane that adjuvants,

---

*References 324, 328-330, 334, 340, 436, 511-515.

**TABLE 6-10** Problems during Induction: Sevoflurane versus Halothane

| | SEVOFLURANE | | | HALOTHANE | | | |
| Problem | No. with Problem | Total | % | No. with Problem | Total | % | References |
|---|---|---|---|---|---|---|---|
| Laryngospasm | 21 | 708 | 3.0 | 20 | 540 | 3.8 | 324, 328, 329, 436, 513, 524, 1916, 1917 |
| Breath holding | 39 | 649 | 6.0 | 46 | 445 | 10.3 | 324, 328, 512, 513, 1916 |
| Coughing | 20 | 477 | 4.2 | 21 | 254 | 8.3 | 324, 328, 329, 340, 514, 1918 |
| Induction excitement | 38 | 375 | 10.1 | 9 | 211 | 4.3 | 324, 328, 513, 1918 |
| Bronchospasm | 2 | 544 | 0.4 | 2 | 379 | 0.5 | 324, 328, 1916 |
| Emergence excitement | 20 | 239 | 8.4 | 51 | 368 | 13.9 | 327, 328, 537, 1917, 1918 |

such as a premedication, concurrent use of nitrous oxide, or other strategies to prevent airway reflex responses, are unnecessary.

Induction of anesthesia with xenon has not been studied in children. In adults, inhalational induction with xenon at equi-MAC with sevoflurane resulted in a more rapid induction with stability of respirations with xenon.[518] These data suggest that xenon may be an excellent induction anesthetic in children, provided its characteristics are upheld in well-designed clinical trials.

There is no single ideal approach to induce anesthesia by inhalation for all children. However, we advocate empowering children as much as possible to minimize fear. After appropriate preoperative preparation (involving premedication or parental presence or distraction techniques), the child is seated on the bed and encouraged to breathe through a face mask scented with a favorite flavor (to disguise the plastic odor of the mask) that is held over the nose and mouth. A fresh gas composed of 70% nitrous oxide in oxygen is breathed (while the pop-off value is completely open for 1 to 2 minutes). As soon as the child becomes "silly" or ceases to respond verbally, 8% sevoflurane is administered. Induction of anesthesia with halothane was performed with stepwise increments in the inspired concentration of 0.5% to 1.0% every three to four breaths until an adequate depth of anesthesia was achieved. This slow increase in the inspired concentration of halothane was thought to attenuate the incidence of airway reflex responses, although this is not evidence based. In fact, when a single breath vital capacity induction was performed in children older than 6 years of age with 5% halothane, the incidence of airway reflex responses was surprisingly small.[515] Initially, sevoflurane was also administered in slow increments of 1% to 1.5% until 8%, but this caused transient agitation and involuntary movement of the extremities, frequently and sometimes violently, particularly in adolescents.[340] This was attributed to an exaggerated excitement phase. To minimize the excitement phase, we recommend that the inspired concentration of sevoflurane be increased as rapidly as possible, from 0% to 8% in a single-step increase.[515] This is based on a study of single-breath induction with 8% sevoflurane and 5% halothane in which the incidence of involuntary movement and need for restraint was significantly less with sevoflurane than it was with halothane.[515] Recently, induction of anesthesia with 12% sevoflurane was reported to be more rapid than with 8%.[519] This is not a surprising finding, although 12% sevoflurane vaporizers should not be used in clinical practice because inspired concentrations of sevoflurane (in a laboratory setting) of 11% in oxygen and 10% in nitrous oxide support combustion.

Although some studies report more rapid induction of anesthesia with sevoflurane than with halothane, others have not. This inconsistency in the relative speed of induction reflects differences in study design that likely failed to take advantage of the 8% sevoflurane vaporizer and the differences in MAC. For children who are unable to perform a single-breath vital capacity induction, a rapid increase in the inspired concentration of sevoflurane has been a very effective alternative, with results comparable to the single-breath technique.[329,513-515]

Sevoflurane does not trigger airway reflex responses either alone or in combination with other agents, such as nitrous oxide. One study suggested that sevoflurane is the least irritating to the airway of all the inhalational anesthetics.[520] Previous studies suggested that airway irritability and excitement during sevoflurane anesthesia were similar whether nitrous oxide was present or absent, although others have disputed these findings.[515,521] The lack of effect of nitrous oxide on the speed of induction in the single-breath study was attributed to its concentration-reducing effect on sevoflurane.[515]

Although halothane has been the preferred agent for induction of anesthesia because of its lack of airway irritability, arrhythmias occur more frequently during halothane than during anesthesia with the ether anesthetics. Halothane-induced arrhythmias occur more frequently during spontaneous ventilation and in association with high levels of circulating catecholamines. Most of these arrhythmias are unifocal or multifocal premature ventricular beats, nodal rhythm, bigeminy, or supraventricular arrhythmias.[330,430,508] Despite their appearance, most of these arrhythmias are benign and preserve the blood pressure; ventricular tachycardia, however, may cause hypotension. Management of arrhythmias during halothane anesthesia includes inflating the lungs with large tidal volumes, hyperventilation to decrease the arterial carbon dioxide tension, increasing the concentration of halothane if there is evidence of "light" anesthesia (i.e., sweating, hypertension), and substituting another inhalational anesthetic for halothane.[430,522] Lidocaine has no role in the treatment of these arrhythmias because the myocardium is not intrinsically irritable. Moreover, a rapid IV bolus of lidocaine (2 mg/kg) may cause profound bradycardia.[523] Arrhythmias are rare during anesthesia with the ether series of anesthetics, but when they occur they are usually nodal in origin.* Arrhythmias during anesthesia with the ether anesthetics are usually self-limiting, resolving spontaneously or with parenteral administration of an anticholinergic. If the arrhythmias persist, then a cardiology consultation should be sought, particularly in a child with a history of congenital heart disease. Both IV and inhalational anesthetics have been used for induction and maintenance of anesthesia in children with congenital heart disease. (See cardiovascular section earlier and Chapter 21 for a more detailed discussion.)

---

*References 330, 426, 427, 505, 508, 515, 524.

Once an adequate depth of anesthesia has been achieved, it is prudent to maintain spontaneous respirations with the maximal inspired concentration of sevoflurane that is tolerated until IV access has been achieved. If hypopnea or apnea occurs, then ventilation should be assisted while avoiding hypocapnia. The reason to recommend this practice is to prevent awareness from occurring in the early induction period.[395,396] Discontinuing or decreasing the inspired concentration of nitrous oxide or sevoflurane individually or together may predispose to awareness, particularly if the child is stimulated at a light plane of anesthesia. This may occur in situations where anesthesia is induced in one location (induction room) and the child is then transferred to another (operating room) without continuously supplying sevoflurane. Appreciating the limited solubility of nitrous oxide and sevoflurane will help to understand how rapidly these anesthetics egress from the body, particularly after a brief exposure. Once IV access is established, some practitioners administer propofol or another IV anesthetic before discontinuing the nitrous oxide to facilitate insertion of a laryngeal mask airway or tracheal intubation. The concentration of sevoflurane can then be decreased.

### Emergence

Emergence or recovery has been arbitrarily divided into early (extubation, eye opening, following commands) and late (drinking, discharge time from postanesthesia care unit or hospital). Although most studies have demonstrated a more rapid early recovery after less soluble anesthetics,[326-328,331,334] few have demonstrated a more rapid late recovery.[324,334,524,525]

The speed of emergence and recovery from anesthesia are discussed above. The incidence of complications, such as airway reflex responses and vomiting during emergence from anesthesia, after mask anesthesia or tracheal intubation, are similar with most inhalational agents.* However, the incidence of airway responses of any severity after desflurane were significantly greater than after isoflurane. Moreover, the incidence of airway adverse responses after removing a laryngeal mask airway (LMA) deep during desflurane anesthesia was significantly greater than was the incidence after removal of an LMA following recovery from desflurane (awake) or after isoflurane anesthesia.[527]

### Emergence Delirium

*Emergence delirium* is defined as a dissociated state of consciousness in which children are inconsolable, irritable, uncompromising, and/or uncooperative (see Videos 46-1, 46-2).[528,529] Children experiencing emergence delirium often demand that all monitors, IV lines, and bandages be removed and that they be dressed in their own clothing. Many of these children fail to recognize and respond appropriately to their parents. Parents who witness this transient state usually volunteer that this behavior is unusual and uncustomary for their child. The core behaviors identified as being associated with emergence delirium after anesthesia in children include nonpurposeful action, and averting eyes or staring.[530]

Emergence delirium is not a new phenomenon, having been reported after the introduction of almost every new anesthetic, including most inhalational anesthetics,† and IV agents, including midazolam, remifentanil, and propofol.[533,534] The incidence of emergence delirium after inhalational anesthesia in children ranges from 2% to 80%.[327,328,331,525,528]

The prevalence of emergence delirium depends on several factors, including the choice of inhalational anesthetic, age of the child, adjuvant medications, presence of pain, and the scale used for diagnosis.[528,529] The prevalence of emergence delirium is similar after desflurane, sevoflurane, and isoflurane, but less after halothane anesthesia.[535,536] The greatest incidence of emergence delirium occurs in children 1 to 5 years of age.[528,537] Fortunately, these episodes usually last only 10 to 20 minutes and resolve spontaneously without sequelae. The mechanism by which emergence delirium occurs remains unknown.

Emergence delirium has been reported in adults as well as infants, although the incidence is much less in both age groups than in children. Diagnosing emergence delirium after anesthesia and surgery has been complicated by our inability to distinguish it from pain. In one study, ketorolac decreased the incidence of emergence delirium threefold to fourfold after myringotomy with either halothane or sevoflurane anesthesia.[526] Because ketorolac does not sedate children, it is likely that pain was confused with emergence delirium. Subsequent studies in children demonstrated that emergence delirium occurs after sevoflurane anesthesia even in the presence of neuraxial blocks.[528,537] The frequency of delirium is independent of the speed of awakening from anesthesia,[538,539] the duration of a deep level of anesthesia,[540] the duration of general anesthesia,[541] and the presence of parents.[536]

The definitive study regarding the incidence of emergence delirium was undertaken in healthy children who required anesthesia for magnetic resonance imaging (MRI) and who did not undergo surgery.[536] The incidence of emergence delirium was twofold greater after sevoflurane than it was after halothane.

However, in most published studies, the metric used to diagnose emergence delirium had not been validated. To address this deficiency, the Pediatric Anesthesia Emergence Delirium (PAED) scale was developed.[529] The threshold PAED score to diagnose emergence delirium was thought to be greater than 10 but more recently a value greater than 12 was suggested.[542] When the PAED scale was compared with two nonvalidated scales,[542] the three appeared to be comparable, although the comparison was biased because the PAED scale was assessed first, followed by the other two scales (Table 6-11).

Pharmacologic interventions to treat emergence delirium were recently summarized in a meta-analysis.[543] Effective inter-

---

**TABLE 6-11** Development and Psychometric Evaluation of the Pediatric Anesthesia Emergence Delirium Scale

1. The child makes eye contact with the caregiver.
2. The child's actions are purposeful.
3. The child is aware of his/her surroundings.
4. The child is restless.
5. The child is inconsolable.

Items 1, 2, and 3 are reverse scored as follows: 4 = not at all, 3 = just a little, 2 = quite a bit, 1 = very much, 0 = extremely. Items 4 and 5 are scored as follows: 0 = not at all, 1 = just a little, 2 = quite a bit, 3 = very much, 4 = extremely. The scores of each item were summed to obtain a total Pediatric Anesthesia Emergence Delirium (PAED) scale score. The degree of emergence delirium increased directly with the total score.
From Sikich N, Lerman J. Development and psychometric evaluation of the pediatric anesthesia emergence delirium scale. Anesthesiology 2004;100:1138-45.

---

*References 327-329, 331, 427, 502, 503, 525, 526.
†References 323, 324, 327, 331, 526, 531-533.

ventions included fentanyl,[544] ketamine,[545] a propofol infusion or a bolus at the end of anesthesia, clonidine,[546,547] and dexmedetomidine.[548] In contrast, a single dose of propofol at induction of anesthesia, midazolam, and flumazenil were not effective.[543,549-553] Additional studies using assessment with a validated delirium scale are needed to clarify the contribution of anesthetics to emergence delirium during pain-free surgery.

### Neuromuscular Junction

All inhalational anesthetics potentiate the actions of nondepolarizing muscle relaxants[554-556] and decrease neuromuscular transmission,[557] the latter, however, only at increased concentrations. The mechanism of the reduced neuromuscular transmission is unknown but is likely attributable to actions of these anesthetics at the synaptic junction rather than PK or CNS effects. The potentiation of action of nondepolarizing relaxants follows the order: isoflurane ~ desflurane ~ sevoflurane > enflurane > halothane > nitrous oxide–opioid technique.[554,558] However, this potentiation may depend on the type of nondepolarizing relaxant studied (longer-acting relaxants are affected to a greater extent than intermediate-acting relaxants)[554,555,559] and the concentration of anesthetic (reduced concentrations may yield small or no differences between anesthetics, whereas greater concentrations may demonstrate substantive differences).[555] In two parallel studies of atracurium infusions in children,[559,560] halothane and isoflurane decreased the atracurium requirements similarly in the first, whereas enflurane markedly decreased the requirements compared with halothane in the second. These observations suggest that inhalational anesthetics potentiate intermediate-acting relaxants as they do long-acting relaxants.

### Malignant Hyperthermia

All potent inhalational anesthetics, except xenon,[561] trigger malignant hyperthermia (MH) reactions in susceptible adults and children.[562-571] Studies indicate that the relative capabilities of the four inhalational anesthetics to augment caffeine-induced contractures in MH-susceptible muscle in vitro are halothane > enflurane > isoflurane > methoxyflurane.[572] Using the surrogate marker of the time interval from administration of anesthesia until a reaction was detected to estimate the relative potency of the modern anesthetics to trigger MH, the order was halothane > sevoflurane > isoflurane ~ enflurane.[573] Currently, all inhalational anesthetics should be avoided in children who are MH susceptible (see Chapter 40).

The wash-out of inhalational anesthetics from anesthetic machines before anesthetizing a child with MH requires an understanding of the PK of these anesthetics in the specific anesthetic workstation. See Chapter 40 for a full discussion.

### Stability and Toxicology of Breakdown Products

Inhalational anesthetics may be degraded via several pathways in the presence of most $CO_2$ absorbents to form several potentially toxic byproducts. Enflurane, isoflurane, and desflurane (but not halothane and sevoflurane) react with desiccated soda lime to produce carbon monoxide. Halothane and sevoflurane react with soda lime to yield several organic compounds that are potentially organ toxic. In contrast, xenon is completely inert with $CO_2$ absorbents, thereby posing no risk from the genesis of metabolites or degradation products in humans.

Two strategies to address the clinical risks associated with the degradation of ether inhalational anesthetics are molecular sieves[574] and new $CO_2$ absorbents.[575-579] While molecular sieves were thought to have great promise, they have not reached the market for clinical use. In contrast, a number of new $CO_2$ absorbents have been developed to absorb $CO_2$ from the breathing circuit without degrading inhalational anesthetics to carbon monoxide and compound A (E-Table 6-2).[575,576] The previous generation of $CO_2$ absorbents differed in their composition and, therefore, in their affinity to degrade inhalational anesthetics. Soda lime contained 95% calcium hydroxide, either sodium or potassium hydroxide, and the balance as water. Baralyme, which is no longer available, contained 80% calcium hydroxide, 20% barium hydroxide, and the balance as water. E-Table 6-2 compares the compositions of the older with the newer $CO_2$ absorbents, which do not contain a strong base. Most recently, Amsorb Plus and Drägersorb Free were formulated for minimal degradation of inhalational anesthetics, as well as to address efficient $CO_2$ absorption.[580]

Carbon monoxide may be produced when a methyl ethyl ether inhalational anesthetic is incubated with a desiccated $CO_2$ absorbent (most commonly soda lime or Baralyme). The absorbent within a $CO_2$ canister may become desiccated if dry fresh gas flows through the canister at a rate sufficient to remove most of the moisture (i.e., more than 5 L/min continuously through the absorbent canister for 24 hours or longer while it is not in service). If the circuit reservoir bag is detached from the canister while fresh gas is flowing, then fresh gas may flow retrograde through the canister and exit primarily where the reservoir bag is normally placed. This cannot occur in anesthetic machines in which the fresh gas enters distal to the inspiratory flow valve. If the fresh gas flows retrograde through the canister for a sufficient time, it desiccates the absorbent and increases the risk of degradation of subsequently administered inhalational anesthetics. If one of the methyl ethyl ether inhalational agents (desflurane, isoflurane, or enflurane) is administered through a desiccated absorbent, carbon monoxide may be generated.[579,581,582] The magnitude of the carbon monoxide production for a specific absorbent follows the order: desflurane = enflurane > isoflurane >> halothane = sevoflurane. Other factors that determine the magnitude of the carbon monoxide concentration produced include the concentration of the inhalational agent, the dryness of the absorbent, the type of absorbent (Baralyme > soda lime > newer absorbents), and the temperature of the absorbent.[581] As the newer absorbents reflect, the removal of the strong alkalis, NaOH and KOH, which are essential for the production of carbon monoxide, virtually eliminates this risk (E-Table 6-3).[583]

Small concentrations of carbon monoxide (up to 18 ppm) have been detected in children who were anesthetized with desflurane or sevoflurane using fresh carbon dioxide absorbent that includes KOH and NaOH.[584] Carbon monoxide concentration correlated well with the fresh gas flow to minute ventilation ratio (less than 0.68) and weakly with the type of anesthetic agent (desflurane) and age.[584] Carbon monoxide has been detected in concentrations up to 3 ppm during and after anesthesia, even spinal anesthesia.[585] One may question whether a minimum fresh gas flow with desflurane and other nonsevoflurane anesthetics is warranted. The presence of carbon monoxide in the exhaled breath has been attributed to heme metabolism, inflammation, and sepsis, although the authors did not use fresh soda lime in their breathing circuits.[585]

Carbon monoxide is not detectable by any freestanding anesthetic agent analyzers, pulse oximetry, or blood gas analyzers (with the exception of co-oximeters), although it is detectable by mass spectrometry. A carbon monoxide analyzer is currently marketed for use during anesthesia. The solution to this problem is prevention: turn off the anesthetic machine at the end of the day, disconnect the fresh gas hose to the absorbent canister, always have the reservoir bag connected to the canister, and avoid passing desflurane, enflurane, and isoflurane through a desiccated absorbent. Others have suggested that high-flow anesthesia should be avoided whenever a circle circuit is used to prevent inadvertent desiccation of absorbent. If the absorbent is desiccated, some have suggested "rehydrating" the absorbent, although this, too, is fraught with potential problems (including clumping of the absorbent).[586] If there is suspicion that the absorbent is desiccated, we strongly recommend replacing the absorbent before introducing an inhalational anesthetic. Alternatives to conventional absorbents, such as the molecular sieve and the newer absorbents, may very well obviate degradation of the ether anesthetics, provided the absorbent is not dessicated.[575,576,578,579] When methyl ethyl ether anesthetics are incubated with desiccated Amsorb, carbon monoxide is not produced, although it may be produced with other desiccated absorbents (see E-Table 6-3).[575,576,579] The incidence of carbon monoxide poisoning during anesthesia remains extremely rare even when soda lime is used as the absorbent. In contrast, the potential for carbon monoxide poisoning is zero if Amsorb or one of the absorbents that does not include strong metal alkali is used.

Halothane is degraded in the presence of carbon dioxide absorbents to the unsaturated vinyl compound, 2-bromochloroethylene, which is lethal in mice.[587] Although 2-bromochloroethylene is potentially nephrotoxic, it poses very little risk in humans, even under low flow conditions, because its maximal concentration in the circuit is less than 3% of its lethal concentration.[588]

Sevoflurane is both absorbed and degraded via the Cannizzaro reaction in the presence of absorbent, resulting in five degradation products.[589,590] Although the degradation of sevoflurane by the absorbent was initially posited to delay its wash-in, evidence suggests that this effect is trivial.[591] Of the five degradation products produced when sevoflurane is degraded in either soda lime or Baralyme, compounds A and B appear in the greatest concentrations. Compound A, fluoromethyl-2,2-difluoro-1-(trifluoromethyl)vinyl ether (also known as PIFE), is nephrotoxic in rats at concentrations of 100 ppm or greater, and has a lethal concentration ($LC_{50}$) of 1100 ppm. Compound B, a methoxyethyl ether compound that is minimally volatile at room temperature, is present in closed circuits at less than 5 ppm and poses no serious risk to animals or humans. The remaining three metabolites, compounds C, D, and E, are present in such low concentrations in the breathing circuit that they are inconsequential. In a low-flow closed circuit model with an inspired concentration of 2.5% sevoflurane, the concentration of compound A peaks at 20 to 40 ppm after several hours of anesthesia.[591-595] In children, compound A concentrations reach 16 ppm after 5.6 MAC hours of sevoflurane in a semi-closed circuit with 2 L/min fresh gas flow.[596] Factors that are known to increase the production of compound A include an increase in the inspired concentration of sevoflurane, Baralyme greater than soda lime, and an increase in the temperature of the absorbent.[590,591] The newer formulation of $CO_2$ absorbents degrade sevoflurane to a lesser degree compared with the previous absorbents (see E-Table 6-2 and E-Table 6-3). As in the case of carbon monoxide production, monovalent bases are important ingredients for the degradation of sevoflurane to compound A and their absence reduced the extent of degradation of sevoflurane.[577,583,597] In rats under low flow

conditions, compound A is nephrotoxic.[598-600] In contrast, studies in humans have been far from conclusive.[592-594,601] Commonly used indicators, such as albuminuria, have yielded inconsistent evidence of renal dysfunction.[592-595,601] One mechanism to explain compound A–induced nephrotoxicity is the β-lyase–dependent metabolism to nephrotoxic fluorinated compounds. However, this has been the subject of intense debate.[602,603] If compound A–associated nephrotoxicity were proven to depend on the β-lyase metabolic pathway, the limited concentration of this enzyme system in the renal cytoplasm and mitochondria of humans would make nephrotoxicity an unlikely outcome. Indeed, the inconsistency in the evidence of nephrotoxicity associated with compound A between rats and humans has been attributed to an 8- to 30-fold greater concentration of β-lyase in rats compared with that in humans.[604] To date, there have been no complications related to compound A and kidney damage in humans.

At the present time, sevoflurane is the only inhalational agent for which authorities have recommended a minimum fresh gas flow when it is administered in a closed circuit with soda lime or Baralyme. The minimal fresh gas flow is 2 L/min, although this has been adopted in a limited number of countries.

## Nitrous Oxide

Nitrous oxide confers several properties that differ substantively from the potent inhalational anesthetics that merit consideration. Nitrous oxide has a very limited solubility in blood, $\lambda_{blood/gas}$ being 0.47. The MAC for nitrous oxide is 104% in adults; MAC has not been determined in children. Its chemical structure is N–N–O.

Nitrous oxide diffuses into gas cavities that are filled with nitrogen more rapidly than nitrogen egresses because it is 34 times more soluble in blood than nitrogen ($\lambda_{blood/gas}$ for nitrogen 0.014). Consequently, the volume of the cavity expands. However, the magnitude of the increase in the volume of the cavity depends, in part, on the concentration of nitrous oxide administered, as determined by the formula $100/(100 - \%N_2O)$. The rate at which the cavity expands also depends on the source of the blood supply: those cavities in which the blood supply decreases as the volume of the cavity increases (e.g., a loop of obstructed bowel) will expand slower and to a smaller overall volume than a cavity in which the blood supply is independent of the cavity volume (e.g., a pneumothorax). By using a model of these conditions the time to double the volume of a loop of obstructed bowel with nitrous oxide was estimated to be 120 minutes, whereas the time to double the volume of a pneumothorax was one tenth, or 12 minutes.[605] Any gas-filled cavities within the body are vulnerable for expansion if nitrous oxide is administered, including obstructed bowel,[605] pneumothorax, gas cavities within the eye, endotracheal tube cuffs,[606] laryngeal mask airways,[607,608] bubbles in veins,[609] and pneumoencephalography.[610] Theoretically, nitrous oxide should be avoided during laparoscopic surgery, to avoid expanding $CO_2$ bubbles that reach the venous circulation (see Chapter 27).

Inhalational anesthetics confer a very low risk for postoperative nausea and vomiting. In contrast, nitrous oxide is considered to be an emetogenic anesthetic. In a large meta-analysis of the impact of nitrous oxide on the incidence of postoperative nausea and vomiting in adults, the authors determined that for emetogenic surgery, eliminating nitrous oxide was salutary (number needed to treat of six) whereas for nonemetogenic surgery there was no benefit from omitting nitrous oxide.[611] Hence, avoiding nitrous oxide in surgery that is emetogenic is reasonable. However, the authors of that study also reported that the number needed to harm, in the form of intraoperative awareness when nitrous oxide was omitted from the anesthetic, was 46, or more than 2%! Hence, omitting nitrous oxide from the anesthetic prescription requires very careful consideration, assessment, and monitoring for awareness.

A number of studies investigated the contribution of nitrous oxide to postoperative vomiting in children. Although there is some evidence that avoiding nitrous oxide reduces the incidence of postoperative vomiting in children,[612] the preponderance of evidence shows no benefit.[613-617] In part, this may be attributed to the multiplicity of factors that contribute to postoperative vomiting, as well as the salutary effects of other factors, such as the use of propofol and/or antiemetics. In none of the studies in which nitrous oxide was omitted in children was awareness reported.

The inclusion of nitrous oxide in remifentanil-propofol anesthesia in children has been associated with a reduction in postoperative hyperalgesia.[618]

## Environmental Impact

Currently, the National Institute for Occupational Safety and Health (NIOSH) recommendations limit the chronic exposure to nitrous oxide to 25 ppm and to inhalational anesthetics to 10 ppm. The basis for these recommendations is uncertain but may be attributed to the risk of teratogenicity and end-organ dysfunction. In pediatric anesthesia, mask anesthesia and/or uncuffed tracheal tubes and laryngeal mask airways in children leak inhalational anesthetics into the environment. As a result there is local exposure to inhaled anesthetics during anesthesia in children that should be considered.

Concern over the pollution of the stratosphere and ozone layer depletion by polyhalogenated anesthetics has raised further questions for the long-term use of these agents and the need to fully recycle or adsorb the waste gases.[619] The polyhalogenated compounds are produced in extremely low concentrations; and although they have a high molecular weight, atmospheric winds likely facilitate their transfer to the stratosphere, where they do harm to the ozone layer. However, the most compelling data of their limited impact on the environment relate to their half-lives. The half-lives of these polyhalogenated anesthetics in the stratosphere are approximately 5 years. Contrast these to nitrous oxide, a compound with a very small molecular weight (in comparison with potent inhalational anesthetics), which is administered in high concentrations (50% to 70%) and which has a half-life in the stratosphere of 120 years! Nitrous oxide is a known greenhouse gas and depletes the ozone layer. The case for banning the polyhalogenated anesthetics pales in comparison with the enormous potential environmental impact of nitrous oxide. Although nitrous oxide is a serious greenhouse pollutant, agriculture and industry account for the vast majority of the nitrous oxide released into the atmosphere, with medical sources accounting for a trivial, unidentified fraction.[620] Highly efficient scrubbers and absorbers are being developed to prevent atmospheric pollution and recycle expensive anesthetics (e.g., xenon) but their use remains experimental at this time. To preserve the ozone layer, all anesthetic practices should limit the fresh gas flow and concentration of polyhalogenated anesthetics and nitrous oxide.

## Oxygen

The concentration of oxygen for each anesthetic should be carefully titrated to the child's needs. Requirements are monitored by inspired oxygen concentration measurement, oxygen-hemoglobin saturation (pulse oximetry), and arterial blood gas determinations. Oxygen is often liberally administered in excess of the child's metabolic needs. However, potential dangers in this excess should be noted,[621] particularly in two areas: (1) Pulmonary oxygen toxicity is well documented; despite the fact that it develops slowly, general recommendations are to use an air/oxygen combination for prolonged procedures when nitrous oxide is contraindicated.[622] (2) Of additional concern is the remote possibility of adverse effects on the immature neonatal retina leading to retinopathy of prematurity (ROP).[623-634] Several cases of ROP have been reported in infants whose only known exposure to supplemental oxygen occurred in the OR; it should be noted that no new cases related to OR management have been reported since 1981![635,636] Many factors contribute to the development of ROP; it has been reported in children with cyanotic congenital heart disease, infants not exposed to exogenous oxygen, and even in stillborn infants.[637,638] A possible relationship of the development of ROP to arterial carbon dioxide variations, hypercarbia, hypotension, candida sepsis, inflammatory response, red blood cell transfusions, corticosteroid therapy, duration of ventilation, elevated blood glucose values, low gestational age, chronic lung disease, a deficiency of insulin-like growth factor, and vascular endothelial growth factor, as well as hypoxemia and fluctuating levels of oxygen, have all been suggested.[639-659] Other factors, such as exogenous bright light, maternal diabetes, maternal chorioamnionitis, and maternal antihistamine use within 2 weeks of delivery, have been found to be risk factors; the evidence for vitamin E deficiency is less convincing.[660-663] The possibility of a genetic predisposition, that is, a genetic polymorphism altering control of neovascularization, has also been proposed.[653,664-666] The use of continuous transcutaneous oxygen tension monitoring was not found to reduce the risk of ROP in infants weighing less than 1000 g, compared with controls.[667] It appears the major risk factor for developing ROP is extreme prematurity; *oxygen therapy represents only part of this complex problem.*[626,627,629] The incidence of ROP is predominantly limited to infants weighing 1000 g or less, but it is a concern in infants with a birth weight less than 1500 g born at less than 28 weeks gestation.[668-670] It should be noted that new treatments may involve systemic administration of propranolol (improves neovascularization) and intravitreal injections of anti–vascular endothelial growth factors are being examined; both these treatments may have anesthetic implications.[671,672] The evidence implicating hyperoxia as contributing to the development of ROP must be recognized but placed in perspective. Although it was thought that tight control of oxygen saturation and minimizing exposure to exogenous oxygen would reduce the incidence of ROP,[673] a multicenter study, the Supplemental Therapeutic Oxygen Prethreshold Retinopathy of Prematurity study (STOP-ROP), failed to support that hypothesis.[674] In fact, the conclusion reached stated, *"Although the relative risk–benefit of supplemental oxygen for each infant must be individually considered, clinicians need no longer be concerned that supplemental oxygen, as used in this study, will exacerbate active prethreshold ROP."*[674] This study suggests that anesthesiologists should take practical precautions to protect an infant's retinas from hyperoxemia without unnecessarily endangering the infant. No comprehensive epidemiologic studies have yet examined anesthetic risk factors, but, given the many cofactors that are associated with this entity, it appears that anesthesia management, although very important, is a small piece of this puzzle.

Bearing in mind the possible role of hyperoxia and hypercarbia, intraoperative management must include careful monitoring of inspired oxygen and expired carbon dioxide concentrations. Maintaining the oxygen saturation at 93% to 95% results in a $PaO_2$ of approximately 70 mm Hg, with values exceeding 80 mm Hg on occasion.[628,675,676] Unfortunately, individual oximeters may vary considerably in terms of their accuracy, so practitioners must be familiar with their equipment.[677] The use of air blended with oxygen can be used to further reduce the inspired oxygen concentration. A transport system equipped with an air–oxygen blender is desirable to continue the titration of oxygen therapy from the OR to the ICU. (When using portable oxygen tanks, a good rule of thumb to determine the capacity of an E-cylinder is as follows: the minutes of oxygen delivery left in the tank = pounds of pressure [in pounds per square inch] × 0.3 divided by gas flow [in liters per minute].) While avoiding hyperoxia, one must never lose sight of the importance of *avoiding hypoxemia; hypoxemia is life-threatening whereas hyperoxia is not.* One cannot be faulted if ROP should occur, provided a reasonable and safe approach to oxygen administration and ventilation has been made.

## Intravenous Anesthetic Agents

The anesthetic effects of IV agents are primarily reflected by brain concentrations; to achieve anesthesia, it is necessary to obtain an adequate cerebral blood concentration. Each drug administered is rapidly redistributed from vessel-rich well perfused areas (brain, heart, lung, liver, and kidneys) to muscle, and finally to vessel-poor less well perfused areas (bone, fat). Thus, termination of the effect of a single drug dose is primarily determined by redistribution. The much slower tertiary distribution to relatively underperfused tissues of the body is noted with long-term drug infusions. Protein binding, body composition, cardiac output, distribution of cardiac output, metabolism, and excretion all alter the PK and PD of IV drugs. Anesthetic depth may be altered if a constant cerebral blood level is not maintained. The changes in body composition and the blood-brain barrier that occur during maturation may also greatly affect the duration of action of IV drugs, especially in neonates. In addition to perinatal circulatory changes (e.g., ductus venosus, ductus arteriosus), there are maturational differences in relative organ mass and regional blood flow while a symptomatic patent ductus arteriosus may also result in differences in distribution. Blood flow, as a fraction of the cardiac output, to the kidney and brain increases with age, whereas that to the liver decreases through the neonatal period.[678] Cerebral and hepatic mass, as proportions of body weight in the infant, are much greater than in the adult.[679] Whereas onset times are generally faster for neonates than adults (a size effect), reduced cardiac output and cerebral perfusion in neonates means that the expected onset time after an IV induction is slower in neonates, although reduced protein binding may counter this observation for some drugs. Offset time is also delayed because redistribution to well-perfused and deep under-perfused tissues is more limited.

### BARBITURATES
#### Methohexital
Methohexital (Brevital) is a short-acting barbiturate for the IV induction of anesthesia (1 to 2 mg/kg). Administered

intravenously as a 1% solution (10 mg/mL), it produces pain at the injection site; hiccups, apnea, and seizure-like activity may also be occasionally observed.[680,681] Methohexital has minimal effects on cardiovascular function (increased heart rate) in children.[682] Methohexital may be contraindicated in children with temporal lobe epilepsy.[680] Slow IV titration averts apnea. A possible advantage of methohexital (clearance 0.76 L/min/70 kg) over thiopental (clearance 0.24 L/min/70 kg) is that its mature rate of metabolism is greater while the volumes of distribution at steady state are similar (170 L/70 kg),[684] suggesting a more rapid recovery when large doses have been administered.[685-687] Anesthesia is achieved at plasma concentrations of 3.12 ± 0.99 mg/L.[688]

Rectal methohexital in a 10% solution (20 to 30 mg/kg) is a safe and atraumatic method of induction with an acceptably small incidence of undesired adverse effects (hiccups 13%, defecation 10%),[689] although this technique is no longer commonly used. It was particularly suited for brief radiologic procedures, such as computed tomographic scans, with a single rectal administration of a 10% solution (100 mg/mL given through a well-lubricated catheter), as well as for minor outpatient surgery.[690,691] Absorption by this route is quite variable and may account for an occasional child with prolonged or rapid onset of sedation.[685,692] This technique and dosage have been used safely in children from 3 months to 6 years of age. It is a useful adjunct to induction of anesthesia in older cognitively impaired children, or in those who are excessively fearful of the anesthesia mask or an IV needle. It is also an alternative for children who are still in diapers and who are not candidates for other premedicants, such as midazolam (e.g., a child taking erythromycin).[693,694]

Oxygen desaturation occurs in approximately 4% of cases and is usually related to airway obstruction; this is generally readily corrected by repositioning the head.[689,695] Methohexital should be administered only under the supervision of a physician trained in airway management to ensure adequacy of the airway and ventilation, because airway obstruction, seizures, or apnea may rarely occur.[696] *Children must not be left unobserved after administration.*

#### Thiopental
The most likely mechanism of action of thiopental is via binding to $GABA_A$ receptors, which increases the duration of GABA-activated chloride channel opening. The median effective dose ($ED_{50}$) of thiopental varies with age: 3.4 mg/kg in neonates, 6.3 mg/kg in infants, 3.9 mg/kg in children aged 1 to 4 years, 4.5 mg/kg in children 4 to 7 years, 4.3 mg/kg in children 7 to 12 years and 4.1 mg/kg in adolescents aged 12 to 16 years.[697,698] Children aged 13 to 68 months given rectal thiopental (44 mg/kg) 45 minutes prior to surgery were either asleep or adequately sedated with plasma concentrations above 2.8 mg/L.[699] The effect-site concentration of thiopental for induction of anesthesia in neonates may be less than that in infants because the neonate has relatively immature cerebral cortical function, rudimentary dendritic arborization, and relatively few synapses.[700]

The hypotensive response in neonates given thiopental appears not as dramatic as that associated with propofol, although it still may occur with reversion to fetal circulation.[701,702] Thiopental has little direct effect on vascular smooth muscle tone. Cardiovascular depression is centrally mediated by inhibition of sympathetic nervous activity and direct myocardial depression through effects on transsarcolemmic and sarcoplasmic reticulum calcium flux. Although doses of 6 mg/kg have been given as premedication before intubation in term infants without physiologic consequences,[703] the mean dose required for satisfactory induction in neonates is less, at 3.4 ± 0.2 mg/kg.[697]

The duration of the clinical effect of thiopental depends primarily on redistribution rather than metabolism (10% per hour). As a result, repeated doses of thiopental may accumulate, causing prolonged sedation. Children 5 months to 13 years of age, however, metabolize thiopental almost twice as rapidly as adults when expressed as per kilogram (see E-Fig. 6-3).[704-706] The elimination half-life of thiopental in neonates is greater than that in adults and children[707,708] because of the reduced clearance in neonates. Clearance, expressed using a ¾ allometric model, at 26 weeks PMA was 0.015 L/min/70 kg and increased to 0.119 L/min/70 kg by 42 weeks PMA.[709] Maturation of the CYP2C19 pathway increases rapidly after birth in term neonates[710] and the mature clearance of 0.24 L/min/70 kg is achieved within 3 months of age.

Acute tolerance to thiopental, well demonstrated in adults, may also occur in children.[711] A total IV dose of 10 mg/kg is generally the upper limit; however, with this dose, it is common to have a prolonged period of sedation after brief surgical procedures. Thiopental is a weak vasodilator and a direct myocardial depressant; both of these effects may cause significant systemic hypotension in the *hypovolemic* state (e.g., dehydration resulting from prolonged fasting or trauma).[712]

Thiopental in a 10% solution (20 to 30 mg/kg) may also be used for induction of anesthesia by rectal instillation when methohexital is contraindicated (temporal lobe epilepsy).[680] The period of sedation may be longer for thiopental than for methohexital, partly because of the reduced rate of metabolism.[713]

Thiopental has also been used in the pediatric critical care setting as a continuous high-dose infusion (approximately 2 to 4 mg/kg/hr) to control intracranial hypertension. Monitoring the blood concentration of thiopental may be useful during such therapy to avoid depressing myocardial function. The elimination half-life of thiopental after a continuous infusion may be markedly prolonged compared with that after a single bolus (11.7 vs 6.1 hours).[705,706] These findings may, in part, be attributed to the underlying illness, intercurrent drug treatment, and zero-order kinetics at higher concentrations (Michaelis constant 28.3 mg/L)[709,714]

## PROPOFOL

Propofol (Diprivan) is a sedative-hypnotic agent useful for both the induction and maintenance of anesthesia.[715] Diprivan is formulated with 1% propofol, 10% soybean oil, 1.25% egg yolk phosphatide (ovolecithin), 2.25% glycerol, EDTA (ethylenediaminetetraacetic acid), and sodium hydroxide to maintain a pH of 7.0 to 8.5. This formulation has a white milky appearance because it is a lipid macroemulsion with average droplet size of 0.15 to 0.3 μmol/L (where 5 to 7 μmol/L is required to pass through capillaries).[716] These droplets remain distinct in suspension owing to the negative surface charges on the phosphate moieties in the ovolecithin phospholipids in the aqueous outer layer. These droplets may coalesce if the negative surface charges on the emulsion droplets dissipate, which is a slow, naturally occurring process, but which may also be precipitated by physical maneuvers (freeze-thawing, high temperatures, or agitation) or by changes in the chemical composition of the emulsion, such as by decreasing pH or the addition of electrolytes (i.e., sodium, potassium, calcium, or magnesium) or medications (i.e., lidocaine [see later discussion]).[716] Soybean oil is composed of

long-chain triglycerides (LCT), defined by the 12 to 22 carbon atoms in their skeletons: linoleic acid (54%), oleic acids (26%), linolenic acid (7.8%), and stearic acid (2.6%). EDTA was added to Diprivan after 1998 as an antimicrobial agent. Generic formulations of propofol are available; these contain sulfites or metabisulfite as the antimicrobial agent.

Propofol is a highly lipophilic drug that is rapidly distributed into vessel-rich organs, accounting for its rapid onset and usefulness as an induction agent. Termination of this effect is achieved by the combination of rapid redistribution and rapid hepatic and extrahepatic clearance.[717-719] The rapidity of the redistribution from vessel-rich organs accounts for its brief action and the need for repeated small boluses or a constant infusion to maintain a stable plane of anesthesia and sedation. PK studies demonstrated a larger Vdss (9.7 L/kg) in children compared with adults, and more rapid redistribution, but a clearance (34 mL/min/kg) that is similar to or greater than that reported in adults.[720-723] Clearance, standardized to a 70 kg person using allometry, is immature in preterm neonates (0.4 L/min/70 kg at 30 weeks PMA); there is rapid maturation around term (1 L/min/70 kg), achieving 90% of mature clearance (1.8 L/min/70 kg) by 5 months postnatal age (see Fig. 6-10).[178,724-727] Clearance is limited by the hepatic blood flow and is consequently reduced in children in low cardiac output states.[728] Although interindividual variability in the PK in neonates is large, the reduced clearance suggests that recovery after propofol in neonates may be prolonged and that repeat doses may not be required as frequently as in older children and adults. Propofol is conjugated to a water-soluble glucuronide in the liver and excreted in the urine.[720] Propofol also undergoes extrahepatic metabolism (in lung, kidney), as evidenced by the similar PK in infants with biliary atresia and healthy controls.[729]

Although measuring the concentration of propofol in blood has been the sole means to assess its disposition in vivo, alternate noninvasive techniques have been sought to provide online measurements. Mass spectrometry of the exhaled breath from adults and children, a technique that is similar to end-tidal gas monitoring of inhalational anesthetics, has proven to provide stable estimates of the concentration of propofol in blood.[730,731] It may soon be possible to guide administration of propofol in the OR by the measurement of expired propofol.[732,733]

In children who have not been premedicated, the dose of propofol required for loss of the eyelash reflex generally increases with decreasing age.[734-738] The ED$_{50}$ for loss of the eyelash reflex in infants (1 to 6 months) is 3 ± 0.2 mg/kg, which decreases in children (1 to 12 years) to 1.3 to 1.6 mg/kg, and increases in older children (10 to 16 years) to 2.4 ± 0.1 mg/kg. A more linear decrease in propofol dosing with increasing age between infants and children 12 years of age was determined in Chinese children.[737] A 10% decrease in the propofol dose for the ED$_{95}$ between children younger than age 2 years, 2 to 5 years, and 6 to 12 years was noted. The ED$_{90-95}$ for loss of eyelash reflex for all age groups is 50% to 75% greater than the ED$_{50}$.[734,735] Larger doses may be required for acceptance of the face mask.[735,739] The dose of propofol in neonates has not been clearly established. In one study, a dose of 2.5 mg/kg permitted tracheal intubation in the majority of neonates, although the exact dose used was not specified.[740] Successful insertion of an LMA in unpremedicated children requires an even larger dose of propofol (5.4 mg/kg [4.7 to 6.8 mg/kg, 95% confidence interval]).[741] After induction of anesthesia with sevoflurane and nitrous oxide, excellent conditions for tracheal intubation are achieved with 1.5 to 2 mg/kg in children.[742-745] Propofol is widely used as a continuous infusion or in intermittent doses in children undergoing brief radiologic procedures, during medical procedures, such as oncology and gastroenterology, and for children with MH.[39,746-749] Although early evidence suggested that 100 µg/kg/min propofol was required after a halothane induction to maintain immobility during MRI,[746] subsequent studies showed that much larger doses are required in unpremedicated children or after sevoflurane inductions.[39] Specifically, initial infusion rates of propofol of 200 to 250 µg/kg/min (12 to 15 mg/kg/hr) or even greater may be required (up to 500 µg/kg/min for the first 15 minutes and then tapered) to prevent nonpurposeful limb movement during scans. The initial rate may have to be increased for younger children (e.g., infants) and for those who are cognitively impaired. Midazolam premedication may reduce the propofol requirements, but it delays emergence after brief procedures. Some advocate intermittent boluses of propofol whereas others advocate continuous infusions. Once movement has abated, the infusion rate of propofol may be titrated approaching 200 µg/kg/min in infants and 150 µg/kg/min in older children. In one study, systolic BP decreased more and the total dose of propofol was greater when continuous infusions were used, compared with intermittent boluses.[749] If minor movement can be tolerated (e.g., medical procedures), then intermittent boluses may be preferred for brief procedures, whereas if immobility is required (radiation oncology and radiologic procedures), then infusions are preferred. In some clinical scenarios, such as radiation oncology, burns, and oncology procedures, repeated sedation with propofol over a prolonged period is required. There is no evidence that tolerance to propofol develops.[750]

Integrated PK–PD studies in neonates are lacking, partly because of a lack of consistent effect measures. The equilibration half-time ($T_{1/2}$keo) for the effect compartment is unknown, but is assumed to be smaller[251] than the 3 minutes described in adults.[751,752] Reduced $GABA_A$ receptor numbers in the neonatal brain may contribute to a reduced target concentration, but this hypothesis remains untested. A circadian night-rhythm effect has been noted in an investigation of infant propofol sedation after major craniofacial surgery,[753] but such an effect is unlikely in neonates who do not have established day–night sleep cycles.[754]

Propofol affects a number of organ system responses in vivo. Systolic BP decreases approximately 15% in children,[721,739,755,756] which is similar to what occurs in adults.[757] Most studies reported similar decreases in BP after propofol and thiopental in children.[756,758] The incidence of apnea after an induction bolus of either propofol or thiopental is similar.[739,755,756,758] The major clinical disadvantage of propofol in children is pain when it is injected intravenously in a small vein.[759] This pain can be diminished by using any one of a number of strategies, including injecting propofol into a large vein; pretreatment with IV lidocaine (0.5 mg/kg), meperidine, nitrous oxide, metoprolol, or tramadol; and combining a small dose of lidocaine (0.5 to 1.0 mg/kg) with the propofol.* The most effective method to eliminate pain is to apply a "mini-Bier block" by manually occluding the IV flow by squeezing the extremity proximal to the IV site for 45 to 60 seconds and injecting IV lidocaine (0.5 to 1.0 mg/kg). As soon as the Bier block is released, the desired dose of propofol is administered painlessly (E-Fig. 6-11). The average number of patients who need to be treated to benefit from this maneuver

to prevent pain (*number needed to treat*) in adults is less than two,[763] indicating that this technique is extremely effective,[759] which should make this a routine practice.[765] Parenthetically, any parenteral form of lidocaine, including those that contain preservative, may be administered intravenously, combined with or before propofol, without triggering an anaphylactoid reaction.

The mechanism by which IV propofol causes pain has been attributed to the nociceptive effects of trace concentrations of propofol (15 to 20 µg/mL) in the outer aqueous layer of the Diprivan soybean-oil micelles. When the concentration of propofol in the aqueous outer layer coating the micelles was reduced (i.e., by increasing the concentration of medium-chain triglycerides in the formulation), irritation of the nociceptive nerve endings in the veins and the severity of the pain during injection were attenuated.[766]

Indicators for recovery from anesthesia, such as time to eye opening and time to extubation, are more rapid in children when anesthesia was induced with propofol compared with thiopental.[767-772] Recovery of psychomotor function is more rapid after a propofol induction and maintenance of anesthesia compared with thiopental–isoflurane anesthesia.[773] Recovery room stay and time to hospital discharge are reduced with propofol.[767,769] Emergence delirium rarely occurs after propofol anesthesia in children.[538,774-777] Propofol reduces the incidence of nausea and vomiting when used as an induction agent or when used for the maintenance of anesthesia.[769,778-784] However, there have been conflicting results for particular procedures, such as strabismus repair and tonsillectomy, and when the drug is combined with opioids.[785-788] Nausea and vomiting may be considered surrogate endpoints for serious adverse outcomes after surgery in children. No studies have demonstrated clinically important abbreviated times to discharge or decrease in overnight admission rate for vomiting and/or dehydration in children treated with propofol. Short-term infusions of propofol for surgical or medical procedures have shown that the depth of sedation is easily controlled by adjusting the infusion rate while still ensuring rapid and complete recovery.[789-793] Compared with thiopental, propofol is less irritating to the airway, which translates into a reduced incidence of laryngospasm.[758,794-796] Insertion of a laryngeal mask airway is substantially easier and more successful after a propofol induction compared with thiopental.[718,741,797,798]

Propofol compromises airway patency and respiration in children; the upper airway narrows particularly in the hypopharyngeal region, but it does remain patent.[799] If airway obstruction occurs, the chin lift maneuver augments the patency of the upper airway.[800,801] Theoretically, collapse of the upper airway increases in parallel with the dose of propofol by direct inhibition of genioglossus muscle activity, as well as an inhibition of centrally mediated airway dilatation and airway reflexes.[802] All of these upper airway changes are reversed on emergence from anesthesia.[803] When propofol is given as an IV bolus, transient apnea may occur.[737,742,756] Concerns over atelectasis and airway obstruction have prompted some to insert a tracheal tube or laryngeal mask airway in children sedated with propofol during medical procedures. However, evidence suggests that the incidence of atelectasis in children who are breathing spontaneously with an unprotected airway is less than in those whose tracheas are intubated.[804]

Diprivan and the current lipid-based generic formulations of propofol must be handled with aseptic techniques, because the lipid is a culture medium.[805] Propofol 1% can support the growth of at least four well-known organisms: *Staphylococcus aureus,*

---

*References 721, 735, 739, 756, 758, 760-764.

*Pseudomonas aeruginosa, Escherichia coli,* and *Candida albicans.*[806-808] When Diprivan was first introduced, it was prepared (as are all lipid emulsions) under strict aseptic conditions, with a layer of nitrogen above the liquid emulsion in each vial.[716] Once opened, external contamination of the vials, however, resulted in severe sepsis and several deaths before antimicrobial agents were mandated to be added to the propofol formulations to prevent or retard bacterial growth. In very small concentrations, EDTA inhibits bacterial growth by chelating vital trace metals without affecting the emulsion droplet size or stability. Other formulations of propofol contain sulfite or metabisulfites, which release sulfur dioxide that prevents bacterial growth. Sulfites are more effective at reduced pH values, but there is a limit to how acidic the emulsion can become because this destabilizes the emulsion droplets. To further prevent any risk of bacterial contamination, all opened vials of propofol should be discarded after 6 hours. These strategies have eliminated concerns of bacterial contamination of propofol and episodes of sepsis.

Long-term propofol infusions were used extensively for sedation in ICUs after recognizing that its favorable PK would facilitate a rapid wake-up.[717] However, a report of five deaths in infants and children (4 weeks to 6 years of age) who were sedated with Diprivan raised serious doubts about the safety of such a practice.[809] The syndrome, now known as propofol infusion syndrome (PRIS), occurs primarily, but not exclusively, in children who are sedated for prolonged periods in ICUs.[809-813] Clinical experience indicates that PRIS is most common when propofol is infused continuously at more than 5 mg/kg/hr (70 μg/kg/min) for more than 48 hours. Manifestations of PRIS include the insidious onset of lipemia, metabolic acidosis, hyperkalemia, and rhabdomyolysis that may precipitously transform into profound myocardial instability and cardiovascular collapse that is refractory to all resuscitative efforts. Manifesting signs may be subtle, with the sudden onset of bradycardia that is refractory to the usual interventions. PRIS was suspected in a 5-year-old undergoing an arteriovenous malformation resection when an unexplained metabolic acidosis was detected after a 6-hour infusion of propofol.[814] When propofol was discontinued, the signs of PRIS abated. In an adult neurosurgical ICU where propofol sedation was used, a retrospective review determined that for every 1 mg/kg/hr that the propofol infusion exceeded 5 mg/kg/hr, the odds ratio of death was 1.93.[815] After a total of at least 28 deaths in children and 14 adults, the FDA cautioned against the use of propofol for long-term sedation. Predisposing risk factors include concomitant catecholamine inotrope infusions or high-dose corticosteroids and sepsis. Mortality currently ranges from 30% to 80%, although early institution of hemodialysis or extracorporeal membrane oxygenation may improve survival.[816]

Unraveling PRIS has proved to be difficult. Early investigations noted that during PRIS, the blood concentrations of malonylcarnitine and C5-acylcarnitine increased. These compounds are known to inhibit carnitine palmitoyl transferase and the transfer of LCT into mitochondria.[817,818] Propofol may also directly inhibit carnitine palmitoyl transferase to impede flux of LCT into the mitochondria. Within the mitochondria, propofol uncouples the β oxidation spiral at complex II in the respiratory chain, which, in turn, inhibits transmembrane flux of LCT into mitochondria, strangling the mitochondria from a much needed source of energy. To reduce the risk of PRIS, new formulations of propofol are being developed that contain less or no LCT. Medium-chain triglycerides are replacing LCTs in propofol. The clinical importance of these developments requires further investigations with multicenter studies.[819]

The safety of propofol in the neonatal period has raised concerns after reports of profound episodes of cardiorespiratory collapse in neonates.[820,821] In these cases, precipitous and severe decreases in systolic BP, heart rate, and oxygenation were observed after a single induction dose of propofol (1 to 7 mg/kg) in neonates without evidence of congenital heart defects or cardiomyopathy. Resuscitation was extremely difficult in all cases despite intervention with both inotropic and chronotropic agents. A myriad of causes of bradycardia associated with propofol administration have been proposed.[822] In a comprehensive review of bradycardia after propofol in children and adults, the authors concluded that "propofol carries a finite risk for bradycardia with potential for major harm."[823] Whether these responses reflect acute right-to-left shunting, a return to fetal circulation, or another, as yet undisclosed, cause in neonates has not been confirmed; caution should be exercised when propofol is used to induce anesthesia in neonates.[702]

Although anaphylactoid reactions have been reported after propofol administration in children, specific causes for the allergic reaction have not been identified.[824] In some instances, the "reactions" were primarily respiratory and attributed to preservatives, such as metabisulfites.[825] However, 13 of 14 adults who developed anaphylactoid reactions after their first exposure to propofol displayed a hypersensitivity response to propofol with at least one test during immunologic testing.[826] Similar findings in children have not been reported. It has been proposed that first exposure reactions suggest a previous sensitization possibly arising from isopropyl epitopes similar to propofol in cosmetics, detergents and cough medicines.

The package insert for Diprivan cautions against its use in all patients with "egg allergy." However, children with egg allergy (including severe allergy) have received measles-mumps-rubella vaccine, which is derived from eggs, without untoward experience,[827-829] although isolated reactions have been reported. In the past 2 decades, no immunologically verified anaphylactic reactions have been reported in children with egg allergy who received Diprivan. In fact, Diprivan contains egg lecithin which is derived from heated egg yolk. Egg lecithin is a phospholipid and has not been reported to trigger allergic reactions, although trace concentrations of egg yolk, of which only 2 of 9 proteins present, Gal d 5 and Gal d 6, are possibly immunogenic. When propofol was given 43 times to 28 children with egg allergy, only one experienced a mild nonanaphylactoid reaction, which led to their recommendation to avoid propofol only in children with documented anaphylaxis to eggs.[830]

Soy protein allergy is primarily a gastrointestinal allergy that dissipates by 5 to 6 years of age because of repeated exposure to soy protein in foods. Very rarely is soy allergy a systemic disease. Although propofol is a soy based emulsion, the Astra-Zeneca web site states that all protein moieties are removed during the manufacturing process rendering soy an exceedingly unlikely epitope to trigger an immunologically based anaphylactic reaction. The reader should note that there is an approximately 5% cross-reactivity between soy and peanut allergy.[831] In children with both soy allergy and peanut anaphylaxis, it may be prudent to avoid propofol, especially if administering generic formulations.

In an effort to divest propofol of its lipid carrier and pain during IV administration, alternate formulations of propofol have been under development for parenteral use. New formulations of propofol must satisfy a number of conditions: easy to administer, stable formulation, no or minimal pain on injection, no infectious risk, and rapid PK. Unfortunately, many of the formulations that have been developed to date have failed in one or more of the above criteria. Most recently, a prodrug (fospropofol [Lusedra]) and nonlipid excipients (cyclodextrin, nanoparticle carriers) have shown promise. Clinical trials with fospropofol for sedation in adults have shown promise.[832,833]

Fospropofol, a phosphate-modified prodrug of propofol, undergoes enzymatic hydrolysis in approximately 8 minutes in blood to remove the phosphate moiety yielding the active form of propofol.[834-838] Fospropofol displays similar kinetics to the parent compound, without pain on injection. With the delayed onset of sedation with this prodrug, the slow increase in blood concentrations should reduce adverse respiratory and cardiovascular side effects, but this also slows induction of anesthesia. This formulation carries a minimal risk of microbial infection because there is no lipid excipient. The release of formaldehyde and formate as metabolites of fospropofol are concerns that require further investigation.[832,839] A frequent adverse effect of fospropofol is transient perianal and perineal pain or burning, for which no preventative measure has been forthcoming.[839] There are no published data with fospropofol in children. Currently, further development of fospropofol by the manufacturer has been suspended.

Regarding the nonlipid formulation using β-cyclodextrins, human studies show a large incidence of pain on IV injection that make it a nonviable alternative.[840] In adults, this formulation produced more pain during injection than Diprivan, rendering this formulation unlikely to reach the marketplace. Another formulation of propofol is Aquafol (Daewon Pharmaceutical Co, Ltd, Seoul, Republic of Korea), a nanoparticle microemulsion that contains two polyethylene glycol–based compounds to stabilize the microemulsion.[841] The PD and safety of Aquafol were similar to those of Diprivan in adults, although differences were noted in the PK. In adults, this formulation yielded more pain during IV administration than Diprivan.[842] Unless this issue is addressed, this formulation is unlikely to be used widely in clinical practice.

Finally, some recommend supplanting long-chain triglycerides in propofol with medium-chain triglycerides to reduce the risk of PRIS and pain during injection. When 1% propofol with long-chain triglycerides was compared with 1% propofol in a mixture of medium and long-chain triglycerides, both with 1 mL of 2% lidocaine, the frequency of pain and its intensity during injection were similar.[843]

## KETAMINE

Ketamine (Ketalar) is a derivative of phencyclidine that similarly antagonizes the $N$-methyl-D-aspartate (NMDA) receptor.[844] Its action is related to central dissociation of the cerebral cortex, and it also causes cerebral excitation. The latter property may be responsible for precipitating seizures in susceptible children and the reason that processed EEG monitoring devices do not work with ketamine sedation or anesthesia.[263-265,845,846]

Ketamine is available as a mixture of two enantiomers; the $S(+)$ enantiomer has four times the potency of the $R(-)$ enantiomer. $(S)$-(+)-ketamine has approximately twice the potency of the other enantiomer. The metabolite norketamine, has a potency that is one-third that of its parent compound. Plasma concentrations associated with anesthesia are approximately 3 µg/mL,[847] whereas concentrations for hypnosis and amnesia during surgery

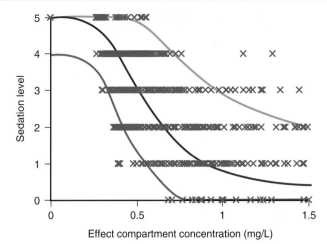

**FIGURE 6-18** The relationship between effect compartment concentration and level of ketamine sedation (*purple line*). The concentration producing 50% of the maximum effect ($EC_{50}$) was 0.562 mg/L. Categorical data are shown as crosses. The *brown* and *blue lines* demonstrate the 5% and 95% confidence intervals. (Reproduced with permission from Herd DW, Anderson BJ, Keene NA, Holford NH. Investigating the pharmacodynamics of ketamine in children. Paediatr Anaesth 2008;18:36-42.)

are reported to be 0.8 to 4 µg/mL; awakening usually occurs at concentrations less than 0.5 µg/mL. Pain thresholds are increased at 0.1 µg/mL.[848] The concentration-response curve for ketamine sedation is steep.[65,849] This means that small serum concentration changes will have dramatic effect on the degree of sedation observed (Fig. 6-18).

Ketamine is very lipid soluble with rapid distribution and the onset of anesthesia after IV administration is approximately 30 seconds. This is usually heralded by horizontal or vertical nystagmus (Video 6-1).[850,851] Studies separating equivalent anesthetic doses of ketamine isomers identified a reduced incidence of side effects, more potent analgesia, and fewer cardiovascular effects with the dextro isomer rather than the levo isomer[850,852-855]; acute tolerance has been reported.[856] Children require greater doses of ketamine (per kilogram) than adults because of greater clearance (per kilogram); however, there is considerable patient-to-patient variability.[262,848,850,852]

Ketamine undergoes N-demethylation to norketamine; metabolized mainly by CYP3A4, although CYP2C9, CYP2B6 also have a role. Elimination of racemic ketamine is complicated by the $(R)$-$(-)$-ketamine enantiomer, which inhibits the elimination of the $(S)$-$(+)$-ketamine enantiomer.[857] Clearance is immature in neonates but matures to reach adult rates (80 L/hr/70 kg, i.e., liver blood flow) within the first 6 months of life, when described using allometric size models.[858] Clearance in neonates is reduced (26 L/hr/70 kg)[859-861] while Vdss is increased (3.46 L/kg at birth, 1.18 L/kg at 4 years, 0.75 L/kg at adulthood).[859] This larger Vdss in neonates contributes to the observation that neonates require a fourfold greater dose than 6-year-old children to prevent gross motor movement.[862]

Bioavailability after intramuscular (IM) administration is approximately 93% in adults and even greater in children.[848,863,864] There is a high hepatic extraction ratio and the relative bioavailability of oral, nasal, and rectal formulations is 20% to 50% (Table 6-12).[864-866] Children presenting for burn surgery had slow absorption (absorption half-time [$T_{1/2}abs$] was 59 min) with large between-subject variability.[865]

**TABLE 6-12** Ketamine Equivalency by Route of Administration*

| Route | Dose (mg/kg) | Approximate Bioequivalence (mg/kg) |
|---|---|---|
| Intravenous | 2 | 2 |
| Intramuscular | 2 | 2.15 |
| Nasal | 2 | 4 |
| Rectal | 2 | 8 |
| Oral | 2 | 11.75 |

Extrapolated from data from Grant IS, Nimmo WS, McNicol LR, Clements JA. Ketamine disposition in children and adults. Br J Anaesth 1983;55:1107-11; Grant IS, Nimmo WS, Clements JA. Pharmacokinetics and analgesic effects of i.m. and oral ketamine. Br J Anaesth 1981;53:805-10; Clements JA, Nimmo WS, Grant IS. Bioavailability, pharmacokinetics, and analgesic activity of ketamine in humans. J Pharm Sci 1982;71:539-42.

*Note that these are estimates and that there is extreme patient-to-patient variability.

Ketamine is an excellent analgesic and amnestic; the recommended dose for induction of anesthesia is 1 to 3 mg/kg intravenously or 5 to 10 mg/kg intramuscularly.[854,867] The duration of action of a single IV dose is 5 to 8 minutes, with an $\alpha$-elimination half-life of 11 minutes, and a $\beta$-elimination half-life of 2.5 to 3.0 hours.[868-870] Further supplementary doses of 0.5 to 1.0 mg/kg are administered when clinically indicated. Atropine or another antisialagogue accompanying the initial dose diminishes the production of copious secretions that occur with ketamine.[871,872] Ketamine may also be administered in very low doses intravenously (0.25 to 0.5 mg/kg) or intramuscularly (1 to 2 mg/kg), either alone or in combination with low-dose midazolam (0.05 mg/kg [50 µg/kg]), along with atropine (0.02 mg/kg) for sedation, for a variety of procedures, such as oncology evaluations, suture of lacerations, or radiologic interventions.[854,867,873-878] If an antisialagogue is not administered, there is a greater risk for laryngospasm,[879] although guidelines for emergency departments suggest that supplementation with atropine or a benzodiazepine may not be necessary with doses of 1 to 1.5 mg/kg.[880,881] Larger doses of ketamine will produce a state of general anesthesia.[882-884] Even after small doses there is potential for apnea or airway obstruction, particularly when combined with other sedating medications.[882,885,886]

Ketamine has also been administered orally, nasally, and rectally, both as a premedication before general anesthesia and for procedural sedation.[683,683,887-902] Oral ketamine administered as a premedicant has also been reported to reduce emergence delirium; there is conflicting evidence regarding the efficacy of ketamine to reduce pain scores after tonsillectomy.[903-905]

There are concerns regarding both rectal and nasal drug administration. Rectal administration can result in very irregular and less predictable times of onset and peak sedation, just as with rectal barbiturates. Nasal drug administration can result in drug entering directly into the CNS by tracking along neurovascular tissue of the nasal mucosa.[906-910] Because the preservative in ketamine has been shown to be neurotoxic, there is the theoretic possibility of CNS toxicity because of the preservative.[911,912] Until better safety information is available, this route of drug administration is not recommended unless preservative-free ketamine is used.

Ketamine has also been administered as a means of providing caudal epidural analgesia.[867,913-918] The same admonition regarding the risk of neurotoxicity during neuraxial administration of ketamine applies here even more importantly: *epidural ketamine must not be administered unless it is preservative free.*

The use of ketamine is increasing for postoperative pain management when administered in small doses as an opioid-sparing drug[854,867,919-922]; although a recent meta-analysis documented reduced pain scores and nonopioid sparing effects, it failed to substantiate its efficacy in opioid-sparing (see later discussion). Ketamine has also been used topically to treat mucositis and other painful conditions.[293,923-929] Ketamine increases heart rate, cardiac index, and systemic BP; it also increases pulmonary artery pressure in adults but has a small effect on respiration.[850,930] In children, there is apparently no effect on pulmonary artery pressure provided that ventilation is controlled.[931] If a child is sedated with ketamine but allowed to breathe spontaneously, increases in end-tidal $CO_2$ could increase pulmonary artery pressures.[932] Ketamine sedation has been shown to maintain peripheral vascular resistance, thus affecting intracardiac shunting less than propofol in children sedated for cardiac catheterization.[933] However, the combination of ketamine and propofol might be superior to either drug alone in this circumstance.[934,935] Ketamine has negative inotropic effects in those who depend on vasopressors.[936] The effect of ketamine on the musculature of the upper airway differs from that of midazolam; in adults, ketamine does not cause airway obstruction, whereas midazolam does.[937] Ketamine has one of the best safety profiles of any anesthetic agent. After unintended overdoses as great as 56 mg/kg IM and 15 mg/kg IV,[938] the duration of sedation persisted for 3 to 24 hours; respiratory depression occurred in four children, whereas tracheal intubation was required in two. When the children who received an overdose were monitored and their airways were maintained, recovery occurred without incident. This report, combined with the minimal effect of ketamine on airway patency, may explain, in part, the successful widespread use of this anesthetic by nonanesthesiologists. However, there remains a small but consistent incidence of adverse airway-related events, such as laryngospasm, apnea, and airway obstruction associated with ketamine, underscoring the need to ensure that the personnel responsible for administering ketamine are trained in advanced airway management. Ketamine also relaxes the smooth musculature of the airway stimulated by histamine[939]; treatment of acute asthma with subanesthetic doses has yielded mixed results.[940-942]

The most common adverse reaction to ketamine is postoperative vomiting, which occurs in 33% of children after anesthesia.[851] Intraoperative and postoperative dreaming and hallucinations occur more commonly in older than in younger children.[851] The incidence of these latter adverse effects may be reduced when ketamine is supplemented with a benzodiazepine.[943,944] One clinical report described two children, each 3 years of age, who had recurrent nightmares and abnormal behavior persisting for 10 months after a single ketamine administration.[945] A soporific environment may reduce the incidence of emergence phenomena.[946]

### Indications

Ketamine is useful for children who are developmentally delayed, or those who become combative because they are too frightened to come to the OR. Ketamine can be used in very low doses (0.25-0.5 mg/kg) for short-term procedures, such as diagnostic spinal punctures and bone marrow aspiration, and in larger doses for angiography and cardiac catheterization. Ketamine may be particularly valuable for burn-dressing changes, suture removal, induction of anesthesia in hypovolemic children, children for whom application of a face mask may prove hazardous (such as with epidermolysis bullosa), and children who require invasive monitoring before induction of general anesthesia.[850,852,947-949] Ketamine has been successfully used even in neonates with less apparent cardiovascular depression than occurs with halothane or isoflurane.[950]

The role of ketamine for postoperative pain has been recently reviewed using meta-analysis. Administration of ketamine in the OR was associated with decreased postoperative pain intensity and nonopioid analgesic requirement in the postoperative care unit, but failed to exhibit a postoperative opioid-sparing effect in the subsequent 6 to 24 hours.[951]

### Contraindications

Ketamine may produce increases in intracranial pressure (ICP) as a result of cerebral vasodilation; it also increases CMRO$_2$. Ketamine may be contraindicated in children with intracranial hypertension.[952,953] This concern regarding ICP has been challenged[954,955]; adult patients whose lungs were mechanically ventilated and who were sedated with a ketamine infusion demonstrated a decrease in ICP after bolus doses of 1.5, 3.0, and 5.0 mg/kg.[956] The caveat is that the tracheas were already intubated, ventilation was controlled, and they were sedated. There may be a use for ketamine sedation in the ICU where there is meticulous attention to airway management and control of ventilation.[955]

A 30% increase in intraocular pressure (IOP) has also been noted; thus, ketamine may be potentially dangerous in the presence of a corneal laceration.[957] In children with active upper respiratory tract infections, copious secretions caused by ketamine may well exacerbate an already irritable airway and result in laryngospasm.[871,879] Ketamine may cause an incompetent gag reflex and thus should not be administered in anesthetic induction doses to children with a full stomach without appropriate airway management. Ketamine may not be useful as the sole anesthetic agent in any surgical procedure in which total control of the child's position is necessary, because purposeless movements frequently occur. Ketamine may be inappropriate in any child with a history of psychiatric or seizure disorder because of its psychotropic and epileptogenic effects.[845,850] In addition, studies in newborn rodents and nonhuman primates correlated ketamine treatment with increased neuronal apoptosis during rapid synaptogenesis.[844,958,959] In neonatal rhesus monkeys, infusions of ketamine (20 to 50 µg/kg/hr) yielded apoptosis after 24 hours but not after 3 hours.[960] At this time, the clinical importance of these findings to humans is unclear, because apoptosis has been studied only in laboratory animals. It is unclear whether these data can be extrapolated from animals to developing humans (see Chapter 23). Similar observations in rodents have been made with isoflurane, nitrous oxide, benzodiazepines, propofol, and other medications commonly used to provide sedation or analgesia and anesthesia to infants. However, current anesthetic practice should not change until rigorous scientific investigations are carried out.[961] Although the administration of ketamine appears simple, its side effects are potentially dangerous. *Ketamine must be administered only by physicians experienced with managing a compromised airway.* We urge that it not be used as a premedication unless given in the presence of continuous supervision by properly trained personnel.

### ETOMIDATE

Etomidate (Amidate) is a steroid-based hypnotic induction agent. It is metabolized principally by hepatic esterases. Concentrations associated with anesthesia are 300 to 500 µg/L. As with most induction agents, offset of effect is by redistribution; clearance is approximately 1000 mL/min/70 kg in children and adults. Children require a 30% increased bolus dose because of an increased V1.[962]

Etomidate is painful when administered intravenously. However, concerns regarding the risks of anaphylactoid reactions and suppression of adrenal function have resulted in most anesthesiologists avoiding this agent in routine cases.[963] Etomidate is very useful in children with head injury and those with an unstable cardiovascular status, such as children with a cardiomyopathy, because of the virtual absence of adverse effects on hemodynamics or cardiac function.[964,965] It is often used by emergency department physicians for management of the airway.[966-968] Commonly used doses include 0.2 to 0.3 mg/kg before administration of a low-dose opioid and a muscle relaxant. Etomidate is often used to facilitate tracheal intubation in critically ill children, that is, those in whom it would seem to offer the most advantage. Because a very large proportion of critically ill children, particularly those resistant to vasopressors, suffer from relative adrenal insufficiency, corticosteroid supplementation may be indicated in such patients in whom etomidate is deemed necessary for their safe airway management.[969,970] (See later discussion, New Drugs in the Pipeline.)

## Neuromuscular Blocking Drugs

### NEUROMUSCULAR MONITORING

The measurement of evoked responses after an electrical stimulus is the standard method for evaluating neuromuscular function. This method allows nearly instantaneous evaluation of the degree of neuromuscular blockade in the unconscious individual. The force of contraction of the thumb, the accelerometer, or the electromyogram may be used to make this assessment.[971] Twitch tension measurements use the force of contraction of the adductor pollicis. This muscle is the only thumb muscle supplied by the ulnar nerve; measurements therefore approach the single-muscle precision of the experimental nerve muscle preparation.[554] The evoked tension of the adductor pollicis in response to stimulation of the ulnar nerve can be recorded by a force displacement transducer (E-Fig. 6-12, *A*). With the electromyogram, the compound muscle action potential is recorded by surface or needle electrodes applied to any muscle, usually the adductor pollicis brevis, the abductor digiti minimi, or the first dorsal interosseous muscle of the hand (see E-Fig. 6-12, *B*). To achieve reproducibility and to ensure full activation of all stimulated nerve and muscle fibers, the stimuli should be supramaximal in intensity, square wave in nature, and no longer than 0.2 millisecond in duration.

Clinically, three types of stimulation are used (E-Fig. 6-13):
1. Single twitch (0.1 to 0.25 Hz [cycles/second])
2. Train-of-four (2 Hz for 2 seconds)
3. Tetanus (50 Hz, usually for 5 seconds)

*Single-twitch* rates are useful whenever there is an observable control response. By comparing the percentage change of twitch tension before and after administration of the neuromuscular blocking agent, one can assess the degree of paralysis. Single stimuli detect relatively high degrees of neuromuscular blockade. In fact, depression of the twitch response can be observed only if more than three fourths of the postsynaptic receptors are blocked.[972]

The *train-of-four* is the most commonly used method for assessing nondepolarizing neuromuscular blockade. It consists of four supramaximal stimuli applied to the ulnar nerve at a frequency of 2 cycles/sec. The ratio of the amplitude of the fourth twitch to the first is an indicator of the degree of neuromuscular blockade. The main advantage of the train-of-four is that it does not require a control measurement. Furthermore, the train-of-four technique can be repeated every 10 seconds, thus allowing rapid changes in neuromuscular blockade to be closely monitored.[554] In general, when the train-of-four is zero, the conditions for tracheal intubation are satisfactory (excellent or good).[973] Preterm infants younger than 32 weeks postconceptional age (PCA) have reduced train-of-four fourth-response values (83% ± 2%) compared with more mature neonates (E-Fig. 6-14).[974] In full-term infants younger than 1 month of age, the height of the fourth evoked response of the train is about 95%.[975] The change to the greater value during the first month of life probably indicates maturation of the myoneural junction. In children 2 months of age and older, all components of the train-of-four are nearly equal (100%).[974]

*Tetanic stimulation* is usually obtained by supramaximally stimulating the nerve for 5 seconds or more. During tetanic stimulation, synthesis of acetylcholine increases; however, this increase is limited. If the duration of stimulation is too prolonged or the frequency of stimulation is too great, fade occurs; that is, a decrement in the height of tetanus is noted. The usual explanation for the occurrence of fade is that during repetitive stimulation, the acetylcholine output-per-impulse wanes. Under normal circumstances, the diminution of acetylcholine output does not affect transmission because of the continuing excess of both acetylcholine and receptors at the myoneural junction (safety factor). During partial receptor blockade with a nondepolarizing relaxant, the progressive diminution of acetylcholine output eventually results in a decreased number of stimulated receptors and a consequent decrease in the amplitude of contraction. An alternative notion holds that fade is not simply the consequence of a spontaneously occurring decrease in the transmitter action but is, in fact, because of a different and separate action of the drug. This suggests that the relaxant has a prejunctional effect.[976] In infants and children anesthetized with halothane, the percent of fade during tetanic stimulation for 5 seconds at 20 cycles/sec is 5% and at 50 cycles/sec it is 9%.[975] These values are comparable to those for adults.[977] If the duration of stimulation is prolonged, an even greater degree of fade may be noted. In small infants, a more than 50% decrement in the height of tetanus has been observed during 15 seconds of tetanic stimulation; this decrement is even more marked in preterm infants.[978,979] These findings suggest that small infants can indeed sustain short periods of tetanic stimulation, but their musculature becomes fatigued more quickly than that of older children.

The integrity of the myoneural junction can also be analyzed by evaluation of posttetanic facilitation. The increased synthesis and release of acetylcholine that occur during tetanic stimulation continue for a short interval after the stimulation has stopped. This increased production normally does not result in facilitation because all the muscle fibers are excited by the stimulus. In the presence of nondepolarizing (competitive) neuromuscular blockade, however, the increased posttetanic acetylcholine release stimulates a greater number of muscle fibers, producing the characteristic posttetanic facilitation.[977]

The posttetanic count has been used to evaluate intense neuromuscular blockade in children.[980,981] This is a measure obtained by applying a 50 cycle/sec tetanic stimulus to the ulnar nerve for 5 seconds, followed by single-twitch stimulation at 1 cycle/sec;

the number of twitches observed in the posttetanic period is known as the posttetanic count (E-Fig. 6-15). Because tetanus and posttetanic responses are indicators of deep neuromuscular blockade, they can usually be elicited during recovery before the reappearance of the train-of-four. At very deep levels of blockade, no tetanus or posttetanic effect can be seen; as the patient recovers, a single posttetanic response eventually manifests itself. The number of posttetanic counts increases as recovery proceeds until, at posttetanic counts of six to seven, the first twitch of the train-of-four reappears. It has been shown that during recovery, the first posttetanic response precedes the first response of the train-of-four by 5 to 10 minutes with intermediate relaxants and by 20 to 30 minutes with long-acting relaxants.[980,981] In a clinical situation in which neuromuscular recording instruments are not available, the number of contractions during train-of-four are counted. This technique depends on the fact that the number of twitches in the train-of-four usually correlates well with the degree of blockade. When the height of the first twitch is about 21% of control, three contractions are usually detected during train-of-four stimulation; at a single-twitch height of 14% of control, two contractions are in evidence, and when the single-twitch height is about 7%, only one contraction is detected.[982] During procedures in which a child's hand is covered by surgical drapes, palpating the number of contractions provides a satisfactory alternative. The number of contractions during train-of-four stimulation thus yields a practical assessment of neuromuscular blockade. For more profound blockade, the posttetanic counts can be used intermittently. However, repeated tetanic stimulation is not ideal because it is painful and can lead to posttetanic exhaustion.

Although twitch monitoring is the standard method of evaluating neuromuscular blockade, the neuromuscular blockade in one group of muscles can differ substantively from that in another. For example, 1.7 times more relaxant is required to block the diaphragm and the vocal cords than the adductor pollicis.[983,984] Nonetheless, recovery of the twitch response is also approximately 50% more rapid in these central muscles. Accordingly, it is conceivable that children could cough or react during intubation in the absence of the twitch response when it is measured peripherally. Perhaps more importantly, when the peripheral twitch response has recovered at the end of the procedure, it is a clear indication that the diaphragm and the vocal cords are in a more advanced stage of recovery. Monitoring the orbicularis oculi contraction (as an estimate of the relaxation of central muscles) to predict whether the conditions for tracheal intubation are suitable, is preferred because it occurs before the twitch response of the adductor muscle of the thumb.[985]

Another method for monitoring neuromuscular blockade is acceleromyography, which uses a piezoelectric sensor to quantitate the movement of the thumb, converting this to an electrical signal. There is considerable disagreement in the published literature as to which of these techniques is most accurate.[986-988] Monitors based on acceleromyography are becoming more commonly available; however, these are not "user friendly" and are difficult to use in infants because of the small arc of the displaced thumb. Some consider this monitor to be more accurate than standard mechanomyography based train-of-four monitors.[989,990] Others think that mechanomyography is more accurate because it is "less influenced by external disturbances," i.e., it does not go out of calibration.[991] Therefore, at present, for clinical purposes in infants and children, mechanomyography still seems to be the simplest and most helpful clinical monitor during the use of nondepolarizing competitive blockers.

## NEUROMUSCULAR JUNCTION

Adult postjunctional acetylcholine receptors possess five subunits—two $\alpha$ and one $\beta$, $\delta$, and $\varepsilon$ subunits. Preterm neonates (less than 31 weeks PMA) have a $\gamma$ subunit instead of an $\varepsilon$ subunit in their neuromuscular receptor.[992] Fetal receptors have a greater opening time than adult receptors, allowing more sodium to enter the cell, with a consequent larger depolarizing potential. The resulting increased sensitivity to acetylcholine is at odds with the observed increased sensitivity to NMBDs, but may compensate for reduced acetylcholine stores in the terminal nerve endings.[993]

Neuromuscular transmission is immature in neonates and infants until the age of 2 months.[975,994] Neonates deplete acetylcholine vesicle reserves more quickly than do infants older than 2 months, in response to tetanic nerve stimulation.[975] Data from phrenic nerve–hemidiaphragm preparations from rats aged 11 to 28 days suggest this is the result of a low quantal content of acetylcholine in neonatal endplate potentials.[243] Neonates display an increased sensitivity to NMBDs. An alternative proposal to explain this increased sensitivity is based on NMBD synergism observations.[995,996] Neonates display poor synergism and this has been explained on the basis that NMBDs occupy only one of the two $\alpha$-subunit receptor sites in neonates as opposed to two in children and adults.[996] If this is true, then neonates may use NMBDs more efficiently than children.

Preterm infants tolerate respiratory loads poorly. The diaphragm in the preterm neonate contains only 10% of the slowly contracting type I fibers. This proportion increases to 25% at term, and to 55% by 2 years of age.[245] A similar maturation pattern has been observed for the intercostal muscles.[245] Type I fibers tend to be more sensitive to NMBDs than type II fibers, and consequently the diaphragmatic function in neonates may be better preserved and recover earlier than peripheral muscles.[984,997-999]

Total body water and extracellular fluid (ECF)[1000] are greatest in preterm neonates and decrease throughout gestation and postnatal life, whereas fat as a percentage of body weight increases with postnatal age. Muscle contributes only 10% of body weight in neonates, and 33% by the end of childhood. Polar drugs, such as depolarizing and nondepolarizing NMBDs, distribute rapidly into the ECF, but enter cells more slowly. Consequently, a larger initial dose of such drugs is required in infants compared with children or adults. Increasing the muscle bulk contributes new acetylcholine receptors. This greater number of receptors requires a greater amount of drug to block activation of receptor ion channels.

## PHARMACODYNAMICS

There is age-related variability in the dose required to achieve a predetermined level of neuromuscular blockade during balanced thiopental–N$_2$O–fentanyl anesthesia. The ED$_{95}$ of vecuronium was $47 \pm 11$ $\mu$g/kg in neonates and infants, $81 \pm 12$ $\mu$g/kg in children between 3 and 10 years of age and $55 \pm 12$ $\mu$g/kg in children aged 13 years or older (Fig. 6-19).[1001]

Similar profiles have been reported for other NMBDs.[984,1002-1005] In addition, duration of neuromuscular blockade is greater in neonates than in children.[1006] The reduced dose requirement in neonates is attributable to immaturity of the neuromuscular junction. The increased Vd from an expanded ECF in neonates means

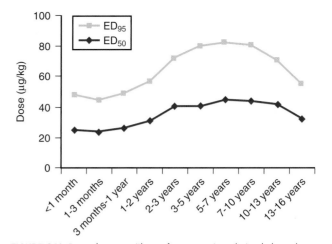

**FIGURE 6-19** Dose changes with age for vecuronium during balanced anesthesia. *ED$_{50}$* is the dose that achieves 50% of the maximum response; *ED$_{95}$* is the dose that achieves 95% of the maximum response. (Data extracted from Meretoja OA, Wirtavuori K, Neuvonen PJ. Age-dependence of the dose-response curve of vecuronium in pediatric patients during balanced anesthesia. Anesth Analg 1988;67:21-6.)

a similar initial dose (per kilogram) is given to neonates and teenagers. Children tend to require larger doses than adults; the reason for the larger dose requirement in children is unclear but it may be the result of increased muscle bulk.

Investigation of concentration–response relationships is more revealing. The plasma concentration required in neonates to achieve the same level of neuromuscular block as in children or adults is 20% to 50% less, consistent with immaturity of the neuromuscular junction.[85,1007-1010] Plasma concentration requirements are reduced by volatile anesthetic agents.[559,1011,1012]

The onset time for NMBDs in neonates is faster than it is in older children and adults. Onset time (time to maximal effect) after vecuronium 70 $\mu$g/kg was most rapid for infants $(1.5 \pm 0.6$ min) compared with that for children $(2.4 \pm 1.4$ min) and adults $(2.9 \pm 0.2$ min).[1006] These observations are similar to those reported for other intermediate- and long-acting NMBDs.[999] The more rapid onset of these drugs in neonates has been attributed to a greater cardiac output seen with the per-kilogram model.[999]

Cardiac output is used as a surrogate measure for muscle perfusion. Onset time is a function of size. An onset time standardized to a 70 kg person using an allometric $\frac{1}{4}$-power model is around 3 minutes for most long acting NMBDs. In children with low cardiac output or decreased muscle perfusion, onset times are prolonged. The onset time of neuromuscular paralysis is proportional to T$_{1/2}$keo. An increase in the T$_{1/2}$keo of *d*-tubocurare with increasing inspired halothane concentration has been demonstrated.[267] The reason for the delayed action of tubocurarine may be that halothane is a negative inotrope[268] and decreases muscle blood flow.[1013]

## PHARMACOKINETICS

The dose of NMBDs at different ages depends on the complex interweaving of PD and PK factors. The Vd mirrors ECF changes and can be predicted using either an allometric $\frac{3}{4}$-power model or the surface area model ($\frac{2}{3}$-power model), both of which approximate ECF changes with weight.[67]

The clearance of *d*-tubocurarine, standardized to an allometric or surface area model, is reduced in neonates and infants compared with older children and adults.[85] These age-related clearance changes follow age-related maturation of glomerular filtration in the kidney,[175] which is the elimination route of *d*-tubocurarine. Total plasma clearance of other nondepolarizing muscle relaxants cleared by renal (alcuronium) and/or hepatic pathways (pancuronium, pipecuronium, rocuronium, and vecuronium) are all reduced in neonates.[1007,1009,1014-1016] In contrast, the clearances of atracurium and cisatracurium are neither renal- nor hepatic-dependent but rather depend on Hofmann elimination, ester hydrolysis, and other unspecified pathways.[1017] Clearance of these drugs is increased in neonates when expressed as per kilogram.[1018-1020] When clearance is standardized using allometric ¾-power scaling, the clearances for atracurium and cisatracurium are similar throughout all age groups. The clearance of succinylcholine, expressed as per kilogram, also decreases as age increases.[209,210] Succinylcholine is hydrolyzed by butyrylcholinesterase. These observations are consistent with that observed for the clearance of remifentanil,[52] which is also cleared by plasma esterases. These clearance pathways are mature at birth.[53]

Conversion of *d*-tubocurarine half-times from chronologic time to physiologic time is revealing. $T_{1/2}\alpha$ increases with age in chronologic time, but in physiologic time it is the same at all ages, as we would expect from a distribution phase standardized by allometry. $T_{1/2}\beta$ decreases with age in physiologic time, consistent with reduced clearance related to the greater Vd in the very young. The $T_{1/2}keo$ is large in neonates and infants, reduced in children, and further reduced in adults, possibly because of increased muscle bulk and concomitant increased muscle perfusion in older children and adults.

## SUCCINYLCHOLINE

Succinylcholine is the only depolarizing relaxant used in children. Infants are more resistant to its neuromuscular effects than adults.[1021] Early studies demonstrated that the degree of neuromuscular blockade achieved by 1 mg/kg IV in infants is about equal to that produced by 0.5 mg/kg in older children.[1022] The increase in dose requirement in younger children is thought to result, in part, from the drug's rapid distribution into the infant's large ECF volume (E-Table 6-4 and Table 6-13).

Succinylcholine remains the NMBD with the most rapid onset. The onset time of a paralyzing dose (1.0 mg/kg) of succinylcholine is 35 to 55 seconds in children and adolescents; the onset time after 3 mg/kg in neonates is faster (30 to 40 sec).[1023] Onset time is dependent on both age and dose; the younger the child and the greater the dose, the shorter the onset time.

As in adults, administration of a continuous infusion of succinylcholine in infants and children can result in tachyphylaxis (increased requirement). In addition, phase II block may be produced, as evidenced by a train-of-four less than 50% (blockade similar to that produced by nondepolarizing muscle relaxants). In children, tachyphylaxis generally develops after administration of about 3 mg/kg of succinylcholine, and phase II block develops during tachyphylaxis after 4 mg/kg.[210,1024]

Succinylcholine is effective when administered by the IM route; in this instance, complete paralysis is achieved in 3 to 4 minutes. Evidence of relaxation of the respiratory muscles, as manifest by decreased positive pressure required to ventilate by face mask, can be detected before the abolishment of the twitch response. A dose of 2 mg/kg IM does not achieve satisfactory relaxation in all children, whereas the higher dose of 3 mg/kg IM produces a mean twitch depression of 85%; 4 mg/kg produces

| TABLE 6-13 | Suggested Standard Intubating Doses of Commonly Used Relaxants in Infants and Children | |
|---|---|---|
| | Infants (mg/kg) | Children (mg/kg) |
| Succinylcholine | 3 | 1.5-2 |
| Cisatracurium | 0.1 | 0.1-0.2 |
| Atracurium | 0.5 | 0.5 |
| Rocuronium* | 0.25-0.5 | 0.6-1.2 |
| Pancuronium | 0.1 | 0.1 |
| Vecuronium | 0.07-0.1 | 0.1 |

(See text for source data.)
*Low-dose rocuronium (0.3 mg/kg) allows tracheal intubation after 3 minutes during inhalational anesthesia in children, but then is easily antagonized in about 20 minutes. Large-dose rocuronium (1.2 mg/kg) may be used as a substitute for succinylcholine for rapid intubation in children.

profound relaxation in all children, but its effects may last up to 20 minutes.[1025] In infants younger than 6 months of age, a dose of 5 mg/kg IM is required to achieve profound relaxation; maximal twitch depression occurred a mean of 3.3 ± 0.4 minutes.[1026] Recovery from the neuromuscular effect of IM succinylcholine is faster in infants than in children. Changes in the heart rate after IM succinylcholine are not pronounced. Consequently, routine IM administration of atropine with IM succinylcholine is not generally indicated.[1027] Succinylcholine has also been administered intralingually.[1028,1029] One study examined the time to clinical apnea in 60 children younger than 10 years of age. Succinylcholine (1.1 mg/kg) resulted in apnea in 75 ± 4 seconds when administered intralingually, in 35 ± 1 seconds when administered intravenously, and in 210 ± 17 seconds when administered intramuscularly.[1029] In that study, 8 of 10 children given intralingual succinylcholine who did not receive concomitant atropine developed an arrhythmia (primarily bradycardia).

In an emergency, an alternate route for administration of succinylcholine (3 mg/kg) when an IV line is not in place should offer a fairly rapid onset of relaxation. Intralingual administration with an onset of 133 sec, is significantly more rapid than after IM injection, 295 sec.[1028] Caution should be exercised, however, when administering sublingual or intralingual medications. To preclude an intralingual hematoma, it is advised that a 25-gauge needle be used and the blood vessels on the undersurface of the tongue identified to minimize the risk of puncture. Sublingual succinylcholine is an alternative to the IV route, but it should be preceded by a vagolytic agent to avoid arrhythmias. The submental approach would seem to avoid the potential for causing bleeding from the tongue.

### Cholinesterase Deficiency

Plasma cholinesterase (pseudocholinesterase) is a circulating glycoprotein that metabolizes succinylcholine into succinylmonocholine. Activity of plasma cholinesterase may decrease as a result of a congenital enzyme variant or an acquired cause. This enzyme codes at the E1 locus of the long arm of chromosome 3. Ninety-six percent of the population is homozygous for the "usual" cholinesterase enzyme and 4% are homozygous or heterozygous for the variant alleles.[1030] Five alleles code for the majority of cholinesterase enzyme: (1) normal cholinesterase enzyme, which is designated by "usual" ($E^u$); (2) decreased cholinesterase activity or quantity, which is designated as atypical ($E^a$) (homozygote in 1:3000 to 1:10,000); (3) fluoride resistant allele ($E^f$)

(homozygote in 1:150,000); (4) silent allele ($E^s$) (homozygote 1:10,000); and (5) the Cynthiana ($C_5$) or Neitlich variant, which is associated with an increase in (or rapid) cholinesterase activity.[1031] Variations on the silent gene have been detected in Eskimo populations with three variants labeled: S for silent, T for trace, and R for residual. The duration of succinylcholine in children who are homozygous for the silent gene may be up to 6 to 8 hours. Additional genetic variants of pseudocholinesterase have been identified, including types H, J, and K, which represent a 60%, 66%, and 30% reduction in enzyme activity, respectively.[1030] Evidence suggests that K variant occurs in 13% of the random population and that K/K homozygous variant may be present in 1:63 population, one of the most common variants with a duration of prolonged blockade of less than 1 hour. Moreover, K variants have occurred in the presence of other mutations suggesting that multiple mutations may be present in the same patient.

Heterozygote atypical ($E^u E^a$), which occurs in 1:30 of the population, may prolong neuromuscular blockade by only a few minutes and may go undetected. In contrast, homozygote atypical ($E^a E^a$), which occurs in approximately 1:3000 population, may cause paralysis for up to 1 hour after a single dose of succinylcholine. Of the genetic variants of cholinesterase, silent gene ($E^s$) confers the least plasma cholinesterase activity and therefore the most prolonged duration of paralysis. Homozygote ($E^s E^s$) occurs in 1:10,000 population and may result in 8 hours of paralysis. Plasma cholinesterase activity is more often diminished when a genetic variant is present, but a number of clinical conditions may also reduce its activity. These include severe liver disease, malnutrition, organophosphate poisoning, severe burns, renal failure, plasmapheresis, and medications (cyclophosphamide, echothiophate iodide, oral contraceptives).[1030,1032,1033] Several conditions are associated with increases in plasma cholinesterase activity, including thyroid disease, obesity, nephrotic syndrome, and cognitively challenged children.[1030,1034-1036]

Plasma cholinesterase activity is determined by the percent inhibition of benzyl choline degradation by the amide local anesthetic dibucaine when it is incubated with a sample of plasma. With the homozygous normal allele ($E^u E^u$), dibucaine profoundly inhibits plasma cholinesterase activity (approximately 80%), whereas with the homozygous atypical allele ($E^a E^a$), it inhibits the activity by only 20%. When fluoride is added to the plasma, fluoride inhibits $E^u E^u$ 60% but inhibits $E^f E^f$ only 36%. Thus, a low dibucaine number indicates a deficiency of plasma cholinesterase.

## Adverse Effects of Succinylcholine

### Temporomandibular Joint Stiffness

IV succinylcholine is infrequently associated with an increase in masseter muscle tone that limits mouth opening (trismus), particularly when given during halothane anesthesia. The incidence of isolated trismus when IV succinylcholine is administered during halothane anesthesia, 0.3% to 1%, is severalfold greater than that after IV thiopental and succinylcholine, 0/4457 (upper 95% confidence of 7/10,000).[1037,1038] The increase in masseter muscle tone after succinylcholine is transient, lasting for only a few minutes and occurring despite abolition of the evoked twitch response in the masseter and peripheral muscles. The increase in masseter muscle tone is usually mild and can be overcome by manually distracting the mandible.[1039] However, on rare occasions, the increase in muscle tone may be so severe that mouth opening is impossible, thus interfering or preventing tracheal

intubation. Whether this increased tone is related to the "trismus" (so-called "jaws of steel") (see Fig. 40-2) encountered in children with MH remains a matter of debate.[1040] Prospective studies designed to evaluate masseter muscle tone have failed to demonstrate a child with a marked increase in masseter tone who later developed evidence of MH.[1041,1042] In several retrospective reports, however, a number of children experienced severe trismus and did develop or have a positive test response for MH.[1043-1045] These studies failed to clarify how best to proceed when severe trismus occurs. Some advocate canceling the surgical procedure, treating the child as susceptible to MH, and recommending a muscle biopsy.[1045,1046] This recommendation is based on a 50% incidence of positive muscle biopsies for MH in children who developed severe trismus after succinylcholine. Others advocate continuing the procedure, avoiding further exposure to triggering agents by changing the anesthetic technique to one that is free of triggers, observing for signs of MH (e.g., increased $CO_2$ production or tachycardia), and, if indicated, initiating arterial and central venous blood gas sampling, as well as early treatment.[1047,1048] Finally, others have advocated continuing with the original triggering anesthetic while monitoring for signs of MH.[1037] For the most part, this entire issue has become moot because sevoflurane has supplanted halothane as the primary inhaled anesthetic in children and the FDA issued a "black box" warning regarding the routine use of succinylcholine for tracheal intubation in children. Curiously, the now widespread use of nondepolarizing relaxants has generated several purported reports of masseter muscle rigidity after use of these agents. Whether these cases actually represent nondepolarizing relaxant–induced masseter spasm or a combination of light anesthesia and incomplete muscle relaxation is unclear.[1049-1051]

### Arrhythmias

The molecular structure of succinylcholine resembles that of two acetylcholine molecules joined by an ester linkage. The consequent stimulation of cholinergic autonomic receptors can be associated with cardiac arrhythmias, increased salivation, and bronchial secretions. Changes in heart rate are frequently observed after treatment with succinylcholine. Heart rate usually increases transiently and this response appears to be more pronounced in the presence of sevoflurane than halothane.[1052] Succinylcholine-associated arrhythmias are rarely a result of ventricular irritability. Prior IV administration of an anticholinergic agent (e.g., atropine) markedly decreases, but does not completely abolish, the incidence of these arrhythmias.[1053] As in adults, the incidence and severity of these irregularities in heart rate increase after a second dose.[1029,1054] Of greater concern is the occasional bradycardia and asystole after a single dose in children.[1053] Accordingly, it is recommended that a vagolytic agent precede the IV administration of succinylcholine unless there is a contraindication to such medications.

### Hyperkalemia

Succinylcholine-induced muscle fasciculation is also associated with mild hyperkalemia, increased intragastric and intraocular pressure, and skeletal muscle pains; rhabdomyolysis and myoglobinemia may occur in those patients suffering neuromuscular disorders. These disorders are not always diagnosable in neonates. Congenital myotonic dystrophy, for example, may present with mild respiratory dysfunction or feeding difficulty in the neonate. The response to succinylcholine in these neonates, however, remains dramatic, with sustained muscle contraction.[1055]

The serum potassium concentration increases 1 mEq/L or less after IV succinylcholine in normal children; this increase does not cause arrhythmias.[1056] However, life-threatening hyperkalemia can occur after a single IV dose of succinylcholine in children with burns (more than 8% body surface area burn), those who are immobile, or who have chronic infections (including intra-abdominal sepsis and *Clostridium*), upper motor neuron lesions (e.g., paraplegia, encephalitis), lower motor neuron lesions (e.g., tetanus, neuropathy complicating nephropathy), crush injuries, and neuromuscular diseases (including Werdnig-Hoffman disease).[1057-1064] In these situations, direct denervation injury or a pseudo-denervation state (immobilization) leads to a proliferation of extrajunctional normal acetylcholine receptors, as well as proliferation of immature (containing γ subunits) and nicotinic (neuronal) acetylcholine receptors, along the muscle membrane, so that the entire muscle becomes capable of releasing potassium during depolarization.[1064] These immature and nicotinic acetylcholine receptors release more intracellular potassium and for a longer period after the channels open, than do the usual acetylcholine receptors. The presence of extrajunctional receptors has been documented within several hours of injury, although clinically significant hyperkalemia does not seem to occur until 1 to 3 days after injury. Thus, administration of succinylcholine to children with these injuries may result in a massive efflux of intracellular potassium, leading to a cardiac arrest.[1065] In contrast to these acquired conditions, children who are born spastic quadriparetic from cerebral palsy or those with a myelomeningocele respond with a normal increase in serum potassium concentration (less than 1 mEq/L) after IV administration of succinylcholine.[1065-1067] The definitive treatment of succinylcholine-induced hyperkalemia is IV calcium (10 mg/kg calcium chloride or 30 mg/kg calcium gluconate or more). This restores the gap between the resting membrane potential of the cardiac cells and the threshold potential for depolarization. Repeated doses of calcium may be required, together with cardiopulmonary resuscitation, epinephrine, sodium bicarbonate, hyperventilation, inhaled albuterol (or intravenous salbutamol), or glucose and insulin, until the arrhythmias abate. Defibrillation of the heart has no role in this circumstance. Successful treatment of hyperkalemia might require a very prolonged resuscitation. Sodium polystyrene sulfonate by nasogastric or rectal administration may be required for leaching potassium after acute redistribution between extracellular and intracellular spaces by the above measures (see Chapters 8, 26, and 39).

### Biochemical Changes

Serum creatine kinase concentrations may increase after administration of succinylcholine in the presence of inhalational agents, especially halothane.[1068] This increase is less pronounced during a thiopental–nitrous oxide anesthetic but more pronounced in children with neuromuscular disease.[1069] After a malignant hyperthermia reaction, creatine kinase reaches its peak 12 to 18 hours after the onset of the reaction. It may also be found in association with a "jaws of steel" response to succinylcholine.

### Rhabdomyolysis

Rhabdomyolysis can occur after halothane or sevoflurane,[1070] even in the absence of succinylcholine as in the case of Duchenne and Becker muscular dystrophy. Isolated rhabdomyolysis or rhabdomyolysis in combination with hyperkalemia as in the case of Duchenne muscular dystrophy, requires hyperhydration with alkalinization of the urine to prevent acute tubular necrosis from deposition of myoglobin.

### *Myoglobinemia*

Myoglobinemia, another sensitive indicator of muscle injury, may occur after succinylcholine treatment, but rarely leads to myoglobinurea (i.e., "cola"-colored urine).[1071] If it occurs, it should be aggressively treated as described previously for rhabdomyolysis.

### *Fasciculations*

Fasciculations are usually observed in adolescents and children but rarely in infants; in children 1 to 3 years old they are described as gross muscle movements.[1068,1072] Pretreatment with small doses of succinylcholine (100 μg/kg), pancuronium (20 μg/kg), fentanyl (1 to 2 μg/kg), or alfentanil (50 μg/kg) may decrease the frequency and intensity of the fasciculations and the consequent rise of intragastric pressure.[1068,1072-1075] This increase in intragastric pressure, however, is offset by the increase in skeletal muscle tone of the crura of the diaphragm, thereby actually increasing the barrier to regurgitation.

### *Intraocular Pressure*

Intraocular pressure increases transiently in children after IV succinylcholine independent of the presence of fasciculations.[1076] The exact mechanism of this increase in IOP is not clear. Initially, the increase in IOP was attributed to tonic contractions of extraocular muscles but it is probably because of the cycloplegic action of succinylcholine, with deepening of the anterior chamber and increased outflow resistance. The IOP usually increases by about 10 mm Hg, peaks in 2 to 3 minutes, and then returns to baseline in 5 to 7 minutes.[1076] It is advisable to perform applanation tonometry before succinylcholine, or wait at least 7 minutes after succinylcholine before performing tonometry in children. Although the use of succinylcholine in children with open eye injuries has not resulted in further damage to the eye,[1077] it is nonetheless prudent to refrain from its use in situations of penetrating ocular wounds unless the eye is not salvageable. High-dose rocuronium (1.2 mg/kg) is a reasonable substitute for succinylcholine rapid-sequence intubation in these circumstances.[1078]

## Clinical Uses of Succinylcholine

The use of succinylcholine for routine surgical procedures in children has been abandoned, primarily because of the rare but life-threatening possibility of cardiac arrest in male children with undiagnosed muscular dystrophy.[1079,1080] On the other hand, succinylcholine does have the most rapid onset and brief duration of action of all currently available muscle relaxants. Consequently, succinylcholine is desirable for rapid-sequence tracheal intubation for brief procedures and for the treatment of laryngospasm.[1023,1081,1082] Because the rapidity of onset is dose related, 1.5 to 2.0 mg/kg IV succinylcholine should be administered to children to depress the neuromuscular twitch 95% within 40 seconds; the smaller dose of 1.0 mg/kg would achieve the same degree of depression in about 50 seconds.[1023,1081] In infants younger than 1 year of age, 3 mg/kg IV would be an appropriate dose because of the larger Vd. These doses provide excellent intubating conditions in all children.[1023] To decrease the incidence of arrhythmias after succinylcholine (particularly after a second dose), atropine 0.01 to 0.02 mg/kg IV should precede the succinylcholine.

In 1993 the FDA issued a "black box" warning against the routine use of succinylcholine in children and adolescents except for emergency airway management. This was based on several case reports of hyperkalemic cardiac arrests, primarily in children with undiagnosed Duchenne muscular dystrophy.[1083] The disturbing observation about this complication was the staggering mortality rate of 55%. Almost all of these cases, however, occurred in male children 8 years old and younger. In many instances the arrhythmias were misdiagnosed as MH and not treated with IV calcium in a timely manner. Subsequently, the FDA and the manufacturer revised the product label (package insert) to read:

*Since there may be no signs or symptoms to alert the practitioner to which patients are at risk, it is recommended that the use of succinylcholine should be reserved for emergency intubation or in instances where immediate securing of the airway is necessary, e.g., laryngospasm, difficult airway, full stomach, of for intramuscular route when a suitable vein in inaccessible.*

In cases in which the child has eaten and is at risk for a hyperkalemic response to succinylcholine, a standard rapid-sequence intubation with equivalent intubation conditions may be performed using high-dose rocuronium (1.2 mg/kg).[1078] The main disadvantage of using a nondepolarizing relaxant is that the duration of the nondepolarizing relaxant may exceed the duration of the planned procedure. A new agent that antagonizes rocuronium (sugammadex) will likely solve the dilemma and allow rapid intubation with rocuronium, even for brief emergency procedures, while avoiding the need to use succinylcholine (see later discussion).[1084-1087]

# Intermediate-Acting Nondepolarizing Relaxants

## ATRACURIUM

Chemically, atracurium (Tracrium) is an imidazoline bisquaternary compound that undergoes spontaneous decomposition into inactive metabolites. At physiologic (alkaline) pH, it undergoes enzymatic hydrolysis independent of plasma cholinesterase (Hofmann elimination), ester hydrolysis, and other unspecified pathways.[1017] In blood and other tissue fluids, the quaternary ammonium compound breaks down primarily into laudanosine and a related quaternary acid (methylacrylate). The elimination half-life of atracurium is similar in infants and children (14 to 20 minutes). The steady state plasma concentration resulting in 50% neuromuscular block ($EC_{50}$) did not differ between infants, children, or adults (363, 444, or 436 ng/mL, respectively).[1008]

For intubating purposes, two to three times the $ED_{95}$ (300 to 600 μg/kg) is given to produce effective blockade in most children.[1088,1089] Such doses provide satisfactory conditions for intubation within 2 minutes. The period of absence of twitch response after an intubating dose of atracurium usually lasts 15 to 30 minutes. Hence, in clinical situations, an intubating dose should provide complete neuromuscular blockade for such an interval, followed by another 20 minutes of intermediate blockade (twitch height 5% to 25%); complete recovery usually occurs within 40 to 60 minutes. Comparison of data from children and adults demonstrate that children require more atracurium per kilogram and generally recover faster. This difference, however, is relatively small and is masked in most cases by the wide range of individual patient responses.

Because atracurium is degraded spontaneously, and its metabolites do not have neuromuscular blocking properties, it can be easily administered by continuous infusion. The infusion requirement to maintain 90% to 99% twitch depression in children is 6 μg/kg/min during isoflurane anesthesia, 7 to 8 μg/kg/min with halothane, and 9 μg/kg/min with a $N_2O:O_2$ opioid technique.[559,560] No significant differences in the Vd, clearance, or half-lives have been detected for atracurium between normal infants and children with impaired hepatic function.[1018] Plasma laudanosine concentrations tend to be greater in children with hepatic impairment than in children with normal hepatic function.[1018]

The side effects of atracurium are minimal. At clinical doses of up to 600 μg/kg, the compound does not significantly alter the heart rate or BP in children. Mild cutaneous flushing reactions are sometimes observed.[1088] Extremely rare instances of anaphylactoid reactions or bronchospasm have been reported.

## CISATRACURIUM

Cisatracurium (Nimbex) is one of the 10 stereoisomers of atracurium (1R-cis, 1'R-cis). Cisatracurium is three times more potent than atracurium, with the same duration of action.[1090] Similar to other nondepolarizing relaxants, its onset can be accelerated by increasing the dose (see E-Table 6-4 and Table 6-13); as with the other relaxants, this will increase the duration of the action. Cisatracurium, like atracurium, is a noncumulative agent with recovery occurring during the elimination phase rather than during the distribution phase.

Cisatracurium has a slightly slower onset of action than atracurium, consistent with its relative potency. Twice the $ED_{95}$ dose (80 μg/kg) of cisatracurium leads to complete suppression of the twitch response in 2.5 minutes. The recovery to 25% and 95% of control response occurs in 31 and 53 minutes, respectively.[1090-1093] Its histamine-releasing effects are minimal; its duration and recovery profile are essentially the same as atracurium.

The distribution and elimination half-lives of cisatracurium in children are 3.5 and 23 minutes, respectively. The Vdss and the total body clearance are greater (expressed as mg/kg, see Fig. 6-4) than in adults, thus explaining the faster recovery in children.[1019] In adults with renal failure, the clearance of cisatracurium is reduced by 13%; plasma laudanosine levels were greater but were only about 10% of those reported with atracurium.[1094] The duration of action of cisatracurium in renal failure patients is not significantly prolonged.[1095] It should be noted that patients receiving chronic anticonvulsant therapy (carbamazepine or phenytoin) can develop a moderate resistance to the action of cisatracurium.[1096]

## VECURONIUM

Vecuronium is the monoquaternary homologue of pancuronium in which the methyl group of the 2β-nitrogen atom is absent. The Vd is greater in infants than in children (357 ± 70 vs. 204 ± 116 mL/kg), whereas plasma clearances are similar (5.6 ± 1.0 vs. 5.9 ± 2.4 mL/kg/min).[1007]

Its primary advantage is the absence of any adverse cardiovascular effects even in doses several times greater than the usually recommended clinical doses (see E-Table 6-4 and Table 6-13).[1097] Vecuronium is primarily metabolized by the liver and excreted in bile.[1098] Dose requirements according to age groups are much more pronounced (more than 50%), with a biphasic distribution of the dose requirement and duration of action; infants younger than 1 year of age are significantly more sensitive to the action of vecuronium than are older children. As adolescence is reached, the requirement diminishes to that of adults.[1001,1006,1099,1100]

However, on rare occasions there may be resistance to vecuronium in neonates.[1101]

Neuromuscular blockers are often administered to critically ill children. Vecuronium has been popular because of the absence of cardiovascular side effects and because its metabolites do not seem to have CNS effects. However, adult and pediatric patients in ICUs have had residual weakness after the discontinuation of vecuronium, possibly contributed by active 3-OH metabolite or its steroid-like structure.[1102-1104] In one study in which the rate of infusion was adjusted by accelerometry, all children recovered within 1 hour. Of note in these children, the requirements of neonates and small infants was 45% less than those of older children.[1105] In this respect, cisatracurium seems to offer an advantage because its recovery from prolonged infusion in children is faster than that of vecuronium.[1106]

## ROCURONIUM

Rocuronium (Zemuron) is a monoquaternary steroidal muscle relaxant similar to vecuronium. It has the fastest onset of action of the intermediate-acting nondepolarizing relaxants because of its low potency and greater dose requirements.[1107] The onset time of rocuronium is 1 to 1.5 minutes following a $2 \times ED_{95}$ dose; this is 20 to 70 seconds faster than vecuronium, although its duration of action is similar.[1108] Rocuronium is eliminated primarily by the liver; the kidney excretes about 10%.[1109-1114] Renal failure does not affect the onset of rocuronium-induced neuromuscular blockade in adults or children. However, it may prolong the duration of action of rocuronium in adults, a finding not shared for children older than 1 year of age.[1109,1111,1114]

Rocuronium has an $ED_{95}$ of 303 µg/kg in children during halothane anesthesia,[1115] with slightly greater doses required during $N_2O:O_2$ opioid anesthesia.[1116-1118] After the administration of 600 µg/kg rocuronium ($2 \times ED_{95}$), 90% and 100% neuromuscular block occurred in 0.8 and 1.3 minutes (see E-Table 6-4 and Table 6-13). At this dose, heart rate increased by approximately 15 beats per minute in children. The mean time to recover to 25% of control was approximately 28 minutes, and recovery to 90% of control was 46 minutes.[1118]

For brief cases in which children are anesthetized with 8% inspired sevoflurane, 0.3 mg/kg rocuronium yields satisfactory intubating conditions within 2 to 3 minutes.[1119] This dose of rocuronium can be antagonized within approximately 20 minutes of administration.[1114] The intubating conditions after rocuronium (600 µg/kg) have been compared with those after vecuronium (100 µg/kg), atracurium (500 µg/kg), and succinylcholine (1 mg/kg). It was found that tracheal intubation could be performed within 60 seconds in all the children who had received rocuronium or succinylcholine, but not until 120 seconds after vecuronium and 180 seconds after atracurium.[1120,1121] The intubating conditions at 60 seconds are improved by increasing the dose[1122]; by increasing the dose to 1.2 mg/kg (3 to $4 \times ED_{95}$), the intubating conditions are similar to those after treatment with succinylcholine.[1078,1118] At the larger doses, heart rate increases transiently, while systolic and diastolic pressures are unchanged.[1115,1123] It is unclear whether this increase in heart rate after rocuronium is the result of pain on injection or an inherent chronotropic effect.[1086] Dosing studies in infants 2 to 11 months of age demonstrated a slightly faster onset of neuromuscular blockade than in older children with the same dose (600 µg/kg). The times to 90% and 100% twitch depression were 37 and 64 seconds, respectively. In infants, the rate of onset of neuromuscular blockade 60 seconds after rocuronium is comparable to that after succinylcholine.[1115,1124] Neonates appear to be more sensitive to rocuronium than older infants.[1125] In neonates, the duration of action of 600 µg/kg is approximately 90 minutes and there is marked patient-to-patient variability. Consequently, 450 µg/kg rocuronium provides adequate intubating conditions, with a duration of action of approximately 1 hour.[1125]

In a PK study, the clearance of rocuronium in infants was less than in children (4 vs 7 mL/kg/min), whereas the Vd was greater in infants. The mean residence time was 56 minutes in infants versus 26 minutes in children, thus explaining the prolonged duration of action of rocuronium in infants compared with children. In a steady-state target-controlled infusion study, the potency of rocuronium was greatest in infants, least in children, and intermediate in adults.[1126] The greater plasma clearance and smaller Vd of rocuronium in children compared with infants and adults result in a markedly smaller mean residence time and a decreased duration of neuromuscular blockade.[1009] Consistent with the dose-response effects of curare and vecuronium in infants, smaller plasma concentrations of rocuronium are required in the effect compartment in infants than in children to produce the same degree of neuromuscular blockade.[85] Sevoflurane markedly potentiates the effects of rocuronium.[1127]

If an IV route is unavailable, the IM route for rocuronium is a reasonable alternative; IM rocuronium (1.8 mg/kg, 3 × the IV intubating dose) provided poor intubating conditions 4 minutes after administration in most children. Neuromuscular blockade (greater than 98%) was achieved in 6 to 8 minutes.[1128] The bioavailability of IM rocuronium at these doses is approximately 80%[1129]; IM rocuronium appears to be a viable alternative to IM succinylcholine although the time of onset of neuromuscular blockade is very slow and may not be appropriate for emergent situations. The duration of IM rocuronium effect (approximately $80 \pm 22$ minutes) is much greater than that after IM succinylcholine.[1128]

## CLINICAL IMPLICATIONS WHEN USING SHORT- AND INTERMEDIATE-ACTING RELAXANTS

Short- and intermediate-acting relaxants have great utility in infants and children because of the large number of brief surgical procedures performed. Because of their short duration of action, these drugs can be given in one intubating dose (atracurium [500 µg/kg]; cisatracurium [200 µg/kg]; vecuronium [100 µg/kg]; rocuronium [600 µg/kg]) and a light anesthetic level maintained throughout the procedure. If more than 45 minutes elapse since the last dose of one of these neuromuscular blockers, one may reasonably assume that neuromuscular function has nearly recovered, but safe practice would recommend confirming *recovery of neuromuscular integrity by clinical signs or by assessment with a neuromuscular blockade monitor. We recommend antagonism in all infants despite clinical signs of recovery.*

The benzylisoquinoliniums and organosteroidal NMBDs are acidic compounds (pH 3 to 4) that can precipitate thiopental (pH 10 to 11) if admixed.[1130] Consequently, when these drugs are administered in tandem, the IV tubing should be thoroughly flushed between the thiopental and these relaxants. Vecuronium and rocuronium are painful when administered intravenously in a small vein during the light stages of anesthetic. This pain is usually demonstrated by withdrawal of the hand. Pain can be attenuated by deepening the level of anesthesia or pretreating with fentanyl, lidocaine, or ketamine.[1131,1132]

## Long-Acting Nondepolarizing Relaxants

For almost half a century the mainstay of muscle relaxants was curare (d-tubocurarine). After the development of intermediate relaxants, its use diminished because its duration of action was too great for most surgeries, and large doses released histamine. Curare is no longer available.

Following curare, several long-acting relaxants with minimal adverse effects were developed. These included metocurine, pipecuronium, and doxacurium, which are two, four, and ten times as potent as curare, respectively. The only long-acting relaxant that is still used in some institutions is pancuronium.

### PANCURONIUM

Pancuronium bromide (Pavulon) is a bisquaternary ammonium steroidal compound with nondepolarizing neuromuscular blocking properties. Pancuronium undergoes partial (15% to 20%) hepatic deacetylation to produce 3-OH, 17-OH, and 3,17-di-OH metabolites. A prolongation of effect can be expected in patients with renal or hepatic failure because a major proportion of pancuronium is excreted in the urine (40% to 60%) and in the bile (11%). Vd ($203 \pm 36$ mL/kg) and plasma clearance ($1.7 \pm 0.2$ mL/kg/min) of pancuronium (0.1 mg/kg) are associated with a long elimination half-life ($103 \pm 23$ min) in children (3 to 6 years) under halothane anesthesia.[1133] It is more potent than curare, metocurine, and gallamine, with a slightly shorter duration of action.[1134] It induces mild tachycardia by blocking presynaptic noradrenaline uptake (increased cardiac output in infants) but has no histamine-releasing properties. As a result, systolic BP tends to increase.[1135] Pancuronium (100 µg/kg) provides satisfactory conditions for tracheal intubation in 70% to 90% of infants and children within 150 seconds of administration. Increasing the initial dose to 150 µg/kg provides satisfactory intubating conditions in all children within 80 seconds (see E-Table 6-4 and Table 6-13).[1081,1136]

Pancuronium is frequently advocated for cardiac surgery and other high-risk procedures in infants and children. The anesthetic technique of combining a high-dose opioid with air–oxygen–pancuronium is well tolerated by infants, from a cardiovascular perspective. The vagolytic effect (tachycardia) of pancuronium counteracts the vagotonic effect (bradycardia) of potent opioids, and its relaxant properties counteract opioid-induced chest wall and glottic rigidity.[1137] Pancuronium has been used to facilitate ventilation in preterm infants in neonatal ICUs.[1138] Because pancuronium increases the heart rate, BP, and plasma epinephrine and norepinephrine levels in neonates, there is some concern that it may contribute to the risk of an intracerebral hemorrhage.[1139] Accordingly, it would seem prudent to administer pancuronium with either general anesthesia or with adequate sedation, to blunt adverse cardiovascular responses. Vecuronium may offer an advantage over pancuronium because it does not significantly increase the BP.[1140-1144] Nasotracheal intubation or intratracheal suctioning in neonates who are paralyzed with pancuronium results in smaller increases in intracranial pressure than in neonates who are not paralyzed.[1144,1145] By abolishing fluctuations in cerebral blood flow through the use of muscle relaxants, the incidence and severity of intraventricular hemorrhages should theoretically be reduced.

## Antagonism of Muscle Relaxants

### GENERAL PRINCIPLES

In children and especially infants, oxygen consumption is greater than it is in adults. Therefore, a slight diminution in respiratory muscle power may lead to hypoxemia and $CO_2$ retention. Consequently, it is very important that neuromuscular function is returned to normal at the end of the surgical procedure. Neonates are at greater risk for residual neuromuscular blockade than adults for several reasons, including (1) immaturity of the neuromuscular system, (2) greater elimination half-life of relaxants, (3) the reduced number of type I muscle fibers in the ventilatory musculature (thus being more susceptible to fatigue [see Chapter 12, Fig. 12-11]),[245] and (4) the closing lung volume of a neonate overlaps with the tidal volume (i.e., airway closure occurs at the end of expiration).[1146] If respiration is mildly impaired as a result of residual muscle paralysis, even more alveoli will collapse. The result may be hypoxemia as well as hypercarbia and acidosis, which may potentiate and prolong the duration of action of the muscle relaxant, thus creating a vicious cycle.

When monitoring neuromuscular blockade in infants and children, train-of-four monitoring of the adductor pollicis overestimates the degree of neuromuscular blockade in the diaphragm.[984] Larger doses of muscle relaxants are required to block the diaphragm than the adductor pollicis train-of-four would suggest. Therefore, if the train-of-four of the adductor has fully recovered, one can assume that the diaphragm has fully recovered.

Clinical evaluation of the adequacy of antagonism in infants is more difficult than in children or adults. Neither grip strength nor voluntary head lifting can be elicited; rather, it is important when working with infants to observe the clinical conditions preoperatively (muscle tone, depth of respiration, vigor of crying) and to aim for a comparable level of activity in the postantagonism period. Useful clinical signs that the neuromuscular blockade has been antagonized include the ability to flex the hips, flex the arm, lift the legs, and the return of abdominal muscle tone.[1147] Inspiratory force may be measured; a negative force of −25 cm $H_2O$ or greater indicates adequate antagonism.[1148] A crying vital capacity greater than 15 mL/kg indicates an adequate respiratory reserve. The train-of-four is a valuable aid because it can be used in the smallest of infants in whom the force of contraction can easily be palpated (four equal contractions indicating adequate antagonism).

Although edrophonium may establish a faster onset of effect, final recovery is invariably greater with neostigmine, which is why the latter is recommended for routine pediatric practice.[1149,1150] The distribution volumes of neostigmine are similar in infants (2 to 10 months), children (1 to 6 years), and adults (Vdss 0.5 L/kg), whereas the elimination half-life is less in children.[1151] Clearance decreases as age increases (13.6, 11.1, 9.6 mL/min/kg in infants, children, and adults 29 to 48 years, respectively).[1151] The dose requirement of anticholinesterase agents to antagonize neuromuscular blockade in children is less than adults.[1151] However, the speed of antagonism depends on the extent of neuromuscular blockade at the time of the antagonism, as well as the type and dose of antagonizing agent. In the presence of train-of-four responses with fade, 20 to 25 µg/kg of neostigmine, preceded by 10 to 20 µg/kg of atropine or 5 to 10 µg/kg of glycopyrrolate, is sufficient to achieve full recovery of muscle strength. This dose of neostigmine can be repeated if required (up to 70 µg/kg).

Doses of neostigmine in excess of 100 μg/kg may induce a paradoxical weakness from excessive acetylcholine at the neuromuscular junction. The dose of edrophonium for children is greater than it is for adults; at least 0.3 mg/kg is needed, but 0.5 to 1.0 mg/kg is most common.[1150,1152-1155]

Some have suggested that it is not necessary to antagonize intermediate-acting relaxants, particularly if a lengthy time interval has elapsed since the last dose. With the advent of reliable neuromuscular monitors and their use in conjunction with clinical observations and measurements of respiratory adequacy, clinicians are more confident that antagonism was not always required. This may be particularly appropriate for the short- and intermediate-acting relaxants, particularly atracurium or cisatracurium, which are hydrolyzed in plasma. Children have the additional advantage of recovering from neuromuscular blockade more rapidly than adults.[1154,1155] In infants, the elimination of all muscle relaxants might be delayed, necessitating antagonism of any neuromuscular blockade. Most importantly, if there is any concern that some degree of neuromuscular blockade persists, then the blockade must be antagonized.

Hypothermia potentiates the action of most nondepolarizing muscle relaxants and delays their elimination.[1156] This effect can create a special problem at the end of a surgical procedure when the children attempt to resume spontaneous respirations. Shivering increases oxygen consumption and augments the load on the respiratory system. If the respiratory muscles are unable to match this increased load, hypoxemia and $CO_2$ retention may occur, which, in turn, may lead to acidosis, which, again, may potentiate the relaxant. To avoid the extra cardiorespiratory load in a postsurgical infant, it is reasonable to warm the infant if the temperature is less than 35° C (95° F). Once the core temperature is above this level, antagonism of neuromuscular blockade may be attempted.

Theoretically, all antibiotics have neuromuscular depressing properties when administered in association with relaxants.[1157] Among the antibiotics, aminoglycoside derivatives, such as gentamicin, tobramycin, and neomycin, have the greatest effect. A single clinical dose of antibiotic will likely have minimal effect on the neuromuscular blockade.[1158] This factor alone does not rule out the possibility that large concentrations of antibiotics, especially in the presence of other potentiating factors, may augment the neuromuscular blockade. The clinical importance of the interaction of antibiotics with muscle relaxants to prolong neuromuscular blockade has diminished with the introduction of intermediate-acting neuromuscular blocking agents.

### SUGAMMADEX

Sugammadex (Org 25969), a member of the cyclodextrin family, is a cyclic oligosaccharide[1159] with hydrophobic molecules within the center (Fig. 6-20).[1160,1161] This compound encapsulates rocuronium, and vecuronium to a lesser degree, and forms a stable complex that prevents further action of the relaxants; the complex is then excreted unchanged by the kidneys. The chemical encapsulation decreases the plasma concentration of rocuronium, thus promoting the dissociation of rocuronium from the acetylcholine receptor, speeding recovery of muscle strength. As more rocuronium dissociates from the receptor, it, too, is encapsulated, thus reversing even very intense neuromuscular blockade from rocuronium. Three minutes after 0.6 mg/kg rocuronium produced profound neuromuscular block in adult volunteers, a single dose of sugammadex, 2 mg/kg or greater, reversed the neuromuscular block within 2 minutes.[1162] An early sugammadex study in children suggests that sugammadex, at 2 mg/kg, reverses a rocuronium-induced moderate neuromuscular blockade in infants, children, and adolescents.[1085] The average time to recover a train-of-four ratio of 0.9 at the time of appearance of the second twitch response was 1.2, 1.1, and 1.2 minutes in children, adolescents, and adults, respectively. If further clinical trials confirm the safety and efficacy of this new concept, and studies in children demonstrate safety and efficacy, then sugammadex may be effective in antagonizing large doses of rocuronium rapidly, efficiently, and soon after the onset of neuromuscular blockade.[1163-1167] Sugammadex rapidly antagonizes even intense neuromuscular blockade in adults, in whom no twitches were observed.[1164,1168] The rapidity of the reversal depends on both the intensity of the block and the dose of sugammadex.[1084,1086,1169] Under these circumstances, rocuronium might then supplant succinylcholine in many circumstances, including rapid-sequence intubations for brief procedures in children.[1087,1170]

However, two impediments have prevented the widespread use of sugammadex. First, there is some evidence that sugammadex may trigger allergic or anaphylactic reactions.[1171] This has halted the approval of sugammadex in North America. Second, sugammadex is not used for routine reversal because it is extremely expensive. This is quite unfortunate, as the incidence of hyperkalemia or MH induced by succinylcholine would likely have decreased to near zero if we could routinely substitute high-dose rocuronium without fear of prolonged neuromuscular blockade. The expense of sugammadex has put this medication out of financial practicality for routine use in nearly every healthcare facility in the world.[1172] Table 6-14 illustrates the approximate cost for reversal of various levels of blockade for several weight ranges. In contrast, reversal with current medications costs very little compared with the expense for similar antagonism with sugammadex. This renders sugammadex a rescue drug only. Data suggest that this drug could be used for rescue of a cannot-intubate/cannot-ventilate situation after administration of a rapid intubating dose of rocuronium (1.2 mg/kg) within 2 minutes, compared with the time for the effects of succinylcholine to abate.[1087,1164]

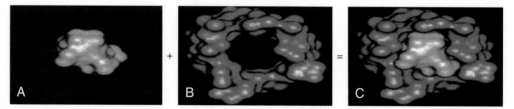

**FIGURE 6-20** X-ray crystallography of (**A**) the rocuronium molecule (shown in *blue*) and (**B**) sugammadex (*green ring*). **C,** The 3-D conformation of the rocuronium molecule complements the conformation of the inner ring of sugammadex. The rocuronium–sugammadex complex is stable, without a dissociation constant, and is excreted unchanged via the kidneys. (Redrawn from Gijsenbergh F, Ramael S, Houwing N, van IT. First human exposure of Org 25969, a novel agent to reverse the action of rocuronium bromide. Anesthesiology 2005;103:695-703.)

**TABLE 6-14** Approximate Cost (USD) for Sugammadex Reversal of Rocuronium by Weight and Density of Block*

| Depth of Block | WEIGHT (kg) | | | |
|---|---|---|---|---|
| | 3 | 10 | 20 | 70 |
| Mild (4 twitches with fade) 2 mg/kg | $1.46 | $9.75 | $19.50 | $67.90 |
| Moderate (1-2 twitches) 4 mg/kg | $1.95 | $19.50 | $39.00 | $135.80 |
| Profound (no twitches) 8 mg/kg | $3.90 | $39.00 | $78.00 | $271.60 |
| Wasted drug (single patient use profound blockade) | $93.60 | $58.50 | $19.50 | $68.03† |

(Personal communication from Neil Morton, MD. UK prices converted to USD as of June 2011.)
*This drug is not yet approved by the US FDA, so price is determined on UK basis.
†Assumes one large vial and one small vial for complete dosing.

In another application of the use of sugammadex, two recent reports describe its effectiveness to stop anaphylactic reactions to rocuronium that were resistant to standard treatment.[1173,1174]

If neuromuscular blockade must be reinstituted after administration of sugammadex, the dose of rocuronium that would be required for neuromuscular blockade is unclear. Although this is feasible,[1133] it would seem much more prudent to switch to a benzylisoquinolinium muscle relaxant that is unaffected by the presence of sugammadex.

## Relaxants in Special Situations

Of the many drug combinations possible, that of succinylcholine after a halothane induction seems to be most likely to trigger MH[1175] (see Chapter 40). The use of depolarizing neuromuscular blocking agents in combination with halogenated agents should be avoided in children at risk for this syndrome.[1176] The safest general anesthetic technique for children at risk for MH is an opioid plus $N_2O$ plus $O_2$ combination, together with benzodiazepines, propofol, and a nondepolarizing relaxant. Nondepolarizing agents devoid of cardiovascular side effects may offer an advantage in not causing tachycardia, an early sign of MH.[1177] There has been some concern of the potential association between mitochondrial disease and MH. A major review, along with evidence from pathology specimens from patients who had a family member with MH, suggest that this is not at all clear and may be a case of "fortuitous association."[1178] Because many of these children are bedridden, it would seem prudent to avoid succinylcholine, although there are *"inadequate data to support the recommendation … that the anesthetic plan for patients with mitochondrial disease should routinely include MH precautions."*[1179]

The use of NMBDs in children with neuromuscular and mitochondrial diseases has been the subject of debate.[1180] Rhabdomyolysis has been reported after succinylcholine in children with Duchenne and Becker muscular dystrophy (see Chapters 22 and 40). It is prudent to avoid succinylcholine in any child with

a suspicious neuromuscular or mitochondrial disease (see earlier). The response of children with neuromuscular disease to nondepolarizing relaxants is variable. Most are relatively sensitive to the NMBDs, particularly those with muscular dystrophy, because of muscle wasting.[1181,1182] The duration of neuromuscular blockade is often prolonged. Rarely, resistance may be evident as a result of chronic immobilization. Of all the nondepolarizing relaxants, we recommend cisatracurium because of its multiple sites of degradation that are independent of organ function.[1183-1185] The dose requirement of atracurium in children with Duchenne muscular dystrophy is similar to that in unaffected children, although the duration of action may be prolonged.[1183] The dose response of rocuronium in children with Duchenne muscular dystrophy shows marked prolongation of both the onset and recovery times (two to three times normal).[1186] Thus, NMBDs should be administered with caution in children with severe preexisting respiratory dysfunction, because even a small dose of a NMBD may cause profound muscle weakness and the need for ventilatory support. Similarly, it is important to antagonize any residual neuromuscular blockade at the end of surgery. *If there is any doubt about the competence of the neuromuscular junction, the trachea should remain intubated until muscle strength has recovered.*

Succinylcholine can cause hyperkalemia in children with burns, which may cause a cardiac arrest.[1187] The more extensive the burn, the more likely and the greater the hyperkalemic response. An 8% burn is the smallest burn that has been associated with hyperkalemia. Although most instances of cardiac arrest have occurred 20 to 50 days after the burn injury, exaggerated increases in the plasma concentration of potassium after succinylcholine can occur within a few days of the burn. However, hyperkalemia after succinylcholine has not been reported in the first 24 to 48 hours after a burn. Hyperkalemia is thought to result from the upregulation of acetylcholine receptors along the surface of the muscle membrane in the postburn phase (see Chapter 34).[1188]

Children with burns may require two to three times the usual IV dose of nondepolarizing relaxants. This resistance peaks about 2 weeks after the burn, persists for many months in those with major burns, and decreases gradually as the burns heal. The degree of resistance appears to correlate with both the extent of the burn and the period of healing. The resistance can be explained, in part, by an increase in the Vd of the relaxant (including binding to an increased plasma concentration of α1-acid glycoprotein) and an increase in number, sensitivity, and type of extrajunctional acetylcholine receptors (see Chapter 34).

## Opioids

### MORPHINE

Morphine is the most frequently used opioid to treat postoperative pain in children and is the standard against which all other opioids are compared. Morphine's main analgesic effect is by supraspinal $\mu_1$-receptor activation. The $\mu_2$-receptor in the spinal cord plays an important analgesic role when the drug is administered by the intrathecal or epidural route.[1189] Morphine is soluble in water, but lipid solubility is poor compared with other opioids. Morphine's low oil–water partition coefficient of 1.4 and its pKa of 8 (10% to 20% un-ionized drug at physiologic pH) contribute to delayed onset of peak action, with slow CNS penetration. The $T_{1/2}keo$ for morphine is approximately 17 minutes in adults[1190] and is estimated to be 8 minutes in the full-term neonate.[1191]

Target analgesic plasma concentrations are thought to be 10 to 20 ng/mL after major surgery in neonates and infants.[1192,1193] The large PK and PD variability suggests that morphine be titrated to effect using small incremental doses (0.02 mg/kg) in neonates and infants suffering postoperative pain.[1194]

Morphine is primarily metabolized by the hepatic enzyme UGT2B7 to morphine-3-glucuronide (M3G) and morphine-6-glucuronide (M6G); both have pharmacologic activity. Sulfation and renal clearance are minor pathways in adults but are more dominant in neonates. Contributions to both the desired effect (analgesia) and the undesired effects (nausea, respiratory depression) of M6G are the subject of clinical controversy.[1195] It has been suggested that M3G antagonizes morphine and contributes to the development of tolerance.[1196]

Clearance increases from 3.2 L/hr/70 kg at 24 weeks PMA to 19 L/hr/70 kg at term, reaching adult values (80 L/hr/70 kg) at 6 to 12 months (see Fig. 6-10).[57] These developmental factors for morphine metabolism explain in part the prolonged duration of action in neonates. The maturation profile also suggests that older infants are able to exceed the reported clearance (in L/hr/kg) of morphine in adults (see Fig. 6-4). Clearance is perfusion-limited, with a high hepatic extraction ratio. Oral bioavailability is approximately 35% because of this first pass effect. The metabolites are cleared by the kidney and, in part, by biliary excretion. Impaired renal function leads to M3G and M6G accumulation. Clearance is reduced in critically ill neonates compared healthier cohorts and in those undergoing cardiac surgery (Fig. 6-21).[57-59,1192]

Morphine PK parameters show large interindividual variability contributing to the range of morphine serum concentrations observed during constant infusions. Protein binding of morphine is small in preterm neonates and has minimal impact on the disposition changes with age.

Although morphine is usually administered intravenously to neonates, other routes have been used. A large variability in the analgesic effect of morphine has been observed after rectal administration; this is a major disadvantage of this route. Although this route is used,[1197] delayed absorption with multiple doses causing respiratory arrest has been reported.[1198] Morphine (25 to 50 µg/kg) can also be given via the caudal route and subarachnoid spaces (see Chapters 41 and 43).[1199,1200,1200-1209] Although systemic absorption is slow, morphine spreads within the CSF to the brainstem where it may cause respiratory depression lasting from 6 to more than 18 hours.[1195]

Morphine may be administered intravenously by intermittent bolus, continuous infusion, or patient-controlled analgesia (see Chapter 43).[1210-1212] The usual initial IV dose is 0.05 to 0.2 mg/kg. A reduced dose is indicated in children who are critically ill, are receiving supplemental analgesics or hypnotics, and/or have nocturnal hemoglobin desaturation during obstructive sleep apnea.[1213-1215]

The major risk associated with opioid use in infants and children is respiratory depression.[234,1182] Morphine infusion rates of 10 to 30 µg/kg/hr provide adequate postoperative analgesia without respiratory depression.[1216] Postoperative analgesia is achieved at reduced infusion rates in infants 4 weeks of age or older (~5 µg/kg/hr for neonates, ~8.5 µg/kg/hr at 1 month, ~13.5 µg/kg/hr at 3 months, ~18 µg/kg/hr at 1 year, and slightly less than 16 µg/kg/hr for 1- to 3-year-olds).[233] Respiratory depression may occur at concentrations of 20 ng/mL in infants and children,[231] but concentration-response relationships in neonates, particularly preterm neonates prone to physiologic apnea, are

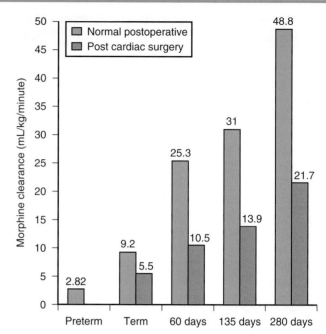

**FIGURE 6-21** Morphine clearance versus postconceptional age in normal postoperative infants and infants undergoing cardiac surgery. Note that there is a rapid increase in an infant's ability to metabolize morphine in the first several weeks of life and that some infants achieve adult values by 1 month of age. Also note that after cardiac surgery infants have a marked impairment of morphine metabolism, which may reflect the use of vasopressors and/or decreased cardiac output to the liver. There is extreme patient-to-patient variability at all ages; preterm infants have the lowest clearance of any age group. (Data from Lynn A, Nespeca MK, Bratton SL, et al. Clearance of morphine in postoperative infants during intravenous infusion: the influence of age and surgery. Anesth Analg 1998;86:958-63 and Mikkelsen S, Feilberg VL, Christensen CB, Lundstrom KE. Morphine pharmacokinetics in preterm and mature newborn infants. Acta Paediatr 1994;83:1025-8.)

unknown. When respiratory depression from morphine occurs, it results from both diminished tidal volume and respiratory rate. Whether morphine causes a parallel shift in the $CO_2$ response curve or a change in the slope, as well as a parallel shift, has not been clearly established. Morphine appears to depress respiration in neonates to a greater extent than meperidine,[1217] although the mechanism behind this is uncertain and may relate to altered PK, an immature blood-brain barrier,[223] altered regional blood flow, or an increased cerebral uptake. In neonatal rats, the brain uptake of morphine is two to three times that in adult rats.[223] This may explain the fivefold reduced $LD_{50}$ of morphine in neonatal versus adult animals.[221-223] This immaturity of the blood-brain barrier may account, in part, for the increased sensitivity of the neonate to morphine compared with meperidine or fentanyl; because of their lipophilicity, the latter two opioids rapidly cross an adult's or infant's blood-brain barrier, that is, there is essentially no blood-brain barrier.[1219] Alternatively, reduced clearance could lead to drug accumulation in some infants given repeat doses.[171] Another possibility is a maturation of the PD effects on respiration rather than altered PK, that is, a maturation of the sensitivity of the respiratory center to morphine, rather than a change in brain equilibrium.[1220] Whether one or more of these mechanisms is relevant, morphine must be used with caution in preterm infants and in infants younger than 1 year of age. Significant histamine release may follow a rapid IV bolus of morphine and,

| **TABLE 6-15** Relative Comparison of Commonly Used Oral and Parenteral Opioids in an Adult | | | |
|---|---|---|---|
| Drug | Parenteral Dose (mg) | Oral Dose (mg) | Half-Life (hour) |
| Morphine | 10 | 30-40 | 2.0-3.5 |
| Hydromorphone | 1.5-2.0 | 6.0-7.5 | 2-4 |
| Oxycodone | | 15-30 | 2-4 |
| Methadone | 7.5-10.0 | 15 | 22-25 |
| Meperidine | 75-100 | 300 | 3-5 |
| Codeine | 120-130 | 200 | 3 |
| Fentanyl | 0.1 | 0.1 | 0.5 |

Adapted from Lugo RA, Kern SE. Clinical pharmacokinetics of morphine. J Pain Palliat Care Pharmacother 2002;16:5-18.

on rare occasions, may result in systemic hypotension.[1221] Urticaria over the course of the vein in which morphine was infused is a local, not systemic, allergic reaction.

The incidence of vomiting in postoperative children is related to the morphine dose. Morphine doses in excess of 0.1 mg/kg are associated with a greater than 50% incidence of vomiting in children.[1222,1223] Withdrawal symptoms may be observed in neonates after cessation of a continuous morphine infusion for more than 2 weeks, and after infusion periods less than 2 weeks if the morphine infusion rate is greater than 40 $\mu$g/kg/hr. Strategies to prevent withdrawal from morphine include the use of neuraxial analgesia, nurse-controlled sedation management protocols, ketamine or naloxone mixed with morphine infusion, and the use of alternate agents (e.g., methadone) with lower potential for tolerance.[1224,1225] Table 6-15 summarizes the relative doses of opioids administered via the parenteral and oral routes.

## MEPERIDINE

Meperidine (Pethidine, Demerol) has been traditionally considered a potent opioid to treat severe pain, although in the past decade, meperidine is no longer indicated as an analgesic (because of its side effects and complications), leaving it indicated only for shivering.

Meperidine is a weak opioid, primarily $\mu$-receptor, agonist that has a potency approximately one-tenth that of morphine. The analgesic effects are detectable within 5 minutes of IV administration, and peak effect is reached within 10 minutes in adults ($T_{1/2}$keo of approximately 7 to 8 minutes).[1226,1227] Meperidine is metabolized by N-demethylation to meperidinic acid and normeperidine. Meperidine clearance in infants and children is approximately 8 to 10 mL/min/kg.[1228,1229] Elimination in neonates is greatly reduced, and elimination half-time in neonates who have received meperidine by placental transfer may be 2 to 7 times greater than that in adults.[1230] The elimination half-life of meperidine in children after IV administration is approximately 3 ± 0.5 hours,[1228] with a variable half-life in neonates between 3.3 and 59.4 hours.[1229] The Vdss in infants, 7.2 (3.3 to 11) L/kg,[1229] is greater than that in children 2 to 8 years (2.8 ± 0.6 L/kg).[1228]

In children, meperidine is indicated only to stop shivering, not for analgesia. Although its onset time is more rapid than morphine, the risk of seizures after repeated dosing in children has all but removed it from routine clinical use. The impression that meperidine causes less histamine release than morphine has been questioned.[1231] Meperidine is no more effective for treating biliary or renal tract spasm than comparative $\mu$ opioids.[1232] The

purported benefits of substituting meperidine for morphine in children who are hypovolemic or asthmatic are questionable.

The dose of meperidine is 1 to 2 mg/kg (see Table 6-15), although reduced doses should be used in critically ill children. Peak plasma values after IV, IM, and rectal administration are 5 minutes, 10 minutes, and 60 minutes, respectively.[1233,1234] Rectal administration of meperidine in children results in wide variations in systemic blood values (32% to 81% of administered dose) and is not recommended.[1228]

Respiratory depression in infants after meperidine appears to be less than after morphine.[1217] The $LD_{50}$ of meperidine in the neonatal animal is only 20% less than in the adult animal, corresponding with the human clinical response.[221] This is consistent with the reduced respiratory depression with meperidine compared with the equivalent dose of morphine. As with any opioid, the use of meperidine in very young infants must be accompanied by careful observation for respiratory depression and airway obstruction because the PK vary considerably.[1229] Meperidine was used for a number of years as a component of various "lytic cocktails" that provided sedation. It was administered rectally, orally and intramuscularly. The safety of these admixtures, especially in neonates, is dubious and its use in sedation mixtures has fallen into disfavor.[1235] Meperidine's local anesthetic properties have been found useful for epidural techniques in adults.[1236]

Because repeated doses of meperidine may result in the accumulation of normeperidine, which causes seizures,[1237,1238] this drug has been removed from the formulary in many children's hospitals. We do not recommend the use of this opioid other than for a single dose administration.

## HYDROMORPHONE

Hydromorphone (Dilaudid) is a semisynthetic congener of morphine with a potency of around 5 to 7.5 times that of morphine.[1239] IV and IM dose is 10 to 20 $\mu$g/kg with a continuous IV infusion of hydromorphone of 1-4 $\mu$g/kg/hr. Its bioavailability is about 55% after nasal and oral (30 to 80 $\mu$g/kg every 3 to 4 hours) administration and about 35% after rectal administration (not recommended)[1240-1242]; there is high first-pass metabolism.[1243] A clearance of 51.7 (range, 28.6 to 98.2) mL/min/kg is reported in children, with a half-life of 2.5 ± 0.9 hours.[1240,1244] Hydromorphone is metabolized to hydromorphone-3-glucuronide (95%) and to other metabolites.[1245]

Hydromorphone is commonly used when prolonged analgesia is required.[1246-1249] Morphine is often changed to hydromorphone to reduce the adverse effects or because of concern of accumulation of morphine metabolites, particularly in the presence of renal failure.[1218] Hydromorphone is commonly administered IV, orally, in the epidural space, and more recently through the nasal mucosa.[1239,1246,1247,1250-1253] Hydromorphone is used for chronic cancer pain, and plasma concentrations of around 4.7 ng/mL (range 1.9 to 8.9 ng/mL) relieve mucositis in children given patient-controlled analgesia devices.[1239,1244]

## OXYCODONE

Oxycodone (OxyContin) is another long-acting semisynthetic opioid that is usually administered orally and is available in a controlled-release formulation.[1254-1256] The relative bioavailability in adults of intranasal, oral, and rectal formulations was approximately 50% that of the IV route. The buccal and sublingual absorption of oxycodone is similar in young children.[1244] The bioavailability after various routes is IM, 68%; buccal, 55%; and orogastric, 37%.[1257,1258] Oxycodone may also be administered rectally, with a similar bioavailability, although absorption can be prolonged, so that route is not recommended.[1259] The IV formulation of oxycodone significantly depresses respiration; 0.1 mg/kg in children after ophthalmic surgery caused greater ventilatory depression than other opioids.[1260,1261] As with many medications, interindividual variability in the elimination half-life of oxycodone in the neonate is extreme.[1262,1263] In children, the elimination half-life after IV, buccal, IM, or orogastric administration is 2 to 3 hours.[1257] Mean values for clearance and Vdss were 15.2 ± 4.2 mL/min/kg and 2.1 ± 0.8 L/kg, respectively, in children after ophthalmic surgery.[1260] This opioid is commonly used to transition from patient-controlled analgesia and to treat chronic painful conditions (see Chapters 43 and 44).

## METHADONE

Methadone is a synthetic opioid with an analgesic potency similar to that of morphine but with a more rapid distribution and a slower elimination. Methadone is used as a maintenance drug in opioid-addicted adults to prevent withdrawal. Methadone might have beneficial effects because it is a long-acting synthetic opioid with a very high bioavailability (80%) by the enteral route. It also has NMDA receptor antagonistic activity and this may be beneficial in chronic pain treatment because agonism of this receptor is associated with opioid tolerance and hyperalgesia. Methadone is a racemate and clinical effect is a result of the *R*-methadone isomer. Methadone is 2.5-20 times more analgesic than morphine.[1264]

The primary indication for methadone in children is to wean from long-term opioid infusions to prevent withdrawal, and to provide analgesia when other opioids have failed or have been associated with intolerable side effects. [1224,1225,1254,1264-1271] IV methadone has been shown to be an effective analgesic for postoperative pain relief (the minimum effective analgesic concentration of methadone in opioid naïve adults is 58 µg/L),[1272] and oral administration has been recommended as the first-line opioid for severe and persistent pain in children.[1269] It seems also to be a safe enteral alternative for IV opioids in palliative pediatric oncologic patients.[1273]

Methadone has high lipid solubility with a large Vd of 6 to 7 L/kg in children and adults.[1274-1277] It is metabolized by N-demethylation, and clearance in adults is 2.7 ± 1.7 mL/min/kg with higher rates reported in children 1-18 years.[1277] The clearances of each racemate (*R* and *S*) are similar (approximately 1.4 to 1.7 mL/min/kg) in adolescents.[1278] There are few PK data available for infants under 1 year of age. The few neonatal data on methadone PK show a slow elimination half-life with enormous interindividual variability (3.8 to 62 hours).[1225] In adults, the mean elimination half-life after oral administration is prolonged, 33 to 46 hours.

## FENTANYL

Fentanyl (Sublimaze) offers greater hemodynamic stability than morphine, a rapid onset (T$_{1/2}$keo of 6.6 minutes in adults) a short duration of effect. Its relative increased lipid solubility and small molecular conformation enables efficient penetration of the blood-brain barrier and redistribution. It is the most commonly used opioid during general anesthesia in infants and children. It is particularly effective in the care of high-risk preterm and term neonates, as well as in infants and children during cardiac surgical procedures. High doses of fentanyl (10 to 100 µg/kg) are often administered to maintain cardiovascular

homeostasis.[1137,1279-1289] Fentanyl may be administered intravenously, intramuscularly, as a supplement to epidural analgesia, orally (trans–oral mucosal absorption), and transdermally–both passively and by iontophoresis.[1290-1295]

Fentanyl is metabolized by oxidative N-dealkylation (CYP3A4) into norfentanyl and hydroxylated. All metabolites are inactive and a small amount of fentanyl is eliminated via the kidneys unchanged. Compared with term neonates, the clearance of fentanyl in preterm infants is markedly reduced (mean elimination half-life is 17.7 ± 9.3 hours) contributing to prolonged respiratory depression in preterm neonates. Clearance matures with gestational age; 7 mL/min/kg at 25 weeks PMA, 10 mL/min/kg at 30 weeks PMA, and 12 mL/min/kg at 35 weeks PMA.[1296] The clearance of fentanyl is reduced to 70% to 80% of adult values in term neonates and, when standardized to a 70 kg person, reaches adult values (approx. 50 L/hr/70 kg) within the first 2 weeks of life.[858] Clearance of fentanyl in older infants (more than 3 months of age) and children is greater than that in adults when expressed as per kilogram (30.6 mL/kg/min vs 17.9 mL/kg/min, respectively), resulting in a reduced elimination half-life (68 minutes vs 121 minutes, respectively).[1279,1282,1297-1299]

Fentanyl's Vdss is approximately 5.9 L/kg in term neonates, and decreases with age to 4.5 L/kg during infancy, 3.1 L/kg during childhood, and 1.6 L/kg in adults.[1300] This increased Vdss results in a lower blood concentration after bolus administration in neonates and infants. Administration of fentanyl 3 µg/kg by slow IV push in term infants (1 to 7 months age) intra-operatively neither depressed respiration nor caused hypoxemia in a placebo-controlled trial.[1301,1302] Slow administration and both an increased Vdss and an increased clearance (per kilogram) in this age group contributed to these results. Fentanyl clearance may be impaired with decreased hepatic blood flow (e.g., from increased intraabdominal pressure in neonatal omphalocele repair), although a maldistribution of blood away from regions of concentrated cytochrome enzyme activity in the liver may also play a role.[1303]

Infants with cyanotic heart disease had reduced Vdss and greater plasma concentrations of fentanyl with infusion therapy.[1281] These greater plasma concentrations resulted from a reduced clearance (34 L/hr/70 kg), that was attributed to hemodynamic disturbance and consequent reduced hepatic blood flow.[1304] Hypothermia has also been shown to reduce fentanyl clearance.[1305] Profound hypotension has been reported after a bolus of midazolam in neonates in whom fentanyl was infused and vice versa.[1306] Other drugs metabolized by CYP3A4 (e.g., cyclosporine, erythromycin) may compete for clearance and result in increased fentanyl plasma concentrations.

Fentanyl is a potent µ-receptor agonist with a potency 70 to 125 times greater than that of morphine. A plasma concentration of 15 to 30 ng/mL is required to provide total IV anesthesia in adults, whereas the EC$_{50}$, based on EEG evidence, is 10 ng/mL.[1307,1308] Fentanyl has been shown to effectively prevent preterm neonates from surgical stress responses and to improve postoperative outcome.[1309] Single doses of fentanyl (3 µg/kg) can reduce the physiologic and behavioral measures of pain and stress associated with mechanical ventilation in preterm infants.[1310] Fentanyl has similar respiratory depression in infants and adults when plasma concentrations are similar.[1311]

The PK of fentanyl in critically ill children receiving long-term infusions is also quite variable, with a mean terminal elimination half-life of 21 hours and a range of 11 to 36 hours.[1312] The infusion rates of fentanyl that are required to achieve a similar level of sedation and analgesia may vary as much as 10-fold.[1312] This

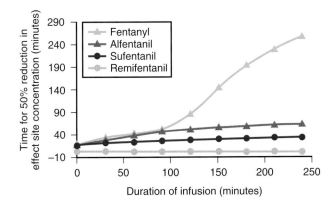

**FIGURE 6-22** This figure is a simulation of the time required for a 50% reduction in the effective site concentration of remifentanil (*yellow circles*), sufentanil (*purple circles*), alfentanil (*brown triangles*), and fentanyl (*blue triangles*) after an infusion (duration of 0 to 240 minutes) designed to maintain a constant effect-site concentration. Note that there is a completely flat curve for remifentanil, suggesting that a plateau effect is rapidly reached with remifentanil compared with the other opioids, such that even after a long infusion, the time to 50% reduction in effect-site concentration is still under 4 minutes. (Redrawn and modified with permission from Westmoreland CL, Hole JF, Sebel PS, et al. Pharmacokinetics of remifentanil [GI87084B] and its major metabolite [GI90291] in patients undergoing elective inpatient surgery. Anesthesiology 1993;79:893-903.)

variability in PK and PD strongly reinforces the need to titrate the dose to effect and to be prepared to provide postoperative ventilatory support as needed. Children who receive a chronic infusion of fentanyl are at risk of rapidly developing tolerance; on discontinuance of the infusion, these children may demonstrate signs of withdrawal. All long-term infusions should be tapered slowly over days rather than discontinuing them abruptly.[1298,1313,1314]

With low-dose fentanyl, the termination of action is primarily a combination of redistribution and rapid clearance by the liver.[1298,1315] The CSHT after a 1 hour infusion of fentanyl is approximately 20 minutes, which increases to 270 minutes after an 8 hour infusion in adults (Fig. 6-22).[38] Although the CSHT is reduced in children, there are no data in neonates.[1299] High-dose fentanyl, accumulates in muscle and fat and is therefore released (recirculated) more slowly, thus accounting in part for the prolonged respiratory depression after high doses. There is no evidence of dose-dependent kinetics; that is, there is no tissue or enzyme saturation in the clinically used ranges.[1315] In some respects, the pharmacology of opioids is very similar to thiopental: at low doses their clinical effect is terminated by redistribution, whereas at high doses their clinical effect is terminated by metabolism.[1311,1316-1319]

The usual initial dose of fentanyl is 1 to 3 μg/kg, a dose that may be supplemented as clinically indicated. Fentanyl is highly lipid soluble and rapidly crosses the blood-brain barrier. This characteristic may, in part, explain why the $LD_{50}$ for fentanyl in neonatal animals is 90% of that in adult animals. Continuous intraoperative and postoperative infusions of fentanyl are common in children of all ages.[1281,1319,1320] Fentanyl is also used to provide patient-controlled analgesia (see Chapter 43).[1321,1322]

Chest wall and glottic rigidity have been reported after IV administration of opioids, although most often after fentanyl. The reason for this is not clear.[1323-1328] Glottic rigidity may account for the inability to ventilate by bag and mask after IV fentanyl.[1328]

This adverse response can be minimized by administering the opioid slowly, and it can be reversed by administering either a muscle relaxant or naloxone. One other concern is the rare association of increased vagal tone with bolus administration; bradycardia may have profound effects on the cardiac output of neonates. Additionally, fentanyl markedly depresses the baroreceptor reflex control of heart rate in neonates.[1329] It is for these reasons that the combination of pancuronium and fentanyl became popular.

Oral transmucosal fentanyl (Fentanyl Oralet) was one of only several medications approved by the FDA for premedication of children, although this formulation is no longer marketed. A new formulation (Actiq) has been approved for adults and children 16 years of age or older, and is currently under investigation in children for the treatment of breakthrough pain.[1330,1331] Fentanyl is rapidly absorbed through the oral mucosa, which bypasses the liver.[787,1291,1292,1332-1336] Nonetheless, approximately half the absorption is gastrointestinal. The bioavailability of this formulation in children (33%) is less than that in adults (50%).[1291,1292] Uptake continues for a period of time after consumption, which potentially can provide analgesia for several hours.[787,1291,1292] The use of this formulation will likely be limited to the treatment of breakthrough pain.

The fentanyl patch was developed to provide an extended release of fentanyl similar to that provided with a continuous IV infusion.[1290,1337-1346] *This formulation was not designed to be administered to treat postsurgical pain, but rather for those who require opioids chronically.* This fentanyl transdermal therapeutic system (TTS) is available with a drug release rate of 12.5 μg/hr and matches the lower dosing requirements of cancer pain control in children.[1347] An approximate conversion factor of 45 mg/day oral morphine to 12.5 μg/hr fentanyl TTS is used for initial dose estimation in children on chronic morphine therapy. This is conservatively low to avoid respiratory depression. In adults, uptake of fentanyl begins within 1 hour and achieves therapeutic levels within 6 to 8 hours and peak levels at 24 hours.[1343,1346,1348] In children, the peak occurs earlier, at about 18 hours.[1349] The skin acts as a reservoir, and even after removal of the patch, uptake continues for several hours, with a consequent apparent elimination half-life of 14.5 ± 6 hours.[1349] Fentanyl uptake is markedly affected by skin blood flow, skin thickness, location of the patch, and adherence to the skin.[1350-1353] Alterations in skin blood flow (e.g., fever) may increase absorption.[1354] Alterations to skin blood flow caused by warming devices (increased absorption) or hypothermia (decreased absorption) during anesthesia should be considered in children with chronic pain who present with TTS fentanyl.

The use of TTS medication should be limited to pain specialists who have familiarity with the unusual PK of this drug delivery system.[1355] One study suggests that the PK of fentanyl by this route in children and adult patients are similar.[1349] A multicenter study in children 2 to 16 years of age reported satisfactory chronic analgesia. However, it should be noted that the data submitted to the FDA revealed plasma concentrations of fentanyl in children 1.5 to 5 years of age that were twice those in adults.[1356] These data are consistent with another study that found a negative correlation between fentanyl concentrations and age, that is, greater concentrations in younger children.[1349] Children may be particularly vulnerable to the rapid drug absorption compared with adults because they have thinner skin and better skin blood flow.[906] Accordingly, it seems prudent to begin with the smallest size patch and gradually increase as indicated (see Chapters 43 and 44). Finally, all patches, including those that have already been used, still contain large amounts of fentanyl that may cause a fatal intoxication if accidentally ingested by a child.[1357,1358] Proper disposal of these opioid-containing patches is required.

Epidural fentanyl is widely combined with an amide local anesthetic for provision of postoperative analgesia, although the use of such combinations continues to be debated. Pruritus, nausea, and vomiting may be exacerbated by the addition of fentanyl. The combination remains popular with bupivacaine as the amide anesthetic, although there is no evidence to support a levobupivacaine combination.[1359] Spread beyond the site of administration is dose-dependent but limited, and respiratory depression is uncommon.[1254,1360]

## ALFENTANIL

Alfentanil (Alfenta) is a fentanyl analogue whose main advantage is its reduced lipid solubility and smaller Vd compared with fentanyl.[1361] It has a rapid onset ($T_{1/2}$keo of 0.9 minutes in adults), a brief duration of action, and one-fourth the potency of fentanyl. A target plasma concentration of 400 ng/mL is used in anesthesia. Metabolism is through oxidative N-dealkylation by CYP3A4 and O-dealkylation and then conjugation to metabolites that are excreted renally.[1362] Studies indicate that brain concentrations of alfentanil are sevenfold to ninefold less, the Vd is four times less, and protein binding is greater than fentanyl.[1363] Alfentanil is more rapidly eliminated from the body than fentanyl, resulting in more frequent dosing. Clearance in neonates (20 to 60 mL/min/70 kg) is one-tenth that in adults (250 to 500 mL/min/70 kg) with rapid maturation.[67] In preterm neonates, the half-life is as long as 6 to 9 hours.[1364,1365] The Vd in children and adults are similar, but increased in preterm neonates (Vd 1.0 ± 0.39 vs 0.48 ± 0.19 L/kg). Clearance is greater in children, expressed as per kilogram (11.1 ± 3.9 mL/kg/min vs 5.9 ± 1.6 mL/kg/min). As a result, the elimination half-life in children is less (63 ± 24 vs 95 ± 20 minutes).[1366-1369] The Vd and elimination half-life in infants 3 to 12 months of age and older children are similar.[1368] Because clearance is markedly diminished in children with hepatic disease, clinical effects are prolonged in those with reduced hepatic blood flow (e.g., children with increased intraabdominal pressure, children receiving vasopressors, and those with some forms of congenital heart disease).[1361,1370,1371] Renal failure has little effect on its elimination.[1372] Because less alfentanil is bound to α1-acid glycoprotein in preterm infants (65%) than in term infants (79%), an increased fraction of alfentanil is available for biologic effect in the former.[78]

The PK and PD of alfentanil suggest potential applications for the rapid control of analgesia and awakening from anesthesia. Alfentanil (10 μg/kg) has been combined with propofol (2.5 mg/kg) for tracheal intubation without a NMBD.[1373] High-dose alfentanil is also used for cardiac procedures. Alfentanil should be used with caution without NMBDs in neonates because of the frequency of chest wall or glottic rigidity.[1229,1374]

## SUFENTANIL

Sufentanil (Sufenta) is a potent synthetic narcotic that in many respects is similar to fentanyl and alfentanil. Sufentanil is 5 to 10 times more potent than fentanyl, with a $T_{1/2}$keo of 6.2 minutes in adults.[1375] A concentration of 5 to 10 ng/mL is required for total IV anesthesia, and 0.2 to 0.4 ng/mL for analgesia. PD differences are suggested in neonates. The plasma concentration of sufentanil at the time of additional anesthetic supplementation to suppress hemodynamic responses to surgical stimulation

was 2.51 ng/mL in neonates, significantly greater than the concentrations of 1.58, 1.53, and 1.56 ng/mL observed in infants, children, and adolescents, respectively.[1376]

Elimination of sufentanil has been suggested by O-demethylation and N-dealkylation in animal studies. As with fentanyl and alfentanil, the CYP3A4 enzyme is responsible for the N-dealkylation.[1377] The majority of studies of IV sufentanil in children have focused on those undergoing cardiac surgery. Evidence has shown age-dependent PK in which neonates have a larger Vdss, reduced clearance, and a greater and more variable elimination half-life than older children and adults (E-Fig. 6-16).[1376,1378,1379] Clearance in neonates undergoing cardiovascular surgery (6.7 ± 6.1 mL/kg/min), is reduced compared with values of 18.1 ± 2.7, 16.9 ± 3.2, and 13.1 ± 3.6 mL/kg/min in infants, children, and adolescents, respectively[1376]; consistent with rapid development of hepatic metabolic pathways.[1378] Clearance maturation standardized to a 70 kilogram person using allometry is similar to that of other drugs that depend on CYP3A4 for metabolism (e.g., levobupivacaine, fentanyl, alfentanil) (see Fig. 6-10).[156] Clearance rates in infants (27.5 ± 9.3 mL/kg/min) were greater, expressed as per kilogram, than those in children (18.1 ± 10.7 mL/kg/min) in another study of children undergoing cardiovascular surgery.[1379] Clearance in healthy children (2 to 8 years) was greater (30.5 ± 8.8 mL/kg/min) than those undergoing cardiac surgery.[1380] Decreased hepatic blood flow reduces clearance.[1380] The elimination of sufentanil is unaffected by renal failure but markedly altered by factors that influence hepatic blood flow; cirrhosis apparently has little effect on its elimination.[1361,1381,1382]

The Vdss was 4.15 ± 1.0 L/kg in neonates; greater than the values of 2.73 ± 0.5 and 2.75 ± 0.5 L/kg observed in children and adolescents, respectively.[1376,1380]

Bradycardia and asystole have been observed after a bolus administration of sufentanil, suggesting that the simultaneous administration of a vagolytic agent (atropine, glycopyrrolate, or pancuronium bromide) may be sensible with rapid administration.[1383,1384] Nasal sufentanil may have a role for sedation in children although data in neonates are lacking and there are concerns about the risk of respiratory depression.[1385-1390] Several studies demonstrated that children are more likely to accept nasal sufentanil compared with nasal midazolam, although there was a greater incidence of vomiting after sufentanil and several children experienced decreased chest wall compliance after or during induction of anesthesia. The dose of sufentanil that is most effective when administered intranasally is 2 to 3 μg/kg.[1386,1388] Epidural sufentanil (0.7 to 0.75 μg/kg) has been effective in children, lasting more than 3 hours, although pruritus can be bothersome.[1391-1393]

## REMIFENTANIL

Remifentanil (Ultiva) is the newest in the family of synthetic opioids.[1394,1395] Its brief elimination half-life of 3 to 6 minutes means that it is usually given as an infusion.[205,1396-1398] This opioid is unique because an ester linkage in the molecule allows rapid degradation to a carboxylic acid metabolite by blood and tissue esterases.[1399] Metabolism is unaffected by hepatic or renal function.[1400] The active metabolite of remifentanil that is eliminated by the kidneys has approximately 1/300th to 1/1000th the opioid activity of the parent compound and, theoretically, could accumulate and cause clinical manifestations in children with impaired renal function.[1401] One study in adults failed to demonstrate any residual opioid effects after a 12-hour infusion in patients with renal failure.[1402] Perhaps the most important

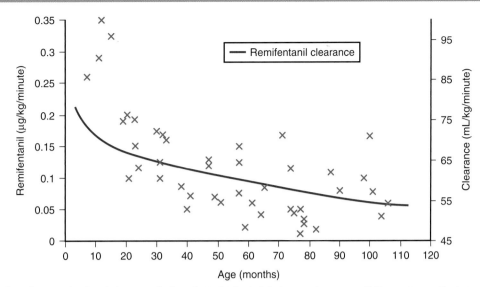

**FIGURE 6-23** The effect of age on the dose (infusion rate) of remifentanil tolerated during spontaneous ventilation under anesthesia in children undergoing strabismus surgery.[257] Superimposed on this plot is estimated remifentanil clearance determined using an allometric model.[12] There is a mismatch between clearance and infusion rate for those individuals still in infancy. The higher infusion rates recorded in those infants can be attributed to greater suppression of respiratory drive in this age group than with the older children during the study; a respiratory rate of 10 breaths per minute in an infant is disproportionately slow compared to the same rate in a 7-year-old child, suggesting excessive dose. (Reproduced with permission from Anderson BJ. Pediatric models for adult target-controlled infusion pumps. Pediatr Anesth 2010;20:223-32; Rigby-Jones AE, Priston MJ, Sneyd JR, et al. Remifentanil-midazolam sedation for paediatric patients receiving mechanical ventilation after cardiac surgery. Br J Anaesth 2007;99:252-61; and Barker N, Lim J, Amari E, Malherbe S, Ansermino JM. Relationship between age and spontaneous ventilation during intravenous anesthesia in children. Pediatr Anesth 2007;17:948-55.)

**TABLE 6-16** Remifentanil Pharmacokinetics by Age

|  | 0-2 Months | 2 Months-2 Years | 2-6 Years | 7-12 Years | 13-16 Years | 16-18 Years |
|---|---|---|---|---|---|---|
| Cmax | 24.2 ± 10.2* | 25.4 ± 3.7* | 34.8 ± 8.2 | 42.5 ± 13.7 | 35 ± 10.2 | 42.7 ± 12.9 |
| Vdss | 452.8 ± 144.7* | 307.9 ± 89.2 | 240.1 ± 130.5 | 248.9 ± 91.4 | 223.2 ± 30.6 | 242.5 ± 109.2 |
| CL (mL/minute/kg) | 90.5 ± 36.8* | 92.1 ± 25.8* | 76 ± 22.4 | 59.7 ± 22.5 | 57.2 ± 21.1 | 46.5 ± 2.1 |
| Half-life (minute) | 5.4 ± 1.8 | 3.4 ± 1.19 | 3.6 ± 1.19 | 5.3 ± 1.4 | 3.7 ± 1.1 | 5.7 ± 0.7 |

Data extracted from Ross AK, Davis PJ, deL Dear G, et al. Pharmacokinetics of remifentanil in anesthetized pediatric patients undergoing elective surgery or diagnostic procedures. Anesth Analg 2001;93:1393-401.

*CL*, Clearance; *Cmax*, peak plasma concentration; *Vdss*, volume of distribution at steady state.

*Significantly different from other groups.

characteristic of remifentanil is its very brief half-life and the associated rapid recovery within about 10 minutes. Clearance in patients with butyrylcholinesterase deficiency is unaffected. The nonspecific blood esterases that metabolize remifentanil are mature at birth.[53]

A target plasma concentration of 2 to 3 μg/L is adequate for laryngoscopy, 6 to 8 μg/L for laparotomy and 10 to 12 μg/L might be sought to ablate the stress response associated with cardiac surgery.[1403] Analgesic concentrations are 0.2 to 0.4 μg/L. The $T_{1/2}$keo is 1.16 minutes in adults,[204] but the neonatal $T_{1/2}$keo has not been reported. Analgesic alternatives should be available for when the short-duration analgesic effect from remifentanil has dissipated. Reports of a rapid development of μ-receptor tolerance with remifentanil are in conflict; activity at δ-opioid receptors may contribute.[1404] Remifentanil clearance can be described in all age groups by simple application of an allometric model.[52] This standardized clearance of 2790 mL/min/70 kg is similar to that reported by others in children[205,1405] and adults.[204,1395] The smaller the child, the greater the clearance when expressed as mL/min/kg. Clearance decreases with increasing age, with rates of 90 mL/kg/min in infants under 2 years of age, 60 mL/kg/min

in children 2 to 12 years of age, and 40 mL/kg/min in adults (Fig. 6-23 and Table 6-16).[52,205,1405] The steady-state Vd was greatest in infants under 2 months age (452 mL/kg) and decreased to 308 mL/kg in children 2 months to 2 years, and to 240 mL/kg in children more than 2 years of age.[205] Elimination half-life appears to be constant, approximately 3 to 6 minutes, independent of dose or duration of the infusion[205,1396]; the CSHT is constant (see Fig. 6-22).[1401] For example, when the infusions of remifentanil differed as much as 20-fold, the time to return to spontaneous respirations varied by only 1 to 3 minutes.[1400,1406] For opioids, its effect on respiration is an excellent reflection of its PD effects.[1407] After 3-hour infusions of alfentanil and remifentanil in adults, the elimination half-lives were 47.3 ± 12 minutes for alfentanil, compared with 3.2 ± 0.9 minutes for remifentanil. The time to recover 50% of the minute ventilation, a PD effect of opioids, was 54.0 ± 48.1 minutes for alfentanil, compared with 5.4 ± 1.8 minutes for remifentanil.[1407]

Although covariate effects, such as cardiac surgery, appear to have a muted effect on PK, cardiopulmonary bypass (CPB) does have an impact. Remifentanil dosage adjustments are required during and after CPB because of marked changes in its Vd.[1408]

Other PK changes during CPB are consistent with adult data in which a decreased metabolism occurred with a reduced temperature[1409] and with reports of greater clearance after CPB (increased metabolism) compared with during CPB.[1405]

Respiratory depression is concentration dependent.[1410,1411] *Vocal cord closure, commonly interpreted as muscle rigidity, remains a concern with bolus doses above 3 μg/kg used for intubation in neonates.*[1412] Induction with propofol (4 mg/kg) and either remifentanil (3 μg/kg) or succinylcholine (2 mg/kg) for intubation were similar, with no bradycardia, hypotension, or chest wall rigidity.[1413] The initial loading dose of remifentanil may cause hypotension and bradycardia[1414] prompting some to target the plasma rather than effect-site concentration when initiating infusion. This hypotensive response has been quantified in children undergoing cranioplasty surgery. A steady-state remifentanil concentration of 14 μg/L would typically achieve a 30% decrease in MAP. This concentration is twice that required for laparotomy, but is easily achieved with a bolus injection. The $T_{1/2}$keo of 0.86 minute for this hemodynamic effect[1415] is less than remifentanil-induced spectral edge frequency changes described in adults ($T_{1/2}$keo of 1.34 minutes).[204,1416]

One theoretical concern that is associated with the long-term administration of remifentanil is the development of acute tolerance. In a study of adult volunteers, the analgesic threshold was one fourth of the peak values within 3 hours.[1417] A study of adolescents undergoing spinal instrumentation for scoliosis has also demonstrated acute tolerance.[1418] These data suggest that the infusion rates should be modified during the infusion of remifentanil to maintain a stable level of analgesia.

Remifentanil has an important role in providing safe analgesia to children of all ages, but, in particular, very sick infants and children.[1419-1422] Its main advantage is the ability to provide an intense opioid effect with cardiovascular stability during the procedure, and then transition to a less intense opioid effect, allowing for early extubation.[1419,1423] *Remifentanil is the only opioid for which there is a greater rather than a reduced clearance (per kilogram) in neonates (see Fig. 6-23), and the reason that it is so valuable in this age group.*[1424-1431] These pharmacologic differences have important clinical implications because they translate into the ability to rapidly titrate the opioid effect, without regard to prolonged sedation. *This opioid should be administered only by continuous infusion. If an IV line becomes interrupted, kinked, or disconnected, the opioid effect will rapidly dissipate and the child will show evidence of pain.* Therefore, this drug should be "piggybacked" into a continuous infusion carrier as close to the IV cannula as possible to provide smooth constant drug delivery. In neonates, a more dilute concentration is useful (e.g., 5 μg/mL). This also means that at the end of a procedure, the anesthetic plan must include a transition to some other form of analgesia, including another longer acting opioid or a regional block.[1432]

Although remifentanil can be administered as a loading dose, 0.1 to 0.25 μg/kg, the risk of hypotension and the rapidity of achieving steady-state analgesia (0.05 to 0.15 μg/kg/min) renders a loading dose unnecessary. However, if a loading dose is used, then the plasma concentration, rather than effect-site concentration, is commonly targeted.[1433] The infusion may be titrated to effect with little fear of producing an "overdose," because of the very favorable PK. As with many synthetic opioids, severe bradycardia and hypotension may occur after bolus administration, especially large doses.[205,1434] Remifentanil may have a direct negative chronotropic effect; therefore, the concomitant use of a vagolytic or pancuronium may prevent this adverse cardiac

response.[1435,1436] However, because the plasma half-life is so brief, there is rarely a need for a bolus, because a steady-state opioid concentration occurs within three to five half-lives. Conversely, this negative chronotropic effect and the concomitant reduction in BP can be used to induce controlled hypotension.[1437,1438]

Remifentanil would seem to be the ideal opioid to provide a deep analgesic effect that allows spinal cord–evoked motor and sensory monitoring.[1439] Nonetheless, anesthesia is not produced by opioids alone. An anxiolytic must be administered to ensure that amnesia occurs. The half-lives of all anxiolytics exceed that of remifentanil, and this needs to be considered during recovery. Remifentanil complements propofol for short-term analgesia during total IV anesthesia for a variety of surgical and nonsurgical procedures, as well as analgesia and sedation in the ICU.* We have commonly used a fixed combination of remifentanil (5 μg/mL) in propofol (10 mg/mL), starting at a propofol infusion rate of 150 μg/kg/min for upper and lower gastrointestinal endoscopic procedures in children under 10 years, and a lower concentration of remifentanil in teenagers (2.5 μg/mL in propofol [10 mg/mL]) because of the hypotension and bradypnea in older children.[1446] Remifentanil seems to cause less respiratory depression in younger children.[1411] For upper endoscopy, tropicalizing the tongue and pharynx with lidocaine helps blunt responses to passing the endoscope through the oropharynx. The infusion rate is adjusted according to the child's responses.

Remifentanil has also been used to supplement propofol to facilitate endotracheal intubation without the use of a muscle relaxant. Two dose-response studies found that about 3 μg/kg of remifentanil combined with 4 mg/kg propofol provided the best intubating conditions. Intubating conditions were the same as with mivacurium or succinylcholine. Resumption of spontaneous respirations after a remifentanil–propofol combination was similar to that after succinylcholine.[1447,1448] It would seem that this combination is a reasonable alternative to succinylcholine to facilitate endotracheal intubation in children in whom succinylcholine is contraindicated, when the duration of intubation is anticipated to be brief, or when spontaneous ventilation is desired.

## BUTORPHANOL AND NALBUPHINE

Butorphanol (Stadol) and nalbuphine (Nubain) are synthetic narcotic agonist-antagonist analgesics that are apparently equianalgesic.[1449-1452] They are effective through κ-receptor agonism and partial μ-receptor antagonism, have 0.5 to 0.7 times morphine's potency, and an antagonist effect 25 times weaker than naloxone. An appealing PD effect is sedation, particularly when compared with midazolam.[1449,1452-1455] Nalbuphine's elimination half-life is significantly shorter in children 1.5 to 5 years of age (0.9 hour) than it was in children 5 to 8.5 years of age (1.9 hours) and in adults 23 to 32 years of age (2.3 hours). A half-life of 4 hours has been reported in neonates, reflecting immaturity of hepatic glucuronide metabolism. The half-life of butorphanol is similar to that of nalbuphine at about 3 hours in adults.[1452,1456,1457] Both of these drugs can be administered orally with bioavailability in young adults of 12% to 17%, but this dramatically increases to about 80% when administered to the nasal mucosa.[1457-1460] The claimed advantage of this family of drugs is adequate analgesia with a ceiling on respiratory depression[1449,1450,1461-1463]; thus, there is some popularity for use in children.[1464-1470] The administration of butorphanol by the nasal

---

*References 1320, 1427, 1428, 1436, 1440-1445.

route may offer particular advantage for children without IV access.[1464,1471-1474] One report suggests a lower rate of postoperative vomiting after butorphanol compared with morphine.[1465] Another describes the use of rectal administration; as expected, the authors found irregular absorption, but peak blood levels were relatively rapidly achieved (25 ± 11 minutes) and the elimination half-life was 2.7 ± 0.7 hours.[1475] We do not recommend the rectal route of administration. What must be remembered is that these agents may reverse μ-receptor–mediated analgesic effects of the more potent opioids and should therefore be used as the initial or the sole opioid.

This family of drugs has had mixed results in reversing or preventing opioid-induced pruritus.[1476,1477] Nalbuphine does not reverse respiratory depression after morphine,[1478] but may be effective after fentanyl.[1479] Butorphanol has also been administered by the caudal epidural route (25 μg/kg).[1480,1481]

## CODEINE

Codeine, or methylmorphine, is a morphine-like opioid with 10% of the potency of morphine. It is mainly metabolized by glucuronidation, but minor pathways are by N-demethylation to norcodeine and O-demethylation to morphine. However, a full accounting of the metabolism of codeine has remained elusive. Approximately 10% of codeine is metabolized to morphine. As the affinity of codeine for opioid receptors is very low, the analgesic effect of codeine is believed to be a result of its morphine metabolite.[1482] Evidence suggests that up to 11% of codeine is metabolized to hydrocodone,[196] which may provide an alternate mechanism of analgesia to its metabolism to morphine. The continued use of this minor opium alkaloid for pediatric analgesia remains baffling and is subject to debate, because it is effectively a prodrug analgesic.[1483]

The primary routes for delivery of codeine are the oral and IM routes, although the rectal route has also been advocated.[1484] The dose of codeine by all three routes is similar, 0.5 to 1.5 mg/kg. IV codeine was used in the past, but serious life-threatening adverse effects, including transient but severe cardiorespiratory depression[1485-1487] and seizures,[1488] led to proscription of this route of delivery.

Codeine's popularity as a perioperative analgesic in children is based in part on its favorable PK. When given orally, it is rapidly and completely absorbed, with 50% undergoing first-pass hepatic metabolism. Bioavailability after oral codeine is 90%, although after surgery the bioavailability may be quite variable.[1482,1489] Blood concentrations after oral codeine reach a peak by 1 hour. Its terminal elimination half-life is 3 to 3.5 hours. When given by the IM and rectal routes, peak blood concentrations are achieved rapidly, within 0.5 hour, with the blood concentrations after the rectal route being less than after the IM route. The duration of action after these two routes of administration is 1 to 2 hours. The elimination half-life after rectal administration in children is approximately 2.6 hours in children, but 4.6 hours in infants,[1490] suggesting the need for a much greater interval between subsequent doses in infants. A Vd of 3.6 L/kg and a clearance (CL) of 0.85 L/hr have been described in adults but there are few data detailing the developmental changes in children.

In vivo, 5% to 15% of codeine is excreted unchanged in the urine. The remaining 85% to 95% undergoes metabolism in the liver by one of three routes: glucuronidation (principal route), O-demethylation, and N-demethylation.[1482] Five percent to 15% of codeine undergoes O-demethylation to morphine. This metabolic pathway depends on CYP2D6, an enzyme responsible for the metabolism of more than 20% of prescribed medications. The N-demethylation pathway depends on the CYP3A enzyme system.

CYP2D6 activity in fetal liver microsomes is either absent or less than 1% of adult values.[1490] O-demethylation begins postnatally with rapid maturation of this enzyme system irrespective of the gestational age at birth, although activity may remain less than 25% of adult values at 5 years of age. Interestingly, CYP2D6 is a noninducible enzyme whose activity, however, may vary with certain disease states, including malignancy, cigarette smoking, and some chronic inflammatory diseases (rheumatoid arthritis).[1482] Glucuronidation is immature at birth but develops throughout infancy, whereas N-demethylation is fully mature at birth. Variability in the clinical response to codeine prompted investigations into genetic variants or polymorphisms of CYP2D6. This enzyme is mapped to chromosome 22 at 22q13.1. Fifty-five polymorphisms of CYP2D6 with a frequency that exceeds 1% of the population have been described.[1491] These include both functional and nonfunctional polymorphisms, as well as gene duplication. The polymorphisms are numbered with *1 being the normal or wild allele (the * denotes an allele). The mutant alleles, *3, *4, *5, *6, and *9, for example, confer no CYP2D6 activity.[1482,1491,1492] The latter polymorphisms account for more than 90% of the poor metabolizers (see later discussion). Variants *2, *10, and *17 have modestly reduced activity and are referred as intermediate metabolizers.[1482] To further complicate the genetic pattern, multiple copies of the same genes[1492] may be present in some individuals, resulting in bizarre phenotypes. The wide array of CYP2D6 polymorphisms of codeine may be summarized into three broad categories: poor metabolizers (PM, negligible morphine produced), extensive metabolizers (EM, normal) and ultraextensive metabolizers (UM, rapid production and large amounts of morphine produced). Up to 10% of Caucasians and 30% of Hong Kong Chinese are PM, rendering codeine an ineffective analgesic for these children.[1482] Alternately, 29% of the Ethiopian and 1% of Swedish, German, and Chinese populations are UM.[1482] Recent evidence suggested that the frequency of CYP2D6 polymorphisms, particularly children who are PM, may be more common and more varied than previously thought. Children with these polymorphisms who also have upregulated opioid receptors as a result of chronic intermittent nocturnal hypoxia may be particularly vulnerable to a mishap after a usual or subclinical dose of codeine.[200,1492a] Consequently, the wide clinical response to a standard (or less than standard) dose of codeine necessitates careful monitoring in those with compromised cardiorespiratory status. Several deaths or near deaths have been reported with "standard" doses of oral codeine in children later found to be UM.[1493,1494,1492a]

Codeine may be effective for pain control, although its limited conversion to morphine likely makes it suitable for only mild and moderate forms of pain. The limited conversion to morphine and fewer adverse effects of codeine has made it popular for infants and young children, particularly when a single dose is involved. There is some evidence that codeine is associated with less nausea and vomiting than morphine.[1495] Codeine is often used in combination with acetaminophen or NSAIDs. The addition of codeine to acetaminophen has been shown to improve postoperative pain relief in infants.[1496] One study found that the analgesic effect of the combination of acetaminophen (10 to 15 mg/kg) and codeine (1 to 1.5 mg/kg) was comparable to that of ibuprofen (5 to 10 mg/kg) in children after tonsillectomy.[1497]

In poor metabolizers, codeine confers little or no analgesia, although adverse effects persist.[1498] In ultra-rapid metabolizers on the other hand, a large incidence of adverse effects might be expected, including apnea, because of large plasma morphine concentrations. Administration (especially of codeine preparations with an antihistamine and a decongestant) in the neonate may cause intoxication.[1499] A mother who ingested codeine while breastfeeding is thought to have transferred morphine in the breast milk, resulting in a fatality in her neonate. The mother, a UM, produced morphine more rapidly from the codeine, which resulted in respiratory depression in the neonate.[1493,1500] Because there is unpredictable variability in the conversion of codeine to morphine, we recommend alternative medications be considered; with codeine, if the child is a PM, they will receive very little analgesia, whereas, if a UM, they could sustain a life-threatening event because of increased conversion to morphine.

### TRAMADOL

Tramadol (Ultram) is a weak opioid with minimal effects on respiration and causes monoaminergic spinal cord inhibition of pain.[1501-1504] This formulation is structurally related to morphine and codeine.[1504] Two enantiomers provide analgesia; one is a opioid $\mu$-receptor agonist, and the other inhibits neuronal reuptake of serotonin and inhibits norepinephrine uptake, thus producing "multimodal antinociception."[1504] It is primarily metabolized into $O$-desmethyltramadol (M1) by CYP2D6, which, because of its extensive polymorphism poses the same concerns as in the case of codeine.[1505] Poor metabolizers have both reduced analgesia and nausea.[1506,1507] The active M1 metabolite has a $\mu$-receptor affinity approximately 200 times greater than tramadol. Tramadol clearance increased from 25 weeks PCA (5.52 L/hr/70 kg) to reach 84% of the mature value (8.58 L/hr/70 kg) by 44 weeks PMA.[1508] A target concentration of 300 $\mu$g/L is achieved after a bolus of tramadol hydrochloride of 1 mg/kg, and can be maintained by infusion of tramadol hydrochloride at 0.09 mg/kg/hr at 25 weeks, 0.14 mg/kg/hr at 30 weeks, and 0.18 mg/kg/hr at 40 weeks PMA.[1508] CYP2D6 activity was observed as early as 25 weeks PCA.[1508] Clearance in children is similar to that in adults, using standardized allometric models.[1509] Tramadol has been shown to be effective for moderate to severe pain in a variety of pediatric populations and may offer some advantage for the treatment of pain after tonsillectomy in children with obstructive sleep apnea.[1510-1518] Tramadol (1.5 to 2 mg/kg) has been administered rectally with peak plasma concentrations occurring at approximately 2 hours.[1519] Tramadol has also been administered in the caudal epidural space[1249] with longer-lasting analgesia than when administered intravenously.[1520] Caudal epidural tramadol (5%, 2 mg/kg) was also compared with caudal epidural bupivacaine (0.25%, 2 mg/kg) and found to provide superior analgesia.[1521] *Caudal administration is not recommended until further clarification of potential neurotoxicity.*[1510,1522] Tramadol has also been very useful as a transition to oral analgesics after IV therapy (see Chapter 43). The low incidence of respiratory depression and constipation, fewer controls on use, and similar frequency of nausea and vomiting (10% to 40%) compared to other opioids make tramadol an attractive alternative.[1523]

## Acetaminophen

Acetaminophen (Tylenol, Paracetamol) is widely used in the management of pain, but lacks antiinflammatory effects.

Prostaglandin $H_2$ synthetase (PGHS) is the enzyme responsible for metabolism of arachidonic acid to the unstable prostaglandin $H_2$. The two major forms of this enzyme are the constitutive PGHS-1 (COX-1) and the inducible PGHS-2 (COX-2). PGHS comprises two sites, a cyclooxygenase (COX) site and a peroxidase (POX) site. The conversion of arachidonic acid to prostaglandin $G_2$, the precursor of the other prostaglandins (E-Fig. 6-17), depends on a tyrosine-385 radical at the COX active site. Acetaminophen acts as a reducing cosubstrate on the POX site. Alternatively, acetaminophen effects may be mediated by an active metabolite ($p$-aminophenol). $p$-Aminophenol is conjugated with arachidonic acid by fatty acid amide hydrolase and exerts its effect through cannabinoid receptors.[1524]

The $ED_{50}$ for rectal acetaminophen to avoid any supplemental opioids after day-stay surgery is 35 mg/kg.[1525] Further studies are required before regular doses greater than 40 mg/kg can be recommended because of concerns about hepatotoxicity,[1525-1527] which can occur even after single doses of 250 mg/kg.[1528] Time delays of approximately 1 hour between peak concentration and peak effect have been reported.[1529,1530] An estimate of a maximum effect was 5.17 (the greatest possible pain relief [VAS 0 to 10] would equate to an Emax of 10 out of 10 pain units) and an $EC_{50}$ of 9.98 mg/L. The $T_{1/2}$keo of the analgesic effect compartment was 53 minutes.[60,1529] A target effect compartment concentration of 10 mg/L was associated with a pain reduction of 2.6/10.[60]

The relative bioavailability of rectal to oral acetaminophen formulations (rectal/oral) is approximately 0.5 in children but the relative bioavailability is greater in neonates and approaches unity.[96] There are two IV paracetamol formulations available, and caution must be exercised with the choice of formulation.[1531] One is an acetaminophen formulation, whereas the other, propacetamol ($N$-acetyl-*para*-aminophenoldiethyl aminoacetic ester), is a water-soluble prodrug of acetaminophen that can be administered intravenously over 15 min. It is rapidly hydroxylated into acetaminophen (1 g propacetamol = 0.5 g acetaminophen).[1532]

The $T_{1/2}$abs of acetaminophen from the duodenum is rapid (4.5 minutes) in children who were given acetaminophen as an elixir.[1533] The $T_{1/2}$abs in infants under the age of 3 months was delayed (16.6 minutes), consistent with delayed gastric emptying in young infants.[96,1533] In contrast, rectal absorption is slow and erratic with large variability. For example, absorption parameters for the triglyceride base were a $T_{1/2}$abs of 1.34 hours (coefficient of variation [CV] = 90%) with a lag time before absorption began of 8 minutes (CV = 31%). The $T_{1/2}$abs for rectal formulations was prolonged in infants less than 3 months (1.51 times greater) compared with those in older children.[1534]

Sulfate metabolism is the dominant route of elimination in neonates, while glucuronide conjugation (via UGT1A6) is dominant in adults. A total body clearance of 0.74 L/hr/70 kg at 28 weeks PMA and 4.9 L/hr/70 kg (CV = 38%) in full-term neonates after enteral acetaminophen has been reported using an allometric ¾-power model.[1534] Clearance increases over the first year of life (see Fig. 6-10) and reaches 80% of that in older children (16 L/hr/70 kg) by 6 months postnatal age.[96,173] Similar clearance estimates are reported in neonates after IV formulations of acetaminophen.[1535,1536] The relative bioavailability of the oral formulation is 0.9.

The Vd for acetaminophen is 49 to 70 L/70 kg. The Vd decreases exponentially, with a $TM_{50}$ of 11.5 weeks, from 109.7 L/70 kg at 28 weeks PCA to 72.9 L/70 kg by 60 weeks, reflective of fetal body composition and water distribution changes over the first few months of life.[96]

The toxic metabolite of acetaminophen, *N*-acetyl-*p*-benzoquinone imine (NAPQI), is formed by CYP2E1, 1A2, and 3A4. This metabolite binds to intracellular hepatic macromolecules to produce cell necrosis and other damage. Infants less than 90 days postnatal age have decreased expression of CYP2E1 activity in vitro compared with older infants, children, and adults,[1537] CYP3A4 appears during the first week after birth, whereas CYP1A2 appears later.[8] Neonates can produce hepatotoxic metabolites (e.g., NAPQI), but the reduced activity of CYP in neonates may explain the rare occurrence of acetaminophen-induced hepatotoxicity in neonates. Nonetheless, two massive 10-fold overdoses of paracetamol were reported in infants and underscore the need for extreme care when administering IV forms of acetaminophen.[1538] Neither infant progressed to acute liver necrosis and both recovered fully.

Acetaminophen is useful as an adjunct to spare opioids.[1525,1539-1545] Acetaminophen can be administered orally before induction of anesthesia to achieve a therapeutic blood concentration at the time of emergence, even after brief surgery, such as myringotomy and tube insertion. For procedures of greater duration, rectal administration of acetaminophen at the beginning of surgery provides therapeutic blood concentrations at the time of emergence and before the child would be likely to tolerate oral medications.[1546] The current maximum 24 hour dosing of oral acetaminophen is 75 to 90 mg/kg/day in children, although dose should be reduced in neonates.[1547] Suppository doses of 35 to 40 mg/kg followed by 20 mg/kg every 6 hours have been proposed for children,[1547] consistent with reduced bioavailability and slower absorption of rectal formulations.[1548]

# Nonsteroidal Antiinflammatory Agents

The nonsteroidal antiinflammatory drugs (NSAIDs) are a heterogeneous group of compounds that share common antipyretic, analgesic and antiinflammatory effects. NSAIDs act by reducing prostaglandin biosynthesis through inhibition of the COX site of the PGHS enzyme (see E-Fig. 6-17).

The prostanoids produced by the COX-1 isoenzyme protect the gastric mucosa, regulate renal blood flow, and induce platelet aggregation. NSAID-induced gastrointestinal toxicity, for example, is likely mediated through blockade of COX-1 activity, whereas the antiinflammatory effects of NSAIDs are likely mediated primarily through inhibition of the inducible isoform, COX-2.

The NSAIDs are commonly used in children for antipyresis and analgesia. The antiinflammatory properties of the NSAIDs have, in addition, been used in such diverse disorders as juvenile idiopathic arthritis, renal and biliary colic, dysmenorrhea, Kawasaki disease, and cystic fibrosis. The NSAIDs indomethacin and ibuprofen are also used to treat delayed closure of patent ductus arteriosus (PDA) in preterm infants.[1549-1551]

NSAID-associated analgesia has been compared to analgesia from other analgesics or analgesic modalities (e.g., caudal blockade, acetaminophen, or morphine) in children. These data confirm that NSAIDs in children are effective analgesic drugs, improving the quality of analgesia, but the effects have not been quantified. Data from adults given ibuprofen after dental extraction suggest a similar Emax to that described for acetaminophen (1.54 on a scale 0 to 3), with an $EC_{50}$ of 10.2 mg/L.[1552] The $T_{1/2}$keo of 28 minutes was less than the 53 minutes reported for acetaminophen.[60] In addition, the slope (reflected by the Hill coefficient, see Fig. 6-5) of the concentration-response curve was steeper than that for acetaminophen (Hill = 2 for ibuprofen, Hill = 1 for acetaminophen) indicating a more rapid onset of analgesia. NSAIDs are rapidly absorbed in the gastrointestinal tract after oral administration in children. The relative bioavailability of oral preparations approaches unity. The rate and extent of absorption after rectal administration of NSAIDs such as ibuprofen, diclofenac, flurbiprofen, indomethacin, and nimesulide, are less than after the oral routes.

The Vd is small in adults (less than 0.2 L/kg) but larger in children. Preterm neonates (22 to 31 weeks gestational age) given IV ibuprofen had a Vd of $0.62 \pm 0.04$ L/kg.[1553] One paper reported a dramatic reduction in ibuprofen central volume after closure of the PDA in preterm neonates (0.244 vs 0.171 L/kg).[1554] The NSAIDs, as a group, are weakly acidic, lipophilic, and highly protein bound. The impact of altered protein binding is probably minimal with routine dosing, because NSAIDs cleared by the liver have a low hepatic extraction ratio.[81]

NSAIDs undergo extensive phase I and phase II enzyme biotransformation in the liver, with subsequent excretion into urine or bile. Renal elimination is not an important elimination pathway for the commonly used NSAIDs. PK parameter variability is large, in part attributable to covariate effects of age, size, and pharmacogenomics. Ibuprofen, for example, is metabolized by the CYP2C9 and CYP2C8 subfamily. Considerable variation exists in the expression of CYP2C activities among individuals, and functional polymorphism of the gene coding for CYP2C9 has been described.[1555] CYP2C9 activity is low immediately after birth (21% of adult values), subsequently increasing progressively to reach a peak activity within 3 months, when expressed as mg/kg/hr.[1556]

Clearance (L/hr/kg) is generally greater in children than it is in adults, as we might expect when the linear per kilogram model is used. Ibuprofen clearance maturation follows the similar pattern to other drugs (Fig. 6-4). Clearance increases from 2.06 mL/hr/kg in extreme preterm neonates 22 to 31 weeks PMA,[1553] to 9.49 mL/hr/kg in preterm neonates 28 weeks PMA,[1554] peaking at 140 mL/hr/kg in preschool children, before decreasing again during late childhood and adolescence (71 mL/hr/kg).[1557] Similar data exist for indomethacin.[1549,1558,1559]

Many NSAIDs exhibit stereoselectivity.[1560] Ibuprofen stereoselectivity is reported in preterm neonates (less than 28 weeks gestation). *R*- and *S*-ibuprofen half-lives were about 10 hours and 25.5 hours, respectively. The mean clearance of *R*-ibuprofen (12.7 mL/hr) was about 2.5-fold greater than that of *S*-ibuprofen (5.0 mL/hr).[1561]

During pregnancy, there is relatively little transfer of NSAIDs from maternal to fetal blood. Very small quantities of NSAIDs are secreted into breast milk. Similarly, infant exposure to ketorolac via breast milk is estimated to be only 0.4% of maternal exposure.[1562]

NSAIDs undergo drug interactions through altered clearance and competition for active renal tubular secretion with other organic acids. A high fractional protein binding has been proposed to explain drug interactions between NSAIDs and oral anticoagulant agents, oral hypoglycemics, sulfonamides, bilirubin, and other protein bound drugs. One paper[1563] showed that warfarin administered with phenylbutazone increased both plasma warfarin concentrations and the prothrombin time in normal volunteers. However, while phenylbutazone displaces warfarin from its albumin binding sites in vitro, this observation does not explain changes in prothrombin time. The increased prothrombin time is a result of increased serum warfarin concentrations attributed to reduced clearance, and not from changes in protein binding.[81] Both warfarin and phenylbutazone compete for similar protein binding sites; they also compete for similar clearance pathways. NSAIDs have the potential to cause gastrointestinal irritation, blood clotting disorders, renal impairment, neutrophil dysfunction, and bronchoconstriction, effects attributed to COX-1/COX-2 ratios, although this concept may be an oversimplification.

Ibuprofen reduces the GFR by 20% in preterm neonates, affecting aminoglycoside clearance, an effect that appears to be independent of gestational age.[1564] No significant difference in the change in cerebral blood volume, change in cerebral blood flow, or tissue oxygenation index was found between administration of ibuprofen or placebo in neonates.[1565] The risk of acute GI bleeding in children given short-term ibuprofen was estimated to be 7.2/100,000 (confidence interval of 2 to 18 per 100,000), a prevalence not different from children given acetaminophen.[1566,1567] The incidence of clinically significant gastropathy in children with juvenile arthritis given NSAIDs is comparable to that in adults given long-term NSAIDs, but the prevalence of gastroduodenal injury may be greater, depending on the assessment criteria applied (e.g., abdominal pain, anemia, endoscopy).[1568,1569] Aspirin- or NSAID-exacerbated respiratory disease (ERD) occurs more frequently in adults, although exacerbations in children and teenagers have been reported. These cases are countered by reports of improvement in the symptoms of asthma when ibuprofen was administered for antipyresis. One study concluded that benefit is likely to occur in younger children with mild episodic asthma and that aspirin-ERD is a concern in one in three teenagers with severe asthma and coexistent nasal disease.[1570] COX-2 inhibitors are reported as safe in NSAID-ERD.[1570]

The commonly used NSAIDs have reversible antiplatelet effects, which are attributable to the inhibition of thromboxane synthesis. Bleeding time is usually slightly increased, but remains within normal limits in children with normal coagulation systems. A Cochrane review has established that even after tonsillectomy, NSAIDs did not cause any increase in bleeding that required a return to theatre in children. There was significantly less nausea and vomiting with NSAIDs compared to alternative analgesics, suggesting their benefits outweigh their negative aspects.[1571] Neonates given prophylactic ibuprofen to induce PDA closure did not have an increased frequency of intraventricular hemorrhage.[1572]

## KETOROLAC

Ketorolac (Toradol) is an NSAID with very potent analgesic properties.[1573-1577] The analgesic properties of ketorolac are similar to those of low-dose morphine for posttonsillectomy analgesia.[1577,1578] The major use in pediatrics is as an adjuvant to opioid analgesia or for treatment of mild to moderate pain where there is a desire to reduce the potential for respiratory depression or for nausea and vomiting.[1575,1579-1584] It is an important adjuvant to the treatment of postoperative pain, especially for children who require prolonged pain management.[1585] It is particularly useful for the transition from IV to oral therapy. Ketorolac may also be administered nasally, although pediatric perioperative data are at present lacking.[1585a,1585b] Data from adult patients (n = 522) given a single oral or intramuscular administration of 10, 30, 60, or 90 mg ketorolac for postoperative pain relief after orthopedic surgery, revealed an Emax of 8.5/10 (VAS of 0 to 10), $EC_{50}$ 0.37 mg/L and $T_{1/2}keo$ 24 min.[1586] This Emax (see Fig. 6-5) is greater than that of acetaminophen or ibuprofen (5.3/10, VAS 0-10).

The PK, standardized using allometry, are similar in adults and children (E-Table 6-5). The terminal elimination half-life in children 4 to 8 years of age is approximately 6 hours, although there is considerable variability.[1587-1589] PK may also be influenced by chronobiology[754] and many NSAIDs exhibit stereoselectivity. Ketorolac is supplied and administered as a racemic mixture that contains a 1:1 ratio of the R(+) and S(−) stereoisomers. Pharmacologic activity resides almost exclusively with the S(−) stereoisomer.[1560,1590] Clearance of the S(−) enantiomer was four times that of the R(+) enantiomer (6.2 vs 1.4 mL/min/kg) in children 3 to 18 years.[1591] Terminal half-life of S(−)-ketorolac was 40% that of the R(+) enantiomer (107 vs 259 min), and the Vd of the S(−) enantiomer was greater than that of the R(+) form (0.82 vs 0.50 L/kg). Recovery of S(−)-ketorolac glucuronide was 2.3 times that of the R(+) enantiomer. Because of the greater clearance and shorter half-life of S(−)-ketorolac, PK predictions based on racemic assays may overestimate the duration of pharmacologic effect.[1591]

One of the major concerns with ketorolac is the inhibition of platelet function through inhibition of cyclooxygenase, and the consequent potential for postsurgical bleeding. Ketorolac has been shown to have minimal effect on prothrombin and partial thromboplastin times but has been shown to cause modest increases in the bleeding time.[1575,1592-1595] Unlike aspirin, the ketorolac antiplatelet effect is reversible and, therefore, the effect is dependent on the presence of ketorolac within the body.[1596] This effect on platelet function has been of most concern in children undergoing adenotonsillectomy.[1597-1600] In the studies reporting posttonsillectomy bleeding, most involved administration of the ketorolac during or at the beginning of the surgical procedure, before hemostasis was achieved. In addition, the increased incidence of bleeding appears to be primarily during the first 24 hours, which corresponds to the several half-lives it would take to eliminate ketorolac from the body. The incidence of bleeding after the first 24 hours does not appear to be different.[1601] It would therefore be reasonable to not administer this medication until the end of surgery, after hemostasis is achieved. Some practitioners eschew this issue altogether and only administer ketorolac when the potential for a life-threatening hemorrhage is less.[1473] Concerns regarding the possibility of postoperative hemorrhage appear to be valid, but the true frequency of life-threatening bleeding due exclusively to ketorolac is quite small.[1583,1602-1605] One paper reported a dose-response relationship for this bleeding propensity; the risk associated with the drug was larger and clinically important when ketorolac was used in higher doses, in older subjects, and for more than 5 days.[1606] Safety assessment showed no changes in renal or hepatic function tests, surgical drain output, or continuous oximetry between groups given placebo, 0.5 mg/kg, or 1 mg/kg at 6 to 18 hours after surgery.[1560,1590] Many clinicians discuss the possible use of ketorolac with the surgeon before administering it and document the conversation in the anesthesia record. Ketorolac can be used to treat pain after congenital heart surgery without an increased risk of bleeding complications.[1603] Ketorolac has been safely used to provide analgesia for preterm and term infants, but the PK in this age group has not been described.[1607]

Another concern is the potential for adverse effects on bone healing, particularly spinal fusion.[1608,1609] Evidence suggests that nonunion of the spine is associated only with large-dose and not low-dose ketorolac. Ketorolac has been used safely to provide analgesia for other types of orthopedic conditions as well.[1610,1611] One other concern is the report of sudden and profound bradycardia after rapid IV administration of ketorolac.[1612] Although the mechanism of this response is unclear, ketorolac should be administered slowly when given intravenously.

# Benzodiazepine Sedatives

These drugs produce anxiolysis, amnesia, and hypnosis. They are commonly used as adjuncts to both local and general anesthesia. Benzodiazepines bind to GABA$_A$ receptors, resulting in increased cellular chloride entry. This renders these receptors resistant to excitation because they are hyperpolarized.

## MIDAZOLAM

Midazolam (Versed) is a water-soluble benzodiazepine that offers significant clinical advantages over diazepam. It is not painful when administered intravenously or intramuscularly. Midazolam is only one of a few medications that are approved as premedicants in children, and is the only benzodiazepine approved by the FDA for use in neonates.

PK–PD relationships have been described for IV midazolam in adults. When an EEG signal is used as an effect measure, the EC$_{50}$ is 35 to 77 ng/mL, with a T$_{1/2}$keo of 0.9 to 1.6 min.[66,1613,1614] The T$_{1/2}$keo is increased in the elderly and in low cardiac output states. PK–PD relationships are more difficult to describe after oral midazolam because the active metabolite, 1-hydroxymidazolam, has approximately half the activity of the parent drug.[1615]

Sedation in children is more difficult to quantify. No PK–PD relationship was established in children, age 2 days to 17 years, who were given a midazolam infusion in the ICU. Midazolam dosing could, however, be effectively titrated to the desired level of sedation, assessed by the COMFORT distress scale.[1616] Consistent with this finding, desirable sedation in children after cardiac surgery was achieved at mean serum concentrations between 0.1 and 0.5 mg/L.[1617-1619] Plasma concentrations of 0.3 to 0.4 mg/L are associated with anesthesia in adults.[1620,1621] A target concentration for sedation (arouses to command) in adults is 0.1 mg/L.[1622]

Midazolam is metabolized mainly by hepatic hydroxylation (CYP3A4).[1623] These hydroxylated metabolites are glucuronidated and excreted in the urine. CYP3A7 is the dominant CYP3A enzyme in utero; it is expressed in the fetal liver and appears to have activity from as early as 50 to 60 days after conception. There appears to be a temporal switch in the immediate perinatal period, and CYP3A4 expression increases dramatically after the first week of life. Hepatic CYP3A4 activity begins to dramatically increase at about 1 week of age, reaching 30% to 40% of adult expression by 1 month.[156] Midazolam has a hepatic extraction ratio in the intermediate range of 0.3 to 0.7. Metabolic clearance depends on both liver perfusion and enzyme activity.

Clearance is reduced in neonates (0.8 to 2.2 mL/min/kg, 60 mL/min/70 kg) (E-Fig. 6-18),[1624-1631] but increases rapidly (Hill coefficient of 3) after 39 weeks PMA,[1628] to reach 90% mature clearance at 1 year of age.[1631] Mature clearance was 523 mL/min/70 kg. The TM$_{50}$ was 73.6 weeks.[1629,1631] Central volume of distribution is related to weight (V1 = 0.591 ± 0.065 L/kg) whereas peripheral volume of distribution remained constant (V2 = 0.42 ± 0.11 L) in 187 neonates weighing 0.7 to 5.2 kg.[1628] It has been suggested that midazolam induces its own clearance.[1617] The latter observation, from infants after cardiac surgery, likely results from the improved hepatic function after the insult of CPB. Neonates have an increase in Vdss during extracorporeal membrane oxygenation therapy (0.8 L/kg to 4.1 L/kg), caused by sequestration of midazolam by the circuitry, although clearance (1.4 ± 0.15 mL/min/kg) was unchanged.[1632]

Clearance may be reduced in the presence of pathology. A reduced clearance of midazolam has been reported after circulatory arrest for cardiac surgery.[1633] Covariates, such as renal failure, hepatic failure,[1619] and concomitant administration of CYP3A inhibitors,[693,694] are important predictors of altered midazolam and metabolite PK in pediatric intensive care patients.[1634] The clearance of midazolam was reduced by 30% in neonates receiving sympathomimetic amines, probably as a consequence of the underlying compromised hemodynamics.[1628]

The suggested infusion rate of midazolam is 0.5 µg/kg/min for preterm infants less than 32 weeks gestational age and 1.0 µg/kg/min for infants more than 32 weeks gestational age. Any factor that impairs hepatic blood flow (e.g., CPB, vasopressors) may decrease midazolam elimination, although cirrhosis only minimally affects its elimination in adults.[1633,1634,1635,1636] Midazolam offers the best PK profile for neonates because the active metabolite has a half-life similar to the parent compound, but with minimal clinical activity.[1299] *Bolus administration to preterm and term neonates has been associated with profound hypotension; the likelihood seems to be greater if the infant is receiving fentanyl.*[1307] *Likewise, a neonate receiving a midazolam infusion is more likely to suffer profound hypotension with a bolus of fentanyl.* Rapid IV and nasal administration have also been associated with seizure-like activity, although it appears that this is myoclonic rather than true seizure activity.[1637] Midazolam has been administered as a continuous infusion, both in the OR as an adjunct to general anesthesia, and in the ICU.[860,1638-1640] Prolonged administration does lead to tolerance, dependency, and benzodiazepine withdrawal.[1641,1642] Long-term infusions, particularly in neonates, should be tapered over days while carefully monitoring for signs of withdrawal (vomiting, agitation, sweating, bowel distention, seizures, change in neurologic status).[1314,1643,1644] A theoretical concern associated with midazolam is benzyl alcohol toxicity with the development of metabolic acidosis and gasping respirations.[1645,1646] The 24-hour dose of benzoyl alcohol in midazolam when administered according to recommended dosing guidelines should not cause toxicity.

Midazolam is the most commonly used benzodiazepine in pediatric anesthesia. It is administered orally, nasally, and rectally, as well as intravenously and intramuscularly.[902,1390,1633,1647-1661] The desired clinical effects include antegrade amnesia (approximately 50%),[1662-1664] as well as sedation and anxiolysis before induction of anesthesia or a medical procedure.* One study suggested that its amnestic properties may be superior to those of diazepam.[1665] The clinical endpoint with midazolam may differ somewhat when compared with diazepam. Midazolam produces a general calming effect with minimal sedation and little effect on speech. In contrast, diazepam frequently causes obvious sedation and slurring of speech. It is important to appreciate the subtle difference between these medications to avoid relative overdose, particularly when using midazolam in combination with other potent CNS depressants.

When midazolam was first introduced, a number of deaths were attributed to respiratory depression. These deaths were probably the result of combining large doses of midazolam with other medications, particularly opioids. An important pharmacologic difference between the benzodiazepines is that the time to

*References 902, 1647, 1648, 1651-1653, 1657, 1658.

achieve peak CNS effect with IV midazolam, 4.8 minutes, is almost threefold greater than with diazepam, 1.5 minutes (see Fig. 47-7).[62,66] This is because of the greater fat solubility of diazepam and therefore a more rapid transit into the CNS.[1666] Accordingly, one must wait sufficient time between doses of midazolam (3 to 5 minutes) to achieve the peak CNS effects before considering supplemental doses or other medications.[1667] IV midazolam depresses the response to hypoxemia, an effect that is exaggerated in the presence of a potent opioid, such as fentanyl. This combination (0.1 mg/kg midazolam and 6 μg/kg fentanyl IV) has been associated with respiratory arrest in an infant.[1668,1669] Children with sleep-disordered breathing who were premedicated with oral midazolam (0.5 mg/kg) experienced only a small incidence (1.5%) of transient desaturation.[1670] However, IV midazolam (0.1 mg/kg) has been shown to cause both central apnea as well as upper airway obstruction, the latter by reducing pharyngeal muscle tone.[1671] In addition, the combination of oral midazolam (0.5 mg/kg) and nitrous oxide (50%) may cause partial upper airway obstruction four times more frequently in children with large tonsils than in those with normal size tonsils.[1672] Interestingly, mouth opening may increase upper airway collapse, thus increasing the airway obstruction in children sedated with midazolam for dental procedures.[1673]

One final concern relates to the administration of drugs that interfere with the cytochrome isoforms that metabolize midazolam (CYP3A4). Examples of such drugs or foods are grapefruit juice, erythromycin, calcium channel blockers, and protease inhibitors.[109,666,667,1652-1655] The net effect is to prolong the duration of action of midazolam.

Midazolam has been used as an induction agent, but is not as satisfactory as other agents.[1654,1674] One author (CJC) has administered as much as 1.0 mg/kg intravenously to a child without producing unconsciousness. The same dose given orally produces sedation and hallucinations. Commonly used doses and routes of administration are presented in Table 6-17. The nasal route has some proponents,[1647] although there is a direct connection with the CNS at that level (see E-Fig. 4-2).[906] Because midazolam is neurotoxic when applied directly to neural tissue,[912] there is the theoretical risk of CNS toxicity.[906] In addition, 85% of children who receive nasal midazolam cry and complain of the bitter aftertaste.[1390,1649] It would seem prudent to avoid this route of administration because the oral route appears to be equally effective and without risk.

### DIAZEPAM

Diazepam (Valium) (0.2 to 0.3 mg/kg) is rapidly absorbed after oral administration, with peak plasma concentrations at 30 to 90 minutes; the absorption rate is more rapid in children than in adults.[1675,1676] It has been used extensively as a premedication,

as an adjunct to balanced anesthesia, and for sedation, amnesia, and control of seizures. Intramuscular administration is painful and results in irregular absorption; plasma concentrations are only 60% of those obtained with a similar oral dose.[1677-1679] Rectal diazepam (0.2-0.5 mg/kg) is used for prehospital treatment of pediatric status epilepticus. The recommended IV dose is 0.1 to 0.2 mg/kg. Diazepam has been administered rectally to children for sedation in doses ranging from 0.3 to 1.0 mg/kg with satisfactory results.[1680-1683] One study found a more rapid uptake during the first 2 hours after administration when administered in liquid rather than suppository form.[1680]

Diazepam is highly plasma bound, with a serum half-life varying from 20 to 80 hours. Its half-life is reduced in younger adults and children (approximately 18 hours).[1680] Hepatic disease may also decrease the elimination of diazepam.[1684] Studies in neonates who received diazepam transplacentally just before delivery demonstrate prolonged drug effects and serum half-lives (40 to 100 hours); a result of immature hepatic excretory mechanisms and reduced hepatic blood flow (see E-Fig. 6-18).[142,1675,1685] Diazepam undergoes oxidative metabolism by demethylation (CYP 2C19). Its active metabolite, desmethyldiazepam, has similar potency to the parent compound and a half-life as long or longer than the parent compound, thus emphasizing that caution is required when administering this benzodiazepine to neonates.[1675,1686,1687]

The preservative benzyl alcohol is present in many formulations of diazepam. This preservative should be avoided in neonates because it is difficult to metabolize, is associated with kernicterus, and can cause a metabolic acidosis.[1688-1690] The amount of benzyl alcohol that accompanies a usual dose of diazepam would likely be insufficient to cause harm to the neonate.[1691] Diazepam has respiratory depressant effects that are quite variable, especially when combined with opioids.[1692]

Diazepam is useful as an oral premedication, although midazolam has overshadowed this role. Its main disadvantage when given intravenously is pain. Administering IV lidocaine before the diazepam and administering the diazepam slowly through a rapidly flowing IV catheter minimizes this pain. Diazepam is avoided in neonates and infants because of the prolonged half-life of the drug and its metabolites. Finally, diazepam should not be administered intramuscularly because of the pain and erratic absorption.

## Other Sedatives

### DEXMEDETOMIDINE

Dexmedetomidine (Precedex), the *dextro* optical isomer of medetomidine, is a pharmacologically selective $\alpha_2$-agonist with sedative, anxiolytic, and analgesic properties. Dexmedetomidine is in the same class as clonidine but differs from clonidine in that its affinity for $\alpha_2$- compared with $\alpha_1$-receptors is eightfold greater. In anesthesia and intensive care, this agent is currently being developed as an IV sedative agent for procedural sedation and as an anesthetic adjunct during surgery. Exploiting dexmedetomidine's greater selectivity for $\alpha_2$-receptors offers a novel and interesting new medication for our pharmacologic armamentarium.

Dexmedetomidine exerts its effects on numerous organ systems via $\alpha$-adrenoceptors. These sympathetic adrenoceptors are categorized as either $\alpha_1$- or $\alpha_2$-receptors, based on receptor selectivity.[1693] The latter are further subdivided into three subtypes: $\alpha_{2A}$-, $\alpha_{2B}$-, and $\alpha_{2C}$-adrenoceptors according to ligand binding. The $\alpha_2$-agonists, such as dexmedetomidine, bind all

**TABLE 6-17** Dosing and Onset Times of Midazolam in Infants and Children (Not Neonates)

| Route | Dose (mg/kg) | Time of Onset (minutes) | Time to Peak Effect (minutes) |
|---|---|---|---|
| Intravenous | 0.05-0.15 | Immediate | 3-5 |
| Intramuscular | 0.1-0.2 | 3-5 | 10-20 |
| Oral | 0.25-0.75 | 5-30 | 10-30 |
| Nasal | 0.1-0.2 | 3-5 | 10-15 |
| Rectal | 0.75-1.0 | 5-10 | 10-30 |

(See text for details.)

three receptor subtypes, although the receptor subtype binding may vary with the dose of dexmedetomidine. The $\alpha_2$-adrenoceptors trigger responses by activating G proteins. The common path for the effector response to dexmedetomidine is sympatholysis (suppression of the sympathetic nervous system). Depending on the specific receptor that is activated, $\alpha_2$-agonists may cause hypotension, bradycardia, sedation, analgesia, attenuation of shivering, and a number of other physiologic responses. Consequently, dexmedetomidine use in neonates and children has expanded to include prevention of emergence delirium, postoperative pain management, invasive and noninvasive procedural sedation, and the management of opioid withdrawal.[747,1694-1702]

The $\alpha_2$-adrenoceptors are located ubiquitously throughout the body. In the CNS, they are located primarily in the locus ceruleus, spinal cord, and autonomic nerves. The CNS manifestations of $\alpha_2$-agonists include sedation and anxiolysis, both of which are mediated through the locus ceruleus. Sedation may also be mediated by $\alpha_2$-agonist inhibition of the ascending norepinephrine pathways. Analgesia is mediated primarily via the spinal cord, although there is evidence that supraspinal and peripheral nerves may contribute to this effect as well. Cardiovascular manifestations of $\alpha_2$-adrenoceptors include actions on the heart and on peripheral vasculature. The primary action of $\alpha_2$-adrenoceptors on the heart is a chronotropic effect in which it slows heart rate by blocking the cardioaccelerator nerves as well as by augmenting vagal activity. In infants, dexmedetomidine-induced bradycardia may be exacerbated by the coadministration of digoxin. Decreasing the dose of dexmedetomidine restores the heart rate to normal values.[1703] The $\alpha_2$-agonist action on the autonomic ganglia includes decreasing sympathetic outflow, which leads to hypotension and bradycardia. Actions on the peripheral vasculature depend on the dose of dexmedetomidine: vasodilatation is the result of sympatholysis, which occurs at low doses, and vasoconstriction is the result of direct action on smooth muscle vasculature at high doses (Fig. 6-24).

In the peripheral nervous system, $\alpha_2$-adrenoceptors are located at both the presynaptic and postsynaptic junctions.[1693] The presynaptic and postsynaptic effects of $\alpha_2$-agonists diminish norepinephrine release and inhibit sympathetic activity. Other manifestations of $\alpha_2$-adrenoceptors include inhibition of shivering as well as promoting diuresis, although their mechanisms remain elusive.[1693,1704]

A plasma concentration in excess of 0.6 µg/L is estimated to produce satisfactory sedation in adult ICU patients,[1705] and similar target concentrations are estimated in postoperative children after cardiac surgery who require sedation in the ICU.[1706] Hypotension has been described in children after cardiac surgery,[1707] and in children presenting for sedation during radiologic procedures. In children sedated with high-dose dexmedetomidine there was a 5% incidence of hypertension and the incidence was greatest in those under 1-year of age and those who required an additional bolus dose to maintain sedation.[1708] These adverse cardiovascular effects of dexmedetomidine generate some concern. Dexmedetomidine also decreases heart rate in a dose-dependent manner in children.[1696,1709-1712] This effect is attributed to a centrally mediated sympathetic withdrawal, which results in unregulated cholinergic activity. With very large doses of dexmedetomidine (2 to 3 µg/kg over 10 minutes followed by 1.5 to 2 µg/kg/hr), 12 children under 6 years of age experienced heart rates less than 50 beats/min although their blood pressures were maintained.[1712] Administration of anticholinergics or other medications to increase the heart rate during dexmedetomidine-induced bradycardia have not been required, but it should be noted that severe and persistent hypertension has been reported when glycopyrrolate was used to treat high-dose dexmedetomidine-induced bradycardia.[1713]

Less favorable results have been noted in the electrophysiology laboratory. Heart rate decreased while arterial BP increased significantly after 1 µg/kg IV over 10 minutes followed by a 10-minute continuous infusion of 0.7 µg/kg/hr. Sinus node

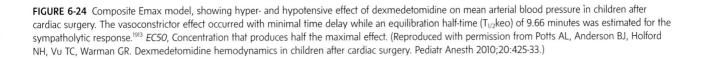

**FIGURE 6-24** Composite Emax model, showing hyper- and hypotensive effect of dexmedetomidine on mean arterial blood pressure in children after cardiac surgery. The vasoconstrictor effect occurred with minimal time delay while an equilibration half-time ($T_{1/2}$keo) of 9.66 minutes was estimated for the sympatholytic response.[1913] *EC50*, Concentration that produces half the maximal effect. (Reproduced with permission from Potts AL, Anderson BJ, Holford NH, Vu TC, Warman GR. Dexmedetomidine hemodynamics in children after cardiac surgery. Pediatr Anesth 2010;20:425-33.)

function was significantly affected and atrioventricular nodal function was also depressed. The use of dexmedetomidine may not be desirable during electrophysiology studies and may be associated with adverse effects in patients at risk for bradycardia or atrioventricular nodal block.[1714]

Population parameter estimates for a two-compartment model were clearance of 42.1 L/hr/70 kg (CV = 30.9%), central Vd of 56.3 L/70 kg (CV = 61.3%), inter-compartment clearance of 78.3 L/hr/70 kg (CV = 37.0%), and peripheral Vd of 69.0 L/70 kg (CV = 47.0%).[1706] Clearance increases from 18.2 L/hr/70 kg at birth in a full-term neonate, to reach 84.5% of the mature value by 1 year postnatal age (see Figs. 6-4 and 6-10). Children given a dexmedetomidine infusion after cardiac surgery had reduced clearance (83.0%) compared with a noncardiac surgical population given a bolus dose.[1706] Similar parameter estimates with reduced clearance in children receiving dexmedetomidine infusion after cardiac surgery have been described by others[1715]; this trait has also been described for morphine, fentanyl, and midazolam.

The preferred route of administration of dexmedetomidine is the IV route, although others have been studied. The PK of dexmedetomidine have also been studied after parenteral (IM), buccal, and oral administration.[1716] Parenteral delivery yielded similar kinetics to IV, buccal yielded an 82% bioavailability, and orogastric yielded only a 16% bioavailability. Data from adults indicate limited effects of renal failure on the kinetics of dexmedetomidine.[1717] Dexmedetomidine is metabolized extensively in the liver (UGT enzymes), with 40% metabolized by CYP2D6 isozyme.[1704] After metabolism to methyl and glucuronide conjugates, 95% of dexmedetomidine is eliminated via the kidneys.[1718] There appears to be no evidence that dexmedetomidine interferes with the PK of other medications that are substrates for CYP2D6 metabolism.[1718] Dexmedetomidine is 93% protein-bound in children.[1704,1711]

Dexmedetomidine is formulated as a concentrated solution in a 2 mL vial (100 µg/mL). After diluting it with normal saline, lactated Ringer's solution, or 5% dextrose in water to an appropriate concentration, dexmedetomidine can be delivered by syringe pump. Current dosing recommendations for dexmedetomidine begin with a loading dose followed by an infusion, although some skip the loading dose during general anesthesia and administer only a constant infusion.[1696,1711,1719] The recommended loading dose is 1 µg/kg dexmedetomidine infused over 10 minutes, although loading doses between 0.5 and 3.0 µg/kg have been reported.[747,1696,1708,1719-1721] The purpose of infusing the loading dose over 10 minutes (as opposed to a rapid IV bolus) is to attenuate the severity of the hypertension that can occur with bolus administration. After completing the loading dose, dexmedetomidine should be infused at 0.5 to 1 µg/kg/hr.[747,1696,1719-1721] (*Note:* dexmedetomidine is infused in *micrograms per kilogram per hour, not micrograms per kilogram per minute.*) In the United States, dexmedetomidine is approved only for infusion up to 24 hours, although data exist attesting to hemodynamic stability even after infusions of greater duration.[1722]

When compared with propofol for sedation during MRI, dexmedetomidine provides adequate sedation during the scan but has a slower recovery profile.[1722,1723] It is our experience and that of others, however, that sedation with the recommended maximal doses of dexmedetomidine will generally require the addition of other sedatives, such as midazolam, in order for a child to remain motionless for a procedure such as an MRI.[747,1724,1725]

One of the major advantages of dexmedetomidine over other sedatives is its respiratory effects, which are minimal in adults and children.[1709-1711,1719,1726-1728] Although dexmedetomidine blunts the $CO_2$ response curve,[1729] it does not lead to extreme hypoxia or hypercapnia. Indeed, respiratory rate, $CO_2$ tension, and oxygen saturation are generally maintained during dexmedetomidine sedation in children.[747,1711,1720] In children without obstructive sleep apnea, increasing doses of dexmedetomidine (1 to 3 µg/kg) result in small changes in the upper airway and do not appear to be associated with clinical signs of airway obstruction. Even though these changes are small, all precautions to manage airway obstruction should be taken when dexmedetomidine is used for sedation.[1730] In children with suspected obstructive sleep apnea, significantly less frequent artificial airway support was required when dexmedetomidine (2 µg/kg/hr) was used for sedation for MRI sleep studies, compared with propofol for sedation.[1731]

Quantifying the MAC-sparing effect of dexmedetomidine has proven to be difficult. Three studies have estimated the MAC of isoflurane or sevoflurane in adults at two doses of dexmedetomidine; high (0.6 to 0.7 ng/mL) and low (0.36 to 0.3 ng/mL) concentration.[1710,1732,1733] The MAC-sparing effect of high-dose dexmedetomidine ranged from 17% to 50% and that of low-dose dexmedetomidine from 0% to 35%. Accordingly, it is difficult to predict the exact MAC-reducing effect of dexmedetomidine on sevoflurane and isoflurane in adults. Similar data in children have not been forthcoming.

Dexmedetomidine provides an interesting quality of sedation that permits arousal with gentle stimulation.[1711] The lack of respiratory depression distinguishes this sedative from opioids, benzodiazepines, and other sedatives. It has been studied for sedation in children for a number of different purposes, including radiologic procedures such as MRI.[747,1696,1719,1720]

Dexmedetomidine provides a modest degree of analgesia, reducing the need for, but not totally supplanting, opioids and other analgesics. Several studies demonstrated that it spares opioid requirements during surgery.[1704,1734,1735]

The CNS effects of dexmedetomidine have been addressed in animals and, in part, in humans.[1736] The data suggest that dexmedetomidine decreases cerebral blood flow directly by vasoconstricting the smooth muscle of the cerebral blood vessels, and indirectly through a reduction in arterial BP and cardiac output. In humans, dexmedetomidine decreases cerebral blood flow 30%, as determined by positron emission tomography, as well as Doppler measurements of the middle cerebral artery. Interestingly, using Doppler measurements of the cerebral blood vessels in adult volunteers, both the $CO_2$ response and autoregulation of cerebral blood flow were preserved. When dexmedetomidine was infused before introducing an inhalational anesthetic, the dexmedetomidine attenuated cerebral vasodilatation induced by the inhalational anesthetic.

Dexmedetomidine depresses sensory-evoked potentials but, for the most part, the potentials are adequate for evaluations.[1737] Similarly, motor-evoked potentials are reduced in a dose-dependent manner during dexmedetomidine infusion but are measurable nonetheless.[1738] There are contrasting reports about the degree of evoked potential suppression, but most report successful spinal cord monitoring during scoliosis surgery.[1739-1742]

Emergence delirium occurs commonly after most inhalational anesthetics in children.[1726] A number of medications have been shown to attenuate the incidence of delirium after anesthesia, including dexmedetomidine.[1699] Dexmedetomidine decreases the incidence of agitation after sevoflurane anesthesia: after an infusion of dexmedetomidine (0.2 µg/kg/hr), recovery was not prolonged,[1743] whereas after a single dose of 0.5 µg/kg, 5 minutes before the end of surgery, emergence was prolonged.[1744] Further studies are required to assess the cost-benefit ratio for this indication.

The interaction between dexmedetomidine and neuromuscular blockade has been studied during balanced anesthesia with propofol and alfentanil.[1745] In adults, dexmedetomidine decreased the twitch response after sevoflurane 7%, although this was not deemed to be clinically important. Current evidence does not substantiate any clinically significant interaction between dexmedetomidine and neuromuscular blockade.

At present, this medication seems to offer specific advantages for awake fiberoptic intubation, awake craniotomy, sedation in the ICU (opioid sparing), and perhaps for reducing the incidence of emergence delirium.[1700,1746-1749] However, high-dose dexmedetomidine is associated with adverse effects on the heart rate and BP, and unpredictable effects with anticholinergics.[1713,1750] Additional research in children is required before recommendations can be made regarding appropriate dosing and drug interactions.[1714,1751,1752] There are conflicting data regarding its safety in children with congenital heart disease.[1714,1753-1755]

### CHLORAL HYDRATE

Chloral hydrate exerts its sedative effect by enhancing the GABA receptor complex, and it does not have analgesic properties. Its primary use in pediatrics is for sedation before noninvasive procedures, or as a premedication. Its principal advantage is that it can be administered orally or rectally, with excellent absorption and relatively good sedation, within 30 to 45 minutes. The usual dose is 20 to 75 mg/kg orally or rectally but total doses up to 100 mg/kg (maximum 2 grams) have been used. It has minimal effects on respiration[1756]; however, chloral hydrate can result in airway obstruction, particularly in children with enlarged tonsils.[1757-1759] In addition, apnea, airway obstruction, bradycardia, and hypotension have been reported in a series of infants younger than 6 months of age who were sedated for echocardiograms; this report emphasizes that this is not the benign drug that many have previously thought.[1760] Deaths after chloral hydrate sedation have been reported.[1237,1761]

Chloral hydrate is the most commonly used sedative for infants undergoing a variety of nonpainful procedures.[1762-1765] Its bitter taste is a disadvantage.[1659] This drug should not be administered on a chronic basis because of the theoretic concern for potential carcinogenicity with metabolites, concerns for producing severe gastritis (possibly related to its metabolism to trichloroacetic acid), and the possibility of accumulation of drug metabolites.[1766,1767] In addition, its use in neonates is not recommended because of its interference with binding of bilirubin to albumin and the potential accumulation of toxic metabolites leading to metabolic acidosis, renal failure, and hypotonia.[1768]

Chloral hydrate is metabolized in the liver and erythrocytes by alcohol dehydrogenase to an active metabolite, trichloroethanol, which has a half-life of 9.7 ± 1.7 hours in toddlers, but 39.8 ± 14.3 hours in preterm infants (see Fig. 47-3).[1769] Trichloroethanol is cleared by UGT (see morphine, acetaminophen, dexmedetomidine), which is immature in neonates. These very long half-lives imply that residual drug effect will be present long after any procedure requiring sedation.[1770,1771] Because of the long half-life, there is a real risk for prolonged sedation or re-sedation after leaving medical supervision.[1772-1775] It is for this reason that *chloral hydrate is not generally recommended for premedication prior to surgery*

and that a prolonged period of observation is recommended after sedation for a procedure. If nitrous oxide is administered to children who have received chloral hydrate, a state of deep sedation or general anesthesia may occur.[1776] Note: Chloral hydrate liquid production ceased in the United States in May 2012. (http://www.fda.gov/drugs/drugsafety/drugshortages/ucm050794.htm Accessed July 25, 2012.)

## Antihistamines

### DIPHENHYDRAMINE

Antihistamines are often used in pediatric anesthesia both for their histamine$_1$-receptor inhibition and for their sedative properties. Diphenhydramine (Benadryl) is one of the more commonly used antihistamines. It is rapidly absorbed when administered orally (at a dose of 1.25 mg/kg) with a duration of effect that lasts anywhere from 3 to 6 hours. Clearance is through CYP2D6 (see codeine). It is often administered as a premedicant or as an in-hospital sedative. Caution is advised for children with respiratory problems because diphenhydramine dries secretions, causing difficulty expectorating. The IV dose to treat an allergic reaction is 0.5 mg/kg.

### CIMETIDINE, RANITIDINE, AND FAMOTIDINE

Cimetidine (Tagamet) was the first generation of potent, highly hydrophilic, competitive inhibitors of histamine$_2$ receptor–mediated histamine reactions, which was later followed by ranitidine and famotidine. This class of drugs increases gastric-fluid pH and reduces gastric fluid residual volume.[1777] Indications for a histamine$_2$-receptor antagonist include a history of gastroesophageal reflux, hiatus hernia, previous esophageal surgery, obesity, or an anticipated difficult intubation that will require prolonged laryngoscopy, as well as, perhaps, high-risk patients (American Society of Anesthesiologists classes 3 and 4). Cimetidine is likely the most studied of this category of drugs, but its use has diminished because of serious drug interactions through its effects on the cytochrome oxidase system. Cimetidine partially inhibits numerous CYP enzymes (CYP1A2, CYP2C9, CYP2C19, CYP2D6, CYP2E1, and CYP3A4), which prolongs the half-lives of many drugs, including phenytoin, phenobarbital, theophylline, cyclosporine, carbamazepine, benzodiazepines that do not undergo glucuronidation, calcium-channel blockers, propranolol, quinidine, sulfonylureas, mexiletine, warfarin, and tricyclic antidepressants, such as imipramine.[1778] Part of its effects on other drugs occurs through reduced hepatic blood flow. The elimination half-life of cimetidine is prolonged in neonates and infants, compared with older children.[1779] The kidney is the primary clearance organ in children. Renal clearance in children 4 to 13 years comprised 70% of total body clearance, more than double that of adults. As expected, children have a higher total body clearance (11.6 mL/min/kg) than do adults (7.0 mL/min/kg), a larger Vd (1.24 vs 0.80 L/kg) and a shorter elimination half-life (83 vs 122 min).[1780]

Although ranitidine (Zantac) also weakly reduces CYP activity, *it does not increase the half-life of other medications significantly* when administered at the usual therapeutic doses.[1781-1784] Ranitidine has been administered by intermittent bolus (2 to 4 mg/kg in four divided doses), or as a loading dose (0.5 mg/kg) followed by an infusion of 0.05 mg/kg/hr.[1785-1787] The peak effect occurs between 2 and 4 hours after administration.[1451] The elimination half-life of ranitidine is 3 ± 1.35 hours. When a dose of 1.5 mg/kg/8 hr was administered, ranitidine maintained the gastric fluid pH greater than 4.[1786] Reduced doses have met with less success in controlling the gastric fluid pH.[1785]

Famotidine (Pepcid) is about eight times more potent than ranitidine and about 40 times more potent than cimetidine.[1788] Famotidine has been well studied, including in neonates. Because famotidine is primarily excreted by the kidneys, dosing depends on the maturity of the renal function. Infants younger than 3 months of age have reduced clearance and require 24 hours between doses (0.25 mg/kg IV or 0.5 mg/kg orally), whereas infants older than 3 months are similar to older children and adults and require 12 hours between doses.[1779,1789,1790] There is some evidence to suggest decreased responsiveness to famotidine (a weaker effect in altering gastric acid pH and volume) with long-term administration.[1791] Famotidine has been shown to increase gastric fluid pH, although it does not reduce gastric residual volumes when administered before anesthesia.[1792]

## Antiemetics

### METOCLOPRAMIDE

Metoclopramide (Reglan) has been used in children for its antiemetic and gastric emptying properties.[1793] The antiemetic properties result from its direct effects on the chemoreceptor trigger zone. Gastric emptying is a result of the antagonism of the neurotransmitter dopamine, which stimulates gastric smooth-muscle activity.[1794,1795] A dose of 0.15 mg/kg at the end of surgery effectively reduces emesis after strabismus surgery and tonsillectomy, although the magnitude of its effectiveness may be limited.[1796] Metoclopramide is less effective than 5-hydroxytryptamine type 3 (5-HT₃) receptor inhibitors, but does offer an alternative rescue medication.[1797,1798] As with many other medications cleared by sulfate and glucuronide conjugation, the elimination half-life in neonates is prolonged compared with older children, thus necessitating a 6 hour interval between oral doses (0.15 mg/kg).[1799]

### 5-HYDROXYTRYPTAMINE TYPE 3–RECEPTOR ANTAGONISTS

Antagonists to the 5-HT₃ receptor include ondansetron (Zofran), granisetron (Kytril), dolasetron (Anzemet), and tropisetron (Navoban). These agents have proven to be an effective preventive and therapeutic measure for postoperative nausea and vomiting (PONV). Notwithstanding their widespread usage, these drugs have been the subject of much debate regarding which is the most effective, which has the better side-effect profile, which lasts the longest, which is best combined with other agents, which costs too much, and so on.[1800-1812] Because ondansetron was the first in this class of serotonergic receptor antagonists that effectively reduced the incidence of nausea and vomiting in children, it forms the basis for discussion of measures to prevent PONV after pediatric surgery.[1813-1822] Some studies report ondansetron 0.1 mg/kg superior to metoclopramide 0.15 mg/kg for the prophylactic control of postoperative vomiting in children undergoing tonsillectomy.[1823] Most pediatric anesthesiologists limit their routine use to children undergoing procedures known to have a substantial incidence of nausea and vomiting, such as strabismus repair, tonsillectomy, or middle ear surgery, and to children with a known history of motion sickness or previous nausea and vomiting after surgery.[1824-1832] Ondansetron is effective in preventing nausea and vomiting, as well as in reducing the severity of established nausea and vomiting. The usual recommended dose is 100 to 150 µg/kg every 6 hours. One clinical trial found efficacy in children as young as 1 month of age, however, the PK were different in the infants younger than 4 months of age, suggesting the need for a longer interval between dosing.[1833] More importantly, the need for anti-emetics at all in children under 1 year of age may be questioned, because postoperative vomiting is infrequent in this age group.[1834] This is unsurprising, given that clearance is by hydroxylation, followed by glucuronide or sulfate conjugation in the liver. A mature clearance of 541 mL/min/70 kg is reported, but ondansetron clearance was reduced by 31%, 53%, and 76% for the typical 6-, 3-, and 1-month-old infant, respectively; clearance matured with a TM₅₀ of 4 months. Simulations showed that an ondansetron dose of 0.1 mg/kg in children younger than 6 months produced exposure similar to a 0.15-mg/kg dose in older children.[1835]

A number of studies in children demonstrated that the antiemetic effect of drugs from this class can be improved if they are combined with dexamethasone or other anesthetic techniques known to reduce vomiting.[1817,1818,1820,1836] An oral disintegrating tablet of ondansetron is also available.[1837]

Other agents in this class (e.g., granisetron, dolasetron, tropisetron) have all been shown to be effective in ameliorating PONV, which is further improved when combined with other antiemetic modalities.[1813,1831,1838-1846]

## Anticholinergics

### ATROPINE AND SCOPOLAMINE

Atropine (0.02 mg/kg) and scopolamine (0.01 mg/kg) both have CNS effects, although the sedating effect of scopolamine is 5 to 15 times greater than atropine. Scopolamine possesses two to three times more potent antisialagogue action than atropine. Atropine and scopolamine decrease the ability to sweat, and thus may cause a slight increase in temperature.[1847] Atropine and scopolamine have equipotent cardiovascular accelerator properties. The dose for both anticholinergics in infants to speed the heart rate is greater per kilogram than adults.[1848] Anticholinergics are appropriate in specific situations, such as to diminish secretions preoperatively, to block laryngeal and vagal reflexes, to treat or prevent the bradycardia associated with succinylcholine, to treat the bradycardia of anesthetic-induced myocardial depression, the muscarinic effects of neostigmine, and the oculocardiac reflex. Atropine is painful when administered intramuscularly. When it is administered as a premedicant, it does not block laryngeal reflexes. Atropine is much more effective in blocking laryngeal reflexes when it is given intravenously. Although some data suggest that children with trisomy 21 are more susceptible to the cardiac effects of atropine,[1849] our clinical experience and that of others do not support this notion.[1850,1851] Because some children with trisomy 21 have narrow-angle glaucoma, atropine must be administered cautiously because it might worsen the glaucoma.[1850,1851] Atropine may be administered orally, rectally, and via the trachea. Oral atropine may blunt the hypotensive response to potent inhalation agents during induction of anesthesia in infants younger than 3 months of age.[1852] When administered via the trachea, atropine is rapidly absorbed, producing physiologic effects.[1853-1856]

Atropine is metabolized in the liver by N-demethylation followed by conjugation with glucuronic acid[1857]; both processes are immature in the neonate. Half the drug is also eliminated by the kidneys. An old technique to diagnose atropine poisoning was to put a drop of the victim's urine into the eye of a cat and observe for mydriasis!

It is anticipated that clearance is reduced in the neonatal age range because of an immaturity of renal and hepatic function, but data remain elusive. Children aged less than 2 years have an increased Vdss (3.2 ± 1.5 vs 1.3 ± 0.5 L/kg) compared to those older than 2 years.[1858] Clearance was similar in those aged less than 2 years (6.8 ± 5.3 mL/min/kg) and those older than 2 years (6.5 ± 1.6 mL/min/kg). The elimination half-life in healthy adults is 3 ± 0.9 hours, whereas that in term neonates is 4 times this.[1858,1859]

PD characterization is similarly lacking in neonates. Infants less than 6 months needed a higher dose to produce an increase in heart rate.[431] A dose of 5 μg/kg had no impact on heart rate. Systolic BP did not change for any dose of atropine (5 to 40 μg/kg) in this neonatal cohort.[431]

In clinical practice, scopolamine is usually limited to those situations in which its sedative effect, combined with that of morphine, will be most advantageous, such as during cardiac surgery. It is also very useful as an adjuvant to ketamine anesthesia because of its antisialagogue and central sedative effects. The central sedative effects of both atropine and scopolamine may be antagonized with physostigmine. Many centers no longer routinely administer anticholinergic medications as part of the premedication because they are painful, the optimal effect may not coincide with induction of anesthesia, and current potent inhalation agents produce fewer secretions and infrequent bradycardia.

Scopolamine is a tertiary amine with greater CNS effects than atropine, causing sedation and amnesia. It has moderate antiemetic activity.[1860] To minimize the relatively high incidence of side effects, the transdermal dosage form has been developed for nausea and vomiting, however its use is generally limited to teenagers so as to avoid potential toxicity.[1861-1863]

Scopolamine has a distribution volume of 1.4 L/kg in adults.[1854] Glucuronide conjugation, sulfate conjugation, and hydrolysis by the CYP3A family are involved in its clearance.[1861] Both glucuronidation and the CYP3A enzyme systems are immature at birth and clearance is anticipated to be reduced.[1854]

### GLYCOPYRROLATE

Glycopyrrolate (0.005 to 0.01 mg/kg) is a synthetic quaternary ammonium compound with potent anticholinergic properties. It offers some advantage over atropine and scopolamine because it minimally penetrates the blood-brain barrier and thus causes few CNS effects. Several studies have demonstrated that glycopyrrolate is superior to atropine because its anticholinergic effects are more prolonged, lasting several hours.[1864,1865] The heart rate changes minimally after IV administration, causing fewer arrhythmias and offering an advantage where tachycardia might be detrimental.[1866,1867] In some children, gastric fluid volume and acidity are reduced after glycopyrrolate administration.[1868,1869] The drug remains popular for antagonizing the parasympathomimetic effects of neostigmine and is as effective as atropine for preventing the oculocardiac reflex.[1870]

There is poor absorption from the GI tract (10% to 25%).[1871] Clearance in infants aged less than 1 year (n = 8) was 1.01 (range of 0.32 to 1.85) L/kg/hr and Vdss of 1.83 (range 0.70 to 3.87) L/kg,[1871] but there are no neonatal data available. However, the renal system accounts for 85% of elimination[1864] and clearance is anticipated to be reduced in neonates because renal function is immature.[175]

## Antagonists

### NALOXONE

Naloxone (Narcan) is a pure opioid antagonist with a greater affinity for the μ-receptor compared with the κ- and δ-receptors. When given intravenously, naloxone has a very rapid onset of antagonism of the opioid receptors (within 30 seconds to 1 minute). Naloxone undergoes glucuronidation in the liver, with minimal bioavailability after oral administration. In adults, the elimination half-life is 1 to 1.5 hours, whereas in neonates it is 3 hours. When administered intramuscularly, the apparent elimination half-life is prolonged from 80 minutes to 6 hours in adults because of the depot effect.[1872]

Naloxone is effective in reversing opioid-induced adverse effects, including respiratory depression, chest-wall and glottic rigidity, nausea and vomiting, pruritus, urinary retention, and constipation. It may be administered via any route, including parenteral, neuraxial, tracheal, and oral. For children who are ventilating and not in extremis, but in whom opioid-induced respiratory depression needs antagonism in the perioperative period, it is reasonable to initiate antagonism with a very small dose of IV naloxone (0.25 to 0.5 μg/kg). This is similar to the dose recommended in one large review, of 10 to 20 μg of naloxone in children in the perioperative period.[1873] If the response is inadequate, the same dose may be repeated until ventilation improves. The same cumulative total IV dose of naloxone can then be administered as an IM injection to ensure that recrudescence of the respiratory depression does not occur. *For children in extremis or in whom a potential opioid overdose has occurred (including neonatal resuscitation), a larger dose of 10 to 100 μg/kg IV of naloxone may be indicated.* The American Academy of Pediatrics simplified the naloxone dosing for infants and children up to 5 years of age, recommending 100 μg/kg, and for children older than 5 years (more than 20 kg), 2 mg naloxone.[1874] This is based, in part, on concerns that smaller doses of naloxone may not be uniformly effective. However, it is equally important to recognize that overzealous dosing of naloxone will not only reverse the opioid analgesic effect but could also lead to profound systemic hypertension, cardiac arrhythmias (including ventricular fibrillation), and pulmonary edema (noncardiogenic).[1875] Evidence suggests that pulmonary edema may not be a dose-dependent response to naloxone, because it has been reported after as little as a single dose of 100 μg. A retrospective review of the management of 195 children and adolescents who received naloxone either postoperatively, in the emergency department or in the pediatric ICU, revealed an IV dosing range of 1 to 500 μg/kg; this resulted in resolution of the respiratory depression, systolic hypertension in 17% of children, and one case (incidence of 0.5%) of pulmonary edema.[1873] A continuous infusion of naloxone may be required to treat severe opioid-induced respiratory depression.[1876] *Any child who receives naloxone for antagonism of opioid-induced respiratory depression must be observed in a monitored environment for a minimum of 2 hours to ensure no recrudescence of the respiratory depression.*

The recommended dose of naloxone during neonatal resuscitation far exceeds that in older children. Doses as great as 400 μg/kg have been used without ill effects.[1877] In a systematic review of naloxone use in neonates, evidence demonstrated that naloxone increased alveolar ventilation, although there was no evidence that outcome, in terms of assisted ventilation or admission to a neonatal ICU, was affected by the use of naloxone.[1878] Caution is recommended when administering naloxone to an infant of a mother who has chronically abused opioids, because seizures have been reported.[1879]

Naloxone has also been administered via infusion at low doses to reverse side effects from opioids, including nausea and vomiting, pruritus, urinary retention, and constipation.[1880] Evidence is mixed regarding the beneficial effect of such a practice,[1881,1882] although a double-blind randomized controlled trial provided a significant reduction in morphine-associated nausea and pruritus during patient-controlled analgesia.[1883] When administered for this indication, there is a need to balance antagonism of the opioid-induced side effects with the antagonism of the pain relief.

### NALTREXONE

Naltrexone (Depade, ReVia) is an oral opioid antagonist that also has a greater affinity for the μ- rather than κ- and δ-receptors. The activity of naltrexone is thought to be a result of both the parent and its 6β-naltrexol metabolite (via hepatic dihydrodiol dehydrogenase). The mean elimination half-lives for naltrexone and 6β-naltrexol in adults are 4 hours and 13 hours, respectively. Naltrexone has a good oral bioavailability, with an elimination half-life of up to 8 hours in children, which is similar to adults.[1884] This opioid antagonist has also been used in the management of autism.[1885] Children displaying self-injurious behavior or hyperactivity have been noted to have high cerebrospinal-fluid endorphin concentrations and decreased pain sensitivity. Some opioid-induced behavior in animals and opioid addicts resembles that seen in autistic children. Naltrexone reduces self-injurious behavior.[1885]

Although Naltrexone reverses opioid-associated adverse effects, its use for this purpose has not become popular.[1878] Naltrexone and its primary metabolite, 6β-naltrexol, are excreted, albeit in low concentrations, in breast milk from a lactating female.[1886] Care should be taken when managing infants of opioid-addicted mothers.

### METHYLNALTREXONE

Methylnaltrexone (Relistor) is the first quaternary ammonium opioid antagonist that has very limited ability to permeate the blood-brain barrier.[1887] It is prepared in an oral as well as in a parenteral formulation for subcutaneous and IV administration. Doses of 0.45 mg/kg have been administered intravenously to adults. At the time of this writing, no pediatric data exist. Because methylnaltrexone does not cross the blood-brain barrier, it is suited to reverse the peripheral adverse side effects of opioids without attenuating the central analgesic effect. Opioid-induced side effects, including gastric emptying, urinary retention, postoperative ileus, and chronic constipation, improve after administration of methylnaltrexone.[1888-1892] If the preliminary adult safety and efficacy data are also demonstrated in children, this drug may offer the benefit of improving our ability to provide opioid-induced analgesia, while eliminating many of the peripheral adverse effects, thus improving the comfort of children.

### FLUMAZENIL

Flumazenil (Romazicon) is a specific $GABA_A$ receptor–competitive antagonist that reverses the effects of benzodiazepines. After a single IV dose, flumazenil shows limited protein binding (40%) with an elimination half-life of approximately 1 hour in adults, owing primarily to rapid and extensive metabolism by hepatic carboxylesterases.[1893-1895] In adults with severe liver disease, elimination of flumazenil is reduced.[1896] In children, the elimination half-life after a single IV dose of 10 μg/kg flumazenil followed by an infusion of 5 μg/kg/min is 35 minutes.[1897] The rectal dose required is higher (e.g., 50 μg/kg). The PK of intranasal flumazenil (40 μg/kg) were determined in healthy children with a median age of 4 years. The elimination half-life was 2 hours.[1898] Oral flumazenil is also available, but its bioavailability is only 16%, owing to the first-pass effect in the liver.[1895]

In adults, a dose of 17 μg/kg of flumazenil has antagonized benzodiazepine-induced sedation; studies in children have found doses of 24 μg/kg to be clinically effective without evidence of re-sedation.[1897] There is a limited role for flumazenil in clinical pediatric anesthesia, although specific indications are warranted, including benzodiazepine overdose, wake-up test during scoliosis surgery, treatment of a comatose child, and paradoxical response to benzodiazepines.[1899,1900] *With its brief elimination half-life, re-sedation after the initial response has been reported in children 1 to 5 years of age, thus necessitating close observation for at least 2 hours after antagonism of benzodiazepine-induced sedation.*[1901,1902] Caution should be taken in administering larger doses of flumazenil, because seizures have been reported.[1903]

### PHYSOSTIGMINE

This tertiary ammonium is a reversible cholinesterase inhibitor used to treat central cholinergic syndrome and delirium, and to antagonize the actions of atropine and scopolamine in the peripheral nervous system and CNS. It is not used to reverse neuromuscular blockade because its nonionized ammonium group facilitates transfer across the blood-brain barrier, causing CNS effects. After an IV dose, its elimination half-life is 20 to 30 minutes, with a duration of action that may exceed 1 hour, depending on the cholinesterase activity. Physostigmine is hydrolyzed at the ester linkage by cholinesterase. The usual single IV dose of physostigmine in children is 10 to 30 μg/kg.[1904] To treat intoxication by long-acting drugs, an infusion of physostigmine may be required at an infusion rate of 30 μg/kg/hr. Side effects of physostigmine include cardiac arrhythmias (bradycardia), cholinergic crisis, and seizures.[1904] Accordingly, physostigmine should be administered with electrocardiographic monitoring.

## Drugs in the Pipeline

Several new drugs are approaching their final stages in development. Their pharmacology is presented below. To date, studies in humans have been limited to adults.

### ETOMIDATE ANALOGUES

At least three qualities limit the use of etomidate in pediatrics: (1) it is not approved for use in children, (2) it has a prolonged half-life, and (3) it suppresses adrenal hormone synthesis. To address these impediments, the molecular structure of etomidate was modified. Figure 6-25 illustrates the molecular structure of the parent compound, etomidate, together with the modified molecules described below.

To address the first problem, investigators added a second ester group to the ester group already present on the etomidate molecule. This bypassed the steric inhibition of esterases by the imidazole group as well as prevented electron sharing between the ester and imidazole groups, rendering methoxycarbonyl-etomidate (MOC-etomidate) vulnerable to nonspecific esterases. MOC-etomidate showed very rapid degradation in vitro as well as in animals (E-Fig. 6-19). In animals, the righting reflex recovers more rapidly after MOC-etomidate treatment than after treatment with the parent compound.[1905]

To address the adrenal suppression, investigators substituted a pyrrole group in place of the imidazole group to preclude the binding of etomidate to 11-β-hydroxylase in the synthesis of adrenal hormones. As a consequence, carboetomidate binds poorly to 11-β-hydroxylase and therefore does not suppress adrenal hormone synthesis (E-Fig. 6-20).[1906]

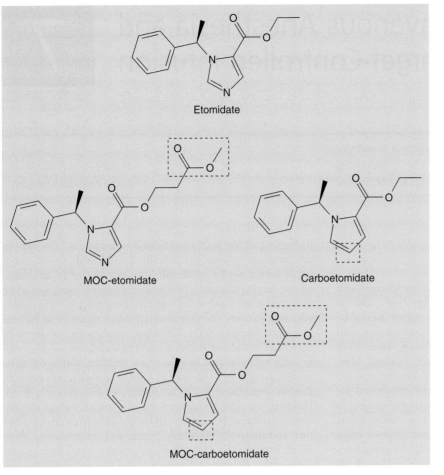

Etomidate

MOC-etomidate

Carboetomidate

MOC-carboetomidate

**FIGURE 6-25** Molecular structures of etomidate (parent compound), methoxycarbonyl-etomidate (MOC-etomidate) (the doubly substituted ester side chain), carboetomidate (the imidazole ring has been replaced by a pyrrole ring) and MOC-carboetomidate (in which both the double ester and the pyrrole-for-imidazole ring substitutions are present). MOC-carboetomidate has a brief duration of action, does not suppress adrenal hormone synthesis, and appears to share similar potency with etomidate. (Reproduced with permission from Pejo E, Cotton JF, Kelly EW, et al. In vivo and in vitro pharmacological studies of methoxycarbonyl-carboetomidate. Anesth Analg 2012;115:297-304.)

To marry these two properties, the investigators combined the two substitutions to create MOC-carboetomidate, which has a very rapid offset because of esterase hydrolysis, as well as virtually no adrenal suppression, while maintaining the potency of the parent compound. Animal studies have verified these findings for the combined molecule.[1907] Given the expected new PK profile and lack of adrenal suppression, we anticipate that MOC-carboetomidate may revolutionize not only sedation but also target-controlled anesthesia, with a safe, cardiovascular-stable anesthetic with no adrenal suppression.

## BUTYFOL

Butyfol (PF0713) is a butylphenol compound that bears similarity to propofol, with substitutions at two sites on the phenol ring that are chiral centers.[1908] These substitutions create optical isomers: the current formulation in humans is the *R,R* stereoisomer of butylphenol. With poor solubility in water, just as in the case of propofol, the current formulation of PF0713 is a 1% aqueous microemulsion. Original studies in animals demonstrated a slower onset and prolonged duration of action compared with propofol, without pain on injection; whether those studies included only the racemic mixture, rather than the stereoisomers, remains unclear. The current formulation, the *R,R* stereoisomer, has not been compared with the racemic mixture in animals or humans. Limited studies to date suggest that a single bolus of the 1% microemulsion of the *R,R* stereoisomer

bears similar properties to propofol, but repeat boluses and infusions have not been reported.

## BENZODIAZEPINE DERIVATIVES

Remi-midazolam (CNS7056) is a new sedative whose molecular structure bears a great similarity to midazolam, but that includes a vulnerable ester group that renders the compound susceptible to degradation by ubiquitous tissue esterases.[1908] As a result, remi-midazolam has a rapid onset, short duration, and rapid offset of sedation. Animal and limited human volunteer studies demonstrated that after a brief (1 minute) infusion, sedation was dose-related, lasting only 10 minutes, one-fourth that of midazolam. In adults, remi-midazolam is approximately one-half as potent as midazolam, with an $ED_{50}$ of approximately 0.15 mg/kg.

JM 1232(–) is a new benzodiazepine agonist that bears little resemblance to the molecular structure of benzodiazepines, but that interacts with the benzodiazepine receptor and is reversible by flumazenil.[1908] The 1% formulation of JM 1232(–) is known as MR04A3. This medication provides effective sedation in human volunteers, with kinetics reflecting a more rapid onset and offset of sedation compared with midazolam. This medication may confer analgesic properties that require further studies.

## REFERENCES

Please see www.expertconsult.com

# Total Intravenous Anesthesia and Target-Controlled Infusion

## 7

### NEIL S. MORTON, FRANK ENGBERS, GRACE LAI-SZE WONG, AND JAMES LIMB

## Total Intravenous Anesthesia

### INDICATIONS

The most common indications for total intravenous anesthesia (TIVA) techniques in children are the following: those at risk for malignant hyperthermia (in whom volatile agents are to be avoided); children with a high risk of postoperative nausea and vomiting; brief radiologic or painful procedures, when rapid recovery is needed (e.g., magnetic resonance imaging, bone marrow aspiration, gastrointestinal endoscopy); frequent repeated anesthesia (e.g., radiation therapy); major surgery to control the stress response; neurosurgical procedures to assist with control of intracranial pressure and for cerebral metabolic protection, spinal instrumentation, and when evoked motor and auditory brain potentials are needed; and children in need of airway procedures (e.g., bronchoscopy).[1-4] Total intravenous sedation and anesthesia are used in pediatric intensive care, but propofol is specifically contraindicated for prolonged use with high infusion rates in very sick or young children, because of the propofol infusion syndrome risk.[5-14]

### DRUGS AND TECHNIQUES

The most commonly used medications include propofol, remifentanil, alfentanil, and sufentanil; ketamine is occasionally used.[15] Delivery can be by a manual infusion scheme (Table 7-1) or by using pharmacokinetic model–driven infusion devices with software developed specifically for use in children. Unfortunately, the commercially available software packages usually limit the applicable age from 1 to 3 years or older, or weight from 10 to 15 kg or greater, and the pharmacokinetic (PK) parameters are derived from studies of a relatively few healthy children. Propofol programs that allow for age-, weight-, and gender-related changes in central compartment volume, clearance, and distribution have been developed and perform well in healthy children.[16,17] However, there are considerable gaps in knowledge for some drugs, for ill children, and for young children, infants, and neonates, so caution is needed when applying such programs to these populations. Therefore, the anesthesiologist can use these preprogrammed devices as a basis for initiating a TIVA technique but must also use skill, knowledge, and experience to titrate the intravenous (IV) agents to avoid awareness, pain, and adverse effects.

### PRINCIPLES

Healthy children often need a relatively high dose of IV agent per unit of body weight, and maintenance infusion rates need to be higher than the weight-corrected dose for adults.[18] Conversely, the immature neonate, the critically ill child, or those with major organ failure need considerably smaller doses of IV anesthetic agents; care is particularly needed in children receiving vasoactive medication and those with congenital heart disease.[19] Titration is advisable to allow for wide interindividual variation in PK and pharmacodynamics (PD). Electronic monitoring of depth of anesthesia (processed electroencephalography) has not been sufficiently well-validated in infants and children, and is yet to be used as the sole guide to dosing. After IV injection, it is assumed that the drug rapidly and evenly distributes throughout the body. However, the drug is delivered into the venous side of the systemic circulation, passes through the pulmonary circulation, and then distributes to the major organs and other tissues, all of which have variable blood flow, metabolic enzyme activity, and composition (in terms of proportions of fat and water). Because regional blood flow, body composition, and body proportions vary during development, the PK and PD of drugs are even more complex in children than in adults.

The apparent volume into which drugs distribute therefore varies among children, within the same individual at different stages of development, and among drugs. A drug that is very lipid soluble will have a very large *volume of distribution* (Vd), as will one that is highly bound to plasma proteins.

*Elimination* of medications and their metabolites commonly occurs by metabolism in the liver and subsequent excretion of water-soluble metabolites via the kidneys. Thus, conditions such as young age and hepatic and renal dysfunction, which are characterized by immature or reduced hepatic and renal functions, will attenuate the elimination of these medications. A measure of elimination of the medication is the *clearance*, which is the volume of blood from which the drug is eliminated per unit of time. Prolongation of the elimination of a drug reflects either an increase in the Vd or a reduction in clearance or both.

For a fixed infusion rate in a single compartment model, it takes five half-lives to reach a steady-state concentration (greater than 96% of the target) in the blood (Fig. 7-1). To more rapidly achieve steady-state conditions, a bolus dose or loading infusion may be administered. This rapidly fills the Vd, after which a new rate of infusion is calculated to maintain the blood concentration (Fig. 7-2). This is the dilemma of manual infusions; this loading dose has to pass the central volume and is usually so large that it will cause adverse effects, hemodynamic instability, and/or toxicity. Even a remifentanil bolus should be administered over several minutes to reduce the risk of bradycardia, hypotension, and/or difficult mask ventilation.

**TABLE 7-1** Manual Infusion Schemes

| Drug | Loading Dose | Maintenance Infusion | Notes |
|---|---|---|---|
| Propofol[26] | 1 mg/kg | 10 mg/kg/hr for 10 minutes, then 8 mg/kg/hr for 10 minutes, then 6 mg/kg/hr thereafter | Adult regimen to achieve blood concentration of 3 µg/mL. Underdelivers to children and achieves lower blood concentration of 2 µg/mL. |
| Propofol[25] | 1 mg/kg | 13 mg/kg/hr for 10 minutes, then 11 mg/kg/hr for 10 minutes, then 9 mg/kg/hr thereafter | Concurrently with alfentanil infusion. |
| Alfentanil[49] | 10-50 µg/kg | 1-5 µg/kg/min | Results in blood concentration of 50-200 ng/mL. |
| Remifentanil[1] | 0.5 µg/kg/min for 3 minutes | 0.25 µg/kg/min | Produces blood concentrations of 6-9 ng/mL. |
| Remifentanil[1] | 0.5-1.0 µg/kg over 1 minute | 0.1-0.5 µg/kg/min | Produces blood concentrations of 5-10 ng/mL. |
| Sufentanil[1,40] | 0.1-0.5 µg/kg | 0.005-0.01 µg/kg/min | Results in blood concentration of 0.2 ng/mL for sedation and analgesia. |
| Sufentanil[1,40] | 1-5 µg/kg | 0.01-0.05 µg/kg/min | Results in blood concentrations of 0.6-3.0 ng/mL for anesthesia. |
| Fentanyl[49] | 1-10 µg/kg | 0.1-0.2 µg/kg/min | |
| Ketamine[49] | 1-2 mg/kg | 0.1-2.5 mg/kg/hr | Smaller dose and infusion rate for analgesia and sedation. Larger dose and infusion rate for anesthesia titrated to effect. |
| Midazolam[49] | 0.05-0.1 mg/kg | 0.1-0.3 mg/kg/hr | |

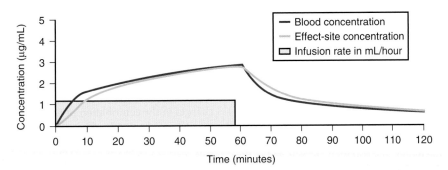

**FIGURE 7-1** Fixed rate infusion of propofol at 10 mg/kg/hr with no bolus dose in a healthy 10-kg, 1-year-old infant. Steady state is not reached after 1 hour. There is a lag of effect-site concentration behind blood concentration both during infusion and after stopping infusion. Effect-site concentration reaches blood concentration at about 1 hour. Context-sensitive half-time is 9 minutes. (Simulated using Tivatrainer. Available at www.eurosiva.org/TivaTrainer/tivatrainer_main.htm)

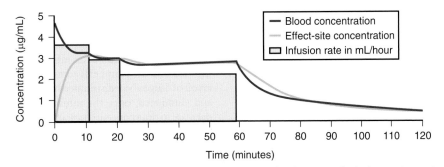

**FIGURE 7-2** Manual infusion in a healthy 70-kg 40-year-old subject. Bolus dose was 1 mg/kg, then 10 mg/kg/hr for 10 minutes, 8 mg/kg/hr for 10 minutes, then 6 mg/kg/hr thereafter until 60 minutes, when infusion is discontinued. Maximum blood concentration is 4.5 µg/mL. Effect-site concentration reaches 3 µg/mL after around 10 minutes but drifts down to around 2.6 µg/mL and then very gradually rises. Context-sensitive half-time after 1 hour is 7 minutes. (Data from the Diprifusor pharmacokinetic data set.)

To more clearly understand the disposition of drugs after an IV dose, it is useful to consider a three-compartment model. The drug is delivered and eliminated from a central compartment, V1 (which includes the blood), but also distributes to and redistributes from two peripheral compartments, one representing well-perfused organs and tissues (fast compartment, V2), and the other representing more poorly perfused tissues, such as fat (slow compartment, V3) (Table 7-2). The transfer of the drug between the central compartment (V1) and the two peripheral compartments (V2, V3), and also the elimination of the drug from the central compartment, is described by a series of clearances indicating the distribution back and forth between paired compartments, such as V1 to V2 and then V2 back to V1. The primary target organ that IV anesthetic agents affect is the brain. Therefore, an additional rate constant (keo) is added to describe the equilibration between the central compartment and the effect site in the brain.

**TABLE 7-2** Nomenclature for TCI Systems

| Term | Meaning | Units |
|------|---------|-------|
| TCI | Target-controlled infusion | |
| Vc or V1 | Central compartment volume | L |
| V2 | Fast compartment volume (vessel rich group) = $V1 \times k_{12}/k_{21}$ | L |
| V3 | Slow compartment volume (vessel poor group) = $V3 \times k_{13}/k_{31}$ | L |
| CL1 | Elimination clearance = $V1 \times k_{10}$ | L/hr |
| CL2 or Q2 | Clearance between V1 and V2 = $V2 \times k_{21}$ | L/hr |
| CL3 or Q3 | Clearance between V1 and V3 = $V3 \times k_{31}$ | L/hr |
| Cp | Blood concentration | |
| Ce | Effect-site concentration | |
| T | Target concentration | |
| CALC | Concentration calculated by TCI software | |
| MEAS | Concentration measured | |
| $k_{10}$ | Elimination rate constant | /min |
| keo | Rate constant for equilibration between blood and effect-site | /min |
| $T_{1/2}$keo | Half-time for equilibration between blood and effect-site $T_{1/2}keo = L_N(2)/keo$ | min |
| $k_{12}$, $k_{21}$ | Rate constants for movement between V1 and V2 | /min |
| $k_{13}$, $k_{31}$ | Rate constants for movement between V1 and V3 | /min |

**TABLE 7-3** Context-Sensitive Half-Times of Opioids in Children

| Opioid | INFUSION DURATION (minutes) | | | | |
|--------|------|------|------|------|------|
| | 10 | 100 | 200 | 300 | 600 |
| Remifentanil | 3-6 | 3-6 | 3-6 | 3-6 | 3-6 |
| Alfentanil | 10 | 45 | 55 | 58 | 60 |
| Sufentanil | | 20 | 25 | 35 | 60 |
| Fentanyl | 12 | 30 | 100 | 200 | |

Data from Absalom A, Struys MMRF. An overview of TCI and TIVA. Gent, Belgium: Academia Press; 2005.

This compartment is not represented by a volume but rather by the time required to equilibrate. Consequently, there is a time lag before changes in the blood concentration are reflected in the effect site (see Figs. 7-1 and 7-2).

A hydraulic model is useful for understanding these concepts. The central compartment is connected to the peripheral compartments and effect site by a series of pipes of different diameters, and also to a drainage pipe to represent elimination (Fig. 7-3, *A* through *F*). The heights of the columns of fluid, which represent concentrations of drug, illustrate the gradient down which drug travels between the central and peripheral compartments, and this can be animated over time to show filling and emptying of compartments relative to each other. The diameter of the interconnecting pipes between the central and peripheral compartments represents the intercompartment clearances, and size of the drainage channel represents elimination. This hydraulic analogy is used in the Tivatrainer PK simulation program.[20]

### Fixed Infusion Rate and a Three-Compartment Model

When a fixed infusion rate is started (see Fig. 7-1), the blood concentration will increase but, almost simultaneously, distribution of drug to the fast compartment and elimination both begin. Distribution of drugs throughout the body contributes more to the removal of drug from blood than elimination for most medications. For remifentanil, extremely rapid esterase clearance dominates. As the concentrations within each compartment equilibrate, the concentration gradient between compartments lessens (slowing drug transfer between compartments) but distribution to the slow compartment continues along with elimination. The net effect is that the blood concentration continues to increase, albeit at a slower rate. As the blood concentration increases toward equilibrium, elimination becomes relatively

more important; Figure 7-1 illustrates how far behind the effect-site concentration lags. Eventually, after several hours (or in some cases, days), a steady state is reached where infusion rate is directly proportional to clearance.

### Bolus and Variable Rate Infusion in a Three-Compartment Model

A loading dose can start to fill the central compartment and ideally should be aiming to create an effect-site concentration at a specific target concentration without overshoot. Then the rate of infusion should decrease in a stepwise manner to maintain a constant effect-site concentration until a steady state is reached. As drug is delivered into the central compartment, it continuously distributes to the peripheral compartments while it is continuously eliminated. The infusion rate must vary because it has to match the changes in the contribution of distribution and elimination with time (Figs. 7-4 and 7-5). When the infusion is stopped, then elimination will continue to drain the central compartment, and drug will continue to distribute to V2 and V3 along concentration gradients from V1 for some time. Equilibrium may be reached, but the drug now begins to move back from the peripheral compartments into the central compartment, maintaining the central compartment drug concentration for a period of time. This can continue for a protracted interval, particularly for highly lipid-soluble drugs that have a very large slow compartment V3 and a reservoir or depot effect (see Fig. 7-3, *F*). Eventually the central compartment concentration will decrease. For most anesthetics, the longer the duration of an infusion, the more the drug has distributed into the peripheral compartments, and the larger the reservoir of drug to be redistributed back into the central compartment and eliminated, once the infusion ceases. The half-time of the decrease in drug concentration in blood, therefore, is related to the duration of the infusion for most drugs (except remifentanil [see later discussion]). This is termed the *context-sensitive half-time* (CSHT), where the context is the duration of the infusion and relates to a pseudo–steady-state maintained by a target-controlled infusion (see later discussion). For an individual drug in an individual patient, CSHT can be plotted against the duration of the infusion (Fig. 7-6, *A* and *B*). The CSHT graph will eventually become parallel to the time axis and this is when the pseudo–steady-state becomes a true steady-state. At that time, the infusion has become context *insensitive*. This pattern is observed for nearly all IV anesthetics. The exception is remifentanil, whose half-time becomes context insensitive almost immediately after initiation of the infusion, because its elimination is rapid and complete; the capacity of the red cell, plasma, and tissue esterase enzyme systems are enormous (Table 7-3). The relevant PK parameters for remifentanil, alfentanil, and sufentanil are summarized in Table 7-4.[1] The

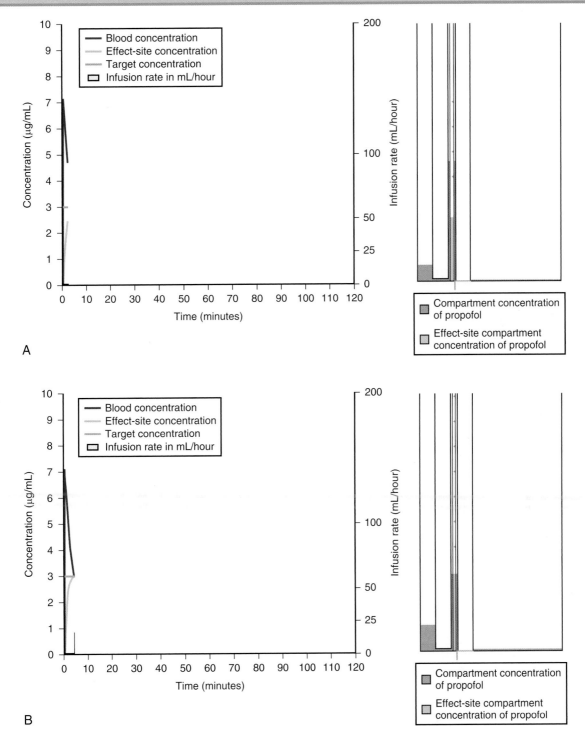

**FIGURE 7-3  A,** Hydraulic model representation of effect-site target-controlled infusion. Compartment volumes (V1, V2, and V3) and intercompartmental clearance values (CL1, CL2, and CL3) for Paedfusor model in a healthy 10-kg, 1-year-old infant: lean body mass 9.0 kg, body surface area 0.46 m², are V1 = 4.6 L, V2 = 9.5 L, V3 = 58.2 L, CL1 = 21.1 L/hr; CL2 = 31.4 L/hr, CL3 = 11.5 L/hr. In the first few minutes the central compartment to effect-site concentration gradient is marked to "overpressure" the transfer of propofol to the effect site. The peak blood concentration is 7.1 μg/mL. Distribution from compartment 1 (C1) to C2 occurs rapidly also, which slows the rise in effect-site concentration and blood concentration. Elimination from C1 and distribution from C1 to C3 is also occurring. **B,** At 4.5 minutes, the effect-site concentration has reached the target of 3 μg/mL and has equilibrated with the concentration in C1. The infusion device, which has been off after the initial loading infusion, now switches back on to maintain the effect-site target concentration at 3 μg/mL.

*Continued*

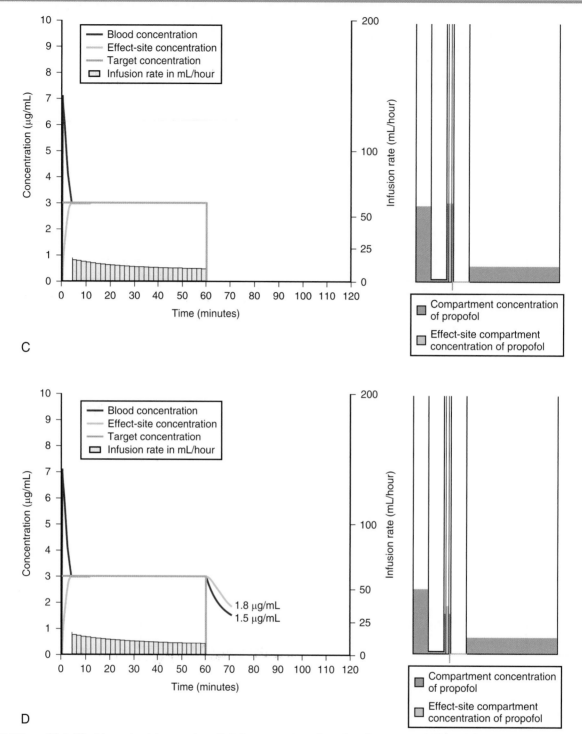

**FIGURE 7-3, cont'd  C,** After 1 hour of maintenance at an effect-site concentration of 3 μg/mL, the target is set to 0 μg/mL and the pump switches off. A total of 14 mL of propofol (1%) has been administered, or 14 mg/kg. There is now a considerable accumulation of propofol in compartment 2 (C2) and C3, while C1 and the effect site are still in equilibrium. **D,** Some 10 minutes after the effect-site target concentration is set to 0, the blood concentration has halved; thus the context-sensitive half-time is 10 minutes. The lag in the decline in effect-site concentration is clearly seen, and there is now a gradient between effect site and C1. There is now also a concentration gradient from C2 to both C1 and C3, and this slows the decline in the concentration in C1.

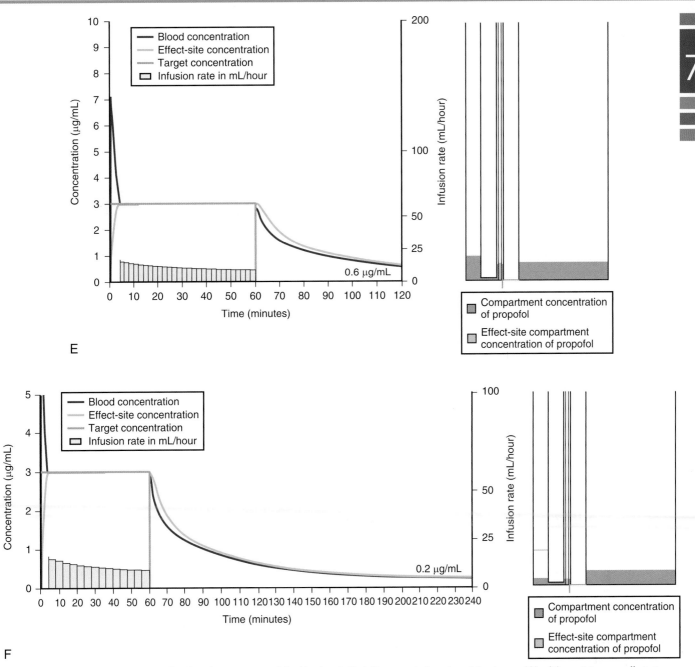

E

FIGURE 7-3, cont'd  **E,** One hour after the infusion is stopped the blood and effect-site concentrations have fallen to one fifth of the maintenance effect-site concentration. There are still considerable quantities of propofol in compartments C2 and C3 that slow the decline of the concentration of C1 and effect-site concentrations. **F,** Even after 4 hours, the depot of propofol in C2 and C3 is considerable, although blood and effect-site concentrations are extremely low. However, these low concentrations may still be exerting significant antiemetic and anxiolytic effects. (Data from the Paedfusor pharmacokinetic data set.)

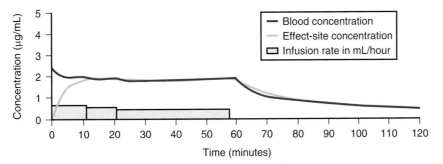

FIGURE 7-4  Manual infusion of propofol in a 1-year-old, 10-kg child. Bolus dose of 1 mg/kg, then 10 mg/kg/hr for 10 minutes, then 8 mg/kg/hr for 10 minutes, then 6 mg/kg/hr thereafter. Infusion stopped at 60 minutes. Effect-site concentration does not equilibrate until 11 minutes. Blood and effect-site concentrations stabilize around 1.8 μg/mL. However, this is unlikely to represent a sufficient depth of anesthesia for surgery. Context-sensitive half-time after 1 hour is 9 minutes. (Data from the Paedfusor pharmacokinetic data set.)

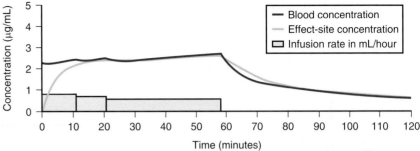

**FIGURE 7-5** Manual infusion of propofol in 1-year-old, 10-kg child. Bolus dose of 1 mg/kg, then 13 mg/kg/hr for 10 minutes, then 11 mg/kg/hr for 10 minutes, then 9 mg/kg/hr thereafter. Infusion stopped at 60 minutes. Effect-site concentration does not equilibrate until 20 minutes. Blood and effect-site concentrations stabilize around 2.4 μg/mL, but gradually rise over the subsequent hour to 2.6 μg/mL. (Data from the Paedfusor pharmacokinetic data set.)

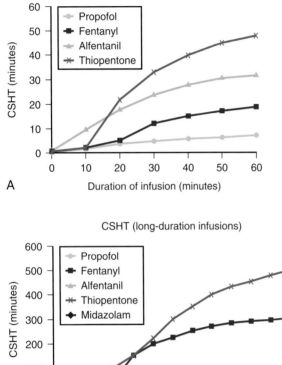

A

B

**FIGURE 7-6 A,** Context-sensitive half-times (*CSHT*s) after short-duration infusions. **B,** CSHTs after longer-duration infusions. For very lipid-soluble drugs such as fentanyl and propofol, V3 is very large compared with V1. Intercompartmental clearance between V1 and V3 is given by the equation $V1 \times k_{13} = V3 \times k_{31}$, which implies that if V1 is much smaller than V3, rapid distribution from V1 to V3 is associated with very slow redistribution from V3 to V1. This is indeed seen with propofol and fentanyl, which have slow offset of effects after prolonged infusion. Propofol has a CSHT that varies from around 3 minutes for a short-duration infusion to 18 minutes after a 12-hour infusion. This is because elimination is quite rapid compared with the rate of redistribution from V3. For alfentanil, the concentration of the un-ionized form is 100 times greater than that of fentanyl (pKa alfentanil 6.4, fentanyl 8.5). Alfentanil therefore has a more rapid onset time and shorter effect-site equilibration half-life, a smaller V1, lower volume of distribution at steady-state, and lower clearance than fentanyl. Fentanyl does, however, have a shorter CSHT than alfentanil after a short-duration infusion lasting less than 2 hours (**A**); but for longer-duration infusions, alfentanil reaches a maximum CSHT after about 90 minutes, whereas for fentanyl, the CSHT continues to increase after 12 hours (**B**). This is because fentanyl has a huge V3, and redistribution back to V1 maintains the blood concentration when the infusion stops. (Simulated using Tivatrainer. Available at: www.eurosiva.org/TivaTrainer/tivatrainer_main.htm.)

**TABLE 7-4** Pharmacokinetic Parameters for Short-Acting Opioids

|  | Remifentanil[50,51] | Alfentanil[52] | Sufentanil[53] |
| --- | --- | --- | --- |
| V1 | $5.1 - 0.0201 \times (age - 40) + 0.072 \times (LBM - 55)$ | Male: $0.111 \times weight$ Female: $1.15 \times 0.111 \times weight$ | $0.164 \times weight$ |
| V2 | $9.82 - 0.0811 \times (age - 40) + 0.108 \times (LBM - 55)$ | 12.0 | $0.359 \times weight$ |
| V3 | 5.42 | 10.5 | $1.263 \times weight$ |
| $k_{10}$ | $2.6 - 0.0162 \times (age - 40) + 0.0191 \times (LBM - 55)/V1$ | 0.356/V1 | 0.089 |
| $k_{12}$ | $2.05 - 0.0301 \times (age - 40)/V1$ | 0.104 | 0.35 |
| $k_{21}$ | $2.05 - 0.0301 \times (age - 40)/V2$ | 0.067 | 0.16 |
| $k_{13}$ | $0.076 - 0.00113 \times (age - 40)/V1$ | 0.017 | 0.077 |
| $k_{31}$ | $0.076 - 0.00113 \times (age - 40)/5.42$ | 0.0126 | 0.01 |
| keo | $0.595 - 0.007 \times (age - 40)$ | 0.77 | 0.12 |

Data from Absalom A, Struys MMRF. An overview of TCI and TIVA. Gent, Belgium: Academia Press; 2005.
Age in years; weight in kilograms; *LBM*, lean body mass.

differences in CSHTs are illustrated in Table 7-3 and Figure 7-6, *A* and *B*. Fentanyl has a small CSHT when given by infusion for a short time, but this dramatically increases as the duration of the infusion increases. Alfentanil's CSHT reaches a plateau after approximately 90 minutes of infusion. Clearances of fentanyl, alfentanil, and sufentanil are reduced in neonates and young infants because of the immaturity of hepatic enzyme systems, whereas clearance of remifentanil is relatively age-independent because esterases are ubiquitous throughout the body and are fully mature in neonates.

Administration of propofol can affect its own distribution and elimination by altering regional blood flow. Both fentanyl and alfentanil increase the volume of V1 and clearance of propofol, whereas propofol and midazolam inhibit the metabolism of alfentanil by the cytochrome P-450 enzyme isoform CYP3A4. Recent evidence in adults suggests that both sevoflurane and remifentanil can significantly increase the plasma concentrations of propofol.[21,22] In addition to these PK interactions there are important synergistic PD interactions between agents that suppress central nervous system activity.[23,24] For TIVA techniques in children, concurrent administration of opioids has a significant "propofol-sparing" effect, while providing analgesia and stress

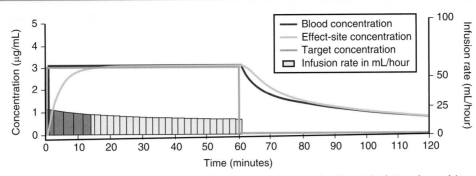

**FIGURE 7-7** Target-controlled infusion modeled using the Paedfusor pharmacokinetic data set. Blood-targeted infusion of propofol in a healthy 1-year-old, 10-kg child. Blood target is 3 µg/mL. Bolus dose of 1.4 mg/kg delivered, then stepwise-reducing infusion of from 19.1 mg/kg/hr to 9.5 mg/kg/hr at 1 hour. Infusion stopped at 60 minutes (i.e., blood target to 0 µg/mL). Effect-site concentration does not reach 3 µg/mL until 15 minutes 44 seconds. Total dose of propofol is 13.6 mg/kg. Context-sensitive half-time is 10 minutes.

control.[24,25] It is especially important to take advantage of this synergism to avoid excessive propofol and long-chain triglyceride load, particularly with concerns about propofol infusion syndrome. *Remifentanil provides the most effective propofol-sparing effect, but fast recovery means alternative techniques of analgesia must be well established before the remifentanil is discontinued.* Fentanyl, alfentanil, and sufentanil are effective in this regard; local and regional analgesia techniques also allow significant propofol dose reduction once the block becomes established. Nitrous oxide and low concentrations of inhalational anesthetics also act synergistically with propofol and opioids.

## MANUAL INFUSION SCHEMES
### Propofol
A simple scheme was devised to maintain a blood concentration of propofol in healthy adults of 3 µg/mL.[26] A bolus IV dose of 1 mg/kg is followed by a continuous infusion of 10 mg/kg/hr for 10 minutes, then 8 mg/kg/hr for 10 minutes, then 6 mg/kg/hr thereafter. When this "10, 8, 6" regimen is modeled and verified using the Marsh model for an adult patient, the estimated blood concentration slightly exceeds 3 µg/mL, but remains reasonably stable.[27] This simple dosing regimen is very effective in adults (see Fig. 7-2). However, when the same regimen is modeled using the "Paedfusor" PK data set for a child 1 year old and weighing 10 kg, the blood concentration achieved is approximately 2 µg/mL, but decreases slowly over time. Thus, this regimen delivers a subtherapeutic blood concentration of propofol in children. The subtherapeutic concentrations of propofol occurred because of a larger central compartment and an increased clearance of propofol in children compared with adults (see Fig. 7-4, Table 7-5). When the Paedfusor is used to calculate the dose of propofol that is required to achieve a blood concentration of 3 µg/mL, the bolus dose needed is 50% greater than in adults (1.5 mg/kg) and the infusion rates needed are approximately "19, 15, 12" each for 10-minute infusion. In addition, it takes approximately 15 minutes for the effect-site concentration to reach 3 µg/mL (Fig. 7-7). These data from the Paedfusor support the notion that the dosing of propofol infusions in young children is approximately twice that in adults. Similar results are predicted using the PK data set of Kataria et al[28] for children 3 to 11 years,[29] and in clinical adaptations of PK models.[30] This increased dose requirement can cause problems, because propofol is formulated in lipid and the lipid load can be considerable, particularly in young patients (Fig. 7-8). Propofol formulations are now available in concentrations varying from 5 mg/mL to 20 mg/mL (0.5% to 2%), and the

| | **TABLE 7-5** Differences between Adult and Pediatric Pharmacokinetic Parameters | | |
|---|---|---|---|
| **Age** | **Vd (mL/kg)** | **Elimination Half-life (minutes)** | **Clearance (mL/min/kg)** |
| 1-3 yr | 9500 | 188 | 53 |
| 3-11 yr | 9700 | 398 | 34 |
| Adult | 4700 | 312 | 28 |

*Notes:* The apparent volume of distribution (*Vd*) of propofol in the child is twice that of adults. The clearance of propofol in young children is twice that of adults and elimination is much more rapid.
Data from Absalom A, Struys MMRF. An overview of TCI and TIVA. Gent, Belgium: Academia Press; 2005.

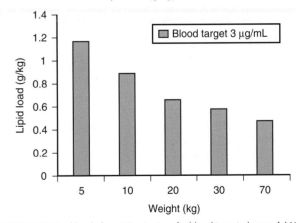

**FIGURE 7-8** Lipid load after 480 minutes of a blood targeted propofol 1% infusion (formulated in a vehicle containing 0.1 g/mL lipid) with target concentration of 3 µg/mL. Note the smaller infants have almost twice the lipid load and so a 2% propofol formulation is recommended to halve the relative lipid exposure; other propofol-sparing and lipid-sparing measures should also be used. (Simulated using Tivatrainer. Available at: www.eurosiva.org/TivaTrainer/tivatrainer_main.htm)

most effective "lipid-sparing" strategy for infusions is to use 20 mg/mL propofol (2%), as this immediately decreases the lipid load.

### Opioids
Simple manual infusion regimens can be used for the opioids fentanyl, alfentanil, remifentanil, and sufentanil. The manual

infusion regimens for these opioids in children are summarized in Table 7-1. Transitioning to maintenance analgesia after infusions of these opioids is a significant issue, and it is important to ensure either adequate regional or local anesthesia techniques are established or that adequate doses of systemic analgesia are given well before the infusion is discontinued. Transitioning is somewhat smoother after sufentanil than after alfentanil or remifentanil in children. The problem of acute tolerance to ultra–short-acting opioids has been noted after use of remifentanil in surgery for pediatric scoliosis.[31]

### Ketamine

Ketamine can be used in a simple basic manual regimen as a loading dose of 1 to 2 mg/kg and a maintenance infusion of 0.1-2.5 mg/kg/hr, depending on whether the target state is analgesia, sedation, or anesthesia (see Table 7-1).

### Midazolam

Slow bolus dosing of up to 0.1 mg/kg followed by an infusion rate of 0.1 mg/kg/hr provides baseline sedation with adjustments and additional bolus doses often needed. Caution is required, with bolus dosing in neonates and infants and in the critically ill because hypotension may occur and the depth of sedation achieved with midazolam is tremendously variable (see Table 7-1).

## Target-Controlled Infusion

A target-controlled infusion (TCI) is controlled by a computer that performs rapid sequential calculations every 8 to 10 seconds to determine the infusion rate required to produce a user-defined drug concentration in the central compartment (which includes the blood) or at the effect site of action of the drug in the brain.[1] *Thus, TCI may be blood targeted or effect-site targeted.* The standard nomenclature for TCI systems is listed in Table 7-2. Modern TCI systems are computer-controlled syringe drivers capable of infusion rates up to 1200 mL/hr, with a precision of 0.1 mL/hr. They incorporate a user interface and display and a range of safety alarms, monitoring functions, and warning systems. For most programs, the user has to choose a drug and its concentration from a menu and one must also select a PK parameter set (referred to as a "model"). The models suitable for use in children are quite limited, and some models are not suitable for all age groups. Others may be suitable but have not been validated in younger children; neonatal and infant models are quite rare. Experience with the various models may be gained by running simulation programs, such as Tivatrainer (www.eurosiva.org/TivaTrainer/tivatrainer_main.htm) or Rugloop (http://www.demed.be/rugloop.htm), on a personal computer. Tivatrainer now allows uploading of new models via a central website and server, and contains details and simulations of pediatric models for propofol, and neonatal and pediatric models for sufentanil, in addition to a wide range of adult models for propofol, alfentanil, remifentanil, fentanyl, ketamine, and midazolam. The simulation shows animated graphs of blood and effect-site concentrations against time, infusion rates, volumes, compartment sizes, and many other features.

The models within TCI systems are derived from studies of small numbers of healthy patients, and are only a guide to drug administration for an individual patient.[17] The accuracy of TCI propofol has been assessed in children.[17,27] TCI propofol has been incorporated into a modified version of the commercial "Diprifusor" device; it is known as the Paedfusor[32] and has been evaluated

**TABLE 7-6** Paedfusor Pharmacokinetic Parameter Set

| 1-12 years | $V1 = 0.4584 \times \text{weight}$; $V2 = V1 \times k_{12}/k_{21}$; $V3 = V1 \times k_{13}/k_{31}$ |
| | $k_{10} = 0.1527 \times \text{weight}^{-0.3}$ |
| | $k_{12} = 0.114$; $k_{21} = 0.055$ |
| | $k_{13} = 0.0419$; $k_{31} = 0.0033$ |
| | $keo = 0.26$ |
| 13 years | $V1 = 0.400 \times \text{weight}$ |
| | $k_{10} = 0.0678$ |
| | (other constants as above) |
| 14 years | $V1 = 0.342 \times \text{weight}$ |
| | $k_{10} = 0.0792$ |
| | (other constants as above) |
| 15 years | $V1 = 0.284 \times \text{weight}$ |
| | $k_{10} = 0.0954$ |
| | (other constants as above) |
| 16 years | $V1 = 0.22857 \times \text{weight}$ |
| | $k_{10} = 0.119$ |
| | (other constants as above) |

*Note:* The $k_{10}$ value in the age group 1-12 years is a negative power function of weight that reflects the increasing clearance values in younger children. Data from [21, 24-26].

$k_{10}$, Elimination rate constant; $k_{12}$ and $k_{21}$, rate constants for movement between V1 and V2; $k_{13}$ and $k_{31}$, rate constants for movement between V1 and V3; *keo*, effect-site equilibration rate constant; *V1*, central compartment volume; *V2*, fast compartment volume; *V3*, slow compartment volume.

**TABLE 7-7** Comparison between Paedfusor and Kataria Parameters for Propofol in Children

| Paedfusor[27,32,35,36] | | Kataria[28] |
|---|---|---|
| V1 | $0.458 \times \text{weight}$ | $0.41 \times \text{weight}$ |
| V2 | $0.95 \times \text{weight}$ | $0.78 \times \text{weight} + 3.1 \times \text{age}$ |
| V3 | $5.82 \times \text{weight}$ | $6.9 \times \text{weight}$ |
| $k_{10}$ | $0.1527 \times \text{weight}^{-0.3}$ | 0.085 |
| $k_{12}$ | 0.114 | 0.188 |
| $k_{21}$ | 0.055 | 0.102 |
| $k_{13}$ | 0.0419 | 0.063 |
| $k_{31}$ | 0.0033 | 0.0038 |
| keo | 0.26* | N/A* |

$k_{10}$, Elimination rate constant; $k_{12}$ and $k_{21}$, rate constants for movement between V1 and V2; $k_{13}$ and $k_{31}$, rate constants for movement between V1 and V3; *keo*, effect-site equilibration rate constant; *V1*, central compartment volume; *V2*, fast compartment volume; *V3*, slow compartment volume.
*This is the value for adults, but Munoz and colleagues[38] have studied these two models to define a more accurate keo for children 3 to 11 years of age, and the values are 0.91 for Paedfusor and 0.41 for Kataria. Jeleazcov[39] has derived age-related keo values by the formula keo = $1.03 \times e^{-(0.12 \times \text{age})}$.

clinically and found to perform well (Table 7-6).[27,33,34] In children undergoing cardiac surgery, the model performed significantly better than the adult model in adults.[32,35,36] Several pediatric propofol models have been validated[17,28] (Table 7-7), but all models have problems.[37] Experience shows that clinicians need to learn how to use each model to optimize levels of anesthesia, to ensure stability during induction and maintenance phases, and to enhance recovery speed and quality. Most pediatric models overestimate the initial Vd[17] which risks too large an initial bolus dose.[17] The Paedfusor model makes an allowance for the steady increase of clearance with age in younger children,

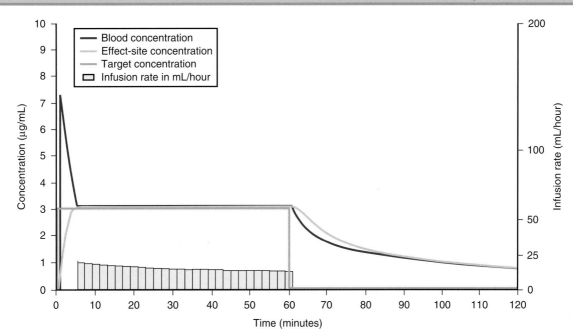

**FIGURE 7-9** Target-controlled infusion modeled using the Paedfusor pharmacokinetic data set. Effect-site–targeted infusion of propofol in a healthy 1-year-old, 10-kg child. Effect-site target is 3 µg/mL. Bolus dose of 3.4 mg/kg is delivered at 45.5 mL/hr to accentuate the gradient from blood to effect site, then infusion switches off for 4 minutes. Peak blood concentration after bolus dose is 7.1 µg/mL. Stepwise-reducing infusion of from 15.7 mg/kg/hr to 9.5 mg/kg/hr at 1 hour was done. Infusion stopped at 60 minutes (i.e., effect-site target is 0 µg/mL). Effect-site concentration reaches 3 µg/mL at 3 minutes 39 seconds. Total dose of propofol is 14 mg/kg. Context-sensitive half-time is 10 minutes 37 seconds.

| TABLE 7-8 | Example of Target-Controlled Infusion (5 µg/mL) Based on Calculated Blood-Concentration Targeting Compared with Calculated Effect-Site Concentration Targeting for a Healthy 1-Year-Old (Weight 10 kg), Using the Paedfusor Pharmacokinetic Parameters | |
|---|---|---|
| | **Blood Concentration Targeting** | **Effect-Site Concentration Targeting** |
| Loading dose | 1.7 mg/kg | 5.7 mg/kg* |
| Maximum blood target reached | 5 µg/kg | 12 µg/kg* |
| Total propofol infused after 60 minutes | 23.2 mg/kg | 23.3 mg/kg |
| Time to achieve effect site target of 5 µg/mL | 17.5 minutes | 4.5 minutes† |

*Potential for hemodynamic changes due to high peak blood concentration from larger bolus dose.
†Very much shorter time to achieve effect-site target.

particularly those below 30 kg in weight (see Tables 7-6 and 7-7, Fig. 7-9). The minimum age and weight limits for each model also differ, with 1 year of age and 5 kg for the Paedfusor system, and 3 years of age and 15 kg for the Kataria system. Below a weight of 12.5 kg and an age of 2 years, the second compartment becomes negative with the Kataria model, which means that model cannot be used clinically in such young patients. For simulation using the Paedfusor parameters, the adult value for keo of 0.26 per minute (T$_{1/2}$keo 2.7 minutes) can be used (see Table 7-7). This means effect-site targeting may be simulated with Paedfusor (Table 7-8), and it may be possible to display a predicted concentration for an effect-site while using a pump in blood-targeted TCI mode, as with Diprifusor. Attempts have been made by Munoz to define a more accurate keo for children,

in an ingenious study using auditory evoked responses with both the Paedfusor and Kataria models.[38] For children 3 to 11 years of age, the median extrapolated keo values for the Paedfusor models was 0.91 per minute (T$_{1/2}$keo 0.8 minutes), and for the Kataria model, 0.41 per minute (T$_{1/2}$keo 1.7 minutes). The bispectral index (BIS) was used to derive a value for the time to peak effect, and hence keo.[39-41] It was concluded that the time to peak effect after a bolus dose was shorter in children than adults, as the extrapolated T$_{1/2}$keo values were considerably smaller, although this extrapolation may be flawed when considering a TCI system.[37] Similar findings were reported by Hahn and colleagues using state entropy monitoring.[42] This has enabled calculation of an age-specific range of values for the keo (Fig. 7-10), which should allow more accurate effect-site targeting using propofol in the future. It must be stressed that compartmental values are highly specific to a single model, and are not interchangeable.[17,37] It can be argued that these calculations and extrapolations are a trick to get around imperfect PK values.[17,37] Integrating PK and PD into models appropriate for use in children is challenging not least because of doubts about the sensitivity and specificity of depth of anesthesia monitoring in children.[42-45]

Effect-site targeting offers the advantages of more rapid achievement of desired depth of anesthesia and less titration of the target depth in practice, but whilst it has been used in research in children, it has yet to become a clinical tool.[46] Table 7-8 shows how the behavior of the TCI differs between blood and effect-site targeted infusion using the adult keo of 0.26 per minute (T$_{1/2}$keo 2.7 minutes). It can be expected that effect-site targeting may have more profound cardiovascular and respiratory effects than blood targeting, because of the larger initial bolus doses and resultant higher peak blood propofol concentrations attained.[46] It is known that slower administration of propofol preserves spontaneous respiration in children.[47] However, use of age-appropriate keo and T$_{1/2}$keo values and careful titration from

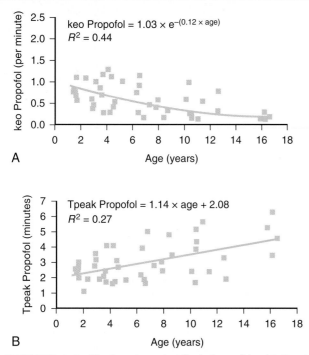

A

B

FIGURE 7-10 **A,** Equilibration rate constant (*keo*) of propofol and **B,** time to peak propofol effect (*Tpeak*) as a function of age. (Data from Jeleazcov C, Ihmsen H, Schmidt J, et al. Pharmacodynamic modelling of the bispectral index response to propofol-based anaesthesia during general surgery in children. Br J Anaesth 2008;100:509-16.)

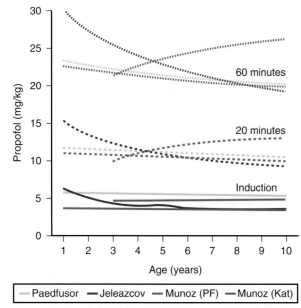

FIGURE 7-11 The predicted propofol doses at induction, 20, and 60 minutes are shown for Paedfusor in plasma-targeted mode, for the Munoz derived keo values in effect-site targeted mode for Paedfusor (*PF*) and Kataria (*Kat*), and for Jeleazcov in effect-site targeted mode. The effect of the variable age-related keo value of Jeleazcov can be seen in the higher bolus and maintenance doses for infants. A propofol target concentration of 5 μg/mL was used for all simulations. (Data from Limb J, Morton NS. Age-specific effect-site TCI in children: modelling using TivaTrainer. Anaesthesia 2010;65:542)

a low initial target value may ameliorate these adverse effects. However, the variable keo of the Jeleazcov dataset, derived from using BIS, means adverse effects may be more marked in infants (Fig. 7-11 and 7-12).[39,46] Although the use of BIS remains uncertain in children,[48] particularly those less than 2 years old, the use

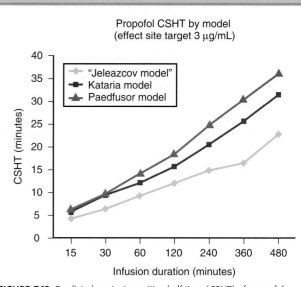

FIGURE 7-12 Predicted context-sensitive half-time (*CSHT*) of propofol depends on the pharmacokinetic model. The Jeleazcov model uses age-appropriate keo values and this results in the shortest predicted CSHTs for all infusion durations. This has clinical importance as it predicts a shorter recovery time for a given target concentration. (Data from Limb J, Morton NS. Age-specific effect-site TCI in children: modelling using TivaTrainer. Anaesthesia 2010;65:542 and Absalom A. A hitch-hiker's guide to the intravenous PK/PD galaxy. Pediatr Anesth 2011;21:915-8)

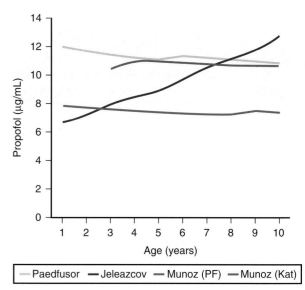

FIGURE 7-13 The peak plasma concentrations attained in simulations in Figure 7-12 for an effect-site target of 5 μg/mL are shown. The high boluses noted in Table 7-8 do not necessarily equate to high peak plasma concentrations because of the variable volumes of distribution in the pediatric models at different ages. (Data from Limb J, Morton NS. Age-specific effect-site TCI in children: modelling using TivaTrainer. Anaesthesia 2010;65:542 and Absalom A. A hitch-hiker's guide to the intravenous PK/PD galaxy. Pediatr Anesth 2011;21:915-8)

of the Jeleazcov model in TCI systems gives the prospect of more accurate and efficient propofol delivery to children.[46] This has safety implications in terms of reducing lipid load and clinical utility by increasing speed of recovery (Fig. 7-13).

## REFERENCES

Please see www.expertconsult.com

# Fluid Management

CRAIG D. McCLAIN AND MICHAEL L. McMANUS

ELECTROLYTE DISTURBANCES ARE COMMON in children because of their small size, large ratio of surface area to volume, and immature homeostatic mechanisms. As a result, fluid management can be challenging. On the ward, in the operating room, or in the intensive care unit (ICU), additional difficulties may result when fluid management is not tailored to the individual or when therapeutic decisions are based on extrapolations from adult data. To better understand the former and to limit the latter, this chapter reviews the basic mechanisms underlying fluid and electrolyte regulation, the developmental anatomy and physiology of fluid compartments, and the management of selected pediatric disease states relevant to anesthesia and critical care.

## Regulatory Mechanisms: Fluid Volume, Osmolality, and Arterial Pressure

Water is in thermodynamic equilibrium across cell membranes, and it moves only in response to the movement of solutes (E-Fig. 8-1). Movement of water is described by the Starling equation:

$$Q_f = K_f[(P_c - P_i) - \sigma(\pi_c - \pi_i)]$$

where $Q_f$ is fluid flow; $K_f$ is the membrane fluid filtration coefficient; $P_c$, $P_i$, $\pi_c$, and $\pi_i$ are hydrostatic and osmotic pressures on either side of the membrane; and $\sigma$ is the reflection coefficient for the solute and membrane of interest. The reflection coefficient gives a measure of a solute's permeability and, consequently, its contribution to osmotic force after equilibration. Across the blood-brain barrier, for example, the $\sigma$ for sodium approaches 1.0,[1] whereas in muscle and other cell membranes, $\sigma$ is on the order of 0.15 to 0.3.[2] Therefore, when isotonic sodium-containing solutions are given intravenously, usually only 15% to 30% of administered salt and water remains in the intravascular space while the remainder accumulates as interstitial edema.[3,4] In contrast, hypertonic solutions permit greater expansion of circulating blood volume with smaller fluid loads and less edema.[5-7]

Both the amount and the concentration of solute are tightly regulated to maintain the volumes of intravascular and intracellular compartments. Because sodium is the primary extracellular solute, this ion is the focus of homeostatic mechanisms concerned with maintenance of intravascular volume. When osmolality is held constant, water movement follows sodium movement. As a result, total body sodium (although not necessarily serum $Na^+$) and total body water (TBW) generally parallel one another. Because sodium "leak" across membranes limits its contribution to the support of intravascular volume, this compartment is also critically dependent on large, impermeable molecules such as proteins. In contrast to sodium, albumin molecules, for example, follow the Starling equilibrium with a reflection coefficient in excess of 0.8.[8] Soluble proteins create the so-called *colloid oncotic pressure*, approximately 80% of which is contributed by albumin.

Although the presence of albumin supports intravascular volume, protein leak into the interstitium (and consequent water movement) may limit its effectiveness. It has been observed, for example, that the reflection coefficient for albumin decreases by as much as one third after mechanical trauma.[9] Furthermore, because of ongoing leakage, a slow continuous infusion of albumen is superior to bolus administration for increasing the serum albumen concentration in critically ill individuals.[10]

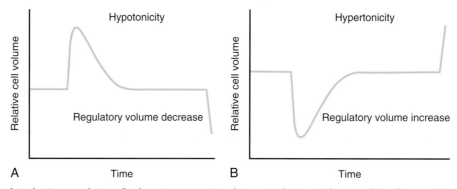

**FIGURE 8-1** Activation of mechanisms regulating cell volume in response to volume perturbations. Volume-regulatory losses and gains of solutes are termed *regulatory volume decrease* (**A**) and *regulatory volume increase* (**B**), respectively. The course of these decreases and increases varies with the type of cell and experimental conditions. Typically, however, a regulatory volume increase mediated by the uptake of electrolytes or a regulatory volume decrease mediated by the loss of electrolytes and organic osmolytes occurs over a period of minutes. When cells that have undergone a regulatory volume decrease (**A**) or increase (**B**) are returned to normotonic conditions, they swell above or shrink below their resting volume. This is due to volume-regulatory accumulation or loss of solutes, which effectively makes the cytoplasm hypertonic or hypotonic, respectively, as compared with normotonic extracellular fluid. (From McManus ML, Churchwell KB, Strange K. Regulation of cell volume in health and disease. N Engl J Med 1995;333:1260-6. ©Massachusetts Medical Society.)

Potassium is the primary intracellular solute, with approximately one third of cellular energy metabolism devoted to $Na^+/K^+$ exchange. Sodium continuously leaks into cells along its concentration gradient, yet it is rapidly extruded in exchange for potassium. As the cell is exposed to varying osmolarity, water movement occurs, causing cell swelling or shrinkage. Because stable cell volume is critical for survival, complex regulatory mechanisms have evolved to ensure that stability is maintained.[11,12] The processes by which swollen cells return to normal size are collectively termed *regulatory volume decrease* processes, and those returning a shrunken cell to normal are termed *regulatory volume increase* processes (Fig. 8-1). With sudden, brief changes in osmolality, regulatory volume increase or decrease processes are activated after small (1% to 2%) changes in cell volume, returning cell volume to normal primarily through transport of electrolytes. If anisosmotic conditions persist, chronic compensation occurs through the accumulation or loss of small organic molecules termed *osmolytes* or idiogenic osmoles (e.g., polyols, sorbitol, myoinositol), amino acids and their derivatives (e.g., taurine, alanine, proline), and methylamines (e.g., betaine, glycerylphosphorylcholine).

Like intracellular volume, circulating blood (intravascular) volume is also tightly controlled. Increases in intravascular volume result from increases in sodium and water retention, whereas decreases in intravascular volume result from increases in excretion of sodium and water. As noted earlier, serum osmolality must be maintained within a very narrow range if serum sodium is to be an effective focus of intravascular volume control. Serum osmolality is usually maintained between 280 and 300 mOsm/L. Changes in osmolality as small as 1% trigger compensatory mechanisms.

Serum osmolality is primarily regulated by antidiuretic hormone (ADH), thirst, and renal concentrating ability. Because the indirect aim of osmolar control is actually volume control, these same osmoregulatory mechanisms are also influenced by factors such as blood pressure (BP), cardiac output, and vascular capacitance.[13,14] In pathologic conditions such as ascites or hemorrhage, intravascular volume preservation takes precedence over osmolality and osmoregulatory mechanisms operate to restore intravascular volume, even at the expense of disrupting physiologic solute balance.

For example, ADH is released from neurons of the supraoptic and paraventricular nuclei in response to osmolar fluctuations in cell size. Solutes that readily permeate cell membranes, such as urea, increase the serum osmolality without triggering the release of ADH. Infusion of solutes with large actual or effective reflection coefficients ($\sigma$) at the cell membrane (e.g., sodium, mannitol) elicits a robust ADH release. ADH release begins when the serum osmolality reaches a threshold of approximately 280 mOsm/L. Rapid increases in osmolality lead to a greater release of ADH than do slow increases. Hypovolemia and hypotension diminish the threshold for ADH release and increase the "gain" of the system by exaggerating the rate of increase in serum ADH concentrations (E-Fig. 8-2). Thus, in a volume-depleted or hypotensive child, brisk ADH release occurs in response to plasma osmolalities as low as 260 to 270 mOsm/L. It has been hypothesized that different populations of vasopressin-secreting cells are responsive to osmotic and baroreceptor-mediated input.

Intravascular fluid volume, salt and water intake, electrolyte balance, and cardiovascular status are interrelated at several levels.[15] For example, as the veins and arteries become replete with fluid and the systemic BP increases, ADH release wanes as both *pressure diuresis* and *natriuresis* commence.[16] The resulting relationship between urine output and arterial pressure is termed the *renal function curve*, and its intersection with salt and water intake determines the *equilibrium point* at which arterial BP ultimately stabilizes (Fig. 8-2). Equilibrium (chronic) BP is influenced only by shifts of the renal function or fluid intake curves. Transient changes in arterial pressure secondary to peripheral vascular resistance changes are always resolved by opposing shifts in total body salt and TBW.

In response to a decreasing arterial pressure, the renin-angiotensin system is also mobilized. With decreased renal perfusion, juxtaglomerular cells release renin, which in turn converts renin substrate (angiotensinogen) to angiotensin I. Angiotensin I is then rapidly converted to angiotensin II by angiotensin-converting enzyme present in lung endothelium. Angiotensin II supports arterial pressure in three ways: (1) direct vasoconstriction, (2) increased salt and water retention (via renal vasoconstriction and decreased glomerular filtration), and (3) stimulation of aldosterone secretion (Fig. 8-3).

ADH, pressure diuresis, and the renin-angiotensin system permit wide ranges in salt and water intake without large fluctuations in BP or volume status. All serve to support the systemic circulation when threatened and complement the more immediate activity of the sympathetic nervous system. In addition to high-pressure sensors such as aortic arch and carotid sinus baroreceptors, intravascular volume information is provided by low-pressure thoracic sensors. For this reason, effective increases or decreases in intrathoracic blood volume may mimic changes in whole-body volume status and produce natriuresis, diuresis, or fluid retention. Intravascular volume may also be sensed as the stretch of atrial muscle fibers, leading to release of atrial natriuretic peptide.[17] Although its complete physiologic role is uncertain, atrial natriuretic peptide may serve to "fine tune" volume status by causing modest vasodilation, gently increasing the glomerular filtration rate (GFR), and decreasing reabsorption of sodium. The combination of complex autoregulatory mechanisms with complementary actions operating on varying time scales, all responding to different, yet interrelated, effector stimuli, yields an elegant system by which the mature individual may maintain circulation amid a variety of challenges. In this context, it is interesting to observe that successful heart transplant recipients, despite general cardiovascular stability, typically manifest fundamental derangements in body fluid homeostasis.[18]

## Maturation of Fluid Compartments and Homeostatic Mechanisms

### BODY WATER AND ELECTROLYTE DISTRIBUTION

Much of our understanding of the development of body water compartments is derived from deuterium oxide dilution studies performed in the 1950s.[19] In a series of 21 neonates, TBW was found to be approximately 78 ± 5% of body weight. Subsequent measurements in fewer subjects showed that TBW decreased to approximately 60% in the second 6 months of life with most of the loss being extracellular. A smaller decrease (to about 57%) is observed late in childhood (Fig. 8-4).

The importance of the extracellular compartment, its relationship to the intracellular space, and much of the chemical anatomy of both were first described by Gamble in educational monographs issued during the first part of the 20th century (E-Fig. 8-3).[20,21] The chemical compositions of mature body fluid compartments are provided in Table 8-1.

### CIRCULATING BLOOD VOLUME

The blood volume in neonates was determined to be 82 ± 9 mL/kg using an iodine 121–labeled human serum albumin technique, although substantial variability may result from the degree of placental-fetal transfusion.[22] In low-birth-weight (LBW), preterm, or critically ill infants, values as high as 100 mL/kg have been measured.[23] Blood volume increases slightly during the first few months of life, reaching its zenith at 2 months of age (approximately 86 mL/kg), then returns to near 80 mL/kg and finally stabilizes at 70 mL/kg by the end of the first year of life. In general, the ratio of blood volume to weight decreases with growth. The most accurate basis for prediction of blood volume is lean body mass, the consideration of which removes any male/female variation even into adulthood.[24] An estimate of the circulating blood volume is presented in Table 8-2.

### MATURATION OF HOMEOSTATIC MECHANISMS

Renal development begins at approximately 5 weeks of gestation and continues in a centrifugal pattern until the full complement of nephrons is in place by about the 38th week. In the outermost regions of the renal cortex, postnatal nephron differentiation may continue for several weeks to months. In the early stages of gestation, renal blood flow is approximately one fifth of normal.

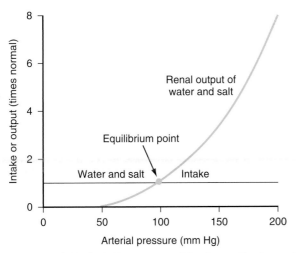

FIGURE 8-2 Analysis of arterial pressure regulation by equating the renal output curve with the salt and water intake curve. The equilibrium point describes the level to which the arterial pressure will be regulated. (That portion of the salt and water intake that is lost from the body through nonrenal routes is ignored in this figure.) (From Guyton AC, Hall JC, editors. Textbook of medical physiology. Philadelphia: WB Saunders; 1996. p. 221-37.)

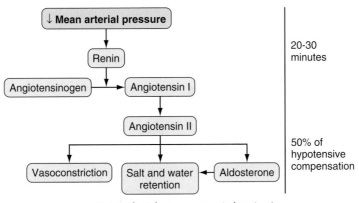

FIGURE 8-3 Physiologic responses to hypotension.

Body Water Compartments

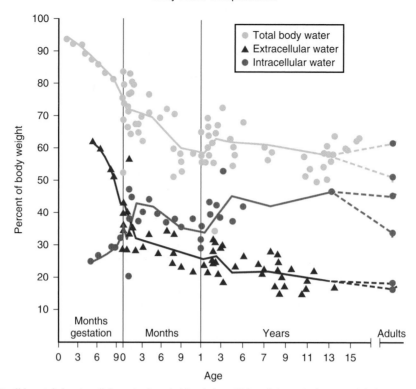

FIGURE 8-4 Total body water (*blue circles*), extracellular water (*purple triangles*), and intracellular water (*orange circles*) as percentages of body weight in infants and children, compared with corresponding values for the fetus and adults. (From Friis-Hansen B. Body water compartments in children: changes during growth and related changes in body composition. Pediatrics 1961;28:169-81.)

**TABLE 8-1 Composition of Body Fluid Compartments**

|  | Extracellular Fluid | Intracellular Fluid |
|---|---|---|
| Osmolality (mOsm) | 290-310 | 290-310 |
| **Cations (mEq/L)** | **155** | **155** |
| $Na^+$ | 138-142 | 10 |
| $K^+$ | 4.0-4.5 | 110 |
| $Ca^{2+}$ | 4.5-5.0 | — |
| $Mg^{2+}$ | 3 | 40 |
| **Anions (mEq/L)** | **155** | **155** |
| $Cl^-$ | 103 | — |
| $HCO_3^-$ | 27 | — |
| $HPO_4^{2-}$ | — | 10 |
| $SO_4^{2-}$ | — | 110 |
| $PO_4^{2-}$ | 3 | — |
| Organic acids | 6 | — |
| Protein | 16 | 40 |

**TABLE 8-2 Estimate of Circulating Blood Volume**

| Age | Estimated Blood Volume (mL/kg) |
|---|---|
| Preterm infant | 100 |
| Full-term neonate | 90 |
| Infant | 80 |
| School age | 75 |
| Adults | 70 |

Initially this is related to structural immaturity, and later it is due to increased renovascular resistance. By 38 weeks of gestation, renal blood flow is approximately one third of normal. High renovascular resistance protects the developing nephron from both pressure and volume overload. The resulting renal contribution to metabolic homeostasis in utero is limited.

As with the pulmonary bed, vascular resistance in the kidney decreases after birth, leading to abrupt increases in renal blood flow and GFR. In utero, despite a low GFR, urine output is brisk, owing to poor reabsorption of salt and water. Plasma renin activity is increased in utero, decreases immediately after birth, and then increases again as excess extracellular water is mobilized and excreted. Aldosterone levels are increased in cord blood and are maintained at this level for the first 3 days of life. The increased aldosterone may be necessary for sodium retention during periods of increased anabolism early in life.

Intrarenal gradients of NaCl and urea are less steep in the immature kidney, and full nephron length has yet to be achieved. Consequently, urine concentrating ability is limited in neonates, with maximum urine osmolality being about half that of the adult (700 to 800 mEq/L versus 1300 to 1400 mEq/L). In part, this also relates to low circulating ADH levels and decreased renal responsiveness to ADH. Although overall ADH production is not impaired, excessive secretion may occur in some disease states. Limited urine-concentrating ability necessitates large urine volumes for elimination of large solute loads.

In the first year of life, renal plasma flow and GFR are approximately one half the adult values of 350 and 70 mL/min/m², respectively.[25] Consequently, serum creatinine is increased in term and preterm infants, yet normalizes in the second month of life. Fractional excretion of sodium ($FE_{Na}$) is markedly increased in preterm infants, decreases somewhat by term, and stabilizes at adult levels by the second month of life. Although the adult kidney may easily achieve $FE_{Na}$ values as low as 0.5%, the 34-week-gestation infant is limited to no less than 2%.

These maturational features make it very difficult for the preterm or young infant to handle fluctuations in fluid and solute loads. Both sodium conservation and regulation of extracellular fluid volume are impaired relative to the older child and adult. Limited GFR makes excretion of a fluid challenge difficult. Excessive urinary sodium loss leads to increased maintenance requirements. Hyponatremia is common. Conversely, diminished concentrating ability increases free water losses during excretion of a solute load, whereas the high ratio of surface area to volume produces increased evaporative water loss. Consequently, fluid requirements are relatively high, and dehydration is common. Any errors in the fluid management are poorly tolerated. As a rule, the most severe impairment exists in preterm infants, and the majority of homeostatic mechanisms are fully developed after the first year of life.

## Fluid and Electrolyte Requirements

Holliday summarized the evolution of contemporary hydration therapy.[20] In 1831, Latta first reported the use of intravenous (IV) fluids in the resuscitation of patients dehydrated by cholera.[26] In 1918, growing information on the subject permitted Blackfan and Maxcy to successfully treat nine infants by intraperitoneal injection.[27] In 1923, Gamble and associates detailed the anatomy of fluid and electrolyte compartments, introducing the use of milliequivalents to clinical practice.[21] This paved the way for the development of the "deficit therapy" regimen of Darrow.[28]

In subsequent decades, various recipes to replace the extracellular and intracellular fluid losses were suggested. For the most part, these failed because of excessive potassium and insufficient sodium content. Hyponatremia was common. When the focus of the treatment shifted to replacing the extracellular fluid deficit, rapid restoration of extracellular fluid volume using solutions with sodium concentrations similar to those in blood became commonplace. This, along with oral rehydration, is the preferred method of treatment today.

The concept of "maintenance fluids" is a complex subject. Although water and salt are required to sustain life, it is fair to say that for an individual child at any particular time, the precise amounts necessary are unknown (and perhaps unknowable). Instead, fluids and electrolytes, like anesthetics, are titrated to effect with general guidelines provided by clinical assessment, basic physiologic principles, and limited published data. The term *maintenance fluids* is often more limiting than helpful, and in all cases it is less precise than other terms familiar to anesthesiologists, such as *minimal alveolar concentration* (MAC) or *median effective dose* ($ED_{50}$).

Holliday and Segar provided calculations for a first approximation of "the maintenance need for water in parenteral fluid therapy" in 1957.[29] Integrating the relevant known physiology at that time, these authors observed that "insensible loss of water and urinary water loss roughly parallel energy metabolism and do not parallel weight." However, because water utilization parallels energy metabolism, energy metabolism follows surface area, and surface area follows weight, it should be possible to estimate water requirement from weight alone. The authors then proceeded under a series of assumptions to extrapolate from limited

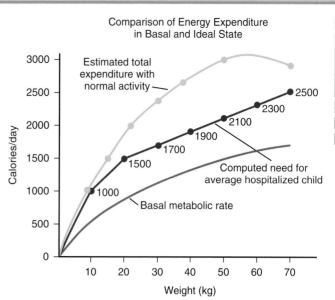

Comparison of Energy Expenditure
in Basal and Ideal State

**FIGURE 8-5** The upper and lower curves were plotted from data from the study by Talbot.[126] Weights at the 50th percentile level were selected for converting calories at various ages to calories related to weight. The computed line for the average hospitalized child was derived from the following equations:
1. 0-10 kg: 100 kcal/kg.
2. 10-20 kg: 1000 kcal + 50 kcal/kg for each kg over 10 kg
3. 20 kg and up: 1500 kcal + 20 kcal/kg for each kg over 20 kg
(From Holliday MA, Segar WE. The maintenance need for water in parenteral fluid therapy. Pediatrics 1957;19:823-32.)

| **TABLE 8-3** Relationship between Weight and Hourly or Daily Maintenance Fluid Requirements of Children as per the 4-2-1 Rule | | |
|---|---|---|
| | **MAINTENANCE FLUID REQUIREMENTS** | |
| **Weight (kg)** | **Hour** | **Day** |
| <10 | 4 mL/kg | 100 mL/kg |
| 10-20 | 40 mL + 2 mL/kg for every kg >10 kg | 1000 mL + 50 mL/kg for every kg >10 kg |
| >20 | 60 mL + 1 mL/kg for every kg >20 kg | 1500 mL + 20 mL/kg for every kg >20 kg |

data to a "relationship between weight and energy expenditure that might easily be remembered."

Assuming energy requirements of "hospitalized patients" to be "roughly midway between basal and normal levels," they constructed a curve of caloric requirement versus weight.[29] This curve could be seen as comprising three linear sections: 0 to 10 kg, 10 to 20 kg, and 20 to 70 kg (Fig. 8-5). Viewing the curve in this manner, the authors reasoned that "fortuitously, the average need for water, expressed in milliliters, equals energy expenditure in calories": 100 mL/kg/day for weights to 10 kg, an additional 50 mL/kg/day for each kilogram from 11 to 20 kg, and 20 mL/kg/day more for each kilogram beyond 20 kg. In anesthetic practice, this formula has been further simplified, with the hourly requirement referred to as the "4-2-1 rule" (4 mL/kg/hr for the first 10 kg of weight, 2 mL/kg/hr for the next 10 kg, and 1 mL/kg/hr for each kilogram thereafter; Table 8-3).

For decades, the simplicity and elegance of the Holliday and Segar formula has made it the starting point for fluid management in healthy children. As recently as 2006, the majority of

**TABLE 8-4** Normal Water Losses for Infants and Children

| Cause of Loss | Volume of Loss (mL/100 kcal) |
| --- | --- |
| Output | |
| Urine | 70 |
| Insensible loss | |
| Skin | 30 |
| Respiratory tract | 15 |
| Hidden intake (from burning 100 calories) | 15 |
| Total | 100 |

consultant anesthetists in the United Kingdom administered hyponatremic glucose-containing solutions intraoperatively and postoperatively to children undergoing elective surgery.[30] However, the uncritical use of these solutions was never intended, and their blind application in the operating room, or in any clinical situation, is unwarranted. Further, as Holliday and Segar have themselves pointed out, their original approach involved hyponatremic glucose-containing solutions rather than near-isotonic solutions such as 0.9% saline or lactated Ringer solution (LR).[30a] In addition, these requirements were assessed at a basal metabolic state and not when the child was acutely ill or under physiologic stress. As the authors cautioned that "understanding of the limitations and of exceptions to the system [is] required. Even more essential is the clinical judgment to modify the system as circumstances dictate." General water losses for infants and children are summarized in Table 8-4.

More recently, Holliday revised the approach to fluid therapy in children that he and Segar enshrined with several caveats.[30b] In a related commentary, Holliday pointed out several problems with applying the original 4-2-1 rule to acutely ill children.[30c] Namely, dysregulation of ADH is a hallmark of critical illness because ADH secretion is affected by a variety of nonosmotic factors such as pain, stress, mechanical ventilation, and many medications. As a result, the choice of intravenous fluid and the rapidity of deficit replacement must be approached with care. The authors recommended a relatively simple strategy for healthy children undergoing elective surgery (including outpatients) to turn off ADH secretion and prevent perioperative water retention and subsequent hyponatremia. When a child (who is without significant heart or kidney disease) presents with marginal to moderate hypovolemia (e.g., after fasting for surgery), 20 to 40 mL/kg of isotonic fluids should be given during surgery and the postanesthesia care unit stay (as rapidly as 10 to 20 mL/kg/hr). Clinical judgment must always allow for modification of these recommendations if indicated for an individual child.[31,32] If hypovolemia is more severe (e.g., after an extensive bowel preparation), 40 to 80 mL/kg may be necessary during the perioperative period.

Postrecovery IV fluid therapy should consist of an isotonic solution infused at half the rate described in the original 4-2-1 fluid regimen (i.e., 2 mL/kg for the first 10 kg, 1 mL/kg for the next 10 kg, and 0.5 mL/kg for each additional kilogram thereafter). If the child does not or cannot tolerate oral intake after 6 to 12 hours, standard maintenance fluid therapy using hypotonic saline (e.g., 0.45% saline) should be initiated to avoid hypernatremia and fluid overload from prolonged administration of the isotonic solutions. This regimen should limit the ADH response and reduce the risk for postoperative hyponatremia and hypernatremia.[31-33] It remains essential, however, to monitor plasma electrolyte concentrations serially on the ward, regardless

of the fluid doctrine followed, to be certain that electrolyte concentrations remain within normal limits.[34,35]

## NEONATAL FLUID MANAGEMENT

In the first few days of life, isotonic losses of salt and water cause the normal neonate to lose 5% to 15% of body weight. Although GFR rises rapidly, urine output is initially low, and renal losses are modest. Day 1 fluid requirements of the wrapped neonate, therefore, are relatively low. Over the next few days of life, losses and requirements increase. In the poorly feeding infant, progression to hypernatremia and dehydration are common. When intake is appropriate, the term infant will regain body weight during the first week of life.

Three distinct phases of fluid and electrolyte homeostasis have been described in LBW[36] and very low–birth-weight (VLBW)[37] infants. In the first day of life, there is minimal urine output, and body weight is stable despite low fluid intake. In the second phase, days 2 and 3 of life, diuresis occurs irrespective of the amount of fluid administered. By the fourth and fifth days of life, urine output begins to vary with changes in fluid intake and state of health.

Prematurity increases neonatal fluid requirements significantly. Fluid requirements are therefore estimated and then titrated to the infant's changing weight, urine output, and serum sodium concentration.

No less important is glucose homeostasis. In the ninth month of gestation, the fetus begins to form glycogen stores at a rate of more than 100 kcal/day. In the unstressed, term infant, hepatic glycogen stores are 5% of body weight. Immediately after birth, glycogenolysis depletes most of these stores within the first 24 to 48 hours. Gluconeogenesis must then proceed to yield glucose at a rate of approximately 4 mg/kg/min.

At birth, fetal serum glucose is 60% to 70% of maternal concentrations. This may decrease within the first hours of life before recovering but should exceed 45 mg/dL to avoid neurologic injury. Symptoms of hypoglycemia may include jitteriness, lethargy, temperature instability, and convulsions. Ten percent dextrose in water ($D_{10}W$) may be given as a bolus of 2 to 4 mL/kg followed by a continuous infusion (through a pump) providing 4 to 6 mg/kg/min. The serum glucose concentration is then analyzed frequently and the infusion adjusted as necessary to prevent hypoglycemia and hyperglycemia. It is important that the amount of glucose being provided be calculated in milligrams per kilogram per minute to avoid errors during fluid changes and to facilitate the diagnosis of persistent hypoglycemia.

Typical *day 1* infant fluid orders call for 70 to 80 mL/kg of $D_{10}W$. Because $D_{10}W$ contains 10 g of glucose per deciliter, this dosage provides

$$10 \text{ g/dL} \times 70 - 80 \text{ mL/kg/day} = 7 - 8 \text{ g/kg/day} = 0.333 \text{ g/kg/hr}$$
$$\cong 5 \text{ mg/kg/min}$$

On *day 2*, fluids are routinely increased to at least 100 mL/kg/day, and sodium is added at 2 to 3 mEq/dL. After urine output is established, potassium is added at 1 to 2 mEq/dL. The final solution, containing 30 mEq $Na^+$ and 10 to 20 mEq $K^+$ per liter, approximates the 0.2% saline "maintenance" solution commonly used previously in older children.

In the neonatal ICU, fluid management focuses on provision of adequate nutrition, maintenance of electrolyte balance, and limitation of fluid overload. The last factor is of particular concern because plasma oncotic pressure is reduced in preterm infants and the whole-body protein reflection coefficient is less than that in adults.[38] VLBW infants are at particular risk for fluid and electrolyte imbalances.[39] Even modest fluid overload may exacerbate pulmonary edema, prolong ductal patency, and more readily produce congestive heart failure. This perspective typically accompanies the infant to the operating room, where the primary considerations are routinely quite the opposite: restoration of circulating blood volume after third space accumulation, maintenance of intravascular volume amid ongoing blood loss, replacement of potentially massive evaporative losses, and maintenance of BP despite anesthetic-induced vasodilatation and increased venous capacitance. During surgery, these concerns must take precedence; yet unnecessary administration of fluid is best avoided.

## Intraoperative Fluid Management

### INTRAVENOUS ACCESS AND FLUID ADMINISTRATION DEVICES

In pediatrics, the first step toward intraoperative fluid management is often the most challenging: that is, gaining IV access. In general, simple procedures in healthy children are successfully approached using a single peripheral IV line. Although preferences vary among anesthesiologists, establishing IV access is most easily accomplished after induction of anesthesia. In young children, anesthesia is often induced by inhalation, and a catheter is inserted by an assistant into a hand or foot vein. In older children, or when IV access is desirable before anesthesia is induced, IV access may be facilitated by the use of topical anesthesia (e.g., EMLA cream, amethocaine, lidocaine infiltration) or sedation or both.

Complex surgeries in sicker children usually require at least two large-bore catheters. In pediatrics, however, "large bore" is a relative term, with 22-gauge catheters typically providing sufficient access in infants. Preferred sites for larger catheters include the antecubital and saphenous veins. In cases in which access to the central circulation is required (as for pressure monitoring, infusion of vasoactive medications, or prolonged access), longer catheters may be placed via the femoral, subclavian, or internal jugular vein (the latter usually via a high, anterior approach).[40] Although secure access may also be obtained via the external jugular vein, it is often difficult to negotiate the J-wire or catheter tip into the central circulation.[41] Peripherally inserted central catheter (PICC) lines are becoming increasingly used in hospitalized children. Although they represent a long-term means of delivering IV fluids and medications in children who require such treatment interventions, there are limitations to their utility intraoperatively. First, practitioners must maintain strict sterile technique when accessing these lines in order to avoid infection. Second, the lines tend to have smaller diameters and are quite long. Therefore, resistance can be significant, even with larger-bore PICC lines. Consequently, bolus and infusion dosing of drugs can be met with high resistance. These lines are not appropriate for large-volume resuscitation, and care should be taken to secure larger-bore IV access if large fluid shifts or significant blood loss is anticipated.

In selecting the appropriate IV catheter, it is useful to consider the relative effects of catheter length and diameter on solution flow rates. Longer catheters offer more resistance to flow than shorter ones and are therefore less desirable when rapid infusion of a large volume of fluids is necessary (see E-Fig. 51-1 and Figs. 51-1, 51-2). In vitro, catheters that were designed for peripheral venous access had 18% to 164% greater flow rates when compared with the same-gauge catheters designed for central venous use. Under pressure, as might be employed during emergent volume resuscitation, rates differed up to 17-fold.[42] Although this seems to suggest that short peripheral catheters should be preferred, in vivo data are more complex. In animal models, overall catheter flow rates are less than in vitro rates, and central access presents somewhat less resistance to flow than peripheral access.[43] Finally, when weighing the risks and benefits of central versus peripheral access, it is also interesting to consider that central administration of resuscitation medications may provide little practical advantage over peripheral administration.[44]

Intraosseous devices are now commonly used in the initial resuscitation of critically ill or injured children (see Fig. 48-6).[45,46] Flow rates via these devices depend less on needle diameter than on resistance in the marrow compartment.[47] In the operating room, the intraosseous route has been used for both induction and maintenance of anesthesia.[48-50] However, onset of drug effect is less predictable, and the device is more easily dislodged than an IV catheter. Potential complications include compartment syndrome[51-53] and, very rarely, damage to the growth plate.[46,54] Such devices are probably best considered an emergency or last-resort option.[49]

To prevent accidental volume overload, the amount of IV fluid available to administer to a child at any one time should not exceed the child's calculated hourly requirement. Particularly in infants, a volumetric chamber should be used to limit the amount of fluid available for infusion. Similarly, a microdrip infusion set limits the rate of fluid administration and permits much greater control. Although a fluid infusion pump provides the most precise mode of regulating the rate of fluid administration (and is therefore very useful in providing supplemental fluids or medications), such devices are impractical on primary access lines because they hinder the ability to administer drugs or fluids rapidly. In addition, the clinician should be mindful that pumps may continue to infuse through dislodged catheters and may give inappropriate reassurance of adequate IV access and fluid administration, providing a false sense of reassurance; administration of a large volume of fluid interstitially will fail to deliver the needed fluid volume (and medications). Moreover, if an identification bracelet of any sort is proximal to the IV insertion site, it may act as a tourniquet, resulting in ischemic digits. Therefore, access to the IV site is important in children, as well as removal of all bracelets that are proximal to ipsilateral IV insertion sites.

In neonates and small infants, when rapid infusion of resuscitation solutions or blood products is anticipated, many practitioners find it helpful to include an in-line stopcock manifold. Additional fluids may be drawn up into syringes and warmed separately; during periods of sudden blood loss, stored syringes may then be inserted into the manifold and a known volume rapidly infused.

Finally, in prolonged surgeries or when volume replacement is great, it is imperative that all IV infusions be adequately warmed. Also, in younger infants and children in whom communication exists between the right and left sides of the circulation (e.g., patency of the foramen ovale), an in-line "bubble" filter is desirable.

### CHOICE AND COMPOSITION OF INTRAVENOUS FLUIDS

In the early 1960s,[55] simultaneous measurements of plasma and extracellular fluid volumes demonstrated that, during surgery, plasma volume is supported at the expense of the extravascular

**TABLE 8-5** Composition of Extracellular Fluid and Common Intravenous Solutions

| | | CATIONS (mEq/L) | | | | | ANIONS (mEq/L) | | |
|---|---|---|---|---|---|---|---|---|---|
| | mOsm/L | Na$^+$ | K$^+$ | Ca$^{2+}$ | Mg$^{2+}$ | NH$_4^+$ | Cl$^-$ | HCO$_3^-$ | HPO$_4^-$ |
| Extracellular fluid | 280-300 | 142 | 4 | 5 | 3 | 0.3 | 103 | 27 | 3 |
| Lactated Ringer solution | 273 | 130 | 4 | 3 | | | 109 | 28 | |
| 0.45% NaCl | 154 | 77 | | | | | 77 | | |
| 0.9% NaCl (normal saline) | 308 | 154 | | | | | 154 | | |
| PLASMA-LYTE A* | 294 | 140 | 5 | | 3 | 1.6 | 98 | 98 | |
| 3% NaCl | 1024 | 513 | | | | | 513 | | |

*PLASMA-LYTE is a trademark of Baxter International Inc., its subsidiaries or affiliates. (Acetate 27 mEq/L and gluconate 23 mEq/L.)

space. At the same time, it was classically observed that isotonic resuscitation fluids temporarily redistribute from the intravascular spaces to what was originally believed to be a third, nonfunctional space. It is now clear that destruction of the endothelial glycocalyx, as caused by surgical trauma, permits fluid to shift from the intravascular to interstitial space. Therefore, the historical "third space" simply represents reversible expansion of the interstitium. Because of the differences in fluid distribution and renal function in infants compared with older children, it was at first unclear that these findings could be extended to infancy. Thus, fluid restriction remained the standard of care until careful studies specifically demonstrated that fluid and electrolyte requirements are often extremely large in neonates who are undergoing major surgical procedures.[56-58]

Although hypotonic fluids are selected for maintenance hydration throughout the hospital (according to the reasoning outlined previously), isotonic solutions are preferred intraoperatively for several reasons. First, most ongoing volume losses are isotonic, consisting of shed blood and interstitial fluids. Second, large volumes of hypotonic solutions may rapidly diminish serum osmolality, producing very low concentrations of electrolytes (in particular, sodium) and undesirable fluid shifts. Indeed, even large volumes of "isotonic" fluids have been shown to significantly decrease serum osmolality in adult volunteers.[59] Third, as discussed earlier, the plasma volume expansion that is necessary in response to diminished vascular tone under anesthesia is difficult to achieve even with isotonic fluids. Finally, increases in ADH and other elements of intraoperative physiology result in free water retention in excess of sodium if inadequate amounts of the latter are provided.

The compositions of commonly used IV solutions are presented in Table 8-5. Assuming normal plasma osmolality of 275 to 290 mOsm/L, it is noteworthy that 0.9% NaCl (normal saline, NS) is slightly hypertonic to plasma and that LR is isotonic (273 mOsm/L), although slightly hyponatremic (130 mEq/L). For dextrose-containing solutions, added osmolality is rapidly dissipated as sugar is metabolized, resulting in increased volumes of free water. Therefore, administration of 5% dextrose in water is ultimately equivalent to administration of free water.

The controversy regarding the perioperative use of colloid versus crystalloid fluid replacement remains an unresolved subject. It is worth noting that aside from 5% albumin, synthetic colloids are gaining popularity among pediatric practitioners. One reason for this is the development of newer synthetic colloids that have a more favorable side effect profile. Hydroxyethyl starches (HES) are synthetic colloids that are simply modified polysaccharides. Circulating amylases quickly break down natural polysaccharides. HES solutions avoid this problem by substituting hydroxyethyl groups for hydroxyl groups at carbon

positions C-2, C-3, and C-6. This results in a soluble molecule that is resistant to hydrolysis. These compounds are characterized by three attributes: average mean molecular weight (MW), molar substitution (MS), and the C2:C6 ratio, which relates to the relative positions of hydroxyethyl groups on the polysaccharide molecule.

HES solutions with a greater MW-to-MS ratio tend to remain in the intravascular space much longer than those with smaller ratios. However, they also are prone to more significant side effects including hypocoagulability. Newer, low MW/low MS solutions have much less effect on hemostatic mechanisms than older, higher MW/higher MS solutions. The exact mechanism of the effect on coagulation remains unclear, although it is thought that the HES compounds interfere with von Willebrand factor, factor VIII, and platelet function. A greater C2:C6 ratio is responsible for the slower degradation of the starch by amylase with fewer side effects.[60] Newer HES solutions (e.g., HES 130/0.42/6:1) are very safe in children scheduled for surgery who have normal renal function; they maintain hemodynamic stability and produce only mild to moderate changes in acid–base status.[61] Synthetic colloids such as these should be considered in surgical patients who demonstrate the need for aggressive intraoperative fluid resuscitation, such as children with large-volume blood loss or excessive insensible losses. Use of these solutions in cardiac surgery remains controversial given the effects on coagulation factors and platelet function induced by the cardiopulmonary bypass circuit.

The routine intraoperative use of glucose-containing solutions has also been a subject of debate. As a rule, operative stress evokes physiologic responses that increase serum glucose. In practice, therefore, hypoglycemia is seldom a problem in healthy children when glucose is omitted from perioperative IV fluids.[62,63] Indeed, the risk should be particularly small if the period of fasting is limited to less than 10 hours.[63] At the same time, rapid administration of dextrose solutions may certainly produce acute hyperglycemia and hyperosmolality.[62,63] Therefore, glucose-containing solutions should not be used to replace fluid deficits, third space losses, or blood losses. However, some populations, such as debilitated infants,[64] children who are malnourished, neonates and infants < 6 months of age[62,64a,64b] and those undergoing cardiac surgery, have been shown to be at risk for intraoperative hypoglycemia,[65,66] and the use of glucose-containing solutions (1% to 2.5% dextrose)[62,64a,67], along with intraoperative glucose monitoring, may be beneficial in these children.

## HYPERALIMENTATION

It is now common practice that critically ill children arrive in the operating room with hyperalimentation solutions infusing. Common contents of hyperalimentation solutions are shown in

| TABLE 8-6 | Common Contents of Parenteral Nutrition Solutions* |
|---|---|

**Carbohydrates**

10%, 12.5%, 20%, 25%, 30% Dextrose

Limited to $D_{10}$ or $D_{12.5}$ if through a peripheral catheter

**Protein**

In the form of amino acids

0.5, 1.0, 1.5, 2.0, 2.5, or 3.0 g/kg/day

**Lipids**

10%, 20% Lipids

**Standard Additives**

Sodium: 30 mEq/L

Potassium: 20 mEq/L

Calcium: 15 mEq/L

Magnesium: 10 mEq/L

Phosphorus: 10 mmol/L

Heparin

*Common contents of parenteral nutrition solutions containing dextrose, protein, lipids, and standard additives such as electrolytes. These values represent standard starting points that may be modified based on individual patient needs.*

Table 8-6. In general, children require 0.5 to 3.0 mg/kg/day of protein, 6 to 9 mg/kg/min of glucose, and 0.5 to 3 g/kg/day of fat. Children receiving parenteral nutrition preoperatively should continue to receive those infusions separately, and a corresponding volume should be deducted from isotonic operative fluids. Hyperalimentation typically consists of two infusions: Intralipid (Fresenius Kabi, Uppsala, Sweden) and a concentrated glucose/protein solution. It is prudent to discontinue the Intralipid solution during surgery; but if that is not possible, then every effort should be made to avoid accessing any ports in the line to reduce the risk of contaminating the Intralipid. Conversely, the concentrated glucose/protein solution should be continued at the same rate (because circulating insulin concentrations have acclimated accordingly). Because of hyperglycemic responses to the stress of surgery and reduced metabolism due to anesthesia and hypothermia, some practitioners routinely decrease hyperalimentation infusion rates by one third to one half. If the latter practice is followed, clinicians should consider checking serum glucose concentrations at regular intervals to monitor for hypoglycemia. Under no circumstances should concentrated glucose solutions (such as $D_{10}$ or $D_{20}$) be abruptly discontinued, because high levels of circulating insulin may cause a precipitous and profound decrease in the serum glucose concentration.

Concerns regarding the routine use of intraoperative dextrose-containing solutions, in large part from recognition that hyperglycemia may exacerbate neurologic injury after an ischemic or hypoxic event, resulted in most clinicians' avoiding such solutions for routine cases. If dextrose-containing solutions are used, appropriate monitoring is advised to avoid serum glucose extremes. Many practitioners administer glucose-containing solutions as a separate piggyback infusion using an infusion pump or other rate- or volume-limiting device to avoid accidental bolus administration. Alternatively, evidence indicates that isotonic solutions that contain reduced glucose concentrations (e.g., 1% or 2.5% versus 5%) are safe alternative solutions for intraoperative use that minimize both hyponatremia and hyperglycemia.[68]

In the United States, several Food and Drug Administration (FDA)-approved solutions containing 2.5% dextrose are available but none in lower concentrations. In Europe, 1% dextrose electrolyte solutions are now available.[64a,68] Because intraoperative administration of solutions containing 5% dextrose ($D_5LR$) frequently causes hyperglycemia, prudent anesthesiologists should selectively administer dextrose-containing solutions to those who are at particular risk for intraoperative hypoglycemia (i.e., neonates, chronic malnourished children, and cachectic children). In these instances, it may be sensible to administer solutions with a reduced dextrose concentration.[60,64a]

## FASTING RECOMMENDATIONS

The goal of fasting is to minimize the volume of gastric contents and thereby lessen the risk of vomiting and aspiration during induction of anesthesia. In children, as opposed to adults, this is of particular concern because in many institutions induction in children is more often accomplished by inhalation than by IV anesthesia and the period of vulnerability to regurgitation is potentially protracted compared with an IV induction.

At issue is the effectiveness of fasting in lowering a child's gastric volume and the benefits of this effect when weighed against the added discomfort and risk of dehydration. Numerous studies of gastric volume and pH have convincingly demonstrated that clear liquids are rapidly emptied from the stomach and the stimulated peristalsis actually serves to decrease gastric volume and acidity. Taking this together with the benefits of improved hydration and mental status, it is clear that prolonged *nil per os* (NPO) status is unwarranted. NPO guidelines currently in use in many institutions are included in Table 4-1.[69] As described earlier, for the vast majority of children, 20 to 40 mL/kg of LR given intraoperatively will provide adequate fluid deficit replacement.

## ASSESSMENT OF INTRAVASCULAR VOLUME

Once the child is anesthetized, many clinical clues to volume status are lost or confounded by operative events. For example, although it is a fairly reliable indicator of volume status in the quietly resting preoperative child, tachycardia may result from any number of factors besides intravascular volume status during surgery. It is the challenge of the anesthesiologist to view the entire clinical picture, consider the possibilities, integrate them into a hypothesis, and then test the hypothesis.

Assessment of intravascular volume begins with knowledge of age-related norms for heart rate and BP (see Tables 2-7 and 2-8). Is the heart rate persistently increased, or does it vary with surgical stimulation? Is the pulse pressure narrow, or, more ominously, is the BP reduced for age? Does it vary with positive-pressure breaths? Are the extremities warm? Is capillary refill brisk? What is the urine output? Are these variables changing? What is the rate of the change? When hypovolemia is suspected, observing the response to a 10- to 20-mL/kg bolus of isotonic crystalloid or colloid may test the hypothesis.

Measurement and continuous monitoring of central venous pressure are often helpful in assessing the status of circulating volume (see Figs. 48-2 to 48-5). In addition to traditional central lines introduced into the superior vena cava or left atrium, animal[70] and limited clinical[71] data suggest that femoral lines that terminate in the abdominal vena cava may also be useful. In infants and children, mean end-expiratory pressure measurements in the right atrial and inferior vena cava differed by less than 1 mm Hg.[71] Assessment of changes in the contour of the arterial waveform may also be helpful in assessing volume status and the response to volume administration (see Fig. 10-11).

### ONGOING LOSSES AND THIRD-SPACING

During all surgical procedures, fluid loss from the vascular space is primarily the result of three simultaneous physiologic processes. First, whole blood is shed at various rates and must be replaced. Second, capillary leak and surgical trauma result in extravasation of isotonic, protein-containing fluid into interstitial compartments (the so-called third space). Third, anesthetic-induced relaxation of sympathetic tone produces vasodilatation (increased capacitance) and relative hypovolemia (a virtual loss). In very small infants, a fourth source of losses, direct evaporation, must also be carefully considered. These ongoing losses are often difficult to quantitate (or even estimate). Although these losses occur in children of all sizes, the small circulating blood volume of an infant (e.g., for a 5-kg infant, 80 mL/kg × 5 kg = 400 mL) leaves little room for error. Faced with uncertainty, the prudent response is constant vigilance and reliance on general principles.

As a rule, 1 mL of shed blood is replaced with 1 mL of colloid (5% albumin or blood) or about 1.5 mL of isotonic crystalloid such as LR.[67,72] Isotonic crystalloid is also used to replenish third space losses. Surgical procedures that involve only mild tissue trauma may entail third space losses of 3 to 4 mL/kg/hr. More extensive surgical procedures involving moderate trauma may require replacement equivalent to 5 to 7 mL/kg/hr to adequately support intravascular volume. In small infants undergoing very large abdominal procedures, the losses may approach 10 mL/kg/hr or more.[56,58] In neonates, fluid requirements for emergent abdominal surgery for necrotizing enterocolitis have been estimated at up to 50 mL/kg/hr.[67] These "losses" result from the vascular compartment and include both evaporation and redistribution of fluid. The latter must be most carefully considered because it is exacerbated by the hemodilution and increased capillary pressures caused by excessive fluid administration.

Although necessary intraoperatively, third space accumulation represents whole-body salt and water overload that will need to be mobilized postoperatively. The price of unchecked fluid administration is generalized anasarca, pulmonary edema, bowel swelling, and laryngotracheal edema. In the healthy child, this relative fluid overload is well tolerated, with most excess fluid excreted over the first 2 postoperative days. In children with impaired pulmonary, cardiac, or renal function, however, such fluid excess may result in clinically important postoperative morbidity.

# Postoperative Fluid Management

## GENERAL APPROACH

Well-planned postoperative fluid management complements the intraoperative plan and accounts for evolving physiology as the child recovers. Replacement of fluid deficits is completed. Ongoing losses are replaced. The child is repeatedly reassessed, and intake is adjusted until normal fluid and electrolyte homeostasis has returned. To aid in decision making, trends in vital signs are identified, all sources of fluid intake and output are quantitated, urine specific gravity is monitored, daily weights are obtained, and serum electrolytes are measured.

In simple outpatient surgeries, discharge is possible after fluid deficits are replaced. In complex cases, replacement fluids may require hourly readjustment that is based on the prior hour's intake and output. Rather than reacting to single pieces of data, such as low urine output, one must discern overall patterns. High urine output and low urine specific gravity may indicate overhydration or diabetes insipidus. Oliguria may suggest hypovolemia when it is accompanied by high urine specific gravity and clinical signs of dehydration or low cardiac output when it is accompanied by signs of poor perfusion. In the well-hydrated child, oliguria may represent renal failure if the urine specific gravity is normal (or dilute) but increased concentrations of ADH if the urine is concentrated. A careful physical examination is necessary; in many cases, certainty in diagnosis requires simultaneous measurement of serum and urine electrolytes.

Frequently, losses via surgical or gastric drains are large in both real and relative terms. For example, a neonate with a nasogastric tube may lose more than 100 mL/kg/day (normally 20 to 40 mL/kg/day) in gastric fluid. Therefore, in determining the volume and composition of replacement fluids, it is sometimes helpful to consider the electrolyte content of various losses (Table 8-7).

## POSTOPERATIVE PHYSIOLOGY AND HYPONATREMIA

Children retain salt and water postoperatively, in part as a result of neuroendocrine activation by stress, continued capillary leak with third space accumulation, non-osmotic stimulation of ADH (fever, stress, opioid administration) and hypovolemia-induced renin secretion. As outlined earlier, intravascular volume depletion is a potent non-osmotic signal for fluid retention and may override osmotic signals under a variety of clinical circumstances.

At the same time, ongoing fluid and electrolyte losses after surgery via chest tubes, nasogastric suction, weeping incisions, and even continued slow bleeding may be substantial. Postopera-

| TABLE 8-7 | Composition of Body Fluids | | | | | |
|---|---|---|---|---|---|---|
| Source | Na⁺ (mEq/L) | K⁺ (mEq/L) | Cl⁻ (mEq/L) | HCO₃⁻ (mEq/L) | pH | Osmolality (mOsm/L) |
| Gastric | 50 | 10-15 | 150 | 0 | 1 | 300 |
| Pancreas | 140 | 5 | 0-100 | 100 | 9 | 300 |
| Bile | 130 | 5 | 100 | 40 | 8 | 300 |
| Ileostomy | 130 | 15-20 | 120 | 25-30 | 8 | 300 |
| Diarrhea | 50 | 35 | 40 | 50 | | |
| Sweat | 50 | 5 | 55 | 0 | Alkaline | |
| Blood | 140 | 4-5 | 100 | 25 | 7.4 | 285-295 |
| Urine | 0-100* | 20-100* | 70-100* | 0 | 4.5-8.5* | 50-1400* |

From Herrin J. Fluid and electrolytes. In: Graef JW, editor. Manual of pediatric therapeutics. 6th ed. Philadelphia: Lippincott-Raven; 1997. p. 63-75.
*Varies considerably with fluid intake.

tively, children often depend entirely on IV fluids for replacement of these and other losses.

Therefore, unless isotonic, sodium-containing fluids are provided, postoperative children are universally at risk for developing hyponatremia.[73,74] In a retrospective review of 24,412 surgical admissions to a large children's hospital, the incidence of significant postoperative hyponatremia was 0.34%, with a substantial mortality rate (8.4%) in these previously healthy children.[75] If this measured incidence were extended to the entire population in the United States, 7448 children would present annually with postoperative hyponatremia and 626 would die from an entirely avoidable cause. Mortality rates as great as 40% to 60% have been reported after hyponatremia, although it may only be a surrogate marker for a disease with a poor prognosis rather than the actual cause of the death.[76,77]

In reviewing the etiology of hyponatremia, two factors stand out: extensive extrarenal loss of electrolyte-containing fluid and IV replacement with hypotonic fluids.[75] In addition, delay in recognition often plays a major role in associated morbidity. The solution seems a simple one: (1) administration of hypotonic fluids without a specific indication should be avoided postoperatively, (2) ongoing losses should be replaced in a timely fashion, and (3) serum electrolytes should be measured routinely in children exhibiting potential symptoms of hyponatremia (see later discussion).

### POSTOPERATIVE PULMONARY EDEMA

Children who receive large volumes of fluid intraoperatively are at risk for development of pulmonary edema as operative fluids are mobilized. Usually, fluid mobilization begins to occur on the second postoperative day and continues through day 3 or 4. Although this is less common in children than in the elderly, it occurs occasionally in children with burn injuries[78] or in pediatric patients receiving large amounts of fluid during resuscitation from trauma or sepsis. In one review,[79] 13 patients (11 adults and 2 children) developed postoperative pulmonary edema; all began to exhibit symptoms within 36 hours after surgery and had total net fluid retention in excess of 67 mL/kg postoperatively.

## Pathophysiologic States and Their Management

### FLUID OVERLOAD AND EDEMA

Edema is essentially a "sodium disease," representing sodium and water overload with excessive fluid residing in the extracellular space. Although intracellular volume changes can sometimes be substantial, prolonged cell swelling represents failure of essential volume regulatory functions and is likely a preterminal event. In fluid-overload states, plasma volume is generally increased unless the balance of Starling forces is disturbed, as in nephrotic syndrome or lymphatic obstruction. Edema formation is opposed by (1) low compliance of the interstitial compartment, (2) increased lymphatic flow, (3) osmotic washout of interstitial proteins, and (4) impedance and elasticity of the proteoglycan gel. The differential diagnosis of fluid overload and edema formation is presented in Table 8-8. Principles of therapy for fluid overload states include the following:

- Fluid restriction
- Salt restriction
- Diuresis, dialysis
- Salt-poor albumin for diminished plasma volume

**TABLE 8-8** Differential Diagnosis of Fluid Overload and Edema Formation

| Condition | Differential Diagnosis |
|---|---|
| Imbalance of intake and output | Salt poisoning |
| | Formula dilution errors |
| | Intravenous infusion errors |
| | Drugs given as sodium salts |
| Steroid excess with normal sodium intake | Congenital adrenal hyperplasia |
| | Exogenous steroids |
| Perceived decreases in effective plasma volume | ↓ MAP → baroreceptors → ↑ sympathetic tone, ADH, renin, aldosterone |
| | Vasodilators |
| | Congestive heart failure |
| | Cirrhosis |
| | Nephrotic syndrome |
| Impaired sodium excretion | Chronic renal failure |
| | Acute glomerular disease (↓ GFR with normal tubular function) |
| | Nonsteroidal antiinflammatory drugs (↓ $PGE_2$ and RBF) |
| Water excess | SIADH |
| | Hypotonic infusion |
| | Stress (↑ ADH) |

*ADH,* Antidiuretic hormone; *GFR,* glomerular filtration rate; *MAP,* mean arterial pressure; $PGE_2$, prostaglandin $E_2$; *RBF,* renal blood flow; *SIADH,* syndrome of inappropriate antidiuretic hormone secretion.

**TABLE 8-9** Clinical Signs and Symptoms for Estimation of Severity of Dehydration in Infants

| Clinical Signs | DEGREE OF DEHYDRATION | | |
| | Mild | Moderate | Severe |
|---|---|---|---|
| Weight loss (%) | 5 | 10 | 15 |
| Behavior | Normal | Irritable | Hyperirritable to lethargic |
| Thirst | Slight | Moderate | Intense |
| Mucous membranes | May be normal | Dry | Parched |
| Tears | Present | Normal to reduced | Absent |
| Anterior fontanel | Flat | Possibly sunken | Sunken |
| Skin turgor | Normal | Slightly increased | Increased |
| Urine output | Normal | Oliguric | Anuric |

Modified in part from Herrin J. Fluid and electrolytes. In: Graef J, editor. Manual of pediatric therapeutics. 6th ed. Philadelphia: Lippincott-Raven; 1997. p. 63-75.

### DEHYDRATION STATES

Dehydration states are common in children. The extent of dehydration is best assessed by weight, because clinical signs such as tachycardia, capillary refill, and skin elasticity,[80] although often reliable, may be influenced by factors other than hydration status. A capillary refill time of 1.5 to 3.0 seconds, for example, suggests a fluid deficit of between 50 and 100 mL/kg, yet this sign is extremely dependent on ambient temperature.[81] Similarly, poor skin elasticity reflects significant volume loss, yet elasticity may be well preserved in children with hypernatremic dehydration.[80] Clinical signs associated with varying levels of dehydration are presented in Table 8-9.

As a first approximation, correction of most dehydration states in older children is most readily achieved with administration of a simple bolus of NS, LR, or PLASMA-LYTE 148 (balanced crystalloid solution). In infants or children with unusual, prolonged, or severe dehydration, however, management must be more precise. A five-point questionnaire to assess the severity of dehydration may help develop an appropriate treatment strategy[82]:

1. *Does a volume deficit exist and, if so, how great is it?*
   As noted previously, assessment of volume deficit is best made by weight, yet rough estimates of 5% (mild), 10% (moderate), and 15% (severe) may be made in infants based on clinical signs (see Table 8-9).

2. *Does an osmolar disturbance exist? Is it acute or chronic?*
   An osmolar imbalance is determined by measuring the serum sodium concentration. The majority of clinically encountered dehydration states (~80%) are isotonic (Na$^+$ = 130 to 150 mEq/L). These isotonic losses are easily managed by almost any strategy.

   Approximately 15% of dehydrated children present with hypertonic dehydration (Na$^+$ > 150 mEq/L). These children are at greatest risk and have usually experienced the greatest fluid losses for a given set of clinical signs.[83] If the condition is chronic, they may require extensive, slow rehydration over much longer periods.[84]

   Five percent of children present with hypotonic dehydration (Na$^+$ < 130 mEq/L). For a given fluid deficit, these individuals are often more symptomatic than others, and their requirement for sodium replacement is greatest. Surprisingly, rapid improvement in clinical condition often results after the first fluid bolus.

   In general, chronic dehydration states must be repaired slowly and acute dehydration states (<24 hours) may be corrected more rapidly. This is because cell volume equilibration occurs acutely through gain or loss of electrolytes (which are moved rapidly) and chronically through gain or loss of organic osmolytes (which are moved more slowly).[11] Reequilibration of brain cell volume during correction of hypertonicity can be very slow, mandating patience in correction of chronic fluid deficits. Similarly, rapid correction of hyponatremic disturbances can be hazardous,[75] even when seemingly safe isotonic solutions are employed.[85]

3. *Does an acid–base abnormality exist?*
   Quantitation of the child's acid–base status gives useful, although limited, information as to the severity of dehydration. When evaluating acid–base status, it is important to recall that bicarbonate reabsorption and urine acidification are limited in preterm and young infants, leaving even the normal infant in a state of mild metabolic acidosis (pH, 7.3; serum bicarbonate 20 to 21 mEq/L [normal 22 to 26 mEq/L]). Although slow, spontaneous correction of acid–base status is typically observed on rehydration, rapid fluid boluses in poorly perfused children may result in a transient "reperfusion acidosis" as returning circulation washes the products of anaerobic metabolism out of the tissues. In this setting, or when renal insufficiency exists, blood-buffering capacity is such that children with serum bicarbonate concentrations lower than 8 mEq/L or pH lower than 7.2 may benefit from administration of supplemental base (sodium bicarbonate) (Fig. 8-6).[82]

   Rapid bedside evaluation of acid–base status utilizes the following general relationships: a pH decrease of 0.1 unit accompanies a base excess (BE) of approximately 6 mEq/L or an increase in carbon dioxide tension (PCO$_2$) of 10 to

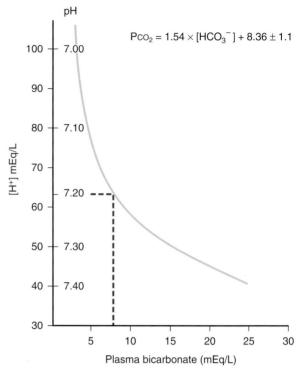

$$PCO_2 = 1.54 \times [HCO_3^-] + 8.36 \pm 1.1$$

**FIGURE 8-6** Data from children with metabolic acidosis[127] were used to depict the displacement of pH as serum bicarbonate declines. The zone of rapid pH displacement (pH < 7.20) has a slope that is several times greater than the zone of gradual pH displacement (pH ≥ 7.20). As the pH moves through the zone of rapid pH displacement, a further decline of serum bicarbonate, of as little as 1 or 2 mEq/L, produces a highly leveraged further decrease of pH. *[H],$^+$* Hydrogen ion concentration; *[HCO$_3^-$],* bicarbonate ion concentration; *PCO$_2$,* carbon dioxide tension. (From Kallen RJ. The management of diarrheal dehydration in infants using parenteral fluids. Pediatr Clin North Am 1990;37:265-86.)

12 mm Hg. The total replacement base required is then determined by the following equation:

$$Dose\,(mEq) = 0.3 \times Weight\,(kg) \times BE\,(mEq/L)$$

Clinically, a smaller sodium bicarbonate dose (1 to 2 mEq/kg) is given initially, the response is verified by blood gas analysis, and the remaining doses are titrated to effect.

4. *Is renal function impaired?*
   Initial evaluation includes the timing of the last urine void and recent urine output, measurement of urine specific gravity, and serum levels of blood urea nitrogen and creatinine. If uncertainty persists, measurement of serum and urine electrolytes for comparison and calculation of the FE$_{Na}$ is indicated (see Chapter 26).

   FE$_{Na}$ values of less than 1% imply prerenal conditions causing renal dysfunction, whereas FE$_{Na}$ values greater than 2% to 3% suggest renal insufficiency. In prematurity, however, values as high as 9% may be seen in otherwise normal infants.

5. *What is the state of potassium balance?*
   Potassium homeostasis is critical to life, and serum potassium levels are generally maintained within a very narrow range. Nonetheless, serum potassium concentrations do not reflect whole-body stores and substantial potassium depletion may exist in the presence of modest changes in serum potassium concentration (K$^+_{serum}$). Gastrointestinal losses or metabolic

acidosis is usually accompanied by a potassium deficit, whereas other dehydration states are not. Rapid fluid boluses or pH correction, or both, may acutely reduce $K^+_{serum}$,[86] and refractory hypokalemia may occur in children deficient in magnesium.[87] In all cases, adequate renal function should be present before administration of potassium, and complete repletion should be accomplished over 48 to 72 hours. Once the nature and severity of dehydration have been determined, the clinician may proceed using any of a variety of correction strategies. In one approach, moderate to severe dehydration deficits may be estimated, as in Table 8-9. Fluid and electrolyte repair may then proceed according to a three-phase approach wherein circulating plasma volume, perfusion, and urine output are restored rapidly using isotonic crystalloid or colloid solution and remaining deficits are corrected over 24 hours as follows[88]:

- Emergency Phase: 20 to 30 mL/kg isotonic crystalloid/colloid bolus
- Repletion Phase 1: 25 to 50 mL/kg over 6 to 8 hours. Anions: $Cl^-$ 75%, acetate 25%
- Repletion Phase 2: remainder of deficit over 24 hours (isotonic) or 48 hours (hypertonic). Include calcium replacement as necessary.

## HYPERNATREMIA AND HYPONATREMIA

As previously detailed, disorders of sodium equilibrium are primarily marked by disturbances of fluid balance and are corrected according to the principles outlined earlier. Serious hypernatremia or hyponatremia is accompanied by neurologic symptoms whose severity is determined by the degree and rate of change of serum sodium concentration ($Na^+_{serum}$).

### Hypernatremia

In contrast to its rareness in adults, acute hypernatremia is common in children. A mortality rate greater than 40% for the acute disorder and 10% for the chronic disorder has been quoted for hypernatremia (serum sodium >160 mEq/L).[76,89] Mortality and permanent neurologic injury are even more common in infants. Depending on degree and duration, neurologic findings include irritability and coma. Seizures may be a presenting symptom, but they are more commonly encountered after the start of therapy. Children with acute conditions are usually symptomatic, whereas those with chronic conditions (acclimated individuals) are typically asymptomatic. General principles for treatment of hypernatremia are as follows:

- In the setting of circulatory collapse, colloid or NS bolus should be administered. Although the assertion is debatable, a colloid bolus provides the theoretical benefit of sustained hemodynamic support with lower fluid load. Saline, in contrast, rapidly reequilibrates, necessitating repeated boluses while adding to the total salt burden.
- Once a stable circulation has been restored, fluid deficit should be assessed as accurately as possible and corrected over 48 to 72 hours. Cautious correction of the serum sodium level is required. The serum sodium concentration and osmolality should be continuously reassessed during fluid administration, aiming for a correction of no more than 1 to 2 mOsm/L/hr. After as little as 4 hours of hypernatremia, idiogenic osmoles (e.g., trimethylamines) appear in the brain to prevent cerebral volume depletion. Rapid administration of free water could induce cerebral edema, seizures, and death. Therefore, free water should be administered slowly. Because of possible

associated hypoglycemia, some solutions should be glucose-containing, and serum glucose levels should be monitored.

- Vigilance for seizures, apnea, and cardiovascular compromise should be maintained, because such complicating factors can be the primary determinants of successful outcome.

### Hyponatremia

Hyponatremia is also common in infants and children. Increasing prevalence due to erroneous formula dilution has intermittently been reported.[90,91] In the practice of anesthesiology, mild hyponatremia is a common postoperative condition after surgery of any severity[92-94]; in neurosurgical patients, hyponatremia may represent cerebral salt wasting or syndrome of inappropriate antidiuretic hormone secretion (SIADH).[95] In general, symptomatic patients are acutely hyponatremic and asymptomatic individuals are chronically hyponatremic.[96] After surgery, acutely hyponatremic children may present with nonspecific symptoms that are often erroneously attributed to other causes. Early central nervous system symptoms include headache, nausea, weakness, and anorexia. Advancing symptoms include mental status changes, confusion, irritability, progressive obtundation, and seizures. Respiratory arrest (or irregularity) is a common manifestation of advanced hyponatremia.

When planning to correct hyponatremia, the presence of symptoms must be considered a medical emergency, whereas asymptomatic children do not require rapid intervention. Chronic hyponatremia must be corrected slowly and by no more than 0.5 mEq/L/hr to avoid neurologic complications that include central pontine myelinolysis.[97] The best treatment for acute hyponatremia is early recognition and intervention. Because hypoxia exacerbates the neurologic injury, the simple ABCs of resuscitation are attended to first, and the airway is secured in the child who has seizures or respiratory irregularity. Hyponatremic seizures may be quieted by relatively modest (3 to 6 mEq/L) increases of serum sodium.[98] In several series,[91,99,100] such limited, rapid correction of symptomatic hyponatremia with hypertonic saline (514 mEq/L NaCl) was found to be well tolerated. It should be emphasized, however, that complete correction is unnecessary and unwise.[101] Initial therapy is aimed at increasing the serum sodium concentration no more than is necessary to stop seizure activity (usually 3 to 5 mEq/L). Further, the correction takes place over several days. Hypertonic saline may be used for the correction until the serum sodium increases to greater than 120 mEq/L. Remembering that TBW may range from 75% in infancy to 60% or less in older children, total sodium deficit is estimated as follows:

Sodium change (mEq/L) × fraction TBW (L/kg) × weight (kg)
= mEq sodium

(Desired $[Na^+]_{serum}$ − observed $[Na^+]_{serum}$) × 0.6 × weight (kg)
= mEq sodium required

For example, in a 25-kg child, to correct a serum sodium concentration of 110 mEq/L to 125 mEq/L using hypertonic saline (514 mEq/L), infuse

$$(125\ mEq/L - 110\ mEq/L) \times 0.6 \times 25 = 225\ mEq\ total$$
*or*
$$225\ mEq/514\ mEq/L = 0.44\ L\ over\ 48\ hours = 9\ mL/hr$$

Because such calculations involve estimates, frequent measurement of the serum sodium concentration is necessary during correction. As with hypernatremia, much of the morbidity and mortality associated with hyponatremia relates to complicating factors such as seizures and hypoxia that may occur during therapy. Therefore, children undergoing therapy should be cared for in a monitored setting. When overzealous correction has occurred, there may be value in acutely relowering Na$^+$$_{serum}$ using hypotonic fluids,[96] although such therapy is not without its own hazards.

General principles for treatment of hyponatremia are as follows:

■ Asymptomatic hyponatremia in and of itself need not be rapidly corrected. Associated cardiovascular compromise due to volume depletion may be addressed by colloid bolus or administration of isotonic saline (1 L/m$^2$/day). Provision of sodium is accompanied by free water restriction.

■ Symptomatic hyponatremia is a medical emergency and may sometimes reflect irreversible neurologic injury. Correction should be rapid, yet limited, as discussed previously. A dose of 2 to 3 mL/kg of 3% saline (514 mEq/L) may be administered over 20 to 30 minutes to halt seizures.

■ Subsequent correction is accomplished through calculation of the sodium deficit and provision of sodium so as to slowly correct at a rate not to exceed 0.5 mEq/L/hr or 25 mEq/L (total) in 24 to 48 hours.

■ If the attendant fluid load is excessive or if oliguria is present, diuretics may be useful.

## DISORDERS OF POTASSIUM HOMEOSTASIS

### Hyperkalemia

Hyperkalemia is occasionally the presenting finding in conditions such as congenital adrenal hyperplasia. More commonly, it results from acute renal insufficiency, massive tissue injury, acidosis, or iatrogenic mishaps. In the operating room, acute hyperkalemia may follow the use of succinylcholine in children with myopathies, burns, upper and lower motor neuron lesions, chronic sepsis, or disuse atrophy and occasionally during massive, rapid transfusion of red blood cells or whole blood (see Chapters 6 and 10).[102] It may occur with rhabdomyolysis or as a late sign in malignant hyperthermia.

Although neurologic status is the main concern for children with abnormal serum sodium levels, cardiac status (rate and rhythm) determines the care of children with hyperkalemia. In children with hyperkalemia, the appearance of peaked T waves is followed by lengthening of the PR interval and widening of the QRS complex until P waves are lost. Finally, the QRS complex merges with its T wave to produce a sinusoidal pattern (Fig. 8-7). Successful treatment traditionally utilizes the following approach:

■ Emergent therapy is first directed toward antagonism of the cardiac effects of potassium by cautious administration of intravenous calcium (calcium chloride [10 to 30 mg/kg] as 0.1 to 0.3 mL/kg of a 10% solution, or calcium gluconate [30 to 100 mg/kg] as 0.3 to 1 mL/kg of a 10% solution) over 3 to 5 minutes to avoid bradycardia. Calcium does not decrease the serum potassium concentration but rather reestablishes the gradient between the resting membrane potential, which is increased in the presence of hyperkalemia, and the threshold potential, which is determined by the calcium concentration. It also increases the refractory period of the action potential, the net effect being the prevention of spontaneous depolarization.

■ Serum potassium is then reduced by returning potassium to the intracellular space. This is done by correcting acidosis

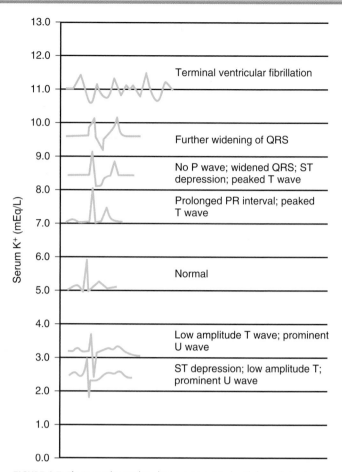

**FIGURE 8-7** Electrocardiographic changes associated with hyperkalemia. (From Williams GS, Klenk EL, Winters RW. Acute renal failure in pediatrics. In: Winters RW, editor. The body fluids in pediatrics: medical, surgical, and neonatal disorders of acid-base status, hydration, and oxygenation. Boston: Little, Brown; 1973. p. 523-57.)

through administration of sodium bicarbonate (1 to 2 mEq/kg), mild to moderate hyperventilation, and administration of a β-agonist.

■ To maintain potassium in the intracellular space, glucose and insulin are administered by infusion (0.5 to 1 g/kg glucose with 0.1 U/kg insulin over 30 to 60 minutes).

■ After stabilization, attention is directed toward removal of the whole-body potassium burden (sodium polystyrene sulfonate [Kayexalate], furosemide, dialysis) and correction of the underlying cause (Fig. 8-8).

The knowledge that β-adrenergic stimulation modulates the translocation of potassium into the intracellular space[103,104] has prompted the consideration of β-agonists in the treatment of acute hyperkalemia.[105-108] In children, a single infusion of an IV β-agonist such as salbutamol (5 μg/kg over 15 minutes) effectively reduces serum potassium concentrations within 30 minutes. Because of the rapidity, efficacy, and safety of salbutamol in children, it has become the first-choice treatment for hyperkalemia.[105] In addition to IV therapy, both salbutamol[109] and albuterol[108] by inhalation effectively reduce the serum potassium concentration. It should be noted that at this time, salbutamol is not available in IV formulations in the United States. The inhalation route has the significant advantages of being readily available in emergency departments and not requiring IV access.

Treatment Algorithm for Hyperkalemia

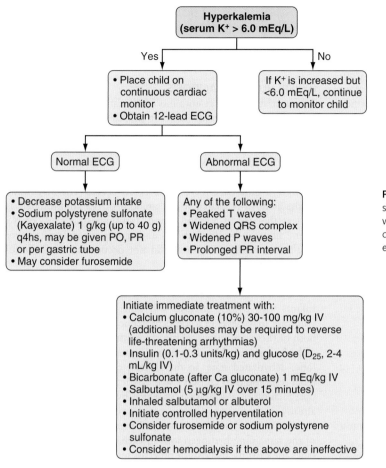

**FIGURE 8-8** Algorithm for treatment of hyperkalemia. After stabilization, attention is directed toward removal of the whole-body potassium burden (Kayexalate, dialysis) and correction of the underlying cause. *D₂₅*, 25% dextrose; *ECG*, electrocardiogram; *IV*, intravenous; *PO*, orally; *PR*, per rectum.

However, the observation that a paradoxical exacerbation of hyperkalemia sometimes occurs on initiation of treatment,[109] together with concerns regarding the possibility of associated arrhythmias,[110] suggests that more experience is required before such therapy can be considered the standard of care. Inhalation of albuterol during such an event in the operating room may speed the reduction in serum potassium while other methods of treatment are instituted.

### Hypokalemia

Hypokalemia is most common in children as a complication of diarrhea or persistent vomiting associated with gastroenteritis. Muscle weakness is the most common sign in hypokalemia and has been correlated with the serum potassium concentration.[111] In the operating room or ICU, hypokalemia may also accompany a wide variety of other conditions, including diabetes, hyperaldosteronism, pyloric stenosis, starvation, renal tubular disease, chronic steroid or diuretic use, and β-agonist therapy. Severe hypokalemia can also be accompanied by electrocardiographic changes, including QT prolongation, diminution of the T wave, and appearance of U waves (see Fig. 8-7).

As noted previously, serum potassium concentrations do not accurately reflect total potassium homeostasis, and low serum concentrations may or may not be associated with significant total body potassium depletion. Indeed, the extracellular fraction of potassium is only a tiny proportion (approximately 3%) of the entire body store. For these reasons, the precise point at which to begin replacement therapy is controversial, and total replacement requirements are impossible to calculate. In general practice, serum potassium values ($K^+_{serum}$) between 2.0 and 2.5 mEq/L are corrected before surgery on the assumption that further decreases may predispose the child to muscular weakness, arrhythmias, and hemodynamic instability.

Potassium replacement is best accomplished orally over an extended period while the underlying cause is evaluated and treated. When IV correction is required, concentrations up to 40 mEq/L should be given slowly *(not to exceed 1 mEq/kg/hr)* in a monitored setting. Because such solutions often cause phlebitis, large-bore or central catheters are preferred. In the setting of hypochloremia and hypokalemia, chloride deficits must first be replaced, usually by administration of normal saline.

### SYNDROME OF INAPPROPRIATE ANTIDIURETIC HORMONE SECRETION

Many non-osmotic factors are capable of stimulating ADH release, and these can occasionally override osmotic control priorities. When this occurs, clinicians have historically deemed the increased ADH concentrations "inappropriate" because control of the serum osmolarity is lost (see Chapter 26). As detailed earlier, however, intravascular depletion is the most potent stimulus for vasopressin release, and it is hardly *inappropriate* that defense of circulation takes priority over defense of serum sodium levels. Pain, surgical stress, critical illness, sepsis, pulmonary disease, central nervous system injury, drugs, and a variety of other factors may all stimulate ADH release above and beyond that necessary to maintain osmolar balance.

SIADH is common in children yet is often overlooked. Minor head trauma, for example, may elicit spikes in ADH levels, although infrequently to the extent that it produces serious hyponatremia and seizures.[112] Urine output after spinal fusion is often reduced because of increased concentrations of ADH, which usually return to normal within 24 hours without therapy.[113] Infants with bronchiolitis and hyperinflated lungs frequently demonstrate markedly increased plasma ADH concentrations and exhibit fluid retention, weight gain, urinary concentration, and plasma hypoosmolality until their illness begins to resolve.[114] Hyponatremia to the point of seizures, however, is only occasionally observed.

The diagnosis of SIADH rests on the identification of impaired urinary dilution in the setting of plasma hypoosmolality. Hyponatremia ($Na^+$ < 135 mEq/L), serum osmolality less than 280 mOsm/L, and urine osmolality greater than 100 mOsm/L in the absence of volume depletion, cardiac failure, nephropathy, adrenal insufficiency, or cirrhosis are generally considered sufficient for diagnosis. Therapeutic principles are similar to those for hyponatremia and depend on the following:

- Restriction of free water
- Repletion of sodium deficits (if present)
- Administration of diuretics to offset the effects of vasopressin

### DIABETES INSIPIDUS

In the operating room and the ICU, diabetes insipidus is most commonly associated with the care of neurosurgical patients.[115-117] Diabetes insipidus is also caused by neuroendocrine failure in brain death, and management may be necessary if organ donation is requested.[118,119] Diabetes insipidus results from decreased secretion of, or renal insensitivity to, vasopressin (see Chapter 26). Manifestations include massive polyuria, volume contraction, dehydration, and plasma hyperosmolality. Dilute polyuria (<250 mOsm, >2 mL/kg/hr) in the presence of hypernatremia ($Na^+$ > 145 mEq/L) with hyperosmolality (>300 mOsm/L) is the hallmark. In central diabetes insipidus, administration of desmopressin concentrates the urine but water deprivation does not. Postoperative diabetes insipidus may initially be difficult to distinguish from mobilization of operative fluids.

Children with craniopharyngioma or a similarly situated pathologic lesion may not manifest vasopressin deficiency early in the disease but become symptomatic preoperatively after steroid administration or intraoperatively during surgical manipulation. Postoperative diabetes insipidus typically begins on the evening after surgery and may resolve in 3 to 5 days if osmoregulatory structures have not been permanently injured. An often-confusing triphasic response may also occur wherein postoperative diabetes insipidus appears to resolve, fluid status normalizes, or SIADH appears and then vasopressin secretion ceases and diabetes insipidus returns. It is hypothesized that this pattern reflects nonspecific vasopressin release from degenerating neurons in the hypothalamic supraoptic and paraventricular nuclei.

Attempts have been made to develop protocols for perioperative management of diabetes insipidus.[120] Because vasopressin is difficult to titrate to urine output, our practice involves maximal antidiuresis and fluid restriction. In this setting, volume status must be monitored closely, because urine output is no longer a marker of renal perfusion. Children who need close perioperative monitoring for the development of diabetes insipidus include those with preexisting diabetes insipidus as well as those who are undergoing resection of craniopharyngiomas or pituitary lesions or other procedures that involve resection or manipulation of the pituitary stalk.[121]

### HYPERCHLOREMIC ACIDOSIS

Administration of large amounts of NS can lead to excess serum chloride.[122] The chloride content of NS is 154 mEq/L. This excess of chloride ions can lead to a hyperchloremic acidosis, which has been categorized as a strong-ion acidosis.[123,124] This type of acidosis results from an excess of strong anions (e.g., lactate, ketoacids, sulfates) relative to the strong cations. As the strong ion difference increases, acidosis occurs. The magnitude of the acidosis is related to the amount of NS administered as well as the rate of administration. Infusions of 35 mL/kg NS over 2 hours in healthy patients undergoing gynecologic surgery resulted in acidosis. Acidosis did not occur with similar infusions of LR.[122]

### HYPOCHLOREMIC METABOLIC ALKALOSIS

Infants with pyloric stenosis and other children with chronic vomiting may develop a hypochloremic metabolic alkalosis. In both of these conditions, chronic vomiting results in large losses of hydrogen and chloride ions and water. This leads to an alkalotic, dehydrated state. In the absence of IV fluid therapy, the renal response is to conserve water by retaining sodium through upregulation of aldosterone, in which hydrogen ions (which are already in short supply because of the vomiting) and potassium ions are excreted in the urine in exchange for sodium. Excretion of the remaining hydrogen ions in exchange for sodium exacerbates the existing alkalosis or prevents resolution of the alkalosis. It also leads to the unusual syndrome of paradoxical aciduria in the presence of a metabolic alkalosis.

The potassium loss leads to hypokalemia. Although hypokalemia between 3.4 and 4.4 mEq/L may appear trivial because the concentration is small, chronic hypokalemia equilibrates throughout all bodily fluids, including the intracellular fluid volume. The intracellular potassium concentration, 135 to 145 mEq/L, is 30- to 40-fold greater than the extracellular concentration. Hence, a chronic decrease of 1 mEq/L in extracellular potassium, which is only 1% to 2% of the total body potassium, may reflect an enormous deficiency in total body potassium stores, on the order of 100 to 200 mEq $K^+$ in an adult. However, potassium loss from the extracellular fluid is not linearly related to the total body potassium (due to interference from $Na^+/K^+$ pumps and other electrolyte-stabilizing mechanisms). With an extracellular $K^+$ concentration of less than 3.5 mEq/L, a small loss in extracellular potassium translates into a huge loss of total body potassium, whereas with an extracellular $K^+$ concentration greater than 4 mEq/L, extracellular potassium losses exert an attenuated effect on the total body potassium.

In infants and children with chronic hypokalemic, hypochloremic, metabolic alkalosis, correction of the electrolyte abnormalities and hypovolemia is optimally achieved using NS with 20 mEq/L $K^+$ infused at a rate of 10 to 20 mL/kg/hr through a peripheral IV access until the potassium level is greater than 3.0 mEq/L, the chloride concentration is greater than 95 mEq/L, and the clinical signs of hypovolemia are resolved. In the case of pyloric stenosis, this may take 24 to 48 hours depending on the severity of the electrolyte and fluid imbalance.

## CEREBRAL SALT WASTING

Cerebral salt wasting (also known as renal salt wasting) is a hyponatremic syndrome of unclear etiology. Most commonly recognized in neurosurgical patients, it is a primary natriuresis probably related to dysregulation of brain or atrial natriuretic peptides. The condition has been increasingly recognized, and an incidence as great as 5% has been reported in children with brain tumors.[125] Cerebral salt wasting can sometimes be difficult to distinguish from SIADH but, unlike the latter, the former is marked by hyponatremia, natriuresis, and *hypovolemia*. Initial therapy consists of fluid resuscitation with isotonic solutions and ongoing correction of intravascular volume depletion with sodium-containing solutions. Although spontaneous resolution is the norm, persistent cases may require mineralocorticoid therapy.

## ACKNOWLEDGMENT

The authors acknowledge the contributions of Letty M. P. Liu to previous editions of this chapter.

## ANNOTATED REFERENCES

Arieff AI, Ayus JC, Fraser CL. Hyponatraemia and death or permanent brain damage in healthy children. BMJ 1992;304:1218-22.
*Much concern has been displayed in recent years about iatrogenic hyponatremia caused by administration of hypotonic solutions. This study highlights the grave consequences of such errors.*
Constable PD. Hyperchloremic acidosis: the classic example of strong ion acidosis. Anesth Analg 2003;96:919-22.
*This review is an excellent description of alternative methods of evaluating acid–base status. The focus of this paper is on the physiology behind the acidosis created by large, rapid administration of normal saline.*
Friis-Hansen B. Body water compartments in children: changes during growth and related changes in body composition. Pediatrics 1961;28:169-81.
*This classic paper is important because it describes the developmental aspects of fluid compartments in children from infants to teenagers.*
Holliday MA, Friedman AL, Segar W, et al. Acute hospital-induced hyponatremia in children: a physiologic approach. J Pediatr 2004;145:584-7.
*This update to the authors' classic 1957 article addresses the problems associated with applying the original formula (4-2-1 rule) to perioperative fluid management. The authors present an alternative approach to perioperative fluid management with a focus on attenuating the antidiuretic hormone response to perioperative stress.*
Holliday MA, Segar WE. The maintenance need for water in parenteral fluid therapy. Pediatrics 1957;19:823-32.
*This classic paper represents the background for basic approaches to fluid management in pediatrics. This article discusses the fluid requirements in healthy children. This approach was not intended by the authors to be applied to perioperative fluid management with balanced salt solutions, although that has certainly been the case.*
Shires T, Williams J, Brown F. Acute change in extracellular fluids associated with major surgical procedures. Ann Surg 1961;154:803-10.
*This classic study from 1961 describes the phenomenon of fluid movement throughout the various compartments during surgical procedures. Specifically, it shows that, during surgery, plasma volume is supported at the expense of extravascular volume. The concept of third spacing of isotonic fluids is also described.*

## REFERENCES

Please see www.expertconsult.com

# Essentials of Hematology

## GREGORY J. LATHAM, MICHAEL J. EISSES, M.A. BENDER, AND CHARLES M. HABERKERN

| | |
|---|---|
| **The Basics** | Idiopathic Thrombocytopenic Purpura |
| Laboratory Values and Diagnostic Tests | **Coagulation Disorders** |
| Guidelines for Transfusion | Screening |
| **Hemolytic Anemias** | Von Willebrand Disease |
| Hereditary Spherocytosis | Hemophilia |
| Glucose-6-Phosphate Dehydrogenase Deficiency | Hypercoagulability |
| Hemoglobinopathies | **Cancer and Hematopoietic Stem Cell Transplantation** |
| **Thrombocytopenia** | Cancer |
| Platelet Disorders and Bleeding | Hematopoietic Stem Cell Transplantation |

HEMATOLOGIC DISORDERS IN CHILDHOOD may manifest in many ways. They may be the primary cause for a surgical procedure, such as hereditary spherocytosis (HS) in a child undergoing splenectomy, or a factor complicating a surgical procedure, such as sickle cell disease in a child undergoing tonsillectomy. Questions about hematologic problems such as anemia, thrombocytopenia, decreased or increased coagulation, childhood cancer, and hematopoietic stem cell transplantation (HSCT) are often raised in the perioperative setting.

In this chapter, we address the hematologic considerations and diseases that are of significant interest to pediatric anesthesiologists. We highlight considerations important to the hematologist that the anesthesiologist should incorporate in the care of a child.

## The Basics

### LABORATORY VALUES AND DIAGNOSTIC TESTS

What is a normal hematocrit or platelet count for an infant or child who comes to the operating room? Red blood cell (RBC), white blood cell, platelet, and coagulation indices evolve in various ways through late gestation, the neonatal period, infancy, and childhood (Table 9-1).

The term neonate has a relative polycythemia, reticulocytosis, and leukocytosis compared with the child. Neonatal platelet counts are similar to those of adults. Although in vitro function may be impaired for the first postnatal month, most in vivo assays of platelet function indicate normal or accelerated function. Preterm and term neonates have prolongation of the prothrombin time (PT) and activated partial thromboplastin time (aPTT) because of a relative deficiency in vitamin K–dependent factors and contact activation factors, respectively; however, concentrations of factor VIII and von Willebrand factor (vWF) are elevated.[1] The international normalized ratio (INR), a normalized PT, has an average value of 1.0 for all age groups. Fibrinogen concentrations are comparable between the term neonate and adult, although neonatal fibrinogen is qualitatively dysfunctional. The plasma concentrations of many anticoagulant factors (i.e., tissue factor pathway inhibitor, antithrombin, vitamin K–dependent glycoproteins, and proteins C and S) are decreased in preterm and term neonates. The quantity and quality of plasminogen are decreased in neonates, a condition that increases the risk for thrombosis, especially in a compromised infant.[1,2] Most of these differences between the neonate and older child or adult persist for 3 to 6 months postnatally.

After the immediate neonatal period, preterm and term infants experience physiologic anemia, presumably due to the downregulating effect of increased oxygen supply in extrauterine life on erythropoiesis and to the dilutional effect of a rapidly increasing blood volume. Preterm infants reach their nadir hemoglobin of 7 to 9 g/dL at 3 to 6 postnatal weeks, and term infants reach their nadir hemoglobin concentration of 9 to 11 g/dL at 8 to 12 postnatal weeks. Most hematologic values reach adult norms by the end of infancy (i.e., first postnatal year), although some continue to change gradually into the second decade. All of these changes underscore the importance of laboratory reports with age-adjusted standards.

There is no ideal single screening test to assess the *bleeding risk* of a child in the perioperative period. *Bleeding time* appears to be greater in the infant and child (and less in the neonate) than it is in the adult, but the range of values is wide and overlapping (see Table 9-1). Although this test is potentially helpful in predicting posttonsillectomy and adenoidectomy hemorrhage,[3] as well as hemorrhage after percutaneous renal[4] and liver[5] biopsy, there is little evidence to support its use as a screening test to predict bleeding in the presence of a careful, inclusive clinical history.[6,7]

The thromboelastogram has been used to investigate the coagulation status of children undergoing spinal fusion,[8] neurosurgical procedures,[9] and cardiopulmonary bypass for cardiothoracic procedures.[10] Although the thromboelastogram may provide useful information in the surgical setting to evaluate fibrinolysis, hypercoagulability, and other coagulation perturbations, its use is usually limited to clinical scenarios with dynamic coagulation changes, such as open heart surgery with cardiopulmonary bypass and liver transplantation. Platelet function analyzer (PFA-100)

**TABLE 9-1** Hematology Values at Different Ages

| Measurement* | Preterm 28-32 Weeks | Preterm 32-36 Weeks | Term Neonate | 1-Year-Old | Child | Adult |
|---|---|---|---|---|---|---|
| Hemoglobin (g/dL) | 12.9 | 13.6 | 16.8 | 12 | 13 | 15 |
| Hematocrit (%) | 40.9 | 43.6 | 55 | 36 | 38 | 45 |
| Reticulocyte count (%) | — | — | 5 | 1 | 1 | 1.6 |
| White blood cell count (/mm³) | 5,160 | 7,710 | 18,000 | 10,000 | 8,000 | 7,500 |
| Platelet count (/mm³) | 255,000 | 260,000 | 300,000 | 300,000 | 300,000 | 300,000 |
| Prothrombin time (second) | 15.4 | 13 | 13 | 11 | 11 | 12 |
| International normalized ratio (INR) | — | 1 | 1 | 1 | 1 | 1 |
| Activated partial thromboplastin time (second) | 108 | 53.6 | 42.9 | 30 | 31 | 28 |
| Fibrinogen (mg/dL) | 256 | 243 | 283 | 276 | 279 | 278 |
| Bleeding time (minute) | — | 3.5 | 3.5 | 6 | 7 | 5 |

Data from Andrew M. The relevance of developmental hemostasis to hemorrhagic disorders of newborns. Semin Perinatol 1997;21:70-85; Andrew M, Vegh P, Johnston M, et al. Maturation of the hemostatic system during childhood. Blood 1992;80:1998-2005; Goodnight SH, Hathaway WE. Disorders of hemostasis and thrombosis, a clinical guide, 2nd ed. New York: McGraw-Hill; 2001. p. 31-8; Ohls RK, Christensen RD. Development of the hematopoietic system. In: Behrman RE, Kliegman RM, Jenson HB, editors. Nelson textbook of pediatrics, 17th ed. Philadelphia: WB Saunders; 2004. p. 1599-1604.
*All values expressed as the mean.

analysis is an additional test that is increasingly used for the assessment of platelet abnormalities, and it has the benefit of avoiding some of the difficulties of obtaining a bleeding time in children. Although several studies suggest PFA-100 analysis is equivalent or superior to the bleeding time for detecting bleeding abnormalities, there is no consensus about its role in preoperative screening.[11] With the increasing use of newer agents that modify platelet function (e.g., platelet G protein–coupled receptor P2Y12 antagonists, glycoprotein GPIIb-IIIa complex antagonists), clinicians must understand that the thromboelastogram, PFA-100, and other methods for assessing platelet function may vary in their ability to monitor the effects of these agents and those of cyclooxygenase inhibitors.[12]

## GUIDELINES FOR TRANSFUSION

Critical analyses of the risks and benefits of transfusions in infants and children in the perioperative period have resulted in fewer transfusions. Even for infants and children in intensive care, a restrictive transfusion threshold (i.e., 7 g/dL) reduces transfusions without increasing morbidity compared with a liberal threshold (i.e., 9.5 to 10 g/dL).[13] Data from the United Kingdom's national audit of clinical transfusion, the Serious Hazards of Transfusion (SHOT), indicate that infants and children younger than 18 years of age are at greater risk for adverse transfusion-related reactions (37 and 18 in 100,000, respectively) than are adults (13 in 100,000). Most events were error related, such as administrative, laboratory, clinical judgment, and handling errors.[14]

Guidelines for RBC transfusion for infants and children in the perioperative setting should be consistent with those established by the American Society of Anesthesiologists Task Force on Blood Component Therapy, which propose that transfusion is not indicated for hemoglobin concentrations higher than 10 g/dL but is indicated for concentrations lower than 6 g/dL.[15] When the concentration is between 6 and 10 g/dL, packed red blood cells (PRBCs) should be transfused based on the child's vital signs, adequacy of oxygenation and perfusion, acuity and degree of blood loss, and other physiologic and surgical factors. When the concentration exceeds 10 g/dL, the decision to transfuse PRBCs to a neonate or infant should be based on the increased baseline concentrations of hemoglobin, increased oxygen consumption,

increased affinity of residual fetal hemoglobin for oxygen, absolute blood volume (i.e., 85 mL/kg for a term neonate and 100 mL/kg for a preterm neonate), and other physiologic and surgical factors applicable to all children. The threshold for transfusing a healthy neonate may be 7 g/dL in some clinical settings, but it may be 12 g/dL or higher for a neonate in other settings, such as significant lung disease requiring mechanical ventilation, chronic lung disease, cyanotic congenital heart disease, or heart failure.[16-18] For a preterm infant, the risks of hypovolemia, hypotension, acidosis, and postoperative apnea are magnified in the setting of operative blood loss and anemia. It is impossible to address all of the guidelines in this chapter, but many pediatric hematology and oncology consultants have clearly defined transfusion thresholds for their patient populations that should be reviewed preoperatively.

Guidelines for platelet transfusion have been published by consensus committees from France, the United Kingdom, and the United States; these reports are based on available evidence that has been gathered and critically reviewed (Table 9-2).[15,19-22] Without evidence that platelet function is significantly different in the healthy infant and child, these guidelines should be applicable to these patients. The decision to transfuse platelets must take into account underlying medical conditions, platelet transfusion history, current medications, surgical bleeding, surgical interventions (e.g., cardiopulmonary bypass), and all other factors that may affect platelet function and turnover.[23-27] Sevoflurane and propofol suppress[28] and enhance platelet aggregation in vitro.[29] Despite these effects on platelet aggregation, no change in the bleeding time has been reported, suggesting that the inhibitory effect does not impair hemostasis in vivo.[30]

Guidelines for the transfusion of other blood products, particularly fresh frozen plasma (FFP) and cryoprecipitate, have been established,[15,26,31] and they are discussed later in the context of coagulation disorders. Indications[32] for transfusing FFP are usually limited to the following:

1. Replacement of documented congenital or acquired coagulation factor deficiency when a specific sterilized or combined factor concentrate is unavailable, especially in the setting of anticipated or active bleeding
2. Acquired coagulopathy resulting from massive transfusion
3. Immediate reversal of warfarin's effect

**TABLE 9-2** Triggers for Platelet Transfusion

| Medical Condition or Procedure | Platelet Count (/mm³) |
| --- | --- |
| Stable hematology-oncology or chronically thrombocytopenic patient | 10,000-20,000 |
| Lumbar puncture in stable leukemic child | 10,000 |
| Bone marrow aspiration or biopsy | 20,000 |
| Gastrointestinal endoscopy in cancer patient | 20,000-40,000 |
| Disseminated intravascular coagulation | 20,000-50,000 |
| Fiberoptic bronchoscopy in hematopoietic stem cell transplantation patient | 20,000-50,000 |
| Neonatal alloimmune thrombocytopenia | 30,000 |
| Major surgery | 50,000 |
| Dilutional thrombocytopenia with massive transfusion | 50,000 |
| Spinal anesthesia | 50,000 |
| Cardiopulmonary bypass | 50,000-60,000 |
| Liver biopsy | 50,000-100,000 |
| Nonbleeding preterm infant | 60,000 |
| Obstetric epidural anesthesia | 70,000-100,000 |
| Neurosurgery | 100,000 |

Data from references 19, 20, 23, 26, 27, 265.

**TABLE 9-3** Indications for Leukocyte-Reduced Red Blood Cell Units

**Prevention of Alloimmunization**

Congenital hemolytic anemias (including sickle cell disease and thalassemia)

Hypoproliferative anemias likely to need multiple transfusions
   Aplastic anemia
   Myelodysplasia/myeloproliferative syndrome
   Plasma cell dyscrasias
   Hematopoietic stem cell transplants
   Hematopoietic malignancies

**Therapy for Preexisting Conditions**

Recurrent, severe febrile hemolytic transfusion reactions

Known HLA alloimmunization

**Possible Uses**

Alternative to cytomegalovirus-seronegative components (see Table 9-5)

Human immunodeficiency virus–infected patients

Modified from Simon TL, Alverson DC, AuBuchon J, et al. Practice parameter for the use of red blood cell transfusions: developed by the Red Blood Cell Administration Practice Guideline Development Task Force of the College of American Pathologists. Arch Pathol Lab Med 1998;122:130-8.

**TABLE 9-4** Indications for Irradiation of Cellular Blood Components

**Well-Defined Indications**

Hematopoietic stem cell transplantation

Actual or anticipated congenital cell-mediated immunodeficiency

Intrauterine transfusion or after intrauterine transfusion

Directed donation from blood relative or HLA-matched donor

Hodgkin disease

Acute lymphocytic leukemia

Immunocompromised organ transplant recipient

**Probable Indications**

Malignancy and organ transplantation treated with immunosuppressive therapy

Exchange transfusion in neonate

Extracorporeal membrane oxygenation in neonate

Low–birth-weight neonate (<1200 g)

Human immunodeficiency virus–infected patient with opportunistic infection

**Possible Indications**

Term neonate (<4 months)

Human immunodeficiency virus–infected patient

Modified from Simon TL, Alverson DC, AuBuchon J, et al. Practice parameter for the use of red blood cell transfusions: developed by the Red Blood Cell Administration Practice Guideline Development Task Force of the College of American Pathologists. Arch Pathol Lab Med 1998;122:130-8; Treleaven J, Gennery A, Marsh J, et al. Guidelines on the use of irradiated blood components prepared by the British Committee for Standards in Haematology blood transfusion task force. Br J Haematol 2010;152:35-51.

4. Coagulation support in disease processes such as disseminated intravascular coagulation and thrombotic thrombocytopenic purpura

5. A source of antithrombin III for children deficient of this inhibitor who require heparin

Cryoprecipitate should be administered only for anticipated or active bleeding in children with congenital fibrinogen deficiencies or von Willebrand disease who are unresponsive to desmopressin acetate (DDAVP) or for patients with acquired hypofibrinogenemia (less than 80 to 100 mg/dL) associated with massive transfusion.

Guidelines have been established by the College of American Pathologists and other transfusion study groups for leukocyte reduction of RBC units,[16] irradiation (x-ray or γ-ray) of cellular blood components,[33] and administration of cytomegalovirus-seronegative RBCs (Tables 9-3 to 9-5).[16] These guidelines are valuable when determining the specific choice of blood components that should be ordered and administered in the perioperative setting. For hematologic patients receiving chronic RBC transfusions, an extended phenotypic crossmatch and leukocyte reduction can decrease the risk of developing alloantibodies and transfusion reactions, especially in children of African descent if the local donor pool is primarily derived from Caucasian populations of Northern European descent.[34] For oncology patients, updated specific requirements for blood products including leukocyte reduction and irradiation are often indicated and should always be reviewed with oncology specialists.

## Hemolytic Anemias

Anemia commonly manifests in the perioperative setting, and primary hemolytic anemias can present unique and challenging problems for the anesthesiologist. Hemolytic syndromes are a group of disorders in which erythrocyte lysis often leads to anemia. Although RBCs in these disorders may be characterized by abnormal morphology and shorter life span, these parameters may be normal at baseline. Clinical signs of a hemolytic syndrome include anemia, splenomegaly, and jaundice, signs that

**TABLE 9-5** Indications for Cytomegalovirus-Seronegative or Leukocyte-Reduced Red Blood Cells for Prevention of Virus Transmission

**Well-Defined Indications**

Low–birth-weight neonate (<1200 g)

Human immunodeficiency virus–infected patient

Recipient of seronegative allogeneic organ or hematopoietic stem cell transplant or prospective recipient

Pregnant woman

Intrauterine transfusion

**Possible Indications**

Hodgkin disease or non-Hodgkin lymphoma

Recipient of immunosuppressive therapy

Candidate for autologous hematopoietic stem cell transplantation

Hereditary or acquired cellular immunodeficiency

**Probable Absence of Indications**

Seronegative term infant

Seropositive pregnant woman

Modified from Simon TL, Alverson DC, AuBuchon J, et al. Practice parameter for the use of red blood cell transfusions: developed by the Red Blood Cell Administration Practice Guideline Development Task Force of the College of American Pathologists. Arch Pathol Lab Med 1998;122:130-8.

may be apparent chronically or only during acute exacerbations of a disease process. Hemoglobinuria may be a late finding if massive hemolysis has occurred. Although not well studied, in theory any hemolytic disorder may alter nitric oxide (NO) metabolism.

Many of the hemolytic anemias that are significant to the anesthesiologist result from intracellular defects and can be classified as erythrocyte membrane defects, such as hereditary spherocytosis (HS); enzymatic defects, such as glucose-6-phosphate dehydrogenase (G6PD) deficiency; and qualitative and quantitative defects of hemoglobin, such as sickle cell disease and thalassemia. Other hemolytic anemias that may be encountered in the operating room are largely extracellularly mediated, such as transfusion-related hemolysis and other immune-mediated anemias (alloimmune or autoimmune); this group of anemias is not reviewed here.

## HEREDITARY SPHEROCYTOSIS

HS, the most common cause of inherited chronic hemolysis in North America and Northern Europe, has a prevalence of approximately 1 to 2 cases per 5000 people, if mild forms of the disease are included.[35-37] First described in 1871, HS is present in many ethnic populations, but rare in African American populations. Because 75% of children inherit the disease in an autosomal dominant pattern, there is often a family history of the disorder, although autosomal recessive mutations, de novo mutations, and incomplete penetrance have been reported.[37]

### Pathophysiology

Abnormalities in any of several erythrocyte membrane proteins, including the β subunit of spectrin, ankyrin, and band 3, can lead to HS. The variety of proteins affected and mutations observed in each gene account for the clinical heterogeneity of the disorder.[36] When the erythrocyte loses surface area, it changes from a biconcave disk to a sphere, which alters its stability and

flow pattern through the capillaries. The deformity leads to a loss of flexibility in the membrane, which makes it vulnerable to rupture, a condition that is worsened if the membrane surface area decreases by more than 3%.[37] Damaged erythrocytes are sequestered in the splenic capillaries, which can lead to splenomegaly. The combination of intravascular and extravascular hemolysis can result in anemia, which induces extramedullary erythropoiesis. The life span of the erythrocyte is reduced from 120 days to just a few days when the RBC membrane has been deformed. If large numbers of damaged erythrocytes are lysed, unconjugated bilirubin is released into the bloodstream, which causes jaundice and possibly gallstones in as many as 60% of children.[36] Membrane fragments from hemolytic reactions can lead to disseminated intravascular coagulation. Pulmonary hypertension may occur in the HS population, presumably as a result of hemolysis-induced alterations in NO metabolism.

### Clinical and Laboratory Features

Children may present at any age with the triad of anemia, splenomegaly, and jaundice, which often is aggravated by concomitant viral infection. Mild, moderate, and severe forms of HS occur and are characterized by variations in laboratory results and clinical correlates. HS can manifest soon after birth and should be considered in infants who are jaundiced after the first postnatal week; resulting hyperbilirubinemia can sometimes necessitate an exchange transfusion. Mild disease occurs in 20% of children with HS; these children only occasionally present with symptomatic bilirubinate gallstones before adolescence. Approximately 5% of children have severe HS characterized by chronic anemic (hemoglobin concentration less than 8 g/dL) and a need for chronic transfusions. The course of this disease may be complicated by viral infections such as parvovirus B19 infection, which can suppress reticulocyte production[37] and precipitate aplastic crises.

HS is most commonly suspected when numerous spherocytes with loss of central pallor appear on a peripheral smear. A complete blood cell count usually reveals a low hemoglobin and elevated reticulocyte count. Osmotic fragility remains the gold standard for the diagnosis of HS, but this test produces age-related results and must be performed by experienced laboratory technicians in a timely fashion. Increasingly, flow cytometry using eosin-5′-maleimide is being employed for diagnosis because it requires little blood and can be performed after overnight storage.[38] As a direct result of chronic hemolysis, unconjugated bilirubin and serum lactate dehydrogenase concentrations increase, and serum haptoglobin concentrations decrease. Thrombocytopenia may develop as a result of hypersplenism.

### Perioperative Considerations

Anemia, thrombocytopenia, and splenomegaly are the major considerations for a child with HS undergoing surgery. The most common disease-related operations performed in children with HS are splenectomy and cholecystectomy, individually or in combination, and these procedures may be performed by laparotomy or laparoscopy.

Splenectomy significantly increases red cell survival in most cases and reduces the severity of the anemia and jaundice. It is usually reserved for more severe cases of HS, characterized by severe anemia that require frequent RBC transfusions, poor growth, chronic fatigue, or evidence of extramedullary hematopoiesis (e.g., frontal bossing). Splenic enlargement in a child interested in participating in contact sports is another indication.[37] Splenectomy is ideally performed after the age of 6 years because of the increased risk of overwhelming infection by encapsulated organisms such as *Streptococcus pneumoniae, Neisseria meningitidis,* and *Haemophilus influenzae* type B in splenectomized younger children.[39] Preoperative vaccination against these organisms is essential unless surgery is required emergently. Guidelines for the indications and duration of postoperative penicillin prophylaxis vary among institutions.[36]

Splenectomies in children are more frequently performed laparoscopically than by open laparotomy because the former is associated with decreased pain, quicker return of bowel function, shorter hospital stay, and improved cosmetic result. Conversion from laparoscopic to open splenectomy is necessary in fewer than 10% of cases.[40] Partial splenectomies are increasingly performed because they allow retention of some immune function against bacterial infections in younger children while reducing the sequestration of spherocytes. However, residual splenic tissue can increase in size and necessitate total splenectomy at a later time.[41,42] If anemia recurs after splenectomy, it may indicate the presence of accessory splenic tissue that was unrecognized initially. Transient postsplenectomy thrombocytosis marked by dramatic increases in platelet counts may also occur in children,[35] in addition to a general increase in the risk of thromboembolic disease.

Gallstones occur in 21% to 63% of children with HS, but cholecystectomy is usually performed only when children are symptomatic with cholelithiasis. Children who undergo splenectomy and who also have radiographically identified gallstones may undergo concurrent cholecystectomy, whether the stones are symptomatic or not.[43-45]

Table 9-6 summarizes the clinical features and important perioperative considerations for the child with HS undergoing incidental or disease-related surgical procedures.

---

**TABLE 9-6** Perioperative Concerns for Patients with Hereditary Spherocytosis

**Preoperative Considerations**

Hemoglobin, reticulocyte count, platelet count

History of transfusions and special blood requirements (e.g., extended phenotypic matching, leukocyte reduction)

History of infections, aplastic crises, and presplenectomy vaccinations

Presplenectomy antibiotic prophylaxis and immunization when indicated

**Intraoperative Considerations**

Appropriate antibiotic coverage

Attention to physiologic effects of laparoscopy on circulatory and respiratory function

Potential for significant blood loss (unusual in splenectomy and cholecystectomy)

Judicious use of regional anesthesia, intramuscular medications, nasogastric tubes, nasal intubation, and other methods when platelet count is low

Limited use of medications with potential bleeding risk (e.g., ketorolac)

**Postoperative Considerations**

Sequential hemoglobin determinations and platelet counts

Potential thrombocytosis: management as recommended by hematology consultants

Infection risk

---

## GLUCOSE-6-PHOSPHATE DEHYDROGENASE DEFICIENCY

G6PD deficiency causes hemolysis in the presence of various oxidative stressors. It is the most common enzyme deficiency in humans, affecting approximately 400 million people worldwide. This enzyme deficiency is inherited in an X-linked, recessive fashion. Although males are most commonly affected, females (heterozygous or homozygous for the gene) may have clinical manifestations of the disease. More than 100 variants have been described, including a relatively mild form that affects about 10% of African American males (i.e., G6PD A−) and a more severe form that affects Italians, Greeks, and other populations in the Mediterranean, African, and Asian regions (i.e., G6PD Mediterranean).[46-48] This deficiency is prevalent in geographic areas where the incidence of malaria is high, presumably because G6PD deficiency may attenuate the severity of malarial infections.

### Pathophysiology

G6PD plays an important role in the hexose monophosphate/pentose phosphate shunt, which is essential for normal energy metabolism in erythrocytes. G6PD generates the reduced form of nicotinamide adenine dinucleotide phosphate (NADPH). NADPH maintains glutathione in the reduced form (GSH), which reduces peroxides and protects cells from oxidative damage in the course of normal biochemical events or in the event of excess free oxygen radical generation. Superoxide ion or hydrogen peroxide, or both, can oxidize hemoglobin, which then precipitates as insoluble membrane inclusions. These inclusions, together with the oxidative damage to cell membranes, lead to cell damage. Erythrocytes are particularly sensitive to oxidative damage because of their lack of synthetic activity. In the presence of oxidants and free radicals (e.g., produced by infection or by ingestion of certain medications and foods), this cascade of events may precipitate hemolysis in the G6PD-deficient child.[46,48]

### Clinical and Laboratory Features

Clinical symptoms of G6PD deficiency may be deceptively variable, and they may occur in the neonatal period or in older age groups as episodic or chronic hemolytic anemia. Presenting signs include anemia and jaundice; in severe cases, these signs can be followed by lumbar and abdominal pain and by renal failure. Acute illness such as diabetic acidosis or ingestion of a variety of substances may precipitate a hemolytic event (Table 9-7). Hemolysis may range from benign and transitory to severe and life-threatening; the latter situation is more likely if the triggering agent is not eliminated or controlled. Laboratory findings include normocytic anemia, increased reticulocyte count and serum bilirubin concentration, and presence of Heinz bodies in the peripheral blood smear.

### Perioperative Considerations

In the perioperative setting, G6PD deficiency does not usually cause problems if the triggering agents are avoided by susceptible children and the precipitating causes are treated or eliminated (Table 9-8). Monitoring for and treatment of possible complications are appropriate; transfusion is rarely required.

Administration of large or excessive doses of medications such as prilocaine, benzocaine, and sodium nitroprusside may trigger hemolysis in G6PD-deficient children in the perioperative setting.[46,48-50] Although these children can reduce methemoglobin that is normally produced by these agents, G6PD-deficient children may not tolerate large amounts of potent oxidizing agents (i.e., superoxide ion and hydrogen peroxide) produced by

**TABLE 9-7** Agents That May Precipitate Hemolysis in Patients with Glucose-6-Phosphate Dehydrogenase Deficiency

**Antibiotics**

Sulfonamides

Trimethoprim-sulfamethoxazole (Bactrim, Septrin)

Dapsone

Chloramphenicol

Nitrofurantoin

Nalidixic acid

**Antimalarials**

Chloroquine

Hydroxychloroquine

Primaquine

Quinine

Mepacrine

**Other Medications**

Aspirin

Phenacetin

Sulfasalazine

Methyldopa

Vitamin C (large doses)

Hydralazine

Procainamide

Quinidine

**Chemicals**

Moth balls (naphthalene)

Methylene blue

**Food**

Fava (broad) beans

---

**TABLE 9-8** Perioperative Concerns for Patients with Glucose-6-Phosphate Dehydrogenase Deficiency

**Preoperative Considerations**

History of hemolysis and precipitating factors

Hemoglobin, reticulocyte count

**Intraoperative Considerations**

Avoidance of triggering agents

Caution in use of high doses of agents that increase methemoglobin, especially in infants

Hemoglobin and urine output in high-risk settings (e.g., cardiopulmonary bypass)

**Postoperative Considerations**

Hemoglobin, reticulocyte count, urine output if hemolysis

---

methemoglobin. Infants may be particularly susceptible to symptomatic methemoglobinemia (because of their low NADPH dehydrogenase activity) and to methemoglobin-induced hemolysis if they are G6PD deficient. Treatment of methemoglobinemia with methylene blue is contraindicated in these infants because the agent itself may precipitate hemolysis.[42] Hemolysis has occurred during cardiopulmonary bypass in G6PD-deficient children,[50,51] and methemoglobinemia has occurred in a child with partial G6PD deficiency after application of EMLA cream, a eutectic mixture of local anesthetics.[52]

## HEMOGLOBINOPATHIES

### Sickle Cell Disease

First identified by Herrick about 100 years ago, sickle cell disease is a group of inherited hemoglobinopathies with a diverse worldwide prevalence. The disease affects about 1 in 375 African American and 1 in 20,000 Hispanic births.[53] The spectrum of the disease includes sickle cell anemia (HbSS), which accounts for about 70% of the American sickle cell disease population; sickle cell/hemoglobin C disease (HbSC), accounting for about 20%; sickle cell/β-thalassemia (HbSβ), accounting for about 10%; and a host of other, uncommon sickle variants whose prevalence is increasing over time.[54] HbSβ includes HbSβ+ and HbSβ0 thalassemias; the distinction depends on whether normal hemoglobin A (HbA) is expressed at all or in only a small concentration. HbSβ0, HbSC, and sickle cell/hemoglobin D disease (HbSD) and additional rare forms have the potential to sickle as severely as HbSS. Sickle cell trait (HbAS), in which approximately 40% of hemoglobin is hemoglobin S, occurs in about 8% of African Americans and in a much smaller percentage of Hispanic and other American subpopulations. The sickle gene is found commonly in Africa, Mediterranean areas, southwestern Asia, and other areas where malaria has been historically endemic and for which the gene is protective. Sickle hemoglobinopathies have many implications for perioperative care because they increase perioperative morbidity and mortality.

### Pathophysiology

Hemoglobin A is composed of two α- and two β-globin chains. Hemoglobin S is caused by a mutant β-globin gene on chromosome 11, which leads to a single amino acid substitution (valine for glutamate at position 6). Replacement of negatively charged and hydrophilic glutamate by noncharged and hydrophobic valine leads to instability of the hemoglobin molecule and decreased solubility of the molecule when deoxygenated. Hemoglobin polymers form, generating long helical strands and inducing a process that leads to hemoglobin precipitation and hemolysis.[55]

Classically, the pathophysiology and clinical complications of sickle cell disease were thought to be related primarily to the accumulation of sickled erythrocytes in the microvasculature in the setting of factors that promote hemoglobin crystallization (i.e., hypoxia, acidosis, and cellular dehydration) and interfere with peripheral perfusion (i.e., dehydration and hypothermia). This accumulation of sickled cells was thought to compromise the microcirculation, producing ischemia and thereby generating a spiral of red cell sickling and end-organ compromise.

The pathophysiologic process in sickle cell disease is much more complex than originally thought.[55-57] Inflammation, vascular endothelial adhesion abnormalities, platelets, and coagulation cascade activation all contribute to vaso-occlusive episodes. The sickle red cell membrane, exposed to the destructive oxidant effects of intracellular iron, develops altered transmembrane ion transport pathways, which lead to altered permeability to sodium, potassium, and calcium, causing dehydration of the cell and irreversible sickling.[58] Membrane abnormalities of phospholipid content also contribute to its deformability, and exposure of phosphatidyl serine facilitates activation of the clotting cascade. These and other factors lead to entrapment of irreversibly sickled red cells in the microcirculation, activation of coagulation and inflammatory pathways, ischemia, and infarction of tissue. At the same time, chronic intravascular hemolysis decreases production of NO, while increased scavenging decreases the bioavailability of NO. The resulting NO deficiency causes endothelial dysfunction and disease complications such as pulmonary hypertension, priapism, and skin ulceration.[58,59]

### Clinical and Laboratory Features and Treatment

Sickle cell disease is a multisystem process involving potentially most organs of the body and often necessitating surgical intervention. Based on data collected in the early 1990s, approximately one third of patients with HbSS disease have progressive disease leading to organ dysfunction and death; about half have significant but less devastating disease; and the remainder have a reasonably stable, slowly progressive clinical course.[60] Therapeutic interventions and genetic factors account in large part for the differences in outcome. Children with persistence of hemoglobin F (which itself protects against the effects of deoxygenation on red cells) and those with HbSC or HbSβ+ have fewer complications than those with HbSS or HbSβ⁰.

Early diagnosis and treatment of sickle cell disease have been facilitated by the widespread use of universal neonatal screening, which was first used in the state of New York in 1975. Most screening programs for sickle cell disease use isoelectric focusing of an eluate from dried blood spot samples, a technique that is also used to screen for other disorders. A few programs use high-performance liquid chromatography. Because a small percentage of children with sickle cell disease are not African American (i.e., Native American, Hispanic, and Caucasian),[53] selective screening may not detect all affected infants. As of 2006, all 50 states and the District of Columbia screen all neonates for sickle hemoglobinopathies. Families of infants diagnosed with sickle trait (HbAS) on neonatal screening may not be made aware of the diagnosis, but these infants rarely develop significant clinical problems in the perioperative period.

Affected children born within the United States before universal neonatal screening and those born outside the United States and not receiving regular health care may not have received a diagnosis and appropriate care before surgery. Notwithstanding the controversy over the utility of nonselective preoperative screening,[61] children at risk whose hemoglobin status is unknown preoperatively should be tested with a sickle-screening test, followed by a hemoglobin electrophoretic evaluation if screening is positive. However, infants younger than 6 months of age may have a false-negative screening test result because of presence of fetal hemoglobin, although electrophoresis is diagnostic at all ages. Children older than 10 years of age with a normal hemoglobin value, standard peripheral blood smear, and unremarkable clinical history are probably at a reduced risk for clinically significant hemoglobinopathy.[62]

Common clinical symptoms of sickle cell disease in children include chronic hemolytic anemia, recurrent vaso-occlusive episodes leading to pain, acute chest syndrome (ACS), infection, renal insufficiency, osteonecrosis, and cholelithiasis. Pulmonary hypertension, priapism, and skin ulcerations are related to the degree of red cell hemolysis.[63] Chronic pulmonary and neurologic disease (e.g., stroke) are additional causes of significant morbidity and mortality.[54] In the perioperative period, the most common complications in sickle cell children include ACS (about 10%), fever or infection (about 7%), vaso-occlusive episodes (about 5%), and transfusion-related events (about 10%).[64]

Chronic hemolytic anemia is a hallmark of HbSS disease. It is characterized by a baseline hemoglobin value of 5 to 9 g/dL (often more than 9 g/dL in HbSC disease), reticulocytosis (5% to 10%), and a distinctive red cell morphology observed on a peripheral smear.[57] Chronic hemolysis is associated with increased red cell turnover and a propensity to form biliary stones. It may be complicated by other anemic events, such as acute splenic sequestration, typically occurring in infants and young children after a viral illness; and acute aplastic anemia, typically associated with parvovirus B19 infection. For some children, chronic and acute severe anemia are managed with RBC transfusions, although these children are prone to develop alloantibodies to RBC antigens, and untreated iron overload can lead to life-threatening cirrhosis and cardiac failure. Hydroxyurea is used to prevent vaso-occlusive episodes and end-organ damage. Most children are maintained on chronic folic acid therapy to prevent megaloblastic erythropoiesis that can result from the increased red cell production.

Vaso-occlusive episodes in sickle cell disease occur as a result of episodic microvasculature occlusions at one or more sites. The occlusive process occurs most commonly in the phalanges (i.e., dactylitis or hand-foot syndrome), long bones, ribs, sternum, spine, and the pelvis; it also can occur in the mesenteric microvasculature, producing abdominal pain that may mimic a surgical acute abdomen. Vaso-occlusive episodes are managed with hydration, warming, acute and chronic pain management (including opioids, antiinflammatory agents, and complementary modalities), and in-hospital care. It is essential to foster an ideal environment for pain control (e.g., calm, pleasant distractions, supportive personnel and objects). For children who have frequent or severe crises, oral hydroxyurea therapy has been effective in decreasing the frequency of events through several mechanisms, including inhibiting hemoglobin precipitation by increasing fetal hemoglobin concentrations, reducing the white blood cell count, modifying the inflammatory response, and facilitating NO metabolism.[59,65,66] Inhaled NO may prove to be effective therapy for vaso-occlusive episodes.[67]

ACS is characterized by acute respiratory symptoms concurrent with a new infiltrate observed on the chest radiograph.[68] ACS frequently occurs 2 to 3 days after a vaso-occlusive episode, and although its clinical presentation varies, it often includes fever, tachypnea, cough, and hypoxemia. The process may be self-limited over a period of a few days, or it may progress to respiratory failure (15%) and even death. The inconsistent presentation in part reflects the complex and variable pathogenesis of ACS. An episode may have a single or multiple causes, including infection (i.e., bacteria [often *Chlamydia* or *Mycoplasma*], viruses, and mixed flora), pulmonary fat embolism, pulmonary infarction, and pulmonary hemorrhage.[69] Acute management includes supportive care and oxygen, antibiotics to cover encapsulated and atypical organisms, bronchodilators, pain control, ventilatory support as needed, and transfusion. Incentive spirometry or continuous positive airway pressure can be helpful, especially in the perioperative setting. Hydroxyurea therapy and chronic transfusion therapy decrease the frequency of ACS, whereas inhaled NO attenuates the process acutely.[59,70-72] Airway reactivity is also common in children with sickle cell disease, in part due to NO deficiency, and it is responsive to bronchodilator therapy.[73,74] In later life, children with sickle cell disease may develop restrictive lung disease and pulmonary hypertension as a result of repeated ACS-induced lung injury and chronic inflammation. NO deficiency, the result of decreased production, increased consumption, or altered metabolism, may also play an important role in these processes.[63,68,75]

Infection is a common problem in this disease because of deficits in the immunologic system and the specific effects of splenic atrophy and dysfunction that occur over the first few years of life.[56] As a result of susceptibility to overwhelming infection by *S. pneumoniae* and *H. influenzae* type B, young children receive penicillin prophylaxis until 6 years of age and bacteria-specific immunizations. A host of infectious organisms have been implicated in ACS, and infection with gram-negative organisms (e.g., osteomyelitis caused by *Salmonella*) is common in older children and adults.[69]

Stroke is a devastating complication that occurs in children with sickle cell disease. A history of overt strokes is elicited in 10% or more of these children, and silent strokes occur in another approximately 15%; one fourth of children are at risk for motor or cognitive deficits at the time of presentation for surgery.[76,77] A child's first stroke often appears as early as 2 to 5 years of age.[78,79] Risk factors include a reduced hemoglobin concentration, increased concentration of HbS, increased leukocyte count, and a history of dactylitis. Strokes may be precipitated by pain episodes, ACS, and infection.[80] Children suffering an acute stroke are managed supportively with exchange transfusion to reduce the concentration of HbS to less than 30% and then chronic intermittent transfusions to minimize the risk of recurrence.[81]

The thrust of the current management of stroke is prevention. Based on the findings of the Stroke Prevention Trials (STOP 1 and 2), children are assessed annually by transcranial Doppler, and children with evidence of cerebrovascular compromise and some of those with magnetic resonance imaging abnormalities are managed with chronic transfusion therapy to minimize the risk of a stroke.[82-84]

Renal abnormalities in sickle cell disease develop from repeated sludging episodes, which may cause thrombosis, progressive infarction, and necrosis of the renal medulla. Proteinuria, hematuria, hyposthenuria, renal tubular acidosis, and other clinical abnormalities occur. Acute and chronic renal failure may develop.[85,86] Renal dialysis and transplantation have been successful therapeutic interventions for this population.[87]

The clinical picture of sickle cell disease is altered to various degrees by concomitant qualitative and quantitative changes of hemoglobin. Sickle cell trait (HbAS) usually is benign, although it may be characterized by hematuria and hyposthenuria,[87,88] and sickling may occur with HbAS under extremely altered physiologic circumstances (e.g., cardiopulmonary bypass).[89,90] There is a small but significant risk of pulmonary emboli and sudden death with extreme exertion by individuals with HbAS, which has led to the mandatory offer of testing to all National Collegiate Athletic Association (NCAA) athletes.[91]

Children with HbSC disease usually have a greater baseline hemoglobin concentration and fewer complications than those with HbSS disease; delayed splenic autoinfarction reduces their risk for infection in early childhood.[62] However, children with HbSC disease are more likely to have proliferative retinopathy and avascular necrosis of bone.[56]

Children with HbSβ⁰ (i.e., one sickle globin allele and one thalassemic allele expressing no β-globin) have a course identical to that of HbSS, whereas those with HbSβ⁺ (i.e., one sickle globin allele and one thalassemic allele expressing β-globin at a reduced level) tend to have a more benign course that is proportional to the amount of normal β-globin expression. The coexistence of hemoglobin S with α-thalassemia produces a variable clinical picture, but it may predispose children to a greater incidence of pain episodes.[62]

In addition to the treatment modalities mentioned earlier, many new and experimental modalities show promise in the treatment of sickle cell disease and its complications. They include induction of hemoglobin F by short-chain fatty acids such as butyrate or demethylating agents such as decitabine; membrane-active medications such as the Gardos channel inhibitors, magnesium; and antiadhesion therapies. New therapeutic targets are being identified, such a BCL11A, a zinc finger protein that plays a key role in the silencing of fetal globin genes. Reduction of BCL11A results in an induction of fetal globin.[92] Hematopoietic stem cell transplantation (HSCT) is increasingly used as a curative intervention for sickle cell disease when instituted before development of organ dysfunction, but its application is limited in part by the lack of suitable donors.[56,93] To circumvent this limitation, gene therapy protocols using a child's own stem cells have been approved for use.

### Perioperative Considerations

Perioperative morbidity and mortality are greater in children with sickle cell disease than in the general population. These children often require surgical procedures; the most common are cholecystectomy[94]; ear, nose, and throat procedures[95]; and orthopedic procedures (especially hip procedures for osteonecrosis).[96] Placement of long-term vascular access for transfusions, antibiotics, analgesia, and other therapies is frequently performed. The Cooperative Study of Sickle Cell Disease reported that 7% of all deaths among children with this disease were related to surgery.[54] Early reviews reported perioperative mortality rates as great as 10% and morbidity rates as great as 50% for children with sickle cell disease.[97-100] Studies published in the 1990s indicated that the 30-day mortality rate was about 1%.[101] In a group of more than 600 patients managed according to standard guidelines of care and prospectively studied, the incidence of any complication was about 30%, and the incidences of ACS and pain crisis were 10% and 5%, respectively.[64] Patient factors (e.g., age, history of pulmonary disease, number of prior hospitalizations) and surgical factors (i.e., invasive or superficial) appear to affect the incidence of complications. The impact of newer interventions and technologies (e.g., laparoscopic and robotically assisted cholecystectomy and splenectomy)[102-104] on perioperative morbidity and mortality rates is unclear.

The principles of optimal perioperative care are based on maintaining optimal physiologic parameters throughout the perioperative period, avoiding factors that may precipitate a sickle crisis, optimizing pain management, and close consultation among hematologists, surgeons, and anesthesiologists (Table 9-9).[105] The child with sickle cell disease who is undergoing surgery should be viewed and managed primarily as a hematology patient whose care is being shared with, rather than assumed by, the surgeon and anesthesiologist during the perioperative period. Avoiding unnecessary and potentially dangerous surgical procedures (e.g., exploratory laparotomy to rule out appendicitis in a child who is experiencing an abdominal pain crisis) and minimizing perioperative complications should be the focus of the multidisciplinary care team. Based on a survey of perioperative management of sickle cell disease among anesthesiologists in North America, most anesthesiologists do consult with hematologists in all cases or on a case-by-case basis.[106]

Although there is no evidence to support or refute many of the long-standing guidelines for perioperative care and individual

**TABLE 9-9** Perioperative Concerns for Patients with Sickle Cell Disease

**Preoperative Considerations**

Screening if unknown status in at-risk children

Primary management by hematology service (in most circumstances)

History of acute chest syndrome, vaso-occlusive pain crises, hospitalizations, transfusions, transfusion reactions

Neurologic assessment (e.g., strokes, cognitive limitations)

History of analgesic and other medication use

Hematocrit

Oxygen saturation (on room air), chest radiograph

Pulmonary function tests (when appropriate)

Echocardiography (when appropriate)

Neurologic imaging (for recent changes)

Renal function studies

Transfusion crossmatch (e.g., antibody-matched, leukocyte reduced, sickle negative)

Transfusion to correct anemia (in most circumstances)

Parenteral hydration for *nil per os* (NPO) status

Pain management

Aggressive bronchodilator therapy

Appropriate antibiotic therapy, including presplenectomy antibiotics and immunizations (as indicated)

**Intraoperative Considerations**

Maintenance of oxygenation, perfusion, normal acid–basis status, temperature, hydration

Availability of appropriately prepared blood (as indicated)

Replacement of blood loss

Anesthetic technique appropriate for procedure and postoperative analgesic requirements

Attention to physiologic effects of laparoscopy on circulatory and respiratory function

Appropriate antibiotic therapy

Judicious use of tourniquets, cell saver, and cardiopulmonary bypass

**Postoperative Considerations**

Management by hematology service

Monitoring for complications, especially acute chest syndrome and vaso-occlusive pain crises

Maintenance of oxygen saturation monitoring and supplementation as needed, including supplemental oxygen the first 24 hours regardless of oxygen saturation

Appropriate hydration (oral plus parenteral)

Appropriate antibiotic therapy

Aggressive pain management

Early mobilization

Incentive spirometry (possibly with continuous or bilateral positive airway pressure) and bronchodilator therapy

---

practices vary widely,[106] it seems appropriate to avoid the specific factors that may promote intravascular sickling: hypoxia, acidosis, hyperthermia, hypothermia, and dehydration.[55] Meticulous attention to pain management is also essential because perioperative vaso-occlusive pain is common and is associated with ACS. Monitoring of vital signs throughout the perioperative period is mandatory, especially monitoring of oxygenation with pulse oximetry. Oxygen saturation as determined by pulse oximetry may underestimate measured oxygen saturation in patients with sickle cell disease, although usually not to a clinically significant degree.[107,108] Because ACS, a common (10%) and potentially life-threatening complication of surgery, occurs 1 to 3 days postoperatively, it is important to extend adherence to guidelines of care into the postoperative period, regardless of the apparent well-being of the child.[64] In light of the renal concentrating defect found in these patients, perioperative hydration is important to maintain and may require in-hospital preoperative care, although overhydration may compromise vulnerable cardiovascular and respiratory physiology.

Transfusion in the perioperative period remains a controversial subject.[109] Transfusion of non-HbS RBCs to a child with sickle cell disease has several beneficial effects: correction of anemia, dilution of HbS red cells, compensation for blood loss, and prevention of some complications (e.g., stroke). However, transfusion is not without risks, including alloimmunization,[34,110] transfusion reactions (about 7% in the perioperative period),[64] infection, iron overload, time, and expense. Although there have been many reports of surgery performed safely in children with sickle cell disease without preoperative transfusion,[111] uncontrolled studies indicate that preoperative transfusion does decrease the rate of perioperative complications.[94,101] The Preoperative Transfusion in Sickle Cell Disease Study Group demonstrated prospectively in 604 operations (70% were cholecystectomies and otolaryngologic and orthopedic operations) that simple transfusion (i.e., correction of preoperative anemia to 10 g/dL with straight transfusion) was as effective as aggressive transfusion (i.e., lowering the preoperative HbS level to less than 30%, often with exchange transfusion) in preventing perioperative complications and was associated with fewer transfusion-related complications in children.[64]

To directly determine if transfusion prevents perioperative complications in the current era of surgical and anesthesia practices, an international randomized trial was initiated, the Transfusion Alternatives Preoperatively in Sickle Cell Disease (TAPS) trial. However, this trial was halted in March 2011 due to an excessive number of complications in the nontransfusion group. Although the final results of TAPS have not been published, it remains prudent to follow prior recommendations for transfusion for moderate and complicated operations in sickle cell patients. It is currently recommended that most children with HbSS undergoing most surgical procedures receive preoperative correction of anemia with simple transfusion to a hemoglobin concentration of about 10 g/dL. Children maintained on chronic transfusion programs (e.g., stroke prevention) should continue such management preoperatively. Recommendations for children with HbSC disease are less clear because these children typically maintain a baseline hemoglobin concentration at about 10 g/dL. For HbSC children who have a history of ACS, frequent pain crises, underlying pulmonary disease, or other complications, it is recommended that they receive selective preoperative exchange transfusion to reduce the HbS concentration without increasing total hemoglobin.[112] Because of the high risk of alloimmunization in the sickle cell population, blood to be administered to these patients should undergo extended phenotype matching, including Rh, Cc, D, Ee, and Kell in addition to ABO[84,113]; leukocyte reduction; and sickle cell screening. Directed donation of blood from family members should be avoided if the child is a hematopoietic stem cell transplant candidate because it can lead to alloimmunization and later graft rejection.

Anesthetic technique does not have a clear effect on perioperative outcomes for children with sickle cell disease.[114] Inhalational anesthetics do not affect the sickling process, although there is some experimental evidence suggesting that halothane may increase the viscosity of sickled blood.[115] Pharmacokinetics of some agents commonly used with general anesthesia such as atracurium may be altered in this population.[116] Regional anesthesia has been associated with an increased risk of postoperative complications in one retrospective study,[101] but it has not been shown to affect perioperative outcome in others.[94,96] Vasodilatory and analgesic properties of regional anesthesia can be effective in the management of vaso-occlusive episodes and priapism and in providing perioperative anesthetic care.[117,118]

Hyperventilation should be avoided because of its potential to reduce cerebral perfusion in children at an increased risk for stroke.[119] The use of a tourniquet in HbSS and HbAS diseases has been questioned.[120-122] However, tourniquets have been applied intraoperatively for up to 2 hours without complication, and the predominance of evidence supports their safe use as long as they are used carefully and selectively in combination with general guidelines of perioperative care (see Chapter 30).[123-126] Intraoperative blood salvage using cell saver devices has been used safely in sickle cell patients,[127] although there is some evidence that the salvage device itself may produce sickling in the processed blood, even sickle trait blood.[128] Cardiopulmonary bypass seems to be an optimal setting in which to induce sickling, given the cold, hypoxic, acidotic, and stagnant environment created. Although there are reports of bypass surgery conducted in children with HbSS or HbAS with standard bypass procedures without transfusion,[129-132] these children usually are managed with aggressive exchange transfusion before or during bypass.

## Thalassemias

Thalassemia disorders are among the most common genetic disorders worldwide, and they are characterized by a perturbation of the normal 1:1 ratio of α to β polypeptide chains, usually due to reduced synthesis of one polypeptide. The clinical severity of the disease in a child is a function of the degree of alteration of the synthetic ratio, ranging from an asymptomatic carrier state to chronic symptomatic hemolytic anemia to fetal death due to hydrops fetalis. α-Thalassemias commonly affect children of Southeast Asian descent and occur in those of African and Mediterranean descent. β-Thalassemias affect primarily children of Mediterranean, African, and Southeast Asian descent. Whereas state neonatal assays screening for HbS can often detect many forms of α-thalassemia, these tests can detect only profound forms of β-thalassemia because of the low levels of adult β chains present in the neonate. The concomitant presence of qualitatively abnormal hemoglobins (e.g., HbS, HbE) affects the clinical course of thalassemia disorders. The primary hemolytic anemia and the therapy used in the treatment of the disease may affect perioperative care.

### Pathophysiology

Anemia in thalassemia is the result of hemolysis and ineffective erythropoiesis; the latter is the result of accelerated cell apoptosis triggered in part by excess deposition of unpaired globin chains in erythroid precursors.[133] Unpaired globin subunits are oxidized and form hemichromes, whose rate of formation determines rate of hemolysis. Precipitation of hemichromes leads to a complex process that includes release of toxic agents and formation of reactive oxygen species; alteration of red cell membranes, causing

cells to become rigid, aggregate, and disintegrate; and activation of the coagulation process. As a result of chronic anemia and ineffective erythropoiesis, bone expansion and extramedullary hematopoiesis may develop in the liver and spleen, and marrow space expansion may occur at sites such as the cranium and paravertebral areas, thereby causing disfiguring bony changes.

### Clinical and Laboratory Features and Treatment

The disease picture in α-thalassemia reflects complete loss of expression of one to four α-globin genes. As a four-gene globin deletion, it is characterized by hydrops and in utero or perinatal death unless diagnosed early and supported with in utero transfusions. As a three-gene deletion, or hemoglobin H (HbH) disease, it is relatively benign, characterized by chronic hemolytic anemia, which may be exacerbated by exposure to stress and oxidants.[134,135] The few patients requiring intermittent transfusion therapy usually have a two-gene deletion along with a hemoglobin Constant Spring (HbCS) mutation. A two-gene deletion alone is characterized by mild, clinically insignificant microcytic anemia. A one-gene deletion is characterized by a silent carrier state with no anemia or microcytosis.

The clinical picture in β-thalassemia reflects partial or complete loss of expression of the β-globin genes. The broad spectrum of disease results from the number of genes affected and the degree to which each is affected. When only one β-globin gene is affected (i.e., β-thalassemia trait), mild microcytic anemia is the primary clinical manifestation. When both β-globin genes are affected, the clinical picture may be mild to moderate (i.e., thalassemia intermedia) or severe (i.e., thalassemia major or Cooley anemia), requiring chronic transfusions. Children with hemoglobin E (HgE)/β-thalassemia have symptoms ranging from very mild to severe, depending on the level of expression of the mutant β-globin gene.

The clinical problems in thalassemia are those associated with chronic anemia: the physiologic response to the need for increased erythropoiesis, transfusions to maintain a hemoglobin concentration greater than 9 g/dL, iron overload from excess transfusions and pardoxical increased iron absorption, and chelation therapy.[134] Clinical problems include transfusion-associated alloimmunization and infection, splenomegaly, bone abnormalities (due to extramedullary hematopoiesis, chelation therapy, and other factors), endocrine dysfunction (including hypogonadism, hypopituitarism, and diabetes mellitus), short stature, pulmonary hypertension, venous thrombosis and thromboembolism, and cardiomyopathy (primarily due to iron overload). Thalassemia patients may be hypercoagulable,[136] a condition that may be exaggerated after splenectomy.[136,137]

Routine therapies used to treat severe diseases and to prevent complications include phenotypic matching and leukocyte reduction of transfused blood, chelation therapy, and hormone and vitamin D therapy. When an appropriate donor is available, HSCT is recommended before severe liver damage occurs because it provides a potential cure for thalassemia. To ameliorate the course of the disease, other therapies are being investigated, including administration of erythropoietin, fetal hemoglobin modifiers (e.g., hydroxyurea, butyrate), and antioxidants. Gene therapy trials are ongoing, and at least one patient has become transfusion independent.[138]

### Perioperative Considerations

Children with moderate or severe thalassemia may require cholecystectomy, splenectomy, and vascular access placement for

**TABLE 9-10** Perioperative Concerns for Patients with Thalassemia

**Preoperative Considerations**

Hemoglobin

Transfusion crossmatch if appropriate (antibody-matched, leukocyte-reduced source for frequently transfused children)

Evaluation for endocrine dysfunction (e.g., diabetes mellitus, hypopituitarism)

Cardiac function, including echocardiogram (when appropriate)

Hepatic function, awareness of risk of cirrhosis and iron or virus-induced damage

Airway evaluation

Presplenectomy antibiotics and immunizations (when appropriate)

Preparation for possible difficult airway

**Intraoperative Considerations**

Careful positioning of demineralized extremities

Attention to cardiovascular function, including postsplenectomy hypertension

Attention to physiologic effects of laparoscopy on circulatory and respiratory function

Prophylaxis for thromboembolism

**Postoperative Considerations**

Monitoring of cardiac function

Prophylaxis for thromboembolism

frequent transfusions.[139] Demineralized long bones may be prone to fracture, and older children may require osteotomies for bony deformities. Bony abnormalities of the maxillofacial area may render securing the airway challenging.[140] Laparoscopic and robotic techniques for cholecystectomy[141] and splenectomy have been used successively in children with thalassemia, although perioperative hypertension may be a common problem in laparoscopic splenectomy.[142,143] Open heart surgery requiring cardiopulmonary bypass with judicious use of sodium nitroprusside therapy has been successfully performed in a patient with HbH disease.[144] Perioperative considerations and concerns for children with thalassemia, especially for those with thalassemia major, are listed in Table 9-10.

# Thrombocytopenia

## PLATELET DISORDERS AND BLEEDING

Platelets are an essential component of hemostatic regulation. Platelets are distributed between the bloodstream (two thirds) and spleen (one third). Their normal life span is 7 to 10 days. In children, the platelet number may decrease due to decreased production or increased consumption, or they may have abnormal function. Bleeding typical of platelet disorders often involves skin and mucous membranes. Although there are many causes of primary and secondary thrombocytopenia in infants and children, this discussion focuses on idiopathic thrombocytopenic purpura (ITP).

## IDIOPATHIC THROMBOCYTOPENIC PURPURA

ITP is the most common cause of acute-onset thrombocytopenia in the otherwise healthy child, and it commonly manifests in the operative setting. ITP has an estimated incidence of about 4 per 100,000 children, and it is usually a benign, self-limited disorder affecting children between the ages of 2 and 10 years.[35] Primary ITP has no clear predisposing cause, but secondary ITP is triggered by a drug or medical disorder. Diagnosis is by exclusion, the differential list is extensive, and response to ITP-specific treatment usually solidifies the diagnosis.

### Pathophysiology

ITP is characterized by antibody-mediated clearance by tissue macrophages, resulting in thrombocytopenia (platelet count less tan $100,000/mm^3$) and shortened platelet survival. Antibodies may also suppress megakaryocytes and platelet development. Platelet autoantibodies may exist alone or as part of immune complexes, and they usually are immunoglobulin G (IgG) in type. They often show specificity for platelet membrane glycoproteins IIb-IIIa and Ib-IX.[145] Thrombocytopenia develops when the reticuloendothelial system, typically the spleen, destroys the antibody-covered platelets.

### Clinical and Laboratory Features and Treatment

Typically, ITP in children is a benign process occurring after a viral illness or immunization that manifests as petechiae of mucosal surfaces or purpura over bony prominences, thrombocytopenia, and a normal to increased mean platelet volume with increased megakaryocytes in the marrow. This process resolves within weeks or months regardless of therapy. ITP is classified as newly diagnosed (less than 3 months), persistent (3 to 12 months), and chronic (more than 12 months).[146]

Although platelet function in children with ITP is usually increased, treatment is often initiated only when the counts are less than 10,000 to $20,000/mm^3$.[145] Observation with avoidance of activity that may lead to head trauma is an increasingly accepted treatment plan. Medical treatment most commonly consists of agents that decrease monocyte/macrophage-mediated destruction of antibody-coated platelets (e.g., steroids, intravenous immunoglobulin, anti-D immunoglobulins, vinca alkaloids). Agents that decrease antibody production (e.g., cyclophosphamide, anti-CD20 antibody) and investigational agents that stimulate the thrombopoietin receptor are reserved for those who demonstrate an inadequate response to initial therapy.[147] Platelet transfusions are recommended only for life-threatening emergencies. Splenectomy removes a major site of platelet destruction and is recommended as an option only in chronic, symptomatic ITP or acute, life-threatening ITP unresponsive to medical treatment.[148,149] This procedure, which is commonly performed noninvasively, has a success rate of about 75%.[150-152]

### Perioperative Considerations

In view of the clinical and laboratory features of ITP, the anesthesiologist providing care for the child with ITP who is undergoing splenectomy or incidental surgery should consider the concerns listed in Table 9-11. A hematologist should be consulted to assess the need for medical therapy, including platelet transfusion, before surgery.

# Coagulation Disorders

Children may present for surgery with a personal or family history suggesting a bleeding disorder. The anesthesiologist must decide expeditiously whether to postpone surgery to further evaluate or treat the child. A careful medical history, physical examination, and family history, followed by laboratory evaluation in consultation with a hematologist, are important elements

**TABLE 9-11** Perioperative Concerns for Patients with Idiopathic Thrombocytopenia Purpura

**Preoperative Considerations**

Hemoglobin, platelet count

History of platelet transfusions

History of corticosteroid use

History of infections

Presplenectomy antibiotic prophylaxis and immunizations (when appropriate)

Discussion with a hematologist regarding medical therapy and platelet transfusion for a platelet count <30,000/mm³

Discontinuation of any platelet-inhibiting medication (e.g., aspirin)

**Intraoperative Considerations**

Appropriate antibiotic coverage

Stress corticosteroid coverage

Medical therapy and platelet transfusion as above (platelets ideally administered after clamping of the splenic artery during splenectomy)

Judicious use of regional anesthesia, intramuscular medications, nasogastric tubes, nasal intubation, and other methods

Limited use of medications with potential bleeding risk (e.g., ketorolac)

Attention to physiologic effects of laparoscopy on circulatory and respiratory function

**Postoperative Considerations**

Hemoglobin, platelet count

Infection

Corticosteroid coverage

Pain management

in screening for, diagnosing, and treating a bleeding disorder in the perioperative setting.

## SCREENING

The clinical history of the child and family is the most essential screening tool. The family history should identify family members who have been labeled as bleeders, who have required blood transfusion unexpectedly during surgery, or who returned to surgery for unexpected postoperative bleeding. A history of maternal menorrhagia may also be significant. Suggestive signs and symptoms in a child's medical history are easy bruising, mucosal bleeding, and in older girls, menorrhagia. Although diagnosing easy bruising is subjective, the clinician should suspect bleeding tendencies if skin bruising occurs in nontraumatized sites (e.g., trunk) or is unusually large without evidence of previous trauma. Mucosal bleeding includes epistaxis and gingival bleeding. Occasional nosebleeds can be common in children, but their clinical significance is enhanced by increased frequency, duration, bilaterality, and coexistence with abnormal bleeding from other sites. Gingival bleeding is common after tooth brushing or flossing, but its clinical significance is enhanced by spontaneous occurrence or chronicity, especially in the presence of good dental hygiene.[153] A history of prolonged or excessive bleeding is important when associated with umbilical dehiscence, dental work (especially extractions), and circumcision. Although mouth injuries can produce impressive blood loss acutely in any individual, recurrent or persistent bleeding from such an injury may indicate an underlying disorder.

Consultation with a hematologist and laboratory evaluation should be considered for children with a clinical history and physical examination result that suggest a bleeding diathesis, especially for children scheduled to undergo procedures associated with large blood loss or that make particular demands on hemostasis, such as tonsillectomy. Laboratory evaluation of all children, regardless of history or type of surgery, may result in false-positive results that lead to costly workups and potentially unnecessary cancellation of operations, both of which can contribute to greater health care inefficiencies and expense. Bleeding due to medications should be distinguished from an actual bleeding disorder.

When a bleeding disorder is strongly suspected, a set of laboratory tests that include a platelet count, PT, INR, aPTT, thrombin time (TT), and fibrinogen concentration should be ordered. The PT test is most sensitive to deficiencies in factors II, V, VII, and X, and it is useful for differentiating a vitamin K deficiency from other causes. The PT is most often used to monitor the anticoagulant effects of warfarin; it is not sensitive to the effects of heparin. The aPTT test is most sensitive to deficiencies in factors VIII, IX, and XI and less sensitive to deficiencies of factor V, factor X, prothrombin, and fibrinogen. The aPTT is also prolonged in deficiencies of the contact or kallikrein/kinin system proteins, factor XII, prekallikrein, and high-molecular-weight kininogen, but these deficiencies are not associated with bleeding. Because aPTT reagents vary in sensitivity for detection of deficiencies of each factor, it is inappropriate to make a general statement about the ability of this test to detect a specific abnormality; abnormal results require discussion with a hematologist or laboratory medicine physician. Although a prolonged aPTT may be caused by a deficiency in one or more factors, it can also result from inhibition by heparin or a plasma inhibitor, such as lupus anticoagulant. Correction of a prolonged aPTT after mixing the child's plasma with normal plasma (1 : 1 mix) suggests a factor deficiency. The TT test, which determines the amount of time it takes for blood to clot, is useful for determining deficiencies or abnormalities in fibrinogen and is very sensitive to heparin contamination. Bleeding time, a thromboelastogram, and platelet function screens (e.g., PFA-100) are probably not appropriate as first-line screening tests.

Children with an upper limit of normal aPTT test result and a strongly suspicious personal or family history for a bleeding disorder may have an abnormality (e.g., von Willebrand disease). These children require further evaluation in consultation with a hematologist. Whether a procedure should be delayed for the consultation depends on several factors, including the patient's history, site and urgency of surgery, potential bleeding risks associated with the planned procedure, and results of previously discussed set of screening tests.

## VON WILLEBRAND DISEASE

von Willebrand disease (vWD) is considered to be one of the most common bleeding disorders, although studies suggest that the prevalence may be as low as 1 case per 10,000 people.[154-157] Initially named *pseudohemophilia* because of an inheritance pattern that is different from that of hemophilia, vWD is the result of an abnormal amount, structure, or function of the vWF.[154]

### Pathophysiology and Classification

The glycoprotein vWF serves two main roles in the coagulation cascade: adhering platelets to damaged subendothelium and carrying factor VIII in plasma. vWF exists as small and large multimers. Large multimers play a more active role in the binding of platelets to subendothelium than do small ones and are therefore necessary for platelet adhesion, whereas binding to factor VIII is independent of multimer size. The two aspects of vWF make it an essential part of primary hemostasis (through platelet binding) and secondary hemostasis (as carrier of factor VIII to sites of injury).

Classification of vWD is essential for understanding and management of this disorder. The current classification was developed by a subcommittee on vWD through the International Society on Thrombosis and Haemostasis.[155,156] The two general types are categorized as quantitative abnormalities (types 1 and 3) or qualitative abnormalities (type 2, including subtypes A, B, M, and N). All types are inherited in an autosomal dominant pattern, except types 2N and 3, which are autosomal recessive.

Because vWD is heterogeneous, clinical definitions have been proposed using categories such as mild, moderate, and severe, categories that are based on bleeding history (i.e., number of bleeding episodes) and laboratory measurement of factor concentration and activity.[157] As the molecular basis of vWD becomes better understood, classification of this disease likely will change to reflect the new data. For example, Rodeghiero and colleagues proposed a practical approach to diagnosing and categorizing patients with vWD to provide optimal management.[157] Their approach includes a standardized bleeding history score, focused laboratory analysis, and a trial infusion of DDAVP in certain subtypes. Categorization of patients with vWD is important for determining how they are managed in the perioperative setting.[158]

### Clinical and Laboratory Features and Treatment

Children with vWD may exhibit many of the clinical features associated with bleeding disorders in general, although there is a notable absence of joint bleeding. The typical symptoms of vWD reflect poor platelet adhesion and include bruising, epistaxis, and menorrhagia.

Children with vWD have traditionally been described as having prolonged bleeding times and aPTTs, but those with mild disease often have normal values. The aPTT is prolonged only if factor VIII activity is at or below a concentration that is determined by the sensitivity of the particular assay at an institution (often below 30% to 35%). The platelet functional assay (PFA-100) has better sensitivity and specificity (both near 90%) for diagnosis of the disease.[159,160] The PFA-100 test, which measures closure time of an aperture on a membrane coated with collagen and adenosine diphosphate (ADP) or epinephrine, depends on vWF activity and platelet function. Because this test has some variability, its interpretation should be used in conjunction with results of other tests.[161] Platelet count is typically normal in all types of vWD except type 2B.

Other laboratory tests used to delineate vWD include vWF antigen (vWF:A), which is a measure of the total level of vWF; vWF activity, often measured as a ristocetin cofactor activity (vWF:R), which is a measure of vWF binding to platelets through GPIb receptors; factor VIII coagulant activity; and vWF multimer analysis. Certain disease states have been associated with "acquired vWD" and include lymphoproliferative disorders or gammopathies (marked by antibodies to vWF), chronic renal failure, hypothyroidism, Wilms tumor, and certain congenital heart diseases, such as aortic stenosis (characterized by proteolysis of vWF multimers).[159]

In consultation with a hematologist, determination of appropriate treatment based on specific diagnosis and response to therapy is necessary before surgery. Treatment focuses on increasing concentrations of endogenous vWF with administration of DDAVP when possible or on replacement of factors with factor concentrates.[162] DDAVP is usually effective in type 1 but less so in types 2A and 2M. DDAVP may have little or even undesired effects in some children: it may increase abnormal vWF in types 2A, 2M, and 2N; it can exacerbate thrombocytopenia in type 2B; and its repeated administration may lead to tachyphylaxis. DDAVP usually is not administered to very young children because of the risk of free water retention, hyponatremia, and central nervous system pathology, including seizures. Similarly, intravenous fluids may need to be limited after its administration to any child. Factor concentrates (including factor VIII and vWF [Humate-P or Alphanate]) typically are required for types 2B, 2N, and 3. Cryoprecipitate may be used when vWF-containing concentrates are unavailable, but it is not recommended as first-line therapy because it is not virus free, and vWF in solvent or heat-treated cryoprecipitate may be abnormal.[153] Because of the complexity of response to therapies in this disease and the ever-changing availability of replacement products, determination of appropriate treatment in a particular child before surgery is crucial.[158,163]

### Perioperative Concerns

The major preoperative concerns in children with confirmed vWD are directed toward appropriate preoperative treatment, avoidance of medications that may interfere with coagulation, and anticipation of intraoperative and postoperative bleeding (Table 9-12).[162,164] All concerns should be addressed in consultation with a hematologist. Although regional anesthesia for these children usually is contraindicated, there are reports of its use without complications.[165]

---

**TABLE 9-12** Perioperative Considerations for Patients with von Willebrand Disease

**Preoperative Considerations**

Consultation with hematologist: establish correct diagnosis and response to desmopressin (DDAVP); administer DDAVP or viral attenuated factor concentrates containing factor VIII and von Willebrand factor (vWF) such as Humate-P for severe vWD or for those types not responsive to DDAVP[161]

Determination of actual and desired factor concentrations and expected duration of postoperative therapy[162]

Discontinuation of any platelet-inhibiting medication (e.g., aspirin)

**Intraoperative Considerations**

Judicious use of regional anesthesia, intramuscular medications, nasogastric tubes, nasal intubation, and other procedures that may cause bleeding

Limited use of medications with potential bleeding risk (e.g., ketorolac)

Coagulation profiles, including platelet counts for more invasive surgeries

Treatment of bleeding with appropriate blood products

Consider use of antifibrinolytic agents (i.e., ε-aminocaproic acid, tranexamic acid)[163]

Possible use of recombinant factor VIIa for severe bleeding episodes in severe vWD type 3 or patients with inhibitors

**Postoperative Considerations**

Follow factor concentrations (i.e., factor VIII and vWF)

Availability of blood products and factors

Appropriate treatment of bleeding episodes

Monitor for thromboembolism in children receiving multiple concentrates or antifibrinolytic agents, or both[161]

**TABLE 9-13** Clinical Manifestations of Hemophilia A

| Clinical Manifestations | Mild (>10%)* | Moderate (2%-10%)* | Severe (<2%)* |
|---|---|---|---|
| Age at first hemorrhage | 3 to 14 years or older | <2 years | <1 years |
| Signs in neonatal period | None | Postcircumcision bleeding | Postcircumcision bleeding, intracranial hemorrhage |
| Musculoskeletal bleeding | Unusual except with severe trauma | Joint and muscle bleeding with minor trauma | Spontaneous |
| Central nervous system bleeding | Rare except with severe trauma | Less prevalent than severe | Prevalence, 3% Mean age, 14 years |
| Postsurgical bleeding | Hematomas and oozing | Wound hematomas and oozing | Usually frank bleeding |
| Trauma-related bleeding | Hematomas and deep bleeding with significant trauma | Muscle and joint bleeding with minor trauma | Common with minor trauma |
| Dental bleeding | Often | Common | Usual |
| Inhibitors present | Rarely | <3% | Prevalence, 15%-20% |

Modified from DiMichele D: Hemophilia A (FVIII deficiency). In: Goodnight SH Jr, Hathaway W, editors. Disorders of hemostasis and thrombosis. New York: McGraw-Hill; 2001. p. 127-39.
*Percent factor VIII activity.

## HEMOPHILIA

Hemophilia was first reported in the *Talmud*, in which there are descriptions of 8-day-old boys exsanguinating after ritual circumcision. Widespread public attention was drawn to this disease after members of Queen Victoria's family developed sequelae from hemophilia in the late 19th and early 20th centuries. The discovery of multiple forms of hemophilia was first made in 1944 when blood from two hemophiliacs was mixed and found to clot. In 1952, hematologists explained their earlier finding by noting that a 10-year-old boy, Stephen Christmas, exhibited a type of hemophilia, factor IX deficiency, which differed from the classic form, factor VIII deficiency.

Hemophilia is a group of congenital bleeding disorders caused by deficiency in factor VIII (i.e., hemophilia A, or classic hemophilia), factor IX (i.e., hemophilia B, or Christmas disease), or factor XI (i.e., hemophilia C). During the 10-year period from 1982 through 1991, the incidence of the more common varieties, hemophilia A and B, was 1 case per 5032 live male births in the United States within a six-state surveillance area; the prevalence of hemophilia A was 10.5 cases per 100,000 male births, and that of hemophilia B was 2.9 cases per 100,000 male births.[166]

Because of X-linked recessive inheritance of hemophilia A and B, family history is very important in establishing the diagnosis. Although boys are usually affected, girls may rarely inherit the disorder if their fathers are affected and their mothers are carriers or in instances of extreme lyonization (inactivation of an X chromosome). The daughter of an affected father is an obligate carrier with a 50% chance of passing it on to any of her sons. De novo mutations are relatively common and suspected in male patients lacking a family history.[159] Hemophilia C is a mild form of hemophilia, affecting primarily Ashkenazi Jews. It is distinguished from the other two forms of hemophilia by an autosomal recessive inheritance pattern (linked through chromosome 4), lack of joint bleeding, and infrequent need for treatment. Affected female patients may notice heavy menses, and affected male patients may have frequent nosebleeds and occasionally have excessive bleeding during surgery.

## Pathophysiology

Normal in vivo hemostasis initiates at sites of endothelial disruption through interaction of activated factor VII (FVIIa) and tissue factor (TF) to form a complex that activates factor IX and factor X directly. Activated factor IX in conjunction with factor VIII further activates factor X, which with factor V converts prothrombin to thrombin. Both factor VIII and factor IX are required for sufficient hemostasis, as evidenced by the severe bleeding that occurs if either is completely deficient. Factor XI activates factor IX, but its precise role in the hemostatic pathway is not completely understood.

### Clinical and Laboratory Features and Treatment

The wide range of clinical features is similar for hemophilia A and B (Table 9-13). The severity of bleeding in these children directly relates to the degree of their deficiency.[159] Children with mild or moderate hemophilia may bleed excessively only after a hemostatic challenge such as trauma or surgery, whereas children with severe hemophilia may bleed spontaneously (e.g., hemarthroses).[167] Female carriers on average have 50% of normal factor concentrations and usually are asymptomatic, although they occasionally present with a clinical picture similar to that of mild cases of hemophilia.[159]

Results of a general coagulation screen are typically normal except for the aPTT, which is prolonged in proportion to the concentration of factors in the blood. The diagnosis is confirmed by measuring the specific factor concentrations.[168] If hemophilia is suspected but there is no family history, testing for vWD is prudent, especially for the types that may mimic hemophilia (i.e., types 2N and 3). Because of the variable sensitivity of the aPTT to specific factor deficiencies, the ability of this test to detect carriers varies between laboratories; diagnosis of a carrier state usually requires specific factor assays.

Hemophilias A and B are treated by replacing the deficient factor concentrations. These factor concentrations should be maintained at specified levels to prevent sequelae (Table 9-14). Exposure to plasma products should be minimized. The duration of treatment should be tailored to the severity of disease. DDAVP may be effective in selected mild cases by increasing factor VIII concentrations through the release of endogenous stores. Because tachyphylaxis limits the prolonged use of DDAVP, it is typically recommended only for minor operations.[167] For most cases, especially for those who require increased factor concentrations to be maintained for effective hemostasis, factor concentrates should be used. Although recombinant forms are preferable because they do not carry infectious risk, substitution with plasma-derived

**TABLE 9-14**  Treatment Targets for Hemophilia A and B

| Bleeding Site | Target Concentrations for Factor VIII or IX (%) | Duration of Treatment (days)* |
|---|---|---|
| Muscle | 30-50 | 1-2 |
| Joint | 50-80 | 1-2 |
| Gastrointestinal tract | 40-60 | 10-14 |
| Oral mucosa | 30-50 | 2-3 |
| Epistaxis | 30-50 | 2-3 |
| Hematuria | 30-100 | 1-2 |
| Retroperitoneal | 80-100 | 7-10 |
| Central nervous system | 80-100 | 14 |
| Trauma or surgery | 80-100 | 14 |

Modified from Brown DL. Congenital bleeding disorders. Curr Probl Pediatr Adolesc Health Care 2005;35:38-62.
*May be reduced depending on clinical circumstances and severity of disease.

**TABLE 9-15**  Perioperative Concerns for Patients with Hemophilia

**Preoperative Considerations**

Consultation with hematologist, establishment of correct diagnosis

Determination and testing of treatment plan, including use of desmopressin or factors (concentrates or recombinant)

Consideration of multiple procedures performed together to reduce factor exposure

Discontinuation of any platelet-inhibiting medication (e.g., aspirin)

**Intraoperative Considerations**

Judicious use of regional anesthesia, intramuscular medications, nasogastric tubes, nasal intubation, and other procedures that may cause bleeding

Limited use of medications with potential bleeding risk (e.g., ketorolac)

Follow coagulation profiles, especially factor levels (factors VIII and IX)

Anticipate and treat bleeding with appropriate blood products

Consider recombinant activated factor VII (rFVIIa) for severe bleeding

**Postoperative Considerations**

Maintain factor concentrations for specified time period as recommended by the hematologist

Ensure availability of blood products and factors from the blood bank

Anticipate and treat bleeding episodes

forms may be needed when supplies are limited.[159,167] For the rare patient with hemophilia C who has excessive surgical bleeding, treatment with recombinant factor XI or FFP may be required. It is essential to consult with a hematologist to determine a customized factor treatment plan for every child with hemophilia.

Children who have developed inhibitors to factor concentrates pose a challenge in the perioperative period. Until recently, they were denied surgery unless it was absolutely necessary, at which point they were often managed with increased concentrations of factors or a desensitization regimen. However, a review that included two randomized, controlled trials and data from the Hemophilia Research Society and the Hemophilia and Thrombosis Research Society reported effectiveness of recombinant factor VIIa (rFVIIa) for most of these patients.[169] Among the randomized trials, one study compared two bolus-dosing regimens (35 versus 90 μg/kg), and the other study compared bolus dosing with continuous infusion; the greater dosing regimen was more effective for major operations. Combining data from these studies and the two Research Society databases, the overall effectiveness rate of rFVIIa in controlling bleeding approached 84%, with a low thrombotic rate of less than 1%. Such evidence is providing more options for these difficult-to-manage patients with inhibitors. Alternatively, partially activated prothrombin complex concentrates, such as factor VIII inhibitor bypass activity (FEIBA, Baxter Healthcare Corp., Westlake Village, Calif.), have been effective for patients with inhibitors undergoing surgery.[170]

### Perioperative Concerns

The perioperative concerns in hemophilia focus on prevention and treatment of bleeding, similar to the management of patients with vWD (Table 9-15). Many consider regional anesthesia to be contraindicated for patients with hemophilia, but there are reports of its use without complications as long as factor concentrations are maintained.[171]

### HYPERCOAGULABILITY

A hypercoagulable state is a condition in which the development of thrombus is favored (i.e., thrombophilia). The condition results in an increased risk for abnormal clot formation and venous thromboembolic events (VTEs), which often are the presenting symptoms at the time of diagnosis. Thrombophilia can be acquired or congenital. The incidence of VTE among children

is less than it is among adults, even in those with known congenital thrombophilic conditions,[172] although neonates and adolescents are at relatively high risk in the pediatric population.[173] Congenital thrombophilic conditions include factor V Leiden disorder, prothrombin gene mutation, protein C and S deficiencies, and antithrombin III deficiency.[174] Risk factors for acquired thrombophilia include the presence of a central venous catheter, infection, malignancy, surgery, or trauma.[173]

Screening of nonoperative children with suspected hypercoagulability is controversial and not recommended for those who are asymptomatic, even those with a positive family history.[172] Evidenced-based guidelines for children are lacking with regard to screening and prophylactic treatment of those with suspected hypercoagulability. Current evidence suggests pharmacologic prophylaxis in the nonoperative setting is recommended only in children on long-term home total parenteral nutrition (TPN) and those with specific complex cardiac lesions (e.g., Fontan patients).[175] However, children who present for surgery with a strong family history of thromboses may benefit from screening and referral to a hematologist for management and consideration of pharmacologic prophylaxis, such as enoxaparin administered postoperatively. The use of nonpharmacologic prophylaxis, including early mobilization after surgery, adequate hydration, and compression stockings, is left to the discretion of individual providers and to institutional practice based on the child's medical history, family history, and risk factors for VTE.

# Cancer and Hematopoietic Stem Cell Transplantation

### CANCER

Cancer is the second and fourth most common cause of death in children younger than 15 and 20 years of age, respectively.[176,177] The most common malignancies affecting children are different from those affecting adults, and they include leukemia, brain tumors, lymphomas, and solid tumors such as sarcomas of soft tissue and bone. Embryonal tumors (e.g., neuroblastoma, Wilms tumor, retinoblastoma, medulloblastoma) are unique to early childhood. Survival rates for most pediatric cancers have improved significantly in the past several decades; more than 80% of children diagnosed with a childhood malignancy will become 5-year survivors of their cancers.[178,179] The great improvements in survival for many malignancies of childhood are directly related to advances in diagnostic modalities and the large percentage of children treated on cooperative clinical trial protocols. Treatment follows these protocols and may include chemotherapy, radiation therapy, biologic modifiers, and HSCT.

Children with cancer typically undergo many surgical procedures that require anesthesia. The procedures may occur before the initiation of cancer therapy, during therapy, years into remission, or during terminal stages of the disease. Certain considerations apply to this population, including the direct effects of the tumor, effects of chemotherapy and radiation therapy, impact of the surgical procedure, pain syndromes, and psychologic vulnerabilities of the child and family. Survivors of childhood cancer experience various long-term sequelae after completion of cancer therapy. Although the broad field of pediatric oncology is beyond the scope of this discussion, some commonalities relating to perioperative care are described.

### Clinical and Laboratory Features and Treatment

The direct effects of tumor, even at the time of diagnosis, may contribute to morbidity and mortality. For example, a childhood tumor may manifest with increased intracranial pressure, pleural or pericardial effusion, or compression of abdominal organs. Lymphoma often manifests with symptoms associated with an anterior mediastinal mass, including respiratory distress and cardiorespiratory collapse under anesthesia.[180,181] Most children with Hodgkin disease or non-Hodgkin lymphoma have mediastinal involvement at diagnosis, and almost one half have respiratory symptoms at presentation (see Chapter 13).[182,183]

Myelosuppression, which manifests with various degrees of anemia, thrombocytopenia, and neutropenia, is a common direct effect of cancer in children. Anemia is common at the time of diagnosis of many pediatric cancers, including 50% to 75% of children with newly diagnosed neuroblastoma, rhabdomyosarcoma, Hodgkin disease, Ewing sarcoma, and osteosarcoma[184] and 80% of children with acute lymphoblastic leukemia (ALL).[185] Thrombocytopenia is typically identified during the diagnosis of children with acute leukemia and is common with tumors causing bone marrow infiltration.[186,187] Neutropenia is usual in children with ALL. Hyperleukocytosis is predominant in children with acute myelogenous leukemia (AML), 20% of whom present with a white blood cell count greater than 100,000/mm³.[185,188] This high concentration of leukemic blasts, especially when the count is greater than 200,000/mm³, may lead to intravascular clumping and the potentially fatal condition of leukostasis.[189] Myelosuppression may be a direct effect of tumor cells and marrow infiltration by tumor cells and may result from radiation therapy and chemotherapy. As a consequence of myelosuppression, children with cancer have a frequent need for transfusion of blood products and are at risk for procedure-acquired and line-related infections and for delayed wound healing after surgical procedures. Frequent hospitalizations and immune compromise predispose them to colonization and infection by nosocomial, community-acquired, antibiotic-resistant organisms

and opportunistic infections. Neutropenia predisposes them to specific infections such as perirectal abscesses and typhlitis.

An uncommon but potentially fatal effect of the tumor itself is tumor lysis syndrome (TLS). TLS is most common with certain hematologic malignancies, especially ALL and Burkitt lymphoma, but it also occurs with other malignancies characterized by a high proliferative rate, large tumor burden, or high sensitivity to cytotoxic therapy. TLS is characterized by rapid and massive destruction of tumor cells and resultant massive release of phosphorus, potassium, nucleic acids, and proteins that is sufficient to cause metabolic derangements and possible renal failure and death.[190,191] TLS can occur spontaneously, especially in children with AML, but it more often manifests in the setting of cytotoxic therapy, radiation therapy, fever, surgery, and anesthesia.[192-197]

Chemotherapy used in pediatric oncology leads to myelosuppression and to a host of important side effects that may be clinically important in the perioperative setting (Table 9-16). These effects of chemotherapy can be synergistic with toxicities of radiation therapy.[198] New chemotherapeutic agents are continuously being introduced, and at academic centers, the use of investigational agents is common. Although it is impossible to provide a comprehensive review of chemotherapeutics, the most common agents that cause toxicities of particular importance to the delivery of anesthesia are briefly mentioned here, and a complete list of toxicities can be found in E-Table 9-1.

Corticosteroids are frequently used and may cause adrenal suppression, hypertension, thromboembolism, and obesity; the latter potentially renders venous access and tracheal intubation difficult. Children who have received corticosteroid therapy have a period of measurable glucocorticoid-induced adrenal suppression of 2 weeks to 8 months after such therapy.[199-205] Because of this variability, administering stress-dose steroids in the first 1 to 2 months after cessation of glucocorticoids is reasonable.[199] However, any child at risk of TLS should not receive corticosteroids without direct discussion with an oncologist.

The anthracycline drugs (e.g., doxorubicin, daunorubicin, idarubicin, and epirubicin) and mitoxantrone cause cardiomyopathy in a dose-dependent fashion, which is aggravated by radiation delivered to the precordial area. About 10% of children who received a cumulative dose of 300 mg/m² or more of anthracycline develop clinically significant cardiomyopathy.[206] Later studies demonstrated clinically significant cardiomyopathy after much smaller doses[207,208] and an increased sensitivity in children with trisomy 21 and leukemia.[209] Children receiving anthracyclines should be evaluated with echocardiography at baseline and intermittently during the course of therapy and for a prolonged period after therapy because anthracycline-induced cardiac failure can take years to fully declare itself.[210,211] Physical examination may miss more than 50% of children with heart failure.[212] A recent echocardiogram should be available preoperatively if a child has received anthracycline therapy and any of the following conditions are met: cumulative dose greater than 240 mg/m², any dose received during infancy, or chest irradiation dose greater than 30 Gy with concomitant anthracycline treatment.[213,214] Although uncommon, radionuclide angiocardiography may be chosen for those with poor echocardiographic windows.[210,215]

Several other chemotherapeutic agents are of interest to the anesthesiologist caring for a child with cancer. L-Asparaginase is associated with a 1% to 2% risk of hemorrhage or thrombosis due to deficiencies in fibrinogen, plasminogen, antithrombin III, and vWF,[216-218] as well as hepatic dysfunction and acute hemorrhagic pancreatitis. Bleomycin can produce acute pneumonitis and

**TABLE 9-16**  Therapy-Related Side Effects and Toxicity

| Drug | Side Effects |
|---|---|
| L-Asparaginase | Hyperglycemia, hypersensitivity, hepatic dysfunction (secondary hypoalbuminemia and coagulopathies), pancreatitis, thrombosis, stroke |
| Bischloroethyl nitrosourea (BCNU) | Encephalopathy, hepatotoxicity, pulmonary toxicity |
| Bleomycin | Anaphylactoid reactions, fever, hyperpigmentation, nausea, vomiting, pulmonary fibrosis |
| Busulfan | Encephalopathy, hepatotoxicity, pulmonary toxicity |
| Carboplatin | Myelosuppression, nausea, vomiting, nephrotoxicity, neurotoxicity, ototoxicity |
| Cisplatin | Nausea/vomiting, nephrotoxicity, ototoxicity, peripheral neuropathy |
| Corticosteroids | Adrenal suppression, avascular necrosis, cataracts, edema, gastritis, hyperglycemia, hypertension, myopathy, osteoporosis, obesity, osteopenia, psychosis |
| Cyclophosphamide (Cytoxan) | Cardiotoxicity, hemorrhagic cystitis, myelosuppression, nausea, vomiting, syndrome of inappropriate secretion of antidiuretic hormone (SIADH) |
| Cyclosporine | Cortical blindness, electrolyte disturbances, encephalopathy, gingival hyperplasia, hemolytic uremia, hepatotoxicity, hyperlipidemia, hypertension, hirsutism, myositis, paresthesias, tremor |
| Cytarabine | Myelosuppression, mucositis, hepatitis, nausea/vomiting, neurotoxicity |
| Dactinomycin (Actinomycin D) | Nausea/vomiting, mucositis, myelosuppression, radiation recall |
| Daunorubicin (Daunomycin) Doxorubicin (Adriamycin) Idarubicin (Idamycin) | Cardiomyopathy, mucositis, myelosuppression, red-orange urine |
| Etoposide | Hypotension, mucositis, myelosuppression, nausea, vomiting |
| Ifosfamide | Hemorrhagic cystitis, myelosuppression, nephrotoxicity, neurotoxicity |
| Melphalan | Mucositis |
| Methotrexate | Hepatotoxicity, mucositis, myelosuppression, renal failure, neurotoxicity |
| Mercaptopurine (6-MP) | Hepatotoxicity, myelosuppression |
| Mycophenolate mofetil (Cellcept) | Electrolyte disturbance, gastrointestinal toxicity, hypercholesterolemia, myelosuppression, rash |
| Procarbazine | Myelosuppression |
| Sirolimus | Hyperlipidemia, myelosuppression |
| Tacrolimus (Prograf) | Anemia, anorexia, back pain, encephalopathy, diarrhea, hyperglycemia, nephrotoxicity, pleural effusion, rash |
| Thiotepa | Neurotoxicity, mucositis |
| Thioguanine (6-TG) | Hepatotoxicity, myelosuppression |
| Total body irradiation | Dental/bony maldevelopment, gastrointestinal toxicity, hepatotoxicity, pulmonary toxicity |
| Vinblastine (Velban) | Myelosuppression, neurotoxicity, SIADH |
| Vincristine (Oncovin) | Neurotoxicity, SIADH |

Modified from Carpenter PA, Mielcarek M, Woolfrey AE. Hematopoietic cell transplantation. In: Irwin S, Rippe JM, editors. Intensive care medicine. 6th ed. Philadelphia: Lippincott Williams & Wilkins; 2008. p. 2150-68.

progression to pulmonary fibrosis. Although the incidence and risk in children are not known, reports suggest that 46% of adults treated with cumulative doses greater than 400 units/m$^2$ develop bleomycin-induced pneumonitis and 3% of these die.[219-221] Studies suggest that high concentrations of inspired oxygen during or soon after bleomycin treatment may promote pulmonary toxicity and lead to postoperative respiratory distress.[222-224] A medical history and physical examination are sufficient to determine whether pulmonary function testing is required preoperatively.[225-227] Cisplatin and ifosfamide may cause renal tubular damage that can lead to Fanconi syndrome with electrolyte wasting. Methotrexate may cause renal failure at large doses (more than 1 mg/m$^2$). Vinblastine and vincristine may cause peripheral neuropathies and seizures. Increasingly, biologic mediators such as retinoids are being used to modify tumor biology, and recombinant antibodies are used to directly attack tumors and modulate the immune response to tumors. The use of investigational agents and novel chemotherapeutics amplifies the importance of reviewing cases with the oncologist.

Toxicity from the effects of radiation therapy to healthy tissues is unavoidable, and the developing tissues of children are particularly susceptible to the acute and late effects of irradiation. The susceptibility of normal tissues depends on the total and fractional dose received, the sensitivity of the tissue to the dose of radiation, the volume of tissue irradiated, and time course of treatment (Table 9-17). Concurrent chemotherapy potentiates toxicity.

Almost every organ system is affected by cancer and its treatment. Nausea and vomiting are common. Nutrition is often compromised, along with skin integrity and bone and tooth mineralization. Mucositis can lead to difficult intubation because of pseudomembrane formation, supraglottic edema, and bleeding from the friable oral mucosa.[228,229] Acute and chronic pain often require complex treatment regimens that may include opioids, nonsteroidal antiinflammatory agents, antidepressants, anxiolytics, and a wide range of complementary and alternative modalities.

## Perioperative Considerations

A retrospective review of 177 children undergoing 3833 radiotherapy sessions with anesthesia reported a complication rate of 1.3%, which is comparable to that for children without cancer

**TABLE 9-17** Late Effects of Radiation Therapy

| Radiation Field | Late Effects | Risk Factors |
|---|---|---|
| Cranial | Neurocognitive deficits | >18 Gy, IV/IT methotrexate |
| | Leukoencephalopathy | >18 Gy with IT methotrexate |
| | Growth hormone deficiency | >18 Gy |
| | Panhypopituitarism | >40 Gy |
| | Large vessel stroke | >60 Gy |
| | Second cancers | Variable |
| | Dental problems | >10 Gy |
| | Cataracts | >2-8 Gy single dose, 10-15 Gy fractionated dose |
| | Ototoxicity | >35-50 Gy |
| Chest | Cardiac disease | |
| | Coronary artery disease | >30 Gy |
| | Cardiomyopathy | >35 Gy, >25 Gy with anthracyclines |
| | Valvular disease | >40 Gy |
| | Pericardial disease | >35 Gy |
| | Arrhythmias | Unknown |
| | Thyroid disease | |
| | Hypothyroidism | >20 Gy local, >7.5 Gy TBI |
| | Hyperthyroidism | >20 Gy local, >7.5 Gy TBI |
| | Thyroid nodules, cancer | Any dose |
| | Pulmonary disease | |
| | Pulmonary fibrosis | >15-20 Gy |
| | Restrictive lung disease | Unknown |
| | Obstructive lung disease | Unknown |
| Abdomen/pelvis | Chronic enteritis | >40 Gy |
| | Gastrointestinal malignancy | Unknown |
| | Hepatic fibrosis/cirrhosis | >30 Gy |
| | Renal insufficiency | >20 Gy |
| | Bladder disease | |
| | Fibrosis | >30 Gy prepubertal, >50 postpubertal |
| | Hemorrhagic cystitis | Enhances cyclophosphamide and ifosfamide effect |
| | Bladder cancer | Unknown |
| | Gonadal dysfunction | |
| | Ovarian failure | 4-12 Gy |
| | Testicular failure | >1-6 Gy |
| Any radiation | Skin cancer | |
| | Musculoskeletal changes | |
| | Bone length discrepancy | >20 Gy |
| | Pathologic fractures | >40 Gy |
| TBI | All the above | |

From Latham GJ, Greenberg RS. Anesthetic considerations for the pediatric oncology patient—part 1: a review of antitumor therapy. Pediatr Anesth 2010;20: 295-304.
*Gy,* Gray; *IT,* intrathecal; *IV,* intravenous; *TBI,* total body irradiation.

anesthetized with propofol.[230] However, it is clear that many children with cancer who present to the operating room are gravely ill and susceptible to relatively small changes to their physiology.

All of the described considerations regarding the possible effects of pediatric cancer and its treatment may influence our strategies in the perioperative period. Children with cancer undergo a host of procedures that require anesthesia during acute and chronic phases of disease. Included among them are diagnostic tumor or lymph node biopsy; tumor resection; placement of peripheral and central venous access for treatment and nutrition; diagnostic and monitoring procedures (e.g., lumbar puncture, bone marrow aspirate and biopsy, lung and liver biopsy, skin biopsy, bronchoalveolar lavage, esophagogastroduodenoscopy); radiologic procedures (e.g., magnetic resonance imaging, computed tomography, nuclear scans, positron emission tomography); radiation therapy; and placement of pain management devices (e.g., indwelling epidural catheters). Splenectomy is performed as part of staging or management of some pediatric malignancies, and the procedure may be associated with increased risk of postoperative infection, postoperative thrombocytosis, and thrombocytopenia.[231]

Surgical intervention may be required for acute and potentially life-threatening emergencies in children with cancer, and the effects of specific tumors can complicate anesthesia care. Wilms tumor may be accompanied by an acquired vWD condition, and anterior mediastinal masses may produce superior vena cava obstruction, pulmonary artery compression, and tracheal obstruction.[181,182] Neuroblastoma may be accompanied by pheochromocytoma-like signs and symptoms (3% of cases),[232] and in advanced stages, it may cause massive hepatic enlargement. Spinal tumors may cause acute spinal cord compression, and tumor or hemorrhage in the brain may cause acute intracranial hypertension. In view of the complexity of pediatric oncologic disease, there are many considerations for the perioperative period,[233] as detailed in Table 9-18.

## HEMATOPOIETIC STEM CELL TRANSPLANTATION

The first attempts to use bone marrow clinically to treat malignancy took place about 50 years ago.[234] HSCT is a potentially curative treatment for a wide range of malignant and nonmalignant pediatric disorders. Throughout the process of HSCT, children are likely to undergo procedures that require anesthesia.

HSCT is used in the treatment of leukemia, lymphoma, solid tumors (e.g., neuroblastoma), myelodysplasia, aplastic anemia, hemoglobinopathies (including sickle cell disease and thalassemia), and congenital immune and metabolism deficiencies.[235,236] Hematopoietic stem cells used in the transplantation can be obtained from bone marrow, "mobilized" peripheral blood, or umbilical cord blood. The source of the cells may be the child (autologous), an identical twin (syngeneic), or another individual (allogeneic). Allogeneic donor cells are commonly derived from HLA-identical siblings (available in about 30% of patients), but advances in matching and supportive care have improved outcomes with HLA-matched unrelated and mismatched donors.[237,238] Accumulative toxicity in HSCT derives from the underlying illness and complications of past therapy, the transplant-conditioning regimen, complications resulting from long-term myelosuppression, and graft-versus-host disease and its treatment.

**TABLE 9-18** Perioperative Concerns in Pediatric Cancer and Hematopoietic Stem Cell Transplantation

**Preoperative Considerations**

Consultation with service primarily responsible for child's care

Complete blood cell count

Serum electrolytes

Echocardiogram or chest radiograph, or both (when appropriate)

Transfusion crossmatch with specifications (e.g., cytomegalovirus seronegativity, leukocyte reduction, irradiation) determined in consultation with oncology service

Determination of blood typing requirements for all stem cell transplant recipients

History of acute and chronic pain medication use

Anxiolytic and analgesic therapy (when appropriate)

Infection prophylaxis with antibiotics

Avoidance of *any* marrow-suppressive medications in stem cell transplant patients

Observation of indicated isolation precautions

Sterile technique with central line access

Use of support services (when appropriate)

**Intraoperative Considerations**

Attention to skin, teeth, eyes, and joints; careful positioning and padding

Sterile technique with central line access

Full-stomach precautions (when appropriate, as in graft-versus-host disease)

Appropriate hydration and maintenance of urine output

Continuation of total parenteral nutrition (and other parenteral fluids with high glucose concentration)

Avoidance of high fraction of inspired oxygen ($FIO_2$) and restriction of hydration if prior treatment with bleomycin

Judicious use of cardiac depressants in patients with compromised cardiac function

Nausea and vomiting prophylaxis

Stress corticosteroids (when appropriate)

Regional anesthesia when safe and indicated

**Postoperative Considerations**

Patient-appropriate opioid and other analgesic administration

Sterile technique with central line access

Observation of indicated isolation precautions

## Clinical and Laboratory Features and Treatment

The process of HSCT involves several steps:

1. The preparative or conditioning regimen, during which high-dose chemotherapy with or without irradiation or immuno-modulating agents eradicates malignancy (where present), clears marrow space for incoming stem cells, and suppresses the recipient's immune system
2. Transplantation through infusion of hematopoietic stem cells
3. Transplant engraftment (more than 30 days after transplantation)
4. Early engraftment (30 to 100 days after transplantation)
5. Late engraftment (more than 100 days after transplantation)

Side effects and toxicities of therapeutic modalities can affect the transplant recipient throughout the process (see Tables 9-16 and 9-17). The incidence of transplantation-related morbidity and mortality depends on the patient's age, primary disease,

comorbidities, and histocompatibility between donor and recipient. Complications contributing to morbidity and mortality are related to infection, regimen-related toxicity, and alloreactivity.[239]

Immunologic and physical host defenses are impaired throughout the transplantation process. Children are vulnerable to a wide range of routine and opportunistic pathogens, including bacteria, fungi, and viruses.

Regimen-related toxicity can involve every organ of the body through the direct and indirect effects of irradiation and chemotherapy (see Tables 9-16 and 9-17 and E-Table 9-1). Mucositis is common and can increase the risk of aspiration and airway compromise.[229,240] Sinusoidal obstruction syndrome (SOS), previously called veno-occlusive disease, occurs in 10% to 40% of children after HSCT. Mortality rates range from 19% to almost 50% due to hepatorenal failure and subsequent multiple-organ failure. SOS is characterized by hepatomegaly, jaundice, and fluid retention; its presence requires careful attention to fluid balance because sodium administration must be minimized, and coagulation abnormalities and refractoriness to platelet transfusions may occur.[241-243] Other gastrointestinal complications include hemorrhage,[244] infection, and opioid-induced abdominal pain and distention (i.e., narcotic bowel syndrome). Acute pulmonary complications occur in 30% to 60% of HSCT patients and include infection, hemorrhage, edema, bronchiolitis obliterans, acute respiratory distress syndrome (ARDS), and idiopathic pneumonia syndrome (IPS), a noninfectious inflammatory lung process.[245-247]

In the early phase after HSCT, significant cardiomyopathy and arrhythmias are uncommon (5%), but sepsis, cardiovascular collapse, and heart failure are common admitting diagnoses of the 10% to 40% of children who require intensive care after HSCT.[247-250] Late cardiac complications depend on the dosage of radiation and cardiotoxic chemotherapeutics used during the conditioning regimen. Acute renal failure occurs in 30% to 50% of children[251,252] and warrants judicious use of fluids in these patients[253]; hemorrhagic cystitis is also common.[254] A process of thrombotic microangiopathy similar to hemolytic uremic syndrome may occur in one fourth of children receiving cyclosporine or the calcineurin inhibitor tacrolimus.[255] Central nervous system complications include infection, hemorrhage, and encephalopathy and peripheral neuropathy due to metabolic and chemotherapeutic effects.[256-260]

Graft-versus-host disease (GVHD) is the clinical manifestation of the recognition of recipient alloantigens by donor T cells. Acute GVHD is a common event (incidence depends on the histocompatibility of the donor and recipient) before day 100 after transplantation, and it is characterized by inflammatory dermatitis, enteritis, and hepatitis. Chronic GVHD occurs in 6% to 50% of pediatric patients and is typically recognized 100 days or more after transplantation. This broad range of incidence depends on the age of donor and recipient, gender matching, and degree of matching between donor and recipient.[261] Chronic GVHD has many features of autoimmune diseases (e.g., sclerodermatous changes, dry mouth and conjunctivae, esophagitis, pulmonary dysfunction including bronchiolitis obliterans, contractures of extremities and soft tissue, alopecia, thrombocytopenia). Opportunistic infections are common during chronic GVHD. Hemolysis is an additional manifestation of alloantigenicity, the result of major and minor blood group incompatibilities between donor and recipient.

In contrast to the myeloablative procedures described previously in the context of malignant disorders, nonablative transplants are increasingly being used, particularly in nonmalignant disorders. Use of these transplants is based on the observation that in some instances, minimal myelotoxicity in conjunction with profound and prolonged immunosuppression leads to successful donor engraftment.[262] This modality is mostly used in children with nonmalignant hematologic conditions, marrow failure, and immunodeficiency syndromes.

## Perioperative Considerations

Surgical and procedural interventions are common throughout the transplantation process and are similar to those described earlier for children with cancer. A surgical procedure that is an integral component of HSCT is harvesting of hematopoietic stem cells from the recipient or another individual. Harvesting of bone marrow in children usually requires general anesthesia, although the procedure can be performed under spinal anesthesia with equivalent safety.[263] The donor is usually placed in a prone position to extract approximately 10 mL/kg (recipient weight) of marrow from the posterior iliac crests. When stem cells are obtained from peripheral blood, placement of vascular access in children usually requires sedation or general anesthesia. There is little evidence to support the avoidance of nitrous oxide for harvesting procedures, a concern raised in the past because nitrous oxide affects methionine synthase activity and DNA synthesis.[264]

In view of the wide range of possible complications, the many issues enumerated earlier for children with cancer must be considered for children undergoing HSCT (see Table 9-18). Radiation, glucocorticoids, mucositis, and chronic GVHD may contribute to an airway that is friable and a neck that is scarred, thereby increasing the risks of airway trauma, dental injury, and difficult tracheal intubation. Chemotherapy and GVHD may affect the skin and make venous access difficult. Chronic GVHD can lead to sclerodermatous changes, which can profoundly restrict range of motion, and sicca syndrome, which may necessitate use of artificial tears. GVHD may alter gut motility and delay gastric emptying. Immune compromise increases the risk of infection from vascular access lines and therefore mandates meticulous technique at all times. Chemotherapy may compromise cardiac and pulmonary function, alter hepatic metabolism of medications, and limit renal excretion of medications and fluids. Immune compromise and modifications resulting from transplantation require special processing of blood components, as recommended by hematology and blood bank consultants (see Tables 9-3, 9-4, and 9-5). Only irradiated, leukocyte-reduced, cytomegalovirus-negative (when the recipient is cytomegalovirus negative) blood components should be administered, and blood typing depends on engraftment of donor antigens. It is critical to coordinate the choice of blood products with the transplant service because often the blood type changes from that of recipient to that of donor.

In summary, hematologic disorders in childhood pose a wide array of challenges for the anesthesiologist caring for children. The considerations described in this chapter also provide many opportunities for collaboration with hematology-oncologists and surgeons to optimize perioperative outcomes for children with these disorders.

## ANNOTATED REFERENCES

Guzzetta NA, Miller BE. Principles of hemostasis in children: models and maturation. Paediatr Anaesth 2011;21:3-9.

*This review article summarizes the fundamentals of hemostasis and highlights the differences in thrombosis and coagulopathy from the preterm neonate through childhood. The impact of disease states on hemostasis are also discussed.*

Key NS, Derebail VK. Sickle-cell trait: novel clinical significance. Hematology 2010;2010:418-22.

*This review discusses sickle cell trait as a risk factor for adverse outcomes, focusing on its impact on exercise, renal function, and venous thromboembolism.*

Latham GJ, Greenberg RS. Anesthetic considerations for the pediatric oncology patient—part 1: a review of antitumor therapy. Paediatr Anaesth 2010;20:295-304.

*This article briefly reviews the current principles of cancer therapy and the general mechanisms of toxicity to the child, focusing on the impact to perioperative care and decision making.*

Latham GJ, Greenberg RS. Anesthetic considerations for the pediatric oncology patient—part 2: systems-based approach to anesthesia. Paediatr Anaesth 2010;20:396-420.

*A systems-based approach is used to assess the impact of the tumor and its treatment on children, and relevant anesthetic considerations are discussed.*

Latham GJ, Greenberg RS. Anesthetic considerations for the pediatric oncology patient—part 3: pain, cognitive dysfunction, and preoperative evaluation. Paediatr Anaesth 2010;20:479-89.

*This paper discusses the psychosocial impact of cancer and pain syndromes that should be considered in the perioperative period. A discussion of preanesthetic testing and evaluation in children with cancer follows.*

Morley SL. Red blood cell transfusions in acute paediatrics. Arch Dis Child Educ Pract Ed 2009;94:65-73.

*The risks and benefits of blood product transfusion in children are considered on the basis of current evidence from adult and pediatric studies.*

Vichinsky EP, Haberkern CM, Neumayr L, et al. A comparison of conservative and aggressive transfusion regimens in the perioperative management of sickle cell disease. The Preoperative Transfusion in Sickle Cell Disease Study Group. N Engl J Med 1995;333:206-13.

*This multicenter study found that a conservative transfusion regimen was as effective as the aggressive strategy in patients with sickle cell disease, and the consevative regimen resulted in one-half as many transfusion-associated complications.*

## REFERENCES

Please see www.expertconsult.com.

# Strategies for Blood Product Management and Reducing Transfusions

# 10

CHARLES J. COTÉ, ERIC F. GRABOWSKI, AND CHRISTOPHER P. STOWELL

DESPITE ADVANCES IN PEDIATRIC SURGERY, the number of infants and children who sustain major operative blood loss remains high. Little information is available about when to expect coagulation defects in the pediatric age group,[1,2] and most studies of massive blood transfusion have involved adult patients.[3]

Judicious blood transfusion is imperative because the supply of blood is limited and because transfusions can cause complications. The risk of these complications varies around the world. In countries with sophisticated health care systems, the most common fatal hazards of transfusion are hemolytic transfusion reactions due to ABO incompatibility (usually as a result of a transfusion error), bacterial infection, or transfusion-related acute lung injury (TRALI). In developing countries, the risk of infectious disease transmission may be substantial because of endemic infections in the population and the technical or logistic limitations of donor screening.

Nothing changed the use of blood products more than the threat of the acquired immunodeficiency syndrome (AIDS).[4-6] Although infection with human immunodeficiency virus (HIV) by blood transfusion has become rare, it was widely publicized in the lay press and is still feared by the public. Implementation of donor education programs, improved health history screening, new tests, and new test technologies (Table 10-1) have markedly altered the spectrum of transfusion-transmitted infectious agents in the developed world. The risks of some of the infectious and noninfectious hazards of transfusion are summarized in Table 10-2.

Despite marked reductions in the transmission of HIV, hepatitis C virus, and hepatitis B virus, transfusions can produce other deleterious effects.[7,8] Every transfusion must be medically justified; benefits must be weighed against the potential infectious, immunologic, and metabolic risks.[9] It is in the child's best interest to transfuse with a clear clinical goal and in the anesthesiologist's best interest to document the reason for each transfusion. It is not acceptable medical practice to administer a transfusion when it is of questionable benefit.

## Blood Volume

The circulating blood volume should be estimated before induction of anesthesia. The blood volume of a preterm infant (90 to 100 mL/kg) constitutes a greater proportion of body weight than that of a term neonate (80 to 90 mL/kg), infants between 3 months and 1 year old (70 to 80 mL/kg), or an older child (70 mL/kg). Consideration must also be given to body habitus. For example, an obese child has a blood volume of 60 to 65 mL/kg. From the estimated blood volume, the initial hemoglobin or hematocrit, and the minimum acceptable hematocrit, an *estimation* can be made of the maximum allowable blood loss (MABL) before red blood cell (RBC) transfusion is indicated.

The minimum acceptable hematocrit varies according to an individual child's need. The balance between oxygen supply and demand depends on a number of factors, including the oxygen content of blood, cardiac output and its regional distribution, and metabolic needs. A child with severe pulmonary disease or cyanotic congenital heart disease probably requires a greater hematocrit than a healthy child to satisfy the metabolic oxygen demands. Preterm infants may require a greater hematocrit to prevent apnea, reduce cardiac and respiratory work, and possibly improve neurologic outcomes,[10] although a Cochrane review suggests that this may not be the case.[11] If there is uncertainty about the need to transfuse these infants, the neonatologist should be consulted.[10,12,13] A healthy child readily tolerates a hematocrit well below 30%. It is our practice not to transfuse otherwise healthy infants up to about 3 months old until their hematocrits have decreased to 20% to 25% and hematocrits of

**TABLE 10-1** Current Blood Screening Tests Used on Donated Blood in the United States

Hepatitis B surface antigen (HBsAg)

Hepatitis B core antibody (anti-HBc)

Hepatitis C virus antibody (anti-HCV)

Nucleic acid amplification testing for HCV RNA

Human immunodeficiency virus type 1 (HIV-1) antibody (anti-HIV-1)

HIV-2 antibody (anti-HIV-2)

Nucleic acid amplification testing for HIV-1 RNA

Human T-lymphotropic virus type 1 (HTLV-I) antibody (anti-HTLV-I)

HTLV-II antibody (anti-HTLV-II)

Serologic test for syphilis (*Treponema pallidum*)

Nucleic acid amplification for West Nile virus (WNV) RNA*

*Trypanosoma cruzi* antibody (Chagas disease)[†]

*This test depends on the incidence in the geographic area.
[†]As of December 2011, at first donation or after residence in endemic area.
From American Association of Blood Banks. Facts about blood and blood banking, 2006. 509 Available at http://www.aabb.org/resources/bct/Pages/bloodfaq.aspx (accessed May 2012).

**TABLE 10-2** Estimated Frequency of Complications per Number of Units Transfused

| Category | Complication | Frequency |
|---|---|---|
| Noninfectious | Allergic (urticarial) | 1:100 |
| | Febrile, nonhemolytic | 1:100 |
| | Transfusion-associated circulatory overload | 1:1000 |
| | Delayed hemolytic | 1:1600 |
| | Transfusion-related acute lung injury | 1:10,000 |
| | Acute hemolytic | 1:50,000 |
| | Fatal acute hemolytic | 1:500,000 |
| Infectious | Hepatitis B virus | 1:250,000 |
| | Hepatitis C virus | 1:1,800,000 |
| | Human T-lymphotropic virus type I | 1:3,000,000 |
| | Human immunodeficiency virus type 1 | 1:2,300,000 |
| | Bacterial contamination of red blood cells | 1:50,000 |
| | Bacterial sepsis of red blood cells | 1:500,000 |
| | Bacterial contamination of platelets | 1:2,000 |
| | Bacterial sepsis of platelets | 1:75,000 |

Data from Davenport RD. Management of transfusion reactions. In: Mintz PD, editor. Transfusion therapy: clinical principles and practice. 3rd ed. Bethesda, Md.: AABB Press; 2011, p. 757-84; Alter HJ, Esteban-Mur JI. Transfusion transmitted hepatitis. In: Simon TL, Snyder EL, Solheim BG, et al., editors. Rossi's principles of transfusion medicine. 4th ed. Oxford: AABB Press, Wiley-Blackwell; 2009, p. 718-45; Barbara JA, Dow BC. Retroviruses and other viruses. In: Simon TL, Snyder EL, Solheim BG, et al., editors. Rossi's principles of transfusion medicine. 4th ed. Oxford: AABB Press, Wiley-Blackwell; 2009, p. 746-59; Park YA, Brecher ME. Bacterial contamination of blood products. In: Simon TL, Snyder EL, Solheim BG, et al., editors. Rossi's principles of transfusion medicine. 4th ed. Oxford: AABB Press, Wiley-Blackwell; 2009, p. 773-90.

**TABLE 10-3** Estimated Predicted Blood Loss and Recommended Monitoring and Equipment

| Predicted Blood Loss | Recommended Monitors or Equipment |
|---|---|
| Less than 0.5 blood volume | Routine monitoring |
| 0.5-1.0 blood volume | Routing monitoring + urine catheter |
| 1.0 blood volume or more | Routine monitoring + urine catheter + CVP + arterial line |
| 1.0 blood volume or more with potential for rapid blood loss | Routine monitoring + urine catheter + CVP + arterial line + large-bore IV line + rapid-infusion device |
| Severe head injury | Routine monitoring + urine catheter + CVP + arterial line + large-bore IV line |
| Major trauma with unknown severity | Routine monitoring + urine catheter + CVP + arterial line + large-bore IV line (preferably in upper extremity or central) + rapid-infusion device |

*CVP*, Central venous pressure; *IV*, intravenous.

adequacy of volume replacement. If a procedure is expected to result in significant blood loss or fluid shifts, the anesthesiologist should strongly consider the use of a urine catheter, a central venous line, and invasive arterial monitoring. The child's size or age should not be a deterrent to the use of a central venous catheter (Table 10-3).

There are three approaches for estimating the MABL: an approximation of circulating RBC mass, a modified logarithmic equation, and a simple proportion.[14,15] All three approaches yield clinically similar estimates of the MABL. The most straightforward method is to estimate the MABL by simple proportion.[14] For purposes of discussion, we use a hematocrit of 25% as the minimum acceptable hematocrit.

$$MABL = \frac{EBV \times (Child's\ hematocrit - Minimum\ acceptable\ hematocrit)}{Child's\ hematocrit}$$

For example, a 10-kg child has an estimated blood volume of 10 (kg) × 70 (mL/kg), or 700 mL. If the child's hematocrit is 42, the MABL is calculated as follows:

$$MABL = \frac{700 \times (42 - 25)}{42}$$
$$= \frac{700 \times 17}{42}$$
$$= 285\ mL$$

These calculations only estimate the MABL. The actual hematocrit varies with the child's preexisting medical conditions, the rapidity of the blood loss, and the rate of concurrent crystalloid replacement.

Initial therapy is directed at replacing fluid deficits and providing maintenance requirements (see Chapter 8). Additional fluid administration is directed at replacing blood loss and third space fluid losses. Although former recommendations for crystalloid replacement of blood loss were 2 to 3 mL per milliliter of shed blood, later studies suggest a smaller volume of replacement, and 1 to 2 mL of isotonic crystalloid or 1 mL of 5% albumin may be adequate.[16-18] The latter type of replacement is expensive, and there is no clear evidence that colloid is superior to crystalloid.[19] New starch volume expanders have been introduced that may hold promise in the future for use in children.

older children have decreased to 20% if there is little potential for postoperative bleeding. *The circulating blood volume must be maintained in every case.* Observing the operative field to estimate blood loss and monitoring the vital signs, hematocrit, urine output, and the central venous pressure (CVP) help to assess the

In a 10-kg child with a 700-mL blood volume and 285-mL MABL, the blood loss can be corrected in one of two ways: 570 mL of isotonic crystalloid or 285 mL of 5% albumin. If blood loss exceeds the MABL, or if the hematocrit decreases to 20% to 25% (particularly if additional blood loss is expected during surgery or in the recovery period), transfusion with packed red blood cells (PRBCs) or whole blood (if available) should be started. If postoperative bleeding is likely to occur (e.g., posterior spinal fusion, open heart operations, burn wound excision and grafting), it is reasonable to transfuse to a level greater than the minimum acceptable hematocrit. This is especially true if a greater hematocrit can be provided without the exposure to additional units of blood by completing only the units that are infusing. If 1 unit of blood has been started, it is reasonable to give the child an additional 5% to 10% rather than a fraction of a second unit postoperatively. It is our practice to administer as much of the unit as can be safely tolerated rather than expose the child to another unit of blood postoperatively. Blood banks often prepare several aliquots from one unit, especially for infants, and they can assign one donor unit to a particular child. One part may be given immediately, whereas the second part may be given later; this reduces the risk of exposure to more than one donor for the child.

There seems to be little danger in replacing the MABL entirely with crystalloid provided that the child is healthy and that postoperative oozing will not exceed the MABL. If correction of lost RBCs is necessary, it is simple to calculate the volume of PRBCs needed to return the hemoglobin to an acceptable value. For example, if a 10-kg child's hematocrit had decreased to 23%, intraoperative or postoperative blood loss is anticipated to continue, and the anesthesiologist elected to increase the hematocrit to 35%, the following calculations can be made:

$$\text{Volume of PRBCs} = \frac{(\text{Desired Hct} - \text{Present Hct}) \times \text{Estimated Blood Volume} (70\ \text{mL/kg} \times 10\ \text{kg})}{\text{Hematocrit of PRCBs}}$$

$$= \frac{(35 - 23) \times (70 \times 10)}{60}$$

$$= 140\ \text{mL PRBCs}$$

Because this volume is less than 1 unit, it may be reasonable to transfuse the child up to a hematocrit of 40% (200 mL PRBCs) to allow an additional margin of safety for postoperative blood loss.

## Blood Components and Alternatives

In countries with well-developed health care systems, most whole blood collected from donors is fractionated into components. A unit of whole blood can provide 1 unit of PRBCs, 1 unit of whole blood–derived platelets, and 1 unit of FFP. Apheresis technology can be used to collect any one of these three components selectively. Separation of the individual components from blood allows each to be stored under conditions that best preserve its function: at refrigerator temperature (4° to 10° C) for PRBC, at less than −18° C for FFP, and at room temperature (20° to 24° C) for platelets. Most children with specific disease states (e.g., anemia, clotting factor deficiencies, thrombocytopenia) require only one of these fractions, which is why use of component therapy is widespread. Many blood banks also separate individual units of blood components into smaller-volume pediatric units, so that multiple RBC transfusions can be administered to an infant from a single adult unit.

**TABLE 10-4** Composition of Compounds Containing Red Blood Cells

| Parameter | CPDA-1 Whole Blood* | CPDA-1 RBC* | Additive Solution RBC† |
|---|---|---|---|
| Storage time (days) | 35 | 35 | 42 |
| Volume RBC (mL) ‡ | 203 | 203 | 203 |
| Residual plasma (mL) § | 248 | 50 | 30 |
| Hematocrit (%)‡ | 40 | 72 | 53 |
| pH | 6.98 | 6.71 | 6.6 |
| Adenosine triphosphate (% of day 1) | 56 | 45 | 60 |
| 2,3-DPG (% of day 1) | <10 | <10 | <10 |
| Total supernatant K+ (mEq) | 5-7 | 5-7 | 5-7 |

*CPDA*, Citrate, phosphate, dextrose, and adenine solution; *DPG*, 2,3-diphosphoglycerate; *RBC*, red blood cell.
*Outdated at 35 days.
†Outdated at 42 days.
‡Based on collection of 450 mL of whole blood with a hematocrit of 45%.
§The concentration of factors V and VIII is reduced to 20% to 50% of normal levels (0.2 to 0.5 units/mL). The other clotting factors are quite stable.

## RED BLOOD CELL–CONTAINING COMPONENTS

Blood components containing RBCs are indicated for the treatment of symptomatic deficits of oxygen-carrying capacity.[20,21] PRBCs are the most widely available RBC-containing blood component, although in settings where the collection facilities do not have the capability of making components, whole blood may be the only component available. Donor whole blood is collected in a preservative-anticoagulant solution that contains citrate, phosphate, dextrose (glucose), and adenine (CPDA) or just citrate, phosphate, and dextrose. In the latter case, the platelet-rich plasma is removed after centrifugation of the whole blood unit, and a solution containing adenine, dextrose, and occasionally mannitol is added to the PRBCs. The additive-solution systems permit storage for 42 days (compared with 35 days for CPDA) and better preservation of 2,3-diphosphoglycerate (DPG) levels. The characteristics of the CPDA and additive-solution PRBCs and of whole blood are shown in Table 10-4. Although the hematocrit is reduced in the additive-solution PRBCs, the red cell mass is the same.

RBCs carry glycoconjugate antigens of the ABH histo-blood group system on the cell surface that are determined by six common alleles on chromosome 9.[19a] During the first year of life, infants begin to elaborate alloantibodies to whichever A or B antigens they lack. These isoagglutinins are invariably present after a few months and constitute a formidable immunologic obstacle to transfusion or transplantation across this ABO barrier. The RBCs for transfusion must be compatible with the ABO isoagglutinins of the intended transfusion recipient. Similarly, components with a large volume of plasma (e.g., whole blood, FFP, apheresis platelets) must be compatible with the A or B surface antigens expressed on the recipient's RBCs. PRBCs must be ABO *compatible* with the recipient, whereas whole blood must be ABO *identical*. Table 10-5 summarizes the permissible combinations.

**TABLE 10-5** ABO Compatibility of Blood Components

| Recipient ABO Group | ACCEPTABLE COMPONENT ABO GROUPS (SECOND CHOICE) | | | |
|---|---|---|---|---|
| | Whole Blood | PRBC | FFP/Cryo | Platelets |
| O | O | O | O (A, B, AB, plasma) | O (A, B, AB) |
| A | A | A (O) | A (AB) | A (AB)* |
| B | B | B (O) | B (AB) | B (AB)* |
| AB | AB | AB (A, B, O) | AB | AB* |

*Cyro*, Cryoprecipitate; *FFP*, fresh frozen plasma; *PRBC*, packed red blood cells.
*Can come from group apheresis platelets (or whole blood–derived platelets for small child) if plasma is removed or replaced.

**TABLE 10-6** Rh(D) Compatibility of Blood Components

| Recipient Rh(D) Type | ACCEPTABLE COMPONENT Rh(D) TYPES (SECOND CHOICE) | | | |
|---|---|---|---|---|
| | Whole Blood or PRBCs | FFP/ Cryo | Apheresis Platelets | Whole Blood–Derived Platelets |
| Positive | Rh positive (Rh negative) | Any | Any | Rh positive (Rh negative) |
| Negative | Rh negative (Rh positive)* | Any | Any | Rh negative (Rh positive)*† |

*Cyro*, Cryoprecipitate; *FFP*, fresh frozen plasma; *PRBCs*, packed red blood cells.
*Depending on inventory, the blood bank may switch to Rh(D) positive, particularly for male patients or postmenopausal females.
†Consider Rh immune globulin for females with childbearing potential receiving whole blood–derived platelets from Rh(D)–positive donors.

Only RBCs express the Rh(D) antigen. Rh(D)-positive patients may receive Rh(D)-positive or Rh(D)-negative RBCs. Rh(D)-negative patients are routinely given Rh(D)-negative RBCs for any elective transfusions, but in the setting of massive transfusion it may be necessary to switch to Rh(D)-positive RBCs to preserve the supply of Rh(D)-negative RBCs. The blood bank usually determines when to make this substitution based on the inventory and does so more quickly for a patient who is a male or a postmenopausal female (Table 10-6). The objective is to avoid exposing a female with childbearing potential to Rh(D)-positive RBCs and possibly triggering the production of the anti-D allo-antibody, which is responsible for the most severe forms of hemolytic disease of the newborn. Table 10-7 shows the common initial volume of PRBCs needed to increase the hemoglobin level by 2 to 3 g/dL.

The changes that occur to RBC during storage under conventional blood bank conditions has been well described.[22] These observations have generated physiologically plausible hypotheses about how such changes may impair the function of the banked RBCs in vivo. The loss of intra-erythrocytic levels of 2,3-DPG and its corresponding decrease in the $P_{50}$ value may reduce the ability of stored RBCs to relinquish bound $O_2$ compared with 2,3-DPG–replete RBCs. The depletion of nitric oxide (NO) may reduce the vasodilatory properties of the RBCs, hence impairing their ability to maintain the patency of the small vessels in the microcirculation and blood flow to the tissues.[23] Numerous changes in the composition and behavior of the RBC plasma membrane, including the loss and oxidation of membrane lipids and proteins and the rearrangement of some membrane constituents,[24] correlate with changes in the shape and elasticity of the

**TABLE 10-7** Common Initial Doses of Blood Components and Expected Effects in Children

| Component | Dose | Effect |
|---|---|---|
| Packed red blood cells | 10-15 mL/kg | Increase hemoglobin by 2-3 g/dL |
| Platelets* | 5-10 mL/kg | Increase platelet count by 50,000-100,000/mm³ |
| Fresh frozen plasma | 10-15 mL/kg | Factor levels increase by 15%-20% |
| Cryoprecipitate | 1-2 units/kg | Increase fibrinogen by 60-100 mg/dL |

*This recommendation may be reduced pending the impact of the prophylactic platelet dose (PLADO) trial, as published for all age groups[40] and for the pediatric age range.[40a]

RBC membrane.[25,26] The loss of elasticity in particular can impede the rapid movement of the RBCs through the microcirculation.

These hypotheses and some supportive data from animal models[27] have led to a number of clinical studies (mostly in trauma, critical care, colorectal surgery, and cardiac surgery) of outcomes after using stored RBCs, but the results have been inconclusive.[28-30] About half of the studies found a statistical association between at an unfavorable clinical outcome measure and the transfusion of RBCs, which had been stored for a longer time. However, no association was seen in one half of the studies, including two that were extensions of previous studies with positive findings. A small number of randomized, controlled trials addressed this issue without statistically significant differences in outcomes between patients receiving RBCs stored for different amounts of time,[31] although two of them were underpowered.[32,33] Knowing that RBCs change during storage raises the question of whether these changes affect the patients in a clinically meaningful way, a question that remains unanswered. Currently, there are four randomized, clinical trials being conducted in North America in populations of especially vulnerable patients: neonates in the intensive care unit, adults in the intensive care unit, and adults undergoing cardiac surgery.[34-37] The results of these trials should help to guide future transfusion practice.

## PLATELETS

Platelets may be obtained from a whole blood donation or collected by apheresis. Whole blood–derived platelets are separated by centrifugation and suspended in 40 to 60 mL of plasma at a concentration that is two to four times greater than in the circulation. Each unit contains a minimum of $5.5 \times 10^{10}$ platelets and is stored at 20° to 24° C with gentle continuous agitation for a maximum of 5 days. One unit of whole blood–derived platelets can be expected to increase the platelet count of a 70-kg adult by 5000 to 10,000/mm³ and increase the count in an 18-kg child by 15,000/mm³.[38,39] A unit of platelets obtained by apheresis contains at least $3 \times 10^{11}$ platelets in 200 to 400 mL of plasma, or the equivalent of approximately 6 units of whole blood–derived platelets. A common dose for pediatric patients is 0.1 to 0.3 unit/kg of body weight, or 10 to 15 mL/kg (see Table 10-7); this dose usually produces an increment of 30,000 to 90,000/mm³. However, a rigorous reassessment of platelet dosing was just carried out in the prophylactic platelet dose trial.[40,41] Doses equivalent to the standard dose of one pheresis pack (or 6 units) per m², half of this dose, and double this dose were compared in 1272 adult and pediatric patients who received at least one platelet transfusion. Blood losses were determined with the World Health Organization (WHO) bleeding scale: grade 0 = no bleeding, grade 1 = petechiae, grade 2 = mild blood loss, grade 3 = gross blood loss, and grade 4 = debilitating blood loss. No differences were observed in bleeding outcomes (WHO grade 2 or greater) among the three doses; this was also true for the subset of 200 pediatric patients. The recommended platelet dose may be reduced in the near future, but this change awaits further discussion by the blood transfusion and hemostasis community.[42-44] This trial did not involve patients undergoing surgical procedures with ongoing blood loss.

In the setting of dilutional thrombocytopenia with ongoing losses or a consumptive coagulopathy (e.g., disseminated intravascular coagulation), larger doses (≥0.3 unit/kg) may be required to boost the platelet count above 50,000/mm³. Because platelets are suspended in plasma that contains the anti-A and anti-B isoagglutinins, they should be ABO compatible with the recipient's RBCs. Some blood donors have high-titer isoagglutinins that can produce hemolysis in transfusion recipients if a large enough volume of plasma is given.[45] The transfusion of plasma-incompatible, whole blood–derived platelets to adult recipients does not produce clinically significant hemolysis because the volume of plasma given is so small relative to the plasma volume of an adult. However, apheresis platelets (and whole blood–derived platelets for small children) should be ABO compatible with the recipient's RBCs. Because platelets do not express Rh antigens, matching for Rh(D) antigen is not necessary for apheresis platelets because they contain virtually no RBCs. However, whole blood–derived platelets may contain enough RBCs to provoke Rh alloimmunization so platelets from Rh(D)-negative donors are given preferentially to Rh(D)-negative recipients with childbearing potential. If a premenopausal female receives whole blood–derived platelets from an Rh(D)-positive donor, Rh immune globulin can be administered within 72 hours to prevent alloimmunization. Platelets should never be withheld in an emergency situation because of Rh(D) incompatibility.

Platelets are essential to hemostasis associated with the vascular injury of surgery and are necessary for the control of surgical bleeding. Platelets are also required for the maintenance of an intact endothelial barrier to spontaneous blood loss. The number of platelets required to provide adequate hemostasis in the surgical setting is much greater than the level needed to provide prophylaxis against spontaneous hemorrhage. A platelet count of 10,000/mm³ is considered adequate to prevent spontaneous bleeding or bleeding from minor invasive procedures (e.g., lumbar puncture, line placement) in an otherwise stable child. If overt signs of bleeding are present or a more significant hemostatic challenge in the form of a surgical procedure is imminent, a level of 30,000 to 50,000/mm³ may be required.[46-50] A target level of 50,000/mm³ is appropriate in the setting of massive transfusion.[47,51-53] Platelets may also be required for children with adequate counts but in whom platelet function is impaired. Many medications (e.g., aspirin; nonsteroidal antiinflammatory agents; dipyridamole; platelet P2Y12 receptor blockers such as clopidogrel or prasugrel; or glycoprotein IIa/IIIb receptor inhibitors such as abciximab, eptifibatide, or tirofiban; serotonin uptake antagonists such as Zoloft) and some conditions (e.g., renal failure with blood urea nitrogen levels above 60 mg/dL) cause abnormal platelet function, which may interfere with surgical hemostasis, in which case it may be necessary to maintain the platelet count at a somewhat greater level, at least until the effect of the medication dissipates or the child's platelets have largely been replaced by banked platelets.[54,55] In a few settings, such as

intracranial, ophthalmic, and otologic surgery, even greater levels (100,000/mm³) are sought.

There is no clear-cut threshold below which the platelet count predicts clinical bleeding in the perioperative period. Each child must be individually assessed by constantly observing the surgical field for evidence of abnormal bleeding.[56] Unfortunately, we lack a well-validated bedside tool to assess platelet function. The utility of the thromboelastogram and other devices to measure platelet function under controlled flow conditions, such as the platelet function analyzer (PFA-100), are being investigated.[57-59] The standard technique for diagnosis and evaluation of thrombocytopathies remains Born-O'Brien platelet aggregometry, but it is not useful in the intraoperative setting.[60] Most commonly, thrombocytopenia rather than a newly acquired platelet function defect is the problem in the operative setting and massive transfusion.

A child occasionally presents for surgery with a previously characterized platelet dysfunction that may be associated with bleeding. If the child has a normal platelet count, it is reasonable practice to ensure that the blood bank has an adequate platelet supply available for the operating room but to withhold transfusion until the child demonstrates pathologic bleeding.

Several additional points should be considered[61]:

1. Not all hospitals have platelets in the inventory. Unless the need is anticipated before surgery, platelets may not be available when required.
2. For children who are thrombocytopenic before surgery, platelets should be infused just before the surgical procedure to ensure the greatest levels during the time of peak demand.
3. Platelets should be filtered only by large-pore filters (≥150 μm) or leukocyte-reduction filters (if indicated). Micropore filters may adsorb large numbers of platelets and therefore diminish the effectiveness of a platelet transfusion.
4. Platelets are suspended in plasma, which may help to replenish coagulation factors other than factors V and VIII, which are labile.
5. Platelets should not be refrigerated or placed in a cooler with ice before administration, because after they are transfused, cold platelets are rapidly cleared from the circulation.

## SPECIAL PROCESSING OF CELLULAR BLOOD COMPONENTS

Leukocytes collected with whole blood donations partition into platelet and PRBC components, and few intact leukocytes are present in FFP. Passenger leukocytes are responsible for most febrile, nonhemolytic transfusion reactions, HLA alloimmunization, and transmission of cytomegalovirus (CMV). To prevent the complications from these leukocytes, they can be very effectively removed (2 to 3 log reduction) by passage through leukocyte-reduction filters that may be done shortly after collection (prestorage leukoreduction) or at the bedside. Leukocyte reduction of RBCs by filtration is a superior technique to washing

**TABLE 10-8** Indications for Leukocyte-Reduced Cellular Blood Components

- To prevent further febrile, nonhemolytic transfusion reactions in a child with a history of such reactions
- To prevent human leukocyte antigen alloimmunization in a child who may require long-term platelet transfusion support (e.g., leukemia, lymphoma)
- To prevent human leukocyte antigen alloimmunization in a transplant recipient
- To prevent cytomegalovirus infection and disease in a susceptible child

or freezing-deglycerolizing, which was used in the past. Table 10-8 provides indications for who may benefit from receiving leukocyte-reduced cellular components (i.e., RBCs or platelets).

CMV transmission can also be reduced by screening donors for CMV exposure (testing for antibody to CMV), although leukocyte reduction is the more widely used approach. Even though primary CMV infection is benign in children with intact immune systems, some pediatric populations are at risk for developing systemic disease and should be protected from CMV transmission by blood. Only patients who have not previously been infected with CMV (i.e., CMV seronegative) are at risk. Children particularly susceptible to systemic CMV infections are listed in E-Table 10-1.

Transfused lymphocytes may mediate a graft-versus-host process in some recipients with impaired cellular immunity. Because this process involves the bone marrow and the usual targets (i.e., skin and gastrointestinal tract), the fatality rate is substantial. Transfusion-associated graft-versus-host disease (GVHD) can be prevented by exposing cellular blood components to gamma irradiation that disables the donor lymphocytes. Children who are considered to be at risk for transfusion-associated GVHD and who should receive irradiated cellular components are listed in E-Table 10-2. This complication can also occur in children with intact immune systems in the unusual circumstance when the transfusion donor is homozygous for an HLA haplotype that is shared with the recipient. In this case, the recipient's immune system, although fully functional, cannot recognize the donor lymphocytes as foreign. The donor lymphocytes mount a GVHD attack on the recipient's tissues, recognizing the mismatched haplotype. This situation is more likely to occur when the donor is a blood relative of the recipient. It is for this reason that blood and HLA-matched platelets donated by family members are routinely irradiated.

## FRESH FROZEN PLASMA

Fresh frozen plasma (FFP) represents the fluid portion of whole blood that is separated and frozen within 8 hours of collection. After thawing at 37° C, which usually requires 30 minutes, it may be administered within 24 hours if stored at 1° to 6° C. The volume of 1 unit varies from 180 to 300 mL and represents 7% to 10% of the coagulation factor activity in a 70-kg patient. It contains all of the clotting factors and regulatory proteins at approximately the native concentration, but after 6 hours at 1° to 6° C, the levels of the labile factors V and VIII begin to diminish.[62] FFP does not provide functional platelets, nor does it contain leukocytes or RBCs.

FFP should be ABO-compatible with recipient red cells because it contains the anti-A and anti-B isoagglutinins. If the recipient's blood type is not known, plasma from a donor with blood type AB, which contains neither anti-A nor anti-B, may be administered. Because the citrate anticoagulant is present in the plasma, rapid administration of FFP is more likely to be associated with citrate toxicity than the transfusion of components with smaller volumes of plasma (e.g., PRBCs).

FFP is frequently administered without justification by evidence-based medicine.[63] One major surgical indication for FFP is to correct the coagulopathy associated with massive blood transfusion (see Table 10-7). Other indications include a prolongation in the prothrombin time (PT) before surgery or in the setting of bleeding, the emergency reversal of warfarin, or the presence of a specific congenital or acquired coagulation protein deficiency for which a factor concentrate or a recombinant factor is not available (e.g., for factor XI deficiency).[64] Administration of vitamin K should not be overlooked in children who are taking warfarin, have hepatic insufficiency, have been exclusively breast-fed,[65-67] who have been on broad-spectrum antibiotics (which often eliminate normal vitamin K–producing gastrointestinal flora), who have been on total parenteral nutrition for inadequate oral caloric intake, or who may have prolonged hospitalizations. Correction of a mild increase in the PT (e.g., international normalized ratio [INR] <1.5) is rarely necessary. Figure 10-1 shows the relationship between the level of coagulation factors and the in vitro clotting times, in this case the PT. Relatively modest levels of coagulation factors can support normal hemostasis, even

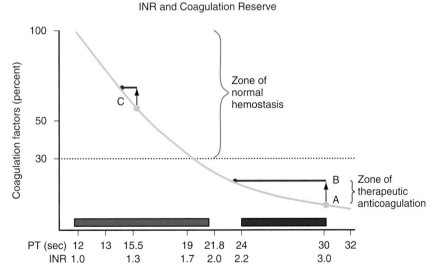

**FIGURE 10-1** Nonlinear relationship between levels of coagulation factor and clotting test results. Decreases in clotting factor levels to about 30% of normal prolong the clotting test times but still support normal hemostasis. Treating an adult or child at point A with fresh frozen plasma to raise the level of coagulation factors to point B has a marked effect on the prothrombin time and the international normalized ratio (INR). The same amount of fresh frozen plasma administered to an adult or child at point C, however, has only a minor effect on the prothrombin time (PT). (Modified from Dzik WH, Stowell CP. Transfusion and coagulation issues in trauma. In: Sheridan RL, editor. The trauma handbook of Massachusetts General Hospital. Philadelphia: Lippincott Williams & Wilkins; 2004. p. 139.)

though the PT is prolonged. When the PT is very prolonged (see Fig. 10-1, point A), the transfusion of 1 unit of FFP, which increases the coagulation factor levels by 7% to 10% in an adult, has a dramatic effect on shortening the PT. When the PT is only mildly prolonged, as at point C, where factor levels are already adequate for hemostasis, the increase in the factor levels by an additional 7% to 10% with 1 unit of FFP (in an adult) has a much smaller effect on the PT. This small effect does not achieve any improvement in hemostasis.

### CRYOPRECIPITATE

Cryoprecipitate is prepared by thawing FFP at 4° to 10° C and expressing most of the plasma, leaving behind precipitated protein that is then resuspended in a small volume of residual plasma (15 to 25 mL) and refrozen. This component contains 20% to 50% of the factor VIII from the original unit of plasma. It also contains von Willebrand factor (vWF), fibrinogen (approximately 250 mg), and factor XIII. It is indicated for the treatment of factor XIII deficiency, dysfibrinogenemia, and hypofibrinogenemia (see Table 10-7).[68-77] It is no longer used for the treatment of von Willebrand disease or hemophilia A. Plasma concentrates of factor XIII and fibrinogen have been available in Europe for several years and recently have been licensed in the United States for use in patients with these congenital deficiencies.

### PLASMA-DERIVED AND RECOMBINANT FACTOR CONCENTRATES

The most commonly administered factor concentrate is factor VIII, used in the treatment of hemophilia A. Children with hemophilia can have many problems related to their disease, including splenomegaly, abnormal liver function, and joint disease related to hemarthrosis. In the past, the use of pooled plasma products was associated with very high rates of transmission of viral hepatitis (especially hepatitis C virus) and HIV.[78-80] The use of more rigorous viral removal and inactivation processes and the introduction of recombinant factor VIII and IX products[81-85] have greatly reduced these problems.[68-75,86] Initial concerns that there may be an increased incidence of inhibitors in children who receive recombinant therapy compared with plasma-derived factor therapy have not been borne out.[87] Mild hemophilia usually responds well to desmopressin (1-deamino-8-D-arginine vasopressin [DDAVP]) therapy.[88,89]

Children with hemophilia B (i.e., Christmas disease or factor IX deficiency) are managed with recombinant human factor IX and highly purified factor IX (preparations with various amounts of factors VII, X, and prothrombin) that are treated to inactivate or remove viruses.[70,71,73,90-103] Careful planning of any surgical procedure for these children includes close communication with the child's hematologist to ensure optimal therapy while reducing unnecessary transfusions (see Chapter 9).

von Willebrand disease is routinely treated with DDAVP or plasma-derived factor VIII concentrates that are also rich in vWF, such as Humate-P, Alphanate, and Koate DVI. In children who have von Willebrand disease and are resistant to DDAVP or for whom DDAVP is contraindicated (e.g., central nervous system [CNS] bleeding, allergic reaction), it is reasonable to withhold treatment with blood-derived products until surgery has begun unless surgery is performed in an area where bleeding is potentially life-threatening, to reduce unnecessary transfusions. These children often do not demonstrate pathologic bleeding. Adjunctive therapies that can further minimize the use of blood products include use of the antifibrinolytic agent ε-aminocaproic

acid (Amicar), which can be administered orally or intravenously, and topical hemostatic agents, including topical collagen and fibrin glues.

### DESMOPRESSIN

DDAVP, a synthetic analogue of vasopressin, can increase the levels of factor VIII:C (i.e., coagulant activity) and factor VIII:vWF in children with mild hemophilia A or von Willebrand disease.[89,104-108] An IV dose of 0.3 μg/kg (maximum 20 μg; a subcutaneous preparation is available in Europe) increases the levels of both factors twofold to threefold within 30 to 60 minutes, with a half-life of 3 to 6 hours.[105] Intranasal DDAVP is also effective, but onset is less rapid. Between 80% and 90% of children with von Willebrand disease are responders,[109,110] and affected children should be tested for their responsiveness to IV DDAVP. This treatment is best suited to bleeding from surgical procedures, which ceases within 2 to 3 days. When bleeding continues beyond this period, as can occur with some orthopedic procedures, daily IV Humate P (or Alphanate or Koate DVI) can obviate possible tachyphylaxis with DDAVP. Products rich in the vWF allow better control over peak levels of factor VIII. When in excess of 200%, factor VIII predisposes to postoperative deep venous thrombosis and pulmonary embolism.

DDAVP has been used to treat the coagulopathy associated with uremia and cirrhosis.[111,112] It may reduce elective surgical bleeding when the potential for blood loss is substantial, such as in cardiac surgery and spinal fusion.[89,113-118] Although initial reports apparently demonstrated a benefit in patients who did not have a preexisting coagulopathy, other controlled studies failed to show an effect despite increases in factor VIII:C and vWF, and its use for these indications has largely been abandoned.[119-121] Because of the potential for hyponatremia from water retention, use of DDAVP is avoided in children younger than 2 years, in children with CNS lesions, including a brain tumor, history of CNS irradiation, or recent neurosurgery or CNS trauma, and in elderly adults.

### ALBUMIN, DEXTRANS, STARCHES, AND GELATINS

Solutions of several high-molecular-weight molecules (i.e., colloids) have been used for volume replacement, although there is no clear advantage to their use over crystalloid solutions. These colloids include albumin, dextrans, starches, and gelatins.

Albumin has the longest track record and the fewest adverse side effects.[122,123] In the past, dextrans (i.e., high- and low-molecular-weight glucose polymers) were administered for volume expansion and hemodilution in children,[124,125] but currently, their primary use is for antithrombosis, although their value for even this indication is questionable.[126]

Starches are branched polysaccharide polymers available in high-, medium-, and low-molecular-weight ranges (480,000 to 70,000 daltons). However, these compounds alter hemostasis by diluting clotting factors and impairing platelet function and the coagulation cascade.[127,128] An additional concern, especially in children, is their accumulation in the reticuloendothelial system and the potential for unknown long-term adverse effects.[129] Several studies have been carried out in children with minor changes in coagulation parameters that occurred when transfusions exceed 20 mL/kg.[130-134] A 6% hydroxyethyl starch (HES 130/0.4) yielded clinical and physiologic profiles similar to those for 5% albumin in volumes up to 16 mL/kg in noncardiac surgery and in volumes up to 50 mL/kg in cardiac surgery, although at smaller cost.[135,136] Several major reviews regarding the use of starches and gels in adult patients who are critically ill have raised significant concerns regarding adverse effects on coagulation[137,138] and renal function,[139,140] and they found inadequate overall safety data, even for the third-generation products.[18,141] If these concerns have been raised in adult populations, we should have even greater concern about their use in children.

Gelatins are polypeptides derived from bovine collagen that seem to have a minimal effect on coagulation and provide reasonable plasma volume expansion. However, a significant number of life-threatening anaphylactic or anaphylactoid reactions have been reported, and their use in children remains somewhat limited.[122,142-146]

## RED BLOOD CELL SUBSTITUTES

Blood substitutes offer the promise of agents with universal compatibility, minimal infectious risks, and prolonged shelf life (years rather than days) to carry oxygen to vital organs.[147] Early efforts to develop these products involved a variety of human, bovine, and genetically engineered hemoglobin polymer solutions, perfluorocarbons, and lipid-encapsulated hemoglobin. Most failed in clinical trials because of severe complications such as renal failure, stroke, and vasoconstriction.[148,149] One formulation, Hemospan (Sangart, Inc., San Diego), is still in clinical trials.[150-152] It is designed to maximize oxygen delivery at the tissue level (i.e., capillary beds with impaired perfusion) rather than maximize oxygen-carrying capacity and have equivalency to hemoglobin.[148,153-157] Further research is needed before these blood substitutes become available for use in children.

## Massive Blood Transfusion

Massive blood transfusion may be defined as replacement of a patient's entire blood volume one or more times. In children, the anesthesiologist must think in terms of percent of blood volumes lost rather than units of blood transfused. The composition of each blood component must be considered to anticipate problems and determine at what stage of a massive transfusion these problems may occur (see Table 10-3). Transfusion of large quantities of blood components may seriously affect coagulation, potassium and calcium concentrations, acid–base balance, body temperature, oxygen-hemoglobin dissociation, and hematocrit (i.e., oxygen-carrying capacity).

Most blood banks should have a system for the expedited release of blood products, often referred to as a *massive transfusion protocol* when there is inadequate time to perform complete serologic testing, including the crossmatch. Type O Rh-negative blood can be transfused into any child without the need for a crossmatch; type O Rh-positive blood may be transfused into male patients. After the blood bank has a sample of the child's blood, it can be switched to type-specific blood and then to blood that has completed standard compatibility testing. Table 10-9 illustrates the process and risks associated with expedited release of RBCs.[158] With massive blood loss, infusing crystalloid solutions alone can only worsen the underlying coagulopathy, such as from trauma-induced bleeding.

## COAGULOPATHY

The coagulation system in children and adults involves platelets, coagulation proteins, and localized tissue factor, which initiate all steps of hemostasis. Figure 10-2 shows that an initial step is platelet adhesion to a wound or site of vessel wall injury, with adhesion being mediated by the vWF through its receptor on

**TABLE 10-9** Approximate Time for Expedited Release of Red Blood Cells

| ABO Group | Crossmatch | Preparation in Blood Bank (min) | Risk of Incompatibility |
|---|---|---|---|
| O | None | 5 | RBC alloantibody |
| ABO specific | None | 15 | RBC alloantibody |
| ABO specific | Abbreviated | 30 | Screen negative = none Screen positive = RBC alloantibody |
| ABO specific | Full | 60 | None |

Modified with permission from Dzik WH, Stowell CP. Transfusion and coagulation issues in trauma. In: Sheridan RL, editor. The trauma handbook of the Massachusetts General Hospital. Philadelphia: Lippincott Williams & Wilkins; 2004. p. 128-47.
*RBC*, Red blood cell.

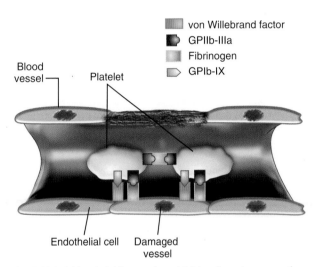

**FIGURE 10-2** A blood clot forms when platelets adhere to one another through the GPIIb-IIIa complex (*purple*), which serves as a receptor for the adhesive protein fibrinogen (*orange*). Platelet interaction with an injured vessel wall requires synergy between the GPIb-IX (*blue*) and GPIIb-IIIa complexes and the adhesive proteins of von Willebrand factor (*green*) and fibrinogen, respectively. In high-velocity gradients, the efficacy of GPIb-IX interaction with the von Willebrand factor is significantly impaired.

the platelet, the glycoprotein Ib–glycoprotein IX complex (GPIb-IX), and fibrinogen through the fibrinogen receptor on the platelet, the glycoprotein IIb–glycoprotein IIIa complex (GPIIb-IIIA). In flowing blood, initial platelet attachment is facilitated by vWF, whereas platelet spreading and more secure (shear stress–resistant) platelet-platelet aggregation is driven by fibrinogen and by the GPIIa-GPIIIa complex. However, there is also evidence that platelets attach even to intact endothelium, which has an activated phenotype, as after inflammatory cytokine exposure or sepsis. Platelets attach to the endothelium through high-molecular-weight von Willebrand multimers. Fibrinogen is attached to endothelium through upregulated integrins and selectins.

Initial platelet hemostasis (i.e., platelet plug formation) is accompanied by local generation of fibrin as the end product of the action of at least three surface-active enzyme complexes. Clotting is initiated by the tissue factor/factor VIIa surface-active enzyme complex and amplified by the factor VIIIa/IXa/X and factor II/Va/Xa complexes. A mural platelet thrombus, which

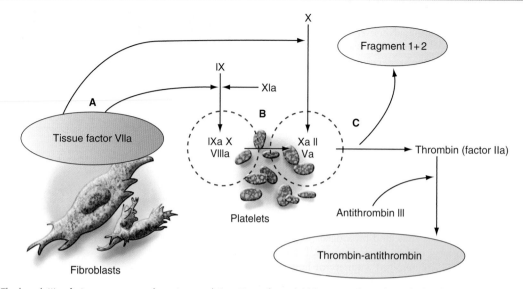

**FIGURE 10-3** The key clotting factor enzyme complexes in coagulation. Tissue factor (A) (shown on the surface of a fibroblast) initiates coagulation, leading to the activation of clotting factors IX and X (shown on the surface of a platelet) and the processing of prothrombin (factor II) to form thrombin (factor IIa). Factor XIa has a contributory role in factor IX activation. Key to this cascade are three surface-active enzyme complexes: (A) the complex of tissue factor and factor VIIa; (B) the complex of factor IXa, factor VIIIa, and factor X; and (C) the complex of factor Xa, factor Va, and factor II (where the letter "a" denotes the activated form of a factor). Prothrombin fragment 1 + 2 and thrombin-antithrombin complexes are markers of the generation of thrombin. Fragment 1 + 2 is an inactive fragment formed during the processing of prothrombin; thrombin-antithrombin complex is formed when antithrombin III binds to thrombin, resulting in the inactivation of thrombin. Not shown in this diagram is the important influence of blood flow; for example, arteriolar and arterial velocity gradients, along with the presence of red cells, promote collisions between platelets and, consequently, platelet aggregation. (Modified with permission from Grabowski EF. The hemolytic-uremic syndrome—toxin, thrombin, and thrombosis. N Engl J Med 2002;346:58-64.)

includes platelets and fibrin, then forms a scaffold on which healing of the vessel wall can take place. The scaffold is removed when no longer needed by means of thrombolysis and the effects of macrophages.

The surface-active enzyme complexes (Fig. 10-3) are active on the phospholipid surfaces provided by platelets, leukocytes, and endothelial cells but not in the bulk of the blood. In this regard, the conventional coagulation cascade shown in Figure 10-4 is oversimplified, although it is a convenient approach to understanding the PT and PTT. All of the steps must be considered in the milieu of flowing blood, such that the high-velocity gradients of arterioles (i.e., mucous membranes of the uterus, gastrointestinal tract, upper respiratory tract, oral cavity, and gums) and arteries favor thrombi with a greater proportion of platelets (i.e., white thrombi), and low-velocity gradient states such as those found in stasis or blood accumulation within a body cavity favor a greater proportion of red cells (i.e., red thrombi). This explains why a patient with von Willebrand disease, characterized by a defect in the protein that allows blood platelets to adhere to a wound, tends to bleed from mucous membranes, sites of high-velocity (arteriolar) gradients, whereas hemophiliacs tend to bleed into joint spaces and muscle planes, sites of low- or near-zero–velocity gradients.

The coagulopathy associated with massive blood transfusions is usually attributable to the dilution of clotting factors or platelets, or both. The point at which the deficiency in clotting factors is sufficient to produce a coagulopathy depends on the volume of blood lost and the type of blood component transfused (i.e., PRBCs or whole blood). Dilutional thrombocytopenia sufficient to cause clinical bleeding depends on the starting platelet count and the volume of blood replaced (Fig. 10-5). In some cases, the cause of bleeding is a consumptive coagulopathy such as fibrinolysis or disseminated intravascular coagulation (DIC).[51,159-179]

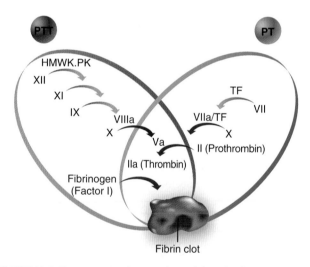

**FIGURE 10-4** The conventional activated partial thromboplastin time (aPTT) is considered to be a measure of the intactness of the intrinsic coagulation system, which includes clotting factors XII, XI, IX, VIII, V, X, II, and I (fibrinogen). The prothrombin time (PT) is a measure of the intactness of the extrinsic coagulation system and encompasses tissue factor–bearing membrane surfaces and microparticles and factors VII, V, X, II, and I. In the PTT test, the blood clots without the need for an exogenous agent and comprises an *intrinsic* or complete clotting system. In practice, an agent such as diatomaceous earth is added to speed the reaction in the laboratory, and the term *activated* is added to the designation (aPTT). In the PT test, the blood clots by virtue of an *extrinsic* activator (i.e., tissue factor). This view in the diagram obscures the central role of tissue factor in clot initiation. Tissue factor circulates in an inactive form in the blood and is no longer considered only an extrinsic factor to the blood itself.

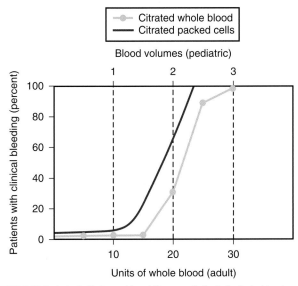

FIGURE 10-5 A study that considered the use of citrated whole blood (*blue line*) in adults found that bleeding in most cases resulted from dilutional thrombocytopenia. The *magenta line* represents estimated points of dilutional clotting factor deficiency if solely citrated packed cells are transfused. (Modified from Miller RD. Transfusion therapy and associated problems. ASA Refresher Courses in Anesthesiology 1973;1:107.)

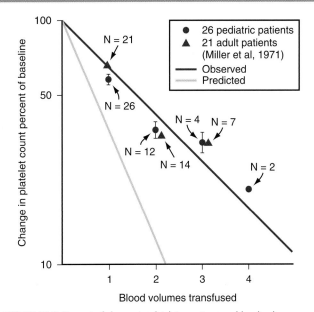

FIGURE 10-6 Percent of change in platelet count versus blood volumes transfused in adults and children.[51,52] The *magenta line* represents observed values, whereas the *blue line* represents calculated values. This difference suggests increased bone marrow production and/or splenic recruitment of platelets during massive transfusion. (From Miller RD, Robbins TO, Tong MJ, Barton SL. Coagulation defects associated with massive blood transfusions. Ann Surg 1971;174:794-801; Coté CJ, Liu LM, Szyfelbein SK, Goudsouzian NG, Daniels AL. Changes in serial platelet counts following massive blood transfusions in pediatric patients. Anesthesiology 1985;62:197-201.)

In other scenarios, bleeding is caused by hypothermia, severe metabolic acidosis, poor tissue perfusion, and the release of tissue factors. Body temperature should be maintained by using efficient blood-warming devices, acidosis should be treated, and normovolemia and cardiac output should be restored to prevent a coagulopathy from developing.[166,180-183]

## DILUTIONAL THROMBOCYTOPENIA

Because of the dearth of published data on the effects of massive blood transfusion in children, we must rely on our clinical experience and data extrapolated from adults to anticipate the effects in children. A study of trauma patients during the Vietnam War reported that the onset of clinical bleeding occurred after about 15 units of whole blood had been transfused. The incidence of coagulopathy was unrelated to an abnormal PT or partial thromboplastin time (PTT) but correlated closely with a platelet count of less than 65,000/mm[3].[51] In a 70-kg adult, the estimated blood volume is approximately 5 L (70 mL/kg × 70 kg = 4900 mL), or approximately 10 units of whole blood. To relate the data in Figure 10-6 to children, assume the 70-kg adult has 5 L of blood, or 10 units of whole blood. If each 10 units of whole blood is one blood volume, some children are expected to develop a coagulopathy after losing about 1.5 blood volumes, but most develop clinical bleeding after losing 2.0 to 2.5 blood volumes. Studies of massive blood loss with *whole blood* replacement appear to support the conclusion that the coagulopathy at these levels of blood loss results from thrombocytopenia rather than a clotting factor deficiency.[51,166-175] Consequently, children should be monitored for thrombocytopenia and possible transfusion of platelets or clotting factor deficiency (see further) after the loss of the first 1.0 to 1.5 blood volumes. After the platelet count has decreased to 50,000/mm[3], it is likely that approximately one platelet dose (i.e., 6 units for an adult or 10 to 15 mL/kg for a child) will be required for each blood volume replaced. If a coagulopathy develops earlier than expected (i.e., before a 1.0-blood volume loss), a search should be initiated for other causes

of bleeding, such as increased arterial or venous pressure in the surgical field or DIC.

Studies of adult and pediatric patients with acute dilutional thrombocytopenia found that clinical bleeding correlated closely with a platelet count of 65,000/mm[3] or less.[51,166-175] Figure 10-6 compares the calculated reduction in platelet count with the observed decline in platelet count in adults and children. The observed decrement differs from the calculated reduction because platelets are mobilized from the bone marrow, lungs, and lymphatic tissues. The platelet count usually does not decrease to concentrations that cause bleeding until 2.0 to 2.5 blood volumes are lost in children, which is consistent with our observations, or until 20 to 25 units of whole blood are transfused in adults.[52,173,184] Clinical bleeding does not usually occur in children whose platelet counts remain above 50,000/mm[3], despite blood losses as great as 5.0 blood volumes (Fig. 10-7, *A*).[52]

The starting platelet count is important for estimating how much blood loss can be tolerated before critical thrombocytopenia occurs. For example, with a starting platelet count of 600,000/mm[3], dilutional thrombocytopenia is unlikely to occur until 4.0 or more blood volumes are lost, whereas with a starting count of 100,000/mm[3], dilutional thrombocytopenia may be expected after 1.0 blood volume has been lost (see Fig. 10-7, *B*). Prophylactic transfusion of platelets typically is not indicated without documented evidence of dilutional thrombocytopenia, visible microvascular bleeding, and ongoing blood loss, although it should be anticipated based on the starting platelet count and the volume of blood lost.[52,56,162,166,185]

Although the primary platelet defect in massive transfusion is thrombocytopenia, some data suggest that platelets may not function normally (i.e., thrombocytopathy) after massive trauma

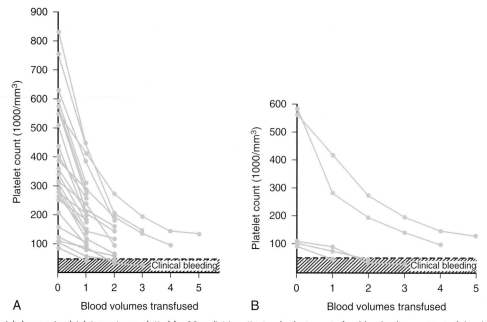

**FIGURE 10-7 A,** Serial changes in platelet counts are plotted for 26 pediatric patients who lost one to five blood volumes. Most of the children suffered from severe thermal injuries, and many had relatively high platelet counts at baseline. Clinically evident signs of coagulopathy appeared when the platelet count decreased below 50,000/mm³. **B,** Platelet counts of five children abstracted from **A.** The baseline platelet count is invaluable in estimating potential platelet needs in relation to blood volumes transfused. A low initial count suggests the need for early exogenous platelet transfusion, whereas a high initial platelet count indicates that exogenous platelets may not be required until several blood volumes have been lost. The three children who developed a coagulopathy began surgery with a relatively low platelet count, whereas the two children with a very high platelet count did not require platelet transfusion despite the loss of four and five blood volumes. (It should be noted that these children received sufficient FFP so as to maintain the PT and PTT within a normal range.) (Reproduced with permission from Coté CJ, Liu LMP, Szyfelbein SK, Goudsouzian NG, Daniels AL. Changes in serial platelet counts following massive blood transfusions in pediatric patients. Anesthesiology 1985;62:197-201.)

or in the presence of hypothermia.[182,186,187] This has not been our experience in the children we studied whose temperature remained within the normal range.[52,167] The only simple test to assess platelet function is the bleeding time. However, this test is also sensitive to thrombocytopenia and its predictive value is of equivocal utility.[162,186,188] The PFA-100 test shows less potential as a rapid screening tool than it once did, because the device uses citrated blood warmed to 37° C and is relatively insensitive to milder defects in platelet-vessel wall interaction, such as that in mild von Willebrand disease. There remains a critical need for a point-of-care device or simple test to assess platelet function. Currently, the platelet count is our best indication for the need for platelet transfusions in situations involving rapid blood loss.[189] Other devices to measure whole blood clotting have been used to guide transfusion therapy, but their efficacy in improving outcomes has not been established.[190]

In several in vitro and animal model systems, recombinant factor VII (rFVIIa) activates factors IX and X on the surface of activated platelets, probably through the binding of rFVIIa to the platelet membrane (from which rFVIIa can also be taken up into storage sites within the platelet) and subsequent recruitment of circulating tissue factor.[191-196] Although this has significantly improved hemostasis for hemophiliacs with inhibitors to factor VIII, there is limited evidence that rFVIIa reduces mortality for off-label use, as in cardiovascular surgery, trauma, and intracerebral hemorrhage. This agent increases the risk of thromboembolism.[197]

Basic clotting studies (e.g., PT, PTT, fibrinogen, platelet count) must be performed before elective surgery when major blood loss can be anticipated to determine the cause of underlying coagulopathies and provide adequate quantities of blood components.

## FACTOR DEFICIENCY

Laboratory assessment of developing deficiencies in clotting factors plays an important part in transfusion decisions in managing massive transfusion. The PT (for the extrinsic system) measures the adequacy of factors VII, X, and V; prothrombin; and fibrinogen,[51] whereas the PTT (for the intrinsic system) measures the adequacy of factors XII, XI, IX, VIII, X, and V; prothrombin; and fibrinogen (see Fig. 10-4). Banked whole blood contains normal plasma concentrations of all of the clotting factors and regulatory proteins, but it has a reduced concentration of factors V and VIII (20% to 50% of normal at the time of outdate). For coagulopathy due to a clotting factor deficiency to develop, factor VIII must be less than 30% of the normal concentration and factor V less than 20% of normal.[167] For these to occur, at least 3.0 blood volumes must be exchanged with *whole blood.* In this scenario, the first coagulation test that is abnormal is the PTT because factor VIII is diluted to less than 30%.[163]

If blood loss is replaced with PRBCs, as is the current practice with blood banking techniques, the amount of plasma that is transfused is minimal because most of it was sequestered in the FFP fraction when it was separated. Massive replacement of blood loss with PRBCs and no other blood products quickly dilutes all of the clotting factors, including fibrinogen (see Fig. 10-4).* Data have confirmed that the PT and PTT are prolonged in children with multiple clotting factor deficiencies (e.g., during massive transfusion) at concentrations of clotting factors that are greater than in children with single clotting factor deficiencies (e.g., congenital coagulopathies).[174,175] This was documented in

---

*References 3, 162-166, 172, 174, 175, 198-200.

| **TABLE 10-10** Changes in Prothrombin and Partial Thromboplastin Times during Massive Blood Transfusions in Children | | | | |
|---|---|---|---|---|
| PT and PTT Times (sec) | Baseline* (N = 26) | 0.5[†] (n = 16) | 0.75[†] (n = 12) | 1.0[†] (n = 10) |
| **Prothrombin Time** | | | | |
| Mean ± SD | 10.9 ± 0.96 | 12.5 ± 0.77 | 13.2 ± 0.76 | 13.6 ± 0.98 |
| Range | 9.3-12.0 | 11.4-14.0 | 11.4-14.2 | 11.9-15.8 |
| **Partial Thromboplastin Time** | | | | |
| Mean ± SD | 31.8 ± 4.4 | 38.0 ± 4.9 | 40 ± 5.4 | 45.1 ± 13.1 |
| Range | 25-45.9 | 28.1-59.6 | 33-51.5 | 25.6-60.0 |

*PRBCs*, Packed red blood cells; *PT*, prothrombin; *PTT*, partial thromboplastin.
*Baseline normal values for blood volume may be greater in infants younger than 3 months.
[†]Blood volume loss. *NOTE:* Not all children in this subset lost a half blood volume or more.

| **TABLE 10-11** Minimal Fresh Frozen Plasma Recommendations according to the Type of Blood Product Transfused and the Volume of Blood Lost | | |
|---|---|---|
| Type of Blood Replaced | FFP Indicated | Volume FFP To Be Transfused |
| Whole blood | After 2.0-3.0 blood volumes lost and each blood volume thereafter | 25%-33% of each blood volume lost |
| PRBCs | After 1.0 blood volume lost and each blood volume thereafter | 1 U FFP / 2 U PRBCs |

*FFP*, Fresh frozen plasma; *PRBCs*, packed red blood cells; *U*, unit.

adult patients who were transfused exclusively with PRBCs and crystalloid. The dilution of multiple clotting factors correlated with the volume of blood and crystalloid transfused.[148] Diluting clotting factors to approximately 30% of normal may be expected replacing 1.0 to 1.5 blood volumes with PRBCs and crystalloid exclusively. Because moderate prolongations of the PT and PTT exist without overt signs of clinical bleeding,[174] the indication for FFP should be onset of clinical coagulopathy. However, to avoid falling behind, the anesthesiologist should anticipate that the clotting factors will be diluted and that FFP should be infused after 1.0 blood volume of blood loss has been replaced with a combination of PRBCs and crystalloid. Documented deficiency of fibrinogen (<80 mg/dL) may also be corrected by transfusing FFP, but marked deficiency, particularly in the presence of a consumptive coagulopathy (e.g., DIC, fibrinolysis), may require the addition of cryoprecipitate (0.2 to 0.4 unit/kg).[3,199,201-203] No published studies have examined massive blood replacement in infants and children using exclusively component therapy.

Our experience with 26 children (12 ± 4 years old, weight of 41.9 ± 15.8 kg; 22 Harrington rod procedures, three tumor excisions, and one Whipple procedure) who did not receive FFP or whole blood during surgery that involved blood losses between 0.5 and 1.0 blood volumes showed that none of the children demonstrated clinical signs of coagulopathy. Slight prolongations of the PT or PTT occurred when blood loss was 1.0 blood volume or less (Table 10-10). Two children who lost 1.5 blood volumes, and one who lost 2.0 blood volumes had prolonged PT and PTT values. The only child who had clinical coagulopathy was the one who lost 2.0 blood volumes, and the coagulopathy could have been ascribed to simultaneous dilutional thrombocytopenia.[204,205]

The magnitude of the change in PT or PTT that predicts a clinical coagulopathy is not well defined. However, the consensus panel of the National Institutes of Health and others suggest that greater than 1.5 times normal (or INR >2.0) should be considered pathologic.[56,169,173,206-209] Our studies suggest that the PT and PTT are prolonged to more than 1.5 times normal when the blood loss is 1.5 or more blood volumes and when the blood loss has been replaced with only PRBCs and crystalloid or PRBCs and 5% albumin.[204,205] Our clinical practice is to initiate FFP after loss of more than 1.0 blood volume has been replaced with PRBCs (Table 10-11). At that point, FFP is administered in a ratio of 1 unit for every 2 units of PRBCs transfused. The indications for and timing of FFP depend on which blood product has been transfused, the volume of that transfusion as it relates to the child's blood volume, and whether the blood loss will continue perioperatively. The PT, PTT, fibrinogen concentration, and platelet count should be determined after each blood volume has been replaced and used to guide the need for additional FFP and platelets.

Recombinant factor VIIa (rFVIIa; NOVO Seven) is approved for use in the United States for hemophiliacs with high-titer inhibitors and for congenital factor VII deficiency. Several anecdotal reports describe its efficacy in controlling hemorrhage in a variety of other settings. However, in randomized clinical trials enrolling patients with partial hepatectomy, liver transplantation, prostate surgery, pelvic (orthopedic) surgery, trauma, or upper gastrointestinal tract bleeding, it conferred little or no benefit.[210-215] In a large randomized clinical trial of intracranial hemorrhage, the patients in the largest-dose group showed a small improvement in hematoma expansion, but 10% also experienced thromboembolic complications. In adults receiving rFVIIa, there is a 1.4% to 10% incidence of major thromboembolic complications, including acute myocardial infarction and stroke.[216] There are anecdotal reports of its successful use in children, but they provide little guidance because of the limited data.[1,2,217-219,219a] Until the results of controlled trials demonstrate a clear benefit for its use, rFVIIa should be used with great caution for off-label indications.[210-215,218,220,221]

Several studies[215,222] have compared different transfusion strategies for treating trauma incurred during combat in the Middle East A consensus conference on massive transfusion concluded that the evidence did not support the up-front use of a 1:1:1 ratio of units of PRBC, FFP, and platelets, but it did support the early use of an antifibrinolytic medication (i.e., tranexamic acid).[222] The consensus conference also recommended an integrated approach to managing massive transfusion that included rapid provision of PRBCs, the use of antifibrinolytics, and a foundation ratio of blood components directed by the results of standard coagulation testing (e.g., PT, PTT, platelet count, fibrinogen) or clot viscoelasticity, or both.[222]

The dilutional coagulopathy associated with massive blood transfusion is reasonably predictable. When using whole blood, dilutional thrombocytopenia usually develops first and may occur as early as after the first blood volume (if the initial platelet count is low) has been replaced. In most cases, clotting factors (particularly factors V and VIII) are not diluted until the blood loss exceeds three blood volumes. On the other hand, when PRBCs are used to replace blood loss, the clotting factors and platelets may be diluted after as little as 1.0 blood volume is lost. However, the predictable coagulopathy of dilution is only an approximate guide. We should monitor the PT, PTT, fibrinogen, and platelet count during massive transfusions and use this information to guide replacement therapy.

## DISSEMINATED INTRAVASCULAR COAGULATION AND FIBRINOLYSIS

DIC and fibrinolysis are frequently associated with shock, trauma, and other forms of tissue damage, with release of procoagulants (e.g., tissue factor) and fibrinolytics (e.g., tissue plasminogen activator). In the presence of massive blood loss, these processes must be differentiated from dilutional coagulopathy. Differentiation may be difficult, because both are associated with pathologic oozing of blood in the surgical field and each may result in prolongation of the PT and PTT, as well as thrombocytopenia.[223,224] With massive replacement using whole blood or PRBCs and *adequate* FFP, the fibrinogen level should remain normal; with uncompensated (acute) DIC, it may be decreased. However, replacing the blood loss with PRBCs, albumin, and crystalloid also leads to a reduction in fibrinogen.

The most helpful test for DIC and fibrinolysis is documentation of a significant increase in the level of D-dimer, a small peptide fragment generated during the digestion of fibrin by ongoing thrombolysis (i.e., through plasmin), along with evidence on the peripheral blood smear of schistocytes and helmet cells (i.e., microangiopathic hemolytic anemia).[195,225,226] Abnormal RBCs and RBC fragments are thought to arise from the slicing action of immobilized fibrin strands in the microcirculation, although the precise mechanism remains unknown. A scoring system used for screening for potential DIC has been devised but not evaluated in the operating room setting.[227] If pathologic oozing in the surgical field is observed and 1.0 blood volume or less has been lost in a child who had a normal platelet count and normal PT and PTT values preoperatively, it should be suspected that the child has developed a consumptive coagulopathy.

The most effective treatment for DIC is to eliminate the cause, such as correcting shock, acidosis, or sepsis. Heparin therapy remains controversial even in children with thrombotic manifestations of DIC and is not advisable in children with active bleeding, especially in the operative setting.[224-226,228]

## HYPERKALEMIA

RBCs leak potassium into the extracellular fluid during storage, particularly as the units age. The concentration of adenosine triphosphate (ATP) decreases, and the ATPase-driven $Na^+/K^+$ pump activity decreases. When the blood is outdated, 1 unit of whole blood or PRBCs has approximately 6 mEq of $K^+$ in the plasma at a concentration that varies considerably (see Table 10-4) because this 6 mEq of $K^+$ is distributed in the plasma and the anticoagulant solution of the stored whole blood and PRBC units. The $K^+$ leak is more rapid from RBCs that have been irradiated.[229-231] To avoid the accumulation of large amounts of extracellular $K^+$, irradiated RBCs are stored for a maximum of 28 days (versus 35 or 42 days for whole blood or PRBCs).

Although extracellular $K^+$ is present in banked RBCs, clinically important hyperkalemia after routine transfusion has not been reported.[232-238] A study of serum potassium in neonates after exchange transfusion with PRBCs documented a decrease in serum potassium concentrations.[239] A retrospective study of children undergoing massive intraoperative transfusion with PRBCs

documented transient, but not life-threatening, hyperkalemia.[240] It appears that clinically important hyperkalemia does not usually occur when PRBCs are administered *at normal, slow infusion rates through peripheral IV access*.[241] This may be explained by of the combination of the small absolute amount of $K^+$ (about 6 mEq per unit); its rapid reabsorption into the potassium-depleted, transfused RBCs; the large volume of distribution; and dilution with crystalloid or albumin during administration. Hyperkalemia in the setting of massive transfusion is usually the consequence of extensive tissue injury or acidemia resulting from inadequate tissue perfusion.

The need to relate the size of the patient to the rate of blood replacement is infrequently a problem in adults, but it is vitally important to consider in an infant or small child. An alert from the Society for Pediatric Anesthesia[242] described 4 deaths among 11 children who developed hyperkalemia during transfusion; 8 were younger than 1 year, and 6 were younger than 6 months old. The Perioperative Cardiac Arrest Registry reported 8 hyperkalemic cardiac arrests related to blood transfusion.[242,243] Hyperkalemia may become a problem when large volumes of whole blood or PRBCs are administered very rapidly in adults (rates ≥120 mL/min) and in infants and children undergoing rapid blood transfusion, particularly through a central venous catheter.[240,244,245] A rapid transfusion rate of 120 mL/min in a 70-kg adult is equivalent to 1.5 to 2 mL/kg/min of blood, which is relatively easy to infuse in an infant or small child using a pressure bag or a rapid-transfusion device. An adult sustained a cardiac arrest and died after receiving Adsol-preserved PRBCs with a supernatant potassium concentration of 24 to 34 mEq/L at a rate of 6.4 mL/kg/min through a rapid infusion device (see Chapter 51).[246] Similar transfusion rates and greater are possible in infants and children without such devices.[240,247,248]

The principle is to avoid falling behind in replacing the blood loss and to avoid a situation in which a rapid and massive infusion of blood is required. Warming the blood and administering it through a peripheral IV line (rather than a central venous catheter) reduce the severe effects of hyperkalemia on the cardiac conduction system. When the rate of infusion of whole blood or PRBCs exceeds 1.5 to 2.0 mL/kg/min, the electrocardiogram must be closely monitored. If ventricular arrhythmias occur with peaked T waves in the setting of hyperkalemia (see Fig. 8-7), appropriate treatment should be instituted (e.g., calcium chloride or calcium gluconate, hyperventilation, sodium bicarbonate, albuterol, glucose and insulin); Kayexalate is the slowest and least effective in this situation and not recommended as an acute intervention.

Rapid, massive transfusion of whole blood or PRBCs to a neonate, particularly blood that has been stored for several weeks, can cause hyperkalemic cardiac arrest. It is common practice to administer RBC-containing components that are relatively young to avoid hyperkalemia in neonates requiring massive blood transfusion. If relatively young units are not available and time permits, it may be possible to wash the PRBCs to reduce the potassium concentration. However, RBC transfusion to an actively bleeding infant should not be delayed to obtain less than 7-day-old PRBCs or to wash the units. Similarly, blood for intrauterine transfusion, exchange transfusion, or neonates is chosen to be relatively young (usually less than 7 days).

These practices are consistent with the recommendations from the Society for Pediatric Anesthesia Wake Up Safe quality improvement initiative, which directs the physician to anticipate the blood loss and transfuse early and cautions that transfusing

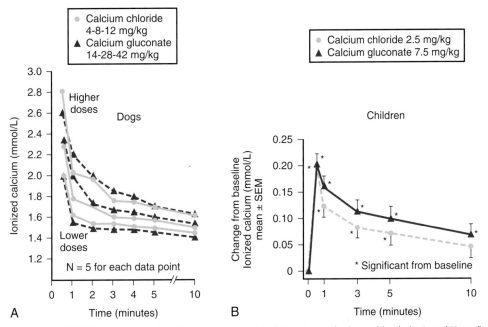

FIGURE 10-8 **A,** Changes in arterial iCa$^{2+}$ levels in dogs after three equal elemental calcium doses of calcium chloride (4, 8, and 12 mg/kg) or calcium gluconate (14, 28, and 42 mg/kg). The rate of change in the iCa$^{2+}$ concentration was identical for each form of calcium at each dose. There was no significant difference between the highest and lowest doses after 2 minutes, suggesting that frequent low doses are equally effective and perhaps safer than large boluses of exogenous calcium. **B,** Changes in arterial iCa$^{2+}$ levels in children who received equal elemental doses of calcium chloride and calcium gluconate. At 30 seconds, both forms of calcium dissociated equally, and these data indicate that hepatic metabolism of the gluconate moiety is not required to liberate ionized calcium from calcium gluconate. (From Coté CJ, Drop LJ, Daniels AL, Hoaglin DC. Calcium chloride versus calcium gluconate: comparison of ionization and cardiovascular effects in children and dogs. Anesthesiology 1987;66:465-470.)

the hypovolemic child should be done slowly and through a peripheral IV catheter rather than rapidly through a central venous catheter.[242] If the infant requires irradiated RBC blood components, it is preferable to transfuse them soon after irradiating the blood.

## HYPOCALCEMIA AND CITRATE TOXICITY

Citrate works as an anticoagulant for stored blood components by chelating ionized calcium (iCa$^{2+}$). As citrate in the blood component is transfused, it is rapidly taken up and metabolized by every nucleated cell in the body, although the primary site of clearance is the liver. During massive transfusion, particularly of whole blood or FFP, the influx of citrate may temporarily overwhelm the capacity to clear it, resulting in its accumulation, which causes the plasma concentration of iCa$^{2+}$ to decrease.[249-253] The plasma fraction in a unit of PRBCs, which contains the citrate, is a much smaller volume than in a unit of whole blood or FFP. Clinically, it is rare for the iCa$^{2+}$ level to decrease unless the transfusion rate is very rapid; in adults, this rate must be 1.0 or more units of whole blood or FFP in 3 to 4 minutes.[249] This effect on the iCa$^{2+}$ concentration has been reported in neonates undergoing exchange transfusion and is more likely to occur in more-premature and lower-weight infants.[253] In adult cardiac surgical patients who received whole blood at 1.5 mL/kg/min, the ventricular function curve did not improve (i.e., cardiac output did not increase although the iCa$^{2+}$ decreased). When a similar volume of heparinized blood was administered at the same rate, the Frank-Starling response to volume loading was normal (i.e., cardiac output increased, but iCa$^{2+}$ level did not change).[254] These findings correlate well with earlier studies in that a decrease in iCa$^{2+}$ concentration of clinical importance (i.e., decreased cardiac

contractility) is expected to occur when the rate of infusion of citrated whole blood exceeds 1.5 to 2.0 mL/kg/min.[249,254]

The change in the iCa$^{2+}$ level after transfusion of large volumes of PRBCs is less than that observed with whole blood or FFP. Although measurable decreases in the iCa$^{2+}$ concentration have been observed during rapid transfusion, they have only rarely been associated with cardiac toxicity in adults. The rates of infusion of citrated whole blood that produce hypocalcemia and hyperkalemia are almost identical, whereas the cardiac electrophysiologic effects produced by hypocalcemia and hyperkalemia are opposite. It is important to observe the electrocardiogram for abnormalities, especially widening of the QRS complex, prolonged QT interval, and peaking of the T wave.[167,255]

Treatment for hypocalcemia and hyperkalemia is administration of exogenous calcium. Evidence from normal animals and children with extensive thermal injuries demonstrated that calcium chloride and calcium gluconate dissociate at a similar rate; hepatic metabolism of the gluconate moiety is not necessary (Fig. 10-8).[256] Other studies during the anhepatic phase of liver transplantation also found equal ionization of calcium chloride and calcium gluconate, establishing that hepatic metabolism is not required to release calcium from gluconate.[257] We recommend using calcium chloride or calcium gluconate to treat acute ionized hypocalcemia, with the caveat that calcium gluconate, which contains one third of the ionizable calcium of calcium chloride (by weight), be administered at a threefold greater dose (milligrams per kilogram) than the latter. Frequent, small boluses are as effective as single large boluses and result in smaller fluctuations in plasma iCa$^{2+}$ values.[256] Ideally, both forms of calcium should be slowly administered through a large peripheral or central vein, because both are sclerosing medications.

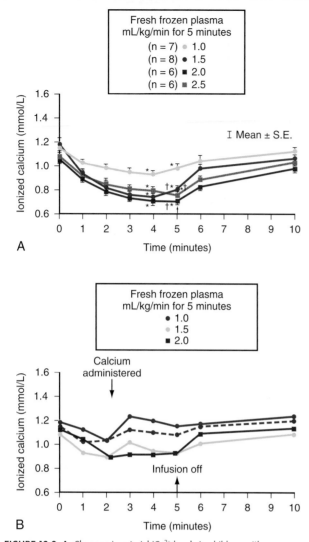

**FIGURE 10-9 A,** Changes in arterial iCa²⁺ levels in children with severe thermal injuries during infusions of fresh frozen plasma at a rate of 1.0 to 2.5 mL/kg/min for 5 minutes through an infusion pump. Notice the dangerous although transient decrease in the iCa²⁺ concentration, with the nadir occurring between the fourth and fifth minute. Ionized hypocalcemia occurs when the infusion rate equals or exceeds 1 mL/kg/min. **B,** Changes in iCa²⁺ levels occurred in four thermally injured children who received calcium chloride (*arrow*) after 2 minutes of fresh frozen plasma infusion. There were no sharp increases or decreases in iCa²⁺ levels. (From Coté CJ, Drop LJ, Hoaglin DC, Daniels AL, Young ET. Ionized hypocalcemia after fresh frozen plasma administration to thermally injured children: effects of infusion rate, duration, and treatment with calcium chloride. Anesth Analg 1988;67:152-60.)

The volume of plasma and therefore the absolute amount of citrate in a unit of FFP are slightly less than the amounts in a unit of whole blood. However, the citrate load can be more rapidly delivered in FFP because it can be infused more rapidly owing to its low viscosity. It is easy to give a large citrate load in a brief period. Caution is urged when FFP or whole blood is rapidly infused, especially if the child already has a low iCa²⁺ concentration or impaired hepatic function (e.g., neonates and children undergoing liver transplantation). Figure 10-9, *A*, shows the changes in iCa²⁺ concentrations that occurred in children who had extensive thermal injuries and who received rapid FFP

infusions at a rate between 1.0 to 2.5 mL/kg/min for 5 minutes. The maximum decrease in iCa²⁺ levels occurred between the fourth and fifth minute. There was no difference in the nadir in the iCa²⁺ concentration among the three largest rates of FFP infusion.[258]

If exogenous calcium is administered *during* rapid FFP transfusion, large decreases in the iCa²⁺ level can be avoided (see Fig. 10-9, *B*). We transfused FFP at a rate of 2 mL/kg/min for 10 minutes (equivalent to an average adult receiving 1400 mL FFP over 10 minutes) in six children with extensive burn injuries and measured very significant decreases in iCa²⁺ levels but observed no consistent adverse cardiovascular events. However, because these children had extensive burn injuries, we presumed they were hypermetabolic and therefore able to rapidly metabolize the excess citrate, which limits our ability to extrapolate these data to children without burn injuries (see Chapter 34).[258]

In dogs anesthetized with halothane, we determined that citrate-induced ionized hypocalcemia caused significantly greater cardiovascular depression as the concentration of expired halothane increased.[259] These findings are consistent with the combined myocardial depression caused by ionized hypocalcemia and the myocardial depressant effects of calcium channel blockade caused by the halothane.[260,261] Although halothane seems to exert the greatest calcium channel blocking activity of the inhalational anesthetics, all inhalational anesthetics depress the myocardium through this mechanism and therefore should augment the myocardial dysfunction associated with citrate-induced hypocalcemia, although similar data with sevoflurane and desflurane have not been forthcoming.[262,263]

The adverse cardiac effects of citrate-induced hypocalcemia may be increased if FFP is rapidly administered through a central venous catheter because there is less time to dilute the FFP and metabolize the citrate before it enters the heart and coronary vessels. FFP may be more safely administered through a peripheral IV site. Calcium should be administered *during* rapid transfusion of FFP (>1 mL/kg/min) to attenuate this transient but dangerous citrate toxicity, especially in the presence of potent inhalational anesthetics.[259-263] Our clinical impression is that neonates and small infants are particularly vulnerable to the developing citrate toxicity because it is easier to administer a relatively large volume of FFP over a brief period to them and because citrate may not be eliminated as rapidly (i.e., first-pass effect through the liver) in infants. In addition to thermally injured patients, children undergoing liver transplantation and cardiac surgery are likely to require FFP and may develop hypocalcemia.[264,265] Liver transplantation recipients are particularly susceptible to decreased iCa²⁺ levels during the anhepatic phase and during the pre-anhepatic phase of surgery because of impaired hepatic metabolism, impaired hepatic blood flow, and the reduced ability to metabolize citrate.[266-270] An IV preparation of calcium should always be available when a major transfusion with FFP is anticipated.

## ACID–BASE BALANCE

Massive transfusions usually occur in one of two situations: severe trauma with shock or major surgery with massive blood loss. In the first situation, severe metabolic acidosis may occur because of low cardiac output and diminished oxygen delivery. Correction of the acidosis with sodium bicarbonate may be a necessary part of the resuscitation, along with blood volume replacement. In this situation, impaired coagulation may occur because of the acidosis.[164,180,271-273] In the operating room, intravascular volume is usually maintained, and because most instances of massive blood loss are anticipated, replacement of acute blood loss is more controlled. Even with repeated massive blood loss, metabolic acidosis is not usually a problem provided severe hypovolemia is avoided.[274-276] Sodium bicarbonate therapy must be governed by the child's acid–base status because metabolic acidosis does not usually occur with massive transfusion unless accompanied by severe hypovolemia, low cardiac output, or hypoxemia.

With massive blood transfusion, the child may develop a moderate to severe metabolic alkalosis due to the large volume of transfused citrate and its conversion to bicarbonate, which causes a metabolic alkalosis within hours of a massive transfusion.[250,265,277-279] If exogenous bicarbonate therapy is superimposed on this endogenous metabolic alkalosis, a leftward shift of the oxyhemoglobin dissociation curve may result. It is important to determine the acid–base status *before* administering sodium bicarbonate to avoid overcorrecting the pH and shifting the oxyhemoglobin dissociation curve further.

### HYPOTHERMIA

Hypothermia may be a significant problem associated with major blood loss and its replacement. Hypothermia decreases oxygen consumption and reduces oxygen demand. It may also increase oxygen consumption if the child shivers and decrease tissue delivery of oxygen by a leftward shift of the oxygen-hemoglobin dissociation curve; severe hypothermia (about 32° C) may induce a refractory ventricular tachycardia.[167,280,281] Hypothermia may also profoundly compromise platelet function and impair the coagulation cascade.[164,180-182,271,272,282,283]

Prevention of hypothermia by all available means is considered an essential part of damage-control resuscitation of trauma patients.[284-287] Banked blood products are stored between room temperature and 4° C, depending on the blood component. In the setting of high-volume transfusions, all blood products should be infused through a blood warmer. No other method should be considered (e.g., storing blood in a warming cupboard, immersing in hot water) because RBCs hemolyze readily with prolonged warming or overheating (>42° C). Warming blood and all other IV infusions with a high-capacity blood warmer, using hot air warming blankets and radiant warmers, placing plastic wrap around extremities, inserting a heated humidifier in the anesthesia circuit, covering the child's head, and maintaining a warm to hot operating room contribute to maintaining thermal neutrality. Rapid-transfusion devices markedly improve the rapidity of transfusion and the thermokinetics involved.[288-294] In one case, one author (CJC) and two nurses transfused more than 50,000 mL of blood products and crystalloid in less than 1 hour, and the child's temperature remained at or exceeded 34.5° C.[288]

### MONITORING DURING MASSIVE BLOOD TRANSFUSION

If massive blood loss can be anticipated, adequate monitoring should be instituted *before* surgery begins so that baseline information can be recorded. Large-bore peripheral IV access is preferable (E-Fig. 10-1) because these catheters have reduced resistance and they avoid giving blood products and drugs directly into the heart, as with a CVP line. If a child arrives in the operating room in shock (e.g., trauma patient), the physician must be careful to differentiate hypovolemia from other causes of shock (e.g., tension pneumothorax, cardiac tamponade) (see Chapters 38 and 39). Invasive monitoring inserted during resuscitation helps with the differentiation. Our philosophy is one of aggressive invasive

monitoring to provide maximum data for evaluation and management of a critically hypovolemic child.

1. Routine monitoring includes an electrocardiogram, blood pressure cuff, stethoscope, temperature, pulse oximetry, and expired carbon dioxide monitoring. The use of a pulse oximeter placed on the tongue may be particularly valuable in special circumstances when a child is vasoconstricted, hypothermic, or without peripheral pulses.[295,296] Hypovolemia may occasionally manifest as pulsus paradoxus, identified by the peripheral pulse oximeter.[297]

2. A urinary catheter allows accurate quantitation of urine output and assessment of organ perfusion and intravascular volume status.

3. An arterial catheter enables continuous blood pressure monitoring, arterial blood gas measurements, and determinations of hematocrit, glucose, calcium, potassium, and clotting parameters. The adequacy of the circulating blood volume may be inferred from the shape of the arterial waveform, presence of the dicrotic notch, and absence of exaggerated respiratory variation (Fig. 10-10).

4. A CVP line may provide useful information, and its ease and safety of insertion have been demonstrated for children of all sizes.[298] The use of ultrasound may improve the success and safety of insertion.[299,300] CVP readings may vary depending on the location of the catheter tip and whether there is rapidly running fluid in the same catheter.[301,302] In the latter case, the infusions should be interrupted intermittently to obtain readings. It is our clinical impression that in healthy, anesthetized,

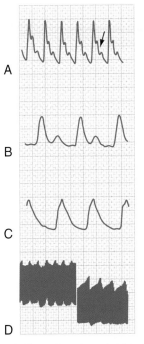

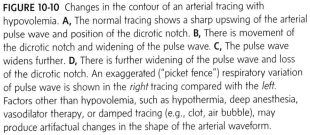

**FIGURE 10-10** Changes in the contour of an arterial tracing with hypovolemia. **A,** The normal tracing shows a sharp upswing of the arterial pulse wave and position of the dicrotic notch. **B,** There is movement of the dicrotic notch and widening of the pulse wave. **C,** The pulse wave widens further. **D,** There is further widening of the pulse wave and loss of the dicrotic notch. An exaggerated ("picket fence") respiratory variation of pulse wave is shown in the *right* tracing compared with the *left.* Factors other than hypovolemia, such as hypothermia, deep anesthesia, vasodilator therapy, or damped tracing (e.g., clot, air bubble), may produce artifactual changes in the shape of the arterial waveform.

supine children, a very small change in CVP (2 to 3 mm Hg) may represent a change of as much as 10% to 15% of a child's blood volume. In most children, right-sided pressures correlate well with left-sided pressures; the right atrial CVP usually is an accurate indicator of cardiac filling pressures of both ventricles. A CVP line provides access for blood sampling and a reliable site for IV administration of medications, fluid, and blood. A CVP line cannot always be relied on as a volume administration line because resistance is large through the long, narrow lumen; a centrally placed introducer is a reliable volume line.

5. Continuous noninvasive cardiac output devices may in the future provide further clinical guidance.

Monitors and the data they generate are helpful, but anesthesiologists must rely on more than numbers. It serves no purpose to have sophisticated monitoring if the data provided cannot be interpreted and related to clinical events. The final monitor is ultimately the anesthesiologist's attention and judgment.

Thromboelastography provides a standardized means of quantitating the rapidity and quality of clot formation and a means for identifying fibrinolysis.[303,304] This device was first used primarily during massive blood transfusion situations related to liver transplantation and now is used in several areas, particularly cardiac surgery.[303-312] Some studies have found that thromboelastographic screening was not useful in predicting bleeding after cardiac surgery and was associated with a large percentage of false-positive results.[313,314] Use of heparinase helps to improve the accuracy of the results by eliminating the effects of heparin, but this requires two machines to simultaneously sample blood (with and without heparinase) to have results within a useful period.[315] This monitor may also be used to guide the effectiveness of antifibrinolytic therapy.[310,311,316] The exact role of thromboelastography in the routine care of pediatric cardiac surgical patients, liver transplant recipients, and children who have had massive blood loss with ongoing coagulopathy has not been established. Tables 10-10 and 10-11 summarize the expected changes in various blood components when administered on a per kilogram basis and the estimated FFP requirement.

### INFECTIOUS DISEASE CONSIDERATIONS

It is important for anesthesiologists to use basic precautions to minimize their risk when administering blood products and contacting body fluids. Blood and body fluids, even in infants, are capable of transmitting hepatitis B, hepatitis C, and HIV through parenteral exposure (e.g., cuts, needlestick), mucous membrane contact, or exposure to nonintact skin.[4,317-326] Accidental needlesticks were the most common means of exposure in the operating room for anesthesiologists. The introduction of safe IV needles, a needleless IV system, the use of stopcocks, and never recapping used needles has reduced the incidence of this problem.[191-193,327] The incidence of HIV seroconversion after needle puncture is estimated to be 0.2% to 0.5% (~1 in 300), although the conversion rate is much greater after a needlestick injury from individuals with hepatitis.[4,194,317,323-325,328]

Anesthesiologists must practice universal blood and body fluid precautions (e.g., gloves, goggles) and should minimize the use of needles and especially the practice of recapping needles. The management of infants may be less than optimal with the use of three-way stopcocks because of the fluid required to flush the system and the ease of introducing air into the IV line. In these infants, single-use needles without recapping or needleless systems are recommended. If an exposure occurs from a known HIV-positive patient or puncture from a needle of unknown origin, consult a specialist immediately to determine the need for immediate institution of prophylactic medical therapy as soon as possible.[327,328] Early institution of drug therapy is recommended to reduce the potential for seroconversion (see Tables 49-6 and 49-7).

## Methods to Reduce Exposure to Allogeneic Blood Components

Public awareness of the infectious hazards of transfusion, particularly from HIV and the hepatitis viruses, has generated considerable interest in developing techniques to avoid allogeneic transfusion. These techniques can minimize transfusions and the attendant risks, at least in some settings, assuaging the fears of patients and sparing the blood supply for patients for whom these options were not suitable. Within the medical community, awareness of the hazards of transfusion prompted a more thoughtful approach to transfusion, greater tolerance of asymptomatic anemia, more attention to medical treatment of anemia, and greater focus on surgical hemostasis. The amount of blood transfused for many surgical procedures has decreased steadily during the past 20 years. During the same period, the risks associated with transfusions have decreased. After the HIV and hepatitis C viruses were identified, sensitive tests, some based on amplification technology for viral RNA, were developed to screen the donor population. Transfusions are associated with other deleterious effects, but two of the most significant risks, bacterial infection and mistransfusion, do not differ materially between banked allogeneic and autologous blood. As the risk differential between allogeneic transfusion and its alternatives narrows, a balanced appraisal of the benefits and untoward effects of each is appropriate.

### ERYTHROPOIETIN

Use of recombinant erythropoietin to promote endogenous RBC production can reduce the need for allogeneic RBC transfusions. This therapy has proved useful in many populations, including preterm infants, children on chemotherapy, children with renal failure, children of Jehovah's Witnesses, and children undergoing elective major reconstructive surgery, spinal surgery, liver transplantation, or cardiac surgery. Coordination with the hematology department, blood banking, and the primary patient care team is required to take full advantage of this form of therapy.[329-347] Although usually well tolerated, erythropoietin should be used with careful monitoring in patients with hypertension. Erythropoietin is available in a lyophilized (freeze-dried form for reconstitution) or in a dilute albumin solution. Some members of the Jehovah's Witness faith who refuse albumin should receive the lyophilized formulation, which is albumin free.

### PREOPERATIVE AUTOLOGOUS BLOOD DONATION

Donation and storage of blood before elective surgery have reduced the use of allogeneic RBCs.[230,330,343,348-361] Banked units of PRBCs may be stored for 35 to 42 days in the liquid state,[362,363] permitting the donation of several units and the time required for the patient (usually teenagers) to regenerate the RBC mass before surgery. Children unable to mount an erythropoietic response to phlebotomy may only succeed in making themselves anemic, so administration of iron, vitamin C, and folate is important, as is monitoring for reticulocytosis to ensure the bone marrow is replenishing the donated RBCs. Autologous donation should not be attempted in children with significant cardiac ischemic disease or those with an active infection because bacteria can seed the collected unit and overgrow during storage. Autologous donation should be discouraged before procedures for which RBC transfusion is unlikely. Donated blood that is not used by the donor must be discarded rather than enter the general blood bank pool.

Patients or family of pediatric patients may wish to obtain blood from family members or friends (i.e., directed donation). Despite the perception that this donor pool may be safer than the pool of volunteer, allogeneic donors, there is no evidence that this is true. Directed donors are considered to be allogeneic donors and are screened and tested in the same manner as any volunteer donor. Because there is a greater risk of transfusion-associated GVHD with cellular components from a donor who is a blood relative, these units are irradiated to eliminate the possibility of this usually fatal complication of transfusion.[364-366]

## INTRAOPERATIVE BLOOD RECOVERY AND REINFUSION: AUTOTRANSFUSION

Recovery of blood from an operative site and reinfusion after some form of processing has been applied to major vascular, cardiac, and multiple trauma situations for many years.[353,358-360,367-377] The common techniques used wash the recovered blood in a centrifuge so the product consists of the child's RBCs suspended in saline at a hematocrit of 50% to 60%.[368,375] Cellular debris, excess citrate or heparin, free hemoglobin, activated clotting factors, and clotted blood are almost completely removed. Autotransfusion avoids the infectious and immunologic risks of allogeneic transfusion and, if reinfusion is carried out in the operating room, minimizes the opportunity for mistransfusion.[367,375,376,378]

Intraoperative blood recovery is not widely used in infants and children.* The equipment is designed for adults, although some manufacturers have adapted standard devices for pediatric use. We have found blood recovery to be a useful adjunct to minimize allogeneic blood transfusion during scoliosis surgery. This technique may also be used in conjunction with preoperative autologous blood donation, further reducing the need for allogeneic RBC transfusions.[358-360,371,372] The capital investment for the devices and the costs for the disposables and a trained operator are significant. However, these expenses can be offset if three fewer units of allogeneic RBCs are transfused. Development of pediatric-sized equipment should make this technique more widely used and more cost-effective even in smaller children.[383]

### Indications

The indications for intraoperative blood recovery and reinfusion include any major surgical procedure in which the use of more than 3 units of banked RBCs is likely or in which massive blood loss is occurring; children with rare blood types; and multiple trauma with major bleeding.

### Contraindications

Major contraindications to blood-recovery devices include contamination of the operative field by bacteria (e.g., bowel trauma, abscess), cancer, and sickle cell disease (e.g., sickling in the device). Recovered blood should not be processed for reinfusion if the surgical field contains topical clotting agents, some topical antibiotics (e.g., Polymyxin, Neomycin), or other foreign materials

(e.g., methylmethacrylate). Surgery for a malignancy is considered to be a relative contraindication because of the (theoretical) concern that malignant cells may be recovered and reinfused; this can be avoided by discarding blood recovered from the operative field while the tumor is being manipulated.[384-386]

## CONTROLLED HYPOTENSION

Controlled hypotension, the intentional reduction of systemic perfusion pressure, has been used to reduce intraoperative blood loss or to provide a relatively bloodless operating field.[329,387-398] Hypotensive anesthesia may be accomplished with several techniques, including continuous infusion of vasodilators, $\beta$-adrenergic blockade, deep inhalational anesthesia, and large-dose opioid infusions (e.g., remifentanil).[388,399-401]

Controlled hypotension is reserved for older children and teenagers undergoing major reconstructive or orthopedic surgery. The choice of technique and the degree of induced hypotension depend on the surgical procedure. For procedures in which a dry surgical field is the end point with little potential for rapid blood loss, a technique that may take some time for recovery is acceptable (e.g., deep inhalational agent with or without $\beta$-blockade). If surgery carries the possibility of rapid or massive blood loss, a technique that is rapidly reversed (e.g., nitroprusside, nitroglycerin, remifentanil) is probably safer. Controlled hypotension with mean arterial pressure (MAP) of 55 to 60 mm Hg is used less in pediatric anesthesia in recent years, although there are insufficient data to categorically state that the risks of controlled hypotension outweigh the purported benefits. Moderate hypotensive techniques with a MAP of 65 to 70 mm Hg are a more common practice and are likely associated with less risk, although no studies have been published in this regard.[347]

### Physiology

All potent inhalational anesthetics decrease the cerebral metabolic rate for oxygen consumption ($CMRO_2$) and increase cerebral blood flow. Isoflurane appears to offer the greatest advantage because it induces the greatest depression of $CMRO_2$, and it has been used as the sole hypotensive agent.[402-408] One of the most important considerations of any hypotensive technique is the effect that it has on cerebral blood flow. Studies of adults demonstrate that little change occurs in cerebral metabolism when the MAP is maintained above 55 mm Hg.[402] There are no comparable data for children. However, experience with children during cardiac bypass suggests that children tolerate cerebral perfusion pressures below this level on an age-related basis. Brain ischemia has been documented when an MAP of 55 mm Hg is combined with hypocarbia; however, no similar pediatric studies have been carried out.[407,408]

Maintenance of normal arterial carbon dioxide tension ($PaCO_2$) is vitally important to ensure adequate cerebral blood flow during induced hypotension. The relationship of cerebral blood flow to $PaCO_2$ is described in greater detail in Chapter 24. To optimize cerebral blood flow, we typically maintain the MAP at 55 mm Hg or greater and the $PaCO_2$ at 35 to 45 mm Hg.

Hypotensive anesthesia may be induced by one of several techniques: direct myocardial depression with inhalational anesthetics alone or in combination with $\beta$-adrenergic blockade,[404,409,410] direct vasodilators, and other medications (e.g., remifentanil). Because hypotensive anesthesia with inhalational anesthetics depresses myocardial function and requires time to wash out, a rapid offset is often difficult to achieve. We advocate alternative strategies (e.g., vasodilating agents, remifentanil) that provide more precise control of blood pressure without

---

*References 329, 330, 359, 360, 371, 372, 375-377, 379-382.

depressing the heart. The rapid offset of action of these latter agents may hold a particular advantage in children who incur rapid blood loss because the systolic blood pressure is quickly restored on termination while fluids are infused to reestablish euvolemia. Remifentanil offers a similar speed of reversal of cardiovascular depression while avoiding the need for high doses of an inhalational agent. Although β-adrenergic blockade decreases the requirements of vasodilators,[411] cardiac arrest can occur with administration to children.[412]

If β-blockade is to be used safely, the clinician must understand the differences in half-lives of anesthetics and the best means for reversing their effects. Esmolol is very short acting, with a half-life in children of approximately 3 minutes.[413] Nonanesthetized children have a greater requirement (μg/kg) than adults.[414] In nonanesthetized children, a loading dose of 500 μg/kg/min is followed by a maintenance infusion at a rate of 25 to 200 μg/kg/min. Because there is limited published experience esmolol in children under anesthesia, a smaller starting dose (25 to 50 μg/kg/min) and titration of dose every 3 to 5 minutes (increase by 12.5 to 25 μg/kg/min) are indicated. Labetalol[410,415-417] and propranolol[418,419] have been used to help induce hypotensive anesthesia; the half-lives, onset of effect, and time to peak effect of these medications are much greater, and the effects are therefore less controllable and not recommended. Acute β-blocker toxicity can be reversed with high-dose IV glucagon (50 μg/kg followed by an infusion of 0.3 to 3.0 μg/kg/min [extrapolated from adult data])[420-422] and possibly with vasopressin.[423]

### Renal System

Renal blood flow autoregulates between an MAP of 80 and 180 mm Hg. However, general anesthesia with inhalational anesthetics profoundly affects autoregulation. Urinary output is a simple method to monitor the adequacy of intraoperative renal perfusion and function. Reducing the MAP decreases renal blood flow, although the effect on renal function, at least in the case of β-blockers, is insignificant. Renal function returns to normal after the period of controlled hypotension.[415,424-427]

### Pulmonary System

An increase in physiologic dead space and intrapulmonary shunting during induced hypotension has been reported in adults and children.[393,395,428-430] This does not seem to be a clinically important problem in children. Their smaller size compared with adults may reduce the gravitational pooling of blood in the lungs. Nonetheless, it is important to measure the arterial blood gases, expired carbon dioxide, and oxygen saturation to assess for this effect.[393,395] An increasing difference between end-expired carbon dioxide values and measured arterial blood gas values suggest the development of a shunt and increased physiologic dead space. Children with severe scoliosis may have significant arterial-to-alveolar gradients for carbon dioxide even before surgery.

### Hepatic System

Catecholamines, $PaCO_2$, circulating blood volume, and anesthetic agents influence the portal circulation.[431] The liver is oxygenated by the arterial circulation but receives most of its blood flow through the portal circulation, and changes in portal blood flow may have profound effects on total hepatic blood flow. Hepatic oxygenation is maintained during periods of induced hypotension during anesthesia if the $PaCO_2$ is within the normal range and an adequate circulating blood volume is maintained.[432]

## Pharmacology

### Sodium Nitroprusside

Sodium nitroprusside has a very rapid onset of action (seconds), brief duration of action (minutes), and minimal side effects when used in the recommended dose range.[433] This agent is extremely potent and is most safely administered by an infusion pump through a separate IV site and with a second pump to provide a continuous, uninterrupted, and stable infusion rate. Its principal mechanism of action is direct vascular smooth muscle relaxation, primarily causing arteriolar dilation and some venodilation.

DOSAGE. The initial infusion rate for sodium nitroprusside is 0.5 to 1.0 μg/kg/min. The rate can be increased as needed to achieve the desired MAP.[434,435] A satisfactory reduction in systemic perfusion pressure can usually be obtained well below the recommended maximum rate of 10 μg/kg/min.

TOXICITY. Cyanide toxicity is characterized by an unexplained metabolic acidosis, increased blood lactate concentrations, and an increased mixed venous oxygen content.[435,436] The nitroprusside radical interacts with the sulfhydryl groups of erythrocytes, releasing cyanide. Nitroprusside contains five cyanide molecules; and as the cyanide is released, it is converted to nontoxic thiocyanate by the rhodanese enzyme system in the liver and is then excreted by the kidneys.[436] If the amount of cyanide released overwhelms the capacity of the rhodanese system, cyanide toxicity (i.e., binding to the cytochrome electron transport system) results. This produces a change to anaerobic metabolism, metabolic acidosis, an increase in mixed venous oxygen content, and eventually death.[435,437-441] Several pediatric anesthetic-related deaths have resulted from cyanide toxicity and its treatment.[438-440]

Three responses to sodium nitroprusside infusion may herald impending cyanide toxicity: more than 10 μg/kg/min required for a response, tachyphylaxis developing within 30 to 60 minutes, and immediate resistance to the drug.[436] If any of these occur, sodium nitroprusside should be discontinued and the child investigated for possible cyanide toxicity. Treatment of cyanide poisoning is directed at reversal of the binding of cyanide to the cytochrome enzymes. This can be accomplished by producing methemoglobinemia with amyl nitrite. Methemoglobin has a greater affinity for cyanide than it does for the cytochrome system, forcing the reaction in the direction of forming cyanmethemoglobin. The breakdown of cyanmethemoglobin is promoted by administering thiosulfate, which reacts with the cyanide to form nontoxic thiocyanate, which is then excreted by the kidneys. Hydroxocobalamin may prevent toxicity by formation of cyanocobalamin.[442]

This treatment is not without hazard. As Posner states, "Overzealous treatment may merely convert a cytotoxic hypoxia to an anemic hypoxia."[442]

The first step in the treatment of toxicity is the *intermittent* administration of amyl nitrite (by inhalation) until sodium nitrite can be administered intravenously. The second step is sodium nitrite administered as a 3% solution (300 mg/mL, 0.2 mL/kg, not to exceed 10 mL [3 g]). Immediately afterward, sodium thiosulfate in a dose of 175 mg/kg (not to exceed 12.5 g) should be administered. One hundred percent oxygen should be delivered continuously. A cyanide poisoning kit is available (Nithiodote, Hope Pharmaceuticals, Scottsdale, Ariz).

Sodium nitroprusside is a safe medication if doses remain well within the guidelines that have been established by various investigators.[443-445] For children, this is a maximum of 50 μg/kg/min for 30 minutes and 8 to 10 μg/kg/min for 3 hours, with frequent blood gas analyses.[435,445] Because of the potential for toxicity and the availability of newer, less toxic vasodilators, this drug has had decreasing popularity for use for controlled hypotension and is now most commonly used for short-term control of blood pressure in special situations.

### Nitroglycerin

The main advantages of nitroglycerin are its relatively rapid onset of action (minutes), lack of tachyphylaxis and toxicity, and brief duration of action (minutes). The major disadvantage of nitroglycerin is the limited reduction in blood pressure achievable.

DOSAGE. Nitroglycerin is administered by an infusion beginning at a rate of 1 µg/kg/min. The dose is increased until the desired response is obtained. Resistance to the hypotensive effects of nitroglycerin may occur in children. However, in view of the reduced potential for toxicity compared with nitroprusside, nitroglycerin appears to be a reasonable alternative.

TOXICITY. Nitroglycerin is relatively free of toxic side effects in the usual doses applied during hypotensive anesthesia.[395,446,447] No toxicities or deaths have been reported with nitroglycerin when it is used for hypotensive anesthesia.[395,446-448] However, several reports have described nitroglycerin-induced methemoglobinemia, and a study of patients undergoing anesthetic procedures using controlled hypotension did not find a relationship between the development of methemoglobin and the dose of nitroglycerin.[449,450] Pulse oximetry may be of value in making the initial diagnosis (i.e., decreased saturation). However, if this occurs, accurate saturation determinations are not possible because of the interference in light absorbance caused by methemoglobin at both ends of the absorbance spectrum used by pulse oximeters.[451,452] The use of other adjuncts (e.g., potent inhalation agents, other vasodilators, β-adrenergic blockade, potent opioid) reduces the total dose of nitroglycerin administered.

### Remifentanil

Remifentanil-induced hypotension is increasing in popularity because of it relative safety, ease of administration, and titratability, particularly if a patient must be awakened during spinal fusion. Administration should be the same as for any other vasoactive anesthetic agent. It requires dedicated IV access, with the infusion as close to the IV catheter as possible and with a separate pump to avoid fluctuations in the rate of administration. The half-life of this drug is so brief that interruptions while changing IVs or boluses when giving other medications need to be avoided. We have found that the combination of a low-dose inhalational agent, low-dose propofol, and a remifentanil infusion provides excellent operating conditions. Systemic arterial pressure can be controlled by the rate of opioid infusion without fear of residual opioid effect at the end of the procedure, and this combination does not significantly interfere with sensory and motor potential monitoring. If an intraoperative wake up is needed, a longer-acting opioid such as fentanyl should be administered before awakening.

DOSAGE. For most children, the starting dose is 0.1 µg/kg/min, which is then increased or decreased depending on the child's response and the degree of surgical stimulus. The anesthesiologist should expect variable opioid requirements during spinal fusions (doses as great as 2 µg/kg/min and as small as 0.05 µg/kg/min). Analgesic doses of a long-acting opioid such as morphine or hydromorphone should be administered approximately 10 minutes before discontinuation to provide adequate analgesia on awakening. This technique often allows a smooth but rapid extubation despite a very long surgical procedure.

### General Concepts of Hypotensive Anesthesia

Before using controlled hypotension, it is important to understand the rationale for using this technique.[453] If it is used to reduce surgical blood loss, the preparation and monitoring of a child are different from the approach in a procedure in which the main objective for reducing the perfusion pressure is to improve operating conditions (e.g., microsurgical techniques). In the former case, direct assessment of circulating blood pressure and volume with an arterial line and central venous catheter is important, whereas in the latter case, only a direct means of measuring blood pressure (arterial line) is needed.

### Anesthetic Management

All inhalational agents, by directly depressing cardiac output, have been used with various degrees of success as a single drug to produce controlled hypotension, but profound cardiovascular depression may be difficult to control and certainly is not readily reversible.[404-406,409,454] We do not advocate hypotensive anesthesia using potent inhalational agents as the sole hypotensive agent because the cardiovascular depression is not rapidly reversed if a problem arises with a relative anesthetic overdose. However, small to moderate concentrations of inhalational anesthetic reduces the amount of vasodilator, β-blocker, or opioid necessary to reduce blood pressure.[455]

The availability of short-acting β-adrenergic blockers offers an alternative method to decrease MAP by directly depressing cardiac output. However, β-adrenergic blockade removes a valuable guide to the depth of anesthesia and volume status. Because the cardiac output in children approximately 2 years old or younger depends on heart rate (see Chapter 16), β-adrenergic blockade is not recommended in this age group. Low-dose, short-acting β-adrenergic blockade may be a reasonable adjunct to hypotensive anesthesia with inhalational anesthetics as a means of reducing the concentration of the anesthetic or as a supplement to reduce the vasodilator requirements.[456] A rapid-acting β-blocker such as esmolol may be the best compromise because its half-life is brief (3 minutes), and it is administered as an infusion. Even with this type of control, serious adverse events have been reported with the use of β-blockers in children.[412]

The safest method to deliver vasodilating agents, ultra-short-acting β-blocking agents, or potent opioids is by using two infusion pumps. The first is used to infuse a continuous and constant flow of fluids through the IV catheter, and the second is used to infuse the hypotensive agent. Use of a separate IV site can minimize an accidental bolus of the hypotensive agent during changes in fluid requirements or during the administration of other medications. The vasodilator, ultra-short-acting β-blocker, or potent opioid should be administered as close to the vein as possible to eliminate dead space and the possibility of accidental bolus administration.

### Monitoring and Management Principles

The following baseline parameters are monitored: oxygen saturation and expired carbon dioxide, electrocardiogram, temperature, hematocrit, blood glucose, arterial blood gases, acid–base status, MAP, and CVP. Arterial pressure is measured using the radial artery.

When the desired MAP has been attained, a new baseline CVP should be measured and maintained at this level or a slightly greater level than the new, reduced CVP value throughout the procedure. To use any hypotensive technique safely, normovolemia is maintained at all times. This means that even small (1 or 2 mm Hg) decreases in the CVP prompt an appropriate fluid response. A small change in cardiac filling pressures in a healthy, supine, anesthetized pediatric patient may represent a significant reduction in circulating blood volume. Even during hypotensive anesthesia, the kidneys should produce 0.5 to 1.0 mL/kg of urine per hour. The failure to detect urine output frequently is caused by obstruction or kinking of the urinary catheter. If the catheter is patent, an IV fluid challenge should be considered. Urine output is one of the best indicators of organ perfusion and renal function during hypotensive anesthesia.

After hypotension has been induced and the surgical field is bloodless, the MAP should be slowly increased in 5- to 10-mm Hg increments until increased bleeding is observed in the surgical field. At that time, the MAP can be again reduced by approximately 5 mm Hg to achieve optimal conditions. With this method, it is sometimes necessary to reduce the MAP only 10% to 20% from baseline to achieve satisfactory hemostasis with hypotensive anesthesia.

POSITION. Make the operative field the highest point of the child's body to take advantage of gravitational forces to help reduce blood pressure. When positioning a child, care must also be taken to minimize any possible impedance to venous drainage that may contribute to blood loss. For example, abdominal pressure from a misplaced roll of sheets can markedly increase venous pressure during spinal instrumentation and completely offset any beneficial effects from reduced arterial pressure.[397,453,457,458] If the head is the surgical site, the arterial transducer must be calibrated at head level rather than heart level to ensure adequate cerebral perfusion pressure.[447,459]

LABORATORY PARAMETERS. Adequate levels of hemoglobin must be maintained to have sufficient oxygen-carrying capacity. Studies have indicated that at normal blood pressures, a hemoglobin value of 5 g/dL is well tolerated in laboratory animals, but ischemia may occur with a reduced hemoglobin concentration.[460] There is some evidence that the combination of hemodilution and hypotensive anesthesia may fail to deliver adequate oxygenation to some vascular beds (e.g., renal, enteric mucosa).[461,462] Although no similar studies have been conducted in children, for additional safety, we maintain the hemoglobin level at 9 to 10 g/dL during controlled hypotensive anesthesia. This is important for children undergoing spinal instrumentation, in which traction on the spinal cord may alter spinal cord blood flow.

Arterial blood gases must be carefully evaluated on a 30- to 60-minute basis to diagnose changes in oxygenation, ventilation, or perfusion or the development of drug toxicity (e.g., nitroprusside) or adverse anesthesia events.[463-465] A large difference between arterial and expired carbon dioxide values may indicate a pulmonary shunt or air embolization. An increase in mixed venous oxygen content may signal cyanide toxicity. Adequate $PaO_2$ must be maintained at all times. Continuous examination of the $PaO_2$ is important during any hypotensive anesthetic technique because cerebral perfusion is directly related to $PaCO_2$.[466,467] Normocarbia should be maintained. The combination of hypocarbia and hypotension should be avoided. The metabolic components of acid–base equilibrium must be monitored; development of acidosis reflects inadequate oxygen delivery or toxicity from the hypotensive agent (e.g., sodium nitroprusside).[433]

Although we do not advocate the routine use of β-adrenergic blockade, blood glucose values should be measured serially if these drugs are part of the chosen hypotensive technique. β-Adrenergic blockade inhibits glycogenolysis and may cause severe, unsuspected hypoglycemia in children.[393,468,469]

### Contraindications

The risks of hypotensive anesthesia are significant.[470] The risk-benefit ratio must always be considered on an individual basis, particularly with neurosurgical patients and those undergoing spinal instrumentation. Any systemic disease compromising the function of a major organ is a relative contraindication to the use of controlled hypotension. Most reported complications are related to the inexperience of the practitioner, inappropriate patient selection, unfamiliarity with the drugs involved, or inattention to details such as blood volume status, pH, $PaCO_2$, or blood glucose or not using infusion pumps to carefully titrate medications.* If a child is healthy and meticulous attention is paid to all the parameters previously detailed, the benefits of improved surgical technique, reduced surgical time, and decreased need for blood transfusion may outweigh the potential risks.

### NORMOVOLEMIC HEMODILUTION

Intentional isovolemic hemodilution is a useful adjunct to an anesthesiologist's strategy for reducing allogeneic blood transfusions.[329,330,353,460,473-480] Two basic methods can be applied:

1. Allow the surgical blood loss to continue until the child's hematocrit value is in the high teens and maintain that hematocrit value until near the end of the procedure. At that time, the hematocrit can be increased to the desired value by transfusing PRBCs. This technique allows surgical bleeding to occur at a reduced hematocrit value, resulting in reduced loss of RBC mass.

2. Blood can be removed from a child at the beginning of the operation while replacing the volume with crystalloid solution (usually) and then returning the blood at the end of the procedure or when significant bleeding occurs.

The latter technique is preferable because it reserves a quantity of the child's own blood, which can be returned at the end of the surgical procedure. For a Jehovah's Witness, this technique often conforms to religious guidelines if direct continuity is maintained with the child's circulation.[460,481-488]

During acute normovolemic hemodilution under anesthesia, the distribution of blood flow improves with the reduced hematocrit. Improved blood rheology is the major compensatory mechanism for maintaining oxygen delivery despite a reduced hematocrit. Oxygen extraction increases in the presence of an inadequate circulating blood volume or when the hematocrit decreases to less than 20%. If the hematocrit decreases to less than 15%, subendocardial myocardial ischemia may develop.[489-492] At this extreme level of anemia, dissolved oxygen begins to assume a more important role in oxygen delivery.[493] In several reports, extreme acute normovolemic hemodilution (hemoglobin as low as 2 g/dL) were well-tolerated,[489,494-497] although we cannot endorse the use of this technique in children because it is impossible to assess the effects of such an extreme hemoglobin concentration on the long-term cognitive ability. Nonetheless, these reports[489,497] indicate that healthy children can tolerate these extreme hematocrit concentrations provided they are anesthetized, normovolemic, slightly hypothermic, and ventilated with 100% oxygen. We limit the absolute minimum hematocrit to

---

*References 393, 438, 439, 453, 457, 471, 472.

15%, but we prefer to maintain the hematocrit closer to 20% at all times.

## Technique and Key Concepts

When blood is collected for normovolemic hemodilution, blood flows directly from the arterial line into sterile blood bags that contain the appropriate anticoagulant. Each bag is weighed before any blood is transferred and then continuously during filling by placing it on a scale. The bag is frequently but gently agitated to ensure an even distribution of the anticoagulant. The total volume of blood to be withdrawn should be calculated preoperatively to reduce the hematocrit to the 20% to 25%. Care must be taken to replace the blood removed with 5% albumin milliliter for milliliter or 1.5 to 2 mL of lactated Ringer's solution for each milliliter of blood removed. Sometimes, an even greater volume of replacement fluid is needed.[479] A reasonable estimate of the adequacy of replacement is to obtain a baseline CVP and then maintain the same CVP as blood is withdrawn and replaced. It is preferable to hemodilute before the surgical incision to monitor changes in hemodynamic indices, although it can be performed during the initial phases of surgery. The major concern is to maintain a normal circulating blood volume and provide adequate oxygen-carrying capacity. It is important to make an educated guess about how much blood loss is anticipated during the surgery so that autologous blood can be reinfused in place of homologous blood. Because a small-pore filter (20 μm) traps many of the platelets that a large-pore filter (≥150 μm) allows to pass, the former is best avoided at this juncture. In many hospitals, use of this small pore filter has been discontinued.

## Indications

Hemodilution may be indicated in any procedure in which blood loss is expected to exceed one half of the child's blood volume.

## Contraindications

Hemodilution is contraindicated in children with sickle cell disease, septicemia, cyanotic cardiac disease, or compromised function of any major organ that may be significantly affected by changes in perfusion and oxygenation. We do not recommend combining extreme hemodilution (hematocrit <25%) with controlled hypotension. Children with moderate anemia are not good candidates because not enough units can be removed to make the technique effective.

## Complications

The major complications of hemodilution are related to blood volume status, hemoglobin content (i.e., removing too much blood), and coagulopathy (i.e., dilution of clotting factors). Anesthesiologists must pay meticulous attention to blood volume replacement. As long as normovolemia is maintained and the hematocrit exceeds 15% (preferably about 20%), problems with organ perfusion or oxygenation should not occur. Sepsis becomes a concern if strict sterile techniques are not followed during the collection process.

## Advantages

The benefits of normovolemic hemodilution are that the units of blood collected at the beginning of the procedure pose no risk of infection (unless contaminated by bacteria during the collection process) or mistransfusion (if they are not removed from the operating room) when they are returned to the child at a later time. It yields a net saving in loss of RBC mass because the surgical losses occur at a hematocrit of 15% to 20% rather than 30% to 45%. The net use of banked RBCs may be reduced if 2 or 3 units can be removed at the beginning of the procedure. This technique can be used only in older children and teenagers, and it is used most frequently in the population undergoing spinal instrumentation.

## The Jehovah's Witness Patient

The children of Jehovah's Witnesses present a particular medical and legal dilemma.[498,499] Transfusion management of anyone with a religious objection to transfusion depends in part on the urgency of the surgical procedure and underlying medical condition of the child. If not emergent, a meeting with the patient (or the parents or guardian if a minor), the patient's spiritual advisor (if the child so chooses), and representatives of the team that will be caring for the child should be held to allow the child to clearly articulate his or her wishes with respect to the refusal of transfusion and its consequences and to discuss possible alternatives, including the use of erythropoietin, iron therapy, acute normovolemic hemodilution, intraoperative cell recovery and reinfusion, and the use of antifibrinolytic medications.[495,496,500-503] Specific inquiries should be made about each child's beliefs regarding the use of albumin, plasma, cryoprecipitate, platelets, and intraoperative cell recovery and reinfusion if the circuit is not continuously connected to the child and, in particular, what the child's response would be if a life-threatening event occurred while he or she was under anesthesia.[481,504] These discussions should be carefully documented in the child's record and informed consent signed beforehand. Not all hospitals or physicians are willing to participate in these cases, in which case arrangements should be made to transfer the child to the care of institutions or physicians who are willing to work within these constraints.

The courts have consistently ruled that the adult patient or emancipated minor has a right to refuse transfusion.[482,505] Physicians have the moral and legal obligations to respect those beliefs if an adult or teenager has made an informed decision and understands that he or she may die or suffer permanent injury without a transfusion if a life-threatening situation occurs. However, in the case of a minor child, the Supreme Courts in the United States and Canada have ruled that the fate of the minor child cannot be determined by the parents' religious convictions. The most important issue is full and open discussion of the effort that will be made to respect the person's religious beliefs and avoid blood transfusions. In the case of minor children about whom a mutual understanding cannot be reached on avoiding blood transfusions, a court order can be obtained to save the child's life. The parents should be informed about this possibility beforehand.[506] The ethics of this issue are discussed in Chapter 5.

## ACKNOWLEDGMENT

The authors wish to thank Richard M. Dsida for his prior contributions to this chapter.

## ANNOTATED REFERENCES

Dzik WH, Stowell CP. Transfusion and coagulation issues in trauma. In: Sheridan RL, editor. The trauma handbook of the Massachusetts General Hospital. Philadelphia: Lippincott Williams & Wilkins; 2004. pp. 128-47.

*This chapter discusses the issues and complications of massive transfusion and provides a practical guide for management of this difficult clinical situation.*

Lacroix J, Hébert PC, Hutchinson JS, et al. Transfusion strategies for patients in pediatric intensive care units. N Engl J Med 2007;356: 1609-19.

*This landmark multicenter clinical trial compared outcomes in pediatric patients randomized to red blood cell transfusion thresholds of 9.5 g/dL or 7 g/ dL. There were no differences with respect to new or progressive multiple-organ failure, mortality, or other clinical outcomes between the two groups, which highlights the capacity of even acutely ill pediatric patients to tolerate anemia.*

Ness PM, Cushing MM. Oxygen therapeutics: pursuit of an alternative to the donor red blood cell. Arch Pathol Lab Med 2007;131:734-41.

*This review provides a comprehensive and balanced summary of the development of synthetic oxygen carriers and the current challenges they face in making the transition from the laboratory to the clinic.*

Slichter SJ, Kaufman RM, Assmann SF, et al. Dose of prophylactic platelet transfusions and prevention of hemorrhage. N Engl J Med 2010; 362:600-13.

*This paper presents new data regarding platelet transfusion for nonoperative but thrombocytopenic patients including 200 children. It is likely that new guidelines will be developed in the near future.*

Steiner ME, Assmann SF, Levy JH, et al. Addressing the question of the effect of RBC storage on clinical outcomes: the Red Cell Storage Duration Study (RECESS) (Section 7). Transfus Apher Sci 2010; 43:107-16.

*There is much controversy regarding the advantages and disadvantages of transfusion with relatively young packed red blood cells. This is one of many studies attempting to address this very important issue.*

## REFERENCES

Please see www.expertconsult.com.

# THE CHEST

# Essentials of Pulmonology

## PAUL G. FIRTH AND T. BERNARD KINANE

| | |
|---|---|
| Respiratory Physiology | Upper Respiratory Tract Infection |
| Preoperative Assessment | Lower Airway Disease |
| Pulmonary Function Tests | Cystic Fibrosis |
| Perioperative Etiology | Sickle Cell Disease |
| and Epidemiology | Summary |

RESPIRATORY PROBLEMS ARE COMMON in children. The anesthesiologist often encounters pulmonary complications ranging from mild acute respiratory tract infections to chronic lung disease with end-stage respiratory failure during perioperative consultations, intraoperatively, or in the intensive care unit. This chapter discusses the basics of respiratory physiology, how to assess pulmonary function, and the practical anesthetic management of specific pulmonary problems. Airway and thoracic aspects pertinent to ventilation are discussed in Chapters 12 and 13; pulmonary issues specific to neonates, intensive care, and various disease states are addressed in the relevant chapters.

## Respiratory Physiology

The morphologic development of the lung begins at several weeks after conception and continues into the first decade of postnatal life.[1] Intrauterine gas exchange occurs via the placenta, but the respiratory system develops in preparation for extrauterine life, when gas exchange transfers abruptly to the lungs at birth.

Development of the lung, which begins as an outgrowth of the foregut ventral wall, can be divided into several stages (Fig. 11-1). During the embryonic period, the first few postconceptional weeks, lung buds form as a projection of the endodermal tissue into the mesenchyme. The pseudoglandular period extends to the 17th week of life, during which rapid lung growth is accompanied by formation of the bronchi and branching of the airways down to the terminal bronchioli. Further development of bronchioli and vascularization of the airways occurs during the canalicular stage of the second trimester. The saccular stage begins at approximately 24 weeks, when terminal air sacs begin to form. The capillary networks surrounding these air spaces proliferate, allowing sufficient pulmonary gas exchange for extrauterine survival of the premature neonate by 26 to 28 weeks. Formation of alveoli occurs by lengthening of the saccules and

thinning of the saccular walls and has begun by the 36th postconceptional week in most human fetuses. The vast majority of alveolar formation occurs after birth, typically continuing until 8 to 10 years postnatally. The neonatal lung at birth usually contains 10 to 20 million terminal air sacs (many of which are saccules rather than alveoli), one-tenth the number in the mature adult lung. Growth of the lungs after birth occurs primarily as an increase in the number of respiratory bronchioles and alveoli rather than an increase in the size of the alveoli.

The abrupt transition to extrauterine gas exchange at birth involves the rapid expansion of the lungs, increased pulmonary blood flow, and initiation of a regular respiratory rhythm. The development of a respiratory rhythm, detectable initially by intermittent rhythmic fetal thoracic movements, begins well before birth and may be necessary for normal anatomic and physiologic lung development. Interruption of umbilical blood flow at birth initiates continuous rhythmic breathing. Amniotic fluid is expelled from the lungs via the upper airways with the first few breaths, with residual fluid draining through the lymphatic and pulmonary channels in the first days of life. Changes in the partial pressures of oxygen ($PO_2$) and carbon dioxide ($PCO_2$) and in hydrogen ion concentration (pH) cause an acute decrease in pulmonary vascular resistance and a consequent increase in pulmonary blood flow. Increased left atrial and decreased right atrial pressure reverse the pressure gradient across the foramen ovale, causing functional closure of this left-to-right one-way flap valve. Ventilatory rhythm is augmented and maintained in part by the increased arterial oxygen relative to the prior intrauterine levels.

Breathing is controlled by a complex interaction involving input from sensors, integration by a central control system, and output to effector muscles.[2] Afferent signaling is provided by peripheral arterial and central brainstem chemoreceptors, upper airway and intrapulmonary receptors, and chest wall and muscle mechanoreceptors.

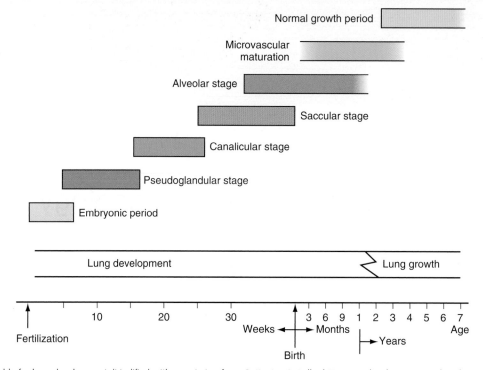

**FIGURE 11-1** Timetable for lung development. (Modified with permission from Guttentag S, Ballard PL. Lung development: embryology, growth, maturation, and developmental biology. In: Tausch HW, Ballard RA, Gleason CA, editors. Avery's diseases of the newborn. 8th ed. Philadelphia: WB Saunders; 2004, p. 602.)

The peripheral arterial chemoreceptors consist of the carotid and aortic bodies, with the carotid bodies playing the greater role in arterial chemical sensing of both arterial $O_2$ tension ($Pao_2$) and pH. The central chemoreceptors, responsive to arterial $CO_2$ tension ($PaCO_2$) and pH, are thought to be located at or near the ventral surface of the medulla.

The nose, pharynx, and larynx have a wide variety of pressure, chemical, temperature, and flow receptors that can cause apnea, coughing, or changes in ventilatory pattern. Pulmonary receptors lie in the airways and lung parenchyma. The airway receptors are subdivided into the slowly adapting receptors, also called pulmonary stretch receptors, and the rapidly adapting receptors. The stretch receptors, found in the airway smooth muscle, are thought to be involved in the balance of inspiration and expiration. These receptors may be the sensors in the Hering-Breuer reflexes, which prevent overdistention or collapse of the lung. The rapidly adapting receptors lie between the airway epithelial cells and are triggered by noxious stimuli such as smoke, dust, and histamine. Parenchymal receptors, also known as juxtacapillary receptors, are located adjacent to the alveolar blood vessels; they respond to hyperinflation of the lungs, to various chemical stimuli in the pulmonary circulation, and possibly to interstitial congestion. Chest wall receptors include mechanoreceptors and joint proprioreceptors. Mechanoreceptors in the muscle spindle endings and tendons of respiratory muscles sense changes in length, tension, and movement.

Central integration of respiration is maintained by the brainstem (involuntary) and by cortical (voluntary) centers. Although the precise mechanism of the neural ventilatory rhythmogenesis is unknown, the pre-Bötzinger complex and the retrotrapezoid nucleus/parafacial respiratory group, neural circuits in the ventrolateral medulla, are thought to be the respiratory rhythm generators.[3] These neuron groups fire in an oscillating pattern, an inherent rhythm that is moderated by inputs from other respiratory centers. Involuntary integration of sensory input occurs in various respiratory nuclei and neural complexes in the pons and medulla that modify the baseline pacemaker firing of the respiratory rhythm generators. The cerebral cortex also affects breathing rhythm and influences or overrides involuntary rhythm generation in response to conscious or subconscious activity, such as emotion, arousal, pain, speech, breath holding, and other activities.[2]

The effectors of ventilation include the neural efferent pathways, the muscles of respiration, the bones and cartilage of the chest wall and airway, and elastic connective tissue. Upper airway patency is maintained by connective tissue and by sustained and cyclic contractions of the pharyngeal dilator muscles. The diaphragm produces the majority of tidal volume during quiet inspiration, with the intercostal, abdominal, and accessory muscles (sternocleidomastoid and neck muscles) providing additional negative pressure. The elastic recoil of the lungs and thorax produces expiration. Inspiration is an active and expiration a passive action in normal lungs during quiet breathing. During vigorous breathing or with airway obstruction, both inspiration and expiration become active processes.

Another effect of age is a change in chest wall compliance. In adults, the end-expiratory volume is equivalent to the functional residual capacity (FRC). In infants, the chest wall is more compliant, so the tendency of the lung to collapse is not adequately counterbalanced by chest wall rigidity. Infants stop expiration at a lung volume greater than FRC, with the inspiratory muscles braking expiration. When this braking mechanism is impaired, as occurs with general anesthesia, the infant has a tendency to develop atelectasis.

# Preoperative Assessment

The preoperative assessment of the respiratory system in a child is based on the history, physical examination, and evaluation of vital signs. Because ventilation is a complex process involving many systems besides the lung, the pulmonary appraisal must also include an assessment of airway, musculoskeletal, and neurologic pathology that might affect gas exchange under anesthesia or in the postoperative period. The potential impacts of esophageal reflux and cardiac, hepatic, renal, or hematologic disease on gas exchange and pulmonary function should be considered. Further investigations, such as laboratory, radiographic, and pulmonary function studies, may be indicated if there is doubt as to the diagnosis or severity of the pulmonary disease.

Because children may be unwilling or unable to give a reliable history, parents or caregivers are often the sole source or an important supplemental source of information during initial evaluation. Risk factors in the history that are associated with an increased risk of perioperative events include a respiratory tract infection within the preceding 2 weeks, wheezing during exercise, more than three wheezing episodes in the past 12 months, nocturnal dry cough, eczema, and a family history of asthma, rhinitis, eczema, or exposure to tobacco smoke.[1,4] Viral upper respiratory tract infections (URIs) are common in children, and the time, frequency, and severity of infection should be established. If wheezing is present, the precipitating causes, frequency, severity, and relieving factors should be determined. Chronic pulmonary diseases often have a variable clinical course, and the details of acute exacerbations of chronic problems should be elicited.

In younger children, the gestational age at birth, the current postmenstrual age, neonatal respiratory difficulties, and prolonged intubation in the neonatal period are particularly important to ascertain. Apneic episodes, subglottic stenosis, and tracheomalacia are possible complications of prematurity and prolonged intubation that may be exacerbated in the perioperative period. Whereas congenital lesions often manifest at birth, symptoms of airway collapse or stenosis may become evident only later in life.

Physical examination begins when you enter the room. Particularly with young children, your best opportunity to observe them before they react to your presence is from across the room, and inspection from a distance can provide useful information. Respiratory rate is a sensitive marker of pulmonary problems, and scrutiny of the rate before a young child becomes agitated and hyperventilates is an important metric. Pulse oximetry is a useful baseline indicator of oxygenation. Nasal flaring, intercostal retractions, and the marked use of accessory respiratory muscles are all signs of respiratory distress. General appearance is also important. Apathy, anxiety, agitation, or persistent adoption of a fixed posture may indicate profound respiratory or airway difficulties, and intense cyanosis can also be detected from a distance. Weight may relate to pulmonary function: Children with chronic severe pulmonary disease are often underweight owing to retarded growth or malnourishment, whereas severe obesity can produce airway obstruction and sleep apnea. Inspection of the chest contour may reveal hyperinflation or thoracic wall deformities.

Closer physical examination adds further information. Atopy and eczema may be associated with hyperreactive airways. Auscultation may reveal wheezes, rales, fine or coarse crepitus, transmitted breath sounds from the upper airway, altered breath sounds, or cardiac murmurs. Chest percussion can provide an estimate of the position of the diaphragm and serve as a useful marker of hyperinflation. Patience, a gentle approach, and warm hands improve diagnostic yield and patient satisfaction.

# Pulmonary Function Tests

Further pulmonary investigations include chest imaging, measurement of hematocrit, arterial blood gas analysis, pulmonary function tests, and sleep studies. Special investigations are not routinely indicated preoperatively and should be reserved for cases in which the diagnosis is unclear, the progression or treatment of a disease needs to be established, or the severity of impairment is not evident. In most cases, a comprehensive history and careful physical examination are adequate to establish an appropriate anesthetic plan. Before requesting a new investigation, the clinician should have a clear idea of the question the test is expected to answer and how the answer will modify anesthetic management and outcome. Many tests are difficult to perform in children who have short attention spans and who cannot sit still for any length of time. Judgment must be exercised when ordering these tests for young children, and due consideration must be given to the child's age and level of maturity and the influence of the parents.

Pulmonary function tests include dynamic studies, measurement of static lung volumes, and diffusing capacity. Pulmonary function tests enable clinicians to (1) establish mechanical dysfunction in children with respiratory symptoms, (2) quantify the degree of dysfunction, and (3) define the nature of the dysfunction as obstructive, restrictive, or mixed obstructive and restrictive.[5] Table 11-1 presents common indications for pulmonary function testing in children.

**TABLE 11-1 Uses of Pulmonary Function Studies in Children**

- To establish pulmonary mechanical abnormality in children with respiratory symptoms
- To quantify the degree of dysfunction
- To define the nature of pulmonary dysfunction (obstructive, restrictive, or mixed obstructive and restrictive)
- To aid in defining the site of airway obstruction as central or peripheral
- To differentiate fixed from variable and intrathoracic from extrathoracic central airway obstruction
- To follow the course of pulmonary disease processes
- To assess the effect of therapeutic interventions and guide changes in therapy
- To detect increased airway reactivity
- To evaluate the risk of diagnostic and therapeutic procedures
- To monitor for pulmonary side effects of chemotherapy or radiation therapy
- To aid in predicting the prognosis and quantitating pulmonary disability
- To investigate the effect of acute and chronic disease processes on lung growth

Modified with permission from Castile R. Pulmonary function testing in children. In: Chernick V, Boat TF, Wilmott RW, Bush A, editors: Kendig's disorders of the respiratory tract in children. 7th ed. Philadelphia: Elsevier Saunders; 2006, p. 168. Reproduced from National Asthma Education and Prevention Program: Full report of the expert panel: guidelines for the diagnosis and management of asthma (EPR-3). Bethesda, Md.: National Heart, Lung, and Blood Institute, National Institutes of Health; 2007.

The dynamic studies, which are the most commonly used tests, include spirometry, flow–volume loops, and measurement of peak expiratory flow. Spirometry measures the volume of air inspired and expired as a function of time and is by far the most frequently performed test of pulmonary function in children. With a forced exhalation after a maximal inhalation, the total volume exhaled is known as the forced vital capacity (FVC), and the fractional volume exhaled in the first second is known as the forced expiratory volume in 1 second ($FEV_1$). Figure 11-2 illustrates a normal pulmonary function test (normal flow–volume loop and spirometry parameters).

An obstructive process is characterized by decreased velocity of airflow through the airways (Fig. 11-3), whereas a restrictive defect produces decreased lung volumes (Fig. 11-4). Examination of the ratio of airflow to lung volume assists in differentiating these components of lung disease. Normally, a child should be able to exhale more than 80% of the FVC in the first second. Children with obstructive lung disease have decreased airflow in relation to exhaled volume. If the volume exhaled in the first second divided by the volume of full exhalation ($FEV_1$/FVC) is less than 80%, then airway obstruction is present (Table 11-2; see Fig. 11-3).

The $FEV_1$ needs to be interpreted in the context of the FVC. A small $FEV_1$ alone is insufficient evidence on which to make a diagnosis of airflow obstruction. Those with restrictive lung disease have both decreased $FEV_1$ and FVC–decreased flow rate and reduced total exhaled volume. Restrictive lung disease is associated with a loss of lung tissue or a decrease in the lung's ability to expand. A restrictive defect is diagnosed when the FVC is less than 80% of normal with either a normal or an increased $FEV_1$/FVC (see Table 11-2 and Fig. 11-4).

Most children with respiratory problems have an obstructive pattern; isolated restrictive diseases are far less common. Asthma

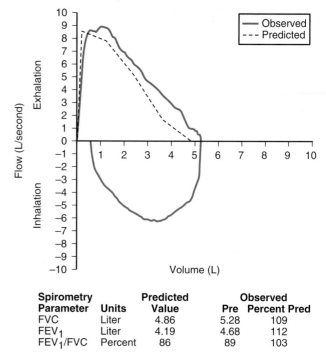

| Spirometry Parameter | Units | Predicted Value | Pre | Observed Percent Pred |
|---|---|---|---|---|
| FVC | Liter | 4.86 | 5.28 | 109 |
| $FEV_1$ | Liter | 4.19 | 4.68 | 112 |
| $FEV_1$/FVC | Percent | 86 | 89 | 103 |

**FIGURE 11-2** Normal pulmonary function test. The normal flow–volume curve obtained during forced expiration rapidly ascends to the peak expiratory flow (highest point on curve), then descends with decreasing volume, following a reproducible shape that is independent of effort. In this normal flow–volume curve, the forced vital capacity (FVC), forced expiratory volume in 1 second ($FEV_1$), and $FEV_1$/FVC ratio are all within the normal range for this child's age, height, gender, and race. The shapes of both the inspiratory and expiratory limbs are normal as well. *Pre*, Prebronchodilator; *Pred*, predicted value.

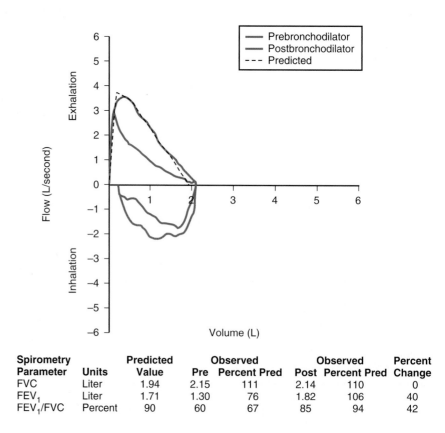

**FIGURE 11-3** This flow–volume curve demonstrates a reversible obstructive defect. The forced expiratory volume in 1 second ($FEV_1$) as a percentage of forced vital capacity (FVC), or total volume exhaled, is decreased in patients with airway obstruction. The observed curve shape before bronchodilator use (*blue curve*) is scooped. After administration of a short-acting bronchodilator, the observed curve shape (*brown*) appears normal, and there is an increase in both $FEV_1$/FVC and $FEV_1$. This child has asthma and demonstrates a marked (40%) increase in $FEV_1$ after treatment with a short-acting bronchodilator. Reversible airflow obstruction is one of the hallmarks of asthma. *Post*, Postbronchodilator; *Pre*, prebronchodilator; *Pred*, predicted value.

| Spirometry Parameter | Units | Predicted Value | Pre | Observed Percent Pred | Post | Observed Percent Pred | Percent Change |
|---|---|---|---|---|---|---|---|
| FVC | Liter | 1.94 | 2.15 | 111 | 2.14 | 110 | 0 |
| $FEV_1$ | Liter | 1.71 | 1.30 | 76 | 1.82 | 106 | 40 |
| $FEV_1$/FVC | Percent | 90 | 60 | 67 | 85 | 94 | 42 |

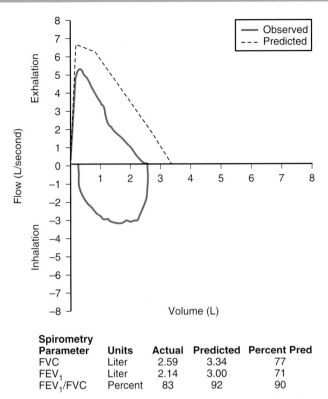

| Spirometry Parameter | Units | Actual | Predicted | Percent Pred |
|---|---|---|---|---|
| FVC | Liter | 2.59 | 3.34 | 77 |
| FEV$_1$ | Liter | 2.14 | 3.00 | 71 |
| FEV$_1$/FVC | Percent | 83 | 92 | 90 |

**FIGURE 11-4** Flow–volume curve demonstrating a restrictive defect. The flow–volume curves in children with restrictive defects are near-normal in configuration but smaller in all dimensions. The ratio of forced expiratory volume in 1 second (FEV$_1$) to forced vital capacity (FVC) is normal, but both FEV$_1$ and FVC are reduced. The curve shape appears normal. This child has interstitial lung disease. *Pred,* Predicted value.

**TABLE 11-2** Characteristics of Obstructive and Restrictive Patterns of Lung Disease

| Measurement | DISEASE CATEGORY | |
|---|---|---|
| | Obstructive | Restrictive |
| FVC | Normal/decreased | Decreased |
| FEV$_1$ | Decreased | Decreased |
| FEV/FVC | Decreased | Normal |

*FEV$_1$,* Forced expiratory volume in 1 second; *FVC,* forced vital capacity.

is the most common obstructive pulmonary disease in children. Rare causes of obstruction include airway lesions, congenital subglottic webs, and vocal cord dysfunction. Restrictive lung disease can arise from limitations to chest wall movement such as chest wall deformities, scoliosis, or pleural effusions or from space-occupying intrathoracic pathology such as large bullae or congenital cysts. Alveolar filling defects (e.g., lobar pneumonia) also reduce lung volume and can be considered as restrictive processes. Although the diseases arise from specific isolated genetic disorders, children with cystic fibrosis (CF) and sickle cell disease (SCD) can have highly variable pulmonary pathologic processes with both obstructive and restrictive components of lung disease. Bronchopulmonary dysplasia may also result in both obstructive and restrictive pathology.

Pulmonary function tests can also be used to differentiate fixed from variable airway obstruction and to localize the obstruction as above or below the thoracic inlet (Figs. 11-5 through 11-7, E-Fig. 11-1). This information can be gleaned from distinctive changes

in the configuration of the flow–volume loop, a graphic representation of inspiratory and expiratory flow volumes plotted against time. A fixed central airway obstruction, such as a tumor or stenosis, may obstruct both inspiration and expiration, flattening the flow–volume curve on both inspiration and expiration (See Video 12-1). The child with tracheal stenosis, for example, has flattening of both inhalation and exhalation curves (see Fig. 11-6). A variable obstruction tends to affect only one part of the ventilatory cycle. On inhalation, the chest expands and draws the airways open. On exhalation, as the chest collapses, the intrathoracic airways collapse. Variable extrathoracic lesions tend to obstruct on inhalation more than exhalation, whereas variable intrathoracic lesions tend to obstruct more on exhalation. This produces the characteristic flow–volume patterns.

In addition to diagnostic uses, spirometry is used to assess the indication for, and efficacy of, treatment. For example, the obstruction in patients with asthma is usually reversible, either gradually over time without intervention or much more rapidly after treatment with a short-acting bronchodilator. An improvement in FEV$_1$ of 12% and 200 mL is considered a positive response. In addition to confirming the diagnosis of asthma, the degree of airflow obstruction, as indicated by the FEV$_1$, is one measure of asthma control. A low FEV$_1$ or an acute decrease from baseline may indicate a child whose asthma is not under good control and therefore who potentially is at greater risk for a perioperative exacerbation (see Fig. 11-3).

Because it measures the amount of air entering or leaving the lung rather than the amount of air in the lung, spirometry cannot provide data about absolute lung volumes. Information about FRC and lung volumes calculated from FRC, such as total lung capacity and residual volume, must be obtained by different means, such as gas dilution or body plethysmography. Gas dilution is based on measuring the dilution of nitrogen or helium in a circuit in closed connection to the lungs, whereas body plethysmography calculates lung gas volumes based on changes in thoracic pressures.

## Perioperative Etiology and Epidemiology

Respiratory problems account for most of the perioperative morbidity in children,[6,7] and cause almost one third of perioperative pediatric cardiac arrests.[8] Adverse events include laryngospasm, airway obstruction, bronchospasm, hemoglobin oxygen desaturation, prolonged coughing, atelectasis, pneumonia, and respiratory failure.[4,9,10] The incidence of perioperative adverse respiratory events in one study of 755 children was 34%,[9] whereas in another observational study of 9297 children it was 15%.[4] The triggers of these problems included airway manipulation, alteration of airway reflexes by anesthetic drugs, surgical insult, and depression of breathing caused by anesthetic and analgesic medications. Various diseases common among children can further affect the frequency of respiratory complications in pediatric anesthesia.

Studies have consistently reported greater respiratory morbidity among younger compared with older children.[4,6,7,11-13] In particular, neonates are sensitive to respiratory problems for many reasons. Although the FRC approaches adult capacity (in liters per kilogram) within days after birth, a persistently large closing capacity increases the likelihood of alveolar collapse and intrapulmonary shunt. Residual patency of the ductus arteriosus can contribute to shunting. The greater metabolic rate of the infant increases oxygen requirements and decreases the time to arterial

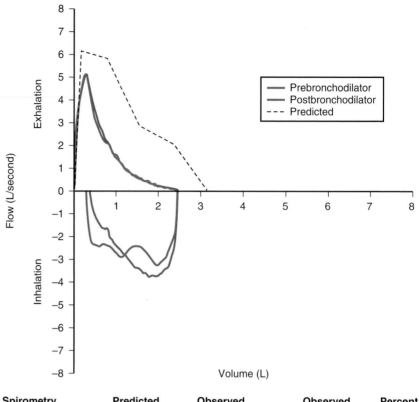

FIGURE 11-5 Pulmonary function test demonstrating a nonreversible obstructive defect. The ratio of forced expiratory volume in 1 second ($FEV_1$) to forced vital capacity ($FVC$) is decreased, as is the $FEV_1$. After administration of a short-acting bronchodilator, there is no significant improvement in the $FEV_1$, in contrast to the pattern in Figure 11-3. This child has cystic fibrosis with a nonreversible obstructive defect. *Post,* Postbronchodilator; *Pre,* prebronchodilator; *Pred,* predicted value.

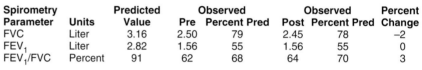

| Spirometry Parameter | Units | Predicted Value | Pre | Observed Percent Pred | Post | Observed Percent Pred | Percent Change |
|---|---|---|---|---|---|---|---|
| FVC | Liter | 3.16 | 2.50 | 79 | 2.45 | 78 | −2 |
| $FEV_1$ | Liter | 2.82 | 1.56 | 55 | 1.56 | 55 | 0 |
| $FEV_1$/FVC | Percent | 91 | 62 | 68 | 64 | 70 | 3 |

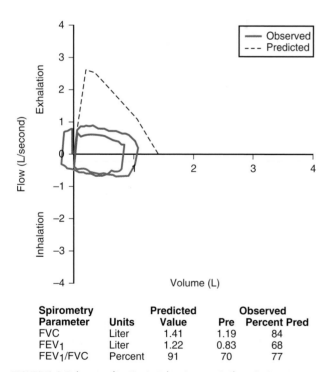

| Spirometry Parameter | Units | Predicted Value | Pre | Observed Percent Pred |
|---|---|---|---|---|
| FVC | Liter | 1.41 | 1.19 | 84 |
| $FEV_1$ | Liter | 1.22 | 0.83 | 68 |
| $FEV_1$/FVC | Percent | 91 | 70 | 77 |

FIGURE 11-6 Pulmonary function test showing an extrathoracic airway obstruction; both the inspiratory and expiratory limbs of the flow–volume curve are flattened. This child has subglottic stenosis that developed at the site of her tracheotomy 2 years after the tracheostomy was removed. *FEV₁,* Forced expiratory volume in 1 second; *FVC,* forced vital capacity; *Pred,* predicted value.

desaturation after an interruption to ventilation and gas exchange. The work of breathing is greater due to high-resistance, small-caliber airways, increased chest wall compliance, and reduced lung parenchymal compliance.

## UPPER RESPIRATORY TRACT INFECTION

Upper repiratory tract infections (URIs) are a common problem among young children. Children are typically infected several times a year, possibly even more frequently if they are in day care. Viruses cause the majority of URIs, with rhinoviruses constituting approximately one third to one half of etiologic species.[14,14a] Other common respiratory viruses in childhood include adenoviruses and coronaviruses.

Although most URIs are short-lived, self-limited infections and are by definition limited to the upper airway, they may increase airway sensitivity to noxious stimuli or secretions for several weeks after the infection has cleared. The mechanisms probably involve a combination of mucosal invasion, chemical mediators, and altered neurogenic reflexes.[14] URIs may also impair pulmonary function by decreasing FVC, $FEV_1$, peak expiratory flow, and diffusion capacity.[15,16]

Compared with uninfected children, children with a recent or current URI have an increased incidence of perioperative laryngospasm, bronchospasm, arterial hemoglobin desaturation, severe coughing, and breath holding (Table 11-3).[4,12,13,17-20] However, most complications can usually be predicted and successfully managed without long-term sequelae by suitably experienced and prepared clinicians.[14,18,20-23] An approach to the child with a URI is to detect the pathologic process and associated

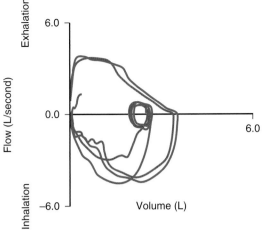

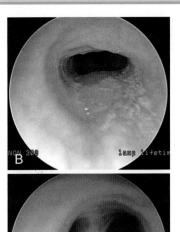

| Spirometry Parameter | Units | Observed Prebron-chodilator | Percent Pred | Observed Postbron-chodilator | Percent Pred | Percent Change |
|---|---|---|---|---|---|---|
| FVC | Liter | 3.53 | 102 | 3.63 | 106 | 3 |
| FEV$_1$ | Liter | 2.63 | 89 | 2.65 | 90 | 0 |
| FEV$_1$/FVC | Percent | 74.7 | | 72.8 | | −3 |

A

**FIGURE 11-7  A,** Pulmonary function test from a child with an intrathoracic airway obstruction (vascular ring). The flow–volume curves suggest a fixed expiratory obstruction. The shape of the inspiratory link is normal; the expiratory flow limb is flattened on both the prebronchodilator (*brown*) and postbronchodilator (*blue*) flow–volume curves. **B,** Slit-like tracheal compression before repair. **C,** Marked improvement in the tracheal lumen after division of the vascular ring. (See E-Fig. 11-1 for a magnetic resonance imaging angiogram of a vascular ring.) (Photographs **B** and **C** courtesy Christopher Hartnick, MD.) *FEV$_1$,* Forced expiratory volume in 1 second; *FVC,* forced vital capacity; *Pred,* predicted value.

**TABLE 11-3**  Incidence of Common Upper Respiratory Tract Infection–Associated Perioperative Adverse Events

| Study | LARYNGOSPASM (%) URI | No URI | BRONCHOSPASM (%) URI | No URI | HEMOGLOBIN DESATURATION (%) URI | No URI |
|---|---|---|---|---|---|---|
| Tait and Knight, 1987[118] | 1.3 | 1.2 | | | | |
| DeSoto et al., 1988[119] | | | | | (<95%) 20.0 | 0* |
| Cohen et al., 1990[11] | 2.2 | 1.7 | | | | |
| Levy et al., 1992[120] | | | | | (<93%) 63.6 | 59.0 |
| Rolf and Coté, 1992[20] | 5.9 | 3.3 | 13.3 | 0.6* | (<85%) 13.3 | 10.5 |
| Tait et al., 1998[121] | 7.3 | | 12.2 | | (<90%) 17.1 | |
| Tait et al., 2001[18] | 4.2 | 3.9 | 5.7 | 3.3 | (<90%) 15.7 | 7.8* |
| von Ungern-Sternberg et al., 2007[13] | 7.6 | 3.1* | | 0.9* | 19.3 | 11.4* |

Data in parentheses under hemoglobin desaturation are the limits for desaturation in each study.
Modified from Tait AR. Anesthetic management of the child with an upper respiratory tract infection. Curr Opin Anaesthesiol 2005;18:603-7.
*URI,* Upper respiratory tract infection.
*P < 0.05 versus corresponding URI group.

comorbidity, establish the acuteness and severity of the URI, and then decide whether to modify the anesthetic technique or postpone surgery (Table 11-4, Fig. 11-8).

The basis for diagnosing a URI is a careful history and physical examination, with further investigations in limited situations. Because they are usually familiar with their child's state of health, the parents or caregivers can provide helpful insight into the presence and severity of a URI. The child should be evaluated for fever (defined as a temperature greater than 100.4° F [38° C]), change in demeanor or behavior, dyspnea, productive cough, purulent sputum production, nasal congestion, rales, rhonchi, and wheezing. A chest radiograph may be considered if the pulmonary examination is questionable, but because the radiographic changes lag behind clinical symptoms, it is typically of limited value. Although laboratory tests may confirm the diagnosis of a viral or bacterial URI, they are not cost-effective or practical in a busy surgical setting.

For children with symptoms of an uncomplicated URI who are afebrile with clear secretions and who are otherwise healthy, anesthesia may proceed as planned, because the problems encountered are typically transient and easily managed.[4,14,18,20-23] Elective surgery is usually postponed for children with more severe symptoms that include at least one of the following: mucopurulent secretions; lower respiratory tract signs (e.g., wheezing) that do not clear with a deep cough; a pyrexia greater than 100.4° F (38° C); or a change in sensorium (e.g., not behaving or playing normally, has not been eating properly).[14,23]

The decision to proceed with surgery becomes much more difficult when the signs of the URI are between the extremes of mild and severe. For these intermediate URIs, other

**TABLE 11-4** Risk Factors for Perioperative Adverse Events in Children with Upper Respiratory Tract Infections

| Study | URI Status | Factors | RR/OR |
|---|---|---|---|
| Parnis et al., 2001[17] | URI and no URI | ETT | |
| | | Child has a "cold" | |
| | | Child snores | |
| | | Passive smoker | |
| | | Anesthetic agent | |
| | | Sputum production | |
| | | Anticholinesterase given | |
| | | Nasal congestion | |
| Tait et al., 2001[18] | URI | Copious secretions | 3.9 RR |
| | | ETT in child <5 years | 1.9 |
| | | Prematurity (<37 weeks) | 2.3 |
| | | Nasal congestion | 1.4 |
| | | Passive smoker | 1.6 |
| | | Reactive airway disease | 1.8 |
| | | Surgery of airway | 1.8 |
| Bordet et al., 2002[12] | URI and no URI | Age <8 years | 1.8 OR |
| | | LMA | 2.3 |
| | | Respiratory infections | 3.7 |
| Mamie et al., 2004[9] | No URI | Nonpediatric anesthesiologist | 1.7 OR |
| | | ENT procedure | 1.8 |
| | | ETT without relaxants | 1.2 |
| von Ungern-Sternberg et al., 2010[4] | URI and no URI | Positive respiratory history | 3.05-8.46 RR |
| | | Symptomatic URI | 2.05 |
| | | URI within previous 2 weeks | 2.34 |
| | | Family history of asthma, atopy, or smoking | |
| | | Anesthetic agent | |
| | | Nonpediatric anesthesiologist | |

Modified from Tait AR. Anesthetic management of the child with an upper respiratory tract infection. Curr Opin Anaesthesiol 2005;18:603-7.
*ENT*, Ear, nose, and throat; *ETT*, endotracheal tube; *LMA*, laryngeal mask airway; *OR*, odds ratio; *RR*, relative risk; *URI*, upper respiratory tract infection.

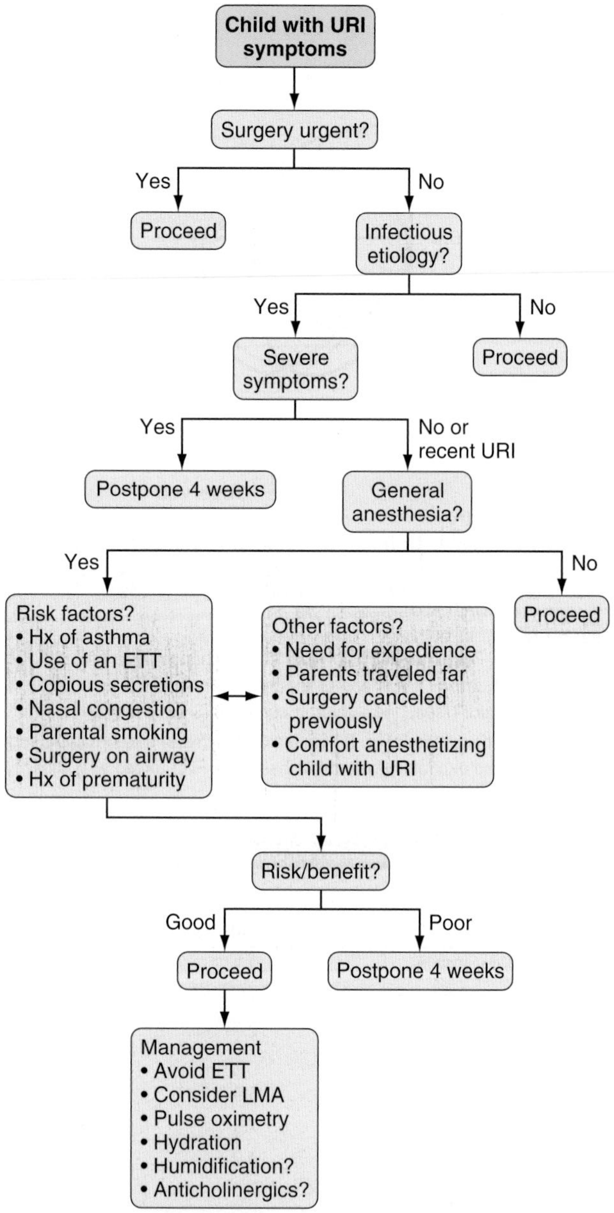

**FIGURE 11-8** Suggested algorithm for assessment and management of the child with an upper respiratory tract infection (URI). *ETT*, Endotracheal tube; *Hx*, history; *LMA*, laryngeal mask airway. (Modified from Tait AR, Malviya S. Anesthesia for the child with an upper respiratory tract infection: still a dilemma? Anesth Analg 2005;100:59-65.)

considerations play a greater role in assessment of the risk/benefit ratio. These include the presence of comorbidities such as asthma, cardiac disease, or obstructive sleep apnea; a history of prematurity; the frequency of URIs; prior cancellations; the type, complexity, duration, and urgency of the surgery; the age of the child; and the socioeconomic implications for the family. The comfort level and experience of the anesthesiologist may also be an underestimated but important factor in the decision to proceed with or postpone surgery, because less experienced anesthesiologists have a greater incidence of complications.[4] The need to admit a child postoperatively because of anesthetic complications or an exacerbation of the URI may expose other children to a contagious illness.

If the decision is to proceed with general anesthesia, management is directed toward avoiding stimulation of the potentially sensitized airway. Use of an endotracheal tube (ETT) should be avoided, if possible, because it increases the risk of complications, especially in younger children.[4,18] Although airway management with a facemask is associated with the smallest frequency of airway complications,[4] it may be inappropriate for certain cases. The laryngeal mask airway (LMA) is associated with fewer episodes of respiratory events than an ETT, but its use may similarly be contraindicated by the type of surgical procedure and the need to protect the airway from pulmonary aspiration of gastric contents.

Whichever airway technique is chosen, it is essential that the depth of anesthesia be adequate to obtund airway reflexes during placement of an airway device. The optimal depth of anesthesia at which to remove an airway device is less clearly defined. Several studies in children with and without URI did not detect a difference in emergence complications between awake and deep extubation,[4,13,18,24] whereas others found a greater incidence of arterial oxygen desaturation or coughing after removal of the ETT or LMA in awake children.[25,26]

The optimal time when an anesthetic can be given after a URI without increasing the risk of adverse respiratory events remains contentious, but most clinicians wait 2 to 4 weeks after the resolution of the URI before proceeding.[4,13,27] This reflects a balance among three critical factors: the time interval to diminish both upper and lower airway hyperreactivity; the perioperative respiratory risk, which includes a recurrence of the URI; and the need to perform the procedure.

Anesthetic techniques may affect complication rates. An observational study of 9297 children reported significantly less laryngospasm after maintenance of anesthesia with propofol than with sevoflurane.[4] This finding might be attributed to a differential effect of propofol versus sevoflurane on airway reflexes.[28] The effect of spraying the cords with lidocaine on the incidence of laryngospasm and bronchospasm is unclear.[4] However, a randomized, controlled trial showed that topical lidocaine gel lubricant applied to the LMA in children with URIs significantly reduced the frequency of adverse airway events.[29] Prophylactic treatment with glycopyrrolate, ipratropium, or albuterol is not effective in preventing URI-related adverse events.[30,31] However, an observational study reported that prophylactic salbutamol was effective in reducing perioperative airway sequelae in children with URIs.[32] Nasal vasoconstrictors (such as phenylephrine or oxymetazoline nose drops) have been recommended for reducing oropharyngeal secretions in children with URIs, but their efficacy remains anecdotal.[23]

## LOWER AIRWAY DISEASE

Acute lower respiratory tract infections in infants and children may result in rapid deterioration necessitating aggressive intervention, including tracheal intubation and ICU admission. Many children are treated with antibiotics on the presumption that the infection is bacterial. However, many may be affected by viruses. In infants and children up to 18 months of age, respiratory syncitial virus is a very serious and common viral infection that infects the lower respiratory tract.[32a] Other viruses include parainfluenza virus, adenovirus, and human metapneumovirus.[32b] Acute inflammation of the small airways may result in bronchiolitis with edema of the small airways leading to desaturation, hypercapnia, and acute respiratory failure. In many instances, bronchiolitis results in several days of tracheal intubation until the acute infection has resolved.

Croup or laryngotracheobronchitis, defined as acute inflammation of the airway (below the vocal cords), has been attributed primarily to parainfluenza virus as well as to adenovirus.

Asthma is one of the most common chronic diseases of childhood, affecting by estimate more than 6 million children in the United States.[33,34] A history of wheezing is associated with an increased risk of perioperative bronchospasm.[4] Rare perioperative complications associated with asthma include anaphylaxis, adrenal crisis, and ventilatory barotrauma such as pneumothorax or pneumomediastinum.[35] An anesthetic approach to children with asthma should include a basic understanding of the disease, an assessment of the child's current state of health, modification

of anesthetic technique as appropriate, and recognition and treatment of complications if they occur.

It is difficult to define asthma with precision, because the exact pathophysiology remains unclear. The word *asthma* derives from the Greek *aazein,* which means "to breathe with open mouth or to pant."[36] A working definition of asthma is a common chronic disorder of the airways that is complex and characterized by variable and recurring symptoms, airway obstruction, inflammation, and hyperresponsiveness of the airways.[33]

Clinical expressions of asthma include wheezing, chest tightness or discomfort, persistent dry cough, and dyspnea on exertion. Severe respiratory distress can occur during acute exacerbations and may be characterized by chest wall retraction, use of accessory muscles, prolonged expiration, pneumothorax, and progression to respiratory failure and death. In some children, the development of chronic inflammation may be associated with permanent airway changes, referred to as *airway remodeling,* that are not prevented by or fully responsive to current available treatments. There is a strong association between asthma and atopy, or immunoglobulin E (IgE)-mediated hypersensitivity.[33]

The diagnosis of asthma can be challenging because cough, wheezing, and bronchospasm may arise from many disease processes. Asthma itself is unlikely to be a single disease entity, and the disease process is markedly modified by various genetic and environmental factors.[33,36] Many young children wheeze, and there is no definitive confirmatory blood, histologic, or radiographic diagnostic test. Given the difficulty with diagnosis, the label "preschool wheezers" may be a more appropriate description for young children with reversible airway obstruction than a diagnosis of "asthma."[36]

The Tucson birth cohort study was the largest longitudinal study in the United States to attempt to differentiate wheezing or asthma phenotypes in children who did not subsequently develop asthma.[37-39] This study examined 826 children at ages 3 years and 6 years from a cohort of 1246 neonates. By the age of 6 years, 48.5% of the children had experienced at least one documented episode of wheezing and were categorized into three groups. "Transient wheezers" were children who wheezed only in response to viral infections, typically during the first 3 years of life. "Non-atopic wheezers" were children who wheezed beyond the first few years of life, often in response to viral infections, but who were less likely to persistently wheeze in later childhood. "Atopy-associated wheezers" were children who had a reversible wheeze together with a tendency toward IgE-mediated hypersensitivity; they had the greatest risk of persistent symptoms into late childhood and adulthood.[37]

The development of asthma is a complex process that probably involves the interaction of two crucial elements: host factors (specifically genetic modifiers of inflammation) and environmental exposures (e.g., viral infections, environmental allergens, pollution) that occur during a crucial time in the development of the immune system.[33] Therefore, the population of young children who wheeze includes a spectrum of disorders rather than one specific pathologic process.

Asthma must be differentiated from other distinct causes that produce similar symptoms (Table 11-5). Tracheomalacia or bronchomalacia may produce wheezing, but this tends to be present from birth (which is unusual for asthma), and the wheezing is commonly of a single pitch heard loudest in the central airways, whereas asthma typically produces polyphonic sounds from the lung periphery. Breathing difficulties due to chronic aspiration are often related to feeding times.

**TABLE 11-5** Causes of Wheezing in Children

**Acute**

| | |
|---|---|
| Bronchiolitis | Pneumothorax |
| Asthma | Endobronchial intubation |
| Foreign body | Herniated ETT cuff |
| Inhalation injury | Aspiration |
| | Anaphylaxis |

**Recurrent or Persistent**

| | |
|---|---|
| Bronchiolitis | Mediastinal mass |
| Asthma | Tracheomalacia/bronchomalacia |
| Foreign body | Vascular ring |
| Bronchopulmonary dysplasia | |
| Cardiac failure | Tracheal web/stenosis |
| Cystic fibrosis | Bronchial stenosis |
| Recurrent aspiration | Roundworm infestation |
| Sickle cell disease | |

*ETT,* Endotracheal tube.

Unremitting wheeze or stridor is often caused by a fixed obstruction or foreign body.

Chronic cough is the most common manifestation of asthma in children. Many children who cough may never be heard to wheeze but still have asthma. A cough with or without wheeze may be caused by a viral infection, whereas a persistent, productive cough may suggest suppurative lung disease such as CF.[35] A positive response of the cough to asthma medications suggests the diagnosis of asthma.

The exact incidence of perioperative complications in the pediatric asthma population is difficult to ascertain because of variations in the definition of asthma, the definition and detection of complications, the presence of coexisting diseases, overlap with adult populations, and changing anesthetic management techniques.

A retrospective review of 706 adult and pediatric patients with a rigorous definition of asthma found an incidence of documented bronchospasm of 1.7% and no instances of pneumonia, pneumothorax, or death.[40] Of 211 children younger than 12 years of age, none developed bronchospasm at the time of surgery. A retrospective review of more than 136,000 computer-based anesthesia records found a 0.8% incidence of bronchospasm in patients with asthma.[41] By contrast, older studies from the 1960s reported that 7% to 8% of asthmatic patients wheezed.[42,43] A blinded, prospective study of 59 asthmatic patients detected transient wheezing after tracheal intubation in 25% of cases; however, most events were brief and self-limited.[44] An observational study of 9297 children reported an overall incidence of 2% for bronchospasm; in the subgroup of 2256 children with a history of respiratory problems, the incidence was 6%.[4,35] An editorial review of the subject of asthma and anesthesia concluded that, although the true incidence of major complications is small, severe adverse outcomes do result from bronchospasm, and children with asthma are at heightened risk for severe morbidity.[45]

Both the severity and the control of asthma must be established preoperatively. These two aspects of the current disease state should be clearly differentiated.[46] For example, asthma may be severe yet well controlled, whereas even mild asthma may be poorly controlled. Both situations may present a heightened potential for perioperative complications, because even the child with intermittent but poorly controlled asthma can have a severe exacerbation.

Severity and control may be assessed by the frequency of symptoms, limitation of effort tolerance, night awakenings, medication use, emergency department attendance, hospitalizations, and need for ventilatory support. An approach to assessment of severity and control in children aged 5 to 11 years is outlined in E-Tables 11-1 through 11-3. A history of a nocturnal dry cough, more than three wheezing episodes in the past 12 months, or a history of past or present eczema is associated with an increased risk of bronchospasm.[4]

Maintenance treatment of asthma is based on a stepwise approach, so that the type of therapy is often an indication of severity. Short-acting inhaled β-agonists are first-line therapy, with inhaled corticosteroids for those patients with persistent symptoms poorly managed by bronchodilators as the preferred second step. Alternative treatments at this step include a leukotriene receptor antagonist, a mast cell stabilizer such as cromolyn sodium or nedocromil, and a methylxanthine bronchodilator such as theophylline. The third step in therapy involves increasing the dose of inhaled corticosteroid or adding an alternative treatment to a smaller dose of corticosteroid; a long-acting β-agonist, a leukotriene receptor antagonist, or theophylline may be considered. Step 4 involves a medium dose of corticosteroid together with a long-acting β-agonist. The final steps of therapy involve a high dose of inhaled corticosteroid or commencing an oral corticosteroid (E-Fig. 11-2).

Most children with asthma have disease that is intermittent or persistent but mild and will be treated with inhaled short-acting β-agonists on an as-needed basis, alone or in combination with low-dose inhaled corticosteroids or an adjunctive therapy. Poor control may relate to poor compliance with medication, inadequate inhaler technique, or incorrect diagnosis. Severe asthma is diagnosed when symptom control is poor despite high doses of corticosteroids (steps 5 or 6 in E-Fig. 11-2). A small group of children have "brittle asthma" that is difficult to control despite optimal therapy and may lead to life-threatening respiratory compromise. A history of severe attacks or admission to intensive care is particularly ominous.

Special investigations are not routinely indicated but may be useful in specific circumstances. A chest radiograph is not usually helpful to assess the severity of asthma but can help diagnose a superimposed infection, pneumothorax, or pneumomediastinum during an acute exacerbation. Pulmonary function tests are important in monitoring long-term responses to therapy but are of little use in the immediate, routine preoperative workup of cases at a stable clinical baseline. Measurements of nitric oxide and various inflammatory markers are primarily of use as research tools at present, but their role in asthma management is evolving.[47]

Although an assessment of disease severity is essential, an important caveat is that many asthma deaths in the community setting occur not in those with severe disease but in those with what was thought to be mild or moderate disease. Asthma is often undertreated,[46] so the sensitivity of medication prescription as a marker of disease activity must be viewed with some caution. Some studies have found a poor correlation between assessment of disease severity and the occurrence of perioperative bronchospasm. However, disease *activity,* as noted by recent asthma symptoms, use of medications for symptom treatment, and recent

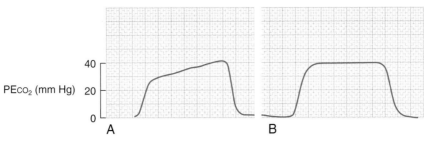

$PE_{CO_2}$ (mm Hg)

A    B

FIGURE 11-9  **A,** Tracing of expired carbon dioxide ($PE_{CO_2}$) in a child with acute bronchospasm. Notice the slowly rising $PE_{CO_2}$ value. **B,** Tracing from the same patient after administration of inhaled albuterol. Note that the $PE_{CO_2}$ waveform now has a flat plateau, indicating relief of the bronchospasm and efficient elimination of $CO_2$ from all areas of the lungs.

therapy in a medical facility for asthma, is significantly associated with perioperative bronchospasm.[40]

Children should continue their regular medications before anesthesia. Midazolam has been reported to be a safe premedication for asthmatics.[48] Corticosteroids may help prevent postintubation bronchospasm in adults,[49] although controlled clinical data to substantiate this practice in children are lacking.[35] Inhaled β-agonists before or shortly after induction of anesthesia attenuate the increases in airway resistance associated with tracheal intubation.[50,51] Ketamine is the traditional choice of intravenous induction agent in children with severe asthma, although its superiority over other agents has not been substantiated in clinical trials.[52,53] Propofol is typically preferred over thiopentone because it causes less bronchoconstriction.[44,54] Desflurane is associated with an increased risk of bronchospasm compared with sevoflurane or isoflurane, and because it can increase airway resistance in children, should be avoided in asthmatics.[4]

Tracheal stimulation is a potent stimulus for bronchospasm.[4] In children with URI, in whom the airways may be acutely hyperactive, the avoidance of tracheal intubation is associated with a reduced incidence of pulmonary complications.[4,17] There are inadequate clinical outcome data on the perioperative management of asthma to make definitive recommendations about airway management. Nevertheless, avoidance of tracheal and vocal cord stimulation by use of a facemask or an LMA instead of an ETT whenever possible seems a sensible approach. If tracheal intubation is mandatory, a deep plane of anesthesia is preferred to blunt airway hyperreactivity. Similarly, unless contraindicated by other factors, deep extubation is preferred for the same reason. Surgical stimulation is another trigger of bronchospasm, and anesthetic depth and analgesia should be adequate to prevent this response.

Intraoperative bronchospasm is characterized variously by polyphonic expiratory wheeze, prolonged expiration, active expiration with increased respiratory effort, increased airway pressures, a slow upslope on the end-tidal $CO_2$ monitor, increased end-tidal $CO_2$, and hypoxemia (Fig. 11-9). Other causes of wheezing must be excluded, such as partial obstruction of the ETT (secretions or herniation of the cuff causing obstruction), mainstem intubation (deep endobronchial intubation), aspiration, pneumothorax, or pulmonary edema. Mechanical obstruction of the circuit or ETT must also be excluded.

First-line treatment for bronchospasm involves removing the triggering stimulus if possible, deepening anesthesia, increasing the fraction of inspired oxygen ($FIO_2$) if appropriate, decreasing the positive end-expiratory pressure (PEEP), and increasing the expiratory time to minimize alveolar air trapping. In severe status

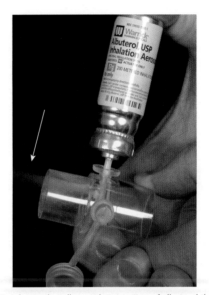

FIGURE 11-10  Adaptor that allows administration of albuterol through an endotracheal tube (ETT) and timing of that dose with inspirations so as to provide maximum delivery; notice that the nebulized albuterol is directed down the ETT (arrow). Use of a long intravenous catheter that extends to the tip of the ETT is an alternative method to further improve drug delivery.

asthmaticus, ventilation strategy focuses primarily on achieving adequate oxygenation, rather than attempting to normalize $PaCO_2$ at the potential cost of inducing pulmonary barotrauma. All children who experience anything more than minor bronchospasm should also receive corticosteroids, if they have not already done so.

Inhaled β-agonists can be delivered by nebulizer or by a metered-dose inhaler down the airway device with specially designed adaptors (Fig. 11-10). Alternatively, a 60-mL syringe can be used to deliver doses of the nebulizer into the breathing circuit (E-Fig. 11-3). However, the efficiency of delivery through an inhaler that is actuated at the elbow of the breathing circuit is poor, especially in small-diameter ETTs.[55] To improve the delivery efficiency of the aerosol in pediatric-size ETTs, the inhaler may be actuated 10 to 20 times at the elbow or once or twice into a narrow-gauge catheter that is passed to the end of the ETT.[55,56]

If intravenous salbutamol is available, the intravenous route is preferred over tracheal administration. In this case, 10 µg/kg IV salbutamol may be repeated, followed by an infusion of 5 to 10 µg/kg/min for the first hour until there is an improvement in the bronchospasm. Thereafter, salbutamol should be infused at 1 to 2 µg/kg/min until the bronchospasm resolves.

**TABLE 11-6** Formal Evaluation of Asthma Exacerbation Severity

| | Mild | Moderate | Severe | Subset: Respiratory Arrest Imminent |
|---|---|---|---|---|
| **Symptoms** | | | | |
| Breathlessness | While walking<br>Can lie down | While at rest (infant—softer, shorter cry, difficulty feeding)<br>Prefers sitting | While at rest (infant—stops feeding)<br>Sits upright | |
| Talks in | Sentences | Phrases | Words | |
| Alertness | May be agitated | Usually agitated | Usually agitated | Drowsy or confused |
| **Signs** | | | | |
| Respiratory rate* | Increased | Increased | Increased | |
| Use of accessory muscles; suprasternal retractions | Usually not | Commonly | Usually | Paradoxical thoracoabdominal movement |
| Wheeze | Moderate, often only end expiratory | Loud; throughout exhalation | Usually loud; throughout inhalation and exhalation | Absence of wheeze |
| Pulse/minute† | Slightly increased | Increased | Tachycardia | Bradycardia |
| Pulsus paradoxus | Absent<br><10 mm Hg | May be present<br>10-25 mm Hg | Often present<br>>25 mm Hg (adult)<br>20-40 mm Hg (child) | Absence suggests respiratory muscle fatigue |
| **Functional Assessment‡** | | | | |
| PEF (% of predicted or of personal best) | ≥70% | Approx. 40%-69% or response lasts <2 hours | <40% | <25% (PEF testing may not be needed in very severe attacks) |
| $PaO_2$ (while breathing room air) | Normal (test not usually necessary) | ≥60 mm Hg (test not usually necessary) | <60 mm Hg: possible cyanosis | |
| $PCO_2$ | <42 mm Hg (test not usually necessary) | <42 mm Hg (test not usually necessary) | >42 mm Hg: possible respiratory failure (see text) | |
| $SaO_2$% (while breathing room air) at sea level | >95% (test not usually necessary) | 90%-95% (test not usually necessary) | <90% | |

Modified from National Asthma Education and Prevention Program: Full report of the expert panel: guidelines for the diagnosis and management of asthma (EPR-3). Bethesda, Md.: National Heart, Lung, and Blood Institute, National Institutes of Health, 2007.

$PaO_2$, Arterial oxygen tension; $PCO_2$, partial pressure of carbon dioxide; *PEF*, peak expiratory flow; $SaO_2$, oxygen saturation.

*Guide to rates of breathing in awake children: at age <2 months, normal rate is <60 breaths/minute; at 2-12 months, <50/minute; at 1-5 years, <40/minute; at 6-8 years, <30/minute.

†Guide to normal pulse rates in children: at age 2-12 months, normal rate is <160 beats/minute; at 1-2 years, <120/minute; at 2-8 years, <110/minute.

‡$PaO_2$ or $PCO_2$ or both may be tested. Hypercapnia (hypoventilation) develops more readily in young children than in adults and adolescents.

The anesthesiologist may be involved in the management of status asthmaticus when consulted to assist a child in the emergency department or on the wards. A drowsy, silent child with a quiet chest on auscultation is in imminent danger of respiratory arrest and requires emergent intubation by an experienced practitioner. Signs and symptoms to assess the severity of an asthma exacerbation are outlined in Table 11-6, and an algorithm for management issued by the American National Heart, Lung and Blood Institute is presented in E-Figure 11-4.

Oxygen is recommended for most children to maintain the oxygen saturation at greater than 90%. Repetitive or continuous administration of short-acting β-agonists is first-line therapy for all children and is the most effective way of reversing airflow obstruction. The addition of ipratropium to a β-agonist may produce additional bronchodilation and may have a modest effect to improve outcome. Systemic corticosteroids should be given to those who do not respond completely and promptly to β-agonists. For severe exacerbations unresponsive to the treatment listed earlier, intravenous magnesium may decrease the likelihood of intubation, although the evidence is limited. Current recommended drug doses are listed in E-Table 11-4.

There is much debate about the role of methylxanthines such as aminophylline in the management of acute exacerbations of asthma. In some countries, aminophylline is considered a first-line treatment in asthma, whereas in others it is considered second-line or used less frequently. The difference in practice may be attributed to its equivocal clinical efficacy in the treatment of acute exacerbations of asthma and to complications from toxicity (including vomiting).[57-60]

Antibiotics are not recommended except for comorbid conditions. Aggressive hydration is not recommended in adults or older children, although it may be indicated in younger children who become dehydrated as a result of decreased oral intake and increased respiratory rate. In general, chest physical therapy and mucolytics are not recommended.

Children with severe atopy-associated asthma are possibly at greater risk of developing anaphylaxis in response to neuromuscular blocking drugs, antibiotics, and latex.[35] Bronchospasm caused by anaphylaxis is differentiated from that due to asthma; it produces additional systemic signs such as angioedema, flushing, urticaria, and cardiovascular collapse.

Adrenal crisis during major surgical stress is a potential complication associated with severe asthma due to iatrogenic suppression of the hypothalamic-pituitary-adrenal axis.[35] Adrenal suppression should be considered in any child who is taking significant doses of corticosteroids for a prolonged period. Short courses of prednisolone used to treat acute flares of asthma may affect function for up to 10 days, but prolonged dysfunction is unlikely. Large doses, prolonged therapy for more than a few weeks, and evening dosing may suppress adrenal function for up to 1 year. Prophylactic corticosteroid administration may be indicated for those receiving prolonged systemic corticosteroids, when their corticosteroid regimen is interrupted by the surgical schedule, or for those who have received high-dose inhaled corticosteroids in the recent past (see Chapter 25).

## CYSTIC FIBROSIS

CF is an autosomal recessive disorder that is caused by one of more than 1200 mutations in the gene coding for the CF transmembrane conductance regulator (located on chromosome 7), a protein that contributes to the regulation of chloride and other ion fluxes at various epithelial surfaces.[61,62] The incidence of CF is approximately 1 of every 2000 births in Caucasian, making it the most common fatal inherited disease in this population.

The disruption of electrolyte transport in the epithelial cells of the sweat ducts, airways, pancreatic ducts, intestine, biliary tree, and vas deferens causes increased sweat chloride concentrations, viscous mucus production, lung disease, intestinal obstruction, pancreatic insufficiency, biliary cirrhosis, and congenital absence of the vas deferens. The clinical outcome is widely variable, even among children with identical mutations at the CF locus. Absence of the gene influences expression of several other gene products, including proteins important to the inflammatory response, ion maturational processing, transport, and cell signaling. These other proteins are potential modifiers of the phenotype and may help explain the substantial differences in clinical severity.

Lung disease is the main cause of morbidity and mortality in CF, and consequently it is the focus of anesthetic concern. The pathophysiology involves mucus plugging, chronic infection, inflammation, and epithelial injury.[63-65] Mucus clearance defends the lung against inhaled bacteria. The mucociliary transport system requires two fully functioning layers to be effective. The base layer of ciliary epithelia bathed in a watery liquid (sol) is overlaid by a more viscous gel (mucus) that is responsible for transporting particles along the tips of the cilia. Normally, mucus is transported at about 10 mm/min, expelling foreign particles and pathogens from the lungs. The efficacy of clearance depends on adequate hydration of the mucus.[66] Lack of regulation of sodium absorption and chloride secretion decreases liquid on the airway luminal surfaces, slows mucus clearance, and promotes the formation of adherent plugs in the airway.[67] Increased secretions, viscous mucus, and impaired ciliary clearance contribute to airway impaction, providing a nidus for infection.

At birth, the lung structure is almost normal.[61] However, chronic and recurrent bacterial infections occur early in life, assisted by the pooling of secretions and impaired neutrophil bacterial killing on airway surfaces.[63,68] Repeated and persistent infections stimulate a chronic neutrophilic inflammatory response,

ultimately destroying the airway walls. Early pathogens include *Staphylococcus aureus* and *Haemophilus influenzae*. *Pseudomonas aeruginosa* typically invade later in life, acquire a mucoid phenotype, and form a biofilm in the lung, an event that is associated with accelerated decline in pulmonary function. The invasion of the lung by antibiotic-resistant pathogens such as certain strains of *Burkholderia cepacia* is often devastating, markedly increasing the death rate from lung disease.

Various insults such as bacteria, viruses, and airborne irritants can cause acute exacerbations of respiratory symptoms of cough and sputum production. This is often accompanied by systemic manifestations such as weight loss, anorexia, and fatigue. These changes from baseline are termed *pulmonary exacerbations.*[69]

Recurrent exacerbations are associated with progressive airway obstruction, bronchiectasis, emphysema, ventilation/perfusion mismatching, and hypoxemia. Growth of blood vessels with advancing bronchiectasis predisposes to hemoptysis. Bronchial hyperreactivity and increased airway resistance are common, whereas bullae formation can lead to pneumothorax.

Pulmonary function abnormalities are commonly obstructive in nature and include increased FRC, decreased $FEV_1$, decreased peak expiratory flow rate, and decreased vital capacity (see Fig. 11-5). Compensatory hyperventilation typically produces a reduced $PaCO_2$, although hypercapnia may supersede in endstage pulmonary pathology. End-stage cor pulmonale may lead to cardiomegaly, fluid retention, and hepatomegaly.

Malnutrition is a common problem in CF that follows from pancreatic insufficiency, failure of enzyme secretion, impaired gastrointestinal motility, abnormal enterohepatic circulation of bile, increased caloric demand due to severe lung disease, and anorexia of chronic disease.[61] Low weight and body mass index are closely associated with, and can predict, poor lung function.

CF-related diabetes arises from progressive pancreatic disease and scarring that compromises the pancreatic islets. More than 12% of CF teenagers older than 13 years of age have insulin-dependent diabetes, and the incidence increases with age. Evidence is accumulating that diabetes contributes to the lung disease and worse outcome.[63-65] In addition, classic diabetic complications occur in older CF patients. Hepatic dysfunction decreases plasma cholinesterase and clotting factors II, VII, IX, and X, whereas malabsorption of vitamin K may also contribute to coagulation issues.[70]

When CF was first distinguished from celiac syndrome in 1938, life expectancy was approximately 6 months. Since then, substantial advances in sustained multidisciplinary supportive care have increased the median survival time to 35 years (E-Fig. 11-5).[61,71] Currently almost half of the CF population are adults.[70] The pillars of treatment include nutritional repletion, relief of airway obstruction, and antibiotic therapy for lung infection. Suppression of inflammation has been a more recent focus of therapy. Organ transplantation, and in particular lung transplantation, has been used in an attempt to improve quality of life and prolong survival, but a clear benefit remains to be demonstrated.[71]

The multisystem nature of the disease and changing demographics mean that children present for a wide variety of surgical procedures. The most common indications for anesthesia in children are nasal polypectomy and ear, nose, and throat surgery, as a result of the frequency of upper airway pathologic processes such as chronic sinusitis and nasal polyps (Table 11-7).[72,73] The investigation or correction of gastrointestinal disorders is the

**TABLE 11-7** Most Frequent Indications for Anesthesia in Cystic Fibrosis

| Neonates | Children/Teenagers | Adults |
| --- | --- | --- |
| Meconium ileus | Nasal polypectomy | Esophageal varices |
| Meconium peritonitis | Intravenous access | Recurrent pneumothorax |
| Intestinal atresia | Ear/nose/throat surgery | Cholecystectomy |
| | | Lung (liver) transplantation |

Modified from Della Rocca G. Anaesthesia in patients with cystic fibrosis. Curr Opin Anaesthesiol 2002;15:95-101.

next most common procedural category that requires anesthesia in the CF population. Other indications for anesthesia include bronchoscopy and pulmonary lavage, gastrointestinal endoscopy, sclerosing injection of varices due to portal hypertension, insertion of venous access devices, and incidental surgical problems.[73-75]

Because of the increasing longevity of this population, the pediatric anesthesiologist may also be involved in the care of adults.[70] Surgical procedures in adults typically include treatment of recurrent pneumothorax, cholecystectomy, and lung or cardiac transplantation. Consultation may also be requested for obstetric cases as increasing numbers of patients survive to adulthood.

Pulmonary disease is the predominant concern when planning anesthesia for these patients. Historically, morbidity and mortality from pulmonary complications were significant, but more recently, the mortality rate has decreased. In 1964, a retrospective study reported a perioperative mortality rate of 27%,[76] but by 1972, this incidence had decreased to 4%.[72] More recent studies confirmed a substantial morbidity rate with a low mortality rate. An observational study of 333 anesthesias for bronchoalveolar lavage reported minor complications (transient worsening of cough or low-grade postoperative fever or both) in 52% of patients; more serious problems, including prolonged intraoperative oxygen desaturation or high fever, occurred in 12% of children.[77,78] A report of 45 bronchoscopies under anesthesia noted a rate of minor intraoperative complications (coughing, desaturation) of 13.3%.[79] A study of 199 anesthesias in 53 patients for ear/nose/throat surgery reported a 5% incidence of minor pulmonary problems and no deaths.[80] A report of 126 anesthesias found no mortality and a CF-specific complication rate of 9% (predominantly pulmonary complications).[73] A 1984 study of 18 patients undergoing anesthesia for pleural surgery concluded that, although the risks for this procedure were great, the anesthetic hazards of CF could be minimized with careful management.[81] In 11 patients undergoing anesthesia for injection of esophageal varices, there were no serious anesthetic complications, but significant deteriorations in pulmonary function tests were detected 48 hours after general anesthesia.[82] It was unclear if these changes persisted past the immediate postoperative period. A larger study found no difference between pulmonary function tests measured 3 months before and 3 months after surgery.[73] Although pulmonary morbidity is a significant problem, mortality is infrequent with modern anesthetic management techniques.

An assessment of the severity, current state, and progression of pulmonary disease should guide anesthetic planning. Fitness is a positive predictor of survival,[61] and exercise tolerance is a useful marker of pulmonary function. The quality and quantity

of secretions, recent and chronic infections, use and effectiveness of bronchodilators, and number of hospitalizations are also important points to elucidate in the history. Examination of the cardiopulmonary systems should aim to detect compromise of cardiac, pulmonary, and hepatic function. Special investigations are not routinely indicated but may quantify organ dysfunction in end stages of the disease. Arterial blood gas analysis, chest radiography, pulmonary function tests, electrocardiography, echocardiography, and liver function tests may assist the planning of anesthetic technique in selected children.[75]

Children are often emotionally vulnerable, not simply because of the usual preoperative anxieties but because of the psychological consequences of progression of an ultimately fatal disease. A preoperative visit should aim to allay distress; oral benzodiazepines have been successfully used as anxiolytics.[73,80] Prophylactic use of osmotic laxatives may be indicated if opioid-induced ileus is anticipated.[75]

Because dehydration of secretions is a central pulmonary issue in CF, general anesthesia poses specific problems. During spontaneous ventilation under normal conditions, inspired gases are warmed to body temperature and saturated with water vapor, reaching this state at the isothermic saturation point just distal to the carina.[83,84] This ensures that the lower airways are kept moist and warm. The alveolar environment in optimal circumstances has a saturated water vapor pressure of 47.1 mm Hg and an absolute humidity of 43.4 g/m$^{-3}$ at 98.6° F (37° C).

The inspiration of cold, desiccated anesthetic gases and vapors can impair the warming and humidification of the airways. The use of any airway device (oropharyngeal airway, laryngeal mask, or ETT) bypasses the nasal and oropharyngeal passages and delivers cold, dry gas farther down the airway.[85] This shifts the isothermic saturation point distally, forcing bronchi that normally function in optimal conditions to take part in heat and gas exchange.[84] These parts of the airway are less adapted to moisture exchange and tend to dehydrate more rapidly, thereby impairing the mucociliary escalator and predisposing to impaction of secretions.[86,87] Direct impairment of mucociliary motion by anesthetic medications, as well as blunting of the cough response and ventilatory drive, can further contribute to the problem.

It is therefore particularly important to minimize mucus desiccation in the perioperative period. Inhalation of hypertonic saline (7% sodium chloride) accelerates mucus clearance, increases lung function, and improves quality of life[88-90]; this is now typically part of the routine maintenance management of CF. Nebulized saline treatments should continue up to the start of anesthesia and recommence after the procedure. Inhaled gases should be humidified, or an artificial "nose" should be inserted into the circuit to conserve airway moisture and minimize inspissation of secretions.

Although removal of pulmonary secretions is considered important in principle, a small prospective trial of intraoperative bronchial wash-out and physical therapy reported an acute increase in airway resistance with no significant long-term benefit in measures of lung function.[91]

At the conclusion of surgery, complete reversal of neuromuscular blockade should be confirmed. Whenever possible, the trachea should be extubated and the child encouraged to breathe spontaneously. A 30- to 40-degree head-up position assists movement of the diaphragm and ventilation. Postoperatively, physiotherapy, airway humidification, close attention to analgesia, and early mobilization should enhance clearance of secretions and minimize atelectasis. The use of regional or local anesthesia, as well as nonopioid analgesics, is useful to avoid respiratory depression. Ambulatory surgery is optimal, if feasible, because it minimizes disruption to the patient's schedule and decreases exposure to nosocomial infection.

## SICKLE CELL DISEASE

SCD is an inherited hemoglobinopathy that results from a point mutation on chromosome 11. The mutant gene codes for the production of hemoglobin S, a mutant variant of the normal hemoglobin A. This leads to widespread and progressive vascular damage.[92,93] Clinical features of the disease include acute episodes of pain, acute and chronic pulmonary disease, hemorrhagic and occlusive stroke, renal insufficiency, and splenic infarction, with mean life expectancy shortened to just over 3 decades.[94] Perioperative problems and management are covered in more detail in Chapter 9, and the discussion here is limited to a brief review of the pulmonary pathology of SCD.

Acute chest syndrome (ACS) is an acute lung injury caused by SCD. Diagnostic criteria include a new pulmonary infiltrate involving at least one lung segment on the radiograph (excluding atelectasis) combined with one or more symptoms or signs of chest pain, pyrexia greater than 101.3° F (38.5° C), tachypnea, wheezing, or cough.[95-97] Precipitants include infection, fat embolism after bone marrow infarction, pulmonary infarction, and surgical procedures.[97-99] Potential risk factors for the development and severity of perioperative ACS include a history of lung disease, recent clustering of acute pulmonary complications, pregnancy, increased age, and the invasiveness of the surgical procedure.[92] A study of 60 laparoscopic surgeries noted that ACS was associated with younger-age patients, reduced body temperature, and greater blood loss.[100]

Minor procedures such as inguinal hernia repair or distal extremity surgery have a reduced risk of pulmonary complications (<5%), whereas intraabdominal or major joint surgery has an ACS rate of 10% to 15%.[99,101,102] Although the overall perioperative mortality from SCD is quite small, <1%,[99] ACS can lead to prolonged postoperative hospitalization, respiratory failure, and death. One study of 604 patients noted that ACS typically developed about 3 days postoperatively and persisted for approximately 8 days; 2 patients died in approximately 60 episodes.[98]

SCD also causes chronic lung damage, known as sickle cell lung disease (SCLD).[103] Because lung function has not yet been assessed longitudinally in a cohort from early childhood to adulthood, the precise pathology of and relationship between the obstructive and restrictive patterns of lung disease is unclear.[104] Children appear to have a predominantly obstructive pattern,[105] whereas adults have more restrictive pulmonary findings.[103,106,107] The later stages of lung damage involve decreased vital and total lung capacities, impaired gas diffusion, pulmonary fibrosis, pulmonary artery hypertension, right-sided cardiomyopathy, and progressive hypoxemia.[103,107] The development of pulmonary artery hypertension, which can precede clinically apparent lung damage, is a particularly ominous sign of disease progression and is associated with a heightened risk of sudden death.[106] Recurrent ACS is an independent risk factor for the development of end-stage SCLD, but subtle evidence of parenchymal and vascular damage commonly precedes clustered episodes of ACS.[103]

Assessment of lung function should include a history of the occurrence, frequency, severity, and known precipitants of ACS and a search for progression of chronic lung damage. A recent chest radiograph can serve as a baseline for comparison if postoperative radiographs are needed and can also delineate lung pathology. Early features of lung damage include decreased distal pulmonary vascularity and diffuse interstitial fibrosis, whereas later stages are characterized by pulmonary fibrosis, pulmonary hypertension, and right ventricular hypertrophy.[103,108] Pulmonary function testing can reveal the need for bronchodilators and the presence of obstructive or restrictive lung disease.

The efficacy of preoperative or intraoperative management techniques beyond basic standards of care has not been clearly demonstrated; well-delivered anesthetic and postoperative care may be the best guarantor of a good outcome.[92,93] Because the effect of perioperative red blood cell transfusion (versus no transfusion) in preventing ACS or other SCD complications has not been tested by an adequately controlled study, the efficacy of prophylactic erythrocyte transfusion is controversial. One guideline suggested that children in low-risk situations should not be transfused prophylactically, but children in high-risk situations may be transfused.[92] A survey of North American pediatric anesthesiologists found that most tend not to transfuse children assessed as being at low risk undergoing minor procedures, whereas a greater number do transfuse those at greater risk (i.e., sicker children undergoing more invasive procedures).[109]

If transfusion is undertaken, exchange transfusion aiming to decrease the concentration of hemoglobin S to 30% is no more efficacious than correction of anemia to a hematocrit of 30% in preventing SCD exacerbations but results in more transfusion-related complications.[98] Consequently, if a decision is made to transfuse in the hope of preventing ACS, the target should be a hematocrit of 30% rather than a specific dilution of hemoglobin S.

The one high-risk group that merits mention are children who have experienced or are at risk for a stroke. Risk factors for strokes include low hemoglobin, hypertension, and male gender as well as three single nucleotide polymorphisms.[110,111] Transcranial Doppler ultrasound and magnetic resonance imaging of the brain have been used serially to detect pathologic changes in blood flow or subclinical strokes, respectively, and in these children transfusion has been effective in reducing subsequent strokes.[112,113] Silent cerebral strokes have been detected in up to 30% of asymptomatic children with SCD.[110] To reduce the risk of stroke, these children are transfused at regular intervals, based on the results of the serial investigations. However, this approach raises concern about iron overload and other complications associated with repeated blood transfusions. A recent study to limit the number of transfusions in those at risk for a stroke had to be stopped prematurely because two strokes occurred despite serial transcranial Doppler monitoring.[114] Chronic hydroxyurea therapy has also been shown to be effective in reducing the risk of stroke.[115]

Children with SCD frequently develop postoperative atelectasis. It is unclear whether this relates to an underlying sickle lung disease, difficulty with analgesia, other causes, or a combination of factors. Pain management can be difficult in these children. Large doses of opioids can depress ventilation and cause atelectasis.[116] ACS tends to involve the lower segments of the lung,[97] suggesting an association between atelectasis and ACS. Incentive spirometry can prevent the development of atelectasis and pulmonary infiltrates associated with ACS.[117] Regional analgesia, supplemental nonopioid analgesics, prophylactic incentive spirometry, early mobilization, and good pulmonary toilet may decrease the incidence of atelectasis and ACS.

Treatment of ACS is focused on supporting gas exchange. Supplemental oxygen, noninvasive ventilatory support such as continuous positive airway pressure, or intubation and mechanical ventilation are indicated by the degree of dysfunction. Bronchodilators, incentive spirometry, and chest physiotherapy may be useful in preventing progression of the disease. In the presence of a significant ventilation/perfusion mismatch, correction of anemia can improve arterial oxygenation. Erythrocyte transfusion increases oxygen-carrying capacity, decreases fractional peripheral tissue extraction, and increases returning venous oxygen levels. Because the mean arterial oxygen content in the presence of a shunt is significantly affected by the oxygenation of blood returning from nonventilated parts of the lung, increasing venous oxygen levels can improve arterial oxygen content. Although transfusion has not been clearly shown to improve outcome, both exchange and simple transfusion can improve oxygenation.[97]

## Summary

Pulmonary complications are a major cause of perioperative morbidity in the pediatric population. Although preexisting pulmonary pathologic processes in children can present significant challenges to anesthetic delivery, a thorough assessment of the problem combined with meticulous anesthetic management allows most children to undergo surgical interventions without long-term adverse sequelae. Consultation with a pediatric pulmonologist is indicated when appropriate for specific problems as outlined in this chapter; a team approach may markedly improve operative and postoperative outcomes.

## ANNOTATED REFERENCES

Bishop MJ, Cheney FW. Anesthesia for patients with asthma: low risk but not no risk. Anesthesiology 1996;85:455-6.

*A thoughtful editorial on the implications, dangers, and practical implications of asthma.*

Davis PB. Cystic fibrosis since 1938. Am J Respir Crit Care Med 2006;173:475-82.

*A succinct discourse on the evolution of management of cystic fibrosis.*

Firth PG, Head CA. Sickle cell disease and anesthesia. Anesthesiology 2004;101:766-85.

*A comprehensive review of anesthetic management of sickle cell disease.*

Huffmeyr JL, Littlewood KE, Nemergut EC. Perioperative management of the adult with cystic fibrosis. Anesth Analg 2009;109:1949-61.

*An updated review of anesthetic implications of advanced cystic fibrosis.*

National Asthma Education and Prevention Program. Full report of the expert panel: guidelines for the diagnosis and management of asthma (EPR-3). Bethesda, Md.: National Heart, Lung, and Blood Institute, National Institutes of Health; 2007.

*An extensive review of current evidence on the pathophysiology, diagnosis, and management of asthma.*

Tait AR, Malviya S. Anesthesia for the child with an upper respiratory tract infection: still a dilemma? Anesth Analg 2005;100:59-65.

*A broad review of the data on perioperative upper respiratory tract infections and suggested approaches to management.*

von Ungern-Sternberg BS, Boda K, Chambers NA, et al. Risk assessment for respiratory complications in paediatric anaesthesia: a prospective cohort study. Lancet 2010;376:773-83.

*A large prospective observational study of perioperative adverse respiratory events and predictive risk factors.*

## REFERENCES

Please see www.expertconsult.com

# The Pediatric Airway

RONALD S. LITMAN, JOHN E. FIADJOE,
PAUL A. STRICKER, AND CHARLES J. COTÉ

THE DIFFERENCES BETWEEN A child's airway and an adult's dictate differences in anesthetic management techniques. Knowledge of normal developmental anatomy and physiologic function is required to understand and manage both the normal and the pathologic airways of infants and children (Video 12-1). Techniques and principles to assist in this management are reviewed in this chapter.

## Developmental Anatomy of the Airway

The classic works by Negus, Eckenhoff, and Fink and Demarest form the foundation of our knowledge about the structure and function of the pediatric and adult airway.[1-3] They suggested that there are five major anatomic differences between the neonatal and the adult airway, which are outlined in this section, although more recent studies suggest that not all of these long-held beliefs are supported by science.[2-4] In addition, the relatively large head of an infant negates the need to place anything under the head to achieve a proper "sniffing position." Older children have airway features that represent a transition between the infant and the adult anatomy.

### TONGUE

In the past, it was thought that an infant's tongue is relatively large in proportion to the rest of the oral cavity and therefore can more easily obstruct the airway, especially in a neonate. However, magnetic resonance imaging (MRI) studies have now demonstrated that there is proportional growth of the tongue and other soft tissues in relation to the bony structures of the oral cavity in children 1 to 11 years of age.[5] Furthermore, the contribution of the tongue to upper airway obstruction with sedation

or induction of anesthesia is relatively minor; much of the obstruction is more likely due to nasopharyngeal and epiglottic collapse, although in a patient of any age the tongue may also contribute to obstruction.[6,7]

### POSITION OF THE LARYNX

An infant's larynx is higher (more cephalad) in the neck, classically described at the level of C3-4, than an adult's larynx, which is at the level of C4-5 (Fig. 12-1). MRI and computed tomography (CT) have confirmed the higher (more cephalad) position of the larynx in children and demonstrated that the hyoid bone is at the C2-3 level in infants and children up to 2 years of age.[8] Consequently, the distances between the tongue, hyoid bone, epiglottis, and roof of the mouth are smaller in infants than they are in an older child or adult.

The proximity of the tongue to the more superior larynx also makes visualization of laryngeal structures more difficult, because it produces a more acute angle between the plane of the tongue and the plane of the glottic opening. It is for this reason that a straight laryngoscope blade, which lifts the tongue from the field of view during laryngoscopy, facilitates visualization of an infant's larynx. This anatomic relationship is further complicated in certain conditions such as the Treacher Collins anomaly and other syndromes associated with mandibular and midfacial hypoplasia that make direct visualization of the glottis difficult and sometimes impossible with standard laryngoscopy (Fig. 12-2). The reason for this difficulty is that with mandibular and midfacial hypoplasia, the base of the tongue is positioned more caudally (known as glossoptosis) and in closer proximity to the laryngeal inlet than normal; the result is an even greater acute angle between the plane of the tongue and the plane of the

Glottic Opening Relative
to Cervical Vertebra (C)

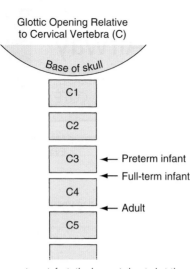

FIGURE 12-1 In a preterm Infant, the larynx is located at the middle of the third cervical vertebra (C3); in a full-term infant, it is at the C3-4 interspace; and in an adult, it is at the C4-5 interspace. (Adapted from Negus VE. The comparative anatomy and physiology of the larynx. Oxford: Butterworth-Heinemann, 1949.)

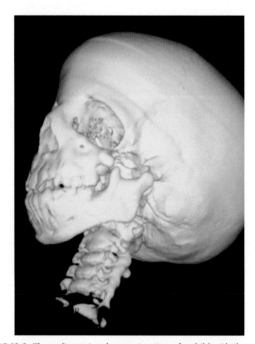

FIGURE 12-2 Three-dimensional reconstruction of a child with the Treacher Collins anomaly demonstrates the retrognathic and more posterior position of the mandible, the midfacial hypoplasia, and the closer proximity and exaggerated angle between the base of the tongue and the laryngeal inlet (almost 90 degrees), which makes direct visualization of the larynx difficult.

laryngeal inlet (often 90 degrees) (Fig. 12-3). In this situation, conventional rigid laryngoscopy provides excellent visualization of the esophageal inlet rather than the laryngeal inlet, necessitating the use of special equipment or special techniques to intubate the trachea.

## EPIGLOTTIS

An adult's epiglottis is flat and broad, and its axis is parallel to that of the trachea (Fig. 12-4), whereas the infant's epiglottis is narrower, omega shaped, and angled away from the axis of the trachea (Fig. 12-5). It is therefore more difficult to lift the infant's epiglottis with the tip of a laryngoscope blade.

## VOCAL FOLDS

In contrast to the adult, in whom the axis of the vocal folds is perpendicular to that of the trachea, the vocal folds (cords) of an infant are angled such that the anterior insertion is lower (caudad) compared with the posterior insertion (compare Fig. 12-4, A, with Fig. 12-5, A). This anatomic feature alters the angle at which the tracheal tube approaches the laryngeal inlet and occasionally leads to difficulty with tracheal intubation, especially with the nasal approach. In the latter case, the tip of the endotracheal tube (ETT) may be held up at the anterior commissure of the vocal folds.

## SUBGLOTTIS

Classic teaching holds that the narrowest part of an infant's larynx is the cricoid cartilage; in an adult, it is the rima glottidis. This teaching was supported by an MRI and CT study in young children (<2 years of age) who were sedated with oral medications and breathing spontaneously.[8] In contrast, a more recent study in children 2 months to 13 years of age undergoing MRI with propofol sedation and spontaneous respirations reported that the narrowest portions of the pediatric larynx were the glottic opening and the immediate sub–vocal cord level and that this finding did not change relative to the dimensions of the cricoid ring throughout childhood.[9] Nonetheless, when a relatively large-diameter tube is inserted into the glottic aperture, the tube passes through the cords but may meet resistance immediately below the cords (e.g., in the subglottic or cricoid ring region). Although these studies demonstrate in vivo physiologic relationships, the cricoid cartilage is *functionally* the narrowest portion of the upper airway.

Growth of the subglottic airway occurs rapidly during the first 2 years of life; thereafter, growth of the airway is linear.[10] At 10 to 12 years of age, the cricoid and thyroid cartilages reach adult proportions, thus eliminating both the angulation of the vocal cords and the narrow subglottic area.

In the adult, the rima glottidis is considered the narrowest part of the airway, and an ETT that traverses the glottis passes into the trachea without resistance. However, in about 70% of adult cadavers, the narrowest portion of the airway was also in the subglottic region.[11] The range in diameter for adult females was 10 to 16 mm, and for adult males it was 13 to 19 mm. The likely reason that ETTs pass easily through the glottic opening into the trachea of an adult is that, overall, the narrowest portion of the airway is still larger than the most commonly used ETT sizes. The apparent subglottic narrowing in adults is generally not evident unless there is the need to pass a larger-diameter ETT such as a double-lumen tube. In contrast, in a child, it is common for an ETT to pass easily through the vocal folds (glottic opening) but not through the subglottic region (Fig. 12-6; see Video 12-1). The larynx in both adults and children should be considered funnel shaped, although this configuration is exaggerated and is of greater import in infants and young children.

The cricoid is the only complete ring of cartilage in the laryngotracheobronchial tree and is therefore nondistensible. Because the mucosa that lines the upper airway is loose-fitting

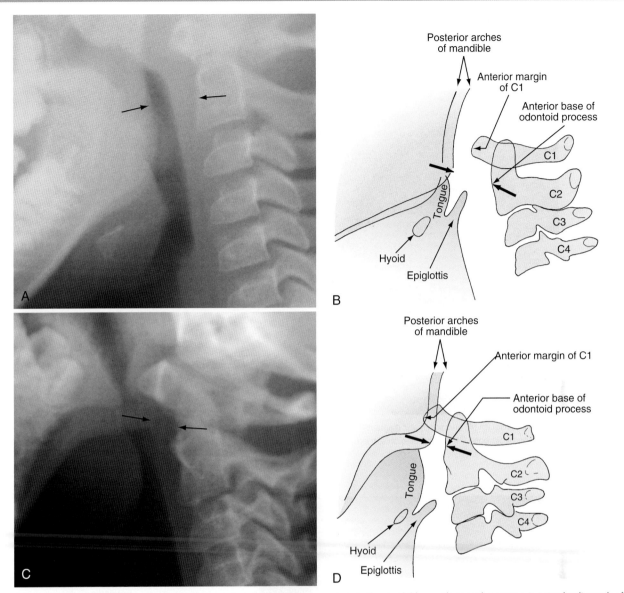

**FIGURE 12-3** The larynx in children with mandibular hypoplasia is located more posteriorly than in children with normal anatomy. **A,** Lateral radiograph of the upper airway including the base of the skull and cervical spine of a normal 7-year-old child; the *arrows* denote the posterior border of the ramus of the mandible and the anterior border of the second cervical vertebra. **B,** Diagrammatic representation of the normal anatomy in **A. C,** The same radiographic projection in a 6-year-old child with Treacher Collins syndrome; the *arrows* again denote the posterior border of the ramus of the mandible and the anterior margin of the second cervical vertebra. **D,** Diagrammatic representation of the anatomy in **C.** Notice the significantly smaller space between the ramus of the mandible and the second cervical vertebra, compared with the normal anatomy; the anterior margin of the first cervical vertebra overlaps the posterior margin of the mandible. This extreme posterior location of the tongue and larynx makes direct visualization of the laryngeal inlet almost impossible in many children with this anomaly because of the acute angulation between the base of the tongue and the laryngeal inlet. (Radiographs courtesy Donna J. Seibert, MD, John A. Kirkpatrick, Jr., MD, and Robert H. Cleveland, MD.)

pseudostratified columnar epithelium, pressure on the mucosa may cause reactive edema that could encroach on the diameter of the lumen. A tight-fitting ETT that compresses the tracheal mucosa at this level may cause inflammation and edema when it is removed, reducing the luminal diameter and increasing the airway resistance at the time of extubation (e.g., postextubation croup). Because the subglottic region in the infant is smaller than in the adult, the same degree of airway edema results in greater resistance in the infant. For example, assuming that the diameter of the cricoid ring in the infant is 4 mm and the diameter

the adult cricoid ring or trachea is 8 mm, 1 mm of edema circumferentially within the airway (i.e., reduction of the diameter of the airway by 2 mm) would decrease the cross-sectional area of the airway in the infant by approximately 75% (to 2 mm), whereas the adult cross-sectional area would decrease by only about 44% (to 6 mm). Physiologically, because the resistance to airflow in the upper airway is turbulent during crying or deep breathing, this reduction in diameter of the upper airway would increase the resistance to flow by the radius to the fifth power, or 32-fold, in the infant, compared with 5-fold in the adult. (Fig. 12-7).[2]

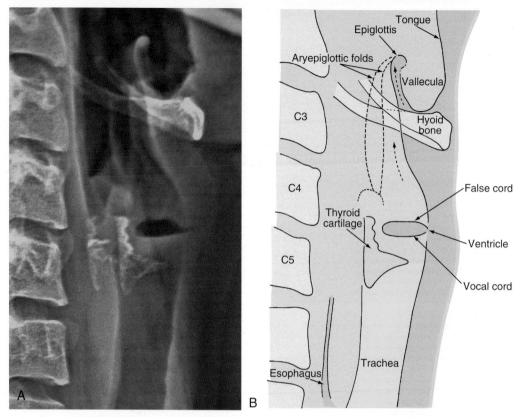

**FIGURE 12-4** Lateral neck xerogram (**A**) and schematic diagram (**B**) of the larynx in an adult. Notice the relatively thin, broad epiglottis, the axis of which is parallel to the trachea. The hyoid bone "hugs" the epiglottis; there is no subglottic narrowing. Also note how the vocal cords are perpendicular to the axis of the trachea.

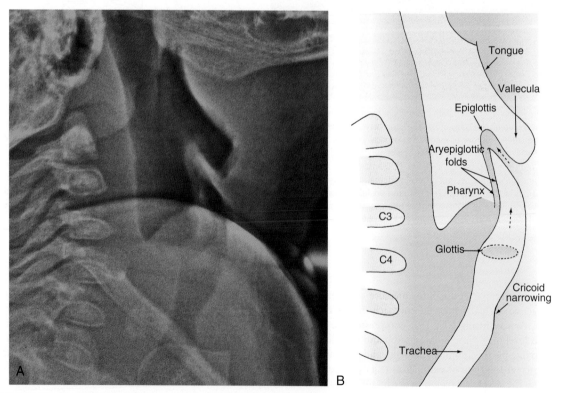

**FIGURE 12-5** Lateral neck xerogram (**A**) and schematic diagram (**B**) of an infant's larynx. Notice the angled epiglottis and the narrow cricoid cartilage. Also note that the vocal cords are angled with a higher attachment anteriorly than posteriorly compared with the perpendicular position of the vocal cords in adults.

# The Larynx

Understanding the anatomy and function of the larynx is critical to knowledgeable, safe, and successful airway management.

## ANATOMY
### Structure
The larynx is composed of one bone (hyoid) and eleven cartilages (the single thyroid, cricoid, and epiglottic cartilages and the paired arytenoid, corniculate, cuneiform, and triticea cartilages). These cartilages are suspended by ligaments from the base of the

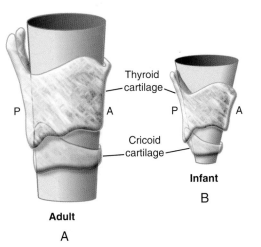

**FIGURE 12-6** Configuration of the larynx of an adult (**A**) and an infant (**B**). Notice that both larynxes are somewhat funnel shaped, but this shape is exaggerated in the infant and toddler. The adult laryngeal structures are of such size that most endotracheal tubes pass easily into the trachea. In infants and toddlers, it is common for the endotracheal tube (ETT) to pass easily through the vocal cords but to become snug at the level of the nondistensible cricoid cartilage. Concern for causing edema at this point resulted in the classic teaching that uncuffed ETTs should be used in young children (see text for more details). *A*, Anterior; *P*, posterior.

skull. The body of the cricoid cartilage articulates posteriorly with the inferior cornu of the thyroid cartilage. The paired triangular arytenoid cartilages rest on top of, and articulate with, the superoposterior aspect of the cricoid cartilage. The arytenoid cartilages are protected by the thyroid cartilage (Fig. 12-8). The triticeal cartilages are rounded nodules of cartilage, approximately the size of a pea in adults, located in the margins of the lateral thyrohyoid ligament.

Tissue folds and muscles cover these cartilages. In contrast to adults, but comparable to most mammals, the cartilaginous glottis accounts for 60% to 75% of the length of the vocal folds in children younger than 2 years of age.[10] Contraction of the intrinsic laryngeal muscles alters the position and configuration of these tissue folds, thus influencing laryngeal function during respiration, forced voluntary glottic closure (Valsalva maneuver), reflex laryngospasm, swallowing, and phonation (Fig. 12-9).

The laryngeal tissue folds consist of the following:
- Paired aryepiglottic folds extending from the epiglottis posteriorly to the superior surface of the arytenoids (the paired cuneiform and corniculate cartilages lie within for support and reinforcement)
- Paired vestibular folds (false vocal cords) extending from the thyroid cartilage posteriorly to the superior surface of the arytenoids
- Paired vocal folds (true vocal cords) extending from the posterior surface of the thyroid plate to the anterior projection or vocal process of the arytenoids
- A single interarytenoid fold (composed of the interarytenoid muscle covered by tissue) bridging the arytenoid cartilages
- A single thyrohyoid fold extending from the hyoid bone to the thyroid cartilage

### Histology
The highly vascular mucosa of the mouth is continuous with that of the larynx and trachea. This mucosa consists of squamous, stratified, and pseudostratified ciliated epithelium. The vocal cords are covered with stratified epithelium. The mucosa and submucosa are rich in lymphatic vessels and seromucus-secreting

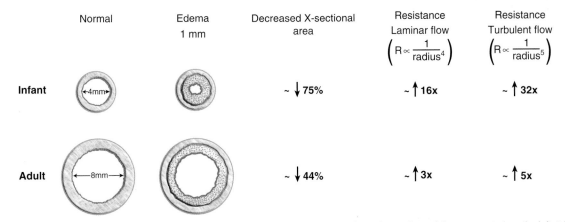

| | Normal | Edema 1 mm | Decreased X-sectional area | Resistance Laminar flow $\left(R \propto \dfrac{1}{\text{radius}^4}\right)$ | Resistance Turbulent flow $\left(R \propto \dfrac{1}{\text{radius}^5}\right)$ |
|---|---|---|---|---|---|
| **Infant** | ←4mm→ | | ~ ↓75% | ~ ↑16x | ~ ↑32x |
| **Adult** | ←8mm→ | | ~ ↓44% | ~ ↑3x | ~ ↑5x |

**FIGURE 12-7** Relative effects of airway edema in an infant and an adult. The normal airways of an infant and an adult are presented on the left. Edematous airways display 1 mm of circumferential edema, reducing the diameter of the lumen by 2 mm. Notice that resistance to airflow is inversely proportional to the radius of the lumen to the fourth power for laminar flow (beyond the fifth bronchial division) and to the radius of the lumen to the fifth power for turbulent flow (from the mouth to the fourth bronchial division). The net result in an infant with a 4-mm diameter airway is a 75% reduction in cross-sectional area and a 16-fold increase in resistance to laminar airflow, compared with a 44% reduction in cross-sectional area and a 3-fold increased resistance in an adult with a similar 2-mm reduction in airway diameter. With turbulent airflow (upper airway), the resistance increases 32-fold in the infant but only 5-fold in the adult.

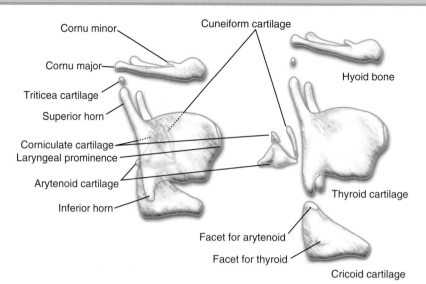

**FIGURE 12-8** Laryngeal cartilages. The natural positions of the laryngeal cartilages are presented on the left, with the individual cartilages separated on the right. (Reprinted by permission from Fink BR, Demarest RJ. Laryngeal biomechanics. Cambridge, Mass.: Harvard University Press, © 1978 by the President and Fellows of Harvard College.)

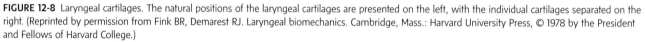

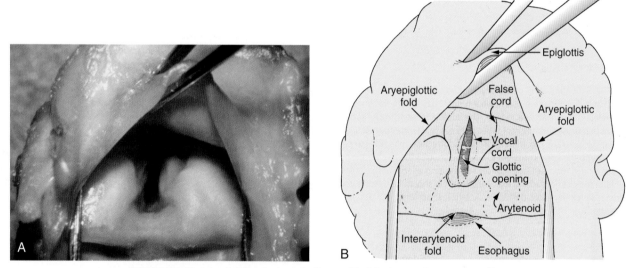

**FIGURE 12-9** Photograph (**A**) and schematic diagram (**B**) of the larynx of a premature infant.

glands, which lubricate the laryngeal folds. The submucosa consists of loose fibrous stroma; therefore, the mucosa is loosely adherent to the underlying structures in most areas. However, the submucosa is scant on the laryngeal surface of the epiglottis and the vocal cords, so the mucosa is tightly adherent in these areas.[12,13] Most inflammatory processes of the airway above the level of the vocal cords are limited by the barrier formed by the firm adherence of the mucosa to the vocal cords.[13] For example, the inflammation of epiglottitis is usually limited to the supraglottic structures, and the loosely adherent mucosa explains the ease with which localized swelling occurs (see Figs. 31-15 and 31-16). In a similar manner, an inflammatory process of the subglottic region (laryngotracheobronchitis) results in significant subglottic edema in the loosely adherent mucosa of the airway below the vocal cords, but it does not usually spread above the level of the vocal cords (see Fig. 31-14, *C*).[12]

**Sensory and Motor Innervation**

Two branches of the vagus nerve, the recurrent laryngeal and the superior laryngeal nerves, supply both sensory and motor innervation to the larynx. The superior laryngeal nerve has two branches: the internal branch, which provides sensory innervation to the supraglottic region, and the external branch, which supplies motor innervation to the cricothyroid muscle. The recurrent laryngeal nerve provides sensory innervation to the subglottic larynx and motor innervation to all other laryngeal muscles.[13,14] Local anesthetic agents injected to block the superior laryngeal nerve result in anesthesia of the supraglottic region down to the inferior margin of the epiglottis and motor blockade of the cricothyroid muscle, which causes relaxation of the vocal cords. Translaryngeal injection of local anesthetic through the cricothyroid membrane or a specific recurrent laryngeal nerve block is required for infraglottic and tracheal anesthesia.[15-17]

## Blood Supply

Laryngeal branches of the superior and inferior thyroid arteries provide the blood supply to the larynx. The recurrent laryngeal nerve and artery lie in close proximity to each other, which accounts for the occasional vocal cord paresis after attempts to control bleeding during thyroidectomy.[18]

## FUNCTION

### Inspiration

During inspiration, the larynx is pulled downward (caudad) by the negative intrathoracic pressure generated by the descent of the diaphragm and contraction of the intercostal muscles. Longitudinal stretching of the larynx results, thus increasing the distance between the aryepiglottic and vestibular folds as well as the distance between the vestibular and vocal folds. When the intrinsic muscles within the larynx contract, the arytenoids move laterally and posteriorly (rocking backward and rotating laterally), thereby increasing the interarytenoid distance and separating as well as stretching the paired aryepiglottic, vestibular, and vocal folds. Overall, inspiration enlarges the laryngeal inlet, both longitudinally (like opening a telescope) and laterally, allowing the passage of greater quantities of air through the airway per unit time.

### Expiration

At the end of expiration, the larynx reverts to its resting position, with longitudinal shortening of the distance between the aryepiglottic, vestibular, and vocal folds (like closing of a telescope). The arytenoids return simultaneously to their resting position by rotating medially and rocking forward, thus decreasing the interarytenoid distance and reducing the tension on the paired aryepiglottic, vestibular, and vocal folds and causing them to thicken.

### Forced Glottic Closure and Laryngospasm

Glottic closure during forced expiration (forced glottic closure or Valsalva maneuver) is voluntary laryngeal closure and is physiologically similar to involuntary laryngeal closure (laryngospasm). Forced glottic closure occurs at several levels. Contraction of the intrinsic laryngeal muscles results in (1) marked reduction in the interarytenoid distance; (2) anterior rocking and medial movement of the arytenoids, causing apposition of the paired vocal, vestibular, and aryepiglottic folds; (3) longitudinal shortening of the larynx that obliterates the space between the aryepiglottic, vestibular, and vocal folds (like complete closing of a telescope). Contraction of an extrinsic laryngeal muscle, the thyrohyoid, pulls the hyoid bone downward (caudad) and the thyroid cartilage upward (cephalad), leading to further closure.[1,3,4,19-22]

Closure of the larynx during laryngospasm is similar to, but not identical to that described for voluntary forced glottic closure. There are two important differences. First, laryngospasm is accompanied by an inspiratory effort, which longitudinally separates the vocal from the vestibular folds. Second, in contrast to forced glottic closure, neither the thyroarytenoid muscle (an intrinsic muscle of the larynx) nor the thyrohyoid muscle contracts; thus, apposition of the aryepiglottic folds and median thyrohyoid folds is minimal. These two differences allow the upper portion of the larynx to be left partially open during mild laryngospasm, resulting in the hallmark high-pitched inspiratory stridor (see Video 12-1).[1,19] Anterior and upward displacement of the mandible (jaw thrust) longitudinally separates the base of the tongue, the epiglottis, and the aryepiglottic folds from the vocal folds, helping to relieve laryngospasm.[20]

### Swallowing

Glottic closure during swallowing is also similar to that which occurs during forced closure of the glottis. Protection of the glottic opening is achieved primarily by apposition of the laryngeal folds and secondarily by upward (cephalad) movement of the larynx. The upward movement of the larynx brings the thyroid cartilage closer to the hyoid bone, resulting in folding of the epiglottis over the glottic opening.[1,19,21,22] With loss of consciousness or deep sedation, the normal protective mechanism of the larynx may be lost or obtunded, thus predisposing to pulmonary aspiration of pharyngeal contents.

### Phonation

Phonation is accomplished by alteration of the angle between the thyroid and cricoid cartilages (the cricothyroid angle) and by medial movement of the arytenoids during expiration.[1,14,23] These movements result in fine alterations in vocal fold tension during movement of air, causing vibration of the vocal folds. Lesions or malfunctions of the vocal folds (e.g., inflammation, papilloma, paresis) therefore affect phonation. Phonation is the only laryngeal function that alters the cricothyroid angle.[1] Therefore, despite significant airway obstruction during inspiration, it may still be possible to phonate.

## Physiology of the Respiratory System

### OBLIGATE NASAL BREATHING

Infants are considered to be obligate nasal breathers.[24,25] Obstruction of their anterior or posterior nares (nasal congestion, stenosis, choanal atresia) can cause asphyxia.[26-28] Immaturity of coordination between respiratory efforts and oropharyngeal motor and sensory input accounts in part for obligate nasal breathing.[29] Furthermore, because the larynx is higher (more cephalad) in the neck of an infant and oropharyngeal structures are closer together, the tongue rests against the roof of the mouth during quiet respiration, resulting in oral airway obstruction.[25] Multiple sites of pharyngeal airway obstruction may also contribute to airway obstruction when the infant attempts to breathe against a partially obstructed upper airway or with relaxation of upper airway muscle tone after sedation or induction of anesthesia.[30-34]

As the infant matures, the ability to coordinate respiratory and oral function increases. The larynx enlarges and moves down lower (more caudad) in the neck as the cervical spine lengthens and the infant begins to breathe adequately through the mouth. This maturation occurs by age 3 to 5 months. Studies have shown that the ability to breathe through the mouth when the nares are obstructed is age dependent: 8% of preterm infants of 31 to 32 weeks postconceptional age were able to breathe through the mouth in response to nasal occlusion, compared with 28% of more mature preterm infants of 35 to 36 weeks postconceptional age[35]; approximately 40% of full-term infants can switch from nasal to oral breathing.[36] However, more recent data contradict these earlier data. Slow and fast nasal occlusion applied to 17 healthy preterm infants (gestational age, 32 ± 1 weeks; postnatal age, 12 ± 2 days) led to a switch from nasal to oral breathing. The authors attributed the difference in findings to the more extended observation period in their study (>15 seconds).[37] The presence of a nasogastric tube may also significantly affect the infant's breathing if the "unobstructed" nasal passage has an existing underlying obstruction.

## TRACHEAL AND BRONCHIAL FUNCTION

Tracheal and bronchial diameters are a function of elasticity and of distending or compressive forces (Fig. 12-10). The larynx, trachea, and bronchi in the infant are quite compliant compared with those in the adult and therefore are more subject to distention and compression forces.[24,38,39] The intrathoracic trachea is subject to stresses that are different from those in the extrathoracic portion.[38] During expiration, intrathoracic pressure remains slightly negative, thus maintaining patency of the intrathoracic

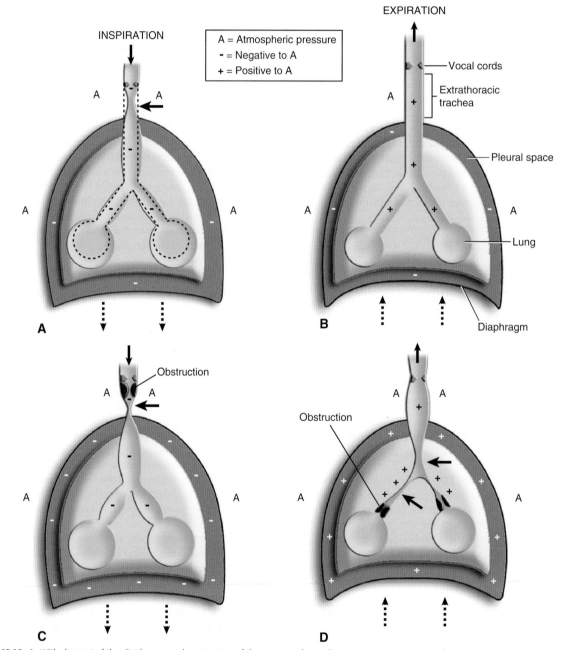

**FIGURE 12-10  A,** With descent of the diaphragm and contraction of the intercostal muscles, a greater negative intrathoracic pressure relative to intraluminal and atmospheric pressure is developed. The net result is longitudinal stretching of the larynx and trachea, dilatation of the intrathoracic trachea and bronchi, movement of air into the lungs, and some dynamic collapse of the extrathoracic trachea (*arrow*). The dynamic collapse is due to the highly compliant trachea and the negative intraluminal pressure in relation to atmospheric pressure. **B,** The normal sequence of events at end-expiration is a slight negative intrapleural pressure stenting the airways open. In infants, the highly compliant chest does not provide the support required; therefore, airway closure occurs with each breath. Intraluminal pressures are slightly positive in relation to atmospheric pressure, with the result that air is forced out of the lungs. **C,** Obstructed extrathoracic airway. Notice the severe dynamic collapse of the extrathoracic trachea below the level of obstruction. This collapse is greatest at the thoracic inlet, where the largest pressure gradient exists between negative intratracheal pressure and atmospheric pressure (*arrow*). (Extrathoracic upper airway obstruction is characterized by inspiratory stridor.) **D,** Obstructed intrathoracic trachea or airways. Notice that breathing against an obstructed lower airway (e.g., bronchiolitis, asthma) results in greater positive intrathoracic pressures, with dynamic collapse of the intrathoracic airways (prolonged expiration or wheezing [*arrows*]).

trachea and bronchi (see Fig. 12-10, *B*). During inspiration, a greater negative intrathoracic pressure dilates and stretches the *intrathoracic* trachea and bronchi.[40] The *extrathoracic* trachea at the thoracic inlet is slightly narrowed by dynamic compression that results from the differential between intratracheal pressure and atmospheric pressure. However, the cartilages of the trachea, along with the muscles and soft tissues of the neck, maintain patency of the airway (see Fig. 12-10, *A*).

Obstruction of the extrathoracic upper airway that can occur with epiglottitis, laryngotracheobronchitis, or an extrathoracic foreign body alters normal airway dynamics. Inspiration against an obstruction results in more negative intrathoracic pressure, further dilating the intrathoracic airways. Clinically, the net effect is a dynamic collapse of the extrathoracic trachea below the level of the obstruction. This collapse is maximal at the thoracic inlet, where the greatest pressure gradient exists between negative intratracheal and atmospheric pressures. As a result, inspiratory stridor is prominent (see Fig. 12-10, *C*, and Video 12-1).[38-45] With intrathoracic tracheal obstruction (e.g., foreign body, vascular ring) (see Video 12-1), stridor may occur during both inspiration and expiration.[46-49] In lower airway obstruction (e.g., asthma, bronchiolitis), significant intrathoracic tracheal and bronchial collapse may occur as a result of the prolonged expiratory phase and greatly increased positive extraluminal pressure (see Fig. 12-10, *D*).[50] In addition, because the airways in children are very compliant, they may be more susceptible to closure during bronchial smooth muscle contraction (e.g., with reactive airway disease). Preterm and term infants may experience airway closure even during quiet respirations.

Avoiding dynamic airway collapse is particularly important. The very compliant trachea and bronchi of an infant or child are prone to collapse, particularly at the extremes of transluminal pressures that may occur when a child is crying vigorously. The susceptibility of a child to these dynamic forces on the airway is inversely related to age, with preterm infants being most susceptible and adults being least susceptible.[51] For this reason, it is essential that children with airway obstruction remain calm. Skill and understanding are required on the parts of the parents, nursing staff, and physicians. *Sedatives and opioids should be used with caution before insertion of an ETT, because they may depress or ablate the life-sustaining voluntary efforts to breathe, resulting in significant morbidity or mortality.*

## WORK OF BREATHING

*Work of breathing* (WOB) may be defined as the product of pressure and volume. It may be analyzed by plotting transpulmonary pressure against tidal volume. The WOB per kilogram body weight is similar in infants and adults. However, the oxygen consumption of a full-term neonate (4 to 6 mL/kg/min) is twice that of an adult (2 to 3 mL/kg/min).[52] This greater oxygen consumption (and greater carbon dioxide production) in infants accounts in part for their increased respiratory frequency compared with older children. In preterm infants, the oxygen consumption related to breathing is three times that in adults.[53]

The location of airway resistance within the tracheobronchial tree differs between infants and adults. The nasal passages account for 25% of the total resistance to airflow in a neonate, compared with 60% in an adult.[25,54] In infants, most resistance to airflow occurs in the bronchi and small airways. This results from the relatively smaller diameter of the airways and the greater compliance of the supporting structures of the trachea and bronchi.[24,55,56]

In particular, the chest wall of a neonate is very compliant; the ribs provide less support to maintain negative intrathoracic pressure. This lack of negative intrathoracic pressure combined with the increased compliance of the bronchi can lead to functional airway closure with every breath.[57-59] In infants and children, therefore, small-airway resistance accounts for most of the WOB, whereas in adults, the nasal passages provide the major proportion of flow resistance.[25,57,58,60-65]

In the presence of increased airway resistance or decreased lung compliance, an increased transpulmonary pressure is required to produce a given tidal volume, and therefore the WOB is increased. Any change in the airway that increases the WOB may lead to respiratory failure. Recall that the WOB (resistance to air flow) is inversely proportional to the fourth power of the radius of the lumen during laminar flow (beyond the fifth bronchial division) and proportional to the fifth power of the radius during turbulent flow (upper airway to the fifth bronchial division). Because the diameter of the airways in infants is smaller than in adults, pathologic narrowing of the airways in infants exerts a greater adverse effect on the WOB. Increase in the WOB may also occur with a long ETT of small diameter, an obstructed ETT, or a narrowed airway. All of these situations increase oxygen consumption, which in turn increases oxygen demand.[66] The increased oxygen demand is initially addressed by an increase in respiratory rate, but the increased WOB may not be sustainable. The end result may be exhaustion, which leads to respiratory failure ($CO_2$ retention and hypoxemia).

The difference in histology of the diaphragm and intercostal muscles of preterm and full-term infants compared with older children also contributes to increased susceptibility of infants to respiratory fatigue or failure. Type I muscle fibers permit prolonged repetitive movement; for example, long-distance runners through repeated exercise increase the proportion of type I muscle fibers in their legs. The percentage of type I muscle fibers in the diaphragm and intercostal muscles changes with age (preterm infants < full-term infants < 2-year-old children) (Fig. 12-11). Any condition that increases the WOB in neonates and infants may fatigue the respiratory muscles and precipitate respiratory failure more readily than in an adult.[67-69]

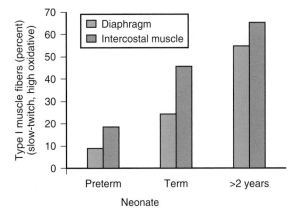

**FIGURE 12-11** Muscle fiber composition of the diaphragm and intercostal muscles related to age. Note that a preterm infant's diaphragm and intercostal muscles have fewer type I fibers compared with term newborns and older children. The data suggest a possible mechanism for early fatigue in preterm and term infants when the work of breathing is increased. (Data from Keens TG, Bryan AC, Levison H, Ianuzzo CD. Developmental pattern of muscle fiber types in human ventilatory muscles. J Appl Physiol 1978;44:909-13.)

## AIRWAY OBSTRUCTION DURING ANESTHESIA

Airway obstruction during anesthesia or loss of consciousness appears to be most frequently related to loss of muscle tone in the pharyngeal and laryngeal structures rather than apposition of the tongue to the posterior pharyngeal wall.[30,31,70,71] The progressive loss of tone with deepening anesthesia results in progressive airway obstruction primarily at the level of the soft palate and the epiglottis.[30,31,34,70,72,73] In children, the pharyngeal airway space decreases in a dose-dependent manner with increasing concentrations of both sevoflurane and propofol anesthesia.[74-76] This reduction in pharyngeal space has been observed mainly in the anteroposterior dimension. As the depth of propofol anesthesia in children increases, upper airway narrowing occurs throughout the entire upper airway but is most pronounced in the hypopharynx at the level of the epiglottis. Extension of the head at the atlantooccipital joint with anterior displacement of the cervical spine (sniffing position) improves hypopharyngeal airway patency but does not necessarily change the position of the tongue. This observation supports the concept that upper airway obstruction is not primarily caused by changes in tongue position but rather by collapse of the pharyngeal structures.[32-34]

Pharyngeal airway obstruction also occurs during obstructive sleep apnea in infants and adults.[29,77] The sniffing position increases the cross-sectional area and decreases the closing pressure of both the retropalatal and the retroglossal space in anesthetized adults with obstructive sleep apnea.[78] The application of continuous positive airway pressure (CPAP) is a common method to overcome such airway obstruction (see Figs. 31-6 and 31-7). During propofol anesthesia in children, CPAP works primarily by increasing the transverse dimension of the airway.[75] This occurs despite the fact that anesthesia obstructs the airway mostly by narrowing the anteroposterior dimension. Chin lift and jaw thrust also improve airway patency in anesthetized children with adenotonsillar hypertrophy.[79-81] Lateral positioning (also known as the "recovery position") dramatically enhances the effects of these airway maneuvers[80,81]; lateral positioning alone improves airway dimensions.[6] Compared with chin lift and CPAP, the jaw thrust maneuver is known to be the most effective means to improve airway patency and ventilation in children undergoing adenoidectomy.[79] (See Video 4-3, *A* and *B*.)

## Evaluation of the Airway

A history and physical examination with specific reference to the airway should be performed in all children who require sedation or anesthesia. In particular, a history of a congenital syndrome or physical findings of a congenital anomaly (e.g., microtia, which has been associated with difficult laryngoscopy[82]) should alert the practitioner to the possibility of difficulties with airway management. In special situations, radiologic and laboratory studies are required to further evaluate and clarify a disorder revealed by the history and physical examination. Although many methods exist for evaluating and predicting the difficult airway (DA) in adults,[83-87] no published studies have assessed the use of any of these techniques in children.[88,89] Routine evaluation of the airway in all children, followed by correlation with any airway problems occurring during anesthetic management, helps the practitioner to develop experience. This experience then may be used to identify in the future children who might have airway difficulties during or after anesthesia.

## CLINICAL EVALUATION

The *medical history* (both present and past) should investigate the following signs and symptoms; a positive history should alert the practitioner to the potential problems that are noted in parentheses.

- Presence of an upper respiratory tract infection (predisposition to coughing, laryngospasm, bronchospasm, and desaturation during anesthesia or to postintubation subglottic edema or postoperative desaturation)[90-94]
- Snoring or noisy breathing (adenoidal hypertrophy, upper airway obstruction, obstructive sleep apnea, pulmonary hypertension)
- Presence and nature of cough ("croupy" cough may indicate subglottic stenosis or previous tracheoesophageal fistula repair; productive cough may indicate bronchitis or pneumonia; chronicity affects the differential diagnosis [e.g., the sudden onset of a persistent cough may indicate foreign-body aspiration])
- Past episodes of croup (postintubation croup, subglottic stenosis)
- Inspiratory stridor, usually high pitched (subglottic narrowing [see Video 12-1], laryngomalacia [see Video 12-1], macroglossia, laryngeal web [Video 12-2], extrathoracic foreign body or extrathoracic tracheal compression)
- Hoarse voice (laryngitis, vocal cord palsy, papillomatosis [see Video 12-1], granuloma [see Video 12-1])
- Asthma and bronchodilator therapy (bronchospasm)
- Repeated pneumonias (incompetent larynx with aspiration, gastroesophageal reflux, cystic fibrosis, bronchiectasis, residual tracheoesophageal fistula, pulmonary sequestration, immune suppression, congenital heart disease)
- History of foreign-body aspiration (increased airway reactivity, airway obstruction, impaired neurologic function)
- History of aspiration (laryngeal edema [Video 12-3], laryngeal cleft)
- Previous anesthetic problems, particularly related to the airway (difficult intubation, difficulty with mask ventilation, failed or problematic extubation)
- Atopy, allergy (increased airway reactivity)
- History of smoking by primary caregivers (increased airway resistance, increased propensity to desaturate)[95]
- History of a congenital syndrome (many are associated with DA management)

The *physical examination* should include the following observations:

- Facial expression
- Presence or absence of nasal flaring
- Presence or absence of mouth breathing
- Color of mucous membranes
- Presence or absence of retractions (suprasternal, intercostal, subcostal [see Video 12-1])
- Respiratory rate
- Presence or absence of voice change
- Mouth opening (Fig. 12-12, *A*)
- Size of mouth
- Size of tongue and its relationship to other pharyngeal structures (Mallampati Score)
- Loose or missing teeth (see Fig. 12-12, *B*)
- Size and configuration of palate
- Size and configuration of mandible
- Location of larynx in relation to the mandible (see Fig. 12-12, *C*)

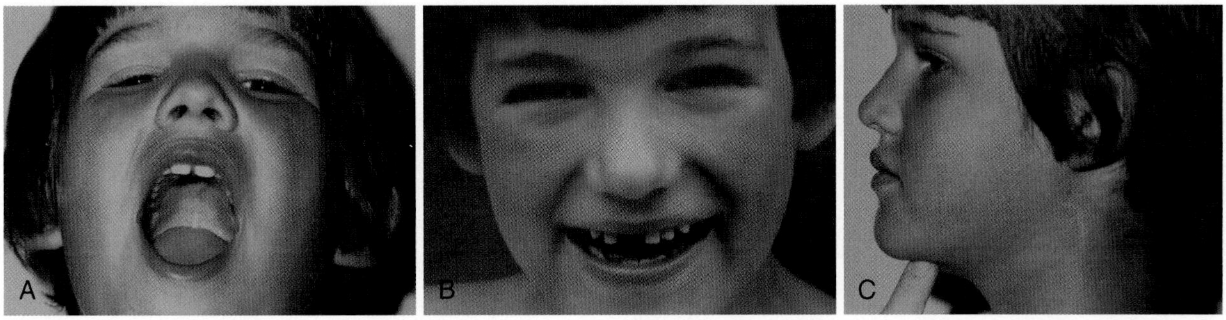

**FIGURE 12-12 A,** How far can a child open his or her mouth? Are there any abnormalities of the mouth, tongue, palate, mandible? **B,** Are any teeth loose or missing? **C,** Is the mandible of normal configuration? How much space is there between the genu of the mandible and the thyroid cartilage? This space is an indication of the extent of the superior and posterior displacement of the larynx; there should normally be at least one finger breadth in a newborn and three finger breadths in an adolescent.

■ Presence of stridor and, if present:
  ■ Is stridor predominantly inspiratory, suggesting an upper airway (extrathoracic) lesion (epiglottitis, croup, extrathoracic foreign body)?
  ■ Is stridor both inspiratory and expiratory, suggesting an intrathoracic lesion (aspirated foreign body, vascular ring, or large esophageal foreign body)? (see Video 12-1)
  ■ Is the expiratory phase prolonged or stridor predominantly expiratory, suggesting lower airway disease?
■ Baseline oxygen saturation in room air
■ Microtia: Bilateral but not unilateral microtia is associated with difficulty in visualizing the laryngeal inlet (grade 3 or 4 in the Cormack-Lehane classification, see Fig. 12-22).[82] Five (42%) of 12 children with bilateral microtia were found to have a difficult laryngeal view, compared with 2 (2.5%) of 81 children with unilateral microtia and 0 of 93 children without microtia.[82] Microtia may represent a mild form of hemifacial microsomia and its associated mandibular hypoplasia. The advantage of understanding this association is that ear deformity is often a more easily recognized clinical finding than mandibular hypoplasia.
■ Global appearance: Are there congenital anomalies that may fit a recognizable syndrome? *The finding of one anomaly mandates a search for others.* If a congenital syndrome is diagnosed, specific anesthetic implications must be considered (see E-Appendix 12-1, which is available online).

### DIAGNOSTIC TESTING

Routine evaluation of the airway usually requires only a careful history and physical examination. In the presence of airway pathology, however, laboratory and radiologic evaluation can be extremely valuable. Radiographs of the upper airway (anteroposterior and lateral films and fluoroscopy) may provide evidence about the site and cause of airway obstruction. When necessary, MRI and CT provide more detailed information.[96-112] *Radiologic airway examination in a child with a compromised airway may be undertaken only if there is no immediate threat to the child's safety and only in the presence of skilled and appropriately equipped personnel able to manage the airway.* Securing the airway through tracheal intubation must not be postponed in order to obtain a radiologic diagnosis when the child has severely compromised air exchange. Blood gas analysis is occasionally of value in assessing the degree of physiologic compromise, especially with chronic airway obstruction and compensated respiratory acidosis. Performing an arterial (or venous) puncture for blood gas analysis, although providing helpful information, is often upsetting to the child and may risk aggravation of the underlying airway obstruction through dynamic airway collapse. Candidates for blood gas analysis must be carefully selected and the procedure skillfully performed.

Endoscopic evaluation (flexible fiberoptic endoscopy) of the airway before tracheal intubation can be useful in infants and in cooperative older children if a glottic pathologic process is suspected or if difficulty is anticipated when visualizing the glottis.

## Airway Management: The Normal Airway

### MASK VENTILATION

Face masks are available in many sizes and shapes. We commonly use the disposable, clear plastic masks with an inflatable cushioned rim. The inflatable rim molds to the contour of the face to provide an atraumatic seal. The use of clear plastic in the cone of the mask allows visualization of humidity (indicating air exchange), secretions, vomitus, or cyanotic lip color. The appropriately sized mask should rest on the bridge of the nose (avoiding the eyes) and extend to the mandible. Although mask anesthesia appears to be easy, it is, in fact, one of the most difficult skills to master. The most common error during mask ventilation is to tightly compress the submental triangle with fingers placed below the mandibular ridge, thereby partially occluding the airway. Minimal pressure is required, and the fingers should rest on the mandible. Another common problem arises when the mouth is completely closed while the face mask is being applied. The upper airway may become completely obstructed, with ventilation becoming impossible both spontaneously and by manual control. In such a circumstance, the fingers should be removed from the mandible and face and a single digit applied to each coronoid process while lifting toward the hairline. This maneuver subluxes the temporomandibular joint, thereby opening the mouth and pulling the tongue and other soft tissues off the posterior pharyngeal wall. A hand should be on the reservoir bag at all times to monitor the effectiveness of ventilation and to provide CPAP if needed to maintain a patent airway. An alternative method is to partially close the adjustable pressure-limiting valve to inflate the reservoir bag and provide CPAP. Insertion of an oral airway may also facilitate gas exchange.

Admonitions against extreme positions of the infant's head during bag-and-mask ventilation are intended to minimize the

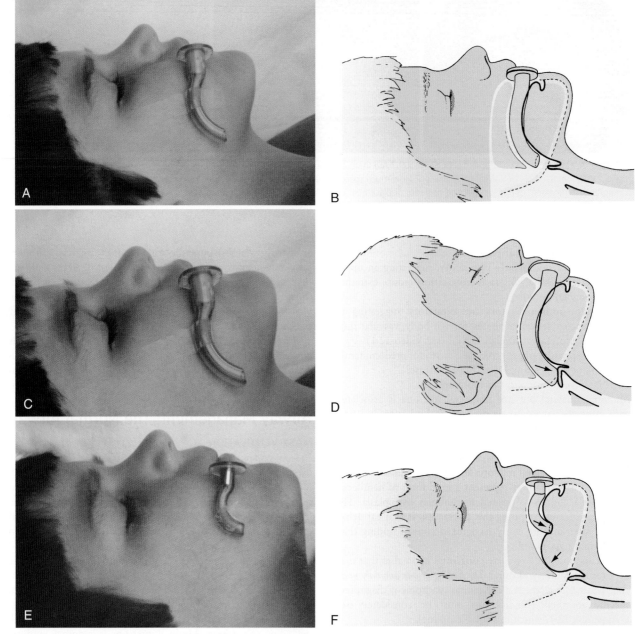

**FIGURE 12-13** Correct airway selection. An artificial airway of proper size should relieve airway obstruction caused by the tongue without damaging laryngeal structures. The appropriate size can be estimated by holding the airway against the child's face: the tip of the airway should end just cephalad to the angle of the mandible (**A**). Use of the correct size should result in proper alignment with the glottic opening (**B**). If too large an oral airway is inserted, the tip will line up posterior to the angle of the mandible (**C**) and obstruct the glottic opening by pushing the epiglottis down (**D,** *arrow*). If too small an oral airway is inserted, the tip will line up well above the angle of the mandible (**E**) and exacerbate airway obstruction by kinking the tongue (**F,** *arrows*).

risk of stretching and thus narrowing and obstructing the very compliant infant trachea. However, a study of 18 healthy, full-term infants younger than 4 months of age showed that the tracheal dimensions did not change when the head position changed.[113] Therefore, stretching of the trachea may not result in narrowing of the tracheal lumen in otherwise healthy infants (Video 12-4). However, this study did not examine the effects of these head positions on the supraglottic airway or in the preterm infant. It is possible that these maneuvers (head extension) could result in supraglottic airway obstruction in some children.

## OROPHARYNGEAL AIRWAYS

An infant's tongue may obstruct the airway during induction of anesthesia or loss of consciousness. An oropharyngeal airway of appropriate size (or a supraglottic airway [SGA] such as the laryngeal mask airway [LMA; LMA North America, San Diego]) may be inserted to relieve the obstruction. By holding the oral airway as shown in Figure 12-13, one can estimate the appropriate size for the child; airways one size larger and one size smaller should be readily available as well. A tongue depressor may be inserted over the tongue to facilitate insertion of the oral airway by preventing downfolding of the tongue, which could impair venous and lymphatic drainage, causing tongue swelling and airway obstruction. If the airway device is too long, it may push the epiglottis into the glottic aperture, creating an additional site of airway obstruction or causing traumatic epiglottitis, or the tip may impinge on the uvula, causing uvular swelling and airway obstruction (see Fig. 12-13, *C, D*).[114,115] If the airway device is too short, it may rest against the base of the tongue, forcing it posteriorly against the roof of the mouth and further aggravating airway obstruction (Fig. 12-13, *E, F*). Oral airways should not be considered panaceas for upper airway obstruction. Care must be taken to avoid trauma to the lips and tongue, which may be caught between the teeth and the flange of the airway. An oral airway is also used to protect an ETT from compression by the child's teeth, and it serves to separate the mandible and maxilla to facilitate oropharyngeal suctioning.

## NASOPHARYNGEAL AIRWAYS

Nasopharyngeal airways are occasionally used in children to relieve upper airway obstruction; the distance from the naris to the angle of the mandible approximates the proper length. Commercial airways are available in sizes 12F to 36F (Rüsch Inc., Duluth, Ga.). Some have an adjustable flange that enables manipulation of the airway to the appropriate length. Alternatively, for infants and small children, a shortened ETT may be used, although this is not as soft and pliable as a commercially available nasopharyngeal airway and may be more likely to cause trauma on insertion. The nasopharyngeal airway may be better tolerated in the lightly anesthetized child than an oropharyngeal airway. Nasopharyngeal airways are usually avoided to prevent trauma to, and bleeding from, hypertrophied adenoids, and they are more commonly used to relieve residual airway obstruction on emergence from anesthesia.

## TRACHEAL INTUBATION
### Technique

As previously discussed, because of differences in anatomy, there are differences in techniques for intubating the trachea of infants and children compared with adults.[1-4,20-22,101,116,117] Because of the smaller dimensions of the pediatric airway, there is increased risk of obstruction with trauma to the airway structures. A technique to be avoided is that in which the blade is advanced into the esophagus with laryngeal visualization achieved during withdrawal of the blade. *This maneuver may result in laryngeal trauma when the tip of the blade scrapes the arytenoids and aryepiglottic folds.*

There are several approaches to exposing the glottis in infants with a Miller blade. One approach consists of advancing the laryngoscope blade under constant vision along the surface of the tongue, placing the tip of the blade directly in the vallecula, and then using this location to pivot or rotate the blade to the right to sweep the tongue to the left and adequately lift the tongue to expose the glottic opening. This technique avoids trauma to the arytenoid cartilages. Lifting the base of the tongue lifts the epiglottis, exposing the glottic opening. If this technique is unsuccessful, the epiglottis may be lifted directly with the tip of the blade (see Video 12-1). Another approach is to insert the Miller blade into the mouth at the right commissure over the lateral bicuspids/incisors (paraglossal approach). The blade is advanced down the right gutter of the mouth, aiming the blade tip toward the midline while sweeping the tongue to the left. Once the blade is under the epiglottis, the epiglottis is lifted with the tip, exposing the glottic aperture. By approaching the mouth

over the bicuspids/incisors, dental damage is obviated. This is a particularly effective approach for the infant or child with micrognathia. Whichever approach is used, care must be taken to avoid using the laryngoscope blade as a fulcrum through which pressure is applied to the teeth or alveolar ridge. If there is a substantive risk that pressure will be applied to the teeth, a plastic tooth guard may be applied to cover the teeth at risk (the central incisors of the maxilla).

Optimal positioning for laryngoscopy changes with age. The trachea of older children (≥6 years) and adults is most easily exposed when a folded blanket or pillow is placed beneath the occiput of the head (5 to 10 cm elevation), displacing the cervical spine anteriorly.[118] Extension of the head at the atlantooccipital joint produces the classic "sniffing" position.[101,119,120] These movements align three axes: those of the mouth or oral (O), pharynx (P), and trachea (T). Once aligned, these three axes permit direct visualization of laryngeal structures. They also result in improved hypopharyngeal patency.[32,34,70,78,119,120] Figure 12-14 demonstrates maneuvers for positioning the head during airway management. In infants and younger children, it is usually unnecessary to elevate the head because the occiput is large in proportion to the trunk, resulting in adequate anterior displacement of the cervical spine; head extension at the atlantooccipital joint alone aligns the airway axes. If the occiput is displaced excessively, exposure of the glottis may actually be hindered. In neonates, it is helpful for an assistant to hold the patient's shoulders flat on the operating room table with the head slightly extended. Some practitioners have adopted the practice of placing a rolled towel under the shoulders of neonates to facilitate tracheal intubation. This technique may be disadvantageous if the laryngoscopist stands but may be advantageous if he or she is seated.

The validity of the three-axis theory (alignment of the O, P, and T) to describe the optimal intubating position in adults has been challenged.[121-124] Some authors question the notion that elevation of the occiput improves conditions for visualization of the laryngeal inlet based on evidence from both MRI and clinical investigations.[121,123] However, one MRI study in children with an LMA in place found that slight head extension improved the alignment of the glottic and pharyngeal axes but worsened the alignment of the pharyngeal and laryngeal axes.[125] In a study of adults, neck extension alone was adequate for visualization of the larynx in most patients, but for obese patients and those with limited neck extension, an optimal intubating position was not determined.[121] Others favor the sniffing position but with varying support for the three-axis theory.[126-132] Even if the tracheas of only a few patients are intubated more easily when placed in the sniffing position compared with simple head extension, the current routine application of the sniffing position appears to be the best clinical practice.

Laryngoscopy can be performed while the child is awake, anesthetized and breathing spontaneously, or anesthetized and paralyzed. Most tracheal intubations in children who are awake are performed in neonates, an approach that is not usually feasible or humane in older awake and uncooperative children. Awake intubation in the neonate is generally well tolerated if it is performed smoothly and rapidly; however, an international consensus group and others have cautioned against this practice unless intravenous (IV) access is not available or there is a life-threatening situation.[133-136] Data suggest that preterm and term infants are better managed with sedation and paralysis to minimize adverse hemodynamic responses.[137-141]

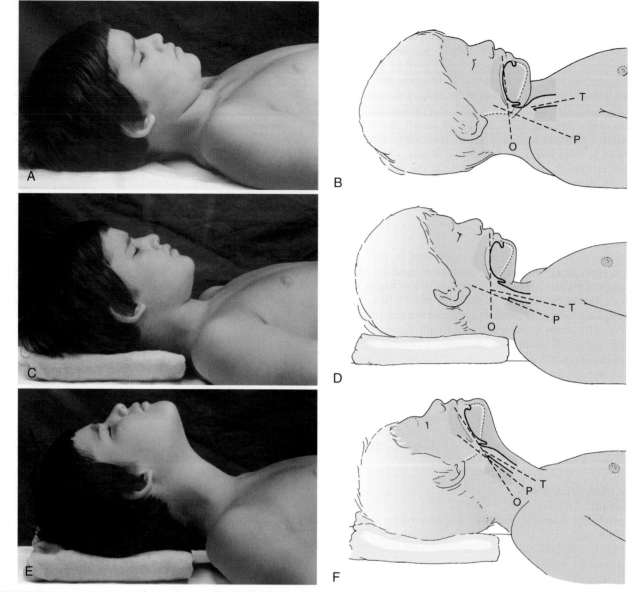

FIGURE 12-14 Correct positioning for ventilation and tracheal intubation. When a patient is lying flat on the bed or operating table (**A**), the oral (*O*), pharyngeal (*P*), and tracheal (*T*) axes pass through three divergent planes (**B**). A folded sheet or towel placed under the occiput of the head (**C**) aligns the P and T axes (**D**). Extension of the atlantooccipital joint (**E**) results in alignment of all three axes (**F**).

### Selection of Laryngoscope Blade

A straight blade is generally more suitable for use in infants and young children than a curved blade because it better elevates the base of the tongue to expose the glottic opening. Curved blades are satisfactory in older children. The blade size chosen depends on the age and body mass of the child and the preference of the anesthesiologist. Table 12-1 presents the ranges commonly used.

### Endotracheal Tubes

Since 1967, all materials used in the manufacture of ETTs have been subjected to rabbit muscle implantation testing in accordance with the standards promulgated by the Z79 Committee.[141a] If the material causes an inflammatory response in the rabbits, it cannot be used in the manufacture of ETTs. This has resulted in the elimination of organometallic constituents, which were used in the manufacture of red rubber ETTs.

**TABLE 12-1** Laryngoscope Blades Used in Infants and Children

| Age | BLADE SIZE | | |
| --- | --- | --- | --- |
| | **Miller** | **Wis-Hipple** | **Macintosh** |
| Preterm | 0 | — | — |
| Neonate | 0 | — | — |
| Neonate-2 years | 1 | — | — |
| 2-6 years | — | 1.5 | 1 or 2 |
| 6-10 years | 2 | — | 2 |
| >10 years | 2 or 3 | — | 3 |

Selection of the proper size of an ETT depends on the individual child.[142] The only size requirement for a manufacturer is a standardized inner diameter (ID). The external (outer) diameter (OD) varies among manufacturers, depending on the material from which the ETT is constructed. This diversity in OD

**TABLE 12-2** Endotracheal Tubes (ETTs) Used in Infants and Children

| Age | Size (mm ID) Uncuffed | Size (mm ID) Cuffed |
|---|---|---|
| Preterm | | |
| 1000 g | 2.5 | |
| 1000-2500 g | 3.0 | |
| Neonate-6 months | 3.0-3.5 | 3.0-3.5* |
| 6 month-1 year | 3.5-4.0 | 3.0-4.0 |
| 1-2 years | 4.0-5.0 | 3.5-4.5 |
| >2 years | (age in years + 16)/4 | (age in years/4) +3 |

*ID*, Inner diameter.
*In some neonates, a cuffed ETT may not have a leak below 30 cm H$_2$O, and therefore an uncuffed ETT may be more appropriate.

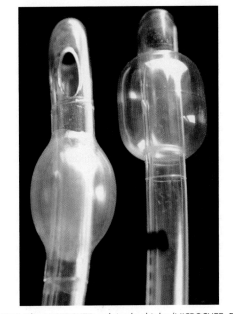

**FIGURE 12-15** The MICROCUFF endotracheal tube (MICROCUFF, PET, I-MPEDC; MICROCUFF GmbH, Weinheim, Germany) (*right*) is designed with an ultrathin polyurethane (10 μm) high-volume/low-pressure cuff that has a more distal position along the shaft of the tube to better accommodate pediatric anatomy. In contrast to more traditional pediatric cuffed endotracheal tubes (*left*), the elimination of a Murphy eye allows a more distal position of the upper cuff border. The location of the cuff on the shaft of the tube helps to ensure cuff placement below the subglottis—perhaps with the advantage of less risk for endobronchial intubation or intralaryngeal cuff position. An anatomically based depth mark on the surface of the tube helps to guide correct placement.

mandates checking for proper ETT size and leakage around the tube. An appropriately sized uncuffed ETT may be approximated according to the child's age and weight (Table 12-2).[143]

ETTs one-half mm ID greater or less than the anticipated size should be available because of variability in the size of the airway. Use of the diameter of the terminal phalanx of either the second or fifth digit is unreliable.[144] Children with Down syndrome often require an ETT with a diameter smaller than anticipated.[145] After tracheal intubation and stable cardiorespiratory indices are obtained, a sustained inflation to 20 to 25 cm H$_2$O (short-term intubation perhaps as high as 35 cm H$_2$O) should be applied to detect an audible or auscultatory air leak over the glottis. If no leak is detected, the ETT should be exchanged for one with an ID 0.5 mm smaller. An air leak at this pressure is recommended because it is believed to approximate the capillary pressure of the adult tracheal mucosa. If lateral wall pressure exceeds this amount, ischemic damage to the subglottic mucosa may occur.[146] Be aware, however, that if the trachea has been intubated without muscle relaxants, laryngospasm around the ETT may prevent any gas leak and mimic a tight-fitting ETT.[147] If such a situation is suspected, the anesthetic depth should be increased, and an air leak may become evident. Changes in head position may also increase or decrease the leak.[147] These maneuvers are important for making the occasional diagnosis of unrecognized subglottic stenosis (see Fig. 36-3, and Videos 12-1 and 12-5).

Traditional teaching has advocated the use of uncuffed ETTs for children younger than 8 years, because an uncuffed ETT with an air leak exerts minimal pressure on the internal surface of the cricoid cartilage and thus poses potentially less risk for postextubation edema (croup).[143,146,148] An uncuffed ETT also allows insertion of a tube with a larger ID, resulting in less airway resistance, although this holds relevance only for a spontaneously breathing child.[149] However, more recent clinical data and clinical practice have challenged these assumptions[150-158]; a number of studies demonstrated no differences in the incidence of postextubation complications after cuffed and uncuffed tubes.[150,155] Cited advantages of cuffed ETTs include decreased numbers of laryngoscopies and intubations to determine the appropriate size for the ETT, reduced subglottic pressure, reduced operating room pollution and costs of anesthetic agents, decreased risk of aspiration, accurate control of carbon dioxide tension (PCO$_2$), better ability to accurately measure the sophisticated physiologic respiratory functions of modern ventilators, absolute ability to deliver increased airway pressures in children with restrictive lung disease,

the ability to control cuff pressure, and no increased risk of postextubation stridor.[150-156,159-161]

A drawback of cuffed tubes is the greater variability in functional OD compared with uncuffed tubes because of differences in cuff shape, size, and inflation characteristics.[162] In general, if a cuffed ETT is inserted, an ETT with a smaller ID should be selected to compensate for the ETT cuff. One study found a 99% rate of appropriate cuffed tube size selection for full-term infants through children 8 years of age using the following formula[155]:

$$ID\,(mm) = (age/4) + 3$$

To overcome the shortcomings of the many pediatric cuffed tubes, the MICROCUFF ETT (MICROCUFF, PET, I-MPEDC; MICROCUFF GmbH, Weinheim, Germany, distributed by Kimberly-Clark USA) was designed with a high volume/low pressure cuff that is more distally placed along the shaft of the ETT to better accommodate the anatomy of the airway in infants and children (Fig. 12-15).[163] The ultrathin polyurethane cuff (10 μm) allows tracheal sealing at low pressures and provides a uniform and complete surface contact with minimal formation of cuff folds.[157,159,163-166] At 20 cm H$_2$O inflation pressure, the cuffs have a cross-sectional cuff area of approximately150% of the maximal internal tracheal cross-sectional area. Uninflated, the cuff adds only a minimal amount to the OD of the ETT. Shortened cuffs and the elimination of a Murphy eye allow a more distal position of the cuff, thereby theoretically reducing the risk of pressure being applied to the cricoid ring and adjacent mucosa.[167] The location of the cuff on the shaft of the tube helps to ensure cuff placement below the subglottis, perhaps with the advantage of less risk for endobronchial intubation or intralaryngeal cuff position. An anatomically based depth mark on the surface of the tube helps to guide correct placement.

An investigation of this specially designed ETT for children used the following guidelines to select cuffed ETT sizes[159]:

- For children ≥2 years, ID (mm) = (age/4) + 3.5
- For children 1 to 2 years of age, ID 3.5 mm
- For neonates ≥3 kg and infants ≤1 year, ID 3.0 mm

Use of these formulas resulted in the need to reintubate to change tube size in 1.6% of children (6/500).[159] The incidence of postintubation croup was 0.4% (2/500 children). In a randomized, multicenter study in 2246 young children (mean age, 1.9 years), investigators reported a similar findings for cuffed (MICRO-CUFF) and uncuffed tubes: postextubation stridor, 4.4% and 4.7%, respectively, and ETT exchange, 2.1% and 30.8%.[161] However, in a cost/benefit analysis of the MICROCUFF tube (three to six times that of standard ETTs), the reduction in anesthetic cost offset the cost of the MICROCUFF ETT.[160]

As a rule, if a cuffed ETT is chosen, the cuff should be inflated to the minimal pressure that seals the air leak; with the MICRO-CUFF ETT, this appears to be approximately 10.6 cm $H_2O$.[159,161,168,169] This air leak must be reevaluated during the anesthetic procedure if nitrous oxide is used, because the gas may diffuse into the cuff, producing excessive tracheal mucosal pressure.[168-170] In fact, the MICROCUFF ultrathin polyurethane ETT cuff has greater permeability for nitrous oxide than conventional polyvinyl chloride cuffs and therefore may increase the cuff pressure more rapidly than other cuffed tubes. However, with the cuff of the MICROCUFF ETT sealing the air leak at approximately 10 cm $H_2O$ in children, the time interval to reach 25 cm $H_2O$ cuff pressure was greater than with a conventional cuffed ETT.[171] Routinely checking cuff pressure or filling the cuff with nitrous oxide is recommended.[172] A pressure relief valve that can be connected to the pilot balloon of a cuffed ETT to limit cuff pressures to 20 cm $H_2O$ when nitrous oxide is used has been described.[173]

### Endotracheal Tube Insertion Distance

The length of the trachea (vocal cords to carina) in neonates and children up to 1 year of age varies from 5 to 9 cm.[40] In most infants 3 months to 1 year of age, if the 10-cm mark of the ETT is placed at the alveolar ridge, the tip of the tube rests above the carina. In preterm and full-term infants, the distance is less. In children 2 years old, 12 cm is usually appropriate. An easy way to remember these lengths is 10 for a newborn, 11 for a 1-year old, and 12 for a 2-year old. After 2 years of age, the correct length of insertion (in centimeters) for oral intubation may be approximated by formulas based on age or weight (Table 12-3)[174-177]:

$$[Age\ (yr)/2] + 12$$
$$[Weight\ (kg)/5] + 12$$
$$ID\ of\ ETT \times 3$$

Some practitioners suggest using anatomic markers to choose the appropriate depth for the tube in the trachea in neonates.[178,179] An advantage of anatomic measurements is that the infant's weight may not be available immediately after birth or in sick neonates who present to the emergency department with urgent respiratory or cardiac compromise. One study that used chest radiographs to evaluate final ETT position determined that the length of the foot was as accurate as weight-based formulas to determine the depth of insertion for a nasotracheal tube (44% versus 56% rate of optimal placement, and 83% versus 72%

**TABLE 12-3** Distance for Insertion of an Oral Endotracheal Tube by Patient Age

| Age | Approximate Distance of Insertion (cm) Even with Alveolar Ridge |
| --- | --- |
| Preterm <1000 g | 6-7 |
| Preterm 1000-2000 g | 7-9 |
| Term newborn | 9-10 |
| 1 year | 11-12 |
| 2 years | 12-13 |
| 6 years | 15-16 |
| 10 years | 17-18 |
| 16 years | 18-20 |
| 20 years | 20-22 |

satisfactory placement).[179] Alternatively, the nasal-tragus length (the distance from the base of the nasal septum to the tip of the tragus) or the sternal length (the distance from the suprasternal notch to the tip of the xiphoid process) predicted the depth of insertion of the ETT. Either distance plus 1 cm accurately estimated oral ETT tube insertion distance; either distance plus 2 cm accurately estimated nasotracheal tube insertion distance.[178] Both measurements compared favorably with weight-based formulas when tube position was verified by chest radiography.

After the ETT has been inserted and the first strip of adhesive tape has been applied to secure it, one must observe for symmetry of chest expansion and auscultate for equality of breath sounds in the axillae and apices (not on the anterior chest wall). The anterior chest wall in the child is not used to verify tracheal intubation because breath sounds may reverberate across the precordium in small children, precluding the diagnosis of an endobronchial intubation. A $CO_2$ monitor confirms intratracheal positioning but does not confirm that the tip of the ETT is not in an endobronchial position. A capnogram that diminishes during the first few breaths suggests an esophageal intubation. Unexpectedly increased airway pressures, persistent desaturation, and asymmetrical chest wall movement all suggest an endobronchial intubation. Visible humidity on the walls of the ETT during expiration also confirms tracheal placement, but the humidity may not be visible in younger infants. It is also important to auscultate over the stomach and to observe for desaturation or cyanosis. Once satisfactory position is achieved, a second strip of tape ensures secure fixation (Fig. 12-16).

We have observed a number of children whose ETT moved into a main stem bronchus after initial correct position during repositioning for the surgical procedure; this manifested as a slight but persistent decrease in oxygen saturation (e.g., from 100% to a range of 93% to 95%). Several studies have demonstrated that simple flexion or extension of the neck can move the ETT sufficiently to cause an endobronchial intubation or dislodgement of the tube from the trachea, respectively.[180-182] *When a small but persistent change in oxygen saturation is noted, rather than increase the inspired oxygen concentration ($FIO_2$), one must first investigate the cause and reassess the position of the ETT.*[183]

### Complications of Tracheal Intubation
#### Postintubation Croup
Perioperative postintubation croup (also referred to as postextubation croup) occurs in 0.1% to 1% of children.[156,159,184,185] Factors associated with increased risk of croup include an ETT with an

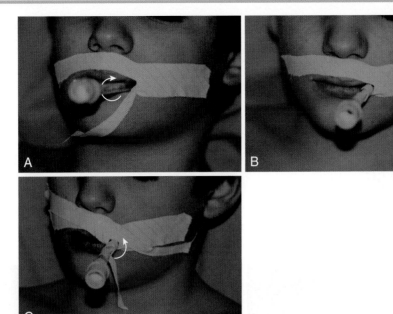

**FIGURE 12-16** Securing the endotracheal tube (ETT). After insertion of the oral ETT and examination for proper position, the area between the nose and upper lip and both cheeks is coated with tincture of benzoin. **A,** After the benzoin is dry, tape that has been split up the middle is applied to the cheek, and the ETT is placed at the division of the split tape. **B,** One half is wrapped circumferentially around the tube, and the other half is applied to the space above the upper lip. **C,** A second piece of tape is applied in similar fashion from the opposite direction. A nasal ETT may also be secured with this technique.

OD that is too large for the child's airway (no leak at >25 cm H₂O pressure or resistance at the time of insertion), changes in position during the procedure, a position other than supine, repeated attempts at intubation, traumatic intubation, patient age between 1 and 4 years, duration of surgery greater than 1 hour, coughing on the ETT, and previous history of croup.[171,172] Concurrent upper respiratory infection has been variously reported as a risk factor and as unrelated.[90,185]

Treatment of postintubation croup consists of nebulized epinephrine and dexamethasone. The rationale for this treatment is based primarily on experience with the treatment of infectious croup.[186-195] Caution should be exercised when translating treatments from one type of croup to another, because the two types of croup are not identical processes, and efficacy of the interventions for the treatment of postintubation croup has not been proved in controlled trials. Studies that examined the effect of dexamethasone given before extubation in children with prolonged intubation are conflicting.[196-199] Methylprednisolone given intramuscularly for the same indication has been reported to reduce postintubation stridor.[200]

### Laryngotracheal (Subglottic) Stenosis
Ninety percent of acquired subglottic stenoses are the result of tracheal intubation, particularly prolonged intubation (see Videos 12-1 and 12-2).[201-205] The incidence of subglottic stenosis after prolonged intubation in preterm neonates is reduced because the cricoid cartilage is relatively immature. At this age, the cartilage structure is hypercellular and the matrix has a large fluid content, making the structures more resilient and less susceptible to ischemic injury.[206]

The pathogenesis of acquired subglottic stenosis is ischemic injury secondary to lateral wall pressure from the ETT. Ischemia results in edema, necrosis, and ulcerations of the mucosa. Secondary infection results in exposure of the cartilage. Within

48 hours, granulation tissue begins to form within these ulcerations. Ultimately, scar tissue forms, resulting in narrowing of the airway (Fig. 12-17).[207-209] Specimens obtained from partial cricotracheal resection in children were found to have severe and sclerotic scarring with squamous metaplasia of the epithelium, loss of glands and elastic mantle fibers (tunica elastica), and dilation of the remaining glands with formation of cysts.[210] Also, the cricoid cartilage was affected on the internal and external side, with irreversible loss of perichondrium on the inside and resorption by macrophages of cartilage on both sides.[194]

Factors that predispose to subglottic stenosis include use of an ETT that is too large, laryngeal trauma (e.g., traumatic intubation, chemical or thermal inhalation, external trauma, surgical trauma, gastric reflux),[211-213] prolonged intubation (particularly greater than 25 days), repeated intubation, sepsis and infection, chronic illness, and chronic inflammatory disease.[204,214,215]

### LARYNGEAL MASK AIRWAY
The LMA has become a standard alternative for airway management during general anesthesia.[216-221] A variety of types have been introduced into practice since the development of the original LMA, which is now called the LMA Classic (Fig. 12-18). These include the disposable LMA Unique, the ProSeal LMA (PLMA, described later), the Flexible LMA, the LMA Supreme (discussed later), and the intubating LMA Fastrach. The Fastrach is available in sizes 3, 4, and 5 and has been described for use in children who weigh more than 40 kg.[222] The LMA Classic is made of medical-grade silicone and consists of a large-bore tubular structure (barrel) that has a 15-mm adapter at its proximal end and an elliptical, mask-like device that fits over the laryngeal inlet at its distal end. All masks are inflated by means of a valved pilot tube and balloon. The LMA Classic and the PLMA can be sterilized for reuse up to 40 times. The LMA Classic is available in eight sizes. Guidelines for selecting the appropriate mask for

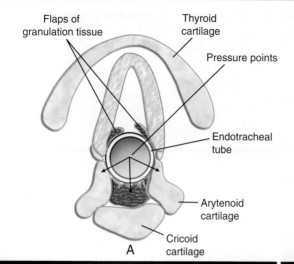

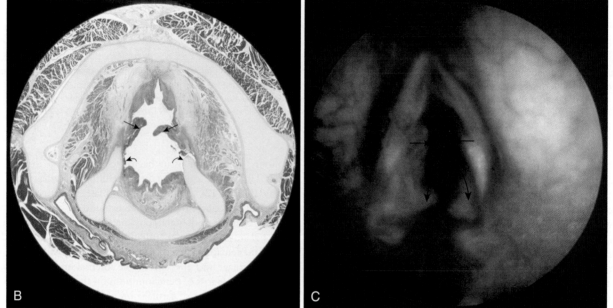

**FIGURE 12-17** The pathogenesis of intubation injuries. **A,** Schemata of a cross section through the glottis. Pressure necrosis causes ulcerations at the vocal processes of the arytenoids with exposed cartilage. Flaps of granulation tissue are present anterior to these ulcerations. **B,** Cross section of the glottis at this same level; *straight arrows* indicate flaps of granulation tissue, and *curved arrows* indicate the absence of mucosa and ulcerations with exposed cartilage on the vocal processes of the arytenoids. **C,** Intubation injury to a 2-month-old infant; *straight arrows* indicate granulation tissue, and *curved arrows* indicate area of ulcerations (*white area*). The most severe area of injury is usually at the level of the cricoid cartilage, resulting in subglottic stenosis. (Reproduced with permission from Holinger LD, Lusk RP, Green CG. Pediatric laryngology and bronchoesophagology. Philadelphia: Lippincott-Raven; 1997.)

children are based on weight (Table 12-4). A number of other manufacturers have developed similar devices; however, there is a dearth of comparative data available for children.

The LMA has been used for many different surgeries.[223] Some suggest that an LMA can be used for any case in which spontaneous ventilation is appropriate or any case that might reasonably be managed by face mask. Advantages of the LMA over the facemask are that it frees the anesthesiologist's hands for other tasks and that it may be associated with less operating room pollution compared with mask ventilation.[224,225] The use of controlled ventilation with the LMA Classic has also been described.[226,227] However, this practice is more controversial than its use in spontaneously breathing children because of the risk of insufflation of ventilated gas into the stomach and resultant regurgitation.[228-230] Insufflation of gas into the stomach is more likely if high ventilating pressures are used or required (i.e.,

pressures greater than the pressure that produces an audible air leak).[226,231] Clinically undetected LMA Classic malpositioning has been reported to be a significant risk factor for gastric air insufflation in children between 3 and 11 years of age undergoing positive-pressure ventilation, especially at peak inspiratory pressures greater than 17 cm $H_2O$.[232] Controlled ventilation with an LMA (with or without neuromuscular blockade) is easily accomplished when there is a relatively good seal and lung inflating pressures are less than about 17 cm $H_2O$.

The PLMA was designed to improve sealing pressures and to provide a conduit for evacuation of stomach contents; these features make it more appealing for use with positive-pressure ventilation. In sizes 3 and larger, there is a second dorsal cuff to increase the seal pressure of the glottic mask. The dorsal and ventral cuffs communicate, allowing simultaneous inflation by a single pilot balloon. In the smaller sizes, there is no second dorsal

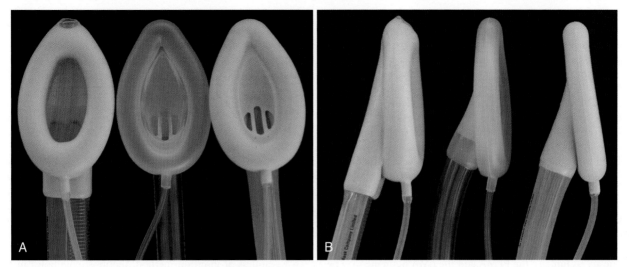

**FIGURE 12-18** Three types of laryngeal mask airway (LMA) are available in pediatric sizes: the reusable LMA Classic, the disposable LMA Unique, and the ProSeal LMA (PLMA). Displayed are pediatric size 2 LMAs of each type. **A,** The transparent material of the disposable LMA Unique (*center*) is medical-grade polyvinylchloride (PVC), whereas the reusable PLMA (*left*) and LMA Classic (*right*) are made of medical-grade silicone. Notice the differences in structure. The drainage tube outlet of the PLMA can be seen at the most distal tip of the cuff. The PLMA uses the drain tube to elevate the epiglottis away from the larynx, whereas the Classic and Unique have aperture bars. In contrast to the Classic and Unique LMAs, the PLMA cuff is softer, has a special shape, and has a deeper mask bowl. These features of the PLMA allow for improved sealing for positive-pressure ventilation. **B,** In profile, the distinct shape of the PLMA (*left*) can be appreciated. The dual-tube structure (drainage and airway lumens) creates a larger tube profile that incorporates a bite block and improves stability.

**TABLE 12-4** Size Selection and Recommended Cuff Volumes for the Laryngeal Mask Airway (LMA)

| Mask Size | Patient's Weight | Maximum Cuff Volume (mL) | Largest Endotracheal Tube (ID, mm), LMA Classic | Largest Endotracheal Tube (ID, mm), LMA Unique* | Largest Endotracheal Tube (ID, mm), ProSeal LMA* |
|---|---|---|---|---|---|
| 1 | Neonate/infants up to 5 kg | 4 | 3.5 | 3.5 | N/A |
| 1.5 | Infants 5-10 kg | 7 | 4.0 | 4.0 | 4.0, some manufacturers 3.5 |
| 2 | Infants/children 10-20 kg | 10 | 4.5 | 4.5 | 4.0 |
| 2.5 | Children 20-30 kg | 14 | 5.0 | 5 | 4.5 |
| 3 | Children/small adults 30-50 kg | 20 | 6.0, cuffed | 5.0, cuffed | 5.0 |
| 4 | Adolescents/adults 50-70 kg | 30 | 6.0, cuffed | 5.5, cuffed | 5.0, cuffed |
| 5 | Large adolescents/adults 70-100 kg | 40 | 7.0, cuffed | 6.0, cuffed | 6.0, cuffed |
| 6 | Anyone >100 kg | 50 | 7.0 cuffed | N/A | N/A |

*ID,* Inner diameter; *LMA,* laryngeal mask airway; *N/A,* not applicable.
*These sizes differ from the manufacturers' recommendations but have been found by the authors to be the better alternatives to ensure easy passage of the endotracheal tube through the LMA. In some cases the tubes listed are smaller; in some cases a cuffed alternative is given as an option rather than an uncuffed tube.

cuff but the profile of the mask has been altered to improve sealing. The PLMA is reported to be easy to insert, to allow greater airway pressures with positive-pressure ventilation, and to provide better protection against gastric insufflation.[233,234] A number of studies support the efficacy of the PLMA for use in children for both spontaneous and controlled ventilation.[234-238] In children, the PLMA is reported to be similar to the LMA Classic in ease of insertion, confirmation of proper position by fiberoptic visualization, and frequency of mucosal trauma. The advantage is that oropharyngeal leak pressure is greater and gastric insufflation is less common with the PLMA.[234,236,238] In children, the ability to provide pressure support ventilation with the PLMA during anesthesia also improves gas exchange and reduces WOB compared with the application of CPAP.[239,240] The greater sealing pressure may also protect against aspiration, as was reported in a 5-year-old child after inguinal hernia repair.[241]

Pediatric gastroscopy is reported to be quicker and to involve fewer airway complications when performed around the PLMA compared with nasal cannulas and with a conventional approach utilizing an anesthetic technique in which children breathed a sevoflurane-air-oxygen mixture spontaneously with 1-mg/kg IV boluses of propofol.[242]

Flexible diagnostic and therapeutic bronchoscopy, radiation therapy, radiologic procedures, ear/nose/throat surgeries, and ophthalmologic procedures are the most commonly described pediatric indications for the LMA.[221,223,243-246] An advantage of the LMA for securing the airway in ophthalmologic surgery is that it is associated with no increase in intraocular pressure, in contrast to endotracheal intubation.[247] The advantage of the LMA for diagnostic and therapeutic flexible bronchoscopy is that it provides a conduit for oxygenation and ventilation while allowing a larger bronchoscope to be used than can be passed through an age-appropriate ETT.[244,245,248,249] It also allows visualization and evaluation of the laryngeal structures. Some LMAs may provide better bronchoscopic conditions than others due to their material or preconfigured shape.[250] For children requiring frequent anesthesias over a short period, as in radiation therapy, the LMA provides a secure airway without the trauma of repeated intubation.[221] The LMA has also been advocated for use in place of intubation in children who are at increased risk for bronchial airway reactivity (e.g., upper respiratory tract infection, history of reactive airway disease).[251-254] However, caution is required in children with an upper respiratory tract infection because the risk of laryngospasm remains substantive.

The LMA has also become an important tool in the management of the DA, particularly in neonates (see later discussion) (Video 12-6). However, it should be noted that the LMA is an SGA device and, as such, does not reliably protect against pulmonary aspiration of gastric contents.[228-230] Because of their gastric access lumens, the PLMA and the LMA Supreme may be better alternatives in this setting, but formal study in children has not been done.[255]

The recommended insertion technique for the LMA is the same for children as for adults (see Video 12-6). The correct technique mimics deglutition or swallowing of food.[256] The cuff is completely deflated, and the posterior surface of the mask is well lubricated. These actions mimic lubrication of a food bolus with saliva and formation of a soft, flattened, wedge-shaped bolus. The child is placed in the age-appropriate intubating position. Induction may proceed by inhalation of halothane or sevoflurane or by IV propofol (3 to 5 mg/kg).[223,257] The nondominant hand is used to extend the head and flex the neck (sniffing position). This head position mimics the elevation of the larynx, neck flexion, and head extension that occurs with swallowing. The LMA is inserted with the mask aperture facing anteriorly (toward the tongue). The index finger of the insertion hand should be placed in the cleft between the mask and the barrel. With the index finger, the LMA is pushed upward and backward, toward the top of the child's head. This flattens the mask against the palate. Continued backward pressure (toward the top of the child's head) guides the LMA along the palate and down into the upper esophageal sphincter. It is essential that pressure be applied to force the LMA against the roof of the mouth. The mask is advanced along the palate until some resistance is felt. These actions mimic the propulsion of a food bolus into the hypopharynx caused by tongue pressure, first upward and backward, then downward in an arc. When resistance is felt, air is injected into the mask cuff (see Table 12-4 for size recommendations and maximum recommended inflation volumes).

Inflation of the cuff causes the end of the airway to move out of the mouth about 1 cm and forms a loose seal around the esophageal inlet, thereby directing gas flow into the trachea. *If no outward movement is observed with inflation of the mask, the LMA may not be properly positioned.* Proper position can be ascertained further by auscultation of breath sounds, movement of the anesthesia bag, measure of expired $CO_2$, the ability to provide gentle assisted ventilation, and, if necessary, by direct visualization with rigid or fiberoptic laryngoscopy. If the lungs cannot be gently ventilated (peak airway pressure <20 cm $H_2O$) or no breath sounds are heard, the LMA must be immediately removed because it has not been properly positioned, or the child's airway might be obstructed. After proper placement is confirmed, the LMA may be secured with tape and a soft bite block (e.g., a rolled gauze) inserted.

Several reports claim that when the traditional insertion technique is used in children, the LMA frequently hangs up in the posterior pharynx, making proper positioning difficult.[258,259] Therefore, other insertion techniques have been described. The rotational or reverse technique for children has been advocated to be simpler and more successful than the traditional placement technique.[260] The LMA is placed in the mouth with the cuff facing the hard palate (the opposite of the traditional technique). It is then advanced and rotated into position simultaneously (Video 12-7).[258,259,261] A partial mask inflation technique has also been advocated as more successful than the traditional (mask deflated) technique.[261-264] The LMA is left partially inflated to smooth the edges of the mask and then is inserted in the usual manner,[262,263] or in a lateral manner and then rotated and advanced,[264] or with a complete 180-degree rotation.[261] For placement of the PLMA, the rotational technique was found to have no advantage over the standard technique in children.[265] A jaw thrust maneuver and the use of a rigid laryngoscope have also been advocated to assist in placement of the LMA Classic.[266]

Regardless of insertion method, the most common cause of failure is use of a wrong size LMA. An LMA that is too large will not pass beyond the posterior pharynx. An LMA that is too small will pass easily but may not seal against the laryngeal inlet. Another common mistake when using the traditional insertion method is to try to press the LMA *down* into the pharynx. Pressure should be directed *back,* toward the pharyngeal wall, so that the airway will follow the natural curve of the pharynx and seat correctly in the esophageal sphincter without kinking. Attempting to place the LMA when the child is inadequately anesthetized may make advancement impossible or result in laryngospasm.

LMA use can result in injuries to upper airway structures[267-269] and in damage to the recurrent laryngeal[270] or the hypoglossal nerves.[271] The incidence of sore throat may be equal to or greater than that seen with tracheal intubation.[272-274] LMA use in infants requires special caution. A review of the use of the size 1 LMA in 50 infants found that the LMA sometimes migrated over time, even after apparent correct initial placement; delayed airway obstruction occurred in 12 infants after apparent successful placement.[275] Vigilance is required to prevent loss of the airway.

LMA placement has been used successfully for neonatal resuscitation[276-278]; it may be an easier skill to acquire than bag-and-mask ventilation.[279,280] Given the recent recognition[280a] that chest compressions are the most important factor in successful outcomes after cardiac arrest and the need to avoid interrupting compressions during cardiopulmonary resuscitation, the LMA may assume a greater role in airway management in cardiac arrest in the neonate. The LMA has also been used to deliver surfactant to neonates with respiratory distress syndrome,[281] for longer-term intensive care management of neonates with DAs,[282-284] and for intrahospital transport of neonates with DAs.[285]

The LMA Fastrach was specifically designed to allow the blind passage of an ETT in an emergent situation in which direct laryngoscopy is not possible or in patients with cervical spine immobilization.[178,286-288] This is a rigid device with a fixed angulation designed primarily for adults (available in sizes 3, 4, and 5). It requires special, flexible ETTs with an ID of 6.0 to 8.0 mm.

The timing for removal of the LMA in children is controversial. Experts have advocated both "awake" and "deep" removal.[289-294] Awake removal ensures return of protective reflexes but with the attendant problems of airway reactivity. Deep removal avoids excessive airway reactivity and potential laryngospasm but may increase the risk of aspiration or airway obstruction (or both) as the child emerges from anesthesia later in the recovery room. One author suggested leaving the cuff inflated until the child

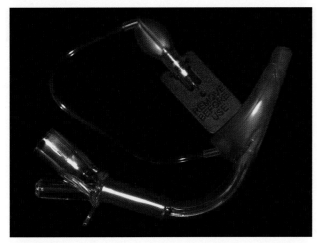

**FIGURE 12-19** The LMA Supreme offers the advantages of a built-in suction port and a built-in bite block. This design may be particularly useful for tonsillectomy, because the ventilating tube is molded in a caudad direction and the bite block offers protection against distortion by a mouth gag or the child's biting on it during emergence.

| TABLE 12-5 | Size Selection and Recommended Cuff Volumes for the Laryngeal Tube | | |
|---|---|---|---|
| **Tube Size** | **Body Size** | **Recommended Cuff Volume (mL)** | **Connector Color** |
| 0 Newborn | <5 kg | 10 | Clear |
| 1 Infants | 5-12 kg | 20 | White |
| 2 Children | 12-25 kg | 35 | Green |
| 3 Adults: small | <155 cm | 60 | Yellow |
| 4 Adults: medium | 155-180 cm | 80 | Red |
| 5 Adults: large | >180 cm | 90 | Purple |

begins swallowing or is able to open the mouth on command as a means for reducing the potential for laryngospasm. The proposed mechanism is that secretions are swept away from the larynx, reducing the stimulus for larygospasm.[294] Lubrication of the cuff with 2% lidocaine jelly or the addition of an intravenously administered opioid to the anesthetic may reduce coughing and laryngeal stimulation on emergence.[262]

The LMA Supreme is a single-use, curved laryngeal mask with an elliptical airway tube and an integrated drain tube that extends to the tip of the mask bowl. The proximal end of the airway tube consists of a bite block, which should lie between the teeth when the mask is properly positioned. A fixation tab allows the mask to be secured to the face. The deflated mask is held at the fixation tab and is inserted along the palate into the pharynx in a fashion similar to that used for the LMA Classic. Once in place, the cuff is inflated and the mask position is confirmed to be appropriate with the use of simple confirmatory tests (Fig. 12-19). An appropriately positioned mask forms a leak-free seal with the glottis, and the mask tip is embedded in the upper esophageal sphincter. A simple test to confirm the position of the mask is the suprasternal notch test, wherein a small amount of water-soluble lubricant is applied to the drain tube of the airway. Application of slight pressure in the suprasternal notch should result in a slight up-and-down movement of the applied lubricant on the drain tube. This confirms that the drain tube is contiguous with and adequately sealed in the upper esophageal sphincter. The ability to easily place a gastric tube through the drain tube further confirms correct positioning of the airway. Suction should not be applied to the gastric tube until it has been advanced into the stomach; this prevents collapse of the drain tube and potential injury to the upper esophageal sphincter. The LMA Supreme is now available in all pediatric sizes. A study comparing the LMA Supreme with the PLMA and the Classic LMAs in a neonatal manikin model demonstrated higher inflation pressures and shorter insertion times with the LMA Supreme.[295] Although the LMA Supreme has been found to be effective in adult populations,[296-299] there are currently no human evaluations of the pediatric sizes.

## OTHER SUPRAGLOTTIC AIRWAY DEVICES

Many other manufacturers have created their own versions of a SGA device similar to the LMA Classic. Some of these devices have design features that make them better conduits for tracheal intubation than the LMA Classic. Some have larger-diameter airway tubes that allow passage of larger (and cuffed) ETTs, lack glottic aperture bars (which can impede ETT advancement during an intubation attempt), and shorter airway tubes. Some devices also offer advantages in terms of cost.[300-302] Those SGAs that have a different design and different mechanism for maintaining the airway are discussed next.

### The Laryngeal Tube

The Laryngeal Tube (LT; VBM Medizintechnik GmbH, Sulz, Germany) is designed to secure a patent airway during either spontaneous breathing or controlled ventilation. This device is available with a single lumen for ventilation only or with a double-lumen tube that also allows suction of gastric contents. This system seals the esophagus at the distal end with a small cuff attached at the tip (distal cuff), and a larger balloon cuff at the middle part of the tube (proximal cuff) stabilizes the device and blocks the oropharynx and nasopharynx. The two openings that lie between the cuffs are positioned so that the more distal opening faces the glottis. The cuffs are inflated through a single pilot tube and balloon, through which cuff pressure can be monitored. There are three black lines on the tube, near a standard 15-mm connector, that indicate adequate depth of insertion when aligned with the teeth. The nondisposable device is made of silicone (latex free) and is reusable up to 50 times after sterilization in an autoclave. There are four variations: (1) standard single-lumen, reusable (LT); (2) single-lumen, disposable (LT-D); (3) double-lumen with drain tube, reusable (LT-suction II, or LTS II); and (4) double-lumen with drain tube, disposable (LTS-D) (E-Fig. 12-1).[303] It is available in six sizes, suitable for neonates up to large adults (Table 12-5).

The LT should be inserted while the child's head and neck are placed in the sniffing or neutral position. The tip of a well-lubricated LT is placed against the hard palate behind the upper incisors. The device is then slid down the center of the mouth until resistance is felt or the device is almost fully inserted. After connection to the anesthesia circuit, proper placement is confirmed by assessing ease of ventilation. Some adjustment (usually slight withdrawal) may be required to provide optimal ease of ventilation. Care should be taken not to push the tongue backward into the posterior pharynx. Ease of insertion of the standard LT is reported to be comparable to that of the LMA Classic, although the LT may require more readjustments of its position to obtain a clear airway.[304,305] The incidence of complications with the two devices appears to be similar.[304] The LT may provide a better seal than the Classic LMA.[306] Compared with the PLMA, the LT may be less effective and more difficult to insert.[307-309]

Although the LT-suction device may have similar success to the PLMA,[310] there are scant data in children.[311-316] An initial report of its use in children ages 2 to 12 years found a successful placement rate of 96% (77/80 children). Complications occurred in two children; one had laryngospasm that resolved with deepening of the anesthetic, and the other complained of mild difficulty with swallowing postoperatively.[312] A study comparing the LT with the LMA found it to be less effective for either spontaneous or assisted ventilation and for fiberoptic evaluation of the airway in children younger than 10 years of age.[311] A study of 70 children using sizes 0 to 3 reported failure to place the LT in 12% of children. Failures were caused by inability to ventilate, hypoxemia, gastric insufflation, cough, and laryngospasm or stridor, particularly for children weighing less than 10 kg; therefore, the LT was not recommended for children of this size.[313] Although the manufacturer states that a flexible fiberoptic bronchoscope (FOB) may be passed through the device, the openings are of insufficient size to permit passage of an ETT.

### The Cobra Perilaryngeal Airway

The Cobra Perilaryngeal Airway (CobraPLA; Engineered Medical Systems, Indianapolis, Ind.) is a disposable SGA that is marketed for the same indications as the LMA Classic but creates a seal more cephalad in the hypopharynx using a cylindrical inflatable cuff. The distal end of the device sits over the larynx, but the distal end is not inflatable (E-Fig. 12-2).[301,317,318] An initial report comparing the CobraPLA with the LMA Classic found that insertion time, airway adequacy, and number of repositioning attempts were similar. Peak airway sealing pressure was significantly greater with the CobraPLA; the authors concluded that the CobraPLA has better airway sealing capabilities than the LMA Classic.[319] A more recent group of investigators studying the CobraPLA in adults raised concerns about both the design and the safety of this device, particularly during controlled ventilation. After studying 29 patients, investigations were suspended and later stopped after two cases of significant pulmonary aspiration occurred in patients while using the CobraPLA.[320] The device is available in eight sizes and can be used in infants as small as 2.5 kg (Table 12-6).[317] The distal grill has a long center slit that is specifically designed to allow passage of a fiberoptic bronchoscope (FOB) and ETT (the size 0.5 neonate CobraPLA allows easy passage of a 3.5 uncuffed ETT). In a pediatric study, the orientation of the larynx as viewed through the CobraPLA using video was obtained in 45 infants and children. An acceptable view of the airway was obtained in all subjects, but the laryngeal view was almost obstructed or completely obstructed by the folding of the epiglottis over the glottic opening in 77% of children weighing less than 10 kg. (A similar problem was encountered in approximately 80% of children managed with the LMA Classic as well.[321]) The investigators suggested extra vigilance to prevent airway obstruction in small children. Also, because the grill bars of the CobraPLA were closely apposed to the epiglottis and supraglottic structures in almost all subjects, it was suggested that removal of the device in a deeper plane of anesthesia may minimize laryngeal stimulation. Further study of this device in children, particularly infants, is needed to define its role compared with the LMA.[322-324]

### The i-gel

The i-gel SGA (Intersurgical, Liverpool, N.Y.) consists of a dual-channeled, noninflatable laryngeal mask made from a gel-like thermoplastic elastomer (Fig. 12-20). It has a built-in bite block and is available in sizes 1, 1.5, 2, 3, 4, and 5 (Table 12-7). One

**TABLE 12-6** Suggested CobraPLA Size, Weight, Cuff Volume, and Endotracheal Tube Sizes

| Size | Patient Weight (kg) | Cuff Volume (mL) | Inner Diameter (ID, mm) | Maximal Size of Endotracheal Tube (mm ID) |
|---|---|---|---|---|
| 0.5 | >2.5 | <8 | 5.0 | 3.0 |
| 1 | >5 | <10 | 6.0 | 4.5 |
| 1.5 | >10 | <25 | 6.0 | 4.5 |
| 2 | >15 | <40 | 10.5 | 6.5 |
| 3 | >35 | <65 | 10.5 | 6.5 |
| 4 | >70 | <70 | 12.5 | 8.0 |
| 5 | >100 | <85 | 12.5 | 8.0 |
| 6 | >130 | <85 | 12.5 | 8.0 |

**TABLE 12-7** Suggested i-gel Supraglottic Device Size, Inner Diameter, Endotracheal Tube Size, and Nasogastric Tube Size

| Size | Patient Weight (kg) | ID (mm) | Maximal Size of Endotracheal Tube (mm ID)* | Maximal Size of Nasogastric Tube (French) |
|---|---|---|---|---|
| 1 | 2-5 | 5.6 | 3 | |
| 1.5 | 5-12 | 6.8 | 4 | 10 |
| 2 | 10-25 | 8.8 | 5 | 12 |
| 2.5 | 25-35 | 10.2 | 5 | 12 |
| 3 | 30-60 | 11.2 | 6 | 12 |
| 4 | 50-90 | 12.3 | 7 | 12 |
| 5 | >90 | 12.5 | 8 | 14 |

ID, Inner diameter.
*May depend on outer diameter specifications of endotracheal tube manufacturer.

channel functions as the airway tube while the second channel exits at the tip of the device and provides gastric access when seated properly. The lubricated posterior surface of the i-gel is inserted along the palate into the posterior pharynx. An observational study in 50 children reported easy insertion in all patients with a mean leak pressure of 25 cm $H_2O$; gastric access was successfully obtained in all children.[325] A study that compared the i-gel to the Ambu AuraOnce laryngeal mask (Ambu, Glen Burnie, Md.) showed higher leak pressures and longer insertion times with the i-gel. The authors noted a tendency for the i-gel to slide out and recommended taping to prevent dislodgment intraoperatively.[326]

### Summary

A variety of SGAs are currently available. Some are imitators of the LMA Classic but available at a reduced cost, whereas others are completely new designs. There are many new devices with various designs to assist in the management of normal and DAs in children, but there are insufficient data to clearly state that one device or one manufacturer is superior to another.

## Airway Management: The Abnormal Airway

### CLASSIFYING THE ABNORMAL PEDIATRIC AIRWAY

It is important to recognize circumstances that may cause airway obstruction or difficult laryngoscopy. Conditions that predispose

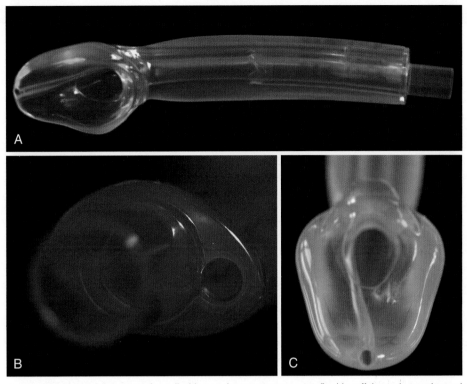

**FIGURE 12-20** The i-gel supraglottic device (**A**) consists of a malleable non–latex-containing, noninflatable cuff that is designed to seal over the laryngeal inlet after insertion. The stem of the i-gel contains a "buccal cavity stabilizer" which is designed to resist accidental rotation after insertion and is made from a hard polymer that resists biting. The i-gel also contains a gastric suction channel next to the 15-mm connector (**B**), with which practitioners may evacuate gastric contents when the device is in the correct inserted position. **C,** The distal position of the suction port.

to airway problems may be grouped according to anatomic location and may result from congenital, inflammatory, traumatic, metabolic, or neoplastic disorders. Tables 12-8 and 12-9 list the more common pediatric airway problems according to anatomic location. E-Appendix 12-1 lists the more common pediatric syndromes and associated anesthetic considerations; more complete information may be obtained elsewhere.[327-330]

## MANAGEMENT PRINCIPLES

For any laryngoscopy, but especially for a DA, the proper array of equipment must always be available. We advocate the creation of a DA cart stocked with equipment useful in the management of the DA for children of all sizes and ages. Suggestions for contents are listed in Table 12-10. The approach to a DA, as described earlier, must include a careful history and physical examination and, when indicated, radiologic evaluation. In the past, lateral neck xerograms have been useful in delineating anatomic aberrations; however, ultrasound, MRI, and CT imaging have replaced this modality.[97-99,101-112,120,331-336] In addition to the airway pathology, the pathophysiology of the congenital syndrome or associated disease process must be fully evaluated.

The safest approach to managing a DA is to formulate a plan that includes several contingencies for failure or loss of the airway and to have skilled help available, especially a surgeon who is experienced in performing pediatric bronchoscopy and tracheostomy. To maximize success and safety, a skilled assistant should help to position the child, facilitate airway management, and observe the monitors and the child's vital signs. To direct an assistant, there should be clear communication about the airway management plan and specific details about maneuvers needed

to facilitate the process. Familiarity with DA algorithms and DA management reviews can help the practitioner formulate a reasonable plan and ensure that no viable management options are missed.[337-343]

Certain principles apply to the care of any child in whom difficulty with airway management is anticipated. In most circumstances, an awake or mildly sedated approach would be the primary management strategy for the anticipated DA if airway concerns were considered in isolation. However, often the practitioner who is caring for a child is restricted from choosing an awake approach because of difficulty obtaining the child's cooperation. Assisted spontaneous ventilation during general anesthesia is the preferred technique when abnormal airway anatomy is present and difficulty with patient cooperation is anticipated; it provides adequate oxygenation while the airway is evaluated for the appropriate approach to tracheal intubation. Therefore, the first choice for management of a potential DA, whether the child is sedated or under general anesthesia, is to *maintain spontaneous ventilation.*[338,343] There are two reasons for maintaining spontaneous gas exchange. First, neuromuscular blockade may result in total airway obstruction due to loss of tone of the tongue, pharyngeal and laryngeal muscles, and suspensory ligaments. This obstruction may not be easily alleviated with manual ventilation of the lungs. Neuromuscular blockade should not be used if airway obstruction or the potential for airway obstruction exists.[34] Second, if a child is paralyzed, the loss of spontaneous breath sounds eliminates a valuable guide to locating the glottis. For example, in children with craniofacial anomalies or cervical burn contractures, one may be able to visualize only the tip of the epiglottis with standard rigid laryngoscopy. In such cases, if specialized airway management equipment is unavailable, shaping

**TABLE 12-8** Pediatric Airway Pathology Related to Anatomic Site

| Anatomic Site | Etiology | Clinical Condition |
|---|---|---|
| Nasopharynx | Congenital | Choanal atresia, stenosis,[26,27,576-578] encephalocele[579-584] |
| | Traumatic | Foreign body, trauma[585-587] |
| | Inflammatory | Adenoidal hypertrophy,[585,588] nasal congestion[28] |
| | Neoplastic | Teratoma[589-591] |
| Tongue | Congenital | Hemangioma, Down syndrome |
| | Traumatic | Burn, laceration, lymphatic/venous obstruction[114,115,585,592-597] |
| | Metabolic | Beckwith-Wiedemann syndrome,[504,598-603] hypothyroidism, mucopolysaccharidosis,[541,604-621] glycogen storage disease,[622-630] gangliosidosis,[631-634] congenital hypothyroidism |
| | Neoplastic | Cystic hygroma,[635-637] cystic teratoma |
| Mandible/ maxilla | Congenital hypoplasia | Pierre Robin syndrome,[413,488,490,517,638-651] Treacher Collins syndrome,[356,489,505,652-663] Goldenhar syndrome,[336,409,530,664-670] Apert syndrome, achondroplasia,[492,671-675] Turner syndrome,[676-679] Cornelia de Lange syndrome,[680-682] Smith-Lemli-Opitz syndrome,[683-686] Hallermann-Streiff syndrome,[687] Crouzon syndrome[688] |
| | Traumatic | Fracture,[689] neck burn with contractures[597,690] |
| | Inflammatory | Juvenile rheumatoid arthritis[691-697] |
| | Neoplastic | Tumors, cherubism[698,699] |
| Pharynx/ larynx | Congenital | Laryngomalacia (infantile larynx) (see Video 12-1),[585,700,701] Freeman-Sheldon syndrome (whistling face),[702-713] laryngeal stenosis,[585,714] laryngocele,[700] laryngeal web,[700,715-717] hemangioma[718] |
| | Traumatic | Dislocated/fractured larynx,[585,719-726] foreign body,[46,47,585,727-735] inhalation injury (burn),[592-595,597,690,736] postintubation edema/granuloma/stenosis,[737-747] swelling of uvula,[114] soft palate trauma, epidermolysis bullosa[748-756] |
| | Inflammatory | Epiglottitis,[42-44,757-760] acute tonsillitis,[588] peritonsillar abscess,[761,762] retropharyngeal abscess, diphtheritic membrane, laryngeal polyposis[763-768] |
| | Metabolic | Hypocalcemic laryngospasm[39] |
| | Neoplastic | Tumors |
| | Neurologic | Vocal cord paralysis, Arnold-Chiari malformation[769-772] |
| Trachea | Congenital | Vascular ring,[48,49] tracheal stenosis or complete tracheal rings (Video 12-8), tracheomalacia (see Video 12-1)[700,714,747,773,774] |
| | Inflammatory | Laryngotracheobronchitis (viral),[41,44,45,185,775-777] bacterial tracheitis |
| | Neoplastic | Mediastinal tumors: neurofibroma,[778] paratracheal nodes (lymphoma) |

**TABLE 12-9** Cervical Spine Anomalies*

| Etiology | Clinical Condition |
|---|---|
| Congenital | Down syndrome,[779-785] Klippel-Feil malformation,[786] Goldenhar syndrome,[336,409,530,664-670] torticollis |
| Traumatic | Fracture, subluxation,[719-723,787] neck burn contracture |
| Inflammatory | Rheumatoid arthritis[691-697] |
| Metabolic | Mucopolysaccharidosis (Morquio syndrome)[604-619,788] |

*Abnormalities of the cervical spine may limit extension and flexion, thereby contributing to the difficulties of airway management; a significant percentage of infants with Down syndrome have atlantoaxial instability.[787]

the ETT tip into a 90-degree angle with a stylet (Fig. 12-21), placing the tip behind the epiglottis (or the center of the base of the tongue if the epiglottis is not visible), and then listening for breath sounds with the ear near the proximal end of the ETT often allows the practitioner to "blindly" locate the glottic opening and trachea.

If the child is able to cooperate while mildly sedated, there are several options for airway management. An opioid-benzodiazepine combination will blunt airway reactivity, decrease discomfort, and provide anxiolysis and amnesia. These combinations, particularly fentanyl and midazolam, are effective for sedation of adolescents and mature preteens.[344] Dosing is based on weight and is guided by clinical parameters, including preexisting medical conditions. However, benzodiazepine-opioid sedation may not suffice for a frightened young child, because the dose requirement for sedation may exceed the dose that causes apnea. Alternatively, ketamine, which provides both hypnosis and analgesia, may be used alone or in conjunction with midazolam.[344] Ketamine usually preserves adequate spontaneous ventilation and upper airway patency[345] while preventing laryngeal reactions to airway manipulation. Ketamine and midazolam should be slowly titrated to effect so as to avoid oversedation and apnea.[346] Midazolam takes almost 5 minutes to achieve peak electroencephalographic effects, necessitating adequate time between incremental doses (see Fig. 47-12).[347,348] Ketamine is usually titrated in doses of 0.25 to 0.5 mg/kg IV every 2 minutes. Although there is a large incidence of psychomimetic emergence reactions in adults, these reactions are less common in children, particularly if ketamine is combined with midazolam. Ketamine may increase secretions that enhance airway reactivity and interfere with video-based airway management. Antisialagogue administration may mitigate these effects. In addition, the anticholinergic effect of atropine or glycopyrrolate will blunt reflex bradycardia that can occur with airway manipulation. Dexmedetomidine may be administered as the sole sedating agent or combined with reduced doses of other sedatives or opioids to be effective for sedation while maintaining spontaneous respiration during fiberoptic intubation in adults and children.[349-356]

Topical anesthesia may be used in conjunction with sedation or general anesthesia to blunt airway reactivity in those children in whom spontaneous ventilation is preserved. Useful methods for providing topical anesthesia to the airway include (1) nebulized lidocaine; (2) topical application of local anesthetic sprays,

**TABLE 12-10**  Items to Consider for an Emergency Intubation Cart

| Drawer 1 | Lens paper |
|---|---|
| LMA Classic (disposable)—sizes 1, 1.5, 2, 2.5, 3, 4, 5 | Surgical lubricant |
| LMA ProSeal (disposable)—sizes 1.5, 2, 2.5, 3, 4, 5 | 2% Lidocaine jelly* |
| LMA Fastrach—sizes 3, 4, 5 | 4% Lidocaine solution* |
| ETTs for Fastrach—sizes (mm ID) 6, 6.5, 7, 7.5, 8 | Atomizer to spray topical lidocaine |
| ETT stabilizers for Fastrach | Suction catheters—sizes 8, 10, 14F |
| Size or weight charts for LMA | Yankauer suction tubes—pediatric and adult sizes |
| | Defogger |
| **Drawer 2** | Silicone spray |
| Transtracheal jet-ventilation catheters* (VBM)—infant (16 gauge), child (14 gauge), adult (13 gauge) | Halogen light bulb |
| | Disposable teeth guards |
| Emergency Transtracheal Airway Catheter (Cook) | |
| Magill forceps—adult and pediatric sizes | **Drawer 4** |
| Aillon tube bender | Facemasks—neonate, infant, toddler, child, adult (small/medium/large) |
| Miller blades—sizes 0, 1, 2, 3, 4 | Frie endoscopy mask—infant, child, adult |
| Macintosh blades—sizes 1, 2, 3, 4 | Bronchoscopy airways*—infant, child, adult |
| Phillips blades—sizes 1, 2 | Bite blocks—infant, child, adult |
| Wis-Hipple blades—sizes 1, 1.5 | Ovassapian airways (2) |
| Oxyscope blades—sizes 0, 1 (with oxygen tubing) | Nasal trumpets*—sizes 2 to 34F |
| Handles (medium and short) | Oral airways—sizes 90, 80, 70, 60, 50, 00, 000 |
| C batteries × 2 | |
| Oxygen Y-connector | **Drawer 5** |
| Albuterol adapters for metered-dose administration (3) | Ambu bag with reservoir |
| Syringes (5 each)—5 mL, 10 mL | Enk Oxygen Flow Modulation set (Cook) |
| Intravenous catheters, 10 of each commonly used sizes (24g, 22g, 20g, 18g, 16g)* | Jet ventilator |
| | Stylets—pediatric and adult |
| Swivel adapters (Portex, Sontex) | ETT exchange catheters with both Luer-Lok and 15-mm OD adapters—sizes (mm OD) 3, 4, 5, 7 |
| No. 3 straight connectors × 2 | Retrograde catheter with extra guidewire |
| **Drawer 3** | Extension cord with converter from Hubble to three-prong plug |
| Preparation forceps or tongue-grabbing forceps | Other equipment to consider: lighted stylets and optical stylets (see text). |
| Safety glasses | |

Modified from Department of Pediatric Anesthesiology. The difficult airway cart. Children's Memorial Hospital, Chicago.
*Cook*, Cook Critical Care, Bloomington, Ind.; *ETT*, endotracheal tube; *F*, French; *ID*, inner diameter; *LMA*, laryngeal mask airway, LMA North America, San Diego; *OD*, outer diameter; *VBM*, VBM Medizintechnik GmbH, Sulz, Germany.
*Items with outdates.

jellies, or ointments; (3) translaryngeal delivery of lidocaine (Video 12-9); (4) "spray as you go" with lidocaine injected onto the surface of the larynx and vocal cords through the channel of an FOB usually used for suctioning or administering oxygen; and (5) superior laryngeal nerve block.[344] Caution is required to avoid delivering a toxic dose of local anesthetic. Maximum doses of the local anesthetic are based on the patient's weight and should be calculated in advance (see Table 41-2). Lidocaine seems to have the best safety profile; we limit our maximum dose to 5 mg/kg. We do not recommend the use of benzocaine (Cetacaine) local anesthetic spray in children weighing less than 40 kg, because it is associated with methemoglobinemia, and it is difficult to titrate or limit the administered dose.[88,357]

Many techniques and devices for managing a DA have been recommended; these are reviewed in detail later. Previous experience in normal airways can render these devices valuable adjuncts in DA management.

*If one is unable to secure tracheal intubation, it is important to recognize the limits of one's ability. Do not hesitate to seek assistance from a colleague or request the surgeon to perform a tracheostomy or*

*bronchoscopy. As an alternative, the child can be awakened and referred to a major pediatric center. In an urgent, life-threatening situation, placement of an SGA device or percutaneous cricothyroidotomy can be lifesaving* (see "The Unexpected Difficult Intubation").[218,248,249,358,359]

### Documentation

Documentation of the DA and its management is essential to provide useful information for the next time that the child requires sedation or anesthesia. A note in the anesthesia record should clearly address the following issues:

1. Whether mask ventilation was attempted, and if so, whether there was any difficulty
2. Special maneuvers that were required for successful mask ventilation
3. Special maneuvers that were not helpful with mask ventilation
4. Any difficulty with tracheal intubation
5. Special techniques that were required for successful intubation
6. Special techniques that were not helpful for intubation

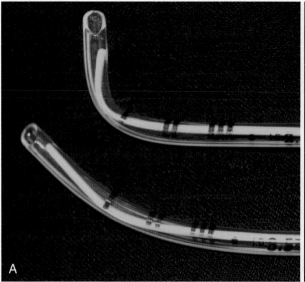

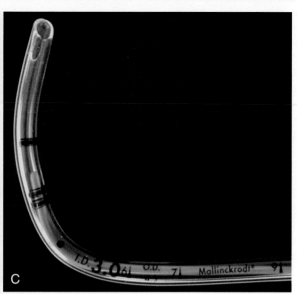

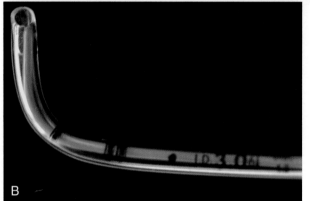

**FIGURE 12-21** A stylet placed within an endotracheal tube (ETT) often facilitates placement. **A,** The "hockey-stick" configuration. **B,** In children with midfacial hypoplasia syndromes, in which the anatomic relation of the base of the tongue to the laryngeal inlet is abnormal, a stylet with a 90-degree bend 1 to 2 cm from the tip allows placement of the ETT behind the epiglottis and at the laryngeal inlet. Breath sounds audible at the 15-mm connector confirm appropriate location. **C,** Maintaining the position of the stylet while advancing the ETT frequently allows successful "blind" endotracheal intubation around the base of the tongue even without the use of special airway equipment.

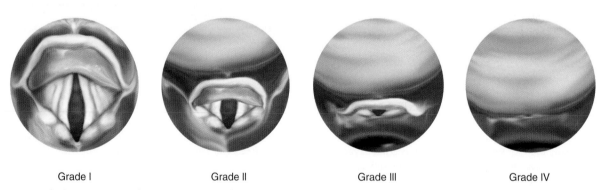

Grade I          Grade II          Grade III          Grade IV

**FIGURE 12-22** The laryngoscopic grading system of Cormack and Lehane offers a reasonable means of describing visualization of the larynx. It is useful to grade the degree of visualization during laryngoscopy and how that visualization was achieved (e.g., external cricoid pressure or laryngeal manipulation, the size and configuration of the laryngoscope blade). This provides useful information for the next person attempting laryngoscopy so that he or she has some degree of knowledge regarding what to expect. Grade I is visualization of the complete laryngeal opening; grade II, visualization of just the posterior area; grade III, visualization of just the epiglottis; and grade IV, visualization of just the soft palate. (Reproduced with permission from Cormack RS, Lehane J. Difficult tracheal intubation in obstetrics. Anaesthesia 1984;39:1105-11.)

7. Grade of laryngoscopic view of laryngeal structures during direct laryngoscopy (Fig. 12-22)

In addition to discussion with the family and the child (when age appropriate), a letter should be given to the family and child outlining the difficulties with the airway, describing how the airway was managed, and referring them to the MedicAlert Foundation registry.[320] This should be copied and circulated to the

medical record and to the MedicAlert registry. In the United States, the MedicAlert registry for difficult airway/difficult intubation can be reached by telephone at 1-888-633-4298. Similar registries are also being formed internationally.[360] The MedicAlert registration form asks for clinical details about the type of airway difficulty as well as which maneuvers were successful in management and which were not. Any practitioner who provides airway

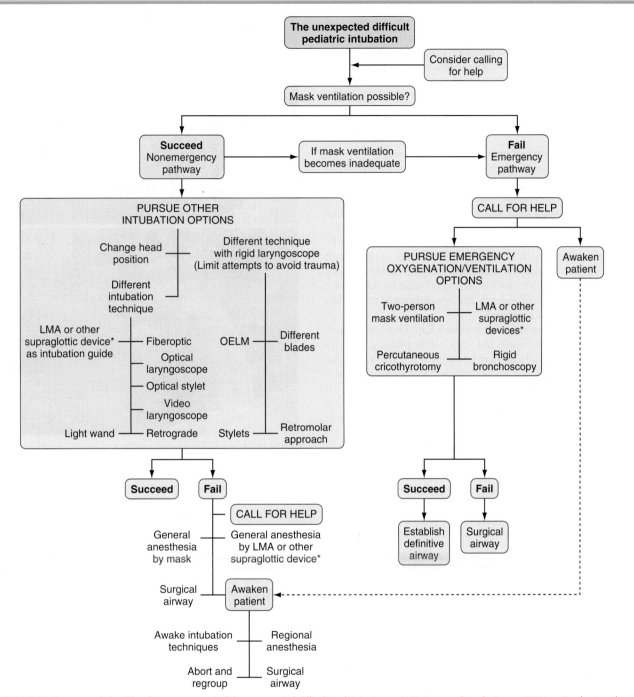

**FIGURE 12-23** A proposed algorithm for management of the unexpected difficult pediatric airway. *LMA*, Laryngeal mask airway; *OELM*, optimal external laryngeal manipulation; *PLMA*, ProSeal LMA. *Consider using PLMA if the child is at risk for aspiration or if high inflation pressures are needed. (Modified with permission from Wheeler M. Management strategies for the difficult pediatric airway. Anesth Clin North Am 1998;16:743-761.)

management to the registered patient can update this information at any time. Although scoring systems used in adults[83-87] have not been thoroughly investigated in all age groups,[88,361] it is useful to describe in detail the view of the larynx that was achieved and how it was achieved (e.g., blade type, size, external laryngeal manipulation).

### The Unexpected Difficult Intubation

With careful preoperative evaluation and planning, the unexpected pediatric DA should be a rare occurrence. However, the

practitioner should always be prepared for this potentially life-threatening event. Because the unexpected DA occurs after the anesthesia (plan A) has been initiated, many of the management decisions required for the anticipated DA have already been made. Of primary importance is maintaining adequate oxygenation while a definitive course of action is pursued (i.e., plan B, plan C, and so on). A reasonable decision tree, based on the DA algorithm of the American Society of Anesthesiologists (ASA), is presented in Figure 12-23. An important difference between infants and adults should be noted in this scenario.

Because infants have an increased metabolic rate and decreased functional residual capacity, the time between the loss of the airway and resultant hypoxemia with potential secondary neurologic injury is significantly diminished compared with adults.[362] In a mathematical model, the approximate time to zero oxygen saturation from an $FIO_2$ of 90% is 4 minutes in a 10-kg child, whereas the same process in a healthy 70-kg adult takes almost 10 minutes.[360,363]

### Extubation of the Child with the Difficult Airway

Preparation for extubation begins shortly after the airway is secured. Equipment used to secure the airway should be rechecked, quickly returned to functional status, and then left in the operating room until successful safe extubation. Children who had prolonged attempts at intubation or who will have procedures that may lead to airway edema may benefit from IV dexamethasone (0.5 to 1 mg/kg, up to 20 mg). If significant airway edema is suspected, consider leaving the child intubated postoperatively until it resolves. The child must be fully awake and have full return of strength and adequate ventilatory effort before extubation is attempted.

A Cook airway exchange catheter with Rapi-Fit adapter (Cook Critical Care, Bloomington, Ind.) is a hollow plastic guide with holes on its distal end that may be useful as a bridge to extubation because the adapter on its proximal end allows the placement of either a Luer-Lok connector for connection to a jet ventilator or a 15-mm adapter for connection to a standard anesthesia ventilating system (E-Fig. 12-3).[364-367] It is available in a variety of sizes to allow the exchange of ETTs with 3.0 mm ID or larger. This can be used for oxygenation and ventilation and as a guide to reinsertion of the ETT if the child's ventilatory efforts are inadequate or if airway obstruction occurs.[368] However, caution is required when using this device for jet ventilation, because significant barotrauma has been reported.[369,370]

An alternative to jet ventilation is the Enk Oxygen Flow Modulation set (Cook Critical Care), which allows flow from a standard low-pressure flow meter to be adjusted by occluding holes in the delivery system with the thumb and forefinger (E-Fig. 12-4, *A*). As a potential substitute for the Enk device, one could cut a side hole in the plastic oxygen delivery tubing to create a similar low-pressure oxygen delivery system (see E-Fig. 12-4, *B*). Pneumothorax, pneumomediastinum, and deaths have occurred when jet ventilation was used with an airway exchange catheter.[371] One report suggested that only insufflation or gentle manual ventilation should be used initially and that jet ventilation should be reserved for situations in which these techniques are ineffective. These authors also recommended that the optimal management was reintubation.[372]

If the child will remain intubated for a prolonged period of time after surgery, it is advisable to return the child to the operating room for extubation. A surgeon who is prepared to perform rigid bronchoscopy and tracheostomy and an anesthesiologist who is familiar with the techniques used for the previously successful airway management should be in attendance.

### SPECIAL TECHNIQUES FOR VENTILATION
#### Multi-handed Mask Ventilation Techniques

Multi-handed mask ventilation techniques can provide an effective temporizing measure until the airway is secured or the child is awakened. One person uses both hands to maintain an adequate mask fit, and a second person compresses the reservoir bag

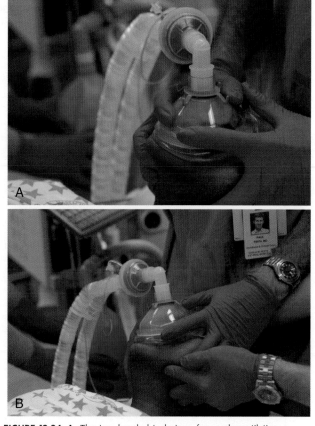

**FIGURE 12-24 A,** The two-handed technique for mask ventilation may be useful to improve mask fit and therefore ventilation when the traditional technique is inadequate. One person holds the mask while a second person squeezes the ventilation bag. **B,** Occasionally, a third person is required to perform a two-handed jaw thrust (see text for details).

(Fig. 12-24). This can also be accomplished by having a single provider use two hands on the mask while the anesthesia ventilator is activated.[373] Occasionally, a second person is required to perform a jaw thrust with one hand while compressing the anesthesia bag with the other. Rarely, a third person may be required to compress the anesthesia bag with two hands (in order to generate a greater peak inflation pressure) while the first person holds the mask with two hands and the second person performs a two-handed jaw thrust.[373]

#### Laryngeal Mask Airway

The LMA has revolutionized DA management in children. Numerous case reports and extensive clinical experience attest to the value of the LMA for establishing an airway when both ventilation and intubation are extremely difficult or impossible.[340,374-376] The LMA has been described as a tool for use in both the nonemergency pathway (cannot intubate, can ventilate) and the emergency pathway (cannot intubate, cannot ventilate [CICV]) of the ASA DA algorithm.[338,340] Use has been described in the awake child (LMA insertion in awake infants with Pierre Robin syndrome [Robin sequence])[377] (Video 12-10) and in the anesthetized child with a known or suspected DA. It can be used as the definitive airway in some circumstances, as a conduit for intubation, or as a temporizing airway while other options are pursued (e.g., a surgical airway). There are now many other SGA devices reported to be useful in the management of the child with a DA, but comparative studies in pediatrics are lacking.[255,378]

## Percutaneous Needle Cricothyroidotomy

In 1992, the American Heart Association changed its recommendations for emergency airway management to a percutaneous needle cricothyroidotomy over a surgical cricothyroidotomy because it was believed that the former entails less risk of injury to vital structures such as the carotid arteries or jugular veins, particularly in the hands of nonsurgical trained practitioners. In addition, most practitioners can more rapidly perform the percutaneous procedure. However, the cricothyroid membrane has a relatively small width in infants and children. Attempts at cricothyroidotomy may readily damage cricoid and thyroid cartilages, resulting in laryngeal stenosis and permanent damage to the speech mechanism. Therefore, this procedure should be reserved for use only under emergency circumstances.[379,380]

Because percutaneous needle cricothyroidotomy is rarely used, it is recommended that experience be gained with patient simulators or in animal models, because success in the hands of the inexperienced is not assured.[381,382] A schema of this procedure is presented in Figure 12-25. A commercial product called the Jet-Ventilation-Catheter (VBM) is available in three sizes: 16, 14, and 13 gauge. It consists of a slightly curved puncture needle within a Teflon, kink-resistant cannula nearly identical to an IV catheter (Fig. 12-26, *A*). This cannula has two lateral eyes at its distal end and a combined Luer-Lok and 15-mm adapter at its proximal end (see Fig. 12-26, *B*). It also has a fixation flange and foam neck tape to secure the airway.

*Percutaneous needle cricothyroidotomy provides only a means for oxygen insufflation and does not reliably provide adequate ventilation.* In the spontaneously breathing patient, simple delivery of intratracheal oxygen (1 to 2 L/min) may be sufficient in the short term, because hypercarbia is generally well tolerated by healthy children.[379,383,384] A number of children with arterial $CO_2$ values well above 150 mm Hg have survived neurologically intact when adequate oxygenation was maintained.[384] Therefore, simple oxygenation without attempts at ventilation may be all that is required to sustain life (Fig. 12-27). For the child without respiratory effort, there is a need to provide ventilation in addition to oxygenation. An Ambu bag with the pop-off disabled can provide limited ventilation through a percutaneous catheter, but these devices will be ineffective at standard pop-off pressures.[379,385] Extremely high ventilating pressures are required, but midtracheal pressures are significantly lower (10 to 16 cm $H_2O$).[379] A percutaneous cricothyroidotomy catheter can also be used with a jet ventilation system. Jet ventilation via a catheter passed through a narrow glottic opening has been described.[386-389]

If upper airway obstruction is present (e.g., after multiple unsuccessful attempts at rigid laryngoscopy), there will be a limited pathway for the egress of air and oxygen, and barotrauma may result from insufflation of oxygen or attempts at ventilation. Very serious morbidity and mortality may result from massive subcutaneous emphysema or tension pneumothorax.[390,391] Therefore, jet ventilation must be used with extreme caution in infants and children.[392]

Another IV catheter–type emergency airway device is the Emergency Transtracheal Airway Catheter (Cook Critical Care), which consists of a 6-F reinforced catheter that is advanced over a 15-gauge needle similar to the devices described earlier

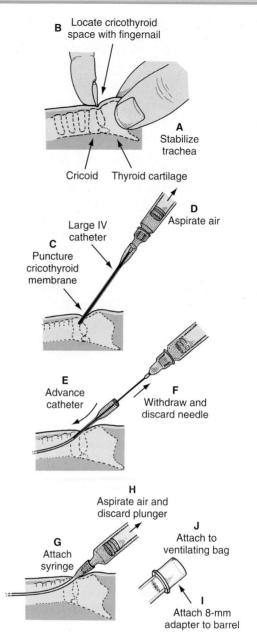

**FIGURE 12-25** Percutaneous cricothyroidotomy. Extend the head in the midline with a rolled towel or folded sheet beneath the shoulders. **A,** Standing to the left of the child, stabilize the trachea with the right hand. **B,** The cricothyroid membrane is located with the index fingertip of the left hand between the thyroid and cricoid cartilages. This space is so narrow (1 mm) in an infant that only a fingernail can discern it. The trachea is then stabilized between the middle finger and thumb of the left hand while the fingernail of the index finger marks the cricothyroid membrane. **C,** A large intravenous (IV) catheter (12 to 14 gauge) is then inserted through the cricothyroid membrane, and air is aspirated (**D**). The catheter is advanced into the trachea through the membrane, and the needle is discarded; an intraluminal position is reconfirmed by attaching a 3-mL syringe (**E**) and aspirating for air (**F**). A 3-mm adapter from a pediatric endotracheal tube can be attached to any intravenous catheter (**G**). Ventilation is accomplished by attaching to a breathing circuit with a standard 22-mm connector (**H**). An alternative would be to leave the barrel of the 3-mL syringe attached to the intravenous catheter, insert an 8-mm endotracheal tube adapter to the syringe barrel (**I**), and then attach to a ventilating system with a standard 22-mm adapter (**J**). (From Coté CJ, Eavey RD, Todres ID, Jones DE. Cricothyroid membrane puncture: oxygenation and ventilation in a dog model using an intravenous catheter. Crit Care Med 1988;16:615-619, © by Williams & Wilkins.)

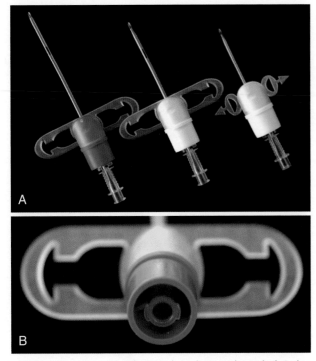

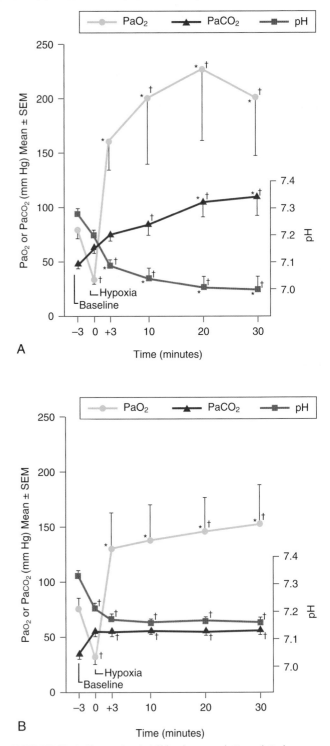

**FIGURE 12-26 A,** The Jet-Ventilation-Catheter (VBM Medizintechnik GmbH, Sulz, Germany) is available in three sizes: From left to right: 13 gauge (adult), 14 gauge (child), and 16 gauge (infant). It consists of a slightly curved puncture needle within a Teflon, kink-resistant cannula. The procedure for insertion is similar to that described in Figure 12-25. **B,** This cannula has two lateral eyes at its distal end and a combined Luer-Lok and 15-mm adapter (surrounding the Luer-Lok) at its proximal end, allowing either jet or standard ventilation. It also has a fixation flange and foam neck tape to secure the airway.

(E-Fig. 12-5). One study simulated use of the Enk Oxygen Flow Modulation set with a variety of IV cannulae and the Emergency Transtracheal Airway Catheter. The investigators concluded that the device worked best when all holes on the Enk device were occluded simultaneously and that minimum flow should never be less than 1 L/min. They also suggested that initial fresh gas flow be set to 1 L/min and then adjusted up or down to effect.[393] Successful ventilation with uncuffed devices may depend on the patency of the upper airway (i.e., the greater the patency, the less the effectiveness of ventilation in the nonbreathing patient).[394] None of these devices has been examined in controlled trials to confirm efficacy, in part because these events are so rare. Therefore, we recommend training on simulators so that each practitioner can determine what device is best in his or her hands.

A number of percutaneous emergency airway devices are available that use a short but large-diameter needle or a needle, guidewire, and dilator to aid insertion of a percutaneous airway.[381,395-397] The Quicktrach (Rüsch) is a device that consists of a tapered 2- or 4-mm catheter with a fixation flange for securing with cloth tape. A removable plastic stopper is designed to limit the depth of needle insertion. This device requires several steps: puncture of the skin, aspiration for air, removal of the stopper, removal of the needle/syringe, and attachment to standard 22-mm connector. A flexible connector is also provided (E-Fig. 12-6). A rabbit model to simulate infant cricothyroidotomy found success in all attempts but 2 of 10 attempts resulted

**FIGURE 12-27 A,** Changes in arterial blood gases and pH are plotted over time for six dogs with spontaneous ventilation; baseline values in room air are plotted at time −3; values after 2 to 3 minutes of hypoxemia as a result of airway obstruction are plotted at time 0. Marked, sustained increases in arterial oxygen tension (*PaO₂*) follow cricothyroid membrane puncture with delivery of only 1.0 L/min oxygen. **B,** Changes in arterial blood gases and pH are plotted over time for five dogs that were not making spontaneous ventilatory efforts. Both oxygenation and ventilation were achieved with a self-inflating bag introduced through the cricothyroid membrane. *PaCO₂*, Carbon dioxide tension; *SEM*, standard error of the mean; *Sig.*, significant difference. (From Coté CJ, Eavey RD, Todres ID, Jones DE. Cricothyroid membrane puncture: oxygenation and ventilation in a dog model using an intravenous catheter. Crit Care Med 1988;16:615-619, © by Williams & Wilkins.)

in fracture of the cricoid cartilage and 1 resulted in damage to the mucosa of the posterior tracheal wall.[398] Conversely, this device has been shown to allow more rapid establishment of an airway than other devices that use a Seldinger technique.[399,400] A larger, cuffed adult model is now available (E-Fig. 12-7).

Other devices that use the Seldinger technique (i.e., needle, guidewire, scalpel incision of the skin, and passage of a dilator and tracheostomy tube) are the Arndt and Melker devices (Cook Critical Care).[401] These devices provide a 3.0-mm ID airway that is sufficient for ventilation as well as oxygenation (E-Fig. 12-8). However, the time required to insert such devices may be longer than for simpler devices and may be inappropriate for immediate rapid establishment of an airway.[381,399,400] In contrast, a porcine cadaver study found greater comfort with this technique compared with a scalpel technique.[402] These devices are useful for elective percutaneous tracheostomy.[403]

Another device, Pertrach (Engineered Medical Systems, Indianapolis, Ind.), uses a split needle on a syringe to puncture the cricothyroid membrane (E-Fig. 12-9). A skin incision is made, and an introducer with tracheostomy tube (3.0-mm ID) is directed into the trachea, splitting the needle, which is removed. The introducer is then removed, and the airway is secured with tracheostomy tape. There are no case reports in the literature to determine the ease or difficulty of insertion in children, but the multiple steps required suggest that it may be a device for elective tracheostomy rather than emergent establishment of a surgical airway.

Another percutaneous tracheostomy device is the Bivona Pedia-Trake kit (Smiths Medical, St. Paul) (E-Fig. 12-10). A skin incision is made with a scalpel, and a large needle is introduced with a skin dilator, which in theory opens the incision sufficiently to allow passage of an obturator and a 3.0-, 4.0-, or 5.0-mm ID tracheostomy tube (with or without cuff). This device appears sufficiently complicated so as to not be useful in a CICV emergency; it might be better suited when there is an urgent need to establish surgical access to the airway.

Other devices with limited pediatric use[395] are kits designed to place a full-sized tracheostomy tube, such as the Nu-Trake (International Medical Devices, Northridge, Calif.) and Abelson (Gilbert Surgical Instruments, Bellmawr, N.J.) devices. They may potentially cause tracheal or laryngeal injury in small patients because of the relatively large size of the needle; again, little experience in children has been published.[396,397,404]

### Laryngeal Mask Airway versus Percutaneous Needle Cricothyroidotomy and Transtracheal Jet Ventilation

The LMA Classic has proved to be an extremely useful device in airway emergencies. In contrast to percutaneous needle cricothyroidotomy, it is an effective device for ventilation as well as a conduit for intubation. The LMA is easily inserted and requires a relatively low level of skill, as demonstrated in numerous studies comparing this technique with other airway management skills (e.g., mask ventilation, endotracheal intubation). More importantly, in contrast to transtracheal jet ventilation, the complication rate with the LMA Classic is exceedingly low.[405] However, this is an SGA device. If glottic or subglottic obstruction to ventilation is present, it will be ineffective, and a surgical airway with or without transtracheal jet ventilation is still the emergency technique of choice. Since the introduction of the LMA, clinical experience suggests that if glottic or subglottic pathology is not suspected, LMA placement to establish ventilation may be appropriately attempted first.[340]

### Surgical Airway

Establishing a surgical airway emergently requires great technical skill. It is difficult to perform quickly, and other methods to provide oxygenation should be pursued first. In nonemergent airway management for children, a tracheostomy is preferred to a cricothyroidotomy because of fewer long-term complications and better results with later decannulation of the airway.[381,406]

### Anterior Commissure Scope and Rigid Ventilating Bronchoscope

Two pieces of equipment used by otolaryngologists that can assist in visualizing the larynx and providing a method of ventilation are the anterior commissure scope and the rigid ventilating bronchoscope. The anterior commissure scope is a rigid, tubular, straight-blade laryngoscope with a light at the tip. The technique to place the anterior commissure scope and the advantages for visualization are similar to those described later for the straight blade used with the retromolar approach.[407]

### SPECIAL TECHNIQUES FOR INTUBATION
### Rigid Laryngoscopy

The rigid laryngoscope is the most familiar and most universally available piece of airway equipment; therefore, it is critical for the practitioner to become facile in its use and to know a variety of techniques. Some suggestions are reviewed here. It is reasonable to take a second look with the rigid laryngoscope after an unexpected failed intubation; however, a good rule is to always change something about the approach that may improve visualization. In the past, awake rigid intubation was the traditional approach to the problematic neonatal airway, but this approach should be used only in an extreme emergency or when IV access is not available.[133-136] Some anatomic features are completely unfavorable for success with the rigid laryngoscope, regardless of technique. Repeated unsuccessful attempts should be avoided, because this can lead to airway trauma and edema. Because infants and children already have smaller airway structures, they are uniquely susceptible to a rapid progression from "cannot intubate, can ventilate" to the CICV scenario.

Whether the child has a normal or an abnormal airway, it is essential to ensure correct positioning and to use age-appropriate equipment. The following maneuvers have been found to be helpful in achieving successful intubation of the child with a DA.

#### Optimal External Laryngeal Manipulation

Pressure can be applied externally to the larynx during the intubation to maximize visualization of the larynx.[408] Optimal external laryngeal manipulation (OELM) is particularly helpful for children with immobile or shortened necks and for infants. Either an assistant or the laryngoscopist can perform OELM. When the laryngoscopist performs the maneuver, the assistant either can pass the ETT into the glottis while the laryngoscopist maintains OELM or OELM can be assumed by the assistant to allow the laryngoscopist to pass the ETT.[408] OELM may also be used in conjunction with other, more advanced airway devices such as the GlideScope (discussed later).[409-411]

#### Intubation Guides

Intubation guides include plastic-coated, flexible metal stylets and the gum elastic bougie. These can be used for blind placement of the ETT under the epiglottis. A flexible stylet is placed inside the ETT and preformed to shape the ETT tip to one that will optimize intubation success (see Fig. 12-21). A hockey-stick

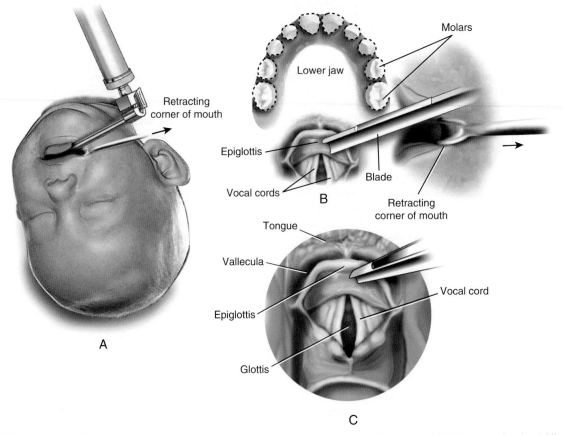

**FIGURE 12-28** **A** through **C,** The retromolar, paraglossal, or lateral approach to rigid laryngoscopy utilizing a straight blade. Notice that the child's head is turned to the left and that the laryngoscope blade is inserted over the molars toward the glottic opening (see text for details).

configuration is frequently useful, particularly if only the epiglottis or the most posterior portion of the glottis can be visualized. The gum elastic bougie has a preformed, angled tip. It is placed alone and then the ETT is threaded over it and into the trachea (E-Fig. 12-11). When the bougie is successfully placed in the trachea, one can detect the subtle "bumpy" feel of the bougie making contact with the anterior tracheal rings. This device may also be used to facilitate intubation through an LMA or as an adjunct to other airway devices.[412-415]

### Oxyscope
The Oxyscope (Heine Optotechnik, Herrsching, Germany) is a Miller 1 laryngoscope blade with an insufflation channel along its length so that it may be attached to an oxygen source. An Oxyscope provides increased $FIO_2$ and is particularly useful for intubation in spontaneously breathing neonates with high oxygen consumption in whom desaturation may rapidly develop (E-Fig. 12-12).[416-418]

### Dental Mirror
The authors of one report used a short-handled dental mirror (no. 3, Storz Instrument Company, Manchester, England) to assist in the indirect visualization of the larynx of a 10-week-old infant. Laryngoscopy was impossible with a Miller no. 1 blade. The infant was returned to spontaneous ventilation, a Macintosh no. 1 blade was used to expose the pharynx, and the mirror was used to visualize the larynx. A styleted ETT was then passed into the glottis under indirect vision.[419]

### Retromolar, Paraglossal, or Lateral Approach using a Straight Blade
Use of a straight blade in a retromolar approach may allow glottic visualization when the classic rigid intubation technique fails, particularly if the difficulty is secondary to a large tongue or small mandible (Fig. 12-28)[407,410,413,420-424] With the child's head turned slightly to the left, a no. 1 Miller blade is introduced into the extreme right side of the mouth. It is advanced in the space between the tongue and the lateral pharyngeal wall; the tongue is swept completely to the left and is essentially bypassed. It is very helpful to have an assistant pull back the right corner of the mouth with a small retractor (e.g., Senn retractor) to increase the space for ETT placement. The blade is advanced while staying to the right, overlying the bicuspids and lateral incisors until the epiglottis or the glottis is visualized. When the epiglottis comes in view, it is lifted with the blade tip to expose the glottic opening. It is extremely unlikely that pressure from the laryngoscope blade on the bicuspids and lateral incisors could loosen these teeth, because they have double roots or longer roots than the central incisors.

At this point in the laryngoscopy, it may be possible to move the proximal end of the blade toward the midline of the mouth to increase room for ETT placement and manipulation, although care must be taken to avoid applying pressure on the central incisors of the maxilla, lest they become loosened. If the glottis is not visualized, the head can be rotated farther to the left and the blade can be kept lateral to improve visualization. The ETT should be styleted and formed into a 90-degree bend configuration to assist in placement (see Fig. 12-21), particularly if the view of the glottis is only partial. A shorter-length blade (usually a Miller no. 1, even in older children) than that used in the traditional midline approach is chosen because the distance to the glottis with this method is greatly shortened.

Several mechanisms are responsible for the improved view of the glottis with the retromolar approach to laryngoscopy. First, there is a reduced need for soft tissue displacement and compression because the lateral placement of the blade bypasses the tongue. This approach to an improved view of the glottic opening is particularly useful for children with micrognathia.[410,413,421,423,424] In such children, the space available to displace the tongue is reduced compared with the traditional midline approach to rigid laryngoscopy. Second, there is an improved line of visualization because the incisors and maxillary structures are bypassed by lateral blade placement and by shifting of the head to the left. Third, the use of a straight blade avoids the possible intrusion of a curved blade into the line of site.[407,420-422] Finally, both the angle and the distance from the insertion of the straight blade at the right commissure of the mouth are reduced, facilitating an easier view of the glottic opening, particularly during a difficult intubation, compared with inserting the blade in the midline.

### Fiberoptic Laryngoscopy

An advantage of using the FOB for intubation of the child with a DA is that it does not require extensive head or neck manipulation and is therefore useful in children who have cervical inflexibility (Klippel-Feil syndrome) or cervical instability (Down syndrome, achondroplastic dwarfism, trauma) (Video 12-9 and 12-11). The technique is also versatile because the flexible instrument conforms to a variety of abnormal airways; it is well tolerated by the sedated, spontaneously breathing child.[344]

Its disadvantage is that the fiberoptic bundle is small, permitting only a limited field of vision. For this reason, the presence of blood or copious secretions may render the FOB ineffective. In addition, use of the FOB requires extensive experience and practice in normal airways first. Our experience suggests that each size of available FOB should be used in at least 20 normal airways before use is attempted in an abnormal airway.[425] Practice with all available sizes of FOBs is important because the manual skills required for each size differ somewhat. Also, FOBs are fragile and expensive. Great care must be taken when using and storing FOBs to prevent breakage of the fiberoptic bundles and the adjustable tip mechanism. They must also be sterilized between uses to maintain the patency of the working channel and clear, bright vision through the fiberoptic bundles and to avoid transmission of infection.

### Equipment

FOBs with directable tips are available in various sizes; the smallest, 2.2 mm in diameter (Olympus LFP; Olympus, Tokyo), can fit through a 2.5-mm ID ETT with or without the 15-mm adapter removed. However, unlike most of the larger FOBs, this scope has no working channel for suctioning or administration of oxygen or topical anesthesia. Newer FOBs with the light source incorporated into the body of the scope are now available. These increase the portability of the instrument, making its use both outside and inside the operating room more simple and convenient.

### Ancillary Equipment

Endoscopy masks can be used to provide oxygen to the spontaneously breathing child and to ventilate the paralyzed child during fiberoptic laryngoscopy. The Frei endoscopy mask (E-Fig. 12-13) and the Patil-Syracuse endoscopy mask are commercially available.[426,427] Patil-Syracuse masks are available in a child size but are too large for most children younger than age 4 years.[88] The Frei mask configuration allows the FOB to be placed in a central position, overlying the nose and mouth, which is more favorable for tracheal intubation. The clear membrane with the hole for the bronchoscope can be rotated to allow either oral or nasal approaches. Alternatively, a disposable facemask can be combined with a bronchoscopic swivel adapter.[428] The FOB can then be passed through the diaphragm of the adapter while ventilation is maintained via the anesthesia circuit. There are two types of commercially available adapters. One type attaches directly to an anesthesia mask. The other type is designed to attach to the ETT and can be modified to fit on the anesthesia mask by the use of a 15- to 22-mm adapter.

Commercial oral airways designed for use in bronchoscopy are available for pediatric patients (IMD Inc., Park City, Utah); however, there are only three sizes (infant, child, and adult), and no studies have evaluated their usefulness in assisting fiberoptic intubation in children. Guedel airways can also be modified for use as oral intubation guides.[428] A strip is cut from the convex surface of the airway to create a channel for placement of the FOB. This modified airway may be used to maintain a midline approach to the glottis; however, it is ineffective as a bite block.

### Direct Technique

The optimal position of the child for fiberoptic bronchoscopy is different from the position for rigid laryngoscopy. The head should be flat on the table and slightly extended at the atlantooccipital joint to prevent the epiglottis from obstructing a view of the glottic opening.[429] If an oral approach is selected, it is vital that the FOB pass in the midline. A nasal approach may make midline placement simpler and avoids the risk of the child's biting the FOB or ETT. One useful technique is to apply oxymetazoline to the naris, place a lubricated nasal trumpet into the nares, and then insert a 15-mm connector from a tracheal tube into the nasal trumpet. This allows oxygen and inhalation agent to be delivered to the child while performing standard fiberoptic laryngoscopy (see Videos 12-9 and 12-11). However, the oral approach offers several advantages over the nasal approach, including avoidance of shearing adenoidal tissue and nasal bleeding. The oral approach may also be less stimulating and better tolerated than the nasal approach. If nasal intubation is chosen in a young child, a topical vasoconstrictor will reduce the risk of bleeding. With both approaches, an assistant should perform a jaw thrust to open the posterior pharyngeal and supraglottic spaces. Alternatively, a bite block or intubating airway may be used. Occasionally, the best view is obtained by direct traction on the tongue, which optimally opens the posterior pharynx. This can be accomplished by grasping the tongue with a gauze, plastic forceps, a stitch through the tongue, or application of high suction to the underside or tip of the tongue (Fig. 12-29).[430]

The tip of the FOB should be introduced behind the tongue and gradually advanced in the midline under direct vision until a recognizable structure is observed. It is essential that the FOB be kept rigid so that when the direction of the tip is altered it remains in the same plane as the handle of the FOB. When the FOB is rotated, the tip should be slightly bent to provide a panoramic view. In general, the tip of the FOB is passed into the trachea before any attempts are made at passing the ETT through the nose or oropharynx. Because the distances in the oropharynx

Suction Flexible fiberoptic
tube bronchoscope

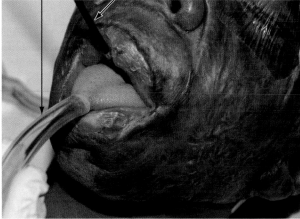

**FIGURE 12-29** Suction can be applied to the tip of the tongue to facilitate pulling it forward to improve glottic visualization. This technique is particularly useful when the tongue is slippery due to secretions or if the mouth opening is small and prevents direct grasping of the tongue with a dry gauze.

in children are less than in adults, the most common initial error when using this technique is to advance the FOB too deeply and into the esophagus. To avoid this pitfall, the FOB should be advanced only toward identifiable airway structures.

Once the FOB is introduced into the airway, a common problem is resistance to passage of the ETT. To minimize this occurrence, the ETT should be loaded onto the scope with the bevel facing down (Murphy eye up) for oral intubation and bevel facing up for nasal intubation.[431,432] This can be remembered by the mnemonic *UNDO*: bevel **U**p for **N**asal intubation, **D**own for **O**ral intubation (see Video 12-10).[433] If persistent resistance is encountered while attempting to pass the ETT past the glottic opening, the ETT should be rotated 90 to 180 degrees to place the bevel in a more favorable orientation for passage through the vocal cords. The depth of anesthesia or sedation as well as oxygen saturation (pulse oximetry) must be carefully monitored throughout the procedure. Arrhythmias may be avoided by providing an adequate depth of analgesia/anesthesia and ensuring a patent airway.

Fiberoptic laryngoscopy techniques should be perfected on manikins and on children with normal anatomy before such techniques are attempted on children with pathologic airway anatomy.[434-440] In a study that compared the time to intubation and complications in 40 infants with the Miller no. 1 laryngoscope or the Olympus LFP FOB, the time to intubation was slightly greater with the FOB (22.8 versus 13.6 seconds), whereas the complication rate was similar.[441] The authors concluded that routine use of the FOB for intubation in normal infants is a safe and reasonable method to gain and maintain skills with this technique.[441] For children, video-assisted fiberoptic intubation appears to offer advantages over fiberoptic intubation using a traditional eyepiece. These include faster mastering of this skill and an overall improved success rate when compared with the traditional method.[425,442]

### Staged Techniques

Staged methods of fiberoptic intubation can be used in infants and small children when the available FOBs are too large to pass through the appropriately sized ETT.[443] One method requires an

FOB with a working channel and a cardiac vascular catheter with guidewire. The guidewire is passed through the working channel of the FOB to within 1 inch of its tip. The FOB is then introduced into the mouth and positioned above the vocal cords. The guidewire is advanced under direct observation through the glottis into the trachea. The FOB is removed, leaving the guidewire in place. The lungs are ventilated by mask while an assistant passes the cardiac catheter over the guidewire (to stiffen the guidewire and facilitate passage of the ETT). The ETT is threaded over the catheter/guidewire combination, which is then removed, leaving the ETT in place.[443-445] Some authors have found that threading of the cardiac catheter over the guidewire is unnecessary. A modification of this technique when the FOB has no working channel has also been described.[446] The authors used an 8-F red rubber catheter attached by waterproof tape to the insertion cord of the FOB proximal to the flexible tip. The larynx was visualized with the FOB, and a guidewire was threaded through the rubber catheter into the trachea. With the guidewire in position, the FOB (with the red rubber catheter) was withdrawn, and an ETT was passed over the guidewire into the trachea.

Another alternative for intubation when the FOB is too large to pass through the appropriately sized ETT is intubation under fiberoptic observation.[447-449] The FOB is introduced through one naris to visually aid the placement of the ETT that is passed through the other naris and manipulated into the glottis. Alternatively, if the observed ETT is not easily passed into the glottis, a small catheter may be more easily manipulated into the glottis and used as a stylet to pass the ETT into the trachea. Spontaneous ventilation is preserved, and oxygen can be administered via the ETT during the intubation. This technique was used successfully in two neonates, one with congenital fusion of the jaws and a second with Dandy-Walker syndrome associated with Klippel-Feil syndrome, micrognathia, hypoplasia of the soft palate, and anteversion of the uvula.[447,448] More recently, an adult video-FOB was used to intubate the trachea of a toddler with temporomandibular joint ankylosis.[450]

If the available FOB is both too large and lacks a working channel, another staged fiberoptic intubation technique can be used. The FOB is loaded with an ETT that is larger than the larynx of the infant. The larynx is visualized with the FOB, and the ETT is advanced and positioned just above the vocal cords. The FOB is then removed, and an ETT changer or catheter is advanced into the trachea through the larger ETT. The larger ETT is then removed, and the appropriately sized ETT for the child is threaded over the tube changer or catheter into the trachea. This technique was used successfully in a 6-month-old infant whose operation had previously been canceled because of failure to intubate.[451]

### Lighted Stylet

A lighted stylet (light wand) is a useful adjunct for managing the pediatric DA (E-Fig. 12-14).[452-456] A number of these devices are available: Trachlight (Laerdol Medical Corporation, Wappingers Falls, N.Y.), Surch-Lite Lighted Intubation Stylet (Aaron Medical Industries, St. Petersburg, Fla.), Light Wand (Vital Signs, Totowa, N.J.), and Trachlite (Rüsch, Tuttlingen, Germany). These devices essentially comprise a malleable stylet with a high-intensity light at the tip; the stylet is shaped into a curve similar to that anticipated for successful passage into the laryngeal inlet (45 to 90 degrees). To begin, an ETT is passed over a well-lubricated lighted stylet. The tip of the stylet should remain within the tip of the ETT to minimize the potential for airway trauma. The room lights should be dimmed at this time to ensure that the stylet is visible when the wand is in the mouth. The lighted stylet is then introduced into the mouth while the proximal end of the stylet is flat against the cheek. As the stylet is inserted into the mouth, the proximal end of the handle is rotated counterclockwise until it is upright. The stylet continues to pass through the oropharynx, following the curvature of the tongue. If the tip of the lighted stylet is not in the proper position (e.g., in the esophagus), a diffuse light or no light will be observed on the surface of the neck. Proper position is usually ensured when a sharp, well-defined, bright circle or cone of light is observed transilluminating the neck directly in the midline at the level of the cricothyroid membrane (see E-Fig. 12-14). Once proper position is ensured, the ETT is gently advanced and the stylet is removed.[455,457]

This technique is useful in those children in whom there is no intrinsic laryngeal or airway pathology but in whom visualization is anticipated to be difficult. The light wand may also be of value in children with a fracture of the cervical spine, because tracheal intubation can be accomplished with minimal movement of the neck.[458] The hemodynamic response to intubation with this technique is similar to that observed with rigid laryngoscopy.[454] The limitations of this technique are that it is a blind technique, the diameter of the device limits it use to larger-sized ETTs, and it may require multiple attempts; however, the success rate markedly increases with experience.[455,457] The most common cause of difficulty in passing the ETT is that the tube hangs up on the epiglottis. When this occurs, the lighted stylet may be withdrawn and its position slightly adjusted more posterior to allow passage behind and beyond the epiglottis. Alternatively, the ETT can be rotated along the long axis of the stylet so that the bevel is facing up. Our advice for using this technique is similar to that for bronchoscopy: it should be used in children with normal anatomy to gain the necessary experience required for managing children with abnormal airway anatomy. This adjunct has also been combined with an LMA to guide the stylet into the trachea.[459]

## Bullard Laryngoscope

The Bullard laryngoscope is used for direct visualization of the laryngeal inlet in children with airway pathology (E-Fig. 12-15). It is available in three sizes: adult, pediatric, and pediatric long. This instrument combines fiberoptic bundles and mirrors. It is positioned within the larynx like a laryngoscope blade, and the direction of force used to displace the tongue is similar to that used with a standard laryngoscope, although this is not intuitively obvious from its configuration. It is designed to provide visualization around a 90-degree bend at the tip (i.e., around the base of the tongue). This configuration may be helpful for direct visualization of the larynx in children with mandibular hypoplasia syndromes (e.g., Robin sequence, Treacher Collins syndrome,[460] Goldenhar syndrome, cervical fracture restricting motion), when the acute angulation of the base of the tongue to the glottic opening is exaggerated, and in children with congenital trismus (Hecht syndrome).[461] The technique used in children is different from that used in adults. Once the laryngeal inlet is visualized, a styleted ETT, with a bent configuration similar to the curve of the Bullard laryngoscope (see Fig. 12-21, *B*), is inserted just to the side of the Bullard laryngoscope blade and advanced under direct vision into the trachea. Success with this instrument is directly proportional to the experience of the anesthesiologist, because the perspective seen through this laryngoscope, the method of

visualization, and the indirect method of ETT placement are so different from standard laryngoscopy.[462,463]

Despite the availability of pediatric Bullard layngoscopes,[464] adult scopes have also been successfully used in children.[465,466] Although tracheal intubation in children 1 to 5 years of age with a Bullard laryngoscope takes more time than with a Wis-Hipple 1.5 blade, the adult Bullard laryngoscope complements the Wis-Hipple 1.5 blade. Occasionally, the Bullard laryngoscope provides a superior laryngeal view and thus allows successful intubation when a failure with the Wis-Hipple blade occurs. When multiple passes of the tube off the adult Bullard laryngoscope were required, this is usually because of contact with the right aryepiglottic fold or anterior vocal cord. The latter appears to be more problematic when the adult laryngoscope is used in children.[465,466]

Additional limitations of the Bullard laryngoscope are that the ETT can partially obstruct the view of the larynx during insertion and that it can be used only for oral intubation.[464] An advantage is that there appears to be minimal motion of the cervical spine in patients with cervical spine disarticulations.[467-469]

## Retrograde Wire-Guided Intubation

The technique of retrograde wire-guided intubation utilizes transtracheal passage of an IV catheter through the cricothyroid membrane into the larynx and retrograde passage of a guidewire from a Seldinger vascular cannulation set to create a guide for intubation.[470-477] A commercial kit is available for use with ETTs that are 5 mm ID or larger (Cook Critical Care). This technique is rarely used in children because of the greater compressibility of the trachea and the increased risk of posterior tracheal wall perforation by the catheter in children compared with adults.

## Video and Indirect Intubating Devices

Advances in technology have led to the reduction in size of video cameras and optical lenses. The integration of these devices into various laryngoscopes and stylets has produced several enhanced tools for securing the airway in children.[478] Several of these new scopes improve visualization during laryngoscopy[412,479-485] and perform better than traditional laryngoscopy in children with difficult direct laryngoscopy.[486-492] However, they are often associated with prolonged time to intubation compared with direct laryngoscopy, and their utility is limited in the presence of blood and secretions. These new devices can be categorized as (1) video laryngoscopes, which incorporate a video camera into the tip of the device; (2) optical laryngoscopes, which use a series of mirrors, prisms, or both to transmit the image from the tip of the device; and (3) optical stylets, which incorporate video or optical systems into a rigid or malleable stylet.

### Video Laryngoscopes

GLIDESCOPE. The GlideScope (Verathon, Bothell, Wash.) (E-Fig. 12-16) consists of a hypercurved blade that incorporates a high-resolution camera with a built-in antifog system. It is available in six sizes (0, 1, 2, 2.5, 3, 4) that accommodate all sizes of patients, including as small as approximately 1 kg. Before clinical use, the GlideScope is switched on to allow the antifog system to warm up. A styleted ETT is necessary for successful intubation, and the stylet's curvature should mimic that of the selected GlideScope blade. The manufacturer markets a GlideScope-specific rigid stylet, but a standard malleable stylet has been shown to be equally effective.[493] Unlike traditional direct laryngoscopy, sweeping the tongue to the left of the blade is unnecessary because of the distally located camera. The GlideScope blade is ideally placed in the midline or slightly to the left in the pharynx (Video 12-12). This position maximizes the space available for introduction of the ETT. The blade tip is placed in the vallecula, and slight elevation of the blade exposes the glottis. The epiglottis may be elevated if placement of the blade tip in the vallecula does not result in optimal visualization. A poor view may occur if the blade size is inappropriate or if the blade is inserted too deeply in the pharynx. OELM may also be used to facilitate laryngeal visualization.[479,494]

Once the best view is obtained, the styleted ETT is inserted under direct vision alongside the GlideScope blade until it just passes the palatoglossal arches and is in full view on the GlideScope monitor. The technique of sequentially visualizing the ETT directly and then on the monitor and creating space by inserting the GlideScope slightly to the left in the pharynx helps minimize the risk of injury to the soft tissues of the airway during advancement of the ETT.[495-499] When the ETT is visible on the monitor, the tip is directed into the glottic inlet. The stylet should be pulled back once the ETT tip is inserted through the cords, because this facilitates the advancement of the ETT down the trachea. Difficult ETT insertion despite a good view of the glottic opening is an occasional problem encountered with the GlideScope and other video and optical laryngoscopes. This is because of the indirect approach to intubation and the need for good hand–eye coordination. These skills can be acquired by frequent use of the device in children with normal airways.[500,501] The GlideScope Cobalt was successfully used for intubation in a cohort of 121 infants. The average intubation time was 30 seconds, and 95% of the intubations were successful on the first two attempts.[502] It has also been used to facilitate intubation in children with craniofacial abnormalities.[409,503-505]

STORZ VIDEO LARYNGOSCOPE. The Storz Video Laryngoscope (Karl Storz GbmH, Tuttlingen, Germany) integrates a camera into Miller- and Macintosh-type blades. This design allows the operator to perform laryngoscopy in the traditional fashion as the Miller-type blade with the video view available if necessary. The video view has been shown to provide a single Comack-Lehane grade improvement over the direct line-of-sight view because of the angulation of the video camera at the tip.[506] It has no antifog mechanism, so use of an antifog solution is needed for unimpaired visualization. Intubation with the Miller video blade can be performed without a stylet, although a styleted ETT with a slight bend at the tip facilitates intubation (E-Fig. 12-17). The Storz Video Laryngoscope is inserted in a similar fashion to the GlideScope. The tip of the blade can be placed in the vallecula; however, because of the magnified lens of the camera, the epiglottis often obstructs the camera view. If this occurs, the blade tip is best utilized to lift the epiglottis to expose the glottis. Once optimal visualization is obtained, the ETT is placed directly along the shaft of the video blade, which guarantees immediate visualization of the ETT in the magnified field of view of the camera and avoids injury to airway soft tissues.

When the Storz Video Laryngoscope was compared with the GlideScope in a pediatric manikin model with normal and DA configurations, the times to intubation and the visual analogue scale scores for field of view and ease of use of the two devices were similar.[507] In another infant manikin study, the Storz Video Laryngoscope was associated with better views, more successful intubations, and similar intubation times as the standard Miller laryngoscope.[506] The Storz Video Laryngoscope has been successfully used to intubate infants and newborns with difficult and

normal airways.[506,508] As with all video laryngoscopes, good hand–eye coordination is necessary for successful intubation. In addition, the operator has to develop the skills necessary to manipulate the ETT indirectly and on a magnified scale. This magnification effect makes subtle movements of the ETT appear large on the video monitor and adds an additional challenge to intubation with these devices. Practice on children with normal airway anatomy is recommended before use on children with abnormal airways.[478]

MULTIVIEW SCOPE. The MultiView Scope (Medical Products International, Tokyo) is a recently introduced video laryngoscope system that integrates a camera into Miller- and Macintosh-style blades (E-Fig. 12-18). The handle of the device has a mounted video screen that displays the image from the blade tip. The image from the screen can be transmitted to an external monitor wirelessly, using a manufacturer-supplied attachment (AirView). Aside from being magnified, the direct line-of-sight view is identical to the camera view, making this an ideal tool for teaching direct laryngoscopy. The MultiView Scope also comes with a malleable stylet attachment that provides the ability to insufflate oxygen through the mounted ETT.

### Optical Laryngoscopes

AIRTRAQ. The Airtraq (Prodol Meditec S.A., Vizcaya, Spain) is a single-use, curved plastic laryngoscope that utilizes lenses and prisms to transmit the image from its distal tip to an eyepiece. It may reduce the incidence of esophageal intubation and may offer greater success rates, particularly in the hands of the inexperienced laryngoscopist.[509] It has a molded channel into which the ETT is inserted (Fig. 12-30), thereby eliminating the need to manipulate the ETT independently during intubation as is required with the GlideScope, Truview, and Storz Video Laryngoscope. The manufacturer offers a wireless monitor for use with the device. The device should be turned on 30 seconds before use to allow the built-in antifog system to warm up. A disadvantage is that a minimum mouth opening of 16 mm is required for insertion of the Airtraq.

The selected ETT and guide channel of the Airtraq are lubricated, and the cuff of the ETT is fully deflated to avoid cuff damage during advancement of the tube in the channel.[510,511] The appropriately sized ETT is loaded into the guide channel of the device, and the child's head is placed in a neutral position. The Airtraq is inserted in the midline in the pharynx and is advanced along the tongue base into the vallecula (Video 12-13). The epiglottis may be elevated to optimize the view, if necessary. Once in position, the Airtraq is gently lifted to obtain optimal glottic exposure, the glottis is centered in the viewfinder by rotating the entire device slightly clockwise or counterclockwise as necessary, and the ETT is advanced after the optimal centered view is obtained. On occasion, the ETT is directed below the glottic opening; if this occurs, the Airtraq should be withdrawn slightly and the advancement attempted again. The guide channel deflects the ETT slightly leftward (an effect that is more pronounced in infants and neonates); this tendency may be countered by rotating the device slightly clockwise as needed.[512,513] Once the trachea is intubated, the Airtraq is separated from the ETT by holding the tube at the mouth and moving it laterally from the guide channel. The Airtraq is then rotated gently out of the oropharynx.

A suboptimal view with the Airtraq is often a result of inserting the device past the glottis. If this happens, the device should be withdrawn slowly until the larynx comes into view. As with

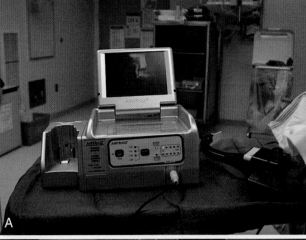

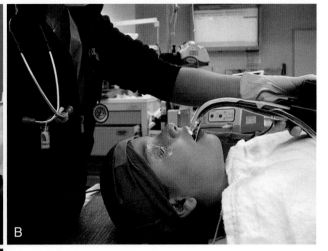

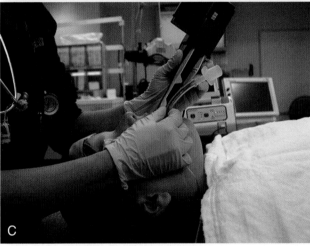

**FIGURE 12-30 A,** The Airtraq optical laryngoscope (Prodol Meditec S.A., Vizcaya, Spain) is a plastic, curved laryngoscope with a distal video camera that allows improved laryngeal views. It is supplied with a portable monitor. **B,** The Airtraq with the endotracheal tube (ETT) loaded into the molded channel is inserted in the midline of the pharynx. **C,** The ETT is held laterally from the Airtraq after intubation, and the Airtraq is then rotated away from the operator and out of the pharynx.

other optical and video-enhanced laryngoscopes, the Airtraq has been associated with airway soft tissue injury. A tonsillar injury in a 4-year-old child was attributed to the width of the guide channel of the device.[514] Care should be taken when using the device in small children, given its size relative to the pharyngeal space. An Airtraq devoid of the guide channel is available for nasal intubations; the intubation may be facilitated with the use of Magill forceps or a gum elastic bougie.[515] The Airtraq has been successfully used for intubation in children with normal and difficult airways; however, despite its having a guide channel, some reports have noted difficulty with directing the ETT in neonates and infants.[412,480-482,516-518] The Airtraq is easily learned and used.[519,520] As with many optical and video devices, there remains a learning curve to using the device,[521] particularly the manipulation of the tracheal tube into the glottis in small patients.[478]

TRUVIEW. The Truview EVO2 Infant (Truphatek International Ltd., Netanya, Israel) is an optical laryngoscope with an angulated, stainless steel blade that transmits a magnified image from the tip of the device to an eyepiece using lenses (E-Fig. 12-19). A camera is available for connection to the eyepiece to allow the image to be viewed on a monitor. A side port is integrated into the blade to allow oxygen insufflation to clear the lens during intubation; however, caution should be exercised when insufflating oxygen in neonates and infants because of the risk of pneumothorax and gastric rupture.[522-524] Because of the indirect

view afforded by the device, a stylet is necessary for successful intubation; a preformed stylet is available from the manufacturer. As with the GlideScope, the ETT should be shaped in a curve similar to the Truview blade. The blade is placed centrally along the tongue in the pharynx to the vallecula, and slight elevation should expose the vocal cords. The ETT is then passed alongside the device, taking care to look in the mouth during initial insertion to make sure the airway soft tissues are not injured. The Truview EVO2 has been compared to laryngoscopy with a Miller blade in children, with results showing improved views of the larynx but longer intubation times.[484] If the head is in the neutral position as for cervical spine instability, application of OELM will improve the view.[525] A study in adults found an improved laryngeal view compared with standard laryngoscopy without the need to align the tracheal, pharyngeal, and oral axes.[526] Once again, there is a learning curve with this device, and practice should shorten intubation times and minimize injury to soft tissues.[478]

### Optical Stylets

Use of optical stylets, unlike FOB intubation, allows the operator to visualize the ETT as it enters the glottis. This is because the stylet is located just within the distal tip of the ETT, providing the operator with a view of the leading edge of the ETT. This view allows immediate recognition of impediments to ETT advancement such as the right arytenoid and enables negotiation of the stylet around these obstacles. The Shikani and the Bonfils are two optical stylets available for pediatric use. Secretions, fogging, and airway soft tissue can impede intubation with optical stylets because of their small lenses and limited depth of view. Impairment of visualization by airway soft tissue can be addressed by combining these devices with direct laryngoscopy. The direct laryngoscope allows the creation of space for visualization with the optical stylet but may require two operators for successful intubation. Optical stylets may be easier to learn and maneuver than FOBs, although some have questioned the utility of these devices in the pediatric population, particularly in the presence of copious secretions.[527,528]

SHIKANI OPTICAL STYLET. The Shikani Optical Stylet (SOS; Clarus Medical, Minneapolis) is a malleable, J-shaped fiberoptic stylet that transmits the image from its distal tip to an eyepiece (E-Fig. 12-20). It has an adjustable tube stop to secure the tube and a port for oxygen insufflation, which should be used with caution in small children.[524,529] The nondominant hand is used to perform a jaw thrust, elevating the epiglottis from the posterior pharyngeal wall, and the stylet is then inserted in the midline in the pharynx (Video 12-14). The tongue base, uvula, and epiglottis are visualized in succession, and the tip is placed just above or just into the glottic inlet. The ETT is then advanced while the SOS is held steady. The SOS is a useful adjunct in the management of the pediatric DA.[530,531]

STORZ BONFILS OPTICAL STYLET. The Bonfils Optical Stylet (Karl Storz) is a rigid fiberoptic stylet with a fixed 40-degree curvature (E-Fig. 12-21). It delivers a higher-quality image than the SOS but is not malleable. Although the manufacturer recommends a retromolar approach to intubation, a midline approach similar to that of the SOS has been found to be successful in children.[532] The Bonfils is available in pediatric and infant sizes and can be coupled to a portable monitor (available from the manufacturer). The use of an antisialagogue and suctioning greatly improves visualization when intubating with optical stylets. When the Bonfils was compared with direct laryngoscopy in a cohort of children with normal airways, the Bonfils was associated with better views but had a greater incidence of intubation failure.[527,528,533]

SHIKANI VERSUS STORZ BONFILS OPTICAL STYLETS. Both of these devices consist of a metal stylet containing a fiberoptic illumination fiber and a fiberoptic vision fiber that are connected to an eyepiece or a video monitor. The light source may be external or battery powered and attached to the housing at the base of the eyepiece; the latter version allows easy transport in an emergency outside the traditional operating room location (see E-Figs. 12-20 and 12-21).[534,535] These devices are described for use either with or without rigid laryngoscopy. There are slight differences between them. Both provide an adapter to hold the ETT that allows delivery of oxygen through the tip of the ETT, but the SOS requires removal of the 15-mm adapter, whereas the Storz Bonfils device uses the 15-mm adapter to hold the tube in place. The pediatric SOS is slightly malleable and can accommodate a 3.0-mm ID ETT; a 2.5-mm ID ETT fits but is tight. The Storz device is not at all malleable but readily accommodates a 2.5-mm ID ETT.[530,534,536,537] One further difference is that the quality of light (on battery mode) seems a bit brighter with the Storz device.

## Laryngeal Mask Airway as a Conduit for Intubation
Numerous case reports affirm the usefulness of the LMA as a conduit for intubation. Several methods for placing the ETT through the LMA have been described: blind, FOB assisted, stylet or bougie assisted, and retrograde assisted.[359,538-544] Because of the high occurrence in children of the epiglottis overlying the laryngeal inlet,[321] even with apparently correct placement as judged by ability to ventilate, a visual technique for ETT placement (i.e., FOB assisted) may be the best method. However, because the LMA and conventional ETTs have similar lengths, all intubation methods are complicated by the inability to stabilize the ETT position as the laryngeal mask is withdrawn; that is, LMA removal over the ETT may cause simultaneous withdrawal of the ETT.[545-548] Proposed solutions are leaving the LMA in place,[548-550] splitting the LMA,[286] cutting and shortening the LMA,[547,551,552] and using longer ETTs,[553] but each technique has disadvantages. Leaving the LMA in place makes securing the ETT difficult and precarious. Modifying the LMA may adversely affect its function, and removing a split LMA can easily dislodge the ETT. Longer ETTs may not be readily available. When an FOB is used to place the ETT, the LMA may be withdrawn first over the scope. The ETT is then grasped, passed through the LMA, and threaded over the FOB into the trachea.[541,554,555] An alternative is to telescope two identical ETTs end to end or to use two that differ in size by 0.5-mm ID, either larger or smaller (E-Fig. 12-22 and Video 12-15).[556-558] These ETTs are then threaded onto the FOB. The upper tube is used to maintain the lower tube in position as the LMA is withdrawn.[375,559] The upper ETT is then removed, the 15-mm adapter is replaced on the lower tube, and the correct position is confirmed by exhaled $CO_2$ and auscultation. The apnea time from insertion of the fiberscope into the LMA until the ETT has been advanced into the trachea can be minimized by using continuous ventilation through a swivel adapter attached to the LMA or ETT.[545,560,561]

It has been suggested that smaller-sized, cuffed ETTs should be used for easier passage and then the cuff can be inflated to eliminate leaks. However, the pilot balloon of a cuffed ETT does not pass through the internal lumen of pediatric LMA sizes of 1.0 to 2.5 (Video 12-16). In larger LMAs, the ETT pilot balloon connection may be too short, so that the pilot balloon can become stuck within the LMA during withdrawal.[562] The largest ETT that will pass through each size of LMA is listed in Table 12-4. For the pediatric-sized LMA Unique and PLMA, even smaller ETTs must be used. The LMA Fastrach is available only in sizes 3, 4, and 5.

### The air-Q
The air-Q Masked Laryngeal Airway (Mercury Medical, Clearwater, Fla.) is an oval shaped laryngeal mask with a shortened, wide, hypercurved airway tube (Fig. 12-31). The air-Q intubating laryngeal mask is available in smaller sizes for younger children and offers some advantages over traditional laryngeal masks when used as an intubation conduit in children. It has a wider airway tube that accommodates cuffed ETTs, and its length is shorter, facilitating removal of the mask after tracheal intubation. The air-Q performs well as a conduit for tracheal intubation and has been successfully used in children with DAs.[563-567] The air-Q is supplied with a red tag attached to the pilot balloon of the mask. This tag equalizes the pressure in the mask to atmospheric pressure, and the mask should be inserted with the tag attached. The manufacturer recommends light lubrication of the back of the mask and the tip of its inner surface.

The air-Q is held in the operator's dominant hand by its airway tube and is inserted into the pharynx at an angle (Video 12-17). The mask is advanced along the tongue base until slight resistance is encountered; a jaw thrust is then performed with the

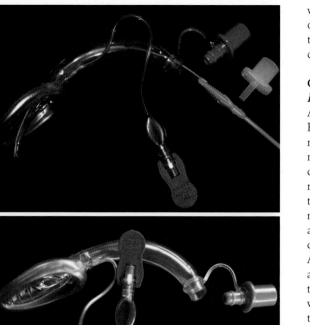

**FIGURE 12-31 A,** The air-Q Intubating Laryngeal Airway (Mercury Medical, Clearwater, Fla.) offers some advantages over traditional laryngeal masks when used as an intubation conduit in children. It has a wider airway tube that accommodates cuffed endotracheal tubes (ETTs), and its length is shorter, which facilitates removal of the mask after tracheal intubation. Before the intubation attempt, one should check that the ETT and its cuff will easily pass through the laryngeal airway size to be used. The 15-mm adapter of the air-Q is removed, the trachea is intubated with a bronchoscope, and the ETT is advanced into the trachea. **B,** When correct tracheal position is assured, a special stylet (coudé-tip Tracheal Tube Introducer, available in three sizes for pediatric-sized ETTs) is inserted into the lumen of the ETT, the cuff of the air-Q is deflated, and with slight advancing pressure the ETT is held in place while the air-Q is gently withdrawn.

nondominant hand, and the mask inserted slightly farther until it becomes seated in the airway. When the air-Q is used as a conduit for intubation, the ETT and its cuff should be checked before the intubation attempt to be sure they will easily pass through the size to be used. The external surface of the ETT should be liberally lubricated. The 15-mm adapter of the air-Q is removed, the trachea is intubated with a bronchoscope, and the ETT is advanced into the trachea. When correct tracheal position is assured, a special stabilizer (available in three sizes for pediatric-sized ETTs) is inserted into the lumen of the ETT. The cuff of the air-Q is deflated, and with slight advancing pressure the ETT is held in place while the air-Q is gently withdrawn (Video 12-17). Proper ETT position is then reconfirmed, and the ETT is taped in place.

The air-Q was compared with the LMA Unique in a cohort of 50 children aged 6 to 36 months. The air-Q had higher airway leak pressure and superior fiberoptic grade of view than the LMA Unique.[568] In another study that evaluated the air-Q as a conduit for tracheal intubation in infants, the mean oropharyngeal leak pressure was $18.5 \pm 1.8$ cm $H_2O$, and the mean insertion time

was $13.3 \pm 3.9$ seconds; tracheal intubation was successful in 19 of 20 infants.[569] The successful use of the air-Q as a conduit for tracheal intubation has also been reported in infants with difficult direct laryngoscopy[567,570]

### Combined Techniques

#### *Retrograde Wire and the Flexible Fiberoptic Bronchoscope*

A case series reported the use of a combined retrograde wire and FOB technique in 20 children aged 1 day to 17 years.[571] Equipment required includes: a ventilating endoscopic mask, equipment for retrograde wire intubation, an FOB with a working channel, and grabbing forceps. The technique begins similarly to retrograde wire-guided intubation. A venous cannula is passed through the cricothyroid membrane in a cephalad manner. The needle is removed, and lidocaine is injected to provide topical anesthesia. Aspiration is done first; detection of air confirms correct placement of the cannula within the lumen of the trachea. A guidewire of suitable length is passed through the cannula and advanced cephalad into the pharynx until it can be retrieved with the forceps from the mouth. The wire is then passed into the working channel of an FOB in a retrograde manner starting at the tip of the FOB (some FOBs may require removal of tip components to allow the wire to pass). An appropriately sized ETT should already be threaded onto the FOB. The FOB is then advanced along the wire while the laryngoscopist looks for familiar anatomic structures. After placement of the FOB tip below the vocal cords is confirmed, the wire is removed in the caudad direction from the IV cannula. The FOB is further advanced to the midtrachea, and the ETT is threaded into place.

Tips for success with this technique are to preserve spontaneous ventilation and to remove the guidewire in the caudad direction, because this tends to pull the FOB farther into the airway rather than out of the airway, which might occur if it is removed in the opposite direction. This technique may improve success over retrograde techniques alone, because the FOB allows direct visualization and is a stiffer guide for the ETT than the wire alone. It also may improve success over the FOB alone, because the glottis is more readily identified even in the presence of blood or secretions.

#### *Rigid Laryngoscopy and the Flexible Fiberoptic Bronchoscope*

The rigid laryngoscope blade may be used to facilitate exposure so that an FOB can be used to visualize the larynx.[572]

#### *Flexible Fiberoptic Bronchoscope Used in a Retrograde Manner*

An FOB was used in a retrograde manner in a 4-year-old child with Nager syndrome who presented for tracheocutaneous fistula closure after decannulation of a tracheostomy. After failed attempts at rigid and direct fiberoptic ETT placement, a FOB was placed in a retrograde fashion, using direct vision, through the fistula, past the vocal cords, into the nasopharynx, and out the naris. It was then used as a stylet for ETT placement.[573] The clinical scenario was unusual, but the technique was successful for this child.

### ACKNOWLEDGMENTS

We wish to thank Melissa Wheeler for her prior contributions to this chapter and I. David Todres posthumously.

Many manufacturers have graciously provided us samples of airway devices so that we could illustrate examples of commonly available equipment. There is insufficient room to illustrate all available devices. Lack of illustration of a device should not be construed as lack of efficacy, nor should illustration of a device be interpreted as endorsement. Practitioners are encouraged to use all equipment available and to make their own educated decision about what devices provide the greatest safety and efficacy in their hands.

## ANNOTATED REFERENCES

Crawford MW, Arrica M, Macgowan CK, Yoo SJ. Extent and localization of changes in upper airway caliber with varying concentrations of sevoflurane in children. Anesthesiology 2006;105:1147-52.

Crawford MW, Rohan D, Macgowan CK, Yoo SJ, Macpherson BA. Effect of propofol anesthesia and continuous positive airway pressure on upper airway size and configuration in infants. Anesthesiology 2006;105:45-50.

*These two papers by Crawford and colleagues clarify how anesthetics produce airway obstruction in children. Airway obstruction during anesthesia or loss of consciousness appears to be primarily related to loss of muscle tone in the pharyngeal and laryngeal structures rather than apposition of the tongue to the posterior pharyngeal wall. This reduction in pharyngeal airway space decreases in a dose-dependent manner with increasing concentrations of either sevoflurane or propofol anesthesia.*

Evans KN, Sie KC, Hopper RA, Hing AV, Cunningham ML. Robin sequence: from diagnosis to development of an effective management plan. Pediatrics 2011;127:936-48.

*This is a recent comprehensive review of the care of newborns with Robin sequence.*

Fiadjoe FE, Stricker P. Pediatric difficult airway management: current devices and techniques. Anesthesiol Clin North Am 2009;27:185-95.

*This review paper is a comprehensive summary of the newer devices and techniques with which to manage the difficult pediatric airway.*

Litman RS, McDonough JM, Marcus CL, Schwartz AR, Ward DS. Upper airway collapsibility in anesthetized children. Anesth Analg 2006;102:750-4.

*This study used an innovative method to measure the propensity of the upper airway to collapse and demonstrated that halothane is a better anesthetic agent than sevoflurane for keeping the upper airway patent during general anesthesia.*

Litman RS, Wake N, Chan LM, et al. Effect of lateral positioning on upper airway size and morphology in sedated children. Anesthesiology 2005;103:484-8.

*This study used cross-sectional magnetic resonance images of the upper airway to demonstrate that when sedated children are placed in the lateral position, upper airway patency improves, mainly at the level of the epiglottis.*

Litman RS, Weissend EE, Shibata D, Westesson PL. Developmental changes of laryngeal dimensions in unparalyzed, sedated children. Anesthesiology 2003;98:41-5.

*This study used magnetic resonance images of the upper airway in children of all ages and developed the relationship between age and laryngeal dimensions. It demonstrated that there is no change in relative dimensions of the subglottic structures from birth through adolescence.*

Practice guidelines for management of the difficult airway: an updated report by the American Society of Anesthesiologists. Task Force on Management of the Difficult Airway. Anesthesiology 2003;98: 1269-77.

*The most recent guidelines from the American Society of Anesthesiologists for management of the patient with a difficult airway, whether anticipated and unanticipated. Although geared for adult anesthesia, the approach outlined in the algorithm may be applied to children.*

Rolf N, Coté CJ. Diagnosis of clinically unrecognized endobronchial intubation in paediatric anaesthesia: which is more sensitive, pulse oximetry or capnography? Paediatr Anaesth 1992;2:31-5.

*This paper determined that pulse oximetry is more sensitive than capnography in detecting endobronchial intubation. It recommends that when a small but persistent change in oxygen saturation is noted, rather than increase the inspired oxygen concentration, one must first investigate the cause and reassess the position of the endotracheal tube.*

Weiss M, Dullenkopf A, Gysin C, Dillier CM, Gerber AC. Shortcomings of cuffed paediatric-tracheal tubes. Br J Anaesth 2004;92:78-88.

*This paper compares the physical characteristics of the most commonly available pediatric endotracheal tubes (ETTs). It also underscores the shortcomings in ETT design that may affect airway-related patient complications and that should be considered in choosing ETTs for children.*

Wheeler M. Management strategies for the difficult pediatric airway. Anesth Clin North Am 1998;16:743-61.

*A discussion of the management issues specific to children with a difficult pediatric airway. This article expands on the ideas supported by the American Society of Anesthesiologists Task Force on Management of the Difficult Airway as they apply to children.*

Wheeler M, Roth AG, Dsida RM, et al. Teaching residents pediatric fiberoptic intubation of the trachea: traditional fiberscope with an eyepiece versus a video-assisted technique using a fiberscope with an integrated camera. Anesthesiology 2004;101:842-6.

*Lack of proficiency using fiberoptic equipment for pediatric airway management remains a concern. This paper supports two important points: (1) one can achieve a satisfactory proficiency with a pediatric fiberoptic system with relatively few intubations, and (2) a video system can both improve the speed of skill acquisition and shorten the time required for successful intubation.*

## REFERENCES

Please see www.expertconsult.com

# Anesthesia for Thoracic Surgery

GREGORY B. HAMMER

| General Perioperative Considerations | Techniques for Single-Lung Ventilation in Infants and Children |
| Ventilation and Perfusion during Thoracic Surgery | Surgical Lesions of the Chest |
| Thoracoscopy | **Summary** |

## General Perioperative Considerations

A thorough preoperative evaluation is essential when caring for the child who is scheduled for thoracic surgery. Appropriate imaging and laboratory studies should be performed according to the lesion involved. Guidelines for fasting, choice of premedication, and preparation of the operating room (OR) are the same as for other infants and children scheduled for major surgery. After induction of anesthesia, placement of an intravenous (IV) catheter, and tracheal intubation, arterial catheterization should be considered for children undergoing thoracotomy as well as those with severe lung disease having thoracoscopic surgery. For thoracoscopic procedures of relatively brief duration in children without significant lung disease, an arterial catheter may not be required. The arterial catheter facilitates monitoring of systemic blood pressure during manipulation of the lungs and mediastinum as well as arterial blood gas tensions during single-lung ventilation (SLV). Placement of a central venous catheter is generally not indicated if peripheral IV access is adequate for projected fluid and blood administration.

Inhalational anesthetic agents are commonly administered in 100% $O_2$ during maintenance of anesthesia. Isoflurane may be preferred owing to less attenuation of hypoxic pulmonary vasoconstriction compared with other inhalational agents, although this has not been studied in children.[1] Nitrous oxide is avoided. IV opioids have a sparing effect on the concentration of inhalational anesthetics required, and therefore may limit the impairment of hypoxic pulmonary vasoconstriction. Alternatively, total IV anesthesia may be used.

A variety of approaches have been described to prevent and treat pain after videoscopic procedures. Bupivacaine infiltration at incision sites before skin incision has been shown to decrease postoperative pain.[2,3] Bupivacaine infiltration was found to be superior to IV fentanyl or tenoxicam for reducing postoperative pain.[4] The combination of general anesthesia with regional anesthesia that also contributes postoperative analgesia, is particularly desirable for thoracotomy, but may also be beneficial for thoracoscopic procedures. This is especially true when thoracostomy tube drainage, a source of significant postoperative pain, is used after surgery. In addition, regional blockade for postoperative analgesia facilitates deep breathing and coughing, which may limit atelectasis and pneumonia. A variety of regional anesthetic techniques have been described for intraoperative anesthesia and postoperative analgesia, including intercostal and paravertebral blocks, intrapleural infusions, and epidural anesthesia (see Chapters 41, 42, and 43).

### VENTILATION AND PERFUSION DURING THORACIC SURGERY

Ventilation is normally distributed preferentially to dependent regions of the lung, so that there is a gradient of increasing ventilation from the least to the most dependent lung segments. Because of gravitational effects, perfusion normally follows a similar distribution, with increased blood flow to dependent lung segments. Therefore ventilation and perfusion are normally well matched. In infants, however, ventilation is normally distributed to the nondependent areas of the lung and perfusion is more evenly distributed because of their smaller anteroposterior distance that mitigates the effect of gravity. These two effects result in increased ventilation/perfusion ($\dot{V}/\dot{Q}$) mismatch. During thoracic surgery, several factors act to further increase $\dot{V}/\dot{Q}$ mismatch. General anesthesia, neuromuscular blockade, and mechanical ventilation may cause a decrease in functional residual capacity of both lungs. Compression of the dependent lung in the lateral decubitus position may cause atelectasis. Surgical retraction and/or SLV collapse the operative lung. Hypoxic pulmonary vasoconstriction, which acts to divert blood flow away from underventilated lung, thereby minimizing $\dot{V}/\dot{Q}$ mismatch, may be diminished by inhalational anesthetic agents and other vasodilating drugs. These factors apply equally to infants, children, and adults. The overall effect of the lateral decubitus position on $\dot{V}/\dot{Q}$ mismatch, however, is different in infants compared with older children and adults.

In adults with unilateral lung disease, oxygenation is optimal when the patient is placed in the lateral decubitus position with the healthy lung dependent ("down") and the diseased lung nondependent ("up").[5] Presumably, this is related to an increase in blood flow to the dependent, healthy lung and a decrease in blood flow to the nondependent, diseased lung because of the hydrostatic pressure (or gravitational) gradient between the two lungs. This phenomenon promotes $\dot{V}/\dot{Q}$ matching in the adult patient undergoing thoracic surgery in the lateral decubitus position.

In infants with unilateral lung disease, however, oxygenation is improved with the healthy lung "up."[6] Several factors account for this discrepancy between adults and infants. Infants have a soft, easily compressible rib cage that cannot fully support the underlying lung. Therefore functional residual capacity is closer to residual volume, making airway closure likely to occur in the dependent lung even during tidal breathing.[7] When the adult is placed in the lateral decubitus position, the dependent diaphragm has a mechanical advantage because it is "loaded" by the abdominal hydrostatic pressure gradient. This pressure gradient is reduced in infants, thereby reducing the functional advantage of the dependent diaphragm. The infant's small size also reduces the hydrostatic pressure gradient between the nondependent and dependent lungs. Consequently, the favorable increase in perfusion to the dependent, ventilated lung is attenuated in infants.

Finally, the infant's increased oxygen requirement, coupled with a small functional residual capacity, predisposes to hypoxemia. Infants normally consume 6 to 8 mL of $O_2$/kg/min compared with adult rates of 2 to 3 mL of $O_2$/kg/min.[8] For these reasons, infants are at an increased risk of significant hemoglobin desaturation during surgery in the lateral decubitus position.

A modest increase in $PaCO_2$ may be beneficial in children during thoracoscopic procedures. In a study of 12 children undergoing video-assisted thoracoscopic surgery for patent ductus arteriosus closure, hypercapnea targeting $PaCO_2$ values between 50 and 70 mm Hg increased cardiac output, central venous and arterial oxygen tension.[9]

## THORACOSCOPY

With the miniaturization of instruments, progress in video technology, and growing experience among pediatric surgeons, video endoscopic surgery of the chest, or thoracoscopy, is being performed for an increasing number of pediatric surgical indications (Table 13-1). Advantages of thoracoscopy include smaller chest incisions, reduced postoperative pain, and more rapid postoperative recovery compared with thoracotomy (Table 13-2,

| TABLE 13-1 Thoracoscopic Procedures in Infants and Children |
| --- |
| Diagnostic inspection |
| Lung biopsy |
| Lobectomy |
| Sequestration resection |
| Cyst excision |
| Lung decortication |
| Foregut duplication resection |
| Thymectomy |
| Patent ductus arteriosus ligation |
| Thoracic duct ligation |
| Esophageal atresia repair |
| Sympathectomy |
| Aortopexy |
| Mediastinal mass excision |
| Anterior spinal fusion |

| TABLE 13-2 Advantages of Thoracoscopic versus Open-Chest Surgery |
| --- |
| Improved surgical visualization |
| Decreased pain |
| Decreased surgical stress |
| Decreased ileus/earlier return to feeding |
| Quicker return to normal activity (parents and child) |
| Shorter hospitalization |
| Fewer long-term complications |
| Cosmetically superior |

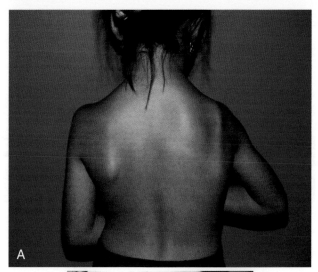

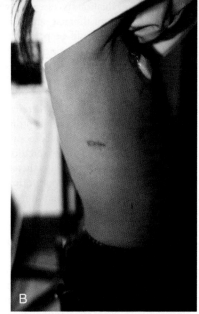

**FIGURE 13-1 A,** Significant chest deformity may occur with growth after thoracotomy. **B,** Smaller incisions associated with thoracoscopic surgery result in minimal musculoskeletal changes.

Fig. 13-1).[10,11] Endoscopes that can be passed through a needle and trocar system are now manufactured, and digital video signals can be electronically modified to yield sharp, detailed, color images with a minimum light intensity. Digital cameras are designed to maintain an image in an upright orientation regardless of how the telescope is rotated. They are also equipped with an optical or digital zoom to magnify the image or give the illusion of moving the telescope closer to the object of interest. The smallest of telescopes use fiberoptics and are less than 2 mm in diameter (Fig. 13-2). Two-millimeter disposable ports, mounted on a Veress needle, are used for introduction of these small instruments. Larger instruments and ports are used in larger children and for more complex cases.

A second area of major advance in video endoscopic surgery is the development of the endoscopic suite, in which all necessary cables and wiring are located within equipment booms, ceilings, and walls. The manipulation of digital images is controlled by

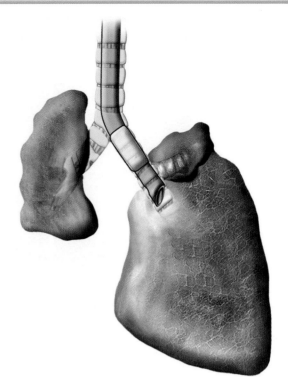

**FIGURE 13-3** Placement of a single-lumen endotracheal tube (ETT) for left-sided single-lung ventilation results in obstruction of the upper lobe orifice if the distance from the proximal cuff to the tip of the ETT is longer than the main-stem bronchus.

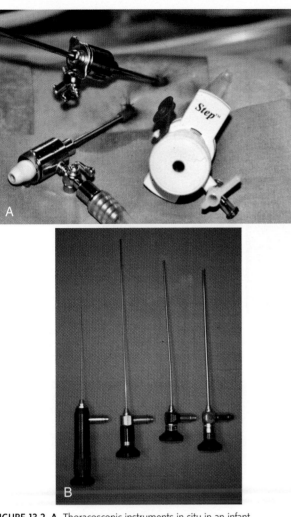

**FIGURE 13-2 A,** Thoracoscopic instruments in situ in an infant.
**B,** Telescopes for use in infants range from 1.2 to 4.0 mm in diameter.

voice or touchscreen command either from the operative field or at a conveniently located station nearby. High-quality digital images are displayed on flat panel monitors that can be positioned within a comfortable viewing range. Remote-controlled cameras can direct any view in the room to any of the monitors or to a remote site. Digital radiographs can be routed from the radiology department to the OR, and consultants in remote locations can be viewed on monitors in the OR so that the surgeon can see to whom he or she is speaking. An additional feature of newer endoscopy suites is voice-controlled bed positioning. Robotic tools can be vocally directed to position telescopes in the surgical field for optimal viewing; these surgical "telemanipulators" facilitate microsurgery in confined spaces, even for small infants. Other endoscopic robots are being developed for a wide range of surgical applications.

Thoracoscopy can be performed while both lungs are being ventilated using $CO_2$ insufflation and placement of a retractor to displace lung tissue in the operative field. However, SLV is extremely desirable during thoracoscopy because lung deflation improves visualization of thoracic contents and may reduce lung injury caused by the use of retractors. There are several different techniques that can be used for SLV in children.

## TECHNIQUES FOR SINGLE-LUNG VENTILATION IN INFANTS AND CHILDREN
### Use of a Single-Lumen Endotracheal Tube
The simplest means of providing SLV is to intentionally intubate the ipsilateral main-stem bronchus with a conventional single-lumen endotracheal tube (ETT).[12] When the left bronchus is to be intubated, the bevel of the ETT is rotated 180 degrees and the child's head is turned to the right.[13] The ETT is advanced into the bronchus until breath sounds on the operative side disappear. A fiberoptic bronchoscope (FOB) may be passed through or alongside the ETT to confirm or guide placement. Alternatively, fluoroscopy may be used to guide and position the ETT.[14] When a cuffed ETT is used, the distance from the proximal cuff to the tip of the ETT must be less than the length of the main-stem bronchus so that the upper lobe orifice is not occluded (Fig. 13-3).[15] This technique is simple and requires no special equipment other than a FOB. This may be the preferred technique of SLV in emergency situations, such as airway hemorrhage or contralateral tension pneumothorax.

Problems can occur when using a single-lumen ETT for SLV. If a smaller, uncuffed ETT is used, it may be difficult to provide an adequate seal of the intended bronchus. This may prevent the operative lung from adequately collapsing or fail to protect the healthy, ventilated lung from contamination by purulent material or blood from the contralateral lung. One is unable to suction the operative lung using this technique. Hypoxemia may occur as a result of obstruction of the upper lobe bronchus, especially when the short right main-stem bronchus is intubated.

Variations of this technique have been described, including intubation of both bronchi independently with small ETTs.[16-19]

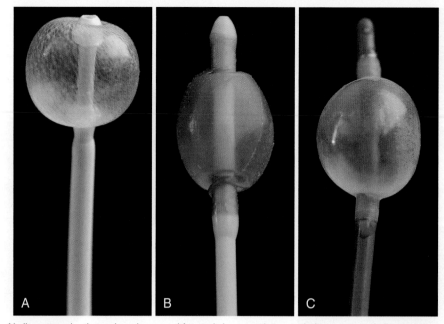

FIGURE 13-4 A variety of balloon-tipped catheters have been used for single-lung ventilation, including an Arrow balloon wedge catheter (**A**) (Arrow International, Inc., Reading, Pa.), a Cook pediatric bronchial blocker (**B**) (Cook Medical, Inc., Bloomington, Ind.), and a Fogarty embolectomy catheter (**C**). (Photographs by Michael Chen, MD.)

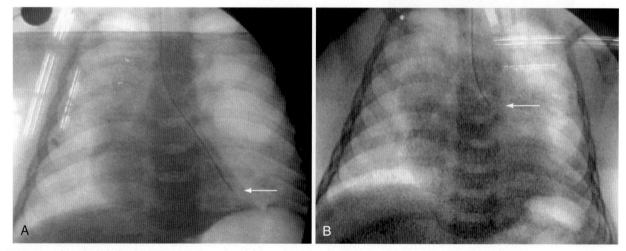

FIGURE 13-5 A bronchial blocker (*arrow*) is placed in a distal left bronchus (**A**) and withdrawn into the proximal left main-stem bronchus (**B,** *arrow*) under fluoroscopic guidance.

One main-stem bronchus is initially intubated with an ETT, after which another ETT is advanced over a FOB into the opposite bronchus. The disadvantages of these techniques include technical difficulties and trauma to the tracheal and bronchial mucosa. Even after successful bilateral bronchial intubation, the inner diameters of the tubes will be small, limiting gas flow and impeding suctioning of the airways.

### Use of Balloon-Tipped Bronchial Blockers

A Fogarty embolectomy catheter or an end-hole, balloon wedge catheter may be used for bronchial blockade to provide SLV (Fig. 13-4).[20-23] Placement of a Fogarty catheter is facilitated by bending the tip of its stylet toward the bronchus on the operative side. An FOB may be used to reposition the catheter and confirm appropriate placement. Various techniques for placing an end-hole catheter outside the ETT have been described. Using one such method, the bronchus on the operative side is initially

intubated with an ETT.[20] A guidewire is then advanced into that bronchus through the ETT. The ETT is removed and the blocker is advanced over the guidewire into the bronchus. An ETT is then reinserted into the trachea alongside the blocker catheter. The catheter balloon is positioned in the proximal main-stem bronchus under fiberoptic visual guidance. Alternatively, if an FOB small enough to pass through the indwelling ETT is not available, fluoroscopy may be used (Fig. 13-5). With an inflated blocker balloon the airway is completely sealed, providing more predictable lung collapse and better operating conditions than with an ETT in the bronchus.

One potential problem with this technique is dislodgement of the blocker balloon into the trachea, blocking ventilation to both lungs and/or preventing collapse of the operative lung. The balloons of most catheters currently used for bronchial blockade have low compliance properties (i.e., low volume, high pressure). They require 1 to 3 mL of air or saline to fully inflate.

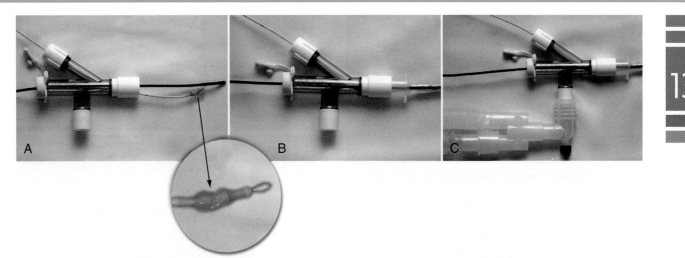

**FIGURE 13-6** The Cook 5F endobronchial catheter is shown inserted in the multiport adapter. **A,** The adapter has four ports for connection to the breathing circuit, fiberoptic bronchoscope (FOB), endobronchial catheter, and endotracheal tube. After the FOB and endobronchial catheter have been inserted through the multiport adaptor, the FOB is placed through the monofilament loop at the distal end of the catheter (*arrow*). The multiport adaptor is then attached to the indwelling endotracheal tube (**B**) and the breathing circuit (**C**). The FOB is directed into the main-stem bronchus on the operative side. The catheter is then advanced until the monofilament loop slides off the end of the FOB into the bronchus. (Photographs by Elliot Krane, MD.)

**TABLE 13-3** Single-Lumen Uncuffed Tracheal Tube Diameters

| ID (mm)* | OD (mm) | Equivalent French Size† |
|---|---|---|
| 3.0 | 4.3 | 13 |
| 3.5 | 4.9 | 15 |
| 4.0 | 5.5 | 17 |
| 4.5 | 6.2 | 19 |
| 5.0 | 6.8 | 21 |
| 5.5 | 7.5 | 23 |
| 6.0 | 8.2 | 25 |
| 6.5 | 8.9 | 27 |
| 7.0 | 9.6 | 29 |
| 7.5 | 10.2 | 31 |
| 8.0 | 10.8 | 32 |

*Note:* Cuffed tubes have approximately 0.5-mm additional outer diameter. The external diameter may also vary by manufacturer.
*ID,* Internal diameter; *OD,* outer diameter.
*Sheridan tracheal tubes (Hudson RCI, Arlington Heights, Ill.).
†French (F) size is 3 × OD (mm).

Overdistention of the balloon can damage or even rupture the airway.[24] A recent study, however, reported that bronchial blocker cuffs produced lower "cuff-to-tracheal" pressures than double-lumen tubes.[25] When closed-tip bronchial blockers are used, the operative lung cannot be suctioned and continuous positive airway pressure (CPAP) cannot be provided to the operative lung if needed.

When a bronchial blocker is placed outside the ETT, care must be taken to avoid injury caused by compression and resultant ischemia of the tracheal mucosa. The sum of the catheter diameter and the outer diameter of the ETT should not significantly exceed the tracheal diameter. Outer diameters for pediatric-size ETTs are shown in Table 13-3. These numbers provide an estimate of the predicted tracheal diameter, which should approximate the size of the uncuffed ETT predicted to produce a seal in the trachea.

Recently, adapters have been developed that facilitate ventilation during placement of a bronchial blocker through an indwelling ETT.[26,27] Use of a 5F endobronchial blocker that is designed for use in children, and has a multiport adapter and FOB, has been described (Cook Medical, Inc., Bloomington, Ind.).[28] The balloon is elliptical so that it conforms to the bronchial lumen when inflated. The blocker catheter has a maximum outer diameter of 2.5 mm (including the deflated balloon), a central lumen with a diameter of 0.7 mm, and a distal balloon with a capacity of 3 mL. The balloon has a length of 1.0 cm, corresponding to the length of the right main-stem bronchus in children approximately 2 years of age.[29] The blocker is placed coaxially through a dedicated port in the adapter, which also has a port for passage of a FOB and ports for connection to the anesthesia breathing circuit and ETT (Fig. 13-6). The FOB port has a plastic sealing cap, whereas the blocker port has a Tuohy-Borst connector that locks the catheter in place and maintains an airtight seal. Because oxygen can be administered during passage of the blocker and FOB, the risk of hypoxemia during blocker placement is diminished, and repositioning of the blocker may be performed with fiberoptic guidance during surgery.

When a FOB is used to guide the placement of a bronchial blocker, both the blocker catheter and FOB must pass through the indwelling ETT. The smallest ETT through which the catheter and FOB can be passed must be larger than the sum of the outer diameters of the catheter and the FOB. The 5F Cook bronchial blocker and an FOB with a 2.2-mm diameter, for example, may be inserted through an ETT with an internal diameter as small as 5.0 mm; for children with an indwelling ETT smaller than this, a blocker catheter can be positioned under fluoroscopy (see Fig. 13-5).[30]

## Use of a Univent Tube

The Univent tube (Fuji Systems Corporation, Tokyo) is a conventional ETT with a second lumen containing a small blocker catheter that can be advanced into a bronchus (Fig. 13-7).[31,32] A balloon located at the distal end of this small tube serves as a blocker. Univent tubes require a FOB for successful placement. Univent tubes are now available in sizes with internal diameters as small as 3.5 and 4.5 mm, for use in children older than 6 years of age.[33] Because the blocker tube is firmly attached to the main

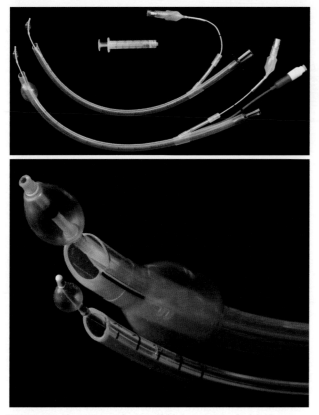

**FIGURE 13-7** The Univent tube is available in a variety of adult sizes, as well as 3.5 mm internal-diameter and 4.5 mm internal-diameter sizes for use in children (*top*). The adult tubes have a tracheal cuff and an end-hole bronchial blocker, allowing administration of oxygen and suction (*bottom*). The pediatric tubes are uncuffed and have a closed-tip blocker. (Photographs by Michael Chen, MD.)

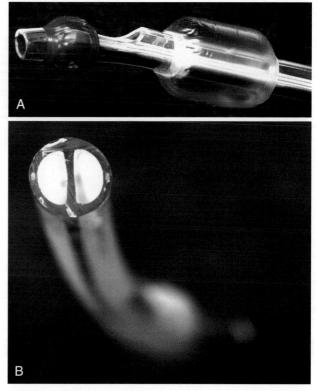

**FIGURE 13-8** Although the bronchial lumen of a double-lumen tube appears to be round (**A**), both the bronchial and tracheal lumens are D-shaped, as evident in a cross-sectional view (**B**). Their actual lumens have restricted limiting diameters. (Photographs by Michael Chen, MD.)

| TABLE 13-4 Univent Tube Diameters | |
|---|---|
| **ID (mm)** | **OD (mm)*** |
| 3.5 | 7.5/8.0 |
| 4.5 | 8.5/9.0 |
| 6.0 | 10.0/11.0 |
| 6.5 | 10.5/11.5 |
| 7.0 | 11.0/12.0 |
| 7.5 | 11.5/12.5 |
| 8.0 | 12.0/13.0 |
| 8.5 | 12.5/13.5 |
| 9.0 | 13.0-14.0 |

*ID*, Internal diameter; *OD*, outer diameter.
*Sagittal/transverse.

ETT, displacement of the Univent blocker balloon is less likely than when other blocker techniques are used. The blocker tube has a small lumen that allows egress of gas and can be used to insufflate oxygen or suction the operated lung.

One disadvantage of the Univent tube is the large cross-sectional area occupied by the blocker channel, especially in the smaller size tubes. Therefore Univent tubes have a large outer diameter with respect to their inner (luminal) diameters (Table 13-4). Smaller Univent tubes have a disproportionately high resistance to gas flow.[34] The Univent tube's blocker balloon has

low-volume, high-pressure characteristics, so mucosal injury can occur during normal inflation.[35,36]

## Use of Double-Lumen Tubes

All double-lumen tubes (DLTs) are essentially two tubes of unequal length molded together. The shorter tube ends in the trachea, and the longer tube ends in the bronchus (Fig. 13-8). DLTs for older children and adults have cuffs located on the tracheal and bronchial lumens. The tracheal cuff, when inflated, allows positive-pressure ventilation. The inflated bronchial cuff allows ventilation to be diverted to either or both lungs and protects each lung from contamination from secretions, purulent material, or blood originating from the contralateral side.

Marraro described a bilumen tube for infants.[37] This tube consists of two separate uncuffed tracheal tubes of different lengths attached longitudinally. This tube is not available in the United States. The smallest cuffed DLT commercially available in the United States is a 26F size (Teleflex Medical, Research Triangle Park, N.C.). This DLT may be used in children as young as 8 years old. DLTs are also available in sizes 28 and 32F (Nellcor brand [Covidien, Mansfield, Mass.]); these are suitable for children 10 years of age and older. Numerous manufacturers produce clear, disposable, PVC Robertshaw-design DLTs, which are available in sizes 35 to 41F (Table 13-5). Essentially, they consist of similar features with small modifications in cuff shape and location. A colored bronchial cuff, commonly blue, permits easy identification by fiberoptic bronchoscopy. In general, the cuffs used in DLTs are high-compliance cuffs that are designed to exert less pressure on the tracheal and bronchial mucosa compared with low-compliance cuffs. For right-sided DLTs, the

**TABLE 13-5** Double-Lumen Tube Dimensions

| Size (F) | Main Body OD (mm) | Limiting Diameter Tracheal Lumen (mm) | Limiting Diameter Bronchial Lumen (mm) |
|---|---|---|---|
| 26* | 8.7 | N/A | N/A |
| 28† | 9.4 | 3.1 | 3.2 |
| 32† | 10.6 | 3.5 | 3.4 |
| 35† | 11.7 | 4.5 | 4.3 |
| 37† | 12.4 | 4.7 | 4.5 |
| 39† | 13.1 | 4.9 | 4.9 |
| 41† | 13.7 | 5.4 | 5.4 |

*Note:* The limiting diameters correspond to the largest suction catheter or fiberoptic bronchoscope that can be placed via the lumen under ideal circumstances (e.g., adequate lubrication). Comparing the data in this table to that in Table 13-3, the OD of the DLTs corresponds to the following tracheal tubes: 26F DLT is equivalent to that of a 6.0-6.5 mm ID tracheal tube; a 28F is equivalent to a 6.5-7.0 mm ID; and a 32F is equivalent to an 8.0 mm ID. Cuff thickness is 0.049 mm; therefore cuff adds 0.10 mm to overall OD of tube.
*DLT,* Double-lumen tube; *ID,* internal diameter; *OD,* outer diameter.
*Teleflex Medical, Research Triangle Park, N.C.
†Covidien, Mansfield, Mass.

endobronchial cuff is donut shaped and allows the right upper lobe ventilation opening to be positioned at the right upper lobe orifice. Despite this design, right upper lobe occlusion may occur because of the shorter length of the right main-stem bronchus.[1,38] Therefore right-sided DLTs are used infrequently.

DLTs are inserted in children using the same technique as in adults, and left DLTs are almost exclusively used.[39] The tip of the tube is inserted just past the vocal cords, and the stylet is withdrawn. The DLT is rotated 90 degrees to the appropriate side and then advanced into the bronchus. After intubation, the tracheal cuff is inflated first and equal breath sounds should be confirmed. To prevent mucosal damage from excessive pressure applied by the bronchial cuff, the cuff is inflated with incremental volumes to seal air leaks around the bronchial cuff into the trachea. Inflation of the bronchial cuff seldom requires more than 2 mL of air. After inflation of the bronchial cuff, bilateral breath sounds should be rechecked to confirm that the bronchial cuff is not herniating across the carina to impede contralateral lung ventilation. Fiberoptic bronchoscopy can be used to directly visualize the proximal edge of the bronchial cuff in the left bronchus, just distal to the carina. One simple way to verify that the tip of the bronchial lumen is located in the designated bronchus is to clamp the tracheal lumen at the level of the connector and then observe and auscultate left and right lungs. Usually, inspection will reveal unilateral movement of the ventilated hemithorax. With the tracheal lumen clamped, auscultation of the chest will demonstrate air entry in the left lung and no ventilation in the right lung. After auscultation and release of the tracheal clamp, the bronchial lumen is clamped and the tracheal lumen is ventilated to confirm movement and breath sounds of the right lung. Whenever a right-sided DLT is used, ventilation of the right upper lobe must be verified. This can be accomplished by careful auscultation over the right upper lung field or, more accurately, by fiberoptic bronchoscopy. When a left-sided DLT is used, the risk of occluding the left upper lobe bronchus by advancement of the bronchial tip into the distal left main bronchus should be considered.

DLTs may be malpositioned in up to 48% of cases despite careful inspection and auscultation.[40] The simplest way to

evaluate proper positioning of a left-sided DLT is to perform fiberoptic bronchoscopy through the tracheal lumen. The carina is then visualized, and only the proximal edge of the bronchial cuff should be identified just distal to the carina. Herniation of the bronchial cuff over the carina to partially occlude the contralateral main-stem bronchus should be excluded. Fiberoptic bronchoscopy should then be performed via the bronchial lumen to identify the patent left upper lobe orifice. When a right-sided DLT is used, the right upper lobe bronchial orifice must be identified while the bronchoscope is passed through the right upper lobe ventilating slot.

The use of FOB to facilitate positioning of DLTs in children is dependent on the availability of small instruments. FOBs with an external diameter of 3.6 mm are commonly available and will pass through a 35F DLT. Smaller FOBs are needed when 26F, 28F, and 32F DLTs are used (see Table 13-5 for "limiting diameters").

In the adult population, the depth of insertion of the DLT is directly related to the height of the patient.[41] No equivalent measurements are available as yet in children. Fortunately, there are very few reports in children of airway damage from DLTs.

The high-volume, low-pressure cuffs should not damage the airway, provided the cuffs are not overinflated with air or distended with nitrous oxide. Alternatively, saline may be used to inflate the cuffs.

A disadvantage of DLTs is the need to change the DLT to a single-lumen ETT if mechanical ventilation is required after surgery. This is a particular problem for children in whom tracheal intubation was difficult initially because of anatomic or functional limitations. Even when an airway was not classified as difficult preoperatively, it may become difficult secondary to facial and supraglottic edema, the presence of secretions and/or blood in the airway, and laryngeal trauma from the initial intubation. The use of an ETT exchange catheter may facilitate the exchange of a DLT for a single lumen ETT.[42] These devices are commercially available in a variety of sizes (Cook Medical, Inc., Bloomington, Ind.) and allow oxygen insufflation and jet ventilation (see E-Fig. 12-3, *A-H*).

Several important caveats should be considered before using an ETT exchange catheter. First, it must be small enough to pass through the tracheal lumen of the DLT. This should be tested in vitro before the procedure is performed in vivo. Second, it should never be advanced against resistance, and the clinician must always be cognizant of the depth of insertion; perforations of the tracheobronchial tree have been reported.[43] Third, a jet ventilator should be immediately available in case the new ETT does not follow the exchange catheter into the trachea and oxygenation via the catheter is needed. The jet ventilator should be preset to a peak inspiratory pressure of 25 psi (172 kPa) by an inline regulator. When passing an ETT over an ETT exchange catheter, a laryngoscope should be used to facilitate passage of the ETT into the trachea. It should be noted that the tip of the ETT may hang up on the laryngeal inlet and may require 90 degrees rotation clockwise or counter-clockwise to successfully pass, should this occur.

### General Considerations in the Management of Single-Lung Ventilation

Once the ETT, bronchial blocker, or DLT is in place, airway pressures should be confirmed during SLV. If peak airway pressure is 20 cm $H_2O$ during two-lung ventilation with a given tidal volume, inflating pressure should not exceed 40 cm $H_2O$ in SLV when the same tidal volume is delivered during SLV. In general, smaller tidal volumes with increased respiratory rates are used to deliver a somewhat reduced minute ventilation with SLV as with two-lung ventilation. Some degree of permissive hypercapnia is targeted to minimize lung trauma.

After the child has been placed in the lateral decubitus position, proper ETT, bronchial blocker, or DLT position should be reconfirmed, because malpositioning may occur when turning the patient. Two-lung ventilation should be maintained for as long as possible before switching to SLV. When SLV is required, an $FIO_2$ of 1.0 is generally used. Assuming an intact hypoxic pulmonary vasoconstriction response, $PaO_2$ during SLV should be between 150 and 210 mm Hg.[44] The lungs should be ventilated with a tidal volume of 8 to 10 mL/kg at a ventilatory rate that maintains the $PaCO_2$ between 45 and 60 mm Hg, unless this degree of hypercapnia cannot be tolerated because of other physiologic factors (e.g., concomitant metabolic acidosis). Inadequate tidal volumes may lead to atelectasis in the ventilated lung (reduced functional residual capacity), and increased intrapulmonary shunting, resulting in hypoxemia. Large tidal volumes may force blood to the nondependent lung (similar to the application of positive end-expiratory pressure), thereby increasing the intrapulmonary shunt.[45,46]

After the institution of SLV, $PaO_2$ may continue to decrease for up to 45 minutes. Should hypoxemia develop, proper positioning of the indwelling blocker or tube should be reconfirmed by fiberoptic bronchoscopy, if possible. Several techniques can be employed to improve oxygenation. The most effective maneuver for improving $PaO_2$ is the application of CPAP to the nondependent lung.[47] Insufflation of oxygen to achieve a CPAP of 10 cm $H_2O$, for example, produces alveolar inflation and decreases intrapulmonary shunt fraction. This can usually be accomplished without significant expansion of the lung and interference with surgical conditions. If the $PaO_2$ continues to decrease despite the application of CPAP to the deflated lung, a malpositioned bronchial blocker or tube should be considered. This may be signaled by a sudden increase in the inflation pressure, a decrease in tidal volume, and/or a change in the capnogram. When a DLT is in place, the surgeon may aid repositioning. The surgeon can palpate the bronchi and manually occlude the main bronchial lumens, thereby guiding the tip of the DLT into the correct position. When the cause of the hypoxemia and/or hypercarbia cannot be readily identified, the balloon or cuff should be deflated and both lungs should be ventilated after informing the surgeon of the problem.

Guidelines for selecting appropriate tubes (or catheters) for SLV in children are shown in Table 13-6. There is significant variability in overall size and airway dimensions in children, particularly in teenagers. The recommendations shown in Table 13-6 are based on average values for airway dimensions. Larger DLTs may be safely used in large adolescents.

## SURGICAL LESIONS OF THE CHEST
### Neonates and Infants

A variety of congenital intrathoracic lesions for which surgery is required may occur in the neonatal or infancy period. These include lesions of the trachea and bronchi, lung parenchyma, and diaphragm, as well as vascular abnormalities.

*Tracheal stenosis* may be acquired or congenital. Tracheal stenosis occurs most commonly because of prolonged tracheal intubation, often in neonates with infant respiratory distress syndrome associated with prematurity. Ischemic injury of the tracheal mucosa may occur as a result of a tight-fitting ETT at the level

**TABLE 13-6** Tube Selection for Single-Lung Ventilation in Children

| Age (yr) | ETT (ID)* | BB (F) | Univent† | DLT (F) |
|---|---|---|---|---|
| 0.5-1 | 3.5-4.0 | 2‡ | | |
| 1-2 | 4.0-4.5 | 3‡ | | |
| 2-4 | 4.5-5.0 | 5§ | | |
| 4-6 | 5.0-5.5 | 5§ | | |
| 6-8 | 5.5-6.0 | 5§ | 3.5 | |
| 8-10 | 6.0 cuffed | 5§ | 3.5 | 26‖ |
| 10-12 | 6.5 cuffed | 5§ | 4.5 | 26‖-28‖ |
| 12-14 | 6.5-7.0 cuffed | 5§ | 4.5 | 32‖ |
| 14-16 | 7.0 cuffed | 5, 7§ | 6.0 | 35‖ |
| 16-18 | 7.0-8.0 cuffed | 7, 9§ | 7.0 | 35, 37‖ |

*BB*, Bronchial blocker; *DLT*, double-lumen tube; *ETT*, endotracheal tube; *F*, French size; *ID*, internal diameter.
*Sheridan tracheal tubes, Hudson RCI, Arlington Heights, Ill.
†Fuji Systems Corporation, Tokyo.
‡Edwards Lifesciences LLC, Irvine, Calif.
§Cook Medical, Inc., Bloomington, Ind.
‖Covidien, Mansfield, Mass.

of the cricoid cartilage, which becomes scarred and constricted after a period of time. *Subglottic stenosis* may develop, resulting in stridor after tracheal extubation. Reintubation may be required because of oxygen desaturation and hypercarbia.

Tracheal and/or esophageal compression may occur as a result of a variety of lesions in the chest, including vascular rings and slings (see also Chapters 14 and 31).

A FOB is used to evaluate the severity of the stenosis and exclude other causes of stridor (e.g., vocal cord paralysis or laryngomalacia). When general anesthesia is required, inhalational anesthesia may be administered via a face mask, with the FOB inserted through an adapter in the mask and into the nasopharynx. This is usually performed while the infant breathes spontaneously.[48] Noninvasive imaging studies are being increasingly utilized for the diagnosis of a variety of congenital airway lesions, including vascular rings.[48] Bronchography and "virtual" computed tomography (CT) scanning may also be useful.[49,50]

A cricoid split procedure may be performed for infants with acquired subglottic stenosis. After diagnostic bronchoscopy, the infant is either intubated with an ETT or a rigid bronchoscope is left in place during the operation. Anesthesia may be maintained with inhalational agents or an IV anesthetic technique, such as with propofol and remifentanil.[51] Typically, an ETT 0.5 mm larger than the original ETT is placed after the repair.

For infants with severe *congenital tracheal stenosis*, a laryngotracheoplasty may be performed. This procedure involves the placement of a costal, auricular, or laryngeal cartilage graft into the anterior and/or posterior trachea.[52] In some cases, a stent may be positioned within the trachea. These infants may require a tracheal tube and mechanical ventilation for a variable period of time postoperatively. In these cases, sedation, analgesia, and at times neuromuscular blockade are maintained after surgery.

*Pulmonary sequestrations* result from disordered embryogenesis, producing a nonfunctional mass of lung tissue supplied by anomalous systemic arteries. Children may present with cough, pneumonia, and failure to thrive; these signs often occur during the neonatal period, and usually before 2 years of age. Diagnostic studies include CT of the chest and abdomen, and arteriography.

Magnetic resonance imaging may provide high-resolution images, including definition of the vascular supply, which may obviate the need for angiography. Surgical resection is performed once the diagnosis is confirmed. Pulmonary sequestrations do not generally become hyperinflated during positive-pressure ventilation. Nitrous oxide administration may result in expansion of these masses, however, and should be avoided.

*Congenital cystic lesions* in the thorax may be classified into three categories.[53] *Bronchogenic cysts* result from abnormal budding or branching of the tracheobronchial tree. They may cause respiratory distress, recurrent pneumonia, and/or atelectasis because of lung compression. *Dermoid cysts* are clinically similar to bronchogenic cysts but differ histologically because they are lined with keratinized, squamous epithelium rather than respiratory (ciliated columnar) epithelium. They usually manifest later in childhood or adulthood. *Cystic adenomatoid malformations* are structurally similar to bronchioles but lack associated alveoli, bronchial glands, and cartilage.[54] Because these lesions communicate with the airways, they may become overdistended as a result of gas trapping, leading to respiratory distress in the first few days of life. When they are multiple and air filled, cystic adenomatoid malformations may resemble congenital diaphragmatic hernias radiographically. Treatment is surgical resection of the affected lobe. As with congenital diaphragmatic hernias, prognosis depends on the amount of remaining lung tissue, which may be hypoplastic because of compression in utero.[55]

*Congenital lobar emphysema* often manifests with respiratory distress shortly after birth.[56] This lesion may be caused by "ball-valve" bronchial obstruction in utero, causing progressive distal overdistention with fetal lung fluid. The resultant emphysematous lobe may compress lung tissue bilaterally, resulting in a variable degree of hypoplasia. Congenital cardiac deformities are present in about 15% of children with congenital lobar emphysema.[57] Radiographic signs of hyperinflation may be misinterpreted as tension pneumothorax or atelectasis on the contralateral side (Fig. 13-9). Positive-pressure ventilation may exacerbate lung

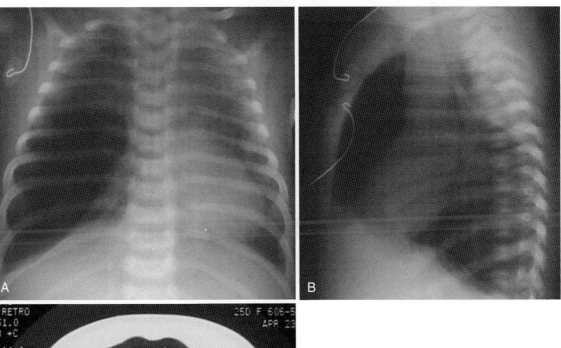
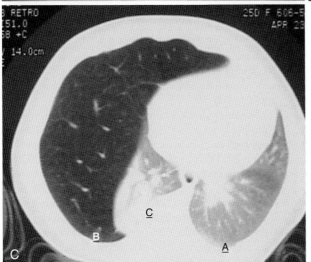

**FIGURE 13-9** Congenital lobar emphysema of the right lower lobe. Plain radiography illustrates hyperlucency of the right lung on the anteroposterior image (**A**) and posterior displacement of the heart and mediastinum on the lateral image (**B**). The computed tomography scan (**C**) demonstrates compression of the left lung (_A_) and right upper lobe (_C_) as well as hyperinflation of the right lower lobe (_B_).

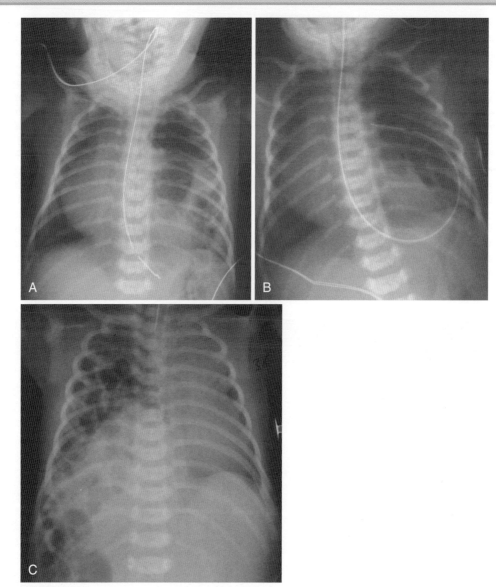

**FIGURE 13-10** The majority of congenital diaphragmatic hernias are left sided. **A,** Chest radiography demonstrates the presence of bowel in the left hemithorax. **B,** A nasogastric tube has been advanced into the stomach. **C,** Congenital diaphragmatic hernias may also occur on the right side.

hyperinflation. Nitrous oxide is contraindicated, and isolation of the lungs during anesthesia is desirable (see also chapter 36).

*Congenital diaphragmatic hernia* is a life-threatening condition that occurs in approximately 1 in 2000 live births. Failure of a portion of the fetal diaphragm to develop allows abdominal contents to enter the thorax, interfering with normal lung growth. In 70% to 80% of diaphragmatic defects, a portion of the left posterior diaphragm fails to close, forming a triangular defect known as the *foramen of Bochdalek.* Hernias through the foramen of Bochdalek that occur early in fetal life usually cause respiratory failure immediately after birth owing to pulmonary hypoplasia. Distention of the gut postnatally with bag-and-mask ventilation exacerbates the ventilatory compromise by further compressing the lungs. The diagnosis is often made prenatally, and fetal surgical repair has been described.[58] Neonates present with tachypnea, a scaphoid abdomen, and absent breath sounds over the affected side. Chest radiography typically shows bowel in the left hemithorax, with deviation of the heart and mediastinum to the right and compression of the right lung

(Fig. 13-10). Right-sided hernias (see Fig. 13-10, *C*) may occur late and manifest with milder signs. In the presence of significant respiratory distress, bag-and-mask ventilation should be avoided and immediate tracheal intubation should be performed (see also Chapter 36).

Because pulmonary hypertension with right-to-left shunting contributes to severe hypoxemia in neonates with congenital diaphragmatic hernia, a variety of pulmonary vasodilators have been used. These include tolazoline, prostacyclin, dipyridamole, and nitric oxide.[59-63] High-frequency oscillatory ventilation has been used in conjunction with pulmonary vasodilator therapy to improve oxygenation before surgery.[64] Occasionally, prostaglandin $E_1$ is used to maintain a patent ductus arteriosus and reduce right ventricular afterload. In cases of severe lung hypoplasia and pulmonary hypertension refractory to these therapies (e.g., $PaO_2$ less than 50 mm Hg with $FIO_2$ of 1.0), extracorporeal membrane oxygenation (ECMO) should be initiated early to avoid progressive lung injury. Improved outcomes have been associated with early use of ECMO followed by delayed surgical repair.[65]

A particularly poor prognosis is predicted if congenital diaphragmatic hernia is associated with cardiac deformities, preoperative alveolar-to-arterial oxygen gradient greater than 500 mm Hg, or severe hypercarbia despite vigorous ventilation.[66,67] Prognosis has also been correlated with pulmonary compliance and radiographic findings.[68,69]

Surgical correction via a subcostal incision with ipsilateral chest tube placement may be performed before, during, or immediately after ECMO.[70,71] In neonates undergoing surgical repair without ECMO, pulmonary hypertension is the major cause of morbidity and mortality. Hyperventilation to induce a respiratory alkalosis and 100% oxygen may be administered to decrease pulmonary vascular resistance. The anesthetic should be designed to minimize sympathetic discharge, which may exacerbate pulmonary hypertension (e.g., a high-dose opioid technique). The lungs of these infants should be ventilated with small tidal volumes and low inflating pressures, to avoid pneumothorax on the contralateral (usually right) side. Both nitric oxide and high-frequency oscillatory ventilation have been used during surgical repair.[72,73] A high index of suspicion of right-sided pneumothorax should be maintained, and a thoracostomy tube should be placed in the event of acute deterioration of respiratory or circulatory function. It is also imperative that normal body temperature, intravascular volume, and acid-base status be maintained. Mechanical ventilation is continued postoperatively in nearly all cases, because lung compliance is markedly reduced after surgery.

Failure of the central and lateral portions of the diaphragm to fuse results in a retrosternal defect, the *foramen of Morgagni*. This usually manifests as signs of bowel obstruction rather than respiratory distress. Repair is usually performed via an abdominal incision (see also Chapter 36).

*Tracheoesophageal fistula* and/or *esophageal atresia* occurs in approximately 1 in 4000 live births. In 80% to 85% of afflicted infants, this lesion includes esophageal atresia with a distal esophageal pouch and a proximal tracheoesophageal fistula.[74,75] The fistula is usually located one to two tracheal rings above the carina. Afflicted neonates present with spillover of pooled oral secretions from the pouch and may develop progressive gastric distention and tracheal aspiration of acidic gastric contents via the fistula. A common association is the VACTERL complex, consisting of vertebral, anorectal, cardiac, tracheal, esophageal, renal, and/or limb defects.[76] Esophageal atresia is confirmed when an orogastric tube passed through the mouth cannot be advanced more than about 7 cm (Fig. 13-11). The proximal pouch tube should be secured and continuous suction applied, after which a chest radiograph is diagnostic (see also Chapter 36).

Mask ventilation and tracheal intubation are avoided before surgery if possible, because they may exacerbate gastric distention and further compromise respirations. Once the trachea is intubated, it is occasionally necessary to occlude the tracheal orifice of the fistula with the tracheal tube. The tip of the tracheal tube is positioned just above the carina by auscultation of diminished breath sounds over the left axilla as the tube is advanced into the right main-stem bronchus, after which the tube is retracted until breath sounds are increased over the left chest (Fig. 13-12, *A*). A small FOB may be passed through the tracheal tube to confirm appropriate placement. Rarely, an emergency gastrostomy is performed because of massive gastric distention. Placement of a balloon-tipped catheter in the fistula via the gastrostomy may be performed under guidance with an FOB, to prevent further gastric distention and/or enable effective positive-pressure

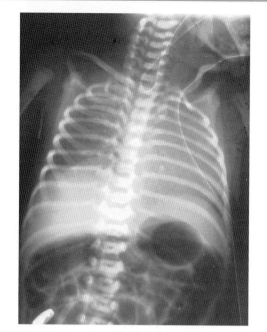

**FIGURE 13-11** Tracheoesophageal fistula with esophageal atresia. Note the feeding tube coiled in the esophageal pouch and the presence of a large volume of gas in the abdomen.

ventilation in cases of significant lung disease (see Fig. 13-12, *B*).[77] "Antegrade" occlusion of a tracheoesophageal fistula has also been reported with a balloon-tipped catheter advanced through the trachea into the fistula (see Fig. 13-12, *C*).[78] Preoperative evaluation should be performed to diagnose associated anomalies, particularly cardiac, musculoskeletal, and gastrointestinal defects, which occur in 30% to 50% of afflicted infants.[79] A poor prognosis for infants with tracheoesophageal fistula and esophageal atresia has been associated with prematurity and underlying lung disease, as well as the coexistence of other congenital anomalies.[80]

Surgical repair usually involves a right thoracotomy and extrapleural dissection of the posterior mediastinum. In most cases, the fistula is ligated and primary esophageal anastomosis is performed ("short gap atresia"). In cases in which the esophageal "gap" is long, the proximal segment is preserved for subsequent staged anastomosis, with or without intestinal interposition.[75] The trachea may be intubated with the infant breathing spontaneously, or during gentle positive-pressure ventilation with small tidal volumes to avoid gastric distention. If a gastrostomy tube is in place, occlusion of the fistula may be confirmed by cessation of bubbling via underwater tubing connected to the gastrostomy or the appearance of $CO_2$ in the end-tidal gas.[55] Alternatively, the tracheal tube may be positioned in the main-stem bronchus, opposite the side of the thoracotomy incision, until the fistula is ligated.

Esophageal atresia without connection to the trachea occurs much less commonly. These lesions are generally diagnosed by radiography after inability to pass an orogastric tube, at which time an absence of gas in the abdomen may be noted (see Fig. 36-4). So-called H-type tracheoesophageal fistula without esophageal atresia is relatively rare. Infants with H-type lesions may present later in childhood or adulthood with recurrent pneumonias or gastric distention during positive-pressure ventilation (see Chapter 36).[81,82]

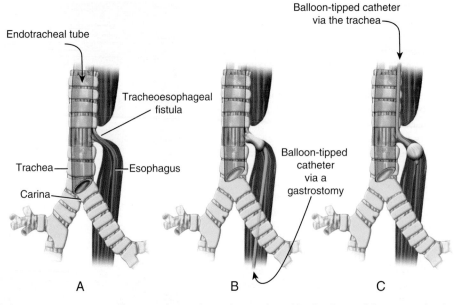

**FIGURE 13-12** Methods for minimizing gastric insufflation in infants with a tracheoesophageal fistula. The tip of the ETT may be placed distal to the fistula in cases in which the fistula is well proximal to the carina (**A**). Alternatively, a balloon-tipped catheter may be placed in the fistula via a gastrostomy (**B**) or via the trachea (**C**).

## Childhood

Some of the lesions described earlier may not be diagnosed until childhood. These include pulmonary sequestration, cystic lesions, and lobar emphysema. Other disorders for which thoracic surgery is performed in children, either for definitive treatment or diagnostic purposes, include neoplasms, infectious diseases, and musculoskeletal deformities.

*Anterior mediastinal masses* include neoplasms of the lung, mediastinum, and pleura. These tumors may be primary or metastatic. Perhaps the most common primary tumors are *lymphoblastic lymphoma*, a form of non-Hodgkin lymphoma, and *Hodgkin disease*. Less commonly, teratomas (germ cell tumors), thymomas, as well as thyroid, parathyroid, and mesenchymal tumors may manifest as anterior mediastinal masses.[83] Signs and symptoms that result from vascular and/or airway compression may include dyspnea, orthopnea, pain, coughing, pleural effusion, and/or superior vena cava syndrome (swelling of the upper arms, face, and neck).[84,85]

Preoperative evaluation should include CT, echocardiography, and flow-volume studies whenever feasible. Tracheal, bronchial, and/or vascular (superior vena cava or pulmonary outflow tract) compression, as detected by CT, is associated with a high incidence of serious complications during induction of anesthesia.[85] However, CT scans are static pictures that may not identify dynamic compression of an airway or vascular outflow tract. These tumors may occur as extrathoracic or intrathoracic, variable obstruction or fixed obstruction. Echocardiography identifies compression of the superior vena cava or pulmonary outflow tract. Flow-volume loops may be effective in detecting dynamic compression of the airways, although their utility in adult patients has been questioned[86] (see Chapter 11 and Fig. 11-6).

Establishing the correct diagnosis often requires a tissue biopsy. More often than not, there is an urgency to secure the tissue for diagnosis, because T-cell type non-Hodgkin lymphoblastic lymphomas, which constitute 30% to 40% of non-Hodgkin lymphoma, have a 12-hour doubling time.[87] A rapid

diagnosis and chemotherapy prescription may prevent widespread dissemination of the tumor. Indeed, today, the 5-year survival of Hodgkin and non-Hodgkin lymphoblastic lymphoma exceeds 80%. Every effort should be made to secure a tissue diagnosis by lymph node or bone marrow biopsy under local anesthesia or sedation, thereby precluding the need for general anesthesia and facilitating early treatment.[88] If peripheral tissue diagnosis cannot be obtained and signs of severe airway and/or circulatory compromise are present, careful consideration should be given to administering a 12- to 24-hour burst of corticosteroids, initiating chemotherapy, and/or treating with limited radiation to decrease the size of the tumor and reduce the risk of life-threatening compression of the airway or major vessels under anesthesia. The risk is that any or all of these interventions may cause involution of the tumor and compromise the tissue diagnosis; thus some oncologists prefer that none of these interventions is used prebiopsy.[89,90] Corticosteroids effect a reduction in tissue mass (i.e., tumor lysis) of lymphomas by inducing apoptosis in the tumor via a number of mechanisms.[91] One study found that four features were predictive of perianesthesia complications in these children: orthopnea, upper body edema, great vessel compression, and main-stem bronchial compression (odds ratio of 5.1 to 8).[92] A second study found that the extent of vascular and airway compression, according to radiologic investigations, was predictive of perianesthesia complications.[88] It must be emphasized that adolescents and adults have different risk factors than small children under the age of 8 years. In adults, for example, intraoperative complications have been associated with pericardial effusions diagnosed by CT scans, whereas postoperative respiratory complications have been associated with greater than 50% tracheal compression on preoperative CT.[92a] Great care must be taken to properly prepare these children and the families for general anesthesia, together with the attendant risks.

Induction of anesthesia in children with anterior mediastinal masses may be associated with severe airway obstruction and

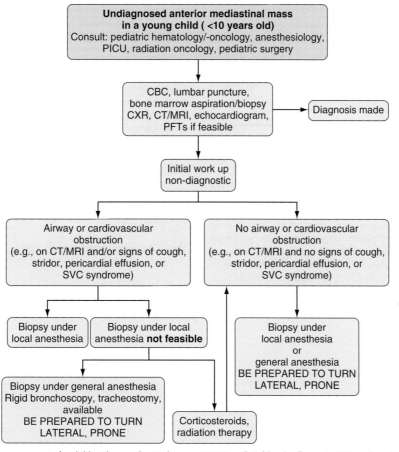

**FIGURE 13-13** Algorithm for management of a child with a mediastinal mass. *CBC,* Complete blood cell count; *CPB,* cardiopulmonary bypass; *CT,* computed tomography; *CXR,* chest radiograph; *LP,* lumbar puncture; *MRI,* magnetic resonance imaging; *PFTs,* pulmonary function tests; *PICU,* pediatric intensive care unit; *SVC,* superior vena cava.

circulatory collapse.[88] This may occur even in children without signs or symptoms of respiratory or cardiovascular compromise.[93,94] Therefore a preoperative assessment of what position provides the most reliable and consistent good gas exchange should be sought from the child or the parents (nocturnal sleep position). Recommended anesthetic techniques for children with anterior mediastinal masses include inhalation induction or a slow IV induction (with ketamine or propofol), with maintenance of spontaneous respiration. The latter offsets the effect of gravity, which pulls the tumor onto the pulmonary artery, superior vena cava, and tracheobronchial tree, causing life-threatening cardiopulmonary consequences.[87,90,95] The use of continuous positive airway pressure while maintaining spontaneous respiration, maintains functional residual capacity that is otherwise reduced under anesthesia.[96] In adolescents and adults, neuromuscular blockade is commonly used to facilitate tracheal intubation and prevent coughing associated with DLT placement. The morbidity associated with neuromuscular blockade appears to be minimal as long as appropriate precautions are taken. The actual risks in young children, however, have not been studied.[92a] Keeping the head of the bed elevated may decrease the deleterious effects of supine positioning, including cephalad displacement of the diaphragm and secondary reduction of thoracic volume.[97] Placing the child in a partial or even full left lateral decubitus position may help to maintain airway patency and reduce cardiovascular and/or tracheal compression.[87] Performing tracheal intubation while deeply anesthetized, without the use of muscle relaxants and

positive-pressure ventilation, preserves the normal transpulmonary pressure gradient and improves flow through conducting airways.[98-100] The loss of negative intrathoracic pressure associated with neuromuscular blockade increases the risk of severe airway compression and reduction in pulmonary blood flow (i.e., cardiac output).[101] As an alternative to tracheal intubation, use of a laryngeal mask airway has been described.[102] The use of a helium-oxygen (70%/30%) mixture has been recommended to decrease the resistance to breathing and to increase hemoglobin saturation when an anterior mediastinal tumor compresses the trachea and/or bronchi (where turbulent gas flow exists).[102] In the event of tracheal or bronchial collapse under anesthesia, lateral or prone positioning and/or rigid bronchoscopy may be lifesaving.[87] Performing a median sternotomy and cardiopulmonary bypass in this situation has been recommended but is quite impractical unless access for partial bypass has been established before induction of anesthesia.[90]

Institutions should have an algorithm in place for the evaluation of children with anterior mediastinal masses that includes a multidisciplinary approach (Fig. 13-13).

## Summary

The anesthesiologist caring for infants and children undergoing thoracic surgery faces many challenges. An understanding of the primary underlying lesion as well as associated anomalies that may affect perioperative management is paramount. Preoperative and intraoperative communication with the surgeon is also essential. A working knowledge of respiratory physiology and anatomy in infants and children is required for the planning and execution of appropriate intraoperative care. Familiarity with a variety of techniques for single-lung ventilation suited to the child's size will provide optimal surgical exposure while minimizing trauma to the lungs and airways.

## ANNOTATED REFERENCES

Capan LM, Turndorf H, Patel C, et al. Optimization of arterial oxygenation during one-lung anesthesia. Anesth Analg 1980;59:847-51.

Rees DI, Wansbrough SR. One-lung anesthesia and arterial oxygen tension during continuous insufflation of oxygen to the nonventilated lung. Anesth Analg 1982;61:507-12.

*These articles describe the maneuvers of choice for increasing oxygenation in patients during single-lung ventilation. Oxygen desaturation is common during single-lung ventilation, especially in children. It is essential that practitioners have an algorithm for addressing this problem promptly during surgery.*

Hammer GB, Harrison TK, Vricella LA, et al. Single lung ventilation in children using a new paediatric bronchial blocker. Pediatr Anesth 2002;12:69-72.

*This article is the first to describe the use of the Cook 5F pediatric endobronchial blocker. This is now the most commonly used bronchial blocker in children. The characteristics of the catheter and the details of the methodology for insertion and proper placement are highlighted.*

Heaf DP, Helms P, Gordon MB, Turner HM. Postural effects on gas exchange in infants. N Engl J Med 1983;28:1505-8.

*Changes in ventilation and perfusion of the lung associated with body position were first described in adults. This paper describes such relationships in infants, highlighting the important differences in this population that have significant clinical relevance during thoracic anesthesia.*

Keon TP. Death on induction of anesthesia for cervical node biopsy. Anesthesiology 1981;55:471-2.

*This was the sentinel article describing death related to administration of anesthesia in a child with an anterior mediastinal mass.*

## REFERENCES

Please see www.expertconsult.com.

# Essentials of Cardiology

14

RALPH GERTLER AND WANDA C. MILLER-HANCE

## Congenital Heart Disease

### INCIDENCE

Congenital heart disease (CHD) represents the most common form of congenital pathology, with an estimated incidence of 0.3% to 1.2% of live births.[1] CHD is a major cause of morbidity and mortality during the neonatal period. However, with advances in medical and surgical management, including significant contributions related to anesthesia care, survival to adulthood is the expectation for most infants and children with CHD.[2-4]

A bicuspid aortic valve (Video 14-1) is the most common cardiac defect, occurring in up to 1% of the population.[5,6] Ventricular septal defects (VSD) (Video 14-2) represent the next most common congenital pathology,[5,7-11] followed by secundum atrial septal defects (ASD) (Video 14-3).[5,12] Among cyanotic lesions, tetralogy of Fallot (TOF) predominates, affecting almost 6% of children with CHD (Fig. 14-1).[13] In the first week of life, D-transposition of the great arteries (Fig. 14-2) is the most frequently encountered cause of cardiac cyanosis; TOF is sometimes not detected until later in life because cyanosis is absent or only mild desaturation is present.

## SEGMENTAL APPROACH TO DIAGNOSIS

Several classification schemes have been proposed to characterize and categorize various congenital cardiac defects.[14-20] The segmental approach to the diagnosis of CHD assumes a sequential, systematic analysis of the three major cardiac segments (i.e., atria, ventricles, and great arteries) to describe the anatomic abnormalities. The principle of this scheme is that specific cardiac chambers and vascular structures have characteristic morphologic properties that determine their identities, rather than their positions within the body.[21] An organized, systematic identification of all cardiac structures or segments and their relationships (i.e., connections or alignments between segments) is carried out to define a child's anatomy.[22]

The initial approach is to determine the cardiac position within the thorax and the arrangement or situs of the thoracic and abdominal organs. The cardiac position can be described in terms of its location within the thoracic cavity (Fig. 14-3) and the direction of the cardiac apex. Although the cardiac position within the thorax may be considered independent of the cardiac base-apex axis, for simplicity the following terms are used: *levocardia* if the heart is in the left hemithorax (as is normally the case); *dextrocardia* if the heart is located in the right hemithorax; and *mesocardia* if the heart is displaced rightward but not completely in the right thoracic cavity. An abnormal location of the heart within the thorax (i.e., cardiac malposition) may result from displacement by adjacent structures or underlying noncardiac malformations (e.g., diaphragmatic hernia, lung hypoplasia, scoliosis).

The visceral situs, or sidedness, of the abdominal organs (i.e., liver and stomach) and atrial situs are considered independently (Fig. 14-4). Visceral situs is classified as *solitus* (i.e., normal arrangement of viscera, with the liver on the right, stomach on the left, and a single spleen on the left), *inversus* (i.e., inversion of viscera, with the liver on the left and stomach on the right), or *ambiguous* (i.e., indeterminate visceral position). Abnormal arrangements or sidedness of the abdominal viscera, heart, and lungs suggests a high likelihood of complex cardiovascular disease. The atrial situs, atrioventricular (AV) connections, ventricular looping (i.e., position of the ventricles as a result of the direction of bending of the straight heart tube in early development), ventriculoarterial connections, and the relationship between the great vessels are then delineated.

Associated malformations are described, including number and size of septal defects and valvar or great vessel abnormalities.

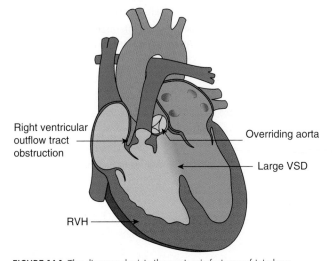

FIGURE 14-1 The diagram depicts the anatomic features of tetralogy of Fallot. The abnormalities consist of right ventricular outflow tract obstruction (typically at any or a combination of valvar, subvalvar, and supravalvar levels), a large ventricular septal defect (*VSD*), aortic override, and right ventricular hypertrophy (*RVH*). Purple aorta indicates desaturation. The small size of the pulmonary artery is indicative of the right outflow tract obstruction.

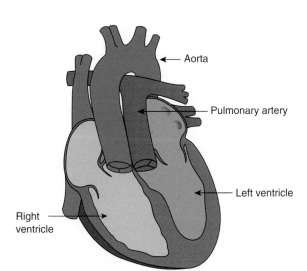

FIGURE 14-2 Discordant ventriculoarterial connections are shown in the diagram of D-transposition of the great arteries. The right ventricle ejects blood into the pulmonary artery and the left ventricle ejects blood into the aorta. Mixing of blood must occur via an atrial septal defect, ventricular septal defect, or patent ductus arteriosus.

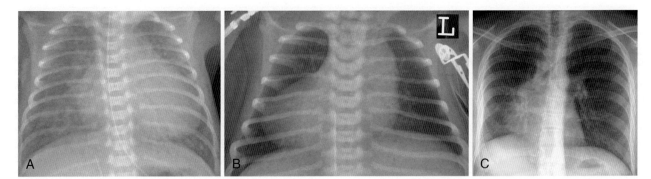

FIGURE 14-3 Chest radiographs demonstrate various cardiac positions within the thorax. **A,** Levocardia (left-sided position). **B,** Dextrocardia (right-sided position). **C,** Mesocardia (centrally located cardiac mass).

Types of visceroatrial situs: atrial localization

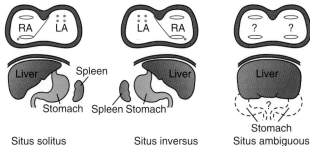

Situs solitus    Situs inversus    Situs ambiguous

**FIGURE 14-4** Three types of visceroatrial situs are shown. *Situs solitus* indicates a normal arrangement of the viscera and atria, with the right atrium (*RA*) on the right side and the left atrium (*LA*) on the left side. The stomach and spleen are on the left, and the liver is on the right. *Situs inversus* indicates inverted arrangement of viscera and atria, with the RA on the left side and the LA on the right side, as in a mirror image of situs solitus. In visceral situs inversus, the stomach and spleen are on the right, and the liver is on the left. *Situs ambiguous* denotes that the visceroatrial situs is anatomically uncertain or indeterminate because the anatomic findings are ambiguous. (From Van Praagh R. The segmental approach to diagnosis in congenital heart disease. In: Bergsma D, editor: Birth defects: original article series. Vol 8. Baltimore: Williams & Wilkins; 1972, p. 23-44. Permission granted by March of Dimes.)

| **TABLE 14-1** Physiologic Classification of Congenital Heart Disease (Representative Lesions) |
| --- |
| **Volume Overload Lesions** |
| Atrial septal defect |
| Ventricular septal defect |
| Atrioventricular septal defect |
| Patent ductus arteriosus |
| Truncus arteriosus |
| **Obstruction to Systemic Blood Flow** |
| Aortic stenosis |
| Coarctation of the aorta |
| Interrupted aortic arch |
| Hypoplastic left heart syndrome |
| **Obstruction to Pulmonary Blood Flow** |
| Pulmonary stenosis |
| Tetralogy of Fallot |
| Pulmonary atresia |
| **Parallel Circulation** |
| D-Transposition of the great arteries |
| **Single Ventricle Lesions** |
| Tricuspid atresia |
| Double-inlet left ventricle |
| Unbalanced atrioventricular septal defect |
| **Intrinsic Myocardial Disorders** |
| Cardiomyopathy |
| Myocarditis |

Whereas many types of congenital defects fall neatly into this classification scheme, others (e.g., heterotaxy syndromes, conditions associated with malposition of the heart and abdominal organs) are often more difficult to precisely define.

## PHYSIOLOGIC CLASSIFICATION OF DEFECTS

The wide spectrum of cardiovascular malformations in the pediatric age group presents a challenge to the clinician who does not specialize in the care of these children. Even for those with a focus or interest in cardiovascular disease, the range of structural defects and the varied associated hemodynamic perturbations can be overwhelming.

A physiologic classification system can facilitate understanding of the basic hemodynamic abnormalities common to a group of congenital or acquired lesions and assist in patient management (Table 14-1).[23,24] Several classification schemes have been proposed, including some that categorize structural defects as simple or complex lesions, consider the presence or absence of cyanosis, or consider whether pulmonary blood flow is increased or decreased.[25-27] The following approach groups pediatric heart disease into six broad categories according to the underlying physiology or common features of the pathologies.

### Volume Overload Lesions

Volume overload lesions typically are caused by left-to-right shunting at the atrial, ventricular, or great artery levels. If the location of the left-to-right shunt is proximal to the mitral valve (e.g., ASDs, partial anomalous pulmonary venous return, unobstructed total anomalous pulmonary venous return), right heart dilation will occur. Lesions distal to the mitral valve (e.g., VSD, patent ductus arteriosus [PDA], truncus arteriosus) lead to left heart dilation. Children with AV septal defects (i.e., AV canal defects) also fit into this category. The magnitude of the shunt and resultant pulmonary-to-systemic blood flow ratio ($\dot{Q}_{pulm}/\dot{Q}_{sys}$) dictate the presence and severity of the symptoms and guide medical and surgical therapies. Diuretic therapy and afterload reduction are beneficial in controlling pulmonary overcirculation and ensuring adequate systemic cardiac output. Transcatheter approaches or surgical interventions may be required to address the primary pathology associated with ventricular volume overload (see Chapter 20).

### Obstruction to Systemic Blood Flow

Several lesions are characterized by systemic outflow tract obstruction. Conditions characterized by ductal-dependent systemic blood flow in the neonate include critical aortic stenosis, severe aortic coarctation, aortic arch interruption, and hypoplastic left heart syndrome. Prostaglandin $E_1$ infusion maintains ductal patency and ensures adequate systemic blood flow until surgical or transcatheter intervention is performed in the first few days of life to relieve the systemic outflow obstruction. Inotropic and/or mechanical ventilatory support are often necessary. Many of these infants also have significantly increased pulmonary blood flow with a high $\dot{Q}_{pulm}/\dot{Q}_{sys}$ ratio, requiring diuretic therapy and manipulation of the systemic and pulmonary vascular resistances to control blood flow.

### Obstruction to Pulmonary Blood Flow

Lesions with pulmonary outflow tract obstruction include those with ductal-dependent pulmonary blood flow. Critical pulmonary valve stenosis and pulmonary atresia with intact ventricular septum, for example, are defects that rely on patency of the ductus arteriosus for pulmonary blood flow. These infants may also require prostaglandin $E_1$ infusions for management of their cyanosis until the pulmonary outflow obstruction is relieved or bypassed.

## Parallel Circulation

In the neonate with D-transposition of the great arteries, the pulmonary and systemic circulations operate in parallel rather than in the normal configuration in series. In this condition, the right ventricle ejects deoxygenated blood into the aorta, and the left ventricle ejects oxygenated blood into the pulmonary circulation. Mixing of blood in this setting may occur at the atrial, ventricular, or ductal levels (see Fig. 14-2). Although prostaglandin $E_1$ therapy maintains ductal patency, balloon atrial septostomy to create or enlarge an existing restrictive interatrial communication and optimize mixing may benefit some infants. Mixing at the atrial level is considered much more effective than at the ventricular or ductal levels.

## Single-Ventricle Lesions

This category is the most heterogeneous group, consisting of defects associated with AV valve atresia (i.e., tricuspid atresia), heterotaxy syndromes, and many others.[28] In some cases, both atria empty into a dominant ventricular chamber (i.e., double-inlet left ventricle), and although a second rudimentary ventricle may be present, the physiology is that of a single-ventricle or univentricular heart. Other cardiac malformations with two distinct ventricles (i.e., unbalanced AV septal defect) may also be considered in the functional single-ventricle category because of associated defects that may preclude a biventricular repair. A common feature of these lesions is complete mixing of the systemic and pulmonary venous blood at the atrial or ventricular level. Another common finding is aortic or pulmonary outflow tract obstruction.

Affected children are a challenge to the practitioner and require careful delineation of their anatomy. An important goal in single-ventricle management involves optimization of the balance between the pulmonary and systemic circulations early in life. This is a critical issue because low pulmonary vascular resistance and limitation of the ventricular volume load represent a prerequisite for later palliative strategies and favorable outcomes in these children. These considerations are also relevant during anesthesia management for noncardiac surgery (see Chapter 21).[26,29,30]

## Intrinsic Myocardial Disorders

Children with primary cardiomyopathies or other forms of acquired heart disease such as myocarditis have heart muscle disease. They frequently have impaired systolic or diastolic ventricular function, and benefit from therapies tailored to their particular disease process.

# Acquired Heart Disease

## CARDIOMYOPATHIES

The term *cardiomyopathy* usually refers to diseases of the myocardium associated with cardiac dysfunction.[31,32] They have been classified as primary and secondary forms. The most common types in children are hypertrophic, dilated or congestive, and restrictive cardiomyopathies. Other forms include left ventricular noncompaction[33-35] and arrhythmogenic right ventricular dysplasia.[36] Secondary forms of cardiomyopathies are those associated with neuromuscular disorders such as Duchenne muscular dystrophy, glycogen storage diseases (i.e., Pompe disease), hemochromatosis or iron overload, and mitochondrial disorders. Chemotherapeutic agents such as anthracyclines may result in

dilated cardiomyopathy.[37] It is important to understand the hemodynamic processes behind the myocardial disease and implications for acute and chronic management.

*Hypertrophic cardiomyopathy* (HCM) is characterized by ventricular hypertrophy without an identifiable hemodynamic cause that results in increased thickness of the myocardium. This accounts for almost 40% of cardiomyopathies in children.[38-41] The condition represents a heterogenous group of disorders, and most of the identified genetic defects exhibit autosomal dominant inheritance patterns.[42,43] This is the most common cause of sudden cardiac death (SCD) in athletes.[44,45] Most children with HCM do not have systemic outflow tract obstruction (i.e., non-obstructive cardiomyopathy). It is unclear whether the few with hypertrophic obstructive cardiomyopathy, previously known as idiopathic hypertrophic subaortic stenosis, are at increased risk for SCD compared with children without obstruction.[44]

Most children with HCM present for evaluation of a heart murmur, syncope, palpitations, or chest pain. Occasionally, an abnormal electrocardiogram (ECG) leads to referral. An accurate family history is essential. An apical impulse is often prominent. Auscultation may reveal a systolic ejection outflow murmur that becomes louder with maneuvers that decrease preload or afterload (e.g., standing, Valsalva maneuver) or increased contractility. The murmur decreases in intensity with squatting and isometric hand grip. A mitral regurgitant murmur may also be present. The ECG meets criteria for left ventricular hypertrophy in most children (Fig. 14-5). In some, the electrocardiographic findings may be striking (Fig. 14-6). A hypertrophied, nondilated left ventricle is a diagnostic feature determined by echocardiography (Video 14-4, *A* and *B*).[45] In many children, the hypertrophy may be asymmetric (Video 14-5, *A* and *B*). Echocardiography is the primary imaging modality for long-term assessment of wall thickness, ventricular dimensions, presence and severity of obstruction, systolic and diastolic function, valve competence, and response to therapy. Other diagnostic approaches such as cardiac catheterization and magnetic resonance imaging (MRI) may add helpful information in some cases.

The care of children with HCM includes maintenance of adequate preload, particularly in those with dynamic obstruction. Diuretics are not indicated and often worsen the hemodynamic state by reducing left ventricular volume and increasing the outflow tract obstruction. Drugs that augment myocardial contractility (e.g., inotropic agents, calcium infusions) are not well tolerated. Patients usually undergo continuous electrocardiographic monitoring (i.e., Holter recording) and exercise testing for risk stratification.[46] β-Blockers and calcium channel blockers are the primary agents for outpatient drug therapy.[47] Therapies range widely and include longitudinal observation with medical management of heart failure and arrhythmias, implantation of cardioverter-defibrillators, surgical myotomy or myectomy, transcatheter alcohol septal ablation, and cardiac transplantation.

*Dilated cardiomyopathy* (DCM), also known as congestive cardiomyopathy, is characterized by thinning of the left ventricular myocardium, dilation of the ventricular cavity, and impaired systolic function.[48-50] The broad number of etiologies range from genetic or familial forms to those caused by infections,[51] metabolic derangements, toxic exposures, and degenerative disorders.[52,53] Chronic tachyarrhythmias can also lead to DCM that may or may not improve after the rhythm disturbance is controlled.[54-56]

Most children with DCM present with signs and symptoms of congestive heart failure (e.g., tachypnea, tachycardia, gallop

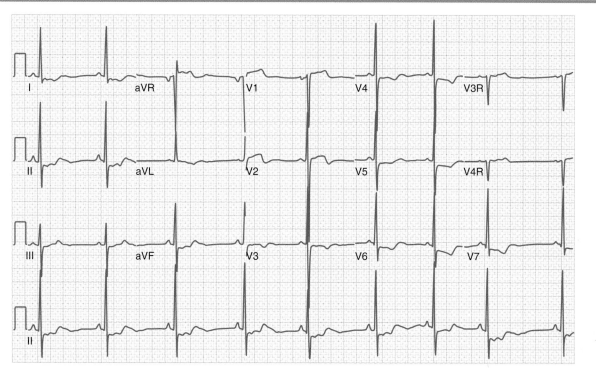

**FIGURE 14-5** The electrocardiogram from an adolescent with hypertrophic cardiomyopathy demonstrates left ventricular hypertrophy (i.e., deep S wave in $V_1$ and tall R waves over the left precordial leads). The ST-segment depression and T-wave inversion over the left precordial leads is related to repolarization changes associated with left ventricular hypertrophy, also known as a *strain pattern*. Reciprocal ST-segment elevation can be seen over the right precordial leads. This recording is consistent with sinus bradycardia (heart rate average of 50 beats per minute).

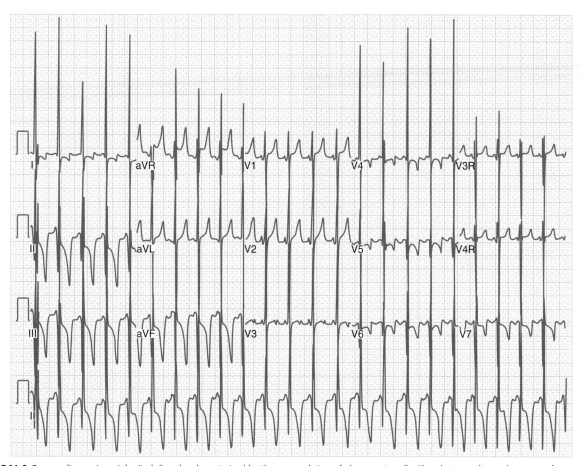

**FIGURE 14-6** Pompe disease is an inherited disorder characterized by the accumulation of glycogen in cells. The electrocardiographic tracing for an infant with this glycogen storage disease and a severe form of hypertrophic cardiomyopathy displays dramatic right and left ventricular voltages, in addition to ST-segment and T-wave abnormalities. The recording is displayed at full standard (10 mm/mV), meaning that the electrocardiogram was not reduced in size to fit on the paper.

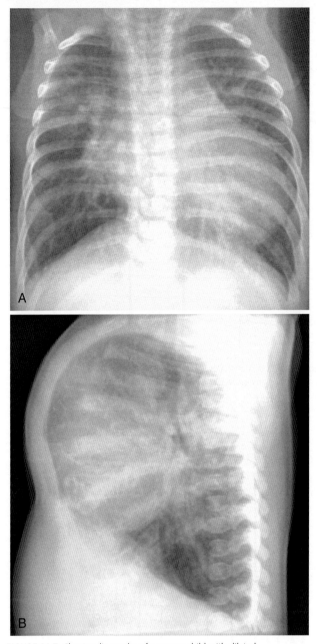

**FIGURE 14-7** Chest radiographs of a young child with dilated cardiomyopathy in the posteroanterior (**A**) and lateral (**B**) projections demonstrate moderate to severe cardiomegaly and pulmonary vascular congestion. The lateral radiograph shows the heart bulging anteriorly against the sternum.

hemodynamic decompensation and cardiovascular collapse. The outcomes of children with dilated cardiomyopathy vary. For most, recovery of left ventricular systolic function occurs, but others eventually require cardiac transplantation.[58] In a subset of children with severe disease, mechanical circulatory support may be necessary as a bridge to recovery or cardiac transplantation (Fig. 14-8) (see Chapter 19).[59-61]

*Restrictive cardiomyopathy* (RCM) is the least common of the major types of cardiomyopathies (5%) and portends a poor prognosis when it manifests during childhood.[62-67] The disorder is characterized by diastolic dysfunction related to a marked increase in myocardial stiffness resulting in impaired ventricular filling. Most cases are thought to be idiopathic. Presenting symptoms are nonspecific and primarily respiratory. Occasionally, the diagnosis is made after a syncopal or sudden near-death event. The physical examination may demonstrate hepatomegaly, peripheral edema, and ascites.

The echocardiographic hallmark of RCM is that of severe atrial dilation and normal- to small-sized ventricles (Video 14-7). The marked diastolic dysfunction leads to increased end-diastolic pressures, left atrial hypertension, and secondary pulmonary hypertension. Children with RCM are prone to thromboembolic complications, and anticoagulation therapy is frequently recommended. This is an important consideration during perioperative care because adjustments in the anticoagulation regimen may be necessary. Atrial and ventricular tachyarrhythmias may also occur. Optimal medical treatment is controversial because no specific agents or strategies have been shown to significantly alter outcomes.[67] Similar to children with HCM, diuretics often cause a decrease in the needed preload with detrimental effects on hemodynamics. Inotropic agents are not indicated because systolic function is preserved and the arrhythmogenic properties of inotropic drugs can induce a terminal event. In many centers, cardiac transplantation has been effectively used.[68,69]

## MYOCARDITIS

*Myocarditis* is defined as inflammation of the myocardium, often associated with necrosis and myocyte degeneration. In the United States, it is most often caused by a viral infection. Over the past 20 years, the spectrum of viral pathogens causing myocarditis has changed, such that adenovirus, enteroviruses (e.g., coxsackievirus B), and parvovirus have become the most frequent causes of fulminant disease.[70-72]

The overall incidence of myocarditis is unknown because it is frequently underdiagnosed and unrecognized as a nonspecific viral syndrome. A large, 10-year, population-based study on cardiomyopathy found an annual incidence of 1.24 cases per 100,000 children younger than 10 years of age; only a fraction of cases represented those with myocarditis.[73] The diagnosis is made using clinical history, physical examination, and imaging modalities. Myocarditis is highly suspected when a child presents with new-onset congestive heart failure or ventricular arrhythmias without evidence of structural heart disease. The ECG typically demonstrates low-voltage QRS complexes with tachycardia, which sometimes is ventricular in origin. Chest radiography often shows cardiomegaly with pulmonary vascular congestion (Fig. 14-9). Echocardiography displays ventricular dilation with decreased systolic function, similar to DCM, and it is useful in the exclusion of alternative diagnoses, such as pericardial effusion or anomalous origin of a coronary artery. Myocarditis is a clinical diagnosis because definitive confirmation requires the analysis of tissue obtained through myocardial biopsy in the catheterization laboratory or the operating room (rarely performed).[74]

rhythm, diminished pulses, hepatomegaly). The chest radiograph typically demonstrates cardiomegaly, pulmonary vascular congestion, and in some cases, atelectasis (Fig. 14-7). The ECG may identify the likely cause of the cardiac dysfunction in those with cardiomyopathy due to rhythm disorders or anomalous origin of the left coronary artery from the pulmonary root (ALCAPA). The echocardiogram can confirm the diagnosis by demonstrating a dilated left ventricle with decreased systolic function (Video 14-6, *A* and *B*).[57] Therapy in the acute setting is supportive and aimed at stabilization. Management may include afterload reduction, inotropic support, and mechanical ventilation. Unlike children with HCM, those with DCM have a volume-loaded, poorly contractile ventricle. Gentle diuresis is beneficial. The infusion of large fluid boluses may be poorly tolerated and result in

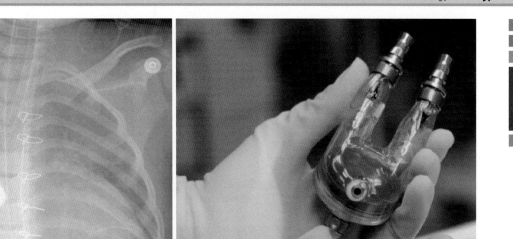

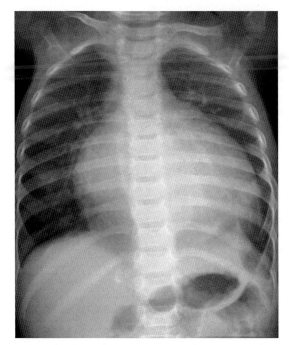

**14**

**FIGURE 14-8** Some children with severe dilated cardiomyopathy (DCM) require mechanical circulatory assist devices. **A,** Chest radiograph of a child with end-stage DCM after placement of a Micromed DeBakey ventricular assist device for circulatory support as a bridge to cardiac transplantation. This miniaturized device includes a titanium pump, inlet cannula placed in the left ventricle, percutaneous cable, flow probe, and outflow graft placed in the aorta (not radiopaque). **B,** The Berlin Heart ventricular assist device allows paracorporeal placement and circulatory support in infants and small children.

**FIGURE 14-9** The chest radiograph of a child with acute myocarditis shows severe cardiomegaly and increased pulmonary vascularity.

Many children with myocarditis have subclinical or mild clinical disease, whereas others progress to overt heart failure or arrhythmias, or both. Among children with heart failure, approximately one third will regain full ventricular function, one third will recover but continue to demonstrate impaired systolic function, and one third will require cardiac transplantation.[75,76] A subset of children, not all of whom initially manifest severe symptoms in the acute period, will progress to have DCM.

Although no specific therapies have been identified to directly treat the myocardial injury, a variety of strategies have been employed.[77-80] The current paradigm includes diuresis and afterload reduction to improve myocardial performance without placing a large burden on an already failing heart.[81] Rhythm disturbances are treated appropriately. Therapy with immune modulation or suppression with intravenous immunoglobulin is the standard of care at many centers.[81-83] Mechanical circulatory support may be required in fulminant disease.[84-89]

## RHEUMATIC FEVER AND RHEUMATIC HEART DISEASE

Acute rheumatic fever and rheumatic heart disease are leading causes of acquired cardiac disease in developing countries and still occur, albeit infrequently, in developed countries.[90] In the United States, the availability of antibiotic therapy for streptococcal pharyngitis has markedly reduced the incidence of this disease, but sporadic cases still occur.[91] In children, the peak incidence occurs between 5 and 14 years of age.

Rheumatic fever results from infection by particular strains of group A β-hemolytic *Streptococcus* or *Streptococcus pyogenes* leading to a multisystemic inflammatory disorder. The incubation period for most strains of group A β-hemolytic *Streptococcus* is typically 3 to 5 days, although some children present with a more remote history of pharyngitis.

The clinical diagnosis of rheumatic fever is based on the modified Jones criteria.[92] Major criteria include carditis, polyarthritis, chorea, subcutaneous nodules, and erythema marginatum. Without a history of rheumatic fever or echocardiographic evidence of typical valvular involvement, the diagnosis in children requires evidence of a prior streptococcal infection along with two major criteria or one major and two minor criteria. Fever and arthritis are common symptoms. The polyarthritis has a migratory pattern, typically affecting large joints. Cardiac involvement or carditis occurs in almost 50% of children with their first attack of rheumatic fever. Rheumatic heart disease represents a sequela of the acute process, and it most frequently affects the mitral and aortic valves.

Primary prevention of rheumatic fever and rheumatic heart disease begins with prompt recognition and appropriate treatment of the initial streptococcal infection.[93,94] Secondary prevention, with ongoing therapy in individuals with a known history of rheumatic fever, has been extremely effective in preventing recurrent attacks. Although there is debate regarding the optimal regimen, intramuscular injections of benzathine penicillin every 3 to 4 weeks appear to be most efficacious.[95]

In a subset of children with severe cardiac involvement, elective or emergent surgery may be required.[96] Valvular disease, rather than global myocarditis, is often the cause of congestive symptoms; medical management therefore has limited efficacy. Valve repair is preferred to replacement.

## INFECTIVE ENDOCARDITIS

### Causes and Treatment

Children with structural or acquired heart disease are at risk for infective endocarditis.[97,98] The risk to a great extent is based on the nature of the cardiac condition. The infection results from deposition of bacteria or other pathogens on tissues in areas of abnormal or turbulent blood flow. The diagnosis of endocarditis is made clinically by applying the modified Duke criteria (Table 14-2).[99,100] Major criteria include demonstration of microorganisms and evidence of pathologic lesions. The presentation of the disease may be acute or subacute. New or changing heart murmurs may indicate the development of regurgitation or obstruction on an affected valve. Among the physical findings may be signs of systemic embolization (i.e., minor criteria). Splinter hemorrhages (i.e., linear streaks under the nail beds), Janeway lesions (i.e., painless macules on the hands or feet), Osler nodes (i.e., small, painful nodules on the fingers), and Roth spots (i.e., retinal hemorrhages with clear centers) may also be present. Inflammatory markers, such as erythrocyte sedimentation rate and C-reactive protein, are typically increased, albeit nonspecific. Microscopic hematuria, as a manifestation of renal involvement, is frequently seen.

Acute bacterial endocarditis is most commonly caused by *Staphylococcus aureus*.[101,102] The clinical presentation includes high fevers, chills, myalgias, fatigue, and lethargy. Some children present in a critically ill state or in shock. Both left- and right-sided endocarditis can occur in children with CHD.[103] Children with indwelling venous catheters have an expanded spectrum of pathogens known to cause acute endocarditis, including coagulase-negative staphylococcal species or other nonbacterial organisms.

Subacute bacterial endocarditis (SBE) often has a more indolent course and presentation. Children present with low-grade fevers, malaise, anemia, and fatigue. Most frequently, one of the *Viridians streptococcus* group and *Enterococcus* species is the underlying pathogen.

Initial evaluation for bacterial endocarditis includes serial blood cultures drawn from separate sites before initiation of

| **TABLE 14-2** Modified Duke Criteria for Infective Endocarditis |
|---|
| **Major Criteria*** |
| *Blood culture positive for infective endocarditis (IE)* |
| Typical microorganism consistent with IE from two separate blood cultures: |
|     *Viridians streptococcus, Streptococcus bovis,* HACEK[†] group of microorganisms, *Staphylococcus aureus,* or community-acquired enterococci without a primary focus |
| *or* |
| Microorganism consistent with IE from persistently positive blood cultures |
| *or* |
| Single positive blood culture for *Coxiella burnetii* or antiphase I IgG antibody titer greater than 1:800 |
| *Evidence of endocardial involvement* |
| Positive echocardiogram for IE: |
|     Oscillating intracardiac mass on valve or supporting structures, in the path of regurgitant jets, or on implanted material in the absence of an alternative anatomic explanation, or abscess |
| *or* |
|     New partial dehiscence of prosthetic valve |
| *or* |
| New valvular regurgitation (worsening of or change in preexisting murmur not sufficient) |
| **Minor Criteria*** |
| Predisposition: predisposing cardiac condition or intravenous drug use |
| Fever: temperature >38.0° C |
| Vascular phenomena: major arterial emboli, septic pulmonary infarctions, mycotic aneurysm, intracranial hemorrhage, conjunctival hemorrhages, and Janeway lesions |
| Immunologic problems: glomerulonephritis, Osler nodes, Roth spots, and rheumatoid factor |
| Microbiologic evidence: positive blood culture that does not meet a major criterion (above) or serologic evidence of active infection with organism consistent with IE |

Modified from Li JS, Sexton DJ, Mick N, et al. Proposed modifications to the Duke criteria for the diagnosis of infective endocarditis. Clin Infect Dis 2000;30:633-8.
*Duke Clinical Criteria for Infective Endocarditis requires two major criteria or one major and three minor criteria or five minor criteria to establish the diagnosis.
†For definition, see http://en.wikipedia.org/wiki/HACEK_endocarditis

antimicrobial therapy. The temporal frequency of cultures depends on the clinical scenario and stability of the child. In up to 20% of children with evidence of endocarditis, a pathogen cannot be isolated (i.e., negative culture), requiring empirical treatment throughout. Transthoracic echocardiography is routinely performed to evaluate evidence of vegetations or other abnormalities.[104] Although visualization of a vegetation establishes the diagnosis, a negative study does not exclude the diagnosis. Depending on how strongly the diagnosis is suspected, further imaging, including transesophageal echocardiography, may be necessary (Video 14-8, *A* and *B*).[105] These imaging modalities are also valuable during follow-up.

Parenteral antibiotics are initiated after blood cultures are collected. Broad-spectrum agents are used initially, and after a pathogen has been identified, the antibiotic regimen is narrowed.[97] Daily blood cultures are obtained until three consecutive cultures remain sterile. A prolonged course of therapy (e.g.,

4 to 6 weeks) is required in all children. This can be facilitated by placement of a peripherally inserted central catheter (PICC) line. Home therapy for endocarditis may be feasible in some patients, but it depends on many factors, including clinical status, initial response to antibiotics, sensitivity of organism to antimicrobial therapy, and ability of infrastructure to support outpatient treatment of a serious infection (e.g., parental or family member's ability, home health care provider).

In addition to medical therapy, some children require surgical intervention. Failure of medical therapy (i.e., inability to clear the bacteremia), abscess formation, refractory heart failure, and serious embolic phenomenon are indications for surgical intervention. Typically, the procedures involve resection of a vegetation, tissue débridement, or repair of consequent cardiac abnormalities. These children should subsequently receive antibiotic prophylaxis for endocarditis before at-risk procedures for the rest of their lives.

A high level of suspicion for endocarditis must be maintained when evaluating a child with known heart disease and with persistent bacteremia (or fungemia) or a fever of unknown origin. The same holds true for any child with foreign material in the heart or vascular tissue, such as indwelling central venous catheters, pacemakers or defibrillators, and closure devices.[106]

### Endocarditis Prophylaxis

The risk for developing endocarditis from transient bacteremia is extremely low in children with normal intracardiac anatomy, however, certain cardiac conditions are predisposed to acquiring endocarditis. The American Heart Association guidelines do not recommend antibiotic prophylaxis based exclusively on an increased lifetime risk of endocarditis, but they propose that it should be restricted to those at greatest risk for an adverse outcome resulting from endocarditis. Children in this category include those with prosthetic cardiac valves, a history of endocarditis, certain congenital heart defects, after specific interventions, and cardiac transplant recipients with valvular disease (Table 14-3).[107]

Transient bacteremia may occur during dental procedures that involve the gingival tissues or the periapical region of teeth or perforation of the oral mucosa. Although several respiratory tract procedures are associated with transient bacteremia, no definitive data demonstrate a cause-and-effect relationship between these procedures and endocarditis. Caution may be warranted for children at high risk undergoing invasive procedures of the respiratory tract that involve incision or biopsy of the mucosa. In contrast to previous guidelines, routine prophylactic administration of antibiotics solely to prevent endocarditis is not recommended for those undergoing genitourinary or gastrointestinal tract procedures. However, for specific clinical scenarios, antibiotic prophylaxis may be considered in these children. Routine endoscopy or transesophageal echocardiography does not merit routine antibiotic administration.[108] Prophylaxis is not considered necessary for cardiac catheterization; and although many practitioners routinely administer antibiotics during transcatheter placement of devices, there is insufficient evidence to support this practice.[109]

The guidelines recommend the administration of antibiotic prophylaxis 30 to 60 minutes before the procedure to achieve adequate tissue levels of antibiotics before bacteremia occurs (Table 14-4).[107] The standard prophylactic regimen for children is

### TABLE 14-3 Cardiac Conditions Associated with the Greatest Risk of Adverse Outcomes from Endocarditis

- Prosthetic cardiac valve
- Previous infective endocarditis
- Congenital heart disease (CHD)*
  Unrepaired, cyanotic CHD, including palliative shunts and conduits
  Completely repaired congenital heart defect with prosthetic material or device, whether placed by surgery or by catheter intervention, during the first 6 months after the procedure†
  Repaired CHD with residual defects at the site or adjacent to the site of a prosthetic patch or prosthetic device (which inhibit endothelialization)
- Cardiac transplantation recipients who develop cardiac valvulopathy

Modified with permission from Wilson W, Taubert KA, Gewitz M, et al., editors. Prevention of infective endocarditis: guidelines from the American Heart Association. A guideline from the American Heart Association Rheumatic Fever, Endocarditis, and Kawasaki Disease Committee, Council on Cardiovascular Disease in the Young, and the Council on Clinical Cardiology, Council on Cardiovascular Surgery and Anesthesia, and the Quality of Care and Outcomes Research Interdisciplinary Working Group. Circulation 2007;116:1736-54.
*Except for the conditions listed, antibiotic prophylaxis is no longer recommended for other forms of CHD.
†Prophylaxis is recommended because endothelialization of prosthetic material occurs within 6 months after the procedure.

### TABLE 14-4 American Heart Association Guidelines for the Prevention of Infective Endocarditis: Antibiotic Regimens

| Situation | Antibiotic | DOSE* Children | DOSE* Adults |
|---|---|---|---|
| Able to take oral medication | Amoxicillin | 50 mg/kg | 2 g |
| Unable to take oral medication | Ampicillin | 50 mg/kg IM or IV | 2 g IM or IV |
| | or Cefazolin or ceftriaxone | 50 mg/kg IM or IV | 1 g IM or IV |
| Allergic to penicillins or ampicillin and able to take oral medication | Cephalexin†‡ | 50 mg/kg | 2 g |
| | or Clindamycin | 20 mg/kg | 600 mg |
| | or Azithromycin or clarithromycin | 15 mg/kg | 500 mg |
| Allergic to penicillins or ampicillin and unable to take oral medication | Cefazolin or ceftriaxone‡ | 50 mg/kg IM or IV | 1 g IM or IV |
| | or Clindamycin | 20 mg/kg IM or IV | 600 mg IM or IV |

Modified from Wilson W, Taubert KA, Gewitz M, et al., editors. Prevention of infective endocarditis: guidelines from the American Heart Association. A guideline from the American Heart Association Rheumatic Fever, Endocarditis, and Kawasaki Disease Committee, Council on Cardiovascular Disease in the Young, and the Council on Clinical Cardiology, Council on Cardiovascular Surgery and Anesthesia, and the Quality of Care and Outcomes Research Interdisciplinary Working Group. Circulation 2007;116:1736-54.
IM, Intramuscular; IV, intravenous.
*Single dose is administered 30 to 60 minutes before the procedure. The total pediatric dose should not exceed the adult dose.
†Alternatively, another first- or second-generation oral cephalosporin is administered in an equivalent pediatric or adult dosage.
‡Cephalosporins should not be used in an individual with a history of anaphylaxis, angioedema, or urticaria to penicillins or ampicillin.

for oral amoxicillin. For the child who is allergic to penicillin or ampicillin, oral alternatives include cephalexin, clindamycin, azithromycin, or clarithromycin. In children who are unable to ingest oral medications, alternative antibiotics include ampicillin, cefazolin, and ceftriaxone by an intravenous or intramuscular route. If the child is allergic to penicillin or ampicillin and unable to swallow oral medications, cefazolin, ceftriaxone, or clindamycin may be used.

Although many health care providers have adopted the updated recommendations, some have been hesitant to alter their practice regarding endocarditis prophylaxis, particularly when caring for patients with CHD undergoing gastrointestinal or genitourinary procedures.[110] Only the American Dental Association has adopted the new guidelines for endocarditis prophylaxis; other associations such as the gastrointestinal and genitourinary groups remain uncommitted to the new guideline.

### KAWASAKI DISEASE

Kawasaki disease (i.e., mucocutaneous lymph node syndrome) represents a fairly common and potentially fatal form of systemic vasculitis of unknown origin.[111-115] It is seen predominantly in infants and young children. The disease can affect the coronary arteries resulting in dilation and aneurysm formation.[116,117]

The diagnosis relies on clinical features. To meet criteria, a child must have persistent fevers and at least four of the following findings[118,119]:

- Polymorphous exanthem
- Peripheral extremity changes (e.g., erythema, desquamation, edema of the hands or feet)
- Bilateral, nonexudative conjunctivitis
- Cervical lymphadenopathy (often unilateral)
- Oral changes (i.e., strawberry tongue; red, dry, or cracked lips)

Nonspecific findings may include irritability, hydrops of the gallbladder, sterile pyuria, arthritis, and aseptic meningitis. Acute-phase reactants and thrombocytosis are usually present.

Intravenous gamma globulin (IVIG) and high-dose aspirin are recommended during the acute phase of the disease. The incidence of coronary artery aneurysms is significantly reduced if IVIG is administered within the first 10 days of the illness.[119] The presence of coronary artery aneurysms is considered diagnostic for Kawasaki disease (Fig. 14-10). In children with coronary artery aneurysms, low-dose aspirin therapy is administered, in some cases in combination with anticoagulants or antiplatelet drugs.[120] Myocardial ischemia and infarction, although uncommon, are important potential complications.[117,121] Anesthetic care in these children requires careful consideration regarding myocardial oxygen demand and supply; on rare occasions, coronary revascularization may be necessary.

### CARDIAC TUMORS

Because cardiac tumors are rare in children, the natural history and optimal treatment strategies are often determined from limited case series.[122-124] Atrial myxomas represent more than 90% of cardiac tumors in adults, but in children, they tend to be rhabdomyomas or fibromas.[125] Less common types include hemangiomas, myxomas (Video 14-9), Purkinje cell tumors, and teratomas. In adults, most tumors are found in the left atrium, but cardiac tumors in children occur in all four cardiac chambers. Malignant primary tumors are rare, and data on their outcomes are limited. Other nonprimary cardiac tumors, such as neuroblastoma, can invade vascular structures and extend into the heart.

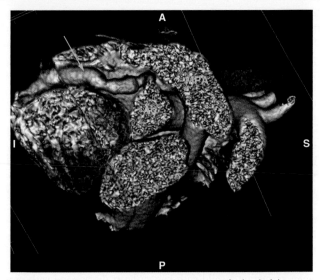

**FIGURE 14-10** Magnetic resonance reconstruction at the level of the great vessels in a child with Kawasaki disease demonstrates a large, fusiform coronary aneurysm (*arrow*). *Ao,* Aorta; *MPA,* main pulmonary artery.

*Rhabdomyomas* are the most common primary cardiac tumors in children. They often involve the ventricular septum and left ventricle and are multiple in most cases.[126] Although they are considered benign, children may present with cardiomegaly, congestive heart failure, arrhythmias, or sudden death. The significance of a rhabdomyoma is determined largely by its size and any obstruction it may cause. Many tumors regress over time or completely resolve; surgery is not indicated unless symptoms are present.[127,128] Many children with cardiac rhabdomyomas have associated tuberous sclerosis.[129,130]

*Cardiac fibromas* are the second most common type of pediatric primary cardiac tumors.[131] They are typically single and involve the ventricular free wall. In a subset of fibromas, the tumor can invade the conduction system.[132] Surgery or cardiac transplantation may be required.[133,134] The tumors can be very large, and complete surgical resection may result in severely depressed cardiac function. Partial resections have been found to result in an arrest in growth with good outcomes while sparing cardiac function.[128]

The primary concerns in the perioperative care of children with cardiac tumors are the impact of the mass on hemodynamics and the associated abnormalities of cardiac rhythm.[135]

## Heart Failure in Children

### DEFINITION AND PATHOPHYSIOLOGY

Heart failure has become a major field of interest and investigation in pediatric cardiology and the subject of various publications,[136] scientific meetings, and several textbooks.[137,138] Pediatric heart failure results from markedly different causes from those reported in adults.[139] The cellular basis of heart failure, compensatory mechanisms, and therapeutic advances represent areas of interest in children.[136-138,140,141] The following discussion highlights key concepts as they relate to anesthetic practice.

Heart failure is considered to be a pump failure and a circulatory failure involving neurohumoral aspects of the circulation.[142] Several conditions may ultimately compromise the ability to generate an adequate cardiac output to meet the systemic circulatory demands. This disease state does not necessarily imply impairment of ventricular systolic function, but diastolic heart failure is an increasingly recognized clinical entity.

## ETIOLOGY AND CLINICAL FEATURES

Causes of heart failure vary with age. In the perinatal period, cardiac dysfunction may be related to birth asphyxia or sepsis or may represent an early presentation of CHD. The neonate with heart failure frequently presents with clinical signs of a low cardiac output state. Causes include left-sided outflow obstruction (e.g., aortic stenosis, aortic coarctation, hypoplastic left heart syndrome), severe valve regurgitation (e.g., Ebstein anomaly), or absent pulmonary valve syndrome.

During the first year of life, most cases of heart failure are caused by structural heart disease. Other causes include cardiomyopathies due to inborn errors of metabolism or acute events such as myocarditis. In infants with heart failure, tachypnea, dyspnea, tachycardia, feeding difficulties, and failure to thrive are prominent symptoms.[143] Physical examination reveals grunting respirations, rales, intercostal retractions, a gallop rhythm, and hepatosplenomegaly. Frequently, a mitral regurgitant murmur is present.

Beyond the first year of life, heart failure is a consequence of previous surgical interventions, unpalliated or unrepaired cardiovascular disease, cardiomyopathies, myocarditis, or anthracycline therapy for a malignancy. Occasionally, a child may present with severe ventricular systolic impairment related to ongoing myocardial ischemia as a result of a coronary artery anomaly or rarely due to acquired pathologies such as Kawasaki disease. Older children with heart failure exhibit exercise intolerance, fatigue, and growth failure, whereas adolescents have symptoms similar to those of adults.

## TREATMENT STRATEGIES

Therapy is tailored to the cause of the cardiac dysfunction and may include supportive care, mechanical ventilation, inotropic support, afterload reduction, prostaglandin $E_1$ therapy to maintain pulmonary or systemic blood flow, maneuvers to balance the systemic and pulmonary circulations, catheter-based interventions, or surgery.[144-148] Maintaining organ perfusion is the main goal of therapy for acute heart failure. Pharmacologic agents include inotropes (used on a very-short-term basis, if necessary) and inodilators. Although the administration of digoxin was the mainstay of chronic therapy in the past, this is no longer the case. Favored agents for use in children include diuretics, angiotensin-converting enzyme inhibitors, and β-blockade.[149,150] Newer agents that have received increasing attention in the management of pediatric heart failure include nesiritide (a recombinant form of human B-type natriuretic peptide)[151-153] and carvedilol (a third-generation β-blocker).[154-156]

## ANESTHETIC CONSIDERATIONS

Anesthesia for children with heart failure can be quite challenging. The severity of the condition and degree of baseline decompensation can influence the likelihood of an untoward event and the potential for hemodynamic instability and a bad outcome. Several publications have addressed the risks associated with anesthesia in this setting.[157-159] It is important to first reexamine the risk–benefit ratio in these patients before going forward with the planned procedure. In most surgical settings, tracheal intubation and mechanical ventilation are indicated. The need for invasive monitoring should be based on the clinical situation,

anticipated nature of the procedure, and impact on hemodynamic state.

# Syndromes, Associations, and Systemic Disorders: Cardiovascular Disease and Anesthetic Implications

Many disorders, including those resulting from chromosomal abnormalities, single-gene defects, gene deletion syndromes, known associations (i.e., nonrandom occurrence of defects), and teratogenic exposure, may manifest as cardiovascular disease. The coexistence of frequently associated multiple organ system comorbidities with cardiovascular disease presents several challenges to the anesthesia care provider.

## CHROMOSOMAL SYNDROMES

### Trisomy 21

Trisomy 21 (i.e., Down syndrome) is the most frequent chromosomal anomaly, occurring with a frequency of 1 case per 800 live births. The incidence increases sharply with advanced maternal age. The syndrome results from trisomy 21 in most children, but it may occur from a balanced or unbalanced chromosome translocation or mosaicism. The phenotypes are indistinguishable. Affected children are typically smaller than normal for age. Craniofacial features include microbrachycephaly, short neck, oblique palpebral fissures, epicanthal folds, Brushfield spots, small and low-set ears, macroglossia, and microdontia with fused teeth. Mandibular hypoplasia and a broad flat nose are typical. A narrow nasopharynx with hypertrophic lymphatic tissue (e.g., tonsils, adenoids) in combination with generalized hypotonia frequently leads to sleep apnea. Other conditions include mental retardation, cervical spine disorders with vertebral and ligamentous instability (i.e., subluxation risk), thyroid disease, leukemia, obesity, subglottic stenosis,[160] and gastrointestinal problems.

Airway issues include the potential for upper airway obstruction due to a large tongue, postextubation stridor,[161] and cervical spine injury.[162-164] Vascular access can be challenging. Subjectively, children have small and abnormal radial vessel sizes,[164a] vascular hyperreactivity, and fragile tissue consistency, and they may suffer from more complications after arterial cannulation.

Cardiovascular defects occur in 40% to 50% of children with Down syndrome, and it has been recommended that they all should undergo screening for CHD in early infancy.[165] The most common lesions include AV septal defects (Video 14-10), VDSs, TOF, and PDA. Bradycardia under anesthesia occurs commonly, although the mechanism is poorly understood.[166,167] Pulmonary hypertension may result from the cardiac pathology or from chronic hypoxemia due to upper airway obstruction (i.e., obstructive sleep apnea) and should be considered in their management.[168] Reduced nitric oxide bioavailability has been reported in patients with Down syndrome, leading to endothelial cell dysfunction[169] and possibly explaining the observed increased pulmonary vascular reactivity.

### Trisomy 18

Trisomy 18 (i.e., Edwards syndrome) is recognized as the second most common chromosomal trisomy (incidence of 1 case per 3500 live births). Most children exhibit microcephaly, delayed psychomotor development, and mental retardation.[170] Characteristic craniofacial features include micrognathia or retrognathia, microstomia, malformed ears, and microphthalmia.[171] These abnormalities can affect airway management.[172,173] Skeletal anomalies include clenched fingers and severe growth retardation. Neurologic problems include developmental delay, hypotonia, and central nervous system malformations. The high mortality rate for children with trisomy 18 is related to cardiac and renal problems, feeding difficulties, sepsis, and apnea caused by neurologic abnormalities.

Cardiovascular disease is present in most children with trisomy 18 and consists primarily of VSDs and polyvalvular disease.[174,175] Implications for anesthesia care include the high incidence of congestive heart failure and aspiration pneumonia.[173] These children may require interventions to address associated gastrointestinal or genitourinary anomalies.

### Trisomy 13

Trisomy 13 (i.e., Patau syndrome) is an uncommon autosomal trisomy with an incidence that ranges from 1 case per 5000 to 12,000 live births. Major features include cleft lip and palate, holoprosencephaly, polydactyly, rocker-bottom feet, microphthalmia, microcephaly, and severe mental retardation.[176,177] Almost all children have associated cardiovascular defects that include PDA, septal defects, valve abnormalities, and dextrocardia.[175] The overall prognosis for these children is extremely poor.

### Turner Syndrome

Turner syndrome is a genetic disorder characterized by partial or complete X chromosome monosomy.[178] The estimated incidence is 1 case per 5000 liveborn female infants. A high degree of spontaneous abortion is seen among affected fetuses. Features of this syndrome include webbed neck, low-set ears, multiple pigmented nevi and micrognathia, lymphedema, short stature, and ovarian failure.[179] Systemic manifestations include cardiac defects (notably aortic coarctation and bicuspid aortic valve), hypertension, hypercholesterolemia, renal anomalies (up to 33%), liver disease, and inflammatory bowel disease. Obesity is common in older children, as is a high incidence of endocrine abnormalities such as hypothyroidism and diabetes.[178,180]

## GENE DELETION SYNDROMES

### Williams Syndrome

Williams syndrome is a congenital disorder with an incidence of 1/20,000 live births. In most cases, the long arm of chromosome 7 is deleted, altering the elastin gene.[181,182] The absence of this gene is detected by fluorescence in situ hybridization (FISH). Features of Williams syndrome include characteristic elfin facies, outgoing personality, endocrine abnormalities (including hypercalcemia and hypothyroidism), mental retardation, growth deficiency, and altered neurodevelopment. Cardiovascular abnormalities can include valvar and supravalvular aortic stenosis (Fig. 14-11) and aortic coarctation.[183,184] This arteriopathy can also involve the origin of the coronary arteries or other vessels. Diffuse narrowing of the abdominal aorta may be associated with renal artery stenosis.

Several reports have described unanticipated events during anesthesia for these children.[185-187] Two conditions can increase anesthetic morbidity and the potential for mortality: coronary artery stenosis leading to myocardial ischemia and severe biventricular outflow tract obstruction. A thorough cardiac evaluation of all children is advisable because the spectrum of disease and the potential devastating implications in affected individuals varies.[188] Children occasionally may require further evaluation

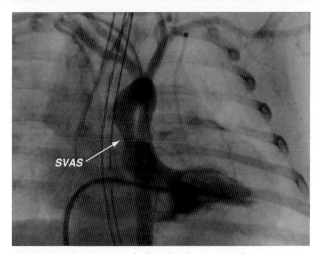

**FIGURE 14-11** The angiogram displays the classic supravalvar aortic stenosis (*SVAS, arrow*) in a child with Williams syndrome.

before undergoing anesthetic care. Even asymptomatic children and those without evidence of clinical cardiovascular disease may be at risk for morbidity and death in the perioperative period.[187] Extreme vigilance and particular attention to signs of myocardial ischemia is warranted, as is a plan of action in the event of acute decompensation. This syndrome is one of the leading causes of cardiac arrest in the Pediatric Perioperative Cardiac Arrest (POCA) registry.[189]

Children with Williams syndrome may exhibit some degree of muscular weakness, and the cautious use and application of muscle relaxants has been recommended.[188] Associated neurodevelopmental delay, attention-deficit disorder, and autistic behavior often requires adequate premedication. Subclinical hypothyroidism has a high prevalence among these children.[190] Renal manifestations include renovascular hypertension, reduced function, and hypercalcemia-induced nephrocalcinosis.

### Chromosome 22q11.2 Deletion Syndrome: DiGeorge and Velocardiofacial Syndrome

The 22q11.2 deletion syndrome, with an estimated incidence of approximately 1 case per 3000 live births, encompasses DiGeorge, conotruncal face, and velocardiofacial syndromes. The syndrome is also known as CATCH 22, a mnemonic for **c**ardiac defects, **a**bnormal facies, **t**hymic hypoplasia, **c**left palate, and **h**ypocalcemia, all of which are commonly present.[191] Cardiac malformations, speech delay, and immunodeficiency are the most common features of the chromosome 22q deletion syndromes. Because no single feature is overwhelmingly associated with the deletion, the diagnosis should be considered for any child with a conotruncal anomaly, neonatal hypocalcemia, or any of the less common features when seen in association with dysmorphic facial features.

Cardiac malformations are often described as conotruncal anomalies; however, outflow tract problems are also frequently seen.[192] The remainder of the cardiac defects encompasses an enormous spectrum of pathologies. Only a few children have a normal cardiovascular system. As a consequence of thymic hypoplasia, children typically have diminished T-cell numbers and function. Their immunodeficiency requires the use of irradiated blood products and strict aseptic precautions during vascular access. Neurodevelopmental features include primarily speech delay and attention-deficit disorders. Psychiatric disorders are well described in these individuals.[193]

## SINGLE-GENE DEFECTS

### Noonan Syndrome

Noonan syndrome, an autosomal dominant syndrome, occurs with a frequency of 1 case per 1000 to 2500 live births. Dysmorphic features include neck webbing, low-set ears, chest deformities, hypertelorism, and short stature.[194] The diagnosis of Noonan syndrome depends primarily on clinical features.[195] In neonates, the facial features may be less apparent; however, generalized edema and excess nuchal folds may be present as in Turner syndrome. The facial features are more difficult to detect in later adolescence and adulthood.

The disorder is associated with a high incidence of CHD (about 50%), and pulmonary valve dysplasia or stenosis is the most common feature.[196] HCM may develop during the first few years of life (10% to 20%).[197] Clinical problems may also include developmental delay and bleeding diathesis.[198]

### Marfan Syndrome

Marfan syndrome is a multisystem disorder with variable expression resulting from a mutation in the fibrillin gene, a connective tissue protein, located on chromosome 15.[199] Clinical manifestations typically involve the cardiovascular, skeletal, and ocular systems.[200,201] Cardiovascular pathology includes mitral valve prolapse and regurgitation, ascending aortic dilation (Fig. 14-12), and main pulmonary artery dilatation. The risk of aortic dissection rises considerably with increasing aortic size but may occur at any point in the course of the disease.[202] Cardiac arrhythmias may be related to valvular heart disease, cardiomyopathy, or congestive heart failure.

β-Blocker therapy and aggressive blood pressure control has been the standard of care in children with aortic root dilation[203]

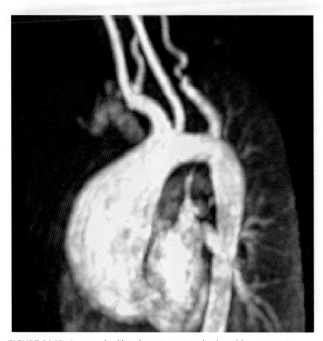

**FIGURE 14-12** A severely dilated aortic root is displayed by magnetic resonance imaging in a patient with Marfan syndrome. There is a marked discrepancy between the diameters of the ascending and descending aorta.

and should be continued perioperatively. Aortic root replacement in Marfan syndrome has been associated with a greater risk of repeat dissection and recurrent aneurysm compared with other children who have undergone similar interventions.[204] It is wise to maintain hemodynamics near baseline values in the perioperative period. After aortic root surgery some individuals may require chronic anticoagulation therapy. Preoperative hospitalization may be necessary to adjust the anticoagulation regimen in anticipation of surgery in these children. In emergency cases, administration of coagulation factors and other blood products may be required. In addition to vascular pathology, children with Marfan syndrome have a predisposition for ventricular dilation and abnormal systolic function.[205,206]

Several factors can result in pulmonary disease in these children.[207] Chest wall deformities and progressive scoliosis can contribute to restrictive lung disease. The fibrillin defect may affect lung development and homeostasis, impairing pulmonary function. Development of a pneumothorax is relatively common.

## ASSOCIATIONS

### Vater or VACTERL Association

VACTERL association is an acronym given to describe a series of nonrandom anomalies that include **v**ertebral, **a**nal, **c**ardiovascular, **t**racheo**e**sophageal, **r**enal, and **l**imb defects.[208,209] Up to three fourths of children with VACTERL association have CHD. The most common lesions include VSDs, ASDs, and TOF. Complex pathology such as truncus arteriosus and transposition of the great arteries occur less frequently.

Vertebral and tracheal anomalies can complicate airway management and regional anesthesia. Approximately 70% of children with VACTERL have vertebral anomalies, usually consisting of hypoplastic vertebrae or hemivertebra and predisposing children to scoliosis. Anal atresia or imperforate anus is reported in about 55% of cases. These anomalies often require surgery in the first days of life. Esophageal atresia with tracheoesophageal fistula occurs in a large number of affected infants. Low birth weight (less than 1500 g) and associated cardiac pathology have been identified to be independent predictors of mortality in infants undergoing surgery for esophageal atresia or tracheoesophageal fistula (see Chapter 36). The presence of a ductal-dependent cardiac lesion further increases perioperative morbidity and mortality.[210] Limb defects occur in most children, potentially affecting vascular access and monitor placement. Renal defects occur in about 50% of children.

### CHARGE Association

CHARGE association is characterized by congenital anomalies that include **c**oloboma, **h**eart defects, choanal **a**tresia, **r**etardation of **g**rowth and development, **g**enitourinary problems, and **e**ar abnormalities. The association is estimated to occur at a rate of 1 case per 10,000 to 12,000 live births. The cause is unknown although many theories have been suggested.[211,212]

Specific genetic abnormalities have also been identified in some individuals.[213,214] Cardiac defects occur in as many as 50% to 70% of children and commonly include conotruncal and aortic arch anomalies.[215] Delayed growth and development usually results from cardiac disease, nutritional problems, and/or growth hormone deficiency. Most children have some degree of cognitive impairment. Anesthetic implications, in addition to those related to the cardiac defects, focus on the airway[216]; a retrospective review of 50 cases reported upper airway abnormalities in 56% of children apart from choanal atresia and cleft lip and palate.[217]

## OTHER DISORDERS

Tuberous sclerosis is a rare genetic disease with an autosomal dominant inheritance pattern and an incidence of approximately 1 case per 25,000 to 30,000 births.[218] In a relatively large number of children, it can be attributed to spontaneous mutations. This systemic disease primarily manifests as cutaneous and neurologic symptoms, but cardiac and renal lesions are frequent findings.

The presence of upper airway nodular tumors, fibromas, or papillomas in affected children may interfere with airway management. Developmental delay, autism, attention-deficit disorder, and aggressive behavior are common. Brain tumors and renal tumors (60% to 80%) may produce significant comorbidities. Cardiac pathology includes cardiac rhabdomyoma in 60% of children and coexisting CHD in 33% of cases.[219-221] Cardiac abnormalities with obstruction to flow, heart failure, arrhythmias, conduction defects, or preexcitation may affect the selection of anesthetic agents. Preoperative evaluation in most cases should include an ECG to assess arrhythmia, conduction defects, or preexcitation.[219] Blood pressure and renal function should also be assessed. Anticonvulsants should be optimized and continued until the morning of surgery. Baseline medical treatment should be resumed as soon as possible because seizures are the most common postoperative complication.[222] A child with mental retardation may require premedication with oral midazolam or ketamine, or both, to facilitate parental separation.

# Selected Vascular Anomalies and Their Implications for Anesthesia

## ABERRANT SUBCLAVIAN ARTERIES

An aberrant or anomalous subclavian artery usually arises from the descending aorta as a separate vessel distal to the usual last subclavian artery in a posterior location. In a left aortic arch, this arrangement is as follows. The first branch is the right carotid artery, followed by the left carotid artery and the left subclavian artery. The aberrant right subclavian artery, rather than arising proximally from the innominate artery as the first arch branch, originates distal to the last (left) subclavian artery as the fourth branch and courses behind the esophagus toward the right arm. This variant is one of the most common aortic arch anomalies. It occurs in 0.4% to 2% of the general population and may or may not be associated with CHD.[223] This anomaly has a high incidence among children with Down syndrome and is associated with VSDs, TOF, and other lesions. In a right aortic arch, the anomalous left subclavian artery originates distal to the origin of the right subclavian artery (Fig. 14-13). This anomaly may be seen in the context of conotruncal malformations. The diagnosis of an aberrant subclavian artery is made by most currently available imaging modalities.

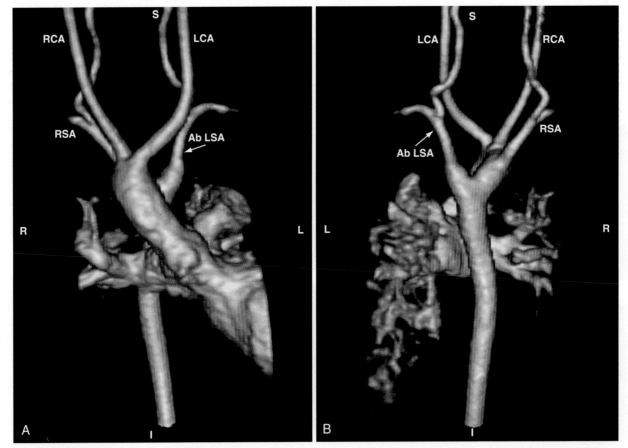

**FIGURE 14-13** Anterior (**A**) and posterior (**B**) magnetic resonance images demonstrate a right aortic arch with an aberrant left subclavian artery (*Ab LSA*). The first arch vessel is the left carotid artery (*LCA*), followed by the right carotid artery (*RCA*), and right subclavian artery (*RSA*). The Ab LSA is the most distal branch originating from the descending aorta and coursing posterior to the esophagus toward the left arm. This vessel may be compressed by a transesophageal echocardiographic probe.

This anomaly has several implications:

- The presence of an aberrant subclavian artery may influence the location of placement of a systemic-to-pulmonary artery shunt.

- This anomaly should be considered in the selection of a site for arterial line placement if transesophageal echocardiography is planned during surgery. The aberrant vessel may be compressed along its retroesophageal course by the imaging probe, resulting in inaccurate recordings.[224] Regardless of the site of arterial line placement, it may be wise to monitor the arm supplied by the anomalous vessel by pulse oximetry or other methods during esophageal instrumentation.

- An aberrant subclavian artery sometimes is part of a vascular ring.

- Rarely, older children with a left aortic arch and aberrant right subclavian artery and without the findings of a complete vascular ring may complain of mild dysphagia (i.e., dysphagia lusorium).

### PERSISTENT LEFT SUPERIOR VENA CAVA TO THE CORONARY SINUS

A persistent left superior vena cava (LSVC) is a form of anomalous systemic venous drainage identified in 4.4% of children with CHD, most frequently those with septal defects.[225] It represents a venous remnant that typically involutes during development. If it persists, it remains patent and drains into the right atrium through an enlarged coronary sinus. Bilateral superior vena cavae may be present (Fig. 14-14), or the right superior vena cava may be absent. Bilateral superior vena cavae may communicate through an innominate or bridging vein. This anomaly has several implications:

- In the absence of an innominate vein, a catheter placed in the left arm or left internal jugular vein and advanced into the central circulation may rest within the coronary sinus, a potentially undesirable location in a small infant. On chest radiography, an unusual course is identified as the catheter courses along the left aspect of the mediastinum and can be mistaken for intracarotid, intrapleural, or mediastinal locations.

- An LSVC may be of relevance during venous cannulation for cardiopulmonary bypass to ensure adequate venous drainage and optimal operating conditions.

- The presence of an LSVC is important in patients with single-ventricle physiology undergoing palliation involving a cavo-pulmonary (Glenn) connection.

- The anomaly may be associated with a dilated coronary sinus. On transesophageal echocardiography, it may be confused with other defects, including an ostium primum ASD (i.e., one that lies in the inferior aspect of the atrial septum) or anomalous pulmonary venous return to the coronary sinus.

- On occasion, an LSVC may drain to an unroofed coronary sinus or directly into the left atrium, in which case a right-to-left shunt is present. It may be identified by injection of agitated saline into a left arm or left neck vein while performing an echocardiogram, and it may be associated with systemic arterial desaturation. This constitutes a risk for paradoxical systemic embolization.

- During cardiac surgery, an enlarged coronary sinus may interfere with the administration of retrograde cardioplegia.

- It may confound placement of a pulmonary artery catheter and cardiac output determinations in the adolescent or adult.

## Evaluation of the Child with a Cardiac Murmur

The finding of an incidental murmur during the perioperative period may result in significant distress to the child or family; may trigger additional diagnostic studies, including a cardiology consultation; and has the potential to delay the scheduled

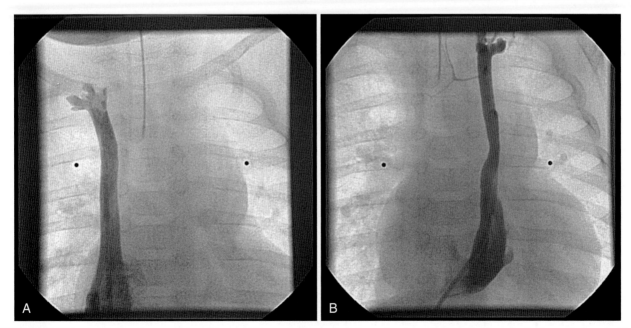

**FIGURE 14-14** Bilateral superior vena cavae may exist separately or may communicate through an innominate or bridging vein. **A,** The angiogram depicts the superior vena cava, normally a right-sided structure, as it drains into the right atrium. **B,** In the same patient, an angiogram shows drainage of a large left superior vena cava into the coronary sinus. The catheter courses from the inferior vena cava into the right atrium, coronary sinus, and left superior vena cava. Contrast into the left superior vena cava demonstrates no innominate vein between the two cavae. The coronary sinus is dilated.

procedure when identified preoperatively. Although cardiac auscultation is a challenging skill that takes many years of practice to master,[226] it is important for the anesthesiologist who routinely cares for children to recognize the main physical findings that may distinguish an innocent cardiac murmur from a pathologic one. Knowledge of several core concepts and red flags can help avoid overlooking potentially important diagnoses.

About 90% of normal children have a murmur at some point in their lives. It is most commonly identified during the neonatal period and early school years. Most murmurs are functional, considered innocent in nature, and require no special treatment. This diagnosis is based on physical findings consistent with the benign nature of the specific murmur.

Although a complete discussion of cardiac murmur evaluation is beyond the scope of this chapter, it is pertinent to review a few key concepts related to the distinction between innocent and pathologic murmurs.[227,228] The basic systematic approach when assessing a heart murmur is the same as when evaluating any child's cardiovascular system. Auscultation with the diaphragm and bell of the stethoscope in the positions of the four primary cardiac valves should occur with the child and environment as quiet as possible. Innocent murmurs of infancy and childhood include pulmonary flow murmur, a Still murmur, physiologic pulmonary branch stenosis, venous hum, and carotid bruit. Innocent murmurs are usually of low intensity (grades I and II of VI) and are associated with a normal cardiovascular examination (e.g., normal precordial activity, first and second heart sounds, peripheral pulses, capillary refill). Innocent murmurs, such as those associated with peripheral pulmonary branch stenosis, right ventricular outflow murmurs, and Still murmurs, tend to be soft, systolic ejection type, and not holosystolic in duration. Physiologic murmurs often resolve by changing the child's hemodynamic state with maneuvers such as lying down or sitting up or with temporal changes such as resolution of fever and improvement in anemia. Diastolic or continuous murmurs are typically abnormal, with the exception of a venous hum. This murmur is thought to be related to turbulent flow of systemic venous return in the jugular veins and superior vena cava and is best heard at the base of the neck. *Murmurs accompanied by a palpable thrill are always pathologic.*

When there is doubt regarding the benign or pathologic nature of a murmur, consultation with a pediatric cardiologist is indicated. A chest radiograph and ECG, although thought by some to add minimal value in the initial diagnostic assessment of a cardiac murmur[229,230] and to not be cost-effective,[231] can be helpful when considering if further consultation is indicated.

## Basic Interpretation of the Electrocardiogram in Children

Despite the increasing applications of imaging modalities in the structural and functional assessment of pediatric heart disease, electrocardiography continues to play a significant role in the diagnosis and management of these children. An ECG is considered an integral part of the evaluation of most children with congenital or acquired cardiovascular pathology.

Although the characteristic features of a normal ECG in infants and children were described many decades ago, it is surprising that it continues to be one of the most often misinterpreted screening tests in pediatric medicine.[232] This is largely because of the developmental changes that occur in the normal individual as he or she progresses from the neonatal period through childhood, adolescence, and adulthood.[233] Normal values for children of various ages have been established.[234] Knowledge of normal configurations and values for various ages of children is essential for accurate interpretation.[233-236] Immediately after birth, there is a predominance of right ventricular forces represented by tall R waves in the right precordial leads (V$_1$ and V$_2$) (Fig. 14-15). Over the first several years, the typical

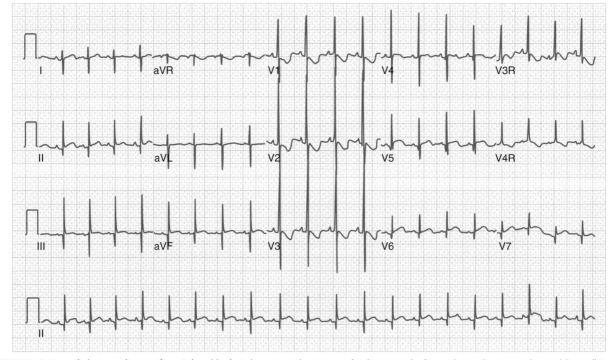

**FIGURE 14-15** Normal electrocardiogram for a 2-day-old infant shows a predominance of right ventricular forces during the neonatal period (i.e., tall R waves over the right precordial leads V$_1$ and V$_2$). The inverted T waves in V$_{1-3}$ are normal for this age.

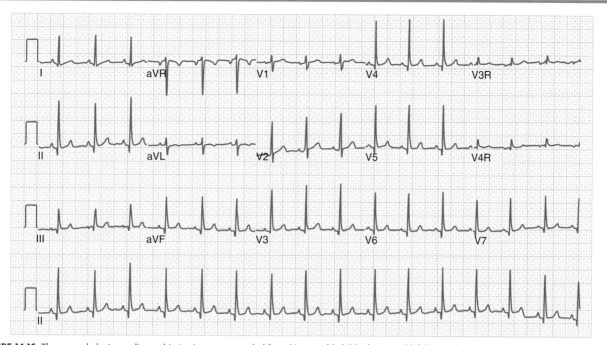

**FIGURE 14-16** The normal electrocardiographic tracing was recorded for a 10-year-old child. The typical left heart–dominant configuration of children this age is characterized by gradual RS progression with tall R waves in the left precordial leads (V$_5$ and V$_6$). This contrasts with the right ventricular–dominant pattern seen during infancy and early childhood. The tracing demonstrates normal sinus rhythm as documented by positive P waves in leads I and aVF.

electrocardiographic changes to a more familiar left heart–dominant configuration with larger S waves in the right precordial leads and a gradual RS progression with tall R waves in the left precordial leads (V$_5$ and V$_6$) (Fig. 14-16). The predominance of right heart forces and the need to evaluate for dextrocardia are the primary reasons that pediatric ECGs should include the V$_3$R and V$_4$R leads, which are not routinely obtained in adult studies. These electrodes are placed in the corresponding V$_3$ and V$_4$ locations over the right precordium.

Clinical information of relevance in the interpretation of an ECG includes the child's age, gender, suspected or documented diagnosis, and indications for the examination. Several requirements are essential for accurate interpretation, including appropriate skin preparation, electrode placement, and an artifact-free recording. The approach to the pediatric ECG should be systematic and organized. Determination of the rate and rhythm, with evaluation of the P-wave vector and the relationship between each P wave and QRS complex, is the first step. It is important to consider the influences of age, autonomic nervous system, level of physical activity, medications, pain, and temperature on the child's heart rate. The P wave should be upright or positive in leads I and aVF, indicating that the sinus node is the pacemaker of the heart (i.e., sinus rhythm) (see Fig. 14-16). Normally, the P wave should precede the QRS complex. Next, the QRS electrical axis should be determined. The QRS frontal plane axis is determined by identifying the most isoelectric lead, which is perpendicular to the direction of ventricular depolarization. Alternatively, the direction of depolarization in leads I and aVF can be examined to roughly estimate the axis. As with all other components of the evaluation, the physiologic changes that occur with growth are responsible for the change in normal values for the QRS axis based on age. Regardless of age, QRS axes that lie in the northwest quadrant (between 180 and 270 degrees with an S-wave–dominant pattern in leads I and aVF) are always abnormal and merit further investigation. This is a

frequent finding in children with AV septal defects. Evaluating the T wave, or repolarization axis, is also important, because a difference of greater than 90 degrees between the QRS and T-wave axes can represent strain on the ventricle, a potential finding in ventricular hypertrophy (see Fig. 14-5).

After the evaluation of rhythm and axes is complete, each component of the cardiac cycle as reflected by the ECG should be examined. The P wave represents atrial systole; and its morphology, with particular interest in leads II and V$_1$, can demonstrate right atrial (P-wave amplitude greater than 2.5 mm or 3.0 mm based on age) or left atrial (P-wave duration greater than 100 to 120 msec based on age) enlargement (Fig. 14-17). The PR interval represents the time required for passage of an impulse from the sinoatrial node until ventricular depolarization and is largely composed of the AV nodal delay. A prolonged PR interval, which is age specific, indicates first-degree AV block. A short PR interval should prompt evaluation of the QRS duration for signs of preexcitation (i.e., Wolff-Parkinson-White syndrome) (Fig. 14-18), although a short PR interval may also reflect a low right atrial pacemaker.

The QRS complex represents ventricular depolarization. The QRS duration should be examined in a lead with a Q wave present (often lead V$_5$ or V$_6$) for signs of conduction delay. Age-dependent normal values are important, because the upper limit of normal QRS duration is only 80 msec in neonates. The presence of a wide QRS complex with an RSR' pattern in V$_1$ indicates a right bundle branch block, whereas a QS pattern in V$_1$ and a tall notched R wave in V$_6$ is consistent with a left bundle branch block. Other conditions associated with prolongation of the QRS duration include ventricular preexcitation and ventricular pacing.

In addition to the QRS duration, the components of the QRS complex should be examined. Q waves are often present in the lateral and inferior leads and in lead aVR, but they should be narrow (less than 40 msec) and shallow (age dependent but usually less than 5 mm deep). Deep or wide Q waves suggest

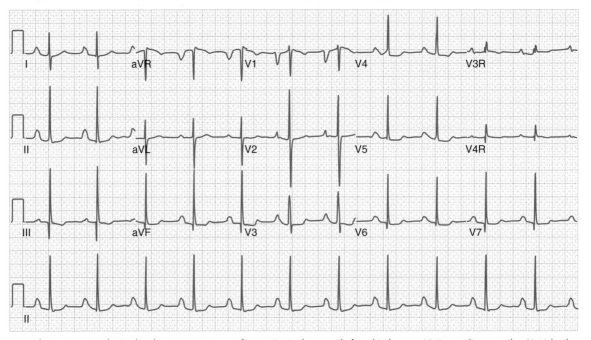

**FIGURE 14-17** The tracing was obtained in the emergency room for a patient subsequently found to have restrictive cardiomyopathy. Biatrial enlargement is established by the tall and wide P waves in leads II and V₁, respectively.

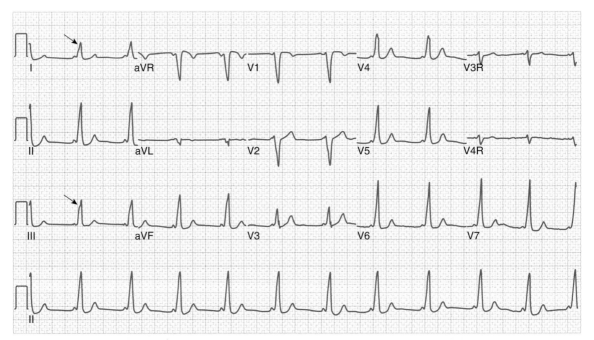

**FIGURE 14-18** The tracing demonstrates the typical electrocardiographic features of the Wolff-Parkinson-White syndrome: short PR interval, delta wave (*arrows*), and prolongation of the QRS interval.

myocardial ischemia and require further evaluation. An uncommon but crucial finding occurs in infants with ALCAPA. Classically, the ECG in this lesion demonstrates deep, wide Q waves in leads I and aVL with ST-segment and T-wave changes in the anterior distribution (V₂ to V₄) consistent with compromised myocardial blood flow (Fig. 14-19). The QRS amplitudes are also important in assessing left and right ventricular hypertrophy. Conditions associated with increased QRS voltages that likely require echocardiographic assessment include HCM, left ventricular noncompaction, and Pompe disease (see Fig. 14-6).

ST segments should be flat and should not be depressed more than 0.5 mm or elevated more than 1 mm in any lead. The major exception to this rule is when there is gradual upsloping of the ST segment in the mid-precordial leads, as seen in early repolarization. T waves represent ventricular repolarization and should all be upright in the precordial leads at birth. Within 1 to 3 days they become inverted, initially in V₁ and eventually in V₂, V₃, and sometimes in V₄. Starting at several years of age, the T waves return to the upright position in the reverse order. In normal adolescents and adults, the T wave in lead V₁ may be upright or

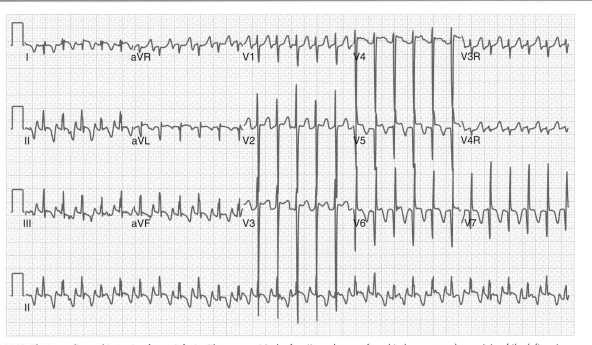

**FIGURE 14-19** Electrocardiographic tracing for an infant with poor ventricular function who was found to have anomalous origin of the left main coronary artery from the pulmonary root. The presence of Q waves in aVL and the diffuse ST-T wave changes suggest ischemia and are classic for this anomaly.

inverted. The only limb lead that typically displays an inverted T wave is aVR.

An aspect of the cardiac cycle that must be examined on any ECG is the QT interval, the time from the onset of ventricular depolarization (marked by the onset of the QRS complex), until the completion of repolarization (marked by the end of the T wave). It represents the duration of electrical activation and recovery of the ventricular myocardium, and it is measured as follows:

$$\text{Corrected QT (QTc)} = \frac{\text{Measured QT interval}}{\text{Square root of preceding R-R interval}}$$

A QTc that exceeds 460 msec is considered abnormal, regardless of age. All QTc values that exceed normal values for age merit further investigation. Medications that prolong the QT interval should be avoided until the child has been evaluated by a cardiologist.

Although a detailed organized approach to interpretation of a pediatric ECG is necessary, there are occasions when particular conditions or circumstances cause global electrocardiographic changes that must be quickly recognized. One such case that may occur in the operating room is related to the electrocardiographic changes associated with hyperkalemia. As the potassium level increases, the T-wave amplitude increases. This is followed by widening of the QRS duration (Fig. 14-20) due to an intraventricular conduction delay and by AV block and arrhythmias, including ventricular tachycardia and fibrillation. Other electrolyte disturbances may result in characteristic changes on the ECG:

■ Hypokalemia: decreased T-wave amplitude, ST-segment depression, and the presence of U waves

■ Hypercalcemia: shortening of the QT interval, sinus rate slowing, and sinoatrial block

■ Hypocalcemia: lengthening of the QT interval

■ Hypomagnesemia: enhanced effects of hypocalcemia

# Essentials of Cardiac Rhythm Interpretation and Acute Arrhythmia Management in Children

Rhythm abnormalities may be identified during the preoperative assessment, in the operating room, or in the postoperative period. Considerations usually include identification of the rhythm disorder, establishing the need for acute therapy, deciding whether to consult a pediatric cardiologist, and conveying pertinent information to the consultant to assist in the characterization of the rhythm disturbance and to establish a management plan. The following principles should be considered in addressing these issues:

1. Operating room, bedside, or transport monitors and strip recordings facilitate the recognition of rhythm disorders, but in most cases, they are inadequate for definitive diagnosis. A 15-lead surface ECG and rhythm strip should be obtained for all children when feasible.

2. Clinicians caring for children should have a basic knowledge of cardiac rhythm interpretation. Although a comprehensive discussion of arrhythmia interpretation is beyond the scope of this chapter, a brief overview of the characteristic features of normal and abnormal cardiac rhythms in the pediatric age group is presented in the following section.

3. The need for acute therapy for a rhythm disturbance should be based primarily on the nature of the disorder, urgency of the situation, and the likelihood that this abnormality would or would not be tolerated beyond the immediate short-term period. The guidelines established by the American Heart Association for Pediatric Advanced Life Support should be followed in all patients.[237] In otherwise healthy children and in contrast to ventricular arrhythmias, supraventricular tachyarrhythmias are rarely life-threatening.

4. The degree of comfort in the characterization and management of pediatric cardiac arrhythmias is likely to be quite

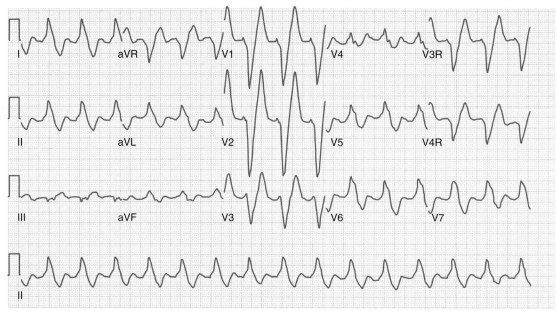

A    25 mm/sec  10 mm/mV  100 Hz

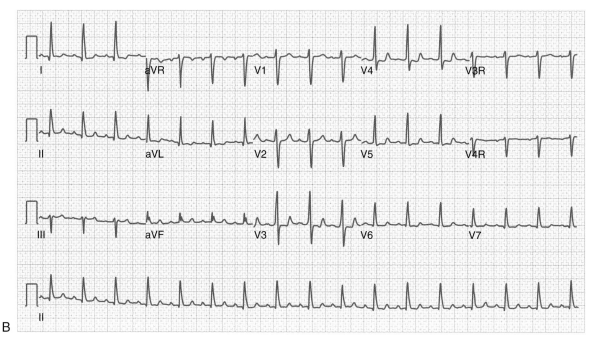

B

**FIGURE 14-20** These electrocardiographic changes may result from hyperkalemia. **A,** Marked widening of the QRS complexes is associated with peaked T waves. If untreated, this condition may progress to ventricular fibrillation and asystole. **B,** A tracing obtained several hours after treatment of electrolyte disturbance in the same patient demonstrates resolution of the electrocardiographic changes.

variable among anesthesia care providers. For arrhythmias caused by respiratory compromise, electrolyte imbalance, or metabolic derangements, consultation with a pediatric cardiologist is probably not required. This is also the case for variants or benign rhythm disturbances such as sinus arrhythmia, low atrial rhythms, or occasional premature atrial beats. Consultation is appropriate for most children with known structural or acquired cardiovascular pathology, in those with a history of a cardiac rhythm disorder under the care of a cardiologist, and in most of those with acute arrhythmias, particularly when initiation of antiarrhythmic drug therapy is contemplated.

5. Information that may be helpful to a consultant includes pertinent details regarding the child's history, clinical diagnosis, nature of the procedure/intervention, relevant laboratory values, description or characterization of the rhythm abnormality, associated hemodynamic parameters, circumstances surrounding the event (including the presence or absence of an intracardiac catheter), review of the pharmacologic agents administered (including anesthetic agents), and other therapies if applicable. The specialist should assist in the characterization of the rhythm disorder, advise about whether further evaluation is indicated, make recommendations for treatment, and facilitate diagnostic/therapeutic interventions as necessary.

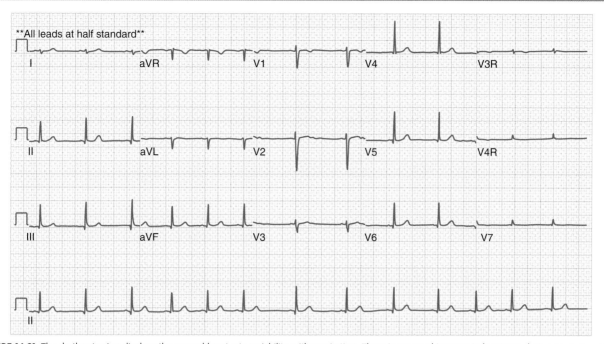

**FIGURE 14-21** The rhythm tracing displays the normal heart rate variability with respiration. There is a normal increase in heart rate during inspiration. This sinus arrhythmia is a natural response and is more commonly seen in children than adults.

## BASIC RHYTHMS
### Sinus Rhythm
Sinus rhythm is characterized by a P wave that precedes every QRS, a QRS that follows every P wave, and an upright P wave in leads I and aVF (see Fig. 14-16).

### Sinus Arrhythmia
Sinus arrhythmia represents cyclic changes in the heart rate during breathing. This is a normal finding in healthy children (Fig. 14-21).

### Sinus Bradycardia
Sinus bradycardia is characterized by sinus rhythm with heart rates below normal for age (see Fig. 14-5). Slow heart rates can be observed during sleep or at times of high vagal tone. When there is significant sinus bradycardia, a slow junctional escape rhythm or a slow atrial rhythm originating from an ectopic focus may be present. Certain forms of CHD may be prone to slow heart rhythms (i.e., heterotaxy syndromes).

In the intraoperative setting, particularly on induction of anesthesia, with laryngoscopy, endotracheal intubation, or tracheal suctioning, sinus bradycardia may occur. Sinus bradycardia may also result from drug administration (i.e., opioids) or increased parasympathetic tone. This type of sinus bradycardia rarely poses significant hemodynamic compromise and, if necessary, can be easily treated with removal of the stimulus, administration of a vagolytic agent (e.g., pancuronium), or with chronotropic drugs such as atropine or epinephrine. Sinus bradycardia may also result from hypoxemia, hypothermia, acidosis, electrolyte imbalance, or increased intracranial pressure. Bradycardia related to hypoxemia should be treated promptly with the administration of supplemental oxygen and appropriate airway management (see Chapter 39). The approach to other secondary forms of sinus bradycardia should focus on addressing the underlying cause. For worrisome slow heart rates, particularly in small infants, or for clinical evidence of compromised hemodynamics,

pharmacologic therapy (i.e., epinephrine, atropine, or isoproterenol infusion) or temporary pacing should be considered.

### Sinus Tachycardia
During sinus tachycardia, sinus rhythm occurs at a heart rate above normal for age (Fig. 14-22). In the perioperative setting this is often the result of surgical stimulation, stress, pain, hypovolemia, anemia, fever, medications (i.e., inotropic agents), malignant hyperthermia, or a high catecholamine state. Treatment is directed at the underlying cause. Prolonged periods of sinus tachycardia may impair diastolic filling time, limit ventricular preload, and compromise cardiac output. Children at risk for hemodynamic decompensation include those with significant degrees of ventricular hypertrophy or diastolic dysfunction, aortic stenosis, Williams syndrome, and HCM.

### Junctional Rhythm
A junctional rhythm is characterized by QRS complexes of morphology identical to that of sinus rhythm without preceding P waves. This rhythm is slower than the expected sinus rate. When this rhythm completely takes over the pacemaker activity of the heart, retrograde P waves and AV dissociation may be seen. Junctional rhythm during cardiac surgery is frequently the result of manipulation or dissection near the right atrium. The central venous pressure contour typically demonstrates prominent v waves (i.e., right atrial pressure wave at the end of systole) due to the loss of AV synchrony (Fig. 14-23). The lack of atrial contribution to ventricular filling may result in decreases in the systemic arterial blood pressure.

## CONDUCTION DISORDERS
### Bundle Branch Block
Incomplete right bundle branch block pattern (rSR′ in right precordial leads with near normal QRS duration) occurs in children with right ventricular volume overload (e.g., those with ASDs). Complete right bundle branch block (QRS complex

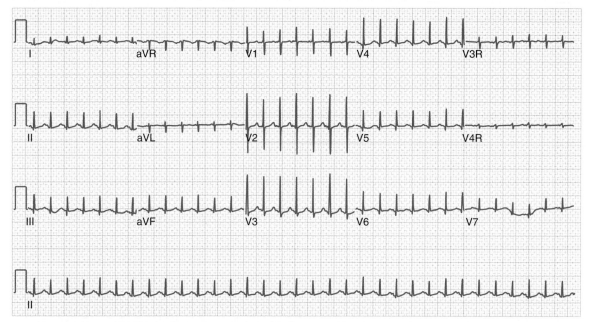

**FIGURE 14-22** Electrocardiogram for a febrile infant with sinus tachycardia, characterized by a heart rate above normal for age and QRS complexes of normal appearance preceded by P waves, which are upright in leads I and aVF.

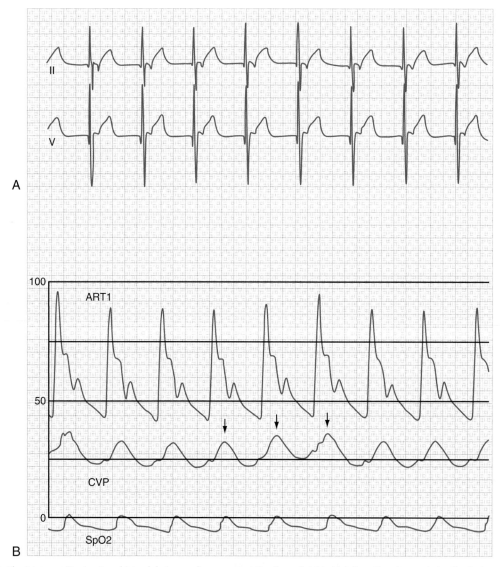

**FIGURE 14-23** The intraoperative tracing obtained during cardiac surgery at the time of right atrial dissection demonstrates the features of a junctional rhythm. Retrograde P waves are identified after the QRS complexes. The central venous pressure (*CVP*) tracing demonstrates prominent v waves (*arrows*) related to the loss of atrioventricular synchrony (scale of 0 to 30 mm Hg for CVP).

greater than 100 msec for infants, 120 msec for older children) is frequently seen in children after surgical procedures that involve the right ventricular outflow tract. This is characterized by an rSR′ wave pattern in $V_1$, an inverted T wave, and a wide and deep S (slurred) wave in $V_6$. Left bundle branch block is an uncommon finding in the pediatric age group that may result from cardiac interventions along the left ventricular outflow tract. Criteria for this conduction disorder include a prominent QS or rS complex in lead $V_1$ and tall, wide, and often notched R wave in leads I, aVL, and $V_6$.

## Atrioventricular Block

### First-Degree Atrioventricular Block
In first-degree AV block, there is prolongation of the PR interval beyond the normal range for age. Each P wave is followed by a conducted QRS. This may be found in healthy individuals but can also be seen in various disease states. First-degree AV block is a benign condition requiring no specific treatment.

### Second-Degree Atrioventricular Block
There are two forms of second-degree AV block: Mobitz type I (Wenckebach) and Mobitz type II. They are characterized by a periodic failure to conduct atrial impulses to the ventricle (i.e., P wave without following QRS complex). In a type I, second-degree AV block, there is a gradual lengthening of the PR interval with eventual failure of conduction of the next atrial impulse to the ventricle. The RR intervals concomitantly shorten. The degree of AV block is expressed as the ratio of P waves per QRS complexes (i.e., 2:1, 3:2). This can occur during periods of high vagal tone or in the postoperative setting. It is usually a benign phenomenon that requires no therapy. In the less frequent type II second-degree AV block, there is a relatively constant PR interval before an atrial impulse that fails to conduct. This is considered a more serious conduction disturbance and merits further investigation.

### Third-Degree Atrioventricular Block
Third-degree (complete) AV block is characterized by total failure of conduction of atrial impulses to the ventricle. It can be congenital or acquired. There is complete AV dissociation, with more atrial than ventricular contractions, and the ventricular rate is usually slow and regular (Fig. 14-24). Temporary pacing may be indicated in the acute setting.

## CARDIAC ARRHYTHMIAS

### Supraventricular Arrhythmias

#### Premature Atrial Contractions or Beats
Isolated premature atrial contractions (PACs) are relatively common in infants and small children. On the ECG, the early P waves exhibit a morphology and axis that are different from those in normal sinus rhythm. Premature atrial contractions may be conducted to the ventricles normally, blocked at the AV node, or conduct aberrantly (i.e., abnormal QRS morphology). They

are usually benign and require no therapy. If a central venous catheter is present, the tip position should be evaluated.

### Supraventricular Tachycardia
Supraventricular tachycardia (SVT) is the most common significant arrhythmia in infants and children.[238,239] It is characterized by a regular tachyarrhythmia (tachycardia heart rate is age dependent but typically more than 230 beats/min in children) with a narrow or usual complex QRS morphology. Supraventricular tachycardia can occur in structurally normal hearts and in various forms of CHD. *Usual complex* implies that the QRS morphology in tachycardia is similar to that in normal sinus rhythm (Fig. 14-25). Occasionally, widening of the QRS in SVT may result from bundle branch block or related to the tachycardia mechanism (i.e., SVT with aberrancy). A wide QRS complex may make the distinction between supraventricular and ventricular tachycardia difficult.

The two types of SVT are automatic and reentrant. They can be differentiated by evaluating characteristics of the tachycardia, usually assisted by the input from a specialist. The evaluation of a tachyarrhythmia should include a surface 15-lead ECG and continuous rhythm strip to document onset and termination. If a medication such as adenosine has been administered, a recording of the response to the drug or pacing maneuvers should be obtained. The management of SVT depends on the clinical status of the child, type of tachycardia, and precise electrophysiologic mechanism. General management principles include the following:

- Hemodynamic stability should be determined. Synchronized direct current cardioversion (0.5 to 1.0 J/kg) should be performed for hemodynamic instability.[237]
- Antiarrhythmic therapy is based primarily on the clinical condition and suspected tachycardia mechanism. Vagal maneuvers may be considered but should not delay treatment. Adenosine is the drug of choice in the acute setting for diagnosis and termination of most supraventricular tachycardias.[240] β-Blockers are most often used for chronic therapy.
- Others measures include treatment of fever if present, sedation, correction of electrolyte disturbance, decreasing or withdrawing medications associated with sympathetic stimulation (i.e., inotropic agents) or with vagolytic properties (i.e., pancuronium).
- In addition to pharmacologic therapy, atrial pacing or cardioversion may be required.

### Ventricular Arrhythmias

#### Premature Ventricular Contractions or Beats
Premature ventricular contractions (PVCs) are characterized by prematurity of the QRS complex, a QRS morphology that is different from that in sinus rhythm, usually a prolongation of the QRS duration for age, abnormalities of the ST segment and T wave, and premature ventricular activity not preceded by a

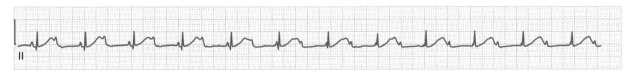

**FIGURE 14-24** Rhythm strip demonstrates independent atrial and ventricular activity (i.e., atrioventricular dissociation) and failure of any atrial impulses to conduct to the ventricles. These features characterize a complete atrioventricular block.

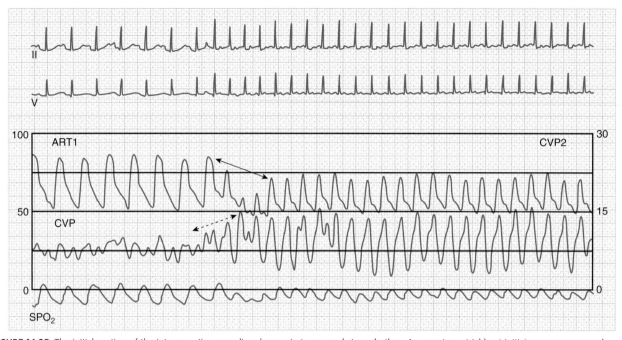

**FIGURE 14-25** The initial portion of the intraoperative recording demonstrates normal sinus rhythm. A premature atrial beat initiates a narrow complex tachycardia (i.e., QRS morphology the same as in sinus rhythm). The supraventricular tachycardia is associated with hemodynamic changes such as a decrease in the systemic arterial pressure (ART 1, scale of 0 to 100 mm Hg) (*arrow*) and increase in the central venous pressure (CVP, scale of 0 to 30 mm Hg) (*broken arrow*). *Spo₂*, Oxygen saturation.

premature atrial beat. PVCs of a single QRS morphology (i.e., uniform), without associated symptoms, and in children with structurally normal hearts are considered benign. An ECG during sinus rhythm should allow careful measurement of the QT interval. Further investigation and consultation are warranted in the presence of PVCs of multiple morphologies (i.e., multiform), if they occur with moderate frequency or in succession (i.e., couplets or runs) and are associated with symptoms or a structurally abnormal heart.

Ventricular ectopy in the perioperative period may be the result of profound hypoxemia, electrolyte disturbances, or metabolic derangements. Other causes include the use of recreational drugs, myocardial injury, poor hemodynamics, and prior cardiac surgical intervention.

### Ventricular Tachycardia

Ventricular tachycardia (VT) is relatively uncommon in children. It is defined as three or more consecutive ventricular beats occurring at a rate greater than 120 beats/min (Fig. 14-26). The QRS morphology in VT is different from that in sinus rhythm, and the QRS duration is typically prolonged for age. ECG features that support this diagnosis include AV dissociation, intermittent fusion (i.e., QRS complex of intermediate morphology between two other distinct QRS morphologies), QRS morphology of VT similar to that of single PVCs, and tachycardia rate in children usually below 250 beats/min.

Acute onset of VT in pediatric patients may be caused by hypoxia, acidosis, electrolyte imbalance, or metabolic problems. Ventricular tachycardia may also occur in the context of depressed ventricular function, halothane anesthesia with or without hypercarbia, poor hemodynamics, prior surgical interventions, cardiomyopathies, myocardial tumors, acute injury (e.g., inflammation, trauma), and prolonged QT syndromes.[241,242]

### Long QT Syndrome

Long QT syndrome (LQTS) (Fig. 14-27) is an electrical cardiac disturbance that can predispose children to arrhythmias that include torsades de pointes ventricular tachycardia (Fig. 14-28), ventricular fibrillation, and bradyarrhythmias, and any of these can result in syncope, cardiac arrest, or sudden death.[243] It occurs with an incidence of 1 case per 2500 births; congenital and acquired forms have been described. The congenital varieties are likely the result of genetic defects in the cardiac ion channels responsible for maintaining electrical homeostasis.[244] Thirteen genotypes have been described on five chromosomes. The cLQT1-3 (Romano-Ward) cases account for 90% of the children. The Romano-Ward syndrome has an incidence of 1 case per 10,000 births and an autosomal dominant pattern of inheritance. The Jervill Lange-Nielsen syndrome has an incidence of 1 case per 1,000,000 births, an autosomal recessive pattern of inheritance, and an association with deafness. Diagnostic criteria proposed for the long QT syndrome include electrocardiographic findings, clinical history (e.g., deafness, syncope), and family history.[245] A frequent feature is prolongation of the QTc on the resting ECG.

An important consideration in the care of children with cLQTS is ensuring adequate β-adrenergic blockade preoperatively and minimizing adrenergic stimulation.[243] Since the introduction of β-adrenergic blockade in patients with cLQTS in 1975, the mortality rate has decreased more than 10-fold. The risk for developing torsades de pointes from the many drugs known to trigger it is almost unpredictable; these drugs have been divided into several groups that are listed and updated online (www.qtdrugs.org).

In a retrospective study of children with cLQTS, three adverse events were reported during emergence from anesthesia immediately after administration of ondansetron and anticholinesterase medications; one was described as torsades de pointes.[244] These

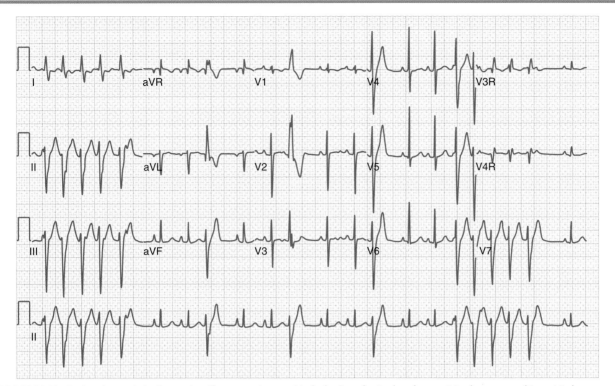

**FIGURE 14-26** The tracing demonstrates frequent, uniform premature ventricular beats and episodes of nonsustained, monomorphic ventricular tachycardia.

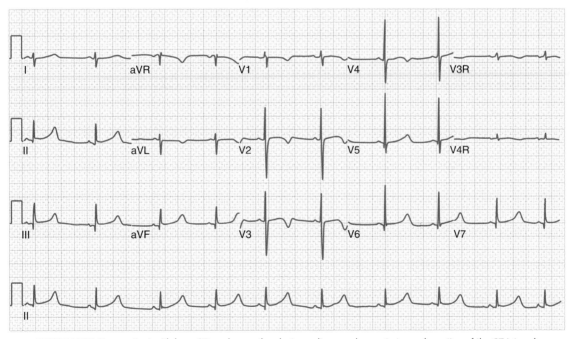

**FIGURE 14-27** For a patient with long QT syndrome, the electrocardiogram demonstrates prolongation of the QT interval.

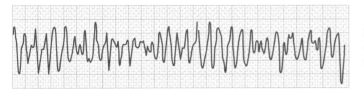

**FIGURE 14-28** The rhythm strip displays positive and negative oscillation of QRS complexes, which is characteristic of torsades de pointes ventricular tachycardia.

arrhythmias resolved quickly with intravenous β-blockers, lidocaine, or the administration of both agents. This report suggests that children with cLQTS are at risk for arrhythmias during periods of enhanced sympathetic activity (i.e., during emergence), particularly in the presence of drugs that prolong the QT interval. Conditions (e.g., hypothermia) and drugs (www.qtdrugs.org) that are known to prolong the QT interval should not be combined if possible. Despite the fact that most intravenous and inhalational medications routinely administered during anesthesia prolong the QT interval, adverse events are rare. This may be attributed in part to the need for a second abnormality beyond a prolonged QT interval to be present to trigger arrhythmias (i.e., increased dispersion of repolarization). Fortunately, most anesthetics do not increase the dispersion of repolarization.

Torsades de pointes is a rare but potentially life-threatening arrhythmia, even in the presence of prolonged QT interval. To trigger torsades de pointes, a second phenomenon must occur (i.e., increased dispersion of repolarization). Dispersion of repolarization refers to the variance in the rate of repolarization; in this case, it is a circumscribed region in the heart muscle (i.e., transmurally from the epicardium to the endocardium). There is much debate over how to quantify an increased dispersion of repolarization from surface ECGs. Some suggest the dispersion is the QTc-max to QTc-min, whereas others recommend measuring the duration of the T wave from its peak to the end; in both instances the upper limit of normal is 65 msec and abnormal values exceed 100 msec.

Prolongation of the QT interval and genesis of torsades de pointes occur more commonly in the presence of several conditions and drugs: electrolyte derangements (e.g., hypokalemia, hypocalcemia, hypomagnesemia), combination drug therapies (e.g., antibiotics, antiarrhythmic agents, class III antiarrhythmics such as amiodarone and procainamide), antipsychotic drugs, cisapride, neurologic or endocrine abnormalities (e.g., hypothyroidism), $5\text{-}HT_3$ receptor–blocking drugs (except palonosetron), neostigmine, stress (including induction of and emergence from anesthesia and laryngoscopy), female sex, bradycardia, and coronary artery disease. Although many anesthetics prolong the QT interval, few affect the dispersion of repolarization (as in the case of sevoflurane),[246] and the risk of torsades de pointes during general anesthesia in children is rare.

Management of torsades de pointes includes the following considerations:

1. Although some atypical forms of supraventricular tachyarrhythmias may mimic VT, a wide QRS tachycardia should always be considered to be of ventricular origin.
2. The initial approach in the setting of an acute ventricular rhythm disturbance consists of prompt evaluation of clinical status and hemodynamic stability. Sustained ventricular arrhythmias are poorly tolerated and require immediate attention. In the unstable child, cardiopulmonary resuscitation should be instituted while preparing for cardioversion. Expert consultation is advisable when advanced drug therapy is contemplated. Potential pharmacologic interventions include lidocaine, amiodarone, and procainamide.[247] The latter two should not routinely be administered during torsades de pointes due to QT prolongation.
3. Magnesium sulfate is considered the first-line treatment of torsades de pointes. Procainamide and amiodarone are contraindicated due to prolongation of the QT interval. Isoproterenol and overdrive pacing may be effective for bradycardia. Electrical cardioversion (1 to 2 J/kg) should be performed only if the arrhythmia is refractory to pharmacologic treatment.
4. cLQTS should be treated with β-blockade (not overdrive pacing); some forms of the cLQTS may require the implantation of a cardioverter-defibrillator.

### Ventricular Fibrillation

Ventricular fibrillation (VF) is an uncommon arrhythmia in children. It is characterized by chaotic, asynchronous ventricular activity that fails to generate an adequate cardiac output. The ECG during VF demonstrates low-amplitude, irregular deflections without identifiable QRS complexes. A loose ECG electrode may mimic these surface electrocardiographic features, and immediate clinical assessment should be performed and adequate pad contact ensured when VF is suspected.

Management of VF includes the following considerations:

1. This is a lethal arrhythmia if untreated.
2. Immediate defibrillation (initial dose of 2 J/kg) is the definitive therapy. Cardiopulmonary resuscitation, beginning with chest compressions, should be immediately resumed and continued for 2 minutes. If defibrillation is unsuccessful, the energy dose should be doubled (4 J/kg) and repeated. Pediatric paddles (2.2 cm in diameter) are recommended for children weighing less than 10 kg. Adult paddles (8 to 9 mm in diameter) are suggested for children weighing more than 10 kg to reduce impedance and maximize current flow.
3. Adequate airway control and chest compressions should be rapidly instituted while preparing for defibrillation or between shocks if several defibrillation attempts are needed. Resuscitative drugs and amiodarone should be considered without delaying defibrillation.

# Pacemaker Therapy in the Pediatric Age Group

## PACEMAKER NOMENCLATURE

Pacemaker nomenclature follows the guidelines of the North American Society of Pacing and Electrophysiology and the British Pacing and Electrophysiology Group[248] (Table 14-5):

- First letter: chambers paced (A = atrium, V = ventricle, D = dual or both, O = none)
- Second letter: chambers sensed (A = atrium, V = ventricle, D = dual or both, O = none)
- Third letter: pacemaker's response to sensing (I = inhibited, T = triggered, D = dual response, O = none)
- Fourth letter: rate modulation (R = rate modulation, O = none)
- Fifth letter: multisite pacing (A = atrium, V = ventricle, D = dual or both, O = none)

## PERMANENT CARDIAC PACING

### Indications

The most recent guidelines for permanent pacing in children, adolescents, and patients with CHD were published in 2008.[249] Indications include symptomatic sinus bradycardia, bradycardia-tachycardia syndromes, congenital third-degree AV block, and advanced second- or third-degree AV block.[249,250]

### Perioperative Considerations

Preoperative evaluation of children with implanted pacemakers should include device interrogation.[251] Familiarity with unit type,

**TABLE 14-5** NASPE/BPEG Generic Pacemaker Codes*

**Position Number and Category**

| I: Chambers paced | II: Chambers sensed | III: Response to sensed event | IV: Rate modulation | V: Multisite pacing |
|---|---|---|---|---|
| A = Atrium | A = Atrium | I = Inhibited | R = Rate modulation | A = Atrium |
| V = Ventricle | V = Ventricle | T = Triggered | | V = Ventricle |
| D = Dual (A + V) | D = Dual (A + V) | D = Dual (I + T) response restricted to dual-chamber devices | | D = Dual (A + V) |
| O = None | O = None | O = None | O = None | O = None |

**Most Common Pacing Modes**

*Single-chamber pacing*

AAI: atrial demand pacing (atrial pacing and sensing, inhibited on sensed beat)
AAIR: atrial demand pacing (atrial pacing and sensing, inhibited on sensed beat), rate responsiveness
VVI: ventricular demand pacing (ventricular pacing and sensing, inhibited on sensed beat)
VVIR: ventricular demand pacing (ventricular pacing and sensing, inhibited on sensed beat), rate responsiveness

*Asynchronous pacing (no sensing)*

AOO: fixed rate atrial pacing
VOO: fixed rate ventricular pacing
DOO: fixed rate AV pacing

*Dual-chamber pacing*

DDD: paces and senses both chambers
DDDR: paces and senses both chambers, sensor-driven rate responsiveness

Modified from Bernstein AD, Daubert JC, Fletcher RD, et al. The revised NASPE/BPEG generic code for antibradycardia, adaptive-rate, and multisite pacing. Pacing Clin Electrophysiol 2002;25:260-4.
*NASPE/BPEG*, North American Society of Pacing and Electrophysiology/British Pacing and Electrophysiology Group.
*The pacemaker mode, specified by a code, describes the mode in which the pacemaker is operating. The most common modes are listed.

settings, date of and indications for implantation, device location, and underlying rhythm is highly recommended. If records are not available and there is no identification card providing details about the unit implanted, a radiopaque marker on a chest radiograph may assist in the identification of the device. Major pacemaker manufacturers can also be contacted at any time because they maintain computerized records of all implanted devices. Results of a recent 15-lead ECG should be reviewed if available.

Reprogramming may be required before the planned procedure to avoid potential problems with pacemaker malfunction related to electrocautery. This represents one of the most common potential sources of electromagnetic interference in children with implanted cardiac devices. Recommendations for the perioperative management of these children include the use of bipolar cautery versus a unipolar configuration if possible, avoidance of cauterization near the generator, and positioning of the indifferent plate for electrocautery away from the pacemaker so that the device is not between the electrocautery electrodes.[252] Devices such as the harmonic scalpel and battery-operated, hot wire, handheld cautery units do not interfere with implanted cardiac devices. Rate-responsive features should be deactivated in most cases.

Chronotropic drugs and alternate pacing modalities should be readily available in the event of pacemaker malfunction and compromising underlying rate. Although insertion of a transvenous pacing system has been advised in children with complete AV block undergoing pacemaker implantation, a 10-year review indicated no benefit to routine preoperative temporary pacing.[253] Capture thresholds can be affected by pharmacologic agents, and this should be considered if pacing is required in the child receiving antiarrhythmic drug therapy.

Perioperative conditions may also influence pacing thresholds. A magnet should be accessible to allow asynchronous pacing if required.[254,255] Most generators respond to magnet application by pacing at a fixed rate asynchronously (i.e., AOO, VOO, or DOO). A potential problem is that the specific magnet rate, as determined by the manufacturer for the particular device, may be different from the desirable or optimal pacing rate. The use of a magnet should not be considered a substitute for preoperative pacemaker interrogation/programming. In addition to perioperative electrocardiographic monitoring, additional modalities that confirm pulse generation during pacing (e.g., esophageal stethoscope for assessment of heart sounds, pulse oximetry, invasive arterial blood pressure monitoring) are strongly encouraged. The device should be tested and reprogrammed after the procedure is completed.

**Transcutaneous Pacing**

Several devices that combine defibrillation and cardioversion capabilities with external pacing features are available. Emergency transthoracic pacing may be considered as a temporizing measure for children with symptomatic bradycardia,[256] but this has not been effective in the treatment of asystole in children.[257] Pacing electrode size should be selected according to patient size (e.g., smaller adhesive pads for weight less than 15 kg). Device settings typically include pacing rate and power output. Sedation may be necessary to tolerate soft tissue discomfort. Prolonged periods of transcutaneous pacing may result in local cutaneous injury. In addition to monitoring for pacemaker capture by ECG, ongoing clinical assessment of the adequacy of cardiac output should be undertaken.

**Implantable Cardioverter-Defibrillators**
The primary goal of an implantable cardioverter-defibrillator (ICD) is the prevention of sudden death. Children with long QT syndrome, HCM, history of near-death events, arrhythmogenic right ventricular dysplasia, and operated CHD with a history of malignant arrhythmias may be considered suitable candidates for device implantation.[250,258,259] The capabilities of these units include pacing and defibrillation. It may be feasible to terminate tachyarrhythmias by pacing.

Over the past several years, more children have been considered for device implantation.[249,259-263] This implies an increasing number of children with these devices who may require anesthetic care. The primary issues associated with intraoperative management of these devices relate to patient monitoring, managing issues with potential for electromagnetic interference, and performing emergent defibrillation, cardioversion, or heart rate support.[252] Perioperative consultation with a cardiologist or electrophysiologist is essential. These devices should be interrogated and likely require programming before and at the conclusion of the planned procedure.

# Diagnostic Modalities in Pediatric Cardiology

## CHEST RADIOGRAPHY
The standard posteroanterior and lateral chest radiographs provide clues to a child's underlying cardiovascular anatomy; however, plain radiographs are an insensitive screening tool for cardiac disease.[264] Children with numerous types of significant CHD may have initially normal-appearing radiographs; alternatively, an infant with a poor inspiratory effort and the presence of a large thymus may give the appearance of cardiomegaly and have normal intracardiac anatomy (Fig. 14-29).

Interpretation of a chest radiograph begins with identification of the patient's name and ensuring that the right-left orientation of the radiograph is correct. All catheters and tubes should be followed to verify their location, course, and likely site of

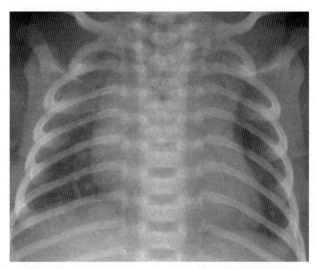

FIGURE 14-29 For a neonate with apneic episodes undergoing evaluation for potential cardiac disease, the radiograph demonstrates a poor inspiratory effort resulting in a large cardiothymic silhouette, making interpretation of cardiac size difficult. No evidence of cardiac disease was identified in this child.

termination. The bones and soft tissues should be inspected for evidence of sternal wires, fractures, vertebral anomalies, or wide intercostal spaces, suggesting a prior thoracotomy. Sidedness, including the location of the gastric bubble, liver, and position and orientation of the cardiac mass, should be observed. The lung parenchyma should be examined for evidence of focal consolidation, such as pneumonia or atelectasis, and for pulmonary vascular markings.

The cardiac silhouette and great vessels should be assessed. In young children, the thymus may obscure the superior portions of the cardiac shadow. Careful inspection of the cardiac silhouette includes an assessment of overall size and evidence of individual chamber or vessel dilation. The size of the main pulmonary artery segment may provide further evidence of the degree of pulmonary overcirculation in children with left-to-right shunt lesions. The tracheal indentation can usually be seen and is useful in determining aortic arch sidedness, although in a young child with a prominent thymus, this can be difficult to assess.

More useful than an individual radiograph as a diagnostic tool are serial chest films obtained to monitor a child's cardiovascular status over time. In a young child with a volume overload lesion, the physical examination and growth parameters coupled with the degree of cardiomegaly and pulmonary overcirculation are more helpful than more advanced imaging techniques. A plain chest radiograph may also guide initiation and titration of pharmacologic therapy and the timing of a surgical intervention.

## BARIUM ESOPHAGRAM
The current applications and uses of barium esophagram (swallow) studies in the diagnosis of CHD are limited. This modality has been largely replaced by MRI and chest tomography.[265-267] In some cases, a barium esophagram is used as an initial screening tool when there is concern about the presence of a vascular ring.[268,269] A double aortic arch represents one of the most common types of vascular rings in young children, but other vascular anomalies such as a right aortic arch with an aberrant left subclavian artery and left-sided ligamentum arteriosus may also cause symptoms. The indentation pattern in the barium column is consistent with the specific vascular anomaly (Fig. 14-30).

## ECHOCARDIOGRAPHY
Echocardiography is the primary diagnostic modality for the initial evaluation and serial assessment in most types of pediatric heart disease.[270,271] Using a variety of transducers, ultrasound is used to acquire real-time images of cardiovascular structures. Various echocardiographic modalities are available, including transthoracic,[272] transesophageal,[273-276] fetal,[277,278] epicardial,[279] intracardiac imaging,[280] and intravascular ultrasound.[281] Each plays an important role in the diagnostic evaluation and management of children with suspected or confirmed cardiovascular disease.

Advantages of echocardiography include its noninvasive nature, provision of excellent temporal and spatial resolution, generation of portable real-time images, cost-effectiveness, and ease of use. As with any type of ultrasound, these waves are transmitted well through homogeneous tissues and fluid but poorly through air and bone. Another limitation of echocardiography is related to limited acoustic windows in certain patient groups, such as those who have undergone multiple cardiothoracic procedures, older individuals, or children with a significant amount of soft tissue or body fat. For this reason, cardiovascular MRI is being increasingly used for noninvasive imaging. Additional challenges of echocardiography include the need to obtain serial two-dimensional tomographic images by sweeping the transducer scan in multiple planes to synthesize these images into three-dimensional structures in one's mind and to achieve expert interpretation. Despite these limitations, echocardiography remains the main diagnostic imaging modality for most children. Many medical and surgical management strategies are primarily based on the findings allowed by this approach.

A standard transthoracic study consists of a two-dimensional examination, M-mode imaging, and Doppler evaluation (i.e., color flow, pulsed-wave, or continuous-wave modalities). Two-dimensional imaging provides structural assessment of the heart and adjacent vasculature. Cross-sectional images are obtained from several windows that allow excellent anatomic detail in multiple planes (Video 14-11). In most cases, this is adequate for a detailed segmental evaluation of the cardiac anatomy as described earlier. M-mode echocardiography allows one-dimensional imaging of the heart with excellent temporal resolution (Fig. 14-31). It is known as an *ice pick view* of the heart in real time and is primarily used in the assessment of ventricular dimensions and function.

Color flow Doppler techniques allow evaluation of directionality and velocity of blood flow. In addition to detecting flow across cardiac valves and great vessels, color flow imaging allows detection of subtle lesions such as small septal defects that can be difficult to identify by standard two-dimensional imaging alone. Traditionally, flow toward the transducer is displayed in red, and flow away is represented as blue. Turbulent blood flow is associated with increased Doppler velocities and can be readily identified as a mosaic of colors; it typically has a greenish tint (Video 14-12).

Pulsed- and continuous-wave Doppler represent spectral modalities that complement the color flow data and provide quantitative information. Pulsed-wave interrogation localizes specific sites of stenosis or turbulence but is limited in the magnitude of velocities it can detect. Continuous-wave Doppler allows quantification of much higher velocities (see Video 14-12). Velocities obtained with pulsed- and continuous-wave Doppler provide estimates of pressures within various cardiac chambers by applying the simplified Bernoulli equation. It states that the difference

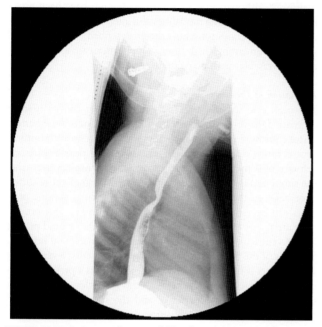

**FIGURE 14-30** Barium swallow in a child with respiratory symptoms demonstrates a filling defect posteriorly in the mid-esophagus, which is consistent with an aberrant subclavian artery.

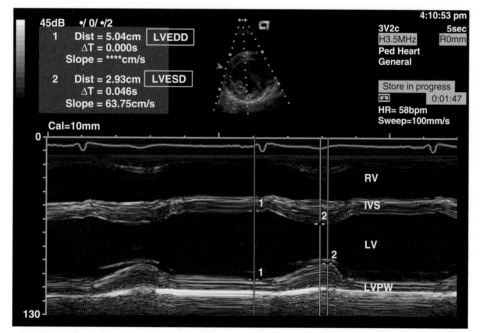

**FIGURE 14-31** An M-mode echocardiogram enables determination of left ventricular dimensions and calculation of shortening fraction. *IVS*, Interventricular septum; *LV*, left ventricle; *LVEDD*, left ventricular end-diastolic dimension; *LVESD*, left ventricular end-systolic dimension; *LVPW*, left ventricular posterior wall; *RV*, right ventricle.

in pressure between two locations is approximately four times the square of the velocity of the jet of flow between them:

$$\text{Pressure gradient (in mm Hg)} = 4 \times v^2$$

The applications of three-dimensional echocardiography in CHD continue to be investigated.[282-284] This approach can provide clear and useful volumetric assessments when the images are adequate. A significant advantage of this modality is that it is able to display cardiovascular structures and their interrelationships in detail, in many cases facilitating the understanding of pathologic conditions over two-dimensional imaging. Three-dimensional echocardiography may also be useful when interventions are planned.

### Interpretation of an Echocardiographic Report
#### *Measurements of Cardiac Chambers and Vessel Dimensions*
Several measurements are routinely performed during an echocardiographic examination. They include ventricular dimensions such as left ventricular end-diastolic (LVED) and left ventricular end-systolic (LVES) dimensions, thickness of the interventricular septum and left ventricular posterior wall, and measurements of valve sizes and great artery dimensions. To determine whether these are appropriate for the child being examined, the measurements are referenced to values obtained in normal children matched for body surface area. This is accomplished by reporting the measured value in addition to a Z score, representing standard deviations of measured values from the mean in a comparative population.

#### *Assessment of Ventricular Function*
Several echocardiographic techniques are able to provide information regarding ventricular performance. Two of the most commonly reported indices of ventricular systolic function are shortening fraction and ejection fraction. Shortening fraction (SF) represents the percent of change in left ventricular diameter during the cardiac cycle. This is calculated using the following equation:

$$\text{SF (\%)} = (\text{LVED dimension} - \text{LVES dimension}/\text{LVED dimension}) \times 100$$

Values range from 28% to 44%, with a normal mean value of 36%. This index, however, depends on ventricular preload and afterload.

Ejection fraction (EF) is the fraction of blood ejected by the ventricle (stroke volume) relative to its end-diastolic volume. This represents the percentage of blood ejected from the left ventricle with each heart beat. Ejection fraction is derived by volumetric analysis of the left ventricle by means of the following equation:

$$\text{EF (\%)} = (\text{LVEDV} - \text{LVESV}/\text{LVEDV}) \times 100$$

In the equation, LVEDV is the left ventricular end-diastolic volume, and LVESV is the left ventricular end-systolic volume. Normal values range between 56% and 78%. A low ejection fraction is associated with systolic functional impairment, but cardiac dysfunction may occur in the presence of a normal ejection fraction. Such may be the case of a child with diastolic heart failure.

Although these functional indices are routinely and easily obtained, they have significant limitations. Estimation of ejection fraction is based on geometric assumptions for the elliptical left ventricle, and this may not be applicable to a systemic right ventricle or other types of ventricular geometries.[285] This accounts

for an escalating interest in alternative approaches that may provide more sensitive and comprehensive information regarding ventricular performance, even in the absence of clinical disease. These techniques include the myocardial performance index (MPI), also known as the Tei index, which combines systolic and diastolic intervals to assess global ventricular function[286-288]; Doppler tissue imaging (DTI), which is used to evaluate intramural myocardial velocities[289]; and strain and strain rate imaging to quantitate the rate of segmental myocardial deformation.[290] Although values in normal children have been established for these imaging modalities and alterations in the presence of pathologic conditions have been described,[291,292] additional studies documenting their clinical applications in specific types of cardiovascular pathology are needed.

#### *Estimation of Pressures*
The peak velocity of a tricuspid regurgitant jet can be used to estimate right ventricular systolic pressure and pulmonary artery systolic pressure in the absence of pulmonary stenosis or outflow obstruction (Video 14-13). For example, if a peak regurgitant velocity of 3 m/sec is recorded across the tricuspid valve using the simplified Bernoulli equation, the pressure gradient or difference between the right atrial and right ventricular systolic pressures can be estimated to be $4 \times 3^2 = 36$ mm Hg. If a normal right atrial pressure is assumed (4 to 6 mm Hg), it would predict a right ventricular systolic pressure of approximately 40 mm Hg. Similarly, if the peak or maximal flow velocity across a ventricular septal defect is measured at 4.5 msec, it predicts a pressure gradient of $4 \times 4.5^2 = 81$ mm Hg between the ventricles, implying that the defect is pressure restrictive and the right ventricular and pulmonary artery systolic pressures are relatively low.

#### *Evaluation of Gradients*
Estimation of a peak instantaneous gradient is the most clinically useful method for quantifying the severity of obstructions across semilunar valves and outflow tracts. It is derived by application of the simplified Bernoulli equation. When obtained across the pulmonary valve, these estimates tend to have a better correlation with catheterization peak-to-peak gradients than those measured across the aortic valve, for which mean gradients (obtained by automated integration of the velocities under a spectral Doppler tracing) have been shown to have a greater correlation.[293] The mean gradient rather than a peak gradient determined by Doppler echocardiography is considered a better indicator of the severity of the obstruction across AV valves and other low-flow venous pathways.

#### *Evaluation of Regurgitant Lesions*
Evaluation of the severity of regurgitant lesions in most pediatric cardiac centers remains largely a qualitative assessment. It is usually characterized as mild, moderate, severe, or a combination thereof when there is overlap among these categories. Serial echocardiographic assessments and comparative data are clinically more meaningful than an isolated report.

### MAGNETIC RESONANCE IMAGING
Cardiovascular MRI-angiography has emerged as a complementary technology to other imaging modalities (Videos 14-14 and 14-15). Benefits have been reported in the assessment of complex pathology,[294-300] delineation of systemic and pulmonary vascular anomalies,[299,300] evaluation of global and regional ventricular function,[301] assessment of myocardial viability,[302] and

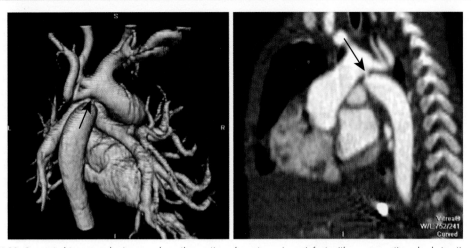

**FIGURE 14-32** Computed tomography images show the aortic arch anatomy in an infant with severe aortic arch obstruction (*arrows*).

characterization of pulmonary blood supply in children with structural alterations of the pulmonary vascular tree.[303] Additional applications that may further expand the utility of cardiovascular MRI include the quantification of left-to-right shunts[304-306] and measurement of blood oxygen saturation.[307] MRI is beneficial for guiding interventions in pediatric heart disease.[308-310]

Although the temporal resolution of MRI is inferior to echocardiography, new sequences and techniques allow real-time acquisition similar to that of fluoroscopy. An important aspect in the acquisition of MRI data with high spatial resolution is the use of cardiac and respiratory gating to allow sampling during only specific portions of the cardiac and respiratory cycles. Slow heart rates and low respiratory rates facilitate this process. MRI, in contrast to computed tomography (CT), does not involve radiation exposure, making it preferable for serial examinations that many young children with cardiovascular pathology require. However, this may be associated with the need for multiple episodes of anesthesia and their inherent risks.

Because of the nature of the magnetic fields generated in MRI, the presence of several types of metal, including pacemakers, ICDs, cerebrovascular clips/coils, or recently implanted intracardiac or intravascular coils and devices, are considered contraindications. Titanium hardware may minimize the artifact produced by the foreign material; stainless steel generates significant artifacts within the study.

An additional limitation of MRI is the need for patient immobility during long examinations for optimal image quality. For small children, this requirement usually necessitates the use of deep sedation or general anesthesia.[311-313] For infants with complex and often cyanotic CHD, specialists are often asked to provide care during the procedures. The severity of the cardiovascular disease and the need for breath holding may add to the challenges presented to the anesthesia care provider in a remote location.[314,315] The lengthy nature of the studies and the significant time requirements to perform postprocessing of the images cause MRI to be much more time intensive for the interpreting physician than other noninvasive imaging modalities.

A significant advantage of this technique is avoidance of harmful radiation inherent to traditional catheterization techniques. As MRI technology improves, with faster scans, increasing availability, and decreasing cost, it will continue to play an increasing role in the diagnosis and longitudinal follow-up of congenital and acquired pediatric heart disease.

## COMPUTED TOMOGRAPHY

Cardiac CT, with or without electrocardiographic gating, has become an option among the various cardiovascular imaging modalities (Fig. 14-32).[294,298,316,317] The major advantage of CT over MRI is the very rapid scan times, and for most children, sedation is minimal or unnecessary. A significant drawback of CT is the large radiation burden, although typically estimated to be similar to or slightly greater than a diagnostic cardiac catheterization, and the likely need for iodinated contrast agents with their concomitant risks.

Cardiac CT is not as accurate as MRI for delineation of intracardiac anatomy, but it provides excellent spatial resolution and information on extracardiac structures. CT has been beneficial in the evaluation of aortic arch anomalies and vascular rings and for defining systemic and pulmonary venous returns. In adult patients, multislice CT provides excellent information on coronary arteries and the presence of atherosclerotic disease; in infants and children with smaller vessels and more rapid heart rates, these images are more difficult to obtain.

## CARDIAC CATHETERIZATION AND ANGIOGRAPHY

Cardiac catheterization involves the invasive measurement of intracardiac and vascular pressures and blood oxygen saturation coupled with angiography to assess cardiac anatomy and hemodynamics (Figs. 14-33 and 14-34). Before the era of two-dimensional echocardiography, cardiac catheterization was frequently used for diagnostic purposes. With the advances in noninvasive imaging, diagnostic procedures represent a relatively small proportion of these studies. Current indications for cardiac catheterization at most centers include the assessment of physiologic parameters such as pressure and resistance data, anatomic definition when other diagnostic modalities are inadequate, need for electrophysiologic testing or treatment, and when interventions are anticipated.

Most catheterizations are performed for interventions, including endomyocardial biopsies; angioplasties and stenting of stenotic vessels, dilation of valves, and conduits; and occlusion techniques for native defects, fistulous connections, and surgically created defects no longer considered necessary (Fig. 14-35, Video 14-16) (see Chapter 20). In some cases, such as critically ill neonates with complex heart disease, catheter-based interventions such as balloon atrial septostomy and other procedures can be lifesaving.

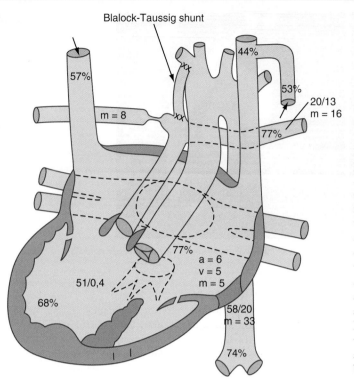

Blalock-Taussig shunt

Weight 3.3 kg

**Diagnosis**
1. Heterotaxy
2. Dextrocardia
3. Complete atrioventricular canal
4. Double-outlet right ventricle
5. Pulmonary stenosis, severe
6. L-Transposition of the great arteries
7. Interrupted inferior vena cava with azygous continuation
8. After innominate to main pulmonary artery shunt
9. Right pulmonary artery isolation

**FIGURE 14-33** A cardiac catheterization diagram is valuable when caring for patients with structural anomalies, such as this child with complex congenital heart disease. Data routinely obtained at cardiac catheterization are shown, including oxygen saturation determinations (in %), pressure measurements (in mm Hg), and hemodynamic calculations. Catheter courses are indicated by *arrows*. The atrial pressures are given for the a wave (*a*), which represents the atrial systole; v wave (*v*), which represents the end of systole (rise in atrial pressure before atrioventricular valve opening); and mean (*m*), all in mm Hg. See section on "Interpretation of a Cardiac Catheterization Report," this page.

In most children, access to the central circulation is accomplished percutaneously through a femoral approach. Most examinations involve hemodynamic evaluation with recording of pressure data through catheters positioned at various sites of interest. Oxygen saturation data are obtained by reflectance oximetry or blood gas measurement from various cardiac chambers and vessels. In contrast to the oxygen saturation calculations derived from a blood gas analysis, reflectance oximetry provides measured values. This allows determination of oxygen content (i.e., total amount of hemoglobin in the blood) and, when combined with values of oxygen consumption, assessment of blood flows and other calculations (e.g., shunts).[318] Additional data that may be obtained include pressure gradients, cardiac output, and parameters for deriving vascular resistances and valve areas.

Fluoroscopy and cineangiography are essential components of most cardiac catheterization studies. Of the two, cineangiography accounts for most of the radiation exposure as images are recorded during the injection of contrast material, typically at 15 or 30 frames/sec.[319] Most angiograms are obtained during biplane imaging by positioning the equipment to obtain optimal views allowing for delineation of the pathology in question (i.e., axial angiography) (Video 14-17, *A* and *B*).[320,321]

Although cardiac catheterization has evolved over the years, providing an improved margin of safety, it remains an invasive procedure involving several risks. They include excessive blood loss, vascular complications,[322,323] infection, arrhythmias, vascular or cardiac perforation,[324] systemic air embolization, myocardial ischemia, and those associated with the administration of contrast agents. These complications are more likely in infants and small children.[325] Interventional catheterizations, by the nature of the procedures, are associated with a greater rate of complications and greater potential for morbidity and mortality. However, as transcatheter interventions become safer and more effective, an increasing number of children may obviate the need for surgery, often undergoing procedures on an outpatient basis.[326] Evolving approaches in this field include percutaneous implantation of valves,[327] strategies that combine cardiac catheterization and surgical intervention (hybrid procedures),[328-330] and catheter-based interventions during fetal life.[331]

### Interpretation of a Cardiac Catheterization Report
*Pressure Data*
Atrial pressure tracings are characterized by several waves (a, c, and v waves) and descents (x and y). Reported values correspond to the a and v waves and the mean pressures. The right atrial pressure is typically a wave dominant. The mean right atrial pressure is normally less than 5 mm Hg. In the presence of significant tricuspid valve regurgitation or a junctional rhythm, the v wave becomes the dominant wave. The left atrial pressure tracing, in contrast to the right atrium, displays v wave dominance, which is accentuated during mitral regurgitation. The mean left atrial pressure rarely exceeds 8 mm Hg.

Ventricular pressures are recorded and reported during systole, at end systole, and at end diastole. For the right ventricle the systolic pressure is normally in the 25 to 30 mm Hg range, with end-diastolic pressure of 5 to 7 mm Hg. The systolic pressure in the left ventricle normally increases with age and should equal the systolic arterial pressure; the end-diastolic pressure is typically less than 10 mm Hg.

The pulmonary artery pressure is reported in terms of systolic, diastolic, and mean pressures. The systolic pulmonary artery pressure in a normal child should be equal to the right ventricular systolic pressure, and the mean pulmonary artery pressure should not exceed 20 mm Hg. The pulmonary artery wedge pressure is obtained by advancing a catheter into a distal vessel until it is occluded, reflecting the left atrial pressure.

The aortic pressure and contour of the tracing depends on the site of interrogation. Typically, there is an increase in the systolic pressure as the catheter navigates toward the peripheral circulation. This phenomenon is known as *pulse wave amplification*.

Pressure gradients, or the pressure differences between two distinct sites, can be measured in several ways (i.e., mean gradient and peak gradient). It is important to consider that several factors may affect their determination. This is significantly influenced by the severity of the obstruction and the ventricular function. Smaller gradients may be seen under sedation or anesthesia.

14

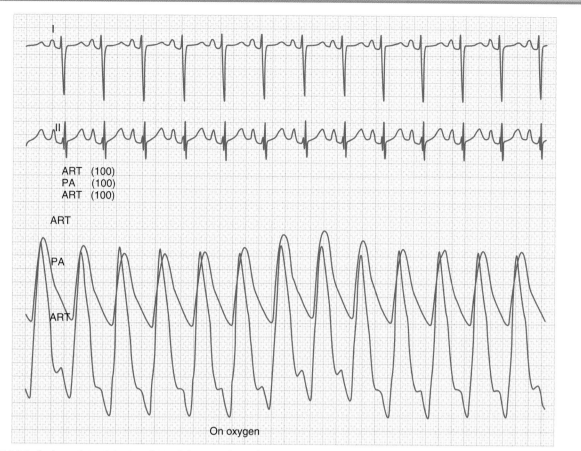

**FIGURE 14-34** In the hemodynamic tracing obtained during cardiac catheterization, notice that the pulmonary artery systolic pressure (100 mm Hg) is at systemic levels in this child with multiple, left-sided obstructions. *ART*, Systemic arterial pressure; *PA*, pulmonary artery pressure.

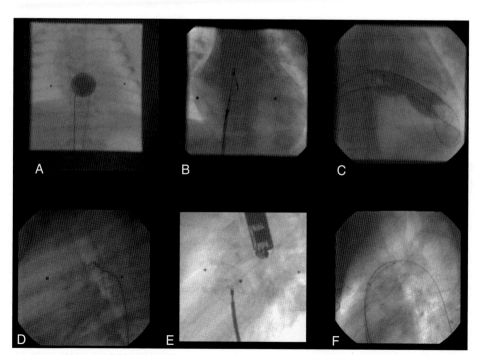

**FIGURE 14-35** Several types of interventions are performed in a pediatric cardiac catheterization laboratory. **A,** Balloon atrial septostomy. **B,** Blade atrial septostomy. **C,** Double-balloon mitral valvuloplasty. **D,** Placement of a ductal coil occluder device. **E,** Transcatheter closure of a secundum atrial septal defect. **F,** Pulmonary artery dilation with stent placement.

*Shunt Calculations*

Shunts are characterized in terms of their direction (e.g., left-to-right, right-to-left, bidirectional) and magnitude. Left-to-right shunts can be quantified based on the pulmonary ($\dot{Q}_{pulm}$) to systemic ($\dot{Q}_{sys}$) blood flow ratio. In the equation, $S_{sys}aO_2$ is the systemic arterial $O_2$ saturation, $S\bar{v}O_2$ is the mixed venous $O_2$ saturation, $S_{pulm}vO_2$ is the pulmonary venous $O_2$ saturation, and $S_{pulm}aO_2$ is the pulmonary arterial $O_2$ saturation.

$$\frac{\dot{Q}_{pulm}}{\dot{Q}_{sys}} = \frac{(S_{sys}aO_2 - S\bar{v}O_2)}{(S_{pulm}vO_2 - S_{pulm}aO_2)}$$

A $\dot{Q}_{pulm}/\dot{Q}_{sys}$ ratio that exceeds 3 to 1 is considered a significant shunt, although smaller ratios may be associated with considerable symptoms.

*Cardiac Output Determinations*

The volume of blood ejected by the heart into the systemic circulation, or cardiac output, can be derived in several ways. Thermodilution measurements use saline as an indicator to measure pulmonary blood flow. In the absence of intracardiac shunts, this is equivalent to cardiac output (expressed as liters per minute). In the Fick method, oxygen is used as an indicator, and cardiac output is obtained by the application of the following formula:

$$\dot{Q}_{sys} \text{ (L/min)} = \frac{\dot{V}O_2 \text{ (L/min)}}{C_{sys}O_2 - C\bar{v}O_2}$$

In the equation, $\dot{V}O_2$ is the oxygen consumption (assumed or measured), $C_{sys}O_2$ is the systemic arterial $O_2$ content, and $C\bar{v}O_2$ is the mixed venous $O_2$ content. The $O_2$ content = $O_2$ saturation $\times (1.36 \times 10 \times$ hemoglobin concentration).

*Vascular Resistances*

Resistance represents the change in pressure in the systemic or pulmonary circulation with respect to flow. It is expressed in Wood units (mm Hg/L/min) and is usually normalized for body surface area. The systemic vascular resistance (SVR) and pulmonary vascular resistance (PVR) are derived as follows:

$$SVR = (\text{aortic mean pressure} - \text{right atrial mean pressure})/\dot{Q}_{sys}$$
$$PVR = (\text{pulmonary artery mean pressure} - \text{pulmonary capillary wedge pressure or left atrial pressure})/\dot{Q}_{sys}$$

# Perioperative Considerations for Children with Cardiovascular Disease

## GENERAL ISSUES

Anesthesia for children with heart disease[332] is challenged by the following factors:

- The remarkable spectrum of disease
- The wide range of congenital lesions and their underlying physiologic consequences
- The numerous interventional and surgical options in CHD (Table 14-6), in addition to their hemodynamic implications
- The fact that many parents are unaware of the full extent or details of the child's lesion or abnormalities

To optimally care for these children, the following objectives should be met:

- Familiarity with the cardiovascular defects
- Understanding of the physiologic abnormalities and available therapies
- Recognition of compensatory mechanisms, signs of limited reserve, and potential perioperative risks[333]
- Ability to identify the potential impact of the proposed intervention/surgical procedure on the child's underlying condition and anticipate how it will be tolerated

This combination of daunting challenges and difficult objectives can be intimidating even for the most experienced clinician. When caring for children with cardiovascular disease, an interdisciplinary approach is recommended, allowing for the formulation and execution of optimal individualized management plans. If available, consultation with the child's cardiologist or primary care physician should include inquiries about the details of the child's disease, overall clinical status, past and current medical treatment, prior catheterization or surgical interventions, and presence of residual pathology. The interaction between members of the perioperative team should allow an exchange of information, discussion of concerns, and recommendations that may facilitate patient care and the development of comprehensive care plans.[334] This is particularly important in the management of children with complex disease.

A complete medical history and focused examination is essential during the preoperative assessment. In addition to evaluating the child's disease processes, overall clinical status, and functional reserve, this allows appraisal of issues that may affect anesthesia management (e.g., limited vascular access, difficult airway, gastroesophageal reflux, manipulations to manage pulmonary and systemic blood flow and pressures). Available diagnostic studies (e.g., ECG, chest radiograph, echocardiogram, Holter monitor, cardiac catheterization) should be reviewed. Depending on the nature of the procedure, complexity of the disease, and potential impact on perioperative outcome, additional evaluation and diagnostic studies may be warranted. In many cases, the anesthesiologist plays a major role in determining whether the available information is adequate.

A fundamental goal in the preoperative evaluation is the identification of children who are at increased risk because of cardiac and pulmonary limitations imposed by their cardiovascular disease. After the preoperative visit, the anesthesiologist caring for a child with CHD should have an understanding of the pathophysiology of the cardiac defect and implications of any previous interventions. Abnormal indices that should raise potential concerns include hypoxemia ($SpO_2$ less than 75%), $\dot{Q}_{pulm}/\dot{Q}_{sys}$ exceeding 3 to 1, outflow tract gradients greater than 50 mm Hg, pulmonary hypertension (i.e., mean pulmonary artery pressure above 30 mm Hg), increased pulmonary vascular resistance index (more than 2 Woods units/m²), or polycythemia (i.e., hematocrit greater than 60%). Several clinical states may place children at significant risk for severe cardiopulmonary decompensation during anesthesia and surgery: recent congestive heart failure, uncontrolled arrhythmias, severe ventricular dysfunction, unexplained syncope, substantial exercise intolerance, or any condition associated with significant functional cardiac or pulmonary impairment. For some children, a planned admission to the intensive care unit (with or without a tracheal tube) should be discussed with the parents, child, and whole care team.

## CLINICAL CONDITION AND STATUS OF PRIOR REPAIR

Children with CHD may present for anesthesia care before or after palliation or for definitive procedures. Corrective

**TABLE 14-6** Surgical Procedures for Congenital Heart Disease

| Procedure | Description | Goal or Result |
|---|---|---|
| Arterial switch (Jatene) operation | Arterial trunks transected above the level of the semilunar valves, relocated to their appropriate respective ventricles, coronary arteries reimplanted into the neoaortic root | Establishes the normal ventricular-arterial connection (right ventricle to pulmonary artery and left ventricle to aorta) in transposition of the great arteries |
| Atrioventriculoseptal defect (atrioventricular canal) repair | Patch closure of atrial and ventricular communications, reconstruction of atrioventricular valves, closure of cleft in left-sided atrioventricular valve | Eliminates the intracardiac shunt |
| Blalock-Taussig shunt | Subclavian artery to pulmonary artery communication; modified implies placement of a graft | Allows or increases pulmonary blood flow |
| Central shunt, Waterston shunt, Pott shunt | Creation of communication between systemic and pulmonary circulations | Allows or increases pulmonary blood flow |
| Closure of septal defects | Patch or primary closure of communications at the atrial or ventricular levels | Eliminates the intracardiac shunt |
| Coarctation repair | Relief of aortic arch obstruction (various approaches) | Establishes patency across the aortic arch |
| Damus-Kaye-Stansel procedure | End-to-side anastomosis of main pulmonary artery onto the aorta; necessitates reestablishing pulmonary blood flow through an alternative route (graft from a systemic artery into the pulmonary artery or a right ventricular to pulmonary artery conduit) | Allows unobstructed systemic outflow in the context of single ventricle associated with obstruction to aortic flow or other settings |
| Division or ligation of a patent ductus arteriosus | Obliteration of the ductus arteriosus | Eliminates shunting at the level of the great arteries |
| Fontan procedure | Connection that directs inferior vena cava blood into the pulmonary circulation | Separates the pulmonary and systemic circulations in patients with single ventricle physiology; usually the final step in the single-ventricle palliation pathway |
| Glenn anastomosis (cavopulmonary connection) | Superior vena cava to pulmonary artery direct anastomosis (bidirectional implies flow from superior vena cava into both pulmonary arteries) | Provides pulmonary blood flow while unloading the single ventricle; may be the first or intermediate step in the single-ventricle palliation pathway |
| Konno-Rastan procedure (aortoventriculoplasty) | Enlargement of the left ventricular outflow tract and aortic annulus; defect created in the ventricular septum to enlarge the outflow tract repaired with a large patch | Alleviates subvalvar and valvar aortic obstruction; when the aortic root is replaced by an autologous pulmonary root, it is referred to as a Ross-Konno procedure. Alternatively, cryopreserved homograft tissue may be used in the form of an extended aortic root replacement. |
| Norwood procedure (stage I palliation) | Involves aortic reconstruction, an atrial septectomy, and placement of a systemic-to-pulmonary artery shunt | Addresses systemic outflow tract obstruction by allowing the right ventricle to eject into a reconstructed aorta. Atrial septectomy provides unobstructed drainage of the pulmonary venous return into the right atrium. The systemic-to-pulmonary artery shunt supplies the pulmonary blood flow. |
| Pulmonary artery banding | Constrictive band placed around the main pulmonary artery | Limits excessive pulmonary blood flow |
| Rastelli operation | Creation of an intracardiac tunnel that allows left ventricular output into the aorta while closing a ventricular septal defect and placement of a right ventricular conduit to pulmonary artery | Allows the left ventricle to eject solely into the aorta, abolishes intracardiac shunting at the ventricular level, and provides unobstructed pulmonary blood flow. The procedure results in separation of the pulmonary and systemic circulations. |
| Sano modification of the Norwood procedure | Placement of graft between the right ventricle and main pulmonary artery as an alternative to a modified Blalock-Taussig shunt in the Norwood operation | Provides pulmonary blood flow |
| Senning or Mustard procedure (atrial switch) | Intraatrial baffle procedure | Allows pulmonary venous blood to be rerouted through the tricuspid valve into the right ventricle (as the systemic chamber that ejects into the aorta). Systemic venous return is channeled across the mitral valve into the left ventricle, which pumps into the main pulmonary artery. |
| Tetralogy of Fallot repair | Closure of ventricular septal defect and relief of right ventricular outflow tract obstruction | Eliminates intracardiac shunting at the ventricular level (cyanosis) and addresses right ventricular outflow tract obstruction (often at several levels) |
| Truncus arteriosus repair | Closure of the ventricular septal defect and establishment of right ventricular to pulmonary artery continuity (usually with a homograft) | Abolishes intracardiac shunting and restores the normal connection between the ventricles and great arteries |
| Valvectomy | Valve excision | Relieves valvar obstruction |
| Valvotomy | Opening of stenotic valve | Relieves valvar obstruction |
| Valve replacement | Placement of bioprosthetic or mechanical valve | Addresses valvar pathology (obstruction and regurgitation) |
| Valvuloplasty | Valve repair | Relieves valvar regurgitation and stenosis |

14

procedures are those that result in a normal life expectancy and full cardiovascular reserve.[335] Children undergoing these interventions usually require no further medical or surgical treatment. In the strict sense, only a few procedures fulfill these criteria: ligation, division, or occlusion of a PDA and closure of an isolated secundum ASD. Other interventions or surgical procedures may result in repair or correction but not necessarily in normal hemodynamics or life expectancy. The clinician should assume some limitation in cardiovascular reserve, a need for close follow-up, further medical management, and potential or additional surgical therapies. In other cases, as in children with palliated CHD, the circulation may still be abnormal. These individuals have been reported to be at greater risk for adverse perioperative events.[336-338] Published data from the Pediatric Perioperative Cardiac Arrest (POCA) Registry examined anesthesia-related cardiac arrests in children with congenital and acquired heart disease.[339] Compared with other children, cardiac arrests were found to occur more frequently in children with heart disease. Causes were primarily cardiovascular in nature. These events occurred more frequently in the general operating room, usually during the surgical maintenance phase. The most common anatomic substrate in this setting was that of a single ventricle, particularly those early in the palliation pathway. The overall mortality rate for children with heart disease was greater than those without heart disease, with the greatest mortality rate occurring in children with aortic stenosis and cardiomyopathy.

The effects of previous procedures on the heart and other systems require careful consideration. Problems may remain or develop after surgical intervention include residual shunts, valvar stenoses or outflow tract obstruction, valvar regurgitation, pulmonary hypertension, arrhythmias, and ventricular dysfunction. Children who require a detailed appraisal of perioperative risks include those with residual significant pathology, suspected or known pulmonary hypertension, or single-ventricle physiology and those after conduit placement or cardiac transplantation (see Chapters 15, 16, and 21).

## Summary

Caring for children with heart disease is a major aspect of pediatric anesthesia practice. The spectrum of cardiovascular disease includes a wide range of structural defects and varied acquired diseases. The ability to provide optimal perioperative care heavily relies on a clear understanding of the basic pathophysiology of the lesions (e.g., how a red cell gets from here to there); familiarity with the commonly used diagnostic modalities and their clinical applications; and medical and surgical treatment options available to affected individuals. In this chapter, we have presented basic concepts in cardiology that can enhance the overall knowledge of the practicing anesthesiologist in pediatric cardiovascular disease.

## ACKNOWLEDGMENT

We wish to thank Timothy C. Slesnick, MD, for his prior contributions to this chapter.

## ANNOTATED REFERENCES

Bai W, Voepel-Lewis T, Malviya S. Hemodynamic changes in children with Down syndrome during and following inhalation induction of anesthesia with sevoflurane. J Clin Anesth 2010;22:592-7.

*The retrospective study evaluated whether children with Down syndrome (n = 96) are at increased risk for bradycardia and hypotension during and after sevoflurane induction. The investigation reported a significantly higher prevalence and degree of bradycardia in children with Down syndrome during and after sevoflurane induction. Despite these findings, there were no differences between Down syndrome and control groups in the prevalence of hypotension or pharmacologic interventions.*

Cordina RL, Celermajer DS. Chronic cyanosis and vascular function: implications for patients with cyanotic congenital heart disease. Cardiol Young 2010;20:242-53.

*This excellent article reviews the effects of chronic cyanosis and associated alterations in blood vessel structure and function, with an emphasis on the endothelium and important implications for patients with cyanotic congenital heart disease.*

Lang RM, Mor-Avi V, Sugeng L, et al. Three-dimensional echocardiography: the benefits of the additional dimension. J Am Coll Cardiol 2006;48:2053-69.

*This article focuses on the benefits of three-dimensional echocardiography; the realistic, unique, and comprehensive views of cardiac valves and congenital abnormalities; and the utility of this method in the intraoperative and postoperative settings.*

Murphy T, Smith J, Ranger M, et al. General anesthesia for children with severe heart failure. Pediatr Cardiol 2011;32:139-44.

*This retrospective study examined the frequency of complications during anesthesia for short noncardiac surgical interventions or diagnostic procedures in children with severe heart failure. Two children (10%) of the 21 who underwent 28 procedures requiring general anesthesia experienced a cardiac arrest, requiring unplanned intensive care admission. In 27 (96%) of the 28 anesthesia procedures, perioperative inotropic support was required. The study authors concluded that general anesthesia for children with severe heart failure was associated with a significant complication rate.*

Pharis CS, Conway J, Warren AE, et al. The impact of 2007 infective endocarditis prophylaxis guidelines on the practice of congenital heart disease specialists. Am Heart J 2011;161:123-9.

*The web-based survey evaluated changes in cardiology practice related to the updated 2007 American Heart Association guidelines on endocarditis prophylaxis for patients with congenital heart disease. The study reported that 28% of respondents thought that the new guidelines left some patients at risk. There remained considerable heterogeneity among cardiologists regarding the prophylaxis of certain cardiac lesions.*

## REFERENCES

Please see www.expertconsult.com

# Anesthesia for Children Undergoing Heart Surgery

**15**

ANGUS McEWAN

## Preoperative Evaluation

In the United States, 40,000 children are born each year with congenital heart disease (CHD),[1] representing an incidence of 6 to 8 cases per 1000 live births.[2] Children with chromosomal abnormalities such as trisomy 21 (i.e., Down syndrome) have a greater incidence of CHD. Having a sibling with CHD increases the risk of CHD, as does the presence of other congenital abnormalities.[3] With improving diagnostic techniques, many children with CHD are diagnosed in the antenatal or early postnatal period. Associated with this improvement in diagnostic ability is a trend in most centers to undertake definitive repair earlier, with many patients undergoing corrective surgery in the neonatal period. Overall, about one half of all children with CHD undergo cardiac surgery in the first year of life, and about 25% undergo surgery in the first month of life.[4,5]

The perioperative management of children with complex cardiac defects requires a dedicated team of surgeons, cardiologists, anesthesiologists, intensivists, perfusionists, and nurses. Anesthesiologists caring for these children are challenged by some of the greatest physiologic aberrations encountered in clinical medicine. The anesthesiologists responsible for the care of these children require a comprehensive understanding of cardiac physiology and pathophysiology. The anesthesiologist must be able to adapt to each nuance of rapidly changing pathophysiology as it is encountered.

In addition to treating children with CHD, the pediatric cardiac anesthesiologist may also be responsible for the care of adults with CHD. This patient population with "grown-up CHD" is expanding as more children with CHD survive to adulthood. Along with CHD, they have some of the comorbidities of older age. The ideal approach for this group of patients is to be cared for in specialist units, but few are available. In the meantime, the care of these patients may fall to the most qualified physicians and the pediatric cardiac anesthesiologist. Some children have acquired rheumatic heart disease, some have cardiomyopathy, and others have undergone heart transplantation and require care from specialists.

For managing children with complex cardiac defects, there is increasing reliance on echocardiography and magnetic resonance imaging (MRI) to acquire diagnostic data. Although fewer children are being subjected to diagnostic angiography, more interventional cardiac catheterization procedures are being performed. Many conditions that would previously have been treated surgically are now treated in the angiography suite by interventional cardiologists, such as atrial septal defects (ASDs), patent ductus arteriosus (PDA), and ventricular septal defects (VSDs). Other interventions include dilating arteries with balloon catheters with and without stents and coiling of aberrant or excessive collateral vessels. The pulmonary artery is commonly balloon dilated and stented, and coarctation of the aorta is treated similarly by balloon dilation. Stenotic valves are also commonly dilated. These procedures have led to the risk being transferred from the angiography suite to the operating room.[6] For the individual child, there has been a dramatic decrease in morbidity as increasing numbers of conditions are treated in the angiography suite, but the risks of complications that occur in the angiography suite have increased as more complex procedures are performed (see Chapter 20).

## THE PREOPERATIVE VISIT AND EVALUATION

The preoperative visit is an important part of the overall management of anesthesia for children with CHD.[7] The preoperative visit has several aims:

- Medical assessment
- Prescribing premedication
- Providing information
- Creating a relationship with the child and family
- Formulating an anesthetic plan

### Medical Assessment

The anesthesiologist must have a clear and detailed understanding of the cardiac pathophysiology, the surgery to be undertaken, and associated congenital abnormalities or medical conditions. The medical assessment includes collation of information from the history, physical examination, and review of imaging and laboratory data. Most diagnostic information is obtained from the medical record. Particular attention should be paid to the echocardiographic, MRI, angiographic, and other imaging data; the chest radiograph; and the electrocardiogram. Many centers have joint cardiac conferences where decisions about treatment are discussed in a multidisciplinary forum. Reports from these meetings are valuable in the preoperative assessment.

In addition to gathering this specific diagnostic information, a directed history and physical examination should be performed to assess the overall condition of the child. Attention should be directed toward assessing the degree of cardiac failure, cyanosis, or risks of pulmonary hypertension and the prior surgical procedures and how this information may alter access to the central circulation and placement of invasive monitors. The general nutritional state of the child should be assessed; poor growth and development may be a sign of severe CHD. Other information should be sought that may have a bearing on the anesthetic plan. For example, is this repeat surgery, and does it require a repeat sternotomy? This has a bearing on line placement because a femoral bypass may be required, and it should be avoided for line placement. The previous use of aprotinin is important because the risk of anaphylaxis is increased in a second exposure and particularly if it has been given in the previous 6 months.[8]

The type of surgery to be performed is important. For example, if a Blalock-Taussig shunt is placed on the left, the arterial line should not be placed in the left arm because the trace will be lost or distorted during subclavian cross-clamping. If a Glenn shunt is planned, a short internal jugular line can be useful to monitor pulmonary artery pressure, but it should be removed early in the postoperative period so as not to risk the formation of thrombosis in the superior vena cava (SVC).

Good veins should be sought and marked for the application of local anesthetic cream. This is useful in sick children even if an inhalational induction is planned because it allows placement of a venous cannula during a very light plane of anesthesia and avoids myocardial depression from high concentrations of inhalation anesthetics.

### Prescribing Premedication

The use of sedative premedication can be useful in cardiac anesthesia, but this practice varies widely. Numerous medications may be used, and numerous recommendations exist. Premedication for infants younger than 6 months of age is usually unnecessary. Premedication for older, healthy children who show little anxiety and with whom good preoperative rapport can be established is often unnecessary. However, older children, particularly those who have undergone previous surgery, have fears about anesthesia and surgery. It is important to address the fears of these children. Sedative premedication may play a pivotal role in achieving adequate anxiolysis for separation from the parents and induction of anesthesia. I prefer to avoid premedication in children with severe congestive heart failure. Cyanotic children such as those with tetralogy of Fallot (TOF) often benefit from sedative premedication because crying and struggling during induction of anesthesia may worsen their cyanosis. However, it is important that these cyanotic children are well supervised after premedication because they have a blunted response to hypoxia.[9] In the United States, supplemental premedication is sometimes administered under the direct supervision of the anesthesiologist in the preoperative facility, providing for a calm child and gentle separation from the parents. In the United Kingdom, where induction of anesthesia takes place in a dedicated anesthesia room, parents are present until after the induction, often making additional premedication unnecessary.

The most common premedication is oral midazolam (0.5 to 1.0 mg/kg).[10] However, the effect of midazolam may be unpredictable and may cause dysphoria. Numerous other medications have been recommended for this purpose, including ketamine, clonidine, temazepam, and chloral hydrate. The use of these drugs is often dictated by local preferences and is not always evidence based.

### Giving Information

Providing information to the parents and to the child if they are capable of understanding is a key element of the preoperative visit. This information includes the use of sedative premedication, the type of induction, fasting times, the type and likely position of invasive lines, the need for a stay in an intensive care unit (ICU) postoperatively, and the expected length of that stay. The use of other monitors such as transesophageal echocardiography (TEE) should be outlined and any contraindications sought, along with the probability of needing a blood transfusion. Questions about the risk of anesthesia and surgery should be addressed to the satisfaction of the parents (see Chapter 4).

### Creating Rapport with the Child and Family

By creating a good relationship with the family, the anesthesiologist can reduce the anxiety of the child and the parents. The family develops a sense of trust, which can improve their hospital experience.

### Formulating an Anesthetic Plan

After assessing the patient, it is possible to formulate a detailed anesthetic plan.

## UPPER RESPIRATORY TRACT INFECTION AND CARDIAC SURGERY

Otherwise healthy children undergoing elective noncardiac surgery in the presence of an upper respiratory infection (URI) are more likely to suffer respiratory complications (Table 15-1). These complications typically are minor, are easily managed, and usually result in minimal morbidity.[11-13] The decision about

**TABLE 15-1** Diagnosis of Upper Respiratory Tract Infection

At least two of the following signs plus confirmation by a parent:
  Rhinorrhea
  Sore or scratchy throat
  Sneezing
  Nasal congestion
  Malaise
  Cough
  Fever >100.4° F (38° C)

Data from Schreiner MS, O'Hara I, Markakis DA, Politis GD. Do children who experience laryngospasm have an increased risk of upper respiratory tract infection? Anesthesiology 1996;85:475-80.

whether to proceed with noncardiac surgery in a child with a URI is made on an individual basis.[14]

The decision to proceed with cardiac surgery in children is difficult. Although children with cardiac failure are prone to multiple URIs, they may also have signs that can mimic URIs. Surgery may be relatively urgent, and postponing surgery exposes the child to an increased risk. Cardiac surgery in children with URIs results in a prolonged stay in the ICU and prolonged ventilation times, although overall hospital stay is not prolonged. There is an increased incidence of pulmonary atelectasis and an increase in postoperative bacterial infections. There appears not to be any statistically significant increase in mortality rates (4.2% with URIs versus 1.6% without URIs) or long-term sequelae in children with URIs who undergo cardiac surgery. The URI group was significantly younger and smaller, which may account in part for the greater but statistically insignificant increased mortality rate.[15] Although this increase in mortality was not statistically significant, it does raise concerns about the risks posed by URIs before cardiac surgery. Children who are scheduled for a Glenn shunt or completion of the Fontan circulation may be at particular risk because an increase in pulmonary vascular resistance (PVR) can adversely affect outcome. It is prudent to postpone surgery in a child with a URI who is scheduled for elective cardiac surgery. If the surgery is urgent, discussion with the surgical team is required to correctly assess the risks and benefits to the child.

## Perioperative Challenges in Pediatric Cardiac Anesthesia

### CYANOSIS
Children with cyanotic cardiac defects compensate for chronic hypoxia with increased erythropoiesis, increased circulating blood volume, vasodilation, and metabolic adjustments of factors, such as circulating 2,3-diphosphoglycerate (2,3-DPG). These changes allow greater tissue delivery of oxygen. The increase in blood viscosity with polycythemia leads to increased vascular resistance and sludging, which may result in renal, pulmonary, and cerebral thromboses, especially in dehydrated children.[16] Long periods without oral intake preoperatively and postoperatively should be avoided in children with polycythemia, unless adequate intravenous hydration is provided.

PVR increases more than systemic vascular resistance (SVR) with an increasing hematocrit, further decreasing pulmonary blood flow in children who already have a compromised pulmonary circulation. Coagulopathies are common in children with cyanotic CHD and may adversely influence surgical hemostasis.[17,18] When the hematocrit exceeds 65%, excessive viscosity impairs microvascular perfusion and outweighs the advantages of increased oxygen-carrying capacity. Reduction of red blood cell volume can correct the coagulopathy and improve hemodynamics when increases in hematocrit are extreme.[19]

### INTRACARDIAC SHUNTING
In CHD, much of the pathophysiology involves communications between chambers or vessels that are normally separate, resulting in shunting of blood between ventricles, atria, the great arteries, or a combination of these, depending on the nature of the lesion. Management of shunting is a major consideration during anesthesia and requires an understanding of the factors that control shunting.

### Restrictive and Unrestrictive Shunts
When communications are small, the size of the defect limits shunting and considerations of relative PVR and SVR become correspondingly less important in determining the amount of shunting. When there is a large pressure differential at the same level of the circulation on either side of a communication, the communication is restrictive. Flow is limited across the defect, and other factors determining shunt flow become less important. This is usually the situation in children with mild heart disease that is asymptomatic or minimally symptomatic, such as small ASDs and VSDs or a small PDA.

### Dependent Shunting during Anesthesia
In children with dependent shunts, the direction and degree of intracardiac shunting are determined by the circulatory dynamics. Control of circulatory dynamics to minimize the shunt is a major goal of anesthesia management. Because shunting depends on the relationship between SVR and PVR, anesthesia management often revolves around control of relative vascular resistances.

In children with dependent right-to-left shunts, the shunt increases when SVR decreases or PVR increases. In children with dependent left-to-right shunts, the shunt increases when SVR increases and PVR decreases. In children with bidirectional or balanced shunting, changes in vascular resistance increase the net shunt away from the side with increased vascular resistance.

For practical purposes, acute increases in left-to-right shunts during anesthesia are of clinical importance in several situations. A substantial steal of systemic blood flow by the pulmonary circulation can occur in conditions such as atrioventricular (AV) canal, truncus arteriosus, and hypoplastic left heart syndrome. Left-to-right shunting is well tolerated, except when pulmonary steal leads to systemic hypotension, increasing acidosis or insufficient coronary perfusion. Shunting from right-to-left, because it is accompanied by at least some degree of arterial oxygen desaturation, is more frequently a problem during anesthesia.

### IMPAIRED HEMOSTASIS
Hemostasis is impaired after bypass in infants and children. This results from a combination of immature coagulation factor synthesis, hemodilution after bypass, and a complex interaction involving consumption of clotting factors and platelets. At birth, the levels of vitamin K–dependent coagulation factors in healthy, full-term neonates are only 40% to 66% of adult values. During the first month of life, these levels increase to 53% to 90% of adult values.[20] However, in children with CHD, especially those

with cyanosis or systemic hypoperfusion, coagulation factors often continue to be depressed due to impaired hepatic protein synthesis. Although antithrombin III levels are also low, true heparin resistance is rare in infants because of parallel decreases in coagulation factors.

At the onset of cardiopulmonary bypass (CPB), the introduction of the prime volume, which is two to three times greater than the child's blood volume, dilutes the factor concentrations, particularly fibrinogen, to 50% of values before bypass and the platelet count to 30% of values before bypass. This degree of dilution occurs even when the pump circuit is primed with whole blood. Greater dilution may occur when packed red cells are used in the priming volume. At the conclusion of neonatal bypass, the activity of clotting factors is often extremely low, the fibrinogen concentration is frequently less than 100 mg/dL, and the platelet count has been reduced to 50,000 to 80,000/mm³.[21,22] In addition to these quantitative changes, functional changes in the platelets occur during bypass. Extracorporeal circulation causes a loss of platelet adhesion receptors, activation of platelets, and formation of leukocyte-platelet conjugates. Platelet adhesion receptors are more depressed in children with cyanotic compared with acyanotic cardiac defects. Heparin also impairs platelet function independent of CPB.[23]

Cardiac surgery is associated with significant activation of the fibrinolytic system.[24] Inadequate heparin levels during CPB may also contribute to postoperative bleeding because inadequate anticoagulation may allow activation of the hemostatic pathways. Activation causes the consumption of platelets and clotting factors. The standard measurement of anticoagulation, the activated clotting time (ACT), shows a poor correlation with heparin levels in children undergoing CPB.[25] In one study, the use of heparin monitoring and heparin titration was associated with larger doses of heparin but smaller doses of protamine for antagonism.[26] Activation of clotting cascades is also reduced, decreasing bleeding in the postoperative period.[26] As a result of this multifactorial coagulopathy, blood loss is a greater problem in children than in adults and is a particular problem in neonates and small infants (see Chapter 17).[27]

### Strategies to Reduce Bleeding after Bypass

In an effort to normalize factors and platelets to effective concentrations, some medical centers use fresh whole blood in the cardiopulmonary circuit prime. In adult patients and an in vitro aggregation study, transfusion of fresh whole blood provided equal or greater hemostatic and functional benefit when compared with transfusion of platelet concentrates. In children, transfusion of fresh whole blood less than 48 hours from harvest is associated with less blood loss compared with transfusion of reconstituted whole blood (e.g., packed erythrocytes, fresh frozen plasma [FFP], and platelets).[28] However, fresh whole blood is often difficult to obtain. The units must be refrigerated for 24 to 48 hours while donor screening is performed, and storage causes significant platelet injury. Insistence on fresh whole blood places tremendous pressures on the transfusion service and donor center to coordinate the matching of donor types with recipient needs.

In practice, individual component therapy is used. In neonates and small infants with dilutional coagulopathy, platelets should be given in combination with cryoprecipitate to correct the defect in clotting. An initial dose of 10 mL of platelets/kg of body weight may need to be repeated. Platelets may be administered if bleeding persists and the platelet count is less than

100,000/mm³.[29] Cryoprecipitate contains high concentrations of fibrinogen, factor VIII, von Willebrand factor, and factor XIII. Fibrinogen and von Willebrand factor are required for platelet adhesion and aggregation to occur. Platelet adhesion and aggregation are the fundamental first steps in primary hemostasis (see Chapter 10). The subsequent step of platelet degranulation switches on the entire coagulation cascade and cannot take place without adhesion and aggregation.[30] Administration of FFP, for which there is no evidence of effectiveness in treating this type of coagulopathy, to the infant may excessively dilute the red cell mass and platelets.[31]

Transfusion guidelines have been described for adults and have been shown to reduce postoperative bleeding and transfusion requirements.[32,33] However, similar guidelines have not been forthcoming for children in whom the practice appears to be more empirical. This is a less than ideal situation, and more work is urgently needed to produce well-validated guidelines. The thromboelastogram and the platelet count may be used to identify which children are likely to bleed after cardiac surgery.

### Antifibrinolytics

The antifibrinolytics used in pediatric cardiac surgery include ε-aminocaproic acid (EACA) and tranexamic acid (TA). In many countries, aprotinin is no longer available, and in other countries, it has only very limited availability after its marketing license was withdrawn due to safety concerns. EACA and TA are lycine analogues that reduce bleeding after cardiac surgery in adults and children.[34,35] They do not exert any antiinflammatory activity. Doses for pediatric cardiac surgery have not been clearly established.

Aprotinin is a serine protease inhibitor that has been studied thoroughly in adults. Early evidence demonstrated that it reduces bleeding, reduces the time taken to extubation, shortens ICU stay, and reduces overall mortality rates.[36] However, subsequent studies have contradicted these earlier findings.[37] The same volume of evidence has not been published for children, although several studies suggest that it is effective in reducing bleeding and that it reduces the time spent on the ventilator and in the ICU.[38-41] An increased risk of renal failure or stroke in adults undergoing revascularization surgery has been reported.[42] The same investigators reported an increase in the 5-year mortality rate for adults after the use of aprotinin in revascularization surgery.[43] Aprotinin has increased the 30-day mortality rate by as much as one third compared with TA or EACA.[37] Comparable data for children have not been forthcoming (see Chapter 18). Aprotinin is available for use in New Zealand, Australia, and Canada. It appears that the early data regarding increased death rates have not been supported by subsequent studies and that the benefits may outweigh risks in specific populations.[44]

### Topical Agents

The use of topical agents to promote clot formation and reduce bleeding in children after cardiac surgery is common. The most commonly used topical agents are fibrin sealants. Fibrin sealants mimic the stages of the blood coagulation process. Unlike the synthetic adhesives, they are biocompatible.[45] Fibrin sealants are usually sourced from plasma components, and most contain virally inactivated human fibrinogen and thrombin with different quantities of factor XIII, antifibrinolytic agents, and calcium.[45] When the fibrinogen and thrombin are mixed during the application process, the fibrinogen is converted to fibrin monomers. This results in the formation of a semirigid fibrin clot.

By mimicking the later stages of the coagulation process, these sealants stop bleeding and assist in wound healing.[45] They have significantly reduced bleeding in children.[46]

### Ultrafiltration

Ultrafiltration is a process that removes ultrafiltrate from a child during and after CPB. It provides many benefits, including increasing the hematocrit, concentrating the clotting factors and platelets, increasing blood pressure, reducing PVR, and removing inflammatory mediators in the ultrafiltrate. It has significantly reduced bleeding after cardiac surgery in children.[47,48]

### Desmopressin

Desmopressin acts by increasing plasma concentrations of factor VIII and von Willebrand factor. It has been effective in reducing bleeding after CPB in adult cardiac surgery.[49] Unfortunately, studies in children failed to demonstrate a similar effectiveness in reducing bleeding or transfusion requirements.[50]

## Anesthesia Management for Surgery Requiring Cardiopulmonary Bypass

### MONITORING

Noninvasive monitoring during pediatric cardiac surgery includes pulse oximetry, five-lead electrocardiography, an automated blood pressure cuff, a precordial or esophageal stethoscope, continuous airway manometry, inspired and expired capnography, anesthetic gas and oxygen analysis, multiple-site temperature measurement, and volumetric urine collection. The pulse oximeter is especially important when managing children with congenital cardiac disease. At least two probes should be placed on different limbs in the event that one fails during the procedure. In children with cyanotic heart disease, conventional pulse oximetry overestimates arterial oxygen saturation as saturation decreases[51]; this error tends to be exacerbated in the presence of severe hypoxemia.[52] When monitoring children with a shunt across the ductus arteriosus, a probe should be placed on a right hand digit to measure preductal oxygenation, and a second probe should be placed on a toe to measure postductal oxygenation (children with a right-sided aortic arch may require the probe to be placed on a left-hand digit). Children undergoing repair of coarctation of the aorta should be monitored with a pulse oximeter on the right upper limb, because it may be the only reliable monitor during the repair, and blood pressure cuffs should be placed before and after the coarctation. These two cuffs may be cycled and the differential documented before and after surgical correction.

Monitoring end-tidal carbon dioxide tension ($PETCO_2$) is of value in most children. However, in children with cyanotic-shunting cardiac lesions, the $PETCO_2$ measurement may be less reflective of $PaCO_2$ because of ventilation-perfusion mismatching.[53] Arterial blood gases are the most accurate measure of the adequacy of ventilation and oxygenation. To provide rapid decision making, it is helpful to have the blood gas analysis machine located in or near the cardiac operating room.[54]

Monitoring ionized calcium concentrations is essential during surgical procedures in which significant quantities of citrated blood are infused rapidly or when entire blood volumes are replaced. Neonates are particularly prone to disturbances in their ionized calcium concentration when citrated whole blood, FFP, or platelets are infused. Those with limited cardiac reserve tolerate ionized hypocalcemia poorly because of their greater sensitivity to the myocardial effects of citrate infusion (see Chapter 10).[55] In isolation, the total serum calcium concentration is misleading.

Temperature monitoring during CPB is a critical guide to adequate brain cooling and to appropriate rewarming before separation from bypass. Because it is not practical to measure brain temperature directly, surrogate measuring sites are used. The tympanic membrane, nasopharyngeal, and rectum have been used; the nasopharyngeal site most closely matches true brain temperature and is the site at which temperature is most often monitored. The tympanic and rectal sites tend to overestimate the brain temperature.[56,57] Measurement of skin temperature gives an indication about peripheral perfusion and provides information about adequate peripheral rewarming.

After induction of anesthesia, an arterial catheter should be placed in children who will undergo CPB. The radial artery may be percutaneously cannulated with relative ease, even in infants. In small infants, the femoral arteries are frequently used for arterial access, and the axillary arteries are commonly used. The brachial artery is avoided because it is an end artery. Catheters placed in the dorsalis pedis or posterior tibial artery often provide inaccurate hemodynamic data, especially after separation from bypass, and it may become difficult to sample blood for laboratory testing. In the rare circumstance that peripheral arterial cannulation cannot be accomplished, the surgeon may place a catheter in the internal mammary artery after sternotomy, and a sterile monitoring line may be passed over the drapes. Ultrasound guidance often is used for insertion of arterial catheters.

Central venous lines can be very useful. For cardiac surgical procedures, there are two commonly used methods of obtaining central access. The decision of which to use may be determined in part by institutional bias. In the first method, the cardiac surgeons expose the heart quickly and have it available for inspection and estimation of filling pressures. Central lines can be readily established from the field and handed off to the anesthesia team. These transthoracic central lines are useful but carry a small amount of risk.[28] In the second method, percutaneous insertion of central venous lines is particularly indicated for long, complex procedures, especially when access to the infant is limited or the heart is not exposed. Percutaneous cannulation of the central circulation through the internal jugular approach or the subclavian approach has been demonstrated to be safe.[29] However, it is important to appreciate that insertion of central venous lines through the internal jugular or subclavian route may fail or may be associated with pneumothorax, hemorrhage, and hematoma formation after puncture of major arteries.[29-31] Cannulation of the external jugular vein may avoid some of these serious complications when the catheter can be successfully threaded into the central circulation.[32] Increasingly, ultrasound-guided techniques are being employed to establish central venous access (see Chapter 48). In the United Kingdom, the use of ultrasound for the placement of these lines is recommended by the National Institute of Clinical Excellence (NICE), and ultrasound is used routinely for the placement of central lines.

In children with unrestrictive VSDs or ASDs, including hearts with a single ventricle or single atrium, central venous pressure is equivalent to left ventricular filling pressure. Cannulation of vessels that drain into the SVC should be approached with caution in children with univentricular anatomy who may undergo the Fontan procedure, because thrombosis of the SVC can be a devastating complication. In such circumstances, the femoral veins may be the preferred sites for venous pressure monitoring.

Pulmonary arterial catheters in children with intracardiac defects usually provide little more information than a simple central line, are difficult to insert without fluoroscopy, and may not provide meaningful measurements of cardiac output. As a result, they are rarely used in pediatric cardiac patients.

### Transesophageal Echocardiography

Use of perioperative echocardiography has become the standard of care in the United States.[58,59] In adult practice, anesthesiologists usually perform the TEE, but in children, the TEE is more commonly performed by a pediatric cardiologist. This may reflect the increased complexity of congenital lesions and the difficulty in accurately assessing these lesions and their repairs. TEE has been cost-effective when used routinely during pediatric cardiac surgery.[60] The use of TEE can have a significant impact on surgical and medical management. In one large study, a second bypass run was undertaken in 7.3% of cases based on the findings of the TEE. There was a surgical alteration in the management of 12.7% and medical alteration in 18.5% of cases. Pediatric cardiac anesthesiologists usually can perform TEE before and after bypass if they have received adequate training.[61]

The introduction of small probes with multiplane capability has greatly increased the use of TEE, even in infants and neonates.[62,63] In 1999, a survey of centers in the United States indicated that 93% used intraoperative echocardiography and that all but one used TEE.[64] The American Society of Echocardiography and the Society of Cardiovascular anesthesiologists have published guidelines for performing a comprehensive intraoperative TEE in adults[65] and children.[66]

Although the use of TEE in children usually is safe, complications do occur and may be more common in small infants.[67] Complications include damage to the mouth, oropharynx, esophagus, and stomach. Other complications include hemodynamic disturbance as a result of compression of the left atrium or other structures. Interference with the airway also occurs in a small number of cases. This includes inadvertent extubation, right main-stem intubation, and compression of the tracheal tube. However, the overall incidence is small, approximately 2%.[68] Information gathered from the TEE examination takes place before and after bypass and may be divided broadly into two categories: hemodynamic assessment with monitoring and structural diagnostic information. Hemodynamic information includes information about ventricular function and filling.[69] Diagnostic information relates to confirmation or otherwise of preoperative findings and assessment of the adequacy of the surgical repair.

### Near-Infrared Spectroscopy

Cerebral near-infrared spectroscopy (NIRS) is becoming widely used during cardiopulmonary bypass in children. This noninvasive monitor is used to determine the degree of brain tissue oxygenation.[70,71] It is likely to lead to improved neurological outcomes after cardiac surgery although there is no clear evidence in humans (see Chapter 51).

### INDUCTION OF ANESTHESIA

In the United Kingdom, induction of anesthesia takes place in an anesthesia room, which is immediately adjacent to the operating room, and the parents are almost always present for induction. Anesthesia is commonly induced while the child is sitting with or being held by a parent. It is possible to involve some parents to the extent that they can hold the mask for the child as he or she is anesthetized. After the child is asleep, he or she is transferred to the anesthetic trolley, where venous and arterial access is secured and the trachea is intubated. This practice differs from most centers in North America, where induction of anesthesia occurs in the operating room.

Induction can be achieved using an intravenous or inhalational technique. Ketamine may be given intramuscularly or orally when intravenous access is difficult and mask induction is refused. The type of induction should be tailored to the child and the cardiac defect. If intravenous access has already been established, an intravenous induction is preferred. If intravenous access has not been achieved, a decision is made about the optimal induction technique. In severely ill children, it is advisable to obtain intravenous access before induction of anesthesia. The use of local anesthetic cream such as EMLA or Ametop Gel helps to reduce the pain of injection. Use of local anesthetic cream is also helpful if an inhalational induction is to be used because it allows insertion of an intravenous cannula during a much lighter plane of anesthesia. This requires that the appropriate veins are selected during the preoperative visit and that clear instructions are given to nursing staff about where the cream should be applied.

The most common inhalational induction agent is sevoflurane. Sevoflurane is very rapid acting and should be used with care in the child with CHD because high concentrations can produce bradycardia, hypotension, and apnea if not titrated carefully. Concentrations should be rapidly reduced after an adequate level of anesthesia is achieved. In children who are cyanotic with a right-to-left shunt and reduced pulmonary blood flow, inhalational inductions are slow. The addition of nitrous oxide can aid an inhalational induction in two ways. First, because it is odorless, it can be started before the introduction of the sevoflurane, allowing the child to be somewhat sedated before the stronger smelling agent is started. Second, it allows a smoother and more rapid induction compared with sevoflurane alone. Concentrations of up to 70% nitrous oxide can be used to smooth induction of anesthesia even in cyanotic children, but the nitrous oxide should be replaced with air and oxygen or 100% oxygen as soon as intravenous access is obtained and a muscle relaxant is given. It is not always necessary to use a mask for an inhalational induction because cupped hands are often more acceptable to the child, particularly one who is frightened of the mask. It is important to tell the child about each event before it happens and to demonstrate the action on yourself, a parent, or toy animal. You should also offer the child the opportunity to hold the mask, or if the child is accompanied by a parent, offer the child the choice of the parent holding the mask. Good premedication often aids this process (see Chapter 4).

For sick children in whom it may be preferable to use an intravenous induction, various options are available. For example, in neonates with coarctation of the aorta or with hypoplastic left heart syndrome who are not ventilated before coming to the operating room, one approach is to administer fentanyl in a dose of 2 to 3 µg/kg, followed by pancuronium and then by a very low dose (i.e., sedative dose) of sevoflurane or isoflurane. Fentanyl obtunds the hypertensive response to intubation, and the pancuronium maintains cardiac output by maintaining the heart rate. The very-low-dose volatile agent provides the sedation or anesthesia. In older children, etomidate is a very good induction agent, providing stable hemodynamics, although it does cause pain on injection. Ketamine is also widely used for intravenous induction in neonates and older children. Ketamine maintains or increases blood pressure, heart rate, and cardiac output. The exact mechanism of these effects of ketamine is unknown; ketamine may stimulate the release of endogenous stores of catecholamines, although it is a negative inotrope in the denervated heart.[72] This negative inotropic effect may make ketamine a poor choice in children in whom catecholamine stimulation may already be maximal, such as in severe cardiomyopathy. It may also be a poor choice if tachycardia is undesirable, such as in the case of aortic stenosis.

Monitoring should ideally be applied before induction begins, but applying monitoring can upset the child, which can be detrimental (e.g., the child with TOF who begins to cry and precipitates a "tet spell"). A pulse oximeter probe may be the only monitor that is applied before induction of anesthesia. Sevoflurane or isoflurane may provide another advantage by offering a degree of ischemic preconditioning to the heart and to other organs, particularly the brain and kidney. In a double-blind study of adult patients undergoing coronary bypass grafting, exposure to 4% sevoflurane for 10 minutes before cross-clamping reduced the degree of myocardial dysfunction and renal damage postoperatively.[73] It is thought that the same effect is observed in children.[74]

## MAINTENANCE OF ANESTHESIA

Maintenance of anesthesia in children with CHD depends on the preoperative status and the response to induction of anesthesia. Whether inhalational agents, additional opioids, or other intravenous agents are used for maintenance depends on the tolerance of the child and postoperative plans for ventilation. If a primary opioid-based anesthetic is chosen, additional opioid should be administered on initiation of CPB to offset dilution from the pump prime and to maintain adequate opioid plasma concentrations. Awareness during adult cardiac surgery has been reported when amnestic agents are not used. Although small children may be unable to describe such events, the potential for awareness during pediatric cardiac surgery should not be underestimated. To prevent awareness, isoflurane may be administered through the membrane oxygenator with an anesthetic vaporizer or intravenous midazolam (0.2 mg/kg) may be administered. Alternatively propofol may be given by infusion during the bypass period to reduce the possibility of awareness.

## INSTITUTION AND SEPARATION FROM BYPASS

Before initiation of CPB, the surgeon requests heparin to be given. After administration of heparin (preferably flushed through a central venous catheter) but *before the initiation of bypass*, the ACT should be determined. The ACT measurement should be at least three times greater than the baseline value. When bypass is started, any additional anesthetic drugs should be administered, and ventilation should cease. Both hypertension and hypotension may complicate bypass. Blood pressure may be controlled within the normal range using α-adrenergic blockers or agonists such as phenylephrine and phentolamine. The child is usually cooled at this stage, using the nasopharyngeal temperature as a guide. If the heart is to be stopped, cardioplegia is given by the perfusionist after the aorta is cross-clamped to provide myocardial protection during the period of ischemia. Cardioplegia is usually repeated every 20 to 30 minutes, although it is not required if the surgery is performed while the heart is beating.

Myocardial damage is related to the duration of the aortic cross-clamping and the effectiveness of the myocardial protection.

At an appropriate time during the surgery, the cross-clamp is removed, and perfusion to the heart is restored. The heart usually starts to beat in normal sinus rhythm, although this is not always the case. In the early phase of reperfusion, it is possible for various degrees of heart block to occur. However, these effects are usually short-lived, and as the effects of cardioplegia wear off, normal sinus rhythm is usually restored. In addition, heart block may result from damage to the conducting system during surgery.

After release of the cross-clamp, any inotropes or vasodilators that are required are usually started. Rewarming may have begun before release of the cross-clamp, but more commonly, the child is rewarmed after release of the clamp.

When the child has adequately rewarmed, as reflected by a normal core and minimal core-peripheral temperature difference, good heart function has returned, the child's lungs are adequately ventilated, and any inotropes required have been started, the child is ready to be separated from bypass. If a TEE probe is in place, the heart should be scanned for the presence of air. If air is present, further de-airing should occur before attempting to come off bypass. In the initial stages after separating from bypass, additional volume can be administered by the perfusionist through the aortic cannula, usually under the direction of the surgeon or anesthesiologist. Many centers institute modified ultrafiltration at this point. This involves taking arterial blood from the aortic cannula and passing it through the ultra-fine filter. This blood, which is oxygenated and warm, is then reinfused into the right atrium. When this process is complete, a thorough TEE examination can be undertaken.

When the team is satisfied with the TEE result, the surgeon asks for protamine to be administered. Before this is done, the perfusionist and the surgical team should be informed that protamine is about to be administered. The surgeons should remove any pump suckers from the field, and the perfusionist should stop all pump suction. This is done to ensure that no protamine enters the bypass circuit in case it is necessary to go back on bypass for any reason. The ACT can be checked along with the blood gas analysis. The ACT should return to levels before bypass. Any blood products required are usually given after the administration of protamine, usually while the surgeons are achieving hemostasis. As soon as the chest is closed, the child can then be transferred to the ICU.

# Control of Systemic and Pulmonary Vascular Resistance during Anesthesia

In some children with hypoplastic left heart syndrome (HLHS) who present for a Norwood procedure, excessive blood flow to the lungs resulting from a relatively low PVR and a relatively high SVR steals blood from the systemic circulation, leading to hypotension, myocardial ischemia, and progressive acidosis. However, when the reverse occurs and the PVR is greater than the SVR, the child develops progressive desaturation. Similar pathophysiology exists with other duct-dependent circulations and to some extent with other shunting lesions. It may prove difficult to manipulate the SVR and PVR predictably because control of PVR is poorly understood, vasoactive drugs usually are distributed on both sides of the circulation, and pharmacologic attempts to modify shunting have produced unpredictable results.[75] Despite these problems, several techniques have proved useful in manipulating the relative PVR and SVR. Potent inhalational anesthetics appear to reduce SVR more than PVR. PVR is decreased in children by increasing inspired oxygen to 100% and by hyperventilation to a pH of 7.6 or greater. Positive end-expiratory pressure, acidosis, hypothermia, and the use of 30% or less inspired oxygen can increase PVR. Because vasoconstrictors such as phenylephrine increase SVR more than PVR, they are effective acutely in reducing right-to-left shunting and increasing left-to-right shunting in the operating room.

During cardiac surgical procedures, a direct method of selectively increasing PVR or SVR is to have the surgeon place partially obstructing tourniquets around pulmonary arteries or the aorta to increase resistance so that flow to the opposite side of the circulation increases. Although these are only temporary measures, they may reestablish a better relative balance of resistances and a more normal physiology in a deteriorating clinical situation.

# Anesthetic Drugs Used in Pediatric Cardiac Anesthesia

## INHALATIONAL AGENTS

### Sevoflurane

Sevoflurane is the induction agent of choice in pediatric anesthesia.[76,77] It is associated with little myocardial depression or dysrhythmias.[78-80] It has specific advantages over halothane when used in children with CHD, particularly in children younger than 1 year of age and in cyanotic children.[81] In contrast to halothane, sevoflurane causes no reduction in heart rate at 1.0 and 1.5 minimal alveolar concentrations (MACs) in healthy children compared with awake values.[82] However, at greater concentrations, it can slow the heart rate and cause respiratory depression. Both features are important in children with CHD because a slow heart rate reduces cardiac output and hypoventilation leads to hypercarbia and hypoxia, which can increase PVR. In the absence of nitrous oxide, sevoflurane causes less depression of myocardial contractility than halothane during induction of anesthesia. Sevoflurane does cause a mild decrease in SVR, but in common with halothane and isoflurane, it does not perturb the shunt between the right and left sides of the heart through an ASD or VSD when it is given in anesthetic concentrations of about 1 MAC in 100% oxygen.[83] Sevoflurane has caused conduction abnormalities in susceptible patients.[84] It should also be used with great caution in children with severe ventricular outflow tract obstruction (see Chapter 6).[85]

### Isoflurane

At equipotent concentrations, isoflurane causes similar hemodynamic depression in neonates and infants compared with halothane. Isoflurane typically is not used for induction of anesthesia because of the high frequency of laryngospasm (greater than 20%).[86] Inadequate ventilation because of laryngospasm or other causes quickly leads to large increases in PVR due to hypoxemia and hypercarbia. This increase in PVR and the resulting pulmonary hypertension is poorly tolerated in small children with heart disease, especially in the presence of right-to-left shunting (see Chapter 6).

### Halothane

In the United States and the United Kingdom, the use of halothane has all but ceased, but it is still widely used in other parts of the world. It is included here for completeness. Uptake of halothane in infants younger than 3 months of age is more rapid than it is in adults. This also is the case for the uptake of halothane by the myocardium.[87] Although the effects of halothane on the human neonatal myocardium are unknown, young rodents have a reduced cardiovascular tolerance for halothane but require greater amounts for anesthesia.[88] Studies have shown a significant incidence of hypotension with bradycardia in infants with normal cardiovascular systems during induction with halothane.[89] During induction of anesthesia in normal infants, halothane decreases the cardiac index to 73% of awake values at 1.0 MAC and to 59% at 1.5 MAC.[90] The MAC for halothane in infants 1 to 6 months of age is the greatest of any age group.[91] This increased anesthetic requirement in infants, combined with the immaturity of their cardiovascular system, explains in part the relative cardiovascular intolerance of halothane by infants. Atropine has been used intramuscularly before induction to partially compensate for the myocardial depression of halothane by reducing bradycardia and hypotension. Although halothane may produce some degree of hypotension, an increase in arterial saturation in children with cyanotic CHD may occur.[92]

A careful induction with sevoflurane is usually well tolerated in children with mild to moderate heart disease. However, large concentrations of potent inhalational agents may be an unwise choice for induction in young infants with severe cardiac disease. In children of any age with marginal cardiovascular reserve and in those with severe desaturation of systemic arterial blood due to right-to-left shunting, inhalational anesthetic-induced myocardial depression and systemic hypotension are poorly tolerated. A more appropriate use of these anesthetic agents in children with severe heart disease is the addition of low concentrations of the inhalational agent to control hypertensive responses after an intravenous induction (see Chapter 6).

### Nitrous Oxide

Nitrous oxide should be avoided for maintenance of anesthesia in children with CHD because of the risk of enlarging intravascular air emboli and the potential to increase the PVR. Nitrous oxide may expand microbubbles and macrobubbles, increasing obstruction to blood flow in arteries and capillaries. In all children with right-to-left shunts, there is a potential for these bubbles to be shunted directly into the systemic circulation and coronaries. Care must be taken to ensure that no air bubbles are accidentally injected into the veins. Adverse outcomes after coronary air embolism are exacerbated by nitrous oxide.[93] The hemodynamic effects of venous air embolism are increased by nitrous oxide, even without paradoxical embolization.[94] In children with preexisting right-to-left shunts, paradoxical air embolism is clearly a potential problem; but even those with large left-to-right shunts can transiently reverse their shunts. This is particularly true during coughing or a Valsalva maneuver, when the normal transatrial pressure gradient is reversed. Several studies have demonstrated right-to-left shunting of microbubbles of air after injection of saline into the right atrium during these maneuvers.[95-97] Because coughing and Valsalva maneuvers may occur during anesthesia induction, even the most rigorous attention to avoiding air bubbles in intravenous lines may not prevent small amounts of air from reaching the systemic circulation. Microbubbles have also been observed after CPB.[98]

Nitrous oxide can increase PVR in adults.[99,100] However, in a 50% inspired concentration, it does not appear to affect PVR or pulmonary artery pressure in infants.[101] Nitrous oxide mildly decreases cardiac output at this concentration.[102] Avoidance of the use of nitrous oxide has been suggested in children with limited pulmonary blood flow, pulmonary hypertension, or depressed myocardial function. In the well-compensated child who does not require 100% inspired oxygen, nitrous oxide (usually at concentrations of 50%) may be used during induction of anesthesia but discontinued before tracheal intubation. If a reduced inspired oxygen concentration is indicated to maintain an appropriate balance between PVR and SVR after tracheal intubation, air may be added to the inspired gas mixture (see Chapter 6).

## INTRAVENOUS INDUCTION AGENTS

### Ketamine

Ketamine is a dissociative anesthetic agent that is a good analgesic. It increases blood pressure, heart rate, and cardiac output. Although the mechanism of the stimulation of blood pressure and heart rate has not been established, it is thought to stimulate the release of endogenous stores of catecholamines. Ketamine exerts a negative inotropic effect on the denervated heart.[103] I think that this combination of effects makes it a poor choice for children in whom sympathetic stimulation may already be maximal, such as in those with severe cardiomyopathy. It is also a poor choice if tachycardia is undesirable, such as in a child with aortic stenosis. Ketamine is thought to have minimal effect on PVR in children with CHD as long as the airway and ventilation are well preserved,[104,105] although it has occasionally increased PVR in children undergoing cardiac catheterization. Ketamine is quite a versatile anesthetic that may be administered intramuscularly and orally when intravenous access is difficult or an inhalational induction is contraindicated. The usual intravenous dose of 2 mg/kg produces a very predictable response, and an intramuscular dose of 8 to 10 mg/kg (combined with 0.1 mg/kg of intramuscular midazolam) is less predictable. The oral dose of ketamine is 5 to 6 mg/kg. The use of ketamine varies greatly from one institution to another, with some units using it extensively and others using it rarely (see Chapter 6).

### Etomidate

Etomidate is a very safe drug, with an $LD_{50}$ to $ED_{50}$ ratio of 26 in animals models.[106] This ratio indicates that the lethal dose (LD) is 26 times greater than the effective dose (ED). It is a short-acting anesthetic with little effect on systemic blood pressure, heart rate, and cardiac output after a single dose in healthy children.[107] Etomidate has a favorable hemodynamic profile even when used in shocked children and appears to have a low risk of clinically important myoclonus or status epilepticus, pain on intravenous injection, and nausea and vomiting.[108,109] The major concern about etomidate is the increased mortality rates reported when it is administered as a continuous infusion. This grave side effect has been attributed to adrenal suppression.[110-112] The inhibition of steroid synthesis occurs after a prolonged infusion and after a single dose of etomidate, and it has created a controversy about its use as an anesthetic agent, particularly in the ICUs in some jurisdictions.[113] However, newer analogues of etomidate have addressed these deficiencies and may lead to a surge in its use in the future (see Chapter 6).

### Propofol

Propofol is a rapidly acting intravenous hypnotic agent that may be administered as a single dose or by continuous infusion. It has no analgesic properties. Propofol has mild antiemetic

properties.[114] Its short duration of action is the result of rapid redistribution and metabolism, which also allows the drug to be given by continuous infusion without accumulation. Induction doses decrease SVR, blood pressure, and cardiac output; the effect on heart rate varies. The $ED_{50}$ for propofol in infants and small children is greater than it is in adults.[110-117] If propofol is given very slowly, smaller doses are required to achieve the anesthetic state, although the induction time increases. A slower infusion also results in more stable hemodynamics.[118] Pain on injection and involuntary movement after intravenous propofol have been concerns that have been overcome (see Chapter 6). Although propofol can be used safely in children with CHD, it is typically avoided as an induction agent in those with severe CHD because of its effects on SVR and blood pressure. It should be avoided in those with a fixed cardiac output such as severe aortic or mitral stenosis because it may cause severe hypotension. It can be used by infusion during CPB to reduce awareness and may be particularly useful if an early extubation is planned (see Chapter 6).

## OPIOIDS

### Fentanyl

As in adults with severe cardiac disease, intravenous fentanyl combined with pancuronium and 100% oxygen or air and oxygen provides an excellent induction technique in very sick children with CHD, although it is not an amnestic. Inclusion of intravenous midazolam or another amnestic agent is strongly urged to avoid awareness. In neonates and infants, the use of high-dose opioid anesthesia provides excellent hemodynamic stability, with suppression of the hormonal and metabolic stress response.[119,120] When fentanyl or other opioids are combined with nitrous oxide, the negative inotropic effects of nitrous oxide may be evident, particularly in sicker children.[121] The high-dose fentanyl technique is effective in preterm neonates undergoing ligation of a PDA.[122] In high-risk, full-term neonates and in older infants with severe CHD, the high-dose fentanyl technique in doses of up to 75 μg/kg, combined with pancuronium maintains stable hemodynamics during induction, tracheal intubation, and surgical incision.[123] Oxygen saturation is well maintained and often improves during induction, even in cyanotic children.[124] The cardiac index, SVR, and PVR in infants given 25 μg/kg of fentanyl do not change significantly.[125] Combining pancuronium with fentanyl is desirable because the vagolytic effects of pancuronium offset the potential vagotonic effects of fentanyl. The hemodynamic stability reported in infants with the combination of high-dose fentanyl and pancuronium may not be replicated when other muscle relaxants are used (see Chapter 6).[126]

### Sufentanil

Sufentanil (5 to 20 μg/kg), an alternative to fentanyl, is 5 to 10 times more potent than fentanyl but has a large margin of safety.[127] It is highly lipophilic and is rapidly distributed to all tissues. It is infrequently used in infants and children with CHD.

### Remifentanil

Remifentanil is an ultra-short-acting opioid that is rapidly metabolized in the plasma and tissue by nonspecific esterases to an inactive metabolite. It has a very brief elimination half-life, with a context-sensitive half-life of only 3 minutes, independent of the duration of infusion. In pediatric cardiac surgery, it is an attractive alternative to fentanyl that provides intense analgesia during the most stimulating parts of surgery but facilitates rapid awakening and weaning from mechanical ventilation without residual opioid effect. Its pharmacodynamics are unaffected by CPB.[128] It provides stable hemodynamic conditions in children, although there is a tendency toward bradycardia and systemic hypotension.[129-131] It has no negative inotropic effect, even in the failing heart.[132]

A significant concern is the development of acute tolerance with increasing analgesic requirements after discontinuing remifentanil.[133-135] Some studies have suggested that this is not clinically important.[136] Strategies to prevent tolerance to remifentanil have included intravenous magnesium infusions as well as nitrous oxide.[137,138] Remifentanil is also used for prolonged sedation of children in the ICU. Many units have moved toward early extubation and discharge from the ICU after cardiac surgery (i.e., fast tracking), and remifentanil is a useful drug in this setting (see Chapter 6). Consideration must be given to transitioning to a longer-acting opioid before discontinuation of remifentanil.

### NEUROMUSCULAR BLOCKING DRUGS

Pancuronium has been studied in depth in children with CHD. When administered over a 60- to 90-second interval, pancuronium maintains heart rate and blood pressure.[140] An intubating bolus dose of pancuronium may produce tachycardia and increase cardiac output. This bolus dose effect is sometimes desirable to support cardiac output in infants in congestive heart failure because their stroke volume is fixed. Pancuronium may be the muscle relaxant of choice when high-dose opioid techniques are used to offset the vagotonic effects of opioids such as fentanyl. Other muscle relaxants are also widely used, particularly if they are to be extubated in the operating room or early in the ICU.

### LONG-TERM NEUROCOGNITIVE-DEVELOPMENTAL OUTCOMES ASSOCIATED WITH ANESTHESIA

Concerns have been raised about the possibility that many of the anesthetic agents such as inhalational anesthetics, propofol, ketamine, and midazolam may cause long-term neurocognitive-developmental problems in neonates and young infants.[139] This effect is thought to result from the neuronal apoptosis caused by these agents. The opioids have not been implicated in these changes, but this may change in time. There is no evidence to directly link anesthetic exposure in infancy to long-term neurocognitive defects. There is much ongoing research in this area (see Chapter 23).

## Regional Anesthesia

The use of regional anesthesia to provide pain relief during and after cardiac surgery in adults also reduces the stress response to surgery and may reduce morbidity and mortality. In adults undergoing cardiac surgery, the benefits of regional anesthesia include earlier extubation, fewer respiratory complications, a reduction in renal failure, fewer strokes, and less myocardial damage after CPB.[141-143] In animals, thoracic epidural anesthesia reduces myocardial damage after coronary occlusion.[144] The same benefits may be achieved by using intrathecal (spinal) analgesia. High spinal anesthesia using bupivacaine reduces the stress response to CPB and β-adrenergic dysfunction and improves cardiac performance after cardiac surgery in adults.[145]

Good research into regional anesthesia and analgesia in pediatric cardiac surgery is limited. Caudal morphine has been used to provide postoperative analgesia and has produced good analgesia for about 6 hours while reducing analgesic requirements for up to 24 hours.[146] Two retrospective studies in children[147,148] included a variety of regional anesthetic techniques. Most children were extubated in the operating room, although ~4% of them required reintubation within 24 hours. Adverse effects included emesis (39%), pruritus (10%), urinary retention (7%), postoperative transient paresthesia (3%), and respiratory depression (1.8%). The rate of adverse effects was less with a thoracic catheter epidural approach compared with various caudal, lumbar epidural, and spinal approaches. Hospital duration of stay was unaffected by the presence of regional anesthesia complications. Although this study appears to indicate that regional analgesia is safe, the numbers in the study are too small to conclude that regional analgesia is safe for pediatric cardiac surgery.

The use of regional anesthesia in cardiac surgery for children remains controversial.[149,150] The main concern is the risk of bleeding and the potential for disastrous neurologic complications. The risks may be greater in children than in adults because of the presence of collateral vessels, increased venous pressure, coagulopathy related to cyanosis, and the use of aspirin. There remain many unanswered questions regarding neuraxial block in children, such as the true incidence of epidural hematoma, the time delay required between placement of the epidural catheter and full anticoagulation, and the correct management of a bloody tap. The estimated risk of epidural hematoma during cardiac surgery in adults is 1 case per 1000 patients and 1 case per 2400 patients for spinal and epidural block, respectively.[151] Whether the risks are similar or greater in children cannot be determined because, the numbers of children involved in studies are too small. A large, randomized, prospective study to evaluate a true risk-benefit ratio without bias is needed; until such data are available, various commentators have advised great caution with the use of regional analgesia for cardiac surgery, and some have suggested that it may not be possible to perform the study required because of ethical considerations.[152]

## Fast Tracking

Fast tracking refers to abbreviating the perioperative period of children undergoing cardiac surgery. It should include every phase of the child's journey from referral and preoperative evaluation to less invasive surgery, early weaning from respiratory support, extubation, and discharge from the ICU and hospital.

Early extubation of pediatric patients after cardiac surgery offers advantages in terms of cost and reduced morbidity associated with longer ICU stays.[153-157] The success of this approach depends on the close teamwork of a multidisciplinary team, with every member of the team working toward the same goal. Successful fast tracking usually requires the development of care pathways to ensure that the quality of patient care is not compromised.[158] Early extubation and discharge from the ICU requires preplanning and the adoption of a technique that facilitates this goal. The use of very large doses of fentanyl is not appropriate; alternative techniques have been used, including smaller doses of fentanyl in combination with inhalational agents[159,160] or the use of remifentanil in combination with inhalational agents or with propofol. Others have advocated regional anesthesia as a means of speeding extubation, but this approach remains controversial. It is important to choose a neuromuscular blocking drug with a shorter duration of action than pancuronium to ensure that it is easy to reverse the neuromuscular block at the end of surgery. Other important considerations to ensure that early extubation is a success include adequate pain relief in the form of intravenous paracetamol (where available), patient-controlled or nurse-controlled analgesia, and antiemetics because nausea appears to be more of a problem in children who are extubated early.

Some clinicians advocate extubating the trachea in the operating room, whereas others advocate waiting until the child is in the ICU. Delaying the extubation until the child is in the ICU may save operating room time and may reduce the risks of cardiovascular instability, bleeding, and hypothermia.[161] Despite these concerns, the tracheas of many children are extubated in the operating room with good outcomes.

## Cardiopulmonary Bypass

Cardiopulmonary bypass is discussed in Chapter 17.

## Stress Response to Cardiac Surgery

Cardiac surgery and CPB are altered physiologic conditions associated with exaggerated stress responses characterized by the release of numerous metabolic and hormonal substances, including catecholamines, cortisol, growth hormone, prostaglandins, complement, glucose, insulin, and β-endorphins.[162,163] The cause of the elaboration of these substances is multifactorial: contact of blood with foreign surfaces, low perfusion pressure, anemia, hypothermia, myocardial ischemia, low levels of anesthesia, and nonpulsatile flow. Other factors that contribute to the increase in stress hormones are delayed renal and hepatic clearance and exclusion of the pulmonary circulation during extracorporeal circulation.[164]

Neonates of all viable gestational ages, older infants, and children have nociceptive systems that are sufficiently developed and integrated with brainstem cardiovascular control centers to trigger humoral and circulatory responses to pain and stress.[165] Substantial humoral, metabolic, and cardiovascular responses to painful and stressful stimulation during surgery have been documented in neonates of all gestational ages and in older infants.[166,167] Hormonal stress responses in neonates subjected to cardiac and noncardiac operations are threefold to fivefold greater than those in adults after similar surgeries. Circulatory responses to stressful stimuli in children include systemic and pulmonary hypertension.

Humoral stress responses are particularly extreme during and after cardiac surgery. These responses are characterized by increases in circulating catecholamines, glucagon, cortisol, β-endorphins, growth hormone, and insulin; circulating concentrations of catecholamines may increase by as much as 400% over baseline preoperative concentrations. This is evidence of a massive activation of sympathetic outflow in response to surgical stimulation. Some of these responses may continue for several days postoperatively.[168]

It has been suggested that such extreme stress responses and neuroendocrine activation may be associated with greater morbidity and mortality. In adults, intraoperative adrenergic activation of 50% above baseline is associated with significant postoperative alterations in β-adrenergic receptor function, including increased β-receptor density and decreased receptor affinity. Mortality among adults with severe congestive failure

is associated with increased levels of hormones regulating cardiovascular function, including aldosterone, epinephrine, and norepinephrine.[169] In neonates undergoing cardiac surgery, increased concentrations of stress hormones may be associated with increased mortality rates.[168]

The metabolic response to stress in children includes increased oxygen consumption, glycogenolysis, gluconeogenesis, and lipolysis. These metabolic responses cause substantial intraoperative and postoperative catabolism. The metabolic responses are usually related to changes in plasma cortisol, catecholamines, and other counterregulatory hormones such as glucagon and growth hormone. The most prominent clinical effects that result from activation of these processes are perioperative hypoglycemia and hyperglycemia, lactic acidemia, and negative nitrogen balance extending well into the postoperative period. Neonates and infants tolerate such metabolic derangements poorly. Their impaired tolerance is the result of a relative lack of endogenous reserves of carbohydrates, proteins, and fats; the large metabolic cost of rapid growth; a high obligate requirement for glucose by the relatively large brain; the immature hormonal control of intermediary metabolism; and the limited functional capabilities of immature enzyme systems in the metabolic organs. Severe stress responses superimposed on the normal neonatal and infant physiology may be poorly tolerated. However, it remains unclear whether these metabolic alterations may provide some beneficial effects for mobilizing the bodily resources to provide a metabolic milieu for healing tissues or they are purely maladaptive, resulting in detrimental effects on postoperative outcome.

Another factor is the potential effect of stress-induced hyperglycemia on the neurologic outcome. Neonates and young infants are capable of substantial rates of glucose production, mainly from glycogenolysis and gluconeogenesis during surgical stress that can result in hyperglycemia. Such hyperglycemic responses may be associated with poorer neurologic outcomes, particularly after a period of cerebral ischemia.[170] The use of high doses of fentanyl (more than 50 µg/kg) has reduced the hormonal stress response and resultant hyperglycemia and may lessen the risk of neurologic injury.[171]

In sufficient doses, opioids can blunt the stress responses in neonates, infants, and adults.[172-174] This blunting results in a more normal, homeostatic humoral and metabolic milieu in the circulation by reducing neuroendocrine activation and levels of regulating hormones. In infants, the use of high-dose opioids for major surgical procedures and postoperative sedation substantially attenuates the neuroendocrine response to surgically induced pain and stress. Catecholamine release that results from intraoperative stress responses may predispose the vulnerable myocardium to dysrhythmias. In neonates with HLHS, sudden ventricular fibrillation occurred in 50% during surgical manipulation under halothane anesthesia. This incidence was dramatically reduced when high doses of fentanyl were introduced as the primary analgesic/sedative.[175] With the use of high-dose opioids, intraoperative ventricular fibrillation has virtually disappeared as a problem in this group of neonates.[176] In several studies, opioids have been shown to increase the ventricular fibrillation threshold in isolated cardiac Purkinje fibers and to alter action potential duration similar to that with class III antiarrhythmic agents.[177,178] Even electrophysiologic events in the neonatal heart, in addition to humoral and hemodynamic responses, may be altered by using high-dose fentanyl anesthesia to attenuate the effects of pain and stress.

## REDUCING THE STRESS RESPONSE TO SURGERY AND BYPASS

### Corticosteroids

Corticosteroids are used in many centers in an attempt to reduce the inflammatory response to surgery and bypass.[179] However, there is a huge variability in the formulation of the corticosteroids used, the doses, the timing of administration, and the indications for their use. The literature lacks adequate evidence for the use of corticosteroids, although several small studies in humans and animals suggest they confer a benefit.[180,181] Many investigators have called for a large multicenter study to determine the benefit of corticosteroids before bypass and the optimal dose and timing.[182]

### Aprotinin

Aprotinin, which was originally used to reduce bleeding after CPB, is now also appreciated to confer significant antiinflammatory effects.[183-187] In adults, it reduces mortality and length of ICU stay.[188] In children, it improves pulmonary function in the postoperative period and reduces the time to extubation and ICU stay. However, aprotinin is no longer available for routine use in the United States or continental Europe. In the United Kingdom, it is available for use on a named patient basis, but its use has been dramatically reduced as a result.

### Allopurinol

Allopurinol is thought to provide protection against oxygen free radicals during reperfusion by inhibiting xanthine oxidase. It reduces oxygen free radical production and may reduce neurologic and cardiac damage after deep hypothermic cardiac arrest.[189] This strategy does not appear to have developed widespread use.

### Ischemic Preconditioning

The heart is capable of short-term rapid adaptation to brief ischemia such that during a subsequent, more severe ischemic insult, myocardial necrosis is delayed. The infarct-delaying properties of ischemic preconditioning have been observed in all species studied. Five minutes of ischemia is sufficient to initiate preconditioning, and the protective period lasts for 1 to 2 hours. Laboratory experiments have demonstrated that the stimulation of adenosine receptors initiates preconditioning and the intracellular signal transduction mechanisms involve protein kinase C and adenosine triphosphate (ATP)-dependent potassium channels, although there may be some differences between species. An analysis of studies of myocardial infarction in humans has demonstrated that some adults who report having had angina in the days before infarction have a better outcome after their infarction in part due to the ischemic preconditioning. More direct evidence has come from an investigation of adults undergoing percutaneous transluminal angioplasty in whom the ST-segment changes induced by balloon inflation were more marked during the first inflation than the second. In adults undergoing coronary artery bypass grafting, the decline in ATP content during the first 10 minutes of ischemia was reduced in those subjected to a brief preconditioning protocol.[190-194]

It may be possible to protect organs other than the heart by ischemic preconditioning. It may even be possible to protect organs remotely by producing a period of ischemia in one area such as a limb, which then confers protection to remote organs.[195]

Cheung and coworkers have demonstrated that the use of a blood pressure cuff to produce short periods of limb ischemia can produce beneficial effects on the heart, lungs, and generalized inflammatory response.[196]

### Glucose-Insulin and Potassium

The use of glucose-insulin and potassium has been advocated for more than 40 years in adult cardiac surgery. It is thought to protect the myocardium from the effects of ischemia caused by aortic cross-clamping.[197-200] Its effects have not been studied in children undergoing cardiac surgery.

# Anesthesia Considerations for Specific Cardiac Defects

Discussion of anesthesia considerations for repair of every form of CHD is beyond the scope of this chapter. However, a brief discussion of the problems that may be encountered during repair of the more common congenital heart lesions is presented. It is useful to group lesions together because the management principles can be applied more generally within groups (Table 15-2).

## SIMPLE LEFT-TO-RIGHT SHUNTS

Simple left-to-right shunts increase pulmonary blood flow. If the shunt is large, blood flow to the lungs can be as much as threefold to fourfold greater than normal, resulting in volume loading of the right heart. This can lead to right atrial enlargement and right

| TABLE 15-2  Classification of Congenital Heart Disease |
| --- |
| **Simple Left-to-Right Shunt: Increased Pulmonary Blood Flow** |
| Atrial septal defect (ASD) |
| Ventricular septal defect (VSD) |
| Patent ductus arteriosus (PDA) |
| Endocardial cushion defect (e.g., atrioventricular septal defect [AVSD]) |
| Aortopulmonary window (AP window) |
| **Simple Right-to-Left Shunt: Decreased Pulmonary Blood Flow with Cyanosis** |
| Tetralogy of Fallot (TOF) |
| Pulmonary atresia |
| Tricuspid atresia |
| Ebstein anomaly |
| **Complex Shunts: Mixing of Pulmonary and Systemic Blood Flow with Cyanosis** |
| Transposition of the great arteries (TGA) |
| Truncus arteriosus |
| Total anomalous pulmonary venous connection (TAPVC) |
| Double-outlet right ventricle (DORV) |
| Hypoplastic left heart syndrome (HLHS) |
| **Obstructive Lesions** |
| Aortic stenosis |
| Mitral stenosis |
| Pulmonary stenosis |
| Coarctation of aorta |
| Interrupted aortic arch |

**TABLE 15-3** Clinical Features of Cardiac Failure in Children

| | |
|---|---|
| Failure to thrive | Cardiac murmur |
| Difficult feeding | Hepatomegaly |
| Breathlessness | Cardiomegaly |
| Recurrent chest infection | Pulmonary plethora |
| Tachycardia | Wheezing |

ventricular enlargement that is perhaps associated with tricuspid and pulmonary regurgitation. This combination results in cardiac failure (Table 15-3).

Medical management of these children is primarily achieved with diuretics. If pulmonary blood flow is large and left untreated, pulmonary vascular disease begins to develop, resulting in pulmonary hypertension. In the early stages, the changes are reversible, but in time, the changes may become irreversible.[201-206] Eisenmenger syndrome refers to severe pulmonary hypertension that leads to suprasystemic pulmonary artery pressures that cause the shunt to reverse, leading to cyanosis. The previous left-to-right shunt reverses to become a right-to-left shunt. At this point, the child's condition becomes inoperable.

Increasingly, definitive surgery is being performed at a younger age to reduce the risk of developing pulmonary vascular disease. If early definitive surgery is not possible, a pulmonary artery band is applied to reduce pulmonary blood flow. This is performed through a sternotomy incision but without the need for CPB. This provides the infant the opportunity to grow, postponing the need for definitive surgery without increasing the risk of developing pulmonary hypertension. In the presence of significantly increased pulmonary blood flow, pulmonary vascular disease is often severe and irreversible by 1 year of age. Definitive surgery should be performed between 3 and 6 months of age to avoid this complication.

### Atrial Septal Defect

ASD is a common heart defect in children, occurring in 1 of 1500 live births and accounting for approximately 10% of all CHD.[207] Several types of ASDs exist.

- Patent foramen ovale (PFO) is a normal fetal communication between the two atria that usually closes soon after birth. The PFO remains patent in up to 30% of people. PFO is usually left untreated in children.
- Primum ASD (Fig. 15-1, *A*) is located in the inferior part of the atrial septum close to the AV valve and may be associated with a cleft mitral valve. This is a variant of AV septal defect (AVSD).
- Secundum ASD (see Fig. 15-1, *B*) is found in the region of the fossa ovalis and results from a deficiency in the septum secundum.
- Sinus venosus ASD (see Fig. 15-1, *C*) occurs high in the atrial septum, often close to the opening of the SVC. It may be associated with partial anomalous pulmonary venous drainage.
- Coronary sinus ASD (i.e., unroofed coronary sinus) is a defect in the atrial wall allows blood to flow from the left atrium to right atrium through the coronary sinus.
- Common atrium has a complete absence of the atrial septum. The AV valves may be abnormal or unaffected.

Many ASDs can be closed using a percutaneous, transcatheter device. PFO and secundum ASDs are most commonly closed using this technique.

#### Anesthesia Considerations

- These children can frequently be extubated on the operating table or early in the ICU, and smaller doses of opioids can be used. Alternatively, short-acting drugs (e.g., remifentanil) administered by infusion and possibly in combination with propofol are useful if early extubation is planned.
- The problems of postoperative pulmonary hypertension are seldom encountered.

### Ventricular Septal Defect

VSD is the most common congenital defect in children, occurring in 1.5 to 3.5 of 1000 live births and accounting for 20% of CHD (Fig. 15-2, *A*).[208] Four types are described: subarterial (5%), perimembranous (80%), inlet (5%), and muscular (10%). If the flow through the VSD is small, it is referred to as *restrictive*, but if the flow is large, it is called *unrestrictive*. It is possible to close a small percent of VSDs using a percutaneous, transcatheter device.

#### Anesthesia Considerations

- Inotropic support may be required postoperatively.
- Postoperative pulmonary hypertension may be a problem if the left-to-right shunt has been significant preoperatively or if the surgery is undertaken late.

### Atrioventricular Septal Defect

AVSDs are also known as AV canal defects or endocardial cushion defects, and they result from a defect in the AV septum. The incidence is about 0.2 cases per 1000 live births, and they account for about 3% of CHD. They are commonly associated with trisomy 21, TOF, and DiGeorge syndrome (Table 15-4). Two common types of AVSD exist:

- Partial AVSD usually consists of a primum ASD with a cleft in the anterior mitral valve leaflet (see Fig. 15-1, *A*).
- Complete AVSD consists of a large septal defect with atrial and ventricular components and a common AV valve (see Fig. 15-2, *B*).

Other descriptions of AVSD refer to balanced or unbalanced conditions, depending on whether the AV valve is stenotic or atretic or some of the valve chordae are straddling (i.e., crossing to the other side of the ventricular septum). The hemodynamic effects associated with AVSD include shunting at the atrial or ventricular level and AV valve regurgitation.

#### Anesthesia Considerations

- If the child has trisomy 21, the anesthesia implications need to be managed.
- Inotropes are frequently required.
- Postoperative pulmonary hypertension may occur.
- TEE is particularly helpful in assessing the repair of the left AV valve.
- Heart block may occur postoperatively.

### Aortopulmonary Window

Aortopulmonary window is a rare CHD defect in which there is a communication between the main pulmonary artery and the ascending aorta, and it accounts for 0.1% of CHD (Fig. 15-3). Four types are classified according to the size and exact position

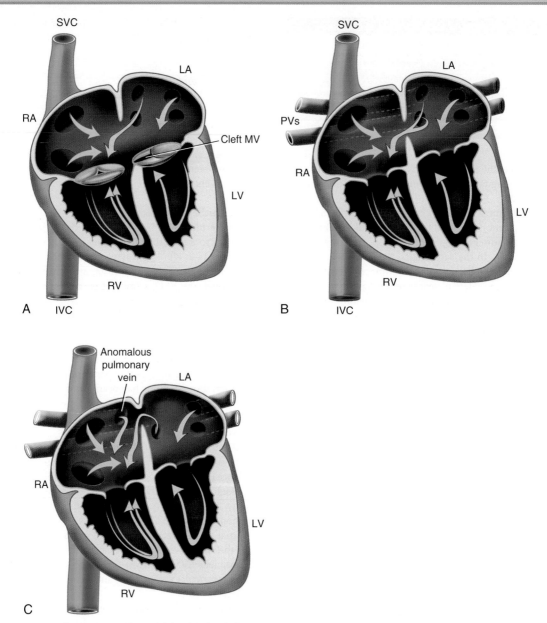

**FIGURE 15-1 A,** Diagram of a primum atrial septal defect (ASD) with the great vessels removed to show the left-to-right shunt through the defect and a cleft of the mitral valve (*MV*), also called a partial atrioventricular septal defect (*AVSD*). **B,** Diagram of a secundum ASD with the great vessels removed to show the left-to-right shunt through the defect. **C,** Diagram of a sinus venosus ASD shows the left-to-right shunt through the defect close to the superior vena cava (*SVC*) and an anomalous pulmonary vein (*PV*) draining to the right atrium (*RA*). *IVC,* Inferior vena cava; *LA,* left atrium; *LV,* left ventricle; *RV,* right ventricle. (Modified from May LE. Pediatric heart surgery: a ready reference for professionals. Milwaukee: Maxishare; 2005.)

of the defect.[209] A left-to-right shunt is usually present. These children present with heart failure and are at risk for pulmonary vascular disease if not treated early. It is frequently associated with other cardiac and noncardiac anomalies:

- VACTERL: *v*ertebral anomalies, *a*nal atresia, *c*ardiac defect, *t*racheo*e*sophageal atresia, *r*enal anomalies, and *l*imb abnormalities
- CHARGE: *c*oloboma of the eye and central nervous system anomalies, *h*eart defects, *a*tresia of the choanae, *r*etardation of growth and development, *g*enital or urinary defects, and *e*ar anomalies
- CATCH-22 association (i.e., mnemonic for DiGeorge syndrome): *c*ardiac defect, *a*bnormal facies, *t*hymic hypoplasia,

*c*left palate, *h*ypocalcemia (velocardiofacial syndrome), with 22q11 chromosome microdeletion (see Table 15-4)

### *Anesthesia Considerations*
- Postoperative pulmonary hypertension may be problematic.
- Inotropes may be required.

### Patent Ductus Arteriosus
The ductus arteriosus, a remnant from the fetal circulation, extends from the descending aorta to the main pulmonary artery and usually closes soon after birth. However, it remains patent in approximately 1 of 2500 live births and accounts for about 10% of all CHD (Fig. 15-4). In the fetus, blood from the right

15

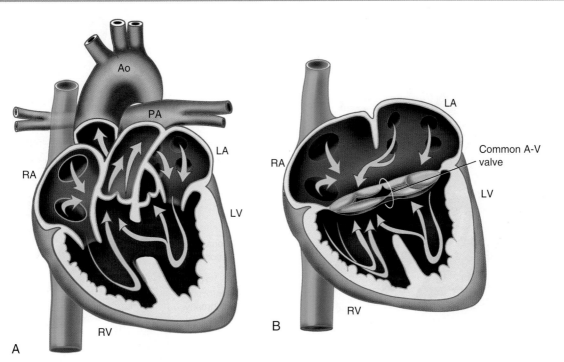

**FIGURE 15-2 A,** Diagram of a ventricular septal defect (VSD) shows a left-to-right shunt. **B,** Diagram of a complete atrioventricular septal defect (AVSD) with the great vessels removed to show the left-to-right shunt through both atrial and ventricular components of the defect and a single common atrioventricular (A-V) valve. *Ao,* Aorta; *LA,* left atrium; *LV,* left ventricle; *PA,* pulmonary artery; *RA,* right atrium; *RV,* right ventricle. (Modified from May LE. Pediatric heart surgery: a ready reference for professionals. Milwaukee: Maxishare; 2005.)

| **TABLE 15-4** | Clinical Features and Concerns of DiGeorge Syndrome |
|---|---|
| Absent or small thymus | |
| T-cell abnormality with associated immunodeficiency | |
| Hypoparathyroidism with associated hypocalcemia | |
| Dysmorphic features, particularly a small mouth | |
| Increased surgical morbidity and mortality | |
| Irradiated blood products needed to prevent graft-versus-host disease | |

ventricle is directed into the pulmonary artery, but because of the high PVR, it flows into the descending aorta. After birth, the PVR decreases, and blood flows from the aorta to the lungs. PDA is common in preterm infants, and its presence may explain an ongoing requirement for mechanical ventilation. In these infants, a left thoracotomy is required to ligate or divide the PDA. It may also occur in older children; but at this age, percutaneous closure by an interventional cardiologist is the preferred approach. The anesthesia implications are similar to those of other lesions described with left-to-right shunts preoperatively.

In many centers, PDA closure in preterm infants who weigh less than 1000 g and who are already mechanically ventilated is undertaken in the neonatal intensive care unit (NICU). This avoids the need to transfer these very small infants to the operating room and the associated problems, particularly hypothermia.

Preoperative requirements include the following:
- Crossmatched blood
- Antibiotics (risk of endocarditis)

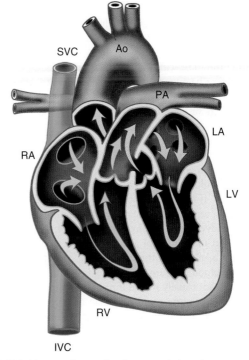
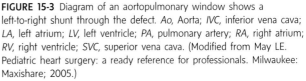

**FIGURE 15-3** Diagram of an aortopulmonary window shows a left-to-right shunt through the defect. *Ao,* Aorta; *IVC,* inferior vena cava; *LA,* left atrium; *LV,* left ventricle; *PA,* pulmonary artery; *RA,* right atrium; *RV,* right ventricle; *SVC,* superior vena cava. (Modified from May LE. Pediatric heart surgery: a ready reference for professionals. Milwaukee: Maxishare; 2005.)

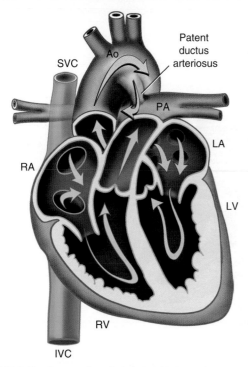

**FIGURE 15-4** The diagram of a patent ductus arteriosus shows a left-to-right shunt. *Ao*, Aorta, *IVC*, inferior vena cava; *LA*, left atrium; *LV*, left ventricle; *PA*, pulmonary artery; *RA*, right atrium; *RV*, right ventricle; *SVC*, superior vena cava. (Modified from May LE. Pediatric heart surgery: a ready reference for professionals. Milwaukee: Maxishare; 2005.)

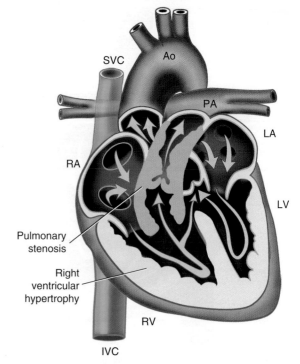

**FIGURE 15-5** The diagram shows the features of the tetralogy of Fallot: ventricular septal defect, overriding aorta, right ventricular hypertrophy, and pulmonary stenosis. Pulmonary and subpulmonary obstructions are shown. The result is right-to-left shunting leading to cyanosis. *Ao*, Aorta; *IVC*, inferior vena cava; *LA*, left atrium; *LV*, left ventricle; *PA*, pulmonary artery; *RA*, right atrium; *RV*, right ventricle; *SVC*, superior vena cava. (Modified from May LE. Pediatric heart surgery: a ready reference for professionals. Milwaukee: Maxishare; 2005.)

- Vitamin K
  Particular perioperative risks include the following:
- Difficulty ventilating or hemoglobin desaturation because of lung retraction
- Tearing the PDA with massive hemorrhage
- Inadvertent ligation of the aorta or pulmonary artery
- Endocarditis
- Paradoxical air embolism

### Monitoring
Monitoring includes the use of all standard monitors, including end-tidal carbon dioxide assessment, and two additional pulse oximeters should be placed, one on the right hand and one on a lower limb. If the pulse is lost from the lower limb during a test clamping of the duct, it may indicate that the aorta has been clamped inadvertently. At my institution, all the requirements are stipulated in a protocol and monitoring and other requirements are in place before the arrival of the operating room team.

Invasive blood pressure monitoring is helpful if already established but is not usually placed if not already in place. Monitors used in non–operating room sites may not be compatible with the electrocautery equipment, resulting in loss of monitoring whenever the cautery is used.

### Anesthesia Considerations
- A dedicated intravenous line for fluids and drugs with a long (100 to 150 cm), low-caliber extension to allow access from a distance (space around the cots in NICU is limited)
- High-dose opioids
- Muscle relaxation

- The tracheal tube should have only a small air leak. A large leak may prevent adequate ventilation during lung retraction (recheck security and correct position of the tip of the tube after repositioning in the decubitus position, before starting surgery).
- Intercostal nerve block by surgeon at the completion of surgery
- Glucose-containing fluids maintained at basal rates

## SIMPLE RIGHT-TO-LEFT SHUNTS
### Tetralogy of Fallot
TOF is the most common cyanotic CHD defect and accounts for 6% to 11% of CHD. It has four features (Fig. 15-5):
- VSD
- Overriding aorta
- Right ventricular outflow tract obstruction (RVOTO)
- Right ventricular hypertrophy

The RVOTO ranges from mild to severe, and the level of the obstruction also varies. Commonly, a dynamic subpulmonary infundibular obstruction is present. Dynamic narrowing of the infundibulum is frequently the cause of hypercyanotic episodes, also known as *tet spells*, in which there is an increase in the shunting of blood from right to left. However, the RVOTO may also be at the level of the pulmonary valve or main or branch pulmonary arteries. Pulmonary atresia may exist as a variant of TOF. Children with pulmonary atresia who have well-developed pulmonary arteries derive their pulmonary blood supply from a PDA, but those with hypoplastic pulmonary arteries derive their pulmonary blood supply from major aortopulmonary collateral arteries.

The right-to-left shunt and cyanosis observed in children with TOF results from a combination of the RVOTO and VSD. The degree of hypoxemia depends on the relationship between the RVOTO and the SVR that determines the degree of right-to-left shunting. TOF may be associated with a large number of other cardiac and extracardiac anomalies. Extracardiac anomalies include DiGeorge syndrome (see Table 15-4) and trisomy 21.

### Hypercyanotic Episodes

Hypercyanotic spells are episodes of cyanosis that occur in 20% to 70% of untreated children. They may be initiated by crying or feeding, and they may occur during anesthesia. The cause of these spells is unclear, but metabolic acidosis, increased $PaCO_2$, circulating catecholamines, and surgical stimulation have all been implicated.

Management of a tet spell requires urgent intervention. Early and aggressive use of a vasoconstrictor is essential. Phenylephrine should be premixed and in a syringe for immediate use in a concentration of 100 µg/mL. The initial dose is 0.5 to 1 µg/kg, which is repeated and doubled in 1-minute intervals until a satisfactory response is observed. Preterm infants may require as much as 30 µg/kg. Management may require any of the following:

- 100% oxygen
- Hyperventilation
- Intravenous fluid bolus
- Sedation or analgesia (e.g., fentanyl, morphine)
- Sodium bicarbonate
- Vasoconstriction
  - Norepinephrine is given as a 0.5-µg/kg bolus and then at a rate of 0.01 to 0.2 µg/kg/min.
  - Phenylephrine is given as a 0.5-µg/kg bolus and doubled at 1-minute intervals until a satisfactory response is achieved; this is followed by an infusion at 1 to 5 µg/kg/min (larger bolus doses may be required in small preterm infants).
- β-Blockers are administered to relax infundibular spasm and reduce the heart rate.
  - Propranolol is given as a 0.1- to 0.3-mg/kg bolus.

### Surgical Management

The optimal surgical management of children with TOF remains controversial. The choice is between initial palliation with a systemic-to-pulmonary shunt followed by a complete repair when the infant is older and complete repair during the neonatal or early infant period. The current trend is toward early complete repair.[210,211] Complete repair involves closure of the VSD and relief of the RVOTO. Relief of the RVOTO most commonly requires a transannular patch that involves a right ventriculotomy. Right ventricular dysfunction is a particular problem after repair, and a degree of pulmonary regurgitation is usually present if a transannular patch has been done. Junctional ectopic tachycardia (JET) is a particular risk after complete correction.

### Anesthesia Considerations

SYSTEMIC-TO-PULMONARY SHUNT. The systemic-to-pulmonary shunt typically is a modified Blalock-Taussig shunt. This is a shunt from the subclavian artery to a branch pulmonary artery.

- The patient is usually a neonate or small infant.
- Sedative premedication is useful to prevent crying during induction, which may provoke a hypercyanotic spell.
- There is a risk of a hypercyanotic spell during induction and surgery.
- Inhalational or intravenous induction is appropriate.
- Surgery is usually performed through a thoracotomy (left or right) but may be through a sternotomy.
- CPB is not usually required.
- Arterial and central venous access is required.
- Tracheal tube should be snug, with no or minimal air leak because lung retraction during surgery makes ventilation very difficult.
- The arterial line should not be in the arm on the side that the shunt will be placed because the subclavian artery will be clamped, and the arterial pressure will be lost.
- Hemodynamic and respiratory disturbance can be problematic during surgery.
- The surgeon may request a small dose of heparin.
- Bleeding may occur after clamps are released; be prepared for a blood transfusion.
- Postoperatively, the pulmonary blood supply predominantly depends on the size of the shunt. If the shunt is too small, the infant may have a low saturation level; if the shunt is too large, the infant may develop heart failure or pulmonary edema and hypotension.
- Pulmonary blood flow also depends on systemic blood pressure; the greater the blood pressure, the more blood flows to the lungs and the higher the saturation.
- Milrinone is often combined with norepinephrine because the norepinephrine increases the low diastolic pressure created by the shunt but does not produce the unwanted tachycardia seen with epinephrine.
- A period of postoperative ventilation may be required.

COMPLETE REPAIR. If the child is scheduled for early complete correction with no systemic pulmonary shunt, the child is likely to be a neonate or small infant. These children remain at risk for hypercyanotic spells. However, if the child has had a shunt placed previously, he or she is likely to be older and much less likely to have a hypercyanotic episode. Some children with less severe disease may not require a shunt and may be operated on when they are a bit older because they remain asymptomatic. Good sedative premedication is important in those at risk for hypercyanotic episodes.

- Both intravenous and inhalational induction agents are appropriate.
- CPB is required.
- Right ventricular dysfunction and pulmonary regurgitation may be postoperative problems.
- Too much of an inotrope may worsen RVOTO postoperatively by dynamic narrowing of the RVOT.
- Milrinone may be particularly useful because it promotes diastolic relaxation of the stiff right ventricle.
- Pyrexia and excessive β-adrenergic stimulation may help precipitate junctional ectopic tachycardia postoperatively.
- Surgeons frequently measure right ventricular pressure to assess the quality of the repair.
- Perioperative echocardiography is useful in assessing repair and right ventricular function.

COMPLEX SHUNTS. In complex shunts (i.e., mixing shunts), there is mixing of pulmonary and systemic blood flow, with resulting cyanosis.

## Transposition of the Great Arteries

Transposition of the great arteries (TGA) is common and accounts for about 6% of all CHD. It frequently occurs as an isolated lesion and is rarely associated with extracardiac anomalies. The operation most commonly performed in these infants is the arterial switch operation (ASO), the short- and long-term results of which have improved to such an extent that children with a good repair can expect a normal life.

TGA refers to the situation in which the aorta arises from the morphologic right ventricle and the pulmonary artery arises from the morphologic left ventricle (Fig. 15-6). In this ventriculoarterial (VA) discordance, the atria are related to the ventricles in the normal way (i.e., AV concordance). This results in two circulations that run in parallel rather than in series, which is the normal anatomic arrangement. Without some mixing of the two circulations, the systemic circulation would remain completely deoxygenated. However, some mixing does occur through the PDA or through a VSD that is present in approximately 25% of cases. If there is no VSD and mixing is inadequate, ductal patency is maintained after birth with an intravenous prostaglandin $E_1$ infusion, and a balloon atrial septostomy is performed urgently in the neonatal period.

In TGA with an intact ventricular septum, the ASO should be performed early in the neonatal period, preferably in the first 2 to 3 weeks of life, because the left ventricle is exposed only to the pressure of the pulmonary circulation. The longer this situation is allowed to continue, the less the left ventricle is able to

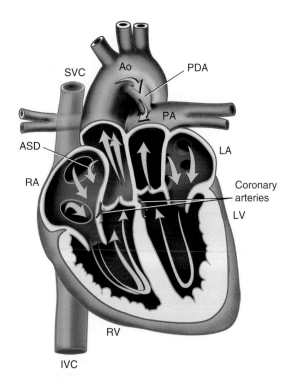

**FIGURE 15-6** Diagram of transposition of the great arteries (TGA) shows an intact ventricular septum. The aorta (*Ao*) arises from the right ventricle (*RV*), and the pulmonary artery (*PA*) arises from the left ventricle (*LV*). The coronary arteries arise from the aorta. These children are cyanotic. *ASD,* Atrial septal defect; *IVC,* inferior vena cava; *LA,* left atrium; *PDA,* patent ductus arteriosus; *RA,* right atrium; *SVC,* superior vena cava. (Modified from May LE. Pediatric heart surgery: a ready reference for professionals. Milwaukee: Maxishare; 2005.)

adapt to the work required to pump blood at systemic pressure after the ASO. However, if there is an unrestrictive VSD, the left and right ventricles are exposed to systemic blood pressure, and the left ventricle is better conditioned to perform the work of the systemic ventricle after the ASO.

If untreated, most infants with TGA die in the first year of life of hypoxia and heart failure. Pulmonary vascular disease develops early and contributes to this high mortality rate.[212,213] The mechanism for the early development of pulmonary vascular disease is complex and not simply related to high pulmonary blood flow. However, the presence of a VSD further accelerates this process. These infants are at risk for pulmonary hypertensive crises in the postoperative period.[214]

### Surgical Options

ARTERIAL SWITCH OPERATION. An ASO is the operation of choice if the intracardiac anatomy is appropriate. The ASO involves transecting the two main arterial trunks distal to their respective valves and switching them to produce VA concordance (Fig. 15-7). It also involves disconnecting the coronary arteries from the "old" aorta and reconnecting them to the neoaorta. This restores anatomic and physiologic normality. The coronary anatomy varies widely in TGA but must be well assessed preoperatively because moving the coronary arteries to the neoaorta is difficult but crucial to a successful outcome. In some cases, the coronary arteries run in the wall of the aorta (intramural), and this poses particular difficulties for the surgeon. Ventricular function after surgery depends largely on unrestricted flow in the coronary arteries.

MUSTARD AND SENNING PROCEDURES. The Mustard and Senning procedures are ASOs. They involve the use of intraatrial baffles to redirect deoxygenated blood from the venae cavae to the left atrium, left ventricle, and pulmonary artery and oxygenated pulmonary venous blood to the right atrium, right ventricle, and aorta. They create AV discordance, restore physiologic but not anatomic normality, and leave the physiologic right ventricle as the systemic ventricle. These procedures were performed as definitive procedures before the arterial switch became successful but are rarely used today as definitive repairs. They are still used as palliation in children with TGA, VSD, and pulmonary vascular disease.[215] In these cases, the VSD is left open.

RASTELLI PROCEDURE. The Rastelli procedure is used in children with TGA, VSD, and left ventricular outflow tract obstruction (LVOTO). The procedure closes the VSD in a way that directs blood from the left ventricle to the aorta. The pulmonary artery is ligated just distal to the pulmonary valve, and a valved conduit is inserted from the right ventricle to the pulmonary artery. The result is continuity between the left ventricle and aorta and between the right ventricle and the pulmonary artery, and the LVOTO (i.e., subpulmonary area) is bypassed. In the past, the Rastelli procedure was performed at 2 to 3 years of age with a Blalock-Taussig shunt performed for palliation in the neonatal period. However, there is a trend toward neonatal Rastelli repair without the need for a shunt.

### Anesthesia Considerations for the Arterial Switch Procedure

- The patient is a neonate in the first few weeks of life.
- Inhalational or intravenous induction is possible.
- Invasive arterial and central venous lines are required. If VSD closure is required, bicaval cannulation may be required for CPB, and because an internal jugular central venous pressure line may interfere with this, a femoral central venous pressure

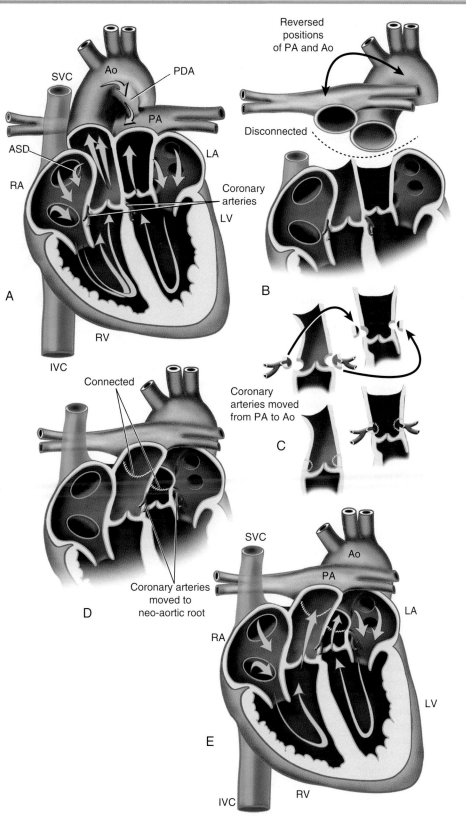

**FIGURE 15-7** Diagram of an arterial switch operation. **A,** The original anatomy. The aorta (*Ao*), pulmonary arteries (*PA*), and coronary arteries are disconnected from their origins. **B,** The PA is moved anterior to the Ao. **C,** The Ao is connected to the left ventricle (*LV*), and the PA is connected to the right ventricle (*RV*). **D,** The coronary arteries are connected to the neoaortic root. **E,** Final configuration. *IVC,* Inferior vena cava; *LA,* left atrium; *RA,* right atrium; *SVC,* superior vena cava. (Modified from May LE. Pediatric heart surgery: a ready reference for professionals. Milwaukee: Maxishare; 2005.)

line may be preferable. If the patient does not have a VSD, a single venous cannula in the atrium can be used for CPB, and the internal jugular vein can be used.

■ Myocardial ischemia occurring after the cross-clamp is removed may be related to coronary air emboli or poor coronary anastomoses. A generous perfusion pressure after removal of cross-clamp encourages flushing air from coronary arteries. If ischemia results from an anatomic problem with the coronary arteries, they may need to be redone with a second bypass run.

■ TEE or epicardial echo is useful in assessing adequate de-airing, myocardial function, and adequacy of coronary anastomoses.

■ Post-CPB myocardial dysfunction may result from one or more of the following:
  ■ An inherently poor left ventricle
  ■ Poor myocardial protection
  ■ Poor coronary transference
  ■ Coronary air

■ The anesthesiologist should anticipate pulmonary hypertension.

■ Inotropes are almost always required. Dopamine or epinephrine can be used, and milrinone is a particularly useful agent in these cases because it is an inodilator.

■ After the repair, the pulmonary artery is anterior to the aorta. Any dilation of the pulmonary artery as a result of pulmonary hypertension can lead to coronary compression and myocardial ischemia.

■ The left ventricle is frequently noncompliant, and volume should be increased with care and in small amounts. Left atrial pressure can rise quickly if fluid is given injudiciously.

■ Coagulopathy after bypass is common.

■ Antifibrinolytics are often used.

### Truncus Arteriosus

Truncus arteriosus is a rare congenital heart defect that occurs in about 0.7 of 1000 live births and accounts for about 1% of all CHD. The basic lesion is that of a common arterial outlet for the aorta and pulmonary artery associated with a single valve and a VSD (Fig. 15-8). The three types depend on how the pulmonary arteries arise from the aorta and on the size of the aorta. Blood mixes at the arterial level with a resultant high pulmonary blood flow. This leads to heart failure and early development of pulmonary hypertension. Surgery must be performed early in life to prevent pulmonary hypertension from becoming irreversible. Truncus arteriosus is associated with DiGeorge syndrome (see Table 15-4). Irradiated blood products should be used and calcium concentrations carefully monitored.

Surgical repair involves separating the systemic from the pulmonary circulation and closure of the VSD. The pulmonary artery or arteries are disconnected from the aorta, and the truncal valve is repaired. The pulmonary arteries are then connected to the right ventricle, usually with a valved conduit. Circulatory arrest may be required. The early postoperative mortality rate is 5% to 25%. Factors that particularly influence mortality are truncal valve stenosis, coronary abnormalities, and low birth weight.

### Anesthesia Considerations

■ The patient is a small neonate in the first month of life.

■ Repair is a high-risk procedure.

■ Heart failure is possible.

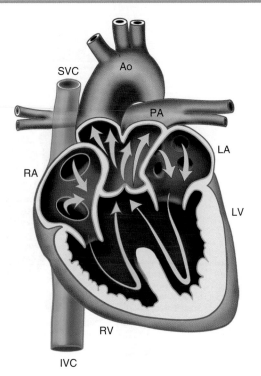

**FIGURE 15-8** The diagram of a truncus arteriosus shows the common truncal valve and mixing of red and blue blood. *Ao,* Aorta; *IVC,* inferior vena cava; *LA,* left atrium; *LV,* left ventricle; *PA,* pulmonary artery; *RA,* right atrium; *RV,* right ventricle; *SVC,* superior vena cava. (Modified from May LE. Pediatric heart surgery: a ready reference for professionals. Milwaukee: Maxishare; 2005.)

■ Risks include a postoperative pulmonary hypertensive crisis.

■ Patients may already be intubated and ventilated and may be on inotropes.

■ If the child is not ventilated, premedication is probably best avoided.

■ Invasive lines are required.

■ Circulatory arrest may be required.

■ Coagulopathy may occur after bypass.

■ Antifibrinolytics are often used.

### Anomalous Pulmonary Venous Connection

Anomalous pulmonary venous connection (i.e., drainage) comprises about 2.5% of CHD and may be total (TAPVC) or partial (PAPVC). In TAPVC, all four pulmonary veins insert into an anomalous site, and in PAPVC, a subset of the veins insert into an anomalous site and the remaining veins insert into the left atrium. Survival is usually good but depends on the site of insertion (e.g., infracardiac survival is poorer than supracardiac and cardiac types) and the size of the venous confluence at the insertion into the left atrium. Three types of TAPVC exist:

■ In supracardiac TAPVC, the pulmonary veins connect to the SVC through an ascending vertical vein (Fig. 15-9, *A*).

■ In cardiac TAPVC, the pulmonary veins connect to the right atrium through the coronary sinus (see Fig. 15-9, *B*).

■ In infracardiac TAPVC, the pulmonary veins connect to the inferior vena cava (IVC) through a common vein, which traverses the diaphragm (see Fig. 15-9, *C*).

Infants with pulmonary venous obstruction, pulmonary hypertension, and reduced pulmonary blood supply usually present early with cyanosis and tachypnea. The degree of

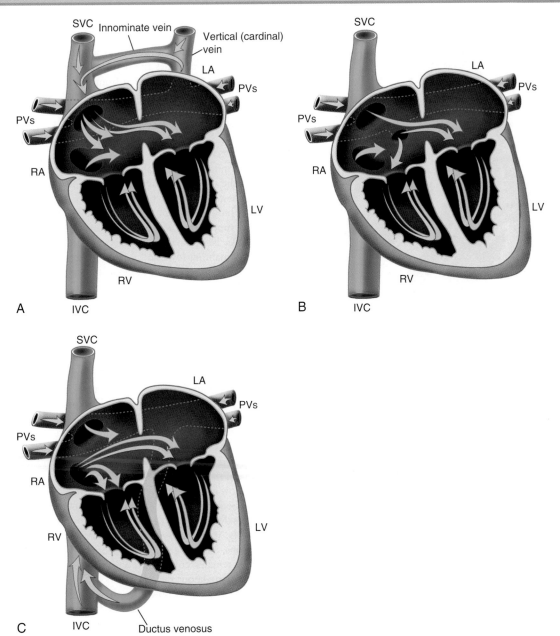

**FIGURE 15-9 A,** In the diagram of a supracardiac total anomalous pulmonary venous connection (TAPVC), the main arteries are removed. The pulmonary veins (*PVs*) drain through the innominate vein to the right atrium (*RA*), and there is an atrial septal defect (ASD). The result is a left-to-right shunt. These children are cyanotic. The veins may also be obstructed, leading to pulmonary hypertension. **B,** In the diagram of an intracardiac TAPVC, the pulmonary veins drain to the RA. There is a ventricular septal defect, and the effect is to create a left-to-right shunt. The veins may also be obstructed, which can lead to pulmonary hypertension. **C,** In the diagram of an infracardiac TAPVC, the PVs drain through the ductus venosus to the RA. An ASD exists, and the circulation results in a right-to-left shunt; the child is blue. The veins may also be obstructed. *IVC,* Inferior vena cava; *LA,* left atrium; *LV,* left ventricle; *RA,* right atrium; *RV,* right ventricle. (Modified from May LE. Pediatric heart surgery: a ready reference for professionals. Milwaukee: Maxishare; 2005.)

cyanosis depends on the size of the ASD and the associated right-to-left shunt and on the degree of mixing of systemic and pulmonary venous blood. Children without pulmonary venous obstruction and pulmonary hypertension usually have few symptoms.

*Anesthesia Considerations*
- The patient may be a neonate.
- Heart failure can occur.
- Pulmonary edema may be present.

- There is a risk of pulmonary hypertension preoperatively and postoperatively; nitric oxide may be required after surgery.
- Circulatory arrest may be used, and profound hypothermia may be required.
- Coagulopathy may occur after bypass.
- Antifibrinolytics are often used.

**Hypoplastic Left Heart Syndrome**
The incidence of HLHS in the United States is about 2 cases per 10,000 live births. In Europe, this figure is probably reduced

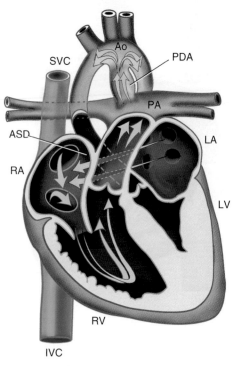

**FIGURE 15-10** Diagram of hypoplastic left heart syndrome shows a very small left ventricle (*LV*), mitral valve, aortic valve, and aortic arch. Pulmonary venous blood drains to the left atrium (*LA*), then through an atrial septal defect (*ASD*) to the right atrium (*RA*), and from there through the right ventricle (*RV*) to the pulmonary artery (*PA*). A patent ductus arteriosus (*PDA*) provides blood to the systemic circulation. *Ao*, Aorta; *IVC*, inferior vena cava; *SVC*, superior vena cava. (Modified from May LE. Pediatric heart surgery: a ready reference for professionals. Milwaukee: Maxishare; 2005.)

because many mothers with a prenatal diagnosis of HLHS opt for pregnancy termination.

The anatomic features of HLHS (Fig. 15-10) include the following:

- Hypoplastic left ventricle
- Mitral stenosis or atresia
- Aortic stenosis or atresia
- Hypoplastic aortic arch
- Duct-dependent circulation

The prognosis for infants who are born with HLHS has improved dramatically. Previously, virtually all of these infants died of this condition, but in some centers, most children now survive at least into childhood.[216] The longer-term outlook has not been fully determined, and many hurdles remain.

The diagnosis of HLHS is usually made in the prenatal period, although it can be difficult and is sometimes missed. At birth, neonates present with tachypnea, tachycardia, and cyanosis, and a systolic murmur can be heard.

### Surgical Palliation

The aim of surgery is to convert the anatomy of the HLHS into a single-ventricle type circulation in which the right ventricle becomes the single systemic ventricle and the pulmonary blood flow is supplied passively from the SVC and IVC (i.e., Fontan circulation). This is done by a series of three operations known as Norwood stage I, Norwood stage II (hemi-Fontan), and Norwood stage III (Fontan).

NORWOOD STAGE I. The Norwood stage I operation is performed in the neonatal period. It involves reconstructing the aortic arch so that it arises from the pulmonary trunk. The pulmonary valve becomes the neoaortic valve. The branch pulmonary arteries are disconnected from the pulmonary trunk, and a new pulmonary blood supply is provided by a shunt from the subclavian artery (i.e., Blalock-Taussig shunt) or from the right ventricle (i.e., Sano modification) (Fig. 15-11).[217] If the ASD is restrictive, it is enlarged.

NORWOOD STAGE II. The Norwood stage II (hemi-Fontan) operation takes place at about 6 months of age. It involves taking down the shunt that was created at the first operation and creating a new connection from the SVC to the pulmonary arteries (i.e., a bidirectional or Glenn shunt). The result is a pulmonary blood supply that is provided by systemic venous blood from the SVC. Flow is passive and depends on pulmonary artery pressures remaining low. The infants remain cyanotic with arterial saturations in the mid-80s because desaturated blood from the IVC continues to flow into the heart and the systemic circulation (Fig. 15-12).

NORWOOD STAGE III. The Norwood stage III (Fontan) operation converts the anatomy into a Fontan circulation. The surgery involves connecting the IVC through an extracardiac or intracardiac conduit to the pulmonary artery. This creates a single-ventricle or Fontan circulation (Fig. 15-13). The single right ventricle pumps blood to the systemic circulation, and the pulmonary blood supply is provided by passive flow by systemic venous blood from the SVC and IVC. The PVR must remain low because any increase will dramatically reduce pulmonary blood flow. It is common for a small hole (i.e., fenestration) to be created between the extracardiac conduit and the right atrium so that if the PVR rises, blood will be directed to the right atrium and allow cardiac output to be maintained. In this situation, the child becomes cyanotic, but cardiac output is maintained, a much safer situation than a state of low cardiac output. Postoperatively, increased systemic venous pressure may cause pleural effusions, an enlarged liver, or protein-losing enteropathy. Later, if PVR remains consistently low, the fenestration can be closed with a transvenous device.

The long-term problem for these children is that the morphologic right ventricle that becomes the systemic ventricle fails over time. The only recourse is heart transplantation.[218,219]

### Anesthesia Considerations

NORWOOD STAGE I.

- The anesthesiologist must understand the anatomy and physiology of HLHS.
- Balance between systemic and pulmonary circulations is maintained by balancing PVR and SVR. If the PVR decreases, blood flow will be directed away from the systemic circulation and the lungs will be flooded. This results in hypotension and hypoperfusion with increasing acidosis. If PVR increases, cyanosis will increase. Before anesthesia, these infants are best managed spontaneously breathing in room air with a prostaglandin $E_1$ infusion to maintain ductal patency. However, if mechanical ventilation is required, it is important to maintain normal to high $PaCO_2$ and very low $FIO_2$, usually with air.
- Air should be available for transfer to the operating room, or a self-inflating bag should be used.
- High-dose opioid technique is preferred.

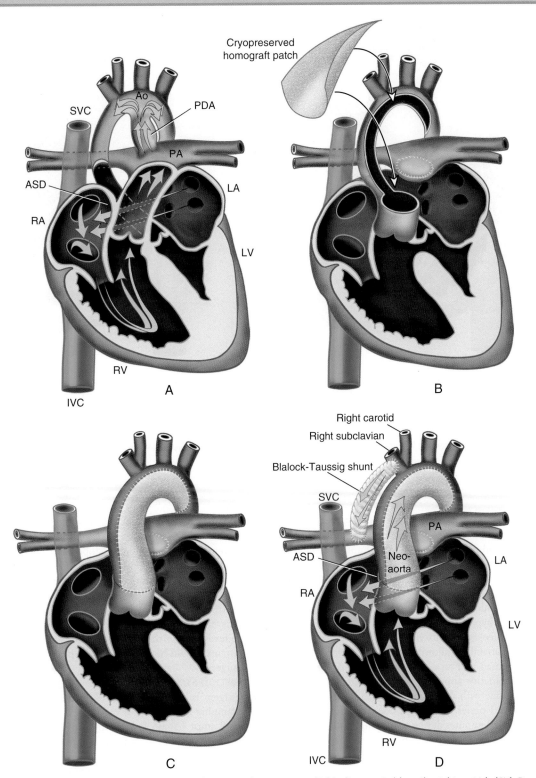

**FIGURE 15-11** Diagram of the Norwood stage I operation. **A,** The main pulmonary artery (*PA*) is disconnected from the right ventricle (*RV*). **B** and **C,** The aortic arch is reconstructed with homograft and connected to the RV, which becomes a single ventricle. **D,** Pulmonary blood is then supplied by a Blalock-Taussig shunt from the subclavian artery to the pulmonary artery. The children remain cyanotic. *Ao,* Aorta; *ASD,* atrial septal defect; *IVC,* inferior vena cava; *LA,* left atrium; *LV,* left ventricle; *PDA,* patent ductus arteriosus; *RA,* right atrium. (Modified from May LE. Pediatric heart surgery: a ready reference for professionals. Milwaukee: Maxishare; 2005.)

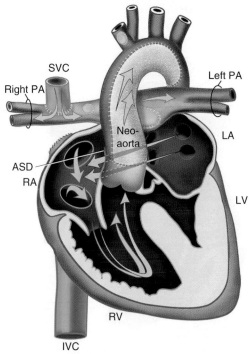

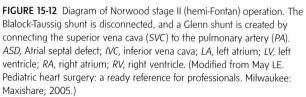

**FIGURE 15-12** Diagram of Norwood stage II (hemi-Fontan) operation. The Blalock-Taussig shunt is disconnected, and a Glenn shunt is created by connecting the superior vena cava (*SVC*) to the pulmonary artery (*PA*). *ASD*, Atrial septal defect; *IVC*, inferior vena cava; *LA*, left atrium; *LV*, left ventricle; *RA*, right atrium; *RV*, right ventricle. (Modified from May LE. Pediatric heart surgery: a ready reference for professionals. Milwaukee: Maxishare; 2005.)

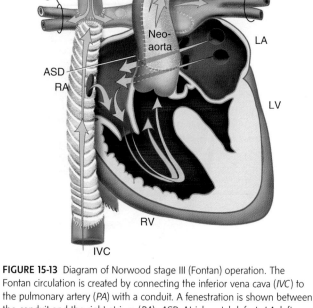

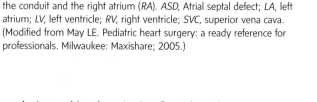

**FIGURE 15-13** Diagram of Norwood stage III (Fontan) operation. The Fontan circulation is created by connecting the inferior vena cava (*IVC*) to the pulmonary artery (*PA*) with a conduit. A fenestration is shown between the conduit and the right atrium (*RA*). *ASD*, Atrial septal defect; *LA*, left atrium; *LV*, left ventricle; *RV*, right ventricle; *SVC*, superior vena cava. (Modified from May LE. Pediatric heart surgery: a ready reference for professionals. Milwaukee: Maxishare; 2005.)

- Venous access is gained through the femoral or umbilical veins. The internal jugular vein is avoided because narrowing of the SVC would jeopardize the Glenn shunt.
- Profound hypothermia may be required.
- Postoperative myocardial dysfunction is common, and inotropes are required.
- Balancing systemic and pulmonary blood flow remains an issue after bypass. Some centers use the long-acting α-adrenergic blocker phenoxybenzamine after bypass to reduce SVR variability, allowing greater concentrations of oxygen to be used and an overall increase in oxygen delivery.[220] The alternative approach is to combine a vasodilator such as milrinone with dopamine or epinephrine to achieve a similar effect. I prefer to deliver a bolus dose of milrinone (25 µg/kg over 20 minutes during rewarming), followed by an infusion of 0.3 µg/kg/min in combination with epinephrine, 0.05 to 0.1 µg/kg/min.
- Coagulopathy may occur after bypass.
- Antifibrinolytics are often used
- The sternum is frequently left open, and closure may be delayed for several days.

NORWOOD STAGE II.
- The procedure is carried out with CPB.
- Cardioplegia is not used. The heart remains beating, and inotropes are seldom required.
- Venous access is achieved through the femoral veins. However, only a single side should be used because femoral bypass is occasionally required. A short temporary cannula is useful in

the internal jugular vein. It reflects the pulmonary artery pressure after anastomosis of the SVC to the pulmonary artery. It is removed early in the postoperative period to avoid any possibility of thrombosis in the SVC.
- This is repeat surgery, and external defibrillator pads should be attached.
- Antifibrinolytics may be used
- The aim is early extubation. Positive intrathoracic pressure reduces flow in the Glenn shunt.
- Infants should be nursed with the head up at 30 degrees after surgery.

NORWOOD STAGE III.
- Surgery is carried out with CPB but usually without cross-clamping the aorta.
- PVR must remain low postoperatively, careful management of the lungs is important to minimize atelectasis, and nitric oxide is occasionally required.[221]
- If an inotrope is required, milrinone is a good choice because of its beneficial effects on PVR.
- Early extubation is beneficial in terms of hemodynamics.
- Large amounts of fluid may be required in the early postoperative period.

## AORTIC STENOSIS

Obstruction to the LVOT can occur at the valvular, subvalvular, or supravalvular area or in various combinations, and it is common, accounting for up to 10% of CHD.[222,223] Congenital valvar aortic stenosis is frequently associated with a bicuspid valve. Severe critical aortic stenosis in neonates occurs in approximately 10% of cases and requires urgent treatment. Supravalvular aortic stenosis may be associated with Williams syndrome.[224]

Despite the many anatomic varieties of aortic stenosis, the resulting pathophysiology remains essentially the same. There is an increasing imbalance between oxygen supply and demand (i.e., impaired coronary blood flow due to low coronary perfusion pressure plus increased workload on the left ventricle leading to subendocardial ischemia), left ventricular hypertrophy, and a risk of left ventricular failure. There is always the risk of sudden death, especially with Williams syndrome. The age at which the child presents is a risk factor; younger children are most at risk. Two thirds of those presenting in the first 3 months of life will require inotropic or ventilatory support before treatment.[225]

### Treatment Options

Treatment options depend on the patient's age and the severity and type of lesion. In neonates with critical aortic stenosis, an urgent valvuloplasty is required. It can be performed surgically using CPB, but it typically is performed using transluminal balloon angioplasty in the cardiac catheterization laboratory.[226] Complications in this age group include ventricular fibrillation, aortic incompetence, or residual aortic stenosis.

In the older child, several surgical approaches may be used, depending on the anatomy. Transluminal balloon valvuloplasty commonly is performed in older patients. The most common complications of valvuloplasty are aortic incompetence and residual aortic stenosis. Valve replacement with a mechanical valve or bioprosthetic valve is delayed as long as possible because of the long-term problems associated with the anticoagulation needed with a mechanical valve and because of the inevitable calcification of the bioprosthetic valve. An alternative surgical option is the Ross procedure, which involves moving the pulmonary valve into the aortic valve position and using a homograft in the pulmonary position. The need for reoperation with the Ross procedure is reduced because the systemic valve (i.e., neo-aortic valve) grows with the child and calcification of the homograft in the pulmonary position is slow. There is no need for anticoagulation.[227-229]

### Anesthesia Considerations

- A crucial aim of anesthesia is to maintain the balance of oxygen supply and demand. This involves maintaining a normal heart rate (no tachycardia or bradycardia), maintaining SVR to preserve coronary perfusion, avoiding hypertension, and avoiding myocardial depression.
- Anesthesia for neonates having surgery with CPB is similar to other neonatal cardiac surgery.
- For transluminal balloon valvuloplasty
  - The catheter crossing the aortic valve and inflation of the balloon can lead to dramatic cardiovascular changes. Cardiac output decreases, myocardial ischemia occurs, and bradycardia is common. In neonates, ventricular fibrillation may occur after passing the wire across the valve. The anesthesiologist must be prepared to resuscitate the neonate quickly, and drugs, particularly epinephrine, should be immediately available.
  - It is possible the child will remain ventilated after the procedure because ventricular function can remain poor for some time.

- Arterial access is needed by the cardiologist for the procedure, but pressure is not always displayed. An independent arterial line is very useful.
- Occasionally, adenosine is given to slow or stop the heart at the time of balloon inflation to prevent damage to the valve by the inflated balloon being expelled through it. However, this practice is not universal.

### Coarctation of the Aorta

Coarctation of the aorta is discrete narrowing of the aorta, and it accounts for about 5% of CHD. The lesion is often isolated with no other associated abnormalities. This type of lesion, however, may occur in association with other cardiac abnormalities such as VSD, aortic arch, or aortic valve abnormalities. The coarctation may be preductal, juxtaductal, or postductal, depending on the relationship to the ductus arteriosus. The most common form presenting in the neonatal period is the preductal type. Preductal coarctation is associated with minimal collateral circulation below the coarctation and requires prostaglandin to maintain ductal patency. Juxtaductal and postductal coarctations are characterized by the development of collateral vessels that supply the area below the coarctation. This is important because the spinal cord is supplied by these collaterals, and these vessels supply the spinal cord during aortic cross-clamping.

In practical terms, children with coarctation of the aorta can be classified in two groups. One group presents in the neonatal period with preductal coarctation with few collaterals and very poor left ventricular function. The second group of children (usually older than 1 year of age) have well-developed collaterals and better left ventricular function. Neonates often present with poor left ventricular function and may be in heart failure. Femoral pulses are often weak, and patients usually have a progressive acidosis. Differences between the systolic systemic blood pressures in the right arm (before stenosis) and left leg (after stenosis) may indicate the presence of a coarctation of the aorta.

### Anesthesia Considerations

NEONATAL REPAIR.

- These infants are sick, with poor left ventricular function. They should be treated very carefully, and the anesthesiologist should not be misled by an infant who looks reasonably well.
- Some infants are already intubated and ventilated, and some may be receiving an inotrope such as dopamine.
- Intravenous access often is established to give prostaglandin $E_1$; this intravenous line can also be used to administer induction agents. I prefer to give incremental doses of fentanyl (up to 5 μg/kg) and then a muscle relaxant and to supplement this with a very low dose of isoflurane (0.3% to 0.5%). This can be omitted if hypotension ensues.
- Inotropes may be required before surgery, and they should be available.
- Ideally, the arterial line should be placed in the right arm to allow blood pressure measurement during arterial cross-clamping. The left subclavian may be partially obstructed during the repair. Some have advocated an arterial line below the coarctation to measure perfusion pressure during cross-clamping, but this may be very difficult in practice because femoral pulses are usually absent.
- A central venous line should be placed.
- Surgery usually takes place through a left thoracotomy without the use of CPB. The lung is retracted, and ventilation may be problematic. The endotracheal tube must fit snugly and have

a minimal leak because a tracheal tube with a large leak may make ventilation very difficult.

- Paraplegia may occur in about 1% of cases and is thought to result from hypoperfusion during aortic cross-clamping.[230,231] To reduce the chance of spinal cord damage, infants should be cooled to 34° C or 35° C before the cross-clamp is applied, although this approach is not evidence based. Normocarbia and upper limb blood pressure should be maintained. Low-dose anticoagulation may be applied. A short cross-clamp time is thought to be important.
- Epidural anesthesia is occasionally used, but I have not adopted this approach.
- Postoperative hypertension may be a problem, and a vasodilator such as sodium nitroprusside may be required.

ANESTHESIA FOR THE OLDER CHILD.

- These children usually are not as sick as the neonates.
- Issues about vascular lines are similar to those in neonatal repair.
- Careful intravenous induction with a combination of fentanyl and an induction agent of choice is standard. Etomidate is a good anesthetic because of its cardiovascular stability.
- Although a collateral blood supply is present, the spinal cord remains at risk during the cross-clamping, and the same precautions taken with neonates should be taken with these children.
- An oral cuffed tracheal tube is useful because early extubation is the norm.
- Postoperative hypertension is a common problem, and good analgesia combined with sodium nitroprusside and β-blockers is usually required. Up to 30% of children eventually develop long-term hypertension that will require therapy.

Some of these children are managed with balloon angioplasty with or without stent placement. Rupture of the aorta is a risk in these patients, and the institution in which the procedure is undertaken should be in a position to deal with this possibility.

### Interrupted Aortic Arch

Interrupted aortic arch is a rare anomaly, accounting for less than 1% of CHD. In this condition, disruption occurs between the ascending aorta and descending aorta (Fig. 15-14). The three types depend on where the disruption takes place. A PDA is present and is required to supply the descending aorta. A VSD is also common. Interrupted aortic arch is frequently associated with a 22q11 deletion and results in the DiGeorge syndrome (see Table 15-4).[232]

These children are often small for gestational age and are started on a prostaglandin infusion to maintain ductal patency. They are often sick with progressive acidosis and poor cardiac output. There is increasing pulmonary blood flow as the duct closes. Surgical repair depends on the presence of associated lesions, particularly a VSD. In the single-stage repair, the arch is reconstructed, and the VSD is closed. The two-stage repair involves repair of the aortic arch and banding of the pulmonary artery to limit blood flow to the lungs. The VSD is closed in a later stage of the procedure. Either way, deep hypothermic circulatory arrest is likely to be employed. Some centers use selective regional perfusion to try and limit neurologic injury.[233] The early and late mortality rates are high. Higher mortality rates correlate with small size, acidosis preoperatively, and associated cardiac lesions.[234]

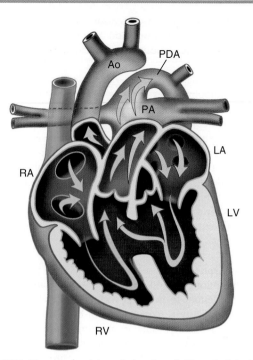

**FIGURE 15-14** Diagram of an interrupted aortic arch. The patent ductus arteriosus (*PDA*) supplies the body below the interruption. *Ao*, Aorta; *ASD*, atrial septal defect; *LA*, left atrium; *LV*, left ventricle; *PA*, pulmonary artery; *RA*, right atrium; *RV*, right ventricle. (Modified from May LE. Pediatric heart surgery: a ready reference for professionals. Milwaukee: Maxishare; 2005.)

### Anesthesia Considerations

- The patient is a small, sick neonate.
- DiGeorge syndrome is identified (particularly hypocalcemia and the need for irradiated blood products).
- High-dose opioid technique is standard.
- Ideally, blood pressure should be monitored above and below the interruption, but this is often difficult in practice.
- Deep hypothermic circulatory arrest may be used.
- An antifibrinolytic is frequently used.
- Coagulopathy may occur after bypass.
- Anticipate poor renal function postoperatively.
- There is a risk of postoperative pulmonary hypertensive crises.

These infants are likely to require repeat operations to deal with recurrent LVOTO, which may occur at any level. Restenosis of the repaired aortic arch can be opened with transluminal balloon dilation.

## Transport and Transfer to a Pediatric Intensive Care Unit

After surgery is completed, cardiac surgical patients need a period of intensive care. The first phase of this care is transport of the children from the operating room to the PICU. This is a potentially hazardous time and requires good organization, teamwork, and appropriate equipment. Guidelines exist for the safe transport of these children.[235]

Transport to the PICU can be defined as a preparatory phase, transport phase, and stabilization phase.[236] During the preparatory phase, the estimated time of arrival in the PICU is communicated with the PICU. The bed space is prepared, ventilator and monitors are configured in an appropriate way, and any additional interventions that may be required are made ready. In my institution, a form is sent to the PICU that indicates the child's age and weight, the ventilator settings that will be required, the number of transducers that will be required, and the infusions that are running. After arrival in the PICU, two basic tasks need to be undertaken: transfer of technology and transfer of information. It is better to allow the technology transfer to occur before the information handover. This includes ensuring that all the monitors are connected and working appropriately, that the ventilator is connected and delivering adequate ventilation, that all infusions are working, and that drains and urinary catheter are all in place with baseline readings documented. After this has been accomplished, a single handover of information should be done with all of the appropriate personnel present, and it should include information given by the anesthesiologist and surgeon. In my institution, a checklist is followed to ensure that no important information is omitted. It is important to avoid a large number of information handovers between individuals rather than a single, comprehensive handover with all the relevant personnel present.

## ACKNOWLEDGMENT

The author wishes to thank Paul R. Hickey, Richard L. Marnach, Dolly D. Hansen, Robert W. Reid, and Frederick A. Burrows for their prior contributions to this chapter.

## ANNOTATED REFERENCES

Arnold DM, Fergusson DA, Chan AK, et al. Avoiding transfusions in children undergoing cardiac surgery: a meta-analysis of randomized trials of aprotinin. Anesth Analg 2006;102:731-7.

*In a meta-analysis of the use of aprotinin in children, these researchers found that most published studies were of poor quality and that there were broad differences in the doses used in children. Although they could not find any convincing evidence for the use of aprotinin in children, they commented that there was an urgent need for further high-quality studies to determine the role of aprotinin in children undergoing cardiac surgery.*

Andropoulos DB, Stayer SA, Diaz LK, Ramamoorthy C. Neurological monitoring for congenital heart surgery. Anesth Analg 2004;99: 1365-75.

*This is a wide-ranging review of cerebral monitoring during cardiac surgery in children. The section on the use of cerebral oximetry is particularly relevant to clinical practice.*

Bettex DA, Pretre R, Jenni R, Schmid ER. Cost-effectiveness of routine intraoperative transesophageal echocardiography in pediatric cardiac surgery: a 10-year experience. Anesth Analg 2005;100:1271-5.

*Bettex and coworkers showed in a retrospective study of 580 pediatric patients undergoing cardiac surgery that the use of routine intraoperative transesophageal echocardiography (TEE) was cost effective. They identified 33 children who required a second bypass run on the basis of the intraoperative TEE. The authors estimate that the savings per child were in the range of $690 to $2130.*

Hoffman TM, Wernovsky G, Atz AM, et al. Prophylactic intravenous use of milrinone after cardiac operation in pediatrics (PRIMACORP) study. Prophylactic Intravenous Use of Milrinone After Cardiac Operation in Pediatrics. Am Heart J 2002;143:15-21.

*In this large, multicenter, prospective, randomized, double-blind study, it was shown that the use of milrinone in high doses (75 µg/kg bolus over 60 minutes, followed by an infusion at a rate of 0.75 µg/kg/min) in infants undergoing complex congenital cardiac operations reduced the incidence of low cardiac output syndrome in the postoperative period.*

Kern FH, Morana NJ, Sears JJ, Hickey PR. Coagulation defects in neonates during cardiopulmonary bypass. Ann Thorac Surg 1992; 54:541-6.

*Kern and colleagues showed that hemodilution is an important factor in the development of post-bypass coagulopathy in neonates. They showed that platelets and coagulation factors were dramatically reduced as soon as the neonate was placed on cardiopulmonary bypass (CPB) and were not significantly reduced further during CPB.*

Malviya S, Voepel-Lewis T, Siewert M, et al. Risk factors for adverse postoperative outcomes in children presenting for cardiac surgery with upper respiratory tract infections. Anesthesiology 2003;98: 628-32.

*These investigators have shown that children with an upper respiratory tract infection at the time of cardiac surgery are at risk for more complications in the postoperative period and have a longer stay in the intensive care unit. These children need very careful assessment before surgery, and the risk-benefit ratio for the child must be considered.*

Mangano DT, Tudor IC, Dietzel C. The risk associated with aprotinin in cardiac surgery. N Engl J Med 2006;354:353-65.

*Mangano and associates reported a large observational study in adult patients undergoing revascularization surgery. They reported an increase in renal failure, myocardial infarction, heart failure, stroke, and encephalopathy. This study has been criticized for not being randomized. These effects have not been shown in children, but it has created an unease about the use of aprotinin in children. It is important that well-designed, independent, large studies are carried out in children to establish the role of aprotinin.*

Naik SK, Knight A, Elliott M. A prospective randomized study of a modified technique of ultrafiltration during pediatric open-heart surgery. Circulation 1991;84(Suppl):III422-31.

*Naik and colleagues were the first to report the use of modified ultrafiltration (MUF) after cardiopulmonary bypass in children. Beneficial effects included reduced total body water, higher hematocrit, higher blood pressure, less postoperative bleeding, and a reduced requirement for inotropes. MUF is now used in many centers worldwide and has a number of benefits.*

## REFERENCES

Please see www.expertconsult.com.

**15**

# Cardiac Physiology and Pharmacology

## ANNETTE Y. SCHURE AND JAMES A. DiNARDO

THE CARDIOVASCULAR SYSTEM plays a dominant role within the human body: a centrally located "powerhouse" provides oxygenation and nutrition via an extensive network of vessels and capillaries throughout the body. All other organ systems depend on its normal development and function. At birth, and especially in the first few hours of life, the heart and the vascular system have to adapt to the extrauterine conditions. Prematurity, congenital defects, complications during labor and delivery, and many other factors can prevent or delay the necessary changes and cause significant morbidity.

A thorough understanding of the fetal circulation, the changes at birth, and the age-specific characteristics is important for the safe management of neonates, infants, and especially the growing number of preterm and small-for-gestational-age (SGA) babies who come to our diagnostic suites and operating rooms. Given the complex embryology and difficult transition from fetal to extrauterine life, it is amazing that more than 90% of neonates are delivered without any special interventions and that congenital heart defects occur in only 7 to 10 of every 1000 live births.[1] (A detailed discussion of the embryologic development is beyond the scope of this chapter; the interested reader is referred to the excellent review by Van Praagh[2] or Langman's classic embryology textbook.[3])

Congenital heart defects are among the most common birth defects. In the United States, approximately 32,000 babies are born every year with congenital heart disease (CHD); a significant number require urgent interventions in the catheterization laboratory or surgical procedures during the neonatal period. In addition, CHD is often associated with other, noncardiac anomalies, and many of these children will present for procedures outside the cardiac operating room. Pediatric anesthesiologists have to be able to classify and recognize the pathophysiologic effects of CHD on the cardiovascular system of the neonate or infant and the potential impact of anesthesia and surgical manipulations.

With recent advances in surgical techniques, critical care, and anesthesia management, 85% of all infants with CHD are now expected to reach adulthood. Anesthesiologists will increasingly encounter children with "repaired" or "palliated" CHD presenting for noncardiac procedures. Chapter 21 addresses specific long-term problems and anesthetic considerations for various repaired heart defects, but a few conditions deserve additional discussion: the basic changes in the exercise physiology of repaired heart defects, the characteristics of the so-called Fontan physiology after single ventricle palliation, and the altered physiologic responses in the transplanted heart.

Many conditions require pharmacologic support with cardiovascular drugs, some of which can have significant age-specific effects. Well-controlled drug studies in infants and children are rare. Dosing is often based on long-standing experience or extrapolation from adult data. Understanding the basic pharmacology of the most commonly used cardiovascular drugs and the special considerations for infants and children is essential for successful perioperative care. This chapter will help the pediatric anesthesiologist to understand the complexity of the neonatal cardiovascular system, the implications of CHD, and basic pharmacologic considerations and will provide the necessary tools to develop a safe management plan.

## Cardiovascular Physiology

### FETAL CIRCULATION

In utero, the placental gas exchange provides the fetus with relatively oxygenated blood; the partial pressure of oxygen ($PO_2$) in the umbilical vein is approximately 30 mm Hg, and in the umbilical arteries it is approximately 16 mm Hg. The fetal lungs are fluid filled and only minimally perfused (10% to 15% of the cardiac output). The normal postnatal circulation can be principally described as a serial circuit: Two pumps, the right ventricle

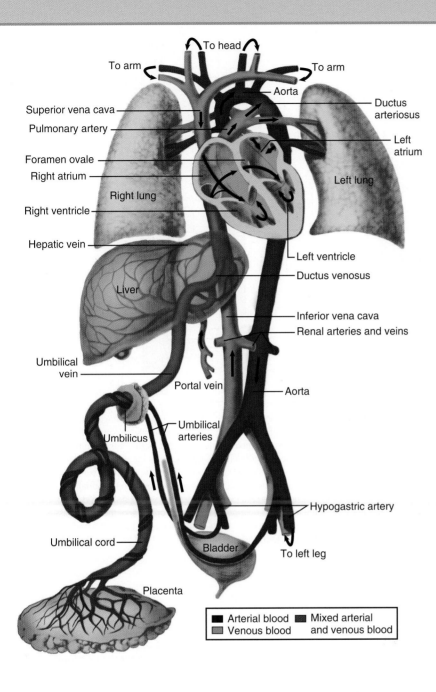

**FIGURE 16-1** Course of the fetal circulation in late gestation. Notice the selective blood flow patterns across the foramen ovale and the ductus arteriosus. (From Greeley WJ, Berkowitz DH, Nathan AT. Anesthesia for pediatric cardiac surgery. In: Miller RD, editor. Anesthesia. 7th ed. Philadelphia: Churchill Livingstone; 2010. Fig. 83-1).

[RV] and left ventricle [LV], support two different resistance systems, the pulmonary and systemic vasculatures, one after the other. In contrast, the fetal circulation is better explained by the concept of a parallel circuit: Both ventricles provide systemic blood flow and a variety of fetal shortcuts or connections allow for mixing of oxygenated and deoxygenated blood (Fig. 16-1).[4,5] Oxygenated blood from the placenta returns via the umbilical vein to the portal venous system, where 30% to 50% of the blood flow is shunted across the *ductus venosus* to the inferior vena cava (IVC), bypassing the liver and thereby maintaining higher oxygenation and velocity. The rest of the umbilical venous blood passes through the hepatic microcirculation into the suprahepatic IVC.

The IVC blood entering the right atrium (RA) is a mixture of bloodstreams with different velocities and saturations: the low-velocity, deoxygenated venous return from the lower body and hepatic veins and the high-velocity, oxygenated umbilical venous blood from the ductus venosus. Valve-like tissue in the RA (eustachian valve) and the Chiari network preferentially direct the high-velocity blood-stream from the IVC across the *foramen ovale* into the left atrium (LA), bypassing the RV and pulmonary vessels. In the LA, the oxygenated blood mixes with the minimal amount of venous return from the pulmonary circulation and is then ejected by the LV into the ascending aorta and the major vessels of the aortic arch. This blood, with a saturation of 65% to 70%, provides the oxygenation for the growing heart and brain.

Most of the venous return from the superior vena cava (SVC) and about 20% of the IVC blood flow (mainly the low-velocity, deoxygenated part) reach the RV and are pumped into the pulmonary artery (PA), where the high pulmonary resistance in the nonexpanded lung redirects 90% of the blood flow into the descending aorta via the *ductus arteriosus*. The bulk of the blood flow in the descending aorta is generated by the RV, with minor

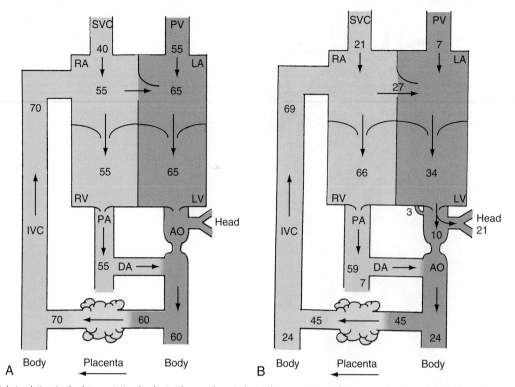

**FIGURE 16-2** Fetal circulation in the late-gestation lamb. **A,** The numbers indicate the percentage of oxygen saturation. Oxygen saturation is greatest in the inferior vena cava (*IVC*), representing flow that is primarily from the placenta. The saturation of the blood in the heart is slightly greater on the left side than on the right side. **B,** The course of the circulation. The numbers represent the percentage of combined ventricular output. Some of the return from the IVC is diverted by the crista dividens in the right atrium (*RA*) through the foramen ovale into the left atrium (*LA*), where it meets the pulmonary venous return (*PV*), passes into the left ventricle (*LV*), and is pumped into the ascending aorta. Most of the ascending aortic flow goes to the coronary, subclavian, and carotid arteries, with only 10% of combined ventricular output passing through the aortic arch (indicated by the narrowed point in the aorta) into the descending aorta (*AO*). The remainder of the IVC flow mixes with return from the superior vena cava (*SVC*) and coronary veins (3%), passes into the RA and right ventricle (*RV*), and is pumped into the pulmonary artery (*PA*). Because of the increased pulmonary resistance, only 7% of the blood passes through the lungs (PV), with the rest passing through the ductus arteriosus (*DA*) to the AO and then to the placenta and lower half of the body. (Modified from Rudolph AM. Congenital diseases of the heart. Chicago: Year Book Publishers; 1974, p. 1-48; and from Freed MD. Fetal and transitional circulation. In: Fyler DC, editor. Nadas' pediatric cardiology. Philadelphia: Mosby-Year Book; 1992. p. 57-61.)

contributions from the LV. The blood has a saturation of only 55% to 60%; two thirds of it returns to the placenta for oxygenation, and the rest is distributed to the intestines, the kidneys, and the lower part of the body (Fig. 16-2).

The fetal circulation has to support a growing fetus in a relatively cyanotic atmosphere (highest oxygen saturation, 65% to 70%). This difficult task is further complicated by the parallel circuit, which creates increased workload for the RV, and the limitations of the fetal shortcuts, which add additional volume load by incomplete shunting of oxygenated and deoxygenated blood. Initially, understanding of the fetal circulation was based mainly on experimental animal data, but recent advances in ultrasound technology have made it possible to assess and monitor fetal cardiovascular parameters, especially stroke volume and cardiac output, under various conditions throughout the gestational period. RV stroke volume has been found to increase from about 0.7 mL at 20 weeks to 7.6 mL at 40 weeks, and LV stroke volume increases from 0.7 mL to 5.2 mL. The combined fetal cardiac output of both ventricles is estimated to be 400 to 425 mL/kg/min, with an RV dominance due to the increased volume load. At 38 weeks, the RV provides approximately 60% of the combined cardiac output (E-Table 16-1).[6-8] Intrauterine growth restriction and placental compromise are associated with redistribution of cardiac output and relative changes in the size

of the foramen ovale.[9] A functional placenta, the fetal cardiovascular high-output state, greater hemoglobin concentrations, and additional alterations in oxygen binding and release (hemoglobin F, increased 2,3-diphosphoglycerate [2,3-DPG]) are all necessary to provide adequate tissue oxygenation for the developing fetus.

Until recently, CHD was thought to be relatively well tolerated in utero, but growing evidence suggests that fetal cardiovascular defects can induce intrinsic autoregulatory changes in cerebral perfusion and thereby compromise brain development.[10,11] Ultrasound and magnetic resonance imaging demonstrate that 30% to 50% of neonates with CHD have neurologic abnormalities before any surgical intervention.[12]

## TRANSITIONAL CIRCULATION

At birth, a variety of humoral, biochemical, and physiologic changes occur abruptly. First, the placental circulation is eliminated shortly after the lungs expand. Second, expansion of the lungs to a normal functional residual capacity (FRC) results in an optimal geometric relationship of the pulmonary microvasculature. Third, air entering the lungs causes the alveolar $PCO_2$ to decrease and the alveolar $PO_2$ to increase. These three factors act in concert to markedly reduce pulmonary vascular resistance (PVR).[5,13,14] The net effect is a considerable increase in pulmonary blood flow, which augments pulmonary venous return to the left heart. Along with elimination of the placenta and the low-resistance umbilical circulation, the LV is suddenly subjected to increased volume and afterload (Table 16-1). Typically, LV end-diastolic pressure, and thus LA pressure, increases enough to exert hydrostatic pressure on the septum primum, resulting in functional closure of the foramen ovale. In contrast to the increased stress for the LV, the RV is relatively unloaded by the transition to extrauterine life.

The three fetal connections (ductus arteriosus, ductus venosus, and foramen ovale) close over a variable period. The ductus arteriosus has functionally (but not anatomically) closed in 58% of normal full-term infants by 2 days of life and in 98% by day 4.[15] Although many substances such as eicosanoids have been implicated, initial constriction probably occurs primarily in response to the increased arterial oxygen tension[16,17] and the reduction in circulating prostaglandins that follow separation of the placenta.[18] The response to oxygen is age dependent: Term neonates usually demonstrate effective constriction of the smooth muscles in the ductal tissue when exposed to oxygen, whereas preterm infants poorly respond and often require medical (prostaglandin inhibitor) or even surgical therapy. Additional catecholamine-induced changes in PVR and systemic vascular resistance (SVR) and other substances such as acetylcholine contribute to ductal closure. Within 2 to 3 weeks, functional constriction is followed by a process of ductal fibrosis, leaving a band-like structure, the ligamentum arteriosum.[19,20] With ligation

of the umbilical vein, the portal pressure falls, triggering functional closure of the ductus venosus. This process rarely requires more than 1 to 2 weeks; by 3 months only fibrous tissue, the ligamentum venosum, is left.

The foramen ovale is functionally closed when the LA pressure exceeds the pressure in the RA, but it remains anatomically patent in most infants, in 50% of children younger than 5 years of age, and in 25% to 30% of adults.[21] Echocardiographic studies have confirmed right-to-left shunting via the foramen ovale in healthy infants emerging from general anesthesia, and this can be a significant cause of persistent arterial desaturation at that time despite ventilation with 100% oxygen.[22]

## NEONATAL CARDIOVASCULAR SYSTEM

Compared with the adult, the neonatal myocardium is immature and incompletely developed (Table 16-2). Differences in cytoarchitecture and metabolism account for many of the functional limitations. The neonatal heart contains fewer muscle cells and more connective tissue than the adult myocardium. Contractile elements add up to only 30% of the total cardiac mass, in contrast to 60% in the adult.[23] The ratio of surface area to mass and that of water to collagen content are larger. There are fewer myofibrils within the muscle cells, and they tend to be less organized (i.e., not parallel to the long axis of the cell). The sarcoplasmic reticulum and the T-tubule network, both important components of rapid and effective calcium regulation, are incompletely developed, and the immature myocardium relies substantially on the calcium flux through the sarcolemma to initiate and terminate contraction.[24-26] One likely practical consequence is a greater degree of contractile dysfunction in the infant exposed to substances that decrease extracellular ionized calcium, such as citrate (blood products) and albumin; there is also increased sensitivity to volatile anesthetics and calcium channels blockers.

Reduced numbers of underdeveloped mitochondria and maturational differences in various signaling pathways and related messenger systems are also characteristic of the neonatal myocardium. Immature mitochondrial enzyme activity for fatty acid transport may explain the primary use of carbohydrates and lactates as energy sources and might be a reason for the greater anaerobic tolerance and faster recovery after periods of

### TABLE 16-1 Hemodynamic Changes at Birth

| Right Ventricle | Left Ventricle |
|---|---|
| Decreased afterload: | Increased afterload: |
| Decreased pulmonary vascular resistance | Placenta eliminated |
| Ductal closure | Ductal closure |
| Decreased volume load: | Increased volume load: |
| Eliminated umbilical vein return | Increased pulmonary venous return |
| Output diminished 25% | Output increased almost 50% |
| | Transient left-to-right shunt at ductus |

### TABLE 16-2 Characteristic Differences between the Immature and the Adult Myocardium

| | Immature Myocardium | Adult Myocardium |
|---|---|---|
| Cytoarchitecture | Fewer mitochondria and SR | Organized mitochondrial rows, abundant SR |
| | Poorly formed T tubules | Well-formed T tubules |
| | Limited contractile elements and increased water content | Increased number of myofibrils with better orientation |
| | Dependence on extracellular calcium for contractility | Rapid release and reuptake of calcium via SR |
| Metabolism | Carbohydrates and lactate as primary energy sources | Free fatty acids as primary source for ATP |
| | Increased glycogen stores and anaerobic glycolysis for ATP | Limited glycogen stores and glycolytic function |
| | Decreased nucleotidase activity, retained ATP precursors | Increased 5'-nucleotidase activity, rapid ATP depletion |
| | Better tolerance to ischemia with rapid recovery of function | Less tolerance to ischemia |
| Function | Decreased compliance | Normally developed tension |
| | Limited CO augmentation with increased preload | Able to improve CO with increased preload and to maintain CO with increasing afterload |
| | Decreased tolerance to afterload | |
| | Immature autonomic innervation: parasympathetic dominance, incomplete sympathetic innervation | |

Data from Mossad EB, Farid I. Vital organ preservation during surgery for congenital heart disease. In: Lake CL, Booker PD, editors. Pediatric cardiac anesthesia. 4th ed. Philadelphia: Lippincott, Williams & Wilkins; 2005. p. 266-90; and DiNardo J, Zwara DA. Congenital heart disease. In: DiNardo J, Zwara DA, editors. Anesthesia for cardiac surgery. 3rd ed. Malden, Mass.: Blackwell Publishing; 2008. p. 167-251.
*ATP,* Adenosine triphosphate; *CO,* cardiac output; *SR,* sarcoplasmic reticulum.

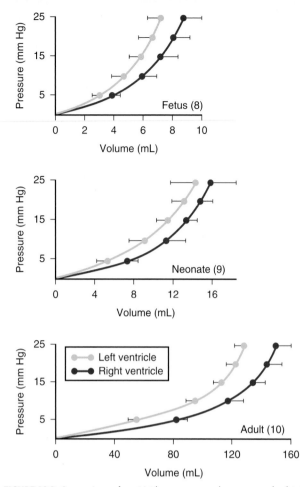

FIGURE 16-3 Comparison of ventricular pressure–volume curves for fetal, neonatal, and adult sheep. Differences between ventricles are significant only in adult sheep. Notice that the right and left ventricles have similar compliance curves in the neonates, making the physiologic relationship between ventricles more intimate (i.e., infants tend to develop biventricular failure). (From Romero T, Covell J, Friedman WF. A comparison of pressure-volume relations of the fetal, newborn and adult heart. Am J Physiol 1972;222:1285-90.)

ischemia. A variety of developmental changes in contractile proteins occur from fetal through early postnatal life, including changes in pH, calcium sensitivity, and adenosine triphosphate (ATP) hydrolyzing activity. The key features of the immature cardiac function are summarized in Table 16-2.

The increased amount of non-contractile tissue in the neonate results in poor ventricular compliance and limited response to increased preload. Compliance of both ventricles progressively increases during fetal life and the postnatal period so that maximal stroke volume occurs at a significantly reduced atrial pressure in the neonate compared with the fetus (Figs. 16-3 and 16-4).[27-29] The extraordinarily high metabolic rate of the neonate (oxygen consumption, 6 to 8 mL/kg/min, compared with 2 to 3 mL/kg/min in the adult) requires a proportional increase in cardiac output. The neonatal heart functions at close to maximal rate and stroke volume just to meet the basic demands for oxygen delivery.[30,31] The cardiac output is commonly described as being primarily heart rate (HR) dependent due to a fixed stroke volume, but echocardiographic studies in human fetuses and neonates clearly demonstrate the capacity to increase stroke volume

(Fig. 16-5).[32] In fact, the neonate employs both tachycardia and stroke volume adjustments simply to meet metabolic demand. On the other hand, neonates exhibit exquisite sensitivity to pharmacologic agents that produce negative inotropic or chronotropic effects. At birth both ventricles are equal in mass and connected via a common septum. Increased pressures in one ventricle lead to a septal shift and decreased compliance of the opposite ventricle, causing a reduction in cardiac output. Neonates and infants often present with biventricular failure as a result of this interventricular dependence.

Immature autonomic regulation of cardiac function persists throughout the neonatal period. Both sympathetic and parasympathetic innervation of the heart can be demonstrated at birth. However, evidence suggests that development of the sympathetic nervous system is incomplete at both the postganglionic nerve-receptor level and the receptor-effector level.[33] The sympathetic system reaches maturity by early infancy, whereas the parasympathetic system reaches maturity within a few days after birth.[34] The relative imbalance of these two components of the autonomic nervous system at birth may account for the clinical observation that neonates are predisposed to exhibit marked vagal responses to a variety of stimuli.

## PULMONARY VASCULAR PHYSIOLOGY

At birth, pulmonary vascular development is incomplete. Lung sections demonstrate diminished numbers of arterioles, and the arterioles exhibit thick medial muscularization (Fig. 16-6).[35-37] The pulmonary vasculature matures during the first few years of life. During this period, arterioles proliferate faster than alveoli, and the medial smooth muscle thins and extends more distally in the vascular tree. PVR continues to decrease as long as pulmonary mechanics and alveolar gas composition remain favorable, with a significant decrease occurring immediately after birth due to lung expansion and oxygenation. Progressive remodeling of the pulmonary vasculature facilitates further decreases in PVR (assuming normal physiology) during the first 2 to 3 months of life; by 6 months of age, the PVR has almost reached the level seen in healthy adults.[37]

The fetal pulmonary vasculature is extremely reactive to a number of stimuli. Hypoxia, acidosis, increased levels of leukotrienes, and mechanical stimulation can cause significant and prolonged increases in PVR (e.g., reactive pulmonary hypertension). On the other hand, acetylcholine, histamine, bradykinin, prostaglandins, β-adrenergic catecholamines, and nitric oxide are strong vasodilators.[35] In the first days of life, many pathophysiologic conditions can trigger severe and sustained increases in PVR[38,39] and prevent the normal adjustment to extrauterine life (E-Table 16-2). The acute load imposed on the RV can induce diastolic dysfunction and promote right-to-left shunting via the foramen ovale. Once PVR exceeds the SVR, a right-to-left shunt develops via the ductus arteriosus and patent foramen ovale. This situation is called *persistent fetal circulation*,[40] and it can result in a life-threatening hypoxemia that may require inhaled nitric oxide,[41-45] sildenafil,[46] or extracorporeal support (i.e., extracorporeal membrane oxygenation)[47,48] (see Chapter 19) to provide oxygenation and sustain life.

*Pulmonary vascular occlusive disease* (PVOD) is a term used to describe structural changes in the pulmonary vasculature after longstanding exposure to abnormal pressures and flow patterns in utero and after birth. Lung biopsies demonstrate thickened muscle layers in the small pulmonary arteries, intimal hyperplasia, scarring, and thrombosis as well as a decreased number of

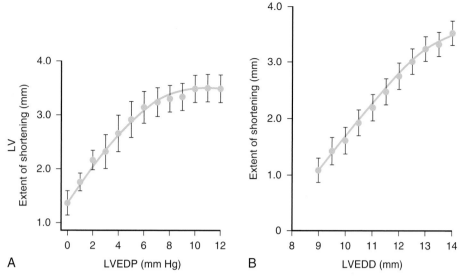

FIGURE 16-4 Frank-Starling relationship in fetal lamb model (gestational age, 135 ± 5 days). **A,** The relationship between left ventricular end-diastolic pressure (LVEDP) and shortening in a chronically instrumented fetal lamb model. Although myocardial performance improves with increasing LVEDP, the effect achieves a plateau at 10 mm Hg. **B,** In the same model, the relationship between left ventricular end-diastolic diameter (LVEDD) and left ventricular shortening. Taken together, these experiments support the capacity, albeit blunted, of the fetal heart to change stroke volume on the basis of volume loading conditions. Each point and vertical bars represent mean ± standard error (SE). (From Kirkpatrick SE, Pitlick PT, Naliboff J, et al. Frank-Starling relationship as an important determinant of fetal cardiac output. Am J Physiol 1976;231:495-500.)

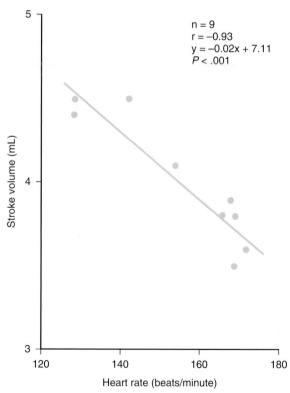

FIGURE 16-5 Doppler echocardiographic comparison of the effect of spontaneous changes in heart rate on stroke volume in a normal human fetus in utero, illustrating decreased stroke volume with increased heart rate. These observations confirm the ability of the fetal heart to change stroke volume under normal physiologic conditions. (From Kenny J, Plappert T, Doubilet P, et al. Effects of heart rate on ventricular size, stroke volume, and output in the normal human fetus: a prospective Doppler echocardiographic study. Circulation 1987;76:52-8.)

distal (intraacinar) arteries.[36] Over time, these changes lead to progressive and finally irreversible obstruction of pulmonary blood flow with increases in PVR and PA pressures. The highly muscularized pulmonary arteries are also extremely reactive to pulmonary vasoconstrictors, which can easily trigger a pulmonary hypertensive crisis.

Many cardiac defects are associated with abnormal pulmonary flow patterns and can be categorized into three basic groups:

- *Exposure of the pulmonary vasculature to systemic arterial pressures and high flow*: The classic example is a large, nonrestrictive ventricular septal defect (VSD) with rapid progression of PVOD.
- *Exposure of the pulmonary vasculature to high flow without increased pressure:* Large atrial septal defects (ASDs) and small, restrictive patent ductus arteriosus (PDA) defects fall into this category. PVOD develops much more slowly in this setting.
- *Obstruction of pulmonary venous drainage resulting in increased PA pressures:* Pulmonary vein stenosis (e.g., total anomalous pulmonary venous return [TAPVR], cor triatrium) or increased LA pressures (e.g., mitral atresia, congenital aortic stenosis, severe coarctation) can cause back pressure in the pulmonary vasculature and induce PVOD.

The muscle tone in the pulmonary arteries is regulated by numerous factors, and various therapeutic interventions can be used to manipulate the PVR (Table 16-3)[14]:

- *Arterial oxygen tension ($PaO_2$):* Alveolar as well as arterial hypoxia increases PVR. A $PaO_2$ value lower than 50 mm Hg, especially when associated with an acidic pH (<7.4), leads to significant pulmonary vasoconstriction. On the other hand, increased inspired oxygen can lead to pulmonary vasodilation.
- *Arterial carbon dioxide tension ($PaCO_2$):* Hypercapnia increases PVR, independent of the blood pH. In contrast, hypocapnia induces alkalosis and thereby decreases PVR. Reliable pulmonary vasodilation can be achieved with $PaCO_2$ of 20 to 33 mm Hg and a pH of 7.5 to 7.6.

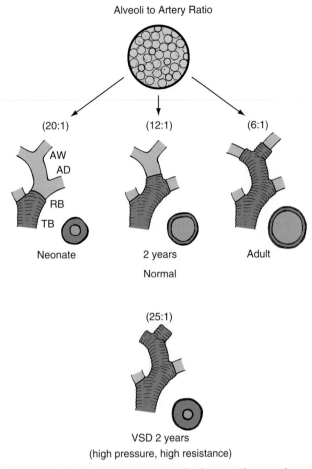

Alveoli to Artery Ratio

VSD 2 years
(high pressure, high resistance)

**FIGURE 16-6** Peripheral pulmonary artery development. The normal pattern of pulmonary vascular development and that of a 2-year-old child with pulmonary vascular changes accompanying a large ventricular septal defect (VSD). Rabinovitch characterized the pulmonary vasculature morphometrically in three respects: vessel thickness, muscular extension, and the ratio of alveoli to arteries seen on lung biopsy specimens. The normal neonate exhibits thick vascular smooth muscle, but this extends only as far as the arterioles accompanying the respiratory bronchiole. In neonates, the alveoli/artery ratio is 20:1. In the first few months of life, the vessels thin substantially and proliferate relative to the alveoli, so that by the age of 2 years, the normal child has an alveoli/artery ratio of 12:1 and thin muscles extending to the arteries associated with alveolar ducts. In the normal adult, the alveoli/artery ratio is 6:1 and muscle extends all the way to the arteries in the alveolar wall. In contrast, in the 2-year-old child with a large VSD, the vessel numbers are markedly diminished (alveoli/artery ratio, 25:1), and persistent neonatal muscle thickness extends all the way to the alveolar wall. *AD*, Artery at alveolar duct; *AW*, artery at alveolar wall; *RB*, respiratory bronchiole; *TB*, artery at terminal bronchiole. (From Steven JM, Nicolson SC. Congenital heart disease. In: Miller RD, series editor. Atlas of anesthesia. vol 7: Pediatric anesthesia [Greeley WJ, volume editor]. Orlando, Fla.: Harcourt Publishers; 1998, p. 6.6; modified from Rabinovitch M, Haworth SG, Castaneda AR, et al: Lung biopsy in congenital heart disease: a morphometric approach to pulmonary vascular disease. Circulation 1978;58:1107-22.)

- *pH:* Respiratory and metabolic acidosis increase PVR; alkalosis reduces PVR.
- *Lung volumes:* PVR is optimized at a lung volume close to the FRC; larger volumes lead to compression of small intra-alveolar vessels, and smaller volumes can cause atelectasis and vascular collapse.

**TABLE 16-3** Manipulations of Pulmonary Vascular Resistance (PVR)

| Increasing PVR | Decreasing PVR |
|---|---|
| PEEP | No PEEP |
| High airway pressures | Low airway pressures |
| Atelectasis | Lung expansion to FRC |
| Low FIo$_2$ | High FIo$_2$ |
| Respiratory and metabolic acidosis | Respiratory and metabolic alkalosis |
| Increased hematocrit | Low hematocrit |
| Sympathetic stimulation | Blunted stress response (deep anesthesia) |
| Direct surgical manipulation | Nitric oxide |
| Vasoconstrictors: phenylephrine | Vasodilators: milrinone, prostacyclin, others |

*FIo$_2$,* Fraction of inspired oxygen; *FRC,* functional residual capacity; *PEEP,* positive end-expiratory pressure.

- *Stimulation of the sympathetic nervous system:* Catecholamine surges from stress, pain, or light anesthesia can trigger significant increases in PVR.
- *Vasodilators:* Most intravenous (IV) agents used for pulmonary vasodilation also affect the systemic circulation and induce hypotension. Alternatively, inhaled substances such as nitric oxide (NO) or prostacyclin can provide a more selective pulmonary vasodilation (see "Cardiovascular Pharmacology").

In summary, the pulmonary vasculature undergoes a complex maturation process that can be influenced by a multitude of external factors and congenital heart defects. Persistent fetal circulation and PVOD are examples of inadequate adaptation and development. In cases of increased PVR, ventilator strategies using greater inspired oxygen concentrations, lung volumes close to the FRC, and interventions aiming for a PaO$_2$ greater than 60 mm Hg, a PaCO$_2$ of 30 to 35 mm Hg, and a pH of 7.5 to 7.6 can improve pulmonary blood flow.

# Incidence and Prevalence of Congenital Heart Disease

CHD can be defined as "a gross structural abnormality of the heart or intrathoracic great vessels that is actually or potentially of functional significance."[49] This definition covers a wide array of defects, which are among the most common congenital malformations. However, the precise incidence of CHD, both collectively and by individual anatomic subset, varies depending on definition, method of case identification, and epoch (E-Table 16-3). Including all categories of CHD, large epidemiologic surveys place the prevalence anywhere between 4 and 50 cases per 1000 live births.[50-53] When stratified according to trivial, moderate, and severe forms, the incidence for moderate and severe forms of CHD is relatively consistent at about 6 per 1000 live births.

Anatomic diagnoses within the population of infants with CHD vary according to the method used to identify cases. In 2002, Hoffman and colleagues compiled 62 epidemiologic studies published after 1955 and investigated the potential causes for the wide variability in the reported incidence of CHD.[54] More recent studies based mainly on prenatal and postnatal echocardiographic screening data often include a large number of trivial lesions (e.g., tiny VSDs, nonstenotic bicuspid aortic valve, "silent" PDA) for which no interventions may be required; other data collections, such as the New England Regional Infant Cardiac Program (NERICP), a registry of children with CHD who died or required catheterization or surgery during the first year of life, are clearly biased toward more severe forms of CHD.[1]

The increasing availability of prenatal diagnostic methods may exert an impact on the relative prevalence of reported lesions as well as their outcome. When fetal echocardiography is used, the apparent shift toward more complex lesions may reflect technical limitations in identifying simple defects.[55] In addition, evaluation in utero skews the results because it includes fatally malformed fetuses that will not survive to term. The prevalence of CHD among spontaneous abortions reaches 20% and remains as large as 10% among stillborn infants.[56] In one study, 50% of women whose children were given a prenatal diagnosis of CHD elected to terminate the pregnancy, particularly when presented with complex heart lesions.[55]

On the other hand, female infants with severe CHD have a 5% lower mortality rate than similarly affected male infants,[1] and with increased survival rates, more females will reach childbearing age. The recurrence risk of CHD for their offspring is about 3% to 4%.[57,58]

A study from Canada examined the changing epidemiology of CHD with respect to prevalence and age distribution in the general population between 1985 and 2000.[59] The prevalence of all categories of CHD in 2000 was 11.89 per 1000 in children (<18 years of age), 4.09 per 1000 in adults, and 5.78 per 1000 in the general population. For the subcategory of severe CHD, the prevalence was 1.45 per 1000 in children and 0.38 per 1000 in adults. In 2000, 49% of all patients with severe CHD were adults, compared with 35% in 1985, and females accounted for 57% of the adult CHD population. The prevalence of CHD increased for both children and adults between 1985 and 2000, although the increase for severe CHD was 85% in adults compared with 22% in children. The median age of all patients with severe CHD was 11 years in 1985 and 17 years in 2000, reflecting the fact that more children with CHD were surviving to adulthood (E-Fig. 16-1). Improved survival may be attributed to improved prenatal care, early diagnostic imaging, and major advances in pediatric cardiac care, particularly for those with severe CHD; these improved outcomes will continue to influence the future demographic profile. The growing number of adolescents and adults with CHD will require long-term follow-up with experienced cardiologists and access to specialized care facilities; this will require a thorough understanding of their underlying pathophysiology by all members of the adult care team, including anesthesiologists.

# Pathophysiologic Classification of Congenital Heart Disease

CHD consists of an almost endless array of anatomic and functional variants. Many different classification systems have been introduced, some using a segmental approach to anatomic features, others by examining the amount of pulmonary blood flow (cyanotic versus acyanotic) or the common physiologic characteristics (e.g., volume versus pressure overload).[60-70] Several of these classifications are discussed in Chapter 14. However, certain defects are better described using the concepts of shunting

(physiologic, anatomic, simple or complex), intercirculatory mixing, and single ventricle physiology, which are presented in the following sections.

## SHUNTING

Shunting occurs when blood return from one circulatory system (systemic or pulmonary) is recirculated to the same system, completely bypassing the other circulation. For example, if deoxygenated blood from the systemic veins flows directly to the aorta, the result is a right-to left shunt with recirculation of deoxygenated blood in the systemic circulation. In contrast, redirection of oxygenated blood from the pulmonary veins to the PA causes a left-to-right shunt with recirculation of oxygenated blood within the pulmonary circulation. The terms *physiologic* and *anatomic* are often used to describe shunting. Basically, any kind of recirculation of blood within one circulatory system is called *physiologic shunting*. In most cases, physiologic shunting is caused by an anatomic shunt (i.e., a communication between the cardiac chambers or the great vessels), but physiologic shunting can also exist by itself, as in the classic transposition physiology.

To really understand the pathophysiology of shunting and its implications, it is important to introduce the concepts of effective and total systemic/pulmonary blood flows. *Effective blood flow* is the quantity of venous blood from one circulatory system that reaches the arterial system of the other circulatory system. Effective *pulmonary* blood flow is the volume of systemic venous blood reaching the pulmonary circulation, whereas effective *systemic* blood flow is the volume of pulmonary venous blood reaching the systemic circulation. Effective pulmonary blood flow and effective systemic blood flow are always equal, no matter how complex the lesions. *Total blood flow*, on the other hand, is the sum of recirculated and effective blood flow and a measure of the workload of the circulatory system. Total systemic and pulmonary blood flows are not equal. Even in healthy patients there is a small amount of normal physiologic shunting (e.g., thebesian cardiac veins, bronchial vessels), but with CHD the difference can be quite significant. Physiologic shunting or recirculation should be viewed as a noneffective, superfluous load added to the essential nutritive blood flow (effective blood flow).

*Anatomic shunts* are communications between the two circulatory systems, either within the heart or at the level of the great vessels. They can be divided into simple and complex shunts, depending on the presence of additional outflow obstructions. In *simple shunts* without any additional outflow obstruction, the size of the communication (the so-called *shunt orifice*) determines the flow characteristics. For small orifices (restrictive shunts) with large pressure gradients across the communication, the size of the opening essentially regulates the amount of shunting. Changes in SVR or PVR have little influence. In contrast, for large orifices or nonrestrictive shunts (also classified as *dependent shunts*), the quantity and direction of blood flow are controlled by the respective outflow resistances (i.e., the ratio of SVR to PVR) (Table 16-4 and Fig. 16-7).

*Complex shunts* are defined by an additional outflow obstruction, which can be at various levels within the ventricle, valves, or great vessels and is often described as subvalvular, valvular, or supravalvular. These obstructions can be fixed (e.g., valvular stenosis) or variable (e.g., dynamic infundibular obstruction by muscle bundles). Shunt flow and direction are determined by the combined resistance across the outflow obstruction and the pulmonary/systemic vascular beds. For severe obstructions

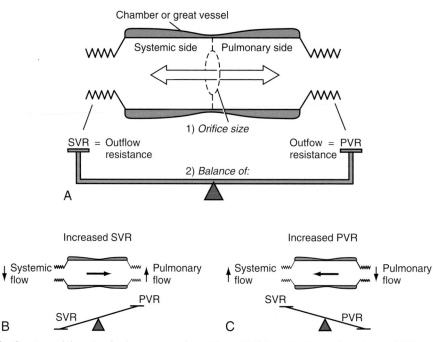

**FIGURE 16-7** Influence of orifice size and the ratio of pulmonary vascular resistance (*PVR*) to systemic vascular resistance (*SVR*) on the magnitude and direction of a simple shunt. **A,** PVR and SVR are balanced, resulting in equal pulmonary and systemic blood flows. **B,** PVR is reduced relative to SVR, resulting in an increase in pulmonary blood flow and a decrease in systemic blood flow. **C,** PVR is elevated relative to SVR, resulting in a decrease in pulmonary blood flow and an increase in systemic blood flow. (Modified from DiNardo J, Zwara DA. Congenital heart disease. In: DiNardo J, Zwara DA, editors. Anesthesia for cardiac surgery. 3rd ed. Malden, Mass.: Blackwell Publishing; 2008. p. 167-251.)

**TABLE 16-4** Characteristics of Simple Shunts (without Additional Outflow Obstruction)

| | Restrictive (Small Shunt Orifice) | Nonrestrictive (Large Shunt Orifice) |
|---|---|---|
| Examples | Small ASD, VSD, or PDA; modified Blalock-Taussig shunt | Large VSD, PDA, CAVC |
| Pressure gradient across shunt | Large | Small or none |
| Direction and magnitude of shunt | Independent of PVR/SVR | PVR/SVR dependent |
| Influence of pharmacologic and ventilatory interventions | Minimal | Large |

Modified from DiNardo J, Zwara DA. Congenital heart disease. In: DiNardo J, Zwara DA, editors. Anesthesia for cardiac surgery. 3rd ed. Malden, Mass.: Blackwell Publishing; 2008. p. 167-251.
*ASD,* Atrial septal defect; *CAVC,* common atrioventricular canal; *PDA,* patent ductus arteriosus; *PVR,* pulmonary vascular resistance; *SVR,* systemic vascular resistance; *VSD,* ventricular septal defect.

**TABLE 16-5** Characteristics of Complex Shunts (with Additional Outflow Obstruction)

| | Partial Outflow Obstruction | Complete Outflow Obstruction |
|---|---|---|
| Examples | TOF, VSD/PS, VSD/ coarctation | Tricuspid or mitral atresia Pulmonary or aortic atresia |
| Shunt magnitude and direction | Relatively fixed | Totally fixed |
| Dependence on PVR/SVR ratio | Inversely related to obstruction | Independent |
| Pressure gradient across shunt | Dependent on shunt orifice and degree of obstruction | Dependent only on shunt orifice |

Modified from DiNardo J, Zwara DA. Congenital heart disease. In: DiNardo J, Zwara DA, editors. Anesthesia for cardiac surgery. 3rd ed. Malden, Mass.: Blackwell Publishing; 2008, p. 167-251.
*PS,* Pulmonary stenosis; *PVR,* pulmonary vascular resistance; *SVR,* systemic vascular resistance; *TOF,* tetralogy of Fallot; *VSD,* ventricular septal defect.

downstream, SVR or PVR will have little influence on the shunt. Tetralogy of Fallot is a good example of a complex shunt lesion. The amount of right-to-left shunt and therefore the amount of cyanosis are influenced by the degree and type of right ventricular outflow tract obstruction (RVOTO). This is especially evident in the setting of a dynamic infundibular obstruction, where changes in preload, contractility, and HR can lead to significant decreases in pulmonary blood flow and increased shunting (Table 16-5).

## INTERCIRCULATORY MIXING

The concept of intercirculatory mixing is often used to explain the unique physiology in children with transposition of the great arteries (TGA). In this cardiac defect, the aorta arises from the RV, transporting deoxygenated blood back to the right heart, and the PA originates from the LV, returning oxygenated blood to the pulmonary circulation (see Fig. 15-6). Unless there is some mixing of blood via an ASD, VSD, or PDA, this defect will result in a complete separation of the two systems, a parallel circulation with 100% physiologic shunting or recirculation of oxygenated and deoxygenated blood that is incompatible with life once the fetal ductus arteriosus has closed. Effective pulmonary blood flow (i.e., deoxygenated blood reaching the pulmonary vascular bed for oxygenation) has to be provided by some form of right-to-left shunt; effective systemic blood flow (i.e., oxygenated blood returning to the systemic circulation) must be achieved by

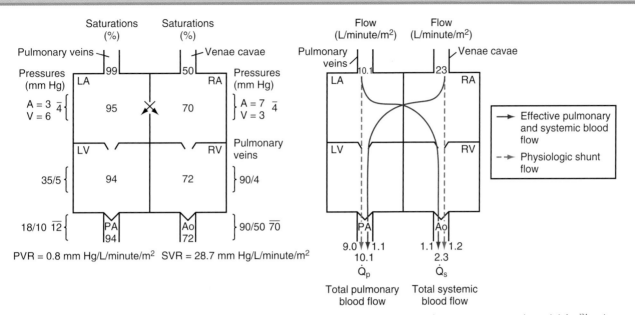

**FIGURE 16-8** Depiction of saturations, pressures, and blood flows in transposition of the great arteries with a nonrestrictive atrial septal defect[134] and a small left ventricular (*LV*) outflow tract gradient. Intercirculatory mixing occurs at the atrial level. Effective pulmonary and effective systemic blood flows are equal (1.1 L/min/m²) and are the result of a bidirectional anatomic shunt at the atrial level. The physiologic left-to-right shunt is 9.0 L/min/m²; this represents blood recirculated from the pulmonary veins to the pulmonary artery (*PA*). The physiologic right-to-left shunt is 1.2 L/min/m²; this represents blood recirculated from the systemic veins to the aorta (*Ao*). Total pulmonary blood flow ($\dot{Q}_p$ = 10.1 L/min/m²) is almost five times higher than the total systemic blood flow ($\dot{Q}_s$ = 2.3 L/min/m²). The bulk of pulmonary blood flow is recirculated pulmonary venous blood. In this depiction, pulmonary vascular resistance (*PVR*) is low (approximately 1/35 of systemic vascular resistance [*SVR*]) and there is a small (17 mm Hg peak to peak) gradient from the LV to the PA. These findings are compatible with the high pulmonary blood flow depicted. *LA*, Left atrium; *RA*, right atrium; *RV*, right ventricle. (From DiNardo J, Zwara DA. Congenital heart disease. In: DiNardo J, Zwara DA, editors. Anesthesia for cardiac surgery. 3rd ed. Malden, Mass.: Blackwell Publishing; 2008. p. 167-251.)

a left-to-right shunt. Intercirculatory mixing is the combined systemic and pulmonary effective blood flow and is only a small portion of the total blood flow. The bulk of the respective systemic and pulmonary total blood flows consists of recirculated blood (Fig. 16-8). Usually the total blood flow and the volume in the pulmonary system are two to three times greater than in the systemic circulation.

The arterial saturation (SaO₂) is influenced by the volumes and saturations of recirculating and effective systemic blood flows and can be calculated with the use of the following equation:

Aortic saturation = [(Systemic venous saturation × Recirculated blood flow) + (Pulmonary venous saturation × Effective blood flow)] ÷ [Total systemic venous blood flow]

Increasing the intercirculatory mixing will improve the arterial saturations, and in severely cyanotic neonates with TGA, intact ventricular septum, and inadequate atrial communication, a balloon atrial septostomy (balloon dilation of an existing patent foramen ovale or small ASD, either echo-guided at the bedside or under fluoroscopy in the catheterization laboratory) can be lifesaving. Additional measures to improve systemic and pulmonary venous saturations (e.g., blood transfusion, inotropic support, ventilatory strategies) can help to stabilize the arterial saturation.

## SINGLE VENTRICLE PHYSIOLOGY

*Single ventricle physiology* defines the circulation present in a wide variety of complex cardiac defects. It is characterized by complete mixing of systemic and pulmonary venous blood return at either the atrial or the ventricular level; the mixed blood is then distributed to both systemic and pulmonary circulations in parallel. The defects can consist of one anatomic single ventricle with severe hypoplasia and inflow or outflow obstruction of the other one (hypoplastic left heart syndrome [HLHS] or pulmonary atresia with intact ventricular septum) or even two well-developed ventricles with atresia of the outflow tract or severe obstruction (tetralogy of Fallot with pulmonary atresia, interrupted aortic arch). In some lesions, a PDA is the only source of systemic or pulmonary blood flow; these are called duct-dependent circulations. In others, intracardiac communications provide adequate blood flow to both circulations (Table 16-6).

Irrespective of the anatomic features, in single ventricle physiology the ventricular output (delivered by one or two ventricles) is the sum of the pulmonary and systemic blood flows. The distribution of the respective flows is directly dependent on the relative outflow resistances into the two parallel circulations. Oxygen saturations in the aorta and PA are equal. The severity and location of anatomic obstructions and the ratio of PVR to SVR determine the balance of flows to the two circulations

The following equation illustrates the various factors that influence the arterial saturation (SaO₂) in a single ventricle physiology:

Aortic saturation = [(Systemic venous saturation × Total systemic venous blood flow) + (Pulmonary venous saturation × Total pulmonary venous blood flow)] ÷ [(Total systemic venous blood flow + Total pulmonary venous blood flow)]

Accordingly, three major variables determine arterial saturation and the initial management options for patients with single ventricle physiology:

**TABLE 16-6** Examples of Single Ventricle Physiology

| Congenital Heart Defect | Aortic Blood Flow from | Pulmonary Blood Flow from |
|---|---|---|
| Hypoplastic left heart syndrome | PDA | RV |
| Neonatal critical aortic stenosis | PDA | RV |
| Interrupted aortic arch | Proximal LV, distal PDA | RV |
| Tetralogy of Fallot with pulmonary atresia | LV | PDA, MAPCAs |
| Pulmonary atresia with intact septum | LV | PDA |
| Tricuspid atresia 1B (VSD and PS) | LV | LV through VSD to RV |
| Truncus arteriosus | LV and RV | Aorta |
| Double inlet left ventricle, no TGA | LV | LV through VSD to bulboventricular foramen |

Modified from DiNardo J, Zwara DA. Congenital heart disease. In: DiNardo J, Zwara DA, editors. Anesthesia for cardiac surgery. 3rd ed. Malden, Mass.: Blackwell Publishing; 2008, p. 167-251.

*LV,* Left ventricle; *MAPCAs,* major aortopulmonary collateral arteries; *PDA,* patent ductus arteriosus; *PS,* pulmonary stenosis; *RV,* right ventricle; *TGA,* transposition of the great arteries; *VSD,* ventricular septal defect.

■ *The ratio of pulmonary to systemic blood flow ($\dot{Q}_{pulm}/\dot{Q}_{sys}$).* With high $\dot{Q}_{pulm}/\dot{Q}_{sys}$, a greater percentage of the blood in the ventricle (or ventricles) is oxygenated because more fully saturated pulmonary venous blood is entering the heart to mix with desaturated systemic venous return. Saturations greater than 85% can be achieved only by significant pulmonary overcirculation. $\dot{Q}_{pulm}/\dot{Q}_{sys}$ can be influenced by careful manipulations of the PVR/SVR ratio.

■ *Systemic venous saturation ($S_{sys}vO_2$):* For a given $\dot{Q}_{pulm}/\dot{Q}_{sys}$ and pulmonary venous saturation ($S_{pulm}vO_2$), any decrease in $S_{sys}vO_2$ causes a decrease in arterial saturation. Oxygen delivery and consumption are the basic determinants for $SvO_2$. Adequate oxygen delivery depends on cardiac output and arterial oxygen content and thus on hemoglobin levels and arterial saturation. All measures that increase oxygen delivery (e.g., transfusion to raise hematocrit levels to between 45% and 50%) or decrease consumption (e.g., adequate analgesia and sedation during painful procedures) improve arterial saturations.

■ *Pulmonary venous saturation ($S_{pulm}vO_2$):* Normally the blood in the pulmonary veins should be fully saturated ($S_{pulm}vO_2$ = 100%) on room air, but lung disease, $\dot{V}/\dot{Q}$ mismatch, or large intrapulmonary shunts can cause significant desaturations. $\dot{V}/\dot{Q}$ mismatch usually responds to therapy with increased inspired oxygen, whereas intrapulmonary shunts are refractory to oxygen therapy. Pulmonary venous desaturation will decrease arterial saturations.

## Special Situations

### EXERCISE PHYSIOLOGY IN THE CHILD WITH REPAIRED CONGENITAL HEART DISEASE

As summarized in E-Table 16-4, children with CHD, including those with lesions considered repaired, exhibit an array of abnormalities elicited during exercise testing consistent with reduced exercise capacity. It is worthwhile to review the various exercise testing abnormalities in order to gain insight into the limitations imposed by the presence of congenital heart lesions.

*Oxygen consumption ($\dot{V}O_2$)* is equal to cardiac output times $O_2$ extraction. $O_2$ extraction is equal to the arterial–venous oxygen content difference. Peak $\dot{V}O_2$ is the greatest measure of $\dot{V}O_2$ obtained during a progressively more difficult exercise test. $\dot{V}O_2$ at rest is defined as 1 metabolic equivalent energy expenditure unit or 1 MET (approximately 3.5 mL $O_2$/kg/min).[71] A typical elite endurance athlete can reach 20 to 22 METs, or 70 to 77 mL $O_2$/kg/min, at peak exercise. Activities of daily living require at least 4 METs or 14 mL $O_2$/kg/min. Peak $\dot{V}O_2$ is the best overall assessment of the capabilities of the cardiovascular system, but determination of normal values is difficult due to the effects of age, gender, effort, and lean body mass versus adipose tissue on peak $\dot{V}O_2$. Nonetheless, peak $\dot{V}O_2$ has been demonstrated to be a reliable predictor of hospitalization and mortality in patients with a wide variety of congenital heart lesions.[72]

During exercise, the HR normally increases linearly with increases in $\dot{V}O_2$. Normal peak HR is generally defined (in beats/min) as 220 minus age in years. In children with chronotropic incompetence, which is defined as the inability to increase HR to greater than 80% of the predicted value at peak exercise, the relationship between HR and $\dot{V}O_2$ is depressed. Chronotropic incompetence is an indicator of poor prognosis and is most commonly the result of sinus node dysfunction. By comparison, well-trained endurance athletes have a normal peak HR and a depressed HR/$\dot{V}O_2$ relationship, because they can generate a larger-than-normal stroke volume increase as exercise progresses. The inability to increase stroke volume (discussed later) during exercise results in an increased HR/$\dot{V}O_2$ relationship as a compensatory mechanism.

The *oxygen pulse* is the quantity of oxygen delivered per heartbeat. The peak $O_2$ pulse is calculated by dividing the peak $\dot{V}O_2$ by the peak HR. Because peak $\dot{V}O_2$ = cardiac output × $O_2$ extraction and because $O_2$ extraction remains remarkably constant over a wide range of exercise, $O_2$ pulse is proportional to stroke volume. Determination of normal peak $O_2$ pulse is hampered by the same factors that confound determination of normal peak $\dot{V}O_2$. In addition, $O_2$ pulse overestimates stroke volume in the presence of erythrocytosis and underestimates it in the presence of anemia or reduced arterial $O_2$ saturation. $O_2$ pulse is reduced in patients with impaired ventricular function, severe valvular regurgitation, or pulmonary vascular disease.[72] It is also uniformly reduced in those with Fontan physiology as a consequence of the inability of this circulation to augment systemic ventricular preload during exercise.[73]

The *respiratory exchange ratio* (RER) is defined as the ratio $\dot{V}CO_2/\dot{V}O_2$ (ratio of the volume of $CO_2$ produced per minute to the volume of oxygen consumed per minute). A normal resting RER is between 0.67 and 1.0, depending on the precise composition of protein, carbohydrates, and fat in the diet. As exercise intensifies, anaerobic metabolism commences and the lactate threshold is reached; buffering of lactic acid with bicarbonate causes the carbon dioxide production ($\dot{V}CO_2$) to increase out of proportion to oxygen consumption ($\dot{V}O_2$), resulting in an increased RER. An RER of 1.09 or greater is thought to indicate the onset of anaerobic metabolism and to be consistent with a good effort.[71,72] Because RER increases only if anaerobic metabolism occurs, exercise limitation and low $\dot{V}O_2$ due to musculoskeletal problems or poor effort are associated with an RER below this threshold.

The *ventilatory anaerobic threshold* (VAT) is used to identify the onset of anaerobic metabolism that occurs before peak $\dot{V}O_2$ and is relatively effort and motivation independent. As aerobic exercise progresses, minute ventilation ($\dot{V}_E$) increases in direct proportion to $\dot{V}CO_2$ and $\dot{V}O_2$. When anaerobic metabolism commences and $CO_2$ production increases as lactic acid is buffered, $\dot{V}_E$ increases accordingly. VAT is the point at which $\dot{V}_E/\dot{V}CO_2$ and $\dot{V}_E/\dot{V}O_2$ diverge, with $\dot{V}_E$ rising in proportion to $\dot{V}CO_2$ but out of proportion to $\dot{V}O_2$. An important characteristic of successful endurance athletes is the ability to reach and sustain effort at an anaerobic threshold that is a large percentage (80% to 85%) of peak $\dot{V}O_2$.

Ventilation efficiency can be assessed with the use of the $\dot{V}_E/\dot{V}CO_2$ slope. This relationship is defined as $863 \cdot \dot{V}CO_2 / [PaCO_2 \cdot (1 - V_D/V_T)]$, where $V_D/V_T$ is the ratio of physiologic dead space to tidal volume.[75] The $\dot{V}_E/\dot{V}CO_2$ slope can be thought of as the number of liters of ventilation required to eliminate 1 L of $CO_2$. Normal children have a $\dot{V}_E/\dot{V}CO_2$ slope of less than 28.[72] In order to maintain a normal $PaCO_2$ during exercise, children with increased $V_D/V_T$ and reduced ventilatory efficiency have a greater than normal increase in $\dot{V}_E$ and therefore a steeper $\dot{V}_E/\dot{V}CO_2$ slope. Increased $V_D/V_T$ is the consequence of either reduced $V_T$ in the setting of a normal $V_D$ or pulmonary flow maldistribution and subsequent $\dot{V}/\dot{Q}$ mismatch that increases $V_D$. The latter is the major source of inefficient ventilation and steepening of the $\dot{V}_E/\dot{V}CO_2$ slope in children with cardiac disease.

In children with PA stenoses such (e.g., repaired tetralogy of Fallot), pulmonary hypertension, or increased LA pressure from any cause (e.g., LV systolic or diastolic dysfunction, mitral valve disease), an increase in the $\dot{V}_E/\dot{V}CO_2$ slope is associated with increased mortality. When pulmonary stenosis is corrected in children with tetralogy of Fallot, the $\dot{V}_E/\dot{V}CO_2$ slope and peak $\dot{V}O_2$ improve.

Children with Fontan physiology also exhibit an increase in $\dot{V}_E/\dot{V}CO_2$ slope. These children have inherent nonhomogeneous pulmonary perfusion at rest due to the lack of pulsatile pulmonary blood flow. In addition, there is poor recruitment of distal pulmonary vasculature during exercise. The presence of a Fontan fenestration further contributes to this increase in the $\dot{V}_E/\dot{V}CO_2$ slope by allowing mixed venous blood high in $CO_2$ to be shunted into the systemic circulation. This produces, via central chemoreceptor stimulation, an increase in $\dot{V}_E$ out of proportion to $\dot{V}CO_2$.[76] Fontan fenestration closure eliminates this right-to-left shunt and reduces the $\dot{V}_E/\dot{V}CO_2$ slope but does not improve peak $\dot{V}O_2$.[76] The reason is that the primary limitation to increases in $\dot{V}O_2$ during exercise in Fontan patients is the inherent inability of the pulmonary vascular bed to substantially increase surface area, flow, and preload delivery to the systemic ventricle.

## FONTAN PHYSIOLOGY

Francis Fontan, a French cardiac surgeon, described a new treatment for complex cardiac malformations with only one ventricle in 1971.[77] To decrease the chronic volume overload for the single ventricle and normalize oxygenation, he separated the systemic and pulmonary circulations by directly connecting the systemic venous return (SVC and IVC) to the PA, without a pumping chamber. This created a circulation wherein pulmonary blood was driven solely by a nonpulsatile pressure gradient across the pulmonary vascular bed, with the single ventricle being the sole source of kinetic energy. All other shunt connections were interrupted. The original indication was tricuspid atresia, but over the years the classic Fontan technique has been modified in many

ways and is now used for various complex cardiac lesions with single ventricle physiology, such as HLHS, double-inlet RV, and pulmonary atresia with intact septum (see also Chapters 15 and 21).[78-82]

It is impossible to create a Fontan circulation at birth; high PVR and small vessel sizes prevent adequate pulmonary blood flow. In the neonatal period, palliative procedures such as stage I Norwood operation with aortic arch reconstruction, atrial septostomy, and aortopulmonary shunts (modified Blalock-Taussig shunt) or the Sano modification of the Norwood procedure (RV-to-PA conduit) aim for balanced systemic and pulmonary blood flows, allowing the baby to grow for several months despite cyanosis and volume load on the ventricle. At the age of 3 to 6 months, an intermediate procedure called the bidirectional Glenn operation or superior cavopulmonary anastomosis, is performed. The SVC is connected directly to the PA, providing nonpulsatile pulmonary blood flow, whereas the IVC remains connected to the heart. As a result, the volume load on the ventricle is significantly reduced, but oxygenated and deoxygenated blood still mix and the saturations remain in the low 80% region. By the age of 1 to 5 years, most of these children are ready for the Fontan circulation. With adequate growth and maturation of the pulmonary vascular bed, the resistance should be low enough to allow the complete separation of the systemic and pulmonary flows. The IVC is now also connected to the PA, most often via a lateral tunnel in the atrium or an extracardiac conduit, with or without a small fenestration (small opening in the baffle or conduit connecting the systemic venous return with the common atrium of the single ventricle). The fenestration can provide a residual right-to-left shunt in case of sudden increases in PVR, maintaining ventricular preload and function. This seems to facilitate the adaptation to the new loading conditions, shorten the recovery time, and decrease the incidence of early complications. The fenestration often occludes spontaneously, or it is closed during a cardiac catheterization and hemodynamic evaluation with a special device (Fig. 16-9; see also Figs. 15-11 through 15-13).[83-86]

The Fontan operation has dramatically improved the mortality rates for children with single ventricles, but the success comes at a price: Chronic systemic venous hypertension and congestion has been implicated in a multitude of potential early and long-term complications, including arrhythmias, residual right-to-left shunts, coagulopathies with increased risk for thrombosis and stroke, lymphatic dysfunction with pleural effusions, and protein-losing enteropathy.[87-92] Late cardiac failure and poor functional outcome remain risks for patients with Fontan circulations. The

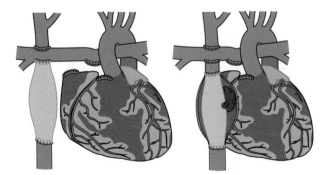

**FIGURE 16-9** Fontan modifications: extracardiac conduit (*left*) and lateral tunnel with fenestration (*right*). (From the Children's Hospital Boston web site. Available at http://www.childrenshospital.org/cfapps/mml/index.cfm?CAT=media&MEDIA_ID=1837)

anatomy of the single ventricle and the type of Fontan connection influence the duration of freedom from complications. Children with systemic RVs and the classic atriopulmonary Fontan (RA directly anastomosed to the PA) tend to have a shorter duration of freedom from complications than those with systemic LVs and newer Fontan modifications (E-Figs. 16-2 and 16-3).[93]

Inherent limitations of the Fontan circulation, such as altered control of cardiac output with decreased hemodynamic response to stress and reduced exercise tolerance, have been documented (Fig. 16-10).[94-102] Even at rest, cardiac output is usually only 70% (range, 50% to 80%) of normal for body surface area. Cardiac output is classically determined by four factors: preload, contractility, HR, and afterload. Over a physiologic range, cardiac output improves with increased preload, contractility, and HR and with decreased afterload. For the Fontan circulation, the determinants of CO are more complex (Fig. 16-11).[97,103] The classic determinants of cardiac output are less effective, while other factors, such as transpulmonary gradient and PVR, must be considered. The following mechanisms regulate cardiac output in children with Fontan physiology.

- *Preload:* The RV usually provides the kinetic energy to distend the pulmonary vasculature and create a preload reservoir for the LV, thereby enabling an increase in cardiac output up to fivefold or greater with exercise.[103,104] The lack of a prepulmonary pump leads to a significant decrease in available pulmonary blood volume and, consequently, reduced or absent LV preload reserve.[97,105,106]
- *Contractility:* During the staged palliation, the single ventricle typically develops from a volume-overloaded and dilated ventricle to a hypertrophied, underfilled ventricle.[107,108] Although the contractile response to β-adrenergic stimulation seems to be preserved, the resulting increase in cardiac output is diminished, most likely due to limited preload reserve.[100,106]
- *Heart rate and rhythm:* Within the physiologic range, atrial pacing at different HRs does not alter cardiac output because there is a simultaneous decrease in stroke volume.[109] Normalization of HR increases the reduced cardiac output associated with severe bradycardia or tachycardia.[110] During exercise testing, Fontan patients demonstrate chronotropic incompetence, a blunted HR response to exercise. This is likely the result of autonomic dysfunction or abnormal reflex control. In contrast to the HR, cardiac rhythm is of utmost importance. Ectopy or loss of atrioventricular (AV) synchronization compromises ventricular filling and decreases the transpulmonary gradient.[111]
- *Afterload:* The Fontan circulation is characterized by increased afterload, which is a physiologic response to decreased cardiac output and occurs because a single ventricle is ejecting into two large resistance beds (systemic and pulmonary vascular) arranged in series.[97,106,112,113] Autonomic regulation and activation of various endocrine systems increase the systemic venous resistance and help to maintain adequate perfusion pressures and venous tone. Because of the limited preload reserve, attempts at afterload reduction often result in significant hypotension. On the other hand, excessive afterload, such as that which occurs with residual aortic arch obstruction, is poorly tolerated.
- *Transpulmonary flow:* Transpulmonary flow is directly proportional to the gradient between the systemic venous pressure (usually between 10 and 15 mm Hg, rarely greater than 20 mm Hg) and the preventricular atrial pressure, which is determined by the functional status of the AV valve, the

ventricle, the rhythm, and the potential presence of outflow obstruction. Transpulmonary flow is inversely proportional to the resistance over the Fontan circuit. This resistance is largely determined by PVR, but mechanical obstruction such as stenosis or thrombosis may also play a role. The geometry of the cavopulmonary connections are also important in that turbulent flow produces energy loss and a reduction in effective driving pressure. It has been suggested that PVR is the key determinant of transpulmonary flow, delivery of pulmonary venous flow to the systemic ventricle, and, consequently, cardiac output (Fig. 16-12).[97,114-124]

In conclusion, the Fontan circulation can be described as a serial circulation with a single kinetic energy pump. Increased systemic venous pressures are necessary to create the transpulmonary pressure gradient that drives flow across the pulmonary vascular bed. Cardiac output depends on adequate preload and low PVR. Decreased cardiac output at rest and limited exercise tolerance are characteristics of the Fontan circulation.

## PHYSIOLOGY OF THE TRANSPLANTED HEART

According to the International Society of Heart and Lung Transplantation (ISHLT), children younger than 18 years of age account for about 12.5% of all heart transplantations. Every year, approximately 450 new pediatric cardiac transplantation cases are reported to this voluntary registry, mainly from centers in Europe and North America.[125] Major indications are cardiomyopathies, CHD, and a growing number of re-transplantations, especially in older children. The average survival time is currently 18 years for infants, 15 years for children (aged 1 to 10 years), and 11 years for teenagers. Ninety-two percent of transplant recipients describe a normal functional status with no limitations during physical activity.[126,127]

As survival continues to improve, more and more children with transplanted hearts will present to operating rooms and sedation suites for diagnostic studies and general procedures. A basic understanding of the physiologic changes in the transplanted heart and the implications of current immunosuppressive therapy are important for safe management.

### Physiology of the Denervated Heart

After transplantation, the function of the surgically denervated heart is primarily dependent on an intact Frank-Starling mechanism and stimulation from circulating catecholamines. The classic Frank-Starling mechanism describes the ability of the cardiac muscle to increase contractility in response to stretch or tension (e.g., increasing cardiac output with increases in venous return). Afferent and efferent denervation has multiple effects on circulatory control mechanisms and leads to significant physiologic changes, including an increase in the resting HR and a blunted response to stress and exercise. Despite excellent physical activity, exercise testing easily demonstrates that heart transplant recipients can usually achieve only 60% to 70% of normal capacity. In the transplanted heart, exercise-induced increase in cardiac output is initially caused by increase in stroke volume, a highly preload dependent process. Tachycardia occurs only later, in response to circulating catecholamines.[128] Further details of the altered physiology are summarized in Table 16-7.[128] The incidence, timing, and extent of sympathetic reinnervation are still being investigated, but the positive effects on cardiac performance have been clearly demonstrated.[129] During standardized exercise testing, transplant recipients with evidence of reinnervation show

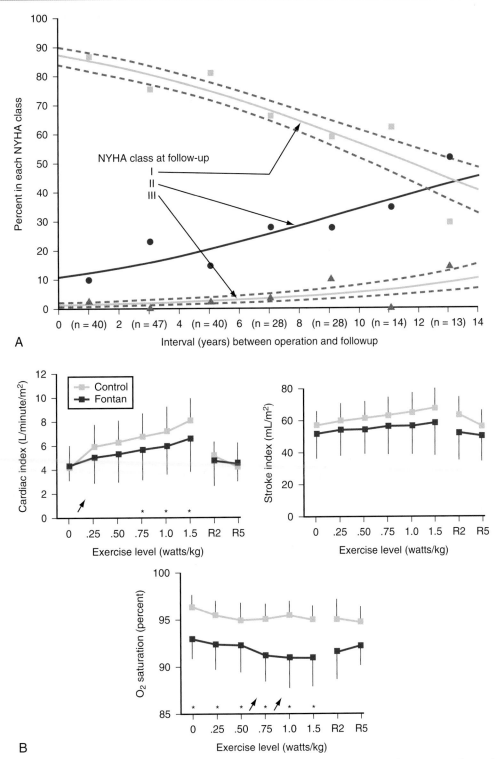

**FIGURE 16-10 A,** Symptomatic outcomes of 334 survivors of Fontan operations who were monitored for 1 month to 20 years. The graph illustrates the changes since surgery in patients assessed as New York Heart Association (NYHA) classification I (*blue squares*), II (*purple circles*) or III (*brown triangles*). Although most children exhibited good functional status (NYHA class I) immediately after surgery, mild functional limitations evolved over time. Broken lines indicate 70% confidence intervals. **B,** Results of exercise studies (cardiac index, stroke index, and oxygen saturation versus exercise level) of 42 children after Fontan operation (*purple squares*) compared with normal control subjects (*blue squares*). Although the protocol was designed to achieve modest targets, significant differences emerged in the capacity of Fontan children to increase cardiac output with exercise, and systemic arterial oxygen saturation remained below normal throughout. The primary reason for the inability to increase cardiac output appears to be an inability to increase pulmonary blood flow and, consequently, systemic ventricular filling. Potential reasons for decreased arterial saturation include intrapulmonary shunting due to arteriovenous malformations and ventilation/perfusion imbalance. *Arrows* indicate a significant difference (*P* < 0.05) in values between consecutive exercise levels. (**A** from Fontan F, Kirklin JW, Fernandez G, et al. Outcome after a "perfect" Fontan operation. Circulation 1990;81:1520-36; **B** from Gewillig MH, Lundstrom UR, Bull C, et al. Exercise responses in children with congenital heart disease after Fontan repair: patterns and determinants of performance. J Am Coll Cardiol 1990;15:1424-32. Reprinted with permission from the American College of Cardiology.)

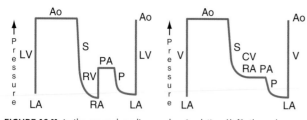

**FIGURE 16-11** In the normal cardiovascular circulation (*left*), the pulmonary circulation (*P*) is connected in series with the systemic circulation (*S*). The right ventricle (*RV*) maintains a right atrial (*RA*) pressure that is lower than the left atrial (*LA*) pressure and provides enough energy for the blood to pass through the pulmonary resistance. In the Fontan circuit (*right*), the systemic veins are connected to the pulmonary artery (*PA*) without a subpulmonary ventricle or systemic atrium. In the absence of a fenestration, there is no admixture of systemic and pulmonary venous blood, but the systemic venous pressures are markedly elevated. *Ao*, Aorta; *CV*, caval veins; *LV*, left ventricle; *V*, single ventricle. (From Gewillig M, Brown SC, Eyskens B, et al: The Fontan circulation: who controls cardiac output? Interact Cardiovasc Thorac Surg 2010;10:428-33.)

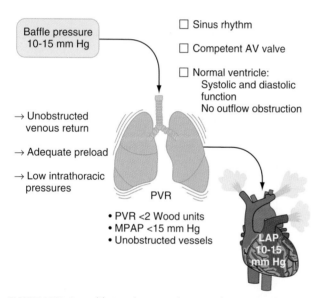

**FIGURE 16-12** Several factors determine the transpulmonary gradient in the Fontan circulation. These include unobstructed venous return, adequate preload, and low intrathoracic pressure on the venous side; low pulmonary vascular resistance (*PVR*) and unobstructed pulmonary vessels; and, on the atrial side, adequate ventricular function, competent atrioventricular valves, normal sinus rhythm, and no evidence of outflow obstruction. *LAP*, Left arterial pressure; *MPAP*, mean pulmonary arterial pressure. (Courtesy A. Schure.)

improved endurance with greater peak HRs and better contractile function.

Chronic denervation also causes an altered response to many medications. Atropine, glycopyrrolate, digoxin, and pancuronium have no chronotropic effect on the denervated heart. Sympathomimetics that act indirectly, such as ephedrine and dopamine, have a blunted response, whereas direct-acting adrenergic agents such as epinephrine, isoproterenol, and dobutamine can cause exaggerated effects and should be carefully titrated.[130] Several case reports have described profound bradycardia and even cardiac arrest after neostigmine used for reversal of neuromuscular

| **TABLE 16-7** Physiology of the Transplanted Heart |
|---|
| Increased filling pressures (LVEDP 12 mm Hg 4-8 weeks after transplantation) |
| Low-normal left ventricular ejection fraction |
| Restrictive physiology (stiff heart) |
| Increased afterload |
| Afferent denervation<br>   No angina during ischemia<br>   Altered cardiac baroreceptors and mechanoreceptors<br>   Less stress-induced increase in systemic vascular resistance<br>   Increased blood volume due to decreased natriuresis and diuresis |
| Efferent denervation<br>   Resting tachycardia (loss of baseline vagal tone)<br>   Impaired chronotropic response to stress (dependent on circulating catecholamines) |
| Altered response to medications<br>   No heart rate response to atropine, glycopyrrolate, and digitalis<br>   Possible severe bradycardia or cardiac arrest with neostigmine<br>   Exacerbated response to calcium channel blockers, β-blockers, adenosine<br>   Exacerbated response to direct acting sympathetic agents<br>   Decreased response to indirect acting agents like dopamine and ephedrine |
| Electrophysiology<br>   High incidence of sinus node dysfunction in immediate postoperative period, normal AV node<br>   Shift to β₂ receptors |
| Possible sympathetic reinnervation: timing and extent variable<br>   Enhanced contractile response and exercise tolerance<br>   Higher peak heart rates during exercise |

Data from Schure AY, Kussman BD. Pediatric heart transplantation: demographics, outcomes, and anesthetic implications. Paediatr Anaesth 2011;21:594-603; and Cotts WG, Oren RM. Function of the transplanted heart: unique physiology and therapeutic implications. Am J Med Sci 1997;314:164-72.
*AV*, Atrioventricular; *LVEDP*, left ventricular end-diastolic pressure.

blockade.[131-134] Neostigmine has been shown to produce an atropine-sensitive, dose-dependent bradycardia in both recent (<6 months) and remote (>6 months) cardiac transplants. Direct stimulation of postganglionic nicotinic cholinergic receptors with denervation hypersensitivity, a direct effect of the old sinoatrial node on the pacemaker cell of the new sinoatrial node, and parasympathetic reinnervation have been postulated as potential mechanisms.[135-137] Avoidance of neuromuscular blockade, use of short-acting neuromuscular blocking agents without reversal, and use of edrophonium for reversal have all been suggested.[133,134] Edrophonium seems to have less effect on the HR in this population than neostigmine.[138]

The denervated heart is also extremely sensitive to adenosine. The magnitude and duration of the effect on the AV node is three to five times greater, and the dose should be reduced by 50%.[139] Calcium channel blockers and β-blockers are associated with exaggerated bradycardia and hypotension. The lack of reflex tachycardia can also lead to profound hypotension with the use of direct vasodilators such as nitroglycerine, nitroprusside, or hydralazine.

### Transplant Morbidity

Children who have undergone cardiac transplantation continue to experience significant morbidity associated with immunosuppressive therapy. Rehospitalization for treatment of infections and episodes of rejection are common, especially during the first year (50%). Acute rejection episodes are a major threat. The incidence decreases from 30% during the first year to 12% after 5 years. Rejection is thought to be associated with the development of cardiac allograft vasculopathy (CAV) or coronary artery disease, which is a major cause of morbidity and graft failure. Indeed, 10 years after transplantation, 34% of children have CAV.[127] Most centers include annual coronary angiography or intravascular echocardiography as a part of regular rejection surveillance. Children with CAV present the same anesthetic challenges as adults with severe coronary artery disease and ischemic heart disease. Aggressive immunosuppressive therapy with induction and maintenance regimens carries its own risks. A detailed discussion is beyond the scope of this chapter, but in general, monoclonal or polyclonal T-cell antibodies (OKT, ATG) and specific interleukin 2 receptor antagonists (basiliximab, daclizumab) are used for the induction phase and various combinations of corticosteroids, calcineurin inhibitors (cyclosporine, tacrolimus, FK506), antiproliferative agents (azathioprine, mycophenolate mofetil), and target of rapamycin inhibitors (sirolimus) for maintenance. Side effects are common and include neurotoxicity with seizures, hypertension, liver and renal dysfunction, hyperlipidemia, diabetes, gingival hypertrophy, hypertrichosis, bone marrow suppression, and posttransplantation lymphoproliferative disease (PTLD).[140]

Several excellent review articles describe the anesthetic management of children with heart transplants (see also Chapter 21).[141-143] A thorough preoperative evaluation with attention to episodes of rejection, presence of coronary artery disease, and organ dysfunction; a detailed medication history with investigation of major side effects; consideration of the denervated physiology; and appropriate choice of anesthetic drugs and other medications are essential components of a sensible anesthetic plan for those with a transplanted heart.

# Cardiovascular Pharmacology

### RATIONAL USE OF VASOACTIVE DRUGS

Many factors influence the selection of appropriate inotropic and vasopressor therapies, including the clinical situation, underlying cardiac abnormalities, and perfusion requirements of other organs. The major goal is to improve tissue oxygenation. Oxygen delivery is principally dependent on cardiac output and oxygen content. In addition to an increased cardiac output (i.e., optimal HR, preload, contractility, and afterload), adequate hemoglobin concentration and oxygen saturation values are often important components. On the other hand, a careful balance of pulmonary and systemic blood flows can be crucial for certain congenital heart defects.

Catecholamines and catecholamine-like agents remain the most commonly used inotropic and vasoconstrictor drugs. It is likely that improvements in cardiac output in neonates in response to drugs such as dopamine or dobutamine are the result of increases in both HR and contractility. Some evidence exists in infants and young children after cardiac surgery that the increases in cardiac output produced by dopamine and dobutamine may be more related to a positive chronotropic effect than to an increase in the intrinsic contractile state.[144-146] With few exceptions, drugs that primarily increase afterload, such as α-adrenergic agonists, have limited use in children. Large increases in afterload without corresponding improvements in contractile state are often poorly tolerated by infants and children,

particularly in the context of significant underlying contractile dysfunction.

### PRACTICAL CONSIDERATIONS FOR THE USE OF VASOACTIVE AGENTS

Commonly used drugs, their doses, and a summary of their effects on selected cardiac functions are presented in Table 16-8. Most of this information has been empirically derived from studies in adults. Limited direct information regarding the effects of commonly used vasoactive drugs in children at different ages and in various pathophysiologic states is available. Neonates, infants, and small children demonstrate unique responses to inotropic and vasoactive drugs due mainly to age-specific pharmacokinetics; differences in receptor types, number, and function; and a high variability in drug delivery. Substantial variations in volume of distribution and measured plasma concentrations have been observed in children receiving inotropic agents. As much as a 10-fold range in plasma concentration has been reported for a given infusion rate.[147-149]

Substantial pharmacodynamic variability (i.e., variability in the serum concentration required to produce the desired effect) can also be observed. Some of these differences are related to receptor maturation and function. For example, it appears that β-adrenergic receptors have a high density in the term neonate and young infant but their coupling to adenyl cyclase may be incomplete.[33,150] In addition to developmental changes, which are to some extent controlled by thyroid hormone, β-receptor and adenyl cyclase activities are diminished in response to sustained administration of exogenous β-agonists and also as a result of increased endogenous catecholamine concentrations, which are often seen as a complication of moderate to severe heart failure and other forms of severe stress (e.g., sepsis).[151-153]

In the neonatal myocardium, chronic catecholamine exposure may upregulate adrenergic receptor number or function, or both, perhaps mimicking the normal developmental program of increasing sympathetic nervous system activity as term approaches.[154] With further maturation in early postnatal life, β-adrenergic receptor density declines. The impacts of various pathophysiologic states on these processes have been incompletely identified. For example, congestive heart failure, cardiopulmonary bypass, and ischemic reperfusion all lead to decreased β-receptor and adenyl cyclase expression and activity.[155-158] On the other hand, the myocardium of infants with tetralogy of Fallot exhibits increased β-receptor density and greater receptor-stimulated adenyl cyclase activity with increased gene and protein expression.[159,160]

One must pay particular attention to technical issues when administering vasoactive infusions to infants. Infusions are often specifically prepared as very concentrated, nonstandardized solutions to minimize the amount of volume infused; hence, the potential for dose or concentration error is substantial. One study at a tertiary care children's hospital demonstrated that the actual concentration of prepared solutions varied significantly.[161] Because of the high concentration of these drugs relative to the child's size, small errors (either in calculation or in infusion pump flow rate) can have a large impact on the actual amount of drug delivered. The extremely small infusion rates can also lead to a delay in drug effect (see Chapter 51). Confirming that the pump drive mechanism is actually delivering drug at the distal end of the infusion tubing, connecting the infusion tubing as close to the child as possible, and using a carrier infusion to "push" the medication at a constant rate are important steps to ensure the

**TABLE 16-8** Inotropics and Vasopressors

| Agent | Intravenous Dose | Comments |
|---|---|---|
| Dopamine | 2-20 μg/kg/min infusion | Primary effects at β₁, β₂, and dopamine receptors, somewhat related to dose; lower doses (2-5 μg/kg/min) can increase contractility and can also have a direct dopaminergic receptor effect to increase splanchnic and renal perfusion; increasing doses increase contractility via β-effects and also increase likelihood of α-mediated vasoconstriction; effects depend on endogenous catecholamine stores. |
| Dobutamine | 2-20 μg/kg/min infusion | Relatively selective β₁ stimulation; also potential β₂ stimulation, tachycardia, and vasodilation, especially at higher doses (>10 μg/kg/min); may be less potent than dopamine, especially in immature myocardium; no significant α-adrenergic effects; tachydysrhythmias perhaps more likely than with dopamine; effects are independent of endogenous catecholamine stores. |
| Epinephrine | 0.02-2.0 μg/kg/min infusion | Primary β-effects to increase contractility and vasodilation at lower doses (0.02-0.10 μg/kg/min); increasing doses (>0.1 μg/kg/min) are accompanied by increased contractility and also increased α-mediated vasoconstriction; may be best choice to augment contractility and perfusion, especially in situations of severely compromised ventricular function, shock, or anaphylaxis. |
| Isoproterenol | 0.05-2.0 μg/kg/min infusion | Pure, nonselective β-agonist; significant inotropic, chronotropic (β₁ and β₂) and vasodilatory (β₂) effects; may be an effective pulmonary vasodilator in some children; tachycardia and increased myocardial oxygen consumption may be dose limiting; tachydysrhythmias may also occur; bronchodilator. |
| Phenylephrine | 1-10 μg/kg bolus, 0.1-0.5 μg/kg/min infusion<br>Preterm and term infants may require as much as 30 μg/kg (see Chapter 15). | Pure α-mediated vasoconstriction; no increase in contractility. |
| Amrinone | 0.75-1 mg/kg repeated twice, maximum 3 mg/kg.<br>Neonates and infants may require loading doses of 2-4 mg/kg and infusions of 10 μg/kg/min. | Increases cyclic adenosine monophosphate by phosphodiesterase inhibition; positive inotropy, positive lusitropy, and smooth muscle vasorelaxation; hypotension; reversible thrombocytopenia. |
| Milrinone | 50-75 μg/kg loading dose, 0.5-1.0 μg/kg/min infusion | Similar to amrinone (antiplatelet effects may be less). |
| Calcium chloride<br>Calcium gluconate | 10-20 mg/kg/dose (slowly)<br>30-60 mg/kg/dose (slowly) | Positive inotropic and direct vasoconstricting effects; inotropy is significant only if ionized calcium is low and/or ventricular function is depressed by other agents; can slow sinus node; increases electrophysiologic abnormalities from hypokalemia and digoxin. |
| Digoxin | Total digitalizing dose (TDD):<br>Premature: 20 μg/kg<br>Neonate (1 month): 30 μg/kg<br>Infant (<2 years): 40 μg/kg<br>Child (2-5 years): 30 μg/kg<br>Child (>5 years): 20 μg/kg<br>Maintenance: 2.5-5 μg/kg q12hr | TDD given in divided doses: ½ TDD followed by ¼ TDD q8-12hr × 2 increases cardiac contractility; slows sinus node and decreases atrioventricular (AV) node conduction; long half-life (24-48 hours) that is prolonged by renal dysfunction; numerous drug interactions; toxicity includes supraventricular tachycardia, AV block, ventricular dysrhythmias; symptoms include drowsiness, nausea, vomiting; toxicity exacerbated by hypokalemia. |

safety and efficacy of drug infusions. The rate of the carrier infusion is also crucial. Most standard infusion setups require rates in excess of 5 mL/hr to effect rapid (less than about 10 minutes) changes in the concentration of drug delivered to the infant and therefore preclude all attempts of fluid limitation.

## VASOACTIVE DRUGS

### Dopamine

Dopamine continues to be the most frequently used inotropic agent in neonates, infants, and children. It has activity at α-, β-, and dopaminergic receptors. Dopamine augments cardiac contractility through two mechanisms. First, it directly stimulates cardiac β₁-receptors and provokes norepinephrine release from cardiac sympathetic nerve terminals. Second, circulating concentrations of endogenous epinephrine and norepinephrine increase significantly during dopamine infusion, leading to the suggestion that at least some of the effects of a dopamine infusion are indirectly mediated via induced release of endogenous catecholamines.[162] Because of its indirect effects, particularly the release of myocardial norepinephrine stores, the response to dopamine may be diminished in children with congestive heart failure or other relatively long-standing forms of hemodynamic stress.

Activity at dopaminergic receptors in the kidney and gastrointestinal tract can lead to improved perfusion of these organ systems. The evidence that dopamine specifically and selectively improves renal perfusion via stimulation of renal dopaminergic receptors (i.e., as opposed to a nonspecific and generalized improvement in cardiac output that might occur with any positive inotrope) is conflicting.[163-167] Regardless of the mechanism, most evidence indicates that renal blood flow and perfusion are increased by dopamine, even at very large doses.

Similar to the situation with other inotropes, pharmacokinetic studies of dopamine have shown wide variability in serum concentration in neonates and children.[168,169] Because of this variability in plasma concentration for a given infusion rate, as well as the wide range of serum concentrations necessary to produce a given effect, doubling or halving a given dopamine infusion rate may be a logical way to approach alterations in therapy. The frequent practice of increasing or decreasing the infusion rate by small proportions (i.e., 5% to 10%) may not be consistent with what is currently known about the pharmacokinetics and pharmacodynamics of most inotropes.

Neonates have classically been considered to have a greater dependence on HR, a reduced myocardial compliance, and a relative resistance to inotropic effects of exogenous catecholamines. Nonetheless, there is substantial echocardiographic evidence of increased myocardial contractility occurring at small dopamine infusion rates (≤5 μg/kg/min) and before significant increases in HR.[170,171] Evidence about the effects of dopamine in sick preterm infants is also somewhat controversial.[164,172-176] There may be a relative dissociation between its effects on the renal and mesenteric beds in these infants, such that a portion of the increase in arterial blood pressure seen with a dopamine infusion is the result of mesenteric vasoconstriction and an actual decrease in mesenteric blood flow.

Although it is generally believed that vasoconstriction is significant when large infusion rates (>10 to 15 μg/kg/min) of dopamine are employed, studies have shown evidence of improved cardiac output and renal blood flow even at very large doses (≥20 μg/kg/min) in neonates and infants.[171a]

The effects of dopamine on PVR are variable. Both minimal effect and increased PVR have been found.[146,177-183] The effects of dopamine on PVR most likely depend on the dose as well as the underlying state of the vascular endothelium and smooth muscle. Vasoconstriction may be more likely after ischemia-reperfusion and in the presence of hypoxia. Conversely, the presence of vasodilators, such as nitroprusside, or α-adrenergic blockers, such as phenoxybenzamine, can prevent increased PVR in response to dopamine.[184,185] Overall, dopamine remains the drug of choice in most infants and children, owing to its beneficial effects on mesenteric and renal blood flow, lesser chronotropic effects than some other agents, and a somewhat reduced arrhythmogenic potential.

## Dobutamine

Dobutamine is a structural analogue of isoproterenol. It was developed to provide relatively selective β-adrenergic receptor stimulation. The inotropic effects are somewhat less potent than those of dopamine, and it has considerably less overall α-adrenergic potential compared with dopamine. Dobutamine does possess significant β2-adrenergic receptor agonist properties, and for this reason it can cause peripheral vasodilation. Substantial vasodilation and tachycardia occur at larger infusion rates (≥10 μg/kg/min).[145,186-189] The tendency toward significant tachycardia and tachyarrhythmia may be greater in neonates than in older children or adults. There is some evidence that the efficacy of dobutamine is reduced in immature animals, perhaps because of greater circulating catecholamine concentrations and alterations in β-receptor expression and function in these immature animal models.[144,145]

Because the actions of dobutamine do not depend on endogenous catecholamine stores, the drug may be more effective in increasing cardiac output in patients with severe congestive heart failure or cardiogenic shock.[190,191] In children with normal LV function, dobutamine has been shown to significantly increase LV relaxation. A decrease in end-systolic wall stress likely contributes to the improved diastolic relaxation caused by dobutamine.[192] As with dopamine, questions of a relative resistance in neonates have arisen, although evidence indicates that dobutamine improves LV contractility in neonates with LV dysfunction.[193] Dobutamine does not selectively improve renal or mesenteric blood flow independently of its effect of increasing cardiac output. The improvement in cardiac output seen with dobutamine is related to both increased contractility and decreased SVR via vasodilation. Pulmonary vasodilation in the presence of increased PVR may also occur.[194]

As was discussed with dopamine, exponential increases in serum concentrations are required to produce linear improvements in cardiac index. There is also substantial pharmacokinetic variability in dobutamine plasma concentrations.[148,195,196] Tolerance may occasionally develop.[197] In one animal study, high-dose dobutamine infusion was associated with significant dysfunction of platelet aggregation after hypoxia and reoxygenation.[198]

## Isoproterenol

Isoproterenol is a pure, nonselective β-adrenergic agonist.[199] It increases HR and contractility and causes vasodilation in mesenteric, renal, and skeletal muscle tissue beds. Isoproterenol is also a fairly effective vasodilator of the pulmonary circulation.[200] Significant tachycardia almost always accompanies its use. The tachycardia and greater contractility cause a significant increase in myocardial oxygen consumption, which is usually well tolerated. However, these changes may be limiting in compromised hearts. The pulmonary vasodilation produced by isoproterenol may be useful in settings in which tachycardia is either unimportant or somewhat beneficial.[201] Systemic vasodilation induced by isoproterenol can be sufficiently profound as to cause systemic hypotension.[182,202] The positive chronotropic effects of isoproterenol may be useful in children with bradycardia.[203] The drug is increasingly used in electrophysiology suites to facilitate the detection of abnormal conduction pathways in infants and children under general anesthesia.[204] Isoproterenol is also a potent bronchodilator. Prolonged use or high doses of isoproterenol and other catecholamines may be associated with the development of myocardial fibrosis.[205]

## Epinephrine

Epinephrine has α-, β1-, and β2-adrenergic agonist effects. Data derived mainly from studies in adults indicate that lower doses of 0.02 to 0.1 μg/kg/min are associated with predominantly β-adrenergic effects. In this range, increases in HR and systolic blood pressure and reduced diastolic blood pressure due to skeletal muscle vasodilation predominate. Doses between 0.1 and 0.2 μg/kg/min have mixed α- and β-effects. At larger doses, α-adrenergic–induced vasoconstriction is significant, and hence there is reduced skin, muscle, renal, and mesenteric blood flow. Compared with pure α-agonists, epinephrine provides significant inotropic effect. The effects of epinephrine do not depend on endogenous tissue catecholamine stores. Based on experience, epinephrine seems to be effective in children who do not respond to dopamine or dobutamine, particularly those with significant dysfunction of the systemic ventricle in the immediate postoperative period. The addition of moderate vasoconstriction to increased contractility may be advantageous to maintain myocardial perfusion and may also increase both systemic and pulmonary blood flow in children with shunt-dependent circulations. Important adverse effects include dysrhythmias (usually ventricular) and, at larger doses, regional ischemia and hypoperfusion due to vasoconstriction. Pharmacokinetic studies have shown a linear relationship between serum concentration and infusion rate, but again there is significant variability in the individual response to a specific concentration.[206]

## Phenylephrine

Phenylephrine is a pure α-adrenergic agonist. As such, its major function is to cause peripheral vasoconstriction. It has no β-adrenergic or inotropic effect and therefore does not increase contractility. It may be temporarily used to improve afterload, systemic blood pressure, and, therefore, critical organ blood flow. But without concurrent inotropic support, an isolated acute increase in afterload is often poorly tolerated, particularly by a compromised ventricle. There are a few situations in which phenylephrine can be extremely useful. For example, it can be given to increase systemic afterload and thereby decrease right-to-left shunting in children with tetralogy of Fallot and dynamic RVOTO ("Tet-spell"). Any additional increase in contractility would worsen the outflow obstruction in this situation. Phenylephrine is also beneficial in cyanotic children who depend on a systemic-to-PA shunt for pulmonary blood flow and adequate oxygenation. The increased afterload may increase flow across the shunt and improve pulmonary blood flow. Treatment of acute hypotension in children with hypertrophic obstructive cardiomyopathy or critical aortic stenosis is another potential indication.[207-210]

## Vasopressin

Arginine vasopressin is a peptide secreted by the pituitary gland. Secretion is promoted by angiotensin II and increased stimulation from hypothalamic osmoreceptors; increased activity from cardiopulmonary baroreceptors and increased levels of natriuretic peptide inhibit the secretion of vasopressin. Vasopressin acts at the tissue level by binding to specific receptors. It causes vasoconstriction via vasopressin$_1$ ($V_{1a}$) receptors and renal reabsorption of water, renal secretion of renin, and synthesis of renal prostaglandins via vasopressin$_2$ ($V_2$) receptors. In addition, vasopressin may mediate vasodilatation via $V_2$ receptors by increasing the release and synthesis of nitric oxide and vasodilating prostaglandins. Vasopressin also sensitizes baroreceptors and therefore may cause vasodilatation by decreasing sympathetic activity. Normally, vasopressin acts primarily via $V_2$ receptors in the kidney to promote water retention. However, during extreme hypotension, vasopressin may act via $V_{1a}$ receptors in the vascular endothelium to induce intense vasoconstriction.

In adults, vasopressin has been shown to be beneficial in the treatment of vasodilatory shock and during cardiopulmonary resuscitation.[211] A few pediatric case reports and small observational studies have demonstrated improved blood pressure and accelerated weaning of inotropic support with low-dose vasopressin.[212-215] However, a multicenter randomized, controlled trial in children with vasodilatory shock could not confirm these findings. Low-dose vasopressin (0.0005-0.002 U/kg/min) had no beneficial effects compared with placebo; there was even a suggestion of increased mortality.[216] Further studies are necessary to establish the effectiveness and safety of vasopressin in children. Currently its role as a "rescue" medication for the treatment of catecholamine-resistant vasodilation during or after congenital cardiac surgery[217,218] and for refractory hypotension in infants with extremely low birth weight[219] is being investigated. A relative deficiency of arginine vasopressin has been reported in some children with CHD who underwent open heart surgery. In a subgroup of children, baseline concentrations of arginine vasopressin were reduced and remained reduced for up to 48 hours after cardiopulmonary bypass. Interestingly, only children with reduced concentrations of vasopressin responded to vasopressin therapy.[220] Extrapolated from adult data, pediatric dosing algorithms currently range from 0.0003 to 0.002 U/kg/min. Careful attention to the infusion rate is important, especially when programming syringe pumps. The literature and common reference tools often cite the doses in U/min, U/kg/hr, U/kg/min or even mU/kg/min, which can be quite confusing and can lead to potential errors.

## Phosphodiesterase Inhibitors

Phosphodiesterase inhibitors, which include amrinone, milrinone, and enoximone, are the most commonly used non–catecholamine-mediated inotropic agents. Their mechanism of action is also relatively straightforward. Phosphodiesterases degrade cyclic adenosine monophosphate (cAMP) to 5′-AMP. Phosphodiesterase inhibitors prevent this degradation and therefore increase levels of cyclic nucleotides, primarily cAMP. The increased concentration of this secondary messenger leads to an increase in calcium availability and thus increased contractility. Because the response is related to an increase in cAMP and not purely to inhibition of phosphodiesterase, the greatest effect occurs if initial levels of cAMP exceed normal values. In this way, synergy exists with β-agonists.[221] The absence of adrenergic stimulation minimizes effects on HR, rhythm, and dependency on endogenous tissue catecholamine stores. In addition to positive inotropic effects, these drugs also have significant lusitropic properties (i.e., diastolic relaxation) and promote peripheral vasodilation.[222-224] Phosphodiesterase drugs may also have substantial antiinflammatory properties that are not well understood at present.[225-227]

## Amrinone

As with all phosphodiesterase inhibitors, there has been an ongoing debate about the relative contribution of systemic vasodilation and afterload reduction versus increased cardiac contractility as the underlying mechanism for improving cardiac output. The bulk of evidence currently indicates that amrinone produces significant increases in myocardial contractility and reduces ventricular afterload.[223,228,229] Evidence of amrinone-induced improvements in cardiac performance in neonates and infants after cardiac surgery has been demonstrated in a number of situations, including postoperatively in children who have undergone the arterial switch procedure and in older children who have undergone the Fontan operation.[224,228,230] Pharmacokinetic data in children suggest that the loading and infusion doses for amrinone need to be approximately twice those reported for adults.[231] In addition to differences in volume of distribution and clearance (both greater in infants), binding of amrinone to the oxygenator membrane may be another factor that needs to be considered if the loading dose is administered during cardiopulmonary bypass.[232] Overall, these data suggest that loading doses of 2 to 4 mg/kg and infusion rates starting in the range of 10 μg/kg/min may be indicated in the neonate and infant.[232] Large bolus doses of amrinone can cause significant systemic hypotension, particularly in the period immediately after cardiac surgery. From a practical standpoint, it may be best to administer the loading dose of amrinone slowly over the period of 1 hour. Caution is also indicated because the elimination half-life of amrinone is large (3 to 15 hours). Other side effects include thrombocytopenia that is reversible, occasional drug-related fever, and increased hepatic enzymes.

## Milrinone

Several studies have demonstrated improved cardiac output and overall efficacy of milrinone after cardiac surgery in neonates and infants and with other states associated with ventricular dysfunction.[233-238] Milrinone has a larger volume of distribution and greater rate of clearance in infants and children compared with adults; adjustments to bolus dosing and infusion rates have therefore been recommended.[233,238] Unlike amrinone, milrinone does not appear to bind to the cardiopulmonary bypass circuit and has less deleterious effect on platelet function. Loading doses of 50 to 100 µg/kg (typically 75 µg/kg) and initial infusion rates of 0.50 to 1.0 µg/kg/min have been recommended.[233,236] Neonates with HLHS who underwent stage I palliation exhibited reduced renal clearance in the immediate postoperative period, and dose adjustments should be considered (i.e., infusion rates of 0.2 µg/kg/min).[239] Milrinone increases cardiac output, reduces cardiac filling pressures, and reduces afterload; its effects are typically not associated with tachyphylaxis and are independent of β-adrenergic receptor density or activity. A recent multicenter, double-blind, placebo-controlled trial demonstrated that prophylactic use of high-dose milrinone significantly reduced the development of low cardiac output syndrome relative to placebo after cardiac surgery in high-risk pediatric subjects.[235] Milrinone is also increasingly used to improve oxygenation in neonates with persistent pulmonary hypertension who are unresponsive to therapy with nitric oxide.[240] Animal studies have shown that IV or inhaled milrinone enhances the response of the pulmonary vasculature to iloprost and prostacyclin.[241,242]

## Enoximone

Enoximone is a phosphodiesterase inhibitor that has been used extensively in Europe but is not currently available in the United States. Its properties are similar to those of the other members of its class.[222,243] Improvements in indirect indices of cardiac function, such as mixed venous oxygen saturation, ventricular filling pressures, and systemic arterial blood pressure, were observed in infants treated with enoximone after cardiac surgery. In addition, the length of hospital stay was reduced.[244] Enoximone was also useful to support cardiac function and potentially reduce PVR in children after cardiac transplantation.[245]

## Digoxin

Digoxin remains the most frequently administered oral inotropic agent. Its efficacy in children with congestive heart failure due to large left-to-right shunts has been questioned. The clinical picture in such children often improved without echocardiographic evidence of increased contractility, and frequently progressive ventricular dilatation was observed.[246,247] Use of digoxin to improve RV dysfunction due to pulmonary hypertension or as part of a multimodel therapy during the interstage phase for infants with single ventricle physiology has also been debated.[248]

Digoxin has both direct and indirect effects. Its direct effects are mediated by inhibition of the membrane sodium-potassium ATPase and thereby outward sodium ion flux. The resulting increased intracellular sodium concentration stimulates the membrane sodium-calcium exchanger, producing increased intracellular calcium and positive inotropic effect. The indirect effects of digoxin are mediated by stimulation of the parasympathetic nervous system. The parasympathetic effects of digoxin result in slowing of atrial and AV node conduction. The drug can also be used to slow down the ventricular response in atrial flutter and atrial fibrillation and to treat supraventricular tachycardia (SVT) (see later discussion).

Because digoxin has a slow distribution phase after oral administration and a long elimination half-life (up to 1 to 2 days in neonates and young infants), a loading dose is usually administered (see Table 16-8). Renal dysfunction can significantly prolong the elimination half-life. Therapeutic digoxin levels are between 0.5 and 2.0 ng/mL. IV and oral dosing regimens are the same, although the onset of electrophysiologic effects from IV dosing is much more rapid (5 to 20 minutes).

Many drugs interact with digoxin and influence its pharmacokinetics. It should be assumed that almost any drug administered along with digoxin can affect the absorption and clearance, usually necessitating a reduction in dose.[249,250] The likelihood of digoxin toxicity increases with serum concentrations greater than 3 ng/mL.[251,252] Symptoms of toxicity include drowsiness, nausea, and vomiting. Various conduction abnormalities and SVT are the most frequent cardiac rhythm manifestations of digoxin toxicity in infants and young children. Older children and adults are more likely to experience AV block, ventricular dysrhythmias, junctional tachycardia, and premature ventricular contractions. Hypokalemia, specifically intracellular potassium depletion (often a result of longstanding diuretic use), exacerbates the proarrhythmogenic effects of digoxin.

## CALCIUM

The role, mechanisms of action, and potential for deleterious consequences of IV calcium continue to be controversial.[253] It is the ionized calcium concentration that is important for myocardial function. Calcium is a positive inotrope, particularly when it is administered in the presence of ionized hypocalcemia. It may also improve ventricular contractility when LV function is depressed by halothane, β-adrenergic blockade, or disease (e.g., sepsis).[254,255] In the presence of a normal myocardium and normal ionized calcium concentrations, the effects of IV calcium on contractility are much more modest.[256] Extracellular calcium levels also play an important role in the regulation of peripheral vascular resistance. A calcium-sensing receptor (CaSR) has been identified on vascular cell walls.[257]

There is evidence in adults that the primary effect of calcium administered after cardiac surgery is to increase SVR and mean arterial pressure with little or no effect on intrinsic myocardial contractility.[253,258] In fact, the increase in afterload, if not accompanied by a corresponding increase in contractility, may only serve to decrease stroke volume and cardiac output. Calcium may cause or exacerbate reperfusion injury and cellular damage by mechanisms that include activation of calcium-dependent proteases and phospholipases and organelle damage due to cellular calcium overload.[259,260] These concerns are particularly relevant in children immediately after cardiac surgery. IV calcium may also attenuate the β-adrenergic effects of concurrently administered epinephrine.[253]

The role of IV calcium administration in neonates and young infants, both alone and after cardiac surgery, is more complicated. Preterm and term neonates have erratic calcium handling and are prone to ionized hypocalcemia.[261,262] The neonatal myocardium is more sensitive to ionized hypocalcemia than the adult myocardium, owing to reduced intracellular calcium stores, immaturity of sarcoplasmic reticulum calcium-handling mechanisms, and greater dependency on transmembrane calcium flux for excitation-contraction coupling.[263] Furthermore, the need to administer

**16**

substantial volumes of citrated and albumin-containing blood products (both of which bind calcium) and other fluids after cardiopulmonary bypass increases the likelihood of ionized hypocalcemia.[264] The most prudent approach includes awareness of the greater dependency of the immature myocardium on extracellular calcium, monitoring of ionized calcium concentrations, and careful administration to maintain normal, or at most mildly increased, ionized calcium concentrations. This approach is particularly needed in neonates and in those with diminished LV function. Administration of large bolus doses of calcium immediately on reperfusion of the heart after a period of ischemia is probably ill advised because of the potential to exacerbate reperfusion injury and even to cause myocardial contracture.

Extravasation of calcium can cause local venous irritation and significant tissue necrosis. Although it has been suggested that calcium gluconate may cause less harm in this regard than calcium chloride, we recommend that both forms be administered via a centrally positioned catheter whenever possible. Both forms of calcium increase ionized calcium concentrations similarly when equal amounts of elemental calcium are administered.[265] Calcium may cause significant slowing of AV conduction and should be administered cautiously in children with sinus bradycardia or junctional rhythm. Care must also be exercised when administering calcium to children who are receiving digoxin, particularly in the presence of concurrent hypokalemia, because IV calcium exacerbates the potential for digoxin-induced dysrhythmias in this setting.

## TRIIODOTHYRONINE

Triiodothyronine hormone ($T_3$) is essential for the maturation of sarcolemmal calcium channels, myosin, actin, and troponin. In addition, hypothyroid rats demonstrate reduced numbers of β-receptors and reduced density of stimulatory secondary messenger protein with an increase in inhibitory secondary messenger protein density. $T_3$ is mostly produced by monodeiodination of thyroxine. This process is inhibited by surgery, hypothermia, catecholamines, propranolol, and amiodarone; therefore, postoperative $T_3$ levels are often reduced.[266-268]

$T_3$ replacement therapy acts via two pathways, intranuclear and extranuclear. Intranuclear effects include an increase in mitochondrial density and respiration, an increase in contractile protein synthesis, and an upregulation in β-adrenoceptors. Extranuclear effects include an improvement in glucose transport, increased stimulation of L-type calcium channels with subsequent calcium mobility, and increased efficiency in calcium reuptake with subsequent improvement in diastolic relaxation.

Endocrine function is compromised after cardiac surgery. Infants younger than 3 months of age with low $T_3$ concentrations on intensive care admission after cardiac surgery have a more complicated intensive care course. Low cortisol concentration is common in the early postoperative period but is not associated with postoperative complications.[269] A randomized, double-blind, placebo-controlled study of $T_3$ administration in children undergoing simple or complex cardiac surgery demonstrated that myocardial function was better and length of stay in the intensive care unit was decreased in the $T_3$ group.[270] $T_3$ improved contractility without any associated increase in oxygen consumption. In addition, the $T_3$ group demonstrated no delay in recovery of thyroid function secondary to exogenous administration. The dose of $T_3$ used was 2 µg/kg on day 1 followed by 1 µg/kg on days 2 through 12. Many of the follow-up studies have been flawed by small numbers and significant patient heterogenicity,

and routine postoperative $T_3$ replacement therapy remains controversial.[271-274]

## CALCIUM-SENSITIZING AGENTS

### Levosimendan

Calcium-sensitizing agents represent a relatively new class of drugs with inotropic properties. Levosimendan is one of the best studied drugs in this class. Although its mechanism of action is not entirely clear, it seems to maintain the calcium-binding site of troponin C in its active conformation. This shifts the calcium binding–concentration relationship toward increased binding (i.e., more binding at reduced intracardiac calcium concentrations). Contraction is thereby enhanced for a given cytosolic calcium concentration. In contrast to other types of inotropic agents, myocardial contractility is greater with minimal increase in oxygen demand. The concept of increasing the sensitivity to calcium rather than the cellular calcium concentration is also attractive because it reduces the deleterious effects of increased calcium concentrations on oxygen consumption, mitochondrial function, and activation of various calcium-dependent proteases and phospholipases (e.g., during ischemia-reperfusion).

Levosimendan has also been shown to stimulate membrane and mitochondrial potassium-sensitive ATP ($K_{ATP}$) channels. The former dilates both the coronary and the peripheral vasculature. Opening mitochondrial $K_{ATP}$ channels is likely to be an important mechanism of pharmacologic (and anesthetic) preconditioning and potential cytoprotection. Interestingly, and for reasons that are not entirely clear, levosimendan has either no effect or a positive effect on lusitropy (diastolic relaxation). At much larger doses than clinically used, it does inhibit phosphodiesterase III. Compared with other inotropic agents (e.g., dopamine, amrinone, milrinone), its efficacy as a positive inotrope is maintained in the depressed myocardium. Both its mechanism of action and experience thus far indicate limited, if any, potential to stimulate arrhythmias.[275]

Clinical effects include improved cardiac output, reduced ventricular filling pressures, and decreased PVR during the acute treatment of adult patients with either stable or decompensated heart failure.[276-279] However, mortality studies failed to show any improvements in short- or long-term prognosis for acute heart failure with levosimendan compared to dobutamine or placebo.[280] Other investigations demonstrated improved cardiac performance after cardiotomy and bypass, including beneficial responses in adult patients who appeared to be poorly responsive to other inotropes.[281-286] Beneficial effects were also found with levosimendan pretreatment directly before bypass.[287]

Current recommendations suggest a 6- to 12-µg/kg loading dose followed by an infusion of 0.05 to 0.2 µg/kg/min. The drug's elimination half-life is approximately 1 hour. There is at least one metabolite that has prolonged (approximately 80 hours) effects, and this may, in part, account for observations of sustained benefit after discontinuation of the drug.[288] There are limited data available regarding its use in children or immature animal preparations.[289-297] One study in a relatively small, heterogeneous group of inotrope-dependent children with acute or end-stage heart failure demonstrated significant reductions in the use of inotropes in both groups and improved ejection fraction in those with acute heart failure.[294] Another study compared milrinone and levosimendan in children after congenital cardiac surgery and concluded that levosimendan is at least as effective as milrinone.[291] These early data and the drug's mechanism of action suggest the need for further study in children and a likely indication for use in infants and children with decreased myocardial performance from a variety of causes, including cardiac surgery, myocarditis, and sepsis.[298]

## B-TYPE NATRIURETIC PEPTIDE AND NESIRITIDE

B-type natriuretic peptide (BNP) and its N-terminal precursor (NTpBNP) are members of the natriuretic peptide family. These peptides are released from the heart in response to pressure and volume overload and play an important role in maintaining fluid balance and hemodynamic stability. BNP is secreted from cardiac ventricles in response to increased stimulation of cardiac stretch receptors and increased wall tension. It acts mainly via natriuretic peptide receptors (NPRs) that are present in large vessels and kidneys. Once stimulated, NPRs promote diuresis, natriuresis, and vasodilation and inhibit the renin-angiotensin-aldosterone system. BNP is used as a marker for heart failure in adults and as a monitor for the response to anticongestive heart failure therapies.[299] These markers are also increasingly used to diagnose cardiovascular disease in neonates, infants, and children. The concentrations of NTpBNP are often markedly increased immediately after birth but decrease during the first week of life. Age-adjusted cut points and reference values have been suggested.[300,301] Currently, it is unclear whether these biomarkers can significantly improve diagnostic accuracy or even serve as a prognostic tool.[302]

Nesiritide is a recombinant form of BNP and therefore acts via NPRs to promote diuresis, natriuresis, and vasodilation. Early investigations in the adult population suggested that nesiritide may be beneficial for patients with decompensated heart failure; it seemed to improve cardiac output, reduce pulmonary capillary occlusion pressure, and dilate arterial and venous vessels with only minimal increase in HR or myocardial oxygen consumption.[303-305] However, a recent multicenter study found no significant advantages of nesiritide and only recommended its use as an individualized case-based therapy.[306] Although nesiritide reduces mean arterial pressure in children after cardiac surgery, more extensive studies are required before its usefulness and safety in children can be determined.[307-313]

## β-BLOCKING AGENTS

There are several indications for the use of β-blockers in children, including control of hypertension (both acutely in a perioperative period and chronically), treatment of cyanotic spells and RVOTO in tetralogy of Fallot, reduction of LVOTO in hypertrophic cardiomyopathy, control of HR in thyrotoxicosis and pheochromocytoma, and control of SVT (see later discussion).[314-318] In contrast to the situation in adults, the use of β-blockers to treat chronic heart failure in children is controversial.[319] Important distinctions include β-receptor subtype selectivity, variability in half-life and metabolism, and intrinsic sympathomimetic activity. Even "selective" β-blockers lose their selectivity at increased plasma concentrations.

### Propranolol

Propranolol is one of the most frequently used β-blockers in children. Typical oral doses start at 0.25 to 0.5 mg/kg every 6 hours, titrated every 3 to 5 days; the usual dose is 2 to 4 mg/kg/day. A sustained-release form is available for older children who are able to swallow pills. IV propranolol is administered at doses of 0.01 to 0.1 mg/kg over several minutes; this may be increased if necessary (maximum dose 1 mg in infants, 3 mg in children). Sinus bradycardia and hypotension can be serious

complications, particularly in infants or after IV administration. Propranolol may also cause conduction disturbances at the level of AV node and worsen pump function in congestive heart failure. Other important adverse effects include fatigue, depression, and lethargy. Interactions with the $\beta_2$-receptor may exacerbate bronchospasm and predispose children to hypoglycemia.[320] Propranolol is primarily metabolized in the liver. Significant population variability in its kinetics has been noted. Metabolism is also affected by factors that alter hepatic blood flow and hepatic metabolic enzyme activity. Its major metabolite, 4-hydroxypropranolol, is also active.[315]

### Atenolol

The use of atenolol has been increasing in children.[318,321,322] Compared with propranolol, it is more selective for the $\beta_1$-adrenergic receptor subtype; the elimination half-life is 8 to 12 hours. There is little hepatic biotransformation, and there are no active metabolites. The typical starting dose is 0.8 to 1.5 mg/kg/day in one or two doses daily, with an upper limit in the range of 2 mg/kg/day. No IV form is available. Atenolol does not cross the blood-brain barrier, so some of the limiting adverse effects common to propranolol are absent. At large doses, $\beta_1$ selectivity is probably lost, leading to the potential to exacerbate bronchospasm and hypoglycemia.

### Esmolol

Esmolol is a relatively selective $\beta_1$-adrenergic blocker with several unique features. Its onset is fast, it can easily be titrated to a desired end point, and its effects are rapidly terminated via metabolism by red blood cell and plasma esterases.[323,324] The drug has been particularly useful for the acute control of perioperative hypertension and for treatment of supraventricular tachyarrhythmia (see later discussion). Loading doses between 100 and 500 μg/kg given over 1 to 5 minutes are followed by maintenance infusions of 50 to 100 μg/kg/min. If the desired response is not achieved, the infusion rate is then typically doubled every 5 minutes until a desired response is achieved.

Specific data on pediatric dosing are limited at present.[325] One study investigated the pharmacokinetics of esmolol therapy after an episode of stimulated or spontaneous SVT. The results were similar to the findings in the adult population.[326] A maximum loading dose of 500 μg/kg and infusion rates of 250 to 300 μg/kg/min are currently suggested. A major potential adverse effect of esmolol is hypotension, particularly during bolus therapy. As noted earlier, esmolol rapidly distributes and has a very small elimination half-life (7 to 10 minutes) that is unaffected by organ blood flow or disease. Therefore, hypotension is usually short-lived, but therapy with vasopressors may occasionally be required until it resolves.[327]

### Labetalol

Labetalol has nonselective β-adrenergic blocking properties and is also a selective α-adrenergic receptor blocker. The ratio of α- to β-blockade efficiency is 1 : 3 and 1 : 7 after oral and IV administration, respectively. The primary use of labetalol in children is to control hypertension. The drug has been given intravenously to treat hypertensive crisis, to control hypertension after aortic coarctation repair, and as an adjunct to induce controlled hypotension during surgery.[328-331] Typical doses are 0.1 to 0.4 mg/kg given every 5 to 10 minutes until the desired effect is achieved with infusions of 0.25 to 1 mg/kg/hr. The elimination half-life of labetalol is 3 to 5 hours.

## Carvedilol

Carvedilol is a newer nonselective β-blocker with additional vaso-dilatory and also some antioxidant properties.[332,333] The ratio $\beta_1$ to $\alpha_1$ blockade is 1.7:1. It is primarily used for the treatment of heart failure. In adults, significant benefit has been demonstrated, including reduced mortality, reduced hospital stay, improved New York Health Association (NYHA) functional class, and a somewhat reduced progression of the clinical disease.[334] However, a randomized, double-blind, placebo-controlled, multicenter study of children and adolescents with symptomatic systolic heart failure found no significant differences in outcome between carvedilol and placebo during an 8-month follow-up period.[335] Carvedilol may have differential effects based on ventricular morphology, and further studies are necessary.[336-339] A retrospective review of the initial experience with carvedilol therapy in children showed that adverse effects—mainly dizziness, headaches, and hypotension—were common (>50%) but well tolerated.[340] The ideal dose in children has not yet been determined. Pharmacokinetic simulation studies suggest that larger doses[341] are appropriate, although clinical experience in small patient populations favors smaller doses.[339]

## VASODILATORS

Vasodilators are used in children to control blood pressure during and after surgery, to treat systemic and pulmonary hypertension, and to decrease afterload on either the systemic or the pulmonary ventricle, thereby improving pump function. Vasodilators are also given during cardiopulmonary bypass to reduce SVR, improve regional perfusion, and facilitate rapid and even core cooling and rewarming.

Vasodilators can be divided in several different pharmacologic groups. Direct-acting nitrosovasodilators such as sodium nitroprusside and nitroglycerin are among the most commonly used cardiovascular medications. These drugs directly relax vascular smooth muscle to cause vasodilation. Hydralazine is another direct-acting smooth muscle vasodilator that is occasionally given to children to reduce blood pressure. Selective α-adrenergic blockers, such as phentolamine and phenoxybenzamine, are occasionally used to reduce blood pressure and SVR in the perioperative period. The classic indication is the treatment of pheochromocytoma, but they are also frequently given during hypothermic cardiopulmonary bypass. Ventricular "remodeling" and long-term blood pressure control is often achieved with angiotensin-converting enzyme (ACE) inhibitors. Prostaglandin $E_1$ (PGE$_1$) is a direct-acting vasodilator primarily used to maintain the patency of the ductus arteriosus in duct-dependent circulations. In contrast, prostacyclin and inhaled nitric oxide are vasodilators with relatively selective effects on the pulmonary vasculature. Commonly used vasodilators and antihypertensive agents are summarized in Table 16-9.

## Sodium Nitroprusside

The primary indication for sodium nitroprusside is the rapid and reliable reduction of afterload and blood pressure before, during, and after a wide variety of procedures. For example, it is used to control intraoperative and postoperative hypertension in children with aortic coarctation and other forms of LVOTO. The reduction in afterload may improve performance of a dysfunctional ventricle, particularly in combination with a positive inotropic agent.[342,343] The ability of nitroprusside to

**TABLE 16-9 Antihypertensives and Vasodilators***

| Drug | Intravenous Dose | Comments |
|---|---|---|
| Propranolol | 0.01-0.1 mg/kg slowly | Nonselective β-blockade; bradycardia, hypotension, worsening of myocardial pump function; atrioventricular block; hypoglycemia; bronchospasm; depression; fatigue |
| Labetalol | 0.1-0.4 mg/kg per dose; 0.25-1.0 mg/kg/hr infusion | Nonselective β-blockade; selective α-blockade; ratio of α- to β-blockade is 1:7 for intravenous form; doses (0.1 mg/kg) can be repeated every 5-10 minutes until desired effect is achieved; side effects are similar to those of propranolol. |
| Esmolol | 100-500 µg/kg loading dose (over 5 minutes); 50-250 µg/kg/min infusion | Relatively selective β-blockade; short elimination half-life (7-10 minutes); hypotension, especially during bolus administration; if less than desired response after 5 minutes, can repeat or double bolus dose, followed by doubling infusion rate; non–organ-based metabolism by plasma and red blood cell esterases; infusion concentrations >10 mg/mL may predispose to venous sclerosis; dilute infusion at high rates increases risk of volume overload. |
| Sodium nitroprusside | Start at 0.5-1.0 µg/kg/min infusion; maximum 6-10 µg/kg/min | Potent direct smooth muscle relaxation; dilates both arteriolar resistance and venous capacitance vessels; hypotension potentiated by hypovolemia, inhalation anesthetics, other antihypertensives; variable pulmonary vasodilation; potential cyanide toxicity; reflex tachycardia; check cyanide and thiocyanate levels if >4 µg/kg/min is infused or drug is used longer than 2-3 days. |
| Nitroglycerin | 0.5-10 µg/kg/min infusion | Direct smooth muscle relaxation; predominantly dilates venous capacitance vessels, modest effects on arterial resistance at larger doses; weak antihypertensive effects; variable pulmonary vasodilation; used to facilitate cooling and rewarming during cardiopulmonary bypass. |
| Phentolamine | 0.05-0.1 mg/kg dose; 0.5-5 µg/kg/min infusion | Selective α-blocker, produces mainly arteriolar vasodilation; some direct vasodilation with mild venodilation. |
| Enalaprilat | 5-10 µg/kg per dose q8-24hr | Long duration of effect; angioedema, renal failure, hyperkalemia; potential problematic hypotension with anesthetic agents (see text) |
| Hydralazine | 0.1-0.2 mg/kg bolus q6hr | Maximum 20 mg/dose; direct-acting smooth muscle (predominantly arteriolar) vasodilation; long effective half-life; tachyphylaxis; reflex tachycardia; lupus-like syndrome; drug fever; thrombocytopenia |
| Prostaglandin E1 | 0.05-0.1 µg/kg/min infusion | Direct smooth muscle relaxation, relatively specific for ductus arteriosus; variable pulmonary and systemic vasodilation; apnea in neonates |

*All drugs should be started in the lower dose range and titrated to effect.

successfully treat pulmonary hypertension is variable and may be age dependent.[344-348]

Sodium nitroprusside is an extremely potent vasodilator that acts directly on smooth muscle to cause dilation.[349,350] Its effects reduce cardiac preload as well as afterload. Onset of effect is fast (within minutes), and offset is similarly rapid; the effect ends within 1 to 2 minutes after termination of the infusion. Because of its potency, it should always be administered via an infusion pump in conjunction with continuous direct arterial pressure monitoring. The starting dosage is 0.5 to 1 μg/kg/min. This can be increased to achieve the desired effect. The hypotensive effects of nitroprusside are potentiated by hypovolemia, inhalation anesthetics, and drugs that inhibit the reflex responses to direct vasodilation (e.g., increase in sympathetic tone, renin release), such as propranolol and ACE inhibitors.

Adverse effects of sodium nitroprusside include cyanide and thiocyanate toxicities, rebound hypertension, inhibition of platelet function, and increased intrapulmonary shunting. Rebound hypertension is most likely caused by activation of the aforementioned reflex mechanisms. It can usually be avoided by slowly tapering the infusion rather than abruptly discontinuing it. Toxicity may occur when more than 10 μg/kg/min of sodium nitroprusside is administered, if tachyphylaxis develops within 30 minutes, or if there is immediate resistance to the drug. A blood cyanide concentration of approximately 500 μg/dL has been associated with death in a child.[351] Cyanide and thiocyanate toxicities are rare but may be more likely in neonates and young infants and in those with impaired hepatic or renal function.[351,352]

Cyanide is produced from the metabolism of sodium nitroprusside. Free cyanide is then conjugated with thiosulfate by rhodanase in the liver to produce thiocyanate. A major mechanism of cyanide toxicity is binding to cytochrome oxidase in the mitochondrial electron transport chain, which prevents mitochondrial respiration and ATP production. Signs of toxicity include tachyphylaxis and an increase in mixed venous oxygen saturation and metabolic acidosis. In children who have received prolonged (>24 hours) or large-dose infusions of nitroprusside and in those with organ dysfunction, it may be advisable to measure blood cyanide concentrations.[353-357] Serum thiocyanate concentrations may also be measured. Thiocyanate concentrations may increase if renal function is abnormal. Central nervous system (CNS) dysfunction can occur when thiocyanate concentrations reach 5 to 10 mg/dL. Treatment of cyanide toxicity consists of IV infusion of sodium nitrite, 6 mg/kg (maximum dose 300 mg) over 5 minutes, and sodium thiosulfate, 250 mg/kg or 7 g/m$^2$ (maximum dose 12.5 g) over 15 minutes. In children with abnormal renal function in whom stimulating the production of thiocyanate from thiosulfate may be contraindicated, administration of hydroxocobalamin has been recommended.[357a,357b]

## Nitroglycerin

Nitroglycerin is primarily a venodilator that acts on venous capacitance vessels. It has a substantially smaller effect on arteriolar smooth muscle, and its ability to attenuate an increased PVR is variable. Compared with nitroprusside, it is a poor antihypertensive agent. It has a short half-life and no significant toxic metabolites. Similar to nitroprusside, it may increase intrapulmonary shunting and cause platelet dysfunction. Nitroglycerin is typically administered in doses of 0.5 to 3.0 μg/kg/min. Effects occur within 2 minutes after nitroglycerin is started and resolve within 5 minutes after discontinuation. Mild decreases in blood pressure may be observed at doses exceeding 2 to 3 μg/kg/min.

In case of prolonged simultaneous infusions of nitroglycerin and nitroprusside, methemoglobin and cyanmethemoglobin levels can accumulate.[358]

Nitroglycerin is frequently used during cardiopulmonary bypass to facilitate rapid and effective cooling and rewarming and to improve tissue blood flow. Nitroprusside and nitroglycerin differ substantially with regard to their effects on the microcirculation. Because nitroprusside primarily reduces arteriolar tone and dilates precapillaries, it decreases microvascular blood flow and tissue perfusion more than nitroglycerin does, particularly in the presence of reduced arterial blood pressure (e.g., during cardiopulmonary bypass).[359] In contrast, nitroglycerin dilates precapillaries and postcapillaries with equal efficacy, thereby maintaining stable or enhanced capillary perfusion.[360,361]

## Phentolamine and Phenoxybenzamine

Both phentolamine and phenoxybenzamine are α-adrenergic blocking agents with little selectively for α-receptor subtypes. Their primary effect is to decrease resistance on the arterial side of the circulation, although both possess weak venodilating capabilities. Phentolamine is usually administered by infusion at 0.5 to 5 μg/kg/min, whereas phenoxybenzamine is administered orally initially 0.2 mg/kg once daily, then slowly increased every 4 days by 0.2 mg/kg/day. The usual maintenance dose is 0.4 to 1.2 mg/kg/day divided in three doses. The elimination half-life of phenoxybenzamine is much greater than that of phentolamine. Some cardiovascular centers have found the potent arteriolar dilating effects of phenoxybenzamine and its prolonged elimination half-life to be advantageous, especially to provide adequate vasodilation during deep hypothermic cardiopulmonary bypass.[362-366]

## Angiotensin-Converting Enzyme Inhibitors

ACE inhibitors are administered to children with increasing frequency.[367-369] In the perioperative setting, they are given to control blood pressure after aortic coarctation repair or to relieve LVOTO. In addition, ACE inhibitors are given on a more long-term basis to reduce afterload on the systemic ventricle and to improve ventricular performance in children with congestive heart failure or single ventricle physiology.[248,370] Among the growing number of ACE inhibitors, captopril, enalapril, and lisinopril are most often used in children, although data in children are scant. Adverse effects common to all ACE inhibitors include angioedema, acute renal failure, and hyperkalemia; case reports of significant complications have been published.[371,372] Cyanosis and coadministration of furosemide were shown to be independent risk factors for acute kidney injury in children undergoing cardiac surgery who were treated with ACE inhibitors.[373]

The contribution of ACE inhibitors to anesthetic-induced hypotension remains controversial.[374-377] Angiotensin receptor–blocking agents such as losartan and lisinopril can produce significant and refractory hypotension with standard anesthetic induction techniques.[378] Because of the potential risk of significant and refractory hypotension, which is usually unresponsive to volume expansion and requires substantial vasoconstrictor treatment, it is our practice to discontinue long-acting ACE inhibitors 1 day before surgery.

### Captopril

Captopril has a relatively brief elimination half-life (<2 hours); it is metabolized in the liver and then excreted by the kidney.[379] Oral dosing in neonates is 0.05 to 0.1 mg/kg every 8 to 24 hours, titrated up to 0.5 mg/kg every 6 to 24 hours. Infants initially receive 0.15 to 0.3 mg/kg every 6 to 8 hours. This can be titrated toward a maximum dose of 6 mg/kg/day in four divided doses. Older children may receive 0.3 to 0.5 mg/kg every 6 to 12 hours. The brief duration of effect, necessitating more frequent dosing, has led to increased use of the longer-acting ACE inhibitors (enalapril and lisinopril) in children.

### Enalapril

Enalapril is metabolized in the liver to its active form, enalaprilat. Enalapril is the only ACE inhibitor currently available in the United States that has an IV formulation. It can be given orally, once or twice daily, with daily doses ranging between 0.1 and 0.5 mg/kg. The IV dose is 0.005 to 0.01 mg/kg/dose, one to three times a day.[367] Both enalapril and lisinopril are eliminated by the kidney. The duration of their hypotensive actions averages 24 hours but can extend to 30 hours.

### Losartan

Losartan blocks selectively angiotensin II type 1 (AT1) receptors. In children, it is used mainly in the treatment of proteinuria and hypertension associated with renal disease and seems to be well tolerated.[380-383]

## Hydralazine

Hydralazine was frequently used in the past for long-term blood pressure control in children, but has been largely replaced by ACE inhibitors. In contrast to its effect in adults, its ability to decrease pulmonary hypertension in children was disappointing.[384] Hydralazine directly relaxes smooth muscle without known effects on receptors. It reduces cardiac afterload but may cause significant reflex tachycardia. With long-term use, it may also cause fluid retention, requiring concurrent administration of a diuretic. Oral dosing is in the range of 0.75 to 1 mg/kg/day divided in two to four doses and is slowly increased over 3 to 4 weeks to a maximum dose of 5 mg/kg/day for infants and 7.5 mg/kg/day for children. In the perioperative setting, it is occasionally used intravenously to control blood pressure and reduce afterload. IV doses are administered as a bolus of 0.1 to 0.2 mg/kg not to exceed 20 mg. The effects of IV hydralazine on PVR are variable.[384,385] Tachyphylaxis to the antihypertensive effects of IV hydralazine may occur. Important side effects include a drug-related fever, rash, pancytopenia, and lupus-like syndrome. The elimination half-life of the drug is approximately 4 hours, but the effective biologic half-life may be substantially longer due to significant binding of the drug to vascular smooth muscle.[386]

## Prostaglandin $E_1$

The major indication for $PGE_1$ is to establish or maintain patency of the ductus arteriosus in infancy. It is best able to reopen a closing ductus in neonates up to 1 to 2 weeks of age but may occasionally be effective even in older infants.[19,387]

Ductal patency is important and often lifesaving for duct-dependent circulations—those in which either the lower body is supplied by right-to-left ductal flow (e.g., interrupted aortic arch, critical aortic stenosis, HLHS) or the PDA is the sole provider of pulmonary blood flow (e.g., pulmonary atresia, tricuspid atresia, severe tetralogy of Fallot). Adverse effects of $PGE_1$ include systemic hypotension, apnea, increased risk of infection, leukocytosis, gastric outlet obstruction, and CNS irritability.[388-390] $PGE_1$ infusions are usually begun at 0.05 µg/kg/min and may be increased to 0.1 µg/kg/min or more. The risk of apnea may be related to the infusion rate. Tracheal intubation and ventilation are often required with infusion rates greater than 0.05 µg/kg/min.[391,392] Prophylactic treatment with aminophylline was found to be effective in reducing the apnea risk.[393] $PGE_1$ has also been used to treat primary or acquired pulmonary hypertension with varying degrees of success.[394-397]

## Inhaled Nitric Oxide

An important development in the treatment of pulmonary hypertension is inhaled nitric oxide gas, which can be delivered directly to the pulmonary circulation. Nitric oxide is an endothelium-derived relaxing factor that acts on guanylate cyclase in vascular smooth muscle.[398] Endogenous nitric oxide is produced by endothelial cell nitric oxide synthase. Nitric oxide synthases convert the amino acid L-arginine into nitric oxide and the byproduct L-citrulline. Nitric oxide then diffuses into the subjacent vascular smooth muscle. It produces relaxation by acting on smooth muscle guanylate cyclase to produce cyclic guanosine monophosphate (cGMP), which acts on a series of protein kinases and reduces intracellular calcium levels to inhibit muscle contraction (see Fig. 36-1 in Chapter 36). Nitric oxide diffusing in the other direction from the endothelial cell into the blood vessel lumen can decrease the adhesiveness of white blood cells and platelets. Nitric oxide in the blood is rapidly bound by oxyhemoglobin, which is then oxidized to methemoglobin. From this reaction, nitric oxide is inactivated and nitrite and nitrate are released in the blood. Red blood cell methemoglobin is subsequently reduced back to hemoglobin. The rapid binding and inactivation of nitric oxide in the blood means that inhaled nitric oxide has a minimal effect on the systemic circulation and functions as a very specific pulmonary vasodilator.

Significant reductions in PVR from inhaled nitric oxide have been demonstrated in adults with mitral stenosis, in neonates with persistent pulmonary hypertension of the neonate, in lung transplant recipients, and in children after surgical repair of a variety of CHDs.[399-403] The efficacy of inhaled nitric oxide is in large part related to the ability to deliver it into the alveolus, which is in close proximity to the pulmonary vascular smooth muscle.

Inhaled nitric oxide has found several indications in children with CHD. In the cardiac catheterization laboratory, it is used to assess the reactivity of the pulmonary vasculature in children with pulmonary hypertension. In this use, it can help distinguish between children with fixed pulmonary vascular obstructive disease and those with a reversible component to pulmonary hypertension, thereby facilitating therapeutic management and operative planning.[404-406]

In the postoperative period after the repair of CHD, nitric oxide can be used to reduce PVR and improve cardiopulmonary performance.[407,408] Experience thus far suggests that children with two ventricles who have increased LA pressure or its pathophysiologic equivalent (e.g., mitral stenosis, severe congestive heart failure, cardiomyopathy, large left-to-right shunt, TAPVR) are more likely to respond to nitric oxide in the postoperative period. On the other hand, children with single ventricle physiology often show no or only minimal improvements in pulmonary blood flow and oxygenation after nitric oxide. Some children who do not respond to nitric oxide immediately after cardiopulmonary bypass in the operating room demonstrate significant reductions in PVR with nitric oxide several hours later. Nitric oxide is administered in concentrations of 1 to 80 ppm in oxygen via a special delivery device attached to the ventilator or oxygen delivery system. Inspired gas is monitored for toxic nitrogen oxides, and during long-term therapy with nitric oxide, blood methemoglobin concentrations should be assessed on a regular basis.[409]

## Prostanoids

Members of the prostacyclin and prostaglandin families are often classified as *prostanoids*. All prostanoids are potent vasodilators and inhibitors of platelet aggregation. Since the 1980s, they have been used in the treatment of PA hypertension and are part of the official treatment guidelines,[410,411] even though they are not selective pulmonary vasodilators. Common side effects include flushing, hypotension, headache, jaw pain, skin rash, nausea and diarrhea, and nonspecific musculoskeletal pains. Tolerance can develop over time, requiring increasing doses.[412] In the United States, only three prostanoids are currently approved by the Food and Drug Administration (FDA): epoprostenol (Flolan), treprostinil (Remodulin), and iloprost (Vantavis). Beroprost is an oral prostacyclin analogue that is licensed in Japan and still being investigated.

### Epoprostenol (Flolan)

Continuous IV infusion of epoprostenol has been used effectively for many years in children with PA hypertension of any cause. It improves hemodynamics by reducing PA pressure, increasing cardiac output, increasing oxygen transport, and improving symptoms such as exercise capacity and dyspnea.[413] It has been used with excellent results in the treatment of primary pulmonary hypertension and irreversible acquired pulmonary hypertension in CHD; in children awaiting heart, lung, or heart-lung transplantation; in children with primary pulmonary hypertension; in neonates with persistent pulmonary hypertension; and in pulmonary hypertensive crises.[414-420] The fact that children who were initially nonresponders may respond after prolonged use of nitric oxide suggests that its mechanism of action involves a degree of remodeling, although no absolute mechanism has been elucidated.

Unfortunately, epoprostenol is chemically unstable at room temperature and has an elimination half-life of only 1 to 2 minutes; it requires continuous IV infusion via a central venous catheter and a specific delivery system. Rapid and unintended decreases in the rate, dislodgments or occlusions of the central venous catheter, or pump malfunctions can lead to severe and life-threatening rebound pulmonary hypertension.[421,422] The infusion is usually started at 1 to 2 ng/kg/min and gradually increased over several months to doses between 30 and 80 ng/kg/min. In patients with pulmonary venous disease, IV epoprostenol can worsen the pulmonary edema; it can also increase the ventilation/perfusion mismatch in patients with pneumonia and thereby negatively affect oxygenation. In the acute setting, epoprostenol is increasingly used in the inhaled form to benefit from the selective pulmonary vasodilation and reduction of ventilation/perfusion mismatch.[412,423-425] Some centers have used inhaled epoprostenol as an alternative to the rather expensive nitric oxide, although the currently available delivery systems are far from ideal and may alter the delivered tidal volumes.[412]

### Treprostinil (Remodulin)

Treprostinil was first introduced in 2002, initially only for continuous subcutaneous infusion, but later also for IV infusion in patients who could not tolerate the pain at the subcutaneous infusion site. The hemodynamic effects are similar to those of epoprostenol, with fewer adverse effects.[426-429] IV infusions of treprostinil are started at 1 to 2 ng/kg/min and slowly increased over several weeks to 40 ng/kg/min, occasionally even higher doses (80-120 ng/kg/min). One pediatric study confirmed the effectiveness of IV treprostinil in children.[430] Since 2009, inhaled treprostinil has been used for long-term outpatient management. Because of the relative short half-life, it must be administered every 6 hours.[431-434]

### Iloprost (Ventavis)

Iloprost, approved by the FDA in 2004, is another prostaglandin $I_2$ analogue that can be delivered intravenously or via an ultrasonic nebulizer. It has a very brief elimination half-life of 15 to 20 minutes and requires frequent nebulized treatments (six to nine times each day). In adult studies, iloprost was shown to be beneficial in patients with PA hypertension of any cause, idiopathic PA hypertension, or chronic thromboembolic pulmonary hypertension. These patients demonstrated improvements in hemodynamics and in subjective parameters such as quality of life scores.[435,436] Studies in children are scarce and have involved only small numbers of patients, although numerous case reports are encouraging.[412,437-443] When iloprost and nitric oxide were compared in children with CHD, the two agents produced similar effects.[444] In one study, combination therapy using both systemic and inhaled prostacyclin analogues showed promise.[445] An animal study in lambs demonstrated an enhanced effect of prostacyclin and iloprost when combined with milrinone.[242]

### Beroprost

Beraprost sodium is an oral prostacyclin analogue that is chemically more stable and has a prolonged elimination half-life but nevertheless requires dosing three to four times per day, reaching its peak blood concentration at 30 minutes. Two double-blind studies showed no significant long-term benefit, but there may still be a role for this drug in combination therapy, because improvements have been observed in the exercise capacity of children with idiopathic PA hypertension.[446,447] Case reports of successful long-term treatment with beraprost and of combination therapy using oral beraprost and inhaled prostacyclin have been published.[445,448-450]

## Endothelin Receptor Antagonists

Endothelin 1 is a potent vasoconstrictor that is thought to be a key factor in the pathogenesis of PA hypertension. There are two known receptors on which it acts: endothelin A and endothelin B. Endothelin A receptors are present on smooth muscle cells, and agonist action causes vasoconstriction; endothelin B receptors are present on endothelial cells, and agonist action causes both relaxation and vasoconstriction through different pathways. In addition, endothelin B receptors are involved in the clearance of endothelin.

Bosentan is an oral, nonselective endothelin-receptor antagonist. Adult studies have shown long-term benefit in patients with PA hypertension. Bosentan can cause abnormal liver function tests, although to date no severe liver dysfunction has been reported in adults.[451-455] Two studies in children showed both short-term reduction in PA pressure and PVR and longer-term improvement in symptoms and stabilization of the disease process.[413,456] In addition, three studies have suggested that the dose for children weighing more than 10 kg could largely follow adult guidelines, with the total daily dosage not exceeding 125 mg. There is growing evidence, although few controlled studies, suggesting that bosentan is an effective and well-tolerated therapy in children. Compared with the results in adult studies, hepatic dysfunction was less frequently reported.[457-459]

## Sildenafil

Sildenafil is a selective inhibitor of phosphodiesterase type 5, the isoform that is responsible for hydrolysis of cGMP in the pulmonary vasculature. By preventing the breakdown of cGMP, sildenafil increases cGMP concentrations and potentiates the pulmonary vasodilation caused by endogenous nitric oxide.[460-462] It has a longstanding track record in the adult population.[463-467] In children, sildenafil is currently used as an adjunctive agent during weaning from nitric oxide and also in the treatment of PA hypertension.[46,468-470] A Cochrane review of the efficiency and safety of sildenafil in the treatment of neonates with persistent pulmonary hypertension found only two eligible trials with a small number of children, prompting a recommendation for further studies.[471,472] Oral therapy begins with 0.25-0.5 mg/kg every 4 to 6 hours with increasing doses as tolerated.[473-475] The IV use of sildenafil for postoperative pulmonary hypertension in children with CHD is currently under investigation.[476] The benefit of combining oral sildenafil with inhaled iloprost for the treatment of severe pulmonary hypertension has also been demonstrated.[477]

## ANTIARRHYTHMIC AGENTS

Antiarrhythmic agents have been traditionally categorized according to the Vaughan Williams classification, which is based on the presumed primary mechanism of action. For example, class I agents are sodium channel blockers. They are also called membrane-stabilizing agents because of their ability to decrease the excitability of the plasma membrane. Class I drugs can be subdivided into class IA, IB, or IC agents depending on their effects on the cardiac action potential (Table 16-10). Many antiarrhythmic drugs have multiple mechanisms of action and are therefore difficult to classify. Commonly used IV antiarrhythmic agents for children are described in Table 16-11.

## Procainamide

Procainamide is one of the most commonly used class IA agents in children. It has sodium channel and moderate potassium channel blocking activities (class III effect). Its major effect is to delay repolarization. This effect is more pronounced at faster HRs. IV procainamide is used to treat SVT associated with the Wolff-Parkinson-White syndrome, atrial flutter, and ventricular dysrhythmias unresponsive to lidocaine.[478-481] It may also be effective in postoperative junctional ectopic tachycardia.[482,483]

Procainamide is the only class IA agent that is still clinically used in children, mainly as a short-term IV therapy. A loading dose of 3 to 10 mg/kg is given over 30 to 60 minutes to infants younger than 1 year of age. Older children receive IV bolus doses of 5 to 15 mg/kg given over 30 to 60 minutes. After the bolus dose, an infusion is usually started at 20 to 80 µg/kg/min. Infusion rates in excess of 100 µg/kg/min are occasionally necessary, particularly in infants. Infusion rates are adjusted to achieve procainamide plasma levels of 4 to 10 µg/mL.[484] The levels should be measured 2 hours after each rate change. It is recommended to stop the infusion if hypotension occurs or the QRS widens by more than 50%. Procainamide can have substantial negative inotropic effects, which may be more pronounced in the ischemic/reperfused or otherwise damaged myocardium.

Procainamide is metabolized in the liver to N-acetyl procainamide (NAPA), which has significant class III antiarrhythmic

**TABLE 16-10** Vaughan Williams Classification of Antiarrhythmic Drugs

| Class | Mechanism | Examples |
|---|---|---|
| I | Sodium channel blockers | |
| IA | Increase length of action potential | Procainamide Quinidine Disopyramide |
| IB | Decrease length of action potential | Lidocaine Mexiletine Phenytoin |
| IC | No effect on length of action potential | Flecainide Propafenone |
| II | β-Blockers | Propranolol Atenolol Metoprolol Esmolol |
| III | Potassium channel blockers | Amiodarone Sotalol Bretylium Ibutilide Dofetilide Dronedarone |
| IV | Calcium channel blockers | Verapamil Diltiazem |
| V | Other or unknown mechanism | Adenosine Digoxin Magnesium sulfate |

Data from Vaughan Williams EM. A classification of antiarrhythmic actions reassessed after a decade of new drugs. J Clin Pharmacol 1984;24:129-47; and Fuster V, Ryden LE, Cannom DS, et al. ACC/AHA/ESC 2006 guidelines for the management of patients with atrial fibrillation: a report of the American College of Cardiology/American Heart Association Task Force on Practice Guidelines and the European Society of Cardiology Committee for Practice Guidelines (Writing Committee to Revise the 2001 guidelines for the management of patients with atrial fibrillation). Developed in collaboration with the European Heart Rhythm Association and the Heart Rhythm Society. Circulation 2006;114:e257-354.

effects.[485] Biotransformation of procainamide and NAPA is based on genetic acetylator status (slow versus fast acetylators). In the past, procainamide and NAPA serum concentrations were added, with a therapeutic goal of 10 to 30 µg/mL. Today, only procainamide plasma concentrations are monitored. Oral procainamide therapy is complicated by unreliable absorption, the need for frequent dosing, potential proarrhythmogenic effects, and a wide spectrum of adverse effects. Typical doses are 15 to 50 mg/kg/day, divided every 4 to 6 hours. A sustained-release form (administered every 8 to 12 hours) is available for older children.

The majority of procainamide-related adverse effects depend on the plasma concentration and the duration of therapy. A systemic lupus erythematosus–like syndrome is common, manifested as fevers, pleural effusions, pericarditis, arthralgias, myalgias, and rashes. A considerable number of children demonstrate positive antinuclear antibodies with chronic therapy, but they do not necessarily require discontinuation of the therapy.

## Lidocaine

Lidocaine is a member of the class IB antiarrhythmic agents, which include mexiletine and phenytoin. Proarrhythmogenia is less common with class IB agents. In addition to blocking fast sodium channels, they also reduce the duration of both the action potential and repolarization.[484] As with class IA agents, the effects of these agents may be greater at faster HRs. Lidocaine primarily affects cells inferior to the AV node. It produces its

**TABLE 16-11** Intravenous Antiarrhythmic Agents

| Agent (Vaughan Williams Class) | Dose | Comments |
|---|---|---|
| Procainamide (IA; sodium ± potassium channel blockade; antivagal effects) | Infant (<1 year): 3-10 mg/kg loading dose over 30 minutes<br>Child (>1 year): 5-15 mg/kg loading dose over 30 minutes<br>All ages, infusion rate: 20-80 µg/kg/min | Used to treat SVT due to WPW, atrial flutter, junctional ectopic tachycardia (with patient hypothermia), lidocaine-resistant ventricular dysrhythmias; hypotension and negative inotropy; lupus-like syndrome. |
| Lidocaine (IB; sodium channel blockade; speeds repolarization) | 1 mg/kg bolus; then 20-50 µg/kg/min | Used for ventricular dysrhythmias; CNS toxicity (apnea, seizures, abnormal sensations). |
| Phenytoin (IB) | 1-3 mg/kg q5min up to 15 mg/kg loading dose, then 5-10 mg/kg divided q6hr | Drug must be infused slowly (>30 minutes) due to potential hypotension; antidysrhythmic profile similar to that of lidocaine; may be useful to treat digoxin-induced dysrhythmias. |
| Propranolol (II; β-adrenergic blockade; sodium channel blockade also) | 0.01-0.1 mg/kg slowly | Nonselective β-blockade; used mainly to treat SVT; bradycardia, hypotension, worsening of myocardial pump function; AV block; hypoglycemia; bronchospasm; depression; fatigue. |
| Esmolol (II; B-receptor blockade) | 100-500 µg/kg loading dose (over 5 minutes); 50-250 µg/kg/min infusion | Used to treat SVT; relatively selective $\beta_1$ blockade; short elimination half-life (7-10 minutes); hypotension, especially during bolus; if less than desired response after 5 minutes, can repeat or double bolus dose, followed by doubling infusion rate; non–organ-based metabolism by plasma and red blood cell esterases; infusion concentrations >10 mg/mL may predispose to venous sclerosis; dilute infusion at high rates increases risk of volume overload. |
| Amiodarone (III; prolongs repolarization; adrenergic and calcium blockade) | 1-2.5 mg/kg bolus over 5-10 minutes (total loading dose up to 5-6 mg/kg); 5-15 mg/kg/24-hour infusion | Used for resistant reentrant atrial and ventricular dysrhythmias; may be useful for postoperative junctional ectopic tachycardia; hypotension with bolus IV administration; bradycardia; AV block; rare proarrhythmia and torsades de pointes; pulmonary fibrosis; hypothyroidism; controversial association with acute perioperative lung injury. |
| Bretylium (III) | 5 mg/kg; then 10 mg/kg q15min (maximum 30 mg/kg total) | Use limited to ventricular tachycardia resistant to other therapies during cardiopulmonary resuscitation; hypotension. (No longer marketed in the United States.) |
| Verapamil (IV; calcium channel blockade) | 0.1-0.3 mg/kg bolus (maximum 5 mg) | Used for SVT in older children and adults; potential for hypotension and asystole contraindicates use in children <1 year of age; bradycardia; AV block; may increase ventricular response rate in some children with WPW. |
| Adenosine | 0.05-0.1 mg/kg rapid bolus followed by flush; may repeat with doses increasing in increments of 0.05 mg/kg q2min (maximum dose 0.25 mg/kg or 12 mg, whichever comes first) | Increases potassium channel flux and inhibits slow inward calcium current; causes transient sinus bradycardia and AV block; transient hypotension; rarely causes ventricular ectopy or atrial fibrillation; bronchospasm; used to terminate SVT; used diagnostically to transiently produce AV block. Reduce dose by 50% in heart transplant patients or if given through a central line. |
| Digoxin | Total digitalizing dose (TDD)*:<br>Premature: 15-25 µg/kg<br>Neonate (<1 month): 20-30 µg/kg<br>Infant (<2 years): 30-50 µg/kg<br>Child (2-5 years): 25-35 µg/kg<br>Child (>5 years): 15-30 µg/kg<br>Child (>10 years): 8-12 µg/kg | TDD given in divided doses: $\frac{1}{2}$ TDD followed by $\frac{1}{4}$ TDD q8-12hr × 2; slows sinus node and decreases AV node conduction; used to slow ventricular response in atrial flutter and fibrillation and may also treat junctional tachycardia or SVT; variable effect on accessory pathways; long half-life (24-48 hours) that is prolonged by renal dysfunction; numerous drug interactions; toxicity includes SVT, AV block, ventricular dysrhythmias; toxicity symptoms include drowsiness, nausea, vomiting; toxicity exacerbated by hypokalemia. |
| Magnesium sulfate | 25-50 mg/kg bolus; maximum single dose 2 g;<br>30-60 mg/kg/24-hour infusion | May be first-line therapy for torsades des pointes; also used for refractory ventricular tachycardia and ventricular fibrillation; hypotension and respiratory depression may accompany IV bolus dosing—IV calcium is an antidote. |

*AV,* Atrioventricular; *CNS,* central nervous system; *IV,* intravenous; *SVT,* supraventricular tachycardia; *WPW,* Wolff-Parkinson-White syndrome.
*Daily maintenance dose varies by age; consult pharmacy or cardiologist.

greatest effects on cells with the longest duration of action potential and thereby balances the ventricular repolarization.

Because of its rapid hepatic metabolism, lidocaine is available only in an IV formulation. It is indicated for the emergency treatment of ventricular dysrhythmias. Lidocaine is initially administered as an IV bolus of 1 mg/kg that can be repeated once within 5 to 10 minutes. Standard lidocaine infusion rates range from 20 to 50 µg/kg/min.

The major side effects of lidocaine administration are well known to anesthesiologists. They primarily consist of CNS toxicity, which typically occurs at plasma concentrations in excess of 6 to 8 μg/mL. Mental status changes, abnormal taste or other sensations, apnea, and seizures may occur. In children with reduced cardiac output and impaired hepatic clearance, lidocaine doses should be reduced. The administration of lidocaine to children with atrial tachydysrhythmias or prolongation of the QT interval can increase the ventricular response rate.[486]

### Phenytoin

Phenytoin shares many similarities to lidocaine in terms of its antiarrhythmic effects, which are also restricted primarily to tissues inferior to the AV node and the bundle of His. Phenytoin primarily binds to sodium channels, maintaining them in the inactivated state. Very large concentrations may also affect calcium channels and automaticity. This drug is useful in treating refractory ventricular arrhythmias and especially digoxin-induced dysrhythmias.[487,488]

IV loading with phenytoin is achieved by a bolus dose of 1 to 3 mg/kg. For treatment of status epilepticus, higher loading doses (10-15 mg/kg) are used. IV maintenance is 5 mg/kg/day divided in two to three doses. IV phenytoin must be administered extremely slowly (>30 minutes) owing to the potential for hypotension. The oral dose in infants and older children is 5 mg/kg/day given every 12 hours, after a total loading dose of 15 mg/kg that has been divided over 6 hours. Other typical adverse effects are well described from its use as an antiepileptic medication and include gingival hyperplasia, aplastic anemia, ataxia, and nystagmus. Phenytoin should be avoided in patients who are pregnant or who may become pregnant because of its significant teratogenic profile (fetal hydantoin syndrome).

### Flecainide and Propafenone

Flecainide and propafenone are class IC agents. As such, they have potent sodium channel blocking activity. In adults, flecainide is used treat various tachyarrhythmias, and it has a special role in the pharmacologic cardioversion of recurrent atrial fibrillation in patients with normal hearts ("pill in a pocket").[489,490] Flecainide has also been extensively evaluated in children.[491-498] It blocks activated slow sodium channels but exerts less of an inhibitory effect on potassium channels. It appears to reduce the refractory time and decrease the automaticity in His-Purkinje cells. In contrast, the duration of the action potential and refractory period is prolonged in ventricular muscle, resulting in a greater duration of the QRS complex.

Oral dosing of flecainide may be more reliable when it is calculated on the basis of body surface area. Typical dosages in infants are in the range of 80 to 90 mg/m²/day, given in two doses (40 to 45 mg/m² every 12 hours). Older children receive 100 to 110 mg/m²/day (50 to 55 mg/m² every 12 hours). Loading doses are not used. Serum elimination half-life is age dependent: approximately 1 day in neonates, 12 hours in infants younger than 6 months of age, and 8 to 12 hours in older children and adults. Therapeutic trough concentrations are believed to be in the range of 200 to 1000 ng/mL. Alterations in diet can markedly affect drug absorption with oral dosing. IV flecainide is available outside the United States. A dose of 1 to 2 mg/kg given over 5 to 10 minutes has been used. Continuous infusions are not given because of its prolonged elimination half-life.

Flecainide has mild to moderate negative inotropic effects. Substantial proarrhythmogenic effects have been observed in children with atrial tachydysrhythmias or significant abnormalities of myocardial anatomy and function. Proarrhythmia was considerably increased in adult patients who received flecainide after myocardial infarction.[499] In children and adults with paroxysmal SVT, a slow but incessant SVT may result on initiation of therapy. As a result, it is recommended to closely monitor these patients when initiating therapy with flecainide. The efficiency and safety of class IC antiarrhythmic agents in children with an abnormal or damaged myocardium are unclear; many pediatric electrophysiologists would avoid these drugs in children with severe myocardial dysfunction, myocardial injury (e.g., immediately postoperatively), right- or left-sided hypertrophy e.g., tetralogy of Fallot), or aortic stenosis.[479,500]

The effects and risks of propafenone are similar to those discussed for flecainide. Propafenone can also control dysrhythmias that arise from automatic mechanisms and can be used to treat postoperative junctional ectopic tachycardia. Oral propafenone is administered at 200 to 600 mg/m²/day divided into three doses (for children under 15 kg, 10-20 mg/kg/day and for children over 15 kg, 7-15 mg/kg/day). IV propafenone is not available in the United States. An IV loading dose of 0.2 to 1.0 mg/kg should be given slowly over 10 minutes. The initial dose may be doubled to achieve a maximum 2 mg/kg total loading dose. Infusion rates of 4 to 7 μg/kg/min have been reported.[501-506]

Significant hypotension can occur with a bolus of propafenone. Hypotension has been attributed primarily to its negative inotropic effects. Like flecainide, propafenone is probably contraindicated in children with significant structural or metabolic myocardial abnormalities, such as those related to severe pressure or volume overload, ischemia-reperfusion, or myocardial infarction. In addition, propafenone has the potential for proarrhythmogenic effects. Propafenone is extensively metabolized in the liver, with significant interindividual variability. Its reported elimination half-life ranges from 4 to 18 hours. Serum concentrations of propafenone do not correlate well with the clinical response.[507]

### β-Blockers

β-Blockers are class II antiarrhythmic agents. Mechanism of action, relevance of subtype selectivity, metabolism, and other features are described in the section on vasoactive drugs. Here we focus on their indications as antiarrhythmic agents. In children, propranolol, atenolol, and esmolol are the most frequently used β-blockers.[318]

#### Propranolol

Propranolol is probably the most widely studied β-blocking agent in children.[508] Its primary indication is the acute control of SVT. In addition to nonselective β-blockade, propranolol has effects on the sodium channels and at high concentrations on calcium channels as well. It seems that conduction tissues of neonates are more sensitive to the drug than those of older children and adults.[488,509]

#### Atenolol

Atenolol is a commonly used, longer-acting β-blocker.[510,511] It has more selective effects on β-adrenergic receptors, although the risk of bronchospasm may not be completely eliminated with this drug. Atenolol does not cross the blood-brain barrier, which may be a reason for its lower incidence of depression, fatigue, and malaise compared with propranolol.[322,512]

#### Esmolol

Esmolol is increasing in popularity for the control of perioperative tachydysrhythmias in children.[479] Esmolol acts predominantly on the sinus and AV nodes. It does not appear to have significant antiarrhythmic effects in the His-Purkinje or ventricular conducting tissues. Pharmacokinetics and the efficacy to terminate SVTs were found to be similar in children and adults.[326]

### Class III Agents

The primary class III agents are amiodarone, sotalol, bretylium, and ibutilide. They prolong depolarization and therefore increase refractoriness. All of these drugs have numerous other properties, including membrane-stabilizing effects, calcium channel blockade, and adrenergic blockade.

#### Amiodarone

In addition to prolonging refractoriness, amiodarone has sodium channel blocking and noncompetitive α- and β-adrenergic receptor blocking properties. It may also interfere with potassium channels and inhibit the release of myocardial norepinephrine. Oral amiodarone is absorbed quite slowly from the gastrointestinal tract and is metabolized in the liver to an active metabolite, desethylamiodarone. Because of its high lipid solubility and large volume of distribution, tissue concentrations are maintained for 2 to 3 months after discontinuation of therapy. There are increasing data demonstrating the efficacy and safety of oral and IV amiodarone for the treatment of dysrhythmias in infants and children.[513-517] In addition to resistant reentrant atrial and ventricular dysrhythmias, amiodarone may be effective in treating postoperative junctional ectopic tachycardia.[518-520] Amiodarone, in a dose of 5 mg/kg IV push, is also indicated for shock-resistant arrhythmias during cardiopulmonary resuscitation in infants and children.[521]

The loading dose for oral amiodarone is 10 to 15 mg/kg/day for 5 to 10 days. After the loading dose, long-term oral dosing is 2 to 5 mg/kg once daily. IV amiodarone is usually given in boluses of 1.0 to 2.5 mg/kg, reaching a total of 5 to 6 mg/kg, with each bolus administered over 5 to 10 minutes. In children with resistant dysrhythmias, the average loading dose was 6.3 mg/kg, with 50% of children requiring a continuous amiodarone infusion of 10 to 15 mg/kg/day.[515,522]

Hypotension is the most significant acute adverse effect of IV amiodarone therapy. The effects of amiodarone may be synergistic with those of other agents that depress sinus node and AV node function. Important cardiac dysrhythmias include bradycardia and AV block. Proarrhythmogenic effects and torsades de pointes may occasionally occur. Long-term oral amiodarone therapy can lead to progressive and irreversible pulmonary fibrosis; these patients are usually monitored with pulmonary function tests at regular intervals.[523,524] The high iodine content of amiodarone can affect thyroid function, resulting in either hyperthyroidism or hypothyroidism. Other effects include drug deposits in the cornea, skin photosensitivity, and chemical hepatitis with increased liver transaminases. Coadministration of amiodarone with other antiarrhythmic agents may result in significant increases in the plasma concentrations of the other drugs.[513,515]

The incidence of perioperative organ dysfunction in children who receive either acute or long-term amiodarone therapy is controversial. A syndrome with similarities to the adult respiratory distress syndrome has been described, particularly in children exposed to high inspired oxygen concentrations who are undergoing thoracic surgery or cardiopulmonary bypass.[525-528] This finding led to the recommendation that amiodarone be discontinued for several weeks before elective surgery.[529]

Subsequent studies failed to demonstrate a significantly increased incidence of injury to lungs or other organs in children undergoing surgery while receiving amiodarone. Because it is most frequently given to children with severe and life-threatening cardiac rhythm disturbances, the current recommendation is to continue amiodarone up to the time of surgery. However, it may be wise to attempt to limit the inspired oxygen concentration and other factors that may predispose the children receiving amiodarone to free radical and inflammatory injury.[530]

#### Dronedarone

Dronedarone is a new, non-iodinated analogue of amiodarone which was developed to reduce the iodine-associated adverse effects of chronic amiodarone therapy. Like amiodarone, it inhibits sodium, potassium, and calcium currents. It is mainly indicated for maintenance of sinus rhythm in patients with atrial fibrillation but is still undergoing investigations regarding its long-term safety profile.[489,531-533] Pediatric data are not yet available.

#### Sotalol

Sotalol, a newer agent available in the United States, is a class III antiarrhythmic that also acts as a nonselective β-blocker. At small doses, the β-adrenergic blocking effects predominate; at larger doses, the class III effects become more significant. Sotalol is indicated for a number of refractory tachydysrhythmias. Current oral dosing recommendations for children start at target doses of 2 and 4 mg/kg in neonates, 3 and 6 mg/kg for children up to 6 years, and 2 and 4 mg/kg, divided into three doses, for children older than 6 years of age.[534] The major adverse effects of sotalol include mild cardiodepression due to its β-blocking ability and prolongation of the QT interval and torsades de pointes due to its class III effects.[535] It should be avoided in children with asthma, heart failure, renal dysfunction, or QT interval prolongation. Sotalol may be used as an alternative to amiodarone in some children who are unable to tolerate the adverse effects associated with amiodarone. Adult studies have shown that sotalol is not as effective for pharmacologic conversion of atrial fibrillation compared to other strategies or medications, but it can be indicated for maintenance of sinus rhythm after an episode of atrial fibrillation, especially for patients with coronary artery disease.[490] It has also been recommended as an alternative to amiodarone for postoperative atrial fibrillation in cardiac patients, but for prophylaxis and rate control pure β-blockers are still preferred.[536-538] The pediatric experience with sotalol is steadily increasing, but most studies have been limited by small numbers.[318,479,539-543]

#### Bretylium

Bretylium has limited use in children, being primarily indicated during cardiopulmonary resuscitation for the treatment of ventricular tachycardia resistant to other therapies.[544] The IV dose of bretylium is 5 mg/kg given as a bolus. Bretylium does have significant hypotensive properties and therefore should be given slowly in children with hemodynamically stable ventricular tachycardia. The total dose should not exceed 30 mg/kg. Bretylium is no longer available in the United States and has been removed from the current advanced cardiac life support algorithms, but it may be available in other countries.

#### Ibutilide

Ibutilide is one of the more recently released intravenous class III antiarrhythmic drugs. It prolongs repolarization by increasing the slow inward sodium current and by blocking the late rectifier current. It can be given intravenously and has a fast onset. Ibutilide is currently indicated for the rapid pharmacologic conversion of atrial fibrillation and atrial flutter, although it may be more efficacious for the latter. As with other class III drugs, ibutilide can prolong the QT interval and can cause associated polymorphic ventricular tachycardia (torsades de pointes, which occur in 5% to 8% of adults).[545,546] Because the elimination half-life of ibutilide is approximately 6 hours, the current recommendation is to observe children for several hours after an IV administration of this drug. Studies to date have used a bolus dose of 10 to 25 µg/kg administered over 10 minutes, which may be repeated once. Ibutilide has been successfully used in children with CHD[547] and in children with accessory pathways.[548]

### Dofetilide

Dofetilide is another new class III antiarrhythmic drug that has been approved for treatment of atrial fibrillation and flutter.[490] It prolongs the effective refractory period by selectively blocking the rapid component of the delayed rectifier potassium current. The major adverse effect is the potential for torsade de pointes due to QT prolongation.[549] Dofetilide is currently available only for oral administration; IV formulations are still under investigation. It has been successfully used in adult patients with CHD, but pediatric data are still missing.[550]

### Verapamil

Verapamil is a member of the class IV antiarrhythmic agents, the calcium channel blockers. Its primary action is depression of sinus node and AV node function.[551] Oral doses range from 4 to 8 mg/kg/day divided into three doses. A sustained-release preparation is available for older children. IV doses range from 0.1 to 0.3 mg/kg with a maximum dose of 5 mg. The most important side effect of verapamil occurs in children younger than 1 year of age, in whom IV administration can cause severe hypotension and asystole.[552] In fact, the drug is now contraindicated in infants (<1 year of age) because of this complication. Other side effects include bradycardia, AV block, and increased ventricular response in some children with Wolff-Parkinson-White syndrome.

Verapamil has been shown to be effective in terminating most SVTs in older children and adults.[479,553,554] Verapamil is also used to relieve outflow obstruction in hypertrophic cardiomyopathy[555] and as an antihypertensive in some children. The negative inotropic and AV conduction effects of verapamil are potentiated by β-blockers and anesthetic agents.[556,557] IV calcium and β-adrenergic drugs such as isoproterenol have been given to reverse the depressive effects of verapamil and other calcium channel antagonists.[558,559]

### Adenosine

IV adenosine has markedly changed the therapy for SVTs. Its electrophysiologic effects are multiple and include increased potassium channel flux and decreased slow inward calcium current. These effects result in sinus bradycardia and transient AV block and are mediated primarily by stimulation of the A1-purinergic receptor subtype. Its onset of action is within 10 to 20 seconds. Bradycardia, AV block, and hypotension last an additional 10 to 30 seconds.

The best response to adenosine is achieved when it is rapidly administered into the central circulation. The initial central venous dose is 50 µg/kg and the initial peripherally administered dose is 100 to 150 µg/kg given as a rapid bolus, followed by a fluid bolus given via a syringe to flush the medication into the circulation. If this is unsuccessful or the effect is not sustained, the procedure can be repeated with a double dose (up to a maximum of 300 µg/kg). In adults, the starting dose is 6 to 12 mg.[560,561] Adenosine can also be used as a diagnostic tool to differentiate between SVT and other dysrhythmias. The slower HR caused by the transient AV conduction block often allows the recognition of specific electrocardiographic features, such as delta waves in Wolf-Parkinson White syndrome.[562]

Other than the noted electrophysiologic changes, the major side effect from adenosine is transient hypotension. In children with an antegrade-conducting accessory pathway, adenosine can induce atrial fibrillation with a rapid ventricular response. Therefore, it should be used only in an appropriate setting with electrocardiographic monitoring and available resuscitation equipment.[563] Dipyridamole and diazepam may inhibit the metabolism or cellular redistribution of adenosine. Either drug can significantly potentiate the effects of adenosine, resulting in more prolonged hypotension and AV node blockade.[564] Children with transplanted hearts can demonstrate prolonged bradycardia and asystole in response to adenosine. The denervated heart is extremely sensitive to the AV node blocking effects. It is recommended that the initial dose be reduced by 50% in these children.[139] This can be very important in the cardiac catheterization laboratory, where wire-induced supraventricular arrhythmias are common during surveillance biopsies. Adenosine has been reported to cause bronchospasm in children both with and without known reactive airway disease. It is usually mild and, if necessary, can be treated with IV aminophylline, which directly counteracts the receptor-mediated effects of adenosine.

### Digoxin

Digoxin has antiarrhythmic as well as positive inotropic effects. Its basic pharmacology and therapeutic dosing were discussed earlier in the section on vasoactive drugs. As an antiarrhythmic agent, digoxin slows both atrial and AV node conduction. It slows the ventricular response in atrial flutter and fibrillation and may be used to treat children with junctional tachycardia and SVT.[318,479] Digoxin can have an unpredictable effect on the refractory period of accessory pathways[565,566] and is therefore relatively contraindicated in children with Wolff-Parkinson-White syndrome or other forms of SVT with accessory pathways. Digoxin easily crosses the placenta and remains the primary treatment for termination of fetal SVT.[567-569]

The dosing of digoxin in infants and children must be undertaken with care. Infants have greater myocellular concentrations of digoxin than adults do.[246,570-572] The dosing schedule of digoxin, based on age, is shown in Tables 16-8 and 16-11. IV and oral dosing are essentially the same. The onset of effect is more rapid with IV dosing (5 to 10 minutes) than with oral dosing (1 to 2 hours). The elimination half-life of digoxin is prolonged, approaching 1 to 2 days in young infants. Significant renal dysfunction and congestive heart failure can extend the elimination half-life. There are no active metabolites of digoxin. Therapeutic digoxin concentrations are 0.7 to 2.0 ng/mL. To properly measure the blood concentration of digoxin, blood should be obtained either just before a dose or at least 6 hours after the preceding dose.

Cardiac injury (e.g., ischemia-reperfusion, myocarditis) may increase the sensitivity to digoxin. Toxicity is more likely in children whose plasma concentrations exceed 3 ng/mL.[251] Signs of toxicity include proarrhythmia, nausea, vomiting, and drowsiness. Infants and young children frequently manifest digoxin toxicity as SVT and AV node conduction disturbances, whereas adults are more prone to ventricular arrhythmias, premature ventricular contractions, AV blocks, and junctional tachycardias. Hypokalemia exacerbates the risk of digoxin toxicity. Many drugs interact with digoxin. As a rule, the administration of other drugs may require a reduction in the digoxin dosing.

## Magnesium Sulfate

Magnesium plays an important role in many biologic processes. The catalytic actions of more than 300 enzymes, including those for ATP and DNA synthesis, depend on the presence of the $Mg^{2+}$ ion, the physiologically active form. Myocardial conduction and contractility, transmembrane calcium flux, potassium transport, vascular smooth muscle tone, coronary reactivity, and nitric oxide synthesis are all regulated by magnesium. Only 1% of the total body magnesium is extracellular; 60% is found in bones and 39% is intracellular, especially in muscle cells. This distribution explains why serum levels of magnesium may be normal despite an underlying intracellular deficiency. Of the extracellular magnesium, 55% is in the active ionized form. Ionized magnesium is a better predictor of the intracellular magnesium status; age-specific reference values have been published.[573-574]

Magnesium sulfate is currently used for the correction of hypomagnesemia, for management of seizures and hypertension, for bronchodilation during status asthmaticus, and in the treatment of life-threatening arrhythmias. It is especially valuable in the treatment of long QT syndromes and torsades de pointes.[575,576] More recently, prophylactic magnesium supplementation during pediatric cardiopulmonary bypass has been advocated to reduce the incidence of postoperative junctional ectopic tachycardia.[577,578] The IV dose is usually 25 to 50 mg/kg over 10 minutes (0.2 to 0.4 mEq/kg), with a maximum single dose of 2 g. This dose can be repeated every 6 to 8 hours depending on renal function and serum concentrations. Because magnesium is excreted solely by the kidneys, renal insufficiency requires increasing the intervals between doses to avoid toxicity. The normal serum concentration of magnesium is 1.5 to 2.5 mEq/L. Levels greater than 5 to 7 mEq/L can lead to increasing CNS and cardiac depression,

initially manifested as loss of deep tendon reflexes and muscle weakness, potentially leading to respiratory depression and cardiac arrest (at levels >15 to 20 mEq/L). IV calcium directly antagonizes magnesium-induced toxicity.

## ACKNOWLEDGMENTS

We wish to thank Avinash C. Shukla, James M. Steven, Francis X. McGowan, Jr., Paul R. Hickey, Robert K. Crone, and Susan L. Streitz for their prior contributions to this chapter.

## ANNOTATED REFERENCES

Baum VC, Palmisano BW. The immature heart and anesthesia. Anesthesiology 1997;87:1529-48.
*Review article describing the developmental changes in the immature heart and the implications for anesthesia on a physiologic, structural, and molecular level.*

Cotts WG, Oren RM. Function of the transplanted heart: unique physiology and therapeutic implications. Am J Med Sci 1997;314:164-72.
*Classic article describing the physiologic changes in the denervated heart.*

Gewillig M, Brown SC, Eyskens B, et al. The Fontan circulation: who controls cardiac output? Interact Cardiovasc Thorac Surg 2010;10:428-33.
*Review article that discusses the fundamental characteristics of the Fontan circulation.*

Hoffman JL, Kaplan S. The incidence of congenital heart disease. J Am Coll Cardiol 2002;39:1890-900.
*Interesting literature review looking into the reasons for the wide range of incidence data on congenital heart disease.*

Kiserud T. Physiology of the fetal circulation. Semin Fetal Neonatal Med 2005;10:493-503.
*Review article with a thorough description of the fetal circulatory physiology and the implications of placental compromise.*

Rhodes J, Tikkanen AU, Jenkins KJ. Exercise testing and training in children with congenital heart disease. Circulation 2010;122:1957-67.
*Original article describing the exercise limitations in children with repaired congenital heart disease.*

## REFERENCES

Please see www.expertconsult.com.

# Cardiopulmonary Bypass and Management

## 17

RALPH GERTLER AND DEAN B. ANDROPOULOS

THIS CHAPTER REVIEWS THE equipment and strategies for cardiopulmonary bypass (CPB) in infants and children, focusing on how they differ compared with CPB in adults. We will review the effects of CPB on the key organ systems and discuss specific management issues that occur in daily practice.

## Basic Aspects of Cardiopulmonary Bypass

The basic principles of CPB remain unchanged from when they were first introduced in the 1950s: the CPB machine assumes the functions of the heart and lungs during the time necessary to complete either an intracardiac or an extracardiac repair. A basic bypass circuit (Fig. 17-1) consists of an oxygenator, heat exchanger, and venous reservoir; pump heads for perfusion, cardiotomy suction, and cardioplegia; and appropriate tubing, cannulas, and monitoring and alarm devices.[1] Major differences exist between pediatric and adult CPB, stemming from anatomic, metabolic, and physiologic differences in these age groups (Table 17-1).

## THE CIRCUIT AND CANNULAS

Unfortunately the circuit size cannot be reduced proportionately to the patient's size; this disproportion commonly leads to hemodilution and dilutional coagulopathies in children. The surgical procedures require extremes of temperature, hemodilution, and changes in flow rates. Because of the smaller size cannulas and higher flow rates (150 to 200 mL/kg/min) in infants and children, cannulas assume a much more important management issue than in adults. Shear stress is significant in small cannulas and is several-fold greater than needed for activation of blood cells and platelets, leading to a disproportionately exaggerated systemic inflammatory response syndrome (SIRS).

### Bypass Circuit

Technical advances in the field of oxygenator construction and size, and reduction of priming volumes to as low as 45 mL for neonatal oxygenators, have allowed marked reductions of circuit volumes over the past decade. Also, tubing sizes can be reduced to $\frac{3}{16}$-inch diameters, which, in combination with shorter length

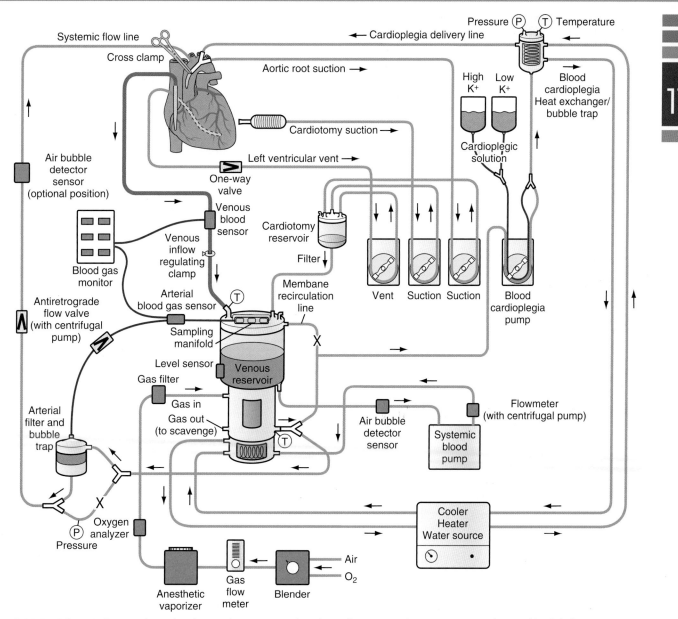

**FIGURE 17-1** Schematic diagram of a cardiopulmonary bypass circuit. This scheme depicts a membrane oxygenator with integral hard-shell venous reservoir and external cardiotomy reservoir. Many circuits have the cardiotomy reservoir, venous reservoir, and oxygenator integrated into one single unit. The systemic blood pump may be either a roller or centrifugal pump. Most pediatric venous cannulations are bicaval with two separate venous cannulas instead of the single venous cannula depicted here. Carbon dioxide can also be added to the inspired gas to facilitate pH-stat blood gas management. *Arrows* indicate direction of flow; *P*, pressure sensor; *T*, temperature sensors; *X*, placement of tubing clamps. (From Hessel EA, Hill AG. Circuitry and cannulation techniques. In: Gravlee GP, Davis RF, Kurusz M, Utley JR, editors. Cardiopulmonary bypass: principles and practice. 2nd ed. Philadelphia: Lippincott Williams & Wilkins; 2000, p. 69-97.)

tubing, allows reduction of priming volumes to the range of 100 to 150 mL for neonates. A summary of the Texas Children's Hospital sizing chart is shown in Table 17-2.

## Heparin Coated Versus Noncoated Circuits

Young children are more susceptible to the adverse effects of CPB than adults, and the inflammatory response to CPB may have serious consequences for neonatal and pediatric patients.[2,3] This is in part related to the surface area of the CPB circuit, which is large relative to the child's blood volume when compared with an adult's blood volume. For example, a 3-kg neonate with a blood volume of 90 mL/kg has a total blood volume of

approximately 270 mL, and with an average priming volume in many centers of 350 mL, the CPB circuit volume thus causes greater than 100% dilution. A 70-kg adult with 70 mL/kg blood volume has an approximately 5000-mL blood volume, and with a CPB circuit prime of 1500 mL, this results in less than 33% dilution. Contact of blood with the surface of the circuit also plays an important role for activation of coagulation and fibrinolysis. Heparin-coated biocompatible bypass systems reduce this activation in children weighing less than 10 kg undergoing CPB.[4] They also have been shown to reduce the activation of factor XII and the complement system.[5,6] This results in less production of kallikrein and bradykinin, which in turn reduces

**TABLE 17-1**  Comparison of Pediatric Versus Adult Cardiopulmonary Bypass

|  | Child | Adult |
|---|---|---|
| Hemodilution | 3-15× adult | Moderate |
| Perfusion pressure | 30-40 mm Hg | Moderate (>50-80 mm Hg) |
|  | Wide flow rates (0-200 mL/kg/min) | Narrow range (CI 2.0-2.4 L/m²/min) |
| Blood gas management | pH-stat ($P_{CO_2}$ 20-80 mm Hg or greater) | α-stat ($P_{CO_2}$ 30-45 mm Hg) |
| Cannulation techniques | Variable | Predictable |
| Aortopulmonary collaterals |  | Uncommon |
| Temperature ranges | Variable | DHCA occasionally |
| Glucose management |  | Predictable |
| Inotropic response | Negative | Positive |
| Perfusion circuit | Per kilogram weight | Standard |
| Parameters | Hematocrit often >55%-60% |  |
|  | $P_{O_2}$ 40-80 mm Hg | ± |
|  | $S_{aO_2}$ 75%-85% |  |
|  | Ultrafiltration (MUF/CUF) | ±Ultrafiltration |

*CI*, Cardiac index; *CUF*, conventional ultrafiltration; *DHCA*, deep hypothermic circulatory arrest; *MUF*, modified ultrafiltration.

**TABLE 17-2**  Cardiopulmonary Bypass Circuit Prime Volume and Constituents at Texas Children's Hospital

| Patient Weight | Prime Volume | Prime Constituents |
|---|---|---|
| <8 kg | 350 mL | Whole blood or PRBC + FFP + crystalloid prime* |
| 8-15 kg | 650 mL | 100 mL albumin 25% ± PRBC + crystalloid prime* |
| 15-25 kg | 900 mL | 100 mL albumin 25% + crystalloid prime* |
| 15-25 kg | 1200 mL | Crystalloid prime* |

*FFP*, Fresh frozen plasma; *PRBC*, packaged red blood cells.
*Crystalloid prime: ½ normal serum + Plasmalyte + $CaCl_2$ + KCl.

the secretion of tissue plasminogen activator from endothelial cells. One study has documented more bleeding with the use of a conventional, non–heparin-coated circuit compared with a heparin-coated circuit.[6] Overall, children operated on while supported with heparin-coated circuits have a significant reduction in inflammatory mediator release and fewer consequences thereof, such as prolonged postoperative ventilation and stay in the intensive care unit (ICU).[7]

## CARDIOPULMONARY BYPASS PUMPS

The two pumps used most commonly for CPB are roller pumps and centrifugal pumps. Roller pumps have the advantages of simplicity, low cost, ease and reliability of flow calculation, and the ability to pump against high resistance without reducing flow.[8] Disadvantages include the need to assess occlusiveness, spallation of the inner tubing surface (potentially producing

particulate arterial emboli), capability for pumping large volumes of air, and ability to create large positive and negative pressures. Compared with roller pumps, centrifugal pumps offer the advantages of less air pumping capabilities, less ability to create large positive and negative pressures, less blood trauma, and virtually no spallation. Disadvantages of centrifugal pumps include higher cost, the lack of occlusiveness (creating the possibility of accidental patient exsanguination), and afterload-dependent flow that requires constant flow measurement. In the setting of short-term CPB for cardiac surgery, it remains uncertain whether the selection of a roller pump over a centrifugal pump, or of any specific centrifugal pump over another, has clinical importance. Pulsatile perfusion may prove to be beneficial in the future, but further outcome data and technical improvements are needed.[9]

## CARDIOPULMONARY BYPASS PRIME

The optimal priming fluid in cardiac surgery is a topic of enduring debate. Crystalloid solutions, colloids, and mixtures of both are used. Children appear to benefit from a colloid prime. If crystalloid is used for priming, it should not contain lactate or dextrose because CPB induces a metabolic acidosis[10] that has been shown to be iatrogenic and not splanchnic in origin.[11] The addition of lactate to the prime increases postoperative serum lactate concentrations and should be avoided.[12] Hyperchloremic metabolic acidosis is the second contributing component of a metabolic acidosis on CPB. This is often only detected by measuring the strong ion difference via the Stewart approach to the acid-base homeostasis.[13] Both acidifying events are attenuated by the dilutional hypoalbuminemia induced by the administration of the pump prime. Because a hyperchloremic acidosis of a mild degree seems to be well tolerated and not associated with a poor outcome, no intervention seems necessary. Understanding the nature of CPB-associated acidosis, however, is likely to prevent unnecessary investigations or interventions.

The avoidance of dextrose is especially important during complex repairs using deep hypothermic cardiac arrest in which the risk of neurologic injury is substantive. The additives in banked blood, namely, glucose in citrate-phosphate-dextrose (CPD) storage solutions, also need to be considered as a source of glucose (together with the increased plasma concentrations of potassium in stored blood). We use a balanced electrolyte solution, such as Plasmalyte, for the crystalloid component of our prime.

The proportionally large volume of the bypass circuit compared with the child's blood volume has a significant impact on the coagulation factors and cellular components. Platelet count decreases and coagulation factors, including fibrinogen, are diluted after bypass; these factors may contribute to a coagulopathy. The fibrinogen concentration at the end of bypass has been shown to correlate with the 24-hour chest drainage in children weighing less than 8 kg.[14] This is seen more frequently in infants and neonates in whom an average decrease in plasma concentrations of hemostatic proteins by 56% immediately on initiation of bypass can be observed.[15] Overall, younger age represents the single most important risk factor for coagulopathy and bleeding complications.[16]

One approach to the just-mentioned problems is the addition of whole blood to the circuit prime. Proponents cite two advantages: (1) improved hemostasis and (2) a decreased SIRS with less edema formation and less organ dysfunction. One study has disproved these perceived advantages; the investigators found that the use of fresh whole blood increased perioperative fluid requirements, leading to a longer duration of mechanical ventilation and ICU stay than in the single component group.[17] The only advantage found by their study was the lesser number of donor exposures, a problem we try to overcome by matching packed red blood cells (PRBCs) and fresh frozen plasma (FFP) from the same donor.[18] In addition, whole blood is frequently not available. An alternative approach is the use of FFP in the prime.[19] Other investigators found that the use of FFP led to greater fibrinogen concentrations at the end of surgery. On average, children in the FFP group needed 1.3 fewer donor exposures and tended to need fewer PRBCs. The lower donor exposure was primarily because of fewer transfusions of cryoprecipitate.[19] FFP may be safely substituted by 5% albumin in the prime in children with less complex repairs and acyanotic lesions.[20] Whenever possible, we prefer fresh blood less than 5 days old. Fresh PRBCs are presumably more balanced metabolically than stored PRBCs; the former contain less potassium, a greater concentrations of glucose, reduced concentrations of lactate, and a greater pH.[21] Also postoperative morbidity increases with increasing age of red blood cells.[22] Pulmonary complications, acute renal failure, and increased infection rates were among the main complications associated with increased red blood cell storage time. As far as potassium levels and acid-base balance are concerned, PRBC priming can be safely performed with stored PRBCs if the priming solution is circulated for 20 minutes before the initiation of CPB.[23]

Depending on the size and age of the child, and the complexity of the repair, a target hematocrit is chosen. Based on the child's blood volume and the prime volume, homologous blood is added using the following calculation:

$$\text{Prime PRBC volume} = [\text{Target hematocrit}] \times \\ [\text{Patient blood volume} + \text{Prime volume}] \\ - [\text{Patient PRBC volume}]$$

The average prime volume of the circuits we use is shown in Table 17-2. Other prime additives are heparin, antifibrinolytics, antiinflammatory agents (corticosteroids), antibiotics, vasodilators, and, sometimes, diuretics (mannitol, furosemide). At the end of the case and before separation from bypass, blood gas analysis is done to ensure that the electrolytes (including calcium and magnesium ions), glucose, and hematocrit are within a desired range. Acid-base changes and sodium concentration are corrected with sodium bicarbonate, and residual lactate is washed out with the help of the hemofiltration.

## ANTIFIBRINOLYTIC AGENTS (SEE CHAPTER 18)
### Aprotinin
Inhibitors of serine proteases regulate and prevent uncontrolled activation of thrombin, coagulation factors, complement products, kallikrein, trypsin, elastase, and cathepsin among others of these potent enzymes. Of the serine protease inhibitors, the broad-spectrum agent aprotinin is the most widely studied in both experimental and clinical settings. Aprotinin is derived from bovine lung. It inhibits plasmin, kallikrein, trypsin, and other proteases, resulting in both antiinflammatory and antifibrinolytic effects and maintenance of glycoprotein homeostasis.

The first use of aprotinin in pediatric cardiac surgery was reported in 1990[24]; a high-dose regimen was administered to 28 children at increased risk of bleeding. This population included those undergoing transposition of the great arteries or reoperations, and children with endocarditis. No reduction in blood loss

or drainage was observed; there were no adverse effects, and chest closure time was reduced.

Despite the high cost of aprotinin, follow-up studies have had more favorable results and its use has been shown to reduce overall costs, with decreased patient charges as a result of reduction in the number of blood products used, operative time, duration of postoperative ventilation, and hospitalization.[25,26] This was confirmed in a recent comparative analysis amongst antifibrinolytic medications.[27] However, this benefit was observed only in complex repairs and the use of a high-dose regimen.[28] The lesser effect of a low-dose regimen may be attributable to the dilutional effects in pediatric surgery compared with the adult population.[29] Pediatric lung transplantation has been studied as a potential target group for aprotinin use.[30] As in most high-risk groups, a significant benefit was found for children with repeat operations (defined as repeat sternotomies or repeat transplantations), either with a high- or a low-dose regimen. This is consistent with our experience. Also, in general, infants younger than 6 months of age and those with repeat sternotomies seem to get a particular benefit from a high-dose regimen of aprotinin[31] compared with reduced doses, despite greater drug costs. Economic studies have shown a cost-effective benefit of aprotinin in repeat cardiac procedures.[25,26]

Aprotinin seems to have an influence on the inflammatory response to CPB in children.[32] Less time mechanically ventilated postoperatively[33] and an improved $PaO_2/FiO_2$ (ratio of arterial oxygen concentration to the fraction of inspired oxygen, or P/F ratio) as an indicator of an attenuated reperfusion injury of the lung with the use of aprotinin have been reported.[34] The clinical relevance of its antiinflammatory action remains unclear but points toward significant antiinflammatory properties.

Although a standard dosing regimen has yet to be defined in children, pediatric studies have demonstrated decreases in operative time post CPB, exposure to donor blood, and postoperative chest tube drainage with the use of aprotinin.[33] In vitro plasma concentrations of aprotinin have been related to antifibrinolytic and antiinflammatory activity at concentrations of 50 to 125 kallikrein inhibitor units (KIU)/mL and 200 KIU/mL, respectively.[25,35,36] Anaphylactic and anaphylactoid reactions may occur with aprotinin, and a test dose should be given before administration of the loading dose or addition of aprotinin to the CPB circuit. In a retrospective review of 681 children, reactions occurred in 1% of first exposures, 1.3% of second exposures, and 2.9% of more frequent exposures.[37]

We used aprotinin for complex neonatal repairs, such as arterial switch operations or Norwood procedures, as well as for most reoperative procedures and organ transplantations.[38,39] Because of safety concerns in adults, the drug is currently unavailable in the USA and Europe. The decision to withdraw the drug was based on data that were obtained entirely from adults, who present with a different profile of complications following cardiac surgery than do children. Aprotinin has been shown to be safe and efficient in the neonate.[40] Furthermore, serious questions have been raised regarding the statistical method used in the sentinel study that questioned the safety of aprotinin. Aprotinin continues to be used in Australia and New Zealand and has been reintroduced for adult coronary artery bypass graft surgery in Canada. Currently, the FDA in the United States is reevaluating the role of aprotinin in anesthesia. Our dosing regimen is weight based, with 60,000 KIU/kg as a loading dose and in the pump prime. Aprotinin is started before the incision and blood levels are maintained with a continuous infusion of 7000 KIU/kg/hour; this is discontinued just before leaving the operating room. Regimens based on body surface area are also used, along with a CPB prime dose based on priming volume designed to achieve a plasma level above 200 KIU/mL. An example is 0.85 to $1.7 \times 10^6$ KIU/m$^2$ loading dose, and into the CPB prime, and 2.0 to $4.0 \times 10^5$ KIU/m$^2$/hour infusion.[25]

### The Lysine Analogues: Aminocaproic Acid and Tranexamic Acid

Despite meticulous surgical technique, it is still frequently difficult to achieve adequate hemostasis after CPB, particularly in neonates. ε-Aminocaproic acid (EACA) and tranexamic acid (TXA) are analogs of the amino acid lysine. They exert their antifibrinolytic effect by interfering with the binding of plasminogen to fibrin, thereby preventing the activation of the active plasmin. TXA may also improve hemostasis by preventing plasmin-induced platelet activation. Both TXA and EACA exercise some antiinflammatory properties but not to the same extent as aprotinin. In one study, the use of EACA reduced bleeding postoperatively in 25 of 71 children undergoing cardiac surgery on CPB and was found to benefit only the children with cyanotic heart disease.[41] The EACA loading dose was 75 mg/kg followed by an infusion of 15 mg/kg/hour; an additional 75 mg/kg was added to the CPB prime. Because the effective dose of EACA is unknown, another study used a regimen of 150 mg/kg bolus followed by an infusion of 30 mg/kg/hour of EACA. Intraoperative blood loss was reduced, but postoperative blood loss was not different between treatment arm and placebo.[42] Blood coagulation measured with a thromboelastograph showed less fibrinolysis with EACA.

EACA compares favorably with TXA; a beneficial effect has been reported only in children with cyanotic heart disease.[43] Those with acyanotic defects or undergoing repeat sternotomies had no benefit from TXA. Their dosing regimen, however, was only 50 mg/kg as a single bolus before incision. In children, the TXA plasma concentration between the post bolus peak and the end of CPB has an 80% decline when a continuous infusion is not used.[44]

In conclusion, though less efficient than aprotinin, TXA and EACA are equally effective in reducing perioperative blood loss in pediatric cardiac surgery.[45] Given their safety profile, they may be even more appealing in the future. Further studies are needed to delineate their pharmacokinetic profiles and their efficacy. We use EACA based on simulation results from a study by Ririe and coworkers.[46] An initial loading dose of 75 mg/kg over 10 minutes and a maintenance infusion rate of 75 mg/kg/hour is used with 75 mg/kg placed in the pump to maintain serum concentrations above the therapeutic concentration (assumed to be 130 μg/mL) in more than 95% of children.

## Special Coagulation and Hematologic Problems

### HEPARIN-INDUCED THROMBOCYTOPENIA

The use of unfractionated heparin for anticoagulation for CPB in adults produces antiheparin antibodies in 25% to 50% of patients within 10 days postoperatively. In a small minority of these patients, high-titer IgG platelet-activating antibodies form and make immune complexes with heparin and platelet factor 4 (PF4).[47] This results in activation of platelets (via their Fc receptors) and formation of procoagulant platelet microparticles,

leading to thrombin generation and thrombosis. Thus, the major problem in heparin-induced thrombocytopenia (HIT) is thrombocytopenia several days after heparin exposure accompanied by thrombosis, often in major vessels or structures. HIT appears to be less common, of milder course, and probably underrecognized in neonates and children. About 1% of children exposed to CPB have PF4 antibodies when tested before their second CPB, and actual HIT is much less common.[48] When HIT is suspected, either PF4 enzyme-linked immunosorbent assay or a functional assay for HIT can be used to make the diagnosis; if positive, no further heparin should be given. If CPB is necessary, alternatives, such as the direct thrombin inhibitors argatroban, lepirudin, and bivalirudin, may be used. None of these agents is approved for use in children for anticoagulation for CPB, but case reports and small series have documented their successful use when HIT is diagnosed.[49-51] The partial thromboplastin time (PTT), activated clotting time (ACT), and a specialized clotting time called the *ecarin clotting time* can be used to follow anticoagulation with these agents, but there is no reversal agent for them. Thus, treatment of post-CPB bleeding involves administration of blood products and coagulation factors as well as recombinant factor VIIa (see later discussion).

### ANTITHROMBIN III DEFICIENCY

Heparin produces anticoagulation by combining in a 1:1 ratio with antithrombin III (ATIII), which then binds to and inhibits thrombin, leading to anticoagulation. Of adult patients, 4% to 13% have a resistance to normal doses of heparin for CPB; most instances occur because of a partial deficiency of ATIII, rendering heparin less effective at producing anticoagulation.[52] In children this is often unknown, and the first suspicion of ATIII deficiency may occur when the standard heparin dose of 300 to 400 units/kg fails to adequately anticoagulate before CPB, that is, the ACT remains less than 300 seconds. The usual response is to apply another dose of heparin from a different vial and remeasure the ACT, but if the ACT is still not adequately prolonged, a diagnosis of ATIII deficiency may be suspected. Infants less than 6 months of age and children with congenital heart disease have decreased ATIII concentrations.[53] Therefore, heparin may not achieve adequate anticoagulation, and disorders in hemostasis and thrombosis and an exaggerated inflammatory response may occur. In this case, blood can be sent for ATIII levels, but to proceed with CPB, the ATIII must be increased. This can be accomplished in two ways: (1) by supplementing ATIII with recombinant ATIII, 75 units/kg, and ensuring that the ACT is adequately prolonged before proceeding with CPB, or (2) by adding FFP (which has ample levels of ATIII) to the CPB prime or administering it to the child.[52,54]

### RECOMBINANT FACTOR VIIa FOR MASSIVE HEMORRHAGE

Recombinant factor VIIa (rFVIIa) was originally approved for use in patients with hemophilia who possess inhibitors to factors VIII or IX, and was shown to be effective at treating bleeding in these patients at doses of 90 μg/kg (see Chapter 10).[55] Endogenous factor VII circulates at low concentrations in the plasma. At a site of tissue or blood vessel injury, tissue factor (TF) is exposed, and the extrinsic coagulation pathway is activated by the binding of factor VII to TF, resulting in the activation of factor X to factor Xa, leading to the generation of thrombin from prothrombin, with further activation of platelets and the coagulation cascade.[56] High concentrations of rFVIIa result in major activation of the extrinsic pathway at the site of injury, theoretically without resulting in systemic hypercoagulability. However, thrombotic complications are increased after its use. rFVIIa also activates platelets, adding to the potential benefit of this agent in significant hemorrhage. Thus, this therapy seems attractive for the treatment of surgical bleeding. A recent analysis of factor VII concentrations during pediatric cardiac surgery recommended that it be used to treat postoperative coagulopathies that were resistant to conventional therapy, when no identifiable surgical cause of bleeding could be determined.[57]

Because of its high cost, and the paucity of data in children undergoing cardiac surgery, rFVIIa should be reserved for life-threatening hemorrhage unresponsive to other measures. A dose of 45 to 90 μg/kg, repeated every 2 hours, can be used. rFVIIa cannot produce hemostasis alone and should only be administered after the transfusion of sufficient amounts of platelets, plasma, and fibrinogen to form the substrate for hemostasis.

## SICKLE CELL DISEASE

Sickle cell disease (SCD), one of the most common hemoglobinopathies among patients of African-American or West Indian origin (with a prevalence of 0.2% to 0.3% in that population), results from the substitution of valine for glutamic acid in position 6 of the β-hemoglobin chain. Normal adult hemoglobin is referred to as HbA, whereas hemoglobin containing the mutant β-hemoglobin chains is referred to as HbS. SCD is represented by a homozygous genotype (HbSS) with fractional concentrations of HbS in the range from 70% to 90%. Sickle cell trait, on the other hand, is a heterozygous manifestation (HbAS) with a prevalence of 8% to 10% in the same population. The definitive diagnosis of any sickle cell hemoglobinopathy is confirmed by hemoglobin electrophoresis (see Chapter 9).

Children with SCD are at a particular risk for perioperative complications.[58,59] Sickling can be triggered by hypoxia, dehydration, acidosis,[60] hypothermia, stress, and infections. Hypoxia induces opening of a $Ca^{2+}$-activated $K^+$ channel (Gardos channel) that causes intracellular dehydration.[61] Chain formation occurs and leads to increased blood viscosity with vaso-occlusion. Opening of the Gardos channel is an important mechanism of sickle cell dehydration, which is temperature dependent, with greater potassium efflux at lower temperatures.[62] Shrinkage of sickle erythrocytes may also result from activation of a $K^+/Cl^-$ cotransport pathway under acidotic conditions.[63] Activation of this pathway can be blocked by increasing the abnormally low level of intracellular magnesium in sickle erythrocytes. The use of magnesium and hydroxyurea in the perioperative period therefore seems to be beneficial.[64]

CPB, particularly for more complex surgical procedures, may involve periods of low flow or even circulatory arrest, as well as hypothermia with consequent local vasoconstriction, hypoxemia, and acidosis. There is some evidence that CPB can be safely undertaken in SCD.[65] Flow conditions are an important determinant of sickle erythrocyte adherence to endothelium. Under low-flow conditions sickle cell adhesion to endothelium increases with contact time in the absence of endothelium activation or adhesive proteins, whereas under venular flow conditions sickle cell adhesion occurs only after endothelial activation. During CPB, both low-flow conditions and endothelial activation may occur. Multiple triggers of sickling are likely to occur during CPB, and close attention should be paid to the conduct of all aspects of bypass.

In the past, routine exchange transfusion has been recommended to prevent these complications.[66] More recent experience provides evidence that not all children require an exchange transfusion.[67] The growing evidence of the harmful effects of blood transfusion adds to the need to carefully reconsider routine exchange transfusion.[68] For uncomplicated bypass surgery without periods of cardiac arrest, the omission of exchange transfusion has led to good outcomes.

Guidelines have been proposed for the perioperative management of children with sickle cell disorders.[67] It is essential to avoid hypothermia using tepid or warm CPB in its stead; blood transfusion only for a decrease in hematocrit to less than 20%; maintenance of intravascular volume and body temperature while on CPB; the avoidance of vasopressors; the use of postoperative multimodal pain therapy; and early incentive spirometry to prevent pulmonary complications.[69] In our practice, we utilize cerebral near-infrared spectroscopy (NIRS) to help determine an acceptable hematocrit for the individual child.

For children undergoing hypothermia, successful management with[70] and without[71] partial or complete exchange transfusion on bypass has been reported. Exchange transfusion can be performed preoperatively or on initiation of CPB.[72] For exchange transfusion during CPB, the extracorporeal circuit is primed with blood and the usual components. When CPB is commenced, the child's blood volume is drained into storage bags and separated. The platelet-rich plasma is reinfused at the end of CPB, and the concentrated sickle cells are discarded. Platelet and plasma sequestration in conjunction with exchange transfusion reduces the need for postoperative transfusion and protects the platelets from the negative effects of CPB.[73]

There seems to be no consensus as to a suitable target HbS level. Reducing the absolute level of HbS may be of greater benefit than achieving a particular ratio of HbA to HbS because the remaining sickle-prone cells are still at risk for sickling.[74] In SCD, exchange transfusion has been shown to favorably affect cerebral tissue oxygenation.[75] Exchange transfusion will decrease both the proportion and absolute amount of HbS, but it does not remove every cell that may sickle; it may also have favorable effects on hypoxic pulmonary vasoconstriction.[75] In this context, these children may benefit from continuous hemofiltration to reduce inflammatory mediators and improve pulmonary recovery.[76] Inhaled nitric oxide also has been suggested as an adjunct for the prevention of sickle cell crisis. It may improve the binding of oxygen, thereby reducing the formation of sickle cells; reduce pulmonary hypertension; and improve pulmonary function without adverse effects on normal hemoglobin.[77]

# A Perspective on Blood Preservation: Cardiopulmonary Bypass in Jehovah's Witness Patients

Jehovah's Witnesses differ from other religious groups in their conscious objection to decline the therapeutic infusion of blood and blood components. They uniformly refuse the transfusion of red blood cells, and some individuals also refuse platelets and plasma, as well as predisposed autologous blood. Individual choices that can be made are the acceptance of fractions of blood, such as albumin and globulins, dialysis, cell savage, and acute normovolemic hemodilution.

Acute isovolumic reduction of hemoglobin down to 5 g/dL is tolerated in healthy individuals under anesthesia and does not appear to reduce tissue oxygenation significantly.[78] Reduction of oxygen delivery to 7 to 8 mL/kg/min under resting conditions does not lead to an oxygen debt and is compensated by increased extraction, an increase in cardiac index, and a subsequent decrease in systemic vascular resistance.[79,80] In a retrospective study of the tolerance of reduced hemoglobin concentration in Jehovah's Witness patients, the hemoglobin concentration of those who died was less than 5 g/dL.[81] A safe limit of hemodilution in children has not been established. One report showed that hemodilution up to 50% in acyanotic children appears to be safe.[82] In cyanotic children, however, the limit was estimated to be around 40%. If this level of hemodilution is exceeded, hemodynamic instability and inadequate oxygen transfer can occur. Evidence suggests that hematocrit levels of 21.5% in infants on CPB leads to significantly worse psychomotor developmental outcome, compared with 27.8%.[83]

The most important and simplest way to avoid transfusion in the setting of cardiac surgery is to limit blood loss. Unnecessary and reduced amounts of blood sampling help to preserve blood.[84] Pharmacologic agents, such as aprotinin and tranexamic acid, reduce the risk of perioperative blood loss.[85] Hormonal stimulation of erythropoiesis with preoperative recombinant erythropoietin is another strategy acceptable to Jehovah's Witnesses. The administration of erythropoietin in the cardiac surgery setting has been shown to reduce the risk of exposure to allergenic blood.[86] However, the associated increase in hematocrit with erythropoietin use may be potentially thrombogenic and could lead to an increase in the incidence of perioperative venous thromboembolism. The cost of using erythropoietin can be large, and cost analysis suggested that its use in cardiac surgery was not cost effective.[87]

Intraoperative recovery of blood with a cell salvage device is also acceptable to many Jehovah's Witnesses. This involves the removal by suction of blood from the operative field followed by washing, filtering, and return of red blood cells to the patient. A randomized controlled trial of intraoperative cell salvage in cardiothoracic surgery has demonstrated a reduction in red blood cell transfusion and an increase in postoperative hemoglobin.[88]

Acute normovolemic hemodilution involves the preoperative removal of a volume of blood from the patient with the simultaneous administration of crystalloid or colloid to maintain circulating volume.[89] The collected blood is then reinfused during the operation. Some Jehovah's Witnesses find this process acceptable, especially if the access line is maintained in continuity with the patient. Acute normovolemic hemodilution has other advantages, including lower costs, because the blood does not need compatibility testing; reduced possibility of administrative error; and a saving in patient time (see Chapter 10). The development of artificial red cell substitutes could potentially abrogate the need for compatibility testing, as well as vastly reduce infection risks, with none of the immunomodulatory side effects of allogeneic blood.[90] Some of these products would also be acceptable to Jehovah's Witness families. Substitutes include perfluorocarbons, hemoglobin solutions, intramolecular cross-linked hemoglobin, and liposome encapsulated hemoglobin. None of these has reached clinical practice. Lastly, autologous retrograde priming has been used in Jehovah's Witness patients and can further reduce the hemodilutional effects of the prime.[89,91]

In the great majority of adult patients, open-heart surgery can be performed without administration of blood or blood components. In children and small infants weighing less than 5 kg, bloodless open-heart surgery is more complicated. Preoperative iron supplementation (6 mg/kg/day) and erythropoietin (200 to 400 U/kg/wk) have been used successfully to augment preoperative hemoglobin levels.[92]

Modern bypass circuits allow the reduction of priming volumes to less than 200 to 300 mL. Main components that are amenable to volume reduction on a regular circuit are the size and length of the lines, small oxygenators and arterial filters, and priming the hemofilter for modified ultrafiltration with blood from the venous line after CPB. Line volumes, for example, may vary from 1.73 mL per 10 cm of a $\frac{3}{16}$-inch tubing to 0.75 mL per 10 cm of a $\frac{1}{8}$-inch tubing. The limiting factor, however, is the necessary flow. For a $\frac{3}{16}$-inch arterial line, a maximum flow of 1.8 L/min was established as the point at which the Reynolds number reaches a value of 1000, indicating a change to turbulent flow. Modified ultrafiltration at the end of CPB through a fluid warmer line to prevent heat loss or continuous ultrafiltration has been used. The venous line and the reservoir are emptied before discontinuation of bypass, the field is suctioned, and all blood is retransfused through the arterial line. Decannulation is achieved and protamine is given as usual. Crystalloid cardioplegia solution should be evacuated from the field by an external sucker to prevent dilution of the pump volume.

Postoperative care involves minimal blood sampling, and only on special indications. Noninvasive monitoring allows uncomplicated weaning from the ventilator.[93] The first report of successful outcomes in Jehovah's Witness children with congenital cardiac defects was in 1985[94]; 110 children older than 6 months of age successfully underwent operation, with a perioperative mortality rate of 5.3%. Only one death was attributed to blood loss. A weight less than 5 kg is considered by some as a contraindication for open-heart surgery and palliative procedures were advocated in the past.[95] For some lesions, however, no palliation is possible. The development of miniaturized circuits, preoperative optimization, use of high-dose aprotinin, vacuum-assisted drainage to allow smaller tubing and cannula sizes, as well as the use of modified ultrafiltration, enabled the safe expansion of surgery into the neonatal population. Individualized heparin level–based anticoagulation management further results in a reduction of coagulation problems, blood loss, and transfusion requirements.[96] The addition of desmopressin, 0.3 µg/kg, also not proven, is thought by some to improve platelet activity and stimulate the release of von Willebrand factor after protamine infusion.

All of the aforementioned considerations are important in approaching the Jehovah's Witness patient; however, at Texas Children's Hospital, Jehovah's Witness children are not treated differently with regard to blood transfusion practice than any other child. Cerebral NIRS is utilized to help determine the safe hemoglobin level for the individual child at all phases of surgery. Consent for blood transfusion in this situation is a complicated issue, because the legal status of children is different from that of an adult. Each institution must develop a legal informed consent process for blood transfusion for Jehovah's Witness children, in consultation with local legal authorities, social work and ethic groups, and representatives of the Jehovah's Witness faith. Currently we have a release of liability form for the parent to sign stating that he or she requests that blood products not be used, but that acknowledges they may be needed to treat his or her child. The parent further agrees to release and hold harmless the physicians and hospital for any liability associated with blood transfusion. This form was developed in conjunction with the local Jehovah's Witness church representatives, and in our practice this has been accepted by more than 95% of parents and has obviated the need for more extreme measures, such as temporary child protective services custody during the perioperative period, which was our former practice.

## Myocardial Protection

Myocardial protection during cardiac surgery has evolved over the years. Melrose and colleagues introduced the concept of chemical cardioplegia in 1955.[97] Before the popular use of chemical cardioplegia, topical cardiac hypothermia was used. In the late 1970s and early 1980s, the concept of cold hyperkalemic blood cardioplegia was introduced.[98] Potassium concentrations in cardioplegic solutions ranging from 12 to 30 mEq/L are typically used to achieve cardiac standstill within 1 to 2 minutes under hypothermic conditions, with higher concentrations (or longer induction times) required for normothermic conditions. Myocardial edema after bypass and global ischemia can be reduced by a number of strategies that involve modifying the conditions of delivery and composition of cardioplegia solutions as they affect the movement of intracellular and interstitial fluid. In contrast to studies in adults, most studies conducted in neonates have shown little difference between blood and crystalloid cardioplegia.[99,100] Hypothermia also decreases myocardial oxygen consumption. The benefits of this approach appear to be optimal at myocardial temperatures between 24° C and 28° C. However, there is growing evidence that warm, intermittent blood cardioplegia may be advantageous to either cold crystalloid or cold blood cardioplegia.[101] The benefits of blood cardioplegia are more pronounced in younger, cyanotic children who require longer aortic cross-clamping. For acyanotic children, the cardioplegic technique is probably not as critical.[102] Avoidance or reduction of myocardial edema occurs by limiting the pressure of cardioplegia infusions and by providing moderately hyperosmolar cardioplegia solutions that contain blood. Buffering the acidosis that results from ischemia is achieved by including tromethamine, histidine-imidazole, or both in the cardioplegia solution. Close management of myocardial calcium balance to avoid extremes of intracellular hypercalcemia or hypocalcemia, especially during reperfusion, is very important.[103,104] The addition of magnesium may solve this dilemma by preventing damage from higher cardioplegic calcium concentrations by its action as a calcium antagonist.[104,105] This prevents mitochondrial calcium overload as a consequence of reperfusion injury. Magnesium also prevents the influx of sodium into the postischemic myocardium, which is exchanged for calcium during reperfusion.

Every cardiac program has its own philosophy regarding cardioplegia and myocardial protection. At Texas Children's Hospital, plain crystalloid cardioplegia is used. The prime blood gas and electrolytes should mimic physiologically the child's arterial blood gas as closely as possible. If whole blood or packed cells are added to the prime, the target hemodilution range should be 28% to 30%; the prime should be recirculated continuously and warmed between 35.0° C and 36.5° C before initiation of bypass. In neonates and infants, albumin is added to the cardioplegic solution to maintain an appropriate colloid osmotic pressure. This may decrease edema formation of the arrested heart. In children undergoing circulatory arrest, long cross clamp times, and large pump suction return cases, 20 mg/kg methylprednisolone is used, up to a maximum of 500 milligrams, to reduce the production of inflammatory mediators that result in myocardial dysfunction. Table 17-3 summarizes the Texas Children's Hospital protocols for cardioplegia and myocardial protection.

## Phases of Cardiopulmonary Bypass

Surgical cases requiring CPB are divided into several basic phases.

### PRE-BYPASS PERIOD

This phase begins with surgical incision and lasts through initial dissection and preparation for cannulation. During this period transesophageal echocardiography (TEE) is performed to confirm the diagnosis and establish a basis for post-bypass comparison.

### CANNULATION AND INITIATION OF BYPASS

After sternotomy and mediastinal dissection, the aorta is cannulated, along with either the right atrium, if single venous drainage is planned, or the superior and inferior venae cavae for bicaval venous drainage. A large dose of heparin (300 to 400 units/kg) is administered intravenously, and the adequacy of anticoagulation is measured using the ACT *before initiating CPB*. The target ACT is usually 480 seconds. High ACTs are maintained during CPB with the addition of heparin to the prime as needed, because larger doses of heparin lead to a reduced degree of consumptive coagulopathy, which translates into reduced blood product therapy requirements.[96] Other methods of measuring anticoagulation include the Hepcon system (a plasma heparin concentration assay), which may allow for more accurate titration of heparin and protamine dosages.[106] The thromboelastogram may also be used as a baseline measure of the coagulation system and then may be repeated during bypass, with heparinase added to more objectively assess each child's anticipated need for coagulation products.[107] An improved preservation of the hemostatic system with subsequent reduction of blood loss and a reduction in transfusion requirements has been demonstrated after maintenance of high heparin levels during CPB.[108] The additional maintenance of high ATIII concentrations may further contribute to a reduction of hemostatic activation.[109]

In most centers, bicaval cannulation is used for all but the smallest children (less than 2 kg) to prevent venous return from interfering with the surgical field. A gradual transition to full CPB is then performed to minimize myocardial stress, using a prime that has essentially the same composition as the child's blood with regard to temperature, pH, calcium, potassium, and hematocrit. CPB flows of 150 mL/kg/min are used for infants weighing less than 10 kg, and 2.4 L/min/m² is used for children weighing more than 10 kg. Flow rates may be reduced during periods of hypothermia (see later), although many centers now prefer to maintain greater flows throughout the bypass period. Misplaced cannulas can lead to significant morbidity. Obstruction of the inferior vena cava (IVC) by a misplaced IVC cannula can lead to increased venous pressure, which causes ascites and decreased perfusion pressure in mesenteric, hepatic, and renal vascular beds. Misplacement of the cannula in the superior vena cava can result in cerebral edema from inadequate venous drainage and a subsequent reduction in cerebral blood flow, potentially resulting in ischemia. Arterial cannula misplacement can also occur. If the cannula inadvertently slips beyond the takeoff of the right innominate artery, preferential perfusion to the left side of the brain can be observed. This can be detected on the NIRS monitor, which may be an important monitor, particularly in pediatric cardiac surgery.[110]

The presence of any anomalous systemic-to-pulmonary shunts can lead to shunting of blood away from the systemic circulation, through the pulmonary circuit, and then through the venous

**TABLE 17-3** Cardioplegia Solution

**Cardioplegia Base Solution (385 mL)**

| Concentration | | Contents | |
|---|---|---|---|
| Sodium chloride BP | 3.54 g/L | Sodium | 23 mmol |
| Anhydrous glucose BP | 6.65 g/L | Potassium | 15 mmol |
| Potassium chloride | 2.92 g/L | Calcium | 0.35 mmol |
| Mannitol | 6.54 g/L | Chloride | 39 mmol |
| Calcium chloride | 135 mg/L | Glucose | 2.52 g |
| | | Mannitol | 2.48 g |
| | | Approximate pH 4.5 | |
| | | 275 mOsm/L | |

**Cardioplegia Buffer Solution**

| Concentration | | Contents | |
|---|---|---|---|
| Sodium carbonate | 9.37 g/L | Sodium carbonate | 0.28 g |
| Sodium bicarbonate | 27.0 g/L | Sodium bicarbonate | 0.81 g |

**Uses of Cardioplegia Solution during Cardiopulmonary Bypass**

*Children weighing <10 kg*

385 mL Cardioplegia base solution

26 mL Cardioplegia buffer solution

100 mL 25% Albumin

Note: This is usually delivered at a pressure of 30 mm Hg for newborns and 30-40 mm Hg for older infants.

*Children weighing >10 kg*

385 mL Cardioplegia base solution

100 mL 0.9% Sodium chloride

10 mL 25% Mannitol

5 mL 8.4% Sodium bicarbonate

Note: This is usually delivered at a pressure of 30-60 mm Hg. A good guide is to note the end-diastolic pressure of each child before bypass. This will be a guide to the normal filling pressure of the coronary arteries. When aortic incompetence is present, the CPS flow may need to be increased.

**Administration of Cardioplegia Solution**

*For all patients:*

| | |
|---|---|
| Temperature | 8° C to 12° C |
| Initial dose | 110 mL/m$^2$/min for 4 minutes |
| Subsequent doses | 110 mL/m$^2$/min for 2 minutes |

Note: Following the initial dose, cardioplegia is to be delivered every 20 minutes during the cross clamp period unless otherwise indicated by the surgeon. The perfusionist will remind the surgeon of the need for cardioplegia and keep track of the time. Because of the nature of the surgical procedure, it may be necessary to deliver cardioplegia directly into the coronary ostia via a hand-held delivery system. In this case the surgeon will direct the perfusionist. Close attention should be paid to the delivery line pressures.

**Examples of Primes**

**Neonate: Whole Blood, If Available, Otherwise Reconstituted**

| | |
|---|---|
| Whole blood | 225 mL |
| Plasmalyte A | 50 mL |
| 0.45% NaCl | 125 mL |
| Heparin | 2500 units |
| NaHCO$_3$ | 5 mEq |
| CaCl$_2$ | 250 mg |

**Pediatric: Packed Red Blood Cells**

| | |
|---|---|
| PRBCs | 250 mL |
| Plasmalyte A | 300 mL |
| 0.45% NaCl | 75 mL |
| 25% Albumin | 100 mL |
| Heparin | 3500 units |
| NaHCO$_3$ | 20 mEq |
| CaCl$_2$ | 300 mg |

**Adult: Crystalloid Prime**

| | |
|---|---|
| Plasmalyte A | 700 mL |
| 0.45% NaCl | 600 mL |
| 25% Albumin | 100-200 mL (volume varies depending on the size of the patient) |
| 5% Dextrose | 40 mL |
| Heparin | 5000 units |
| NaHCO$_3$ | 40 mEq |
| CaCl$_2$ | 300 mg |
| KCl | 2.4 mEq |

*BP*, The material conforms to the specifications and procedures outlined in the British Pharmacopoeia; *CPS*, cardioplegia solution; *PRBCs*, packed red blood cells.

cannula to the CPB machine. Thus, the systemic perfusion is shunted away from the body in a futile circuit back to the CPB machine. Anatomic lesions where such shunting can occur include an unrecognized patent ductus arteriosus and large aortopulmonary collaterals, as found in pulmonary atresia. Bypass flow needs to be increased to compensate for these shunts.

## COOLING PHASE

Systemic cooling is used for nearly every case. Hypothermia is classified as mild (30° C to 36° C), moderate (22° C to 30° C), or deep (17° C to 22° C). In general, lower temperatures are used for more complex operations that carry a greater potential for requiring periods of low-flow bypass or circulatory arrest. Cooling is primarily achieved extracorporeally through the heat exchanger

in the bypass circuit, although some surgeons also request that ice be applied to the head to prevent rewarming during the circulatory arrest.

## AORTIC CROSS CLAMPING AND INTRACARDIAC REPAIR PHASE

The aorta is cross clamped, with the heart then rendered asystolic after infusion of cardioplegia solution into the aortic root.

## DEEP HYPOTHERMIC CIRCULATORY ARREST OR SELECTIVE CEREBRAL PERFUSION PHASE

If circulatory arrest is to be used, it is initiated after a slow cooling period of at least 20 minutes, and an attempt is made to limit the total duration of deep hypothermic circulatory arrest (DHCA) to less than 40 minutes. Special bypass techniques (see later) have been developed to avoid the necessity of using DHCA and may also be performed during this time.

## REMOVAL OF AORTIC CROSS CLAMP AND REWARMING PHASE

After completion of the intracardiac repair and de-airing of the heart, the aortic cross clamp is removed, allowing reperfusion of the myocardium. Optimally, normal sinus rhythm and myocardial contractility are restored during this time, while the child is slowly rewarmed. During rewarming, surgery is completed, inotropic and vasoactive agents are started, and ventilation begins. Hemofiltration and blood transfusion are used to achieve the desired hematocrit. Left atrial and/or pulmonary artery monitoring lines, if indicated, are placed at this time, as are temporary atrial and ventricular pacing wires. If the child is incompletely rewarmed before separation from CPB, a significant afterdrop with precipitous post-bypass reduction in core body temperature can occur. This can lead to vasoconstriction, shivering, increased oxygen consumption, and acidosis. However, postischemic hyperthermia can lead to delayed neuronal cell death.[111] Mild degrees of hypothermia and certainly the avoidance of hyperthermia are essential in the perioperative period.[112] In children, rectal temperature mostly reflects peripheral temperature. One study showed that the temperature of the foot was more sensitive than the temperature of the hand.[113] Another study revealed that for anatomic or physiologic reasons, temperature gradients in the toes develop more readily than those in the fingers.[114] Several endpoints have been proposed, such as nasopharyngeal temperatures greater than 35.0° C, bladder temperature greater than 36.2° C, or skin temperatures greater than 30° C[115,116]; we use an endpoint of 35.5° C rectal temperature.[117]

## SEPARATION FROM BYPASS

The child's core body temperature, hematocrit, and metabolic parameters should be optimized before attempting separation from CPB. Careful observation for left-sided air, confirmation with the TEE, and concurrent inspection of electrocardiogram (ECG) changes should continue throughout the weaning process, with the child in the Trendelenburg position and the aortic root vented. While fluid volume is gradually added to the child by reducing the outflow to the venous reservoir until optimal filling pressures are achieved, CPB flow is then slowly reduced to zero. If inotropic support is anticipated to separate from CPB, infusions should be prepared before beginning separation.

## POST-BYPASS PERIOD

This phase lasts until chest closure and transfer to the ICU have been accomplished. During this time, modified ultrafiltration (MUF) may be performed for 10 to 15 minutes after cessation of CPB. Cardiac function and the quality of the surgical repair are assessed via TEE, and, if found to be satisfactory, protamine is administered to neutralize residual heparin. The usual dose of protamine is 1.0 to 1.3 mg/100 units of heparin given at the onset of bypass. Limiting protamine to this dose prevents an overdose with its associated effects on platelet function (reduction of the interaction of glycoprotein Ib receptor interaction with von Willebrand factor).[118] If the ACT remains increased or prime blood is given back to the child, an additional 25% of the initial dose of protamine is added and the ACT is rechecked. However, particularly in infants, the administration of protamine and the persistent treatment of a suspected incomplete heparin reversal should not distract and delay the treatment of other commonly associated post-bypass coagulopathies, such as thrombocytopenia, platelet dysfunction, and other coagulation factor deficiencies.

Protamine reactions occur much less frequently in children younger than 16 years of age, approximately 1.76% to 2.88%.[119] Independent risk factors are a female gender, a larger protamine dose, and smaller heparin doses. Type I reactions or effects during administration are rare and adding calcium does not change the hemodynamic consequences of injection.[120] Fortunately, severe anaphylactic reactions (type II) or catastrophic pulmonary vasoconstriction (type III) are rare but have been observed by us and others.[121] Administering the protamine over no less than 5 minutes reduces the severity and precipitous nature of any protamine reaction.

Unstable neonates and small infants may have their sternums temporarily left open, with surgical closure planned 24 to 72 hours later when cardiac function has improved and myocardial edema diminished.

Because CPB can have a multitude of adverse physiologic effects, attempts are made to minimize both the duration of CPB and ischemic (aortic cross clamp) time; thus, as much of the surgery as possible is performed outside of these phases. In general, physiologic responses to bypass are more extreme with decreasing age and size of the child. The neonate experiences a greater degree of hemodilution on bypass and colder temperatures on bypass and frequently requires longer aortic cross clamp times, all of which can result in a greater inflammatory response. Table 17-4 summarizes clinical management issues during the major phases of CPB.

# Particular Aspects of Management on Cardiopulmonary Bypass

## pH-STAT VERSUS α-STAT MANAGEMENT

Some degree of hypothermia is used for nearly every cardiac operation to slow the metabolism and oxygen consumption of all organs, particularly the brain and heart.[122] During cooling, the carbon dioxide contained in blood becomes more soluble and its partial pressure decreases. The $PaCO_2$ sensed by the body decreases as body temperature decreases, with the result that at a core temperature of 17° C to 18° C, if pH and $PaCO_2$ have not been corrected for temperature, the body experiences a pH of about 7.6 and $PaCO_2$ of 15 to 18 mm Hg (Fig. 17-2).[123] This very low $PaCO_2$ causes cerebral vasoconstriction, particularly during the cooling phase of bypass, which in turn leads to less cerebral blood flow, less efficient brain cooling, and less cerebral protection at a given temperature.[124] Because blood samples are normally heated to 37° C before measurement of pH, $PaCO_2$, and $PaO_2$, the use of pH-stat management indicates that blood gases are being corrected for the child's actual body temperature by increasing the $PaCO_2$ during bypass, as it is measured at 37° C, so that the body experiences a $PaCO_2$ of approximately 40 mm Hg and a pH of 7.4 at all temperatures. Conversely, α-stat management means not correcting the blood gases for temperature, as if the child's blood was always at 37° C, with the goal of pH 7.4 and $PaCO_2$ 40 mm Hg. In the early days of CPB, pH-stat was used to preserve cerebral blood flow at all ages.[123] Subsequently, in the 1970s and 1980s, randomized controlled studies in adults undergoing CPB confirmed that acute, post-CPB neurologic problems were worse with the use of pH-stat management.[125]

**TABLE 17-4  Checklist for Bypass Management**

**Before CPB**

1. Check temperature; maintain normothermia during induction and preparation.
2. Supplement premedication.
3. Ensure noninvasive monitoring: blood pressure, ECG, pulse oximetry, stethoscope.
4. Perform inhalational induction after preoxygenation; intravenous induction, if cannula is in place.
5. Peripheral intravenous placement(s)
6. Neuromuscular blockade and ventilation
7. Intubation and mechanical ventilation according to shunt lesion ($CO_2$, $O_2$ control)
8. Monitoring:
   a. Arterial line and central venous line
   b. ECG electrodes
   c. Bladder catheter
   d. Temperature probes
   e. TEE probe (in infants >3 kg)
9. Positioning
10. Deepening of anesthetic level
11. Antifibrinolytics and corticosteroids, as indicated
12. Heparin, 300-400 U/kg, before arterial cannulation
13. Check activated clotting time >400 seconds.
14. Supplement anesthetics on initiation of bypass.

**During CPB**

1. Stop ventilation and drips when full flow is reached.
2. Inspect head perfusion.
3. Evaluate quality of perfusion (perfusion pressure, central venous pressure, diuresis, arterial blood gases, temperature gradient).
4. Prepare for separation.
   a. Drips (inotropic drugs, calcium)
   b. Pacemaker
   c. Blood products
5. Set and control temperature and rewarming (heating blanket, room temperature).
6. Zero transducers
7. Check arterial blood gases in preparation for discontinuation of CPB; correct abnormalities.
8. Suction and ventilate.

**After CPB**

1. Separate when
   a. Temperature >35.5° C
   b. Stable rhythm or pacing
   c. Heart contracting well
2. Fine-tune blood pressure; consider direct blood pressure measurement for hypotension at the aortic cannula; volume ± drips.
3. Consider modified ultrafiltration.
4. Check arterial blood gases.
5. Evaluate with transesophageal echocardiography for residual defects.
6. Give protamine, 1-1.3 mg/100 IU of initial heparin.
7. Check activated clotting time and arterial blood gases.
8. Chest closure and recheck arterial blood gases.
9. Transport to the intensive care unit.

*CPB,* Cardiopulmonary bypass; *ECG,* electrocardiogram; *TEE,* transesophageal echocardiography.

α-Stat management was, therefore, adopted for both adult and pediatric CPB. However, studies in a neonatal pig model have challenged this conclusion, proving that neurologic outcomes, both behavioral and neuropathologic, are significantly worse when α-stat management is used in infants.[124,126]

Advantages of pH-stat CPB have been shown to include:

- A decreased brain metabolic rate[127]
- An increased rate of brain cooling and reperfusion,[128] thereby providing better protection through more even and faster cooling and rewarming secondary to increased CBF[128,129]
- Molecular effects of altered $PaO_2$ and pH, including changes in cerebral oxygenation and brain enzyme activity, as well as decreased brain electrical activity[129-131]
- Decreased oxyhemoglobin affinity[132]
- Increased cortical oxygenation before arrest (through hypercapnic capillary vasodilation) and decreased oxygen metabolic rate, providing slower deoxygenation compared with α-stat management (approximately 10 vs. approximately 7 minutes).[124,133] Cortical anoxia occurs at 36 minutes versus 24 minutes for α-stat management.

In cyanotic infants with aortopulmonary collaterals, pH-stat management results in significantly improved brain oxygenation as measured by near-infrared cerebral oximetry.[134] A retrospective study of 16 infants revealed worse neurodevelopmental outcomes with α-stat management.[135] In a randomized prospective trial of pH- versus α-stat management in 182 infants younger than 9 months of age, there was a strong trend toward improved outcomes with pH-stat management, including earlier return of electroencephalographic activity, fewer seizures, and improved psychomotor development index.[136] One study examined the effects of α-stat and pH-stat on developmental and neurologic outcomes after deep hypothermic CPB in infants.[137] Psychomotor Development Index scores of 110 patients did not differ significantly between the groups ($P = .97$). The results of the Mental Development Index scores were dependent on diagnosis. In all but the ventricular septal defect subgroup, the pH-stat group did not have statistically greater Mental Development Index scores. Abnormalities on the electroencephalogram ($P = .77$) and neurologic examination ($P = .70$) were similar with the two methods of blood gas management. The authors concluded that the use of α-stat or pH-stat strategy is not consistently associated with improved or impaired early neurodevelopmental outcomes in infants undergoing deep hypothermic CPB.[137] One reason for the differing results between pediatric and adult studies is that cerebral emboli are more common in the adult population because of the presence of atherosclerotic plaques, which cause microembolic infarcts, and the increased cerebral blood flow produced by pH-stat management, which leads to a greater number of cerebral emboli in adults. Emboli occur much less frequently in children, and the primary cause of neurologic injury from CPB in children is hypoxic-ischemic.[138] Thus, the increased cerebral blood flow observed on CPB with pH-stat management lessens this risk in children. Interestingly, this putative mechanism has been recently challenged by a study involving a controlled microembolic load and DHCA in pigs that revealed that pH-stat was still associated with improved outcomes when compared with α-stat.[139] pH-stat also improves oxygen delivery by counteracting the pH- and hypothermia-associated leftward shift in the oxyhemoglobin dissociation curve. Studies have also revealed a decrease in peak postoperative troponin levels, reduced ventilator dependence, and reduced ICU stays with pH-stat versus α-stat.[140] Most programs specializing in surgery for

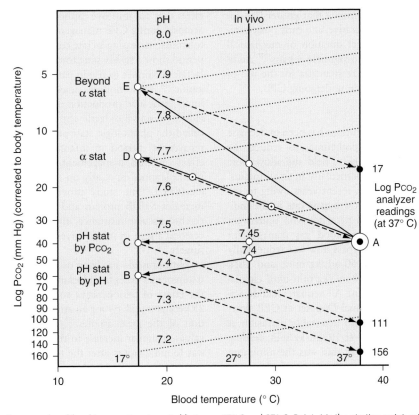

**FIGURE 17-2** pH and $P_{CO_2}$ changes when blood temperature is varied between 17° C and 37° C. Point *A* is the starting point, with pH 7.4 and $P_{CO_2}$ 40 mm Hg at 37° C. Points *B, C, D,* and *E* are the conditions the brain experiences at 17° C with various blood gas management strategies. pH-stat management (correcting the pH and $P_{CO_2}$ for temperature) results in an acid-base environment that is neutral, whereas α-stat management (not correcting for temperature) results in a very alkalotic environment at 17° C. Warming the blood sample (as is done for blood gas measurement) results in very high $P_{CO_2}$ values when pH-stat is used. The pH of blood becomes slightly more alkalotic with cooling, owing to the decreased dissociation of hydrogen ions. (From Jonas RA. Carbon dioxide, pH, and oxygen management. In: Jonas RA, DiNardo J, Lawson PC, et al, editors. Comprehensive surgical management of congenital heart disease. London: Arnold Publishers; 2004, p. 151-60.)

congenital heart defects currently use pH-stat management. This necessitates careful attention to $PaCO_2$ during all phases of bypass, and possibly reducing the sweep gas flow into the CPB oxygenator (to decrease the efficiency of $CO_2$ removal), and often adding inspired $CO_2$ to the sweep gas of the bypass circuit, particularly in small infants.

## HEMATOCRIT ON BYPASS

The relatively small total blood volume in children, along with the volume required to prime the CPB circuit, means that adding blood to the CPB prime is mandatory for small infants. Practice is institution specific; but in many centers adding either whole blood, PRBCs with FFP (for children less than 8 kg), or PRBCs alone (for children less than 12 to 15 kg) is necessary to ensure that the hematocrit on bypass is not less than 20%. As a result of increased transfusion-related concerns from bloodborne viral disease transmission during the 1980s and 1990s, and given that a low hematocrit is thought to be necessary to ensure adequate blood flow through capillary beds (because the blood viscosity increases at low temperatures), hematocrits of 20% or less on CPB with deep hypothermia were frequently tolerated.[141] There is increasing evidence that the practice of extreme hemodilution is detrimental to neurologic outcome in children. In a piglet model, one group of investigators determined that the incidence and degree of hypoxic-ischemic brain injury after a period of DHCA was significantly greater with a hematocrit of 20% versus

one of 30%, regardless of whether pH- or α-stat strategy was used.[142] In another piglet model, using intravital microscopy of pial capillaries during deep hypothermic CPB, a hematocrit of 30% did not impair cerebral microcirculation when compared with a hematocrit of 20%.[143] Finally, in a prospective randomized trial of CPB hematocrit of 20% versus 30% at the Children's Hospital Boston, children in the lower hematocrit group demonstrated significantly reduced psychomotor development index scores 1 year after surgery.[83] In a follow-up study of hematocrit 25% vs. 35%, the same group did not observe a difference in neurodevelopmental outcomes.[144] However, when they combined all children from both hematocrit trials, they found that a hematocrit less than 24% was associated with lower psychomotor index scores 1 year after surgery.[145] The hypoxic-ischemic damage most likely occurs during the cooling and rewarming phases of bypass, when cerebral oxygen metabolism is not suppressed, yet hematocrit and, thus, oxygen delivery, is low. Therefore, many centers are now maintaining higher hematocrits on CPB (at least 25%), which either means using more donor blood products or using hemofiltration to raise the hematocrit during bypass. The current estimate by the American Red Cross of the risk of viral transmission from a single unit of blood is 1 in 205,000 for hepatitis B, 1 in 1.9 million for hepatitis C, and 1 in 2.1 million for human immunodeficiency virus.[146] The risk–benefit ratios therefore favor the greater hematocrit approach, a definitive change from previous practice patterns. Balanced against this practice of a greater hematocrit on CPB is the finding that greater transfusion of blood products in the intraoperative, and early postoperative periods, is associated with longer duration of mechanical ventilation in infants undergoing two-ventricle repairs.[147] Additional studies are required to optimize strategies for the use of blood products in infants and children undergoing CPB.

## FLOW RATES ON BYPASS

The traditional practice in many institutions has been to decrease CPB flows, particularly during hypothermia, to reduce the volume of blood returning to the surgical field and allow more efficient completion of the surgery, particularly in small infants. This concept has been questioned in recent years owing to the inability to determine the safe low-flow bypass rate in the individual child. One report studied 28 neonates who underwent arterial switch operation with α-stat blood gas management during CPB.[148] At 14° C to 15° C, bypass flow was sequentially reduced from 150 mL/kg/min to 50 mL/kg/min, and then further decreased in increments of 10 mL/kg/min until circulatory arrest was begun (to 0 mL/kg/min). All neonates had detectable cerebral blood flow by transcranial Doppler at CPB flows above 20 mL/kg/min, but one had no detectable perfusion at 20 mL/kg/min, and eight had none at 10 mL/kg/min, leading the authors to conclude that 30 mL/kg/min was the minimum acceptable flow in this population. A neonatal pig model determined that, at normothermia, bypass flows of at least 150 to 175 mL/kg/min were necessary to ensure full oxygenation of all end organs and tissues.[149] Clinical studies of a high-flow bypass strategy, which included flows of 150 mL/kg/min at all phases of bypass except during DHCA, minimal use of DHCA, and α-adrenergic receptor blockade with phenoxybenzamine to produce long-duration systemic vasodilation, demonstrated excellent short- and long-term clinical and neurodevelopmental outcomes, with no child scoring outside normal ranges for testing performed at a mean age of 9 years.[150] This strategy also has led to excellent early results for the Norwood operation, with an early perioperative survival of 83% for cases carried out from 1993 to 1999.[151] During the same era, one report documented that 26.7% of arterial switch children had neurologic abnormalities and 55% had at least one abnormal area on neurodevelopmental testing (performed at a mean of 10 years) when DHCA and low-flow bypass had been used.[151]

Vasoconstriction and increased vascular resistance, resulting in uneven regional organ perfusion, are among the undesired side effects of CPB. Endogenous catecholamine production and the alkaline α-stat CPB technique, if used, are responsible for these effects. To be able to run full flow during hypothermic CPB without significant hypertension, vasodilators are often used. Agents currently used to provide systemic vasodilation and more even cooling and rewarming include phentolamine, nitroprusside, or nitroglycerin. Phenoxybenzamine, which is no longer available, was used as part of a treatment strategy after stage 1 palliation for hypoplastic left heart syndrome, and has been associated with improved outcome.[152,153] Phenoxybenzamine was more effective than sodium nitroprusside in improving peripheral circulation, as shown by temperature gradients intraoperatively.[154] Greater CPB flows are associated with an improved oxygen delivery, which can improve patient outcome.[155]

Phentolamine is a nonselective competitive $\alpha_1$ and $\alpha_2$ catecholamine receptor blocker. It has a half-life of 19 minutes and is eliminated mainly by the kidneys. Through postsynaptic $\alpha_1$ and $\alpha_2$ receptor inhibition it has a vasodilating and hypotensive

effect that can improve cardiovascular parameters and metabolic acidosis during CPB management.[156] In children receiving phentolamine, increasing lactate concentrations at the end of the CPB period show a steady state toward the end of the surgery, whereas lactate continues to rise in patients who did not receive phentolamine.[156] These findings suggest that the use of phentolamine limits lactic acid production during the hypothermic period and aids the disposal of lactic acid from tissues. Seelye and associates called the physiologic state after hypothermia the "oxygen debt repayment" period in infants.[157] Although it has a beneficial effect on CPB management, the potential harmful effects of phentolamine, especially on the brain, have still not been fully elucidated. One study provided evidence that phentolamine increases S100B protein and a parameter indicative of altered cerebrovascular resistance, the pulsatility index in the middle cerebral artery, in infants given phentolamine during open-heart surgery.[158]

Nitroprusside has been used as an easily titratable agent with α-adrenergic receptor–blocking capacity. One study examined the effect of perioperative sodium nitroprusside application in 25 neonates undergoing an arterial switch operation for transposition of the great arteries.[159] In comparison to the pre-bypass values, a similar increase in the concentration of S100B protein was found 2 hours after the termination of CPB in the sodium nitroprusside-treated and nontreated neonates, which decreased over the subsequent 48 postoperative hours. However, significantly reduced post-bypass serum levels of S100B protein were found in the sodium nitroprusside-treated group after 24 and 48 hours of treatment.

Nitroglycerin has been used with the same success. The only proven benefit over other agents is its nitric oxide donation capacity.[160] In Japan, high-dose chlorpromazine has been used as part of a low-resistance strategy during CPB for the Norwood procedure.[161]

We routinely use phentolamine, 0.1 to 0.2 mg/kg, to provide normal CPB flow and mean arterial pressure in the range of the diastolic pressure. If hypotension develops during bypass, the flow should be increased up to 150% of predicted; also one should examine the acid-base status in conjunction with cerebral oxygenation and mixed venous saturations. Often, severe hemodilution with oxygen debt is the cause and should be treated as such. After exclusion, we treat the hypotension carefully with vasoconstrictors, knowing that normal systemic pressures will not restore splanchnic hypoperfusion[162] and that vasoconstrictors will often lead to a greater base excess. Excessive α-adrenergic receptor blockade can be antagonized by vasopressin.[163] One study demonstrated that vasoconstrictor treatment results in more sodium bicarbonate to treat the acidosis and is associated with a later time to extubation and return of bowel function.[164] In conclusion, α-adrenergic receptor blockade during bypass should be considered because of its benefits for tissue perfusion, but carefully executed and balanced against potential drawbacks afterwards.

## CONVENTIONAL ULTRAFILTRATION AND MODIFIED ULTRAFILTRATION

Ultrafiltration involves placing a hemofilter (similar to those used for continuous arteriovenous or venovenous hemofiltration in the ICU) in the CPB circuit and has become the standard of care for nearly all programs that specialize in surgery for congenital heart defects.[165] Conventional ultrafiltration (CUF) is performed during CPB, with the filter placed between the arterial and venous sides of the CPB circuit. The hemofilter has thousands of fibers with pores, which allow water, electrolytes, and small molecules to be filtered out of the blood. Suction is applied to the hemofilter on CPB, and an ultrafiltrate of plasma is produced. Advantages of ultrafiltration include the ability to increase the hematocrit, fibrinogen, plasma proteins, and platelet count,[166,167] without necessitating further blood transfusion, the ability to remove excess free water and sodium (which contribute to excess intravascular volume, tissue edema, pulmonary and myocardial edema), as well as the ability to correct acid-base and electrolyte imbalances, and to remove small molecules, such as interleukins and tumor necrosis factor-$\alpha$ (TNF-$\alpha$) in particular,[168] which are involved in the post-bypass inflammatory process.[169,170] This improves systolic and diastolic function of the myocardium and reduces endothelial dysfunction in the systemic and pulmonary vasculature.[170,171] Pulmonary function is better preserved, probably owing to a slight reduction in interleukin 6 (IL-6) and thromboxane $B_2$,[172] even though this is not a consistent finding in the literature.[173,174] Endothelin-1, another mediator of pulmonary damage and hypertension, was not reduced by any filtration method.[174] Clinically, however, any ultrafiltration method seems to benefit children, especially those undergoing complex repairs, neonates, and children with preexisting pulmonary hypertension.[173]

Modified ultrafiltration (MUF) is performed for 10 to 15 minutes immediately after the conclusion of CPB. It can be performed in an arteriovenous manner with a hemofilter placed between the aortic cannula and the IVC cannula, or in a venovenous fashion using bicaval cannulation or an internal jugular venous catheter.[175] It was developed in 1991[176] as an alternative method to reduce the side effects of CPB. CUF during bypass is often limited by the minimal venous reservoir levels and requires the addition of crystalloid or colloid to be able to continuously remove cytokines during ultrafiltration. During MUF, blood passes out of the aorta, through the hemofilter, and is returned through the IVC cannula. The theoretical advantage of MUF over CUF is that only the child's blood volume is filtered, yielding a more efficient system for achieving the goals just outlined. The disadvantages are that the child remains heparinized, and body temperature may decrease during the process (unless the circuit is modified to include the heat exchanger).[177] It also requires extra time, an aortic cannula is needed that can obstruct the aorta in small infants, and acute intravascular volume shifts may occur at a time when the child is prone to hemodynamic instability. Opposite to the expected effects of fluid removal, MUF actually increases arterial pressures despite decreasing filling pressures and improving myocardial performance.[178]

There is increasing evidence that the use of ultrafiltration reduces bypass-related postoperative morbidity. Outcome studies have demonstrated that ultrafiltration improves myocardial and pulmonary function, lessens tissue edema, allows faster weaning from mechanical ventilation, and decreases the need for inotropic support.[179] In that aspect it may be as efficient as the perioperative application of steroids.[180] The reduction of inflammatory transmitters is only temporary, because the levels of cytokines are similar after 24 hours.[181]

Although each method has its proponents, and some centers perform both techniques in the same children, controlled comparative studies revealed no difference in outcome between MUF and CUF.[179,182] We routinely use a balanced ultrafiltration technique for all cases on CPB because it removes fluids and cytokines, as well as reduces lactate, which can aggravate reperfusion injury.[183]

## Pre-Bypass Anesthetic Management

The objectives of the anesthetic management of children before bypass include maintenance of normal sinus rhythm and ventricular function and avoidance of extreme increases in heart rate, ventricular contractility, and pulmonary vascular resistance (PVR). The duration of the pre-bypass period varies greatly, particularly in children who have had previous surgeries, and maintaining hemodynamic stability for prolonged periods of time can often be challenging. Adequate anesthetic depth should be ensured to avoid increases in sympathetic stimulation and hypercyanotic spells, and temperature homeostasis should be maintained to avoid cardiac arrhythmias, especially when the duration of the pre-CPB surgical dissection is protracted. For children undergoing repeat sternotomy, blood products with an appropriate-capacity blood warmer should be readily at hand in case of emergent need.

Neonates and children who have been receiving total parenteral nutrition preoperatively receive an infusion of 5% or 10% dextrose before CPB, with frequent monitoring of glucose concentrations to avoid hypoglycemia or hyperglycemia. Older children receive Plasmalyte, a balanced electrolyte solution, at a reduced maintenance rate, allowing the administration of 5% albumin, if necessary, for volume augmentation.

The placement of purse-string sutures before cannulation, as well as the actual cannulation of the great vessels before CPB, can often precipitate arrhythmias, hypotension, and arterial desaturation, especially in small infants and children. It is common for volume replacement to be necessary during placement of the cannula; if the aortic cannula is already in place, it is our practice to coordinate the administration of fluid volume between the anesthesiologist and perfusionist while the surgeon completes cannulation. Calcium chloride (10 mg/kg) is also frequently useful to support hemodynamics at this time.

## Anesthesia on Cardiopulmonary Bypass

### CHANGES IN PHARMACOKINETICS

The initiation of CPB introduces additional volume to the intravascular space (hemodilution). This greatly affects drug distribution, plasma concentrations, and elimination. The major factors responsible for this are hemodilution and altered plasma protein binding,[184] hypotension, hypothermia,[185] pulsatility,[186] isolation of the lungs from the circulation, and uptake of anesthetic drugs by the bypass circuit.[187,188] Drugs in the blood exist in the free (unbound and therefore the active form) or plasma bound (inactive form bound to protein, e.g., albumin) forms and therefore are subject to marked changes with alterations in plasma protein levels. CPB alters all these factors, which makes description of pharmacokinetic parameters during CPB problematic. The greatest changes occur within 5 minutes of initiation of CPB. The addition of the prime volume immediately reduces the protein concentration, and the ratio of bound-to-free drug in the circulation changes. A reduction in red blood cell concentration occurs, and this reduces the free drug concentrations. This will reduce the amount of drug available for interaction with the receptors. Most studies show a reduction in total drug concentration in plasma with little change in unbound drug concentration over time, whereas on CPB other than the transient (less than 5 minutes) reduction at initiation of CPB[189] it would appear that the greatest risk for unwanted "lightening of anesthesia" is within this time frame, and additional doses of fentanyl, muscle relaxant, and midazolam are generally administered just before or with the onset of CPB. The explanation for why unbound drug concentrations are sustained during CPB is that the volume of distribution for most anesthetic agents is large relative to the volume of the CPB prime and serves as a huge reservoir for drug after intravenous administration. A decrease in the plasma concentrations of medications as a result of hemodilution shifts drugs down their concentration gradient from tissue to plasma. Hypothermia contributes to the changes in plasma concentrations primarily by depressing enzyme function and slowing the metabolism of medications. Drug metabolism is diminished during hypothermia; enzyme activity is approximately halved for every 10° C reduction in temperature. This may increase the free drug available for binding. When normothermia is reestablished, reperfusion of tissues might lead to washout of drug sequestered during the hypothermic CPB period. This may explain the secondary increases in plasma concentrations of opioids reported during the rewarming phase. pH-stat management also affects the degree of ionization and protein binding of certain medications, leading to increased unbound drug. During CPB, the lungs are out of circuit and medications that are taken up by the lungs (e.g., opioids) are sequestered during CPB. These medications are released when systemic reperfusion is established and concentrations are transiently increased. The volume of distribution of many drugs is expanded because of the priming volume of the bypass circuit, especially with neonates and small infants, where the priming volume is often greater than the child's blood volume. Finally, medications may be taken up by various components of the CPB circuit itself.

### CHANGES IN PHARMACODYNAMICS

The pharmacodynamic effects of anesthetic agents are affected primarily via the central nervous system, which undergoes major changes during CPB. For example, hypothermia during CPB reduces anesthetic requirements. Hypothermia causes a host of other effects, including decreases in receptor affinity (e.g., decreased opioid receptor affinity[190] and nicotinic acetylcholine receptor sensitivity[191]), enhanced effects of neuromuscular receptor blocking drugs at the neuromuscular junction,[192,193] and alterations in tissue blood flow that may affect the response to catecholamines.[194]

CPB also affects the degree of ionization and protein binding (hence free or unbound drug concentrations) of weak acids and bases, as well as the electrolyte balance achieved by the blood gas management strategy used during CPB. Plasma concentrations of calcium, magnesium, and potassium decrease during CPB,[195,196] and these changes may lead to muscle weakness, dysrhythmias, and digitalis toxicity. The number of receptors available for interaction with a ligand will determine the subsequent magnitude of a drug effect. A reduction in the number of cardiac receptors has been observed in congestive heart failure, and defects in receptor transduction, as well as impairment of synthesis and reuptake of norepinephrine occur.

Administration of β-adrenergic agonists in this condition has been associated with further reductions in β-receptor numbers, with diminished pharmacologic effect. Removal of β-adrenergic blockade may lead to β-adrenergic receptor upregulation and increased adrenergic responsiveness.[197] Changes in receptor density and function may occur very quickly and have been observed to occur during cardiac surgery. Many perfusionists, under the direction of the anesthesiologist, can also administer

inhalation agents via a separate vaporizer mounted on the bypass machine. Anesthetic requirements decrease with systemic hypothermia,[198] but as rewarming is initiated, additional anesthetic drugs, including a benzodiazepine, are added to the pump to ensure that amnesia is maintained. Further work is required to elucidate the mechanisms and clinical implications of these acute changes in receptor density and function.

## Special Techniques

### MANAGEMENT OF DEEP HYPOTHERMIC CIRCULATORY ARREST

In the early days of cardiac surgery and CPB, hypothermia was used to improve intracardiac surgical exposure. In 1950, Bigelow and colleagues were the first to show that hypothermia decreases the metabolic rate.[199] Since then, we have discovered other advantages of hypothermia, including decreases in the inflammatory response of CPB,[200] decreases in blood loss,[201] myocardial protection,[202] and neuroprotection.[203] The last effect relates primarily to the decrease in the metabolic rate (by approximately 64%) that is achieved by cooling from 37° C to 27° C. The disadvantages of DHCA include a prolongation of CPB and a greater tendency toward postoperative bleeding.[204] Postoperative recovery, however, is not prolonged by hypothermia.[205] The rate of wound infection is uninfluenced by hypothermic bypass.[206]

Hypothermia during cardiac surgery gained widespread acceptance only after the development of a heat exchanger that could be integrated into the CPB machine in 1959.[207] Deep hypothermic circulatory arrest involves cooling the child's body temperature during CPB to 17° C to 18° C, stopping the bypass machine, draining the blood from the child into a venous reservoir, and removing the cannulas from the heart. After the first reports of DHCA in the 1960s, this technique gained popularity in the 1970s and 1980s because the bloodless field it provided, thus facilitating complex intracardiac and aortic repairs in neonates and small infants,[208] as well as reducing myocardial edema. However, it soon became evident that DHCA was associated with neurologic morbidity. Choreoathetosis, seizures, coma, and hemiparesis were all noted, especially with prolonged (>60 min) DHCA. The incidence of these acute morbidities seemed to increase when α-stat management became the accepted standard in many centers. Long-term adverse neurodevelopmental outcomes have also been associated with long periods of DHCA, including abnormalities in mental development and in fine and gross motor skills.[209] The Boston Circulatory Arrest Study is a remarkable achievement in which 155 neonates undergoing the arterial switch operation from 1988 to 1992 were studied, with follow-up complete to 8 years of age.[210] The CPB protocol in those years included α-stat management, routine hemodilution to a hematocrit of 20%, and the absence of an arterial filter on the CPB circuit. A DHCA time of greater than 40 minutes was associated with a significant increase in adverse long-term neurologic outcomes (Fig. 17-3). Although the 40-minute cutoff is now well-accepted in surgery for congenital heart defects, a number of changes have subsequently been made to bypass protocols. Results from animal experiments using a neonatal pig model of DHCA, as well as data from the Boston Circulatory Arrest Study, led to the following recommendations for increasing the child's safety margin when using DHCA:

- Hematocrit of 30% should be the target.[83]
- Systemic hypothermia should be achieved slowly, over no less than 20 minutes.[211]

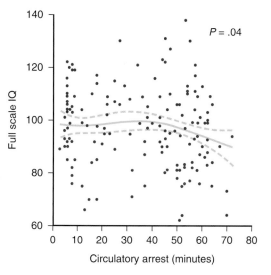

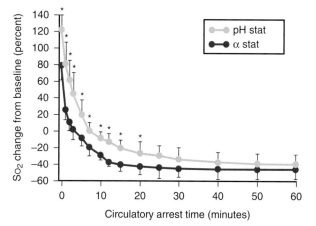

| Variable | Cut-point estimate (minutes) | 95% lower confidence limit (minutes) |
|---|---|---|
| Full-scale IQ | 42 | 27 |
| Verbal IQ | 41 | 23 |
| Performance IQ | 47 | 31 |
| Average achievement | 43 | 4 |
| Grooved pegboard | 35 | 13 |
| Mayo test for apraxia | 40 | 29 |
| Combined analysis (overall six outcomes) | 41 | 32 |

**FIGURE 17-3** Safe duration of circulatory arrest. From the Boston Circulatory Arrest Study, 155 8-year-olds underwent arterial switch operation for D-transposition of the great arteries as neonates. Bypass protocol used α-stat pH management, with hematocrit of 20% and temperature of 18° C. Above 40 minutes DHCA, both mental and physical performance test scores decreased significantly. (From Wypij D, Newburger JW, Rappaport LA, et al. The effect of duration of deep hypothermic circulatory arrest in infant heart surgery on late neurodevelopment: the Boston Circulatory Arrest Trial. J Thorac Cardiovasc Surg 2003;126:1397-403.)

**FIGURE 17-4** Cortical oxygen saturation ($So_2$) during deep hypothermic circulatory arrest in pH-stat and α-stat groups. The cortical $So_2$ half-life during arrest was significantly greater in the pH-stat than in the α-stat group. Mean ± SD, eight animals per group. *$P < .05$ between groups. (From Kurth CD, O'Rourke MM, O'Hara IB. Comparison of pH-stat and alpha-stat cardiopulmonary bypass on cerebral oxygenation and blood flow in relation to hypothermic circulatory arrest in piglets. Anesthesiology 1998;89:110-8.)

- pH-stat blood gas management should be used, at least for cooling (Fig. 17-4).[124,126]
- Core body temperatures of 17° C to 18° C should be used, and ice bags should be applied to the head.[212]
- DHCA should be divided into periods of less than 20 minutes, allowing a reperfusion period of at least 2 minutes between each segment of DHCA, to improve neurologic outcome.[213]
- Low-flow CPB is better than DHCA. Selective regional cerebral perfusion may be better than full body low-flow CPB.[214]
- Normoxemia should be maintained to decrease exacerbation of brain injury after DHCA.[215]

Neurologic monitoring (see later discussion) may be useful in the individual child to aid in determining the safe duration of DHCA.[124,216]

Although there are situations in which DHCA must be used, many surgeons are avoiding it whenever possible, minimizing its duration and dividing the periods of its use, or using alternate methods, such as selective cerebral perfusion (see the following discussion).

## REGIONAL CEREBRAL PERFUSION

To avoid the use of DHCA, several novel CPB techniques have been developed. The purpose of these techniques is to allow perfusion of the brain during critical periods of surgery, such as aortic reconstruction during the Norwood operation.[217,218] These techniques are collectively referred to as selective cerebral perfusion. Regional cerebral perfusion (RCP) is one variation in which a small Gore-Tex graft of 3 to 4 mm is sewn onto the innominate artery before initiation of CPB and is then used as the aortic cannula during CPB (Fig. 17-5). During aortic reconstruction, snares are placed around the brachiocephalic vessels and CPB flow is decreased, with only the brain receiving perfusion via the right carotid artery during this period. In this way, a bloodless operative field is achieved, just as if DHCA was being performed, yet the brain is still receiving blood flow and oxygen, theoretically increasing protection from hypoxic ischemic brain injury. Another potential advantage of this technique occurs in neonates, who frequently have extensive arterial collaterals between the proximal branches of the aorta and the lower body via the internal mammary and long thoracic arteries. In this instance, the use of selective cerebral perfusion also provides some blood flow to the lower body, protecting renal, hepatic, and gastrointestinal systems from hypoxic damage as well.[219] This protection is, however, incomplete and RCP at 25° C is no more protective than DHCA.[220] Also, the ongoing perfusion prolongs the effective bypass time, leading to more cytokine release and capillary leakage, with worse pulmonary function, more weight gain, and decreased right ventricular function.[221]

Despite the theoretical advantages of selective cerebral perfusion and a study demonstrating that selective cerebral perfusion does provide oxygenated blood flow to both cerebral hemispheres,[222] no long-term outcome studies have been performed that prove it is superior to standard techniques. This may in part be related to the novelty of this procedure. Neurologic monitoring has been used to determine the flow rate that is necessary during RCP.[222,223] We use 40% to 50% of full flow and adjust it according to brain saturation or Doppler measurements,

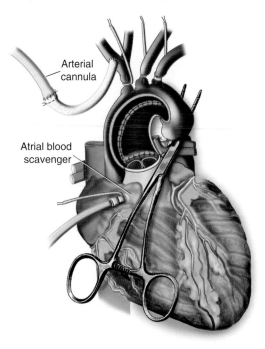

**FIGURE 17-5** Selective cerebral perfusion for the Norwood stage I palliation for hypoplastic left heart syndrome. Arterial inflow for bypass is provided by a small polytetrafluoroethylene graft sewn to the right innominate artery. Instead of deep hypothermic circulatory arrest, flow is provided to the brain at low rates, while the brachiocephalic vessels and descending thoracic aorta are snared, providing a bloodless operating field. (From Pigula FA, Nemoto EM, Griffith BP, Siewers RD: Regional low-flow perfusion provides cerebral circulatory support during neonatal aortic arch reconstruction. J Thorac Cardiovasc Surg 2000; 119:331-339.)

maintaining baseline saturation before the onset of RCP. If a left radial arterial line or a femoral arterial line (or umbilical arterial line) is in place, an abdominal perfusion pressure of about 12 mm Hg, which correlates with radial artery pressures of 25 to 30 mm Hg, is the goal.[222]

# Effects of Cardiopulmonary Bypass

## CARDIAC EFFECTS

In addition to myocardial ischemic injury secondary to aortic cross clamping, several other factors can contribute to perioperative myocardial dysfunction. The first is entrainment of air into the coronary arteries, which frequently occurs during weaning from bypass.[224] Despite meticulous de-airing of the heart, air may enter the right coronary artery, producing ischemia that is heralded by a pale myocardium, poor contractility, and ST-segment elevation of the ECG. Should this occur, appropriate management involves remaining on CPB, increasing perfusion pressure, and "milking" the air through the coronary arteries, allowing time for recovery of the ECG and ventricular function before attempting to wean from bypass. Surgical factors, such as reimplantation of coronary arteries with possible resultant ischemia or residual surgical defects, can also occasionally contribute to myocardial dysfunction.

The inflammatory response to CPB (see later discussion) has important implications for cardiac function.[225] This systemic response results in a capillary leak syndrome, which in turn leads to accumulation of edema fluid in interstitial and extravascular

spaces, including the myocardium.[226] Myocardial edema can contribute to post-CPB myocardial dysfunction by impairing diastolic function and causing mechanical limitation of cardiac filling and outflow in small infants whose sternums have been closed. Additionally, myocardial edema has been implicated as a causative factor in the frequent decline in myocardial function that occurs 6 to 12 hours after conclusion of CPB. Inflammatory mediators also affect the responsiveness of the myocardium to catecholamines by interfering with their binding to the cell surface receptors,[227] rendering exogenously administered drugs, such as dopamine and epinephrine, as well as the child's endogenous catecholamines, less effective at increasing cardiac output in the perioperative period.

Mechanisms for prevention and treatment of myocardial dysfunction include the use of ultrafiltration and antiinflammatory drugs, such as corticosteroids and aprotinin.[228,229] The prophylactic use of noncatecholamine inotropic agents, such as milrinone, has also been shown to prevent low cardiac output syndrome in infants, even if cardiac function is adequate in the immediate postoperative period.[230]

## SYSTEMIC AND PULMONARY VASCULATURE EFFECTS

The inflammatory response to CPB often produces mediators that directly increase pulmonary and systemic vascular resistance. These include interleukins, leukotrienes, and endothelin.[231] Indeed, when pulmonary artery pressure is measured directly, it is often significantly increased immediately after bypass, even if surgical results are optimal. This increase can be extremely detrimental in children with large left-to-right shunts, those undergoing cardiac transplantation secondary to dilated cardiomyopathy, and those undergoing bidirectional cavopulmonary anastomosis, where right ventricular output depends on maintaining low PVR. Prevention and treatment of increases in PVR include maintaining an adequate depth of anesthesia, ventilating with 100% oxygen, and judicious use of hyperventilation. Milrinone will increase right-sided heart output via its actions as both an inotropic agent and a pulmonary vasodilator. When PVR is significantly increased, inhaled nitric oxide is often used to assist in the early postoperative period.[232] Although effective, its cost is not inconsequential, and because PVR almost always decreases with time, nitric oxide is generally reserved for selected cases of pulmonary hypertension. Other simpler, less expensive treatments include oral or intravenous sildenafil[233,234] and inhaled nebulized prostacyclin.[235]

## PULMONARY EFFECTS

The lungs are not ventilated during CPB and are usually totally collapsed by intention, with the ventilator circuit disconnected, especially in small infants. This leads to significant atelectasis. The lungs are also at least partially ischemic during the bypass period, resulting in decreased production and alveolar levels of surfactant after CPB.[236] In addition, reperfusion injury (pulmonary edema or hemorrhage after a sudden increase in pulmonary flow) can also occur after creation of a systemic-to-pulmonary artery shunt or pulmonary artery unifocalization. Inflammatory mediators liberated by the bypass run, also predispose to increases in smooth muscle tone and resistance, and can result in bronchospasm.[237]

In addition to complement, endotoxins and certain cytokines can also activate neutrophils and attract them toward sites of inflammation.[238] In animal studies, endotoxin-induced lung injury can lead to rapid (within 45 minutes) accumulation of

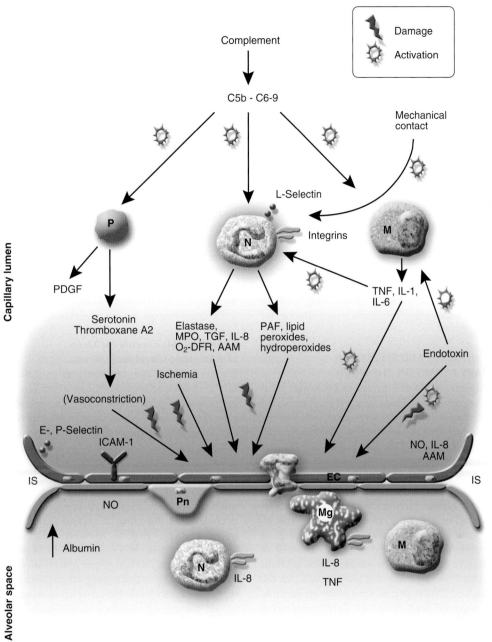

**FIGURE 17-6** Leukocytes, endothelial cells (*EC*), and humoral inflammatory mediators have been shown to play an important role in the cardiopulmonary bypass-induced lung injury. Complement (*C*) activation and complement-independent mechanical injury activates leukocytes, which, in their turn, secrete several inflammatory mediators, such as proteases and cytokines. Complement, cytokines, and ischemia-reperfusion also activate endothelial cells. Endotoxin, probably released from intestinal bacteria, exerts similar effects on leukocytes and endothelium. This process leads to disruption of endothelial and epithelial integrity and allows albumin, plasma, and activated leukocytes to enter the interstitial and alveolar space, causing tissue edema and reducing pulmonary compliance and blood oxygenation. *AAM,* Arachidonic acid metabolites; *ICAM-1,* intercellular adhesion molecule 1; *IL,* interleukin; *IS,* interstitial space; *M,* monocyte; *Mg,* macrophage; *MPO,* myeloperoxidase; *N,* neutrophil; *NO,* nitric oxide; *O₂-DFR,* oxygen-derived free radicals; *P,* platelet; *PAF,* platelet-activating factor; *PDGF,* platelet-derived growth factor; *Pn,* pneumocyte; *TGF,* tumor growth factor; *TNF,* tumor necrosis factor. (From Asimakopoulos G, Smith PL, Ratnatunga CP, Taylor KM. Lung injury and acute respiratory distress syndrome after cardiopulmonary bypass. Ann Thorac Surg 1999;1107-15.)

neutrophils within lung capillaries. Activation of neutrophils, with upregulation of adhesion molecules, neutrophil adhesion to the endothelium of lung vessels, and endothelial damage through proteases, appears to be the main step of the underlying pathophysiologic mechanism (Fig. 17-6). Macrophages play an important role in the evolution of the inflammatory acute lung injury through the secretion of cytokines, cytotoxic metabolites, and chemoattractants for leukocytes. At the clinical level, acute respiratory distress syndrome (ARDS) is often only one part of multiorgan failure, and lung injury should be seen as part of a more general state of systemic inflammation. The reported prevalence of ARDS after CPB in adults is 0.5% to 1.7%; the incidence in children is unknown. Interestingly, general hypothermia at 28° C failed to prevent the loss of ATP and the accumulation of lactate in lungs.[239] Other methods that aim to protect the lungs during CPB, such as continuous lung perfusion, pneumoplegia, and nitric oxide ventilation at lung reperfusion, prevent more severe hemodynamic deterioration and preserve reactivity of the pulmonary vasculature, but fail to prevent pulmonary dysfunction.

The severity of pulmonary dysfunction after CPB can be measured via changes in the alveolar-arterial oxygenation gradient, intrapulmonary shunt, degree of pulmonary edema, pulmonary compliance, and PVR. Treatment of pulmonary atelectasis includes careful reinflation of the lungs when weaning from bypass (by administering several vital capacity breaths), gentle but thorough suctioning of the tracheal tube, and prophylactic use of inhaled bronchodilators before separation from CPB. Using these measures, pulmonary function has been shown to improve immediately in most children with large left-to-right shunts, with the duration of CPB seemingly having little effect on pulmonary outcomes.[240] Thus, CPB itself has little effect on pulmonary function in most children. There is still an occasional child, however, who experiences classic "pump lung" ARDS, caused by the factors noted earlier. Treatment is supportive as for anyone with ARDS.

## NEUROLOGIC MONITORING AND EFFECTS OF CARDIOPULMONARY BYPASS ON THE BRAIN

Cerebral monitoring can help to detect those children who are at risk for neurologic sequelae after bypass, promptly recognize and treat changes in cerebral blood flow/oxygenation, evaluate the effect of therapeutic interventions on cerebral physiology, optimize brain protection during the vulnerable periods of CPB, and potentially improve short- and long-term neurologic outcomes.[241]

The cerebral NIRS monitor measures brain tissue oxygenation. This device noninvasively measures the cerebral tissue oxygen saturation and displays a numerical value for the cerebral regional oxygen saturation ($rSO_2$), the ratio of oxyhemoglobin to total hemoglobin in the light path. $rSO_2$ is a measure of local microcirculatory oxygen supply-and-demand balance and is reported on a scale from 15% to 95%. It has been assumed from anatomic models that 75% of the cerebral blood volume in the light path is venous and 25% is arterial. One study verified this in children with congenital heart disease by directly measuring the jugular venous bulb and arterial oxygen saturations and comparing these with the cerebral oxygen saturation measured with NIRS.[242] The actual ratio in children varied widely, but on average the venous to arterial ratio was 85 : 15. All devices measure both the arterial and venous blood oxygen saturations. Accordingly, this device does not provide a measure of the jugular venous bulb oxygen saturation ($SjvO_2$). A corollary of this is that maneuvers that increase arterial oxygen saturation (e.g., increasing $FIO_2$) increase cerebral oxygenation as measured by these devices, although the $SjvO_2$ may remain unchanged. In a study of 40 infants and children with congenital heart disease who were undergoing cardiac surgery or catheterization, NIRS correlated poorly with $SjvO_2$ measurements, except in infants younger than 1 year of age.[243] In contrast, in a study of 30 children undergoing cardiac catheterization, NIRS correlated very well with $SjvO_2$ ($r = .93$).[244] These data suggest that NIRS is a useful indicator of trends in cerebral oxygenation in individual infants and children. NIRS values also correlate with long-term neurodevelopmental outcomes in infant heart surgery. In a prospective study of 104 two-ventricle repairs, low $rSO_2$ in the intraoperative period did not correlate with death or major morbidity.[245] However, when these children underwent neurodevelopmental testing at 1 year of age, lower average and minimum $rSO_2$ in the 60 minute period immediately after CPB correlated with worse psychomotor development index scores. Low $rSO_2$ also correlated with remote ischemic changes on brain MRI at 1 year of age.[246]

### Neurologic Monitoring for Low-Flow Hypothermic Bypass

Transcranial Doppler (TCD) ultrasonography has been used to determine the threshold of detectable cerebral perfusion during low-flow CPB. *TCD velocities reveal trends or changes in cerebral blood flow and not absolute values.* One report studied 28 neonates undergoing the arterial switch operation using α-stat blood gas management.[148] Their study suggested that NIRS and TCD may be useful to determine the minimum acceptable bypass flow rate for an individual neonate during low-flow hypothermic bypass. Blood flow becomes insufficient at bypass flow rates less than 30 mL/kg/min.[148,247] Inadequate blood flow to the brain during this technique could be undetected without such monitoring, and low-flow bypass may confer no advantage to the brain over DHCA in some children. Long-term outcome studies of this monitoring strategy are not available.

### Neurologic Monitoring for Deep Hypothermic Circulatory Arrest

Despite clinical and experimental evidence that periods of DHCA that exceed approximately 40 minutes are associated with an increased risk of adverse long-term neurologic and developmental outcomes, this technique is still widely used in surgery to correct congenital heart defects. Recent recommendations for improving outcome after DHCA, based on both animal and clinical studies, were described previously. During DHCA, $rSO_2$ predictably decreases to a nadir 60% to 70% (relative change) below baseline values obtained before bypass. The nadir is reached at 10 to 20 minutes, after which there is no further decrease.[248] At this point, it appears that there is no additional oxygen uptake by the brain. Several studies suggest the potential for near-infrared cerebral oximetry to determine the safe conduct and duration of DHCA in the individual child. In a study of infants and children undergoing surgery with bypass and DHCA, three children with low $rSO_2$ developed acute postoperative neurologic changes—seizures in one, and prolonged coma in two.[248] In these three children, the increase in $rSO_2$ after the onset of CPB was much less (average 3% relative increase vs. 33% increase in children without neurologic deficit) and the duration of cooling before DHCA shorter than in the remaining 23 children who did not develop neurologic changes. In a neonatal pig model, the timing of the nadir of $rSO_2$ values during DHCA correlated with neurologic outcome: a more prolonged period without oxygen uptake by the brain correlated with a greater incidence of adverse neurologic outcome. The maximum safe duration at 17° C without additional brain oxygen uptake was 30 minutes.[142] Interestingly, this time period correlates with clinical and experimental studies, suggesting that 40 minutes is the safe duration for circulatory arrest (see Fig. 17-3). When circulatory arrest is initiated at greater temperatures (e.g., 25° C), the $rSO_2$ decreases more rapidly, and the nadir is achieved sooner, than at lower temperatures.[249] Reperfusion results in an increase in $rSO_2$ to levels observed at full bypass flow before DHCA, with a subsequent decrease during rewarming. Based on these data, our current practice is to reperfuse after the NIRS nadir has been reached for a period of 20 to 25 minutes.

### Neurologic Monitoring for Regional Cerebral Perfusion

RCP (also known as selective cerebral perfusion or antegrade cerebral perfusion) uses a polytetrafluoroethylene (PTFE) graft or a small aortic cannula as arterial inflow to the right innominate artery for neonatal aortic surgery, such as the Norwood stage operation or aortic arch advancement. The other brachiocephalic vessels and descending thoracic aorta are snared, resulting in a bloodless operating field. The brain is perfused through the right innominate and right vertebral arteries only. This approach significantly reduces or eliminates the use of DHCA for these operations and preserves brain perfusion, potentially improving neurologic outcome. Initial descriptions of this technique used the pressure in the radial artery or a predetermined bypass rate of 25 to 30 mL/kg/min as an estimate for the bypass flow during RCP without neurologic monitoring. When flow rate was estimated on the basis of NIRS monitoring in individual children, it was determined that 20 to 25 mL/kg/min was required.[217] However, NIRS was applied only to the right side of the skull (i.e., brain), the same side as the sole arterial inflow. Using a pH-stat blood gas strategy for RCP, we noted that the majority of our children had an $rSO_2$ of 95% (the maximum reading on the $rSO_2$ scale) when we used the left radial artery pressure of 20 to 25 mm Hg as the target for bypass flow. These children were theoretically at risk for excessive cerebral perfusion. Therefore, we performed a study using both NIRS and TCD of the right cerebral hemisphere, to determine if TCD could be used as a guide to RCP flow rate.[222] Bypass flow rate was adjusted to achieve a cerebral blood flow volume within 10% of baseline (e.g., TCD was used to determine necessary flow). The estimated flow rate, 63 mL/kg/min (range, 24 to 94 mL/kg/min), proved to be significantly greater than that estimated in the earlier studies. This flow rate did not correlate with the pressure in the right or left radial artery. The $rSO_2$ was well maintained in all children, leading us to conclude that TCD was a useful monitor to ensure adequate but not excessive cerebral blood flow during RCP. Because RCP perfuses the brain through a single arterial inflow vessel, questions have arisen about the adequacy of cerebral blood flow and oxygenation to the left cerebral hemisphere. Although the circle of Willis is expected to be intact without stenoses in neonates, 10% of healthy full-term neonates exhibit deviations from normal flow patterns. Two studies concluded that although cerebral blood flow and oxygenation were adequate to both cerebral hemispheres in neonates during RCP, bilateral monitoring, at least of NIRS, may be warranted.[222,250]

### SYSTEMIC INFLAMMATORY RESPONSE SYNDROME

In cardiac surgery, SIRS is thought to result from four main sources of injury: (1) contact of the blood components with the artificial surface of the bypass circuit, (2) ischemia-reperfusion injury, (3) endotoxemia, and (4) operative trauma. Inflammatory cytokines, together with endothelial activation and endothelial-leukocyte interactions, appear to play an important role in the induction of this systemic inflammatory response.

Exposure of blood to the artificial materials in the bypass circuit—plastics, polypropylene oxygenator fibers, and metal suction devices—initiates a cascade of inflammatory responses, including activation of the complement system, the kallikrein system, and the coagulation system.[226] As a result, interleukins, tumor necrosis factor, endotoxin, heat shock protein, and many other inflammatory mediators are released into the circulation. Leukocyte activation also results in secretion of inflammatory mediators, such as proteases and cytokines (e.g., TNF-α and

IL-1), which are secreted early in the evolution of the inflammatory process. This chemokine-mediated increased leukocyte activation constitutes an important link in the chain of the propagation of the inflammatory response (see Fig. 17-6).

This inflammatory response is counterbalanced by a complex system of inhibitors, such as IL-10 and soluble cytokine receptors.[251] Also, the inflammatory response of the neonate may be more exaggerated than that of the infant or older child,[252] justifying a more aggressive approach to its modulation in the neonate (see later discussion).

A number of novel treatments have been studied, including monoclonal antibodies for inflammatory products, such as complement, endotoxin, and tumor necrosis factor. Although theoretically attractive, no clinical difference has been noted with any of these treatments.

Effective treatments used every day in the operating room and ICU include:

- Use of corticosteroids[253]
- Ultrafiltration[228] (see earlier discussion)
- Aprotinin[229] (see earlier discussion)
- Leukocyte depletion[254]: leukocyte-depleted blood in prime and in-line arterial filter; initiate bypass using normoxic management ($FIO_2$ of 21%) in severely cyanotic infants.

Corticosteroids interrupt the inflammatory response at several levels by entering cell nuclei and changing the rate of transcription of inflammatory molecules. Increasing evidence suggests that glucocorticoids act by regulating transcription or translation of antiinflammatory cytokines, such as IL-10, and altering expression of other proteins, such as endothelin-1 and inhibitor NF-κβ.[255,256] Because these processes take time to develop, the effects of corticosteroids are not immediate, taking up to several hours.[257] Thus, the common practice of adding corticosteroids to the CPB prime will not fully prevent the inflammatory response[258]; to be effective, corticosteroids may need to be administered 4 or more hours before the onset of CPB.[259]

Despite these theoretical advantages of using corticosteroids to modulate the inflammatory response, a recent large discharge database review of over 46,000 infants and children, in which 54% did receive corticosteroids, demonstrated no difference in mortality. Using propensity score matching the authors concluded that corticosteroids were associated with greater length of hospital stay, greater rate of infection, and greater use of insulin. There was no difference in duration of ventilation. Steroids conferred no significant benefit; conversely in the simpler surgery categories, there was increased morbidity with these drugs.[260] Although inflammatory activation from CPB definitely occurs, and it would seem intuitive that this would lead to worse outcomes in those patients with excessive inflammation, in contemporary practice, the correlation of the magnitude of this response and length of ICU stay and blood product administration, is statistically significant, but clinically modest, accounting for only 4% to 9% of the difference in these variables, in a large study of infants undergoing two-ventricle repairs.[261]

### COAGULATION EFFECTS

Blood coagulation is frequently abnormal after CPB for several reasons. The inflammatory cascade activates the coagulation system, resulting in factor consumption and fibrinolysis, which, in turn, breaks down existing blood clots, leading to increased bleeding.[16] Treatment is adequate heparinization, reversal with protamine, and the use of an antifibrinolytic to inhibit fibrinolysis and improve platelet function.[33] In addition, the smaller the child, the greater the dilution of clotting factors by the bypass prime, and the greater the risk for low concentrations of clotting proteins and fibrinogen postoperatively. Platelets are also degranulated and consumed by the CPB circuit, leading both to low platelet counts and nonfunctioning platelets.[16] The smaller the infant, the greater the duration of bypass, and the more complicated the surgery, the greater the incidence of coagulopathy after bypass. Efforts to minimize the post-bypass coagulopathy in infants includes priming the CPB circuit with fresh whole blood for small infants, if available, or packed cells plus fresh frozen plasma (FFP) if fresh whole blood cannot be obtained.[19,262] Treatment involves administration of platelets to small infants as the first line of therapy, followed by the replacement of fibrinogen and FFP to replace clotting factors. If these factors are not effective after correcting coagulation parameters, such as platelet count, prothrombin/PTT, fibrinogen, and thromboelastogram, then surgical bleeding may be the cause and surgical reexploration may be warranted.[263] Factor VIIa has also been used as a last resort in children who have significant post-bypass bleeding unresponsive to standard measures.[56]

### HEPATIC, RENAL, AND GASTROINTESTINAL EFFECTS

The liver, kidneys, and gastrointestinal tract, like the brain and heart, may be rendered ischemic by prolonged CPB, DHCA, or low cardiac output syndrome. Renal function is compromised on CPB. This is manifested by the appearance of proteinuria and impaired tubular cellular function immediately after CPB. Renal dysfunction from ischemia is also common. Low urine output may occur secondary to secretion of antidiuretic hormone, a response to surgical stress. However, the latter appears to be transitory and usually resolves spontaneously.[264] The incidence of acute renal dysfunction after surgery with bypass to correct congenital heart defects is 17%, ranging from 0.7% for arterial septal defect closure to 59% for arterial switch operations.[265] Deep hypothermic cardiac arrest subjects the kidney to additional ischemia reperfusion injury.[266] Acute renal failure after CPB is uncommon in children, with fewer than 3% requiring dialysis perioperatively.[265,267] Infants who undergo cardiac surgery routinely receive diuretics or a peritoneal dialysis catheter, the latter prophylactically in some instances.[268,269] Although some have attributed the improved survival with early peritoneal dialysis to the prevention of fluid overload, others have attributed it to a more rapid clearance of CPB-induced proinflammatory cytokines.[270] Further study is required to clarify the mechanism of action of early peritoneal dialysis. In our center, neonates and children with a complex heart defect usually receive peritoneal dialysis immediately postoperatively to prevent fluid overload.

Recovery of hepatic and gastrointestinal function follows hemodynamic recovery, but may require several days. Therapy is mainly supportive. Splanchnic and renal perfusion can be monitored noninvasively using somatic oximetry. Somatic oxygenation may predict renal dysfunction and predict organ failure. Interventions based on the somatic NIRS may improve outcome.[271]

### IMMUNE SYSTEM EFFECTS

Leukocytes are activated by the CPB circuit, although their numbers may be depleted by leukocyte filters, which are sometimes used to attenuate the inflammatory response. Despite the theoretical possibility that this may increase the risk of infection or neutrophil dysfunction, this has not been observed in published studies or clinical practice.[272]

### ENDOCRINE SYSTEM EFFECTS

The magnitude of the inflammatory and endocrine responses after cardiac surgery depends in part on the duration of the surgical procedure and CPB.[273] In children undergoing brief operating times, postoperative blood concentrations of cortisol, adrenocorticotropic hormone, and β-endorphins are significantly greater than those in children undergoing prolonged operation times. In contrast, the serum concentrations of the proinflammatory cytokines IL-6, IL-1β, and TNF-α are similar in the two groups. Adrenocorticotropic hormone and cortisol concentrations correlated positively with the blood concentrations of IL-1β, IL-6, and TNF-α in the group of children with prolonged operation times.

The plasma concentrations of both epinephrine and cortisol increase after cardiac surgery.[274] In children, pre- and post-bypass cortisol and norepinephrine increase significantly during isoflurane anesthesia when 2 μg/kg of fentanyl is used rather than 25, 50, 100, or 150 μg/kg.[275] No significant increase in the blood concentrations of these hormones occurred with any of the fentanyl doses of 25 μg/kg or greater. In addition to cardiovascular stability, continued use of larger doses of opioids during bypass minimizes the stress responses and stabilizes hemodynamics during and after bypass, but may delay recovery.[276] Also, growth hormone, glucose and insulin, lactate, glutamate, aspartate, and free fatty acid concentrations increase after cardiac surgery, whereas total triiodothyronine concentrations decrease.[277] Limiting the amount of opioids balances the negative effects of inflammation and stress with the opportunity to fast-track children's recovery after surgery for congenital heart disease.[278,279]

## Transport to the Intensive Care Unit

Extreme vigilance is required during transfer of the child from the cardiac operating room to the ICU. Monitoring of ECG, arterial, venous, and atrial pressures, and end-tidal $CO_2$ and pulse oximetry must be maintained continuously; the battery charge of the monitor and the infusion pumps should be checked beforehand to prevent monitor failure and interruption of the infusions of vasoactive medications. Resuscitation drugs, airway equipment, and blood products should accompany the child to the ICU. Before leaving the operating room, a report should be given to the ICU staff. Children who are transported with tracheal tubes in situ are usually ventilated manually during transport via a Jackson-Rees circuit, with either 100% oxygen or, for those who require a $FIO_2$ less than 1.0, an oxygen-air blender. For children who require nitric oxide, a respiratory therapist should assist with transport to ensure that no interruptions in therapy occur and that a smooth transfer occurs in the ICU as well. On arrival in the ICU, vital signs are confirmed, all monitoring devices are transferred sequentially to the ICU monitors and rechecked to ensure they are in working order, and a detailed report is given to the ICU staff.

## Summary

Cardiopulmonary bypass is a necessary technique for intracardiac and major extracardiac surgery on the great vessels. CPB induces a multitude of physiologic and inflammatory derangements, but, through extensive experience and research, these ill effects can be largely mitigated by a number of evidence-based strategies. Therefore, outcomes after CPB have improved dramatically, and CPB is no longer a barrier to accomplishing complex surgery to correct congenital heart defects, even in neonates.

## ANNOTATED REFERENCES

Andropoulos DB, Stayer SA, McKenzie ED, Fraser CD Jr. Regional low-flow perfusion provides comparable blood flow and oxygenation to both cerebral hemispheres during neonatal aortic arch reconstruction. J Thorac Cardiovasc Surg 2003;126:1712-7.

*Regional cerebral perfusion (RCP), a technique designed to avoid deep hypothermic circulatory arrest, was studied in 20 neonates undergoing the Norwood stage I palliation or aortic arch reconstruction. When RCP flow is guided by transcranial Doppler ultrasound flow velocity, and near-infrared cerebral oximetry, both right and left cerebral hemispheres have comparable flow velocity and oxygenation values; therefore, this technique can support the whole brain when adequate bypass flows are used.*

du Plessis AJ, Jonas RA, Wypij D, et al. Perioperative effects of alpha-stat versus pH-stat strategies for deep hypothermic cardiopulmonary bypass in infants. J Thorac Cardiovasc Surg 1997;114:991-1000.

*In this study, 182 neonates and infants were randomized to pH-stat or α-stat CPB strategy. Important trends or statistically significant improved outcomes were seen with pH-stat management for deaths, EEG seizures, return of EEG activity, acidosis, hypotension, inotropic support, and length of mechanical ventilation. These improvements were most significant for arterial switch operation patients.*

Jonas RA, Wypij D, Roth SJ, et al. The influence of hemodilution on outcome after hypothermic cardiopulmonary bypass: results of a randomized trial in infants. J Thorac Cardiovasc Surg 2003;126:1765-74.

*One hundred thirteen infants randomized to a target hematocrit of 20% (actual 21.5%) versus 30% (actual 28%) on CPB had lower neurodevelopmental outcome scores at 1 year of age: 82 on the Psychomotor Development Index of the Bayley Scales of Infant Development with lower hematocrit versus 90. The children with lower target hematocrit also had a greater incidence of scores more than 2 SD below the mean (29% vs. 9%).*

Miller BE, Mochizuki T, Levy JH, et al. Predicting and treating coagulopathies after cardiopulmonary bypass in children. Anesth Analg 1997;85:1196-202.

*This is the classic article describing the reasons for post-CPB bleeding in infants and children. Platelet defects are the most important cause and the first blood product to administer; hypofibrinogenemia is the second most important, and fibrinogen is the next most important blood product, with fresh frozen plasma ineffective or possibly worsening bleeding.*

Newburger JW, Jonas RA, Soul J, et al. Randomized trial of hematocrit 25% versus 35% during hypothermic cardiopulmonary bypass in infant heart surgery. J Thorac Cardiovasc Surg 2008;135:347-54.

*Perioperative hemodynamics during hypothermic cardiopulmonary bypass and developmental outcome and brain magnetic resonance imaging at 1 year were evaluated. Hemodilution to hematocrit levels of 35% compared with those of 25% had no major benefits or risks overall among infants undergoing two-ventricle repair. Developmental outcomes at 1 year of age in both randomized groups were below those in the normative population.*

Wypij D, Newburger JW, Rappaport LA, et al. The effect of duration of deep hypothermic circulatory arrest in infant heart surgery on late neurodevelopment: the Boston Circulatory Arrest Trial. J Thorac Cardiovasc Surg 2003;126:1397-403.

*Neurodevelopmental outcomes were assessed with a battery of 6 tests in 155 8-year-olds who had a neonatal arterial switch operation using a-stat bypass management, hematocrit of 20% on bypass, and varying duration of DHCA at 18° C. Neurodevelopmental outcomes were not adversely affected for the group as a whole until the DHCA time exceeded 41 minutes (95% lower confidence limit 32 minutes).*

Wypij D, Jonas RA, Bellinger DC, et al. The effect of hematocrit during hypothermic cardiopulmonary bypass in infant heart surgery: results from the combined Boston hematocrit trials. J Thorac Cardiovasc Surg 2008;135:355-60.

*In this combined review of 271 infants, analysis was undertaken of the effects of hematocrit level at the onset of low-flow cardiopulmonary bypass. A hematocrit level at the onset of low-flow cardiopulmonary bypass of approximately 24% or higher was associated with higher Psychomotor Development Index scores and reduced lactate levels.*

## REFERENCES

Please see www.expertconsult.com.

# Medications for Hemostasis

## PHILIP ARNOLD AND ADAM SKINNER

BLEEDING IS AN INEVITABLE CONSEQUENCE of surgery and trauma. Provided the coagulation processes are normal, a meticulous hemostatic surgical technique is usually adequate to achieve hemostasis for most surgical procedures. If, however, the degree of injury is more extensive, major blood loss can occur, particularly if there is a coexistent deficiency of the normal coagulation process. It has been appreciated since the early part of the 20th century that transfusion of fluids and human (allogeneic) blood can prevent many of the adverse effects of blood loss. Despite this, it is important to appreciate the risks and limitations of transfusion; red cell concentrates alone will fail to correct any existing coagulopathy and the immunologic and pathophysiologic adverse effects of exogenous stored blood products are now well known.

This chapter will examine specific treatments aimed at correcting coagulopathy and at reducing the requirement for transfusion of blood products by encouraging hemostasis. Although similar, these objectives are not the same. During many types of surgery, in vitro tests may only demonstrate mild coagulation defects, and yet the use of hemostatic medications may reduce blood loss and obviate the need to transfuse red cells.[1,2] In the absence of these medications, bleeding itself is often unlikely to be life-threatening. In comparison, severe coagulopathic bleeding is, by its nature, life-threatening. Transfusion of blood products cannot be avoided and the hemostatic medications used are often the blood products themselves. Fundamentally, the equation of risk and benefit is very different in these two situations. In the former case, benefit will occur if the risk reduction associated with the avoidance of blood products is greater than any risk from the medication itself. In the latter case, the use of medications that carry a high risk of causing adverse effects is more acceptable if the aim is to prevent death from uncontrolled bleeding. As an example of this, aprotinin has been largely rejected for use during adult cardiac surgery as a strategy to reduce transfusion,[3] whereas use of recombinant factor VIIa (almost certainly a more "hazardous" drug) is still considered appropriate for the treatment of life-threatening bleeding.

Avoidance of transfusion of human blood products seems to be a fundamentally good notion. However, many common ideas about the potential harm of transfusion may be mistaken. A national audit of the serious hazards of transfusion (SHOT) in the United Kingdom reported 3239 adverse events over a 10-year period; this is only 0.013% of all blood transfusions.[4] These adverse events were more common in infants, but were only reported in 0.037% of infants given transfusions. The true incidence of events is likely to be more common because of underreporting, though many of these "events" were procedural errors not associated with actual harm. It is clear that the risk of immediate harm directly attributable to transfusion is exceptionally low. The risk of direct transmission of infection (the most feared risk in the public perception) is particularly small; the risk of transmission of HIV from transfusion of blood in the UK is 1 in 5 million, and no child has contracted a viral infection from transfusion in the last 4 years.[4] The greatest hazard of immediate harm is of a mistake leading to transfusion of incompatible blood.[5] However, subtle negative effects of transfusion on children's outcomes may be considerably more important.[6] Transfusion of blood may lead to deterioration in pulmonary function and immunologic effects that predispose children to infection. In addition, if the objective of transfused red cells is to boost tissue oxygenation by improving oxygen carrying capacity, then transfused blood is less effective than the child's own blood for this function.[7] Additional considerations include the increasing costs of transfused blood products, the logistical difficulties of maintaining a secure blood supply (in both well-resourced and less well developed health systems), substantially greater risks of transfusion (in poorly developed health systems), and the possibility of new, unrecognized infective agents entering the blood supply.

There are 2.3 million transfusions each year (37 per 1000 population) in the UK; 4.2% are given to children under 18 years of age (7.1 per 1000) and 1.7% to infants (52 per 1000). An audit of pediatric blood transfusion from Australia revealed 41% of blood transfused was given perioperatively,[8] and blood was transfused during 6.3% of instances of anesthesia. The majority of units were used during heart surgery (58% of perioperative use) while a very small minority, 4% were used during major trauma surgery. Heart surgery (on and off bypass), craniosynostosis surgery, and liver transplantation were all commonly associated with blood transfusion. The epidemiology of major bleeding is less certain. Reports of blood use may be misleading (e.g., neonates undergoing cardiac surgery to correct congenital defects may receive few blood units despite significant bleeding), and blood is also used for purposes such as priming the bypass circuit. Observational studies have reported very heavy blood loss associated with heart surgery in children, with increased (per kg) blood loss in smaller children and more complex surgery.[9,10] Cardiac surgery can probably be considered the main cause of major blood loss in children and will account for most severe bleeding events in children less than 1 year of age.

In this chapter we review the physiology of normal coagulation and how this is deranged in situations likely to be encountered by the pediatric anesthesiologist, particularly during cardiopulmonary bypass and massive transfusion situations. We will demonstrate the importance and limitations of newer physiologic models of coagulation for the understanding of bleeding. The management of major bleeding (with the exception of the off-label use of factor VIIa) has been largely unchanged for many years. Newer approaches are now emerging, although at the time of this writing, robust evidence of risk and benefit is not available.

## Physiology of Coagulation

The understanding of coagulation has shifted greatly in the last few years. The "traditional" model, which emphasizes the importance of a cascade of proteolytic enzymes has given way to the "cell based" model of coagulation that emphasizes the importance of cellular elements in coagulation and presents coagulation as a complex web of interactions rather than a linear process.[11,12]

To achieve effective hemostasis, a platelet plug must form at the site of vessel injury. In addition, the procoagulant factors need to remain localized to the injured site to avoid widespread clotting activation. This is achieved through changes at the cell surface and localization of the procoagulant reactions on the surfaces of specific cells. Different cells possess different procoagulant and anticoagulant properties; these are incompletely understood, but platelets and cells bearing tissue factor (TF) are central to the process. Intact endothelium is also vital to normal control of coagulation, as it keeps these different procoagulant components apart and modifies coagulation through expression of inhibitory proteins such as thrombomodulin. The described phases of coagulation are overlapping and involve initiation, amplification, and propagation.[12]

### INITIATION

Coagulation is initiated by a membrane-bound lipoprotein called tissue factor. This is usually expressed on subendothelial

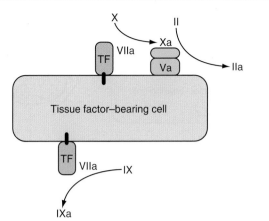

**FIGURE 18-1** Initiation. The TF/VIIa complex on the tissue factor–bearing cell activates factors IX and X. The factor Xa/Va complex, known as the "prothrombinase" complex, forms small amounts of thrombin (factor IIa). (Reproduced from Hoffman M. Remodeling the blood coagulation cascade. J Thromb Thrombolysis 2003;16:17-20.)

TF-bearing cells, such as stromal fibroblasts; in the absence of vessel injury it is separated from the vessel lumen. After injury, a complex is formed between TF and factor VIIa (TF/VIIa), which activates factors IX and X. Factor Xa, in association with cofactor Va, forms "prothrombinase" complexes on the surface of the TF-bearing cell, which activates a small amount of thrombin (factor IIa)[12] (Fig. 18-1). The purpose of this small generation of thrombin and Xa is to activate platelets and factors V and VIII.

Tissue factor pathway inhibitor (TFPI) and antithrombin III (ATIII) provide a localizing function on factor Xa by inhibiting any factor Xa that becomes dissociated from the TF-bearing cell. Factor IXa is not localized to the cell in the same way.

Low levels of IX and X activation occur in the absence of tissue injury without causing clot formation. The process only leads to amplification when damage to the vasculature allows intravascular platelets and a complex formed by factor VIII and von Willebrand factor (VIII/vWF) to adhere to the extravascular TF-bearing cells.[11]

### AMPLIFICATION

Small quantities of thrombin are generated on the TF-bearing cells. This sets up the subsequent propagation phase, during which thrombin is generated in large quantities (Fig. 18-2). This thrombin has many major functions:

- Activation of platelets, exposing receptors and binding sites for clotting factors
- Activation of cofactors V and VIII on the activated platelet surface, thereby releasing vWF to mediate additional adhesion and aggregation at the injury site
- Activation of factor XI to XIa[13]
- Activation of factor XIII (fibrin stabilizing factor) and promotion of fibrin crosslinking
- Cleaving fibrinopeptides A and B from fibrinogen (forming fibrin)

### PROPAGATION

Propagation occurs on the surface of activated platelets that are recruited to the site in large numbers. Activated factor IX (from both initiation phase and provided by factor XI on the platelet) binds to VIIIa. The resultant IXa/VIIIa complex activates factor X on the platelet surface. This factor Xa associates with factor Va

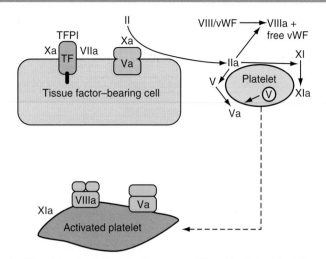

**FIGURE 18-2** Amplification. Small amounts of thrombin (factor IIa) set the stage for large-scale generation of thrombin in the propagation phase. Small amounts of thrombin activate platelets, as well as other important coagulation enzymes and cofactors. (Reproduced from Hoffman M. Remodeling the blood coagulation cascade. J Thromb Thrombolysis 2003;16:17-20.)

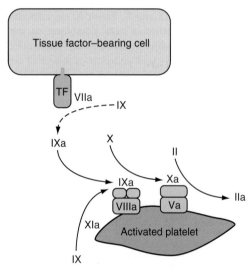

**FIGURE 18-3** Propagation. Factor Xa is formed locally by the VIIIa/IXa complex on the surface of the activated platelet. The resulting Xa/Va prothrombinase complex causes a burst of thrombin (factor IIa) generation. (Reproduced from Hoffman M. Remodeling the blood coagulation cascade. J Thromb Thrombolysis 2003;16:17-20.)

and forms the prothrombinase complex. The prothrombinase complex causes a "burst" of thrombin generation to cause clotting via fibrinogen (Fig. 18-3).[11]

This sequence explains why children with hemophilia bleed despite having a normal TF/VIIa complex; the factor Xa during the initiation phase is broken down by ATIII and TFPI if it dissociates from the TF-bearing cell. It is therefore unable to activate the "burst" of thrombin generation that normally occurs in this propagation phase. The factor Xa needs to be generated on the platelet itself via the IXa/VIIIa complex.[11]

Of note, an alternative pathway is initiated by contact factors (XII, XI, prekallikrein, and high-molecular-weight kininogen [HMWK]). It is of no physiologic importance in terms of coagulation activation; however, it provides important acceleration

loops through feedback activation of factors VIII, IX, and XI[14] and is important in fibrinolytic and inflammatory pathways.[15]

## CLOT INHIBITION

The clot is confined to the site of injury by direct and indirect thrombin inhibitory systems. The direct system comprises ATIII, $\alpha_2$-macroglobulin, and heparin cofactor II (HCII). ATIII and HCII activities are accelerated in the presence of heparin.

Several indirect systems inhibit thrombin, such as the protein C–protein S–thrombomodulin (TM) and the TFPI systems. Thrombin binds to TM on the surface of intact endothelial cells and can no longer cleave fibrinogen to form fibrin. The TM/thrombin complex is neither able to activate platelets nor activate factors V and VIII. Instead, this complex activates protein C, which binds to the cofactor protein S and inactivates factors Va (on the surface of endothelial cells and platelets) and VIIIa.[11,14] TFPI bound to endothelial surfaces can form complexes with factor Xa that inhibit factor VIIa. Thrombin generation is therefore inhibited.[14]

## FIBRINOLYSIS

Fibrinolysis (the breakdown of fibrin into soluble degradation products) is mediated by the proteolytic enzyme, plasmin. Plasmin is formed from an inactive zymogen, plasminogen, which is produced in the liver. This process is controlled by activators and inhibitors. The principal plasminogen activators are tissue plasminogen activator (tPA) and urokinase (uPA). Although overlap exists between the functions of these activators, they have distinct physiologic roles. uPA is primarily involved in a wide variety of extracellular processes, including remodeling of tissues. tPA is the major intravascular activator of fibrinolysis and is discussed in more detail later.[16] The main inhibitory proteins are plasminogen activator inhibitor-1 (PAI-1), antiplasmins ($\alpha_2$-PI and $\alpha_2$-macroglobulin), and thrombin activated fibrinolysis inhibitor (TAFI)[17] (Fig. 18-4).

As well as cleaving fibrin, plasmin metabolizes a number of other proteins, including the platelet receptor for fibrinogen (glycoprotein IIb/IIIa) and fibrinogen.[18] In addition, plasmin accelerates its own production by metabolizing the conversion of single chain plasminogen activators to more active two-chain versions. The action of plasmin on fibrin produces a series of degradation products some of which convey anticoagulant properties; this effect is achieved by preventing polymerization of fibrinogen and by inhibition of platelet function.

tPA is released by vascular endothelium of small blood vessels. Release is increased in the presence of stimuli such as trauma, endotoxins, ischemia, or normal exercise. This effect is mediated via contact activation (through the kallikrein system) and also by a series of other substances, including thrombin. Once released, tPA is rapidly metabolized by the liver with a half-life of approximately 5 minutes.[17] Fibrin binds both plasminogen and tPA and greatly accelerates the conversion of plasminogen to plasmin (facilitating its own degradation, but also localizing the process to areas of clot). An alternative mechanism for plasminogen activation by tPA exists through binding to receptors expressed by certain cells (endothelium, white cells and some tumor cells); the importance of this in health or disease is unclear.

Excessive fibrinolysis can directly result from excess production of fibrin, as in disseminated intravascular coagulation. This is termed secondary hyperfibrinolysis and in this context the fibrinolysis is considered beneficial because it prevents

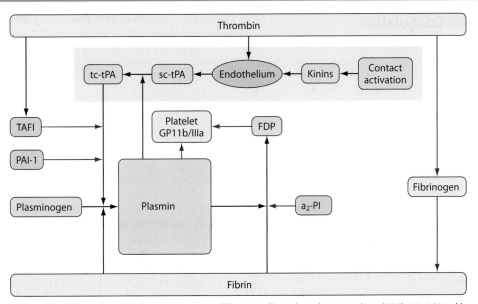

**FIGURE 18-4** The main fibrinolytic pathway, leading to the breakdown of fibrin into fibrin degradation products (*FDP*). It is initiated by release of tissue plasminogen activator (*tPA*) from endothelial cells in response to contact activation (*shaded area*). Plasminogen needs to be bound to fibrin in order to allow conversion to plasmin. *sc-tPA* and *tc-tPA* refer to single- and (more active) two-chain tPA, respectively. Endogenous fibrinolysis inhibitors are shown in *blue boxes: TAFI* is thrombin activated fibrinogen inhibitor, *PAI-1* is plasminogen activator inhibitor, and $\alpha_2$-*PI* is $\alpha_2$ plasmin inhibitor. Interactions with the coagulation system are shown by *red arrows.*

widespread vascular occlusion. Therapy is directed at replacement of consumed clotting factors, inhibition of excessive coagulation, and treatment of the underlying cause. Primary hyperfibrinolysis can occur during cardiac bypass, massive blood loss, trauma, and liver transplantation.[19] During the anhepatic stage of liver transplant surgery, there is hyperfibrinolysis because of failure to metabolize tPA. On reperfusion of the liver, a further surge of tPA occurs that can take several hours to return to normal. In coagulopathic patients, reduced thrombin formation may lead to reduced production of TAFI (important in inhibition of membrane bound plasmin), whereas conversion of single- to two-strand tPA by plasmin may further sustain the process. Individual susceptibility is likely to be important and may have a genetic component.[20,21]

Two groups of drugs are used clinically to inhibit fibrinolysis:

1. Synthetic lysine analogues, e.g., tranexamic acid (TXA) and ε-aminocaproic acid (EACA).
2. Protease inhibitors (e.g., aprotinin).

Synthetic lysine analogues are fairly specific inhibitors of plasminogen activation, working by competitively binding to lysine-binding sites on the plasminogen molecule (Fig. 18-5). This blocks the binding of plasminogen to fibrin; a required step for the conversion of plasminogen to plasmin by plasminogen activators.[22] At larger doses, they may have additional effects through direct inhibition of plasmin; this includes inhibition of the plasmin mediated effects on platelets.

Aprotinin is a less specific inhibitor of proteolytic enzymes; it has actions on the kallikrein–kinin (contact) system, as well as enzymes involved in coagulation and fibrinolysis. In addition, aprotinin may be associated with greater preservation of platelet function, as well as an antiinflammatory effect. This wider spectrum of effects from aprotinin may have additional benefits over the antifibrinolytic lysine analogues. Some additional effects may not necessarily be of benefit; for example, the contact system may have protective effects against ischemic reperfusion injury that are inhibited by aprotinin.[15]

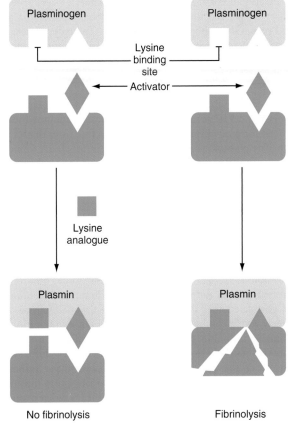

**FIGURE 18-5** Diagrammatic representation of the mode of action of the synthetic lysine analogues tranexamic acid and ε-aminocaproic acid. (Reproduced from Mahdy AM, Webster NR. Perioperative systemic haemostatic agents. Br J Anaesth 2004;93:842-58.)

# Developmental Coagulation

The hemostatic system in the neonate rapidly matures towards that of the adult (see also Chapter 9).[23-25] One must consider how the coagulation system matures in the child to interpret coagulation tests and use appropriate modalities to manipulate hemostasis in vivo.

All fetal coagulation factors are produced independently of the mother; fibrinogen starts to be formed as early as 5.5 weeks gestation, and blood can clot at 11 weeks. The introduction of microassays in the 1980s allowed for the determination of reference ranges for the coagulation factors beginning at 19 weeks gestational age.[14,23,24] In general, there are four fundamental differences between the coagulation systems in the infant and the adult[26]:

■ Concentrations of components of the hemostatic system
■ The turnover rate of various components of the coagulation cascade
■ The rate of synthesis
■ Differences in the overall ability to generate and regulate the key enzymes: thrombin and plasmin

Despite the upregulation of coagulation factors at birth, the vitamin K–dependent factors II, VII, IX, and X in the neonate are only 50% of adult values; this leads to a slightly prolonged prothrombin time (PT) or international normalized ratio (INR).[14] The contact factors HMWK, prekallikrein, and factors XI and XII are also approximately 50% of adult values.[14,26] The reduced contact factors account for a disproportionally prolonged activated partial thromboplastin time (aPTT). The reduced concentration of factors at birth is probably explained by the reduced synthesis of factors by the liver; however, concentrations increase rapidly, reaching approximately 80% of adult values by 6 months of age.[14,27]

In contrast, the plasma concentrations of fibrinogen and factors V and VIII at birth are similar to those in adults, although the fetal form of fibrinogen differs in structure from that of the adult. The physiologic significance of this is not clear.[28] Concentrations of vWF in the first 2 months of life are greater than those in adults.[29]

The inhibitor systems of coagulation also differ from adults. At birth, plasma protein C and S are 35% of adult values, although the fetal forms of the proteins differ from the adult forms. The concentration of protein C does not reach adult values until adolescence. Neonatal concentrations of ATIII and HCII are 50% of adult values; they reach adult concentrations by 6 months of age. The $\alpha_2$-macroglobulin value, however, is increased at birth and remains increased throughout childhood; it is postulated that this may be one of the mechanisms that protects young children from thromboembolic complications.[30]

Finally, thrombin generation in vitro is reduced in children to approximately 75% of adult values,[30] but there is difficulty in interpreting the apparent discrepancy between the sufficient hemostasis seen in vivo and these in vitro laboratory thrombin generation assays. It still remains to be clarified whether neonates and children are more susceptible to bleeding[14]; however, the risk of thromboembolic complications appears to increase with age.[30]

Despite reduced plasma concentrations of many procoagulant and anticoagulant proteins in infants, there still appears to be an effective hemostatic balance; healthy fetuses, neonates, and children do not suffer excessive hemorrhage in the presence of minor challenges. This is consistent with the thromboelastogram (TEG) studies of healthy children younger than 2 years of age; no defects in coagulation were noted using this test compared with adults, indicating an intact hemostatic system.[31] Another TEG study reported that infants younger than 1 year of age with complex congenital heart disease have an intact and balanced coagulation–fibrinolytic system but at a "lower level" than healthy children. This has been interpreted as a reduction in hemostatic potential with less reserve.[32]

## GENETICS OF BLEEDING

The hemophilias are a group of genetic diseases that cause excessive bleeding, often in response to minor trauma. von Willebrand disease and hemophilia A are the most common variants (see also Chapter 9), associated with low levels of von Willebrand factor and factor VIII respectively. A wide range of single gene defects resulting in deficiencies of single clotting proteins or regulatory proteins have now been described. A further group of single gene disorders may result in thrombophilic disorders, associated with abnormalities of inhibitory proteins.

Unexplained variation has been observed in bleeding between apparently similar patients in the absence of specific factor deficiency. The causes of this variation are likely to be multifold according to nuances of surgical technique and subtle difference in disease process and therapy. It might appear counterintuitive that genetic factors have a significant role in acquired bleeding resulting from surgery; however, recently there has been increased interest in the interplay of genetic and environmental factors in the progress of acquired diseases. The genetics of most clotting proteins has been described, and common variations within populations have been revealed for some. Of these, a common polymorphism of PAI-1 has been well described. PAI-1 is an important endogenous inhibitor of fibrinolysis, and deficiency is associated with increased bleeding.[33] The $G5/G5$ polymorphism is common (about 20% in European populations) and is associated with lower levels of PAI-1. It has been linked (though not consistently) to bleeding after heart surgery and to increased benefit from use of antifibrinolytics.[20,21] Should these findings be substantiated, then PAI-1 may still be an exceptional example. In general, the influence and consequences of genetic determinants of bleeding are likely to be more subtle. In infancy an additional factor in the mix may be the relationship between developmental and genetic factors. Many clotting proteins are present in infants as isoforms distinct from those in adults. This implies a different gene expression in the young. It is possible that understanding genetically determined variations in bleeding will increase our understanding of bleeding and, perhaps, allow us to guide therapy for the individual patient. The practical applications of such techniques, however, remain speculative.

# Coagulopathy and Major Surgery

Bleeding is an inevitable consequence of invasive surgery. Severe bleeding can be associated with derangement of coagulation, which may increase the severity of bleeding or, alternatively, may put the child at risk for thrombosis. These two adverse events are not mutually exclusive: patients who bleed more and who demonstrate coagulopathic bleeding may also be at increased risk of thrombosis.

Coagulation changes during major surgery and bleeding are complex[34] and depend on the clinical context in which bleeding occurs. Coagulation changes that occur in surgical patients have some similarities to those who present after severe trauma; however, the balance of pathophysiologic factors is likely to be very different. The factors underlying these coagulation changes include:

- *Dilution.* Components of the coagulation system are lost in shed blood. The volume of blood lost is then replaced by crystalloid, colloid, or blood products lacking these components, leading to progressively smaller concentrations of these coagulation components. To some degree such changes are balanced, as the concentration of coagulation inhibitors also falls. In addition, coagulation components may be produced or released in response to trauma, which limits the reduction in concentration. To complicate this issue, a reduction in the concentration of one component of the coagulation system may not have the same clinical effect as the same reduction of another component. For example, substantial decreases in the concentration of many clotting proteins will not result in severe bleeding, while even modest decreases in platelet numbers or in the fibrinogen concentration may be significant (see also Chapter 10).
- *Effect of tissue damage.* Extensive interactions occur between inflammatory and coagulation pathways. Inflammation following trauma to tissues can be linked to excess activation of fibrinolytic pathways (resulting in excess bleeding) and to activation of procoagulant pathways (resulting in increased risk of thrombosis).
- *Physiologic derangement associated with blood loss.* Acidosis, hypothermia, and hypocalcemia are associated with excess bleeding.[35] Hypothermia will result in a general slowing of proteolytic enzyme activity, reduced fibrin synthesis, and reduced platelet function. These effects are largely reversible on rewarming. Acidosis is associated with a marked reduction in activity of coagulation proteins.[36] These effects are not fully reversed by correcting acidosis. The degree to which coagulation changes reflect acidosis itself or reflect other underlying factors is unclear. During major bleeding, calcium ion concentration should be monitored and replaced as needed.
- *Effects of treatment.* The use of some synthetic colloids may worsen bleeding to an extent greater than might be expected by dilution. The use of hydroxyethyl starch leads to increased risk of coagulation abnormalities and of acute kidney injury when compared to albumin, gelatins, or crystalloids. Whether differences exist in coagulation effects between different starches is controversial.[37-39] Caution should be exercised in the use of starches in children at risk of coagulation problems, and in larger volumes.
- *Use of specific techniques during surgery.* The important effects of cardiac bypass and anticoagulation are discussed later. Liver transplant surgery (see also Chapter 29) and major trauma (see also Chapter 38) are discussed in detail elsewhere in this book.

## Alterations in Hemostasis during Pediatric Cardiac Surgery

### ROUTINE ANTICOAGULATION

#### Heparin

Heparin remains the most effective anticoagulant used to facilitate cardiopulmonary bypass (CPB).[40] The binding of heparin to lysine sites on ATIII causes a conformational change in ATIII. This results in an increase in ATIII potency; the inhibition of thrombin and factors IXa, Xa, XIa, and XIIa are increased by a factor of 1000.[41,42] In infants ATIII levels are low until 3 to 6 months of age and other heparin cofactors, in particular, $\alpha_2$-macroglobulin may have greater importance. However neonates requiring surgery for congenital heart disease have unusually reduced concentrations of all major heparin cofactors, and this may explain the greater concentrations of thrombin production in these patients.[43]

Heparin therapy is most frequently guided by the activated clotting time (ACT). The ACT is an inexpensive and rapid on-site test in which a small sample of blood is mixed with a coagulation activator, such as Celite, kaolin, or diatomaceous earth. The ACT is the time to produce a stable clot, with a normal value being between 80 and 140 seconds. A number greater than 400 seconds is required for CPB.

There are limitations to the use of the ACT; first, the ACT is altered by hypothermia, hemodilution, platelet activation, activation of the hemostatic system, and aprotinin therapy.[44,45] Accordingly, it does not accurately reflect the heparin concentrations. One study found that as soon as children go on CPB, the heparin concentrations decreased by 50% as a result of hemodilution, even though the ACT doubled.[46] Second, in the bleeding child, the ACT is unable to differentiate between bleeding resulting from excess heparin or from other acquired hemostatic defects.[46] The gold standard for measurement of heparin concentration is considered to be the antifactor Xa assay; however, this test remains too cumbersome for routine clinical use. A further method is protamine titration, which has been available as a point-of-care test for some years (Medtronic Hepcon HMS Plus, Medtronic, Minneapolis, USA). In adult patients, use of this system has been shown to lead to reduced thrombin formation[47]; however, the accuracy of the device has been questioned.[48] Reduced bleeding and reduced thrombin generation in children has been demonstrated with the use of this system, whereas other studies have demonstrated reduced thrombin formation[22,49] in infants. A trial in small infants was terminated early when increased bleeding and increased length of stay was demonstrated in children in whom the Hepcon device was used.[49] The device underestimated heparin concentration in this group, leading to excess dosing of heparin and inadequate reversal with protamine. After modification of their protocol, use of the device demonstrated reduced bleeding, length of stay, and reduced thrombin formation compared to standard treatment.[49] Agreement between protamine titration, measures of heparin concentration, and laboratory measures has been demonstrated, but the Hepcon devices tended to underestimate heparin concentrations in infants.[50]

A common feature of the pediatric studies using the Hepcon device is increased heparin use compared to regimes based on units/kg dosing or ACT. This is consistent with other studies of traditional dosing regimes. Using common pediatric heparin regimens (300 units/kg before CPB, then 100 units/kg to keep the ACT above 450 sec), 50% of children on CPB had low levels of heparin (less than 2 units/mL).[46] It is suggested that reduced heparin concentrations during CPB is a major factor responsible for activation of coagulation and fibrinolysis. It is likely that widely used regimens for dosing of heparin in children lead to inadequate dosing, and that units/kg dosing fails to allow for important pharmacokinetic (PK) and pharmacodynamic (PD) differences in children.

Even effective dosing of heparin does not completely abolish the production of thrombin. Low-grade ongoing thrombin production leads to ongoing activation of the coagulation cascade, platelets, fibrinolysis, and the endothelium. The continued thrombin generation and activity during CPB reflects the inability of the heparin–ATIII complex to inactivate fibrin-bound thrombin or to inhibit thrombin-induced platelet activation.[51] Theoretically, direct thrombin inhibition may be free of these limitations. Practically, the use of the current generation of thrombin inhibitors (such as hirudin and bivalirudin) is limited because of a lack of effective monitoring and reversal. Currently few reports exist of the use of hirudin in children, although it would be indicated in children in whom heparin use is not possible.[52]

Adverse effects of heparin are uncommon; hypotension can result from a reduction in calcium ions or, rarely, anaphylaxis. A benign transient decrease in the platelet count can occur. Heparin-induced thrombocytopenia is a rare but life-threatening pro-thrombotic condition.

### Reversal of Anticoagulation with Protamine

Protamine is a positively charged polypeptide derived from salmon sperm. It neutralizes heparin by forming an ionic bond with heparin. The resultant complex is removed by the reticulo-endothelial system. The most appropriate dosing regimen has yet to be determined. Current dosing used in pediatric practice fails to take into account the range of concentrations of heparin that occurs in infants and children.[40,49] The administered heparin dose is often used to guide the dose of protamine; however, it is unclear how this should be modified by various factors, such as additional doses of heparin administered (to prime or during bypass), duration of bypass, techniques (e.g., ultrafiltration), or developmental coagulation differences in children.[53]

Excessive protamine has been associated with catastrophic pulmonary hypertension and hemorrhagic pulmonary edema. It is also known that protamine can be associated with coagulation abnormalities; an increasing ACT occurs at a protamine-heparin ratio of 2.6 : 1, and platelet aggregation occurs with a minimal excess in protamine.[54] Although some studies on titrating protamine regimens in adults demonstrated encouraging results in terms of reduced bleeding,[55] others failed to demonstrate differences in transfusion requirements.[56]

The clearance of protamine is greater than that of heparin, and "heparin rebound" is described as tissue-bound heparin redistributes.[40] The diagnosis of residual heparin effect or heparin rebound is challenging. The ACT is not a specific measure of excessive heparin and is also poor at detecting heparin at low concentrations (less than 0.5 unit/mL).[57] The aPTT and PT are similarly nonspecific and may be increased after CPB in the absence of heparin.[58] An unmodified TEG does not reliably detect heparin rebound if the heparin concentration is small.[59] The sensitivity of these tests may be improved by performing similar tests in parallel and comparing the results, such as a reptilase time (unaffected by heparin), or by eliminating residual heparin in vitro with heparinase or protamine. Protamine titration can be used to guide protamine dose in children; however, in infants protocols will require modification (50% higher than calculated dose).[49] In practice most anesthesiologists continue to give protamine empirically at a protamine-heparin ratio of between 1 and 1.3 to 1.

### FAILURE OF HEMOSTASIS ASSOCIATED WITH CARDIAC SURGERY

Complex abnormalities occur in the coagulation system in cardiac surgery, owing to the profound surgical insult, hypothermia, acid-base disturbance, blood transfusion, anticoagulants, CPB

| TABLE 18-1 Causes of Excessive Bleeding after Pediatric Cardiac Surgery |
| --- |
| **Preoperative Causes** |
| Liver immaturity |
| Congenital coagulopathy |
| Poor nutrition |
| Cyanotic congenital heart disease |
| Drugs: prostaglandin $E_1$, aspirin, clopidogrel |
| **Intraoperative Causes** |
| *Surgical Insult* |
| Inadequate surgical hemostasis before bypass |
| Inflammatory cascade, fibrinolysis, etc. |
| *Cardiopulmonary Bypass* |
| Inflammatory cascade |
|   Ongoing fibrinolysis |
|   Increased vascular permeability |
|   Capillary damage |
| Hemodilution |
|   Platelet reduction |
|   Clotting factor reduction |
|   Fibrinogen reduction |
| Complement activation |
| Platelet abnormality |
| Fibrinogen reduction |
| Disseminated intravascular coagulation |
| **Post Cardiopulmonary Bypass** |
| Inadequate surgical hemostasis |
| Acidosis |
| Hypothermia |
| Hypocalcemia |
| Excessive blood transfusion and clotting factor dilution |
| Inadequate reversal of heparin with protamine |
| Excess protamine |
| Inadequate reversal of heparin in transfused pump blood |

(contact activation, platelet dysfunction, and hemodilution), and in some cases, deep hypothermic cardiorespiratory arrest. In addition children and infants with congenital heart disease may have preexisting coagulation defects or be taking medications that affect coagulation before surgery (Table 18-1).

Antiplatelet drugs such as aspirin or clopidogrel may exacerbate bleeding. The clinician must balance the risk of perioperative bleeding against the risk of drug discontinuation when deciding if and when to withhold the drug before surgery. In most cases aspirin can be safely discontinued 5 days before surgery. Prostaglandin $E_1$ can inhibit platelet aggregation, acting in synergy with endothelial cell–derived factors (nitric oxide and prostacyclin) at clinically relevant concentrations,[60] although this effect was too subtle to detect in vitro using the TEG.[32] It is usually not possible to stop the prostaglandin $E_1$ infusions, because neonates are dependent on its use to maintain ductal patency. For elective surgery in children on oral anticoagulant therapy, it is usually possible to transfer to heparin before surgery. An INR of less than 1.5 is usually considered acceptable for surgery. If urgent correction of anticoagulants is required, prothrombin complex concentrates, together with vitamin K, are more effective than FFP.[61] FFP should only be used if prothrombin complex concentrates are not available.

In the child with cyanotic congenital heart disease, hemostasis is further impaired because of polycythemia, low platelet count and altered function, reduced factors V, VII, and VIII, and increased fibrinolysis.[32,62] The degree of derangement is related to the degree of cyanosis.[63] Preexisting coagulopathy may also occur in children with severe underlying illness or poor nutritional status.

Despite improvements in design and materials of the CPB circuit, abnormal activation of the coagulation and fibrinolytic systems persist. The normal balance of coagulation and fibrinolysis is particularly delicate in children, and more susceptible to exogenous perturbations.[64] Shortly after CPB is established in children, all hemostatic protein concentrations are decreased (to a variable degree) as a result of dilution.[65] Because of the relative volume of the circuit in relation to the size of the child, it is not surprising that the magnitude of the effect of hemodilution is greater than in adults.[46]

Reductions in coagulation factor concentrations after cardiac surgery contribute to bleeding in adult cardiac patients,[66] and a reduction in platelet count is well described on initiation of bypass. In adults, the platelet count is reduced on CPB by approximately 50%.[67] This is also attributed primarily to dilution, although other factors include organ sequestration, mechanical disruption, and adhesion to the circuit.[68] A relatively greater reduction will occur in smaller children, although newer combined filter and oxygenators should considerably reduce the circuit volume and, hence, the degree of dilution. Significant platelet dysfunction also occurs.[46,69] Low platelet counts have been strongly associated with increased bleeding.[10,31,70]

Further activation of platelets and denaturing of plasma proteins will occur at interfaces between blood and air, or on contact with extravascular tissue. CPB pump suction and spilling of blood into the pericardium will further contribute to coagulopathy. Greater coagulopathy is also seen during prolonged bypass and when deep hypothermic circulatory arrest is employed.[71]

The major mechanism for activation of the coagulation cascade during CPB is thought to be the "extrinsic" TF pathway, which is activated as a result of surgical trauma and inflammation.[42,72,73] Inflammatory mediators such as tumor necrosis factor (TNF) and interleukin-1 induce expression of TF on endothelial cells and monocytes. The "intrinsic" coagulation system is also activated when factor XII is adsorbed onto the surface of the CPB circuit, causing activation of complement, neutrophils, and the fibrinolytic system via kallikrein.[42] Although the intrinsic system has little role in initiating coagulation, activations of kinins will lead to increased fibrinolysis and inflammation.[15]

The blood loss in the first 24 hours after cardiac surgery can vary between 15 and 110 mL/kg, although the risk of excessive blood loss is greatest among those weighing less than 8 kg, younger than 1 year of age, and children undergoing complex surgery.[10] The common preoperative and intraoperative risk factors for excessive bleeding are summarized in Table 18-2.

Blood loss and transfusion requirements in pediatric cardiac surgery vary inversely with age; neonates bleed more and receive more products per kilogram than any other age group.[74] There are some correlations between coagulation tests before and during CPB and postoperative blood component transfusion requirements, although the sensitivity and specificity of the tests are not sufficient to justify routine coagulation tests while on CPB. Of all the tests, a platelet count of less than 108,000/mm$^3$ while on CPB yielded the greatest sensitivity (83%) and specificity (58%) for predicting excessive blood loss.[70]

| **TABLE 18-2** Common Predictive Factors for Bleeding | |
|---|---|
| **Preoperative** | **Intraoperative** |
| Age <1 year or weight <8 kg | Individual surgeon |
| High hematocrit | Complex surgery |
| Congestive heart failure | Low platelet count during CPB |
| Repeat sternotomy | Prolonged CPB |
| Congenital and preoperative acquired coagulopathy | Duration of hypothermia on CPB |
| Cyanotic congenital heart disease | Deep hypothermic cardiac arrest |

Williams GD, Bratton SL, Ramamoorthy C. Factors associated with blood loss and blood product transfusions: a multivariate analysis in children after open-heart surgery. Anesth Analg 1999;89:57-64.
CPB, Cardiopulmonary bypass.

## Medications Used for Hemostasis

The pathophysiology of coagulopathies and bleeding in children during surgery are complex, and the etiology is multifactorial (see Table 18-1). No single blood component or drug treatment can reverse the abnormal clotting profile. Initially an attempt should be made to identify causes of bleeding that can be remedied by surgical interventions. The anesthesiologist should attempt to ensure adequate reversal of heparin and restore normal physiologic variables, such as body temperature, serum [Ca$^{2+}$], and acid-base balance. In the postoperative period, platelets, and other blood products, such as fresh frozen plasma (FFP) and cryoprecipitate, remain the mainstay of treatment for excessive bleeding.[75] Blood products (see also Chapter 10) are briefly discussed here, primarily within the context of pediatric heart surgery.

### BLOOD PRODUCTS

Frequently it is necessary to administer blood products on a largely empirical basis; laboratory tests describe only parts of the coagulation process[32] and are practically too slow to direct the anesthesiologist in real time as to the requirement for blood components. The TEG is a dynamic whole-blood test that is frequently used as a near-patient test to assess clot elasticity properties and, hence, more precisely delineate the bleeding and homeostasis profile. The role of TEG during pediatric heart surgery has been recently reviewed.[76] The use of treatment algorithms based on TEG can limit transfusion of blood products in adults[77-81] and children.[82] In children, it may not be appropriate to use protocols originally designed for adults. An alternative approach has recently been proposed.[76]

### PLATELETS

Platelet dysfunction and thrombocytopenia are common after cardiac bypass in infants. Hence, in the presence of bleeding, transfusion of platelets is logical. Coagulation variables that relate to platelet number and function (such as TEG maximum amplitude) are corrected by infusion of platelets, and clinical experience indicates that platelet transfusion reduces bleeding. This has been confirmed in a small study of children after cardiac surgery.[31] A platelet count of less than 108,000/mm$^3$ has been identified as a predictor of bleeding, whereas clot strength measured by TEG reduces steeply at platelet counts below 120,000/mm$^3$. The current recommendation of targeting a platelet count of approximately 100,000/mm$^3$ appears to be logical. It would also appear reasonable to use platelets for the initial treatment of presumed coagulopathic bleeding (in the absence of specific clotting tests).

## FRESH FROZEN PLASMA

The case for use of fresh frozen plasma (FFP), either as empirical treatment of bleeding, or guided by coagulation tests, is considerably weaker than for platelets. The use of FFP in cardiac surgery is based on the observation that the concentration of clotting factors are often low in bleeding patients, especially in the period following bypass. The PT (with its derived measure, INR) is the most common test used to detect the presence and gauge the severity of clotting factor–deficient coagulopathy. Unfortunately, observation studies have shown that the PT correlates poorly with clinical bleeding, and that transfusion of plasma often achieves no measurable change in the INR, nor is of any known clinical benefit (particularly if the INR was only marginally raised to less than 1.7).[83] Despite this, FFP is frequently transfused in the absence of either bleeding or significantly raised PT.[84] Administration to patients with higher PT values will be more effective in correcting clotting tests, however large volumes may be required,[83] even in the absence of ongoing loss of clotting factors. The situation is further complicated, in that coagulation tests that are initially normal will deteriorate during severe bleeding.

A systemic review of the use of FFP to treat or prevent bleeding resulting from acquired coagulopathy failed to demonstrate benefit, although the trials examined were small, used a wide range of outcomes, and were conducted in heterogeneous populations.[85] In a small observational study of children undergoing heart surgery, a number of patients had coagulopathic bleeding after transfusion of platelets; if these patients were then given FFP, the bleeding increased, whereas if cryoprecipitate was given bleeding decreased.[31]

It is possible that the lack of efficacy may be related to the dose of FFP used. The dose of FFP most frequently recommended (10 to 15 mL/kg)[84,86] may be inadequate to restore factor concentration.[83] Of note, dosage of plasma is inexact. Hence, interinstitution practices differ considerably in defining both a threshold INR for prophylactic plasma administration and the actual dosage of plasma prescribed.[87]

Modeling of FFP administration in major trauma suggests that larger doses (30 to 40 mL/kg) may be required to increase or maintain factor concentrations[88]; however, administration of such a large volume is often undesirable in the absence of severe ongoing bleeding. Addition of FFP to the bypass circuit or during modified ultrafiltration may allow administration of much larger doses; benefit appears to be confined to younger children.[89,90] It is always important to document the specific reasons for FFP administration.

## CRYOPRECIPITATE

Not all coagulation factors are of equal importance during bleeding. Fibrinogen is present in much greater concentrations than other clotting factors, and while other factors are mainly involved in initiating or amplifying thrombin formation, fibrinogen is a substrate for the production of fibrin. Deficiencies of fibrinogen are reflected in reduced strength of clot and are associated with increased bleeding.[91] Cryoprecipitate is the most concentrated fibrinogen replacement widely available, with a fibrinogen concentration 4 to 8 times that of FFP; however, a unit of cryoprecipitate contains less fibrinogen than a unit of FFP, and multiple cryoprecipitate units will be required in larger patients. One

cryoprecipitate unit for each 10 kg should raise fibrinogen concentration by 0.5 to 1.0 g/L. As well as fibrinogen, cryoprecipitate is a source of von Willebrand factor and factors VIII and XIII, although the clinical significance of this to bleeding is unclear. Cryoprecipitate has been effective in treating bleeding resistant to platelet concentrates alone during pediatric heart surgery.[31]

## FRACTIONATED HUMAN BLOOD PRODUCTS

Products such as FFP or cryoprecipitate can be considered as only crudely purified blood products. It is possible to produce more refined products containing high concentrations of only a single clotting protein or relatively standardized concentrates of selected proteins. Examples of these are prothrombin complex concentrates and fibrinogen concentrate (e.g., Riastap, CSL Behring, King of Prussia, Pa., USA; Haemocomplettan P, CSL Behring, Marburg, Germany). These products are human blood products produced from pooled plasma; they are presented as a powder requiring reconstitution for use. They do not require freezing or cross matching, which simplifies their supply, storage, and administration. Risk of viral transmission should be low[92] because of sourcing of plasma from low-risk populations, pooling of plasma from many individual donors (reducing viral load resulting from a single infected donor), and pasteurization. Although the effect of pasteurization on prion infection is less certain, the risk of transmission would be expected to be similarly low. Recombinant factor concentrates (as opposed to factor concentrates of human origin) are increasingly available and avoid cross infection. One such agent, recombinant activated factor VII (rVIIa), is discussed later in this chapter (see also Chapter 10). Although the agents discussed in this section are used in a similar way to traditional factor supplementation to reestablish near physiologic concentrations, rVIIa is used very differently to produce factor levels greatly in excess of "normal."

Prothrombin complex concentrates (PCCs) are mixtures of factors II (prothrombin), VII, IX, and X, plus the coagulation inhibitors Protein S and C. They are indicated when urgent reversal of oral anticoagulation (with warfarin or related drugs) is required. Dose is specific for each make of PCC, and is dependent on the child's INR and the target for correction (generally an INR of 1.5). Older reports of lack of efficacy or risk of thrombosis probably relate to older brands of PCCs with low levels of factor VII or of inhibitors.[93] PCCs are more efficacious than FFP for warfarin reversal.[61] They have also been used in other causes of acquired coagulopathy and bleeding, including after adult heart surgery.[94,95] Potentially these products are superior to FFP in such situations; however, routine use for treatment of acquired bleeding in children (other than reversal of warfarin) cannot be recommended until further evaluation is conducted. Dosing in this situation is also uncertain.

The importance of fibrinogen depletion in coagulopathy and bleeding has been increasingly appreciated.[96,97] It has also been recognized that traditional cut-off values for supplementation of fibrinogen during bleeding (1.0 g/L) are likely to be too low and that further advantage can be gained from higher targets; possibly as high as 2.0 g/L. This may be difficult to achieve with traditional blood products. FFP contains only physiologic concentrations of fibrinogen and only modest increases may be achieved, while cryoprecipitate will require administration of product from several donors to achieve significant increases in fibrinogen concentration (especially in larger patients). Human fibrinogen concentrate has been available in continental Europe for some time and has recently been licensed within the United Kingdom and the United States for treatment of congenital fibrinogen deficiency. Unlike cryoprecipitate, they contain only fibrinogen and a direct comparison in other forms of coagulopathy has not been made. Recent reports have demonstrated advantages to its use in adult cardiac surgery and other causes of bleeding.[98,99] Reports of its use in children with acquired coagulopathy are limited. Combining use of fibrinogen concentrates with rapid measurement of fibrinogen concentration (using modified TEG) is an attractive approach.[100]

The most obvious use for fibrinogen concentrates is as an alternative to cryoprecipitate. Their apparent safety and ease of administration may, however, make other applications possible. A small randomized study comparing prophylactic administration of fibrinogen concentrate to placebo in adult cardiac patients demonstrated a reduction in bleeding.[99] Alternatively, it has been proposed that targeting larger fibrinogen concentrations with these agents may reduce the requirement for platelet transfusion. Animal work has demonstrated the effectiveness of this approach in models of bleeding and thrombocytopenia.[101] The product of fibrinogen concentration and platelet count may be a better predictor of bleeding in children than either measure alone.[91] If the concentration of fibrinogen is high, the amplitude of TEG recordings can be normal, even in the absence of platelets. In vivo, it would be expected that there are limits to this phenomenon; at some point, platelets are required for formation of clot. Such an approach requires proper clinical evaluation before being more widely adopted. Recombinant fibrinogen in fibrin sealants is currently undergoing phase II trials, although widespread availability of systemic recombinant fibrinogen is still some years away.[102] With proper assessment, recombinant fibrinogen has the potential to greatly alter the management of severe bleeding and coagulopathy.

Deficiency of factor XIII during and after cardiopulmonary bypass has been described, although the importance of this finding is uncertain.[103-105] Supplementation with human or recombinant factor XIII has been demonstrated to reduce bleeding after adult heart surgery, although possibly only in the presence of factor deficiency.[104,106,107] The action of factor XIII is to catalyze the formation of cross bridges between fibrin molecules. It also has a wider function in promoting fibroblast proliferation, and it has been used in the treatment of chylothorax after pediatric heart surgery (with possibly only minor benefit).[108] Recombinant factor XIII is currently being considered for approval by the FDA, and wider availability may lead to greater use of this agent. Evidence to support widespread use is currently not available.

## PHARMACEUTICAL AGENTS TO REDUCE BLEEDING

Blood products are, in most cases, effective at treating coagulopathic bleeding, but may be associated with deleterious effects on the patient. Drug use is aimed at reducing bleeding and blood product requirements. These drugs are principally the two classes of antifibrinolytics:

1. Synthetic lysine analogues, such as EACA and TXA (see Fig. 18-5)[106]
2. Protease inhibitors (aprotinin)

More recently rVIIa has been employed as a rescue therapy for severe bleeding unresponsive to traditional therapy using blood products. Desmopressin has also been used in the past and is discussed later.

### The Effectiveness of Synthetic Antifibrinolytics during Pediatric Heart Surgery

A meta-analysis comparing TXA and placebo in children undergoing heart surgery[2] concluded that antifibrinolytics reduced bleeding and that TXA was as effective as aprotinin. Figure 18-6 shows a summary of the studies included in this meta-analysis[109-116]; the figure has been updated to include a more recent trial.[115] There were 1061 children entered into nine studies, and results demonstrated a mean reduction in bleeding of approximately 14 mL/kg (95% confidence interval [CI] of 12.7 to 15.6 mL). This is a clinically useful reduction in blood loss. The meta-analysis also demonstrated a small reduction in transfusion of red blood cells with use of TXA.

Data concerning more clinically important outcomes (e.g., reexploration or "life-threatening" hemorrhage) are lacking.

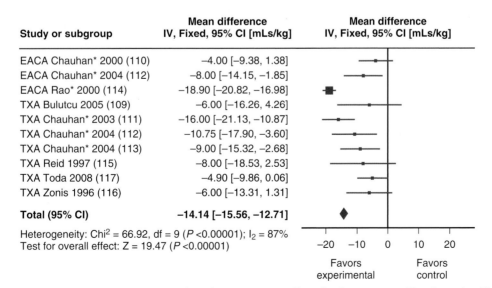

| Study or subgroup | Mean difference IV, Fixed, 95% CI [mLs/kg] | Mean difference IV, Fixed, 95% CI [mLs/kg] |
|---|---|---|
| EACA Chauhan* 2000 (110) | −4.00 [−9.38, 1.38] | |
| EACA Chauhan* 2004 (112) | −8.00 [−14.15, −1.85] | |
| EACA Rao* 2000 (114) | −18.90 [−20.82, −16.98] | |
| TXA Bulutcu 2005 (109) | −6.00 [−16.26, 4.26] | |
| TXA Chauhan* 2003 (111) | −16.00 [−21.13, −10.87] | |
| TXA Chauhan* 2004 (112) | −10.75 [−17.90, −3.60] | |
| TXA Chauhan* 2004 (113) | −9.00 [−15.32, −2.68] | |
| TXA Reid 1997 (115) | −8.00 [−18.53, 2.53] | |
| TXA Toda 2008 (117) | −4.90 [−9.86, 0.06] | |
| TXA Zonis 1996 (116) | −6.00 [−13.31, 1.31] | |
| **Total (95% CI)** | **−14.14 [−15.56, −12.71]** | |

Heterogeneity: $Chi^2$ = 66.92, df = 9 ($P$ <0.00001); $I_2$ = 87%
Test for overall effect: Z = 19.47 ($P$ <0.00001)

**FIGURE 18-6** A forest plot of trials of synthetic antifibrinolytic drugs (ε-aminocaproic acid [*EACA*] and tranexamic acid [*TXA*]) to reduce bleeding during pediatric heart surgery. Number in parentheses after each study refers to reference from main text. *Study is from The All Indian Institute of Medical Science. (Forest plot generated using Review Manager (RevMan) Version 5.1. Copenhagen: The Nordic Cochrane Centre; The Cochrane Collaboration, 2011.)

Analyses have a high degree of statistical heterogeneity ($I^2$ = 78%), indicating differences in the populations, interventions, or study methodology.[115-117] This makes pooling of results less valid and makes it impossible to exclude factors that could introduce bias to conclusions. The patients and protocols are clinically variable with differing drugs, dosing regimens and patient populations. Only 163 of the patients did not have cyanotic heart disease; data on 6-hour blood loss was available for 144 of these children and did not demonstrate a significant reduction in bleeding (mean reduction 1. 8 mL/kg, 95% CI of –0.8 to 4.5 mL/kg).[115-117] The majority of studies come from a single institution (The All Indian Institute of Medical Science),[111-114] and these patients represented a specific population undergoing relatively late correction of cyanotic disease. Polycythemia, and presumably severe cyanosis, was common, with a mean hemoglobin concentration of 19 g/dL.

Another feature of the studies[115-117] is that only one study recruited infants less than 2 months of age.[116] The mean age of patients was 40 months. This may be important, because the fibrinolytic system in neonates differs from adults; plasminogen levels are about 50% of adult values, plasminogen activation occurs more slowly, and levels of inhibitor (PAI-1) are normal.[25] This may make neonates relatively resistant to fibrinolysis. In turn, this may mean that antifibrinolytic medication is less effective, although in vitro experiments using neonatal plasma do not demonstrate a difference in the ability of synthetic antifibrinolytics to inhibit fibrinolysis.[118,119]

In conclusion, current pediatric data support the use of synthetic antifibrinolytics in cyanotic children older than 2 months of age, but data supporting more widespread use are unclear. While there is substantial evidence to support the use of these drugs in adults,[120] extrapolation of conclusions to children is uncertain and has implications with regard to drug development.[121] If it can be demonstrated that there are similarities for both the disease process (e.g., hyperfibrinolysis as a contributor to hemorrhage) and drug effect at different age groups (e.g., hyperfibrinolysis reduction), then adult data for efficacy could more reliably be used in children. Hyperfibrinolysis is most likely part of an inflammatory response to cardiopulmonary bypass and would be expected to occur in children (other than neonates) in a similar way to adults. It would also be expected that antifibrinolytic drugs function in a similar way in children and adults. It seems reasonable to extrapolate adult data of efficacy to children. A more difficult question is whether this reduction in bleeding is worthwhile when balanced against adverse effects (discussed later). Small children have more bleeding (relative to body weight) compared to adults. This does not in itself imply that an intervention to reduce bleeding will have greater effect in children. It has been suggested that factors other than fibrinolysis make a greater contribution to bleeding in children.[91]

## SYNTHETIC ANTIFIBRINOLYTIC MEDICATIONS

There is considerable uncertainty about the dose of these drugs. A recent survey of pediatric cardiac anesthetists in the UK demonstrated a 50-fold variation in TXA dose used during surgery (from a single dose of 5 mg/kg to a cumulative dose of 250 mg/kg).[122] In the studies summarized in Figure 18-6 there was also wide variation.

Rational dosing of a drug is determined by its PK and how the resulting plasma (or tissue) concentration translates to a clinical effect (PD). TXA has a volume of distribution (Vd) of 9 to 12 L in adults. The drug is water soluble and poorly protein bound. Most of the drug is excreted unchanged by the kidneys, so the dose should be reduced in renal failure. The terminal elimination half-life is about 2 hours,[123] although CPB will affect this. In adults a loading dose of 12.5 mg/kg followed by 6.5 mg/kg/hour with 1 mg/kg added to the pump prime maintains the concentration of TXA greater than 52.5 µg/mL.[124] However, neonates and infants will be expected to have a relatively larger Vd and a greater change in Vd with initiation of CPB. In addition, clearance will be reduced in neonates because of renal immaturity. The effects of the surgical insult, CPB, hypothermia, ultrafiltration, and fluid resuscitation on the PK and PD of TXA remain to be established.

The target concentration of TXA is not clear. A plasma concentration of greater than 100 µg/mL will produce complete inhibition of fibrinolysis in vitro, however a concentration of 30 µg/mL accounts for most of the pharmacologic effect of the drug.[125] It is difficult to translate these in vitro effects into clinical dosing recommendations. Dosing regimens that involved multiple doses were more effective than a larger single bolus at the start of cardiac surgery, in terms of sternal closure time, blood loss, and blood product requirement, despite similar total doses.[113] The administration of a loading dose (50 mg/kg repeated on bypass) in addition to an infusion of 15 mg/kg/hour achieved mean tranexamic concentrations above 100 µg/mL, although concentrations may be below this concentration after bypass.[126] This dosing regimen reduced bleeding compared with placebo, and greater tranexamic concentrations were associated with less bleeding (although this does not demonstrate causality). Dosing regimens using a smaller total dose (30 to 50 mg/kg in divided doses) have also been effective. A detailed PK study of TXA in children undergoing heart surgery is currently under way and may help to improve decision making about dosing.

The use of EACA during surgery to correct a congenital heart defect was first described in 1969.[127] The dose of EACA is based on a small PK study in children undergoing heart surgery.[128] Most of the drug is excreted unchanged by the kidneys, while about 35% of EACA undergoes hepatic metabolism. The terminal elimination half-life is 1 to 2 hours.[129] Children have a greater weight-adjusted clearance and Vd compared with adults before, during, and after CPB. Consequently, larger doses are used in children: 75 mg/kg over 10 minutes, 75 mg/kg in the CPB circuit, and 75 mg/kg/hour as an infusion. This regimen maintains concentrations of EACA above the presumed "therapeutic" concentration of 260 µg/mL.[128] While the target concentration is not clear, this triple-dosing regimen appears to be clinically effective in children. One study (using three doses of 100 mg/kg EACA before, during, and after CPB) demonstrated a reduction in postoperative blood loss, reduced blood and platelet transfusion requirements, and reduced reexploration rate compared with control subjects.[114] The PK have not been studied in infants and neonates.

### Adverse Effects of Synthetic Lysine Analogues

As with any drug used to promote hemostasis, the most worrisome complication is thrombosis. This is likely to be a particular concern in cardiac surgical patients because of vascular anastomoses, conduits, and indwelling lines. Thrombosis is also a potential concern for those patients on extracorporeal support.

Patients following any major surgery or trauma can be hypercoagulable and at risk of thrombosis. Unlike aprotinin, the lysine analogues (TXA or EACA) have not shown an increased risk of renal, cardiac, or cerebral events in adult cardiac surgery patients.[130]

Several meta-analyses in adults concluded that prophylactic lysine analogues in cardiac surgery did not increase the incidence of thromboembolic complications.[120,131,132] However, thrombosis has been reported in nonsurgical hypercoagulable states.[133] Despite occasional anecdotes, there is no clear-cut evidence that the incidence of thrombosis is increased with either of the lysine analogues. Both TXA and EACA appear to have a very low incidence of other serious adverse effects, such as anaphylaxis.

The most common acute adverse effect of EACA is hypotension, usually associated with rapid intravenous (IV) administration. Rash, nausea, vomiting, weakness, retrograde ejaculation, myopathy, and rhabdomyolysis have been less frequently reported and are associated with longer-term use.[123] EACA is teratogenic and therefore contraindicated in pregnancy.

Rapid IV administration of TXA can cause hypotension. Oral administration can be associated with gastrointestinal adverse effects. In an adult study, prolonged infusion was associated with renal dysfunction.[134] There is a possible association between TXA and seizures (without any neurologic injury). TXA is found in the cerebrospinal fluid following IV administration (though at concentrations much lower than in plasma),[135] and when applied directly to an animal's brain can initiate seizures. Two observational studies (one in children) have reported an association with seizures[136,137]; however, the incidence of seizures (in both those treated and not treated) was much greater than that which occurred at the authors' institutions. The significance of this association is unclear.

## SERINE PROTEASE INHIBITOR: APROTININ

The use of aprotinin has become a source of considerable controversy since publication of data that appeared to demonstrate increased morbidity and mortality with its use in adults undergoing heart surgery.[3,130] This is discussed further, later, but has lead to a reduced availability of the drug in most countries. If aprotinin remains available, the decision to continue to use it must rest on a balance of the benefits (principally reduction in bleeding) and uncertain risks. More precisely, one must consider how this risk–benefit balance compares with that of the synthetic antifibrinolytics, which have more certain risk profiles.

### Effectiveness of Aprotinin for Reducing Bleeding

Two meta-analyses demonstrated that aprotinin reduces bleeding and volume of red cell transfusion in children undergoing heart surgery.[2,138] However, similar difficulties arise for studies of synthetic antifibrinolytic drugs: statistical heterogeneity, suboptimal methodology, varied dosing regimes, different study populations, and small, underpowered studies. In particular, most studies are extremely small: 12 of these studies (67%) had less than 50 children in total and only one study had more than 100 children. A meta-analysis of studies in adult patients detailed 107 studies and a total of 11,000 patients.[120] There were 94 trials (just less than 10,000 patients) that examined aprotinin use in cardiac surgery. Risk of blood transfusion, volume of blood transfused, volume of blood loss, and requirement for reexploration were all reduced. As with lysine analogues, similar caveats exist with extrapolation of adult data to pediatrics. It appears a reasonable conclusion that aprotinin is effective at reducing blood loss during cardiac surgery and that this conclusion also applies to children. Importantly, there is evidence for efficacy in neonates, where a controlled trial demonstrated reduced blood loss, exposure to allogeneic blood products, and reexploration after arterial switch procedures.[139] A further randomized trial of aprotinin in neonates was terminated early (because of the concerns about toxicity in adults), but it failed to show any advantage in indices of bleeding or postoperative recovery.[140]

### Secondary Benefits of Aprotinin

While synthetic antifibrinolytics are selective inhibitors of fibrinolysis, aprotinin is a less specific inhibitor of proteolytic enzymes.[15] Proteolytic enzymes are important mediators of inflammation via contact activation and the compliment system; it is postulated that aprotinin may exert a beneficial antiinflammatory effect. A number of studies have demonstrated a reduction in markers of inflammation; however, other studies have failed to demonstrate this effect.[141] A recent trial demonstrated reduced inflammatory markers postoperatively in infants treated with aprotinin in comparison to infants treated with TXA.[142] A further small study in older children undergoing mainly low complexity surgery failed to demonstrate any effect of aprotinin on a series of inflammatory markers compared to control.[143] There are no convincing clinical data to show any benefit from an antiinflammatory action of aprotinin. A trial designed to detect a reduction in ventilation days (as a marker of organ dysfunction) in neonates was terminated before an adequate number of patients had been recruited to identify a significant effect.[140]

### Adverse Effects of Aprotinin

There is great concern about the adverse effects of aprotinin in adult patients. This followed the publication of an observational study in adults with acute coronary syndromes, which concluded that rates of renal failure, serious intravascular thrombosis (myocardial infarction and stroke), and of death (at 5 years) were increased if aprotinin was used.[3,130] The rate of these complications was not increased with the use of synthetic antifibrinolytics, whereas all agents appeared effective for reducing bleeding. This was followed by the early termination of a large randomized trial (BART trial), comparing synthetic antifibrinolytics and aprotinin (in "high risk" adults undergoing heart surgery), when interim analysis showed an increased mortality in the group treated with aprotinin.[144] Excess deaths appeared to result from heart failure and myocardial infarction. Rates of renal failure were not increased in those treated with aprotinin, although an increase in plasma creatinine was common. The relative risk of death in adults treated with aprotinin compared to those treated with either TXA or EACA was 1.53 with a 95% CI of 1.06 to 2.22. Data on bleeding in this study were inconclusive, although they suggested a small benefit for aprotinin for preventing severe bleeding. The conclusion of these papers was that aprotinin should not be used in the patient populations studied. This has lead to differing responses from drug regulators and pharmaceutical companies in different countries. The drug is effectively unavailable in a number of countries; it has remained available in the UK on a restricted, named patient basis.

The implication of these studies for children and young adults with congenital heart disease is controversial. The use of aprotinin has reduced dramatically within the UK.[122] An important large observation series (over 30,000 patients) demonstrated no increased risk of death or dialysis in children,[145] and there was a significant reduction in length of stay for those undergoing reoperation. The main cause of death reported in adult patients was from stroke and myocardial infarction. Although thrombotic complications do occur in children, the pathogenesis and underlying risk factors are very different from those in adults (especially in adults with ischemic heart disease). Renal failure occurs in children after high-risk operations, and may share pathogenic factors with postoperative renal failure in adults; aprotinin accumulates within renal tissue and affects local autoregulation of blood flow in response to ischemia. The evidence is unclear as to whether aprotinin causes any more than temporary derangement of renal function tests in adults or children. A further retrospective series demonstrated no increase in the incidence of renal failure in neonates when corrected for confounding variables.[146]

As with many polypeptides, anaphylactic reactions can occur with aprotinin. The reported incidence of adverse reactions in children varies, but the largest reported experience with aprotinin found 1 reaction from 2202 primary exposures (0.05%) and 6 reactions from 453 reexposures (1.3%). There have been no severe reactions to aprotinin since 1998 and this is attributed to the elimination of its use in recently exposed patients.[147,148] Studies report the incidence and severity of reaction to be less than that of adults. This may be due to the immature neonatal immune system.[149] It has been recommended that:

- Test dose and initial loading dose are not given until it is possible to rapidly initiate CPB (package insert).
- Aprotinin is avoided within 12 months of previous exposure (FDA recommendation).

### Dosing of Aprotinin

The lack of clarity regarding the efficacy of aprotinin in children may reflect differing doses used in clinical studies. Aprotinin rapidly redistributes into the extracellular space after IV administration. It is metabolized in the proximal renal tubules and eliminated in a biphasic pattern: a distribution half-life of 40 minutes and an elimination half-life of 7 hours.[129,150] A PK study of aprotinin in children undergoing CPB examined aprotinin concentrations after administration of weight-based dosing (25,000 KIU/kg bolus pre-CPB, 35,000 KIU/kg in CPB prime, and 12,500 KIU/kg/hour infusion).[151] Although there was considerable variation in plasma concentration of aprotinin, there was a correlation between concentration and weight at 5 minutes after administration and 5 minutes after cardiopulmonary bypass. This study can provide one possible explanation as to why there are such inconsistent results from aprotinin trials in children. Using a dose-per-weight regimen, the smaller children may fail to achieve therapeutic concentrations of aprotinin, in terms of plasmin inhibition and the possible antiinflammatory effects (a low concentration of aprotinin, e.g., less than 200 KIU/mL, would be insufficient to inhibit contact activation on the CPB circuit). This is consistent with greater clearance (expressed as per kilogram) in children (see also Chapter 6, Fig. 6-4). To achieve target concentrations, aprotinin should be given according to nonlinear functions (e.g., body surface area or an allometric $\frac{3}{4}$-power model; see Chapter 6), as opposed to the linear dose per kilogram. This would result in a 2.5 times greater dose in neonates than would otherwise be given.[48] A recent qualitative literature review suggested that an initial loading dose of at least 30,000 KIU/kg is required, followed by an infusion. The pump prime dose should be based on the volume of the pump rather than the weight of the child.[149]

### WHICH ANTIFIBRINOLYTIC DRUG FOR PEDIATRIC CARDIAC SURGERY?

A meta-analysis of trials in adult patients demonstrated no difference between EACA and TXA. Aprotinin was more effective than either TXA or EACA, and although that effect appeared

marginal, only aprotinin was demonstrated to reduce the risk of reoperation.[120] Direct comparison between TXA and EACA has demonstrated no difference in children.[112,152] Low-dose aprotinin (10,000 KIU/kg followed by 10,000 KIU/kg/hour) has been compared with EACA (100 mg/kg on induction, 100 mg/kg in the pump prime and 100 mg/kg on weaning CPB).[110] There was a reduction in postoperative blood loss and in transfusion requirements in both groups compared with control but no significant difference between the two drugs. These data are difficult to interpret because substantially larger doses of aprotinin are frequently used in current practice. More recently, TXA (100 mg/kg before, during, and after CPB) was compared with aprotinin (30,000 KIU after induction, 30,000 KIU in the pump, and 30,000 KIU after weaning off bypass). There was a reduction in the time to sternal closure, transfusion requirements, and blood loss compared with control, but no significant difference between the two drugs. When the two drugs were combined at the same doses, they showed no additional benefit.[109] A recent retrospective study confirmed these findings.[153]

There remains uncertainty about the comparative effectiveness of lysine analogues and aprotinin; data suggest that there are no differences or only marginal differences. The choice of antifibrinolytic will, therefore, depend on the adverse effect profiles and cost. The incidence of important adverse effects is also uncertain. Both mechanistically and from the available data it would appear that the recent "safety" concerns about aprotinin in adults may not be applicable to children. A more certain risk of aprotinin is anaphylaxis with repeated exposure. This is a concern because many pediatric cardiac patients (and a large proportion of those at a increased risk of severe bleeding) will undergo repeat surgery. The greater cost of aprotinin will also be difficult to justify in the absence of clear advantage over lysine analogues. In the absence of further studies, it is the authors' conclusion that if an antifibrinolytic is indicated, lysine analogues are preferred over aprotinin.

### USE OF ANTIFIBRINOLYTIC DRUGS IN NONCARDIAC SURGERY

A recent trend has been towards increased use of antifibrinolytic drugs (especially TXA) during noncardiac surgery; principally major orthopedic surgery (e.g., spinal instrumentation, see also Chapter 30) and craniofacial surgery (see also Chapter 33). Aprotinin is less commonly used because of reduced availability and the safety concerns discussed previously.

There are 27 trials that have examined the use of TXA during orthopedic surgery in adults[120]; they report a 50% reduction in the relative risk of requiring a blood transfusion. There was a reduction in the incidence of total blood loss of over 400 mL in 20 of these trials. Almost all these studies were conducted in adults undergoing major joint replacement surgery. In one study of adults (n = 147) undergoing posterior spinal fusion, TXA reduced total blood loss by 25%; however, the reduction in blood products transfused was not statistically significant.[154] The popularity of antifibrinolytic use during scoliosis surgery in children and adolescents is reflected in two surveys, which show use in 70% to 80% of hospitals.[155,156] It is unclear whether this use is mostly confined to higher-risk cases; however, in the authors' institution TXA is currently used during all scoliosis surgery as part of a program aimed at reducing the use of blood products. Two meta-analyses have examined this question (looking at 6 and 7 studies, respectively); no individual study had more than 45 patients.[2,157] These meta-analyses conclude that antifibrinolytic drugs reduce bleeding and volume of red cells transfused. To date there has been no single prospective trial that compares different antifibrinolytics. A retrospective comparison of TXA and EACA appeared to show superiority of TXA; however, doses used were not comparable.[158] The two meta-analyses failed to establish any difference between the drugs.[2,157] It is also not possible to determine whether reported benefits hold for all children undergoing scoliosis repair. Bleeding is greater in children with secondary scoliosis (including patients with Duchenne muscular dystrophy),[159] those with hemostatic disorders, and in those undergoing more extensive surgery; these might, therefore, be expected to see a greater advantage in terms of bleeding reduction. At least one study examined children with idiopathic scoliosis and demonstrated a reduction in blood loss with use of aprotinin (see also Chapter 30).[160] As with cardiac studies there is a considerable range in the dose of drug used; in a survey of practice in the UK, TXA dose ranged from three- to fivefold, whereas in published trials, the dose varied 10-fold.[155]

Antifibrinolytics are also used widely in craniosynostosis surgery. In a survey of North American practice, they were used in 20% of hospitals for strip craniotomy, rising to 30% for more complex repairs.[161] Four small trials (total 141 children) have addressed the use of these agents for this indication; three using TXA[162-164] and one using aprotinin.[165] All of these trials have demonstrated reductions in blood transfused and in bleeding. A recent publication demonstrated a greater than 50% reduction in the volume of blood transfused and in the proportion of children transfused (70% vs. 37%).[162] Although all these studies were relatively small, it would appear likely that antifibrinolytics produce a useful reduction in blood loss for craniosynostosis surgery.

## ANTIFIBRINOLYTIC MEDICATION AND TRAUMA

There is no evidence in children concerning the use of antifibrinolytic medications to treat massive hemorrhage following trauma. The CRASH 2 study (a blinded randomized control trial of over 20,000 patients) demonstrated a reduction in mortality with TXA in adult trauma patients with, or at risk of, significant hemorrhage; mortality was reduced from 16% to 14.5%.[166] Mortality due to bleeding was reduced from 5.7% to 4.9%. No difference was seen in rates of vascular occlusive events. Despite the size and complexity of the study, it appears to have been properly randomized and blinded. It is difficult to see an explanation for the reduction in mortality, other than a reduction in bleeding. It is therefore likely that TXA can be efficacious in the treatment of established bleeding (at least in the context of trauma). Ideally, further studies would be required to establish the effectiveness of TXA in the treatment of established bleeding of other causes in children; however, it is unlikely a controlled trial of pediatric trauma would be large enough to be adequately powered. In the absence of such studies, and in the absence of definite evidence of toxicity, it would be reasonable to consider TXA as part of the treatment of established *severe* bleeding resulting from trauma or surgery. Some caution is required, and given the uncertainty concerning dosing, it would be premature to recommend the widespread use of the drug in young children. When used, it should be reserved for severe bleeding; for example, bleeding requiring treatment with non–red cell blood products. An important caveat to this is that administration greater than 3 hours after injury appeared to increase mortality.[167] The significance of this is unclear; however, such late administration should be avoided.

## AUTHORS' RECOMMENDATIONS FOR USE OF ANTIFIBRINOLYTICS

There are 2260 children and more than 25,000 adults who have been recruited into trials that investigated antifibrinolytics during surgery. As a result, we can conclude that these drugs reduce bleeding during a variety of surgeries. However, the dose remains uncertain, important adverse effects unclear, the choice of drug open to question, and their effectiveness in different patient subgroups and clinical situations debatable. Further studies should be designed very carefully to address these questions. Establishing the safety of interventions, in particular with respect to uncommon but devastating complications, is a particular challenge. In the absence of this data it is not possible to make solid recommendations. One of the author's current practice is as follows:

- Antifibrinolytics are used routinely during heart surgery in children with cyanotic heart disease; especially in the presence of polycythemia, reduced saturations for a prolonged period, or iron deficiency.
- Antifibrinolytics are used during other cardiac procedures in children to help reduce the use of blood products. Greater benefit is likely (but not proven) in children with greater tendency to bleeding, including smaller children (when prolonged bypass times are anticipated) and repeat surgery.[115,168]
- Consideration is given to use of antifibrinolytics during other major noncardiac procedures in children to help reduce the use of blood products
- Synthetic antifibrinolytics are used in preference to aprotinin, outside of well-conducted trials.
- TXA is used in high dose: 50 mg/kg bolus followed by 15 mg/kg/hour infusion (plus if cardiac bypass is used an additional 50 mg/kg to the CPB pump). Infusion is continued until significant bleeding has stopped up to 4 hours postoperatively.
- EACA is not used by the authors, however, an appropriate dose would be 75 mg/kg bolus followed by 75 mg/kg/hour (plus, if cardiac bypass is used, an additional 75 mg/kg to the CPB pump).
- Synthetic antifibrinolytics are administered during severe bleeding, in the doses given previously; however, in the case of traumatic hemorrhage, they are not given more than 3 hours after the initial injury.

## DESMOPRESSIN

Desmopressin acetate (1-desamino-8-D-arginine; DDAVP) is a synthetic analogue of vasopressin. The production of desmopressin involves alteration in the chemical structure of naturally occurring vasopressin. In the process, the antidiuretic effect is enhanced and the vasopressor effect is virtually eliminated. Desmopressin is more resistant to enzymatic cleavage, and hence the duration of action is prolonged to 6 to 24 hours.[123] Desmopressin potently causes endothelial release of factor complexes VIII/protein C and VIII/vWf. It has been used in mild hemophilia, von Willebrand disease, coagulopathy of uremia, liver failure, and in adults undergoing cardiac and spinal fusion surgery (see also Chapter 10).

During the early phase of coagulation, platelets bind via the glycoprotein receptor Ib to vWf on the damaged endothelium. IV desmopressin releases vWf, thus enhancing the binding of platelets to damaged endothelium. The maximum effect of desmopressin is observed at a dose of 0.3 µg/kg. It must be given *after* cessation of the extracorporeal circuit to prevent unwanted platelet activation.[48]

18

Several meta-analyses of its use in adults have been published, the most recent showing that desmopressin was associated with a small reduction in blood loss, but no benefit in terms of repeat sternotomy, proportion of patients requiring transfusion, or mortality.[131] It was also associated with a 2.4-fold increase in risk of myocardial infarction.

In children, desmopressin at 0.3 μg/kg failed to demonstrate any benefit for both non–high-risk[169] and high-risk cardiac surgery.[170] Younger children are not as capable of releasing vWf from endothelial storage sites as are older children, and the maximal release of vWf caused by the operative stimulus cannot be enhanced by desmopressin.[171] Potential adverse sequelae from desmopressin include fluid retention, hyponatremia, tachyphylaxis, tachycardia, and mild hypotension.[172] Desmopressin is not currently recommended in pediatric surgery,[64] although one could postulate that it could be reserved for those with ongoing bleeding with evidence of platelet function abnormalities, such as prolonged bleeding time or decreased maximum amplitude values on a TEG.[173]

## FACTOR VIIA

Recombinant activated factor VII (rVIIa) is known to be safe and effective for treatment and prevention of hemorrhage in children with hemophilia who have circulating inhibitors to replacement factors (see also Chapters 9 and 10). It is also used in patients with Glanzmann thrombasthenia refractory to platelet transfusion, and in patients with Factor VII deficiency. Regulatory approval has been granted in Europe and the United States for these conditions.

Off-label use of this drug has grown steadily over the last few years and now accounts for 97% of in-hospital use.[125] This has encompassed a number of indications involving treatment or prevention of acquired bleeding or coagulopathy[174-186] of varying severity. The most common off-label indications are treatment of bleeding related to cardiovascular surgery, trauma, and intracranial bleeds. Off-label use in children is also widespread. One retrospective study recorded 3655 administrations (in 39 U.S. pediatric hospitals over a 7-year period); 46% were in children admitted to a surgical specialty or to a pediatric intensive care unit, over 20% to cardiac surgery or cardiology. Administration was most common in children under 1 year of age.

For rVIIa to exert a beneficial action, it must generate a burst of thrombin at the sight of injury. Two mechanisms are likely to work in synergy to produce this. First, the TF pathway described previously is stimulated to augment generation of factor Xa. Second, high concentrations of rVIIa will bind directly to the surface of activated platelets, again activating factor Xa, leading to thrombin production (Figs. 18-7 and 18-8).[187]

Usually such processes will be confined to the site of injury; however, in markedly proinflammatory states, expression of tissue factor on activated monocytes and platelets increases the risk of thrombosis distant from the injury. For this reason rVIIa is contraindicated in disseminated intravascular coagulation and should be used with caution in children on extracorporeal life support.[188] The importance of this to more routine bypass is unknown. The therapeutic effects of factor rVIIa begin at doses up to 10 times greater than physiologic concentrations of the endogenous factor. It is therefore not simply a "replacement" therapy of a deficient factor.[147]

The action of rVIIa is to produce a surge of thrombin; however, because clots comprise fibrin, platelets, and red cells, it is unlikely that rVIIa will be effective in the absence of these

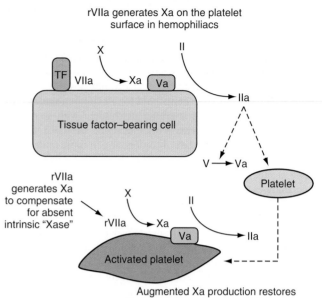

FIGURE 18-7 Schematic representation of the cell-based coagulation model and the proposed mechanism of how recombinant activated factor VII (*rVIIa*) can potentially improve coagulation in hemophiliacs. At supraphysiologic concentrations, rVIIa can bind to the phospholipid membranes of activated platelets, where it activates factor X independent of the tissue factor (*TF*) pathway, causing a large rise in thrombin at the platelet surface. It can therefore compensate for a lack of factor VIII or IX, a possible explanation for its effectiveness in platelet function disorders (From Welsby IJ, Monroe DM, Lawson JH, Hoffmann M. Recombinant activated factor VIIa and the anaesthetist. Anaesthesia 2005;60:1203-12.)

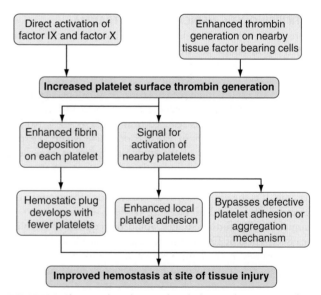

FIGURE 18-8 Theoretical mechanisms by which recombinant activated factor VII could increase thrombin generation and fibrin deposition that may lead to improved hemostasis. (From Welsby IJ, Monroe DM, Lawson JH, Hoffmann M. Recombinant activated factor VIIa and the anaesthetist. Anaesthesia 2005;60:1203-12.)

substrates. Measures should be taken to ensure adequate fibrinogen concentration and platelet numbers before giving rVIIa. In addition, factors such as acidosis and hypothermia will reduce the efficiency of rVIIa (although mild to moderate hypothermia has only minor effects in vitro).[148] Given the expense of rVIIa, in addition to doubts over safety, it would appear to be wise to employ more established measures before its use, along with (as dictated by local agreements) consultation with a hematologist.

Evidence that rVIIa will reduce bleeding comes mainly from case reports. Numerous anecdotes appear to demonstrate dramatic reductions in bleeding in apparently catastrophic situations. Demonstrations of even occasional success, in the face of an otherwise hopeless situation, might itself be taken as a good reason to use the drug. Events are rarely, however, that clear cut and rVIIa is often used on patients at much lower risk of bleeding to death. Reported cases of off-label use in anesthesiology and surgical practice range from truly prophylactic use (in high-risk populations before evidence of severe bleeding), to use to control prolonged or severe (but not immediately life-threatening) bleeding, through to compassionate use in immediately life-threatening bleeding after exhaustion of all conventional treatments. The balance of risk and benefit will vary widely within these differing clinical scenarios.

Most controlled trials of rVIIa have focused on prophylaxis use or use in less severe bleeding. There are 26 randomized controlled trials that have examined off-label use of rVIIa, and 5 have focused on surgical use.[150,189-192] A meta-analysis of these trials demonstrated no reduction in mortality and only relatively modest reductions in bleeding and transfusion.[193] A study[190] that examined patients with moderately severe bleeding (more than 200 mL/hr or greater than 2 mL/kg for 2 consecutive hours) following heart surgery in adults reported that although 2619 patients had consented to the trial, only 179 subsequently had sufficient bleeding to be randomized. The results demonstrated a reduction in reexploration, bleeding, and in transfusion requirements. The objective of the trial was to examine the safety of using rVIIa. Unfortunately, the trial was terminated early; although a trend to increased adverse effects was seen, the result was inconclusive. The authors of this study cautioned against wider use before further trials. A single randomized trial (n = 76) that examined prophylactic rVIIa administration (40 µg/kg) in infants undergoing heart surgery,[191] demonstrated neither efficacy nor toxicity in this group. The study was small but larger than several of the adult studies that demonstrated an effect. Whether this demonstrates a genuine difference between adults and infants or is related to the relatively low dose rVIIa used is unclear. The use of rVIIa in children has been recently reviewed.[188]

Concerns about adverse effects of this drug have grown. Two studies have attempted to systematically review the data on toxicity.[194,195] The rate of thrombosis was greater (10.2% vs. 8.7%) in those treated with rVIIa, but this increase was largely confined to the elderly. The second study examined data from observational trials with comparator groups; mortality was not affected by treatment with rVIIa, although the risk of thrombosis was increased in some groups (including adult cardiac patients). Both these reviews combined data from studies on very different patient populations, and some caution is required in their interpretation. The risk of thrombosis in children is uncertain and data inconclusive.[188] Neonates treated with either FFP or rVIIa for similar indications had a similar incidence of thrombosis (7%).[196] Thrombotic complications occurred in 10.8% of children who received off-label rVIIa; the overall mortality in those receiving rVIIa was 34%.[197] It is not possible to know how this was affected by use of rVIIa. It is clear that both thrombotic complications and mortality are common in patients with bleeding serious enough to warrant use of this drug. Use of rVIIa will very likely increase the risk of thrombosis, although the impact

of this (and the benefit of the drug) will vary in different clinical situations.

The dose regimen for off-label use of rVIIa is yet to be firmly established. One of the difficulties is that there is no satisfactory laboratory test to monitor its effectiveness,[198,199] and factor VII activity does not always predict efficacy.[200] Although it is known that the PT, aPTT, and TEG improve after rVIIa is given in liver surgery,[201] they cannot reliably be used to determine a dosing regimen. If the main effect of rVIIa is at the site of injury, clinical observation still remains the best indication of effect.[198] The dose used often closely relates to the dose indicated in hemophilia patients (90 µg/kg), although in practice doses are often rounded to the nearest vial.[201] Although Warren et al. recommended a lower dose of 40 to 60 µg/kg, a dose of 40 µg/kg has been shown to have no effect.[191] Larger doses of 60 to 90 µg/kg may prove more effective.

The justification to use larger doses is supported by differences in PK. In older children with hemophilia, the terminal elimination half-life of rVIIa is less than in adults (1.3 vs. 2.7 hours), and the clearance is greater (67 vs. 37 mL/kg/hour).[202,203] When prophylactic rVIIa at 100 µg/kg was given to 10 preterm infants between 23 and 28 weeks gestational age every 4 hours for 72 hours, two umbilical artery catheter thromboses were reported and no embolic events or increase in intraventricular hemorrhage rate compared with those not given rVIIa.[204] There were no other treatment-related side effects, despite this large repeated dose, which suggests that a large study in neonates is warranted.

Since the previous edition of this book, there have been a considerable number of publications related to the use of rVIIa. Unfortunately, information, especially that concerning specific indications, remains sparse. It would appear that rVIIa can be effective for the treatment of severe bleeding refractory to other treatments, but it is certainly not universally effective. The risk of thromboembolic complications is substantial in those recovering from severe bleeding, and rVIIa is likely to increase this risk. There seems to be no reason to think that these considerations do not apply to children, although the balance of risk and benefit may be very different in children. It is the authors' current view that rVIIa should only be used for treating life-threatening bleeding that has proved refractory to other treatments. Outside of properly conducted trials, it should not be used for prevention of bleeding, treatment of less severe bleeding, or as an alternative to blood products. Its use should not delay surgical reexploration if indicated. Every attempt should be made to ensure an adequate platelet count, adequate fibrinogen concentration, correction of acidosis, and near normothermia before use.

## Summary

We began this chapter by reviewing the mechanism of coagulation and how this alters during normal development and disease. This understanding of coagulation has lead to the development of new treatments, most notably rVIIa.[12] Complex systems such as the coagulation system behave in unanticipated ways and while mechanisms can be found to justify many interventions, not all interventions will bring a clinically useful improvement for the patient. The coagulation model becomes more complicated when we consider the interactions between coagulation and other systems (noticeably the kinin–kallikrein system[15] and other proinflammatory cascades), as well as the effects of transfusion of allogeneic blood products. Mechanistic justifications for use of any treatment are therefore limited. Direct evidence that a specific treatment brings a benefit to the child is required. Although the evidence available is still lacking, and at times appear contradictory, we have aimed to give clear advice to the practicing anesthesiologist when possible.

The problems of research into this subject are demonstrated by aprotinin studies. Despite relatively large numbers of patients (including children) recruited into trials, many important questions remain incompletely resolved. Concerns over safety in an entirely different population have led to the effective withdrawal of what may (or may not) have been a useful medication in children. Beyond moderate reductions in blood loss, few advantages have been convincingly demonstrated for this drug.[2] For therapies aimed at treatment rather than prevention of bleeding, the challenges of conducting well-designed trials are even greater. Currently, several therapeutic approaches are proposed (rVIIa, fibrinogen concentrates, transfusion protocols based on TEG) that differ from traditional treatment. The requirement for well-conducted trials, with meaningful outcome measures, is greater than ever.

## ANNOTATED REFERENCES

Eaton MP. Antifibrinolytic therapy in surgery for congenital heart disease. Anesth Analg 2008;106:1087-100.

*A clear review on the use of antifibrinolytics in children for cardiac surgery. The author illustrates the difficulties in drawing quantitative conclusions from the varied trial designs.*

Guzzetta NA, Miller BE. Principles of hemostasis in children: models and maturation. Paediatr Anaesth [Review] 2011;21:3-9.

*An excellent of review of the changes in coagulation with development, with a particular emphasis of the relevance of this to the use of rVIIa in pediatric practice. This is part of an issue of* Pediatric Anesthesia *themed around topics related to coagulation.*

Hoffman M. Remodeling the blood coagulation cascade. J Thromb Thrombolysis 2003;16:17-20.

*Hoffman explains the difficulties associated with the "old model" of coagulation cascade. The paper contains an excellent step-by-step discussion of the cellular based model of coagulation.*

Mangano DT, Tudor IC, Dietzel C. The risk associated with aprotinin in cardiac surgery. N Engl J Med 2006;354:353-65.

*A frequently cited large observational study on the use of aprotinin, this adult study suggested an increased incidence of thrombotic complications and renal failure. The authors seriously questioned the safety profile of aprotinin in adult cardiac patients. The methodology and interpretation has been questioned by some; we would therefore also like to direct the reader to the correspondence that followed:*

Brown JR, Birkmeyer NJO, O'Connor GT. Aprotinin in cardiac surgery. N Engl J Med 2006;354:1953-7 (Correspondence).

Ferraris VA, Bridges CR, Anderson RP. Aprotinin in cardiac surgery. N Engl J Med 2006;354:1953-7 (Correspondence).

Levy JH, Ramsay JG, Guyton RA. Aprotinin in cardiac surgery. N Engl J Med 2006;354:1953-7 (Correspondence).

Mangano DT. Aprotinin in cardiac surgery. N Engl J Med 2006;354:1953-7 (Correspondence).

Schouten ES, van de Pol AC, Schouten AN, et al. The effect of aprotinin, tranexamic acid, and aminocaproic acid on blood loss and use of blood products in major pediatric surgery: a meta-analysis. Pediatr Crit Care Med 2009;10:182-90.

*A systemic review and meta-analysis of the role of antifibrinolytic drugs during pediatric surgery*

Warren OJ, Rogers PL, Watret AL, et al. Defining the role of recombinant activated factor VII in pediatric cardiac surgery: where should we go from here? Pediatr Crit Care Med 2009;10:572-82.

*A thorough review of the use of rVIIa in pediatric heart surgery.*

Webber TP, Grosse Hartlange MA, Van Aken H, Brooke M. Anaesthetic strategies to reduce perioperative blood loss in paediatric surgery. Eur J Anaesthesiol 2003;20:175-81.

*This is an overview of current strategies for reducing blood loss in children. The authors discuss pros and cons of various techniques, including practical limitations of cell salvage.*

Welsby IJ, Monroe DM, Lawson JH, Hoffmann M. Recombinant activated factor VIIa and the anaesthetist. Anaesthesia 2005;60:1203-12.

*This is a very good overview of the mechanisms and use of rVIIa.*

## REFERENCES

Please see www.expertconsult.com

# Mechanical Circulatory Support

LAURA K. DIAZ

THE NUMBER OF INFANTS and children hospitalized with heart failure resulting from congenital or acquired heart disease continues to increase each year; according to a recent analysis of 15 million pediatric hospitalizations in the United States, this number grew by 25% between 2003 and 2006.[1] Failure of the myocardium, despite maximal medical therapy, to provide sufficient cardiac output for adequate support of end-organ perfusion results in the need for mechanical support of the circulation, either as an adjunct to cardiopulmonary resuscitation (CPR) or as a bridge to myocardial recovery or cardiac transplantation. Data from the Randomized Evaluation of Mechanical Assistance for the Treatment of Congestive Heart Failure Trial (REMATCH) demonstrated prolonged survival and increased quality of life in adult patients with end-stage heart failure who received mechanical cardiac support (MCS).[2] Although the number and type of MCS devices available for children remains comparatively limited, particularly for children weighing less than 20 kg in the United States, the use of extracorporeal life support in this population has continued to grow, with a 32% increase in the use of ventricular assist devices (VADs) between 2003 and 2006.[3] Initiatives by the National Heart, Lung, and Blood Institute (NHLBI) supporting the development of MCS devices for infants and children offer promising future alternatives for children.[4]

## Initiation of Mechanical Circulatory Support

### INDICATIONS AND CONTRAINDICATIONS

Mechanical circulatory support in children is most often necessary due to intrinsic failure of the myocardium. Preoperative cardiopulmonary stabilization may be required in children with profound hypoxemia and/or cardiovascular collapse due to hypercyanotic spells, pulmonary hypertensive crises, obstructed total anomalous pulmonary venous return, occlusion of systemic-pulmonary shunts, or cardiogenic shock (Table 19-1). Extracorporeal membrane oxygenation (ECMO) was used to bridge to surgical repair or palliation in 26 children, with 62% surviving to discharge and no observed differences in outcome between single and biventricular patients.[5] ECMO has also been successful in

stabilizing children with refractory dysrhythmias.[6-8] In a retrospective study, ECMO was used in nine infants with a variety of tachy- or bradydysrhythmias, with all nine surviving to discharge.[9] ECMO has also been used to stabilize children in the cardiac catheterization laboratory, both preemptively before high-risk interventional procedures[10] and as a rescue technique for catheter-induced complications, persistent low cardiac output, or hypoxemia.[11]

Postcardiotomy myocardial dysfunction can manifest as either early (inability to wean from cardiopulmonary bypass [CPB]) or late failure (sustained postoperative low cardiac output syndrome), with poor end-organ function, persistently increased plasma lactate concentrations, low mixed venous oxygen saturations, and escalating inotropic support. To maximize survival, it is essential to rule out the presence of residual surgical lesions, coronary insufficiency secondary to surgical manipulation, and mechanical problems (e.g., cardiac tamponade) before initiating MCS.[12] Both ECMO and left ventricular assist devices (LVADs) have been used for postoperative ventricular support in infants with anomalous origin of the left coronary artery from the pulmonary artery trunk (ALCAPA), either as a bridge to recovery or transplant.[13,14] The routine use of MCS after a Stage I Norwood procedure has also been advocated in order to optimize postoperative cardiac output.[15]

Other cardiac pathophysiologic processes, such as acute myocarditis, coronary ischemia, graft rejection after cardiac transplantation, or end-stage heart failure due to chronic cardiomyopathies, dysrhythmias, or congenital heart defects, may also warrant the use of MCS.[16-18] The steadily enlarging population of adults with congenital heart disease who develop heart failure will pose special challenges due to their complex anatomy and prior surgical palliations.

Noncardiac indications for MCS include severe hypothermia, drug toxicity, and near-drowning. ECMO can also provide short-term respiratory support for tracheobronchial reconstruction in infants and children with critical airways, when conventional mechanical ventilation is not feasible or has not been successful.[19] Although septicemia was initially considered a contraindication to MCS, a recent review of 45 children who required ECMO for hemodynamic support due to septic shock reported

**TABLE 19-1** Indications for Mechanical Circulatory Support

**Preoperative Stabilization**

Severe cyanosis/hypercyanotic spells
Pulmonary hypertensive crises
Myocardial dysfunction
Malignant dysrhythmias
Sepsis

**Postcardiotomy Patients**

Failure to wean from cardiopulmonary bypass
Late postcardiotomy failure (prolonged low cardiac output syndrome)
Stage I palliation for hypoplastic left heart syndrome
After ALCAPA repair
Malignant dysrhythmias

**Bridge to Myocardial Recovery**

Acute myocarditis
Cardiomyopathy
Acute cardiac transplant rejection

**Bridge to Transplantation**

Direct bridge to transplantation
Bridge to bridge (short- to long-term support)

**Noncardiac Indications**

Near-drowning
Severe hypothermia
Drug toxicity
Critical airway (tracheal stenosis)
Sepsis/shock

*ALCAPA,* Anomalous origin of the left coronary artery from the pulmonary artery.

**TABLE 19-2** Suggested Clinical Criteria for Mechanical Cardiac Support Implementation

**Rapid Circulatory Deterioration (CI <2 L/min/m²)**

Inotropic dependence

**Critical Peripheral Perfusion**

Development of metabolic acidosis
Mixed venous oxygen saturation <40%

**Signs of Renal, Hepatic and Respiratory Failure**

Ventilatory support with increasing $FIO_2$

**Critically Impaired Myocardial Function on Echocardiography**

High or rapidly increasing B-type natriuretic peptide

Modified from Hetzer R, Potapov EV, Alexi-Meskishvili V, et al. Single center experience with treatment of cardiogenic shock in children by pediatric ventricular assist devices. J Thorac Cardiovasc Surg 2011;141:616-23; and Potapov EV, Stiller B, Hetzer R. Ventricular assist devices in children: current achievements and future perspectives. Pediatr Transplant 2007;11:241-55.
*CI,* Cardiac index.

a 47% survival to discharge.[20] ECMO can provide a bridge to lung transplantation or retransplantation, and posttransplantation can be used in cases of severe primary graft dysfunction, although survival in these patient groups remains less overall than for other indications.[21-23]

Contraindications to implementation of MCS should be considered on a case-by-case basis and may include advanced multisystem organ failure, significant neurologic damage or intracranial hemorrhage, severe coagulopathy, and/or extreme prematurity. Additionally, the presence of certain chromosomal abnormalities, multiple congenital anomalies, or existing infections may influence decision making. For children who require MCS secondary to a cardiac etiology, due consideration should be given to the likelihood of recovery of myocardial function before instituting support; and if not, whether the child is a suitable candidate for cardiac transplantation.

## TIMING AND PREPARATION FOR THE INITIATION OF SUPPORT

As experience with the use of pediatric circulatory support continues to grow, it has become increasingly evident that early institution of support better preserves end-organ function and maximizes the opportunity for recovery or bridge to transplantation. The following criteria for implementation of MCS have been used in one institution: (1) cardiac index less than 2 with inotropic dependence; (2) poor peripheral perfusion with metabolic acidosis and mixed venous oxygen saturation less than 40%; (3) signs of impending respiratory, renal, or hepatic failure;

and (4) increased or rapidly increasing B-type natriuretic peptide (BNP) concentrations (Table 19-2).[24]

During routine preparation for MCS, baseline laboratory hematologic studies should be obtained, including a complete blood cell count (CBC), platelet count, prothrombin time (PT), activated partial thromboplastin time (aPTT), activated clotting time (ACT), plasma hemoglobin, antithrombin III, fibrinogen, and thromboelastogram (TEG). A minimum of two units of packed red blood cells (PRBCs) should be available (preferably cytomegalovirus-negative, leukocyte-reduced, and irradiated), because all such children should be considered potential cardiac transplant candidates (note that the potassium concentration of irradiated PRBCs may be greatly increased, resulting in acute hyperkalemia if administered rapidly) (see also Chapter 10). In infants, ultrasonography of the head is useful before considering institution of MCS. Anesthesiologists are frequently involved during the cannulation procedure, and all arterial and central venous lines, as well as the tracheal tube, should be well secured and the ventilator easily accessible.

The emergent use of ECMO for children during in-hospital cardiac arrest with failure of conventional resuscitation methods has become increasingly common. An analysis of data from the National Registry of CardioPulmonary Resuscitation (NRCPR) database of outcomes from children less than 18 years of age who received extracorporeal cardiopulmonary resuscitation (ECPR) for cardiac arrest that was refractory to conventional CPR demonstrated a 43.7% survival to discharge. Preexisting conditions of septicemia, pneumonia, and renal insufficiency correlated with an increased risk of mortality. Children with a cardiac disease diagnosis showed slightly improved odds of survival to discharge when compared with children without cardiac disease.[25] In a review of pediatric cardiac patients from the Extracorporeal Life Support Organization (ELSO) registry who received ECPR, single ventricle physiology and a history of more complex cardiac surgery were negative predictors of survival.[26] Renal dysfunction, pulmonary hemorrhage, neurologic injury, and the need for additional CPR during ECMO have also been associated with increased mortality.[27]

Acceptable neurologic outcomes have been described in children after CPR of up to 3 hours in duration before institution of ECMO.[28] The duration of CPR before ECMO cannulation did not differ between survivors and nonsurvivors.[29] Of the children in the ELSO registry who received ECPR, 22% of the 682 developed an acute neurologic injury, with an in-hospital mortality rate of 89%. The risk of neurologic injury in children with cardiac disease in this cohort was reduced.[30]

A dry circuit can be kept ready for rapid deployment, with crystalloid prime used during initiation of support and addition of blood products (PRBCs and fresh frozen plasma) as soon as they become available. During resuscitative efforts before the institution of mechanical support, multiple doses of vasoconstrictors should be avoided, if possible, acidosis should be corrected, and ice may be placed around the head to provide cerebral protection. Ultimately, the restoration of cardiac output, even with a low hematocrit, is the most important factor for successful resuscitation and long-term survival.[31,32]

## Mechanical Circulatory Support Devices

In pediatric practice, the size of the child and the type of support required (cardiopulmonary vs. cardiac) are the most important considerations when choosing an MCS device (Table 19-3). Secondary factors are the indication for, and expected duration of, support and the desired end point: bridge to bridge, procedure (surgery or catheterization), recovery, or transplantation. Certain devices, such as the intra-aortic balloon pump (IABP), ECMO, and centrifugal pump, are best used for short-term support (less than 2 to 4 weeks) and may occasionally serve as a "bridge to bridge" for institution of a long-term mechanical support device.[33]

A VAD may be defined most simply as a mechanical pump attached between the heart and either the aorta or pulmonary artery to circulate blood when one or both ventricles are no longer capable of adequately maintaining circulation. In short, a VAD is a pump supporting a failing ventricle, whether right, left, or biventricular (BiVAD). Isolated ventricular dysfunction with adequate oxygenation, as seen in acute myocarditis, acute rejection after cardiac transplantation, or dilated cardiomyopathy, is the ideal cardiac pathology for VAD support. ECMO, on the other hand, provides full cardiopulmonary support and may be preferable to VAD support for children with pulmonary hypertension, complex congenital heart lesions involving intracardiac shunts, severe hypoxemia, or respiratory failure (Fig. 19-1).

### SHORT-TERM SUPPORT

#### Intra-Aortic Balloon Pump

IABPs are support devices with a balloon ranging from 2.5 to 20 mL in size mounted on a 4.5F to 7F catheter that may be inserted either via the femoral artery or, in infants, via the ascending aorta. The balloon inflates during diastole, forcing blood toward the heart and increasing blood flow to the coronary arteries, and deflates before systole, decreasing ventricular afterload. Cardiac output is augmented by 10% to 20%, whereas left atrial, left ventricular end-diastolic, and pulmonary artery pressures are all decreased.

Anatomic contraindications to the use of an IABP include patent ductus arteriosus, aortic insufficiency, aortic aneurysm, and recent aortic surgery. Technical limitations in children consist of size constraints, the increased distensibility and compliance of the aorta, and the difficulty of synchronizing pump function with an infant or child's rapid heart rate,[34] although use of M-mode echocardiography-timed IABP in infants and children to assist with cardiac synchronization has been described.[35] IABP use in

**TABLE 19-3** Mechanical Circulatory Support Devices: Advantages and Disadvantages

| Device | Advantages | Disadvantages |
|---|---|---|
| ECMO | No patient size limitations<br>Cardiopulmonary support<br>Central or peripheral cannulation<br>Relatively inexpensive<br>Extensive pediatric experience | Short-term support<br>Increased bleeding and thromboembolic complications<br>More complex circuit<br>Nonpulsatile flow<br>No patient mobility<br>Need for trained personnel |
| Centrifugal VAD | No patient size limitations<br>Right, left, or biventricular support<br>Simpler setup than ECMO<br>Less anticoagulation than ECMO<br>Better ventricular unloading than ECMO | Short-term support<br>No respiratory support<br>Nonpulsatile flow<br>No patient mobility<br>Direct cannulation of the heart required |
| Thoratec | Pulsatile flow<br>Right, left, or biventricular support<br>Extubation/ambulation possible | BSA >1.2 m²<br>Sternotomy required for implantation |
| Berlin Heart Excor and Medos HIA-VAD | No patient size limitations<br>Pulsatile flow<br>Right, left, or biventricular support<br>Extubation/ambulation possible<br>Long-term support possible | Not currently available in the United States<br>Sternotomy required for implantation |
| MicroMed DeBakey Child VAD | Noiseless pump<br>No compliance chamber<br>No artificial valves<br>Fewer moving parts<br>Small blood-to-device interface<br>Long-term support possible | BSA >0.7 m²<br>Only left ventricular support |

From Diaz LK, Andropoulos DB. New developments in pediatric cardiac anesthesia. Anesthesiol Clin North Am 2005;23:655-76.
*BSA*, Body surface area; *ECMO*, extracorporeal membrane oxygenation; *VAD*, ventricular assist device.

an adult patient with Fontan physiology and severe ventricular failure has been reported, with improvement in end-organ function and successful weaning.[36] IABP support must be initiated early, while ventricular function is still capable of sustaining adequate cardiac output,[37] because the balloon pump only augments, and does not replace, ventricular output. It can only support the left ventricle.

### Extracorporeal Membrane Oxygenation

Whereas adults generally have isolated left ventricular failure, children more often require cardiopulmonary support due to hypoxemia, pulmonary hypertension, or concurrent right ventricular failure. For infants and children who require short-term or urgent cardiopulmonary support, ECMO remains the modality of choice. Initially reported for the treatment of cardiac failure in children in the 1970s,[38] ECMO was subsequently used for mechanical support during interhospital transport.[39] Since the ELSO registry began in 1989, ECMO has been the MCS

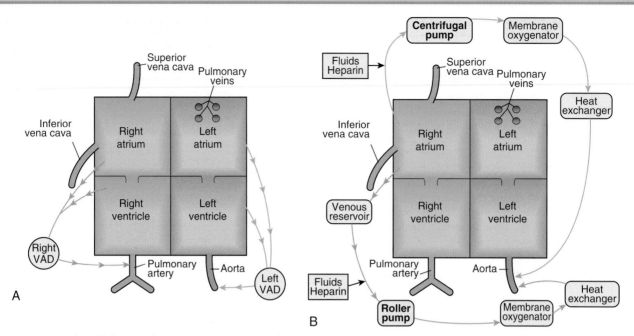

**FIGURE 19-1 A,** Right and left ventricular assist circuits. For biventricular assist, both the right ventricular assist device (*VAD*) and left VAD circuits are used. **B,** Venoarterial extracorporeal membrane oxygenation circuits using either a venous reservoir and roller pump, or a centrifugal pump without a reservoir.

modality with the most pediatric usage, with more than 7500 neonates and children using it for cardiac indications.[40]

A typical ECMO circuit is composed of a pump (either a roller pump with a servoregulatory mechanism for controlling circuit flow or a centrifugal pump); a hollow fiber or membrane oxygenator; a heat exchanger; and cannulas (either venoarterial or venovenous). A modified ECMO circuit composed of a heparin-coated circuit, Bio-Medicus centrifugal pump (Medtronic, Minneapolis), hollow fiber membrane oxygenator, flow probe, and hematocrit/oxygen saturation monitor, allowing the circuit to be set up and primed in 5 minutes for rapid resuscitation, has been described.[41] Most hospitals supporting such a service have readily available trained personnel to assist with implementing and maintaining ECMO therapy. Versatility is one of the advantages of ECMO; venoarterial cannulation in postcardiotomy patients may be either transthoracic via the right atrial appendage and aorta, transcervical via the right internal jugular vein and common carotid artery, or femoral via the femoral artery and vein in larger patients. Heparin-bonded circuitry is often used to minimize surface-induced complement activation, platelet dysfunction, and anticoagulation requirements.[42]

Other advantages of ECMO include the lack of patient size limitations, the ability to institute support either in the pediatric intensive care unit or the operating room without the need for CPB, the ability to provide ultrafiltration or hemodialysis for children during mechanical support, and the ability to provide biventricular cardiopulmonary support even in very small children. In a review of 27 children who underwent venoarterial ECMO for cardiac indications, both nonsurgical and postcardiotomy, the overall survival rate was 59%; of these, 56% were undergoing CPR at the time ECMO support was instituted. Of the latter group, 73% survived.[43] Hemodynamic benefits of ECMO include decreased right ventricular preload and pulmonary artery pressures. Due to reentry of blood into the aorta an increase in afterload often occurs and may require pharmacologic afterload reduction therapy, such as milrinone, nitroprusside, hydralazine, or phenoxybenzamine.

Several management options exist for children with single-ventricle physiology and shunt-dependent pulmonary circulation who require ECMO support. The survival rate of 10 children who underwent single-ventricle palliation and subsequently required ECMO support was greater in those in whom the aortopulmonary shunt was left open during ECMO.[44] Adequate alveolar ventilation must be provided, however, and greater ECMO flow rates are generally required to maintain adequate pulmonary and systemic circulations. In children with low pulmonary vascular resistance, pulmonary blood flow may prove to be excessive and limitation of shunt flow with surgical clips may become necessary. Children with single-ventricle physiology have comparable survival rates after ECMO support compared with other cardiac patients.[43] ECMO has been particularly successful in treating children with single-ventricle physiology who develop acute shunt thrombosis or transient depression of ventricular function.[45] Of 44 children with shunted single-ventricle physiology who required ECMO support, the indication for support was the strongest predictor of survival to discharge, with 81% of those cannulated due to hypoxemia surviving, but only 29% of those cannulated for hypotension surviving to discharge.[46] Patients with Fontan physiology who require ECMO have a significantly greater mortality rate (65%), possibly the result of longstanding ventricular dysfunction that is not easily reversible.[47]

Disadvantages of ECMO include complex circuitry, the need for greater levels of systemic anticoagulation than required by VADs, the necessity for both blood prime and frequent transfusions, and decreased pulmonary blood flow. Compared with other support modalities, ECMO circuitry is complex and requires full-time supervision by trained personnel. Left atrial decompression may occasionally be inadequate, requiring either the placement of a left atrial vent or an atrial septostomy. Inadequate unloading of the left atrium can lead to mitral regurgitation and pulmonary edema or hemorrhage, and can also minimize the chances of myocardial recovery when the left ventricle is not sufficiently unloaded. Moderate levels of ventilatory

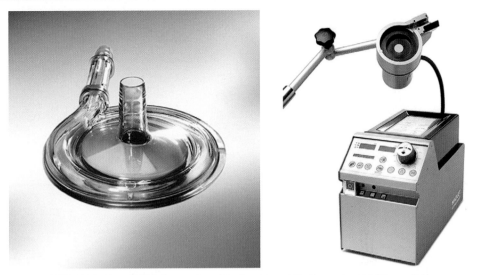

**FIGURE 19-2** Maquet's RotaFlow system. (Courtesy Maquet Cardiovascular, LLC, Wayne, N.J.)

support must be maintained to ensure that well-oxygenated blood is provided to the coronary arteries, and the child must remain intubated and sedated throughout the period of ECMO support.[48]

Although effective for rapid rescue and short-term support, ECMO support is generally maintained only for 1 to 3 weeks before the increasing risk of significant complications limits its usefulness.[49] In children requiring postcardiotomy ECMO support, the need for prolonged support, renal failure, and low pH in the first 24 hours of support have been associated with a higher mortality.[50] A review of combined data between 2004 and 2009 from the ELSO registry and the Organ Procurement Transplant Network database showed that over half the children bridged with ECMO to heart transplant failed to survive to hospital discharge, illustrating that ECMO is not able to reliably provide intermediate to long-term mechanical support to bridge children safely to transplantation.[51] Survivors of ECMO support also have greater rates of neurologic impairment than those supported with VADs, with poorer outcomes noted in younger children with more complex disease.[52]

### Centrifugal Pumps

Currently used centrifugal pumps include the Bio-Medicus Bio-Pump (Medtronic, Minneapolis), CentriMag (Levitronix GmbH, Zurich), RotaFlow (Maquet Cardiovascular, Wayne, N.J.), Capiox (Terumo Cardiovascular Systems Corporation, Ann Arbor, Mich.) and TandemHeart (CardiacAssist, Inc., Pittsburgh). The CentriMag pump is available as an investigational device only in the US. The term *centrifugal pump* is not always synonymous with VAD, because centrifugal pumps may also be used with an oxygenator to construct an ECMO circuit. Without an oxygenator, they may be used for right, left, or biventricular support (except in infants, when size limitations can preclude the presence of two pumps[53]) and offer the advantage of excellent ventricular unloading and decreased wall stress, optimizing the chances of myocardial remodeling and recovery. Unloading the left ventricle can also decrease left ventricular cavity size and improve septal configuration, resulting in improved tricuspid valve function and right ventricular inflow.[54] When used as a VAD without an oxygenator and heat exchanger, reduced systemic anticoagulation is required, compared with ECMO usage.

Centrifugal pumps offer the advantage of decreased trauma to red blood cells and a less pronounced systemic inflammatory response compared with roller pumps.[55] A centrifugal VAD spins, creating a vortex, with negative pressure at the inlet drawing blood into the cone and positive pressure at the outlet allowing nonpulsatile ejection at the base. The RotaFlow pump (Fig. 19-2) has a rotating mechanism that is levitated in three magnetic fields with one point bearing, allowing laminar flow and reducing mechanical friction, heat production and clotting potential compared to the Bio-Medicus pump.[56] Cardiac output from a centrifugal pump depends on preload, afterload, and the rotational speed of the pump. Because increases or decreases in preload and afterload can affect pump flow without changes in rotational speed, a flow probe is necessary. Excessive negative inlet pressures (hypovolemia) must be avoided because air can be entrained into the circuit.

The TandemHeart system is a low-prime centrifugal pump capable of flows of 0 to 5 L/min, with a hydrodynamic fluid bearing supporting the spinning rotor (Fig. 19-3). Although size requirements (greater than 40 kg) preclude its use in most children, it is advantageous in that it can be placed percutaneously through the femoral vessels, with a transseptal extended flow cannula allowing entry from the femoral vein into the left atrium. The arterial cannula may be placed into the femoral artery, or in patients less than 80 kg, a vascular graft to the femoral artery may be cannulated to avoid lower extremity vascular compromise.[57] A pediatric TandemHeart pump with a priming volume of 4 mL for children from 2 to 40 kg is currently undergoing in vitro testing.[58]

Compared with ECMO, centrifugal pumps are less expensive and can be set up more rapidly, they have reduced priming volumes, and reduced anticoagulation requirements. Disadvantages of centrifugal pumps include the potential for circuit thrombus formation, nonpulsatile flow, and limited duration of usage (usually less than 3 weeks). Excellent outcomes with centrifugal VAD support have been reported in children who required postcardiotomy ventricular MCS of limited duration, such as those with ALCAPA, or ventricular failure due to cardiomyopathy.[59] In addition, fewer post-support neurologic complications were noted in children who received VAD support compared with those who received ECMO for similar indications.[60]

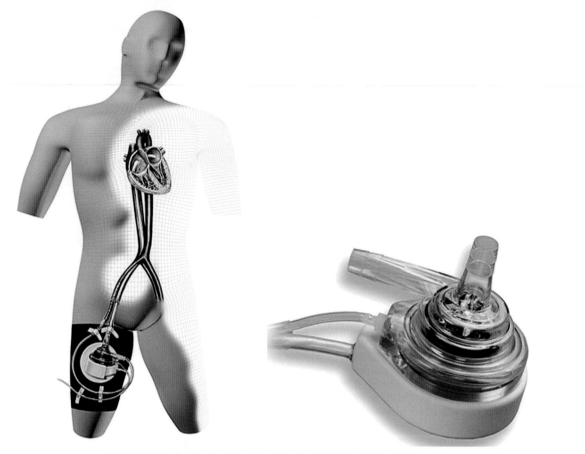

FIGURE 19-3  TandemHeart assist system. (Courtesy CardiacAssist, Inc., Pittsburgh.)

## INTERMEDIATE- TO LONG-TERM SUPPORT
### Pulsatile Pumps
Pulsatile pumps are VADs that facilitate chronic support of the circulation while also allowing tracheal extubation, the use of enteral nutrition, and ambulation for the child. They are paracorporeal and either pneumatically or electromechanically driven. Like centrifugal pumps, pulsatile VADs enjoy several advantages over ECMO: they are simpler in design, less expensive, require lower levels of anticoagulation, and may be used for left, right, or biventricular support of the circulation. Unlike the previously discussed devices, pulsatile pumps are suitable for intermediate- to long-term mechanical circulatory support, but until the advent of the Berlin Heart Excor, their use in infants and children was severely limited by patient size constraints. Internationally, the Berlin Heart Excor and the Medos HIA-VAD pulsatile systems (Berlin Heart GmbH, Berlin, and Medos Medizintechnik AG, Stolberg, Germany, respectively) have been successfully used in children of all ages.[61,62] Insertion of a pulsatile VAD requires the use of CPB and closure of any existing septal defects.

### *Thoratec*
The Thoratec pulsatile ventricular assist system (Thoratec Corporation, Pleasanton, Calif.) is a pneumatically driven pump with a 65-mL blood sac, Björk-Shiley tilting disc valves, and exteriorized inflow and outflow cannulas (Fig. 19-4). Inflow may be from either the left atrium or left ventricular apex, with outflow to the aorta. Pump output, depending on the cannula size and length,

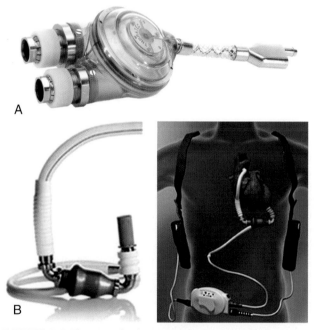

FIGURE 19-4  **A,** Thoratec pulsatile ventricular assist device. **B,** Thoratec HeartMate II axial pump. (Courtesy Thoratec Corporation, Pleasanton, Calif.)

may vary from 5 to 7 L/min.[63] The Thoratec pulsatile VAD may be operated in three modes: synchronized to the child's underlying heart rate, asynchronous, with a set rate programmed into the device, or fill-to-empty, in which the device fills to a set volume before ejection. Although use of the Thoratec has been described in children as small as 17 kg,[64] the risk of thromboembolic events is greater in smaller children, because lower blood flow in the relatively oversized device can lead to stasis and thrombus formation.[65] Children with congenital heart disease and/or left atrial cannulation are at greater risk for neurologic complications during Thoratec support.[66] The use of a fixed-rate mode, with an increased stroke rate of 80 to 90 per minute and partial stroke volumes, is currently recommended because it is associated with fewer cerebrovascular events. Anticoagulation for the Thoratec VAD initially consists of a heparin infusion, whereas long-term protocols generally use warfarin (Coumadin) and aspirin, with maintenance of an international normalized ratio (INR) of 2.5 to 3.5.[67]

The worldwide experience with the Thoratec paracorporeal VAD in 209 children younger than 18 years of age, ranging from 17 to 118 kg and with a body surface area (BSA) of 0.7 to 2.3 m[2], has been summarized. Overall survival to discharge was 68%, but subgroups with cardiomyopathies and myocarditis had greater survival rates than did children with congenital heart disease. Device configuration and the type of support used (LVAD vs. BiVAD) were not correlated with negative patient outcomes.[68]

### Berlin Heart Excor

First used in adults in 1987,[69] the Berlin Heart Excor is a pulsatile, paracorporeal pump currently manufactured in three pediatric sizes (10, 25, and 30 mL) and three adult sizes (50, 60, and 80 mL) (Fig. 19-5, *A*). The pediatric version was first used in 1992[70] and has since been successfully employed in neonates and

infants with a BSA as low as 0.2 m[2].[61] An investigational device exemption trial was begun in the United States in 2007; before this, the Berlin Heart was used nearly 100 times in North America at 29 different institutions, under compassionate use regulations. A recently published review of 73 of these initial patients (weight 3 to 87.6 kg) revealed a 77% success rate in bridging to either transplant or recovery, with a median support time of 1.6 months. Younger age and the need for BiVAD support were risk factors for increased mortality.[71]

The Berlin Heart Excor design has not changed since 2001, and consists of a pneumatically driven translucent polyurethane pump, trileaflet polyurethane inlet and outlet valves, and silicone inflow and outflow cannulas. All blood-contacting surfaces, including the polyurethane valves, are heparin-coated (Carmeda AB, Upplands Väsby, Sweden). A flexible diaphragm in three layers divides the pump chamber into an air chamber and a blood chamber (Fig. 19-5, *B*), with the two diaphragm layers facing the air chamber serving as driving membranes and the third seamless blood membrane passively moved by the driving membranes.[72] The Berlin Heart Excor has been successfully used to provide univentricular (left or right) or biventricular support, even in infants, and may be operated in a synchronous, asynchronous, or fill-to-empty mode. A rechargeable battery is available that can provide up to 5 hours of independent power supply for adult-sized pumps, but power requirements are greater for pediatric pump operation, owing to the greater flow resistance with small-diameter cannulas and greater pump rates.[73]

Although initial outcomes were not as favorable in infants and children with congenital heart disease,[74] survival rates of 70% have now been reported for children younger than 1 year of age, even those requiring prolonged support. Improvements in survival have been attributed to the development of optimized

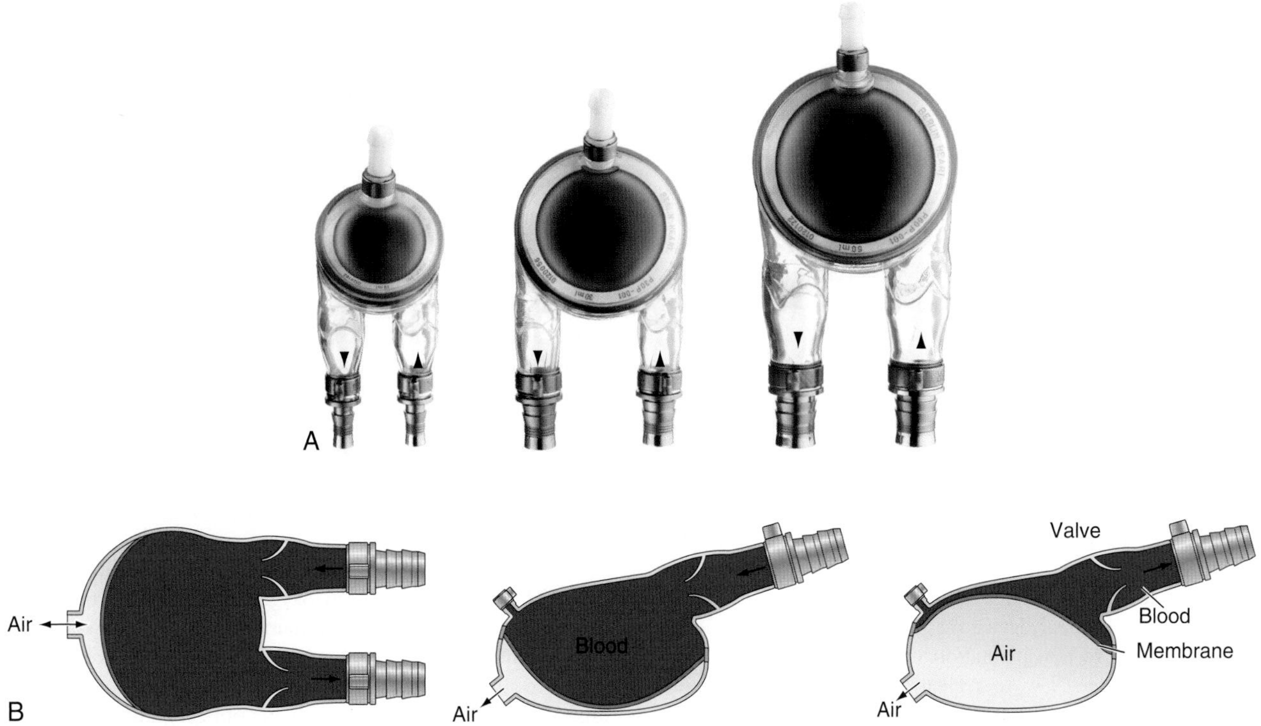

**FIGURE 19-5 A,** Berlin Heart Excor ventricular assist device in pediatric and adult sizes. **B,** A flexible diaphragm in three layers divides the pump chamber into an air chamber and a blood chamber. (From Hetzer R, Potapov E, Stiller B, et al. Improvement in survival after mechanical circulatory support with pneumatic pulsatile ventricular assist devices in pediatric patients. Ann Thorac Surg 2006;82:917-25.)

miniaturized apical cannulas, the addition of heparin-coated tubing allowing lower anticoagulation levels, the use of dipyridamole and aspirin after week 1 of support, and continued experience with surgical and intensive care management with use of TEGs and platelet function tests to guide the modification of anticoagulation.[61] In a single-center review of their Berlin Heart Excor experience, comparing the 1990-to-2001 experience with the current era (from 2002 onward), the percent of infants less than one year of age discharged to home after transplantation or weaning increased from 17% in the early era to 93% in the current era. The majority of children successfully weaned from support had a diagnosis of myocarditis, with no long-term complications after removal of the left ventricular cannula reported. Major causes of mortality in both eras were cerebrovascular accidents and multiorgan failure.[24]

Major benefits of Berlin Heart Excor support include the ability to extubate the trachea of children, encourage enteral nutrition, and optimize patient mobility during chronic support. In addition, the transfusion of blood products during MCS is less in children supported with the Berlin Heart Excor when compared with those supported with ECMO. In a study comparing 30 children receiving Berlin Heart Excor support to 34 children on ECMO support, transfusion requirements for platelets, red blood cells, and fresh frozen plasma were significantly less in Berlin Heart Excor patients. The overall mortality rate was also noted to be lower in Berlin Heart Excor patients.[75] Anticoagulation is currently initiated with unfractionated heparin, maintaining aPTT at 60 to 80 seconds. TEG is also used, along with platelet aggregation tests, to monitor the use of aspirin and dipyridamole. Antithrombin III concentrations are closely monitored and substituted if the concentrations fall below 70%.[72] Low-molecular-weight heparin (LMWH), with monitoring of anti–factor Xa concentrations, has been used since 2007.[24] Pump exchange may be necessary if thrombus formation occurs in the valves, although one group reported no complications from this procedure during 15 years of adult and pediatric experience.[76]

### Medos System
The Medos HIA-VAD was first used for children in 1997.[77] The Medos HIA-VAD is a pulsatile, paracorporeal pump available in several different sizes; it differs from Excor in that the left ventricular pumps offer 10% greater stroke volumes than the corresponding right ventricular pumps.[78] Survival has been reported to be 57% in children (ranging in age from less than 1 year to 16 years) awaiting cardiac transplantation.[79]

### Continuous Flow Pumps
Continuous flow pumps can be either axial or centrifugal, depending on the design of the impeller, and are designed to limit the interaction of moving parts. The MicroMed DeBakey VAD Child (MicroMed Cardiovascular, Inc., Houston) is an axial flow device currently available for use in the United States for children 5 to 16 years of age, through a US Food and Drug Administration (FDA) human device exemption. It was first introduced for use in March 2004, making it the first FDA-approved intracorporeal device for provision of left ventricular MCS as a bridge to transplantation in the pediatric population. Children must have New York Heart Association class IV end-stage heart failure that is refractory to medical management, be currently listed for cardiac transplantation, and have a BSA between 0.7 and 1.5 m$^2$ to be considered candidates for DeBakey VAD Child support. The MicroMed DeBakey VAD Child is placed via median sternotomy using CPB. A titanium inlet cannula is sutured into the apex of the left ventricle via a circular core ventriculotomy, and a 12-mm gel-weave outflow graft is then anastomosed to the ascending aorta.[80] A percutaneous cable containing the pump power and flow probe cables passes through the skin to the clinical data acquisition system. A separate unit, the "VADPAK," contains a pump controller and two 12-volt batteries in a carrying case that can allow 5 to 8 hours of patient mobility.[81]

The Thoratec HeartMate II (see Fig. 19-4, B) is an intracorporeal, axial flow device that has been approved by the FDA for use as bridge-to-transplant and destination therapy in adults. Although recommended for use in patients with a BSA greater than 1.5 m$^2$, its use has been reported in adolescents with a BSA as low as 1.3 m$^2$. The HeartMate II has a low thromboembolic risk compared to other devices, and anticoagulation is managed using vitamin K antagonism and antiplatelet therapy (aspirin and dipyridamole). The portable system controller is also small enough to wear on a belt, allowing unencumbered movement for several hours, and potentially even discharge home.[82] The VentrAssist (Ventracor Limited, Chatswood, Australia) was another small, implantable, continuous-flow device that had been successfully used in patients with a BSA as small as 1.1 m$^2$ for prolonged support, allowing both bridge to recovery and to transplantation.[83] Unfortunately this device is currently unavailable.

Like a centrifugal pump, axial pump function depends on the preload and afterload. Decreases in preload can cause emptying and collapse of the ventricle, whereas increases in afterload initially result in reductions in forward flow and ultimately can lead to regurgitant flow. Axial pumps offer several advantages over pulsatile pumps, including their small blood-to-device interface, the lack of a compliance chamber or artificial valves, and fewer moving parts. They are quieter than pulsatile pumps, which is a decided advantage for the child. Axial pumps can also allow some pulsatile flow to occur as the ventricle recovers, and cardiac output can increase in response to increased patient activity. The major disadvantages for children are the continuing size limitations for placement and the fact that the device provides only left ventricular support.

## OUTCOMES
According to the Healthcare Cost and Utilization Project Kids' Inpatient Database, 187 children underwent VAD implantation in 2006 in 67 different U.S. hospitals. High-volume large teaching hospitals reported significantly greater survival rates and reduced costs compared with other institutions.[3] Regardless of the type of MCS chosen, it has become increasingly clear that the indication for and timing of initiation of support are major factors in determining outcome. Universally, survival has been greater in children who required support secondary to acute myocarditis or dilated cardiomyopathy, as compared with children who received support due to congenital heart defects or postcardiotomy failure.[84]

When feasible, VADs offer several major advantages over ECMO. First, the lack of an oxygenator simplifies the circuit, lessening anticoagulation requirements, as well as trauma to blood elements. Second, ECMO-supported patients have been shown to suffer greater rates of neurologic impairment than those supported with VADs, particularly in younger children with more complex heart disease.[52] Additionally, evidence suggests that VAD support provides superior ventricular decompression and physiologic rest, promoting myocardial recovery in children with acute myocarditis or dilated cardiomyopathy by allowing normalization of ventricular geometry and reverse remodeling.[85-87] A pilot study in children suggests that even short-term LVAD support of 1 to 2 weeks can reverse molecular remodeling.[88]

Children with chronic heart failure awaiting transplantation who experience progressive multiorgan dysfunction have been shown to benefit from the use of pulsatile VADs with potential recovery of pulmonary, renal, and hepatic function.[89] A review of 55 pediatric patients revealed significantly increased survival rates in children who received Berlin Heart Excor support compared with those who received ECMO, despite a mean duration of support that was nearly three times as great in the Excor group.[90] A multiinstitutional study reviewing the outcomes of 99 children bridged to cardiac transplantation with MCS, compared them with 2276 children listed for transplantation during the same era who did not require MCS. Significant findings included a lack of difference in survival rates between VAD-supported and non–VAD-supported children, along with similar survival rates for children who required BiVAD support versus LVAD support. An increasing trend in the number of children undergoing transplantation who required pretransplantation VAD support was also observed, with an increase in the use of long-term MCS devices in the most recent era. Children with long-term devices were significantly more likely to survive to transplantation than those with short-term devices. Ten children were "double bridged" from ECMO to VAD support before transplantation, with nine then undergoing successful transplantation. Not surprisingly, smaller, younger patients and those with congenital heart disease had less successful outcomes.[91]

Use of MCS in single-ventricle patients presents special challenges, particularly in patients with cavopulmonary anastomoses; the reported use of VADs in these patients remains limited compared to ECMO.[47] Ventricular dysfunction in the failing Fontan may be addressed with VAD support of the systemic ventricle as long as pulmonary vascular resistance is not significantly increased.[92] Management of anticoagulation may also prove difficult in this population because of liver dysfunction and coagulation factor abnormalities.[93]

In children with a cardiac etiology for MCS, irrespective of the type of mechanical support employed, if significant improvement in myocardial function has not been observed within 48 to 72 hours of institution of support, the child should be evaluated for potential cardiac transplantation.[94] In the current era, earlier consideration for implementation of mechanical support with a staged approach, first using ECMO installation, with a transition to VAD therapy if necessary, has led to markedly improved survival rates.[24]

# Perioperative Management and Complications of Mechanical Circulatory Support

Successful management of critically ill children on MCS requires the expertise of many groups of practitioners. The Hospital for Sick Children, Toronto, Ontario, developed an Interprofessional VAD Support Team involved in clinical care, education, and family support for patients receiving Berlin Heart MCS. In addition to physicians (cardiac surgeons, cardiac intensivists, heart failure and transplant cardiologists, hematologists and psychiatrists) and nurses (cardiac and critical care), team members include pharmacists, respiratory therapists, dieticians, social workers, physiotherapists, biomedical engineers, and perfusionists.[95] Development of a team approach and use of interdisciplinary guidelines for care of these children can enhance communication, family support, and outcomes.[96]

## HEMODYNAMICS

During ECMO support, central venous pressure should remain low if adequate venous drainage is being achieved. Left atrial pressure should be closely monitored and can be estimated via echocardiographic evaluation of atrial septal position. An increase in left atrial pressure may indicate incomplete unloading of the left atrium and ventricle, potentially requiring a blade and/or balloon atrial septostomy[97] or surgical placement of a left atrial vent. Anatomic issues, such as the presence of aortopulmonary collateral vessels, aortic insufficiency, or a patent ductus arteriosus, can also result in a persistently increased left atrial pressure.

Increased arterial pressures and systemic vascular resistance during ECMO can be due to large pump flows, but other causes, such as unrecognized seizure activity, inadequate pain or sedation management, and hypothermia, should also be considered. High systemic vascular resistance during ECMO support can be pharmacologically managed. In general, mean arterial pressures should be maintained at a level appropriate to the child's size and body weight.

Unlike ECMO support, support of the left ventricle with a VAD requires maintenance of effective right ventricular output to provide adequate left ventricular preload. Right ventricular failure, pulmonary hypertension, and arrhythmias can all limit left ventricular filling and must, therefore, be aggressively treated.[98] Other potential causes of inadequate left ventricular filling include cannula malposition or low intravascular volume. Evaluation of central venous pressure can be used to evaluate volume status, and serial echocardiograms are useful for ongoing assessment of right ventricular function and estimation of right ventricular and pulmonary artery pressures. Clinical signs of right-sided heart failure include increased central venous or right atrial pressures, hepatomegaly, peripheral edema, and decreasing hemoglobin-oxygen saturations. Right ventricular function can be augmented pharmacologically with drugs such as milrinone or isoproterenol. Increased pulmonary artery pressures are best initially treated by ensuring adequate alveolar ventilation, and subsequently by using inhaled nitric oxide, if necessary. Mechanical issues, such as cardiac tamponade, can also negatively affect hemodynamics and can be diagnosed at the bedside with echocardiography. Inadequate left ventricular decompression can cause resultant increases in left atrial and pulmonary artery pressures and may be treated by augmenting LVAD flow; if necessary, biventricular support can be initiated or the child can be placed on ECMO support.[99]

Children on VAD support often require vasodilators to maintain the low systemic vascular resistance necessary for optimal pump function. Frequently used drugs include sodium nitroprusside, milrinone, hydralazine, β-blockers, angiotensin-converting enzyme inhibitors, and clonidine. Left atrial pressure is optimally maintained at 3 to 4 mm Hg, while allowing some ventricular ejection to avoid stasis. Measurement of systemic mixed venous hemoglobin-oxygen saturation, either continuously via in-line monitoring with a centrifugal VAD, or intermittently with a paracorporeal pulsatile VAD, is also useful to ensure that adequate cardiac output is being delivered.

## RESPIRATORY CONSIDERATIONS

Although ECMO can provide full cardiopulmonary support, the trachea should be intubated and the ventilation continued to avoid atelectasis and to optimize oxygenation of blood returning to the left atrium that will provide coronary artery blood flow. Modest ventilator settings are generally recommended: (1) 10 to 12 mL/kg tidal volume, (2) 5 to 10 cm $H_2O$ of positive end-expiratory pressure, (3) a rate of 10 to 12 breaths per minute, and (4) a fractional inspired oxygen value of 0.4 or less to avoid oxygen toxicity. Maintenance of adequate ventilation is particularly important in children with single-ventricle physiology with an open systemic-pulmonary shunt. Because of the complexity of the ECMO circuit, mechanical issues, such as oxygenator malfunction, must be considered when increasing hypoxemia occurs. After ruling out oxygenator failure, ECMO flow may be increased or the membrane size may be increased to improve systemic oxygenation.

Children on VADs receive only cardiac support. In the case of centrifugal VAD support, the trachea generally remains intubated and the lungs mechanically ventilated. Paracorporeal pulsatile VADs and implantable VADs, on the other hand, allow children to be weaned to extubation. Anatomic issues, such as an atrial septal defect, should be recognized as potential causes of hypoxemia due to right-to-left shunting.[100] Children who receive left ventricular support via either a centrifugal or pulsatile VAD may also require inhaled nitric oxide to decrease pulmonary vascular resistance and improve right ventricular function.

## HEMATOLOGIC CONSIDERATIONS

Managing the anticoagulation continues to be one of the most challenging clinical issues in caring for children who require MCS, because of the risk of hemorrhage and/or thromboembolic complications.[101] Ongoing hemorrhage around cannulation sites is frequent, particularly for those on ECMO. Of greater concern is hemorrhage in the gastrointestinal tract, the lungs, or, more devastatingly, intracranial hemorrhage; infarctions or thromboembolic events may also occur. Serial ultrasonography of the head may be used to monitor for intracranial bleeding in infants and neonates, and, when possible, computed tomography may be used in older children.

Although ECMO protocols vary at individual centers, ACTs are generally maintained between 180 and 200 seconds via use of a heparin infusion at 10 to 50 units/kg/hour. The use of heparin-bonded tubing can reduce the need for greater ACTs. The hematocrit is generally maintained between 40% and 50%, although efforts are made to limit transfusions, because most such children are potential candidates for cardiac transplantation. When necessary, leukocyte-reduced, cytomegalovirus-negative, irradiated red cells are administered. Platelet counts greater than $100,000/mm^3$ and fibrinogen concentrations greater than 100 mg/dL are maintained to minimize bleeding complications.[102] In the presence of continued bleeding, cryoprecipitate and/or fresh frozen plasma may be added to the circuit prime and TEG may be helpful in assisting with appropriate use of blood products. In cases of persistent hemorrhage refractory to blood component administration, recombinant activated factor VII has been shown to significantly decrease bleeding and aid in normalizing the TEG profile,[103-105] although disastrous clotting of circuitry has also been reported with its use.[106] Hemolysis may be monitored by measurement of plasma-free hemoglobin, with increasing concentrations potentially representing the development of thrombus in the circuit.

Without an oxygenator in the circuit, anticoagulation requirements are not as stringent for children on VADs, and their ACTs may be maintained between 140 and 180 seconds. After placement of a Berlin Heart Excor, unfractionated heparin infusions are initially used with a target aPTT of 60 to 70 seconds. The use of argatroban has been described in children with heparin-induced thrombocytopenia type II.[107] Longer term anticoagulation includes the use of LMWH with anti–factor Xa activity monitoring.[108,109] After normalization of the platelet count and function, aspirin and dipyridamole are started, with monitoring via TEG and platelet aggregation tests, with a target activation of 30%. Once a child is tolerating enteral feedings, a transition to warfarin may occur. Although embolic and bleeding complications remain problematic, with this management strategy a marked increase in survival has been noted in children undergoing Berlin Heart Excor support compared to earlier regimens.[110]

Although hemolysis and thrombosis may be less frequent with continuous flow devices, the frequent development of acquired von Willebrand syndrome has been described in adult patients, most likely occurring secondary to the shear stress of the pump, with unfolding and cleavage of the high-molecular-weight multimers of von Willebrand factor. This is also thought to account for the increased incidence of gastrointestinal bleeding noted in these patients, though not all patients with documented acquired von Willebrand syndrome display increased bleeding tendencies.[111,112]

## PREVENTION OF INFECTION

Infection is a constant concern, particularly in children requiring intermediate- to long-term VAD support. Devices with larger surface area and areas of turbulent flow have been correlated with greater infection rates due to increased adherence of blood-borne pathogens; therefore, smaller, fully implantable devices and devices with improved flow dynamics may continue to facilitate decreases in the incidence of infection.[113,114] Devices, such as the Berlin Heart Excor, that facilitate removal of tracheal tubes, indwelling catheters and intravenous lines, and minimize the need for blood transfusions, also offer advantages in minimizing the risk of device-related infections.[75,115] Deep wound complications of inflow and outflow cannulas have been successfully treated with vacuum-assisted wound closure systems.[116]

The use of mechanical support devices can result in immunologic dysfunction, further increasing infection risk.[117] Signs and symptoms of infection can be subtle, and a need for increasing inotropic support to maintain mean arterial pressure can often be a harbinger of infection. Endogenous reactions to infection can also result in activation of the coagulation cascade, increasing the difficulty of anticoagulation management.[118] Many children prophylactically receive antibiotics with gram-positive coverage, as well as oral nystatin for fungal prophylaxis.

## ANESTHETIC CONSIDERATIONS

In preparing for the anesthetic care of infants and children, when ECMO or VAD support is being used or when implementation of MCS is imminent, initial planning centers on two main areas of concern: the child's current status and the location of the proposed procedure (Table 19-4). The need for emergency surgery, the child's condition at the time of surgery, the presence of preoperative multiorgan failure, and the need for CPB with cross-clamping of the aorta have all been shown to increase perioperative risk.[119]

**TABLE 19-4** Anesthetic Considerations

**Preoperative Assessment**

*History*

Etiology and duration of cardiac failure
End-organ dysfunction
Pulmonary
Renal
Hepatic
Neurologic
Medications
Inotropic/vasoactive support
Angiotensin-converting enzyme inhibitors
Antiarrhythmic therapy
Anticoagulation protocols
Sedative drugs
Antibiotics
Planned surgical procedure
Timing of procedure: elective/urgent/emergent

*Laboratory*

Complete blood cell count
Electrolytes
Liver function studies
Blood urea nitrogen, creatinine
Coagulation studies
Platelet count
Prothrombin time/partial thromboplastin time
Fibrinogen concentration
Activated clotting time
Thromboelastogram
B-type natriuretic peptide concentration

*Physical examination*

Airway
Vascular access, both existing and available
Neurologic status
Evidence of ongoing hemorrhage
Assessment of intravascular volume status

**Intraoperative Management**

*Availability of blood products*
*Monitoring*

Standard monitors: electrocardiogram, noninvasive blood pressure, end-tidal $CO_2$, temperature, peripheral oxygen saturation
Assess need for invasive monitoring, arterial or central venous
Urine output

*Transesophageal echocardiography*

Presence of septal defects
Aortic insufficiency
Mitral stenosis
Cardiac de-airing
Ventricular function

*Management principles*

Avoid abrupt decreases in preload
Support right ventricular function, reduce pulmonary vascular resistance
Adequate ventilation
Inotropic support: milrinone, prostaglandin $E_1$
Nitric oxide availability
Maintain adequate intravascular volume/preload for ventricular assist device
Hypotension can be treated with volume or α-adrenergic agonists

**Postoperative Issues**

Transport to intensive care unit
Control of ongoing hemorrhage
Timing of extubation

A comprehensive preoperative evaluation of the child is essential, with knowledge of the underlying etiology necessitating MCS and the length of the child's illness, along with evaluation of other potential multiorgan dysfunction, including neurologic, hematologic, renal, hepatic, and pulmonary issues. Review of current drug therapy, particularly the duration and degree of current inotropic support, anticoagulation protocols, sedation regimens, cardiac function, intravascular volume status, and the presence and degree of preoperative hemorrhage, is also necessary. Physical examination should encompass the airway and both current vascular access, as well as the availability of sites for potential vascular access.

Preoperative laboratory evaluation should include CBC with platelet count, electrolytes, blood urea nitrogen and creatinine concentrations, PT and partial thromboplastin time, and liver function tests. Concentrations of BNP, produced in the myocardium, serve as a marker of ventricular overloading and have been shown in adult and pediatric patients with congenital heart disease to correlate with the degree of ventricular dysfunction.[120,121] Serial BNP concentrations in pediatric patients supported with ECMO have also been used to predict clinical outcomes, with greater BNP concentrations noted after termination of ECMO support in nonsurvivors than in children who ultimately survived.[122]

Useful preoperative coagulation data includes recent TEG results, fibrinogen concentrations, and platelet function tests, if available. The most recent echocardiography data and chest radiograph should be reviewed. Blood products, including PRBCs, platelets, cryoprecipitate, and fresh frozen plasma, should be available at the bedside or in the operating room, with provision for continuing supply of products as needed. Appropriate antibiotic prophylaxis should be discussed with the surgeon.

Standard American Society of Anesthesiologists monitoring should be employed before induction of anesthesia. Depending on the child's condition and the type of surgery planned, use of arterial and central venous lines should be considered. In children who have been in the intensive care unit for a prolonged time, or those undergoing current resuscitation, the placement of additional vascular access lines can be quite challenging and may occasionally require surgical assistance. For children already on a mechanical support device, it is important to be aware that VAD ejection is usually asynchronous with the child's underlying heart rate, yielding a discrepancy between the observed electrocardiographic and the arterial line waveform. Multiple peripheral intravenous lines are useful for the administration of volume and blood products. If right VAD support is in place special care must be taken not to entrain air if the great veins are accessed.

For patients undergoing placement of a VAD, etomidate is generally an advantageous drug for induction of anesthesia because it does not result in myocardial depression at clinically relevant concentrations, even in children with severely compromised ventricular function.[123] Judicious doses of opioids and benzodiazepines may be added, while the choice of a neuromuscular blocking agent is often determined by the presence of compromised hepatic or renal function. Adequate depth of anesthesia should be ensured before tracheal intubation, to avoid abrupt increases in pulmonary vascular resistance, particularly in children with marginal right ventricular function. In children undergoing device placement, induction drugs should be given incrementally, because the onset time may be abnormally slow owing to depressed ventricular function. Children may exhibit decreased responsiveness to β-adrenergic agonists due to depletion of myocardial catecholamines.[124] Hypotension on induction of anesthesia and decreased responsiveness to catecholamines may also be observed in children who have been chronically receiving angiotensin-converting–enzyme inhibitors for afterload reduction preoperatively.[125-127] Opioids, benzodiazepines, and neuromuscular blocking agents are generally used for anesthetic maintenance before ECMO cannulation or initiation of CPB for VAD implementation, with the express goal of maintaining adequate cardiac output and resultant systemic perfusion to end organs. Trends in serum lactate concentrations, mixed venous hemoglobin-oxygen saturations, and the presence or absence of metabolic acidosis are useful indices for evaluating the adequacy of cardiac output.

Unless contraindicated by patient size or the presence of gastrointestinal bleeding, a transesophageal echocardiographic (TEE) probe should be placed after the induction of anesthesia, for use throughout the procedure. Initial TEE examination is important for determining the presence of any intracardiac shunts that would require closing before initiation of MCS. The competence of the aortic valve should also be evaluated, because more than trivial insufficiency can result in recirculation of blood through an LVAD. The mitral valve should also be examined for significant stenosis that could limit left ventricular inflow. After device placement, TEE helps in ensuring that adequate cardiac de-airing has occurred, as well as in ongoing evaluation of ventricular function. TEE is also useful after device placement for monitoring the orientation of intracardiac cannulas and decompression of the left atrium and ventricle after pump activation.

For children undergoing placement of an LVAD, as the venous line from the CPB circuit is occluded, the pump speed will be gradually increased. If LVAD flow (and rate when fill-to-empty mode is used) is less than desired, the major areas of concern are hypovolemia or poor right ventricular function. The right ventricle should be monitored closely for signs of dysfunction or failure. In children with preexisting right ventricular dysfunction, pulmonary vasodilatory agents, such as milrinone, prostaglandin $E_1$, or nitric oxide, should be aggressively used to optimize right-sided heart function. Children with low pressures and signs of vasodilatory shock may require infusions of vasopressin, epinephrine, or norepinephrine for circulatory support. In addition, adequate volume loading and VAD output should be ensured.

Tracheal extubation is not an option for those undergoing ECMO or centrifugal VAD support, but children receiving pulsatile VADs or axial pumps may be considered candidates for extubation. Timing of extubation will depend on the child's preoperative condition, degree of preexisting pulmonary dysfunction, duration of the surgical procedure, extent of postoperative bleeding, and maintenance of appropriate hemodynamic parameters.

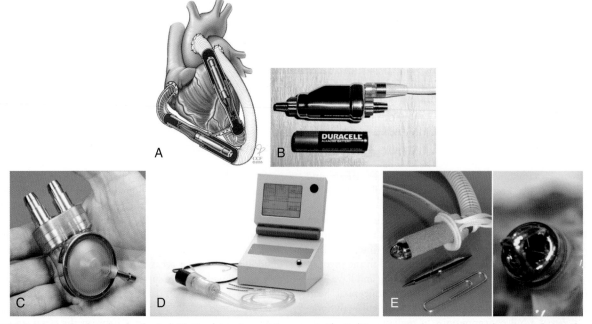

**FIGURE 19-6** Devices developed under the Pediatric Circulatory Support Program. **A,** The PediPump ventricular assist device showing application for biventricular support. **B,** PediaFlow ventricular assist system. **C,** Penn State infant pediatric ventricular assist device. **D,** Ension's Pediatric Cardiopulmonary Assist System with prototype controller console. **E,** Infant-size pediatric Jarvik 2000 showing thrombus-free bearings after 5 weeks in a lamb animal model. (From Baldwin J, Borovetz H, Duncan B, et al. The National Heart, Lung, and Blood Institute Pediatric Circulatory Support Program: a summary of the 5-year experience. Circulation 2011;123:1233-40.)

Not surprisingly, with the steadily increasing use of VAD support in infants and children, a growing demand for anesthesia for noncardiac surgeries during the period of support has also occurred. Transport and care of these children often requires the assistance of respiratory therapists and the availability of a pump specialist. Temporary conversion from warfarin or LMWH to unfractionated heparin infusion should be discussed with the team caring for the patient, including the hematologist, before surgery, and appropriate blood products should be ordered. For children on VAD support, appropriate pump function will continue independently of the induction drugs used, as long as adequate preload is maintained and no acute decrease in systemic vascular resistance occurs. In a series of children with in situ Berlin Heart Excor support undergoing noncardiac surgeries, anesthetic induction with ketamine was found to be less likely to induce hypotension requiring treatment with fluid bolus or α-adrenergic agonists.[128] Inspection of the pump chamber for wrinkling of the membrane assists in deciding whether the use of a fluid bolus or an α-adrenergic agonist is more appropriate. In children who are only on LVAD support, care should be taken to avoid increases in pulmonary vascular resistance, as the likeliest cause of decompensation in such patients is right ventricular failure. Nitric oxide and appropriate vasoactive drugs should be readily available for use if needed. When possible, the use of spontaneous ventilation is thought to improve venous return and hemodynamic stability.[57,129]

## Future Directions

The Pediatric Circulatory Support Program (PCSP) of the NHLBI was established to foster development of circulatory support devices suitable for children from 2 to 25 kg. Five contracts were awarded in early 2004 and concluded in 2009, with devices under development including a next-generation ECMO system (Pediatric Cardiopulmonary Assist System, Ension, Inc., Pittsburgh), an implantable VAD (PediPump, The Cleveland Clinic Foundation, Cleveland), an intraventricular pump (Pediatric Jarvik 2000, Jarvik Heart Inc., New York), a pulsatile VAD (Pediatric Ventricular Assist Device, The Pennsylvania State University, Hershey, Pa.), and a miniaturized blood pump (PediaFlow VAD, University of Pittsburgh) (Fig. 19-6). In 2008 the NHLBI requested proposals for the Pumps for Kids, Infants, and Neonates (PumpKIN) program, with three of the five contractors from the NHLBI PCSP program receiving program awards in January 2010. Clinical trials are anticipated to begin in 2013.[130]

## ANNOTATED REFERENCES

Adachi I, Fraser C. Mechanical circulatory support for infants and small children. Semin Thorac Cardiovasc Surg Pediatr Card Surg Annu 2011;14:38-44.

*This is a review article summarizing currently available devices for support of children with acute heart failure.*

Almond C, Singh T, Gauvreau K, et al. Extracorporeal membrane oxygenation for bridge to heart transplantation among children in the United States: analysis of data from the Organ Procurement and Transplant Network and Extracorporeal Life Support Organization Registry. Circulation 2011;123:2975-84.

*The authors review data from two major databases, evaluating outcomes of children undergoing ECMO as a bridge to heart transplantation in the United States between 1994 and 2009.*

Baldwin J, Borovetz H, Duncan B, et al. The National Heart, Lung, and Blood Institute Pediatric Circulatory Support Program: a summary of the 5-year experience. Circulation 2011;123:1233-40.

*This paper presents a summary of the progress made and devices under development in the United States from the Pediatric Circulatory Support Program.*

Barrett C, Bratton S, Salvin J, et al. Neurological injury after extracorporeal membrane oxygenation use to aid pediatric cardiopulmonary resuscitation. Pediatr Crit Care Med 2009;10:445-51.

*This is a retrospective cohort study of data from the Extracorporeal Life Support Organization registry, evaluating neurologic injury in children undergoing ECPR.*

Blume E, Naftel D, Bastardi H, et al. Outcomes of children bridged to heart transplantation with ventricular assist devices: a multi-institutional study. Circulation 2006;113:2313-9.

*This paper presents a multi-institutional review of children undergoing heart transplantation, evaluating outcomes in those who required VAD support as bridge to transplantation.*

Hetzer R, Potapov E, Alexi-Meskishvili V, et al. Single-center experience with treatment of cardiogenic shock in children by pediatric ventricular assist devices. J Thorac Cardiovasc Surg 2011;141:616-23.

*The authors offer a review of management strategies and outcomes in 94 patients with Berlin Heart EXCOR support, between 1990 and 2009.*

Jefferies J, Price J, Morales D. Mechanical support in childhood heart failure. Heart Fail Clin 2010;6:559-73.

*This is a comprehensive review of indications for MCS and currently available devices for children of all ages.*

Mossad E, Motta P, Rossano J, et al. Perioperative management of pediatric patients on mechanical cardiac support. Paediatr Anaesth 2011; 21:585-93.

*The authors review the demographics of children requiring MCS and perioperative management concepts for their care.*

## REFERENCES

Please see www.expertconsult.com.

# Interventional Cardiology

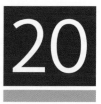

GEOFFREY K. LANE AND ADAM SKINNER

THE USE OF CATHETERIZATION in the care of children with congenital heart disease (CHD) was first described by Dexter and colleagues in 1947.[1] It has evolved from a physiologic assessment tool to a technique to define anatomic relationships and has become a therapeutic modality. The first interventional procedure, balloon atrial septostomy, was described by Rashkind and Miller in 1966,[2] and since then, the discipline of interventional cardiology has continued to evolve.

As echocardiography and magnetic resonance imaging (MRI) diagnostic capabilities have increased, the need for purely diagnostic cardiac catheterization has declined.[3,4] However, technologic advances and more sophisticated equipment have increased the scope for interventional procedures, and the patient population has changed as more children with CHD are surviving longer. As the surgical management of CHD has evolved, it has introduced a new spectrum of surgical complications. Some surgical operations have been replaced altogether by interventional procedures, and some interventional procedures have facilitated more complex heart surgery.[5] The shifts in practice and population have affected the anesthetic management of these children.[6] Procedures are more diverse, and patients can vary from moribund neonates to healthy adolescents. There are no simple anesthesia recipes for all children and all heart conditions; the type of anesthesia must fit each child and each procedure.

In this chapter, we outline the main procedures performed in interventional cardiology, describe the potential issues and complications faced by anesthesiologists, and address the principles and details of anesthetic techniques.

## Types of Procedures Performed

### DIAGNOSTIC CATHETERIZATION

Diagnostic catheterization allows accurate documentation of pressure and oxygen content from all regions of the circulation. Interpretation of these hemodynamic data allows quantification of the degree of intracardiac shunting and calculation of the vascular bed resistances. This information is necessary to assess the suitability of a child to undergo palliative or reparative surgery for congenital heart lesions. Expected values for hemodynamic variables are listed in Table 20-1. There are no absolute values for these variables, and they vary according to the age of the child. The use of angiocardiography to define anatomy is waning because of the widespread use of noninvasive imaging modalities such as echocardiography, computed tomography, and MRI.

### INTERVENTIONAL CATHETERIZATION

At many centers, interventional catheterization accounts for more than 60% of cardiac catheterization cases.

#### Atrial Septostomy

Atrial septostomy improves mixing of oxygenated and deoxygenated blood at the atrial level in neonates with D-transposition of the great vessels. Children with this disorder are born with ventriculoarterial discordance. The right ventricle pumps deoxygenated blood to the aorta, and the left ventricle pumps oxygenated blood to the main pulmonary artery. Enlargement of the foramen ovale by atrial septostomy improves mixing of oxygenated and deoxygenated blood, resulting in increased systemic oxygen saturation. This procedure can be performed in the catheterization laboratory with fluoroscopic guidance, or it can be easily and safely undertaken at the bedside in the intensive care unit using echocardiographic guidance.[7] A femoral venous or umbilical venous approach can be used. The drawback with the umbilical venous route is the often-encountered difficulty in traversing the ductus venosus to secure access to the inferior vena cava. The major risks with this procedure are vessel injury, paradoxical embolism, arrhythmia, and cardiac perforation.

### Atrial Septal Defect Closure

With the development of specifically designed closure devices, atrial septal defect (ASD) closure has become one of the most commonly performed endovascular procedures. The technique is intended for closing secundum ASDs, which are defects located in the region of the fossa ovalis. Defects falling outside this area, such as sinus venosus and primum ASDs, are not suitable for percutaneous closure.

To warrant closure, children need to demonstrate clear evidence of volume loading of the right heart structures and a defect that is unlikely to close spontaneously in the short to medium term. The choice of closure device depends on the size and the margins of the defect. The two types of closure devices have either a centering or a noncentering design (Fig. 20-1). The choice of one design over another is based more on the clinician's preference than scientific performance, although the Amplatzer Septal Occluder (AGA Medical Corporation, Golden Valley, Minn.) can close a wider range of defect sizes.[8-10] Daily aspirin in

a dose of 3 to 5 mg/kg is recommended for a minimum 6 months after implantation of either type of device. The main complications associated with ASD closure include vessel injury, cardiac arrhythmia, cardiac perforation, and device embolization.[11] Atrial septal closure devices have also been used to close surgically created fenestrations between the atrium and venous conduits after a Fontan operation. This is undertaken only when the fenestration is no longer required.

### Ventricular Septal Defect Closure

Ventricular septal defect (VSD) closure presents a technically greater challenge than ASD closure and is associated with a greater risk. The VSDs most suitable for device closure are those in the midmuscular septum or those closer to the apex.[12] With further refinement of the implantation technique and equipment, this approach has been undertaken with perimembranous defects.[13,14]

During device closure of VSDs, a snare is placed in the right side of the heart to capture a guidewire that has been passed across the VSD from the left ventricle. The guidewire is brought outside the body to form an arteriovenous rail. The delivery sheath for the VSD device is then advanced over the wire to approach the VSD from the right side of the heart. For anterior and high muscular defects, the wire is best snared and exteriorized through a femoral vein approach, whereas for defects in the middle to low muscular septum, the wire is best snared and exteriorized through a jugular venous approach (Fig. 20-2). Complications include dysrhythmias, blood loss, valve dysfunction, and device embolization.[15,16] At our institution,[17] device closure of perimembranous VSDs with the Amplatzer Membranous VSD Occluder had an unacceptable incidence of complete heart block and is therefore not currently performed. However, other medical units have continued to undertake this intervention, and alternative devices are being developed with the goal of implantation that does not cause complete heart block.

### Patent Ductus Arteriosus Closure

Closure of patent ductus arteriosus (PDA) was the second specific intervention developed for children with CHD, and it continues to be a common procedure performed using techniques that are similar to the original methods pioneered by Rashkind and

| TABLE 20-1 Normal Values in Diagnostic Cardiac Catheterization | |
|---|---|
| Structure | Value (mm Hg) |
| Right atrium | 3-5 (mean) |
| Right ventricle | 20-25/3-5 (systolic/end-diastolic) |
| Pulmonary artery | 12-15 (mean) |
| Left atrium | 7-10 (mean) |
| Left ventricle | 65-110/3-5 (systolic/end-diastolic) |
| Aorta | 65-110/35-65 (systolic/diastolic) |

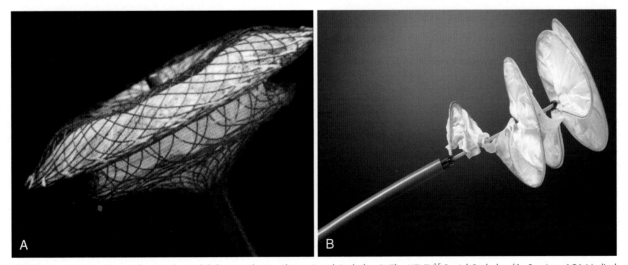

**FIGURE 20-1** Devices for closure of an atrial septal defect. **A,** The Amplatzer Septal Occluder. **B,** The HELEX[1.5] Septal Occluder. (**A,** Courtesy AGA Medical Corporation, Golden Valley, Minn. **B,** Courtesy W.L. Gore & Associates, Flagstaff, Ariz.).

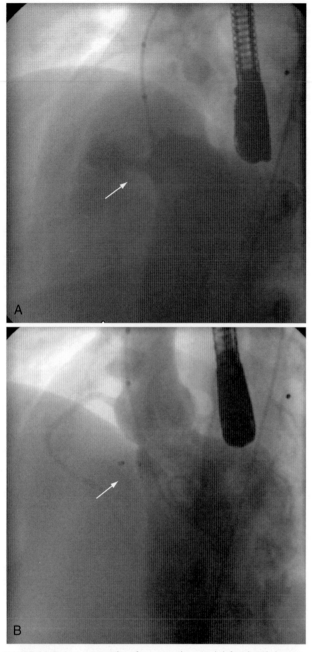

FIGURE 20-2 **A,** Angiography of a ventricular septal defect (VSD) device before deployment. Contrast agent passes through the perimembranous VSD (*arrow*). **B,** Appearance of same region (*arrow*) after deployment of the device.

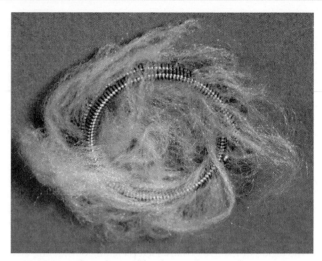

FIGURE 20-3 The coil is used for closure of a patent ductus arteriosus.

associates.[18] The customary approach is to perform an aortogram to define the size and geometry of the PDA. Based on this information, a choice is made between using a stainless steel coil or an occluder device.[19] Most interventional cardiologists implant a stainless steel coil to close a small PDA (no greater than 3 mm) using a retrograde or antegrade approach.[20] To lessen the chance of coil embolization during implantation, several techniques can control release of the coils.[21-23] For the larger PDA, most interventional cardiologists implant an occluder device because it lessens the risk of a significant residual shunt. The major risks associated with this procedure are vessel injury and device or coil embolization. Coils are also used to close major aortopulmonary collateral vessels (Figs. 20-3 and 20-4).

## Balloon Dilation and Stent Implantation

Balloon angioplasty techniques are used to dilate stenotic aortic, mitral, tricuspid, and pulmonary valves and stenotic segments of the aorta or of the pulmonary arteries. In neonates, membranous atresia of the pulmonary valve may be crossed with the stiff end of a guidewire[24] or with radiofrequency catheters.[25] After both techniques, the valve is dilated with a balloon that is approximately 120% the size of the annulus. Balloon angioplasty of stenotic pulmonary valves in children beyond infancy is often a curative procedure, whereas balloon valvuloplasty of critical pulmonary stenosis in the neonate often requires intervention again in later infancy. The potential hemodynamic behavior of the child depends on the nature of the lesion. A neonate with duct-dependent critical stenosis and little antegrade flow can tolerate balloon dilation well because there is little disruption of the cardiac output, whereas neonates and infants with less critical stenosis can suffer significant reductions in cardiac output when the balloon is inflated, especially if the ductus arteriosus is not patent. Older children tend to tolerate balloon valvuloplasty surprisingly well,[26] and life-threatening hypotension is uncommon.[27]

In contrast to pulmonary balloon valvuloplasty, aortic balloon valvuloplasty is usually only a palliative procedure, with most children eventually requiring surgery. Balloon dilation of aortic stenosis in the neonate is a high-risk procedure. These infants often present in a low cardiac output state requiring ventilation, inotropic support, and prostaglandin $E_1$ ($PGE_1$) infusion to maintain ductal patency. Catheterization can be complicated by arrhythmias (including asystole), the development of significant aortic regurgitation (which may require surgical intervention), and sudden death due to acute coronary ischemia.[26] The complication rate in older children is less than in younger children, and transient hypotension, bradycardia, and left bundle branch block are commonly reported.

Stents are sometimes implanted across focal areas of persistent stenosis in the systemic and pulmonary circulations. The technique of stent implantation requires great precision in positioning the stent, and the cardiac interventionalist needs to take into account the inevitable shortening that occurs with stent implantation when selecting a device for a particular lesion. The major complication encountered with stent implantation, in addition to those of balloon angioplasty, is stent malposition with the

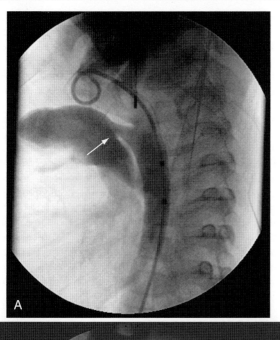

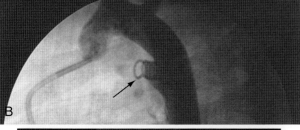

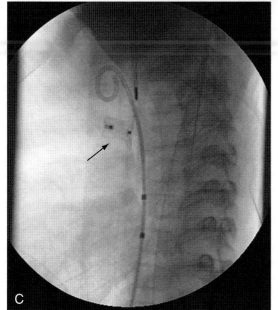

**FIGURE 20-4 A,** Lateral angiography demonstrates a patent ductus arteriosus (PDA) (*arrow*). The PDA lies between aorta and pulmonary artery (*arrow*). The angiography catheter is in the proximal aorta. **B,** Lateral angiography after closure of the PDA with a coil (*arrow*). **C,** Lateral fluoroscopy after closure of the PDA with the Amplatz Duct Occlude device. The device (*arrow*) is in the PDA.

potential for dislodgement. Rarely, late aneurysm formation has been reported after stenting the aorta for coarctation.

### Nonsurgical Pulmonary Valve Replacement

It is more than a decade since Bonhoeffer and colleagues[28] first described the technique of replacing a dysfunctional valve in a right ventricle to pulmonary artery conduit with a catheter-implanted valve. The technology used has matured, and the Melody Valve (Medtronic Inc, Minneapolis, Minn.) is available for use in Europe and is undergoing clinical trials in the United States. The Edwards Sapien Transcatheter Heart Valve (Edwards Lifesciences LLC, Irvine, Calif.) has also been used but is currently not licensed for this indication. Other results[29] have confirmed a high procedural success rate and satisfactory short-term valve function with implantation of the Melody Valve. The need for careful patient selection and for adequate relief of right ventricular outflow tract obstruction at the time of valve implantation are paramount in achieving results comparable to those of surgical replacement of dysfunctional conduits. Unfortunately, most children after tetralogy of Fallot repair with a transannular patch are currently unsuitable for implantation of a stented valve because of an aneurysmal right ventricular outflow tract.

Alternative devices are being sought to overcome these problems and to reduce the size of the delivery systems to enable use of these technologies in younger and smaller children. A novel use of Melody devices in an animal model that replicates the clinical situation of an aneurysmal right ventricular outflow tract has been reported.[30] Implantation of Melody Valves in branch pulmonary arteries appears to favorably reduce the regurgitant fraction in this animal model.

### ELECTROPHYSIOLOGIC CATHETERIZATION

Endocardial catheters that record an electrocardiogram first became available in the early 1960s. Endovascular techniques were developed as an alternative to surgery for certain forms of tachycardia. These therapies initially used direct current energy and subsequently have made use of radiofrequency energy and localized freezing techniques. Tachycardia may be treated by this technique in children with structurally normal hearts and those who have dysrhythmias after surgery for CHD.[26] Ablative procedures account for about 20% of all cardiac catheterization procedures.

The technique requires specialized equipment, specially trained staff, and use of multiple catheters to measure the electrical signals within the heart at any given time. These procedures are often more time consuming than other catheterization procedures. The success of the therapy depends on the mechanism of the tachycardia, the location of the aberrant pathway, and the technique for interrupting the aberrant pathway. Ablation of ectopic foci has a good success rate and small complication rate.[31,32] The main risks with this procedure are heart block, cardiac perforation, vessel injury, and stroke.

### CHOICE OF VESSEL ACCESS

The most common approach for cardiac catheterization is the femoral route. Femoral venous catheterization avoids the risk of pneumothorax, and the vein is easier to access than the internal jugular vein in the unanesthetized child. In children who are likely to have a cavopulmonary shunt placed surgically for palliation, avoiding routine cannulation of the internal jugular vein can decrease the risk of compromising the superior vena cava. However, internal jugular vein access sometimes is required, such as during VSD closures, investigation of cavo-pulmonary connections in children, and when the cardiac interventionalist is unable to obtain access through the femoral veins. In neonates, the umbilical vein may be used, although it can sometimes be difficult to cross the ductus venosus. Patency of the ductus venosus can be assessed by ultrasound before the procedure to avoid unnecessary manipulation of the umbilical vein. An alternative is transhepatic puncture. This route has been used for temporary access during catheterization and for long-term vascular access.[33]

# Complications and Limitations of Procedures

Interventional cardiology can be associated with significant morbidity and mortality. Complications attributable to the procedure or the physiology of the child occur far more frequently than purely anesthesia-related problems. An important prerequisite for providing quality anesthesia care is understanding the diagnosis and management of anticipated complications. Complications such as tamponade, dysrhythmia, embolism, and rupture may occur suddenly and without warning. The anesthesiologist must be vigilant and maintain communication and rapport with the cardiologist throughout the procedure. The availability of backup from surgeons, cardiologists, and anesthesiologists is preferable, and standard procedures for emergencies should be in place. Some clinicians advocate the availability of cardiopulmonary bypass or extracorporeal membrane oxygenation (ECMO) for children with unanticipated difficulties.[16] Although this type of therapy is available in major referral hospitals, it may not be an option in some centers. Institutions must develop policies regarding the procedures that can be undertaken locally (based on experience and infrastructure) and those that require referral of children to centers that are better equipped to address more complex procedures.

## OVERALL MORTALITY
Despite the increased complexity of interventional procedures, the mortality rate is steadily decreasing. A report from the early 1960s found an overall mortality rate (neonates through to adulthood) of 0.44%,[34] but more recent data show overall mortality rates of 0.08%,[35] 0.14%,[36,35] and 0.39%.[27] All reviews describe a relatively high mortality rate among infants and neonates in particular.[27,36,37] Explanations include a reduced physiologic reserve, presence of uncorrected or partially palliated congenital heart defects, increased risk of obstruction to great vessels and cardiac chambers, and greater susceptibility to catheter-induced damage in infancy.[27] However, neonatal mortality rates are diminishing; one institution reported a decrease from 6.7% to 0.9% during a span of 20 years.[36] The explanations cited for this decrease were noninvasive imaging that reduced the number of neonates who required cardiac catheterization, improved management of the critically ill child, correction of metabolic abnormalities, use of $PGE_1$, and use of improved catheters and better support equipment such as temperature control.[36]

## OVERALL MORBIDITY
Complications are frequently categorized as major, minor, and incidental.[27,37] Major complications are potentially life-threatening events that require surgical intervention or are significant permanent lesions resulting from the procedure (e.g., cerebral infarct).

Minor complications are transient and resolve with specific treatment (e.g., transient arterial thrombosis, temporary loss of a pulse or decreased perfusion after arterial puncture). An incidental complication has no effect on the patient's condition and requires minimal or no treatment (e.g., transient hypotension responding to volume infusion, catheter-induced arrhythmia). The incidence of major complications is between 1.4%[37] and 2.6%,[38] and the incidence of minor complications is between 6.8%[37] and 7.5%.[38] The overall complication rate has remained stable for the past 20 years.[38]

Three groups of children are at substantial risk for complications: those who are young, those with low weight, and those undergoing interventional rather than diagnostic procedures; balloon interventions are associated with the greatest risk.[36-38] The incidence of vascular access complications after interventional procedures is three times greater than the rate for diagnostic procedures[36]; this may reflect the use of larger-diameter catheters during interventional procedures than during purely diagnostic procedures. Closure of a PDA and balloon atrial septostomy carries a small overall risk.[27,36]

## VASCULAR COMPLICATIONS
Vascular complications are the most common and broadest category of complications.[36] They may be acute, leading to unexpected hemodynamic instability, or delayed, leading to longer-term morbidity. Many factors contribute to unexpected hemodynamic instability, including the child's condition, blood loss, dysfunction of a valve, arrhythmias, tamponade, vessel rupture, balloon dilation, catheter-induced interruptions in blood flow or coronary perfusion, and device malposition.

### Arterial Thrombosis and Occlusion
Femoral artery occlusion due to thrombosis is a common complication after femoral cannulation.[36] The true incidence of arterial compromise is unknown,[39] although 32% of infants had compromised blood flow to the leg as measured by Doppler after femoral arterial cannulation in one study.[40] The clinical incidence of arterial compromise is 2.4% to 3.7%.[36,37] Infants undergoing dilational interventional procedures are at a greater risk.[41] The incidence of these complications can be reduced by minimizing the size of the sheath, use of systemic heparinization, and avoidance of arterial entry by using alternative techniques to enter the left side of the heart.[36] Despite the widespread use of intravenous heparin for prophylaxis against arterial occlusion, there is no agreement on the appropriate dosage. Commonly, 50 to 100 IU/kg heparin is used, but schedules vary.[26] Larger doses than these do not reduce the incidence of arterial compromise.[39]

In most cases where the pulse is reduced or absent after catheterization, the occlusion either spontaneously resolves or is managed with anticoagulation or thrombolytic therapy.[36,37,41] Guidelines are available for the management and prevention of femoral artery thrombosis, but advice should be sought from a pediatric hematologist.[42] Although surgical intervention is rarely required, it is most commonly indicated for an arterial tear or avulsion, arterial thrombosis (including iliac arteries), and arterial pseudoaneurysm.[41] Occasionally, despite medical therapy and a well-perfused lower limb, a pulse may be persistently reduced. There is little evidence to predict how and when a reduced pulse may cause delay in limb growth,[36] although cases have been reported.[41] Although femoral cannulation for balloon intervention is associated with vascular compromise of the superficial femoral artery, one small study (43 children between 1 day and

15 years of age) failed to demonstrate significant limb growth discrepancy after a median follow-up of 3.5 years.[43]

## Venous Thrombosis and Occlusion

Although venous thrombosis is a well-known complication of central venous access, the incidence after cardiac catheterization is unclear. Isolated cases of femoral or iliofemoral venous occlusions with limb edema have been published as part of large series,[36,37] in which the incidence of symptomatic venous occlusion was less than 0.3%. All of these children responded to heparin therapy without the need for further intervention.[37] As in arterial thrombosis, the use of smaller catheters and heparin prophylaxis during catheterization procedures may reduce the incidence of venous thrombosis.

## Vessel Rupture, Perforation, and Dissection

Vessel rupture can occur at the site of vessel entry or at the site of intervention. It is a rare but potentially catastrophic event. One death due to intraabdominal hemorrhage after rupture of a femoral vein in a neonate was reported in a series of 4454 catheterizations.[27] Arterial or venous perforation was responsible for four major complications and six minor complications in a series of 4952 procedures, and significant groin hematoma occurred in 25 cases.[36] Femoral artery injuries may require surgical consultation and exploration.

Vessel perforation has occurred at the site of intervention, particularly during balloon interventions. Ruptures have been reported most often after balloon dilation of branch pulmonary arteries,[4,26] but they also have occurred along the ascending aorta and arch after balloon dilation of the aortic valve. Depending on the site of the tear, rupture may cause hemopericardium or hemothorax, or both.[41] Intrapulmonary hemorrhage is usually self-limited. If rupture or hemorrhage occurs, hypertension should be avoided, the trachea should be intubated (if the airway is not already secured), and any circulating heparin should be reversed. Pulmonary artery disruption after balloon dilation may manifest as hemoptysis. Increased blood flow after balloon dilation of pulmonary vessels may lead to unilateral pulmonary edema, which may also present as hemoptysis. Occasionally, arterial dissection,[41] aneurysm, and pseudoaneurysm formation may occur.

## CARDIAC TAMPONADE AND PERFORATION

Cardiac tamponade is an uncommon complication of cardiac catheterization, but when it occurs, it can be responsible for significant morbidity and mortality. The incidence of cardiac tamponade in three large series was 0.1%,[36] 0.04%,[27] and 0%.[37] In one series of 4952 patients, tamponade was responsible for two deaths: one neonate after a balloon atrial septostomy and one 4-year-old child after a recent Fontan procedure for stent insertion in a branch pulmonary artery.

Although tamponade is uncommon, perforation is not. The atrial appendage and right ventricular outflow tract are the sites most commonly perforated,[41] whereas the left ventricle has been punctured less commonly.[42] Perforation of the heart is described during many procedures, including balloon and blade atrial septostomy, balloon dilation of the mitral valve,[4] and attempted radiofrequency perforation of membranous pulmonary atresia.[5]

Signs that suggest a perforation include wires appearing in unexpected places, atypical contrast appearance, lack of a return to baseline blood pressure after catheter-induced tachycardia, and hemodynamic instability. Echocardiography should always be immediately available to confirm any suspicion of perforation or tamponade. If it occurs, a cannula can be placed in the pericardium to remove blood that can then be returned to the child through the femoral venous catheter. If the tamponade is not controlled with catheter drainage, the cardiac surgeons should be notified and an operating room prepared.

## DAMAGE OR DYSFUNCTION OF A VALVE

Damage to a valve is not particularly common, although it is more likely to occur with a balloon valvuloplasty procedure than with other procedures.[41] The primary complication is creation of excessive regurgitation. The hemodynamic consequences of such a defect are more significant on the systemic side of the circulation than on the pulmonary side.[5,41] The mechanism of injury is most commonly leaflet avulsion during dilation, although the leaflet can be inadvertently perforated by the guidewire, and there is the likelihood of significant further damage to the leaflet with advancement and inflation of the angioplasty catheter. Emergency repair is occasionally required.[41] Injuries to the atrioventricular valves have rarely been reported. Placement of wires and large sheaths across atrioventricular valves and septal defects can cause severe hemodynamic disturbance. This is particularly true during implantation of VSD occlusion devices.[15,26] ASD and PDA occlusions are less likely to produce significant hemodynamic disturbance.[26] Rarely, the implanted ASD and VSD devices adversely affect the functioning of an atrioventricular valve.

## BLOOD LOSS

Blood loss may be sudden with rupture of vessels, but more often, it is slow and insidious due to multiple blood samples and blood loss associated with catheter exchanges. Anemia may be difficult to detect in a dark room and a covered child. Significant loss is more likely to occur during insertion of a closure device. Blood transfusion was required in 54% of 86 VSD closure devices in one early study.[15] Because interventions have the potential for blood loss, it is reasonable to have a unit of blood and blood administration equipment in the cardiac catheterization laboratory.

## DYSRHYTHMIAS AND THE CATHETERIZATION LABORATORY

Transient dysrhythmias are common during cardiac catheterization.[27] Most dysrhythmias are mechanically induced, and repositioning the wire or catheter usually resolves the dysrhythmia. Other causes of rhythm abnormality include coronary air embolism, electrolyte imbalance, and hypercarbia. Although they are usually minor complications, dysrhythmias are one of the most common causes of major complications, with a frequency of 2.6%[36] to 3.6%.[37] Infants have the greatest incidence of rhythm disturbance. A defibrillator, a pacing device, and antiarrhythmic agents must be present in the cardiac catheterization suite. Doses of any unfamiliar antiarrhythmic drugs should always be double-checked or determined before the procedure with the cardiologist.

### Types of Dysrhythmias

Dysrhythmias may be atrial or ventricular in origin or involve degrees of heart block. Atrial arrhythmias such as supraventricular tachycardia or atrial flutter frequently resolve spontaneously, but persistent atrial dysrhythmias can be treated pharmacologically or with overdrive pacing. They rarely progress to major events.[36,37]

Atrioventricular block occurs in 0.4% of cases, of which one fourth required pacing, although all children were in sinus rhythm by the time of discharge from hospital.[37] First- or second-degree atrioventricular block is well tolerated at all ages. When complete heart block occurs, it usually resolves shortly after the procedure and rarely persists.[36] Device closure for VSD has a high incidence (10.5%) of severe junctional bradycardia or complete heart block, and almost half of these children require pacing or isoproterenol.[15] Transient left bundle branch block has been reported after dilation of the aortic valve.[26]

Overall, the incidence of ventricular tachycardia or fibrillation is approximately 0.2%.[36,37] However, 30% of children who underwent VSD device placement had serious dysrhythmias and hypotension requiring catheter withdrawal, and 8.5% of them had ventricular arrhythmias requiring lidocaine or cardioversion.[15] Even relatively low-risk procedures are associated with dysrhythmias. Balloon atrial septostomy is frequently accompanied by rhythm disturbances. Typically, they are transient, but rarely, they can be permanent or even fatal.[4]

### Cardioversion

Atrial, supraventricular, and ventricular tachyarrhythmias; bradycardias; atrioventricular block; and bundle branch blocks have been described after cardioversion. Factors that influence the incidence of tachyarrhythmias include the underlying rhythm disturbance and cardiac disease, metabolic derangement, drugs (e.g., digoxin), and the strength of shock. Histologic injury to the myocardium is rare when the starting power for cardioversion is set at 0.5 J/kg.[26] Systemic and pulmonary emboli are rare in children compared with adults, for whom the incidence is 1% to 2%. Children with pacemakers are becoming more common, and these patients may require defibrillation. This can be done safely if the electrode pads are placed a distance from the generator and the pacemaker circuits and programming mode are checked afterward.

### CYANOSIS

When cyanosis occurs in the catheterization laboratory, it may be respiratory or circulatory in origin. A transesophageal echocardiographic (TEE) probe can cause desaturation by compressing the bronchi or vessels, pressing on the trachea, or precipitating bronchospasm. These events are more common in children weighing less than 10 kg.[26] Pneumothorax is rare but documented.[37] Hypercarbia, acidosis, excessive positive-pressure ventilation, contrast media, and hypoxia can increase pulmonary vascular resistance, which may lead to increased shunting and cyanosis. Hypercyanotic episodes are frequently observed,[36] particularly in infants with uncorrected tetralogy of Fallot. In one study, 12% of children with tetralogy of Fallot exhibited a hypercyanotic episode within 12 hours of catheterization despite adequate hydration, sedation, and the use of nonionic contrast media.[37]

### EMBOLIZATION

Misplaced devices, fragments of catheters, devices and balloons, thrombi, and air can result in embolization.

### Device and Balloon

In a 1998 report of 1457 interventional cases, 18 devices embolized; 3 required surgical removal, 8 were removed in the catheterization laboratory, and 7 were of no hemodynamic consequence and were left in situ.[36] Devices that embolized included coils, duct umbrellas, an atrial defect occlusion device, and endovascular stents.[36] Improvements in device design have reduced the risk for embolization; for example, for ASD devices the risk has decreased from 11.1% to less than 1.1%.[4,44]

Balloon rupture was common in the past, although it rarely produced intimal damage or embolic phenomena.[41] Balloon fragmentation has become uncommon because of technologic improvements in materials and design. To minimize this risk, an inflation device with an attached manometer is recommended to ensure that the pressure does not exceed the burst pressure of the balloon.

### Thrombus or Dislodged Material

Thrombus may be dislodged from devices or catheters, and balloon dilation may dislodge calcium, intimal lining from conduits, and thrombus from surgical systemic-pulmonary shunts.[4]

### Air

Gas emboli may occur in sheaths and catheters, burst balloons, or anesthetic infusion lines. Air embolus (as well as blood loss) is a known risk during interventional procedures in which there are many wire and catheter exchanges.[26] Balloons are dilated with a weak contrast mixture, and in view of the occasional balloon rupture, it is important to ensure all gas bubbles are eliminated from the contrast mix syringe and catheter before dilation is undertaken. Balloons used for flotation tip catheters should be filled with carbon dioxide rather than air to minimize the potential embolic effect if the balloon bursts. All intravenous lines, injections, and infusions must be free of air bubbles because these sources can cause embolic occlusion of arterial vessels, producing cerebral or myocardial ischemia in children with right-to-left mixing. Nitrous oxide should be avoided because it may expand any air embolism.

### CONTRAST TOXICITY

Adverse reactions to intravascular contrast are relatively uncommon, but the anesthesiologist must diagnose and manage a contrast-mediated reaction early in order to minimize morbidity or mortality. Reactions are often classified as idiosyncratic (i.e., unpredictable reactions independent of dose or concentration such as anaphylaxis) or chemotoxic (i.e., related to dose and physiologic characteristics such as osmolality). The pathophysiology of most reactions, however, is complex.[45]

There is reasonable evidence that severe anaphylactoid reactions to contrast media are not immunoglobulin E (IgE) mediated, but this does not explain the increased risk among atopic and asthmatic individuals. Many mechanisms have been proposed, including direct mast cell activation and degranulation, complement activation, inhibition of various enzyme systems, and binding to plasma proteins with conformational change.

### Acute Reactions

Acute reactions to contrast agents can vary from mild to severe. Flushing, nausea, pruritus, vomiting, headache, and urticaria occur in 1% to 3% of patients receiving nonionic contrast.[46] These reactions are usually mild and self-limiting, requiring no specific treatment. Intermediate effects can manifest as moderate hypotension and bronchospasm and as more severe degrees of the mild reactions. Severe reactions can include convulsions, laryngeal edema, dysrhythmias, and cardiac arrest.

The likelihood of reaction varies with the type of contrast material; low osmolar (nonionic) solutions have considerably reduced risk. The incidence of severe reactions to high osmolar (ionic) contrast is 0.2% to 0.06%, whereas reaction to low osmolar contrast is five times less common.[45] Reactions are more common when contrast medium is given through an arterial access compared with a venous access. Acute reactions should be managed according to anaphylaxis protocols (i.e., oxygen, intravenous fluid, epinephrine, corticosteroids, and histamine$_1$- and histamine$_2$-antagonist therapy). Prophylaxis with corticosteroids and antihistamines should be considered only if there is a well-documented history of acute reaction to a nonionic contrast material. If there is a history of reaction to nonionic contrast material, other imaging modalities, such as MRI, should be strongly considered. Occasionally, staining of the myocardium by contrast material has been observed, although this does not appear to confer any significant consequences.[37]

### Delayed Reactions

Delayed reactions to ionic and nonionic media are well described, with an incidence in one study of 8%.[47] Manifestations of these reactions include flulike illness, parotitis, nausea and vomiting, abdominal pain, headache, and rashes. The pathophysiology is unknown. Reactions (e.g., seizures, cerebral edema, electrolyte imbalance) to high- or low-osmolar solutions are possible if given in excessive doses.

### Renal Adverse Reactions and Prevention

The term *contrast media nephrotoxicity* (CMN) refers to an increase in serum creatinine concentration by more than 25% or 0.5 mg/dL within 3 days of receiving intravenous contrast media in the absence of another cause.[45,47] The underlying mechanism of the renal injury is unclear, although it is thought that contrast agents can reduce renal perfusion and are toxic to the tubular cells.

CMN occurs almost exclusively in children with preexisting renal damage. Children with CHD undergoing coronary angiography with low-osmolar contrast media may develop limited glomerular effects and reversible tubular dysfunction, but no long-term effects have been demonstrated. However, any child with reduced renal perfusion (e.g., dehydration, cardiac failure) should be regarded as at risk for CMN. It has been suggested that infants and children who receive more than 5 mL/kg of nonionic contrast agent are at increased risk for CMN.[48]

Many interventions have been given prophylactically to prevent CMN, including normal saline/half-normal saline hydration, administration of *N*-acetylcysteine (NAC), mannitol, theophylline, calcium channel blockers, diuretics, dopamine, dopamine$_1$ (D$_1$) receptor antagonists, endothelin receptor antagonists, atrial natriuretic peptide, angiotensin-converting enzyme inhibitors, and PGE$_1$.[49,50] Although preliminary studies with NAC have been promising, no interventions have been more effective than normal saline hydration. To minimize the risk of CMN, the minimal dose of contrast agent should be used.[49,50] When possible, potentially nephrotoxic drugs should be stopped at least 24 hours before the procedure.[51]

Gadolinium-based contrast materials are considered nonnephrotoxic in the normal MRI dose of up to 0.3 mmol/kg.[51] However, there is some evidence that the increased doses required for cardiac angiography may confer adverse renal effects.[52]

### NEUROLOGIC EVENTS

Central and peripheral neurologic damage can occur as a complication of the catheterization procedure. In one prospective study, 0.38% children suffered a neurologic complication, and the incidence is significantly greater after interventional procedures than diagnostic procedures.[53]

### Central Nervous System

An ischemic cerebrovascular event may occur as a result of embolization, damage to the carotid artery, or acute low cardiac output states causing hypoxic-ischemic encephalopathy.[37,53] Thrombotic emboli may originate from any site in which there is endovascular or endocardial damage from the inner surface of the catheter or an implanted device. Factors that increase the risk during interventional procedures include large catheter size, more numerous vascular punctures, and procedures of increased duration.[53] However, embolic strokes also can follow an unremarkable catheterization procedure. The most common complications after an embolic stroke are convulsion and hemiplegia. Children with this type of stroke usually recover fully.[53] Seizures have been associated with lidocaine toxicity.[54] The outcome is more guarded after hypoxic-ischemic encephalopathy that occurs after a period of reduced cardiac output.[53]

### Peripheral Nervous System

As with any prolonged procedure under general anesthesia, it is crucial to consider pressure areas and traction forces on nerves such as the brachial plexus. Reduced cardiac output states associated with cardiac catheterization can augment the risk. Frequently, the arms are extended above the head to improve the lateral views of the heart. Brachial plexus injury is a risk in these circumstances[26,55] and is an important cause of malpractice lawsuits.[56]At-risk positions should be accepted only if the cardiologist clearly indicates it is required. If it is necessary to bring the arms above the head, the elbows should be flexed and elevated at least 15 cm above the level of the table to minimize traction on the brachial plexus. Head rotation should be minimized.[55,57] Passive movement may help to reduce injury, but it increases the risk of dislodging monitoring equipment or the airway. If such a position is required, it should be documented in the anesthesia record that this was the demand of the cardiologist.

### RADIATION

Radiation poses a risk to the patient and staff. Radiation overexposure can lead to scarring and skin injury, cellular injury, gene mutation, cell death, leukemia, bone cancer, thyroid cancer, and birth defects.[58] The principle with regard to radiation exposure is expressed by the acronym ALARA (or ALARP) which means as low as reasonably achievable (or practical). This principle must be applied in the context of obtaining adequate diagnostic images.

### Radiation Exposure of Patients

Radiation exposure is a particularly important for children because of their greater radiosensitivity compared with adults. Moreover, a greater proportion of their body is irradiated during procedures. Complex interventional procedures require long fluoroscopy times with multiple angiographic or fluoroscopic acquisitions.[59] Children undergoing electrophysiologic studies are particularly at risk for long fluoroscopy times.

When estimating the lifetime risk of cancer from radiation exposure, the child's age and weight need to be considered along with the duration and effective dose of radiation exposure. The risk for adult coronary angiography is 6% per sievert (Sv), and the average dose is about 10 mSv, which gives an increased risk of 0.06%.[60] In contrast, infants require smaller exposures due to their reduced body weights, but they have an increased sensitivity. An infant has a lifetime cancer risk of 11% to 15% per sievert. If an infant is exposed to approximately 20 mSv (e.g., 1 hour of fluoroscopy and seven digital acquisition runs), the lifetime cancer risk is estimated as 0.03%.[60]

### Radiation Exposure of Staff

Most exposure comes from scatter from the beam entry point on the patient. Lesser amounts come from the x-ray tube and intensifier. The need for staff protection is well established and is accomplished by wearing lead aprons and by using thyroid shields, goggles, and suspended mobile glass lead screens for the head and neck. Operators should have monitoring devices to assess exposure, and only essential personnel should be present in the unprotected area.

## HYPOTHERMIA AND HYPERTHERMIA

The procedure is often prolonged, increasing the need for close temperature monitoring. Children may become hypothermic, which can exacerbate blood loss or dysrhythmias, or they may become hyperthermic, which may exacerbate any neurologic injury. For any procedure that is expected to last more than 1 hour, a forced-air warming device should be used. Central temperature should be measured.

## ENDOCARDITIS

Antibiotic prophylaxis against endocarditis for routine diagnostic cardiac catheterization varies among medical centers. All children scheduled for insertion of implantable devices should receive prophylactic antibiotics during the procedure, and most centers continue to recommend endocarditis prophylaxis for a minimum of 6 months after implantation. Although most centers do not routinely administer antibiotics for angioplasty procedures, there is usually a residual flow disturbance after the procedure that warrants ongoing endocarditis prophylaxis.

## OVERCOMING LIMITATIONS

The main limitation in the use of catheterization techniques in younger or smaller children has been the delay in development of equipment of appropriate size. To overcome this difficulty, clinicians have developed hybrid procedures to permit current catheter-based techniques to be used in infants and small children. Examples of this collaborative approach between surgeon and interventional cardiologist include perventricular closure of muscular ventricular septal defects[61] and hybrid stage 1 palliation for hypoplastic left heart syndrome (i.e., off-pump placement of a PDA stent and creation of an unrestricted ASD).[60]

The next great challenge is to develop equipment and techniques that can be used in conjunction with MRI.[62] This would minimize radiation exposure to children and staff. However, there are significant technical obstacles that need to be overcome before this approach can fully replace catheterization laboratories using ionizing radiation.

# Anesthesia

## WHO AND HOW?

The aims of anesthesia care for pediatric interventional cardiology are to ensure the child is not distressed, to provide optimal conditions for accurate diagnostic measures and successful completion of any intervention, and to manage the complications and significant derangements that may occur in the child's cardiovascular physiology during the procedure. These aims may require general anesthesia or occasionally may be met with deep sedation.

The care of these children may be provided by a nurse anesthetist, general pediatric anesthesiologist, or specialized cardiac pediatric anesthesiologist, depending on the complexity of the child's condition and qualifications of the practitioner. Because deep sedation can easily merge into general anesthesia, current guidelines sensibly suggest that deep sedation should be supervised by someone skilled at providing anesthesia and sedation.[63] This person should be skilled at resuscitation of children with CHD and must not be the proceduralist. The choice of sedation or general anesthesia and the seniority of anesthesiologist should match the procedure and the child.

Increasingly, there are fewer diagnostic procedures and more interventional procedures. This change is reflected in a shift from sedation to general anesthesia and the expanding role of specialized cardiac pediatric anesthesiologists.[64] Anesthesia providers for these children must have a high level of experience in pediatric anesthesia and a thorough understanding of pediatric cardiology and CHD. They must understand the physiology, the procedure, and the potential complications.

## PREPROCEDURAL ASSESSMENT AND MANAGEMENT

Children scheduled for elective interventional cardiology are often admitted to the hospital on the day of the procedure. Ideally, all children should have an anesthesia assessment at the same time as their preprocedural cardiologic workup. An efficient and complete anesthesia assessment requires good coordination and communication between cardiology and anesthesia units. The anesthesia preoperative assessment should establish the cardiac anatomy and function and determine details of the planned procedure or intervention.

Up to 25% of children with CHD have syndromes or other anomalies that may affect their anesthesia care and require a thorough assessment of all relevant systems. The children might have had previous cardiac surgery or several other interventions. Obtaining intravenous access may be very difficult in some of them. Children with CHD are likely to have undergone anesthesia several times in the past, and the family may be well informed about the child's condition, hospital process, and anesthesia. During the preoperative assessment, it is important to have a discussion about the sedative premedication, parental presence, and the mode of induction of anesthesia (see Chapters 1 and 4).

Interventional cardiology procedures may involve considerable physiologic trespass, and some children may have limited cardiac reserve. They should be in optimal health whenever possible. Intercurrent illness or infection may bias cardiorespiratory diagnostic values, increase the risk of endocarditis, and increase the risk of anesthesia complications such as laryngospasm. The urgency of the procedure, the cardiovascular status of the child, and the extent of the procedure should be considered carefully before proceeding in a child with an intercurrent illness.

## ANATOMY AND FUNCTION

When assessing the anatomy and function, answers to four primary questions may affect anesthesia management:

- Where does the blood go?
- What is the ventricular function?
- How reactive is the pulmonary circulation?
- Is there a fixed or dynamic stenosis?

Answers to these and other questions can help the anesthesiologist determine the optimal approach to management:

- How well is hyperoxia or hypoxia tolerated?
- What will be the effect of increased sympathetic stimulation, vasodilation, or reduction in myocardial contractility?
- What are the likely causes of cardiovascular collapse, and how should they be managed?

Most primary questions can be answered from the record, details of previous surgery, and recent echocardiographic results. Very poor function may be easily discovered in the history and physical examination, but moderate levels of dysfunction may not be offered or easily detected clinically.

Blood should be taken for a hematocrit evaluation and crossmatched for possible rapid transfusion. Premedication may consist of paracetamol for postprocedural analgesia and, if needed, sedation with oral midazolam (0.5 mg/kg) or ketamine (up to 5 mg/kg). Larger doses of sedative premedications may be used to provide more reliable or greater sedation if heavy sedation is mandatory, but large doses may cause delayed recovery or significant sedation after the procedure.

Care should be taken that these children do not become excessively dehydrated. Fasting times should be adequate but not excessive, and in selected children, a preprocedural intravenous line should be started. Topical anesthesia creams can be used if an intravenous induction is planned. To plan optimal anesthesia, the anesthesiologist must understand exactly what the cardiologists are hoping to achieve and what conditions the cardiologist needs.

## THE ENVIRONMENT

Cardiac catheterization laboratories are often remotely located from the main operating room complex, limiting availability of immediate assistance and increasing transport times to and from central recovery areas. Ideally, cardiac catheterization laboratories should be located adjacent to cardiac theaters to facilitate rapid management of complications. For some cases, ECMO and cardiopulmonary bypass circuits should be nearby and immediately available. Blood gas analysis should be rapidly available, and blood should be immediately available for urgent transfusion for interventional procedures such as balloon dilation and device insertion.

The cardiac catheterization laboratory is a hostile environment for anesthesiologists. Access to the child may be limited by the anteroposterior and lateral x-ray cameras, sterile drapes, and radiation protection devices. The x-ray cameras are bulky and may be unexpectedly moved for oblique views, different fields, or greater magnification. The lighting is often subdued to enhance viewing of the radiographs (Fig. 20-5).

Great care must be taken to secure all monitoring and airway devices before draping begins or the x-ray cameras are positioned. Access to the child during the procedure is limited and hazardous. Blind manipulation under the drapes can dislodge monitors or the tracheal tube. Moving cameras are a hazard to the anesthesiologist and may also dislodge anesthesia monitors, the tracheal tube, and the airway circuit.

## THE CARDIAC PATIENT

The management of anesthesia for children with CHD is discussed further in Chapters 15 to 17. Important considerations include the potential for myocardial dysfunction and poor ventricular function reserve. This may be a particular problem in children with hypertrophied right ventricles operating at near-systemic pressures or with volume-loaded dilated ventricles.

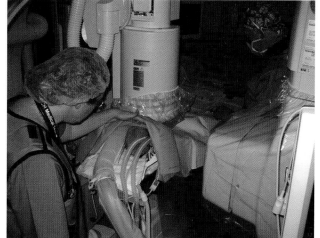

**FIGURE 20-5** Typical setup of a catheterization laboratory, showing limited access to a child.

Another important consideration is pulmonary hypertension and the reactivity of the pulmonary circulation. Pulmonary resistance is particularly important in several situations:

- Patients may have increased reactivity, such as in neonates or children with primary pulmonary hypertension.
- Children may have chronically increased pulmonary artery pressures and minimal right ventricular reserve.
- Children may have balanced circulations, such as after a Norwood procedure, in which increases or decreases in pulmonary vascular resistance may lead to spiraling hypoxia or systemic ischemia and acidosis.
- Children may have low-pressure pulmonary circulations, such as cavopulmonary shunts or after Fontan surgery.

## CHOICE OF ANESTHESIA

The choice of anesthesia should be determined by the three factors linked to the aims stated earlier. The ideal anesthesia prescription should achieve the following:

- Ensure the child is not distressed
- Provide optimal conditions for accurate diagnostic measures or successful completion of any intervention
- Minimize any risk inherent in children with abnormal cardiovascular physiology

Many anesthetic agents and techniques have been used in pediatric interventional cardiology. To some extent, the choice is determined by the procedure and the pathology.

### Sedation

The difference between deep sedation and general anesthesia is imprecise and controversial, especially for small children in whom consciousness and memory are harder to measure (see Chapters 45 and 47). When considering the suitability of sedation or general anesthesia, several issues are important:

- Does immobility need to be guaranteed?
- What will be the level of stimulation?
- Do oxygen and carbon dioxide tensions need to be controlled?
- What will be the cardiovascular effects of the anesthetic agents?
- How likely is significant physiologic trespass?
- What will be the duration of the procedure?

Sedation is associated with a degree of movement that may make some procedures difficult or potentially dangerous, such as in device placement or balloon dilation. Stimulating procedures such as balloon dilation may make smooth sedation difficult. Sedation is poorly tolerated if the arms need to be placed above the head for long periods or if the procedure is prolonged. As for any other procedure, sedation for interventional cardiology is unwise if the child has obstructive sleep apnea or airway abnormalities. If significant cardiovascular complications are likely due to the procedure or the status of the child, control of the airway with general anesthesia may be safer. For all children, if sedation is used, there must be provision for rapid and expert transition to general anesthesia.

Sedation techniques have evolved over the past 2 decades, resulting in much more effective and titratable strategies today. Since the 1950s, the classic lytic cocktail, consisting of intramuscular meperidine, promethazine, and chlorpromazine, has been the standard for sedation.[65] However, this cocktail has a high incidence of failure and oversedation, and is associated with sterile abscess formation.[66] Oral ketamine and midazolam provide more reliable sedation, but occasionally, respiratory support is required.[67] In theory, intravenous ketamine is an excellent choice for sedation because it provides a stable or increased heart rate and blood pressure and has little or no effect on pulmonary vascular resistance. However, prolonged recovery, vomiting, and dysphoric reactions may be problematic.[68] Intravenous ketamine has been successfully used alone or in combination with midazolam[69] or propofol.[70] Propofol is also widely used for sedation, but compared with ketamine, it causes a greater reduction in systemic blood pressure and systemic vascular resistance, with no effect on pulmonary vascular resistance. This may increase a right-to-left shunt, or in diagnostic procedures, it may attenuate the gradient across a stenosis, making the decision to dilate the stenosis more difficult.[68,71,72] Compared with propofol sedation, a combination of ketamine with propofol produces similar sedation with less cardiovascular depression.[73] Dexmedetomidine has been proffered for sedation of children undergoing cardiac catheterization, although it may not provide sufficient sedation by itself.[74] When combined with ketamine, dexmedetomidine was inferior to propofol and ketamine.[75]

In sedated children, local anesthesia with the use of a topical cream may facilitate venous access.[76] Spinal anesthesia has been described as an alternative to sedation or general anesthesia in high-risk infants younger than 6 months of age when the procedure is expected to take less than 90 minutes.[77]

Sedation is often used to avoid the potential effects of general anesthesia on diagnostic measures. However, as the diagnosis shifts to intervention, this argument assumes less relevance. Deep sedation may be associated with significant respiratory changes[67,78] and hypoxia[72] in some children. These changes can have as much effect on the circulation as general anesthesia, limiting the theoretical advantage of sedation. General anesthesia and sedation may alter hemodynamics and intracardiac shunts.[67,72]

## General Anesthesia

If general anesthesia is required for diagnostic procedures, the aim should be to maintain normal levels of inspired oxygen and arterial carbon dioxide, a low intrathoracic mean pressure, and minimal direct hemodynamic effects. Positive-pressure ventilation more easily maintains the target carbon dioxide concentrations than spontaneous ventilation, but it decreases preload to the pulmonary and systemic atria, increases afterload on the right ventricle, and decreases afterload on the left ventricle; especially if the mean intrathoracic pressure is increased. If the child can maintain adequate oxygenation and normal carbon dioxide tension during sedation or general anesthesia, spontaneous ventilation is often preferred.

No general anesthetic agent is definitely superior to others. Using physiologic and theoretical arguments, there is evidence for and against inhalational and intravenous anesthesia, but no outcome studies have provided strong evidence for either technique. Great care should be taken to avoid myocardial depression or vasodilation associated with excessive doses of inhalational or intravenous anesthetics. For this reason, some argue against inhalational induction, although it can also be argued that the use of total intravenous anesthesia is unwise given the wide variability in children's responses. Nitrous oxide should be avoided if there is an element of reversible pulmonary hypertension and to avoid expansion of gas bubbles.

Etomidate may have a role in children with significant compromise because it has little hemodynamic effect on systemic or pulmonary pressures or resistances.[79] Remifentanil may offer an advantage in cardiac procedures because of the short, context-sensitive half-time that allows rapid awakening on completion of the procedure, although it is an opioid and lacks the sedation qualities of other medications. Concerns remain about the possible risks of bradycardia, hypotension, and chest wall rigidity with this opioid.[80,81] In some cases, postprocedural sedation may offer an advantage in reducing patient movement, thereby reducing the risk for dislodging a clot on the catheter or at the catheterization site.

Opioids are not usually needed for postoperative analgesia after interventional cardiology procedures, and they may contribute to postanesthesia nausea and vomiting. Adequate infiltration with local anesthesia around the femoral vessels can significantly limit the degree of stimulus and should not impair ease of vessel access. However, earlier reports of local anesthetic toxicity in children undergoing cardiac catheterization led to a moratorium on the use of local anesthetics in the cardiac catheterization laboratory in some centers.

Radiofrequency ablation procedures may be protracted and require an immobile child. They may also precipitate arrhythmias, requiring defibrillation. For these reasons, general anesthesia is preferred. General anesthetic agents have effects on conduction that may affect the generation of preexcitation and automatic tachycardia. Good clinical data are scant; however, it appears that for preexcitation, isoflurane and sevoflurane have little effect at less than 1 minimal alveolar concentration (MAC), whereas propofol and opioids have no demonstrable effects at any dose. In contrast, automatic tachycardia may be suppressed by large doses of opioids, propofol or dexmedetomidine.[82] In a prospective, randomized trial, isoflurane- and propofol-based anesthesia resulted in a similar duration of anesthesia and effectiveness of ablation.[83] Because of the protracted time course of these procedures, a forced-air warming device is indicated to maintain thermal homeostasis. Esophageal ulceration and atrioesophageal fistula have been reported in up to 3% of patients undergoing these procedures, particularly when excessive energy is applied during ablation (e.g., more than 25 W for extended periods).[84] We recommend using energy levels less than 25 W during the ablation and to monitor the esophageal temperature by inserting an esophageal temperature probe to the level of the mid-esophagus. Position of the stethoscope may be verified by injecting contrast dye in the bulb of the stethoscope.

**20**

## Principles of Technique

Attention to detail is essential for providing safe anesthesia for children with reduced ventricular reserve and critical pulmonary circulations. The most frequent error precipitating adverse events is providing inadequate anesthesia. Hemodynamic consequences of light anesthesia, such as hypoxia due to laryngospasm, are poorly tolerated in children with pulmonary hypertension. Hypoxia or hypercapnia may lead to increasing pulmonary vascular resistance, which may increase the shunt and further worsen the hypoxia. Increased pulmonary hypertension may also lead to significant decreases in pulmonary compliance, further increasing hypoxia and precipitating a downward spiral.[85] Another cause of adverse outcomes is the use of unfamiliar anesthesia techniques. For example, it is imprudent to use remifentanil for the first time in a child with primary pulmonary hypertension. Although there are theoretical grounds to support the use of one drug or another, the most important principle of anesthesia in children with CHD is to carefully use techniques that are reliable and familiar. This reinforces the need for these children to be anesthetized only by those with sound knowledge and experience with the physiology of the CHD and the planned procedures. Careful anesthesia entails attention to preprocedural anxiolysis, fluid management, full monitoring, expert assistance, and taking extra time to deliver anesthetic drugs slowly or in incremental doses to avoid overpressure or excessive blood levels. A useful approach is to transduce the cardiologist's arterial access onto the anesthesia monitor. This can be accomplished with a slave connection or by adding a second stopcock to the system with a second transducer for the anesthesia monitor.

The procedures often involve long periods of very little painful stimulation with occasional painful moments such as a sheath change or balloon dilation. These moments can be anticipated if good communication is maintained between the cardiologist and the anesthesiologist. During dilation of the aortic arch or aortic valve, it is prudent to have an arterial line (preferably a right radial line) to allow continuous blood pressure monitoring. Dilation of arterial or venous vessels is quite painful and may cause coughing or significant discomfort if the child is only sedated.

TEE is increasingly used as part of diagnostic procedures or during device placement. Because TEE can be painful, it requires a deeper plane of anesthesia with the addition of opioids or neuromuscular blockade, or both. TEE requires a tracheal tube to provide a patent airway, and care must be taken to hold the tube securely during manipulations of the TEE probe because the manipulations and gel required can easily dislodge the tracheal tube.

Coughing and straining on extubation may increase the risk of bleeding. For this reason, deep extubation may be preferred. The advantages of deep extubation must be balanced with the risks of hypoxia and hypercapnia and loss of airway control or laryngospasm that may ensue if the tracheal tube is removed before the child is fully awake. Postoperative delirium and restlessness can increase the risk of bleeding. Children should have sufficient analgesia to prevent postoperative distress. This is usually provided with paracetamol and local anesthetic infiltration.

Reliable intravenous access is essential in these children to provide rapid resuscitation. Using leg veins may not be ideal if the femoral veins are occluded with thrombosis or catheters. Similarly, pulse oximetry and noninvasive blood pressure cuffs should not be placed on the legs.

## FUTURE OF ANESTHESIA IN INTERVENTIONAL CARDIOLOGY

Anesthesia for interventional cardiac catheterizations will become more challenging as new interventions are developed for sicker children and as more cardiology procedures are performed in combination with open surgery or MRI. More children are likely to need anesthesia instead of sedation, and specialist pediatric cardiac anesthesiologists will be spending an increasing proportion of their time in interventional cardiology suites.

## ANNOTATED REFERENCES

Arnold PD, Holtby HM. Anesthesia for the cardiac catheterization laboratory. In: Andropoulos DB, Stayer SA, Russell IA, editors. Anesthesia for congenital heart disease. Malden, MA: Blackwell Futura; 2005. p. 407-26.
*The article is a good, readable source for information about anesthesia for congenital heart disease.*
Bennett D, Marcus R, Stokes M. Incidents and complications during pediatric cardiac catheterization. Paediatr Anaesth 2005;15:1083-8.
*This paper describes the complications in pediatric cardiac catheterization.*
Cassidy SC, Schmidt KG, Van Hare GF, et al. Complications of pediatric cardiac catheterization: a 3-year study. J Am Coll Cardiol 1992;19:1285-93.
*The complications of pediatric cardiac catheterization are described.*
Feltes TF, Bacha E, Beekman III RH, et al. AHA scientific statement: indications for cardiac catheterization and intervention in pediatric cardiac disease. Circulation 2011;123:2607-52.
*The American Heart Association has provided a comprehensive overview of the subject.*
Friesen RH, Alswang M. Changes in carbon dioxide tension and oxygen saturation during deep sedation for paediatric cardiac catheterization. Paediatr Anaesth 1996;6:15-20.
*The authors review a significant issue for sedation techniques.*
Reddy K, Jaggar S, Gillbe C. The anaesthetist and the cardiac catheterisation laboratory. Anaesthesia 2006;61:1175-86.
*This is a good review of anesthesia for adult and pediatric cardiac catheterization.*
Taylor CJ, Derrick G, McEwan A, Haworth SG, Sury MRJ. Risk of cardiac catheterization under anaesthesia in children with pulmonary hypertension. Br J Anaesth 2007;98:657-61.
*This investigation examined the important high-risk subgroup of patients with pulmonary hypertension.*
Vitiello R, McCrindle BW, Nykanen D, et al. Complications associated with pediatric cardiac catheterization. J Am Coll Cardiol 1998;32:1433-40.
*This important paper describes the complications in pediatric cardiac catheterization.*

Video 20-1
Closure of a patent ductus arteriosus with the Amplatzer Septal Occluder.

Video 20-2
Retrograde coil occlusion of a patent ductus arteriosus.

## REFERENCES

Please see www.expertconsult.com.

# Anesthesia for Noncardiac Surgery in Children with Congenital Heart Disease

## 21

WANDA C. MILLER-HANCE

ADVANCES IN THE PAST SEVERAL DECADES have dramatically altered the natural history of congenital heart disease (CHD). These refinements have resulted in decreased morbidity and mortality for affected children and improvements in quality of life. As life expectancy continues to increase and survival rates further improve, an escalating number of children with CHD will need to undergo noncardiac surgery or other procedures unrelated to their heart disease. Because the trend continues to be for earlier cardiac surgery, children with CHD who have undergone palliative treatment or repair represent the main patient group that an anesthesiologist is likely to encounter during elective or emergent noncardiac surgery. In some cases, children may require noncardiac surgery before undergoing procedures to address their cardiovascular disease. In others, the condition may not require or be amenable to surgical intervention. The care of children with CHD is becoming more common in all diagnostic and surgical settings.

A wide spectrum of extracardiac anomalies has been described in children with CHD.[1-5] A great incidence of chromosomal syndromes and genetic disorders is associated with CHD, and the reported prevalence of associated malformations ranges between 10% and 33%.[6-8] The organ systems most often affected include musculoskeletal, central nervous, renal-urinary, gastrointestinal, and respiratory. Although many extracardiac malformations are relatively minor and have limited or no clinical implications, many children with CHD have significant noncardiac comorbidities.[9] These pathologic and disease processes may necessitate surgical intervention. Other routine ailments and conditions may affect these children and require diagnostic procedures and surgical care.

The challenges of caring for children with CHD are magnified by the diversity of structural malformations, each with specific physiologic perturbations, hemodynamic consequences, and severity. This is further complicated by the variety of medical and surgical management strategies available. Most children require an individualized approach to anesthetic care.[10-12]

Clinical outcomes for CHD depend on the nature of the anatomic abnormalities and the possibility of successful palliation or correction.[13] The primary goal of palliative surgery is to favorably influence the natural history of the defect and decrease the likelihood of the severe consequences of the disease. However, children continue to have abnormal cardiovascular anatomy and physiology, and their abnormal circulation is associated with an increased risk of perioperative adverse events.[14-17]

Reparative, corrective, or definitive procedures are expected to improve hemodynamics and cardiac function while minimizing long-term ill effects of an abnormal circulation, improving the overall clinical outcome. Although the pathology might have been surgically treated, the cardiovascular system should not be considered normal. True surgical correction may be the exception rather than the rule in CHD, and repair of a congenital cardiac lesion should not be equated to a cure for most children.

Despite these considerations, for children with good hemodynamic results, the risks associated with noncardiac surgery may not be significantly different from those of others without CHD. These children are considered to be doing well clinically, have a good functional status, require few or no medications, have no exercise restrictions, and undergo routine surveillance. They require minimal or no adjustment in perioperative care compared with that provided to children without CHD. In others, however, residual abnormalities exist. In some who are less fortunate, a pathologic process may remain or develop after cardiac surgery that is related to the primary disease or therapy. This may lead to severe cardiovascular or pulmonary impairment. These residua and sequelae may necessitate further medical or surgical interventions and may increase perioperative morbidity during noncardiac surgery.[18] Management of these children is influenced by several factors but to a significant extent by the residual problems of the disease and treatment and associated hemodynamic perturbations.[19,20]

Many publications have examined the implications of anesthesia for children and adults with CHD undergoing noncardiac surgery.[10,19-33] However, only a limited number of studies have provided data on perioperative outcomes.[34-38] In contrast to the extensive literature regarding perioperative cardiac assessment and risk stratification during noncardiac surgery in adults with heart disease and the development of guidelines aimed at improving clinical outcomes, the lack of rigorous scientific data on this subject for the pediatric age group has made an equivalent effort challenging.[39]

In this chapter, general principles of anesthesia practice are reviewed as they pertain to the care of children with CHD undergoing noncardiac surgery. Unique perioperative considerations and issues applicable to high-risk patient groups are described. Anesthesia management for these children is significantly influenced by factors such as structural abnormalities, pathophysiologic consequences of the defects, functional status, potential residua, sequelae, and long-term outcome.

## Preoperative Assessment

A detailed preoperative evaluation is indispensable for identifying and anticipating factors that may place a child with CHD at increased risk during anesthesia (Table 21-1).[40,41] An important goal of this assessment is to gather information regarding the nature of the cardiovascular disease and prior therapeutic interventions. A determination of functional status is based on clinical data. The history and physical examination, in addition to the laboratory data and ancillary tests, provide complementary information about anatomic or hemodynamic status, enabling an overall risk assessment. Based on this clinical assessment and

**TABLE 21-1** Factors That Place Children with Congenital Heart Disease at Increased Risk during Anesthesia for Noncardiac Surgery

Anticoagulation therapy

Arrhythmias

Congestive heart failure

Emergent surgery

History of implanted device (pacemaker or defibrillator)

Hypoxemia

Long-standing cyanosis

Major noncardiac surgery

Older age at the time of cardiac intervention

Older type of cardiac surgical procedure

Pulmonary hypertension/pulmonary vascular disease

Significant outflow tract obstruction

Significant sequelae or residua

Single-ventricle physiology or complex defects

Syncope

Unrepaired pathology

Ventricular dysfunction

Young age (infancy)

consideration of the major pathophysiologic consequences of a particular condition, a systematic, detailed, organized plan should be formulated for anesthesia and perioperative management. In some cases, the preoperative evaluation may establish the need to delay or defer elective noncardiac surgery, other interventions, or diagnostic procedures.

### HISTORY AND PHYSICAL EXAMINATION

As for all children undergoing anesthesia, the history and physical examination results are essential components of a thorough preoperative evaluation. In addition to the specifics regarding the present illness and planned procedure, the history should focus on the status of the cardiovascular system. Relevant information includes the type of cardiovascular disease and comorbid conditions, medications, allergies, prior hospitalizations, surgical procedures, anesthesia experiences, and complications. Symptoms, including tachypnea, dyspnea, tachycardia, rhythm problems, and fatigue, should be sought. Feeding difficulties and diaphoresis may represent significant symptoms in infants, whereas decreased activity level or exercise intolerance may be a concern for older children. Palpitations, chest pain, and syncope should be characterized. The history should include an assessment of growth and development because these may be affected in children with CHD. Failure to thrive suggests ongoing cardiorespiratory compromise. Those with decompensated disease, complex pathologies, associated genetic defects, or other syndromes may be particularly vulnerable. Recent illnesses such as intercurrent respiratory infections or pulmonary disease may increase the potential for perioperative complications and require careful appraisal of the risk/benefit ratio in elective cases.[42,43]

The physical examination should include the child's weight and height. Vital signs, including heart rate, respiratory rate, and blood pressure, should be documented. If the child is known or suspected to have or has been treated for any form of aortic arch obstruction or has had any systemic-to-pulmonary shunt, upper and lower extremity and the right and left upper extremity blood pressure recordings and palpation of the quality of pulses should be documented. This assessment provides information about the patency of arterial beds and helps in the selection of blood pressure monitoring sites. The examination should explore suitable sites for venous and arterial access and identify potential difficulties. Emphasis should be given to the airway and cardiovascular system, with particular attention to any changes from previous examination findings.

General assessment should include the child's level of activity, breathing pattern, level of distress (if any), and presence of cyanosis. Respiratory evaluation should include the quality of the breath sounds and indicate the presence or absence of labored breathing, intercostal retractions, wheezing, rales, or rhonchi. Abnormalities may suggest congestive symptoms or a pneumonic process. Cardiac auscultation should include assessment of heart sounds, pathologic murmurs, and gallop rhythms. The presence of a thrill, representing a palpable murmur, should be documented. The abdomen should be examined for the presence of hepatosplenomegaly. Assessment of the extremities should include examination of pulses, overall perfusion, capillary refill, cyanosis, clubbing, and edema. Noncardiac anomalies or pathology that may affect anesthesia care (e.g., specific syndrome complex, potentially difficult airway, gastroesophageal reflux) should be recorded.

An important objective of the preoperative evaluation is to identify children with functional cardiopulmonary limitations imposed by their cardiovascular disease. Symptoms and signs consistent with congestive heart failure, cyanosis, hypercyanotic episodes, and compromised functional status (i.e., significant exercise intolerance or syncopal episodes) should raise concerns about potential perioperative problems. The pediatric cardiologist should obtain information about the nature and severity of the cardiovascular pathology, describe the child's overall clinical status, and assess prior complications. The cardiologist should assist in the identification of children at great risk and optimize their preoperative clinical condition. The perioperative care teams should be alerted to any particular concerns that may affect the care of the child. The anesthesiologist should have a detailed understanding of the child's cardiac defect, pathophysiologic consequences, nature of the medical and surgical therapies applied, functional status, and implications for perioperative management. Although the surgical team may not have an in-depth understanding of the child's cardiovascular disease, by sharing the details of the surgical plan and likely perioperative issues with the anesthesiologist, problems may be anticipated and proactively addressed.

## ANCILLARY STUDIES AND LABORATORY DATA

The baseline systemic arterial saturation value should be determined by pulse oximetry ($SpO_2$) when the child is calm and, in most cases, while breathing room air. Acceptable values depend on many factors, including the specific cardiovascular defects, whether the child has a two- or a one-ventricle circulation, the preoperative versus postoperative status with respect to the cardiac pathology, and the stage in the palliative pathway for those undergoing such a strategy. Children who have undergone definitive procedures should be expected to have normal to a near-normal $SpO_2$ value (at least 95%). After palliative interventions, $SpO_2$ values typically range between 75% and 85%.

The extent of preoperative laboratory testing largely depends on the status of the patient and the type, anticipated duration, and complexity of surgery. Studies most commonly obtained include hematocrit, hemoglobin, electrolytes, and coagulation

tests. In cyanotic children, a complete blood cell blood count allows determination of polycythemia, microcytic anemia, and thrombocytopenia. Prothrombin time, partial thromboplastin times, and international normalized ratio (INR) provide an indication of clotting ability. Cyanotic children usually have increased red blood cell mass and relatively small plasma volumes. The collection of specimens for coagulation tests requires sampling tubes that adjust the amount or concentration of citrate to prevent artifactual prolongation of the values. For those receiving diuretic therapy, digoxin, or angiotensin-converting enzyme inhibitors, the determination of a basic metabolic panel may be useful. Blood typing and crossmatching should be performed depending on the anticipated need for blood administration.

A recent electrocardiogram (ECG) should be reviewed for any changes from prior studies (particularly regarding criteria consistent with chamber dilation or ventricular hypertrophy), the presence of rhythm abnormalities, and findings suggesting myocardial ischemia. If an arrhythmia is identified, further evaluation is warranted because it may reflect an underlying hemodynamic abnormality that may affect the perioperative course. A continuous ECG recording (i.e., Holter monitor) and further evaluation may be indicated in the child with a history of rhythm disturbance, palpitations, or syncope or with an ECG suggesting significant ectopy or arrhythmia. An exercise tolerance test or treadmill study may be warranted if there is concern about myocardial ischemia, as may be the case for the child with aortic stenosis, coronary artery anomalies, or exercise-induced arrhythmias.

Review of a recent chest radiograph, including a lateral view, provides information regarding cardiac size, chamber enlargement, and pulmonary vascularity. Prior studies such as echocardiograms, cardiac catheterizations, electrophysiologic procedures, and magnetic resonance imaging should be reviewed. In some cases, it may be necessary to obtain further diagnostic information before proceeding with the planned procedure if there are symptoms that merit additional investigations or issues of concern. These evaluations should be coordinated with the child's cardiologist. It is also important to consider whether the child may benefit from cardiac catheterization for diagnostic or interventional purposes to address significant structural, functional, or hemodynamic abnormalities before the anticipated procedure. In addition to providing potentially helpful information, the clinical status of the child can be substantially improved in many cases by catheter-based interventions. This may be of significant benefit when the anticipated procedure is considered to be major.

One of the goals of the preoperative evaluation is to obtain the most diagnostic information with the fewest tests and the least risk, discomfort, and expense for the child. The anesthesiologist is particularly suited to determine which tests are appropriate for optimal perioperative planning and whether additional data are needed.

## INFORMED CONSENT

The physicians involved in the care of the child should meet with the patient and family to discuss the anesthetic plan and answer any questions. The preoperative consultation provides the opportunity to alleviate patient and parental anxiety. At the same time, the benefits and risks involved should be discussed. Although surgery in children with CHD, particularly in those with uncorrected defects, may carry an increased risk, it may not be possible to define the specific contribution of each factor to the overall risk.

## FASTING GUIDELINES

Although the optimal period of fasting for children before surgery has been the subject of some debate, most centers follow established guidelines to reduce the risk of aspiration.[44-47] The same guidelines are applicable to children with CHD with a few additional considerations. Intake of clear fluids or the intravenous administration of maintenance fluids may be required in some children to ensure adequate hydration if the fasting period is prolonged. This is particularly important in small infants and in patients with obstructive lesions, cyanotic disease, or single-ventricle physiology. Maintenance of adequate hydration and ventricular preload may limit potential detrimental hemodynamic changes associated with anesthesia and surgery.

## MEDICATIONS

Children with CHD may be receiving medications such as digoxin, diuretics, vasodilators, anticoagulants, antiarrhythmics, or immunosuppressant agents. Although there may be an occasional exception, such as diuretic or anticoagulation therapy, there is usually no need to discontinue chronic medications before surgery. It is often important to continue these drugs until the time of surgery, and in most centers, children are allowed to take scheduled oral medications with small sips of water preoperatively.

## Intraoperative Management

Anesthesia and surgery impose additional stresses on the cardiovascular system and provoke compensatory mechanisms to maintain homeostasis. It is important to assess the child's physiology and cardiovascular reserve to anticipate his or her ability to increase cardiac output to meet metabolic demands. This information, along with the nature and complexity of the surgery, can help to decide the extent of monitoring required. This information can be used to choose anesthetic agents and techniques that least affect the child's cardiovascular system. Prompt intervention is imperative if decompensation occurs. Good communication among the surgeon, cardiologist, anesthesiologist, and nursing teams during the entire perioperative period is essential in treating children with complex disease.

### GENERAL CONSIDERATIONS
#### Anesthesia Care Provider

Anesthesia care should be provided by an experienced individual who is familiar with children with CHD, the planned operative procedure, and the surgeon's usual approach. The most important factor that an anesthesiologist can offer a child with CHD is a comprehensive understanding of the anatomic abnormalities, pathophysiology of the cardiac malformation, and how this may be affected by the anesthetic and surgical procedure. Familiarity with the most likely residua and sequelae is essential.[18] Adequate communication among all physicians involved enhances the likelihood of the best possible outcome.

#### Premedication

The use of premedication to provide sedation and anxiolysis is routine before most surgical procedures because some degree of fear or anxiety is expected. This facilitates parental separation, entry into the operating room, placement of monitors, and induction of anesthesia. The cardiorespiratory effects of premedication in children may be influenced by the underlying systemic disease.[48-52]

Commonly used premedications include oral or intravenous benzodiazepines, opioids, and small amounts of hypnotic agents. Drugs such as barbiturates and ketamine are occasionally used. Alternative routes for premedication include intramuscular, intranasal, and rectal methods. Children with hemodynamic decompensation may require little or no premedication. Caution should also be exercised for those with a history of cardiovascular pathology associated with significant increases in pulmonary artery pressure or pulmonary arteriolar resistance because hypoventilation and hypoxemia may be detrimental. Conversely, children susceptible to hypercyanotic episodes or those with catecholamine-induced arrhythmias may benefit from heavy premedication. In selected children (e.g., infants and children with cyanotic heart disease), oxygen saturation monitoring after premedication and the administration of supplemental oxygen is recommended.[50]

### Intravenous Access

Secure intravenous access is mandatory for administration of fluids and medications during anesthesia care. In most children with CHD, intravenous access is established after an inhalational induction. In those considered at great risk, such as children with severe outflow tract obstruction, moderate to severe cardiac dysfunction, pulmonary hypertension, or potential for hemodynamic compromise, consideration should be given for placement of intravenous access before induction of anesthesia or very early in the induction. The size of the intravenous catheter should be determined by the anticipated fluid requirements. If peripheral access is poor, central venous access may be necessary, particularly if there is potential for large intravascular volume shifts and to allow monitoring of central venous pressure. Placement of a central venous catheter may be assisted by audio Doppler or two-dimensional ultrasound guidance (see Chapter 48). In the small infant with single-ventricle physiology, central venous cannulation with catheter placement in the superior vena cava may be undesirable in view of concerns about potential vascular complications that may affect pulmonary blood flow or subsequent surgical palliation. In these children, a small catheter or alternative approach (e.g., femoral venous access) should be considered. In children with an existent or potential right-to-left shunt, all air must be removed from intravenous infusion tubing. Air filters may be difficult to use in the operating room because they may restrict the rate at which intravenous fluids or blood may be administered in emergency situations. They may be more useful in the preoperative and postoperative periods.

### Emergency Drugs

In view of the potential for hemodynamic instability in some children with CHD that may occur under any circumstance and at any time, drugs for emergency situations should be prepared or immediately available to the anesthesiologist providing care.

## MONITORING

A basic principle of intraoperative monitoring is to use techniques or devices that provide useful information to help with clinical decision making and to avoid monitors that are distracting or redundant. Basic monitoring involves observation of the child, including skin color, capillary refill, respiration, pulse palpation, events on the surgical field, and color of shed blood. Standard noninvasive monitors used during most surgical interventions include oscillometric blood pressure assessment, electrocardiography, pulse oximetry, capnography, and temperature monitoring. A precordial stethoscope can be extremely helpful for monitoring changes in heart tones that may suggest early hemodynamic compromise. In the child with CHD, relatively sophisticated and invasive monitoring may be needed.

### Arterial Blood Pressure Assessment

Basic blood pressure monitoring begins with pulse palpation. An automated blood pressure cuff is used in most children. The selection of monitoring site may be influenced by vascular anomalies (e.g., aortic arch pathology, aberrant origin and course of aortic arch vessels) or prior surgical interventions (e.g., Blalock-Taussig shunt, arterial cutdown). Direct systemic blood pressure monitoring by an indwelling arterial catheter may be necessary for beat-to-beat assessment and for blood gas analysis. In children, this is usually accomplished after induction of anesthesia. Arterial cannulation can be achieved percutaneously in most circumstances with a reduced risk of complications (see Chapter 48). Use of the radial arteries is preferable, particularly in the neonate, to minimize catheter-related vascular problems. Ultrasound guidance with Doppler or two-dimensional imaging may facilitate cannulation. The decision regarding the need for invasive monitoring is largely based on the child's clinical condition and nature of the surgical procedure.

### Electrocardiography

An ECG is used to monitor heart rate, cardiac rhythm, and ST-segment analysis. One or multiple leads typically are displayed. Most systems use two leads: standard lead II for arrhythmia monitoring plus inferior ischemia detection and precordial lead $V_5$ for lateral ischemia detection. Arrhythmias may occur as a result of hypoxia, electrolyte imbalances, acid-base abnormalities, intravascular or intracardiac catheters, and surgical manipulations near or around the thorax. Ischemia may be evident on direct examination of the ECG or ST-segment analysis.[53] Although in the adult population this is associated with worsened outcome, the implication for children is unknown.[54,55]

### Pulse Oximetry

Placement of an oximeter probe is well tolerated, even by uncooperative children, and it is typically one of the earliest monitors applied during induction of anesthesia. Monitoring arterial oxygen saturation is particularly useful in infants, cyanotic children, and those with complex anatomy or significant hemodynamic compromise. In addition to providing continuous assessment of oxygen-hemoglobin saturation and heart rate, the pulse oximeter waveform may indicate the adequacy of peripheral perfusion and cardiac output.[56,57] Other parameters that may be reflected by the $SpO_2$ include intracardiac or great artery–level shunting and pulmonary blood flow.

### Capnography

Capnography can confirm proper endotracheal tube placement, help to assess the adequacy of ventilation, and aid recognition of pathologic conditions such as bronchospasm, airway obstruction, and malignant hyperthermia. In spontaneously breathing, sedated children receiving supplemental oxygen through a nasal cannula, capnography monitors the end-tidal or exhaled carbon dioxide ($PETCO_2$) concentration. A prospective, observational study in children undergoing cardiac catheterization with sedation administered by nonanesthesiologists found that monitored $PETCO_2$ values provided a reasonable estimate of arterial blood $CO_2$ values.[58] Although the absolute value for $PETCO_2$ may not be as reliable as in the presence of an endotracheal tube, the capnograph waveform confirms the presence or absence of respirations and air exchange. End-tidal $CO_2$ monitoring also provides a gross index of pulmonary blood flow. In children with cyanotic heart disease, $PETCO_2$ values may underestimate arterial carbon dioxide tension ($PaCO_2$) measurements due to altered pulmonary blood flow and ventilation/perfusion mismatch.[59,60]

### Temperature Monitoring

Temperature should be routinely monitored during most procedures. Although temperature swings are usually not profound, some children, particularly small neonates, may become significantly hypothermic because of the large body surface area to body weight ratio and decreased amount of subcutaneous tissue. This may influence oxygen delivery (i.e., increased oxygen consumption) and emergence from anesthesia, cause detrimental changes in hemodynamics, and affect hemostasis.

### Urinary Output Measurements

The production of urine is a useful index of the adequacy of renal perfusion and cardiac output. Urine output is usually monitored during cases involving major fluid shifts or blood loss or when the surgical procedure is expected to be prolonged. No specific value for urine output is necessarily predictive of good renal function in the postoperative period.

### Transesophageal Echocardiography

Numerous publications have documented the utility of transesophageal echocardiography as a monitoring device in high-risk adults undergoing noncardiac procedures.[61-72] Sporadic reports have demonstrated the utility of this imaging approach in children undergoing noncardiac surgery.[73-78] However, the contribution or application of this modality in the pediatric age group in this particular setting has not been well defined and requires further investigation.

## SELECTION OF TECHNIQUES AND AGENTS

Several anesthetic regimens have been used in children with CHD undergoing noncardiac surgery and studies or procedures that require deep sedation or immobility. Although no single formula or recipe is recommended, the anesthetic techniques and agents used for a particular situation should be selected in consideration of the procedure, the child's disease process and functional status, and the impact of the hemodynamic effects of the anesthetic and procedure on the pathophysiologic process. Factors such as age, physical characteristics, and preferences of the anesthesiologist must be taken into consideration. The primary goals of anesthesia management with respect to the cardiovascular system are to optimize systemic oxygen delivery, maintain myocardial performance within expected parameters for the patient, and ensure the adequacy of cardiac output. A potentially limited cardiovascular reserve, reduced tolerance for perioperative stress, and detrimental alterations of the balance between pulmonary and systemic blood flow during anesthesia and surgery should be considered. A carefully titrated anesthetic, regardless of the specific agent, is optimal.

### Anesthesia Technique

General anesthesia has the advantages of wide acceptance, ease of application, and relative certainty of effect. It is the appropriate choice for most children undergoing noncardiac surgery. Disadvantages include a greater potential for wide fluctuations in the hemodynamics and a prolonged recovery period. The intravenous route allows for rapid induction of anesthesia. If intravenous access is not available, inhalational induction may be performed. Inhalational anesthetics dilate vascular beds and reduce sympathetic responsiveness. These are desirable goals for most children, even those with heart disease, because adequate myocardial function and a reactive sympathetic nervous system are usual. However, children with ventricular dysfunction may require an increased resting sympathetic tone to maintain systemic perfusion. Potent inhalational agents in this setting may further impair myocardial function, decrease sympathetic tone, and potentially cause cardiovascular decompensation. These children and others with a relatively fixed cardiac output may require a technique that combines several medications (i.e., balanced technique) to achieve anesthesia while minimizing the risk of hemodynamic compromise. A potent opioid, amnestic agent, and muscle relaxant technique minimizes myocardial depression and tends to leave sympathetic responsiveness intact while providing analgesia, amnesia, and immobility.

Regional anesthesia has been safe and effective in children with CHD (see Chapters 41 and 42).[76-79] Advantages of regional anesthesia, such as epidural and spinal techniques, include an effect largely limited to the surgical site, decreased number of systemic medications, a potentially brief recovery period, and usually a more pleasant experience for the child. Use of these techniques, however, may not always be effective. Regional anesthesia retains the potential for hemodynamic compromise, particularly in hypovolemic children or those with a fixed cardiac output. It is also contraindicated in those with coagulation defects. The administration of agents such as local anesthetics, opioids, or other adjuvants (e.g., clonidine) into the caudal space may attenuate the sympathetic outflow associated with surgical manipulation and noxious stimuli and facilitate postoperative pain management.

The choice of technique affects termination of the anesthesia and emergence. Anesthesia performed with fewer agents is inherently simpler and usually easier and more predictable to terminate. The availability of ultra-short-acting opioids (e.g., remifentanil) and other agents (e.g., dexmedetomidine) has avoided the need for postoperative ventilation solely related to residual effects of depressant drugs. Ventricular function and the presence of intracardiac shunts can significantly affect uptake and distribution of inhalational anesthetics and the kinetics of intravenous medications (see Chapter 6).

### Inhalational Agents

The use of inhalational anesthetics has been at the forefront of pediatric anesthesia practice for many years.[80,81] Sevoflurane was introduced in the mid-1990s, replacing halothane for induction of anesthesia in many centers. A study on the safety and efficacy of inhaled agents in infants and children with CHD during cardiac surgery demonstrated twice as many episodes of hypotension, moderate bradycardia, and emergent drug use in those who received halothane compared with those who received sevoflurane.[82] These data and those from other studies that demonstrated the potential benefits of sevoflurane on hemodynamic stability and minimal impact on myocardial performance led to sevoflurane becoming the preferred anesthetic agent for children, particularly those with heart disease.[83-88] Nonetheless, in some jurisdictions and under some conditions, halothane may remain the primary anesthetic for children.

### Intravenous Agents

*Propofol* is one of the most frequently used medications for intravenous sedation and general anesthesia. It has been used in children with CHD in numerous settings.[89-92] The hemodynamic effects of propofol have been investigated in children with normal hearts and in those with cardiovascular disease. An echocardiographic study in infants with normal hearts undergoing elective surgery demonstrated that propofol did not alter heart rate, shortening fraction, rate-corrected velocity of circumferential fiber shortening, or cardiac index after intravenous induction.[93] However, this medication decreased arterial blood pressure to a greater extent than thiopental, an effect attributed to a reduction in afterload. A comparison of propofol and ketamine during cardiac catheterization found that propofol caused a transient decrease in mean arterial pressure and mild arterial oxygen desaturation in some children.[94] In view of the significantly faster recovery, it was concluded that propofol was a practical alternative to ketamine for elective cardiac catheterization in children.

Another investigation in 30 children with CHD undergoing cardiac catheterization demonstrated significant decreases in mean arterial blood pressure and systemic vascular resistance during propofol administration.[89] No changes in heart rate, mean pulmonary artery pressure, or pulmonary vascular resistance were observed. In children with intracardiac shunts, the net result of propofol was a significant increase in the right-to-left shunt, a decrease in the left-to-right shunt, and decreased pulmonary-to-systemic blood flow ratio, resulting in a statistically significant decrease in the $PaO_2$ and arterial oxygen saturation ($SaO_2$), as well as reversal of the shunt direction from left-to-right to right-to-left in two patients. It was also shown that propofol could lead to further hemoglobin desaturation in children with cyanotic heart disease.

The effects of propofol have been examined in children undergoing electrophysiologic testing and radiofrequency catheter ablation for tachyarrhythmias. The drug has no significant effect on sinoatrial or atrioventricular node function or accessory pathway conduction in Wolff-Parkinson-White syndrome.[95,96] However, a study documented that ectopic atrial tachycardia may be suppressed during propofol administration in children.[97]

Collectively, these data suggest that the judicious use of propofol may be a reasonable option in children with adequate cardiovascular reserve who can tolerate mild decreases in myocardial contractility and heart rate and mild to moderate decreases in systemic vascular resistance. The effects of propofol on the direction and magnitude of intracardiac shunts may be an important consideration in children with cyanotic heart disease and may influence the hemodynamic assessment of those undergoing evaluation of pulmonary-to-systemic blood flow ratios in the cardiac catheterization laboratory.

*Thiopental*, a rapid-acting barbiturate, was used for many years for induction of anesthesia. Several investigations have documented the cardiovascular responses to this agent in the pediatric age group. In children with normal hearts, the cardiac index remains unchanged, although the shortening fraction decreases and alterations in load-independent parameters of contractility occur.[93] The myocardial depressant properties of barbiturates are well established, as are its effects on venodilation and blood pooling in the periphery. These data suggest that a subset of children who receive thiopental may be at risk for hemodynamic instability. It has been suggested that thiopental should be used with caution, particularly in those with limited reserve or increased sympathetic tone. Thiopental is not available for use in the United States.

*Etomidate,* a carboxylated imidazole derivative, has anesthetic and amnestic properties but no analgesic effects. This agent demonstrates favorable qualities over other intravenous drugs due to its lack of effect on hemodynamics.[98,99] This, combined with laboratory and clinical data that support minimal effects on myocardial contractility, makes this drug a particularly desirable agent in critically ill children and in those with limited cardiovascular reserve.[100] Despite these benefits, several undesirable adverse effects are associated with etomidate, including pain on intravenous administration, myoclonic movements that may mimic seizure activity, and inhibition of adrenal steroid synthesis perioperatively.[101,102] Although used primarily as an induction agent, etomidate has been administered for sedation of children during cardiac catheterization and in other settings.[103-105] A concentrated form of this medication is available in Europe but not in the United States.

*Ketamine* is a dissociative anesthetic agent administered by the intravenous, intramuscular, and oral routes. In view of its sympathomimetic effects that result in an increased heart rate, blood pressure, and cardiac output, this drug has been widely used in children with heart disease, particularly in younger children. The effects of this agent on systemic vascular resistance make it a suitable choice in children with right-to-left shunts because pulmonary blood flow is enhanced. This contrasts with inhalational agents, which by causing systemic vasodilation may decrease pulmonary blood flow in the presence of an intracardiac communication and potentially worsen the degree of cyanosis. In clinical use, however, oxygen saturation typically increases with both agents. Additional favorable properties include intense analgesia at subanesthetic doses and a lack of respiratory depressant effects.

Several investigations have addressed the concern of potential detrimental changes in pulmonary vascular tone resulting from ketamine although no significant effects have been reported on pulmonary arterial pressures and pulmonary vascular resistance at the usual clinical doses.[106-109] Regarding its effect on myocardial performance, in-vitro investigations have shown a direct myocardial depressant effect in animal species and the failing adult human heart. This is considered to be the result of inhibition of L-type voltage-dependent calcium channels in the sarcolemmal membrane and may be a consideration in critically ill infants with severely impaired cardiac reserves. Additional undesirable effects of ketamine include emergence reactions, excessive salivation, vomiting, and increased intracranial pressure.

*Dexmedetomidine* is a selective $\alpha_2$-adrenergic agonist agent being increasing used in the pediatric age group. Compared with clonidine, the drug exhibits greater specificity for the $\alpha_2$-adrenergic receptor over the $\alpha_1$-adrenergic receptor. Favorable effects of the drug include sedation, anxiolysis, and analgesia. This medication provides hemodynamic stability, although adverse effects have been reported, including bradycardia, hypertension, and hypotension. A study of the hemodynamic effects in children undergoing dexmedetomidine sedation for radiologic imaging demonstrated modest decreases in heart rate and blood pressure. These changes in response to moderate doses were independent of age, required no pharmacologic interventions, and did not result in any adverse events; however, high dose dexmedetomidine can be associated with significant bradycardia.[110,110a] In addition, treatment of dexmedetomidine-induced bradycardia with glycopyrrolate (5 µg/kg) has been associated with severe persistent hypertension.[110b]

Dexmedetomidine is used as a premedication agent, during diagnostic studies and procedural sedation, to reduce emergence delirium, in the treatment of symptoms associated with opioid withdrawal, and as an adjuvant agent in the operating room and postoperative settings.[111] In children with CHD, its benefits have been reported during monitored anesthesia care, diagnostic and interventional cardiac catheterization, intraoperative sedation, after cardiac and thoracic surgery, as a primary agent during invasive procedures, and in the treatment of perioperative atrial and junctional tachyarrhythmias.[112-119] This medication has also been used in children with pulmonary hypertension with good results.[120,121]

The effects of dexmedetomidine on cardiac electrophysiology have been examined in children; the drug significantly depresses sinus and atrioventricular nodal function.[122] Other findings included a reduction in the heart rate and increases in arterial blood pressure. Hammer and colleagues concluded that this medication should be considered undesirable for electrophysiologic studies and that it could be associated with adverse effects in patients at risk for bradycardia or atrioventricular block.[122] In contrast, another study concluded that dexmedetomidine was not associated with any significant or any atypical ECG interval abnormalities, except for a trend toward a decrease in heart rate in children with CHD.[123] Until additional data are available, it may be prudent to exercise caution when considering the use of dexmedetomidine in children with conduction abnormalities.

Although the experience suggests an overall safety profile in children with CHD, fragile patients may not tolerate the heart rate and blood pressure fluctuations associated with dexmedetomidine administration. Significant adverse effects have been described that include severe bradycardia progressing to asystole.[124]

*Opioids* and *benzodiazepines* are widely used medications in pediatric anesthesia practice. Opioids attenuate the neuroendocrine stress response associated with anesthesia and surgery.[125,126] After repair of CHD, these medications have been shown to blunt the stress response in the pulmonary circulation elicited by airway manipulations.[127] Morphine administration may be associated with histamine release and hypotension. The synthetic opioids are devoid of these effects and provide excellent hemodynamic stability with minimal changes in heart rate and blood pressure in children with CHD.[128] The primary concern about opioid administration is their central respiratory depressant effects because their primary cardiovascular manifestations are minimal. Benzodiazepines provide sedation and amnesia during the perioperative period. Midazolam administration may allow a reduction in the inspired concentration of inhalational anesthetic agents, which is a desirable feature in children with labile hemodynamics or in those considered at great risk for the myocardial depressant properties of inhalational anesthetics. Studies of the effects of benzodiazepines in children with CHD are limited.[129]

*Neuromuscular blocking drugs* facilitate endotracheal intubation and prevent reflex movement during surgery if the anesthetics alone are insufficient. All inhalational anesthetics potentiate the effects of nondepolarizing muscle relaxants. These medications have various onsets and durations of action and diverse hemodynamic effects. The cardiovascular and autonomic effects of muscle relaxants have been characterized mainly in adults with acquired cardiovascular disease[130-133] (see also Chapter 6). Drug selection is based on the need to facilitate endotracheal intubation and surgical relaxation, hemodynamic side effects, and the anticipated duration of surgery.

## INDUCTION OF ANESTHESIA

Induction of anesthesia in children with CHD most commonly can be accomplished using the inhaled or intravenous route. The intramuscular route (i.e., ketamine administration) may be preferable in some cases, particularly in an uncooperative, developmentally delayed, or combative child. Less common induction techniques include subcutaneous, intranasal, and rectal administration of agents. These various approaches may also be used in combination (see Chapter 4).

An intravenous induction may be preferable in some children in view of its potentially greater safety margin. In addition to the ability to titrate medications and rapidly correct hemodynamic alterations, other benefits include the speed of effect, although this may be slowed in children with large left-to-right shunts due to recirculation of the drug in the lungs. Left-to-right shunting results in a less concentrated amount of anesthetic agent reaching the brain and delayed onset of action. Right-to-left shunts speed intravenous induction because a significant portion of the medication bypasses the lungs (where it is degraded) and directly enters the systemic circulation, reaching the brain more rapidly than an intact circulation.

If intravenous access is not available, an inhalational induction is performed in most cases. A carefully titrated inhalational induction and early placement of an intravenous catheter usually is safe even in children with moderate hemodynamic disturbances, particularly after premedication has been given. This produces loss of consciousness, with acceptable conditions for establishing intravenous access. Inhalational induction may be delayed in cyanotic children and those with right-to-left shunts, particularly for anesthetics with reduced blood solubility, because the decreased pulmonary blood flow limits the rate of increase in the concentration of the anesthetic in the systemic arterial blood. The rapidity of an inhalational induction is increased in the presence of a reduced cardiac output because the anesthetic partial pressure in the alveoli increases more rapidly as less anesthetic is removed by the smaller pulmonary blood flow (see Chapter 6). Left-to-right intracardiac shunts have limited effects on the speed of induction of inhaled anesthetics.

## MAINTENANCE OF ANESTHESIA

After induction, anesthesia can be maintained using an inhalational, intravenous, or combined inhalational and intravenous technique. In children with CHD, anesthesia may result in hemodynamic changes regardless of the technique, agents, or experience of the anesthesiologist. Some children may not tolerate even minor alterations in hemodynamics. Factors that may lead to cardiovascular collapse in the marginally compensated child include hypovolemia, relative anesthetic overdose, increased vagal tone, positive-pressure ventilation, hypoxemia, airway obstruction, alterations in $Paco_2$ or other factors that influence the balance between systemic and pulmonary blood flow, myocardial ischemia, arrhythmias, and anaphylaxis. The anesthesiologist should be prepared to manage these rare but occasionally unavoidable occurrences.

## EMERGENCE FROM ANESTHESIA

Most children undergoing noncardiac surgical interventions are expected to awaken immediately at the completion of the procedure or shortly thereafter. This usually involves reducing and then discontinuing intravenous or inhalational anesthetics, antagonizing neuromuscular blockade, and extubating the trachea. Ensuring the return of protective reflexes and monitoring the adequacy of the airway and respirations are important considerations.

## Postoperative Care

The postoperative management of the child with CHD involves many of the same physiologic principles applicable to intraoperative care. The extent of the postoperative care, optimal place for recovery, and need for monitoring and hospitalization depend in large part on the child's clinical condition and type and extent of the procedure. Immediately after surgery, most children awaken from anesthesia and recover from muscle relaxants, which may impose various stresses and hemodynamic changes. Adequate oxygenation and ventilation along with airway protection must be ensured and may need to be provided if the child cannot manage these functions on his or her own. Significant hypoventilation must be avoided during this time because it may negatively affect pulmonary vascular tone and overall hemodynamics in vulnerable children with CHD. Adequate pain control and, sometimes, sedation are important postoperatively. This may be a challenging issue for the child who requires noncardiac surgery soon after a prolonged hospitalization in view of the increased likelihood for tolerance to analgesic and sedative drugs.

Observation and physical examination provide much information about the child's respiratory status, cardiac function, and systemic perfusion during the postoperative period. Adequacy of oxygenation and ventilation can also be assessed with noninvasive monitoring and blood gas analysis. Monitoring urine output may be helpful.

Hemoglobin or hematocrit values are monitored as a measure of oxygen-carrying capability in cases in which significant blood loss or the administration of fluids might have occurred. Serum electrolytes are screened if fluid shifts have taken place during the surgical and postoperative periods. Although digoxin is now used less frequently, particular attention should be given to the avoidance of hypokalemia in children receiving this drug. Serum glucose levels should be followed in neonates and small infants and dextrose-containing fluids administered as appropriate. Determination of ionized calcium ($iCa2^+$) levels may be indicated for patients with a history of DiGeorge sequence because of a propensity for hypocalcemia. The required fluid replacement is dictated by the child's heart defect, type of surgery performed, and volume losses (see Chapters 8 and 10).

## Perioperative Problems and Special Considerations

Several potential perioperative problems related to multiple factors may be encountered while caring for children with CHD who require noncardiac interventions. Because it is not feasible to detail all possible problems and potential concerns, this section highlights the more common issues to serve as a framework.

### HYPOTENSION

Hypotension may be related to hypovolemia due to prolonged fasting, volume loss, arrhythmia, anesthetic agents, myocardial dysfunction, or mechanical influences associated with the operative procedure. A practical diagnostic approach to the hypotensive patient is to consider factors that may affect ventricular preload, contractility, afterload, and the assessment of cardiac rhythm. Although the management of hypotension should be guided primarily by the causative factor, acutely increasing blood pressure by the administration of volume and an appropriate vasopressor, if indicated, often restores adequate perfusion while definitive therapy is instituted. Ensuring adequate intravascular volume with a fluid challenge often helps to restore perfusion and blood pressure, especially in hypovolemic patients. A pure α-adrenergic agent such as phenylephrine increases systolic blood pressure without further increases in heart rate. Some children are unable to tolerate any degree of myocardial depression or reduction in sympathetic outflow and require continuous inotropic support or vasopressor infusions throughout and after the operative procedure.

## CYANOSIS

Cyanosis is a common finding in children with defects characterized by limited pulmonary blood flow or intracardiac mixing. As surgical management strategies evolve to target the youngest of infants, the effects of cyanosis may be limited in these children. However, in those requiring delayed surgery, palliation, or staged correction of their defects, the effects of cyanosis may be long lasting. Chronic hypoxemia affects all major organ systems. Compensatory mechanisms that attempt to provide adequate systemic oxygen delivery in the presence of chronic hypoxemia include polycythemia, increases in blood volume, alterations in oxygen uptake and delivery, and neovascularization. Despite the favorable effects of the adaptive responses, these alterations may be detrimental. Polycythemia, the most significant compensatory response, is associated with increases in blood viscosity and red cell sludging. The common occurrence of iron-deficiency anemia in cyanotic children further enhances hyperviscosity and the unfavorable consequences of this condition. Several hemostatic abnormalities (e.g., thrombocytopenia, altered platelet function, and clotting factor abnormalities) have been documented as a result of hypoxemia and erythrocytosis that may affect the coagulation system and increase perioperative risks.[134-139] This is compounded by increased tissue vascularity, with a large number of blood vessels per unit of tissue.

The increased blood viscosity in children with cyanosis is associated with stasis and a risk for thrombotic events.[140] If the hematocrit exceeds 65% preoperatively, some clinicians advocate phlebotomy to reduce the hematocrit to 60% to 65%. This limits sludging of red blood cells and increases oxygen delivery to tissues. If blood is removed by preoperative phlebotomy, it may be saved for autologous transfusion in the perioperative period.

During the perioperative period, adequate hydration should be maintained in children with cyanotic CHD, and care should be taken to avoid prolonged venous stasis. Cyanotic children are at risk for paradoxical embolic events, mandating meticulous attention to intravenous lines during fluid or drug administration. This is a reasonable routine approach for all children with CHD, regardless of the nature of the structural abnormalities. The addition of air filters to intravenous tubing should not replace vigilance.

## TETRALOGY SPELLS

Hypercyanotic episodes may result from further decreases in pulmonary blood flow in children with tetralogy (i.e., tet spells) and significant dynamic right ventricular outflow tract obstruction. Tet spells are rare during noncardiac surgery, probably because general anesthesia attenuates the triggers. Occasionally, however, increased cyanosis may occur without warning in response to obscure stimuli. Whatever the cause, worsening

cyanosis implies increases in dynamic obstruction and exacerbation of ventricular-level right-to-left shunting. Factors that decrease systemic blood pressure and systemic vascular resistance, such as hypovolemia and extreme vasodilation, should be avoided. Therapy consists of increasing blood volume and systemic vascular resistance, the latter using either phenylephrine 5 μg/kg IV initially and then 1 to 5 μg/kg/min by continuous infusion or norepinephrine 0.5 μg/kg IV initially and then 0.1 to 0.5 μg/kg/min by continuous infusion. Increasing the inspired oxygen concentration and reducing inspiratory ventilatory pressures may also produce clinical improvement. Additional therapies include increasing the level of sedation or anesthetic depth and β-adrenergic blockade (esmolol [50 μg/kg/min] has largely replaced propranolol in this setting) (see also Chapters 15 and 16). Pulmonary vascular resistance does not play a major role in the physiology of hypercyanotic episodes in tetralogy of Fallot.

## HEART FAILURE

In infants, congestive heart failure is most often due to ventricular volume overload resulting from communications at the ventricular level or between the great arteries. Heart failure may also result from severe valvar regurgitation or obstructive lesions. Structural defects may lead to heart failure as a result of poor myocardial contractility, compromising cardiac output and not meeting the systemic demands.

In children with significant pulmonary vascular congestion, positive-pressure mechanical ventilation may be necessary before and after surgery. In cases of elective surgery, it may be of significant benefit to optimize medical therapy or address the particular defects before the planned procedure.

In a retrospective review of 21 children with severe heart failure who underwent 28 general anesthetics, 10% had a cardiac arrest requiring unplanned postoperative admission to the intensive care unit, and 96% required perioperative inotropic support. The investigators concluded that general anesthesia for children with severe heart failure is associated with a significant complication rate.[141]

## VENTRICULAR DYSFUNCTION

Children with CHD may have ventricular dysfunction involving the right heart, left heart, both sides of the heart, regional cardiac tissue, or global cardiac tissue. It may be temporary or permanent. In systolic dysfunction, contractile function is primarily impaired. Diastolic dysfunction is associated with abnormal relaxation or ventricular compliance. Some children have systolic and diastolic dysfunction. Ventricular dysfunction may result from factors such as age at the time of the operation and chronicity of the cardiac workload (pressure or volume); may be caused by the primary disease, myocardial hypertrophy, ischemia, or cyanosis; or may occur as a direct effect of surgery (e.g., ventriculotomy, cardiopulmonary bypass, ischemic time, circulatory arrest). Diseases that affect cardiac muscle (e.g., myocarditis, dilated cardiomyopathy) may be associated with congestive symptoms, whereas others (e.g., restrictive cardiomyopathy) may lead to diastolic heart failure.

In children with cardiomyopathy that was accompanied by severe ventricular dysfunction, general anesthesia for noncardiac procedures was associated with an increased frequency of complications.[142] They often required hospital support before and after the procedure that in many cases included intensive care management. Hospital stay was prolonged for children with severe ventricular dysfunction compared with those with a lesser degree of impairment. Based on these findings, early consideration of perioperative intensive care support was recommended for monitoring and optimization of cardiovascular therapy.[142]

## VENTRICULAR VOLUME OVERLOAD

Ventricular volume overload, which manifests as increased left atrial pressure, left ventricular end-diastolic pressure, and stroke volumes, is a common feature in many children with unoperated CHD. Long-standing volume overload results in atrial enlargement, ventricular dilation, and cardiomegaly. In the postoperative child, residual valvar regurgitation may be associated with altered loading conditions that, if significant, may result in congestive symptoms and ventricular dysfunction. The palliated single-ventricle patient may be particularly vulnerable to conditions associated with ventricular volume overload (e.g., systemic-to-pulmonary artery shunts).

## VENTRICULAR PRESSURE OVERLOAD

Pressure overload in the postoperative patient typically results from residual or recurrent muscular, valvar, or distal outflow obstruction or from increased pulmonary artery pressure or vascular resistance. In children with abnormal distal pulmonary arterial beds, for example, the hypoplastic vessels may not be amenable to surgical repair or other intervention, although associated defects may be satisfactorily addressed. This results in increased proximal pulmonary artery and right ventricular pressures and compensatory myocardial hypertrophy. Right ventricular pressure may exceed systemic values and compromise left ventricular function because septal shift may impair left ventricular filling or result in obstruction to systemic outflow. Abnormal pressure loads to the right ventricle may also result from progressive conduit stenosis after procedures that involve outflow tract reconstructions. Because of the anticipated need in children for successive conduit replacements, these surgical interventions are delayed as much as possible. This implies long-standing pressure loads on the myocardium with associated wall hypertrophy and potentially some element of ischemia until the criteria for surgical intervention have been fulfilled.

Whether the altered loading conditions affect the right or left ventricle primarily, the result is an increased demand due to the increased wall tension. This implies an increased susceptibility of the ventricular myocardium to the supply-and-demand relationship, a reduced tolerance for factors that may alter this fine balance, and an increased risk of ischemia.

## MYOCARDIAL ISCHEMIA

Several factors can cause myocardial ischemia in children with CHD. They include chronic hypoxemia, increased systolic and diastolic wall stress, and decreased coronary perfusion due to reduced diastolic pressures in the presence of large systemic-to-pulmonary shunts. The effects of cardiopulmonary bypass, aortic cross-clamping, and surgery itself cannot be ignored. Other conditions with a propensity for myocardial ischemia include congenital coronary artery lesions and the increased blood viscosity associated with cyanosis. The deprivation of myocardial perfusion may result in ventricular dysfunction and subsequent development of myocardial fibrosis.

## ALTERED RESPIRATORY MECHANICS

Chronically increased pulmonary blood flow and pulmonary artery pressures may result in progressive pulmonary vascular changes, increases in pulmonary vascular resistance, and alterations in lung mechanics. The primary effects on respiratory mechanics are related to increased airway resistance and decreased lung compliance. These alterations may have detrimental respiratory consequences in children with inadequate palliation or residual shunts. In some children, left atrial dilation may lead to respiratory compromise (e.g., air trapping, atelectasis) due to bronchial compression.

## PULMONARY HYPERTENSION

Pulmonary hypertension is a relatively common feature of unoperated CHD. It usually is the consequence of an increased pulmonary blood flow. One of the benefits of early correction is a reduction in pulmonary artery pressures and the incidence of pulmonary vascular reactivity after cardiac surgery. However, in some cases, pulmonary hypertension may persist or develop after an intervention.

A less common entity is increased pulmonary vascular resistance, which may be reactive or fixed. The diagnosis is formally determined at cardiac catheterization and involves pulmonary vascular reactivity testing. Pulmonary hypertension and increased pulmonary vascular resistance represent risks for major perioperative complications in children, regardless of cause.[143,144]

Acute increases in pulmonary vascular tone, also known as pulmonary hypertensive crisis, may result in cardiac arrest. In the presence of an intracardiac communication that allows for shunting, acute increases in pulmonary artery pressure may manifest as arterial desaturation, bradycardia, and systemic hypotension. In the absence of an intracardiac communication, the acute increase in right ventricular afterload may lead to unfavorable leftward shifting of the interventricular septum, compromising left ventricular filling and decreasing cardiac output.

Several factors can increase pulmonary vascular tone (Table 21-2). Therapy should be aggressive in the acute setting, aimed at reducing pulmonary artery pressures with interventions such as additional sedation, hyperventilation, hyperoxygenation, and treatment of acidosis. The use of selective pulmonary vasodilators (e.g., inhaled nitric oxide, other agents) and inotropic support of the right ventricle may be indicated. Manipulation of pulmonary hemodynamics is challenged by the difficulty of directly measuring these parameters in children. Management of critical situations requires a thorough understanding of the pathophysiologic process and experienced clinical judgment. Because of the significant morbidity and potential periprocedural mortality for children with a history of severe pulmonary hypertension, an in-depth evaluation of the risk/benefit ratio of the planned procedure and its impact on the overall quality of life is essential.

## ENDOCARDITIS PROPHYLAXIS

The latest guidelines of the American Heart Association for the prevention of infective endocarditis indicate that routine antibiotic prophylaxis is no longer needed for most children

| **TABLE 21-2** Factors Associated with Increased Pulmonary Vascular Tone |
| --- |
| Acidemia |
| Atelectasis |
| Hypercarbia |
| Hypothermia |
| Hypoxemia |
| Stress response, stimulation, light anesthesia, pain |
| Transmitted positive airway pressure |

with CHD (see Table 14-4).[145] In contrast to earlier guidelines, the administration of antibiotics solely to prevent endocarditis is not recommended for children undergoing genitourinary or gastrointestinal tract procedures, although neither of these subspecialty professional bodies have fully adopted the new guidelines. It is important to discuss the need for prophylaxis with the responsible physician.

The guidelines target individuals at increased risk for a poor outcome if they develop endocarditis (see Chapter 14). Preventive antibiotics for dental procedures are recommended for children with the following conditions:

- Prosthetic cardiac valve
- History of infective endocarditis
- Unrepaired cyanotic CHD, including palliative shunts and conduits
- Completely repaired congenital heart defect with prosthetic material or a prosthetic device, whether placed by surgery or by catheter intervention, during the first 6 months after the procedure
- Repaired CHD with residual defects at the site or adjacent to the site of a prosthetic patch or prosthetic device (which inhibit endothelialization)
- Cardiac transplant recipients who develop cardiac valvulopathy

## SYSTEMIC AIR EMBOLIZATION

Intracardiac shunts in children with CHD allow for the possibility of right-to-left shunting and paradoxical systemic air embolization. This risk is further enhanced by the increased right-sided pressures associated with many cardiovascular malformations. Because this may lead to catastrophic consequences, it is imperative to ascertain the presence of or likelihood for intracardiac or vascular shunting or to assume that this may be the case in most children and consider appropriate precautions.

## ANTICOAGULATION

Anticoagulants, antiplatelet drugs, and thrombolytic agents are increasingly being used in children, particularly in those with CHD.[146-150] Decisions regarding management are primarily influenced by the nature of the procedure, urgency of the intervention, specific drug therapy, and expected effects or laboratory data. The major concern is the potential for bleeding. Recommendations for the management of children taking warfarin (Coumadin) vary widely.[151-153] The proposed strategies are quite heterogeneous, and the lack of consensus reflects the paucity of randomized trials addressing this issue. The problem is further complicated by the lack of guidelines specific to pediatric practice.[154]

If the indications for anticoagulation are for native valve disease or atrial arrhythmias, the risk of a major thromboembolic event is considered to be relatively small, and warfarin may be discontinued 1 to 2 weeks before the day of surgery. In those with mechanical prosthetic valves, the risk of thromboembolic events is greater. Many recommend discontinuing the oral anticoagulant a few days before surgery and allowing the prothrombin time to return to within 20% of normal.[151] Administration of parenteral vitamin K or clotting factors, including fresh frozen plasma (FFP), may be required to restore the prothrombin time within an acceptable range, especially in those with liver disease and in emergency cases. Some experts advise preoperative hospitalization, particularly in high-risk individuals such as those with mitral or combined valve prostheses, to discontinue warfarin therapy and to initiate a heparin infusion, which is continued up until a few hours before surgery. Others suggest that low-molecular-weight heparin may be the better option instead of unfractionated heparin because the perioperative conversion from warfarin therapy to heparin can be accomplished without the need for hospitalization.[152]

Anticoagulation is usually reinitiated after 24 hours in children with valvular prostheses, and this may be achieved with a continuous heparin infusion or intermittent subcutaneous injections. The advantage of heparin is the ability to rapidly reverse the drug effect with protamine sulfate if bleeding complications occur. Oral anticoagulants are reinitiated 2 to 3 days after surgery if there are no bleeding concerns and the child is able to swallow oral medications. Although it has been suggested that there is no need to discontinue anticoagulation therapy for minor procedures, such as dental or ophthalmologic surgery in adults, guidelines for children are less clear.

The risk of bleeding from the surgical intervention versus the risk of a thromboembolism from a reduced anticoagulant dose determines to what extent and for what duration the anticoagulant therapy should be reduced. In some cases, the cardiologist and surgeon may decide to temporarily use aspirin therapy before and after surgery. There is disagreement regarding whether antiplatelet therapy is preferable to anticoagulation in children with prosthetic aortic valves or after certain surgical interventions.[155-158]

## CONDUCTION DISTURBANCES AND ARRHYTHMIAS

Acute rhythm disturbances may occur with the use of any anesthetic agent or technique and may be related to several factors. The administration of agents with vagolytic or sympathomimetic properties requires consideration in patients with prior history of or pathology associated with arrhythmias. Bradycardia may occur during induction of anesthesia, laryngoscopy, and endotracheal intubation, particularly in infants and in children with Down syndrome.[159-161] In most cases, bradycardia is self-limited and requires no therapy.

Certain lesions may be associated with rhythm abnormalities and the potential for acute hemodynamic deterioration, increasing perioperative risks. Conduction system disorders and rhythm disturbances may occur after cardiac surgery as a direct result of the procedure or may develop due to the inadequacy of the palliation or repair. Because cardiac arrhythmias are more prevalent among specific surgical subgroups, anticipation for their occurrence and planning for management are advocated.

## PACEMAKERS AND IMPLANTABLE CARDIOVERTER-DEFIBRILLATORS

An in-depth discussion of perioperative considerations related to implanted pacemakers or defibrillators can be found in Chapter 14. Consultation with a cardiologist or electrophysiologist is essential when caring for children with implanted devices. Unit interrogation and programming are required in most cases. The main goal is to avoid problems with hardware malfunction related to electromagnetic interference (i.e., electrocautery). Chronotropic agents and backup pacing modalities (e.g., transvenous, epicardial, transcutaneous) should be readily available and carefully considered in the event of pacemaker malfunction associated with an inadequate underlying heart rate. A magnet should be accessible to enable asynchronous pacing if required. Perioperative ECG monitoring is essential, as well as the use of modalities that can confirm pulse generation during pacing. Implanted devices should be interrogated and reprogrammed after the procedure.

## NERVE PALSIES

Surgery for CHD may be associated with transient or permanent injury to the recurrent laryngeal and phrenic nerves. Recurrent laryngeal nerve injuries may result in abnormal phonation or airway difficulties and lead to aspiration, particularly in small infants. Diaphragmatic palsies resulting from phrenic nerve injuries are associated with abnormal lung mechanics and limited pulmonary reserve, both of which may account for perioperative complications.

## EISENMENGER SYNDROME

Eisenmenger syndrome is characterized by irreversible pulmonary vascular disease and cyanosis related to reversal in the direction of an intracardiac or arterial level shunt.[162,163] This is unlikely to occur in the current surgical era, but it may occasionally occur in older children, adolescents, or adults with CHD. Morbidity is linked to problems associated with chronic cyanosis and erythrocytosis. Other problems include hemoptysis, gout, cholelithiasis, hypertrophic osteoarthropathy, and decreased renal function. Variables associated with poor outcome include syncope, increased right ventricular end-diastolic pressure, and significant hypoxemia (i.e., systemic arterial oxygen saturation less than 85%). Life expectancy is significantly reduced.[164] Most succumb suddenly, probably from ventricular tachyarrhythmias. Surgical modalities that have been advocated in selected patients include combined heart and lung transplantation[165] and lung transplantation alone.[166]

Despite the overall poor prognosis and the extremely high risk of a bad outcome, several reports have documented successes with a variety of anesthetic techniques and agents.[167-171] Nevertheless, it is vital that the family and patient, if of appropriate age, understand these risks before undertaking any procedure requiring anesthesia or deep sedation.

## CARDIAC TRANSPLANTATION

Cardiac transplantation may be considered the best option in end-stage cardiac pathology as a result of congenital or acquired disease.[172,173] A major consideration in the care of these children is the lack of external nerve supply of the transplanted heart. The physiology of the denervated heart implies that the usual autonomic regulatory mechanisms are not operational, increasing the vulnerability of transplanted children to hemodynamic alterations.[174] Compensatory responses may be delayed, further increasing the potential for compromise.

In the child with a transplanted heart, the resting heart rate is greater than normal due to the loss of parasympathetic inhibition. Critical determinants of cardiac output include the systemic venous return and maintenance of an adequate heart rate. During the early posttransplantation period, the heart rate is supported by exogenous chronotropes or pacing. Subsequently, the heart rate is driven by circulating catecholamines. Regardless of the time interval from transplantation, medications with chronotropic properties should be available, as should drugs with direct action on the myocardium and vasculature and access to emergent cardiac pacing modalities.

Chronic immunosuppression in children who have undergone cardiac transplantation presents several issues during noncardiac surgery. First, administration of multiple medications, particularly immunosuppressant agents, throughout the perioperative period is a concern. The potential need for stress-dose corticosteroids is a controversial subject. Second, immunosuppressive therapy is associated with adverse effects that may impact various organ systems. Cyclosporine administration, for example, increases systemic arterial blood pressure, potentially influencing hemodynamics. The drug is also responsible for renal dysfunction. Anesthesia management must consider potential alterations in hepatic and renal function. Third, strict aseptic technique is needed in managing a child with a compromised immune system.

An additional concern is the potential for graft vasculopathy (i.e., small-vessel coronary artery disease). Because older children or adolescents with ongoing myocardial ischemia may not experience anginal symptoms, it is reasonable to assume that most of these children are at risk for ischemic events, particularly those who are several years after transplantation.

## PERIOPERATIVE STRESS RESPONSE

The typical physiologic response to painful stimuli in normal children consists of an increase in heart rate and blood pressure and a transient decrease in $PaO_2$. These normal patterns, however, may be detrimental to children with CHD. Tachycardia may shorten diastolic filling time and diminish cardiac output, and hypertension increases ventricular afterload. The reduced ability of the postoperative child with CHD to increase cardiac output in response to stimulation and their limited maximal exercise capacity have been well documented for several cardiac malformations.

# Outcomes of Noncardiac Surgery

Limited data regarding the risks of noncardiac surgery and anesthesia in children with CHD raises concerns. A review of 110 children with CHD who underwent 135 anesthesias over a 1-year period found a 47% incidence of adverse events and more than one adverse event in a significant number of children.[34] Continuous monitoring of perioperative rhythm abnormalities in 70 children with CHD and a history of ventricular arrhythmias documented a 35% and 87% incidence of intraoperative and postoperative ventricular arrhythmias, respectively.[175] Other studies have reported cyanosis, treatment for congestive heart failure, poor health, and young age as risk factors.[35] A retrospective review of a large number of children documented that these risks involved major and minor interventions.[37]

Data from the Pediatric Perioperative Cardiac Arrest (POCA) registry shed further insight into this subject. Anesthesia-related cardiac arrests in children with congenital and acquired heart disease were examined. Causes of cardiac arrest were primarily cardiovascular in nature, occurring more frequently in those with heart disease than those without. Events occurred more frequently in the general operating room, usually during the maintenance period. Among children who suffered a cardiac arrest, the most common type of CHD was a single ventricle (i.e., Fontan physiology), particularly those managed early with palliation. The overall mortality rate for children with heart disease was greater than for those without heart disease, and children with aortic stenosis (i.e., Williams syndrome) and cardiomyopathy have the greatest mortality rate.[176]

# Specific Congenital Heart Defects

The anesthetic care of children with CHD undergoing noncardiac surgery is strongly influenced by the particular nature of the cardiovascular malformations, pathophysiology of the lesions, operative state (e.g., unoperated, prior palliative, definitive procedure), complications associated with the primary pathology or treatment, and other comorbidities.[12]

This section addresses relevant anatomic features, hemodynamic consequences of selected cardiac defects, and treatment strategies. Potential residua, sequelae (Table 21-3), and long-term outcomes of the lesions are discussed, focusing on their implications for perioperative care.

## ATRIAL SEPTAL DEFECTS
### Anatomy and Pathophysiology

Defects in the interatrial septum, or atrial septal defects (ASDs) (see Fig. 15-1), are among the most common congenital cardiac anomalies (30% to 40% of CHD) in childhood. ASDs occur in 1 of 1500 live births. Based on their location, several types of defects have been identified:

1. *Ostium secundum or fossa ovalis defect,* the most common type (75%), results from a deficiency in the region of the fossa ovalis (see Fig. 15-1, *B*). These defects may be associated with mitral valve prolapse or mitral regurgitation.[177-179]

2. *Ostium primum defect,* a form of atrioventricular septal (canal or endocardial cushion) defect (see Fig. 15-1, *A*),[180] is characterized by a deficiency in the inferior portion of the interatrial septum. They account for 15% to 20% of ASDs. They frequently are associated with a commissure or cleft in the anterior leaflet of the mitral valve and various degrees of regurgitation.

3. *Sinus venosus defect,* which occurs in 5% to 10% of ASDs, typically is located at the superior aspect of the interatrial septum, below the region where the superior vena cava joins the right atrium (i.e., sinus venosus defect of the superior vena cava-type) (see Fig. 15-1, *C*).[181] It is frequently associated with anomalous pulmonary venous drainage.[182]

4. *Coronary sinus defect* is uncommon and consists of a communication between the left atrium and mouth of the coronary sinus. It is commonly associated with an unroofed coronary sinus and persistent left superior vena cava that drains directly into the left atrium, resulting in a right-to-left shunt.[183]

5. *Other entities* that may allow interatrial shunting include a patent foramen ovale (PFO) at one end of the spectrum and a common atrium at the other. A PFO has been identified in as many as 25% of individuals. This communication may have implications for perioperative care because it has the potential for right-to-left shunting and paradoxical emboli.[184,185] In a common atrium, there is complete or near-total absence of the interatrial septum. This may be found in complex CHD.

An atrial communication allows mixing of the pulmonary and systemic venous returns. A left-to-right shunt allows pulmonary venous blood to enter the right atrium. The magnitude of shunting correlates with the size of the defect, relative ventricular compliances, and pulmonary artery pressures. A clinically significant defect results in right-sided volume overload. A pulmonary-to-systemic blood flow ratio ($\dot{Q}_{pulm}/\dot{Q}_{sys}$) that exceeds 2 to 1 and the potential detrimental effects of chronic right ventricular volume overload are indications for intervention.

### Treatment Options, Residua, Sequelae, and Long-Term Outcomes

Surgical closure of secundum ASDs in childhood provides excellent results, almost normal long-term survival, and negligible mortality.[186-189] Normal ventricular function should be anticipated after repair of these defects. Rarely, children may

demonstrate persistent right ventricular dilation and abnormal ventricular septal motion, but this may not be associated with a functional deficit.[190] Atrial arrhythmias and ventricular dysfunction may occur after late repairs as a result of chronic volume overload. Delayed defect closure may be a risk factor for the rare development of pulmonary hypertension or pulmonary vascular disease later in life due to the abnormally increased pulmonary blood flow.[191]

Transcatheter approaches are an alternative to surgery for closure of secundum ASDs in selected children, with excellent success rates for relatively small communications (see Chapter 20).[192-194] Complications are rare and may be associated with the intervention or occur at a later time.[195]

After surgical closure of ostium primum defects, morbidity manifests primarily as mitral valve dysfunction (e.g., mitral regurgitation) and left ventricular outflow tract obstruction.[196-200] In most children, outcomes are favorable after repair at an early age. After closure of sinus venosus defects, potential problems include pulmonary venous obstruction and loss of sinus node function.[201-203] Repair of coronary sinus defects consists of patch closure of the atrial communication at the mouth of the coronary sinus. This leaves a small right-to-left shunt as deoxygenated blood from the coronary sinus continues to drain directly into the left atrium.[204] If a connection between the left superior vena cava and left atrial connection persists, a variety of surgical approaches may allow redirection of the abnormal systemic venous return. For most children with atrial communications, significant postoperative sequelae are unlikely to occur, and outcomes are generally good. In most cases, no major repercussion from the repaired defect should be expected for future anesthesia care.

## VENTRICULAR SEPTAL DEFECTS
### Anatomy and Pathophysiology

Ventricular septal defects (VSDs) are the most common of all congenital cardiac anomalies, comprising 30% to 60% of CHD (excluding a bicuspid aortic valve) and occurring in 2 to 6 cases per 1000 live births (see Fig. 15-2, *A*).[205] VSDs can be found in isolation or in the context of other structural malformations. Large defects require early attention for symptoms related to congestive heart failure or pulmonary hypertension. VSDs have a greater rate of spontaneous closure in childhood—about 75% closure by 6 months to 1 year.[206,207]

Various classification schemes have been proposed for VSDs based on their anatomic location, size, restrictive or nonrestrictive nature, and hemodynamic significance.[208,209] The following scheme categorizes defects as four major morphologic types based on their anatomic location. In some cases, the boundaries of a defect may extend beyond the margin of a particular region of the ventricular septum into another.

1. *Perimembranous defects* (most common type) are located in the membranous region, under the septal leaflet of the tricuspid valve and just below the level of the aortic valve. They are frequently associated with redundant septal tricuspid valve tissue (e.g., aneurysm) that may limit shunting or eventually result in complete defect closure.

2. *Muscular defects* are located anywhere within the trabecular or muscle-bound component of the ventricular septum. Multiple defects give the appearance of a "Swiss cheese" septum, which complicates surgical closure.

3. *Doubly committed, subarterial or supracristal defects* are found within the region of the subpulmonary infundibulum. They

**TABLE 21-3** Potential Issues after Interventions for Selected Congenital Heart Defects

### Atrial Septal Defects

Residual intracardiac shunt

Persistent right ventricular dilation and abnormal motion of interventricular septum

Atrial arrhythmias, ventricular dysfunction if late repair

Pulmonary venous obstruction (sinus venosus defect associated with anomalous pulmonary venous return)

Mitral valve problems, left ventricular outflow tract obstruction (ostium primum defect with cleft mitral valve)

Development of pulmonary vascular disease (rare)

### Atrioventricular Septal Defects

Mitral valve problems (regurgitation, stenosis)

Left ventricular outflow tract obstruction

Residual intracardiac shunts

Atrioventricular block, conduction abnormalities

Prior palliation with pulmonary artery banding might have resulted in inadequate protection of pulmonary vasculature or distortion of pulmonary artery anatomy.

Pulmonary hypertension may persist.

### Coarctation of the Aorta

Systemic hypertension

Residual or recurrent obstruction

Death from untreated pathology related to heart failure, aortic rupture or dissection, infective endarteritis or endocarditis, premature coronary artery disease, or cerebral hemorrhage

Endocarditis risk with concomitant aortic valve disease

### Coronary Artery Anomalies

May go unsuspected for some time

Myocardial ischemia

Ventricular dysfunction

May present as syncope or lead to sudden death

### D-Transposition of the Great Arteries

Residual pathology (e.g., intracardiac shunts, outflow tract obstruction)

After atrial baffle procedure: baffle leak, obstruction of systemic or pulmonary venous pathways, progressive right ventricular dilation or failure, tricuspid regurgitation, sinus node dysfunction, or atrial arrhythmias

After arterial switch operation: aortic root dilation, aortic regurgitation, supravalvar stenosis (pulmonary or aortic), or coronary insufficiency

### Ebstein Anomaly

Progressive tricuspid regurgitation and right-sided volume overload

Right ventricular dysfunction

Atrial tachyarrhythmias (including Wolf-Parkinson-White syndrome)

Potential for paradoxical right-to-left shunting in the presence of an interatrial communication

Valve repair or replacement may be necessary

### Interrupted Aortic Arch

Residual intracardiac defects

Subaortic obstruction

Residual or recurrent aortic arch obstruction

### Left Ventricular Outflow Tract Obstructions

Residual or recurrent obstruction

Aortic regurgitation, aortic root dilation

Risk of endocarditis

Ventricular dysfunction

Potential subendocardial ischemia if ongoing ventricular pressure overload

Coronary ostial stenosis, diffuse arteriopathy (supravalvar aortic stenosis)

Need for reoperation in those with bioprosthetic or mechanical valves or conduits

After Ross procedure: autograft or right ventricular homograft failure, progressive aortic root dilation, or aortic regurgitation

### L-Transposition of the Great Arteries (Congenitally Corrected Transposition)

Residual defects (e.g., shunts, outflow tract obstruction)

Systemic (right) ventricular dilation, dysfunction, failure

Left-sided (tricuspid) valve regurgitation

Atrioventricular block or arrhythmias

### Patent Ductus Arteriosus

Residual or recurrent shunting

Increased pulmonary vascular resistance (now rare)

### Right Ventricular Outflow Tract Obstructions

Residual or recurrent obstruction resulting in ventricular pressure overload

Pulmonary regurgitation may require intervention

After right ventricle–to–pulmonary artery conduit: need for intervention or reoperation related to conduit failure

### Single Ventricle

After aortopulmonary shunt: shunt stenosis with associated hypoxemia, ventricular volume overload, systemic ventricular dilation, distortion of pulmonary artery anatomy, or pulmonary hypertension

After bidirectional Glenn connection or hemi-Fontan procedure: progressive cyanosis due to venous collaterals or other vascular communications, allowing venous pathways to bypass the pulmonary circuit or due to development of pulmonary arteriovenous malformations (more likely with classic Glenn anastomosis)

After Fontan procedure: increased systemic venous pressures, right atrial hypertension (with atriopulmonary connection), sinus node dysfunction, atrial rhythm disturbances, atrioventricular valve regurgitation, hepatic dysfunction, thrombotic complications, coagulation defects, protein losing enteropathy, or progressive systemic ventricular dilation or dysfunction

### Tetralogy of Fallot

Residual or recurrent pathology (e.g., intracardiac shunts, right ventricular outflow tract obstruction, distal pulmonary artery bed abnormalities)

Progressive pulmonary regurgitation with need for repeat intervention (e.g., right-sided heart dilation, dysfunction)

Arrhythmias associated with poor hemodynamics

Syncope or sudden death (arrhythmogenic cause)

Restrictive right ventricular physiology

### Truncus Arteriosus

Residual intracardiac shunting

Revision of right ventricle–to–pulmonary artery reconstruction (for stenosis or regurgitation)

Truncal (aortic) valve stenosis or regurgitation

### Ventricular Septal Defect

Potential residual defects

Risk of endocarditis (diminishes with time after repair)

Aortic regurgitation

Rarely, increased pulmonary vascular resistance may not improve postoperatively may be associated with aortic valve herniation or prolapse into the defect and aortic regurgitation.[210]

4. *Inlet defects* are located in the posterior aspect of the ventricular septum close to the atrioventricular valves. Associated anomalies of the atrioventricular valves frequently coexist.

The characterization of VSDs based on their size and likely hemodynamic significance is extremely useful when caring for children who have not undergone repair:

*Small defect:* The pulmonary-to-systemic systolic pressure ratio is less than 0.3, and the $\dot{Q}_{pulm}/\dot{Q}_{sys}$ is less than 1.4. The defect causes negligible to minimal hemodynamic changes. Normal right ventricular systolic pressure, pulmonary vascular resistance, and left ventricular size are typically found.

*Moderate defect:* The systolic pressure ratio is greater than 0.3, and the $\dot{Q}_{pulm}/\dot{Q}_{sys}$ is 1.4 to 2.2. The defect may be associated with volume overload and congestive symptoms. Some degree of left atrial and left ventricular dilation exists, as well as increased pulmonary artery pressures.

*Large defect:* The systolic pressure ratio is greater than 0.3, and the $\dot{Q}_{pulm}/\dot{Q}_{sys}$ is greater than 2.2. The defect is associated with significant symptoms (e.g., failure to thrive, congestive heart failure). Cardiomegaly and increased pulmonary vascularity are frequent findings.

The physiologic effects of the communications that allow shunting at the ventricular level are determined by the size of the defect, amount of shunting, and relative pulmonary and systemic vascular resistances. Physiologically, isolated defects may be classified as pressure restrictive (i.e., right ventricular pressure less than left ventricular pressure) or nonrestrictive defects (i.e., equal or near-equal ventricular pressures). Restrictive defects often imply limited flow through the communication. This is frequently the case with small VSDs in which the pressure gradient determines the magnitude of shunting. If the defect is large and nonrestrictive, the amount of flow across the orifice depends on the ratio between the pulmonary and systemic vascular resistances. Reduced pulmonary vascular resistance in the context of a nonrestrictive VSD leads to a large left-to-right shunt, increased pulmonary blood flow, pulmonary hypertension, and increased myocardial work, as evidenced by a volume load to the left heart. Nonrestrictive left-to-right shunts result in pulmonary congestion and abnormal respiratory mechanics characterized by decreased lung compliance, increased airway resistance, and increased work of breathing. Increases in alveolar dead space and alveolar to arterial oxygen gradients are to be expected, as well as increases in minute ventilation and potential oxygen requirements.

An important perioperative consideration for children with defects associated with increased pulmonary blood flow is the pulmonary steal phenomenon, which may result from decreases in pulmonary vascular resistance as left-to-right shunting increases at the expense of systemic blood flow. This requires an appraisal of the factors that may influence pulmonary vascular tone to prevent compromises in systemic perfusion.

### Treatment Options, Residua, Sequelae, and Long-Term Outcomes

Surgical closure of VSDs early in childhood results in excellent outcomes, usually without sequelae.[211-213] Surgical intervention in older children may lead to reduced left ventricular function and increased left ventricular mass.[214] Small communications, although regarded as hemodynamically insignificant, may not be benign. This has led to ongoing controversy regarding the need

for definitive intervention. Several young children with moderate defects remain relatively asymptomatic until later life, when gradual decompensation may ensue related to increased end-diastolic volume and ventricular dilation. In these children, defect closure is indicated if the magnitude of the increase in pulmonary vascular resistance is not prohibitive, which is rarely the case. Severely increased pulmonary vascular resistance (more than 7 Wood units per m²) augments the risks associated with the surgical procedure, and it may not return to normal levels after the intervention.[215] If postoperative pulmonary hypertension persists, the prognosis is unfavorable, with the potential for eventual right ventricular failure.[216] Development of Eisenmenger syndrome (i.e., pulmonary vascular obstructive disease and reversal in the direction of the ventricular level shunt) has become rare due to early recognition and management of children with these defects.

Postoperative sequelae after VSD closure include residual or, less commonly, recurrent defects, arrhythmias or other conduction system disturbances, subaortic obstruction, and valvar regurgitation.[217] Although surgical closure is considered the gold standard, transcatheter closure by device placement is feasible for selected muscular and postoperative residual defects defects.[218,219] Early data demonstrate excellent closure rates with reduced rates of complications[220] (see also Chapter 20). Limited experience and follow-up are available with catheter-based interventions for closure of membranous communications.[221-224]

## ATRIOVENTRICULAR SEPTAL DEFECTS
### Anatomy and Pathophysiology

Atrioventricular septal defects (AVSDs), also known as atrioventricular canal defects or endocardial cushion defects, result in deficiency of the atrioventricular septum and altered formation of the atrioventricular valves (see Fig. 15-2, *B*).[225] These rare defects comprise only 4% of CHD cases, although they have a prevalence among patients with Down syndrome of 25%. AVSDs can be classified as follows:

1. The *complete form* (i.e., common atrioventricular canal defect) consists of an ostium primum defect, an interventricular communication at the superior aspect of the inlet or posterior muscular septum, and a common atrioventricular valve. They are frequently associated with various degrees of atrioventricular valve regurgitation.

2. The *partial form* (i.e., incomplete form) is characterized by an ostium primum ASD accompanied by a cleft or commissure in the left-sided atrioventricular valve. Two functionally distinct atrioventricular valvar orifices are usually identified (see "Atrial Septal Defects").

3. The *transitional or intermediate form* is a combination of a partial AVSD with a small, interventricular communication and two distinct atrioventricular valve components.

Complete defects are associated with nonrestrictive intracardiac shunting, excessive pulmonary blood flow, congestive heart failure, and systemic right ventricular and pulmonary artery systolic pressures. Without intervention, they may lead to early pulmonary vascular changes. The severity of atrioventricular valve regurgitation also influences the clinical presentation. Partial AVSDs are less likely to be associated with pulmonary overcirculation of sufficient severity to cause significant heart failure symptoms.

Perioperative concerns similar to those previously described in children with nonrestrictive ventricular communications are applicable, but they also are magnified in those with unrepaired complete defects. In children with increased pulmonary vascular resistance and a reactive pulmonary bed, issues such as airway manipulation, light anesthesia, hypoxemia, or hypercarbia may lead to an increase in pulmonary artery pressures to suprasystemic levels.

### Treatment Options, Residua, Sequelae, and Long-Term Outcomes

The surgical approach for complete defects has evolved from a two-stage intervention (i.e., initial pulmonary artery banding to limit pulmonary blood flow and subsequent complete repair) to a single strategy of primary repair in infancy. For a complete defect, this consists of partition of the common atrioventricular valve, patch closure of the intracardiac communications, and closure of the left-sided valvar cleft. The long-term outlook after repair is generally good, with a small likelihood of residual dysfunction.[226-228]

Postoperative problems include left atrioventricular valve regurgitation or stenosis, residual intracardiac shunting, atrioventricular block, and subaortic obstruction.[199,200] Occasionally, pulmonary hypertension persists or develops postoperatively; it is more likely in children with Down syndrome. In the remote past, uncorrected defects resulted in Eisenmenger physiology, accounting for significant late morbidity and early death.[229] Considerations for noncardiac surgery in children after surgical repair include the residual effects of the prior ventricular volume load, the status of the atrioventricular valve, and patency of the left ventricular outflow tract.

### RIGHT VENTRICULAR OUTFLOW TRACT OBSTRUCTIONS
#### Anatomy and Pathophysiology

Pulmonary valve stenosis is the most common pathology among children with right ventricular outflow tract obstruction.[230] Other lesions that result in obstruction to pulmonary blood flow include infundibular stenosis, muscle bundles within the body of the right ventricle, and anatomic alterations in the pulmonary arterial bed. These pathologies may be found in isolation or occur as part of more complex malformations. Such is the case in tetralogy of Fallot (discussed later), in which multiple anatomic levels of right ventricular outflow tract obstruction are typically encountered (see Fig. 15-5).

Although isolated valvar pulmonary stenosis is congenital in most cases, the disease can be progressive. In the uncomplicated or pure variant, an interatrial communication in the form of a PFO or secundum ASD may be identified, and the ventricular septum is intact.

The magnitude of right ventricular outflow tract obstruction is directly related to the degree of valvar narrowing. This imposes an afterload burden on the right ventricle, resulting in right ventricular hypertrophy, decreased ventricular diastolic compliance, and tricuspid regurgitation. In severe cases, the systolic pressure generated by the right ventricle may exceed that of the left ventricle. Cyanosis in children with pulmonary stenosis usually reflects right-to-left interatrial shunting and reduced pulmonary blood flow. It may be associated with severe right ventricular hypertrophy, fibrosis, or ventricular dysfunction.

Most children with mild to moderate valvar stenosis remain asymptomatic, and the pathology is relatively well tolerated chronically. Severe obstruction in older children is frequently associated with limited exercise tolerance. Subendocardial ischemia is a potential risk in children with a hypertensive, hypertrophied right ventricle. Management is directed at maintaining coronary perfusion and an inotropic state of the myocardium.

### Treatment Options, Residua, Sequelae, and Long-Term Outcomes

Percutaneous balloon valvuloplasty is very effective and currently considered the treatment of choice for valvar pulmonary stenosis, replacing surgical valvotomy in most cases. Outcomes are excellent, and long-term issues are rare.[231-233] Dysplastic valves have a less favorable response to catheter-based interventions, and affected children are more likely to require surgery. Indications for repeat intervention include residual right ventricular outflow tract obstruction and progressive pulmonary regurgitation.[234]

In children with significant right ventricular hypertrophy undergoing noncardiac surgery, adequate ventricular preload and optimization of volume status are recommended. Further increases in right ventricular afterload should be avoided in those with residual or recurrent outflow tract obstruction.

### LEFT VENTRICULAR OUTFLOW TRACT OBSTRUCTIONS
#### Anatomy and Pathophysiology

Left ventricular outflow tract obstruction may occur at the level of the aortic valve, supravalvar region, or subvalvar region. It may take place in isolation or as part of complex cardiovascular disease. A *bicuspid aortic valve* is the most common of all congenital cardiac anomalies, occurring in approximately 2% of the general population.[235] Although it may not necessarily imply valvar stenosis, this abnormality can be associated with progressive obstruction or regurgitation. A bicuspid valve may be found in asymptomatic individuals or within the context of severe left heart obstruction. The prevalence of coexistent defects is relatively large and frequently includes patent ductus arteriosus, VSD, aortic coarctation, and other abnormalities of the aorta and its branches.

Infants with critical aortic stenosis and those with severe obstruction require early intervention in view of ductal dependency, heart failure symptoms, and the degree of ventricular dysfunction. Older children with moderate to severe obstruction may present with decreased exercise tolerance, syncopal episodes, or myocardial ischemia. Impedance to left ventricular ejection in aortic stenosis results in elevation of left ventricular systolic pressure and increased myocardial force. Ventricular hypertrophy is the compensatory response to the increased afterload. Contractile function is normal to increased, but diastolic impairment may occur.

In *supravalvar aortic stenosis,* the narrowing typically occurs at the sinotubular junction. The coronary arteries arise proximal to the area of obstruction and are subjected to increased systolic pressures equal to that of the left ventricle. The arteriopathy found in many of these children may involve the origin of the coronary arteries or other systemic and pulmonary vessels.[236] This malformation may occur as part of Williams syndrome, which is characterized by elfin facies, mental retardation, idiopathic hypercalcemia, and other features. Several reports have described unexpected complications in these children, including death during anesthesia care.[237-240] Affected children should be considered at increased risk for any procedure.

*Subvalvar aortic stenosis* may take a variety of forms, including a discrete fibromuscular ridge or membrane, complex tunnel-like obstruction, or hypertrophy of the interventricular septum (i.e., hypertrophic cardiomyopathy). The association of left ventricular obstructive lesions such as a bicuspid aortic valve, subaortic stenosis, aortic coarctation, and mitral valve inflow obstruction (e.g., parachute mitral valve, supravalvar mitral ring) is referred to as the *Shone complex.*

Hypoplastic left heart syndrome (HLHS) represents an extreme form of left ventricular outflow tract obstruction (see Fig. 15-10). It encompasses a constellation of malformations, affecting left-sided cardiac structures (e.g., mitral and aortic valves, aorta, arch) (see "Single Ventricle").

Common features of the anomalies that result in obstruction to left ventricular output include a pressure gradient across the involved region, increased left ventricular systolic pressure, increased myocardial force, and left ventricular wall stress. With chronic obstruction, the hypertrophied myocardium is at risk for subendocardial ischemia as a consequence of an imbalance in the ratio of myocardial oxygen supply and demand. Factors such as increases in left ventricular afterload, inadequate hypertrophic remodeling, and decreases in myocardial systolic or diastolic performance may compromise stroke volume and contribute to cardiac dysfunction and heart failure in this setting.[241] These issues are relevant for children with more than mild obstruction, and they influence anesthesia care during noncardiac surgery or other interventions.

### Treatment Options, Residua, Sequelae, and Long-Term Outcomes

Individuals with a bicuspid aortic valve may remain asymptomatic for many years but are at risk for aortic stenosis or regurgitation and concomitant hemodynamic alterations. Some of those requiring surgical intervention during childhood undergo reoperation for recurrent stenosis or progressive regurgitation in the next 25 years.[242] Percutaneous balloon valvuloplasty may be a treatment option for critical or severe aortic valve disease.[243] Surgical alternatives include valvotomy, mechanical or bioprosthetic valve placement, and root replacement with homograft or autograft material. In the Ross operation, the native, diseased root is replaced by a pulmonary autograft, and an extracardiac conduit establishes continuity between the right ventricle and main pulmonary artery.[244] Repeat intervention for eventual failure of the right ventricular conduit is anticipated in these children.[245] In addition to surveillance of the right ventricular outflow tract, monitoring for aortic root dilation and concomitant regurgitation is an important component of follow-up.[246,247]

Management of discrete subaortic stenosis remains a challenge, and the timing of surgery is controversial.[248] Postoperative complications include residual or recurrent obstruction and progressive aortic regurgitation. For severe supravalvar obstruction, surgical intervention is recommended, and it results in adequate relief of the obstruction in most cases.[249]

Myocardial fibrosis and ventricular dysfunction may be a feature of severe aortic outflow obstruction in infancy. Although adequate relief of the obstruction results in significant clinical improvement, abolition of congestive heart failure, and myocardial remodeling in most children, ventricular hypertrophy or dilation persists along with various degrees of systolic or diastolic impairment in many. Other problems include myocardial ischemia, ventricular failure, and risk of sudden death.[250,251] Important concerns related to anesthesia and surgery are the potentially limited left ventricular functional reserve and alterations of the fine balance between myocardial oxygen supply and demand. Maintenance of coronary perfusion and ventricular contractile function is key in the care of these children. Pharmacologic agents with vasoactive and inotropic properties should be readily available during anesthesia care.

## PATENT DUCTUS ARTERIOSUS
### Anatomy and Pathophysiology

The ductus arteriosus is a vascular structure connecting the pulmonary trunk and thoracic aorta (see Fig. 15-4). It enables right ventricular output into the descending aorta during fetal life, within the context of typically increased pulmonary vascular resistance. Persistent patent ductus arteriosus (PDA) may be an isolated finding or associated with other forms of heart disease. Prematurity is an important risk factor.

The magnitude and direction of great artery shunting depends on the size of the communication and the pulmonary vascular resistance. In children with moderate or large left-to-right shunts, the physiologic effects are those of increased pulmonary blood flow and left ventricular volume overload.

### Treatment Options, Residua, Sequelae, and Long-Term Outcomes

Children with a tiny or small PDA have a normal life expectancy.[252] Those with hemodynamically significant communications eventually develop symptoms related to left ventricular volume overload. In some cases, this predisposes them to moderate or severe pulmonary hypertension. Although unlikely in the current era, in the past, the long-standing, high-pressure, and high-flow states associated with a moderate or large communication resulted in Eisenmenger syndrome in some children.

Ductal closure can be performed by surgical ligation or division. This is the favored approach in preterm infants and those with large communications.[253] Percutaneous catheter occlusion can also be accomplished with a good success rate[254] (see also Chapter 20). Video-assisted thoracoscopic surgery has been used for ductal ligation.[255,256] Regardless of the approach, interruption of this vascular structure is rarely associated with long-term issues. Children can expect a normal cardiovascular reserve and should be managed accordingly during future anesthesia care.

## COARCTATION OF THE AORTA
### Anatomy and Pathophysiology

Coarctation of the aorta is characterized by narrowing of the aortic lumen in the thoracic region. The constriction may be discrete or diffuse. In infants, a long, narrowed aortic segment often is associated with hypoplasia of the transverse arch and aortic isthmus, in which case other structural cardiac malformations may also exist.[257] Associated defects include a bicuspid aortic valve, VSD, mitral valve abnormalities, and other types of left-sided obstructive lesions.

Hemodynamic consequences result from obstruction to systemic blood flow and increased left ventricular afterload. During infancy, ventricular dilation and heart failure predominate. In older children, arterial hypertension is found proximal to the region of aortic obstruction, and they have some degree of left ventricular hypertrophy. Ventricular function is usually well preserved. Collateral circulation develops with a long-standing pathologic process.

### Treatment Options, Residua, Sequelae, and Long-Term Outcomes

Symptoms associated with severe aortic arch obstruction or concomitant cardiovascular pathology lead to early intervention in some children.[258] Alterations in ventricular systolic function associated with a neonatal presentation usually resolve after relief of the obstruction. Systemic hypertension and a residual gradient that exceeds 25 to 30 mm Hg are regarded as indications for repeat intervention. Various catheter-based and surgical approaches have been applied to the management of this lesion; each has advantages and disadvantages[259] (see also Chapter 20).

Repair at an early age is advocated in view of reduced surgical risks for the younger age group, and early repair minimizes late morbidity.[260] Long-term issues include systemic hypertension (independent of the hemodynamic result) and residual or recurrent aortic arch obstruction.[261] Left ventricular hypertrophy may persist in some children after repair, particularly in those undergoing interventions later in childhood. Abnormalities in diastolic ventricular function have been reported after successful repair.[262] Catheter techniques (i.e., balloon angioplasty with and without stent implantation) have been effective in relieving the obstruction and normalizing blood pressure.[263] This approach may be used as primary therapy or to address residual or recurrent disease.[264] Aortic aneurysms can occur around the area of coarctation or elsewhere in the aorta after surgical intervention or balloon angioplasty. Additional long-term problems result from coexistent defects, such as bicuspid aortic valve and premature development of coronary artery disease. Aortic coarctation has been associated with cerebral aneurysms.

## TETRALOGY OF FALLOT
### Anatomy and Pathophysiology
Tetralogy of Fallot (TOF) is the most common cyanotic cardiac lesion (see Fig. 15-5).[265] This malformation is characterized by right ventricular outflow tract obstruction, an interventricular communication, right ventricular hypertrophy, and aortic override. There is considerable variation in the severity of the disease, accounting for the spectrum of clinical manifestations. The subpulmonary obstruction arises from anterior deviation of the infundibular septum and may have dynamic and fixed components.[266] Pulmonary valve stenosis almost invariably exists, and the main pulmonary artery and distal branches often demonstrate various degrees of hypoplasia. The limitation of pulmonary blood flow and magnitude of ventricular level right-to-left shunting account for the degree of cyanosis.

Pressure overload accounts for hypertrophy of the right ventricular myocardium. The large, nonrestrictive VSD and the outflow obstruction result in a right ventricular pressure at systemic levels, and the pulmonary artery systolic pressure is reduced. Increases in the severity of the right ventricular outflow tract obstruction or decreases in systemic vascular resistance exacerbate right-to-left intracardiac shunting and systemic arterial desaturation, increasing the level of cyanosis. These features characterize hypercyanotic episodes or tet spells.

Several TOF variants are recognized, including the "pink" or mild forms at one end of the spectrum, and complex defects, such as pulmonary atresia with diminutive or discontinuous distal branches, at the other. Associated cardiovascular anomalies in children with TOF include an atrial communication, right aortic arch, multiple VSDs, persistent left superior vena cava to the coronary sinus, complete AVSD, and abnormal origin or course of the coronary arteries. Unoperated TOF is associated with the potential for hypercyanotic episodes and ventricular outflow tract obstruction.

### Treatment Options, Residua, Sequelae, and Long-Term Outcomes
The surgical management of TOF has evolved from a strategy of a staged approach with initial palliation using a systemic-to-pulmonary shunt to a single-stage, definitive repair in infants. Ongoing controversy exists about the favored approach in the neonate or very young infant in need of surgical therapy.[267,268] In selected cases, percutaneous balloon pulmonary valvuloplasty may be performed as a palliative, temporizing measure.[269] The definitive repair of TOF, although a successful operation enabling most children to be free of symptoms, may be associated with significant postoperative residua.[270,271] Volume loads may arise from pulmonary regurgitation, residual shunts, and the presence of aortopulmonary collaterals. Ventricular pressure loads, however, may result from residual or recurrent right ventricular outflow tract or obstruction to the pulmonary artery bed. This situation is associated with right ventricular hypertension, myocardial hypertrophy, and reduced ventricular compliance.

Conditions that may require repeat intervention include pulmonary regurgitation of significant severity, residual or recurrent pulmonary outflow tract obstruction, and residual, hemodynamically significant intracardiac shunts. Catheter-based procedures may be effective in the management of obstruction of the pulmonary vasculature, and they have been applied to rehabilitate the vascular tree in cases of significant underdevelopment. Children who have undergone right ventricle–to–pulmonary artery reconstruction by means of placement of an extracardiac conduit eventually develop conduit failure (i.e., stenosis or regurgitation) requiring reoperation.[272] Aortic root dilation can lead to increasing degrees of regurgitation and the need for surgical intervention.

In the past, most children underwent definitive repair at an older age, consisting of an extensive right ventriculotomy to facilitate resection of the infundibular obstruction and closure of the VSD. Many were also subjected to procedures that included placement of a large patch that encompassed the subpulmonic region, valve annulus, and supravalvar region (i.e., transannular patch). Although effective in relieving the obstruction, this approach invariably resulted in pulmonary regurgitation, which was reasonably well-tolerated but progressed over time.

On late follow-up, pulmonary regurgitation has been identified as a major cause of morbidity, and it may result in progressive right ventricular dysfunction due to significant volume overload, ventricular arrhythmias with their associated disabilities, and even death. In recognition of the long-term morbidity linked to severe pulmonary regurgitation, the surgical strategy for this defect has undergone reappraisal and modification over the years.[273] A current method uses a transatrial approach for closure of the VSD, minimizing the size of an infundibular incision (if one is required) and avoiding or limiting the size of the transannular patch.[274,275]

Although surgical refinements have led to overall improvements in postoperative outcomes, the preoperative evaluation of these children should include inquiries regarding exercise tolerance as an indicator of functional status and an appraisal of right ventricular function, residual pathology, potential rhythm abnormalities, and conduction disturbances. Magnetic resonance imaging is extremely useful in the evaluation of right ventricular systolic function, quantitation of the severity of pulmonary regurgitation, and evaluation of the distal pulmonary vascular bed. Electrophysiologic testing and programmed ventricular stimulation may be indicated to refine antiarrhythmic drug therapy, for ablation of arrhythmia foci, or for implantation of a cardioverter-defibrillator system.

Postoperatively, a subset of children develops a pattern that is characterized by right ventricular diastolic noncompliance, which is known as *restrictive right ventricular physiology*. It is associated with a reduced likelihood of progressive pulmonary regurgitation and right ventricular dilation. In these children, the right ventricle operates at a greater end-diastolic pressure, and the children demonstrate superior exercise performance in addition to a reduced likelihood of developing ventricular rhythm abnormalities.[276]

Perioperative goals for the child with pulmonary regurgitation and right ventricular dysfunction include optimizing right ventricular filling, maintaining or supporting right ventricular function, and minimizing factors that may further increase right ventricular work (e.g., increased pulmonary vascular resistance, increased peak inspiratory pressures). Any detrimental factor that may affect the right ventricle may also negatively affect the left ventricle due to ventricular interdependence. In children with restrictive right ventricular physiology, the myocardial supply-to-demand relationship is of particular importance because the stiff, poorly compliant right ventricular myocardium may not tolerate alterations in this balance and may be vulnerable to decreases in subendocardial oxygen delivery.

## D-TRANSPOSITION OF THE GREAT ARTERIES
### Anatomy and Pathophysiology

In D-transposition of the great arteries (D-TGA), the aorta arises from the anatomic right ventricle, and the pulmonary artery arises from the left ventricle (see Fig. 15-6). This anomaly accounts for the most common cause of cyanotic heart disease in the neonatal period. Associated defects include VSDs, left ventricular outflow tract obstruction, and coronary artery anomalies.

In D-TGA, the systemic and pulmonary circulations operate in parallel rather than in series, resulting in cyanosis. Mixing at the atrial, ventricular, or ductal level is essential for survival. Initial management in most infants includes prostaglandin $E_1$ therapy to maintain ductal patency and to enhance intercirculatory mixing. If restrictive, the interatrial communication may require enlargement by balloon atrial septostomy.

Because most neonates with D-TGA are otherwise healthy, the concerns before surgical correction primarily are those associated with diagnostic procedures or interventions in the cardiac catheterization laboratory. Considerations for anesthetic management primarily are related to cyanosis and heart failure, which are more likely to occur in infants with coexistent large VSDs. An inadequate communication for intercirculatory mixing may account for profound hypoxemia, potentially progressing to metabolic acidosis due to compromised tissue oxygenation. Less commonly, increased pulmonary vascular resistance may account for severe cyanosis despite prostaglandin $E_1$ therapy and an adequate anatomic communication.

### Treatment Options, Residua, Sequelae, and Long-Term Outcomes

Several decades ago, the approach to D-TGA consisted of an atrial baffle (i.e., atrial switch) or redirection procedure (i.e., Mustard or Senning operations). Physiologic correction was accomplished by allowing systemic venous blood to drain into the left ventricle and pulmonary artery while pulmonary venous blood was rerouted through the tricuspid valve into the right ventricle and aorta. The right ventricle remained as the chamber ejecting against systemic afterload. These procedures provided relief of cyanosis and reasonably good survival.[277] In the long term, however, this approach led to complications such as sinus node dysfunction and atrial rhythm disturbances.[278] Progressive right ventricular dilation, tricuspid (i.e., systemic atrioventricular valve) annular dilation, associated regurgitation, and eventual right ventricular dysfunction or failure were causes of major morbidity.[279-281] In addition to the rhythm abnormalities and conduction defects, this problem was thought to account for sudden death in some individuals later in life. Other problems included progressive obstruction of venous pathways and intracardiac shunting through atrial baffle leaks. Abnormal right and left ventricular responses to exercise have also been documented in these patients.[282]

The arterial switch operation (i.e., Jatene procedure) is the standard surgical approach in neonates with D-TGA. The repair establishes a normal, concordant relationship between the ventricles and their respective great arteries, achieving anatomic correction. The procedure involves transection of the arterial trunks above the level of the semilunar valves, anastomotic connections to their appropriate outflows, translocation of the coronary arteries to the neoaortic root, and closure of any intracardiac communications (see Fig. 15-7, *A-E*). Normal physiology is restored, enabling the left ventricle to function as the systemic pump. This procedure can be performed with good results, and long-term outcomes usually are very favorable.[283-286] Potential postoperative problems include supravalvar pulmonary or aortic obstruction. Neoaortic root dilation and aortic regurgitation may be identified on follow-up. Ventricular function is normal in most cases.[287]

Anesthetic management of most children after the arterial switch operation should be the same as in those without structural or functional abnormalities. However, there is some concern about coronary complications in these children that may not be evident clinically or identified by routine surveillance methods. Investigations have demonstrated postoperative regional left ventricular wall motion abnormalities, evidence of myocardial perfusion defects, and pathologic changes in the coronary vasculature, suggesting a risk for coronary insufficiency.[288-292]

## CONGENITALLY CORRECTED TRANSPOSITION OF THE GREAT ARTERIES
### Anatomy and Pathophysiology

Congenitally corrected transposition of the great arteries, also known as L-transposition of the great arteries (L-TGA), is characterized by malposition of the great vessels and ventricular inversion (i.e., atrioventricular and ventriculoarterial discordance). In this anomaly, the right atrium empties into an anatomic left ventricle, which then contracts into the pulmonary trunk. The left atrium opens into an anatomic right ventricle, which ejects into the aorta. The aorta is typically oriented in a leftward and anterior position with respect to the pulmonary artery.

Cyanosis is absent because the circulations are physiologically corrected. The anatomic right ventricle functions as the systemic pump. Associated defects are frequently present and include pulmonary outflow tract obstruction, a ventricular communication, and tricuspid (left-sided) abnormalities. In some individuals, this lesion may remain undetected until the onset of arrhythmias or syncope due to complete atrioventricular block or the effects of concomitant pathology.[293]

## Treatment Options, Residua, Sequelae, and Long-Term Outcomes

Without associated defects, children with corrected transposition may do well for many years. Development of complete atrioventricular block is common with increasing age.[294] Selected children, particularly those at a young age or with coexistent defects that maintain left ventricular pressure at systemic levels, may be suitable candidates for a surgical intervention that restores the left ventricle as the systemic chamber.[295] This complex repair, known as the double-switch operation or a variation thereof, combines redirection of the systemic and pulmonary venous flows in an atrial baffle procedure with the arterial switch operation. This strategy, however, may not affect mortality compared with conservative management.[296]

Issues that require long-term surveillance in children with congenitally corrected transposition include right ventricular performance and tricuspid valve competency.[297] The overall long-term survival of individuals with this condition is substantially reduced compared with age-matched controls.[298,299]

## TRUNCUS ARTERIOSUS
### Anatomy and Pathophysiology

Truncus arteriosus is characterized by a single arterial trunk that gives rise to the aorta, pulmonary root, and coronary arteries (see Fig. 15-8). A ventricular communication usually exists underneath the single arterial root or truncal valve. Various anatomic types are identified according to the origin of the pulmonary arteries from the arterial trunk.[300,301] Associated pathology includes a right aortic arch, aortic arch interruption, abnormalities of the truncal valve (e.g., abnormal number of cusps, stenosis, regurgitation), and coronary artery anomalies. Approximately one third of children with truncus arteriosus have DiGeorge syndrome (see Chapter 14).

Clinical features of the neonate with this defect largely depend on the status of the pulmonary vasculature. If the resistance is increased, the infant is well compensated. The normal decrease in pulmonary vascular resistance leads to symptoms related to pulmonary overcirculation and congestive heart failure, accounting for the need for surgical intervention early in life. Truncus arteriosus is one of the structural malformations associated with a significant risk for adverse events before correction, because balancing the pulmonary and vascular resistances may be quite challenging.[302] The physiology that characterizes a reduced pulmonary vascular resistance and a significant runoff setting is that of an increased arterial oxygen saturation, reduced diastolic arterial pressures (potentially leading to myocardial ischemia), systemic hypotension, impaired cardiac output, and hypoperfusion of distal beds.

## Treatment Options, Residua, Sequelae, and Long-Term Outcomes

Surgery for truncus arteriosus consists of detaching the main pulmonary artery segment from the truncal root, repairing the ensuing aortic wall defect, closing the VSD to allow left ventricular output through the arterial root, and placing an extracardiac right ventricle–to–pulmonary artery conduit. Alternative approaches to establishing this continuity have been performed without the use of conduits.[303]

Neonates undergoing truncus arteriosus repair have excellent survival rates.[304-307] Late complications include conduit failure, residual or recurrent pulmonary artery obstruction, and truncal valve problems. Truncal valve dysfunction may require repair or replacement. The main issues of concern are the status of the right ventricle–to–pulmonary artery conduit and truncal root, consequences related to semilunar valve problems, and biventricular function.

## EBSTEIN ANOMALY
### Anatomy and Pathophysiology

The classic findings in Ebstein anomaly for the tricuspid valve include a large sail-like anterior leaflet and apically displaced septal and posterior leaflets.[308,309] This configuration commonly results in an atrialized portion of the right ventricle and tricuspid regurgitation. Some degree of right ventricular dysplasia is common. An interatrial communication is a frequent finding, and it may produce right-to-left shunting and clinical cyanosis. The spectrum of disease ranges from minimal or no symptoms to intractable congestive heart failure.[310] A neonatal presentation implies a major clinical problem and usually portends a poor prognosis. Symptoms in older children include cyanosis, palpitations, dyspnea, and exercise intolerance. Initial symptoms may be related to supraventricular tachycardia.

## Treatment Options, Residua, Sequelae, and Long-Term Outcomes

Children with Ebstein anomaly may require only conservative management and follow-up. In most cases, however, surgery is indicated for tricuspid regurgitation, closure of interatrial communications, or other associated problems. Procedures to ablate arrhythmias may be indicated. In contrast to adults, children are less likely to require valve replacement.[311] A cavopulmonary or Glenn connection may be performed in some cases as part of a so-called one and a half ventricle approach to limit the right-sided volume load associated with severe tricuspid valve regurgitation.[312,313] One report indicated good functional outcomes and long-term survival after surgery for Ebstein anomaly.[314] Atrial arrhythmias (including Wolf-Parkinson-White syndrome) are common before and after surgery.

## INTERRUPTED AORTIC ARCH
### Anatomy and Pathophysiology

Interrupted aortic arch is an uncommon malformation characterized by discontinuity between the ascending and descending thoracic aorta (see Fig. 15-14). Ductal patency is essential for systemic perfusion beyond the area of interruption. This anomaly is classified in terms of the site of interruption. It is type A if it occurs distal to the left subclavian artery, type B if between the left carotid and left subclavian arteries, and type C if between the carotid arteries. Type B interruption is the most common variant, followed in frequency by types A and C.

Interrupted aortic arch is typically associated with a posteriorly malaligned VSD, resulting in subaortic obstruction. Other defects include a right aortic arch, aberrant origin of a subclavian artery, and truncus arteriosus. Many children with this anomaly have DiGeorge syndrome.

Neonatal presentation of interrupted aortic arch is related to ductal closure in the setting of aortic arch obstruction (e.g., congestive heart failure, poor perfusion, cardiovascular collapse, shock) and occasionally to differential cyanosis. Stabilization of the infant and initiation of prostaglandin $E_1$ therapy is critical.

The site of interruption and presence of coexistent anomalies can influence the selection of sites for blood pressure monitoring and pulse oximetry. An adequate response to prostaglandin $E_1$ therapy implies no significant gradient between the areas proximal and distal to the obstruction and an oxygen saturation differential (i.e., increased values in beds supplied proximal to the interruption, reduced values distally).

### Treatment Options, Residua, Sequelae, and Long-Term Outcomes

Surgical intervention is necessary for interrupted aortic arch during the first few days of life. The goal is to establish aortic arch continuity and to address coexistent defects. The current approach favors a one-stage repair.[315-317] Survival in uncomplicated cases is excellent.[318] Problems after repair mainly involve the left ventricular outflow tract.[319] Reoperation may be required and in some cases may consist of left ventricular outflow tract enlargement (i.e., Konno procedure). Eventual aortic root or valve replacement or a Ross-Konno procedure may be necessary.

## CONGENITAL ANOMALIES OF THE CORONARY ARTERIES

### Anatomy and Pathophysiology

Congenital anomalies of the coronary arteries include an abnormal origin of one of the main branches, aberrant vascular course, or pathologic communications that involve the coronary circulation.[320,321] The most common anomalies detected during childhood include anomalous origin of the left main coronary artery from the pulmonary artery (ALCAPA), coronary artery–to–pulmonary artery fistulas, and coronary cameral fistulas (i.e., connection between a coronary artery and cardiac chamber). Although rare, anomalous origin of a coronary artery from the incorrect (contralateral) sinus of Valsalva may occur in asymptomatic children and adolescents.[322] In some instances, a major coronary artery courses between the great arteries. This situation may be associated with compromised coronary blood flow and myocardial ischemia during exercise, presumably related to dilation of the arterial roots to accommodate the increased stroke volume.

The clinical presentation varies according to the nature of the anomaly. Infants and young children with ALCAPA may exhibit severe ventricular dysfunction and mitral valve regurgitation, which are largely ischemic in nature. Children with fistulous coronary artery connections may present with a heart murmur or evidence of ventricular volume overload. Significant symptoms may indicate congestive heart failure. Other coronary artery anomalies may manifest as myocardial ischemia, causing exertional syncope or chest pain, and in some cases, arrhythmias may lead to a near-death event.

### Treatment Options, Residua, Sequelae, and Long-Term Outcomes

After surgical intervention for ALCAPA, most children demonstrate significant recovery of myocardial function. Others continue to exhibit alterations in myocardial performance and may develop dilated cardiomyopathy; if it is severe, they may require cardiac transplantation. A few children reach adulthood without symptoms or any intervention. Coronary artery fistulas resulting in congestive symptoms may be referred for catheter-based or surgical interventions. Anginal complaints, myocardial infarction, and sudden death are risks when an aberrant coronary artery courses between the arterial trunks. The risk is greater when the left coronary artery originates from the right sinus of Valsalva and courses between the aorta and the right ventricular outflow tract. Sudden death is most likely to occur during or immediately after strenuous exercise. The implications of anesthesia for coronary artery anomalies primarily are related to the underlying potential for myocardial ischemia, effects of ventricular volume overload, and ventricular dysfunction.

## SINGLE VENTRICLE

### Anatomy and Pathophysiology

The single-ventricle (i.e., univentricular heart) spectrum encompasses several congenital cardiac defects. They are characterized by abnormalities such as ventricular hypoplasia (i.e., HLHS), atrioventricular valve atresia (i.e., tricuspid atresia), or abnormal atrioventricular connections (i.e., double-inlet left ventricle). Pathologies with two distinct ventricles may also be considered in the functional single-ventricle category due to associated defects that preclude a biventricular circulation (i.e., unbalanced AVSD).

Single-ventricle physiology is characterized by complete mixing of the systemic and pulmonary venous circulations at the atrial or ventricular levels. Aortic or pulmonary outflow tract obstruction is a common feature in these pathologies. An important management strategy early in the palliation pathway involves optimizing the balance between the pulmonary and systemic circulations.

### Treatment Options, Residua, Sequelae, and Long-Term Outcomes

Surgical interventions available for children with functional single-ventricle physiology include the following:

#### Aortopulmonary Shunt

Infants with limited or ductal-dependent pulmonary blood flow require the creation of a connection between the systemic and pulmonary circulations. This most commonly takes the form of an aortopulmonary shunt, which is achieved by placement of a Gore-Tex graft between the right subclavian and right pulmonary arteries (i.e., modified right Blalock-Taussig shunt). This procedure augments or allows pulmonary blood flow. Potential problems include shunt malfunction associated with reductions in pulmonary blood flow and congestive heart failure related to excessive pulmonary blood flow. Several factors determine blood flow across an aortopulmonary shunt, with systemic arterial pressure playing a major role.

#### Pulmonary Artery Band

Pulmonary artery banding results in limitation of pulmonary blood flow in children with minimal or no restriction. This procedure protects the pulmonary vascular bed from increased flow and excessive pressure, an essential requirement for subsequent strategies in the child with a functional single ventricle.

Distortion of the proximal branch pulmonary arteries may result from pulmonary artery band placement. The primary considerations for these children are the presence of an intracardiac communication, associated shunting, ventricular volume load, the consequences of ventricular hypertrophy developed as a response to the mechanical limitation of pulmonary blood flow, and issues associated with coexistent defects. In a few children, pulmonary artery banding may lead to ventricular dysfunction and the development of or an increase in the severity of atrioventricular valve regurgitation.

## Norwood Procedure

In infants with HLHS, its variants, and other lesions with similar hemodynamic consequences, systemic blood flow largely depends on patency of the ductus arteriosus. Cerebral and coronary blood flow is provided in retrograde fashion across a typically hypoplastic transverse aortic arch. A key strategy in the management of these infants before cardiac surgery is to optimize systemic perfusion and the balance between the pulmonary and systemic circulations. Alteration of this balance may manifest with signs of inadequate systemic output (e.g., hypotension, lactic acidosis, decreased urine output) within the context of high systemic arterial oxygen saturation, reflecting the relatively excessive pulmonary blood flow.

In this setting, maneuvers that increase pulmonary vascular resistance are indicated to improve hemodynamics. Measures employed include limiting inspired oxygen concentrations, the administration of subambient gas mixtures, and increasing the partial pressure of carbon dioxide ($PCO_2$) by hypoventilation or the administration of inspired carbon dioxide. A comparison of hypoxia versus hypercarbia in infants with HLHS under conditions of anesthesia and paralysis demonstrated that although $\dot{Q}_{pulm}/\dot{Q}_{sys}$ decreases in both conditions, inspired $CO_2$ was more effective than hypoxic gas mixtures at increasing parameters associated with improved systemic output.[323] The administration of inspired $CO_2$ may be favored over hypoventilation as a means of increasing pulmonary vascular resistance and improving the overall clinical condition.

The Norwood procedure is considered the first step among the three stages in the palliative pathway for infants with HLHS or similar cardiac malformations.[324] The intervention, also referred to as stage I single-ventricle palliation or reconstruction, is typically performed within the first few days of life. Surgery consists of aortic reconstruction or creation of a neoaorta, establishing continuity between the native main pulmonary artery and aortic arch to provide for unobstructed systemic outflow from the right ventricle; the creation of an unrestricted atrial communication by means of an atrial septectomy; and establishing a source of pulmonary blood flow (see Fig. 15-11). For many years, pulmonary blood flow was established by fashioning a modified Blalock-Taussig shunt. Currently, a right ventricle–to–pulmonary artery conduit (i.e., Sano modification and similar variations) is used as an alternative to provide pulmonary blood flow. Although the potential benefits of one approach over the other have been elucidated, additional studies, some with long-term follow-up, are required to provide further information.[325-331]

Another approach, a hybrid stage I strategy, has been applied to selected neonates. In this procedure, a median sternotomy is performed, and both branched pulmonary arteries are banded. A stent is then delivered across the ductus arteriosus under fluoroscopic guidance,[332,333] and the interatrial communication is then enlarged.

Outcomes after the Norwood procedure vary; good results imply operative survival for 85% to 90% of infants.[334] Immediate postoperative problems include systemic hypoxemia, decreased myocardial performance, and excessive pulmonary blood flow. Monitoring of mixed venous oxygen saturation and cerebral near-infrared spectroscopy are helpful in balancing the pulmonary and systemic circulations in this setting. Occasionally, aortic arch obstruction occurs, and less commonly, the atrial septum becomes restrictive. Interstage mortality accounts for attrition among Norwood survivors.[335] Among infants who have undergone placement of a right ventricle–to–pulmonary artery conduit,

stenosis of the conduit associated with progressive cyanosis may account for significant interstage morbidity and often requires intervention or early second-stage palliation.[336,337]

The anticipated arterial oxygen saturation after stage I surgery is expected to be in the range of 75% to 85%. During perioperative care, blood pressure monitoring should consider the potential presence of a Blalock-Taussig shunt that may compromise ipsilateral subclavian artery flow. In these infants, the right ventricle ejects into the pulmonary and systemic circulations. Although this is a more stable arrangement compared with that before the Norwood procedure, it remains a relatively fragile parallel circulation. These infants display little tolerance to even the most common childhood conditions, and ailments such as dehydration, febrile illnesses, or other stresses that may have catastrophic consequences. Despite these challenges, successful outcomes have been reported during noncardiac surgery for a variety of procedures, including those that may be associated with significant hemodynamic perturbations, such as laparoscopic surgery.[338]

### Glenn Anastomosis or Hemi-Fontan Procedure

A cavopulmonary connection or Glenn procedure (i.e., stage II palliation) consists of the creation of a direct anastomosis between the superior vena cava and one of the pulmonary artery branches (see Fig. 15-12). This is considered an intermediary step in the sequential diversion of the systemic venous blood into the pulmonary vasculature in children with single-ventricle physiology. The original or classic operation consisted of an end-to-end anastomosis of the transected superior vena cava onto a disconnected right pulmonary artery, and it was complicated by increasing desaturation that was attributed in many cases to the development of pulmonary arteriovenous fistulae.[339] The current approach is to attach the superior vena cava to the right pulmonary artery in end-to-side fashion, preserving pulmonary artery continuity (i.e., bidirectional cavopulmonary anastomosis [BCPA] or bidirectional Glenn connection). Depending on the specific anatomic abnormalities, right, left, or bilateral BCPAs may be indicated.

An alternative approach in second-stage palliation is a hemi-Fontan procedure. It entails anastomosis of the superior vena cava to the pulmonary artery confluence and placement of a patch between the cavopulmonary anastomosis and common atrium. The patch allows systemic venous return from the superior vena cava to be diverted into the pulmonary circulation rather than enter the heart directly. Ligation of the systemic circulation–to–pulmonary artery connection (shunt or conduit) is performed as part of stage II palliation, whether a BCPA or hemi-Fontan procedure is undertaken.

The second-stage intervention requires a reduced pulmonary vascular resistance because of the passive nature of the pulmonary blood flow. This approach provides adequate palliation to a significant number of infants at an early age while conferring favorable hemodynamic benefits.[340] Diverting a portion of the systemic venous return directly into the pulmonary bed reduces the output requirements of the single ventricle while decreasing the ventricular volume load and myocardial work.

One study demonstrated a 12% rate of interstage attrition between BCPA and the Fontan procedure in children with HLHS palliation.[341] Risk factors included tricuspid valve regurgitation and low weight at the time of the BCPA. These factors may affect the anesthesia-related risks for noncardiac procedures required between these two stages of palliation.

Considerations include the passive nature of the pulmonary blood flow, the importance of maintaining adequate intravascular volume (i.e., minimal fasting) to enhance pulmonary blood flow, and limiting significant increases in pulmonary vascular tone. Pulmonary blood flow and systemic arterial oxygenation are significantly influenced by the interplay between pulmonary artery pressure (i.e., equal to the pressure in the superior vena cava), pulmonary venous pressure, and pulmonary vascular resistance. The expected systemic arterial oxygen saturation ranges between 75% and 85%. Although factors that increase pulmonary vascular resistance may negatively influence pulmonary blood flow, the observation has been made that early after BCPA, moderate hypercapnia with respiratory acidosis improves arterial oxygenation and reduces oxygen consumption, enhancing overall oxygen transport in these children.[342] Hyperventilation can decrease cerebral oxygenation and should be avoided.[343] Postoperative issues include hypoxemia related to the development of collateral vessels that bypass the pulmonary circulation, atrioventricular valve regurgitation, and impaired ventricular function.

### Fontan Procedure

The Fontan procedure is the final step (i.e., stage III reconstruction) in the separation of the pulmonary and systemic circulations in children with a functional single ventricle. This intervention allows passive blood flow from the inferior vena cava into the pulmonary vascular bed while bypassing the heart and achieves a circulation in series (see Fig. 15-13). A fenestration, or communication, between the systemic venous pathway and physiologic common atrium may be created in some cases. It allows right-to-left shunting, which provides cardiac output that is not solely dependent on pulmonary blood flow. It also alleviates potential problems associated with chronically increased systemic venous pressures. Common features of the numerous Fontan modifications are separation of the pulmonary and systemic circulations and relief of hypoxemia.[344] Pulmonary blood flow occurs without an intervening ventricular chamber. It depends critically on the transpulmonary pressure gradient (or driving pressure across the pulmonary bed) and is influenced by pulmonary vascular resistance. This blood flow determines cardiac output, emphasizing the importance of adequate hydration and maintenance of central venous pressure.

Several anatomic and hemodynamic variables influence Fontan physiology. Critical factors include unobstructed systemic venous return, status of the pulmonary vasculature, reduced intrathoracic pressures, systemic atrioventricular valve competency, systemic ventricular function, unobstructed systemic outflow, and atrial contribution to ventricular filling.[345] Long-term problems are related to sinus node dysfunction, loss of atrioventricular synchrony, atrial arrhythmias, atrioventricular valve regurgitation, ventricular dysfunction, venous pathway obstruction or thrombotic complications, and symptoms resulting from a chronic reduced cardiac output state.[346] Long-standing increases in systemic venous pressures in children after the Fontan procedure can produce hepatic dysfunction, coagulation defects, protein-losing enteropathy, and rhythm disturbances. The quality of life after the Fontan operation may be compromised by a late decline in functional status, reoperations, arrhythmias, and thromboembolic events.[347-352] Decreased exercise tolerance in most children represents limited cardiopulmonary reserve, which manifests as an inability to increase cardiac output to meet the metabolic demands associated with increased work.

In some cases, surgical revision to a more hemodynamically favorable Fontan modification is indicated.[353,354]

Several considerations are important in the perioperative care of children with Fontan circulation.[355-357] Even mild alterations in factors that influence cardiac output, such as ventricular preload, atrioventricular synchrony, contractile function, afterload, and stress response, may adversely impact hemodynamics. Ensuring the adequacy of hydration, preserving sinus rhythm, and limiting the stress response are key goals. Maintenance of adequate ventricular function may require the administration of inotropic or vasoactive agents perioperatively. Because systemic venous pressures are typically increased, the potential for bleeding and its effects on ventricular filling should be considered. The likelihood of blood loss with ensuing hemodynamic instability is exacerbated by the coagulation defects in these children.[358] The potential for end-organ dysfunction related to chronically decreased organ perfusion, particularly in the renal and hepatic systems, should be considered, and problems may require interventions to minimize perioperative morbidity. Drugs or devices appropriate for cardiac rhythm or arrhythmia management should be accessible.

Some principles apply to airway and ventilatory management after the Fontan operation. Although spontaneous ventilation favors phasic pulmonary flow patterns in these children, controlled ventilation is preferable in most cases. This approach minimizes the detrimental effects of factors such as hypoventilation, atelectasis, hypoxemia, hypercarbia, and respiratory acidosis on pulmonary vascular resistance during spontaneous ventilation, limiting passive drainage of systemic venous blood into the pulmonary circulation. The pH and $PCO_2$ should be maintained within the normal range, and arterial oxygen saturation should remain close to baseline. The saturation level may depend on the presence or absence of a fenestration and the degree of right-to-left shunting. Mechanical ventilation with large lung volumes may impair pulmonary blood flow as increases in mean intrathoracic pressures transmitted to the pulmonary vascular bed increase pulmonary artery pressures and decrease systemic venous return. Judicious use of mechanical ventilatory support is therefore warranted. Suggested parameters include smaller than usual tidal volumes and reduced positive end-expiratory pressures, allowing delivery of the smallest mean airway pressure possible and normal to relatively small inspiratory times (i.e., normal to slightly prolonged inspiratory-to-expiratory ratios). Although adequate minute ventilation may require increases in the respiratory rate, the potential detrimental effects of very fast rates should also be considered. The goals are to maintain adequate lung volumes, functional residual capacity, and optimal gas exchange.

## Summary

Noncardiac surgery in children with CHD can usually be accomplished in a safe and effective manner. A comprehensive understanding of the child's cardiovascular anatomy and physiology is essential to guide appropriate perioperative management and to achieve the best possible outcomes. Many children with CHD have undergone complete repair in infancy, with resultant normal or near-normal hemodynamics at the time of noncardiac surgery. Routine care is likely to be well tolerated by these children. Special attention must be paid to identify children at increased risk, particularly those with unrepaired defects or those who have undergone palliative interventions. Factors such as congestive heart failure, cyanosis, pulmonary hypertension, young age, or significant residual or sequelae increase the potential for perioperative problems.

An important objective in caring for children with a history of CHD is to diminish cardiac-related morbidity and minimize the likelihood of an adverse outcome. An interdisciplinary approach is much preferred to accomplish this goal. Application of perioperative strategies that may limit the risks of anesthesia and surgery should be a combined effort by all health care providers involved. Anticipation of these risks can decrease the likelihood of complications and facilitate prompt and appropriate treatment when difficulties are encountered. Good communication among the perioperative team members is essential.

## ANNOTATED REFERENCES

Baum VC, Barton DM, Gutgesell HP. Influence of congenital heart disease on mortality after noncardiac surgery in hospitalized children. Pediatrics 2000;105:332-5.

*The investigation evaluated the incremental risk of congenital heart disease on mortality after noncardiac surgery in children. Short-term and 30-day mortality rates were increased for these patients. Mortality rates were also increased for children with congenital heart disease in the two youngest age groups for the 100 most common operations and for 10 relatively minor operations. Children with more severe forms of heart disease had greater mortality rates than those with less serious cardiac diagnoses.*

Carmosino MJ, Friesen RH, Doran A, Ivy DD. Perioperative complications in children with pulmonary hypertension undergoing noncardiac surgery or cardiac catheterization. Anesth Analg 2007; 104:521-7.

*A retrospective review of medical records was conducted of children with pulmonary hypertension who underwent anesthesia or sedation for noncardiac surgical procedures or cardiac catheterizations. Two hundred fifty-six procedures were performed in 156 patients. The study concluded that children with suprasystemic pulmonary artery pressures have a significant risk of major perioperative complications, including cardiac arrest and pulmonary hypertensive crisis.*

Coté CJ, Wax DF, Jennings MA, et al. End-tidal carbon dioxide monitoring in children with congenital heart disease during sedation for cardiac catheterization by nonanesthesiologists. Pediatr Anesth 2007; 17:661-6.

*This prospective observational study compared end-tidal carbon dioxide values with blood gas carbon dioxide measurements in children sedated by nonanesthesiologists during cardiac catheterization. End-tidal carbon dioxide monitoring provided a reasonable reflection of blood carbon dioxide values if the expired gas-sampling catheter was taped in place after ensuring a good waveform.*

Galantowicz M, Cheatham JP, Phillips A, et al. Hybrid approach for hypoplastic left heart syndrome: intermediate results after the learning curve. Ann Thorac Surg 2008;85:2063-70; discussion 2070-71.

*The authors reported intermediate results in a prospective data collection study enrolling children with hypoplastic left heart syndrome who were managed by an initial hybrid approach (n = 40). This strategy yielded acceptable intermediate results that were comparable to those with the traditional Norwood procedure. Proposed advantages of the hybrid approach over conventional management included the avoidance of circulatory arrest and a delay in the major surgical intervention until later in life.*

Ohye RG, Sleeper LA, Mahony L, et al. Comparison of shunt types in the Norwood procedure for single-ventricle lesions. N Engl J Med 2010;362:1980-92.

*The two strategies (modified Blalock-Taussig and right ventricle–pulmonary artery shunt) that allow for pulmonary blood flow in infants with hypoplastic heart syndrome or related anomalies were compared in infants undergoing the Norwood procedure. Infants (n = 555) at 15 North American centers were randomized to surgery that included one type of shunt or the other. For these children, transplantation-free survival at 12 months was better with the right ventricle–pulmonary artery shunt than with the modified Blalock-Taussig shunt. After 12 months, however, the data demonstrated no significant difference in transplantation-free survival between the two groups.*

Ramamoorthy C, Haberkern CM, Bhananker SM, et al. Anesthesia-related cardiac arrest in children with heart disease: data from the Pediatric Perioperative Cardiac Arrest (POCA) registry. Anesth Analg 2010;110:1376-82.

*This is a report from the Pediatric Perioperative Cardiac Arrest (POCA) registry on anesthesia-related cardiac arrests, with a focus on children with heart disease. The data was provided by a large number of North American institutions. Children with heart disease who suffered a cardiac arrest were sicker that those without heart disease and more likely to arrest from cardiovascular causes. Mortality rates were greater for those with heart disease. The events were more likely to occur in the general operating room compared with the cardiac setting. The subset of children with a single ventricle was the most common category of heart disease to suffer cardiac arrest. Children with aortic stenosis and cardiomyopathy had the greatest cardiac arrest–related mortality rates.*

Williams GD, Maan H, Ramamoorthy C, et al. Perioperative complications in children with pulmonary hypertension undergoing general anesthesia with ketamine. Paediatr Anaesth 2010;20:28-37.

*This is a retrospective study in children with pulmonary arterial hypertension to determine the nature and frequency of periprocedural complications and to assess whether ketamine administration was associated with complications. In this cohort (68 children), the incidence of cardiac arrest was 10% for major surgery, 0.78% for cardiac catheterization, and 1.6% for all procedures. There was no procedure-related mortality. Ketamine administration was not associated with an increased rate of complications.*

## REFERENCES

Please see www.expertconsult.com.

Children with cerebral palsy require neuroimaging to confirm the diagnosis and underlying cause of the condition. Although some centers use oral sedation (i.e., midazolam or chloral hydrate) for neuroimaging, many children require general anesthesia. They may require multiple anesthesias throughout their lifetimes because of the associated comorbidities (i.e. respiratory, gastrointestinal, neuromuscular, and orthopedic), common surgical conditions, and problems unique to cerebral palsy that require treatment.[19]

Many of the comorbid conditions can affect anesthesia management. Understanding the pathophysiology and comorbidities of cerebral palsy allows anesthesiologists to anticipate and prevent perioperative complications.

## Multisystem Comorbidities

Most children with cerebral palsy have clinically significant oromotor dysfunction, and when associated with gastroesophageal reflux, it may lead to recurrent aspiration, decreased respiratory reserve, esophageal stenosis, and malnutrition.[20] Frequently employed procedures include fundoplication, gastrostomy, and esophageal dilation treatment.[12] Immobility, underhydration, and poor diet predispose patients to bowel stasis and constipation, which may become severe, with fecal impaction occurring occasionally. Malnutrition may depress immune responses, and electrolyte imbalance and anemia are common. Preoperative assessment of these parameters is essential.

Pulmonary complications are common causes of death in cerebral palsy. Aspiration associated with gastroesophageal reflux is the leading cause, and it may be exacerbated by excessive oral secretions, bulbar dysfunction, recurrent respiratory infection, and chronic lung disease.[21,22] Scoliosis may also restrict pulmonary function, with cardiopulmonary involvement depending on the curve pattern and the severity of the curve (see Chapter 30).[12]

Orthopedic operations are the most frequently performed procedures in children with cerebral palsy.[12] Procedures include tendon releases to ease contractures, femoral osteotomy, and hip adductor and iliopsoas releases.[23] The trend in orthopedic surgery is to perform multiple procedures involving tenotomies or osteotomies at different levels of all extremities during a single general anesthesia, rather than staging them during multiple operations.[12,19] Scoliosis often requires surgery to prevent further deterioration in lung function and to stabilize the spine to facilitate ambulation and sitting. Spinal fusion is considered in all children with progressive curves greater than 40 to 50 degrees.[24]

Botulinum toxin is commonly used to reduce muscle spasticity in afflicted children, and it may be injected with or without sedation or, more commonly, under general anesthesia. The need for repeated treatments (every 3 to 6 months) and the use of a nerve stimulator to confirm correct placement of the needle should be taken into consideration when assessing the child's need for sedation or anesthesia.

Approximately 30% of children with cerebral palsy have epilepsy. It is more common in spastic hemiplegia and less common in the ataxic and choreoathetotic forms. Generalized and focal seizures frequently occur. Anticonvulsants should be maintained until the surgery date (given the morning of surgery) and restarted as soon as possible in the postoperative period.[12,25]

## Anesthesia Considerations for Cerebral Palsy

The many multisystem comorbidities and therapies specific to children with cerebral palsy must be understood to minimize perioperative complications. Risk factors include an inability to walk, severe neurologic deficit, major cognitive dysfunction, severe scoliosis, malnutrition, and the presence of a gastrostomy or tracheostomy.[19] Severely compromised children can be optimally managed postoperatively with admission to the pediatric intensive care unit to provide analgesia with comprehensive monitoring, maximum support, and aggressive respiratory care, and after they are stabilized, they can be transferred to a setting with less intense monitoring.

All medications that the child is receiving should be reviewed; they may include anticonvulsant, antireflux, and antispasticity agents. Baclofen should not be discontinued abruptly because it can produce acute withdrawal symptoms. Oral dantrolene has also been used to reduce spasticity. Because baclofen and dantrolene cause weakness, the dose of neuromuscular blocking drugs may need to be reduced because these antispasticity drugs can delay the return of adequate respiratory effort during emergence from anesthesia.

Most of these children have above-average intelligence. They have the same emotional and cognitive concerns as others about undergoing anesthesia, including preoperative anxiety that may require premedication. Children with contractures, especially in the upper extremities, may present a challenge for establishing intravenous access. If gastroesophageal reflux is not controlled, consideration should be given to rapid-sequence induction. Although these children have a neuromuscular disorder, intravenous succinylcholine yields only a normal release of potassium,[26] despite evidence of proliferation of extrajunctional acetylcholine receptors.[27] Maintenance of and emergence from anesthesia requires special considerations, including the possibility of a reduced minimal alveolar concentration (MAC),[28] resistance to neuromuscular blocking agents,[29] and reduced bispectral index (BIS) measurements.[30] If vomiting is likely to occur, the airway must be protected.

These children have normal responses to pain, which should be managed as if they were unaffected by cerebral palsy. Caudal or epidural analgesia may be a reasonable approach for perioperative pain management if the child does not have a ventricular-peritoneal shunt. Management and assessment of perioperative pain in children with neurocognitive impairment is addressed in Chapter 43.

## MALFORMATIONS OF THE NERVOUS SYSTEM

Malformations are common in pediatric neurologic practice and a frequent cause of early mortality. The appearance of the neural plate shows that the central nervous system (CNS) develops very rapidly in the 2-week embryo and continues until several years after birth. The cause of CNS malformations is largely uncertain, but timing appears to be more important than the nature of the insult in producing the specific type of malformation. Causative agents include maternal drugs such as sodium valproate, which is associated with neural tube defects (NTDs); infections such as cytomegalovirus, which can cause various cerebral lesions, depending on the time in gestation of the infection; toxins such as alcohol; vitamin deficiency (e.g., folic acid), and genetic disorders. Historically, because diagnostic investigation was limited, postmortem examination was required to demonstrate the neuropathologic changes causing the clinical disorder. MRI now can provide adequate images to enable a diagnosis in many instances (e.g., cortical dysplasia).[31]

### Neural Tube Defects: Cranial and Spinal Dysraphism

The prevalence of NTDs in the United States is about 6 in 10,000 live births. NTDs are a group of birth defects presumed to have a common origin in failure of the neural tube to develop properly during the embryonic stage. NTDs include anencephaly, encephaloceles, and spina bifida.

The cause of NTDs is multifactorial, with genetic and environmental factors being the most important. Approximately 10% of NTDs are caused by chromosomal abnormalities such as trisomies (i.e., 18, 13, and 21), triploidy, and Turner syndrome. Preconceptual folic acid supplementation has reduced the prevalence of NTDs by 30% to 50%.[32] Along with antenatal ultrasound examination, screening is done for increased maternal serum levels of α-fetoprotein, reduced human chorionic gonadotropin levels, and reduced unconjugated estriol levels; termination of pregnancy in cases that test positive has further reduced the prevalence of NTDs.[33]

*Anencephaly* is a lethal disorder that results from failure of the neural tube to form. This leads to disorganization of neural elements and the absence of skull formation.[31] Some deep cerebral structures may remain intact, and the brainstem may develop normally. With the latter, normal respiration and cardiovascular functions may develop, enabling the infant to survive for hours or days after birth. Other structures in the head and brain, including the eyes, face, and pituitary gland, may not develop normally.

*Encephalocele* is a herniation of neural tissue and meninges out of the skull through deficient skin and bone (see Fig. 24-11, *B*). They are frequently associated with other cerebral malformations, such as agenesis of the corpus callosum. Encephaloceles found anteriorly are associated with underlying brain, orbital structures, or pituitary gland anomaly. Posteriorly, encephaloceles are associated with cerebral or cerebellar tissue that herniates through a bony defect in the posterior cranium. Intranasal encephaloceles may be difficult to detect. These defects carry a poor prognosis for long-term survival. Most infants die, and in survivors, severe neurodevelopmental disability is common. Most of these children have hydrocephalus.[34]

*Spina bifida* refers to a group of conditions in which there is abnormal or incomplete formation of the midline structures over the back (see Fig. 24-11, *A*, in Chapter 24).[31] Skin, bony, and neural elements may be involved singly or in combination. Congenital malformations of the spinal cord may exist in isolation or in association with brain anomalies. These defects may present at birth, as in the case of the more severe and open lesions (i.e., spina bifida) or be identified later in childhood if the skin overlying the spinal defect is intact (e.g., spina bifida occulta). Those who develop a Chiari malformation may present with cervical cord or bulbar deficits, placing them at risk for respiratory embarrassment (see Figs. 24-12 and 24-13). Children with spinal cord lesions are at increased risk for sensory deficits, making meticulous skin care and positioning essential to prevent pressure sores and damage to neuropathic joints.

*Spina bifida occulta* occurs in the absence of herniation of neural tissue or coverings so that the overlying skin appears to be intact and normal. In many cases, a hairy patch or a dermal sinus (i.e., sacral dimple) may communicate with the meninges or attach to the spinal cord or a lipoma that causes a fatty swelling overlying the bony defect. The spinal cord may be tethered by internal connection to such structures, making it vulnerable to trauma at surgery and during growth, especially at puberty. The spinal cord may be abnormally formed, with cartilaginous or bony spurs that damage or divide the cord during growth as the neural tissue grows at a slower rate than the surrounding bone (i.e., diastematomyelia). These infants may not be candidates for a caudal block because the spinal cord may end at an unusually low position.

*Spina bifida cystica*, which is the most common type of spinal dysraphism, manifests as an obvious lesion on the back. The defect may be diagnosed antenatally or at birth. The abnormally developed spinal cord may be covered by a layer of meninges (i.e., meningocele) or remain uncovered (i.e., myelomeningocele). Myelomeningoceles need to be repaired within a few days of birth to prevent infection and further damage to the neural tissues. A cerebrospinal fluid (CSF) leak or frank dural rupture may develop, leading to intravascular volume and electrolyte abnormalities that should be treated preoperatively.

When the defect is identified at birth, it is optimally managed in a specialist center by a multidisciplinary team (i.e., pediatrician, neurologist, neurosurgeon, orthopedic surgeon, and others) who can anticipate, prevent, and treat complications and assist in the child's long-term care. Children with dysraphism often develop postoperative hydrocephalus because of disrupted CSF flow and require a ventricular-peritoneal shunt. Long-term complications, including paraparesis, neurogenic bladder and bowel, renal insufficiency, trophic limb changes, pressure sores, joint contractures, and scoliosis, may require surgical repair and future intervention. These children are also at risk for latex allergy. From the outset, all children with NTDs should be considered latex sensitive and undergo management in a latex-safe environment. The anesthesia considerations for NTDs are presented in Chapter 24.

### Chiari Malformation

Chiari malformations of the nervous system may coexist with other anomalies and manifest in the neonatal period or later in the early decades of life (Table 22-3).

**TABLE 22-3** Chiari Malformations

| Type | Main Features | Associated Abnormalities | Neurologic Features |
|---|---|---|---|
| Chiari I | Downward displacement of cerebellar tonsils; elongation of fourth ventricle and lower brainstem | Platybasia, basilar impression, syringomyelia, hydrocephalus | Later onset (> age 12 years), cervical cord signs: tetraparesis, sensory deficits of upper limbs |
| Chiari II | Downward displacement of cerebellar vermis or tonsils alongside cervical cord, kinking of cord at C2-3 level | Myelomeningocele in most, brainstem anomalies, aqueduct stenosis | Present in neonate, macrocephaly, increased intracranial pressure, cranial nerve palsies, cord signs |
| Chiari III | Downward displacement of cerebellum into posterior encephalocele; elongation of fourth ventricle | Posterior defects: cervical spina bifida ± cranium bifidum | Present in neonate with signs of hydrocephalus ± brainstem and cervical cord signs |
| Chiari IV | Cerebellar hypoplasia | Usually none | ± Ataxia |

±, With or without.

## Syringomyelia

Syringomyelia results from a glial cell–lined cavitation within the spinal cord. Diagnosis has been greatly simplified by the use of MRI, which provides images of the spinal cord and the tubular fluid-filled space within.[31] The pathogenesis of syringomyelia remains unclear. It complicates several conditions, such as rare familial cases, congenital malformations, trauma, and meningeal infection. It has been reported as a coincidental finding in normal individuals.

Syringomyelia manifests with dissociated sensory loss, usually in the upper limbs, causing loss or impairment of pain and temperature sensation, which may cause trophic changes in the fingers and neuropathic joints. It may progress to paralysis and hyporeflexia later in life. The lower limbs may exhibit pyramidal signs; some lesion may extend upward (i.e., syringobulbia) and produce lower brainstem signs, such as stridor and laryngospasm (i.e., vocal cord palsy). Spinal deformity causes scoliosis at an early stage.

Treatment is controversial, especially if the lesion is asymptomatic. Management may focus on associated disorders because syringomyelia may progress slowly or not at all.

## Hydrocephalus

Hydrocephalus results from overproduction or impaired drainage of CSF from the brain.[34] In practice, overproduction is an uncommon source of hydrocephalus; these cases most often result from tumors of the choroid plexus. Obstructed CSF drainage is the far more common basis. Causes of hydrocephalus include intraventricular hemorrhage, Arnold-Chiari malformation, brain tumor, congenital obstruction, and myelomeningocele.

Children typically present with a headache and irritability, but signs and symptoms can progress to lethargy, seizures, vomiting, and ophthalmoplegia as pressure within the brain increases. If left untreated, it may lead to a reduced level of consciousness, oculomotor palsies, sluggish pupillary light reactions, bradycardia, and eventually respiratory arrest. Diagnosis of hydrocephalus is confirmed by neuroimaging, often with computed tomography (CT) in the acute situation, followed by MRI.

Surgical treatment for hydrocephalus involves insertion of a drainage system to shunt CSF from the brain to another site in the body (see Fig. 24-10). The anesthesia considerations for treating hydrocephalus are discussed in Chapter 24.

## DISORDERS OF VENTRAL INDUCTION

Holoprosencephaly is a cephalic disorder in which the forebrain of the embryo fails to develop into discrete hemispheres with normal connections.[31] There are three types:

1. Lobar: There is almost complete separation of the hemispheres, and the corpus callosum is almost absent.
2. Semilobar: The two hemispheres are divided posteriorly, with interhemispheric connections present anteriorly. The corpus callosum is absent anteriorly, and the thalami are fused in the midline.
3. Alobar: An undivided and small forebrain with a dorsal sac may contain some cortex. Severe facial defects may include cyclopia (i.e., single orbit with fused globes), cebocephaly (i.e., single nostril), and a midline cleft lip.

Associated malformations (e.g., congenital heart disease, scalp deficits, polydactyly) are common. Chromosomal anomalies may be identified, and a complex syndromic disorder may occur in some of these children. The diagnosis rests on a careful description of the external and internal morphology using MRI, followed by genetic assessment. Complications include hydrocephalus, endocrine deficits, epilepsy, and severe complex disability, usually with a shortened life expectancy.

## DISORDERS OF CORTICAL DEVELOPMENT

Malformations of the cerebral cortex are many and varied. Although uncommon, development of lissencephaly or agyria (i.e., smooth cortex), pachygyria (i.e., thickened cortex), and polymicrogyria (i.e., multiple, small gyri) depends on the stage of embryogenesis affected.[31] MRI has advanced the identification of these features and their classification.

Environmental agents and genetic abnormalities have been identified for many of these malformations, and genetic derangements can produce a multisystem syndrome. Intrauterine insults in early pregnancy have been implicated in cases coming to autopsy. Clinical effects vary, and the severity depends on the site and extent of the lesion. Survivors may have no symptoms or have profound, complex neurodisability. Children may have learning disabilities, epilepsy, focal neurologic deficits, motor dysfunction, and other system involvement.

# Progressive Neurologic Disorders

## PRIMARY BRAIN TUMORS

The incidence of primary brain tumors is 2.6 per 100,000 children, and they account for more than 20% of all childhood malignancies. One third of these tumors occur before 5 years of age, and 75% occur before 10 years of age.[35] Two thirds are located infratentorially and one third supratentorially (Table 22-4).[36]

Pathologic classification, which is based on the cell of origin and degree of malignancy, extends from grade I (benign) to grade 4 (malignant).[37] The patient's presentation depends on the site of the tumor. Infants typically display irritability, failure to thrive, and macrocephaly, whereas older children develop headache, nausea, vomiting, seizures, gait disturbances, and visual deficits. If the lesion is rapidly expanding and is accompanied by significant cerebral edema or obstructs CSF drainage, the intracranial pressure (ICP) will increase. Occasionally, hemorrhage may occur into the tumor, causing a dramatic progression of signs and symptoms, mandating emergency treatment. Ultimately, brainstem decompensation and death ensue if the lesion is not treated.

Diagnosis of a primary brain tumor is usually confirmed with MRI and magnetic resonance spectroscopy (MRS). Tissue diagnosis by a biopsy is always desirable, although not always achievable. Microscopy of CSF may yield tumor cells and facilitate the diagnosis. Image-guided biopsy may be possible and is preferred for appropriately sited lesions.

Surgery is the mainstay of treatment and is usually combined with radiotherapy or chemotherapy, or both. Preoperatively, cerebral edema should be treated with corticosteroids to reduce ICP, alleviate symptoms and signs, and enable correction of fluid and electrolyte abnormalities. Seizures require anticonvulsant therapy. Nutrition may be poor and necessitate aggressive management with enteral and parenteral feedings. Operative intervention for raised ICP may require CSF diversion by shunting internally or externally. Depending on the tissue diagnosis and location, total resection of the tumor may be indicated, although the timing of the surgery may depend on whether the tumor should first be treated with radiation therapy or chemotherapy. Aggressive surgery with the intent of completely resecting the tumor

**TABLE 22-4** Common Central Nervous System Tumors in Childhood

| Tumor Type | Percentage of All Childhood CNS Tumors | Clinical Features | Treatment | Prognosis or Survival |
|---|---|---|---|---|
| Medulloblastoma | 14-20 | Acute ataxia<br>↑ Intracranial pressure | Surgical excision + radiotherapy or chemotherapy in children <2 years old | 75% at 5 years<br>50% at 10 years |
| Cerebellar astrocytoma (80% cystic) | 15-20 | Subacute-chronic ataxia<br>Head tilt<br>± ↑ Intracranial pressure | Surgical excision | 100% at 5 years, if totally excised |
| Posterior fossa ependymoma | 6-10 | Cranial nerve palsies<br>Stiff neck ataxia<br>↑ Intracranial pressure | Surgical excision<br>Radiotherapy | 40% at 5 years but 14% if <5 years old |
| Brainstem glioma | 6-16 | Cranial nerve palsies<br>Long tract signs<br>↑ Intracranial pressure late | (Stereotactic) biopsy if possible.<br>Radiotherapy ± chemotherapy: depends on age and cell type | Survival variable and depends on cell type |
| Craniopharyngioma | 6-10 | Endocrine disorders<br>↑ Intracranial pressure<br>Visual impairment | Surgery<br>Hormonal therapy | Survival variable |
| Visual pathway glioma | 3-5 | Proptosis, ↓ vision<br>Associated disorders (e.g., neurofibromatosis type I) | Controversial and individualized | Variable |
| Pineal region tumors | <2 | ↑ Intracranial pressure<br>Loss of upward gaze | Surgery ± radiotherapy | Variable |
| Hemisphere glioma | 25-30 | α Location: ↑ intracranial pressure, seizures, focal neurologic deficit | Surgery ± radiotherapy ± chemotherapy | Depends on cell type |
| Meningioma | <2 | ↑ Intracranial pressure<br>Seizures | Surgery | Variable |
| Ganglioma and dysembryoplastic neuroepithelial tumor (DNET) | 1-5 | Focal epilepsy | Surgery | Good<br>May cure epilepsy |
| Primitive neuroepithelial tumor (PNET) | 1-2 | ↑ Intracranial pressure, focal neurologic deficit | Surgery + radiotherapy | Poor |
| Intraventricular tumors, various cell types | 5 | ↑ Intracranial pressure: hydrocephalus | Shunting and surgical excision | Variable |
| Basal ganglia tumors, various cell types | 5 | Hemiparesis, dystonia | Stereotactic biopsy<br>Radiotherapy if malignant | Depends on cell type |

*CNS,* Central nervous system; ±, with or without; ↓, decreased; ↑, increased.

improves the prognosis for many tumor types but carries with it significant risks of residual neurologic deficits.

The 5-year survival rate of greater than 60% for primary brain tumors largely reflects improved imaging, aggressive surgery, and evidence-based therapy.[38] Unfortunately, children who survive CNS tumors frequently have permanent neurologic deficits, including epilepsy, learning disabilities, visual or hearing impairment, and growth and endocrine disorders. Short-term and long-term follow-up evaluations by specialist teams are required, along with careful emotional and social support for children and their families. Some children have genetic predispositions for CNS tumors, such as neurofibromatosis (i.e., schwannomas of the spinal cord, peripheral nerve tumors, skeletal deformities, carcinoid syndrome, and multiple endocrine neoplasia, including pheochromocytoma) and tuberous sclerosis (i.e., brain tumors, cardiac rhabdomyomas, renal abnormalities, and hepatoma), and they require genetic analysis and long-term follow-up.

Tumors of the spinal cord are rare in childhood. They may be benign or malignant and sited within the cord (intramedullary) or outside (extramedullary). Symptoms and signs may initially be nonspecific and vague, especially in young children. This may delay the diagnosis and increase the risk of spinal cord compression. Delayed relief of compression may cause vascular compromise, which may lead to total and irreversible paralysis of the limbs, bladder, and bowel and permanent, severe disability. Diagnosis is best made by MRI of the cord, which provides details of the lesion and adjacent structures without the risk of further decompensation, a problem raised by the use of myelography in the past.[36]

Treatment usually involves surgery to decompress the cord and excise or biopsy the lesion. For intramedullary tumors, excision may be impossible, and biopsy may risk further damage to the spinal cord. Cell type may be determined by CSF examination. Follow-up treatment with radiotherapy may be indicated. Children with established neurologic deficits require a program of rehabilitation.

## METABOLIC DISEASE
Inborn errors of carbohydrate, protein, or fat metabolism usually are genetic in origin. The molecular defects of many of these metabolic disorders have been identified.

**TABLE 22-5** Neurometabolic Disorders

| |
| --- |
| Lysosomal diseases |
| Mucolipidoses, sialidoses, disorders of glycoprotein metabolism |
| Peroxisomal disorders |
| Amino acid disorders |
| Organic acid disorders |
| Neurotransmitter disorders |
| Urea cycle disorders |
| Disorders of vitamin metabolism |
| Lactic acidosis |
|    Respiratory chain disorders |
|    Mitochondrial fatty acid β-oxidation defects |
| Disorders of cholesterol metabolism |
| Disorders of copper metabolism |
| Miscellaneous disorders |

These diseases may cause a static encephalopathy but more often produce a progressive course with loss of physical and intellectual skills. Epilepsy, especially myoclonus, is common, as is loss of vision, neuropathy, deafness, or involvement of other organ systems (particularly cardiac). Some neurometabolic diseases are associated with intellectual deficits and some with physical deficits; systemic features may be prominent, and neurologic signs are common (Table 22-5).

There are three main groups of neurometabolic diseases[39]:

1. Those with a known enzymatic defect, including disorders of amino acid metabolism (e.g., phenylketonuria), peroxisomal disorders (e.g., adrenoleukodystrophy), and lysosomal storage disorders (e.g., Tay-Sachs disease)
2. Those with abnormal storage accumulation in CNS cells, including lysosomal storage disorders and mucopolysaccharidoses
3. Those with no identified biochemical defect (e.g., Cockayne syndrome), a heterogeneous group that is shrinking as research identifies the biochemical defects

There is considerable overlap among the three groups. All of these disorders are rare, and although some are treatable, most are relentlessly progressive and associated with early death. Many patients show a steady decline, with a gradual increase in symptoms and loss of function or a stepwise deterioration with bouts of acute illness leading to a sudden loss of function.

Treatment is available for only a few of the diseases and consists primarily of dietary strategies, although some pharmacologic treatments are used. Started early, especially in the presymptomatic phase, treatment may prevent neurologic complications. An example is phenylketonuria, a disorder of amino acid metabolism. The prevalence varies by population, with an incidence of 1 case per 100,000 people in the United States. Screening occurs in the neonatal period, and affected children are begun on a special diet. Those who have good dietary management throughout life may develop relatively few problems, although close monitoring by a specialist team of physicians and dieticians is essential to ensure metabolic stability. Unfortunately, treatments may be of questionable benefit for many children.

Disorders that cause lactic acidosis are the most common of these diseases, although many individuals who harbor the genetic substrate for one of these disorders may not express it or may come to diagnosis very late in life.[40] The features of these diseases are extremely varied, and although the neuropathologic, biochemical, and imaging abnormalities are well recognized, a precise diagnosis may remain elusive.

### Anesthesia Considerations for Progressive Neurologic Disorders

The risks associated with general anesthesia for children with progressive neurologic disorders include problems posed by fasting and by the need to keep the patient's metabolism stable during a period of stress. Meticulous planning with the child's metabolic specialist is essential before elective procedures. In the case of emergency surgery, the children and parents should be aware of or have written instructions regarding the preferred management of nutrition and metabolic indices, or they should have a resource person to call for specific advice.

## Neuromuscular Disorders

Neuromuscular disorders are caused by an abnormality of any component of the lower motor neuron system: anterior horn cell in the spinal cord, axon, neuromuscular junction, or muscle fiber (Fig. 22-1).[41] The cardinal features are weakness of skeletal muscles that is proximal, distal, or generalized in distribution, hypotonia, and reduced deep tendon reflexes. True fatigability suggests a defect of the neuromuscular junction. Neuropathy is characterized by distal weakness and sensory deficit. Joint contractures, scoliosis, and respiratory and cardiac involvement are common complications, and some conditions are associated with cognitive deficits.

### DISORDERS OF THE ANTERIOR HORN CELL
#### Spinal Muscular Atrophies

The spinal muscular atrophies (SMAs) are a group of disorders in which there is progressive degeneration of the anterior horns of the spinal cord and death of motor neurons. They are inherited as an autosomal recessive trait. The type of SMA (I, II, or III) is determined by the age of onset and the severity of symptoms.[41] The diagnosis is a clinical one, but confirmation by molecular testing for the survival of motor neuron gene (*SMN*) in a blood sample is now possible, and electrophysiology and muscle biopsy are no longer necessary.[42] Curative treatment is not available, but much can be done to improve duration and quality of life, especially for mildly affected children.

Type I SMA (i.e., Werdnig-Hoffmann disease) manifests at or soon after birth in most cases. The infant may appear neurologically normal at first, but the typical picture soon emerges. Parents may first notice an abnormal breathing pattern as the intercostal muscles are affected, and the respiratory pattern becomes diaphragmatic, with a bell-shaped chest observed clinically and radiographically. The infant is usually very alert and interactive but severely weak and floppy. There is good facial expression and normal eye movements, but the tongue fasciculates, and the tendon reflexes are absent. There is no cardiac involvement. Weakness, hypotonia, and bulbar involvement lead to progressive respiratory insufficiency and swallowing dysfunction, which are frequently complicated by episodes of aspiration. Most children die within the first 2 years of life, mainly due to respiratory complications. Management is essentially palliative, with gentle physiotherapy to keep the limbs flexible and special care with feeding. Noninvasive nocturnal ventilation is increasingly used, but invasive ventilation through a tracheostomy is not considered appropriate in most medical centers. This issue has provoked considerable debate in the literature.[43]

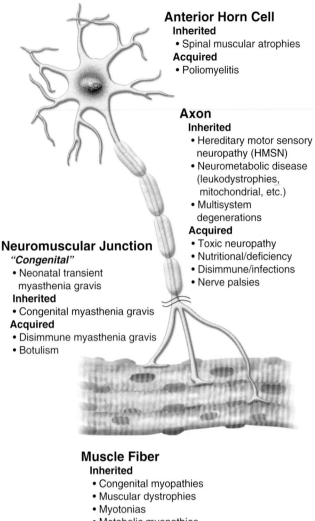

**Anterior Horn Cell**
**Inherited**
• Spinal muscular atrophies
**Acquired**
• Poliomyelitis

**Axon**
**Inherited**
• Hereditary motor sensory neuropathy (HMSN)
• Neurometabolic disease (leukodystrophies, mitochondrial, etc.)
• Multisystem degenerations
**Acquired**
• Toxic neuropathy
• Nutritional/deficiency
• Disimmune/infections
• Nerve palsies

**Neuromuscular Junction**
*"Congenital"*
• Neonatal transient myasthenia gravis
**Inherited**
• Congenital myasthenia gravis
**Acquired**
• Disimmune myasthenia gravis
• Botulism

**Muscle Fiber**
**Inherited**
• Congenital myopathies
• Muscular dystrophies
• Myotonias
• Metabolic myopathies
**Acquired**
• Disimmune myopathies (dermatomyositis)
• Endocrine myopathies
• Toxic (e.g., drug-induced [steroid])

**FIGURE 22-1** Diagram of a lower motor neuron. (Modified from Dubowitz V. Muscle disorders in childhood. Philadelphia: WB Saunders; 1978. Courtesy A. Moosa, MD.)

Type II SMA is an intermediate form, and it is the most prevalent. Because the weakness is milder, many children survive for years with meticulous multidisciplinary therapy, orthopedic and respiratory management, and care with nutrition. Onset occurs at 6 to 18 months of age. The clinical signs are similar to those of type I SMA, and the children are bright, intelligent, and particularly verbal. Type II patients usually achieve independent sitting at some stage, but these children never bear weight or walk. Respiratory infections are a particular problem, and noninvasive nocturnal respiratory support (i.e., biphasic or continuous positive airway pressure) with a facemask and portable ventilator is well tolerated by children and parents. This improves well-being and enables remarkably full activity despite weakness.[44,45]

Joint contractures are almost inevitable, as is progressive scoliosis, which usually appears early, and management is difficult in the very young child. Operative correction and stabilization with instrumentation is delayed as long as possible to prevent the complications of pubertal growth with a fixed spine; children usually tolerate the procedure well if they are carefully prepared and managed.

Some children with type II SMA develop feeding difficulties because of weakness of bulbar musculature or as a complication of chronic nocturnal hypoventilation. Good nutrition is essential for health, and supplementation and gastrostomy feeding may be required.[46]

Type III SMA (i.e., Kugelberg-Welander disease) is a mild variant with similar signs of flaccid and areflexic weakness of lower more so than upper limbs and with proximal predominance. These children attain independent walking, although it may be later than normal and tenuous. There is often deterioration around the time of puberty, when the growth spurt causes the previously precariously balanced muscle groups to become dysfunctional. Obesity and joint contracture also may affect the situation. Aggressive measures to keep the child walking are often effective and delay or prevent scoliosis and lower limb contracture.[47] Respiratory support may be necessary for nocturnal hypoventilation. Prognosis for long-term survival is good.

Other SMA variants exist in childhood. A rare type (SMA with respiratory disease) has severe diaphragmatic involvement and respiratory failure in infancy.[48] Some variants have associated features such as cerebellar atrophy, distal involvement, or additional myopathic features.

### Anesthesia Considerations for Spinal Muscular Atrophies
Children with SMA present for a variety of surgical procedures, including gastrostomy placement, tracheostomy, and spinal surgery, and they may also require anesthesia for diagnostic evaluation.[49] Rigorous preanesthesia evaluation is essential; perioperative care needs to be tailored to each child's needs, and postoperative respiratory support may be required. A variety of anesthesia techniques have been used successfully with and without muscle relaxants. Various degrees of sensitivity to nondepolarizing relaxants have been described, and it seems prudent to avoid or reduce the dose of these agents. If they are used, neuromuscular function should be assessed continuously and the effect of the relaxant antagonized at the conclusion of surgery. Spinal and epidural anesthesia and postoperative epidural analgesia have been used without adverse effects; however, the potential for respiratory depression may be increased with the addition of neuraxial opioids.

### Poliomyelitis
Poliomyelitis is a highly contagious, infectious disease caused by poliovirus, a human enterovirus. Most poliovirus infections are asymptomatic. If symptomatic, it occurs in two phases: an acute, nonspecific, febrile illness followed by aseptic meningitis and acute, flaccid, lower motor neuron paralysis. It typically manifests asymmetrically and may affect any muscle group. In children with respiratory involvement, lifelong ventilation may be needed. Fortunately, this situation is almost unheard of in the Western world because polio has been almost eradicated by immunization.[50]

## AXONAL DISORDERS
### Hereditary Neuropathies
Hereditary neuropathies are a group of inherited disorders that affect the peripheral nervous system. There are four main subcategories: hereditary motor and sensory neuropathy (most common

is Charcot-Marie-Tooth disease),[51] hereditary sensory neuropathy, hereditary motor neuropathy, and hereditary and autonomic sensory neuropathy.

Clinical presentation depends on the subtype and can occur at any age. Children usually present with disorders of gait or foot deformity, or they may come to the attention of a neurologist or geneticist through an affected parent. Clinical signs are usually confined to the lower limbs in the early years and may lead to orthopedic intervention before diagnosis. Some neuropathies are associated with multisystem involvement, including cardiac, autonomic, and respiratory systems, and a complete preoperative assessment of these children is essential.[52]

Peripheral neuropathy is a component of various neurometabolic disorders in which there is involvement of other parts of the nervous system or of other organs. For example, in the leukodystrophies, demyelination affects central and peripheral axons, giving a clinical picture of combined upper and lower neuron features. There are many neurometabolic disorders (e.g., mucopolysaccharidoses, sphingolipidoses, urea cycle disorders, organic disorders, amino acid disorders) with many variants, and presentation can occur at all ages from birth to adulthood. In children with mitochondrial diseases, peripheral neuropathy is often found, along with myriad other features.[53]

Multisystem degenerations are often genetically determined disorders of the nervous system that rarely begin in childhood.[52] Features may include dementia, epilepsy, extrapyramidal signs, brainstem dysfunction, vision and hearing impairment, anterior horn cell involvement, and peripheral neuropathy. They tend to have a progressive course.

### Acquired Disorders of the Peripheral Nerves

Acquired disorders of the peripheral nerves are rare in childhood. In clinical practice in the developed world, neuropathies complicating metabolic or nutritional disorders and treatment for cancer are the most common forms. In underdeveloped parts of the world, nutritional deficiencies, especially of vitamins E, $B_1$, $B_6$, $B_{12}$, niacin, and thiamine, are important. The neuropathic features may be overshadowed by the other characteristics of the disease.

### Guillain-Barré Syndrome

Guillain-Barré syndrome is an acute demyelinating disorder that causes progressive weakness usually 2 to 4 weeks after an illness with features of a viral infection or after immunization.[33] The inflammatory lesions in the peripheral nerves typically are associated with loss of myelin. In severe cases, the axons are damaged, a feature that is also seen in some acute cases without significant demyelination. The precise pathologic process has not been delineated, but various antibodies, immune complexes, and complement components have been found, suggesting causal heterogeneity.

The disorder is rare in children younger than 3 years of age, and the onset is usually sudden, although subacute presentations have been reported. The first sign is weakness in the lower limbs, which characteristically ascends the body, next affecting the trunk, the upper limbs, and occasionally the cranial nerves. It causes a flaccid paralysis, usually sparing sensory function but causing pain and areflexia at all levels. Autonomic neuropathy may develop, causing instability of blood pressure and cardiac arrhythmias. Involvement of respiratory muscles may produce acute respiratory failure or apnea that necessitates tracheal intubation.

Guillain-Barré syndome is diagnosed clinically, and the diagnosis is reinforced by finding an increased protein concentration in the CSF (despite a normal cell count) and abnormalities on nerve conduction studies. The studies may confirm demyelination by showing lowered nerve conduction velocity with distal delay, axonal involvement by low-amplitude action potentials, and in early cases, abnormality or absence of the H reflex, indicating absence of the spinal reflex arc. MRI of the spine may show thickening and contrast enhancement of the nerve roots and cauda equina.[54]

Patients with very mild symptoms that do not interfere with activities of daily living can be observed for deterioration without treatment. Corticosteroids are ineffective and may delay recovery. Intravenous immunoglobulin and plasmapheresis are the current treatment options.[53]

Supportive care in the intensive care unit may be needed for children with severe bulbar or respiratory weakness.[55] Children with axonal neuropathies are usually slower to recover motor function than those with demyelination, and our impression is that early treatment with intravenous immunoglobulin may alter the course.

### Chronic Inflammatory Demyelinating Polyneuropathy

Chronic inflammatory demyelinating polyneuropathy is extremely rare in childhood, and it is usually confined to older age groups. It manifests in a subacute or relapsing and remitting pattern with prominent sensory involvement. diagnostic investigations are similar to those for acute Guillain-Barré syndrome. Corticosteroids, intravenous immunoglobulin, and plasma exchange have been effective.[55] Although these treatments may be effective in the short term, recurrences may take place, and the usual pattern is that of a chronic, disabling, and relapsing and remitting condition that does not threaten longevity but interferes significantly with the quality of life.[56]

### Nerve Palsies

Like neuropathies, nerve palsies are uncommon in childhood.[51] The most common palsy encountered in children is neonatal or congenital facial nerve palsy. Cranial nerve palsies, especially those that involve the eye muscles, are usually related to intracranial disease such as increased ICP in children, but they may also be isolated findings that result from viral infections. In the latter instances, recovery is the norm.

Peripheral nerve palsies such as carpal tunnel syndrome have been reported in childhood.[57] They may complicate severe juvenile arthritis[58] or storage disorders such as mucopolysaccharidoses. Because symptoms may be difficult to elicit from children at the best of times, identifying palsies may be problematic in severely learning disabled children. Specialist care may require routine assessment of nerve conduction and possible surgical decompression. Concern has been expressed regarding the emergence of carpal tunnel syndrome as a type of repetitive strain injury in children due to excessive use of video games.[59] Case reviews refer to other types of repetitive strain injury, such as basketball training and skiing, as etiologic factors.[60]

## DISORDERS OF THE NEUROMUSCULAR JUNCTION
### Myasthenia Gravis

Myasthenia gravis is a disorder of the neuromuscular junction. The autoimmune disorder is characterized by one of several lesions of acetylcholine-mediated transmission.[61] Weakness results from antibodies that block acetylcholine receptors, inhibiting the excitatory effects of acetylcholine at the neuromuscular junction. This reduction in the number of acetylcholine receptors results in a characteristic pattern of progressively reduced muscle strength with repeated use and recovery of muscle strength after a period of rest.

### Neonatal Transient Myasthenia Gravis

Neonatal myasthenia gravis is caused by placental transfer of antibodies to acetylcholine receptors from an affected or previously affected mother. The infant may present with feeding difficulties or respiratory dysfunction.[62] Treatment, which involves anticholinesterase medications, must be tailored to the nature and severity of the weakness, and intensive support occasionally is required. This form of myasthenia gravis is a transient disorder for which treatment is temporary and the risk of recurrence small. It should be anticipated in the offspring of any woman who has active myasthenia gravis or a history of the disorder, because cases have been described in infants of mothers in remission from myasthenia gravis.

### Congenital Myasthenic Syndromes

Congenital myasthenia gravis represents several genetically determined defects of the neuromuscular junction that have in common an exercise-induced weakness of skeletal muscle.[63] Fourteen genetic mutations have been identified, but many cases of congenital myasthenia gravis do not have an identified mutation. Inheritance of mutations usually follows an autosomal recessive pattern.

Although rare, congenital myasthenia gravis should be considered in the differential diagnosis of any neonate or infant who presents with motor problems (e.g., weakness, hypotonia, fatigability), eye signs (e.g., ptosis, ophthalmoplegia, pupillary abnormalities), and respiratory insufficiency (e.g., recurrent apneas, ventilator dependence). Late-onset muscle weakness has been reported in adolescence or early adulthood. Diagnosis may be difficult because the classic features of myasthenia gravis, including responses to anticholinesterase medications, may be absent.[64] A Tensilon test, electromyography with repetitive nerve stimulation, a muscle biopsy, and molecular analysis in a specialist center should be sought to confirm the diagnosis.

### Juvenile Myasthenia Gravis

Juvenile myasthenia gravis, like the adult version of the disease, is an immunologic disorder that may be associated with enlargement of the thymus gland and the presence of circulating antiacetylcholine receptor antibodies. Occurring at any age, fatigable weakness suggests the diagnosis, which may be confirmed by electromyography and by antiacetylcholine receptor antibody analysis.

Treatment of myasthenia gravis varies with the type and biochemical characteristics. Careful titration of pyridostigmine is needed. Corticosteroids and surgical thymectomy are indicated for patients with immunologic abnormalities.[65]

### Anesthesia Considerations for Myasthenia Gravis

The anesthesiologist may become involved in the management of children with myasthenia gravis for several reasons[66]:

- Children may suffer a crisis requiring mechanical ventilation or when large-bore central access is attempted to facilitate plasma exchange transfusion.
- They may require thymectomy.
- They may undergo elective or emergency surgery unrelated to their myasthenia.

The severity of the muscle weakness and the muscle groups affected by the disease should be documented preoperatively,

focusing on respiratory and bulbar function. Myasthenic patients' responses to muscle relaxants depend on the type of relaxant. Decreased density of acetylcholine receptors at the motor end plate means that children with myasthenia may require up to four times the calculated dose of succinylcholine to establish a depolarizing muscle block. Because succinylcholine is metabolized by acetylcholinesterase, its metabolism is reduced and duration of action prolonged in the setting of chronic acetylcholinesterase inhibition. For this reason, succinylcholine is best avoided in these children.

The activity of nondepolarizing muscle relaxants is increased as their duration of action is increased. Unfortunately, the degree to which the sensitivity is increased is somewhat unpredictable and depends on an interaction between the severity of the disease (e.g., level of acetylcholine receptor antibodies) and the efficacy of treatment. Inhalational anesthetic agents inhibit neuromuscular transmission, and these effects may be exaggerated in myasthenia gravis patients. However, no clinically significant postoperative neuromuscular depression has been demonstrated with isoflurane, sevoflurane, or desflurane. These potential neuromuscular effects are not shared by propofol, making total intravenous anesthesia (TIVA), in theory at least, the technique of choice for these children. For all but the most minor surgery in the patient with stable myasthenia gravis without significant respiratory or bulbar compromise, a tracheal tube and intermittent positive-pressure ventilation are likely to be required. If possible, intubation of the trachea should be performed without the use of muscle relaxants. Tracheal intubation with inhalational anesthetics alone or propofol with a short-acting opioid has been described in these children.[67]

### Myasthenia-like Syndrome

The toxin of *Clostridium botulinum* produces a myasthenia-like syndrome that may occur through two mechanisms: ingestion of food contaminated by *C. botulinum* toxin, including contaminated honey, and wound infection by *C. botulinum*. Features include blurring of vision with ptosis, dilated and unresponsive pupils, cranial nerve palsies, limb paralysis with areflexia, feeding difficulty, and respiratory insufficiency. Diagnosis depends on clinical suspicion, identification of the toxin in residual food, and electromyography.

Treatment is supportive, and recovery may take weeks to months.[68] Succinylcholine is contraindicated in children with infections that affect the neuromuscular junction, including botulism and tetanus.[69]

## DISORDERS OF MUSCLE FIBERS
### Myopathies
#### Congenital Myopathies

Congenital myopathies are rare disorders that have extreme variations in the type and severity of features (Table 22-6).[70] The myopathies may manifest at any age, but in many cases, they become apparent only in adulthood, challenging the *congenital* designation.[71] In infancy, the usual features are weakness and hypotonia (i.e., the floppy baby).[72] Although these are inherited disorders, there is often no family history, and because many cases are autosomal dominant or X-linked recessive, the carrier parent may have subclinical signs of a myopathy.

Children usually present with ptosis, facial weakness, limb weakness (proximal more than distal), and there may be evidence of respiratory muscle weakness and cardiomyopathy. In some cases, the extraocular muscles may be affected with external

**TABLE 22-6** Common Congenital Myopathies

| Disorder | Genetics |
|---|---|
| Central core disease | 19q13, *RYR1*, ryanodine receptor |
| Multicore or minicore disease | 1p36, *SEPN1* |
| Nemaline myopathy | 2q21.2-q22, *NEB*, nebulin |
| Desmin myopathy | 2q35, *DES*, desmin |
| Myotubular or centronuclear myopathy | Xq27.3-q28, *MTM1*, myotubularin 1 |

Data from http://neuromuscular.wustl.edu/syncm.html (accessed June 2012); http://www.genenames.org (accessed June 2012).

**TABLE 22-7** Metabolic Myopathies

Channelopathies
Mitochondrial myopathies
Glycogenoses
Lipid myopathies

22

ophthalmoplegia. Joint contractures and scoliosis can also develop. Infants often have characteristic facies, with a long and narrow face, prominent ears, and a narrow, high-arched palate. Deep tendon reflexes are reduced or absent. The diagnosis usually is confirmed by characteristic findings on muscle biopsy. Molecular analysis is available for many of these myopathies in specialist laboratories.[73]

Paralleling the clinical features, the course of congenital myopathies varies greatly. Many individuals are mildly affected and may come to diagnosis only if a more severely affected child is diagnosed. All parents, even those without symptoms, must be carefully examined by a neurologist with expertise in neuromuscular disease to detect very mild weakness of particular muscles. For a parent who demonstrates weakness, it may help to perform a muscle biopsy and molecular testing to confirm the diagnosis. For many children with congenital myopathy, there is little or no deterioration in muscle strength as the child ages, and many children experience gradual improvement in muscle strength and a reduction in symptoms. However, weakness is severe in some cases, and clinical complications, including deglutition difficulties and respiratory failure, limit survival, although these features are not specific to congenital myopathies.[74,75]

Support of respiration and nutrition may be necessary. Minimally invasive methods such as noninvasive nocturnal ventilation by facemask are indicated to assist with management at home. Regular passive movements and careful management of posture and positioning to prevent contractures, especially scoliosis, is essential. Meticulous care of skin, joints, bowels, and teeth help to avoid the need for more invasive management. A complete evaluation of cardiovascular and respiratory status is required before anesthesia and surgery.[76]

Malignant hyperthermia (MH) is a disorder of skeletal muscle that manifests in response to anesthetic triggering agents. Central core disease is a myopathy closely associated with MH (see Chapter 40), with extreme variation in the severity of its features. MH and central core disease are primarily disorders of calcium regulation in skeletal muscle. Genetic testing identifies mutations in the ryanodine receptor gene (*RYR1*) in most affected individuals, accounting for their susceptibility to MH.[77] The *RYR1* gene encodes the channel that controls calcium release from the sarcoplasmic reticulum in skeletal muscle and to a lesser extent in other organ systems. *RYR1* abnormalities alter the channel kinetics for calcium inactivation, and calcium buildup causes excessive skeletal muscle contraction due to disinhibition of the normal actin-myosin interaction. The level of adenosine triphosphate (ATP) decreases, leading to anaerobic and aerobic metabolism and to acidosis. Other effects of MH include heat production, sympathetic nervous system activation, hyperkalemia, tachycardia,

muscle rigidity, tachypnea, disseminated intravascular coagulation, fever, myoglobinuria, and multiorgan dysfunction and failure.

The in vitro contracture test (IVCT) was developed to confirm susceptibility to MH by studying the contracture of muscle fibers in response to triggers such as caffeine and halothane.[78] This is an invasive and expensive investigation because an open muscle biopsy is required, and very few specialized centers perform this procedure. Most individuals with central core myopathy may be susceptible to MH, as demonstrated by IVCT, which has been the only means to confirm MH susceptibility until the emergence of molecular testing.[79] DNA analysis can provide a fairly reliable test for susceptibility to MH for 60% of affected individuals who have had an IVCT but for only 20% of those who have not had an IVCT (see Chapter 40).[80] However, the complexity of the situation is such that assessment and advice by a specialist is recommended rather than immediately embarking on DNA analysis so that the child and family may benefit from appropriate investigation and interpretation. Any individual with central core disease and his or her family should be informed about the clinical situation, diagnosis, and possible risks and complications, including MH, and should be offered a specialized investigation. An individual who may be susceptible to MH should carry information to inform medical staff in an emergency.[81] Any elective operative procedure must be meticulously planned in advance with the full involvement of the anesthesiologist.

### *Metabolic Myopathies*

Metabolic myopathies (Table 22-7) are uncommon and complex. Most affected children have multisystem involvement of sufficient severity to mask the myopathic features. The most important concerns for the anesthesiologist are the risk of metabolic instability during surgery and the need for close liaison with the child's pediatrician to plan fluid and electrolyte balance and nutritional management.[81,82]

### *Mitochondrial Disorders Underlying Myopathies*

Mitochondrial disorders are a common cause of inherited neurologic disease in children, occurring in 1 of 5000 live births. They are caused by mutations in mitochondrial or nuclear DNA. The respiratory chain is under bigenomic control: nuclear DNA codes for 85% of the proteins, and mitochondrial DNA codes for 15%. Nuclear DNA is inherited along mendelian inheritance patterns, whereas mitochondrial DNA follows maternal inheritance patterns in a ratio of 9 to 1. Most mitochondrial disorders in children are determined by nuclear DNA, whereas those in adults are determined by mitochondrial DNA. The organs involved by mitochondrial disease are determined by the presence of defective nuclear or mitochondrial DNA in the embryo. The relative amount of defective DNA in affected tissues determines the severity of the disease. Disruption of the most fundamental cellular energy process, the mitochondrial respiratory

**TABLE 22-8**  Clinical Mitochondrial Syndromes in Childhood

| Syndrome | Features |
|---|---|
| Alper-Huttenlocher, neuronal degeneration | Catastrophic onset of epilepsy, paralysis, ataxia, dementia, visual impairment, liver disease; death usually in months |
| Leigh encephalomyeloneuropathy | Brainstem signs predominant; relapsing/remitting or steadily progressive to death |
| Infantile myopathy and lactic acidosis | Hypotonia in infancy, feeding difficulties, respiratory problems, cardiomyopathy; fatal and nonfatal forms |
| Leber hereditary optic neuropathy (LHON) | Progressive visual loss in childhood, cardiac arrhythmias, dystonia |
| Kearns-Sayre (KSS) | Progressive external ophthalmoplegia, pigmentary retinopathy, deafness, heart block, choreoathetosis and ataxia, myopathy, endocrine disorders |
| NARP | Neuropathy, ataxia, retinitis pigmentosa |
| MELAS | Mitochondrial encephalomyopathy, lactic acidosis, stroke-like episodes, dementia |
| MERFF | Myoclonic epilepsy, myopathy with ragged red fibers (muscle Gomori trichrome stain), ataxia |
| MNGIE | Myoneurogenic gastrointestinal encephalopathy |

chain, results in a diverse and variable group of multisystem disorders known collectively as mitochondrial disease. Involvement of the brain, nerves, and muscles can occur in isolation or in combination.

Diagnosis relies on characteristic clinical features, an understanding of mitochondrial genetics, and a logical, informed approach to investigations. Abnormalities of the mitochondrial genome are extremely common, and they can cause devastating phenotypes or be completely subclinical. Assessment and diagnosis are challenging.[5]

Neurologic symptoms and signs are common. However, they tend to be varied and include myopathy, neuropathy, strokelike episodes, ataxia, dementia, epilepsy, migraine, sensorineural deafness, and pigmentary retinopathy. The more common clinical scenarios in childhood are outlined in Table 22-8. Involvement of other organ systems, such as diabetes mellitus, gastrointestinal disease, and cardiomyopathy, may coexist or dominate the clinical picture. Evidence of mitochondrial dysfunction, such as lactic acidosis, increased CSF protein, and ragged red fibers on muscle biopsy, may or may not exist. Assessment of the child with atypical and otherwise unexplained features should include a search for evidence of mitochondrial abnormalities. The clinical details determine the investigative plan, which should include cerebral imaging with MRI and MRS (to detect lactate peaks), blood biochemistry (i.e., creatine kinase, lactate, and glucose levels), tests of urinary amino and organic acids, cardiologic assessment (i.e., chest radiography, electrocardiogram, and echocardiogram), electroencephalography, and exercise testing and neurophysiology, leading to mitochondrial studies of blood and muscle tissue. Muscle biopsy investigations include histopathology, electron microscopy, respiratory chain enzymology, and molecular analysis of mitochondrial DNA. Further investigation with respiratory chain enzymes and molecular genetic analysis is indicated in some cases.[83]

Treatment of mitochondrial disorders includes management of specific features such as antiepileptic therapy and efforts to maintain stability of metabolic pathways. Vitamins and other supplements such as coenzyme $Q_{10}$ (i.e., ubiquinone), riboflavin, thiamine, and carnitine are referred to as the *mitochondrial cocktail* and are used in most of the mitochondrial disorders. Use of the cocktail is largely based on the assumption that higher doses of these agents may improve mitochondrial energy generation.[84] Arginine has been used in the treatment of patients with mitochondrial encephalopathy with lactic acidosis and stroke-like episodes (MELAS).[85]

### Anesthesia Considerations for Myopathies

The challenge for the anesthesiologist is to maintain metabolic stability and prevent complications. In children prone to lactic acidosis, intravenous fluids that contain lactate should be avoided, whereas administration of glucose-containing solutions is essential in any but the shortest of procedures to avoid hypoglycemia.[82] In all children with mitochondrial disorders, the preoperative fasting period should be kept to a minimum to avoid hypovolemia and depletion of glucose stores. Stresses that may provoke increased energy requirements, such as perioperative pain, hypothermia, or hyperthermia, must be minimized. Children with Kearns-Sayre syndrome must have adequate assessment and perioperative monitoring because they may have cardiac conduction abnormalities as well as myopathy, diabetes, proximal renal tubular acidosis, and other multisystemic abnormalities.[84]

Inhalational and intravenous forms of anesthesia have been used successfully in children with mitochondrial disorders. Few serious complications have occurred, and none related to anesthesia were reported in two retrospective reviews of perioperative complications after general anesthesia in children with mitochondrial myopathies.[82,86] Inhalational anesthetics have been used without consequences in these children, and there is no evidence that this population has a greater susceptibility to MH than normal children.[87] However, mitochondrial disorders result from a variety of molecular changes and have varied responses to anesthetics.[88]

All inhalational anesthetics and propofol depress mitochondrial function at several levels. It has been suggested that children who develop metabolic acidosis and myocardial failure after propofol infusions for extended periods (more than 5 mg/kg/hr for more than 48 hours) have a subclinical form of a mitochondrial disorder. Although propofol infusion syndrome (PRIS) impairs mitochondrial oxidation and transport of free fatty acids in a manner not unlike that in mitochondrial myopathies, there is no evidence that the two disorders are linked. In a review of 61 patients with PRIS, seven (four children and three adults) developed PRIS during anesthesia.[89] Impaired tissue perfusion (as seen in sepsis) may be a common underlying mechanism. Propofol interferes with fatty acid metabolism and the respiratory chain, in much the same manner as other anesthetics and medications, suggesting that its use during general anesthesia for children with mitochondrial myopathies is reasonable, and it has been used widely.[90,91] Evidence suggests that any anesthesia technique may be used in children with mitochondrial myopathies.

**TABLE 22-9** Muscular Dystrophies

| Disorder | Genetics |
|---|---|
| **Myotonic dystrophy** | |
| DM1 (98%), autosomal dominant | 9q13.3, *DMPK* or *DM1*, dystrophia myotonica |
| DM2 (2%), autosomal dominant | 3q21, *CNBP* (formerly *ZNF9*) |
| **Congenital Muscular Dystrophies** | |
| Autosomal recessive | |
| Fukuyama type | 9q31-q33, *FKTN*, fukutin |
| Walker-Warburg | 9q34.1, *POMT1* |
| Merosin negative | 6q22-q23, *LAMA2* |
| Merosin positive | 21q22.3, *COL6A1, COL6A2* |
| Ulrich | 2q37, *COL6A3* |
| X-linked recessive dystrophinopathies | |
| Duchenne and Becker types | Xp21.2, *DMD*, dystrophin |
| Emery-Dreifuss muscular dystrophy | |
| X-linked recessive | Xq27.3-q28, *EMD*, emerin |
| Autosomal dominant | 1q22, *LMNA*, lamin A/C |
| Limb girdle muscular dystrophies | |
| Autosomal recessive | 12 currently characterized |
| Autosomal dominant | 7 currently characterized |
| Facioscapulohumeral muscular dystrophy | 4q35, *FSHMD1A* |
| Autosomal dominant | |
| Distal myopathies | 5q31.2, *MATR3*, matrin 3 |
| Oculopharyngeal | 14q11.2, *PABPN1* (formerly *PABP2*) |

Data from http://neuromuscular.wustl.edu/syncm.html (accessed June 2012); http://www.genenames.org (accessed June 2012).

Sensitivity and resistance to nondepolarizing neuromuscular blocking agents have been reported in children with these myopathies. To ensure appropriate dosing, the drugs should be titrated judiciously while neuromuscular blockade is monitored.

## Muscular Dystrophies

Muscular dystrophies represent a group of more than 30 inherited disorders of muscle that may occur in infancy, childhood, or adulthood (Table 22-9). The word *dystrophy* implies a destructive progressive process, and although this is the characteristic clinical course for many of those afflicted with muscular dystrophies, the course is extremely slow or has no muscle strength deterioration for others.[92]

This area of neurology has advanced greatly due to developments in molecular genetics and to a lesser extent in muscle pathology. Duchenne muscular dystrophy was the first inherited disorder for which the causative gene and defective protein were identified.[92] Characterization of defective proteins leads to advances in immunohistochemistry that can assist diagnosis using a muscle biopsy. Detection of genetic mutations enables the diagnosis to be determined using a blood specimen in most instances, removing the need for muscle biopsy in many children. The mutated gene and molecular site of the defect have been identified for most of the common disorders, enabling much more focused management and informed counseling of families.[93]

The characteristic clinical features of muscular dystrophy include muscle weakness, the distribution of which varies from type to type; contractures, sluggish deep tendon reflexes, and involvement of respiratory and heart musculature. Other features, including learning disabilities, deafness, and ophthalmologic disorders, often exist. The creatine kinase level may be normal or increased to a minor or major degree; it provides an important marker for some disorders, such as the dystrophinopathies, in which it is raised on the order of 100 times normal. Diagnosis rests on careful clinical assessment, creatine kinase determination, molecular analysis, and muscle biopsy. Although there is no specific curative treatment for any of these disorders, advances in understanding the molecular genetic defect and proteins responsible for a disease have focused the search for an effective pharmacologic treatment to reverse the clinical signs and symptoms.[94,95]

For an infant who presents with severe weakness and hypotonia, signs of facial weakness, reduced alertness, and reduced respiratory effort raise the possibility of a congenital myotonic dystrophy (DM1), which is usually inherited from the mother in an autosomal dominant fashion. Clinical suspicion of DM1 may be confirmed by molecular testing for the affected gene (*DMPK*), which codes for myotonic dystrophy protein kinase. This protein is expressed predominantly in skeletal muscle, and the gene is located on the long arm of chromosome 19. This information negates the need for a muscle biopsy. A similar infant with good facial muscle movement, alertness, areflexia, and a diaphragmatic respiratory pattern indicating intercostal weakness is most likely to have SMA. The molecular test for the survival motor neuron is indicated to avoid the need for a muscle biopsy. Similar principles may be applied to children who present later in childhood. For example, a boy with gait abnormalities and a creatine kinase level 10 to 100 times normal is most likely to have a dystrophinopathy, and targeted molecular genetic testing can avoid the need for a biopsy.[96]

### Myotonic Dystrophy

Myotonic dystrophy is the most common inherited neuromuscular disorder in the general population, and many cases remain subclinical or undiagnosed.[4] All degrees of severity are possible, from the almost immobile infant with the congenital variant to the elderly adult with minimal motor weakness. Severity of the muscle weakness correlates with the molecular defect.

These children are susceptible to prolonged recovery from anesthesia, and care should be taken with the use of sedative medications and neuromuscular blocking agents.[97] Sensitivity to succinylcholine is increased, and maximal use of regional nerve blocks or local infiltration with local anesthetic agents should be employed whenever possible to minimize the need for opioids.

Most children with congenital or later-onset myotonic dystrophy have some degree of learning difficulties, which may be severe. One or the other parent is affected to a greater or lesser extent. In congenital cases (DM1), the mother is always the affected parent and, in most instances, is not aware of the disorder, the diagnosis is made by the pediatrician or pediatric neurologist who sees the child.[98] The infant does not demonstrate signs of myotonia, and a muscle biopsy is not helpful for the diagnosis at this age. The finding of facial weakness and clinical myotonia in the mother strongly suggests this disorder in a weak and floppy neonate.[99] The neonatal literature suggests that shaking the maternal hand (i.e., mother is unable to easily release her grip) may be sufficient to allow the pediatrician to make this diagnosis.[100] However, because it is possible to confirm the diagnosis by molecular testing of blood from the infant and mother, it is no longer necessary to rely on clinical expertise in muscle strength testing. Genetic counseling is essential and should be offered to the wider family circle. It is not unusual to uncover a large kindred with previously unsuspected disease in this situation.

These infants may require intensive care in the neonatal period, including respiratory support, but they tend to improve with age. However, significant learning disability is the rule, and the input of the multidisciplinary child development team followed by special schooling is the norm. Specific conditions requiring surgery include scoliosis and joint contractures, and perioperative care must be carefully planned.[98]

### Dystrophinopathies

The next most commonly encountered dystrophies are the dystrophinopathies. Duchenne muscular dystrophy (DMD) is the more severe phenotype, and Becker muscular dystrophy (BMD) is the milder phenotype. Both dystrophies are inherited in an X-linked recessive pattern and affect boys almost exclusively.[101] These disorders are caused by a deficiency of dystrophin (i.e., less than 3% of the normal content in DMD), a muscle membrane protein essential to the skeletal and cardiac muscle cytoskeleton and to neural tissue. Dystrophin reinforces the inner strength of the myocyte during lateral stretching and is involved in signal transduction (Fig. 22-2). DMD occurs as a result of mutations, mainly deletions in the dystrophin gene (*DMD*, locus Xp21.2).[96]

In affected children, muscle strength deteriorates between the ages of 2 and 8 years, and use of a wheelchair is usually required before adolescence. Respiratory, orthopedic and cardiac complications emerge with increasing age. By 8 to 10 years of age, serial echocardiograms should be performed to document cardiomyopathy. Because the lack of dystrophin affects the integrity of neural tissue, progressive cognitive dysfunction may occur. The absence of dystrophin predisposes the muscle to tearing from normal use or from use of drugs such as succinylcholine. Additional damage to skeletal muscle cells appears to stem from increased intracellular calcium concentrations, which may result from a defect in the sarcoplasmic reticulum. Upregulation of acetylcholine receptors has also been reported in these children. Without intervention, children with DMD usually die by a mean age of 19 years.

Coordination of clinical care is a crucial component of DMD management. Care is best provided in a multidisciplinary setting in which the individual and family can collaborate with specialists about the required multisystem management of DMD. Depending on local services, coordinated clinical care can be provided by a wide range of health care professionals including neurologists or pediatric neurologists, rehabilitation specialists, neurogeneticists, pediatricians, and primary care physicians. The person responsible for coordination of clinical care must be aware of the available assessments, tools, and interventions to proactively manage all potential issues for the child with DMD.

For children with DMD, glucocorticoids are the only available medication that slows the decline in muscle strength and function, which reduces the risk of scoliosis and stabilizes pulmonary function.[102] Cardiac function may also improve; the limited data indicate a slower decline in echocardiographic measures of cardiac dysfunction.[103,104] Prednisone is commonly used,

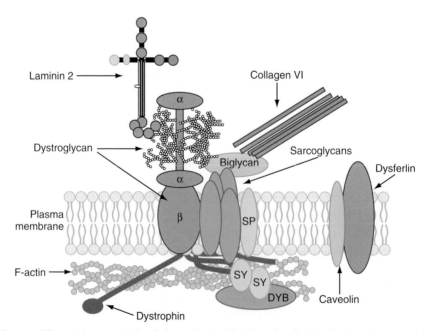

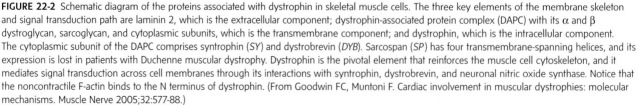

**FIGURE 22-2** Schematic diagram of the proteins associated with dystrophin in skeletal muscle cells. The three key elements of the membrane skeleton and signal transduction path are laminin 2, which is the extracellular component; dystrophin-associated protein complex (DAPC) with its α and β dystroglycan, sarcoglycan, and cytoplasmic subunits, which is the transmembrane component; and dystrophin, which is the intracellular component. The cytoplasmic subunit of the DAPC comprises syntrophin (*SY*) and dystrobrevin (*DYB*). Sarcospan (*SP*) has four transmembrane-spanning helices, and its expression is lost in patients with Duchenne muscular dystrophy. Dystrophin is the pivotal element that reinforces the muscle cell cytoskeleton, and it mediates signal transduction across cell membranes through its interactions with syntrophin, dystrobrevin, and neuronal nitric oxide synthase. Notice that the noncontractile F-actin binds to the N terminus of dystrophin. (From Goodwin FC, Muntoni F. Cardiac involvement in muscular dystrophies: molecular mechanisms. Muscle Nerve 2005;32:577-88.)

although deflazacort is an alternative used in some countries and is probably just as effective. The most effective prednisolone regimen appears to be 0.75 mg/kg/day. International guidelines for initiation of steroids and other pharmacologic agents and the implementation of multidisciplinary care are clearly outlined in a Consensus Statement on Standard of Care for Congenital Muscular Dystrophies.[105]

If lower limb contractures exist despite range-of-motion exercises and splinting, surgery can be considered in some scenarios.[106] The approach must be strictly individualized.[105] Surgical intervention is frequently used to treat lower limb contractures and enable rehabilitation in long leg orthoses so that the ambulatory phase may be prolonged.[107] This is usually indicated for children between 8 and 12 years of age, and it is well tolerated and successful if supported by a specialist team, but it may increase the burden of care for parents and families.[108]

Patients not treated with glucocorticoids have a 90% chance of developing significant progressive scoliosis[109] and a small chance of developing vertebral compression fractures due to osteoporosis. Although glucocorticoids can reduce the risk of scoliosis,[110,111] the risk of vertebral fracture is increased.[112,113] Spinal care should involve an experienced spinal surgeon and comprises scoliosis monitoring, support of spinal and pelvic symmetry, and spinal extension by the wheelchair seating system. Children receiving glucocorticoids should be monitored for painful vertebral body fractures. Corrective spinal surgery improves posture and seating options, eliminates pain due to vertebral fracture from osteoporosis, and slows the rate of respiratory decline.[109,114] The procedure is fraught with difficulty due to postoperative respiratory weakness and possible cardiac dysfunction.[114] Careful preparation and liaison among the pediatrician or neurologist, surgeon, and anesthesiologist is essential; a plan for postoperative management, including the provision of intensive care, should be made.[81]

Facioscapular muscular dystrophy is less often encountered in childhood, and specific surgical and anesthesia issues are limited. There are several phenotypes in childhood, including a severe neonatal form and a variably progressive childhood type that may be associated with sensorineural deafness. Irregular alignment between phenotype and genotype implies inconsistent expression of the molecular defect.[115,116] These children may benefit from surgery to fix the scapulae, which improves functionality of the upper limbs.[117,118]

Limb girdle syndromes (no longer a single entity; see Table 22-9) occur infrequently. Some have cardiac and respiratory implications and require preoperative assessment. In Emery-Dreifuss muscular dystrophy (EDMD), a syndrome in which cardiac conduction defects and dysrhythmias are common, syncope is usually the presenting complaint. These children are followed by a specialist team that includes a cardiologist.[81]

### Anesthesia Considerations for Muscular Dystrophies

The anesthesia implications for muscular dystrophies are dictated by the age of the child and severity of the disease. In early childhood, those affected by DMD undergo destruction of skeletal muscle, and when exposed to triggers that include succinylcholine and inhalational anesthetics, they have presented with severe rhabdomyolysis and hyperkalemia that resulted in cardiac arrest. Some children who were not known to have muscular dystrophy had a cardiac arrest during inhalational anesthesia as the first sign of the disorder. In contrast, during adolescence and adulthood, progressive cardiac and respiratory failure are the major concerns.

The severity of DMD usually is greater than that of BMD and EDMD.

Despite extensive documentation that inhalational anesthetics or succinylcholine, or both, can trigger life-threatening rhabdomyolysis in children with muscular dystrophy, this problem persists.[119-121] Case reports have described rhabdomyolysis, hyperkalemia, and cardiac arrest with or without the use of succinylcholine in children with DMD. No single inhalational anesthetic appears to be without blame.

The defect in dystrophinopathies results from the lack of the membrane-stabilizing protein dystrophin. It has been suggested that the addition of another destabilizing agent, such as an inhalational anesthetic, predisposes these children to mild or severe rhabdomyolysis, hyperkalemia, and death. Those most at risk for these complications are younger children, some of whom are undiagnosed until the perioperative rhabdomyolysis develops and establishes the diagnosis. Adolescents in whom muscle breakdown has waned and muscle mass has been lost and replaced by fatty infiltration have had uneventful perioperative courses when exposed to inhalational anesthetic agents and succinylcholine. Although succinylcholine is infrequently used today, the mortality rate associated with a succinylcholine-induced cardiac arrest is 30%.[122]

Although there is insufficient evidence to contraindicate inhalational anesthetics in children with muscular dystrophy, total intravenous anesthesia (TIVA) has emerged as an alternative to inhalational anesthetics in them.[108] In the absence of a compelling reason, it seems prudent to avoid inhalational anesthetics in children with DMD.[121,123] At the same time, without knowledge of the minimum concentration of inhalational anesthetic that triggers muscle breakdown, there is little justification for cleaning anesthetic workstations as in cases of MH. However, in certain clinical situations, such as a child with DMD and a difficult airway for whom an intravenous technique may be contraindicated or who refuses establishing IV access awake, brief exposure to an inhalational anesthetic to secure the airway seems reasonable. The anesthesia technique could then be converted to TIVA. The child should be carefully monitored for the signs of rhabdomyolysis (i.e., serum $K^+$ level) and the urine for myoglobin to detect a subclinical reaction, even if the risk is low, to avoid sequelae.[123]

Rhabdomyolysis caused by anesthetic agents may mimic MH.[124] The risk of MH in DMD children is the same as in the general population.[125] Hyperkalemic arrhythmias are most effectively reversed by rapid intravenous administration of calcium (10 mg/kg of calcium chloride), which may be repeated until the arrhythmias abate. Other therapies, including hyperventilation, administration of bicarbonate, albuterol, and insulin and glucose, are also recommended. The hyperkalemia associated with acute rhabdomyolysis may be refractory to the usual treatments and may require a prolonged resuscitation (see Chapter 8).

Boys with undiagnosed DMD have been anesthetized with inhalational agents and developed rhabdomyolysis. To minimize the risk of this complication, clinicians should question family members about any history of dystrophinopathies during the preoperative evaluation, mild signs of hypotonia, and motor weakness and delayed motor milestones. However, at least 30% of children represent a new mutation and therefore lack a positive family history. A brief developmental and neuromuscular history should be obtained, and if there is any question or suspicion, it is reasonable to measure a random blood creatine phosphokinase concentration preoperatively.

### Undiagnosed Myopathy

The child with a possible myopathy (e.g., floppy, hypotonic, motor developmental delay) but without a definitive diagnosis can pose a problem to the anesthesiologist.[126] A careful history and physical examination should be carried out. Blood creatine kinase and lactate concentrations should be evaluated, and the child's pediatrician or pediatric neurologist contacted for advice. If a progressive muscular dystrophy cannot be excluded (in the presence of an increased creatine kinase level), it may be prudent to avoid inhalational anesthetics, although their careful use for induction may be considered. An increased creatine kinase level in an asymptomatic infant or child may suggest a progressive muscular dystrophy, and inhalational anesthetics should be used with caution unless DMD or BMD are excluded.

# Epilepsy

Epilepsy is a common disorder in childhood, with a prevalence of 0.5% to 1% in the school-aged population. It is defined as the tendency to have recurrent spontaneous seizures. A seizure is a sudden, excessive, uncontrolled electrical discharge of cortical neurons.[127]

Any part or all of the cerebral cortex may be involved, and the manifestations of seizures are numerous. The first and most important step in managing epilepsy is to establish a correct diagnosis by determining whether the episodes are epileptic, classifying the episodes, and identifying the epilepsy syndrome that matches the clinical features (Table 22-10).

Diagnosis of seizures is largely a clinical process, with investigations providing information to determine cause (imaging) or seizure syndrome (electroencephalography). The cause may be a cerebral lesion of any type, in which case neurologic deficits may coexist, such as in cerebral palsy, or it may be a genetic disorder with no other neurologic features.

---

**TABLE 22-10** Epilepsy

**Classification of Seizure Types**

Self-limited seizures
  Generalized
  Focal
Continuous seizures
  Status epilepticus

**Epilepsy Syndromes in Childhood**

Neonatal seizures

Early infantile epileptic encephalopathy (Ohtahara)

Early myoclonic encephalopathy

Benign familial convulsions

Infantile spasms (West)

Febrile seizures

Benign myoclonic epilepsy of infancy

Primary generalized epilepsy
  Absence seizure syndromes
  Generalized tonic clonic seizure syndromes
  Juvenile myoclonic epilepsy (Janz)

Benign focal epilepsy syndromes (centrotemporal or occipital)

Lesional focal epilepsy

Data from the International League against Epilepsy. Available at http://www.ilae.org (accessed June 2012).

---

After a diagnosis of seizures has been made, the next step is to determine the epilepsy syndrome. This is achieved by reviewing the following:

- Seizure type
- Age
- Associated features
- Electroencephalographic features
- Interval since the last seizure
- Current medication, timing of the last dose, and blood levels

The details of the epilepsy syndrome can guide further investigations, help to plan treatment, and educate the family regarding the prognosis.[128]

Management is directed at treating the cause if possible and in preventing seizures using antiepileptic drugs. Medication is chosen according to the seizure type and epilepsy syndrome, taking into account the age of the child, associated disorders, and other maintenance medications[129] Most of the current antiepileptic drugs are licensed for use in childhood, although there are limitations for some drugs, especially in younger children. The aim of the treatment is to eliminate all seizures with the least number of antiepileptic drugs at the minimum doses. The American Epilepsy Society guidelines and practice parameters are available at www.aesnet.org, and the U.K. Epilepsy guidelines are available at www.nice.org.uk/CG020.

For children with epilepsy who are undergoing surgical procedures under anesthesia, the main problems are provocation or increased frequency of seizures, which have several causes:

- Anti-seizure medication missed due to perioperative fasting
- Epileptogenic anesthetics (e.g., enflurane)
- Hypoxia
- Electrolyte disturbance (e.g., hyponatremia)
- A direct effect of neurosurgery on the brain
- Cerebrovascular instability
- Coincidental exacerbation of severe epilepsy
- Postoperative ileus resulting in poor drug absorption

Certain disorders that cause epilepsy may be associated with other medical conditions, such as cardiorespiratory deficits, nutritional difficulties, and learning disabilities.[130]

Preparation for surgery should include a thorough review of the child's clinical status, including consultation with the physician who manages the child's epilepsy. For most minor elective procedures, there is no need to miss or omit any medication in the perioperative period, and parents should be advised to give regular medications as usual on the morning of surgery and anesthesia. Careful scheduling of the time of surgery may facilitate this because many children receive antiepileptic drugs on twice-daily regimens, with doses given at 8 AM and 8 PM. If surgery is scheduled for late morning or early afternoon, no medication need be missed. For children with complex epilepsy, such as those undergoing neurosurgery for the epilepsy itself, careful preoperative assessment is imperative.[131] In managing surgery and anesthesia in children with epilepsy, the aim is to prevent seizures and enable smooth and effective treatment (Table 22-11).

# Summary

Neurologic disease is common in childhood. Many severely disabled children are living longer but with increasingly complex medical and social needs. The challenges for surgeons and anesthesiologists in treating them include consent, complications of anesthesia, and issues related to long-term outcomes. The key to

**TABLE 22-11** Perioperative Medication Management for Children with Epilepsy

**Preoperative Management**

Liaise with child's pediatrician or neurologist.

Clarify usual seizure types, frequency, and trigger factors.

Review and document regular medication regimen (ideally twice daily).

Check antiepileptic drug level (phenobarbitone, phenytoin, or carbamazepine only).

Review rescue medication regimen.

Check drug allergies and adverse reactions.

**Management for Minor or Day Surgery**

Schedule for early afternoon.

Allow usual morning medication.

Avoid prolonged fasting.

Aim for evening medication as usual.

**Management for Major Surgery**

Ensure regular medications up to fasting.

Use intravenous preparations of regular drugs (phenytoin, phenobarbitone, valproate, benzodiazepine), if possible; use same doses two or three times daily.

If regular drugs not possible, administer the following:
Phenytoin: Give intravenous load of 20 mg/kg (maximum, 1 g) and then give twice-daily maintenance dose of 2.5-5.0 mg/kg.
Benzodiazepine: Give intravenously as rescue.

If enteral administration is possible, reestablish regular maintenance and wean intravenous phenytoin dose.

effective management is good basic neurologic and pediatric care with careful preparation, including close liaison with parents and the child's usual clinicians.

## ANNOTATED REFERENCES

Aicardi J. Diseases of the nervous system in childhood. 3rd ed. London: Mac Keith Press; 2009.
*This is a superb, comprehensive textbook that is well illustrated and extensively referenced.*
Dubowitz V, Sewry CA. Muscle biopsy: a practical approach. 3rd ed. Philadelphia: WB Saunders; 2007.
*This textbook provides a comprehensive review of neuromuscular conditions and associated pathology in children.*
Emery AELH. The muscular dystrophies. Oxford: Oxford University Press; 2002.
*This textbook provides a supplementary review of the muscular dystrophies, along with the molecular genetics and advances in management.*
Hoffmann GF, Johannes Zschocke J, Nyhan WL. Inherited metabolic disease: a clinical approach. Berlin: Springer-Verlag; 2010.
*This textbook provides an excellent review of an extremely complex subject.*
Klinger W, Lehmann-Horn F, Jurgat-Rott K. Complications of anaesthesia in neuromuscular disorders. Neuromuscul Disord 2005;15:195-206.
*The article reviews the topic for anesthesiologists.*
Neuromuscular Disease Center, Washington University at St. Louis, St. Louis. Available at http://neuromuscular.wustl.edu (accessed June 2012).
*This is a web-based review of all childhood neuromuscular disorders.*

## REFERENCES

Please see www.expertconsult.com.

# Surgery, Anesthesia, and the Immature Brain

## 23

ANDREAS W. LOEPKE AND ANDREW J. DAVIDSON

MILLIONS OF CHILDREN UNDERGO SURGERY with anesthesia every year.[1] During the perioperative period they are exposed to a multitude of stressors capable of interfering with normal brain development. Pain, stress, inflammation, hypoxia, and ischemia have all previously been shown to adversely affect the immature central nervous system. However, recent findings from animal studies have indicated that sedatives and anesthetics—the very drugs used to reduce pain and stress—may themselves undesirably influence brain development by triggering structural and functional abnormalities. There is now an extensive body of work, mostly based on laboratory research, that has defined this phenomenon and explored mechanisms and protective strategies. However, translating these laboratory findings to humans in clinical settings is laden with uncertainties and questions.

Human epidemiologic studies have found mixed evidence for an association between surgery (and anesthesia) in childhood, and subsequent neurodevelopmental delay. Some studies identified more learning disabilities in children after surgery with general anesthesia early in life, whereas others have not. Although surgery or comorbidities may play a central role in these abnormalities, emerging laboratory data regarding the deleterious effects of anesthesia without surgery has forced clinicians to consider the possibility that anesthetics may play a role in this

phenomenon. However, similar to the uncertainties surrounding animal studies, the interpretation of the human data is fraught with substantial limitations.

Any discussion of the long-term effects of anesthetics on the developing brain is further complicated by the fact that anesthetic drugs may be neuroprotective under certain conditions, and may indeed mitigate brain damage that is due to inflammatory responses, hypoxia-ischemia, or other insults that might occur during the perioperative period.

It is currently impossible to provide any definitive statements about the effects of anesthesia on neurodevelopment. This chapter provides an overview of the current laboratory and clinical data concerning the affect of sedatives, anesthetics, and analgesics on the immature brain.

## Background

About 160 years ago, William T. G. Morton conducted the first public demonstration of a drug-induced, reversible coma, later termed anesthesia, at the Massachusetts General Hospital and instantaneously revolutionized the field of surgery. After witnessing Morton's demonstration, Oliver Wendell Holmes coined the name for what he saw from the greek words "an" (without) and "esthesia" (sensibility). The inscription on Morton's tombstone, "Inventor and Revealer of Inhalation Anesthesia: Before Whom, in All Time, Surgery was Agony; By Whom, Pain in Surgery was Averted and Annulled; Since Whom, Science has Control of Pain," represents a powerful testament to the tremendously positive impact that anesthesiology has made on the field of medicine. This positive impact is now tempered by the possibility that anesthetics may impede normal brain development in the young. During the first century of their use, general anesthetics quickly became ubiquitous during surgery, although they were also regarded with serious concern because they were combustible and they depressed the hemodynamic and respiratory systems. Accordingly, up until 25 years ago, general anesthesia was rarely used in critically ill neonates because of the fear of myocardial depression and hemodynamic instability. Perioperative drug regimens were limited by some to neuromuscular blocking drugs and nitrous oxide. However, with the realization that unopposed pain exerted deleterious effects on the developing brain, that dramatic stress responses to painful stimulation can be detected even in preterm infants, and that modern anesthetics and analgesics can abolish these responses without substantial hemodynamic compromise, pediatric anesthesia, for the past two decades, has afforded critically ill neonates the benefits of amnesia, analgesia, and immobility during increasingly invasive surgery. These surgical interventions have helped to save lives and preserve the quality of life in one of the most vulnerable of patient populations. All the while, the powerful effects of general anesthetics on the brain were thought to be limited to the duration of immediate exposure, and no serious long-term adverse effects were expected following emergence from anesthesia. This notion of safety is now being seriously questioned, because apoptosis (defined as programmed cell death, see later) has been detected in neonatal animals during and immediately after anesthesia, and long-term learning defects have been reported in animals and children that were exposed to anesthesia at a young age.

## Normal Brain Development

The human brain undergoes a complex and extended process of enormous growth in cell number, synapses, and connections. Combined with this expansion of cells and connections, massive regressive processes also occur during normal brain development. These expanding and regressive processes allow the brain to fully develop and eventually execute complex tasks, such as talking, walking, reading, writing, calculating, acquiring social skills, perfecting fine motor dexterity, and planning and executing long-term objectives, while at the same time maintaining all life-sustaining functions. In order to accomplish these tasks, several specialized cells populate the brain. These cells are commonly divided into two large groups: neurons and glial cells, the latter subdivided into astrocytes and oligodendrocytes. Neural development starts with proliferation from a neural stem cell, followed by migration of that cell to its final place, differentiation into a specialized neuron, outgrowth of synapses during synaptogenesis to integrate into neural networks, and, finally, myelination of axons. In humans, many of these specialized processes occur in utero, but will also continue for an extended period of time postnatally. Indeed, some brain regions exhibit lifelong neurogenesis.

In utero and during the early postnatal period, the human brain initially undergoes a rapid growth in size and cell number, and is then pared back to achieve the efficient network of about 100 billion neurons of the adult brain. At birth, the size of the immature brain is one-third that of the adult brain, doubling in size within the first year of life, and reaching 90% of its eventual size by 6 years of age.[2] This dramatic growth spurt coincides with a remarkable overabundance of neurons and neuronal connections. In fact, less than half the neurons generated during development survive into adulthood.[3,4] Superfluous neurons that lose in the competition for a limited amount of trophic factors are removed by programmed cell death. Also called apoptosis, this cellular suicide program is built into every mammalian cell. Apoptotic cells enter a well-orchestrated, stepwise, and energy-consuming destruction process that involves a cascade of enzymes called caspases and ultimately leads to the breakdown of cellular proteins and DNA.[5] This process is heavily used during development, such as during embryonal deletion of the interdigital mesenchymal tissue to separate fingers and toes. Similar to the clotting cascade, the apoptotic cascade remains active throughout life and is held in check by antiapoptotic factors, whereas proapoptotic factors promote its execution. Neurons are protected from apoptosis by neurotrophic factors. Conversely, noxious stimuli, such as pain, hypoxia, and ischemia, can increase the level of proapoptotic factors and activate the apoptotic suicide program, leading to neuronal cell death.

In addition to an overabundance in the total number of neurons generated during early development, the mammalian brain also forms an excess of neuronal connections, or synapses, during this period. Depending on brain region, synaptic density reaches its maximum in infants and young toddlers between 3 and 15 months of age, and will undergo a progressive reduction by about half into adulthood.[6] Connections that are active with continued electrical and chemical signals are sustained, whereas those with little or no activity are lost.

In summary, brain architecture changes rapidly and dramatically throughout life. Neuronal density is greatest during fetal life, and excess neurons are eliminated via apoptosis, predominantly in utero, during the neonatal period and throughout infancy.[7] Rapid growth of dendrites and synaptic connections occurs during infancy and early childhood, and unneeded dendrites and synapses are trimmed back, predominantly during later childhood and adolescence.[6,7]

Accordingly, the first several years after birth represent a critical period of development for many brain regions. Recent findings in animals suggest that exposure to anesthetics or sedatives may interfere with proper neuronal development, brain architecture, and subsequent function. Although the exact molecular mechanisms by which anesthetics afford their therapeutic properties of amnesia, analgesia, and immobility are only incompletely understood, their interaction with a wide variety of ion channels, such as sodium, calcium, and potassium channels, as well as several cell membrane proteins, including the receptors for γ-aminobutyric acid (GABA), glycine, glutamate (and N-methyl-D-aspartate [NMDA]), acetylcholine, and serotonin, make it conceivable that anesthetics could interfere with normal electrical and chemical activity in the developing brain. In fact, both GABA and NMDA play critical roles as trophic factors and in regulating neuronal maturation and programmed cell death. During brain development, GABA directs cell proliferation, neuroblast migration, and dendritic maturation.[8] Developmental NMDA receptor stimulation fosters survival and maturation of some neurons.[9,10] It is therefore not implausible that anesthetics might interfere with these developmental processes.

# Effects of Anesthetic Exposure on the Developing Brain

Concerns regarding neurologic abnormalities following general anesthesia in young children were first raised more than half a century ago, when postoperative personality changes were observed following the administration of vinyl ether, cyclopropane, or ethyl chloride for otolaryngologic surgery.[11] However, these abnormalities were felt to be psychological in nature because they were alleviated by the timely administration of preoperative sedative drugs.[11,12] Approximately two decades later the focus of research shifted to examine the effects of anesthetics in animal models that represented occupational exposure in pregnant healthcare workers.[13-16] Delayed synaptogenesis and behavioral abnormalities were observed in neonatal rats born to dams that were chronically exposed to subanesthetic doses of halothane during their entire pregnancy. However, interest in the effects of anesthetics on children did not elicit widespread interest until publications began to appear 10 years ago. In a seminal study in neonatal rat pups, widespread neuronal degeneration was observed after repeated injections of ketamine.[17] This led to numerous editorials and review articles, and more than 200 publications in which structural brain abnormalities and/or functional impairment were demonstrated after a wide variety of immature animal species (including chicks, mice, rats, guinea pigs, swine, sheep, and rhesus monkeys) were exposed to almost every sedative and anesthetic in clinical use.[18-65] However, no discussion about the effects of drug exposure on the developing brain would be complete without examining the effects of opioid analgesics in the developing brain.[54,55] Accordingly, this chapter will examine the various specific effects of sedatives, anesthetics, and analgesics in the immature brain.

## APOPTOTIC CELL DEATH

The most widely studied deleterious consequence of exposure to sedatives or anesthetics in immature animals is apoptosis, or programmed cell death. Although neuronal apoptosis eliminates approximately 50% to 70% of neurons throughout the brain during development, at any particular time, this natural process affects only a small fraction of cells. Exposure to anesthetics or sedatives briefly, but dramatically, increases the number of apoptotic neurons (Fig. 23-1). Some studies demonstrated up to a 68-fold increase in the density of degenerating neurons after a combination of anesthetics in neonatal rats, compared with control animals, although it remains unclear what fraction of the entire neuronal population these degenerating neurons represent. Unpublished data from one of the authors' laboratory suggest

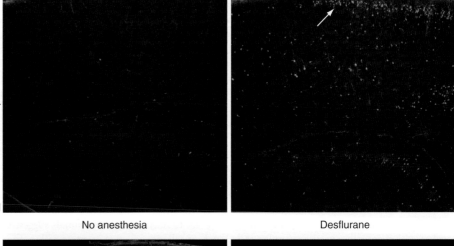
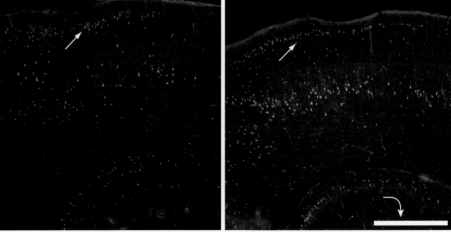

**FIGURE 23-1** Prolonged exposure to anesthetics causes widespread apoptotic cell death in the developing animal brain. Representative photomicrographs of brain sections from 7- to 8-day-old mice exposed to 6 hours of equipotent doses of 7.4% *desflurane*, 1.5% *isoflurane*, 2.9% *sevoflurane* in 30% oxygen, respectively, or fasted, unanesthetized litter mates in room air (*no anesthesia*). These doses were previously determined to represent 0.6 minimum alveolar concentration for the respective anesthetics. *Arrows* mark clusters of cells in layer II/III of neocortex that are dying from programmed cell death and are therefore labeled for the apoptotic marker, activated caspase 3 (bright green). Scale bar = 500 μm. (*curved arrow*) (From Istaphanous GK, Howard J, Nan X, et al. Comparison of the neuroapoptotic properties of equipotent anesthetic concentrations of desflurane, isoflurane, or sevoflurane in neonatal mice. Anesthesiology 2011;114:578-87.)

No anesthesia            Desflurane

Isoflurane            Sevoflurane

that a 6-hour exposure to a clinically relevant dose of isoflurane triggers apoptotic cell death in 2% of neurons in the superficial cortex of neonatal mice, whereas less than 0.1% of neurons undergo physiologic apoptosis in this region in unanesthetized litter mates (Loepke, personal communication). Interestingly, dying neurons are immediately adjacent to seemingly unaffected neighboring cells (Fig. 23-2), and the exact mechanism and selectivity of the cell death process remains unknown. Increased neuroapoptosis has also been observed following either in vitro or in vivo, exposure to a wide variety of sedatives and anesthetics, including chloral hydrate, clonazepam, diazepam, midazolam, nitrous oxide, desflurane, enflurane, halothane, isoflurane, sevoflurane, ketamine, pentobarbital, phenobarbital, propofol, and xenon, as well as opioid receptor agonists, in a wide variety of species, including chicks, mice, rats, guinea pigs, piglets, and rhesus monkeys (E-Table 23-1). Cell death–selective stains, such as cupric silver and Fluoro-Jade (EMD Millipore, Billerica, Mass.), have confirmed the cellular demise in neurons that positively stain for activated caspase 3, the central executioner enzyme of the apoptotic cascade.

Apoptosis represents an inherent, energy-consuming process using a cascade of enzymes called caspases. Apoptosis is highly conserved among species and culminates in self-destruction and elimination of cells, even under physiologic conditions, when these cells are functionally redundant or potentially detrimental to the organism.[208] Apoptosis involves an orderly breakdown of the cell that includes chromatin aggregation, nuclear and cytoplasmic condensation, and partitioning of cytoplasmic and nuclear material into apoptotic bodies for subsequent phagocytosis, without an extensive inflammatory response. That contrasts with the features observed during necrosis, which include energy failure, cellular swelling, membrane rupture, and release of cytoplasmic content into the extracellular compartment, followed by an inflammatory response.[208] Accordingly, apoptosis has also been termed cellular suicide and is extensively used during tissue homeostasis, endocrine-dependent tissue atrophy, and normal embryogenesis (e.g., ablation of tail tissue as part of tadpole metamorphosis in amphibians). Similarly, brain cells are also produced in excess during normal brain development, and up to 50% to 70% of immature neurons are eliminated during normal brain maturation in rodents, nonhuman primates, and humans.[3,4] Accordingly, physiologic apoptotic cell death is critical to establish proper brain structure and function, and any disruption of this process can lead to massive brain malformations and intrauterine demise.[209] However, in addition to this intrinsic pathway of physiologic, developmental apoptosis, cell death can also be triggered by pathologic, extrinsic factors, such as hypoxia and ischemia.[210] It currently remains unknown whether anesthesia-induced neuroapoptosis accelerates physiologic programmed cell death or whether it eliminates cells not destined to die, as in pathologic apoptosis.

Animal studies have identified a narrow window of maximum susceptibility to neuronal cell death induced by several anesthetic drugs, such as the NMDA antagonist ketamine, the GABA agonist isoflurane, or ethanol (a combined NMDA antagonist and GABA agonist). Ketamine-induced neuronal demise occurs in neonatal rodents between 5 and 7 days of age, or before 6 days of age in monkeys, but not in older animals.[17,69,139] Similarly, neurotoxicity was not detected after isoflurane anesthesia in 1-day-old animals or in those more than 10 days of age, whereas neuroapoptosis reached a maximum effect at 7 days of age.[87] However, preliminary data from the laboratory of one of the

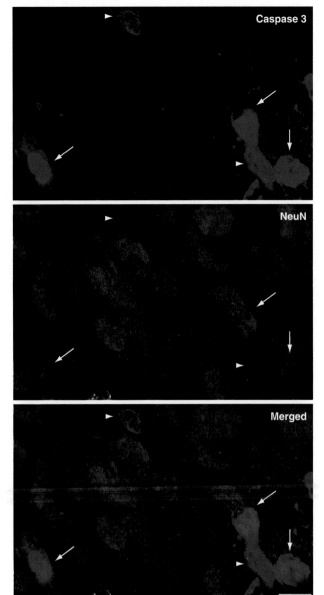

**FIGURE 23-2** Neurons affected by apoptotic cell death following anesthetic exposure are surrounded by seemingly unaffected cells. Representative photomicrograph from a 7-day-old mouse following a 6 hour exposure to 1.5% isoflurane, showing neocortical cells stained for the apoptotic cell death marker activated caspase 3 (*blue, top*), the neuronal marker NeuN (*red, middle*), and a merged image of the two stains (*bottom*). The majority of dying cells are identified as postmitotic neurons, as indicated by the purple cells coexpressing activated caspase 3 and NeuN in the bottom (*arrows*), whereas some cells expressing caspase 3 are NeuN-negative (*arrowheads*). Importantly, cells affected by anesthetic-induced neuroapoptosis are surrounded by numerous, seemingly unaffected neurons. Scale bar = 10 µm. (Image courtesy the Loepke Laboratory.)

authors challenges the notion that anesthetic-induced neuroapoptosis is limited to this age range (Loepke and associates, unpublished data). Conversely, intrauterine exposure to clinical doses of isoflurane in prenatal rats may actually decrease physiologic apoptosis and improve subsequent memory retention,[96] whereas only supraclinical doses of isoflurane induced neuroapoptosis in this setting.[112]

## LONG-TERM BRAIN CELLULAR VIABILITY, NEUROLOGIC FUNCTION, AND BEHAVIOR

In order to answer the important question whether anesthetics simply hasten physiologic apoptosis or whether they induce pathologic apoptosis, long-term neuronal density and neurologic function have to be assessed in adult animals exposed to anesthesia as neonates. If exposure to anesthetics or analgesics only temporarily accelerated physiologic apoptosis, one would expect normal cell counts and function in adult animals. Conversely, a permanent neuronal cell loss and long-term neurocognitive impairment after anesthetic exposure early in life would suggest that anesthesia-induced neuronal apoptosis may be pathologic in nature. However, this would only be true if the organism was unable to compensate for the neonatal cell loss by increasing neuronal plasticity and repair. To answer these questions, several studies measured neurologic function, assessed behavior, and/or determined neuronal density in adult animals after they were exposed to anesthesia in the neonatal period. Unfortunately, results from these studies are conflicting. Several studies reported long-term neurocognitive or behavioral abnormalities after exposure of neonates to enflurane, halothane, isoflurane, sevoflurane, propofol, or ketamine, or to a combination of isoflurane, nitrous oxide, and midazolam.* Importantly, however, many of these studies only observed abnormalities in very specific tests or subsets of neurocognitive batteries, whereas many other neurobehavioral domains remained intact. For example, a 6-hour exposure to midazolam, isoflurane, and nitrous oxide in neonatal rats led to transient impairment in a water maze learning task in young adulthood and in older animals, whereas, in the same animals, several other tests of behavior and learning, including acoustic startle response, sensorimotor tests, spontaneous behavior in an open field, and learning and memory in the radial arms maze, remained unimpaired.[85] Similarly, after a 4-hour exposure to the minimal alveolar concentration (1 MAC) of isoflurane in 7-day-old rats, long-term memory retention was abnormal at two time points, whereas performance at several other time points, as well as in other tests of learning and memory, remained intact.[107] Accordingly, the relevance of these limited learning deficits remains uncertain. Similar to humans, performance of rodents and primates in learning tasks depends to a great extent on maternal behavior and rearing conditions, making them strong confounders during neurocognitive testing.[105,211-213] Moreover, another obvious and important factor in neurocognitive testing is the verification of similar degrees of motivation when comparing separate groups of animals. For example, a 24-hour exposure to ketamine sedation early in life impaired subsequent performance of rhesus monkeys in learning and memory tests, in addition to decreasing their motivation to perform these tasks.[158]

Studies of prolonged opioid administration in immature animals have also found evidence for long-term impairment in learning tasks,[174-176,179-181] as well as altered pain responses in adult animals after exposure to morphine, fentanyl, heroin, or methadone early in life.†

Conversely, several other investigations have observed no neurologic abnormalities after administration of midazolam, isoflurane, sevoflurane, or ketamine, even when using complex neurologic tests in neonatal animals.* It remains to be determined whether these differential findings are attributable to the anesthetic doses, exposure times, species, or related to the type or timing of the neurologic tests performed. Interestingly, escalating exposure times of isoflurane in neonatal rats caused neuronal apoptosis beginning at 2 hours of anesthesia, but no evidence of long-term neurologic abnormalities until 4 hours of anesthesia.[106] In another study, a 6-hour exposure to isoflurane caused significant apoptosis immediately after exposure in neonatal mice, but resulted in no measurable long-term deficit in performance of complex neurologic tests as adult animals.[105] Moreover, in brain regions significantly affected by the neonatal neuroapoptosis, adult neuronal density was not diminished compared with unanesthetized litter mates.[105] These findings could either suggest that isoflurane may only accelerate physiologic apoptosis or that the developing brain's plasticity and capacity for repair could compensate for a pathologic insult early in life. Conversely, a study in similarly aged rats observed a permanent elimination of neurons, as well as neurologic abnormalities in adult animals, after exposure to isoflurane, nitrous oxide, and midazolam as neonates, suggesting that either the specific combination of anesthetic drugs (isoflurane alone vs. the combination exposure) or species differences (rats vs. mice) could affect any relationships between neonatal neuroapoptosis and long-term function and neuronal density.[97] Alternatively, these conflicting results may be explained by the dissimilar testing environment, because neurocognitive tests are easily transferable among laboratories.[214] On the other hand, neonatal apoptosis may not be causally linked to adult neurocognitive performance at all, as evidenced by substantial apoptosis immediately after carbon dioxide–induced hypercarbia in neonatal rats without long-term neurologic sequelae.[107]

## EFFECTS ON NEUROGENESIS AND GLIOGENESIS

The generation of new neurons, or neurogenesis, as well as new astrocytes, or gliogenesis, is most active in the immature brain in utero or soon after birth. Accordingly, anesthetic exposure during this critical period may interfere with neuronal proliferation, or even eliminate neuronal precursor cells, thereby portending permanent reductions in neuronal density and long-term neurologic impairment. To test this relationship, several studies have investigated the effects of anesthetic exposure, primarily isoflurane, on progenitor viability and rates of neurogenesis. Although isoflurane did not cause neural progenitor cell death in vitro, 3.4% isoflurane for 4 hours did decrease the rate of neuronal proliferation and increased neuronal fate selection.[108] These findings were recently confirmed in vitro, where 2.8% isoflurane for 6 hours resulted in no effects on neural stem cell viability and larger doses inhibited cell proliferation.[121] Similarly, morphine has been found to decrease DNA synthesis in cerebellar neuronal precursors without affecting cell survival.[170]

Isoflurane also impairs the growth of immature astrocytes and delays their maturation after 24 hours of 3% isoflurane, although this enormous exposure had no effect on cell viability.[119] Morphine, although increasing apoptosis in neurons and microglia, did not affect astrocytes in a study involving human fetal cell cultures.[173]

## ALTERATIONS IN DENDRITIC ARCHITECTURE

The immature brain accumulates an overabundance of neuronal connections in infancy, and the number of dendrites and

---

*References 13, 14, 74, 76, 85, 103, 106, 107, 113, 118, 129, 130, 142, 144, 158, 196, 198, 202
†References 77, 81, 82, 161, 162, 177

---

*References 72, 96, 105, 106, 115, 117, 132, 141, 145, 166, 196

synapses dramatically decreases after the first year of life. Several studies have examined the effects of propofol, isoflurane, sevoflurane, desflurane, midazolam, and ketamine on dendritic arborization and synaptic architecture.* A common theme in these studies is that anesthetics can affect dendritic arborization and synaptic density, and that the direction of this change, whether it is an increase or a decrease in the number of dendritic spines, depends on the age at which the animals were exposed to anesthetics, and therefore the developmental state of the brain. During the first 2 weeks of life, the evidence indicates that anesthetic exposure leads to a decrease in synaptic and dendritic spine density in small rodents, while causing an increase in the number of dendrites beyond that age.[110,197] However, the permanence of these changes remains controversial, with some studies only observing a transient effect after ketamine, midazolam, or isoflurane anesthesia early in life.[120,153]

### DECREASE IN TROPHIC FACTORS
Isoflurane- or propofol-based anesthesia in the neonatal animal has been associated with a decrease in brain-derived neurotrophic factor (BDNF),[91,109,198] a protein integral to neuronal survival, growth, and differentiation. The cellular mechanism involves a reduction in tissue plasminogen activator and plasmin, which converts proBDNF to BDNF. Accordingly, isoflurane triggered proBDNF/p75[NTR] (p75 neurotrophin receptor) complex–mediated apoptosis in neonatal mice.[109] Moreover, prolonged exposure to opioid receptor agonists early in life has also been found to alter nerve growth factors in the immature brain.[66,164]

### DEGENERATION OF MITOCHONDRIA
Ultrastructural morphologic abnormalities have been reported in mitochondria of pyramidal neurons in the subiculum of 7-day-old rats after 6 hours of isoflurane, nitrous oxide, and midazolam.[126] A morphometric analysis demonstrated mitochondrial enlargement, impaired structural integrity, and decreased mitochondrial density, indicative of a protracted injury to the mitochondria after anesthetic exposure. Moreover, ultrastructural examination of pyramidal neurons of anesthetized animals by electron microscopy revealed evidence for increased autophagy, a form of cell death.

### ABNORMAL REENTRY INTO CELL CYCLE
Ketamine induces reentry of postmitotic neurons into cell cycle in immature rats.[155] Neuronal progenitor cells enter cell cycle during proliferation, but mature neurons lose this ability, and if they are forced to reenter cell cycle they will follow a path to apoptotic cell death.

### DESTABILIZATION OF THE CYTOSKELETON
The integrity of the cellular cytoskeleton is critical for proper neuronal morphology and function. Actin is one of the major components of the cytoskeleton of all eukaryotic cells, and participates in important cellular processes, including cell signaling, motility, and cell division. It is also essential in the formation of dendritic spines. Isoflurane can lead to depolymerization of actin in neurons and astrocytes, initiating cytoskeletal destabilization, impairment of astrocyte morphologic differentiation and maturation, as well as neuronal apoptosis.[119,123]

---

*References 70, 109, 110, 120, 136, 140, 152, 153, 165, 197

### EFFECTS ON THE DEVELOPING SPINAL CORD
Most animal studies have focused on the effect of general anesthetics and sedatives on the developing brain. However, it is important to also consider the developmental impact of anesthetics on the spinal cord. After 6 hours of 0.75% isoflurane with 75% nitrous oxide in 7-day-old rats, neuroapoptosis increased in the lumbar region of the spinal cord.[100] Similar results were reported after 6 hours of isoflurane in a similar model, although 1 hour of isoflurane or spinal bupivacaine resulted in no neuroapoptosis.[124] Intrathecal ketamine causes neuroapoptosis in the developing spinal cord of 3-day-old rats, but not at 7 days of age.[157] Preservative-free ketamine was associated with long-term alterations in spinal cord function and gait disturbances,[157] whereas, in a separate study, even high-dose intrathecal morphine produced no signs of spinal cord toxicity.[215]

## Putative Mechanisms for Neurotoxicity

The exact mechanisms that trigger the above responses to anesthetics and sedatives in the immature brain remain unresolved. Elucidating these mechanisms is critical in order to establish the relevance of these findings for pediatric anesthesia and neonatal critical care medicine, as well as to develop mitigating interventions, if necessary. The current, overarching hypothesis is that anesthetics and sedatives interfere with normal $GABA_A$ and NMDA receptor–mediated activity, which are the putative targets for unconsciousness, amnesia, and immobility,[216] but are also essential for mammalian central nervous system development.[9,217] Some have suggested that administering $GABA_A$-receptor agonists and/or NMDA-receptor antagonists may cause abnormal neuronal inhibition during a vulnerable period in brain development, triggering apoptosis in susceptible neurons, which in turn leads to neurocognitive impairment and decreased neuronal density in adults.[22,60,85,97] Other lines of evidence suggest that the NMDA receptor–blocking properties of ketamine may upregulate NMDA receptors, rendering the neurons more susceptible to excitotoxic injury caused by endogenous glutamate immediately after ketamine withdrawal.[135,139] However, several observations violate both hypotheses; neuronal cell death has been reported during exposure to anesthetics and not only after their discontinuation. Moreover, several anesthetics with minimal NMDA-receptor interaction, such as propofol and barbiturates, have demonstrated robust neurotoxic properties, whereas the neurotoxic potency of the NMDA-antagonist xenon is limited, therefore casting doubt on receptor upregulation being the sole mechanism for anesthetic neurotoxicity. In terms of abnormal neuronal inhibition being the main trigger for apoptosis in developing neurons, $GABA_A$-receptor stimulation indeed decreases neuronal activity in the mature brain; however, it also causes excitation in developing neurons,[218] thereby contradicting the inhibition hypothesis. In immature neurons, intracellular chloride ($Cl^-$) concentration is high, thus GABA-induced opening of $Cl^-$ channels allows this anion to exit the cell, leading to membrane depolarization. On the other hand, the intracellular $Cl^-$ concentration is low in mature neurons. When anesthetics open $Cl^-$ channels in mature neurons, ions enter the cell, thereby hyperpolarizing the membrane. This reversal of the cellular $Cl^-$ gradient occurs as a result of a switch from the immature $Na^+$-$K^+$-$2Cl^-$ cotransporter 1 (NKCC1) to the mature brain form, $K^+$-$Cl^-$ cotransporter 2 (KCC2).[219] Along these lines, studies in neonatal rats demonstrated excitatory properties in the brain and episodes of epileptic seizures during sevoflurane anesthesia in neonatal rats.[204] Isoflurane has also been shown to cause an excessive release of $Ca^{2+}$ from the endoplasmic reticulum via over-activation of inositol 1,4,5-trisphosphate receptors (InsP3Rs) in neonatal rats in vivo and in vitro.[220] A similar mechanism may be linked to the production of Alzheimer-associated increases in β-amyloid protein levels after anesthesia.[221] Moreover, whereas xenon and hypothermia cause neuronal inhibition, they do not appear to exacerbate isoflurane-induced neuronal cell death, as expected by cumulative neuronal inhibition, but rather significantly reduce it.[94,101,207]

Importantly, evidence indicates that equianesthetic concentrations of the three contemporary inhalational anesthetics cause similar degrees of neuroapoptosis, suggesting that it is the anesthetic depth and not the doses of the anesthetics that determines the cytotoxic potency.[71] However, other studies have failed to link the anesthetic and the apoptotic mechanisms. Specifically, although racemic ketamine and (S)-ketamine both elicit their anesthetic effects via NMDA-receptor blockade, (S)-ketamine induces up to 80% less cell death in vitro when compared with equipotent doses of racemic ketamine.[154] Moreover, concomitant administration of the GABA_A-receptor antagonist gabazine did not attenuate neuroapoptosis induced by the GABA agonist isoflurane, whereas the α₂-agonist dexmedetomidine did.[73] Decreases in anesthetic-induced neuronal activity may therefore be less important than the disruption of the neuronal balance of excitation and inhibition, as demonstrated by a series of studies that examined anesthesia-induced dendritic morphologic changes in mice.[70,152] Whereas simultaneous blockade of excitatory and inhibitory activity with tetrodotoxin did not lead to structural changes during synaptogenesis as would have been expected from a causative relationship between neuronal inhibition and structural damage, the administration of either GABA_A-agonistic or NMDA-antagonistic compounds alone altered synaptogenesis.[152]

It is not entirely clear at this time whether cytotoxicity is a direct effect of the anesthetic itself, or of anesthetic byproducts, or by the metabolic acidosis and respiratory derangements that have been observed during anesthesia in small rodents.[105,107,222] Hypercarbia can trigger widespread neuroapoptosis, even in unanesthetized neonatal rats exposed to increased partial pressures of carbon dioxide. Whereas apoptotic cell death was quantitatively indistinguishable from neurodegeneration in isoflurane-treated litter mates, which were also hypercarbic, adult neurocognitive impairment was only observed in the isoflurane-treated animals.[107]

Lastly, experimental models of neurodegeneration have implicated reentry of postmitotic neurons into the cell cycle, leading to cell death. Ketamine exposure has been found to induce aberrant cell cycle reentry, leading to apoptotic cell death in the developing rat brain.[155]

# Specific Anesthetic and Sedative Agents

In order to provide a succinct overview of the available laboratory data, we briefly review the effects of each class of anesthetics separately. Although the effects of some anesthetics, such as ketamine and isoflurane, have been extensively studied on the developing brain, the effects of others, such as xenon and desflurane, have not. However, the current data suggest that all anesthetics exert deleterious effects to some degree, on the developing animal brain (see E-Table 23-1). It is important to appreciate that although the MAC values for inhalational anesthetics are fairly constant across species, equipotent dosing of intravenous (IV)

medications is not. That is, the dose of most IV medications to effect sedation or anesthesia in animals is approximately 6- to 10-fold greater than that in humans. The dosing is further complicated by the different routes by which drugs are administered in neonatal animals, which include the subcutaneous and intraperitoneal (IP) routes, as opposed to the oral or IV routes in humans. The possible importance of the interspecies differences in the pharmacology of IV medications on neuroapoptosis and cognitive dysfunction has not been addressed.

## KETAMINE

Possibly the most frequently studied anesthetic is ketamine, an antagonist of the NMDA and glutamate receptor that also interacts with other cell membrane proteins, such as muscarinic and opioid receptors, as well as voltage-gated calcium channels. Ketamine's properties, which include potent analgesia, dissociative anesthesia, and relative hemodynamic stability, have made it a popular choice for procedural sedation in children, as well as for induction of anesthesia in children with critical congenital heart disease or pulmonary hypertension.[223-225] However, about 10 years ago, a seminal study that examined the effects of repeated IP injections of ketamine on the brain of neonatal rats observed widespread apoptosis.[17] Seven injections of 20 mg/kg of ketamine, administered over a 9 hour period in evenly divided intervals, to 7-day-old rat pups caused a 3- to 31-fold increase in degenerating neurons, depending on brain region. This led to speculation that these changes might contribute to neuropsychiatric disorders.[17] These initial findings for ketamine have been confirmed in more than fifty studies in small rodents, as well as nonhuman primates, both in vitro and in vivo (see E-Table 23-1). Several of these studies have identified relationships between neurodegeneration and dose, duration of treatment, as well as animal species and age during exposure. Single doses of up to 75 mg/kg or multiple IP injections up to 17 mg/kg/hr for 6 hours were not neurotoxic to neonatal rat brains,[128] whereas single doses between 20 and 50 mg/kg were neurotoxic to neonatal mice brains.[74,134] Six or seven repeated injections of 20 to 25 mg/kg consistently cause apoptosis in neonatal rat brains.[17,128,131,149,150] Although the doses of ketamine in these small-animal models appeared to be excessive and plasma concentrations in the rodents were up to 7 times greater than those in humans,[131] these increased doses are consistent with the requirements for IV anesthesia in small animals (refer to later section on interspecies comparison). Coadministration of midazolam, diazepam, propofol, or thiopental compounded the neuronal injury caused by ketamine.[74,134,142] Studies in rats, mice, and nonhuman primates suggest that the susceptibility to ketamine-induced neurotoxicity is limited to a brief period after birth, with a maximum impact between 3 and 7 days of age in small rodents and less than 35 days of age in monkeys.[17,139] Beyond these ages, ketamine-induced neuroapoptosis subsides. In addition to apoptosis, both small rodents and nonhuman primates that were anesthetized with ketamine have exhibited impaired learning tasks later in life.[129,130,158]

In summary, ketamine is the most frequently studied anesthetic, in terms to its neurotoxic effects, and has repeatedly been shown to cause widespread apoptosis (an effect that is exacerbated by the coadministration of other anesthetics), as well as neurologic impairment in adult animals exposed early in life. Importantly, long-lasting learning impairment has been demonstrated in nonhuman primates, the closest animal model to humans.[158] However, these animals were anesthetized with ketamine for 24 hours to produce this effect, a duration that exceeds the usual clinical scenario. Furthermore, it is unclear whether the observed learning abnormalities could not be explained by a reduction in motivation to perform the learning tasks.[158]

## INHALATIONAL ANESTHETICS

The second most commonly studied class of drugs is the inhalational anesthetics (see E-Table 23-1). The anesthetics desflurane, sevoflurane, isoflurane, enflurane, and halothane exert their anesthetic properties predominantly by their agonistic effects on the GABA$_A$ receptor, but also by differing degrees on glycine, NMDA, acetylcholine, serotonin (5-HT$_3$), α-amino-3-hydroxy-5-methyl-4-isoxazolepropionic acid (AMPA), and kainate receptors. Whereas GABA represents the main inhibitory neurotransmitter in the adult central nervous system, it has excitatory properties in the developing brain,[218] which may have implications for neurotoxicity, as discussed previously. Most studies of inhalational anesthetics examined either isoflurane alone or a combination of midazolam, isoflurane, and nitrous oxide. This combination of GABA agonists and NMDA antagonists has been repeatedly found to cause widespread increases in brain cell degeneration in neonatal animals.[85,87,91,92] In addition to the immediate deleterious effects on brain structure, long-term abnormalities in spatial learning tasks and decreased neuronal cell density in adult rats have been observed after exposure to this anesthetic combination early in life.[85,97] One MAC of isoflurane administered as the sole anesthetic for 4 hours to neonatal rats led to neurocognitive deficits in rats when they matured to adults,[106,107] whereas up to 0.6 MAC for 6 hours in neonatal mice, while causing widespread neuronal degeneration immediately after exposure, failed to cause neurocognitive deficits or decreases in neuronal density in adulthood.[105,115] These inconsistent findings raise the question of whether neonatal neuronal apoptotic cell death is linked directly to behavioral and learning abnormalities in adulthood. Neuronal cell death has also been observed in neonatal rhesus monkeys after 5 hours of 0.75% to 1.5% isoflurane,[114] although long-term neurologic studies in this species have not yet been published.

Similar to isoflurane, sevoflurane has also been shown to induce neuroapoptosis in neonatal mice,[71,115,202] although the long-term effects on learning and behavior are conflicting.[72,115,202] To date, few studies have examined desflurane in this context. Desflurane causes age- and species-dependent neuronal cell death in 7-day-old mice, but not 16-day-old rats.[70,71]

Few studies have compared the neurotoxicity of contemporary anesthetics. At equianesthetic concentrations of desflurane, isoflurane, and sevoflurane in neonatal mice, the degree of neuronal degeneration in the superficial neocortex, a brain region significantly affected in this model, is similar.[71] These results contrast with those from a study of lower concentrations of sevoflurane and isoflurane, in which cell death was less after the former than the latter, but without differences in neurocognitive performance in adult rats.[115] In another comparative mouse study, desflurane caused a greater degree of neurodegeneration than isoflurane and sevoflurane, and long-term neurologic impairment only occurred after desflurane.[72] The significance of these differential findings remains unknown, but could be related to methodologic differences.

Although largely phased out from clinical pediatric anesthesia practice, halothane and enflurane have been shown to induce brain abnormalities. These anesthetics were studied in models of intermittent or chronic occupational exposure during pregnancy, and caused subsequent delayed synaptogenesis and behavioral and learning abnormalities in rats after fetal exposure.[13-16,76]

In summary, inhalational anesthetics represent one of the most frequently used classes of anesthetics in pediatric anesthesia, and their neurotoxic properties have been extensively studied. Consistent findings include widespread apoptosis immediately after exposure in a wide variety of animal models, including nonhuman primates. However, neurologic impairment in adult animals exposed early in life to anesthesia has not been a consistent finding, and in fact some studies have found no neurologic impairment at all. Therefore long-lasting learning impairment has not been convincingly linked to neonatal neuroapoptosis. Primate studies on long-term neurocognitive outcomes after inhalational anesthesia early in life have not yet been published.

## NITROUS OXIDE

Nitrous oxide, an NMDA antagonist, is the oldest anesthetic in clinical use, although its low potency (MAC of 115% in adult humans) necessitates the coadministration of other anesthetics to provide surgical anesthesia. Anesthetic combinations with nitrous oxide often include the GABA agonist midazolam, and the mixed GABA-agonist/NMDA-antagonist isoflurane.* In rats, nitrous oxide alone did not induce neuronal apoptosis,[85,87,94] whereas in an in vitro study, it did cause neuronal cell death in mouse hippocampal slices.[94] When administered in combination, however, nitrous oxide has been shown to exacerbate neuronal cell death induced by isoflurane, and also to contribute to long-term neurologic abnormalities in rats when combined with isoflurane and midazolam.[85]

## XENON

Due to the cost differential between other inhalational anesthetics and this rare, colorless, and odorless noble gas, xenon has not reached widespread clinical anesthesia practice, despite its NMDA-antagonistic, anesthetic properties.[226] Xenon has a relatively low anesthetic potency, with a MAC measuring between 65% and 70% in adults[227,228]; its low blood-gas solubility speeds emergence from anesthesia.[229] Xenon's effects on neuronal apoptosis have been examined by two groups, with slightly differing results. Although 75% xenon for 6 hours did not cause neuronal apoptosis in 7-day-old rat pups,[94] 70% xenon for 4 hours did increase neuroapoptosis in 7-day-old mice.[207] Interestingly, both studies demonstrated that xenon decreased the neurodegeneration induced by isoflurane anesthesia,[94,207] which may have relevance to the phenomenon's putative mechanism, as discussed.

## BENZODIAZEPINES

Benzodiazepines, such as clonazepam, diazepam, and midazolam, have been investigated regarding their effects on the immature brain, either alone or in combination with other drugs. These GABA agonists are frequently used in toddlers and older children for preoperative anxiolysis, but infrequently in neonates and infants. Studies have shown that they increase neuronal degeneration in small-animal models, depending on the dose, region of the brain, species, and age of the animal. Although single doses of 5 mg/kg of diazepam or 9 mg/kg of midazolam IP did not increase neuronal cell death in neonatal rats,[68,85] 5 mg/kg

---

*References 79, 85, 87, 91, 92, 97, 98.

subcutaneous diazepam did cause neuronal cell death in some brain regions in mice, though this was not associated with learning deficits in adults.[74] In these studies, the neuroapoptosis associated with diazepam was significantly augmented by the coadministration of other sedatives, such as ketamine.[74] Studies have consistently reported increased neuroapoptosis in neonatal rats after diazepam in doses of 10 mg/kg or greater,[68,69] an effect that was prevented by the coadministration of the benzodiazepine-antagonist flumazenil in one study.[68] Two studies reported no neurocognitive learning disabilities in adult mice after they were sedated with diazepam or midazolam as neonates.[74,166]

## CHLORAL HYDRATE

The sedative chloral hydrate, a chlorination product of ethanol that is a GABA agonist as well as NMDA antagonist, has been largely supplanted by barbiturates and benzodiazepines in pediatric clinical practice. However, it is still being used in doses of up to 120 mg/kg for sedation for radiology studies,[230] and its neurotoxic properties have been investigated. Preliminary results indicate that it causes neuroapoptosis in the cerebral cortex and the caudate-putamen complex in immature mouse pups in doses of 100 mg/kg or greater.[67] The neurofunctional outcome in adult mice, however, has not as yet been investigated.

## BARBITURATES

Barbiturates act largely via the $GABA_A$ receptor, but also exert effects via nicotinic acetylcholine, AMPA, and kainate receptors. Thiopental alone, in doses of 25 mg/kg subcutaneously in neonatal mice, did not induce apoptosis, although when doses of 5 mg/kg were administered in conjunction with 25 mg/kg of ketamine subcutaneously, neuronal degeneration occurred and was associated with long-term impairment of learning and memory.[142] Pentobarbital and phenobarbital have been shown to induce neurodegeneration in mouse and rat pups. Furthermore, after receiving these sedatives as neonates, long-term alterations in brain protein expression and learning and memory have been observed,[103,184,186] although in one study these long-term alternations may be attributed in part to hypoxia and hypercarbia during the neonatal sedation.[184] Interestingly, estradiol has been shown to attenuate phenobarbital-induced neuroapoptosis.[68,185]

## PROPOFOL

In recent years, propofol has supplanted the barbiturates as the IV induction agent of choice in children. Propofol predominantly acts via GABA and glycine receptor–agonistic properties, but also weakly on nicotinic, AMPA, and NMDA receptors, and has been repeatedly studied regarding its neurotoxic profile, both in vitro and in vivo. The overall consensus of this body of literature is that propofol, in a dose- and exposure time–dependent fashion, has dramatic effects on the developing brain in animals. Propofol has consistently caused neuroapoptosis after doses exceeding 50 mg/kg (subcutaneous or IP) or repeated doses exceeding 20 mg/kg/hr for 4 to 5 hours in neonatal small rodents.[142,148,191,196] Interestingly, lithium protected from propofol-induced neuroapoptosis in neonatal mice.[148] However, after 24 hours of IV anesthesia with propofol (6 mg/kg/hr) and fentanyl (10 µg/kg/hr), there was no evidence of apoptosis.[192] Apart from overt neuronal cell death, propofol decreases the GABAergic enzyme glutamic acid decarboxylase,[188] decreases nerve growth factors,[194,198] and causes neurite growth cone collapse in tissue culture.[190] In addition, propofol alters dendritic spine architecture in developing rats, depending on the age at the time of anesthetic exposure.[197] For example, dendritic spine density decreased if the rat was anesthetized during week 1 of life, but it increased spine development if exposure took place during week 3 of life; the mechanism of these differing responses remains elusive.[197]

## DEXMEDETOMIDINE

Unlike other anesthetics and sedatives, dexmedetomidine is a sedative and analgesic that does not interact with GABA, NMDA, or opioid receptors, but rather acts by stimulating presynaptic $\alpha_2$-adrenergic receptors. Given this different mechanism of action, it is interesting that dexmedetomidine, administered in three IP injections of 1 to 25 µg/kg at 0, 2, and 4 hours to 7-day-old rat pups, did not cause neuronal apoptosis, but attenuated isoflurane-induced neuroapoptosis. Even a dose of 75 µg/kg dexmedetomidine (75-fold greater than the median effective dose needed for sedation), did not cause apoptosis in this model. Furthermore, dexmedetomidine prevented the long-term cognitive impairment from isoflurane.[73]

## OPIOID ANALGESICS

To date, only one study investigated neurotoxic properties of opioids in relation to an inhalational anesthetic regimen. Mechanically ventilated, neonatal pigs, sedated with an IV bolus of 30 µg/kg fentanyl followed by 15 µg/kg/hr for 4 hours, exhibited significantly less neuroapoptosis in several regions of the brain, compared with an intramuscular injection of 1 mg/kg of midazolam, followed by 4 hours of 0.55% isoflurane and 75% nitrous oxide.[79] These initial findings are interesting, although future neurotoxicity studies that include opioid infusions need to also include adjuvants that produce amnesia, as is customary in pediatric anesthesia practice. Moreover, when comparing different anesthetic regimens regarding their neurotoxic potential, equianesthetic potency should be established during the study.

Importantly, however, the long-term consequences of opioid administration to the immature brain needs to be further elucidated before recommending such a regimen as an alternative strategy. Similar to GABA and NMDA receptors, opioid receptors are also intimately involved in early brain development and synaptogenesis,[231,232] which would make it plausible that opioids could similarly affect brain development during the critical period of synaptogenesis. Increased neuronal cell death and decreased neuronal density after perinatal exposure to opioid receptor agonists, such as morphine and heroin, have been observed in developing animals.[82,83,233] Chronic buprenorphine and methadone treatment early in life have been found to diminish concentrations of nerve growth factors in the immature brain.[66,164] Moreover, immediate and permanent reductions in µ-opioid receptor density have been observed after perinatal exposure to morphine,[168,169] and may be associated with long-term impairment of memory and cognitive function in small animals,[171,174-176,179-181] as well as exaggerated nociceptive responses to a pain challenge later in life.[177,182] Stimulation of the κ-opioid receptor may amplify neuronal cell death induced by proapoptotic agents.[234] High-dose fentanyl has been shown to significantly exacerbate white-matter brain lesions induced by glutamatergic overstimulation in mice.[78] All these animal data suggest that prolonged perinatal exposure to opioids may have immediate and long-term effects on the developing brain and may amplify proapoptotic stimuli, although the effects of a brief or single dose exposure to opioids is not well understood.

These data suggest that further studies into the interactions of opioid analgesics and anesthetics in the developing brain are warranted.

## Exposure Time, Dose, and Anesthetic Combinations

Neuronal injury depends on the anesthetic dose and/or duration of anesthesia for inhalational anesthetics, and the dose, route of administration, and the number of doses for injectable anesthetics. Moreover, combinations of several anesthetics and sedatives have, in general, caused more neuroapoptosis and long-term cognitive changes than have single drugs. For example, combinations of midazolam, nitrous oxide, and isoflurane cause a much greater degree of neuroapoptosis in neonatal rats than isoflurane alone, even when the latter is administered at a greater inspired concentration.[85] In the case of ketamine, its neurodegenerative potency is amplified when coadministered with thiopental or propofol.[142] Anesthetic combinations of mixed GABA agonists and NMDA antagonists demonstrate exaggerated effects. This evidence supports the notion that a deeper level of anesthesia increases the neuroapoptotic injury. However, two anesthetics, xenon and dexmedetomidine, which actually attenuate the neurotoxic effects of isoflurane anesthesia,[73,94,207] do not lend support to this notion.

## Deleterious Effects of Untreated Pain and Stress

Given the evidence for deleterious effects of anesthetics and analgesics on the developing brain and the paucity of complete anesthetics devoid of cytotoxicity, would children fare better by withholding potentially toxic drugs and allowing them to experience the pain and stress of surgery? Of course such a practice would be unethical, and there is a plethora of evidence of the deleterious effects caused by the stressful conditions of exposing the immature nervous system to recurrent painful stimulation. Noxious stimulation in the neonate has been associated with subsequent hyperalgesia or hypoalgesia, depending on the type and severity of injury.[235] Repetitive painful skin lacerations for procedures as minor as blood draws in neonates have been found to lead to long-term, local sensory hyperinnervation.[236] In addition to these local responses, repetitive, inflammatory pain early in life has been found to result in hyperalgesia and lasting changes in nociceptive circuitry of the adult dorsal horn.[237] Repeated painful injections into the paws of rat pups resulted in a generalized thermal hypoalgesia.[235] In addition to altered pain processing and sensory perception, repetitive or persistent pain in the neonate alters behavior and cognitive function in adulthood, decreases pain thresholds, and increases vulnerability to stress and anxiety disorders or chronic pain syndromes later in life.[141,238-241]

In addition to painful stimulation, early adverse emotional experiences can also induce long-lasting abnormalities, such as imbalances of the inhibitory nervous system,[242] impairment of normal development of the nociceptive system, long-term behavioral changes,[243] and persistent learning impairment.[179] Therefore fetuses, neonates, and infants subjected to pain and stresses associated with invasive procedures without adequate anesthesia and analgesia may be at risk for long-term adverse outcomes.

Accordingly, preemptive administration of analgesics and sedatives, such as morphine or ketamine, has been found to ameliorate the deleterious effects of neonatal pain in some of the animal studies.[141,179,241] However, either the presence of painful stimulation or 5 days of morphine administered to neonatal mice independently impaired adult rewarded behavior, although the combination did not.[179]

Clinical reports have also demonstrated that human neonates and infants can mount a metabolic and endocrine response to perioperative stress and painful stimulation, which include surges in catecholamine, cortisol, β-endorphin, insulin, glucagon, and growth hormone levels.[244-246] Some of these markers, such as cortisol, remain increased for more than a year after the insult, possibly as a result of cumulative stress related to multiple painful procedures early in life.[247] Inhalational anesthetics, opioid analgesics, as well as regional anesthesia, inhibit intraoperative stress and improve postoperative outcomes.[245,248,249] Moreover, adequate perioperative anesthesia reduced the incidence of other complications, such as the incidence of sepsis and disseminated intravascular coagulation, that led to a decrease in overall mortality.[250] Even less invasive procedures, such as circumcisions performed without analgesia in young boys, can exaggerate responses to painful challenges (e.g., immunizations) later in life.[251] Conversely, topical or regional anesthesia for circumcision blunts not only the immediate humoral stress response during the procedure,[252] but also pain-induced, long-term hyperalgesia.[251] In preterm neonates, painful stimulations early in life have also been associated with subsequent diminished cognition and motor function.[253] In a retrospective study of children greater than 1 year of age who were born at less than 32 weeks gestational age without significant neonatal brain injury or major sensorineural impairment, the more skin-breaking procedures from birth to term (including heel sticks, intramuscular injections, chest tube placements, and central line insertions) predicted poorer subsequent cognitive and motor development (as assessed using the Bayley Scales of Infant Development II) when compared with term controls. Importantly, after controlling for severity of illness, duration of morphine administration, and exposure to postnatal dexamethasone, gestational age at birth was not significantly associated with cognitive or motor outcome. These findings suggest that repetitive pain-related stressful experiences and not prematurity per se was responsible for the poor neurodevelopmental outcome.[253] Although this study did not examine the effects of anesthetic or analgesic administration during painful stimulation on subsequent outcome, a small, retrospective study suggested an improvement in outcome after administering anesthesia during painful stimulation.[254] Painful stimulation during reduction of herniated bowel without anesthesia in infants suffering from gastroschisis tended to more frequently lead to serious adverse events, such as bowel ischemia, need for total parenteral nutrition, and unplanned reoperation, than in infants undergoing the same procedure with general anesthesia.[254] However, despite persistently large numbers of painful and stressful procedures performed in vulnerable neonates, data indicate that the majority of these procedures are still not accompanied by adequate analgesia or anesthesia.[255]

Together, the data from animals and humans suggest that pain-related stress experienced early in life is deleterious to the developing nervous system, that pain in children remains undertreated, and that analgesics and/or anesthetics may alleviate many of the degenerative effects of unopposed pain and improve outcome. If anesthetics protect from the deleterious effects of painful stimulation, but confer their own cytotoxic adverse effects, the major question remains whether other compounds can alleviate these adverse effects.

## Potential Alleviating Strategies

Whereas the translational relevance of anesthetic-induced neurotoxicity in neonatal animals to humans remains unresolved, several laboratory studies have tested strategies to alleviate some of the deleterious effects of anesthetics and sedatives in animals. These have been directed at both the immediate effects after anesthesia, such as neuronal cell death, as well as long-term abnormalities, such as neurocognitive impairment. Importantly, many studies administered adjuvants immediately before or during anesthesia, thereby maintaining an adequate level of anesthesia and analgesia to avoid the deleterious effects of unopposed pain.

The sedative dexmedetomidine and the anesthetic xenon possess very limited neurotoxic potencies themselves, but dramatically reduce isoflurane-induced neuroapoptosis.[73,94,207] In addition, the coadministration of dexmedetomidine prevents long-term memory impairment after 6-hour isoflurane exposure in rats.[73] Interestingly, neuroprotective preconditioning has been demonstrated in pheochromocytoma PC12 cells in which pretreatment with a small concentration of isoflurane prevented the neurotoxic response to a subsequent greater dose.[95] In in vitro studies, the inositol triphosphate–receptor antagonist xestospongin C, tissue plasminogen activator, plasmin, inhibition of the neurotrophic receptor p75[NTR] and the RhoA receptor, or prevention of cytoskeletal depolymerization with either jasplakinolide or TAT-Pep5 significantly attenuated isoflurane-mediated neuroapoptosis.[104,109,123] In addition, L-carnitine attenuated neuronal apoptosis after 6 hours of isoflurane and nitrous oxide in 7-day-old rat pups.[102] Supplementation with the naturally occurring hormones β-estradiol or melatonin prevented the deleterious effects on neuronal survival of a prolonged exposure to midazolam, isoflurane, and nitrous oxide.[87,91] Similarly, coadministration of β-estradiol significantly reduced phenobarbital-induced neuroapoptosis.[68,185] The only potentially protective agent that has been unsuccessfully tested in published studies is the GABA antagonist gabazine.[73] On the other hand, pilocarpine reduces neuroapoptosis induced by the GABA agonists isoflurane and midazolam, while augmenting the damage after administration of the NMDA antagonist phencyclidine, based on preliminary results from neonatal mice.[93] Preliminary data from the same laboratory also suggest that whole-body hypothermia with a targeted brain temperature of less than 30° C may protect from the neuroapoptotic ramifications of a 4-hour exposure to 0.75% isoflurane or to 40 mg/kg of IP ketamine in neonatal mice.[41,101] Another therapy that has been successfully tested in mouse pups that received 40 mg/kg of ketamine or 100 mg/kg of propofol was lithium, 3 to 6 mEq/kg subcutaneously, which abolished the anesthetic-induced neuroapoptosis in cortex and the caudate-putamen complex.[148]

Because the applicability and extent of anesthetic neurotoxicity has not been established in humans, it is obviously premature to recommend any of these protective strategies for children. Moreover, the safety of many of these drugs and interventions has not been established in human neonates and infants. Tissue plasminogen activator and plasmin promote fibrinolysis and may not be first-line treatments during invasive surgical procedures. The sex hormone β-estradiol may not be a feasible adjuvant in prepubescent boys. The safety of pilocarpine in young children

may be hampered by its proconvulsant activity observed in animal studies.[256,257] Lithium has been labeled harmful to the human fetus and may cause neurocognitive impairment in young children.[258-260] Whole body hypothermia below 30° C may not be a clinically feasible modality because even mild perioperative hypothermia, at least in adults, has been causally linked to numerous complications, including increased blood loss and transfusion requirements, morbid myocardial outcomes, prolonged postanesthetic recovery and hospitalization, thermal discomfort, as well as an increased risk of surgical wound infections.[261] Therefore hypothermia to treat anesthesia-induced neurotoxicity is unlikely to play a substantive role during routine pediatric anesthesia, but may have a role in infants undergoing hypothermic cardiopulmonary bypass for heart surgery to treat congenital defects. Unfortunately, the latter population often presents with neurocognitive abnormalities before anesthesia.[262] Although xenon's scarcity renders it a very expensive anesthetic, dexmedetomidine's wider availability and increased usage in pediatric anesthesia makes it a more attractive option for further research into protective strategies.[263,264]

## Anesthetic Neuroprotection

Even relatively brief periods of inadequate oxygen or blood flow to the brain may lead to neuronal injury and long-term neurologic impairment, because of the limited tolerance of the brain to ischemia. Importantly, animal studies have repeatedly confirmed the protective properties of anesthetics when administered during episodes of brain hypoxia-ischemia. However, most of these studies have been conducted in adult animals.[265] In immature animal models, anesthetics have also been found to reduce neurologic injury and improve functional outcome after brain ischemia. Desflurane alleviates neuronal cell death and early neurologic dysfunction in a model of the neonatal pig during hypothermic cardiopulmonary bypass and deep hypothermic circulatory arrest.[266,267] Isoflurane treatment before hypoxia-ischemia protects the brain and improves survival in neonatal rats and mice.[268-270] Both xenon and sevoflurane protect the immature brain during simulated hypoxia-ischemia in an in vitro model.[271] Furthermore, sevoflurane may be protective in a neonatal mouse in vivo model.[272] These findings in immature animals suggest that critically ill human neonates could potentially benefit from these protective properties during clinical scenarios of neurologic injury, such as cardiopulmonary bypass, neurologic surgery, or perioperative cardiocirculatory arrest; these potential benefits need to be weighed against the potential neurotoxic properties of the current anesthetics.

## Critical Evaluation of Animal Studies and Interspecies Comparisons

To determine whether the findings from animal studies should guide clinical practice, it is important to rationally evaluate how well animal studies represent the human clinical scenario.*

To date, no animal model has been developed that covers all aspects of human physiology and pathophysiology during surgical procedures. The task of modeling potential vulnerabilities of the developing human brain in animals is complicated by the

---

*References 2, 22, 85, 105-107, 158, 273-278

fact that human CNS development is much more protracted than that of any of the model species. However, human neurocognitive performance is also much more complicated compared with lower animals, and therefore a potential injury might have a greater impact in such a complex system.

## DURATION OF EXPOSURE

In order to elicit toxic effects, the designs of many animal studies include durations of anesthesia from 1 to 24 hours. Accordingly, some of these times may extend well beyond the average time of routine pediatric anesthesia. However, expressing the duration of anesthesia as a fraction of a subject's life span, thereby equating a 6-hour anesthetic in mice to a 2-week or greater anesthetic in humans, is probably an oversimplification. The duration of neurodevelopment may not be immediately relevant when considering the likelihood of injury at a cellular level. Nonetheless, the extent of the injury and its functional implications may potentially be related to the duration of the entire brain developmental period, even though the mechanism of anesthetic-induced neurodegeneration is unknown. Because human brain development occurs at a much slower pace than in any of the other species, similar exposure times could have different effects on potential susceptibility and the ability for postexposure repair among species. For example, the brain reaches adult size at 20 days of age in rats, 3 years of age in rhesus monkeys, 7 years of age in chimpanzees, and not until 15 years of age in humans.[2,279,280]

Exposure to anesthesia during a larger proportion of the period of development could be expected to have a greater impact on total development and maturation. Similarly, given the plasticity of the developing brain, it seems conceivable that brains with slower growth rates possess more time for repair.[281,282] Conversely, in complex organisms, such as humans, relatively minor degrees of injury in crucial areas and at crucial times during development could have relatively profound long-term effects.

## ANESTHETIC DOSES

In all animal studies, doses needed for injectable anesthetics to cause neuronal degeneration were greater, sometimes by orders of magnitude, when compared with weight-based doses commonly used in human clinical practice. However, to produce immobility, small animals also required significantly greater doses of IV anesthetics than larger animals. Due to their smaller size, greater metabolic rate, and shorter physiologic time, drug doses in animals significantly differ from those used in humans.[283] Using a process called allometric scaling, which takes these species differences into account, animal drug doses comparable to human doses have been estimated to be approximately three-, six-, or twelvefold greater, respectively, for monkeys, rats, or mice (see also Chapter 6).[283,284] Whereas drug doses used in anesthetic neurotoxicity studies frequently still exceed these doses calculated using allometric scaling, they do not include a significant safety margin (Fig. 23-3). Moreover, using allometrically scaled

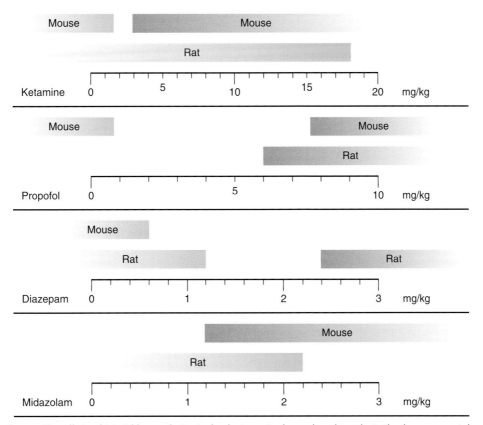

**FIGURE 23-3** Neurodegenerative effects of injectable anesthetics in developing animals are dose-dependent. *Blue bars* represent doses of the respective anesthetics not causing neurodegeneration in rats and mice; *pink bars* represent doses causing neurodegeneration in animals. Figure includes only studies using single injections of anesthetics and doses used in animals were scaled to doses for children by using an allometric scaling technique, based on calculations outlined in reference 284. Neurotoxic data are based on experiments described in references 17, 68, 69, 74, 85, 128, 131, 134, 139, 142, 151, 194.

doses, plasma concentrations for ketamine, for example, were approximately 3 to 10 times greater in small rodents and monkeys than those observed during clinical human practice.[131,139] This suggests that the neurotoxic properties observed with large doses of injectable anesthetics, such as ketamine, would only have direct applicability to humans if the anesthetic and the neurotoxic effects were based on the same molecular mechanism, which has yet to be verified. Otherwise, animal studies would expose subjects to much greater plasma concentrations of a neurotoxicant than those used during anesthesia in humans, thereby leading to an overestimation of the neurotoxic effects of IV anesthetics in laboratory studies.

Doses for inhaled anesthetics generating immobility in animals, on the other hand, are much closer to clinically used doses. Moreover, similar to human anesthesia, potency of inhaled anesthetics increases with subject age, necessitating larger doses in younger animals,[71,222,285] which could suggest closer applicability of laboratory data to humans.

## EXPERIMENTAL VERSUS CLINICAL CONDITIONS

Another important distinction between laboratory studies in animals and clinical studies in humans is the presence of significant comorbidities, such as the presence of stress and pain associated with the underlying disease that require the administration of anesthetics and analgesics. Very few of the laboratory studies to date have included the presence of surgical stress that may increase or decrease the degree of anesthesia-induced neurotoxicity. Tail clamping or injection of caustic substances are used as a model for surgical stress. Results from these studies varied: one study reported no influence of the painful stimulus on anesthesia-induced apoptosis,[206] whereas a second reported that painful stimulation increased anesthetic-induced neuroapoptosis.[127] In contrast, therapeutic effects have been demonstrated with concomitant administration of small doses of analgesics or sedatives, compared with no analgesia or sedative when pain was induced.[141,179]

When studies measured metabolic and respiratory effects of anesthetic exposure in small rodent species, several demonstrated significant differences from pediatric anesthesia practice, such as extensive hypercarbia, metabolic acidosis, and hypoglycemia observed in the small rodents.[105,107,222] Tracheal intubation and mechanical ventilation do not seem to completely obviate these abnormalities.[222] In stark contrast to anesthesia in children, administering clinical doses of anesthetics for as little as 2 to 4 hours can be lethal for more than 20% of small rodents,[105] even when intermittent painful stimuli were applied.[107] Moreover, rearing conditions after anesthesia have a profound impact on the brain's repair mechanisms after injury. Environmental enrichment and exercise dramatically increase neurogenesis in rodents and therefore may facilitate plasticity and repair after anesthesia, compared with regular cage housing conditions.[286,287] Children face daily cognitive challenges in their "enriched" environment, different from laboratory animal housing,[79,114,139,158] that could attenuate the postulated neurocognitive effects of anesthesia. This is highlighted in a recent study in which environmental enrichment reversed the deleterious effects of anesthesia on subsequent neurologic performance in rats, resulting in performance similar to environmentally enriched, unanesthetized animals and superior to unenriched control and anesthesia-exposed animals.[206] This study suggests that neurobehavioral outcome depends on multiple factors and that anesthesia may be only one minor insult compared with the many other more significant events in childhood.

## COMPARATIVE BRAIN DEVELOPMENT

A major obstacle in translating animal data to humans centers on the difficulties of matching up brain maturational stages in model animals with the equivalent stages of the immature human brain. The ongoing discussion regarding these comparisons is somewhat reminiscent of the cliché of 1 "dog year" being equivalent to 7 "human years." Because animal studies have suggested that anesthesia-induced neuroapoptosis may be limited to very defined, early stages of development, such as from 3 to 10 days of age in small rodents,[17,87] it becomes imperative to identify the equivalent period during human brain development, in order to assess human applicability of the animal data and to adequately plan clinical studies.

Brain architecture and development, however, are not easily compared among mammalian species. Small rodents, such as mice and rats, have a smooth (or lissencephalic) brain surface, whereas humans and monkeys exhibit the typical fissured, gyrencephalic brain surface of gyri and sulci. Overall brain size and number of neurons are vastly different between humans and animal species. Moreover, brain development varies dramatically in terms of timing and duration. Whereas considerable brain development takes place postnatally in rodents, most critical steps in humans occur in utero.[273] It has generally been accepted that mice and rats are born at relatively earlier stages of brain maturity compared with humans, but that neurodevelopment in small rodents rapidly catches up with humans, mostly during the first 2 to 3 weeks of the rodent's life. Older data based on simple estimations of brain cell numbers and degree of myelination have been interpreted to mean that the first week of life in small rodents, when the peak of vulnerability to anesthetic neurotoxicity occurs, equates to an extended time span in humans, from the third gestational trimester all the way to the third year of life.[2,22,274] However, more contemporary approaches, including computational models, have approximated the 7-day-old rat to be closer in brain maturity to human fetuses at 20 to 22 weeks gestation, and the immature rhesus monkey to approximate the immature human brain closer to term (Fig. 23-4).[275-277,288] According to these models, stages of brain maturity equivalent to term human neonates are not reached until after postnatal day 14 in rats or mice (online calculator available at http://www.translatingtime.net, accessed January 23, 2012). Therefore it remains questionable whether rodent models hold relevance to routine pediatric anesthesia in term neonates and infants, or whether they more closely correspond to brain maturational states during fetal surgery in midgestation. Nonhuman primates, on the other hand, exhibit brain maturation more comparable to human brain maturation at birth and could be more applicable to neonatal anesthesia. Interestingly, a recent study in rhesus macaques corroborates the greater fetal susceptibility by demonstrating a higher degree of neuroapoptosis after ketamine anesthesia in utero compared with postnatally.[160] However, major differences in brain development still exist between humans and nonhuman primates. In general, brain development progresses at a much slower pace in humans and developmental stages are up to 50% longer. Even on a cellular level, remarkable differences exist between humans and animals; cell cycle duration during cortical neurogenesis is approximately 17 hours in mice, 28 hours in macaque monkeys, and 36 hours in humans.[282] All these differences indicate that it is not sensible to directly apply observations of anesthetic effects in the developing animal brain of any species to human clinical anesthesia practice.

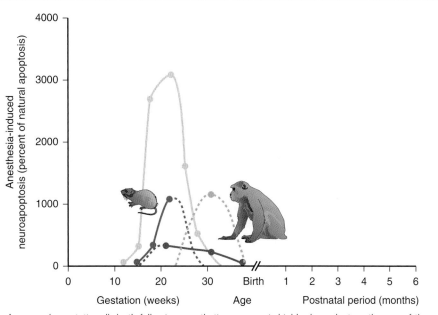

**FIGURE 23-4** The degree of neuronal apoptotic cell death following anesthetic exposure is highly dependent on the age of the animal during exposure. Graphs demonstrate the percent increase of apoptotic cell death compared with natural apoptosis following an exposure to an isoflurane/nitrous oxide–based anesthetic in immature rats (*dark gray*) or very young macaque monkeys (*dark brown*) or prolonged exposure to ketamine in immature rats (*light gray*) or macaque monkeys (*tan*). *Solid lines* connect the available data points; *interrupted lines* represent extrapolations of the available data. Neurotoxicity data were derived from references, 17, 91, 114, 139. To infer the potential age of anesthetic vulnerability in humans, respective brain maturity in the animal species during exposure were equated to the corresponding state of the developing human brain, and relative human ages for each data point were plotted accordingly, using the mathematical model outlined in references, 276, 277, 288 and available in the online calculator at http://www.translatingtime.net.

## ASSESSING NEUROBEHAVIORAL OR COGNITIVE OUTCOMES

Translating neurodevelopmental outcomes from animals to humans is difficult. Human cognitive performance includes the vast capacity for learning, the ability for abstract thinking, the aptitude for solving complex mathematical equations, and even the capability of inventing and operating complex machinery. Cognition is a complex process that includes such diverse processes as perception, attention, working memory, long-term memory, executive function, language, and social cognition. These brain functions are all difficult to model in animals.[278] It is therefore imperative to critically evaluate any animal models attempting to replicate human cognitive performance. Moreover, it is important to assess the validity of these models in the context of the critical period for human brain development that they are trying to represent. Current assessment of neurocognitive performance after developmental exposure largely relies on hippocampal-dependent tests administered to adult animals following anesthetic exposure early in life.[85,105-107,158] However, it remains unclear whether these are the same domains that may potentially be targeted in children during anesthesia. Brain regions maximally affected by anesthesia may change with the age of the animal and developmental state of the brain.[79,160] Accordingly, subsequent neurobehavioral abnormalities may vary depending on the age at which anesthesia was administered.

This discussion, however, does not entirely discredit the results from small animal studies, but rather seriously limits the generalizability of their findings to clinical pediatric anesthesia practice. More closely resembling clinical pediatric anesthesia practice, several large-animal models have used tracheal intubation and mechanical ventilation.[79,114,160] However, none of these large-animal studies included surgical stimulation during the anesthesia.[79,114,139,158]

## Long-Term Outcome in Children Exposed to Anesthesia and Surgery

The difficulties in translating animal data to clinical anesthesia in human infants increases the importance of identifying potential clinical evidence for or against neurologic abnormalities in children after otherwise uneventful anesthesia early in life. Unfortunately, this question is not easily answered.

There is evidence for an association between surgery with anesthesia in early childhood and subsequent altered neurodevelopmental outcome.[37] Some human cohort studies have demonstrated an association between major surgery in the neonatal period and poor neurodevelopmental outcome.[289] Children born with esophageal atresia had a lower IQ and more frequently suffered from depression, emotional, and behavioral problems compared with the general population.[290] Children with congenital diaphragmatic hernia repair also have a high rate of neurologic sequelae.[291] Extremely premature, low–birth-weight neonates who underwent laparotomy had poorer neurodevelopmental outcomes compared with matched controls.[292] A cohort of infants who underwent major surgery did not perform as well in school as a matched control group of healthy infants or with infants who had major nonsurgical medical conditions.[293] In a randomized trial of indomethacin treatment in 426 infants less than 1000 g at birth, neurologic impairment was present in significantly more of the 110 children who had undergone surgery (53%) compared with that in the 316 children who had received medical therapy (34%).[294] In a study of extremely preterm infants, the IQ of those who had undergone surgery was lower at 5 years of age and exhibited more sensorineural disability than those who had not undergone surgery.[295]

These studies all included infants with major confounding factors, such as congenital malformations or very preterm birth, which might increase the risk of poor neurodevelopmental outcome independent of surgery and anesthesia. Moreover, surgery itself can lead to poor outcome as a result of the perioperative neurohumoral and inflammatory response, or the hemodynamic instability associated with major surgery. Severity of illness may have also been greater in surgical patients compared with their respective control groups. Thus, whereas these studies suggest that some infants undergoing major surgery are at increased risk of poor neurodevelopmental outcome, none of the studies provide conclusive evidence that surgery or even anesthesia is the cause of the increased risk of poor neurodevelopmental outcome.

Several recent cohort studies have focused primarily on the effects of anesthesia. In an established population–based, retrospective birth cohort, Wilder and colleagues studied the association between anesthetic exposure before 4 years of age and the subsequent development of learning disabilities.[296] Regression was used to calculate hazard ratios for anesthetic exposure as a predictor of learning disability, with adjustment for gestational age at birth, sex, and birth weight. Of 5357 children in the cohort, 593 had been exposed to general anesthesia before 4 years of age. Compared with those not exposed to anesthesia, a single exposure was not associated with an increased risk of learning disability (hazard ratio = 1.0; 95% confidence interval [CI] of 0.79 to 1.27). However, children who underwent two separate episodes of anesthesia had an increased risk of a learning disability (hazard ratio = 1.59; 95% CI of 1.06 to 2.37) and those who underwent 3 or more separate episodes of anesthesia had an even greater risk (hazard ratio = 2.60; 95% CI of 1.60 to 4.24). The association between learning disability and multiple episodes of anesthesia remained after adjusting for American Society of Anesthesiologist physical status. The risk for a learning disability also increased according to the cumulative duration of anesthesia. However, this study suffered from several deficiencies. Because the study reported anesthetics administered between 1976 and 1982, the most common anesthetic treatment was halothane and nitrous oxide, and none of the children were monitored with pulse oximetry or capnography. It is not possible to determine in how many of these children excessive hyperventilation or unrecognized desaturation had occurred. Furthermore, the maternal birth histories were not described (e.g., magnesium may cause neuroapoptosis or be neuroprotective). Three different learning disabilities were considered with equipoise in the final analysis, and these disabilities were not tested in all children, but only when a teacher or parent requested testing. These questions limit the external validity of these data.

To reduce the impact of confounding factors, using the same population-based, retrospective birth cohort, the same group conducted further studies with a matched cohort design.[297] The researchers matched 350 children exposed to anesthesia before the age of 2 to 700 children not exposed to anesthesia. The matching was based on several known risk factors for learning disabilities: gender, mother's education, birth weight, and gestational age at birth. Outcomes of interest were: learning disability, need for individualized education program for an emotional or behavioral disorder, and group-administered achievement tests. In the analysis, an adjustment was also performed for burden of illness. The primary finding was that children exposed to two or more occurrences of anesthesia (but not a single occurrence) were at increased risk for having a learning disability (hazard ratio = 2.12 with 95% CI of 1.26 to 3.54), and an amplified need for individualized education programs for speech and language impairment. However, there was not an increased need for a

program for emotional or behavioral disorders. The authors also detected an association between multiple exposures to anesthesia and lower mathematical scores. The same criticisms apply to this study as to the earlier study from this institution.[296]

To investigate a potential association between perinatal exposure to general anesthesia during cesarean delivery and subsequent diagnosis of learning disability,[298] the risk of a learning disability was compared in the 193 children delivered via cesarean section under general anesthesia, the 304 delivered via cesarean section under regional anesthesia, and 4823 delivered vaginally without any anesthesia. The association between mode of delivery and learning disability was adjusted for sex, birth weight, gestational age at birth, exposure to anesthesia before 4 years of age, and maternal education. The risk of disability was similar between children delivered by vagina with no anesthesia, and cesarean delivery under general anesthesia, but risk of disability was less in children delivered via cesarean under regional anesthesia than by vagina with no anesthesia (hazard ratio = 0.64, 95% CI of 0.44 to 0.92; $P = 0.017$). The results implied that brief exposure to general anesthesia during delivery was not associated with subsequent learning disability, but the reason why the risk was less with regional anesthesia compared with no anesthesia is unclear, although this may suggest the possibility of substantial confounding influences. To explore the possibility that the regional blockade was protective, the authors subsequently compared those born without general anesthesia by vaginal delivery, with and without regional analgesia, and found no difference in risk of learning disability.[299]

Using the same epidemiologic cohort, the same research group detected an increased prevalence of attention deficit hyperactivity disorder (ADHD) in children who had undergone repeated surgical procedures with anesthesia, compared with none or only one exposure.[299a] Kalkman and associates performed a small pilot study to test the feasibility of using a cohort of children who had urologic surgery, in order to test the association between age at surgery and neurobehavioral outcome (measured with the Child Behavior Check List).[300] In their sample of 314 children, they found no evidence for an association between timing of surgery and neurobehavioral outcome.

DiMaggio and colleagues performed a retrospective cohort analysis using the New York State Medicaid records.[301] The researchers matched 383 children who underwent hernia repair before 3 years of age to 5050 children who did not undergo inguinal hernia repair. After adjustment for sex, age, and complicating birth conditions (such as low birth weight), children who had hernia repair were more than twice as likely to have a subsequent diagnosis of a developmental or behavioral disorder (hazard ratio = 2.3, 95% CI of 1.3 to 4.1).

To reduce environmental confounding effects, the authors then proceeded to use the data from the New York State Medicaid program to construct a retrospective sibling birth cohort.[302] Once again, they assessed the association between exposure to anesthesia in children less than 3 years of age and the subsequent risk of diagnosis of developmental or behavioral disorders. A total of 10,450 siblings were identified; 304 of whom underwent surgery before 3 years of age, without any history of behavioral or developmental disorders before the surgery, and 10,146 children who did not undergo surgery. The association of exposure to anesthesia with subsequent developmental or behavioral disorders was assessed with both proportional hazards modeling, and pair-matched analysis. As with their previous study, they found evidence for an association between surgery and poor neurodevelopmental outcome. The incidence of developmental or behavioral disorders was 128.2 diagnoses per 1000 person-years for those that had surgery and 56.3 diagnoses per 1000 person-years for those that did not. This association persisted when adjusted for sex, history of birth-related medical complications, and clustering by sibling status; the estimated hazard ratio of developmental or behavioral disorders associated with any exposure to anesthesia was 1.6 (95% CI of 1.4 to 1.8). The risk increased from 1.1 (95% CI of 0.8 to 1.4) for one operation to 2.9 (94% CI of 2.5 to 3.1) for two operations and 4.0 (95% CI of 3.5 to 4.5) for three or more operations. The number of siblings available for a matched analysis was relatively small. There were only 138 sibling pairs. In the pair-matched analysis there was no evidence for an association between surgery and poor outcome, with a relative risk of 0.9 (95% CI of 0.6 to 1.4); however, the small numbers may limit the power of this analysis.

Even better than sibling studies, investigations involving identical twins may further reduce confounding environmental and genetic influences. Performing such a study, Bartels and associates examined the possible association between anesthesia exposure before 3 years of age and school performance in 1143 monozygotic twin pairs.[303] In the identical twins who were discordant for exposure to anesthesia (one twin was exposed to anesthesia and the other was not), their school performance was identical. This would suggest that surgery with anesthesia may not be the cause of poor school performance. Interestingly, the school performance in both the discordant pairs and the pairs where both twins underwent surgery was poorer than that for concordant twin pairs where neither twin was exposed to anesthesia. This finding could imply that there may exist an unknown genetic factor that increases the risk of both the need for surgery and poor school performance.

The Western Canadian Complex Pediatric Therapies Follow-up Group recently published a prospective follow-up study of 95 infants at 2 years of age who underwent surgical correction for congenital heart disease at the Alberta Children's Hospital from April 2003 to December 2006.[304] A multiple logistic regression analysis of variables associated with developmental delay found that only more days of ventilatory support postoperatively and older age at surgery were associated with significant developmental delay. There was also no evidence for an association between the sedation variables and significant motor delays. However, the use of two neurocognitive assessment tools during the study period precluded an analysis of the cognitive and motor scores as continuous variables, which may have been a more sensitive way to detect subtle impairment.

Hansen and colleagues used a very large Danish birth cohort to compare academic performance in 2689 children that had inguinal hernia repair in infancy with 14,575 children who were randomly selected as an age-matched sample from the general population.[305] Those who had hernia repair performed worse at school, but there was no evidence for any association between surgery and school performance after adjustment for likely confounding variables. In contrast to the studies of DiMaggio and Wilder, this study detected no evidence for an association between surgery and poor neurobehavioral outcome.

Lastly, in a recent study using the Western Australian Pregnancy Cohort (Raine), Ing and colleagues found an association between language and abstract reasoning deficits in 10-year-old children who were exposed to one or more anesthetics prior to age 3, compared with previously unexposed children. After adjustment for confounders, any anesthetic before age 3 increased the risk ratio of disability in receptive, expressive, or total language as measured by the Clinical Evaluation of Language

Fundamentals (CELF) test, as well as abstract reasoning (Raven's Colored Progressive Matrices) to between 1.7 and 2.1 of unexposed controls, whereas other tests of vocabulary, behavior, and motor function were unaffected by exposure.[305a]

## Outcome after Exposure to Anesthesia Outside of the Operating Room

The operating room is not the only area where anesthetic neurotoxicity may be relevant. Ketamine and benzodiazepines are frequently administered in the emergency room, and in neonatal and pediatric intensive care units. These drugs may be administered for a protracted period of time, increasing their theoretical risk of neurotoxicity.[53,55]

Unfortunately, determining the clinical relevance of any neurotoxicity in intensive care patients is even more difficult than for the operating room. The total number of children that can be examined is smaller, they tend to be a very heterogeneous population, and most importantly, these children often have multiple significant confounding comorbidities, including exposure to anesthesia, which could significantly affect neurologic outcome. To date, there is mixed evidence that exposure to anesthetic or sedative drugs is associated with poorer neurobehavioral outcome. A Cochrane review found some evidence for worsened short-term outcome in neonates who had prolonged exposures to midazolam infusions.[306] In contrast, after correction for severity of illness, another study (using the EPIPAGE cohort) found no evidence for an association between prolonged sedation exposure and adverse neurologic outcome.[307] In that study, however, many children received opioids for sedation rather than benzodiazepines.

## Limitations of the Available Clinical Studies

There are numerous reasons why the clinical data on neurobehavioral outcomes after anesthesia are difficult to interpret, and it is perhaps not surprising that clinical studies return conflicting results. None of the currently available clinical studies are prospective randomized trials. Due to their retrospective nature, several of these studies require mathematical adjustments, such as multiple logistic regression analyses for confounding variables. However, this limits the findings to known or suspected confounders, and does not address as yet unknown variables that may be more important to the outcome.

Epidemiologic studies are generally unable to separate the effects of surgery, or the need for surgery, from the potential anesthetic effects. As previously discussed, surgery may result in significant neurohumoral stress and/or inflammatory responses that may influence neurocognitive outcome, in addition to metabolic, hemodynamic, and respiratory events that occur perioperatively. Data collection for several of the epidemiologic studies occurred before continuous pulse-oximetry and capnography monitoring were standard, and at a time when inhalational anesthetics with profound adverse cardiovascular effects, such as halothane, were used.[296-297] Prospective studies of capnography and pulse oximetry have demonstrated that the very population considered to be at risk (those under 2 years of age) had the greatest incidence of desaturation events, hypercarbia, and hypocarbia.[308-310]

Children undergoing surgery or diagnostic procedures early in life may suffer more frequently from concomitant chromosomal and genetic abnormalities or comorbidities, such as prematurity, which have been linked to abnormal neurobehavioral outcomes. For example, children with cyanotic congenital heart disease often have abnormal neurocognitive development before any surgical or anesthesia intervention.[262] The indication for surgery or for a diagnostic procedure requiring anesthesia, such as injury or infection, may artificially increase the incidence of neurodevelopmental abnormalities in the anesthetized cohort.[262] On the other hand, it has been argued that subjects suffering from underlying abnormalities adversely affecting neurodevelopment that do not receive the required surgery may be introduced into the pool of unanesthetized children, and therefore mask potentially toxic effects of anesthesia.[57]

Further complicating the interpretation of retrospective data is the substantial gap in time between exposure and neurologic assessment. The advantage of performing neurologic assessments in school-age children includes the increased precision and greater predictive value of such assessments compared with neurobehavioral testing performed for children under 2 years of age, for both prospective and retrospective studies.[311] However, especially in retrospective studies that cannot adequately control for confounders, the protracted time interval between surgery and the neurocognitive assessment may introduce even more "noise" into the study by increasing the time for negative influence of other environmental confounders of brain development or, conversely, the positive effects of repair mechanisms and plasticity to affect neurologic outcome.

Current animal studies do not provide sufficient guidance on the specific dose or duration of the anesthetic exposure that may lead to long-term impairment, the individual neurocognitive domains that may be affected, or the particular age at which the human brain may potentially be most susceptible to the neurotoxic effects of anesthetic exposure.

No consensus exists, even in the animal literature, concerning what duration of anesthesia exposure is required to induce long-lasting injury. Although the anesthetic exposure may represent a much larger fraction of an animal's life than a humans, at the cellular level apoptosis is likely to be triggered by a more similar duration of exposure. However, cell cycle duration and also the developmental period of the brain are considerably greater in humans than in rodents. It is therefore plausible, if an anesthesia-induced increase in apoptosis does occur in humans during a few hours of exposure, that it may be functionally less important than the same increase in apoptosis over the same period of time in a rodent. Similarly, the plasticity and capacity for recovery may differ between species. On the one hand, it can be argued that the period of development in humans is greater than it is in animals, and hence there may be more time for recovery, but on the other hand, human development is far more complex and humans may therefore be more vulnerable. Moreover, injuries during critical periods of development may have an exaggerated effect compared with the same injury outside of these periods.[273,312] Accordingly, studies that find no evidence of association with shorter exposures may not be generalizable to all applications of anesthesia, and studies that find evidence for an association with greater exposure times may not be applicable to short exposures.

As children grow they develop additional skills and abilities, and wider arrays of psychometric tests can be applied to evaluate these more extensive neurobehavioral domains. However, we currently lack adequate information on which specific domains to examine in humans following anesthetic exposure, complicating the interpretation of human cohort studies. Many of these studies use summary scores, such as IQ or average school grades. These outcome measures may miss subtle effects confined to specific neurobehavioral domains. Similarly, a diagnosis of developmental delay or behavioral problems may also miss more subtle changes in particular areas. In contrast, broad batteries of detailed tests are increasingly likely to find at least one association purely by chance.

The vulnerable period in humans, if it exists, has not been clearly identified. Animal data seem to suggest that anesthetic exposure may be most relevant during pregnancy or in early infancy, but it could be possible that the period of vulnerability may extend beyond infancy and young age. These critical uncertainties not only complicate the interpretation of published studies, but make the design of future, prospective studies very difficult.

Lastly the possible neuroprotective effects of anesthesia complicate this conundrum even further. Infants undergoing surgery who experience major intraoperative adverse events, such as cardiopulmonary arrest, are generally expected to suffer from abnormal neurologic outcomes, irrespective of their anesthetic exposure. Neurologic abnormalities observed after an otherwise uneventful procedure are considered neurotoxic effects of anesthesia. However, because anesthetics may also, at least partially, protect from the harmful metabolic, immunologic, and humoral responses to surgery and pain,[245] an alternative explanation may be that inadequate levels of anesthesia, insufficient postoperative pain relief, or unabated inflammation may be the culprit for the observed neurodevelopmental abnormalities. It is also possible that anesthetics may protect in major adverse settings, but may be deleterious in the absence of toxic stimuli, causing injury during minor procedures, but ameliorating injury during major surgery, such as complex heart surgery involving cardiopulmonary bypass.

In summary, there is mixed evidence for an association between anesthesia exposure in early childhood and poor neurobehavioral outcome in human studies. Collection of more definitive data supporting a deleterious role for anesthetics during brain development are complicated by uncertainties regarding the toxic threshold dose for anesthetics, the lack of information about the age of maximum susceptibility, and ambiguity related to the most appropriate neurobehavioral domains to examine. On the other hand, any positive association between anesthetic exposure and learning abnormalities may be spurious because of sampling bias in selecting children in need of early-life surgery and the inability to separate anesthetic effects from those of surgery and related comorbidities. Currently, clinical studies have not established causation between exposure to anesthesia in young children and adverse neurobehavioral outcomes, but at the same time, they do not rule out that possibility.

## Future Research

Further animal data will continue to provide information on the mechanisms of and susceptibility to anesthetic neurotoxicity. Understanding the mechanisms will be critical in translating the animal findings to clinical settings. Moreover, future animal work may also assist in determining which domains of neurobehavioral outcome are most likely to be affected, and this would assist in the design of human clinical trials. If neurotoxicity is found to be clinically relevant, animal data will also guide in devising prevention strategies.

Further human clinical studies must also be performed. Cohort studies will better identify children most at risk and characterize the neurobehavioral changes that occur. Because of the multiple confounding factors, cohort studies will always have great difficulty determining if the outcomes are a result of the surgery, the comorbidities, or the anesthetic exposure. Finding evidence for a lack of neurologic abnormalities in certain populations would provide some reassurance that laboratory studies in animal models lack immediate clinical relevance, however, it is important to note that such findings may not be automatically generalizable to all clinical settings.

Future clinical studies will need to take into account unique human functions, such as language skills. Moreover, ongoing and future research will have to better delineate the effects of early life exposure to surgery with anesthesia on specific neurologic domains. Preliminary results presented at the British Journal of Anaesthesia Special Workshop on Anesthesia, Neurotoxicity, and Neuroplasticity (Salzburg, Austria, June 2012) indicate that infant anesthesia may subsequently affect certain forms of recognition memory more than others and may also have differential effects dependent on gender. (Greg Stratmann, MD, PhD, personal communication).

To definitively answer this important health concern, clinical trials provide the strongest evidence. However, such trials are difficult to perform, as randomization to anesthesia or no anesthesia is impossible. It is, however, feasible to randomize to different types of anesthetic agents or approaches, such as regional versus general anesthesia. Even when using this approach, the appropriate outcome measure still has to be better defined. To perform a meaningful neurobehavioral assessment requires that the child is at least 2 years of age, if executive function is to be assessed, and 5 years of age or older would be preferable.

Even if anesthesia-induced neuroapoptosis is found to be clinically irrelevant, it is still important to recognize that there is a strong association between major surgery in neonates and abnormal neurobehavioral outcome. Thus the questions become which other factors may be causing the poor outcome and which perioperative interventions could be performed by anesthesiologists to improve outcomes in these children.

## Recommendations for Clinical Practice

The currently available laboratory data are not sufficient to make recommendations for clinical pediatric anesthesia practice. As outlined above, numerous laboratory studies have unequivocally documented deleterious effects of anesthetic exposure on the developing animal brain. Although these results should not be easily dismissed, the problems in translation from animal to human are substantial. Epidemiologic studies in children are also contradictory and can neither rule out nor confirm anesthetic-related neurotoxicity. Accordingly, the U.S. Food and Drug Administration (FDA) and the International Anesthesia Research Society (IARS) state that "dangers to infants and children from anesthesia remain unproven at this point" (http://www. smarttots.org/familyResourceCenter.html).

Pediatric surgery is never entirely elective, and in neonates may be required in order to preserve life, such as for critical congenital heart disease, necrotizing enterocolitis, or congenital diaphragmatic hernia. Accordingly, calls to postpone infant surgery are not easy to accommodate. Delaying surgery is also problematic, as no vulnerable or safe period has been identified in animal studies to guide this practice. Accordingly, the FDA and IARS have stated, "Currently, there is no scientific basis for delaying essential surgery" (http://www.smarttots.org/familyResourceCenter.html). It might be reasonable to delay purely elective surgeries; however, these only represent a very small fraction of surgeries performed in children.

It is well documented that neonates are at an increased risk for respiratory and cardiovascular complications during anesthesia, which influences the choice of anesthetic technique and drugs used in this population. It would be very unwise to change practice based on concerns over anesthetic neurotoxicity, while potentially increasing the risks of cardiovascular or respiratory complications. Similarly, it must be stressed that insufficient anesthesia and analgesia are definitely associated with poor neurologic outcomes.

Lastly, when discussing the risks and benefits of anesthesia with parents, pediatricians, and surgeons, anesthesiologists need to be cautious not to cause undue alarm, while taking the matter of potential toxicity seriously and not hastily dismissing any parental concern.

## ANNOTATED REFERENCES

Ikonomidou C, Bosch F, Miksa M, et al. Blockade of NMDA receptors and apoptotic neurodegeneration in the developing brain. Science 1999;283:70-4.

*This paper represents the first study to examine the effects of anesthetic exposure early in life on brain structure, demonstrating widespread neuronal degeneration following repeated administration of ketamine in newborn rats.*

Istaphanous GK, Howard J, Nan X, et al. Comparison of the neuro-apoptotic properties of equipotent anesthetic concentrations of desflurane, isoflurane, or sevoflurane in neonatal mice. Anesthesiology 2011;114:578-87.

*This is the first study in animals to compare the neurodegenerative properties of equipotent doses of the contemporary inhaled anesthetics with each other, finding no significant differences in the degree of apoptotic neuronal cell death among the agents.*

Jevtovic-Todorovic V, Hartman RE, Izumi Y, et al. Early exposure to common anesthetic agents causes widespread neurodegeneration in the developing rat brain and persistent learning deficits. J Neurosci 2003;23:876-82.

*This is a seminal study into the brain structural and long-term functional effects of a combined exposure to isoflurane, nitrous oxide, and midazolam in newborn rats, showing both increased neuroapoptosis immediately following exposure, and long-term learning impairment.*

Paule MG, Li M, Allen RR, et al. Ketamine anesthesia during the first week of life can cause long-lasting cognitive deficits in rhesus monkeys. Neurotoxicol Teratol 2011;33:220-30.

*This is the first study in nonhuman primates to link a prolonged exposure to ketamine very early in life to long-term neurobehavioral abnormalities.*

Wilder RT, Flick RP, Sprung J, et al. Early exposure to anesthesia and learning disabilities in a population-based birth cohort. Anesthesiology 2009;110:796-804.

*The authors provide one of the earliest epidemiologic studies to suggest an association between repeated exposure to surgery with anesthesia early in life to long-term neurobehavioral abnormalities in children.*

## REFERENCES

Please see www.expertconsult.com.

# Pediatric Neurosurgical Anesthesia 24

CRAIG D. McCLAIN, SULPICIO G. SORIANO, AND MARK A. ROCKOFF

CHILDREN REQUIRING NEUROSURGICAL PROCEDURES present unique challenges to pediatric anesthesiologists. In addition to addressing problems common to general pediatric anesthesia practice, anesthesiologists must consider the effects of anesthesia on the developing central nervous system (CNS) of children with neurologic disease. This chapter reviews the age-dependent physiology of the CNS of children undergoing neurosurgical procedures requiring anesthesia.

## Pathophysiology

### INTRACRANIAL COMPARTMENTS

The skull can be compared to a rigid container with almost incompressible contents. Under normal conditions, the intracranial space is occupied by the brain and its interstitial fluid (80%), cerebrospinal fluid (CSF, 10%), and blood (10%). In pathologic states, space-occupying lesions such as edema, tumors, hematomas, or abscesses alter these proportions. The Monro-Kellie hypothesis, elaborated in the 19th century, states that the sum of all intracranial volumes is constant. An increase in volume of one compartment must be accompanied by an approximately equal decrease in volume of the other compartments, except when the cranium can expand to accommodate a larger volume. Gradual increases in intracranial volumes, such as a slow-growing tumor or hydrocephalus, can be compensated by the compliant nature of open fontanelles and sutures in young children; increasing head circumference can result.[1] However, herniation can occur in children with open fontanelles if large increases in intracranial pressure (ICP) develop acutely. In the nonacute situation, the brain can compensate for pathologic increases in intracranial volume by intracellular dehydration and reduction of interstitial fluid.[2-4]

Under normal conditions, CSF exists in dynamic equilibrium, with absorption balancing production. The rate of CSF production in adults is approximately 0.35 mL/min or 500 mL/day.[5] The average adult has 100 to 150 mL of CSF distributed throughout the brain and subarachnoid space. Children have correspondingly smaller volumes of CSF, but the rate of CSF production is similar to that of adults.[5,6]

Production of CSF is only slightly affected by alterations of ICP and is usually unchanged in children with hydrocephalus.[6] Some drugs, including acetazolamide, furosemide, and corticosteroids, are mildly effective in transiently decreasing CSF production.[1,7,8] There is an inverse relationship between the rate of CSF production and serum osmolality; an increase in serum osmolality causes a decrease in CSF production. Choroid plexus papillomas causing overproduction of CSF are rare but are more likely to occur during childhood.

Absorption of CSF is not well understood, but the arachnoid villi appear to be important sites for reabsorption of CSF into the venous system. One-way valves between the subarachnoid space and the sagittal sinus appear to open at a gradient of about 5 mm Hg. Some resorption may occur from the spinal subarachnoid space and from the ependymal lining of the ventricles. Resorption increases with an increase in ICP. However, CSF absorption is decreased by pathologic processes that obstruct arachnoid villi or interfere with CSF flow, such as intracranial hemorrhage, infection, tumor, and congenital malformations.[9]

### INTRACRANIAL PRESSURE

Increased ICP causes secondary brain injury by producing cerebral ischemia and ultimately causing herniation. Ischemia occurs when ICP increases and cerebral perfusion pressure (CPP) decreases. As cerebral blood flow (CBF) and the supply of

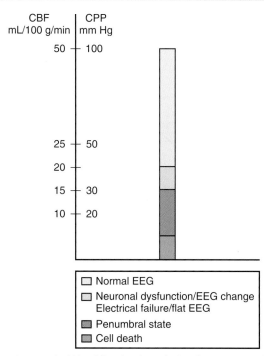

FIGURE 24-1 Cerebral blood flow (*CBF*), cerebral perfusion pressure (*CPP*), and brain ischemia. Changes in CBF and CPP affect neuronal synaptic function and cellular integrity. When CBF decreases to 15 to 20 mL/100 g/min, there is distinct neuronal dysfunction on the electroencephalogram (*EEG*). At 15 mL/100 g/min, the EEG is essentially flat, and electrical activity ceases to function. At 6 to 15 mL/100 g/min, a penumbral state occurs in which there is energy for cellular integrity but insufficient energy for synaptic function. Neuronal survival is unlikely if this low CBF is allowed to persist for more than an ill-defined but critical period. At less than 6 mL/100 g/min, there is no energy for cellular membrane integrity. Infarction occurs at this stage unless reperfusion is accomplished immediately.

nutrients are curtailed, cell damage and death occur, leading to increased intracellular and extracellular water and further increases in ICP. When ICP increases, CPP can decrease, the brain can become ischemic, and cell death can ensue (Fig. 24-1).[10]

### Herniation Syndromes

Several herniation syndromes exist. The most common is *transtentorial* herniation, in which the uncus of the temporal lobe is displaced from the supratentorial to the infratentorial space. Compression of the third cranial nerve and brainstem results in pathognomonic signs of pupillary dilatation, hemiparesis, and loss of consciousness. If this compression is not promptly relieved, apnea, bradycardia, and death occur.

In *cerebellar* herniation, the cerebellar tonsils herniate through the foramen magnum from the posterior fossa to the cervical spinal space. This can lead to obstruction of CSF circulation and ultimately to hydrocephalus. Compression of the brainstem results in cardiorespiratory failure and death.

### Signs of Increased Intracranial Pressure

The clinical signs of increased ICP vary in children. Papilledema, pupillary dilation, hypertension, and bradycardia may be absent despite intracranial hypertension, or these signs may occur with normal ICP.[9,11] When associated with increased ICP, they are usually late and dangerous signs.[12] Chronic increases in ICP are

often manifested by complaints of headache, irritability, and vomiting, particularly in the morning. Papilledema may not be present even in children dying as a result of intracranial hypertension.[13] A diminished level of consciousness and abnormal motor responses to painful stimuli are frequently associated with an increased ICP.[9] Computed tomography (CT) or magnetic resonance imaging (MRI) can reveal small or obliterated ventricles or basilar cisterns, hydrocephalus, intracranial masses, and midline shifts. Diffuse cerebral edema is a common finding when increased ICP is associated with closed-head injury, encephalopathy, or encephalitis.

### Monitoring Intracranial Pressure

Techniques to monitor ICP in adults have been successfully used in children.[14-16] Ventricular catheters are generally accepted as the most accurate and reliable means of measurement, permitting removal of CSF for diagnostic or therapeutic indications. The major risks of intraventricular catheters are infection and hemorrhage; although rare, they can lead to devastating complications. These catheters may be difficult to insert precisely when they are needed most, as in a patient with severe cerebral edema with small ventricles. Compared with intraventricular catheters, subarachnoid bolts can be placed even when the ventricles are obliterated. This procedure minimizes trauma to brain tissue and poses less risk of serious infection and hemorrhage. The major disadvantages are that subarachnoid bolts may underestimate ICP, particularly in areas distant from their insertion site, and they are difficult to stabilize in infants with thin calvaria.

Epidural monitors that do not require a fluid interface can be implanted outside the dura, avoiding the risks of CSF contamination and the limitations of fluid-dependent systems.[17,18] Most epidural systems correlate well with intraventricular measurements, but they cannot be recalibrated after insertion. Epidural monitors have also been secured noninvasively to the open anterior fontanelle of infants and appear to reflect changes in ICP. Fiberoptic catheters with self-contained transducers can also be used to measure ICP from intraventricular, subarachnoid, or intraparenchymal sites. These monitors avoid some of the problems of external fluid-filled transducers, but like epidural transducers, they cannot be recalibrated after insertion.

The normal ICP in children is less than 15 mm Hg. In term neonates, normal ICP is 2 to 6 mm Hg; it is probably even less in preterm infants. Children with intracranial pathology but normal ICP values occasionally exhibit pressure waves, which are considered abnormal.[9] In children with open fontanelles, the ICP may remain normal despite a significant intracranial pathologic process; increasing head circumference may be the first clinical sign. Bulging fontanelles may not develop, especially when the process evolves slowly.

### Intracranial Compliance

The absolute value of ICP does not indicate how much compensation is possible. If the ICP increases significantly, compensatory mechanisms have failed. However, pathologic states may be present despite an ICP within the normal range. Intracranial compliance (i.e., the change in pressure relative to a change in volume) is a valuable concept. Figure 24-2 is a schematic diagram of the relationship between the addition of volume to intracranial compartments and ICP. The shape of the curve depends on the time over which the volume increases and the relative size of the compartments. At normal intracranial volumes (point 1), ICP is low, but compliance is high and remains so despite small

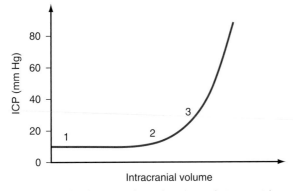

**FIGURE 24-2** Idealized intracranial compliance curve for intracranial pressure (*ICP*) plotted against intracranial volume.

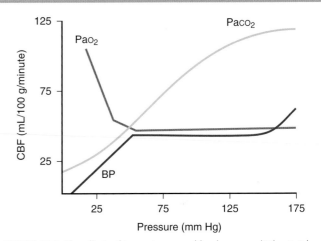

**FIGURE 24-3** The effects of increasing mean blood pressure (*BP*), arterial partial pressure of oxygen (*PaO$_2$*), and arterial partial pressure of carbon dioxide (*PaCO$_2$*) on cerebral blood flow (*CBF*) in the normal brain. (From Shapiro HM. Intracranial hypertension: therapeutic and anesthetic considerations. Anesthesiology 1975;43:447.)

increases in volume. If volume increases rapidly, compensatory abilities are surpassed, and further increases in volume are reflected as increases in pressure. This can occur when the ICP is still within normal limits but the compliance is low (point 2). If the ICP is already increased further volume expansion causes a rapid increase in ICP (point 3). In clinical practice, compliance can be evaluated with a ventriculostomy catheter or by observing the response of ICP to external stimulation (e.g., tracheal suction, coughing, agitation).

Several physiologic and mechanical factors such as a greater percentage of brain water content, less CSF volume, and greater percentage of brain content to intracranial capacity contribute to a relatively decreased intracranial compliance in children compared with adults.[2] Children may be at increased risk for herniation compared with adults when similar relative increases in ICP have occurred. However, infants faced with a slowly increasing ICP may have a greater compliance due to their open fontanelles and sutures.

### CEREBRAL BLOOD VOLUME AND CEREBRAL BLOOD FLOW
In addition to CSF, cerebral blood volume (CBV) represents another compartment in which compensatory mechanisms influence ICP. Although the CBV occupies only 10% of the intracranial space, changes related to dynamic blood volume occur, often initiated by anesthesia or intensive care procedures. As with other vascular beds, most intracranial blood is contained in the low-pressure, high-capacitance venous system. Increases in intracranial volume are initially met by decreases in CBV. This response is apparent in hydrocephalic infants, in whom venous blood shifts from intracranial to extracranial vessels, producing distended scalp veins.[19]

In the normal adult, CBF is approximately 55 mL/100 g of brain tissue per minute.[20-22] This represents almost 15% of the cardiac output for an organ that accounts for only 2% of body weight. Estimates of CBF are less uniform for children. Normal CBF in healthy awake children is approximately 100 mL per 100 g of brain tissue per minute, which represents up to 25% of cardiac output.[23,24] CBF in neonates and preterm infants (approximately 40 mL/100 g/min) is less than in children and adults.[25,26] In infants, CBF is subject to modification by sleep states and feeding.[27]

CBF is regulated to meet the metabolic demands of the brain. In adults, the cerebral metabolic rate for oxygen consumption (CMRO$_2$) is 3.5 to 4.5 mL O$_2$/100 g/min; in children, it is greater.[23] General anesthesia reduces CMRO$_2$ by as much as 50%.[28] Coupling of CBF and CMRO$_2$ is probably mediated by the effect of local hydrogen ion concentration on cerebral vessels. Conditions that cause acidosis (e.g., hypoxemia, hypercarbia, ischemia) dilate the cerebral vasculature, which augments CBF and CBV. A reduction in brain metabolism (i.e., CMRO$_2$) similarly reduces CBF and CBV. When autoregulation is impaired, CBF is determined by factors other than metabolic demand. If the CBF exceeds metabolic requirements, luxury perfusion or hyperemia exists. Many pharmacologic agents act directly on the cerebral vasculature to alter CBF and CBV.

### CEREBRAL PERFUSION PRESSURE
CPP is a useful and practical estimate of the adequacy of the cerebral circulation, because CBF is neither easily nor widely measured. Defined as the pressure gradient across the brain, CPP is the difference between the systemic mean arterial pressure (MAP) at the entrance to the brain and the mean exit pressure (i.e., central venous pressure [CVP]). When ICP is increased, it replaces CVP in the calculation of CPP. In supine children, the mean CPP is the difference between the MAP and the mean ICP (CPP = MAP − ICP). If the brain and heart are positioned at different heights, all pressures should be referenced at the level of the head (e.g., external auditory meatus).

### CEREBROVASCULAR AUTOREGULATION
#### Effects of Blood Pressure
In adults, CBF remains relatively constant within a MAP range of 50 to 150 mm Hg (Fig. 24-3). Autoregulation enables brain perfusion to remain stable despite moderate changes in MAP or ICP. Autoregulation is partially mediated by myogenic control of arteriolar resistance. When CPP decreases, cerebral vessels dilate to maintain CBF, thereby increasing CBV. When CPP increases, cerebral vasoconstriction occurs, maintaining the CBF with a reduced CBV. When ICP and CVP are low, MAP normally approximates CPP. Beyond the range of autoregulation, CBF becomes pressure dependent. In children with chronic hypertension, the upper and lower limits of autoregulation are increased. Cerebral autoregulation can be abolished by acidosis, medications, tumor, cerebral edema, and vascular malformations, even at sites far removed from a discrete lesion.[20]

The limits of autoregulation are not known for normal infants and children, but autoregulation probably occurs at lower absolute values than in adults.[29] Although the lower limit of autoregulation in adults is approximately 50 mm Hg, this blood pressure may be beyond that of the neonate. Intact autoregulatory mechanisms have been demonstrated within lower blood pressure ranges in newborn animals compared with mature animals.[30] Cerebral autoregulation may also be abolished in critically ill humans.[31]

### Effects of Oxygen

CBF is constant over a wide range of oxygen tensions. When the partial pressure of arterial $O_2$ ($PaO_2$) decreases to less than 50 mm Hg, CBF increases exponentially in adults; for example, at a $PaO_2$ of 15 mm Hg, CBF is doubled compared with normal (see Fig. 24-3).[32] The resulting increase in CBV increases ICP when intracranial compliance is low; the lower limit for $PaO_2$ is probably less in neonates. Oxygen delivery is more important than the actual $PaO_2$. Evidence suggests that hyperoxia decreases CBF. Kety and Schmidt demonstrated a 10% decrease in CBF in adults breathing 100% $O_2$, although decreases of 33% have been reported in neonates.[33,34]

### Effects of Carbon Dioxide

The relationship between the arterial partial pressure of carbon dioxide ($PaCO_2$) and CBF typically is linear (see Fig. 24-3). In adults, a 1-mm Hg increase in $PaCO_2$ increases CBF by approximately 2 mL/100 g/min.[33] The direct effect of changes in $PaCO_2$ on CBF and the consequent effect on CBV are the basis for the fact that hyperventilation reduces ICP. Likewise, increases in $PaCO_2$ increase the CBF, although the limits at which this occurs in neonates differ from those in adults. In lambs and monkeys, CBF does not seem to change in response to decreased $PaCO_2$.[35] There are no data to suggest what the limits of $PaCO_2$ are in human infants and children. Similarly, there is little information about the extent and duration of cerebrovascular responsiveness to hyperventilation in brain-injured and critically ill children. Moderate hyperventilation has been used to reduce ICP immediately, but several reports have demonstrated worsening cerebral ischemia in children with compromised cerebral perfusion.[36-38]

Autoregulation of CBF is impaired in areas of damaged brain.[39] Blood vessels in an ischemic zone are subject to hypoxemia, hypercarbia, and acidosis, which are potent stimuli for vasodilation. These vessels develop maximally reduced cerebrovascular tone or vasomotor paralysis. Small, localized lesions may impair autoregulation in areas far removed from the site of injury.[20] The extent of autoregulatory impairment varies in brain-damaged children.

## Management of Anesthesia

### PREOPERATIVE EVALUATION

#### History

Preoperative evaluation of infants and children is discussed in Chapter 4. Children who are scheduled for neurosurgery might have been healthy until the onset of their symptoms, might have been developmentally delayed from birth, or may have impaired neuromuscular function. The anesthetic plan, including postoperative care, needs to consider the particular issues of each child and the disease state.

A history of food or drug allergies, eczema, or asthma may provide warning of an adverse reaction to the contrast agents frequently used in neuroradiologic procedures. Special attention

should be given to symptoms of allergy to latex products, such as lip swelling after blowing up a toy balloon or tongue swelling after insertion of a rubber dam is into the mouth by a dentist, because latex anaphylaxis has been reported in some children who have undergone multiple operations, especially those with a meningomyelocele.[40] Latex allergic children may also report allergies to fruits (e.g., kiwi, banana, avocado, strawberry, and others).

Concurrent pediatric diseases and symptoms of neurologic lesions may influence the conduct of anesthesia. Protracted vomiting, enuresis, and anorexia due to intracranial lesions should prompt evaluation of hydration and electrolytes. Diabetes insipidus or inappropriate secretion of antidiuretic hormone is common. A history of the use of aspirin or aspirin-containing remedies for headaches or respiratory tract infections is information that is not usually forthcoming but may have important implications for operative and postoperative bleeding. Corticosteroids are often initiated at the time of diagnosis of intracranial tumors, and they should be continued and a pulse dose administered during the perioperative period. Therapeutic concentrations of anticonvulsants should be verified preoperatively and maintained perioperatively. Children receiving long-term anticonvulsants may develop toxicity, especially if seizures are difficult to control; this is frequently manifested as abnormalities in hematologic or hepatic function, or both. Children receiving chronic anticonvulsant therapy may also require increased amounts of sedatives, nondepolarizing muscle relaxants, and opioids because of enhanced metabolism of these drugs (see also Chapters 6 and 22).[41-43]

### Physical Examination

The physical examination should encompass a brief neurologic evaluation, including level of consciousness, motor and sensory function, normal and pathologic reflexes, integrity of the cranial nerves, and signs and symptoms of intracranial hypertension. Examination of pupillary size and responsiveness can detect benign anisocoria. Preoperative respiratory assessment should include the effects of motor weakness, impaired gag and swallowing mechanisms, and evidence of active pulmonary disease, such as aspiration pneumonia. Muscle atrophy and weakness should be documented, because upregulation of acetylcholine receptors may precipitate sudden hyperkalemia after administration of succinylcholine and induce resistance to nondepolarizing muscle relaxants in the affected limbs.[44]

### Laboratory and Radiologic Evaluation

In all but the most minor procedures, laboratory data should include a hematocrit determination. Blood typing and cross-matching should be performed for any major procedure. The need for additional studies, such as evaluation of coagulation parameters, serum electrolyte levels and osmolality, blood urea nitrogen and creatinine values, arterial blood gas analysis, chest radiography, or electrocardiography (ECG), is determined on an individual basis. Liver function tests and a hematologic profile should be obtained if not recently reviewed in children on long-term therapy with anticonvulsants. Specific neuroradiologic studies are usually obtained by the neurosurgeon and should be reviewed by the anesthesiologist. For example, the anesthesiologist should know which children with a ventriculoperitoneal shunt have "slit ventricles," because these children have special risks in the perioperative period[45] (see "Hydrocephalus"). Information on the amount of sedation needed to perform radiologic studies may also be helpful in planning the induction of anesthesia. Preoperative neurophysiologic studies, including electroencephalography (EEG) and evoked potentials, may provide a baseline for comparison of intraoperative and postoperative evaluations.

## PREMEDICATION

Sedation is usually withheld from pediatric neurosurgical patients until they arrive in the preoperative area to allow titration of drug to desired effect while under direct supervision. Opioids are usually withheld preoperatively because they may cause nausea or respiratory depression, especially in children with increased ICP, and sedatives alone usually are adequate to relieve anxiety.

Sedatives are administered in the parents' presence to facilitate a smooth separation and induction. Midazolam (0.5 to 1.0 mg/kg) may be given orally; it usually requires 10 to 20 minutes to take effect. Incremental doses of intravenous midazolam (0.05 mg/kg) may also be useful in children who tolerate intravenous placement.

## MONITORING

Minimal monitoring for pediatric neuroanesthesia requires a stethoscope (precordial or esophageal), electrocardiograph, pulse oximeter, sphygmomanometer, capnograph, and thermometer. Neuromuscular blockade monitoring is also important, but nerve stimulators may give misleading information about the extent of relaxation if applied to a denervated extremity. If the child has paresis, nerve stimulation should be at a site of normal neurologic function. Precordial Doppler ultrasound is recommended in children undergoing craniotomy, especially in the head-up position, because the relatively large head size of children places them at increased risk for air emboli. Monitoring devices for ICP are used for the same indications as in adults. Intraoperative EEG and electrophysiologic monitoring require advanced coordination among the neurosurgeon, anesthesiologist, and neurophysiologist. Urinary output should be measured during prolonged procedures, in cases with anticipated large blood loss, and when diuretics or osmotic agents are administered.

An arterial catheter is placed for craniotomies in which there is a potential for sudden and severe hemodynamic changes. Small child size should not preclude the use of invasive monitoring and may actually be an indication for a more aggressive approach. An increase in the paradoxical arterial pressure waveform with positive-pressure ventilation is often an excellent indication of intravascular volume deficiency and the need for fluid replacement (see Fig. 10-10). Intraarterial catheters can be placed percutaneously in the radial, dorsalis pedis, or posterior tibial arteries even in small infants, and it is rarely necessary to resort to surgical cutdown. The arterial transducer should be zeroed at the level of the head if the head and heart positions are different so that CPP can be accurately assessed. The lateral corner of the eye or the external auditory meatus approximate the level of the foramen of Monro, and either is a convenient landmark. In the first days of life, the umbilical artery and the umbilical vein can be cannulated. These catheters should be discontinued as soon as alternative access is established because of the potential for serious complications.

Percutaneous central venous cannulation (i.e., external or internal jugular, femoral, or subclavian veins) using the Seldinger technique is possible even in the smallest infants (see Chapter 48). However, in children undergoing neurosurgical resections, consideration should be given to sites other than neck veins, such as the femoral vein, thereby avoiding the Trendelenburg position during catheter insertion and the risk of accidental carotid artery puncture and hematoma formation, which may compromise CBF and intracranial venous drainage. If there is no issue with ICP, the subclavian vein is a reasonable alternative. Cannulation of antecubital veins may provide central venous access, but threading the catheter into the inlet of the right atrium may be technically difficult in small children. When rapid blood loss is a consideration in a small child in whom adequate peripheral venous access is difficult to obtain, a single-lumen, large-bore catheter is most commonly inserted in a femoral vein. Catheters inserted into the femoral veins usually are accessible to the anesthesiologist during most neurosurgical procedures. Multiple-lumen central venous catheters are inadequate for rapid blood transfusion. All central catheters should be removed as soon as possible after the procedure to minimize the risk of venous thrombosis.

## INDUCTION

For children with intracranial hypertension, the primary goals during induction are to minimize severe increases in ICP and decreases in blood pressure. Most intravenous drugs decrease $CMRO_2$ and CBF, which consequently decreases ICP.[46] Historically, sodium thiopental (4 to 8 mg/kg) was the default induction agent for neurosurgical cases. However, sodium thiopental is no longer available in the United States, although it remains available in other countries. In the United States, propofol has become the intravenous induction agent of choice for most children. Propofol (2 to 4 mg/kg) appears to have similar cerebral properties and an antiemetic effect; however, its antiemetic effect is usually not relevant for lengthy procedures. Etomidate, a possible neuroprotective agent, can be used if hemodynamic stability is a concern.[47-49] Ketamine should be avoided because of its known ability to increase cerebral metabolism, CBF, and ICP. Sudden increases in ICP have been reported after ketamine administration, especially in infants and children with hydrocephalus.[50,51]

Other measures to reduce ICP during induction include controlled hyperventilation and administration of fentanyl and supplemental hypnotics before laryngoscopy and intubation. Lidocaine (1.5 mg/kg) limits the increase in ICP when administered intravenously just before laryngoscopy.[52]

Sevoflurane has replaced halothane for inhaled inductions because of its more rapid onset, acceptability for pediatric patients, and hemodynamic stability. Similar to isoflurane in its cerebral physiologic effects, sevoflurane with hyperventilation appears to blunt the increase in ICP due to cerebral vasodilation from inhalational anesthetic agents alone.[53-55] Sevoflurane offers an additional advantage because it causes less myocardial depression compared with halothane.[56] However, sevoflurane when combined with hyperventilation produces epileptiform activity as measured by EEG. This may occur even in children with no history of clinical seizure activity (see Chapter 6).[57]

A common presentation is an uncooperative toddler who has an intracranial tumor and moderately decreased intracranial compliance and is agitated and resistant to separation from parents. Some clinicians would argue that a crying, agitated child has demonstrated a tolerance to increased ICP and that an intravenous induction is safer. Fortunately (for the anesthesiologist, although not for the child), children who have severe intracranial hypertension typically have a decreased level of consciousness, and it becomes easier to insert an intravenous catheter in those situations when it is most necessary.

## AIRWAY MANAGEMENT AND INTUBATION

Airway management must be effective and smooth to avoid the ICP-increasing effects of hypoxemia, hypercarbia, and coughing. Opioid administration and supplemental hypnotics before intubation improve cerebral compliance and minimize increases in ICP caused by laryngoscopy and intubation.

Either oral or nasal intubation may be appropriate. Nasotracheal intubation offers the advantage of increased stability and increased comfort for children when postoperative intubation is necessary. Nasotracheal tubes are often used for children who will be in the prone position (e.g., for a posterior fossa craniotomy), children whose airway will be inaccessible during the surgical procedure, and for smaller children.

Contraindications to nasal intubation include choanal stenosis, possible basilar skull fracture, transsphenoidal procedures, and sinusitis. If nasotracheal intubation is planned, it is advantageous to prepare the nares with topical vasoconstrictors, recognizing that systemic hypertension can occur in response to nasally administered vasoconstrictors. Placing a few drops of 0.25% phenylephrine (Neo-Synephrine) or oxymetazoline on cotton-tipped applicators and positioning them in the nares against the nasal mucosa can prevent overdosage and help to gauge the patency of the nasal passage when anesthesia has been induced. It may also be useful to use a red rubber catheter or a nonlatex nasal trumpet to gently dilate the nares and minimize the risk of bleeding.[58] Whichever route is chosen for intubation, it is important to secure the tracheal tube with care because loss of airway intraoperatively in a prone child in pins or a child with limited airway access can result in disaster.

In prolonged, combined neurosurgical and craniofacial reconstructions, the tracheal tube may be sutured to the nasal septum or wired to the teeth. A nasogastric or orogastric tube is inserted after intubation to decompress the stomach and evacuate gastric contents; leaving it open to gravity drainage during the case can prevent positive pressure from building up in the stomach if air leaks around an uncuffed tracheal tube. The child's eyes should be closed and covered with a large, clear, waterproof dressing.

## NEUROMUSCULAR BLOCKING DRUGS

Because of its rapid onset and brief duration of action, succinylcholine is frequently used to facilitate intubation in children with a full stomach. The intubating dose is 1 to 2 mg/kg given intravenously or 4 to 5 mg/kg given intramuscularly.[59] In children, it may be safest to precede this with atropine (0.01 to 0.02 mg/kg) to prevent bradycardia. Succinylcholine does not significantly increase ICP in humans,[60] and any effect may be minimized by pretreatment with a nondepolarizing muscle relaxant.[61] However, this may make succinylcholine less effective, even when the dose of succinylcholine is increased. Succinylcholine is contraindicated when it may induce life-threatening hyperkalemia in the presence of denervation injuries due to various causes, including severe head trauma, crush injury, burns, spinal cord dysfunction, encephalitis, multiple sclerosis, muscular dystrophies, stroke, or tetanus.[62]

Alternatively, nondepolarizing muscle relaxants such as rocuronium, pancuronium, cisatracurium, or vecuronium may be used, but all have a slower onset of action than succinylcholine. However, when rocuronium is administered in sufficiently large doses (1.2 mg/kg), the onset of action is comparable with that of succinylcholine, with equivalent intubating conditions achieved in less than 1 minute.[63]

## POSITIONING

Positioning is an especially important consideration in pediatric neuroanesthesia. Children with increased ICP should be transported to the preoperative holding area and operating room with the head elevated in the midline position to maximize cerebral venous drainage.

After the child is in the operating room, the neurosurgeons and anesthesiologists must have adequate access to the child. In infants and small children, slight displacement of the tracheal tube can result in extubation or endobronchial intubation. During prolonged procedures, it is important for the anesthesiologist to be able to visually inspect the tracheal tube and circuit connections and to suction the tracheal tube when necessary. Using proper draping and a flashlight, the operator can usually create a "tunnel" to ensure access to the airway. All but very small children are placed in pins in a Mayfield head holder. The direction of the tube exiting the nares should be adjusted to remove pressure and avoid the risk of ischemia, particularly for cases that will continue for several hours. Neonates and small infants have thin calvaria, so head-pinning systems are often avoided. Instead, there are a variety of non–pin-based headrests available for these children. Adequate padding should be used in such situations (Figs. 24-4 and 24-5). Extreme head flexion can cause brainstem compression in children with posterior fossa pathology, such as

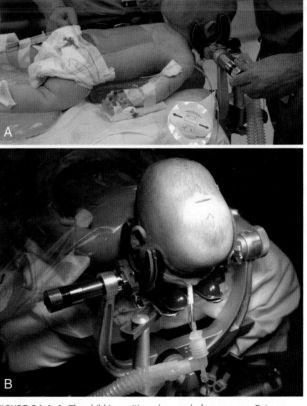

**FIGURE 24-4 A,** The child is positioned prone before surgery. Extreme head extension was needed for correction of craniosynostosis, but the equipment for securing the head was the same as that used for a prone craniotomy. **B,** This particular frame uses gel pads to support the chin, ears, and forehead.

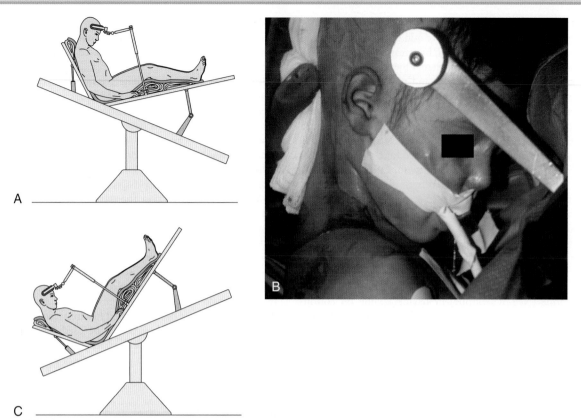

**FIGURE 24-5** Resuscitation from the modified standard sitting position. The normal operative position (**A** and **B**) is compared with the resuscitation position (**C**). The position can be expeditiously changed by one control of the operating table.

a mass lesion or Arnold-Chiari malformation. Extreme flexion can also cause high cervical spinal cord ischemia and tracheal tube kinking and obstruction.[64]

Extremities should be well padded and secured in a neutral position (i.e., palm supinated or neutral to avoid ulnar nerve compression). It is important to avoid stretching peripheral nerves and to prevent skin and soft tissue pressure injury because of direct contact with surgical accessories such as instrument stands and grounding wires (see Fig. 24-5). It is also important to ensure that extremities that are not directly visible to the anesthesiologist (e.g., those on the opposite side of the operating room table) cannot fall off the table during surgery, even if the table is rotated. In older children and adolescents undergoing prolonged procedures, deep vein thrombosis prophylaxis should be considered using compression or pneumatic stockings.[65,66]

### Prone Position

The prone position is commonly used for posterior fossa and spinal cord surgery. The torso should be supported to ensure free abdominal wall motion because increased intraabdominal pressure may impair ventilation, cause vena cava compression, and increase epidural venous pressure and bleeding. This is achieved most easily by placing silicone rolls or rolled blankets laterally on each side of the child's chest running from the shoulders toward the pelvis. A separate silicone roll or rolled blanket under the pelvis may occasionally be necessary in larger children. These rolls must not press into the flexed hips or compress the femoral nerve or genitalia. Placing the rolls in this position should also allow a precordial Doppler monitor to be easily placed on the anterior chest without undue pressure.

The head position depends on the surgical procedure. If surgery is limited to the lower spine, the head may be rotated and supported by padding, with care taken to avoid direct pressure on the eyes and nose and to keep the ears flat. For posterior fossa surgery, the head usually is suspended in pins to maintain central alignment of the head and maximal flexion. For infants and toddlers, a cerebellar head frame is another alternative when the cranium is too thin for pins. In this situation, the child's forehead and cheeks rest on a well-padded head frame, and the eyes are free in the center of a horseshoe-shaped support. Ensure that the tracheal tube is properly positioned (after taping) and does not migrate to a main-stem position while positioning the child prone. This can be confirmed while the child is still supine by flexing the child's head onto the chest and auscultating air entry bilaterally. Tape used to fix other tubes (e.g., gastric, esophageal) should not adhere to the tracheal tube tape so that accidental dislodgement of these tubes does not cause an extubation. An emergency plan should be formulated to turn the child supine if it suddenly becomes necessary.[67]

Significant airway edema may develop in a child who is in the prone position for an extended period. Oral airways are best avoided because they can cause edema of the tongue. Alternatively, a folded piece of gauze can be inserted between the teeth to prevent the tongue from extruding. Rarely, prophylactic postoperative intubation may be necessary if a great deal of facial swelling has developed during a prolonged surgery. Postoperative vision loss has been linked with prolonged spine surgery in the prone position and significant blood loss.[68] Avoidance of direct pressure on the globe of the eyes, staged procedures to decrease surgical time, and maintenance of stable hemodynamics with avoidance of excessive intraoperative fluid administration should be ensured in prone children.[69]

## Modified Lateral Position

Insertion or revision of ventriculoperitoneal shunts may require that the child be rotated from the supine to the semilateral position. This is achieved by placing a roll under the child's dependent axilla (to prevent a brachial plexus injury). The knees should be supported in a slightly flexed position and the heels padded. This position is also used for some temporal and parietal craniotomies.

## Sitting Position

The sitting position is now used less commonly in pediatric neurosurgical procedures and is rarely used in children younger than 3 years of age. However, this position may be used for morbidly obese children who cannot tolerate the prone position due to excessive intrathoracic and abdominal pressures. When it is used, precautions to prevent hypotension and air embolism must be followed. The lower extremities should be wrapped in elastic bandages. The head must be carefully flexed to avoid kinking the endotracheal tube, advancing it into a bronchial position, or avoid compressing the chin on the chest, which can block venous and lymphatic drainage of the tongue. Extreme flexion can also result in brainstem or cervical spinal cord ischemia, or both. As in the prone position, nasotracheal tubes are often used because they are more secure. The child's upper extremities are supported in the child's lap. Control levers to lower the head position should be easily accessible to the anesthesiologist and unencumbered by wires and drapes (see Fig. 24-5).

## LOCAL ANESTHESIA

Local anesthetic should be injected subcutaneously before a skin incision to provide analgesia, and epinephrine is included in the local anesthetic to reduce cutaneous blood loss. If 0.25% bupivacaine with 1:200,000 epinephrine is used, the dose should be limited to 0.5 mL/kg. When greater volumes are required, the solution can be diluted with normal saline. This dilute solution is still effective for vasoconstriction and provides a prolonged sensory block postoperatively. Specific blocks of supraorbital and supratrochlear nerves can provide analgesia from the frontal area to the midcoronal portion of the occiput.[70] Blockade of the great occipital nerve provides analgesia from the posterior of the occiput to the midcoronal area of the occiput, whereas block of the supraorbital nerve provides analgesia to the front of the occiput (see Figs. 41-9 and 41-10).[71,72]

## MAINTENANCE OF GENERAL ANESTHESIA

General anesthesia is required for most therapeutic and many diagnostic procedures in pediatric neurosurgery. Ventilation is controlled if intracranial hypertension is a concern. Although spontaneous ventilation provides another indication of brainstem function, its disadvantages (eg., hypoventilation, increased potential for air embolism) are usually outweighed by the safety of controlled ventilation.

Maintenance of general anesthesia can be accomplished using inhalational anesthetics, intravenous infusions, or a combination of these drugs. Anesthetics that decrease ICP and $CMRO_2$ and maintain CPP are most desirable (Table 24-1). The commonly used inhalational agents uncouple CBF and $CMRO_2$ such that CBF increases while $CMRO_2$ decreases. All potent inhalational agents are cerebral vasodilators, which increase the CBF and ICP. Low concentrations of isoflurane, sevoflurane, or desflurane, combined with ventilation to maintain normocarbia, minimally affect CBF and ICP.[53,54,73] Isoflurane is often the inhalational agent of choice for maintenance of neuroanesthesia. At two times the minimal alveolar concentration (MAC), this dose of isoflurane induces a level of anesthesia that is associated with an isoelectric EEG while, unlike several other inhalational agents, maintaining hemodynamic stability. Enflurane is no longer used

| Agent | MAP | CBF | CPP | ICP | $CMRO_2$ | CSF Production | CSF Absorption | SSEP Amplitude | SSEP Latency |
|---|---|---|---|---|---|---|---|---|---|
| Nitrous oxide | 0-↓ | ↑↑↑ | ↓ | ↑↑↑ | ↓↑ | ↑↓ | ↓↑ | ↓ | ↑-0 |
| **Inhalational Anesthetics** | | | | | | | | | |
| Halothane | ↓↓ | ↑↑↑ | ↑↑ | ↑↑ | ↓↓ | ↓↓ | 0-↓ | ↓ | ↑ |
| Enflurane | ↓↓ | ↑↑ | ↑↑ | ↑↑ | ↓↓ | ↑ | ↓ | ↓ | ↑ |
| Isoflurane | ↓↓ | ↑ | ↑↑ | ↑ | ↓↓↓ | ↓↑ | ↑ | ↓ | ↑ |
| Sevoflurane | ↓↓ | ↑ | ↑ | ↑ | ↓↓↓ | ↑ | ↓ | ↓ | ↑ |
| Desflurane | ↓↓ | ↑↑ | ↑ | ↑ | ↓ | ↑↓ | ↑ | ↓ | ↑ |
| **Hypnotics** | | | | | | | | | |
| Thiopental | ↓↓ | ↓↓↓ | ↑↑↑ | ↓↓↓ | ↓↓↓ | ↑↓ | ↑ | ↓ | ↑ |
| Propofol | ↓↓↓ | ↓↓↓ | | ↓↓ | ↓↓↓ | ↑↓ | ↑ | ↑ | ↑ |
| Etomidate | 0-↓ | ↓↓↓ | ↑ | ↓↓↓ | ↓↓↓ | ↑↓ | ↑ | ↑ | ↑ |
| Ketamine | ↓↓ | ↑↑↑ | ↓ | ↑↑↑ | ↑ | ↑↓ | ↓ | ↑ | 0 |
| Benzodiazepine | 0-↓ | ↓↓ | ↑ | 0-↓ | ↓↓ | N/A | ↑ | ↓ | 0-↑ |
| Opioids | 0-↓ | ↓ | ↑↓ | 0-↓ | ↓ | ↑↓ | ↑ | ↓ | ↑ |
| Droperidol | ↓↓ | N/A | ↑ | ↓ | 0-↓ | N/A | N/A | N/A | N/A |

*CBF,* Cerebral blood flow; *$CMRO_2$,* cerebral metabolic rate for oxygen; *CPP,* cerebral perfusion pressure; *CSF,* cerebrospinal fluid; *ICP,* intracranial pressure; *MAP,* mean arterial pressure; *N/A,* not applicable; *SSEP,* somatosensory evoked potential; ↑, increased; ↓, decreased; *0,* no change.
*NOTE:* The relative number of arrows refers to the degree of effect on the noted parameter. For example, $CMRO_2$ is decreased much more with isoflurane than opioids. In cells with up and down arrows, there are conflicting reports on the effect of the drug.

and may be epileptogenic, especially when combined with hyperventilation.[74] Other studies have demonstrated a similar effect with sevoflurane and hyperventilation, but the clinical implications of this are yet to be defined.[75]

Practitioners debate the routine use of nitrous oxide for intracranial neurosurgical procedures. Opponents cite the increased risk of postoperative nausea and vomiting (PONV) with nitrous oxide in a surgical population already at greater risk for PONV.[76] Proponents cite studies that failed to demonstrate an increased risk of PONV.[77] Nitrous oxide can increase CBF in humans in a dose-dependent fashion through cerebral vasodilatation.[78,79] This increase in CBF can lead to an increase in ICP, which can be deleterious if the child already has reduced intracranial compliance.[80] Nitrous oxide can also affect somatosensory and motor evoked potentials, especially when concentrations in excess of 50% are used.[81-83] Animal data have shown that nitrous oxide can counteract the protective effects of thiopental in a model of cerebral ischemia.[84]

Proponents of the use of nitrous oxide for intracranial procedures cite the long track record of safety. There are no outcome studies in humans showing a difference between using nitrous oxide or not. It is often of great clinical interest to obtain a neurologic assessment immediately after the conclusion of an intracranial procedure, and some practitioners prefer the use of nitrous oxide to aid in achieving this goal. Studies have demonstrated the safety of using nitrous oxide in a variety of combinations with other agents during intracranial procedures.[85] Nitrous oxide is relatively contraindicated, however, if the child has undergone a craniotomy within the past few weeks because air can remain in the head for prolonged periods after previous neurosurgery.[86]

Fentanyl is often administered as part of an opioid-based technique because it is easily titratable with minimal adverse effects. A common loading dose is 5 to 10 µg/kg, with a dose of 2 to 5 µg/kg/hr usually adequate for maintenance. Adverse effects, including hypotension, can be avoided by giving the loading dose incrementally. Practitioners commonly use other opioids such as remifentanil and sufentanil. Dexmedetomidine, an $\alpha_2$-agonist sedative, has also been used in children for neurophysiologic monitoring, for awake craniotomies, to facilitate smooth wake-ups after neurosurgical procedures, and for neuroprotection.[87-90]

## APOPTOTIC NEURODEGENERATION

Several investigators have demonstrated that commonly used anesthesia drugs accelerate programmed cell death (i.e., apoptosis) in the CNS of immature rodents and rhesus monkeys.[91-93] This laboratory observation has provoked a heated debate about its relevance to anesthetizing neonates,[94-97] which has been extended to the lay press.[98] Although these experimental paradigms have yielded some surprising findings, extrapolating these data to the practice of anesthetizing human neonates is questionable (see Chapter 23).

The animal and in vitro studies have significant limitations with respect to the experimental model, agent dosage or concentration, duration of exposure (absolute and compared with human exposures), lack of surgical stimulation, and developmental age and stage. No detectable clinical marker or syndrome is associated with early anesthesia exposure in former neonates who have undergone surgery and anesthesia at birth or in the first several years of life during rapid brain growth (i.e., synaptogenesis). In the only primate study, the degree of apoptosis after 3 hours of a ketamine infusion was similar to that of the control

but significantly less than after a 24-hour infusion.[93] This occurred in the presence of blood concentrations of ketamine that were 10-fold to several hundred-fold greater than those reported after a single dose of ketamine in infants. These findings suggest that in this model, ketamine-associated neurodegeneration is a time-dependent, dose-dependent phenomenon whose limits have not been established.

Despite the confounding effects of prematurity and coexisting congenital anomalies, clearly characterized syndromes have been associated with maternal consumption of alcohol and anticonvulsant drugs. Discrepancies in neurocognitive outcomes exist.[92,99] Most neonatal and infant surgery is urgent, and anesthesia care is essential to proceed safely. Several retrospective database studies suggest that multiple anesthesia episodes are associated with learning disabilities and cognitive dysfunction, but most of these children were anesthetized before pulse oximetry and capnography were a standard of care. Unrecognized episodes of hypoxemia or excessive ventilation with reduced CBF might have contributed. It is also unclear whether children who required more than one surgical procedure when younger than 4 years of age might have had neurocognitive developmental issues that were associated with the pathology requiring surgery and were totally separate from exposure to anesthetic agents.[100-102] One retrospective study demonstrated that identical twins who were discordant for general anesthesia and surgery showed no evidence of cognitive dysfunction in follow-up assessments.[103]

In summary, a growing body of evidence supports the idea that some anesthetic agents are harmful to the developing brain in various species of neonatal animals. There is neither adequate evidence nor a consensus among practitioners that this phenomenon occurs in very young humans, but this remains an area of great interest and research.

## BLOOD AND FLUID MANAGEMENT

Blood loss is difficult to estimate accurately during neurosurgery because most of the losses are absorbed by the operative drapes and the surgical field is difficult for the anesthesiologist to visualize. Accuracy can be improved if all suctioned blood is collected in calibrated containers visible to the anesthesiologist and an overhead camera provides a view of the operative field at all times. Blood loss is usually greatest at the beginning of surgery, when the scalp is incised, and when a large bone flap is removed.

Fluid and blood product management is discussed in Chapters 8 and 10. Disruption of the blood-brain barrier by underlying pathologic processes, trauma, or surgery predisposes neurosurgical patients to cerebral edema, which may be exacerbated by excessive administration of intravenous fluids. Intravenous fluid management during neurosurgical anesthesia involves cerebral perfusion, cerebral edema, water and sodium homeostasis, and serum glucose concentration.

In most cases, blood transfusions are not planned and attempts are made to avoid administration of blood products with their associated risks. Crystalloid solutions are commonly administered. Lactated Ringer solution is not considered a truly isotonic solution because its osmolality is 273 mOsm/L (normal: 285 to 290 mOsm/L). Normal saline, which is slightly hypertonic (308 mOsm/L), is the fluid of choice because reduction of serum osmolality is not desirable. However, rapid infusion of large volumes of normal saline has been associated with a hyperchloremic non-anion gap metabolic acidosis.[104] The clinical significance of this acidosis is not clear. If there are large fluid requirements during surgery, alternating bags of lactated Ringer solution with normal saline can minimize the risk of hypernatremia and acidosis and avoid hypoosmolality.

Inducing dehydration with osmotic and loop diuretics is a useful strategy to minimize cerebral edema and provide an optimal surgical field. However, hypotension and rebound effects may be associated with their use. Rapid administration of hypertonic solutions can cause profound but transient hypotension due to peripheral vasodilation.[105] Glucose-containing solutions usually are unnecessary during neurosurgical procedures because blood glucose concentrations are well-maintained even in small children in the absence of intravenous glucose administration during typical (balanced) neurosurgical anesthetics. However, glucose may be indicated when hypoglycemia is a concern, such as in diabetic children, children receiving hyperalimentation, preterm and full-term neonates, and malnourished or debilitated children. In these situations, glucose solutions should be administered at or slightly below maintenance rates (by constant infusion pump) and serum glucose concentrations should be monitored periodically throughout surgery. The potential association of larger cerebral infarct size with hyperglycemia (i.e., blood glucose values in excess of 250 mg/dL) during ischemia is of particular concern.[106]

Meticulous management of fluids and blood products to minimize cerebral edema is a cornerstone of pediatric neuroanesthesia. Although cerebral hemorrhage is fortunately a rare event, when it does occur, it can be sudden and catastrophic. All children should have secure, large-bore intravenous access, and blood products should be available along with the means for warming the blood.

## TEMPERATURE CONTROL

Because the head accounts for a large proportion of an infant's body surface area, infants are particularly susceptible to heat loss during neurosurgical procedures. Attention should be focused on maintaining normal temperature from the time the child is brought into the operating room, although moderate hypothermia during neurosurgery may be useful to decrease the $CMRO_2$. Ambient room temperature should be increased during positioning, preparation, and draping. Infrared warming lights may be helpful for infants, and warming blankets may be useful for infants weighing less than 10 kg. Forced-air warming remains the most effective means of maintaining body temperature.[107]

## VENOUS AIR EMBOLI

Venous air embolism (VAE) is a potential danger during intracranial procedures. The larger the pressure gradient between the operative site and the heart, the greater the potential for clinically significant entrainment of air into the central circulation.[108] For example, when the operative site is far above the heart (e.g., in a seated craniotomy) or when the CVP is low (e.g., acute blood loss during craniofacial procedures), it creates an environment for a VAE. Intracranial procedures are a particular concern because intracranial venous sinuses have dural attachments that impede their ability to collapse. Other potential air entry sites during neurosurgical procedures include bone, bridging veins, and spinal epidural veins. The sequence of events that should be followed when a VAE occurs is to identify the problem, stop further air entrainment, and support the circulation. Understanding the cause, prevention, and treatment of VAE is crucial because the consequences can be life-threatening.

When air enters the central circulation, it can accumulate in the right atrium or the right ventricular outflow tract. Cardiac output may be reduced, depending on the size of the air lock. If enough air is entrained into the circulation, the preload to the right ventricle decreases, or the right-sided heart afterload increases acutely, which can lead to cor pulmonale, acutely decreasing left ventricular preload and ultimately causing cardiovascular collapse. One study in dogs demonstrated that as little as 1 mL/kg of air could increase pulmonary artery pressure 200% to 300%.[109] Intracardiac shunts such as a patent foramen ovale, atrial or ventricular septal defects, and other congenital cardiac defects may allow air to access the systemic circulation, including the coronaries and brain. The risk of VAE is even greater in infants and children because potential intracardiac shunts exist in many otherwise healthy infants and children. They may become clinically important if pulmonary hypertension develops acutely after a large air embolism. Some clinicians recommend preoperative echocardiographic screening for patent foramen ovale in any child being considered for a sitting craniotomy; others regard a patent foramen ovale to be an absolute contraindication to the sitting position.[110,111]

Although the incidence of VAE is greatest in the sitting position, the lateral, supine, and prone positions are not free of risk. VAE have also been observed during craniotomy for craniosynostosis, even when the operating room table is flat and rarely when the surgery involved endoscopic strip craniectomy, although most occur without clinical sequelae.[112,113] The incidence of VAE in children undergoing suboccipital craniotomy in the sitting position is not significantly different from that in adults, but children appear to have a greater incidence of hypotension and a smaller likelihood of successful aspiration of central (intravascular) air.[114]

Several techniques may be used to detect VAE. Depending on the study design, the usual order of sensitivity of detecting air in the heart is transvenous intracardiac echocardiography (0.15 mL/kg) > transesophageal echocardiography (0.19 mL/kg) = precordial Doppler probe (0.24 mL/kg) > pulmonary artery pressure (0.61 mL/kg) = end-tidal $CO_2$ tension (0.63 mL/kg) = arterial $O_2$ tension > mean arterial pressure (1.16 mL/kg) = arterial $CO_2$ tension.[115,116] Transvenous intracardiac echocardiography is commonly used to guide catheters in cardiac ablation procedures or insertion of foramen ovale occlusion devices, but it is invasive and infrequently used in pediatric anesthesia. A precordial Doppler probe has been traditionally placed over the fourth or fifth intercostal space at the right sternal border to best monitor right heart sounds, although evidence suggests that placing the Doppler probe at the left parasternal border may be at least as sensitive (Fig. 24-6).[117,118] Appropriate Doppler positioning can be confirmed by listening for the characteristic change in sounds after rapid administration of a few milliliters of saline into a venous catheter. The precordial Doppler probe is particularly valuable because it is inexpensive, easy to use, benign, and noninvasive. Although transthoracic or transesophageal echocardiography is the most specific method for detecting small air emboli, it is not easily used intraoperatively, especially in children during neurosurgical procedures.[110,119,120]

Monitoring end-tidal gas tensions is important during neurosurgical procedures. When VAE occurs, there is a ventilation/perfusion mismatch caused by the air blocking passage of blood through the pulmonary circulation, increasing dead space ventilation with a sudden decrease in end-tidal $CO_2$ partial pressure and activation of complement resulting in pulmonary interstitial edema, neutrophil infiltration, and lung injury (Fig. 24-7).[115] The end-tidal $CO_2$ partial pressure remains a useful and cost-effective

## AIR EMBOLISM
### Relative sensitivity

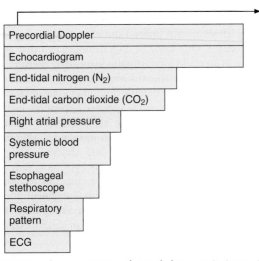

- Precordial Doppler
- Echocardiogram
- End-tidal nitrogen ($N_2$)
- End-tidal carbon dioxide ($CO_2$)
- Right atrial pressure
- Systemic blood pressure
- Esophageal stethoscope
- Respiratory pattern
- ECG

**FIGURE 24-6** Relative sensitivities of air embolism–monitoring modalities. *ECG*, Electrocardiogram.

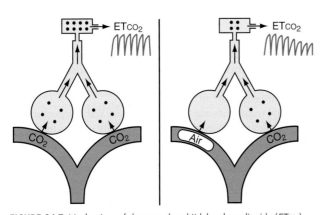

**FIGURE 24-7** Mechanism of decreased end-tidal carbon dioxide (*ETco₂*) after an air embolus. (Courtesy J. Drummond, MD.)

strategy in diagnosing massive VAE, although its sensitivity has been surpassed by other approaches (see Fig. 24-6). An increase in end-tidal nitrogen partial pressure during continuous monitoring is a specific sign of air emboli. Although slightly more sensitive than a decrease in end-tidal $CO_2$, an increase in end-tidal nitrogen is not detected by most infrared analyzers in practice and is usually of such small magnitude that it may be difficult to detect.

Less sensitive or more invasive methods to detect VAE include ECG changes, changes in heart rate, decreases in systemic blood pressure, and increases in right atrial and pulmonary arterial pressures. Right atrial and pulmonary artery pressures increase quickly after the emboli (within 30 seconds). The magnitude of these increases correlates with the size of emboli, although these findings should not be relied on alone for monitoring and diagnosis.

On suspicion or diagnosis of VAE, immediate measures must be taken by the surgeons and anesthesiologists to prevent continued entrainment of air and consequent hemodynamic deterioration. The surgeon should immediately flood the field with saline and apply bone wax to exposed bone edges. The anesthesiologist should discontinue nitrous oxide and place the child in the Trendelenburg position, which has the effect of increasing cerebral venous pressure, stopping entrainment of air, augmenting the child's peripheral venous return, and increasing systemic blood pressure. Occlusion of the internal jugular veins in an attempt to increase cerebral venous pressure should be done with great care because occlusion of the carotid arteries can lead to cerebral ischemia. The application of positive end-expiratory pressure increases CVP but also decreases cardiac filling pressure, cardiac output, and blood pressure; extreme increases in positive end-expiratory pressure are usually unwarranted. Chest compressions, vasopressors, and aggressive fluid resuscitation may be required.

Aspiration of air from a central venous catheter is rarely successful unless massive amounts have been entrained. When central venous catheters are necessary, such as for a child in the sitting position or when massive blood loss is anticipated, an attempt should be made to place the tip at the junction of the superior vena cava and right atrium to provide the optimal location for aspiration of entrained air. More importantly, a central venous catheter is useful to estimate maintenance of circulating blood volume and to rapidly administer fluids and resuscitative medications when necessary. The position of a central venous catheter near the heart should be confirmed by radiograph, by transducing CVPs, or with the aid of ECG monitoring (i.e., biphasic P waves develop in a lead at the tip of the catheter). The threshold for aspirating air may be increased by properly positioning a multiple-orifice central venous catheter using a transvenous intracardiac echocardiography probe.[115] Because erosion of the catheter tip through the heart causing fatal pericardial tamponade has occurred after surgery in small children, soft silicone catheters are recommended.[121,122]

## EMERGENCE
Protecting the brain is a major concern during neurosurgical procedures (Table 24-2). Emergence and extubation should be smooth and controlled to prevent fluctuations in ICP and in venous and arterial pressures.[123] To avoid vomiting during emergence, a multimodal antiemetic approach is advised.[124] Despite this approach, the incidence of PONV is high, which may be attributed to several factors: blood in the CSF is a potent emetic, opioids are often used to treat postoperative pain, and headache itself can precipitate emesis.

Intravenous lidocaine (1.0 to 1.5 mg/kg) given before extubation may help to suppress coughing and straining on the tracheal tube, although fentanyl appears to be equally effective and may be less sedating. Labetalol, an α- and β-adrenergic blocking agent, can be administered incrementally for the control of blood pressure during the acute period of emergence, but this is rarely necessary in children who have received adequate doses of opioids during surgery. For adolescents, intravenous labetalol (0.1 to 0.4 mg/kg given every 5 to 10 minutes until desired effect is achieved) may be necessary, but this usually does not have to be repeated in the postoperative period. Esmolol is used by some practitioners and has been as effective as labetalol in controlling hypertension after intracranial surgery in adults.[125] However, esmolol should be used with caution in infants and smaller children because their cardiac output depends on heart rate. There are no studies evaluating the use of esmolol in children for such an application. Dexmedetomidine may be useful in facilitating a smooth emergence while still allowing evaluation of the child's neurologic status.

**TABLE 24-2** Maneuvers of Neuroprotection

| Goals | Avoid cerebral edema |
| --- | --- |
| | Avoid cerebral hypoxia |
| | Avoid cerebral hypoperfusion |
| | Avoid cerebral hypermetabolism |
| | Avoid neuronal membrane damage |
| **Maneuvers** | |
| Head of bed at 30 degrees in midline | Increases cerebral venous drainage while maintaining CPP |
| Corticosteroids | May improve outcome in spinal cord injury |
| | Decrease vasogenic cerebral edema in children with tumors |
| | Stabilize neuronal membranes |
| | Free-radical scavengers |
| Controlled ventilation | Maintain PaCO$_2$ at normal to slightly low levels: prevents both cerebral vasodilation and increased ICP |
| Muscle paralysis | Avoids coughing, straining, child movement, and other causes of increased ICP |
| Ventricular drainage | Decreases ICP |
| Antihypertensives | Prevent further cerebral edema, ischemia, and cerebral hemorrhage. Severe hypotension can significantly decrease CPP. |
| Anticonvulsants | Prevent seizure activity and increased ICP |
| Hypothermia | Decreases CMRO$_2$ and CMRglu consumption |
| Barbiturate coma | Membrane-stabilizing effect |
| | Decreases CBF and CMRO$_2$ |

*CBF,* Cerebral blood flow; *CMRglu,* cerebral metabolic rate for glucose; *CMRO$_2$,* cerebral metabolic rate for oxygen; *CPP,* cerebral perfusion pressure; *ICP,* intracranial pressure; *PaCO$_2$,* partial pressure of arterial carbon dioxide.

Neuromuscular blockade should be pharmacologically reversed because even the slightest residual weakness is poorly tolerated and may interfere with the neurologic examination. Adequate spontaneous ventilation and oxygenation and an awake mental status are required before extubation. If postoperative intracranial hypertension is possible or if the child does not meet respiratory or neurologic criteria for extubation, the tracheal tube should be left in place, sedation should be administered, and the child should be transported to an intensive care unit.

The child should be as fully alert as possible immediately after the operation to permit repeated neurologic examinations to assess recovery and to detect a deteriorating status. In unconscious children, ICP can be monitored invasively. CT scans can help to evaluate the cause of an increased ICP or deteriorating mental status.

Pain is usually not severe after a craniotomy, but it can be treated with incremental doses of opioids. Ketorolac is best avoided in the early postoperative period because of its effects on platelet function. Acetaminophen may be administered orally, rectally, or intravenously for mild pain.[126]

Diabetes insipidus or inappropriate secretion of antidiuretic hormone may complicate postoperative fluid and electrolyte management, particularly when surgery is in the region of the hypothalamus and pituitary gland. Careful observation of fluid status and repeated laboratory evaluation of blood and urine osmolality and sodium levels are important in this situation. When diabetes insipidus occurs, it can be managed

with a continuous infusion of dilute aqueous vasopressin (1 to 10 mU/kg/hr).[127] In such circumstances, large volumes of hypotonic intravenous solutions must be avoided because they may rapidly decrease the serum sodium level and osmolality. If normal saline is administered in strictly limited volumes, aqueous vasopressin can control the electrolyte and fluid balances of children with diabetes insipidus until they resume oral fluids. At that time, intranasal or oral desmopressin (DDAVP) can be substituted. When diabetes insipidus develops after surgery in the pituitary region (e.g., during resection of a craniopharyngioma), it may only be transient, and it is important to repeatedly assess the need for vasopressin.

Portable EEGs and evoked auditory, somatosensory, and less commonly, visual potentials may be helpful in assessing children who are deeply sedated or paralyzed. Observation in an intensive care unit capable of managing children is essential for the prevention or early detection and treatment of postoperative complications. CT and MRI are often performed 1 or 2 days after a craniotomy or earlier if neurologic deterioration develops.

## Special Situations

### TRAUMA

#### Head Injury

Among children, trauma is the primary cause of death, and head injuries produce most of this mortality and cause much of the morbidity in survivors.[128-130] Motor vehicle accidents continue to be the most frequent preventable cause of head injury, although domestic violence and sports-related head injury are also common in children (see Fig. 38-1). Assaults and suicide attempts have become increasingly common among adolescents.

Children with head trauma may have minimal neurologic abnormalities at the time of initial evaluation. However, increased ICP and neurologic deficits may progressively develop. They develop slowly because brain injuries occur in two stages. The primary insult that occurs at the time of impact results from the biomechanical forces that disrupt the cranium, neural tissue, and vasculature. The secondary insult is the parenchymal damage caused by the pathologic sequelae of the primary insult. These changes can result from hypotension, hypoxia, cerebral edema, or intracranial hypertension. Whereas prevention of primary injuries must be addressed in a sociopolitical forum such as through seatbelt laws, sports injury prevention, and domestic violence legislation, anesthesiologists are instrumental in preventing or minimizing secondary insults (see Chapter 38).

There are significant differences between children and adults in the pattern of CNS injuries. Although intracranial hematomas (i.e., epidural, subdural, or intraparenchymal) are common in adults, they are less common in children. In contrast, diffuse cerebral edema after blunt head trauma occurs more often in children than in adults.[131]

#### Scalp Injuries

One of the most common head injuries in children is the scalp laceration. Most can be managed in the emergency department, but more serious injuries may require the operating room to provide immobility and comfort. Children can lose a significant amount of blood from a scalp injury because a larger fraction of the cardiac output perfuses the head compared with adults. Infants younger than 1 year of age may become hemodynamically unstable from blood loss from a subgaleal hematoma alone, as in a closed scalp injury, and hypovolemia should always be considered and treated before induction of anesthesia. Coexisting intracranial or other injuries must be considered, and a preoperative CT scan may be warranted.

## Skull Fractures

Skull fractures are a common manifestation of head trauma in children. Most are linear and do not require surgical treatment. These fractures are of concern primarily because the force required to produce them may damage the underlying brain and vasculature. A linear fracture over a major blood vessel (e.g., middle meningeal artery) or a large dural sinus may result in intracranial hemorrhage. Most children have an uneventful course after sustaining a simple skull fracture. A few develop a leptomeningeal cyst or growing fracture that eventually requires surgical treatment. Multiple skull fractures in the absence of documented major trauma should always raise the suspicion of child abuse (See Fig. 38-2), which is also referred to as *nonaccidental trauma.*

Depressed skull fractures often require surgical repair. They may occur even in the absence of a scalp laceration. However, displacement of the inner table of the skull requires greater force than that needed to produce a simple linear fracture and has greater potential to damage underlying tissues. Approximately one third of all depressed fractures are uncomplicated, another third are associated with dural lacerations, and the remaining third are associated with cortical lacerations. The extent of cortical injury is the primary determinant of morbidity and mortality. Surgical débridement and elevation of the depressed bone are usually performed as soon as possible after the injury (Fig. 24-8, *A*).

Basilar skull fractures are less common in children. Despite the force needed to produce these fractures, they typically have an excellent prognosis and rarely require surgical intervention. However, the possibility of a basilar skull fracture should be considered when caring for children with altered mental status, seizures, or associated trauma requiring surgery. Findings include periorbital ecchymoses ("raccoon eyes"), retroauricular ecchymosis (i.e., the Battle sign) (see Fig. 38-2, *B*), hemotympanum, clear rhinorrhea, or otorrhea. Unless absolutely necessary (e.g., mandibular wiring), nasotracheal intubation or passage of a nasogastric tube is best avoided because these tubes have inadvertently traversed these skull fractures and entered the cranium.[132-134] Complications of basilar skull fracture include meningitis from a CSF leak, cranial nerve damage, and anosmia.

## Epidural Hematoma

Epidural hematomas most commonly develop in the temporoparietal region due to arterial bleeding from a severed middle meningeal artery. They can also develop in the posterior fossa as a result of bleeding from a venous sinus. Epidural hematomas are not necessarily associated with an overlying skull fracture. The classic natural history in adults is a "lucid interval" between the initial loss of consciousness and subsequent neurologic deterioration. Infants and children may not demonstrate an altered mental status in the early stages after the injury. However, as the hematoma expands, it can lead to a loss of consciousness, hemiparesis, and pupillary dilatation. This deterioration can be quite rapid once a mass effect occurs. Treatment is prompt surgical evacuation because delays are associated with increased morbidity. Medical therapy directed at decreasing ICP should be instituted as soon as a diagnosis is suspected but should not delay surgical repair (see Fig. 24-8, *B*). Children recover well after these

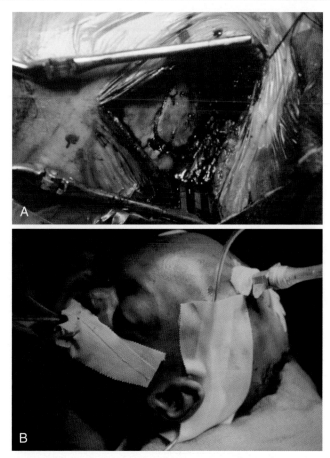

**FIGURE 24-8 A,** This depressed skull fracture required surgical intervention. **B,** Children with severe head trauma (in this case, a shaken baby) may present with marked increases in intracranial pressure.

hemorrhages, although morbidity is usually a reflection of underlying brain injury or lengthy delay in treatment.

## Subdural Hematoma

Subdural hematomas are usually associated with cortical damage resulting from direct parenchymal contusion or laceration of venous blood vessels. Acute subdural hematomas are almost always traumatic and are frequently a result of abuse, such as shaking of small children, particularly those younger than 1 year of age. Shaken baby syndrome occurs when an infant is shaken so vigorously that significant neuronal disruption occurs and tears in the cortical bridging veins cause subdural hematomas.[135-137] These infants suffer significant brain damage complicated by episodes of apnea and further hypoxic insult.

Subdural hematomas occasionally result from birth trauma within the first hours of life. Vitamin K deficiency, congenital coagulopathies, and disseminated intravascular coagulation are considerations in these situations. Great force is required to produce a subdural hematoma, whether by direct impact, laceration of blood vessels, or traumatic separation of the brain and overlying dura. Cerebral edema, uncontrolled intracranial hypertension, and persistent neurologic deficits often characterize the postoperative course. Chronic subdural hematomas or effusions may also develop in infancy, although these children do not usually present with acute symptoms. Children are often diagnosed because they are irritable and vomiting or have an increased head circumference. Chronic subdural hematomas can increase in size, causing slow but significant increases in ICP. Although a craniotomy is sometimes performed, most children undergo some form of hematoma drainage or shunting procedure as definitive treatment.

## Intracerebral Hematoma

Intracerebral hematomas are fortunately rare but have a poor prognosis. Deep parenchymal hematomas are most often extensions of cortical contusions in a child with severe neurologic injury. Rarely, a localized hematoma may be appropriate for surgical evacuation to decompress the brain. However, intraparenchymal hematomas are not evacuated for fear of damaging viable brain tissue. Anticonvulsants are usually administered prophylactically, and it is safest in the initial period after injury to avoid any medications that interfere with coagulation (e.g., ketorolac).

## Spinal Injury

Although isolated cervical spine injuries are uncommon in children, those with severe head trauma should always be managed as if they also have a cervical spine injury.[138,139] Different causes of spinal injuries are associated with specific age groups. Motor vehicle accidents produce the largest number of injuries in older children and adolescents, whereas birth injuries and falls are the most common cause in infants and young children.[140] Spinal cord injury itself may be caused by a variety of forces, including hyperflexion, hyperextension, rotation, vertical compression, flexion rotation, and shearing. The injury may involve bony, ligamentous, cartilaginous, vascular, or neural components of the spine or adjacent structures. The biomechanics and functional anatomy of the pediatric spine depend on the age of the child. Older children and teenagers are more likely to sustain injuries in the thoracolumbar region of the spine, whereas infants and younger children are more likely to suffer injuries in the high cervical region, particularly in the atlantoaxial region. The cervical spine is at greater risk in the infant and younger child because of the relatively weak and flexible neck muscles that support a proportionally large and heavy head, with the atlantooccipital area acting as a pivot point. Atlantooccipital dislocations are major neurologic injuries, leaving children neurologically devastated but not necessarily dead.

As with brain injury, spinal cord injury occurs in two phases. The primary insult results from biomechanical forces and bony fragments directly impacting the spinal cord. The secondary insult results from the pathologic sequelae of the primary insult: edema and ischemia due to cortical compression, hypotension, or hypoxia. Inappropriate manipulation of a child with an unstable fracture can exacerbate primary and secondary injuries. Anesthesiologists who provide care for a child with a potential cervical spine injury should be aware that spinal cord injuries in children commonly occur without actual evidence of spinal bone fractures on plain cervical radiographs. These injuries are known as spinal cord injuries without radiologic abnormality (SCIWORA).[141] Injuries to the cervical spine in particular are often difficult to recognize but may be identified by odontoid displacement or prevertebral swelling on radiographs. As a result, CT is frequently indicated when a spinal injury is initially suspected in a child with trauma. After a child with a potential spinal injury is determined to be medically stable, these studies should be obtained as soon as possible. The child's airway and cardiorespiratory function must be continuously and closely monitored until a spinal cord injury can be ruled out. Sometimes, as with brain injury,

there can be a delay in the onset of neurologic deficits with SCIWORA injuries.[142]

Respiratory failure is the most common cause of death after isolated cervical spine injury. The level of injury determines the degree of impairment. The phrenic nerve originates primarily from C4 but receives contributions of fibers from C3 and C5. Lesions at C5 leave partial diaphragmatic innervation but impair abdominal and intercostal accessory muscles. Lesions between C6 and T7 preserve diaphragmatic innervation but diminish accessory muscle function.

Children with a cervical spine injury may rapidly develop respiratory failure due to decreased vital capacity, increased dead space, retention of secretions, and respiratory muscle fatigue. Resultant hypercarbia and hypoxia aggravate the secondary injury to the brain and spinal cord. Respiratory status may be further impaired by associated trauma to the chest, causing pulmonary contusion or pneumothorax, or by aspiration of gastric contents.

Prompt airway management is essential to avoid hypoxia, ensure adequate respiratory mechanics, preserve neural function, and prevent extension of spinal injury (see Figs. 38-5 through 38-7). The head and neck must be immediately immobilized; restraint of the extremities may also be required. Various tracheal tubes and laryngoscope blades should be available, as well as equipment and personnel for an emergency tracheostomy. Insertion of a laryngeal mask airway may be lifesaving until a more secure airway can be achieved with fiberoptic or other means.[143-148] Small fiberoptic bronchoscopes (2.2-mm diameter) can fit through infant-sized tracheal tubes. Retrograde intubation using a guidewire introduced through the cricothyroid membrane may be useful in older children or adolescents (see Chapter 12). However, an unstable infant or child whose airway cannot be secured by conventional means is probably best managed by an emergency tracheostomy. As a temporizing measure, a cricothyroidotomy can be performed (see Figs. 12-25 through 12-27).[149] This permits oxygenation (although inadequate ventilation) until personnel and equipment for tracheostomy are assembled. An emergent surgical airway can be extremely difficult to perform on a small child or infant, even by experienced and skilled hands.

Hemodynamic instability may be a problem due to hypovolemia from other injuries or severe head trauma. Other sites of bleeding such as long bone fractures and abdominal trauma should be ruled out. Children with spinal shock exhibit loss of vasomotor tone or loss of normal neurocardiac function with associated bradycardia and decreased myocardial contractility; intravenous fluids and vasopressors may be necessary.

Although there are few data for adults and children, corticosteroids are often administered with spinal injuries as soon as possible after the initial trauma in the hope of reducing the neurologic injury. The most commonly used drug is methylprednisolone; 30 mg/kg is administered over the first 15 minutes, followed by an infusion of 5.4 mg/kg/hr for the next 23 hours.[150,151] Methylprednisolone is thought to be effective through multiple mechanisms, including improved spinal blood flow, inhibition of the arachidonic acid cascade, and modulation of the local immune response.[152] Some evidence suggests that $GM_1$ ganglioside, with or without methylprednisolone, may be advantageous in decreasing demyelination and promoting neurologic recovery if administered soon after a spinal injury.[153-159]

If the spinal cord injury is more than 24 hours old, succinylcholine should be avoided because it can result in massive hyperkalemia.[160] Physiologic changes may result from autonomic hyperreflexia, which frequently develops after cervical or high thoracic spinal lesions. Autonomic hyperreflexia can produce severe and life-threatening vasomotor instability with hypertension and arrhythmias.[161,162]

## CRANIOTOMY
### Tumors

Brain tumors are the most common solid tumors in children, exceeded only by the leukemias as the most common pediatric malignancy.[163] Between 1500 and 2000 new brain tumors are diagnosed annually in children in the United States. Unlike those in adults, most brain tumors in children are infratentorial in the posterior fossa. They include medulloblastomas, cerebellar astrocytomas, brainstem gliomas, and ependymomas of the fourth ventricle. Because posterior fossa tumors usually obstruct CSF flow, increased ICP occurs early. Presenting signs and symptoms include early morning vomiting and irritability or lethargy. Cranial nerve palsies and ataxia are also common findings, with respiratory and cardiac irregularities usually occurring late. Sedation or general anesthesia may be required for radiologic evaluation or radiation therapy.

Surgical resection of a posterior fossa tumor presents a number of anesthetic challenges. Children are usually positioned prone, although the lateral or sitting positions are used by some neurosurgeons. In any case, the head is flexed, and the position and patency of the tracheal tube must be meticulously ensured. In the event that the tracheal tube does become dislodged when the child is in a head holder and prone, successful emergent airway management has been described using a laryngeal mask airway.[164]

Arrhythmias and acute blood pressure changes may occur during surgical exploration, especially when the brainstem is manipulated. The electrocardiogram and arterial waveform should be closely monitored. Altered respiratory control may be masked by neuromuscular blocking drugs (NMBDs) and mechanical ventilation. Even when ICP is only marginally increased, intracranial compliance is presumed to have decreased. This warrants precautions against further increases in ICP. If ICP is markedly increased or acutely worsens, a ventricular catheter may be inserted before the tumor is resected. VAE is a potentially serious complication that is not eliminated by the prone or lateral position because head-up gradients of 10 to 20 degrees are frequently used to improve cerebral venous drainage. In infants and toddlers, large head size relative to body size accentuates this problem.

Supratentorial tumors in the midbrain include craniopharyngiomas, optic gliomas, pituitary adenomas, and hypothalamic tumors and account for approximately 15% of intracranial tumors. Hypothalamic tumors (i.e., hamartomas, gliomas, and teratomas) frequently manifest with precocious puberty in children who are large for their chronologic age. Craniopharyngiomas are the most common parasellar tumors in children and adolescents and may be associated with hypothalamic and pituitary dysfunction. Symptoms often include growth failure, visual impairment, and endocrine abnormalities.

Signs and symptoms of hypothyroidism should be sought and thyroid function measured. Corticosteroid replacement (i.e., dexamethasone or hydrocortisone) usually is administered because the integrity of the hypothalamic-pituitary-adrenal axis may be uncertain. Diabetes insipidus can occur preoperatively and is a common postoperative problem. The history usually reveals this condition preoperatively, especially if attention is focused on nocturnal drinking and enuresis. Evaluation of serum electrolytes and osmolality, urine specific gravity, and urine output is helpful because hypernatremia and hyperosmolality, along with dilute urine, are typical findings. If diabetes insipidus does not exist preoperatively, it usually does not develop until the postoperative period because there is an adequate reserve of antidiuretic hormone in the posterior pituitary gland capable of functioning for many hours, even when the hypothalamic-pituitary stalk is damaged intraoperatively.

Postoperative diabetes insipidus is marked by a sudden large increase in dilute urine output associated with an increasing serum sodium concentration and osmolality. Protocols have been developed to guide intraoperative and postoperative management of diabetes insipidus (see Chapter 8).[127] Return of antidiuretic hormone activity a few days postoperatively may cause a marked decrease in urinary output, water intoxication, seizures, and cerebral edema if it is not recognized and fluid administration is not adjusted appropriately.

Transsphenoidal surgery typically is performed only in adolescents and older children with pituitary adenomas. However, it should be treated like other midbrain tumors in terms of monitoring and vascular access. Children are usually intubated orally to give the surgeon optimal access to the nasopharynx, and preparations for an emergent craniotomy should be anticipated in case unexpected massive bleeding develops. Because nasal packs are inserted at the end of surgery, the child should be fully awake before tracheal extubation.

Gliomas of the optic pathways occur with increased frequency in children with neurofibromatosis. Presenting symptoms include visual changes and proptosis; increased ICP and hypothalamic dysfunction are usually late findings. Neurofibromas tend to be highly vascular, and the anesthesiologist should be prepared for significant blood loss.

Approximately 25% of intracranial tumors in children involve the cerebral hemispheres. They are primarily astrocytomas, oligodendrogliomas, ependymomas, and glioblastomas. Neurologic symptoms are more likely to include a seizure disorder or focal deficits. Succinylcholine should be avoided if motor weakness is present because it can cause sudden severe hyperkalemia. Nondepolarizing NMBDs and opioids may be metabolized more rapidly than usual in children who are receiving chronic anticonvulsants. Choroid plexus papillomas are rare but occur most often in children younger than 3 years of age. They usually arise from the choroid plexus of the lateral ventricle and produce early hydrocephalus as a result of increased production of CSF and obstruction of CSF flow. Hydrocephalus usually resolves with surgical resection. When lesions lie near the motor or sensory strip, a special type of somatosensory evoked potential monitoring called *phase reversal* may be used to delineate the locations.[165] If cortical stimulation is planned to help identify motor areas, NMBDs must be permitted to wear off and the anesthetic technique adjusted to achieve immobilization without paralysis.

Stereotactic biopsies or craniotomies present special concerns regarding airway accessibility. Newer head frames have adjustable anterior positions so that the airway is readily accessible (E-Fig. 24-1). They are especially useful for stereotactic neurosurgery. It is more comfortable and less distressing for the child to be anesthetized before the head frame is applied, even though this means the anesthesiologist must induce anesthesia in the radiology suite and then transport the child from the CT scanner to the operating room. The wrench that is used to apply and remove the head frame should be taped to the frame at all times so that it is always readily available if emergent removal of the head frame becomes necessary (e.g., during transport).

## Vascular Anomalies

### Arteriovenous Malformations

Arteriovenous malformations consist of large arterial feeding vessels, dilated communicating vessels, and large draining veins carrying arterialized blood. Large malformations, especially those involving the posterior cerebral artery and vein of Galen, may manifest as congestive heart failure (i.e., high-output heart failure, often with pulmonary hypertension) in the neonate. The prognosis for these types of arteriovenous malformations is quite poor. Saccular dilation of the vein of Galen may manifest later in infancy or childhood as hydrocephalus due to obstruction of the aqueduct of Sylvius. Malformations not large enough to produce congestive heart failure usually remain clinically silent unless they cause seizures or a stroke or until the acute rupture of a communicating vessel results in subarachnoid or intracerebral hemorrhage.[166] Intracranial hemorrhages are the most common presentation in this population, with an associated mortality rate of 25%.

Treatment usually consists of embolization or irradiation of deep malformations, surgical excision (usually of the more superficial ones), or a combination of these modalities. Management for elective embolic procedures involves general anesthesia. Moderate hyperventilation may enhance visualization of abnormal blood vessels that do not respond with vasoconstriction. The anesthesiologist should be knowledgeable about the types of embolic agents that can be used and their potential complications. Anticonvulsant therapy is routine. Neonates in cardiac failure may be receiving inotropic agents. Bleeding, especially from the femoral arterial puncture site (which cannot always be visualized), should always be a consideration. Fluid overload result from the large amount of contrast agents administered, especially in a young infant who may already be in high-output cardiac failure. The anesthesiologist should be prepared for the possibility of an emergency craniotomy if a vessel ruptures.

### Aneurysms

Intracranial aneurysms most often result from a congenital malformation in an arterial wall. Children with coarctation of the aorta or polycystic kidney disease have an increased incidence of these aneurysms. They usually remain asymptomatic during childhood; most ruptures that occur in childhood are fatal. Symptoms of subarachnoid or intracerebral hemorrhage frequently appear suddenly in a previously healthy young adult. When technically feasible, surgical ligation or clipping constitutes the treatment of choice.[167]

Anesthesia for surgical resection of vascular malformations and aneurysms in children presents unique challenges, especially if the diagnosis has been preceded by an intracranial hemorrhage. Blood products should be in the operating room and verified before the start of the procedure. An adequate depth of anesthesia should be ensured before any invasive maneuver to prevent precipitous hypertension. Adequate venous access to respond to sudden and massive blood loss is crucial but can wait until after induction of anesthesia. A blood-warming device, such as a rapid transfusion device, should be immediately available.

Controlled hypotension may be valuable in some situations for brief periods to reduce tension in the abnormal blood vessels and improve the safety of surgical manipulation.[168] It is not clear, however, whether the benefits of controlled hypotension are worth the risks, especially in small children (see Chapter 10). Controlled hypotension should not be used in children with increased ICP because of the risk of decreasing CPP, with resulting ischemia and further increased ICP. Although the absolute limits of acceptable hypotension are unknown, a mean blood pressure greater than 40 mm Hg for infants or 50 mm Hg for older children appears to be safe; teenagers should have a target mean arterial pressure no less than 55 mm Hg. At the conclusion of the procedure, the blood pressure is returned to normal, but before closing the dura, the operative site should be inspected for bleeding.

Hemodynamic stability is important during emergence to avoid bucking, coughing, straining, and hypertension during extubation. Excessive hypertension can result in postoperative bleeding, although in most cases of aneurysm clipping, a slightly increased blood pressure may be desirable postoperatively to minimize the risk of vasospasm. After resection of an arteriovenous malformation, there can be serious postoperative complications due to cerebral edema with increased ICP or hemorrhage. This *normal perfusion pressure breakthrough* is probably caused by hyperemia of the areas surrounding the previous arteriovenous malformation site, where vessels suffer from continued vasomotor paralysis and cannot vasoconstrict. Treatment is controversial but usually involves therapy for increased ICP (e.g., diuretics, moderate hyperventilation, head elevation) in addition to judicious use of moderate hypotension (while maintaining CPP) and moderate hypothermia. When surgery is completed, it is important that children are able to cooperate with a neurologic examination and that there is careful control of blood pressure in the intensive care unit.

### Moyamoya Disease

Moyamoya disease is an anomaly that results in progressive and life-threatening occlusion of intracranial vessels, primarily the internal carotid arteries near the circle of Willis.[169] An abnormal vascular network of collaterals develops at the base of the brain, and the appearance of these many, small vessels on angiography was originally described by the Japanese name *moyamoya*, which roughly translates as "puff of smoke." The congenital form of the disease can involve the systemic vasculature, including pulmonary, coronary, and renal vessels; affected renal arteries are the most commonly identified angiographic lesion. The acquired variety (i.e., moyamoya syndrome) may be associated with meningitis, neurofibromatosis, chronic inflammation, connective tissue diseases, certain hematologic disorders, Down syndrome, or prior intracranial radiation. Some children with neurologic symptoms from sickle cell disease may also have moyamoya.[170] Moyamoya disease appears to be more common among children of Japanese ancestry. Associated intracranial aneurysms are rare in children but may occur in more than 10% of affected adult patients. Abnormal electrocardiographic findings have been described with the syndrome in adults.

Moyamoya disease usually manifests as transient ischemic attacks progressing to strokes and fixed neurologic deficits in children. The attacks may be precipitated by hyperventilation.[171] The morbidity and mortality rates are high if the condition is left untreated. Medical management consists of antiplatelet therapy, such as aspirin, or calcium channel blockers. The most common surgical operation for correction in children is pial synangiosis, which involves suturing a scalp artery (usually the superficial temporal artery) directly onto the pial surface of the brain to enhance angiogenesis (Fig. 24-9).[172]

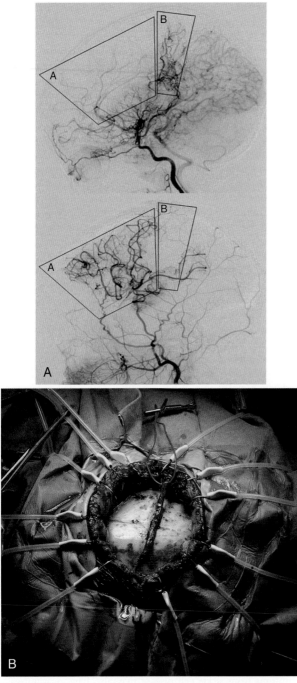

**FIGURE 24-9** Moyamoya disease. **A,** The top angiogram shows the pattern of arterial filling after injection of the internal carotid artery in a child with moyamoya disease before pial synangiosis. *Area A* shows poor filling from the middle cerebral artery as a result of the disease process. *Area B* shows the characteristic hazy collaterals, or moyamoya vessels. The bottom angiogram is from the same child after pial synangiosis. The angiogram was obtained after injection of the superficial temporal artery, and it shows good filling in the middle cerebral artery distribution in *area A.* *Area B* does not fill from the middle cerebral artery. **B,** Pial synangiosis. The superficial temporal artery is prepared to be sutured to the pia of the cerebral cortex. After the craniotomy is completed, this artery can be sewn directly onto the underlying pia mater. The result of this procedure is improvement of blood flow to ischemic areas of the cerebral cortex.

Careful and continuous monitoring of end-tidal $CO_2$ partial pressure is essential in anesthesia management.[173] Children with moyamoya disease have reduced hemispheric blood flow bilaterally, and hyperventilation may further reduce regional blood flow and cause significant EEG and neurologic changes.[174] Normocapnia must be maintained throughout all phases of the procedure, including induction of anesthesia. Adequate hydration and maintenance of baseline blood pressure are indispensable. Most of these children have an intravenous catheter inserted the night before surgery and are given 1.5 times the amount of maintenance fluids to avoid dehydration during the perioperative period. EEG monitoring during these procedures can detect and help to treat ischemia that appears to be a result of cerebral vasoconstriction in response to direct surgical manipulation of the brain.[175] Normothermia is maintained, particularly at the end of the procedure, to avoid postoperative shivering and an exaggerated stress response. As with most neurosurgical procedures, a smooth extubation without hypertension or crying is desirable. Although scant literature exists regarding intraoperative and postoperative complications during moyamoya surgery, it appears that most complications (e.g., strokes) occur postoperatively and are associated with dehydration and crying (i.e., hyperventilation) episodes.[176]

### Seizure Surgery

Epilepsy is one of the most common neurologic disorders of childhood. Despite the development of new drugs and regimens, the prevalence of pharmacologically intractable seizures remains high. Advances in neuroimaging and EEG monitoring provide epileptologists anatomic targets that mediate some medically intractable seizure disorders. Advances in pediatric neurosurgery have exploited these technologies and dramatically improved the outcomes for infants and children.[177]

Children presenting for surgical management of seizures take anticonvulsant medications, which can have serious side effects, including abnormalities of hematologic function such as abnormal coagulation, depression of red or white blood cell production, and decreased platelet counts. Other problems may arise from altered hepatic function. Specific anticonvulsant concentrations should be determined preoperatively to detect subtherapeutic or toxic concentrations. Many anticonvulsants enhance metabolism of nondepolarizing NMBDs and opioids, increasing (up to 50%) the amount of these drugs needed during a surgical procedure. The preoperative evaluation should detect underlying conditions that are causing the seizures and the disabilities that can result from progressive neurologic dysfunction.

A major concern during resection of seizure foci is avoiding harming brain tissue that controls vital functions, such as motion, sensation, speech, and memory (so-called eloquent cortex), especially if a seizure focus is adjacent to cortical areas controlling these functions. Cooperative adolescents and adults can assist in determination of the limits of safe cortical resection if they can be continually assessed during the surgical procedure. The technique of awake craniotomy is often performed in carefully selected adolescents. An awake craniotomy encompasses a wide variety of techniques whose common goal is to allow intraoperative assessment and feedback to determine if the eloquent cortex is at risk during resection.

Children are selected for this procedure on an individual basis. Most children younger than 12 years old and many teenagers cannot tolerate an awake craniotomy. However, selected individuals may do well. The anesthesiologist should have detailed conversations with the child and parents to determine appropriateness before initiating such a procedure.

Some practitioners perform the entire procedure, including line placement, infiltration of local anesthetic, skull and dural opening, and resection, with the child completely awake or with minimal sedation. This particular approach requires an extremely motivated child. A variation on this technique uses short-acting sedatives and analgesics, such as propofol and fentanyl, titrated to induce unconsciousness but maintain spontaneous ventilation for instillation of local anesthetics, insertion of monitoring catheters, placement of head pins, and skull opening.[178] Subsequently, children can be allowed to awaken during surgical resection. They can then have sedatives and opioids reinstituted for the craniotomy closure.

Alternatively, some anesthesiologists use the asleep-awake-asleep technique. It consists of inducing general anesthesia and maintaining airway control with a supraglottic device (i.e., laryngeal mask airway). General anesthesia is maintained for line placement, placement of head pins, and skull and dural opening. The child is then awakened, the supraglottic airway is removed, and the surgeons proceed with resection. At the conclusion of the resection, general anesthesia is again induced and the supraglottic airway reinserted for closure of the dura, skull, and skin. There are several disadvantages to the asleep-awake-asleep approach. One of the major concerns when employing this approach is airway management during emergence and induction while the child is in head pins. If the child coughs or bucks while immobilized, cervical spine injuries or scalp lacerations can occur. Brain swelling is also a concern in a child who is breathing spontaneously under general anesthesia with an inhalational anesthetic and possibly with nitrous oxide.

Regardless of the technique chosen, the anesthesiologist must have an in-depth discussion with the child or adolescent about intraoperative needs and expectations. The preoperative period is the time to decide whether the child is a candidate for an awake craniotomy. There are no randomized, controlled trials comparing the safety or effectiveness of the techniques described.

Younger children (up to 12 years of age) or uncooperative children of any age do not tolerate this approach and require general anesthesia throughout. In these circumstances, intraoperative electrophysiologic studies, such as somatosensory evoked potentials, EEG, and motor stimulation, may be used to help localize and determine the function of the site of planned resection. If EEG studies are to be performed, the anesthetic technique should be adjusted to maximize EEG signals. If direct cortical motor stimulation is planned, NMBDs must be permitted to wear off. Occasionally, a seizure focus is difficult to identify intraoperatively. In these situations, hyperventilation or methohexital (in small doses, 0.25 to 0.5 mg/kg) may be helpful in lowering the seizure threshold and producing EEG seizure activity.[179,180]

In some children, the site of origin of generalized seizures is difficult to determine. When this occurs, evaluation with intracranial EEG monitoring ("grids and strips") may be accomplished with direct electrocorticography (E-Fig. 24-2). The leads are placed on the surface of the cortex after a craniotomy performed under general anesthesia. Intraoperative EEG monitoring is limited during these procedures to ensuring that all leads are functional; monitoring for seizures takes place over the next several days to identify a focus that is amenable to resection. These children need to be observed carefully in the postoperative period because complications can develop from having

intracranial electrodes in place. Because air frequently persists in the skull for up to 3 weeks after a craniotomy,[86] these children should not have nitrous oxide administered for a subsequent procedure (e.g., to resect a seizure focus, to remove the electrocorticography leads) until their dura has been opened to prevent the development of tension pneumocephalus.

When a focal resection is not possible, a lobectomy or corpus callosotomy may be attempted. However, children undergoing the latter procedure are often somnolent for the first few postoperative days, especially if a complete callosotomy is performed. This also occurs in children who have undergone insertion of multiple subdural grids and strips. Occasionally, small children undergo a hemispherectomy because their seizures are attributed to an abnormal hemisphere that is already severely dysfunctional, as when affected by hemiparesis. These can be challenging cases for the anesthesiologist because much blood can be lost (from one half to multiples of the estimated blood volume).[181] This procedure is usually performed when children are very young to permit the other hemisphere to take over the function of both sides. Large-bore intravenous access is necessary in these cases to facilitate rapid replacement of blood, crystalloid solutions, and medications. Arterial pressure monitoring is routine, and many practitioners also use CVP monitoring.

An advance in the treatment of epilepsy has been the development of the vagal nerve stimulator. Although its exact mechanism of action is not well understood, it appears to inhibit seizure activity at brainstem or cortical levels.[182,183] It is becoming a popular form of treatment because it has shown benefit with minimal side effects in many children who are disabled by intractable seizures. Large, randomized trials are being conducted to determine the overall efficacy of this treatment. There are few published series of vagal nerve stimulation in children, but it is estimated that there is a 60% to 70% improvement in seizure control, with the best results achieved in those with drop attacks.[184,185]

The vagal nerve stimulator is a programmable device that is similar to a cardiac pacemaker placed subcutaneously under the left anterior chest wall. Bipolar platinum stimulating electrode coils, which are implanted around the left vagus nerve, are connected to the generator by subcutaneously tunneled wires. The device automatically activates for up to 30 seconds every 5 minutes. Although stimulation of the vagal nerve in this manner may affect vocal cord function, sudden bradycardia or other side effects are uncommon.[186] When children with vagal nerve stimulators return for subsequent operations, it may be appropriate to deactivate the stimulator while the child is under general anesthesia to prevent repetitive vocal cord motion.

## HYDROCEPHALUS

Hydrocephalus is a condition involving a mismatch of CSF production and absorption, resulting in an increased intracranial CSF volume. It can be caused by a variety of pathologic processes, including arachnoid cysts (E-Fig. 24-3). Except for rare instances of excess CSF production, such as in choroid plexus papillomas, most cases of hydrocephalus result from some type of obstruction or an inability to absorb CSF appropriately. Commonly, this is a result of neonatal intraventricular or subarachnoid hemorrhage, congenital problems (e.g., aqueductal stenosis), trauma, infection, or tumors, especially those in the posterior fossa. Hydrocephalus can be classified as nonobstructive/communicating or obstructive/noncommunicating based on the ability of CSF to flow around the spinal cord in its usual manner.

Intracranial hypertension or decreased intracranial compliance typically accompanies untreated hydrocephalus in children. How much intracranial compliance exists and how acutely hydrocephalus develops are both factors in how severe the signs and symptoms of hydrocephalus become. If hydrocephalus develops slowly in the young infant, the skull will expand and the cerebral cortical mantle will stretch until massive craniomegaly (often with irreversible neurologic damage) occurs. However, if the cranial bones are fused or the cranium cannot expand fast enough, neurologic signs and symptoms rapidly become apparent. The child may become progressively more lethargic and develop vomiting, cranial nerve dysfunction (i.e., setting sun sign), bradycardia, brain herniation, and death.

Unless the cause of the hydrocephalus can be definitively treated, treatment usually involves surgical placement of an extracranial shunt. Most shunts transport CSF from the lateral ventricles to the peritoneal cavity (i.e., ventriculoperitoneal shunts). The distal end of the shunt occasionally must be placed in the right atrium or pleural cavity, usually because of problems with the ability of the peritoneal cavity to absorb CSF. Newer shunt systems with programmable valves are being tried to reduce the need for shunt revisions.[187]

The use of a percutaneous flexible neuroendoscope through a burrhole in the skull has provided an alternative to extracranial shunt placement.[188,189] During these procedures, a ventriculostomy may be made to bypass an obstruction (e.g., aqueductal stenosis) by forming a communicating hole from one area of CSF flow to another using a blunt probe inserted through the neuroendoscope (Video 24-1). Common locations for a ventriculostomy are through the septum pellucidum (allowing lateral ventricles to communicate) or through the floor of the third ventricle into the adjacent CSF cisterns. Complications such as damage to the basilar artery or its branches or neural injuries can be life-threatening when they occur, and the anesthesiologist should be prepared for an emergency craniotomy during these procedures. Hemodynamic instability may occur intraoperatively if excessive cold irrigating solutions or large volumes are infused through the endoscope.

The anesthetic plan for a child with hydrocephalus should be directed at controlling ICP and relieving the obstruction as soon as possible. Children with an increased ICP are at risk for vomiting and pulmonary aspiration. Rapid-sequence induction and tracheal intubation should be performed. Ketamine is avoided in these children because of its potential to cause sudden massive intracranial hypertension.[190] Despite this concern, there is some evidence that ketamine may ameliorate the increased intracranial pressure in children.[191,192] In infants, hydrocephalus often produces large, dilated scalp veins, and they can be used for induction of anesthesia if necessary. If intravenous access cannot be established, induction with sevoflurane and gentle cricoid pressure may be an alternative, although less desirable, method of induction.[193] This method results in venodilation and usually facilitates establishment of intravenous access. After an intravenous catheter is inserted, the child may be paralyzed, the lungs ventilated, the trachea intubated, and the inhalational agent decreased or discontinued. The possibility of VAE during placement of the distal end of a ventriculoatrial shunt should always be considered. Postoperatively, children should be observed carefully because an altered mental status and recent peritoneal incision place them at increased risk for pulmonary aspiration after feeding begins. Analgesia may be provided with a variety of easily performed blocks of the head (see Figs. 41-15 and 41-16).

Anesthesiologists should be familiar with a few special situations involving shunts. Children who develop a shunt infection usually have the entire shunt system removed and external ventricular drainage established. They return to the operating room for insertion of a new shunt several days after the infection has been treated with antibiotics. While an external drain is in place, the operator must be careful not to dislodge the ventricular tubing. The height of the drainage bag should not be significantly changed in relation to the child's head to avoid sudden alterations in ICP. For example, suddenly lowering an open drainage bag can siphon CSF rapidly from the head, resulting in collapse of the ventricles and rupture of cortical veins. When transporting children with CSF drainage or when moving them from a stretcher to an operating room table, it is best to close off the ventriculostomy tubing during these brief periods.

Anesthesiologists should be aware of the condition known as slit ventricle syndrome (Fig. 24-10). This situation develops in 5% to 10% of children with CSF shunts and is associated with overdrainage of CSF and small, slitlike, lateral ventricular spaces. Children with this condition do not have the usual amount of intracranial CSF to compensate for alterations in brain or intracranial blood volume. Special attention should be paid when CT scans identify this condition. It is probably safest to avoid the administration of excess or hypotonic intravenous solutions in these situations in the intraoperative and postoperative periods to minimize the potential for brain swelling. Some of these children cannot accommodate to situations that otherwise healthy children can easily tolerate. Episodes of postoperative cerebral herniation have been reported after uneventful surgical procedures.[45]

## CONGENITAL ANOMALIES

Congenital CNS anomalies typically occur as midline defects. This dysraphism may occur anywhere along the neural axis, involving the head (i.e., encephalocele) or spine (i.e., meningomyelocele) (Fig. 24-11, *A*). The defect may be relatively minor and affect only superficial bony and membranous structures, or it may include a large segment of malformed neural tissue.

### Encephalocele

Encephaloceles can occur anywhere from the occiput to the frontal area. They can even appear to be nasal polyps if they protrude through the cribriform plate. They are rarely filled with so much CSF that the defect can be almost as large as the head itself (see Fig. 24-11, *B*). Large defects may present challenges to tracheal intubation. Blood loss can be severe, especially if venous sinuses are involved. Adequate intravenous access should be ensured and blood products readily available. If hemodynamic instability is anticipated, an arterial catheter is indicated.

### Myelodysplasia

Defects in the spine are known as *spina bifida*. Meningoceles are lesions containing CSF without spinal tissue. When neural tissue is also present within the lesion, the defect is called a *meningomyelocele*. Open neural tissue is known as *rachischisis*. Hydrocephalus is usually present and is often associated with a type II Chiari malformation.

Most children with a meningomyelocele present for primary closure of the defect within the first 24 hours of life to minimize the risk of infection. Many are now scheduled electively before birth for repair because the defect is usually apparent on prenatal ultrasonography. Many neurosurgeons prefer to insert a

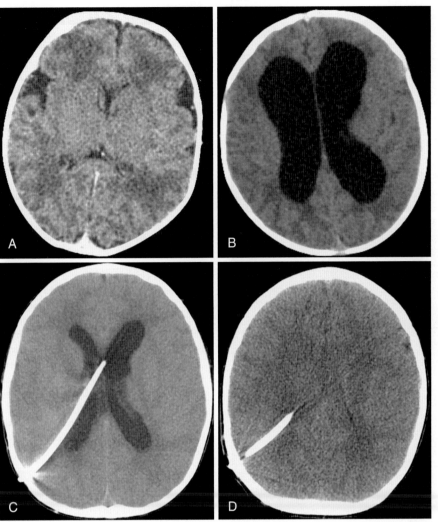

**FIGURE 24-10** Computed tonographic scans of children with normal-sized ventricles (**A**), untreated hydrocephalus (**B**), hydrocephalus treated with a ventricular shunt (**C**), and hydrocephalus treated with a ventricular shunt, resulting in slit ventricles (**D**). (Courtesy Ellen Grant, MD.)

ventriculoperitoneal shunt at the time of initial surgery. Alternatively, a shunt may be inserted a few days later or is occasionally deferred if there is no evidence of hydrocephalus at birth.

A major anesthesia consideration is positioning the neonate for induction at surgery. In most cases, tracheal intubation can be performed with the infant in the supine position and the uninvolved portion of the child's back supported with towels (or a donut ring) so there is no direct pressure on the meningomyelocele. For very large defects, it is occasionally necessary to place the infant in the left lateral decubitus position for induction and tracheal intubation. Succinylcholine is rarely needed for tracheal intubation, although it is not associated with hyperkalemia because the defect develops early in gestation and is not associated with muscle denervation.[194] Airway management, mask fit, and intubation may be difficult in infants with massive hydrocephalus or very large defects. In such cases, awake intubation after preoxygenation and administration of atropine occasionally may be the safest alternative. Blood loss may be considerable during repair of a larger defect when skin is undermined to cover the defect.

Children with myelodysplasia are at high risk for latex sensitivity and possibly anaphylaxis.[40] This likely results from repeated exposure to latex products encountered during frequent bladder catheterizations and multiple (usually more than five) surgical procedures, during which latex gloves have been in contact with large mucosal surfaces. These children should be managed in a latex-free environment from birth to minimize the chances for sensitization.[195] Latex allergy should be suspected if signs and symptoms of anaphylaxis develop during surgery. Suspected anaphylaxis should be treated with intravenous epinephrine in a dose of 1 to 10 μg/kg, as required. Many hospitals have replaced most or all of their latex-containing supplies with nonlatex alternatives; this has resulted in complete elimination of latex anaphylactic reactions during anesthesia in some institutions.[196] Children who develop latex allergy exhibit cross-reactivity with some antibiotics[197,198] and foods, especially tropical fruits such as avocados, kiwis, and bananas.

Postoperatively, respiratory status should be carefully assessed. Pulse oximetry is valuable during recovery from anesthesia because breathing difficulties may occur after a tight skin closure and the ventilatory responses to hypoxia and hypercarbia may be diminished or absent when a Chiari malformation coexists.[199] Intrauterine surgery has been advocated as a way of diminishing the degree of damage caused by myelodysplasia.[200-202]

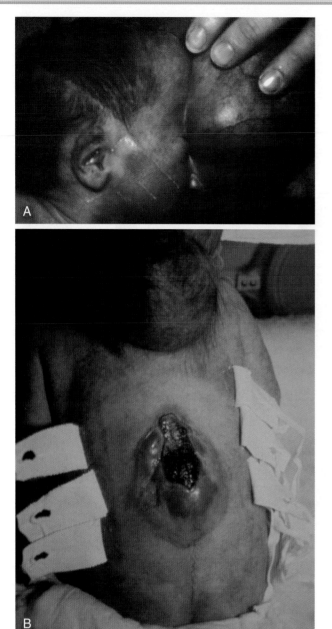

**FIGURE 24-11 A,** An infant with an anterior encephalocele. **B,** An infant with a posterior encephalocele and myelomeningocele defects. Notice the large exposed surface areas that make this child prone to dehydration. Difficulty may be encountered in positioning for induction of anesthesia, and significant loss of blood and cerebrospinal fluid during surgical correction should be anticipated.

### Chiari Malformations

There are several types of Chiari malformations (Table 24-3). The Arnold-Chiari malformation (type II) usually coexists in children with myelodysplasia. This defect consists of a bony abnormality in the posterior fossa and upper cervical spine with caudal displacement of the cerebellar vermis, fourth ventricle, and lower brainstem below the plane of the foramen magnum. Medullary cervical cord compression can occur (Figs. 24-12 and 24-13). Vocal cord paralysis with stridor and respiratory distress, apnea, abnormal swallowing and pulmonary aspiration, opisthotonos, and cranial nerve deficits may be associated with the Arnold-Chiari malformation and usually manifests during infancy. Children

**TABLE 24-3** Types of Chiari Malformation

| Type I | Caudal displacement of cerebellar tonsils below the plane of the foramen magnum |
| --- | --- |
| Type II (Arnold-Chiari; associated with myelomeningocele) | Caudal displacement of the cerebellar vermis, fourth ventricle, and lower brainstem below the plane of the foramen magnum |
| | Dysplastic brainstem with characteristic kink, elongation of the fourth ventricle, beaking of the quadrigeminal plate, hypoplastic tentorium with small posterior fossa, polymicrogyria, enlargement of the massa intermedia |
| Type III | Caudal displacement of the cerebellum and brainstem into a high cervical meningocele |
| Type IV | Cerebellar hypoplasia |

with vocal cord paralysis or a diminished gag reflex may require tracheostomy and gastrostomy to secure the airway and to minimize chronic aspiration. Children of any age may have abnormal responses to hypoxia and hypercarbia because of cranial nerve and brainstem dysfunction.[199,203] Extreme head flexion may cause brainstem compression in otherwise asymptomatic children.

Type I Chiari malformations can occur in healthy children without myelodysplasia. These defects also involve caudal displacement of the cerebellar tonsils below the foramen magnum, but children usually have much milder symptoms, sometimes manifesting only as headache or neck pain.[204] Surgical treatment usually involves a decompressive suboccipital craniectomy with cervical laminectomies.

### Other Spinal Defects

Other spinal anomalies (e.g., lipomeningoceles, lipomyelomeningoceles, diastematomyelias, dermoid tracts) may manifest as tethered cords. Skin defects, typically over the lower lumbar region, may occur as dural sinus tracks or lipomeningoceles. Midline hair tufts, skin dimples, or fat pads may be associated with spinal defects. These anomalies sometimes manifest when toilet training or ambulation is observed to be abnormal or later in childhood when children complain of back pain. Children who have had a meningomyelocele repaired after birth may also develop an ascending neurologic deficit from a tethered spinal cord during growth. Early detection of a tethered cord is easily diagnosed with MRI. Prophylactic surgical untethering is common.

Anesthesia management for surgical release of a tethered cord usually entails monitoring the innervation of the lower extremities and bowel and bladder with nerve stimulators and rectal electromyelograms or manometry. Muscle relaxants should be avoided or permitted to dissipate before intraoperative assessment.

### NEURORADIOLOGIC PROCEDURES

Many neuroradiologic procedures are performed in children. Anesthetic considerations for neurodiagnostic procedures (e.g., CT, MRI) are discussed elsewhere in this book (see Chapters 45 and 47), but certain therapeutic neuroradiologic procedures are addressed here.

To improve intraoperative navigation during intracranial procedures, the concept of intraoperative MRI was introduced in the mid-1990s. The technology has advanced to include a variety of operating room suite designs that encompass MRI machines (E-Fig. 24-4). These procedures present special challenges for

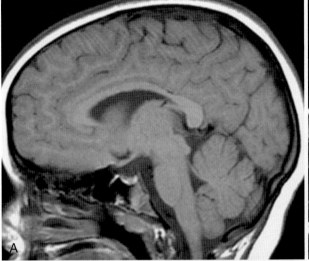

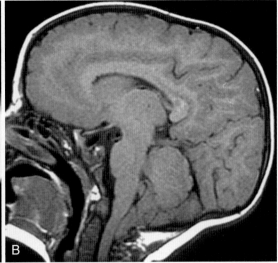

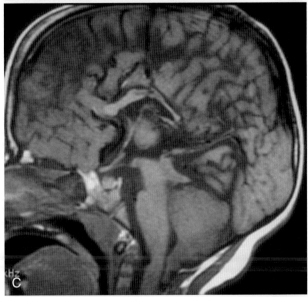

FIGURE 24-12 **A,** Sagittal, T1-weighted magnetic resonance imaging (MRI) of a normal child. **B,** Sagittal, T1-weighted MRI of a child with a Chiari I malformation, which consists of caudal displacement of the cerebellar tonsils at least 5 mm into the upper cervical spinal canal, often with no clinical symptoms. **C,** Sagittal, T1-weighted MRI of a child with a type II Chiari malformation, which is characterized by caudal displacement of the cerebellar tonsils, additional brain anomalies, and a meningomyelocele deformity. (Courtesy Ellen Grant, MD.)

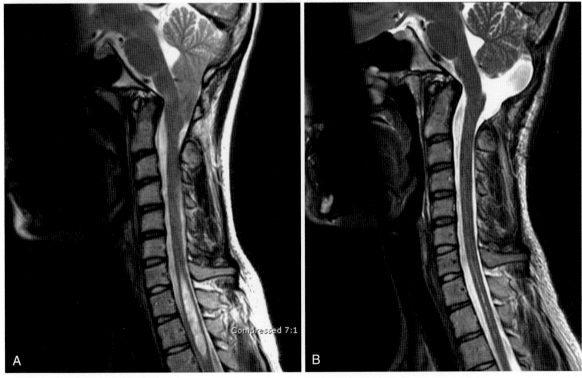

FIGURE 24-13 The images show the posterior fossa in a child with a Chiari II malformation before and after posterior fossa decompression. **A,** Notice the downward herniation of the cerebellar tonsils. **B,** Resolution of cerebellar tonsillar herniation after posterior fossa decompression.

neurosurgeons and anesthesiologists.[205-209] As with anesthesia for diagnostic MRI scans, special monitors, infusion pumps, and an MRI-safe or MRI-conditional anesthesia machine are required. It is challenging to do surgical procedures in this environment, especially because these procedures may take many hours, they may be associated with significant blood loss, and access to the child is severely limited. Some monitoring equipment found in conventional operating rooms (e.g., precordial Doppler ultrasonography, core temperature probes, fluid warmers) is not MRI safe or conditional. Nevertheless, numerous neurosurgical procedures have been safely performed in children in these MRI operating rooms, and the equipment for these procedures is rapidly evolving.

## ACKNOWLEDGMENTS

The authors wish to thank Veronica Miller, MD, and Elizabeth A. Eldredge, MD, for their prior contributions to this chapter.

## ANNOTATED REFERENCES

Coles JP, Fryer TD, Coleman MR, et al. Hyperventilation following head injury: effect on ischemic burden and cerebral oxidative metabolism. Crit Care Med 2007;35:568-78.

*Hyperventilation has a detrimental effect on brain tissue at risk after head injury. The authors refute the often-taught dogma regarding routine hyperventilation, especially after a traumatic brain injury. This article and several others on the same subject should give the anesthesiologist pause when hyperventilating children with intracranial pathology.*

Cox RG, Levy R, Hamilton MG, et al. Anesthesia can be safely provided for children in a high-field intraoperative magnetic resonance imaging environment. Paediatr Anaesh 2011;21:454-8.

*This case series demonstrates the safety of intraoperative MRI for neurosurgical procedures in children. As this technology becomes more prevalent, pediatric neuroanesthesiologists need to be aware of the challenges in caring for patients in this unique environment.*

DiMaggio C, Sun LS, Li G. Early childhood exposure to anesthesia and risk of developmental and behavioral disorders in a sibling birth cohort. Anesth Analg 2011:113;1143-51.

*This is one of many retrospective cohort studies that have assessed the relationship of early anesthetic exposure in human children to the development of cognitive deficits. This study looks at cognitive differences in a sibling cohort in which one sibling was exposed to general anesthesia before 3 years of age. It is not possible to draw a causal relationship from this or similar studies because of problems with selection bias and difficulty controlling for the myriad confounders with respect to a child's cognitive development. However, these studies are an important step in answering whether general anesthesia can harm the developing child. All pediatric anesthesiologists must be familiar with these data, because parents and other physicians expect their expert advice in weighing the risks and benefits of proceeding with surgery on infants and young children.*

Jevtovic-Todorovic V, Hartman RE, Izumi Y, et al. Early exposure to common anesthetic agents causes widespread neurodegeneration in the developing rat brain and persistent learning deficits. J Neurosci 2003;23:876-82.

*This extremely important paper addresses the controversies surrounding the use of common anesthetic agents in neonates. The authors present compelling animal data showing that commonly used anesthetic agents such as isoflurane cause histologically evident neurodegeneration and cause behavioral and cognition problems. This reference is commonly cited when this discussion arises. However, no human data on this issue exist, and extrapolating these data to the practice of anesthetizing human neonates is questionable.*

Lassen NA, Christensen MS. Physiology of cerebral blood flow. Br J Anaesth 1976;48:719-34.

*This review article discusses the various physiologic mechanisms of control of cerebral blood flow.*

Pollack IF. Brain tumors in children. N Engl J Med 1994;331:1500-07.

*Although this review is from the 1990s, it provides a comprehensive overview of the epidemiology of pediatric brain tumors and treatment approaches. Knowledge of various treatment approaches to different histologic types of tumors can inform the anesthesiologist about the extent of the process behind the procedure and how aggressive the surgery needs to be to achieve a desired outcome.*

Reasoner DK, Todd MM, Scamman FL, Warner DS. The incidence of pneumocephalus after supratentorial craniotomy: observations on the disappearance of intracranial air. Anesthesiology 1994;80:1008-12.

*This well-conceived study evaluates the length of time pneumocephalus persists after supratentorial craniotomy. The take-home message is that air persists in the head for several weeks after craniotomy, and care should be taken not to exacerbate the situation during subsequent administration of anesthetics. Nitrous oxide should be avoided in these children, because tension pneumocephalus could develop.*

## REFERENCES

Please see www.expertconsult.com.

# Essentials of Endocrinology

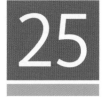

ELLIOT J. KRANE, ERINN T. RHODES, AND JOSEPH I. WOLFSDORF

## Diabetes Mellitus*

The incidence of both type 1 and type 2 diabetes mellitus in children is increasing worldwide.[1-6] The use of insulin pumps and various multicomponent insulin regimens has increased the complexity of perioperative management of children with diabetes. Anesthesiologists must carefully consider the pathophysiology of the disease, as well as each child's specific diabetes treatment regimen, glycemic control, intended surgery, and anticipated postoperative course, when devising an appropriate perioperative management plan. Standardized algorithms for perioperative diabetes management improve care[7-9] without significantly increasing costs[9]; several guidelines and studies of perioperative management of children with diabetes are available in the literature and examples are included.[10-15]

### CLASSIFICATION AND EPIDEMIOLOGY IN CHILDREN
Type 1 and type 2 are the most common forms of diabetes.[16,17] Type 1 diabetes is characterized by absolute deficiency of insulin, which usually results from immune-mediated destruction of pancreatic beta cells.[17] In contrast, type 2 diabetes results from a combination of insulin resistance and a relative deficiency of insulin.[16,17] Children with type 2 diabetes typically are overweight and frequently have a first- or second-degree relative with type 2 diabetes.[16] However, the increasing prevalence of obesity in children[18] has made distinction between type 1 and type 2 diabetes, at times, rather difficult. Children with phenotypic characteristics of type 2 diabetes may have pancreatic autoimmunity,[19-21] and approximately 35% of children with diabetes who require exogenous insulin at diagnosis are overweight or obese,[22,23] consistent with the prevalence of childhood overweight and obesity in the general U.S. pediatric population.[24] Other forms of diabetes may be less commonly encountered (Table 25-1). Additional modifications to the perioperative treatment regimen may be necessary when diabetes is associated with genetic syndromes and/or other endocrinopathies, such as adrenal insufficiency (see later discussion).

Although the worldwide incidence of type 1 diabetes is quite variable,[25] the incidence is increasing in almost all populations throughout the world.[4] In the United States, the SEARCH for Diabetes in Youth Study, which began in 2000, provides the most comprehensive estimates of the prevalence and incidence of type 1 and type 2 diabetes among youth less than 20 years of age in the United States.[26-30] Type 1 diabetes remains the most common form of diabetes observed among youth in the United States, with the greatest prevalence (2 per 1000) among non-Hispanic Caucasians.[29] The epidemic of obesity has also contributed to a

*Modified from Rhodes ET, Ferrari LR, Wolfsdorf JI. Perioperative management of pediatric surgical patients with diabetes mellitus. Anesth Analg 2005;101:986-99.

**TABLE 25-1** Classification of Less Common Forms of Diabetes Mellitus

**Genetic Defects of Beta Cell Function**

Monogenic diabetes (formerly referred to as maturity-onset diabetes of the young [MODY])
Permanent neonatal diabetes
Mitochondrial disorders

**Disease of the Exocrine Pancreas**

Cystic fibrosis–related diabetes

**Drug-Induced Diabetes**

Steroids
Chemotherapeutic agents

**Genetic Syndromes**

Prader-Willi syndrome
Down syndrome
Turner syndrome
Wolfram syndrome

**Endocrinopathies**

Autoimmune polyglandular syndrome
Cushing syndrome

Modified from Rhodes ET, Ferrari LR, Wolfsdorf JI. Perioperative management of pediatric surgical patients with diabetes mellitus. Anesth Analg 2005;101:986-99.

**TABLE 25-2** Insulin Preparations Classified according to Their Pharmacokinetic Profiles*

| | Onset (hours) | Peak (hours) | Duration (hours) |
|---|---|---|---|
| **Rapid-Acting[†]** | | | |
| Insulin lispro (Humalog)[‡] | <0.25 | 0.5-2.5 | ≤5 |
| Insulin aspart (Novolog)[‡] | <0.25 | 1-3 | 3-5 |
| Insulin glulisine (Apidra)[‡] | <0.25 | 0.5-1.5 | 3-5 |
| **Short-Acting[†]** | | | |
| Regular (soluble) | 0.5-1 | 2-4 | 5-8 |
| **Intermediate and Long-Acting[†]** | | | |
| NPH (isophane) | 1-2 | 2-8 | 14-24 |
| Insulin glargine (Lantus)[‡] | 2-4 | No peak | 20-24 |
| Insulin detemir (Levemir)[‡] | 1-2 | 3-9 | Up to 24 |

Adapted from Rhodes ET, Ferrari LR, Wolfsdorf JI. Perioperative management of pediatric surgical patients with diabetes mellitus. Anesth Analg 2005;101:986-99.
*NPH*, Neutral protamine Hagedorn.
*Times of onset, peak, and duration of action vary within and between patients and are affected by numerous factors, including dosage, site, depth of injection, dilution, temperature, and other factors.
[†]Premixed combinations of intermediate-acting and either rapid- or short-acting insulins are available whose pharmacodynamic profiles have a bimodal pattern reflecting the two insulin components.
[‡]Insulin analogue developed by modifying the amino acid sequence of the human insulin molecule.

progressive increase in the incidence and prevalence of type 2 diabetes in U.S. children.[1] In the SEARCH study, the prevalence of type 2 diabetes in 10- to 19-year-old youth ranged from 0.18 per 1000 among non-Hispanic Caucasian youth to 1.45 per 1000 among Navajo youth, and the incidence ranged from 3.7 per 100,000 per year among non-Hispanic Caucasian youth to 27.7 per 100,000 per year among Navajo youth.[29,30] Increases in the incidence and prevalence of type 2 diabetes have been noted in other parts of the world.[2,3,5,6,31-34]

## GENERAL MANAGEMENT PRINCIPLES

Understanding both the pharmacokinetic and pharmacodynamic properties of different insulin preparations and antihyperglycemic medications is critical to developing an appropriate perioperative plan.

Type 1 diabetes always requires treatment with insulin. However, an increasing number of insulin preparations (Table 25-2) and delivery systems are available. The least complex insulin regimens consist of two or three insulin injections per day. They incorporate a combination of an intermediate-acting insulin (e.g., neutral protamine Hagedorn [NPH]) and/or a long-acting insulin (e.g., insulin detemir [Levemir] or insulin glargine [Lantus]) for basal coverage with a short- or rapid-acting insulin (e.g., regular, insulin aspart [NovoLog], insulin lispro [Humalog], or insulin glulisine [Apidra]) to provide prandial glycemic coverage. More intensive insulin regimens are being used with greater frequency and typically consist of insulin glargine, a long-acting insulin, which provides a relatively constant 24-hour basal concentration of circulating insulin without a pronounced peak, to simulate basal insulin secretion,[35] in conjunction with rapid-acting insulin administered with food. Some studies have demonstrated superior glycemic control with such regimens as compared with regimens using NPH insulin and regular insulin,[36] although the ideal insulin regimen for children with type 1

diabetes remains controversial.[37] Another long-acting insulin, insulin detemir, may also be used in intensive insulin regimens and has demonstrated more predictable glucose-reducing effects than both NPH insulin[38-40] and insulin glargine.[38]

Many children with type 1 diabetes are managed with an insulin pump,[41,42] a device that administers a continuous subcutaneous infusion of insulin (typically a rapid-acting insulin, see Table 25-2) at a basal rate that is supplemented by bolus doses of insulin given with meals and snacks and to correct hyperglycemia. In appropriately selected children, pump therapy has shown superiority over injection regimens.[43-46] Standard insulin preparations are U100, meaning that there are 100 units of insulin per milliliter. However, very young patients with type 1 diabetes may require diluted insulin (e.g., U10) to achieve accurate dosing.[47] Parents of toddlers with type 1 diabetes should be specifically questioned about their use of diluted insulin.

Most children with type 2 diabetes are managed with insulin and/or oral metformin, the only oral agent approved for use in children with diabetes in the United States.[48-50] Metformin's primary action is to decrease hepatic glucose production and, secondarily, to increase insulin sensitivity in peripheral tissues. Occasionally, other oral agents, including sulfonylureas, which promote insulin secretion, and thiazolidinediones, which increase insulin sensitivity in muscle and adipose tissue, are used in adolescents.[48,51] Nutritional therapy is always included in the management of children with type 2 diabetes. Studies, such as the Treatment Options for Type 2 Diabetes in Adolescents and Youth (TODAY) trial,[52,53] are evaluating the optimal treatment for type 2 diabetes. Monotherapy with metformin was associated with durable glycemic control in approximately half of children and adolescents with type 2 diabetes. The addition of rosiglitazone, but not an intensive lifestyle intervention, was superior to metformin alone.

New medications introduced to manage adults with diabetes may eventually become available for use in children. Incretins, including glucose-dependent insulinotropic polypeptide and glucagon-like peptide-1 (GLP-1), are gastrointestinal hormones released after eating that stimulate insulin secretion and are necessary for normal glucose tolerance.[54,55] GLP-1 acts through a G protein–coupled receptor to promote glucose-dependent insulin secretion, suppression of glucagon secretion, slowing of gastric emptying, and reduction in food intake.[54] Exenatide (Byetta) is a GLP-1 receptor agonist widely used in adults with type 2 diabetes as an adjunctive therapy for those taking metformin and/or a sulfonylurea.[56] Inhibitors of dipeptidyl peptidase-IV,[57] the enzyme that degrades GLP-1, are also increasingly being used for the treatment of type 2 diabetes in adults, but have not been approved for use in children. Pramlintide acetate (Symlin) is a synthetic amylin receptor agonist that can be used as an adjunct to insulin therapy in adults with type 1 or type 2 diabetes.[58-61] Amylin, a 37-amino acid polypeptide islet hormone cosecreted with insulin from beta islet cells,[54] has three effects: delays gastric emptying, inhibits glucagon secretion, and modulates satiety.[54]

## METABOLIC RESPONSE TO SURGERY

Trauma of any kind, and surgery in particular, causes a complex neuroendocrine stress response, including suppression of insulin secretion and increased production of counter-regulatory hormones (frequently called "stress hormones" in the anesthesiology literature), particularly cortisol and catecholamines.[62,63] Insulin is the primary anabolic hormone that promotes glucose uptake in muscle and adipose tissue while suppressing glucose production (glycogenolysis and gluconeogenesis) by the liver.[64] The counter-regulatory hormones, which include epinephrine, glucagon, cortisol, and growth hormone, exert the opposite effects, resulting in resistance to insulin action[65-67] and an increase in blood glucose concentration by: (1) stimulating glycogenolysis and gluconeogenesis in the liver, (2) increasing lipolysis and ketogenesis, and (3) inhibiting glucose uptake and utilization in muscle and fat. Glucagon, secreted by alpha cells in the pancreatic islets, suppresses insulin secretion while stimulating hepatic glycogenolysis, gluconeogenesis, and ketogenesis.[64,65] Epinephrine, which acts via $\beta_2$- and $\alpha_2$-adrenergic receptors, stimulates glucagon production, increases glycogenolysis and gluconeogenesis, stimulates lipolysis, decreases insulin secretion, and decreases glucose utilization in insulin-sensitive tissues.[64] Cortisol stimulates gluconeogenesis, proteolysis, and lipolysis, and decreases glucose utilization.[65,68] Growth hormone augments glucose production, decreases glucose utilization, and accelerates lipolysis.[69] Pro-inflammatory cytokines may further stimulate secretion of counter-regulatory hormones and alter insulin receptor signaling.[67] These changes increase catabolism, as evidenced by increased hepatic glucose production and breakdown of protein and fat. In the diabetic patient with absolute or relative insulin deficiency, the enhanced catabolism resulting from surgical trauma can lead to marked hyperglycemia and even diabetic ketoacidosis.[70] These metabolic effects may be exacerbated by a prolonged fast before and during surgery.

## METABOLIC RESPONSE TO ANESTHESIA

Although adequate analgesia is essential to minimize the neuroendocrine stress response to surgery, some anesthetics may also independently contribute to perioperative hyperglycemia.[10,71] Inhalation anesthetics, such as isoflurane, may cause hyperglycemia by inhibiting insulin secretion[72,73]; the hyperglycemia results from both impaired glucose uptake and increased glucose

production.[71] In contrast, epidural analgesia with local anesthetics prevents this hyperglycemic effect[74,75] through an inhibitory effect on endogenous glucose production.[71] Similarly, intravenous (IV) anesthesia with opioids mitigates the hyperglycemic response of surgery[71,76,77] through its apparent neutral effect on endogenous glucose production but decrease in glucose clearance.[71] Although these differences are important to consider, the metabolic effects of anesthesia are relatively minor compared with the direct effects of surgery.[10]

## ADVERSE CONSEQUENCES OF HYPERGLYCEMIA

Hyperglycemia can impair wound healing by hindering collagen production, which may decrease the tensile strength of the surgical wound.[78] Hyperglycemia may also have adverse effects on neutrophil function, including decreased chemotaxis, phagocytosis, and bactericidal killing.[79-82] Evidence from controlled experimental studies in rabbits demonstrated that these effects may be reversed, in part, by glycemia-independent effects of insulin.[83] However, the overall benefits of intensive insulin therapy, including a reduction in mortality, were derived mainly from maintenance of normoglycemia, whereas glycemia-independent actions of insulin exert only minor, organ-specific effects.[83]

Clinical studies in humans have not consistently supported the relationship between perioperative glycemic control and short-term risk of infection or morbidity.[84,85] However, several studies in diabetic adults undergoing surgery have shown an association between postoperative hyperglycemia and infectious complications.[86,87] A meta-analysis showed that patients in surgical intensive care units (ICUs) appear to benefit from intensive insulin therapy, whereas patients in other ICU settings do not.[88] These outcomes have contributed to confusion regarding specific glycemic targets and the means for achieving them in both critically and noncritically ill patients. A recent consensus statement[89] recommended that an insulin infusion should be used to control hyperglycemia in the majority of critically ill patients in the ICU setting, with a starting threshold of no greater than 180 mg/dL. Once IV insulin therapy has been initiated, the glucose level should be maintained between 140 and 180 mg/dL. With no prospective, randomized controlled trial data for establishing specific guidelines in noncritically ill patients treated with insulin, pre-meal glucose targets should generally be less than 140 mg/dL and random blood glucose values less than 180 mg/dL, as long as these targets can be safely achieved. To avoid hypoglycemia, one should reassess the insulin regimen if blood glucose levels decline below 100 mg/dL. Modification of the insulin regimen is necessary when blood glucose values are less than 70 mg/dL, unless the event is easily explained by other factors (such as a missed meal).[89]

The single pediatric trial to date demonstrated shorter length of stay, attenuated inflammatory response, and decreased mortality in patients randomized to targeting of age-adjusted normoglycemia.[90] However, the rate of severe hypoglycemia (less than 40 mg/dL) in that study was too frequent, at 25% of the total cohort, making the implementation of this approach ill-advised without further evidence from ongoing multicenter pediatric trials. Other retrospective studies of critically ill children managed in pediatric ICUs have also demonstrated associations of hyperglycemia with morbidity and mortality.[91-94] In the 1980s and 1990s the dogma of tight glucose control replaced an era in which the mantra of caring for diabetic surgical patients was "keep them sweet," but in more recent years glucose control has become controversial and is unresolved, with conflicting evidence;

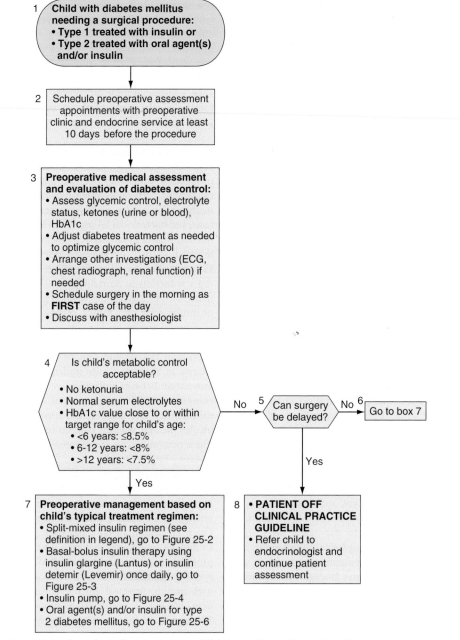

**FIGURE 25-1** Clinical practice guideline for perioperative management of diabetes mellitus. Split-mixed insulin regimen refers to a regimen combining multiple daily injections of intermediate- or long-acting insulins (e.g., neutral protamine Hagedorn [NPH] or insulin detemir [Levemir]) and multiple injections of rapid- or short-acting insulins (regular, insulin lispro [Humalog], insulin aspart [NovoLog], or insulin glulisine [Apidra]). *ECG*, Electrocardiogram. (Modified from Rhodes ET, Ferrari LR, Wolfsdorf JI. Perioperative management of pediatric surgical patients with diabetes mellitus. Anesth Analg 2005;101:986-99.)

a systematic review of the literature concluded that there are insufficient data regarding the best strategy or regimen to attain target blood glucose levels in ambulatory surgical patients with diabetes mellitus.[95] The recommended practice for subspecialties, such as cardiac, neurosurgical, and solid organ transplant surgical patients, requires still more study, and it must be highlighted that few of the published investigations and meta-analyses have focused specifically on the pediatric age group.

## PREOPERATIVE ASSESSMENT

When feasible, children with diabetes should not undergo elective surgery until they are metabolically stable (Fig. 25-1, *box 4*);

that is, there is no ketosis, serum electrolytes are normal, and the glycated hemoglobin (HbA1c) value is close to or within the ideal range for the child's age. Although there is no consensus regarding the ideal metabolic targets for control of diabetes in children,[96] the American Diabetes Association recommends an HbA1c less than or equal to 8.5% for children younger than 6 years of age; less than 8% for children 6 to 12 years of age; and less than 7.5% for 13 years of age or older, with a more stringent target of less than 7% to be considered in this last age group, for children in whom this can be achieved without excessive hypoglycemia,[96] as well as for those with type 2 diabetes.[16] The preoperative consultation to assess the adequacy of metabolic control should be scheduled at least 10 days before the procedure (see Fig. 25-1, *box 3*). If metabolic control is poor, surgery should be delayed if possible. Both the endocrinology and anesthesiology services should participate in this assessment. Whenever possible, surgery for children with diabetes should be scheduled as the first case in the morning so that prolonged fasting is avoided and diabetes treatment regimens may be most easily adjusted.

Children who present for emergent surgery, for example, because of trauma or acute surgical conditions, require a multidisciplinary preoperative assessment with collaborative involvement of both the endocrinology and anesthesiology services. In these situations, surgery often cannot be delayed even if metabolic control is poor, as in the case of a child requiring emergent surgery who presents in diabetic ketoacidosis. This has implications for the intraoperative management of such children, as described later under "Special Surgical Situations."

## PREOPERATIVE MANAGEMENT

The regimen for managing diabetes before, during, and after a surgical or diagnostic procedure that requires the child to fast should aim to maintain near-normoglycemia, that is, blood glucose levels of 100 to 200 mg/dL. In this blood glucose range there will be a reduced risk of osmotic diuresis, dehydration, electrolyte imbalance, metabolic acidosis, infection, and hypoglycemia in the sedated child who may be unaware of hypoglycemia or unable to communicate with staff.[97] The child need not be admitted before the day of surgery, but rather early on the same morning as the surgery or procedure. Parents should receive explicit written instructions regarding appropriate modifications of their child's diabetes regimen before and for the day of surgery. On admission to the hospital, metabolic control should be assessed, including a preoperative determination of glucose concentration. On the morning of surgery, no rapid- or short-acting acting insulin should be administered *unless* the blood glucose level exceeds 250 mg/dL. However, admission to the hospital before *major* surgical procedures in children[10] and adults has been recommended if the metabolic status needs to be optimized preoperatively.[65] If the surgery must be delayed for any reason, frequent blood glucose monitoring is mandatory to prevent perioperative hypoglycemia or hyperglycemia.

If the blood glucose exceeds 250 mg/dL, a conservative dose of rapid-acting insulin (e.g., insulin lispro or insulin aspart) or short-acting insulin (regular) is administered to restore near-normoglycemia. This is achieved using the child's usual sliding scale or a "correction factor." The insulin "correction factor" is the decrease in the blood glucose concentration expected after administering 1 unit of rapid- or short-acting insulin. This can be calculated using the "1500 rule": divide 1500 by the child's usual total daily dose (TDD) of insulin. For example, if a child typically receives 30 units of insulin daily, this child's "correction factor" would be 1500 ÷ 30 = 50. Therefore 1 unit of rapid- or short-acting insulin would be expected to decrease the child's blood glucose concentration by approximately 50 mg/dL. Various correction factors have been described, including a "1500 rule" for short-acting insulin (regular) and an "1800 rule" for rapid-acting insulin, such as insulin lispro.[91,98] For simplicity and because of insulin resistance stimulated by surgical stress, the "1500 rule" is appropriate in this setting, even with the use of a rapid-acting insulin. To then calculate an appropriate corrective dose of insulin to restore near-normoglycemia, the anesthesiologist should aim for a target blood glucose concentration of 150 mg/dL.

The "correction factor" rather than a sliding scale is used to manage a child with hyperglycemia and restore the blood glucose concentration to 150 mg/dL. For example, if the child has a correction factor of 1 unit of rapid- or short-acting insulin to reduce the blood glucose concentration by about 50 mg/dL, and the current blood glucose value is 300 mg/dL, to reduce the blood glucose concentration from 300 mg/dL to 150 mg/dL, a total dose of (300 − 150)/50 or 3 units of insulin would be required. At the start of the procedure, the "correction" dose may be administered subcutaneously (using rapid-acting insulin) or IV using short-acting (regular) insulin in those children who will be managed with an intravenous insulin infusion during the procedure. For children with type 2 diabetes who do *not* require insulin (but who are, by definition, insulin resistant), an insulin dose of 0.1 unit/kg of rapid-acting insulin may be administered subcutaneously to correct a blood glucose concentration greater than 250 mg/dL.

More detailed preoperative recommendations must be based on the individual child's usual treatment regimen. For most children with diabetes undergoing minor outpatient surgical procedures, insulin can be provided perioperatively with subcutaneous injections. In adults, especially those with type 2 diabetes, this practice is commonly,[97] although not universally, preferred.[99] Others routinely recommend insulin infusions even for minor outpatient surgical procedures in children.[10] Several reports suggest that better glycemic control can be achieved in the perioperative period with a continuous intravenous infusion rather than subcutaneous insulin administration.[12,100,101] However, these studies were conducted before the availability of rapid-acting insulins whose rapid and reproducible effects after subcutaneous administration[102] may more closely match the ability to titrate IV-administered short-acting insulin. Subcutaneous insulin lispro has been shown to be as efficacious as regular IV insulin for treatment of uncomplicated diabetic ketoacidosis in children.[103] Whatever the management strategy for the diabetes, it is most important that it is coordinated between the anesthesiology and endocrinology services, and the modifications to the child's diabetic regimen at home needs to be communicated clearly and in a timely manner to the family.

Split-mixed insulin regimens involve two to three injections per day with a combination of NPH or insulin detemir plus a rapid- or short-acting insulin. For children who use such a regimen, 50% of the usual morning dose of NPH or the full usual dose of insulin detemir should be administered on the morning of the procedure (Fig. 25-2). For the child whose basal insulin is once-daily insulin glargine or insulin detemir, no additional insulin is given on the morning of the surgery if the child received a dose in the evening of the previous day (Fig. 25-3). However, if insulin glargine or detemir is typically administered in the morning, the full dose should be administered on the morning of the procedure to prevent ketosis.

Management of the child on an insulin pump depends on the duration of the surgical procedure (Fig. 25-4). Those undergoing minor procedures expected to last less than 2 hours can continue to receive their usual basal rate via their insulin pump. However, this approach requires that the anesthesiologist is familiar and comfortable with the use of the pump in the operating room. Other protocols include transitioning patients who use an insulin pump to IV insulin infusion or subcutaneous insulin glargine.[65] For procedures longer than 2 hours, children should be transitioned to an IV insulin infusion, as described in the next section.

**25**

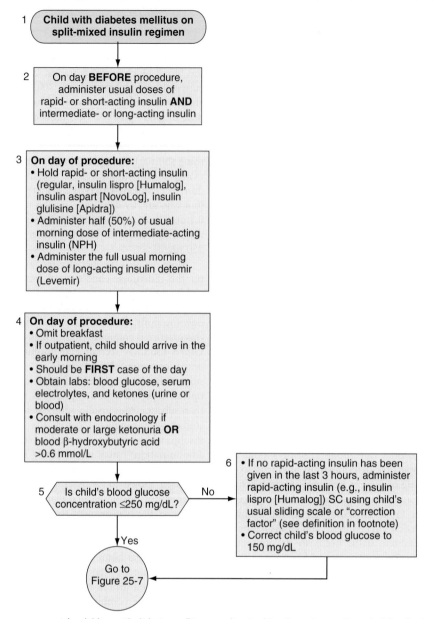

**FIGURE 25-2** Preoperative management for children with diabetes mellitus on split-mixed insulin regimens. The calculation for insulin "correction factor" is as follows:

1. Divide 1500 by child's total daily dose (TDD).
2. If daily dose varies (i.e., use of sliding scales), use the *average* daily dose in the past week to determine TDD.
3. Example: if TDD = 50 units, then insulin correction factor is 1 unit insulin lispro (Humalog) to reduce blood glucose by 30 mg/dL.

*NPH*, Neutral protamine Hagedorn; *SC*, subcutaneous. (Modified from Rhodes ET, Ferrari LR, Wolfsdorf JI. Perioperative management of pediatric surgical patients with diabetes mellitus. Anesth Analg 2005;101:986-99.)

## MAJOR SURGERY AND INTRAVENOUS INSULIN INFUSIONS

For children who require major surgery, especially procedures anticipated to last more than 2 hours, an IV insulin infusion is the preferred perioperative diabetes management plan (Fig. 25-5). Studies in children[12] and adults[7] have demonstrated that glycemic control is superior with infusions of IV insulin compared with subcutaneous injections. These children should receive their usual doses of insulin on the day before the procedure. On the morning of the procedure, an IV infusion of 5% dextrose in half-normal saline should be started at a maintenance rate, and an IV insulin infusion should also be provided to accommodate the dextrose infusion to maintain blood glucose in the target range of 100 to 200 mg/dL (see Fig. 25-5). The maintenance rate for IV fluids in a child depends on body size and can be calculated either based on body weight (4 mL/kg/hr for the first 10 kg body weight, 2 mL/kg/hr for 11 to 20 kg, and then 1 mL/kg/hr for each kg over 20 kg) or body surface area (1.5 L/m$^2$/day). The insulin dose varies with the child's pubertal status; prepubertal children are relatively more sensitive to insulin than pubertal adolescents.[104] In prepubertal children with type 1 diabetes, after the remission (honeymoon) period, the insulin requirement is typically 0.6 to 0.8 unit/kg/day, whereas in adolescents, the

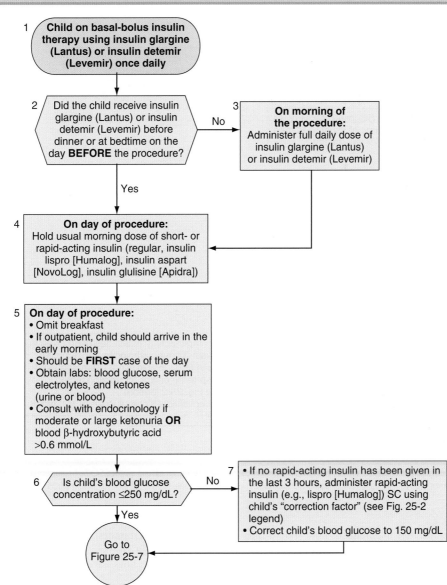

**FIGURE 25-3** Preoperative management for children with diabetes mellitus on once-daily insulin glargine (Lantus) or insulin detemir (Levemir) regimens. Note that insulin glargine and insulin detemir should not be mixed with any other insulin. *SC,* Subcutaneous. (Modified from Rhodes ET, Ferrari LR, Wolfsdorf JI. Perioperative management of pediatric surgical patients with diabetes mellitus. Anesth Analg 2005;101:986-99.)

requirement is 1 to 1.5 units/kg/day.[105,106] Children with type 2 diabetes may require even greater doses of insulin because of their insulin resistance. With IV insulin, a suitable initial ratio of insulin to dextrose may be estimated from the child's usual or average total daily insulin dose (TDD) using the formula 500 ÷ TDD. For example, if the child typically receives 50 units of insulin daily, then 500 ÷ 50 = 10. Therefore, in this example, 1 unit of insulin would be administered via a "piggyback infusion" for each 10 g of dextrose contained in the maintenance IV infusion to prevent hyperglycemia. Note that a maintenance IV solution of 5% dextrose contains 10 g of dextrose in every 200 mL. Only regular insulin should be used for IV infusions.

## SPECIAL CONSIDERATIONS FOR PREOPERATIVE MANAGEMENT OF TYPE 2 DIABETES

Children with type 2 diabetes may require insulin or one of several oral antihyperglycemic agents (Fig. 25-6). Metformin should be discontinued 24 hours before a procedure because of

its long half-life and the risk of lactic acidosis in the presence of dehydration, hypoxemia, or poor tissue perfusion.[107] Other oral agents, such as sulfonylureas and thiazolidinediones, may be discontinued on the morning of the procedure. Figure 25-6 outlines additional recommendations for children with type 2 diabetes who use a split-mixed or basal-bolus insulin regimen. Adjustments for other insulin regimens or oral hypoglycemic agents in type 2 diabetes should be determined in consultation with an endocrinologist or diabetologist.

## INTRAOPERATIVE MANAGEMENT

The insulin and fluid regimen during and after surgery depends on the duration of the procedure. If the procedure is likely to be brief (e.g., ≤1 hour) and one can reasonably anticipate that the child will be able to drink soon after the procedure, it may not be necessary to start a glucose-containing IV infusion. If the duration of fasting is likely to be more prolonged, an IV infusion should be started at a maintenance rate as described

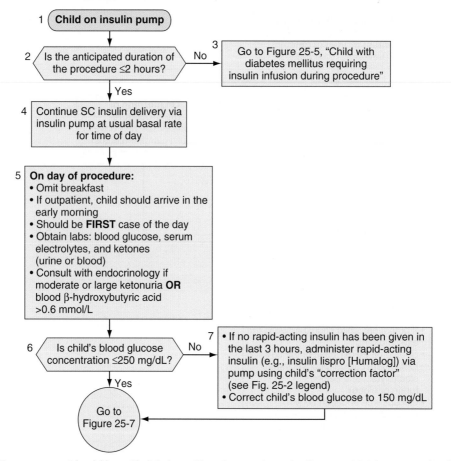

**FIGURE 25-4** Preoperative management for children with diabetes mellitus who are using an insulin pump. *SC*, Subcutaneous. (Modified from Rhodes ET, Ferrari LR, Wolfsdorf JI. Perioperative management of pediatric surgical patients with diabetes mellitus. Anesth Analg 2005;101:986-99.)

earlier (Fig. 25-7). Intraoperative maintenance fluid should then be replaced with a comparable glucose-containing solution. Replacement of insensible losses and intravascular volume owing to blood or other body fluid losses should be with an appropriate isotonic solution (e.g., lactated Ringer's solution or normal saline).

Although some protocols include potassium chloride in the maintenance IV fluid solution,[10,65,97] this practice should generally be avoided because of the danger of inadvertent intraoperative administration of large quantities of potassium during fluid resuscitation. Children undergoing a brief procedure with a baseline normal serum potassium concentration and well-controlled diabetes have a small risk of hypokalemia. Those undergoing more prolonged surgeries or emergent surgeries during which metabolic decompensation is more likely, require intraoperative assessment of electrolytes and appropriate adjustment of the electrolyte composition of their IV solution. *In all cases, blood glucose concentrations should be measured hourly and either insulin or dextrose adjusted, as necessary, to maintain blood glucose in the target range of 100 to 200 mg/dL.* If the blood glucose exceeds 250 mg/dL, urine or blood ketones should also be measured (see Fig. 25-7). Either an increase in the rate of continuous insulin infusion or subcutaneous administration of a rapid-acting insulin analog is used to correct intraoperative hyperglycemia. Intraoperative IV bolus of regular insulin is not recommended because this causes a rapid supraphysiologic increase in serum insulin concentration, which, owing to insulin's short half-life

(approximately 5 minutes), will have a short-lived effect on blood glucose levels. In contrast, subcutaneously administered rapid-acting insulin analogs have a typical and reproducible pharmacologic profile.

## POSTOPERATIVE MANAGEMENT

As soon as the child is able to resume drinking and eating normally, the usual diabetes regimen, including insulin and/or oral agents, may be reinstituted and the dextrose infusion discontinued, if applicable (Fig. 25-8). One exception to this approach is for children with type 2 diabetes who take metformin; metformin should be held for 48 hours and renal function must be within normal limits before its resumption. For children who are unable to eat or drink, IV dextrose and electrolyte solution should be continued until oral intake is restored. An infusion of IV short-acting insulin (regular) or intermittent subcutaneous rapid-acting insulin should be administered, not more than every 3 hours, to maintain blood glucose in the target range of 100 to 200 mg/dL. Frequent blood glucose monitoring and monitoring blood or urine ketones is essential because of the variable effects of surgical trauma, inactivity, pain, anxiety, nausea and/or vomiting with poor oral intake, medications, and postoperative infection. At the time of discharge from the hospital, children and their parents or care providers should be given appropriate guidelines regarding these issues. Those who are admitted to the hospital overnight after surgery should be managed in consultation with the

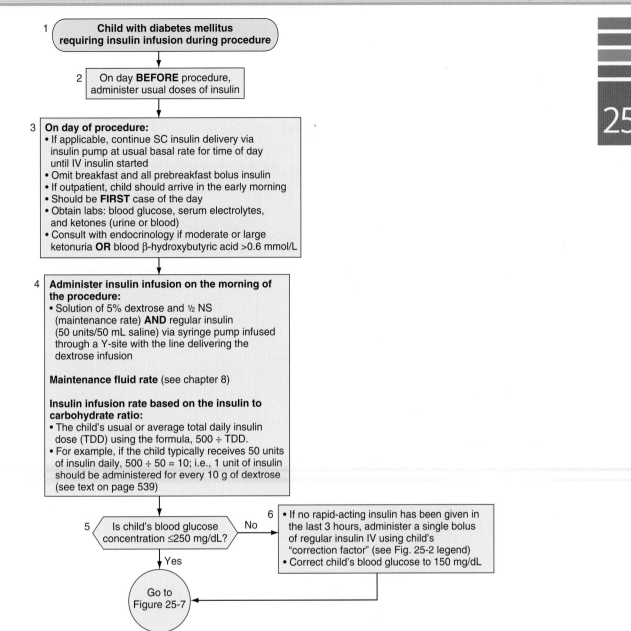

**FIGURE 25-5** Preoperative management for children with diabetes mellitus who require insulin infusions during surgery. *IV,* Intravenous; *NS,* normal saline; *SC,* subcutaneous. (Modified from Rhodes ET, Ferrari LR, Wolfsdorf JI. Perioperative management of pediatric surgical patients with diabetes mellitus. Anesth Analg 2005;101:986-99.)

endocrinology service, if possible, to coordinate appropriate scheduling and subsequent dosing of insulin.

### SPECIAL SURGICAL SITUATIONS

Children with diabetes who need urgent surgery must have a full clinical and biochemical assessment. Frequently, the problem necessitating surgery may have led to metabolic decompensation that must first be corrected and stabilized, unless the need for surgery is immediate. These children are often dehydrated; in addition to administering insulin, rehydration and electrolyte replacement is critical to address their metabolic derangements and restore normal glomerular filtration rate and renal function. In most cases, these children require emergent surgery that should be managed with an IV infusion of insulin as described

earlier (see Fig. 25-5). Children with diabetic ketoacidosis require close collaboration between the anesthesiology and endocrinology services.

## Diabetes Insipidus

Children undergoing neurosurgical procedures for tumors in or near the pituitary gland, especially craniopharyngioma, often require management of diabetes insipidus (DI), as do children with known DI who require anesthesia for surgical or radiologic procedures. The perioperative management of these children is frequently complicated by either overhydration or underhydration and electrolyte disturbances.

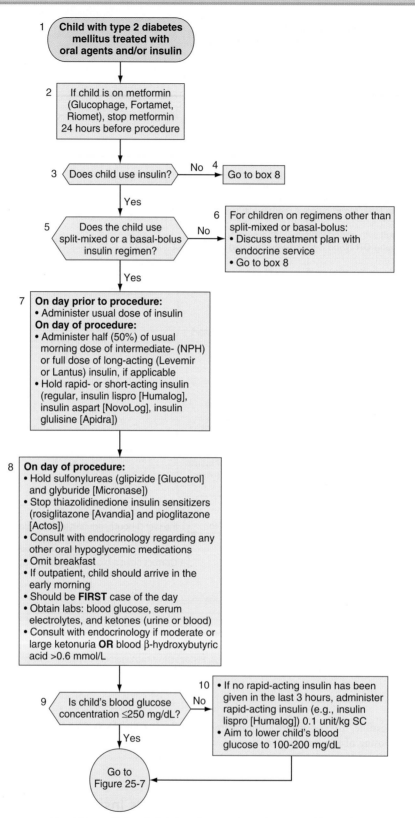

**FIGURE 25-6** Preoperative management for children with type 2 diabetes who are using oral agents and/or insulin. *NPH,* Neutral protamine Hagedorn; *SC,* subcutaneous. (Modified from Rhodes ET, Ferrari LR, Wolfsdorf JI. Perioperative management of pediatric surgical patients with diabetes mellitus. Anesth Analg 2005;101:986-99.)

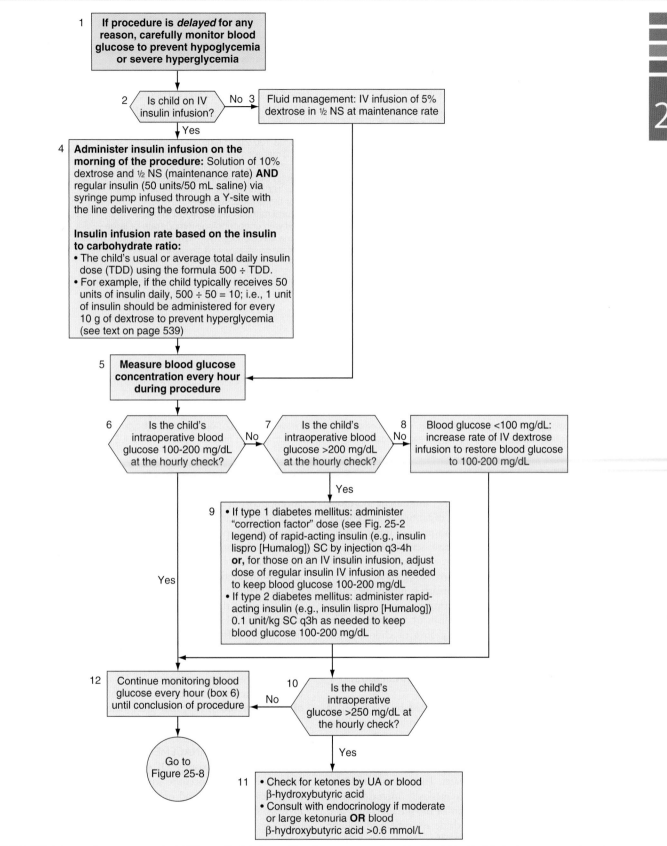

**FIGURE 25-7** Intraoperative management of children with diabetes mellitus. The management goal for the child with diabetes is near-normoglycemia (100-200 mg/dL). Maintenance fluid rate calculation is 4 mL/kg/hr for the first 10 kg of body weight, 2 mL/kg/hr for body weight between 11 and 20 kg, and 1 mL/kg/hr for every kg of body weight over 20 kg. *IV*, Intravenous; *NS*, normal saline; *SC*, subcutaneous; *UA*, urinalysis. (Modified from Rhodes ET, Ferrari LR, Wolfsdorf JI. Perioperative management of pediatric surgical patients with diabetes mellitus. Anesth Analg 2005;101:986-99.)

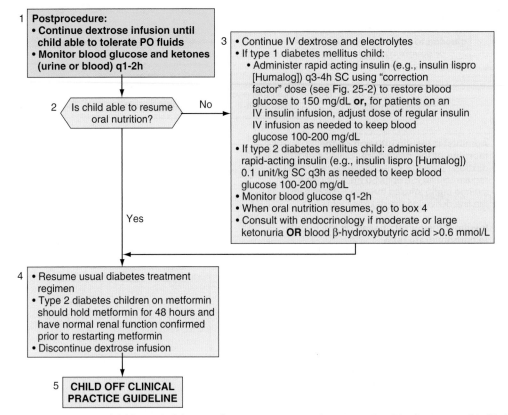

FIGURE 25-8 Postoperative management of children with diabetes mellitus. *IV*, Intravenous; *PO*, postoperative; *SC*, subcutaneous. (Modified from Rhodes ET, Ferrari LR, Wolfsdorf JI. Perioperative management of pediatric surgical patients with diabetes mellitus. Anesth Analg 2005;101:986-99.)

DI is caused by a deficiency of the antidiuretic hormone arginine vasopressin, which acts on the distal tubule and collecting duct of the kidney to promote reabsorption of water. Central (hypothalamic, neurogenic, or vasopressin-sensitive) DI can be caused by disorders of vasopressin gene structure; accidental or surgical trauma to vasopressin neurons; congenital anatomic hypothalamic or pituitary defects; neoplasms; infiltrative, autoimmune, and infectious diseases affecting vasopressin neurons or fiber tracts; and increased metabolism of vasopressin. The etiology is unknown in approximately 50% of children with central DI.

### DIAGNOSIS OF NEUROSURGICAL DIABETES INSIPIDUS: THE TRIPLE-PHASE RESPONSE

It is important to distinguish polyuria caused by the onset of acute postsurgical central DI from polyuria resulting from diuresis of fluids given during surgery. In both cases, children may have a large volume (exceeding 200 mL/m$^2$/hr) of dilute urine. Serum osmolality will be increased in DI but will be normal in the child excreting excess salt and water. The normal child who excretes excess salt and water has a markedly increased urine osmolality. A meticulous examination of the intraoperative and postoperative records and careful bedside assessment of volume status (jugular venous distention, capillary refill) will help to distinguish between these two entities.

Of special interest is the triphasic pattern of vasopressin secretion, often, but not always, observed after neurosurgical procedures that interfere with the supraoptic-hypophyseal tract.[108] After surgery, an initial phase of transient DI may be observed,

lasting between 12 hours and 2 days. This may be explained by local edema that interferes with normal vasopressin secretion. If significant vasopressin-secreting cell damage has occurred, release of stored vasopressin from damaged neurons leads to a second phase that involves water retention. The syndrome of inappropriate antidiuretic hormone secretion (SIADH) may last up to 10 days. Finally, a third phase, permanent neurogenic DI, may follow if more than 90% of vasopressin cells are destroyed. Pronounced SIADH in the second phase generally portends permanent DI in the final phase of the triple response. In children with vasopressin and cortisol deficiency (e.g., in combined anterior and posterior hypopituitarism after neurosurgical treatment of craniopharyngioma), symptoms of DI may be masked because cortisol deficiency impairs renal free water clearance. Institution of glucocorticoid therapy may precipitate polyuria, leading to the diagnosis of DI (Fig. 25-9).

### PERIOPERATIVE MANAGEMENT OF MINOR PROCEDURES

Children with preexisting DI who are scheduled for a minor procedure, i.e., a procedure without significant blood loss and not followed by a period of further fasting or fluid shifts (e.g., myringotomy, radiologic imaging, peripheral orthopedic procedures) are treated differently from those undergoing a more major procedure associated with blood loss or fluid shifts and delayed postoperative resumption of fluid intake (see Fig. 25-9).

Children undergoing minor procedures under anesthesia should receive their usual morning dose of desmopressin (DDAVP) (Table 25-3). The anesthetic technique is tailored to the procedure (e.g., IV sedation for MRI, general endotracheal

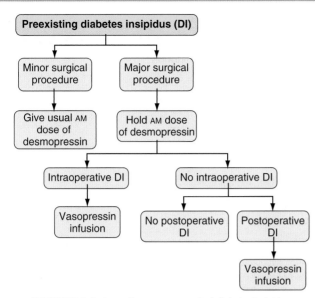

**FIGURE 25-9** Perioperative management of diabetes insipidus.

| **TABLE 25-3** Medications for Management of Central Diabetes Insipidus | |
|---|---|
| Desmopressin acetate (100-, 200-µg tablets; nasal tube 10 µg/0.1 mL; nasal spray 10 µg/0.1 mL: delivers 0.1 mL/spray) | |
| Oral | Dose: 100-400 µg q12h <br> Oral doses are 10-20 times intranasal doses of desmopressin <br> Onset of action: ~15-30 minutes <br> Duration: 8-12 hours <br> May develop tachyphylaxis |
| Intranasal | Dose: ~10-20 µg/dose q12-24h <br> Onset of action: 5-15 minutes <br> Duration: 8-12 hours |
| Vasopressin (Pitressin) (20 units/mL; 0.5-mL, 1-mL, and 10-mL vials; conversion: 1 unit = 2.5 µg) | |
| Intravenous | Dose: 1.5 milliunits/kg/hr <br> Onset of action: minutes <br> Half life: 5-10 minutes |

anesthesia for tonsillectomy). Arterial and urinary catheters are not required, and recovery takes place in the postanesthesia care unit (PACU). Once the morning dose of desmopressin has been administered, intraoperative and postoperative fluids should be restricted to the rate of 1 L/m²/24 hours, i.e., to match insensible free water losses and obligatory urine output. Oral fluids may be offered once the child is awake. Although modern PACU policies often no longer require successful fluid intake before discharging the ambulatory patient, discharging the child with DI should be delayed until the child is able to freely take oral fluids without vomiting. Subsequent doses of desmopressin should be administered according to the child's usual preoperative schedule.

## PERIOPERATIVE MANAGEMENT OF MAJOR PROCEDURES

A major surgical procedure is defined as an operation associated with the potential for significant blood loss; intraoperative or postoperative hemodynamic, neurologic, or respiratory instability; entry into a body cavity (e.g., craniotomy, abdominal surgery,

thoracic surgery); craniofacial or airway surgery; major orthopedic surgery (e.g., spine surgery, tumor resection or amputation, major osteotomies); and/or surgery followed by delayed resumption of unrestricted fluid intake. The child with DI should be scheduled as the first case of the day. On the day before the procedure, the child treated with desmopressin should receive the usual morning dose, but only 50% of the usual evening or bedtime dose (see Fig. 25-9). On the morning of the procedure, desmopressin is withheld. The child undergoing a major procedure should receive general anesthesia with conventional monitoring, as well as insertion of arterial and urinary catheters, and after surgery is admitted to the ICU. A central venous catheter for monitoring central venous pressure, although not indicated solely for the management of DI, is useful in the postoperative period.

At the start of the procedure, an infusion of aqueous vasopressin (20 units/1000 mL to yield a final concentration of 20 milliunits/mL) should be started at 1.5 milliunits/kg/hr (0.0015 unit/kg/hr). IV fluids, using normal saline with 5% dextrose, should total 1 L/m²/24 hours to approximate insensible losses and obligate urine output. Additional IV saline, isotonic fluid, or blood products may be given, as needed, to correct blood and surgical fluid loss, to correct third space fluid loss, and to maintain hemodynamic stability. Urine output should not routinely be replaced in the child receiving a vasopressin infusion.

### NEW PERIOPERATIVE DIAGNOSIS

The new diagnosis of intraoperative or postoperative DI is based on clinical and laboratory findings, including serum sodium level greater than 145 mmol/L, polyuria (greater than 4 mL/kg/hr) for 30 minutes or more, increased plasma osmolality (greater than 300 mOsm/kg) in association with hypotonic urine (less than 300 mOsm/kg), and after excluding the presence of glycosuria and diuretic or mannitol administration as possible causes of polyuria.

When DI occurs, an infusion of aqueous vasopressin (20 units/1000 mL) is initiated at 1.5 milliunits/kg/hr (0.0015 unit/kg/hr) and the dose is doubled after 15 to 30 minutes if the child does not respond, until urine output decreases to less than 2 mL/kg/hr. Once a urine output of less than 2 mL/kg/hr is achieved, the vasopressin infusion is maintained at a constant rate.

IV desmopressin should *not* be used in the acute management of postoperative central DI because it offers no advantage over aqueous vasopressin and because its long half-life (8 to 12 hours) compared with that of vasopressin (5 to 10 minutes) increases the risk of water intoxication and precludes dose titration.

### POSTOPERATIVE MANAGEMENT

The child with DI should be cared for in an ICU after major surgery. Fluid input and output, serum electrolytes and osmolality are monitored closely (hourly if necessary) in the intraoperative and postoperative periods. Until stability is achieved, it is important to have a urinary catheter in place to distinguish postoperative urinary retention from oliguria. The vasopressin infusion initiated intraoperatively is continued in the ICU. Fluid administration is *not* adjusted according to urine output; however, fluid deficits are replaced and blood pressure supported until antidiuresis (urine output of less than 2 mL/kg/hr) is clearly established. Total (oral and IV) maintenance fluids should not exceed insensible plus obligatory urinary losses of 1 L/m²/24 hours. In the postoperative period, appropriate maintenance fluid is generally 5% dextrose in half-normal saline with

**25**

0 to 40 mEq/L of potassium chloride (depending on the serum potassium concentration). Blood loss should be replaced with normal saline, 5% albumin, or blood products, as appropriate.

Aqueous vasopressin at a dose of 1.5 milliunits/kg/hr results in a supranormal blood vasopressin concentration of approximately 10 pg/mL, twice that needed for full antidiuretic activity.[109] The effect of vasopressin is maximal within 2 hours after starting an infusion.[109]

After hypothalamic, but not trans-sphenoidal surgery, greater initial concentrations of vasopressin are occasionally required to treat acute DI. This may be attributed to the release of a substance related to vasopressin from the damaged hypothalamo-neurohypophyseal system, which acts as an antagonist to normal vasopressin activity.[110] Much greater rates of vasopressin infusions, resulting in plasma concentrations greater than 1000 pg/mL, should be avoided because they may cause cutaneous necrosis,[111] rhabdomyolysis,[111,112] and cardiac rhythm disturbances.[112]

### POST–INTENSIVE CARE UNIT MANAGEMENT

Children treated with vasopressin for postneurosurgical DI should be switched from IV to oral fluid intake at the earliest opportunity. With an intact thirst mechanism and access to free water, the patient will better regulate blood osmolality. Once oral intake has been resumed without nausea and vomiting (often by the morning of the day after surgery), the vasopressin infusion should be stopped; all IV infusions should be stopped to avoid iatrogenic fluid overload, and oral fluids are permitted freely. Desmopressin is reinstituted (nasally or orally) in the child with preexisting DI or begun in the child who has new-onset DI (see Table 25-3).

## Syndrome of Inappropriate Antidiuretic Hormone Secretion

SIADH is characterized by hypotonic hyponatremia, urine osmolality in excess of plasma osmolality, natriuresis in the absence of edema and volume depletion, and normal renal and adrenal function.[113] The dilutional hyponatremia of SIADH develops because of persistent detectable or increased plasma arginine vasopressin (AVP; also known as antidiuretic hormone [ADH]) concentrations in the presence of continued fluid intake. Chronic hyponatremia, however, is the result of a combination of water retention and sodium excretion.[114] The major causes of SIADH are neurologic diseases, neoplasia, lung diseases, and medications (Table 25-4).[115] Inappropriate infusion of hypotonic fluids in the postoperative period is among the most common causes.[116] The clinical manifestations are principally neuromuscular (headache, nausea, vomiting, muscle cramps, lethargy, restlessness, disorientation, and depressed reflexes). The severity of symptoms is related to both the absolute serum sodium concentration (most patients with serum sodium greater than 125 mEq/L are asymptomatic) and its rate of decrease, especially if greater than 0.5 mEq/L/hr.

Although ADH secretion impairs water excretion, the mechanisms that regulate volume (renin-angiotensin-aldosterone system and atrial natriuretic peptide) are intact. Volume expansion activates natriuretic mechanisms (decreased proximal sodium reabsorption and decreased aldosterone production), resulting in sodium and water excretion and the restoration of near-euvolemia. With *chronic* SIADH, sodium loss is a more prominent feature

| TABLE 25-4 | Causes of Syndrome of Inappropriate Antidiuretic Hormone Secretion (SIADH) |
| --- | --- |

**Central Nervous System Disturbances**

Head injury
Brain tumor
Subarachnoid hemorrhage
Stroke
Infection (meningitis, encephalitis)
Acute psychosis

**Drugs**

Vasopressin, desmopressin
Carbamazepine, oxcarbamazepine
Cyclophosphamide
*Vinca* alkaloids
Cisplatin
Phenothiazines
Serotonin uptake inhibitors (e.g., fluoxetine, sertraline)
Tricyclic antidepressants
Monoamine oxidase inhibitors
Methylenedioxymethamphetamine ("ecstasy")
Nicotine

**Major Surgery**

Major abdominal or thoracic surgery
Pituitary surgery
Pain
Severe nausea

**Pulmonary Disease**

Pneumonia, tuberculosis
Asthma
Atelectasis
Pneumothorax
Positive-pressure ventilation

**Neoplasia**

Carcinoma of lung (e.g., small cell carcinoma)
Leukemia
Thymoma
Lymphoma
Other tumors

**Infection**

Human immunodeficiency virus

**Hereditary SIADH**

Functional mutations in the gene for vasopressin-2 receptor

than is water retention. Severe hyponatremia increases cell size because of entry of water into the cell along its osmotic gradient, and may be associated with loss of intracellular potassium and other solutes in an attempt to restore cell volume.

### PERIOPERATIVE MANAGEMENT

Many of the causes of SIADH are transient and resolve as the underlying condition is corrected. Treatment of chronic SIADH consists of water restriction; that is, fluid intake is restricted to less than or equal to 1 L/m²/24 hours. Unless sodium intake is adequate, water restriction can lead to volume depletion in children with a sodium deficit. In asymptomatic chronic (more than 3 days) dilutional hyponatremia and in chronic SIADH, specific therapy may not be required.

Hypertonic (3%) saline should be used with caution in children. Rapid correction of chronic hyponatremia can lead to serious, permanent, and even fatal neurologic complications from osmotic demyelination (central pontine myelinolysis).[117] Only children with neurologic symptoms (e.g., altered level of consciousness, coma, or seizures) attributable to acute hyponatremia of less than 3 days' duration require rapid initial correction of the sodium deficit (use 3% hypertonic saline to deliver 5 mEq/kg per hour). The rate of increase of serum sodium concentration in states of chronic hyponatremia should not exceed 0.5 mEq/L/hr (or 8 to 10 mEq/L/24 hours).[118,119] The saline infusion should stop when the absolute concentration of serum sodium reaches 120 to 125 mEq/L. Hypertonic saline is usually combined with furosemide to limit treatment-induced expansion of the extracellular fluid volume.[119] Thereafter, treatment should consist of fluid restriction.

## Thyroid Disorders

Thyroid hormones play an important role in metabolic processes, growth, and development in children.[120] The thyroid gland develops from the embryonic pharyngeal floor and descends along the thyroglossal duct to its final position in the anterior neck. Thyroid hormone production is controlled by the hypothalamic-pituitary-thyroid axis. Two principal thyroid hormones are produced. Although thyroxine ($T_4$) is the predominant circulating thyroid hormone, triiodothyronine ($T_3$), primarily formed by peripheral conversion from $T_4$ by a family of deiodinases, is the major physiologically active thyroid hormone. Serum $T_3$ and $T_4$ concentrations in turn regulate hypothalamic thyrotropin-releasing hormone (TRH) and pituitary thyroid stimulating hormone (TSH) secretion via negative feedback. Thyroid hormones are transported in the blood by carrier proteins, including thyroxine-binding globulin (TBG), prealbumin, and albumin. Protein-bound $T_4$ and $T_3$ are not biologically active. Only 0.03% of circulating $T_4$ and 0.3% of $T_3$ are unbound and active.[121,122]

### HYPOTHYROIDISM

#### Classification and Epidemiology
Hypothyroidism, the most common thyroid disorder in children, can range from subclinical to overt disease. In subclinical hypothyroidism, children maintain a normal $T_4$ level by increasing TSH release. Over time, however, thyroid function can decompensate despite increased TSH stimulation and progress to overt thyroid hormone deficiency.[123-125] Iodine deficiency continues to be the foremost cause of hypothyroidism worldwide.[126] However, in the United States and other regions in which the intake of iodine is adequate, autoimmune thyroid disease is the most common cause of hypothyroidism.[124] Other less frequent causes of hypothyroidism include secondary and tertiary processes resulting from pituitary or hypothalamic insufficiency, respectively, which are relevant in many surgical situations, especially tumors of the central nervous system (CNS).

#### Biochemical Tests of Thyroid Function
In general, measurement of serum TSH and either total $T_4$ or free $T_4$ suffices for assessment of thyroid function. However, several conditions exist in which thyroid hormone levels appear abnormal yet the individual is clinically euthyroid. These conditions may lead to erroneous diagnosis and inappropriate treatment for hypothyroidism or hyperthyroidism. TSH is the most sensitive test for diagnosing primary thyroid disorders and generally

precedes noticeable changes in total $T_4$ and $T_3$ levels. Thyroid function can also be assessed by measurement of unbound or free $T_4$. When the total $T_4$ level is reduced but free $T_4$ and TSH values are normal, TBG deficiency is the most likely diagnosis. No treatment is required for TBG deficiency because these individuals have normal concentrations of free T4 and are euthyroid. Likewise, medical intervention is unnecessary for familial dysalbuminemic hyperthyroxinemia, which manifests with increased total $T_4$ levels but normal free $T_4$ and TSH values.[127]

Importantly, if the hypothalamic-pituitary axis is not intact, TSH becomes a useless measurement of thyroid function. Therefore, in cases of secondary or tertiary (central) thyroid disorders, diagnosis and treatment is based solely on serum $T_4$ levels and clinical signs. During times of stress or acute illness, increased conversion of $T_3$ to a metabolically inactive form (reverse $T_3$) occurs. In addition, $T_4$ and TSH values may both be reduced, reflecting a decreased metabolic state. Individuals are considered euthyroid based on non-elevated TSH values but the differential diagnosis includes central hypothyroidism, a distinction that often cannot be made by laboratory evaluation. Controversy still exists regarding possible benefits of using $T_4$ or $T_3$ to treat euthyroid sick syndrome, in which there are abnormal thyroid tests in the setting of a nonthyroid illness, such as a critical illness. Typically, children with euthyroid sick syndrome have a reduced $T_4$ level with a normal or low-normal TSH level, indicating a decreased metabolic state.[128-131]

#### Clinical Manifestations
Because thyroid hormone affects all metabolically active cells, hormone deficiency leads to a wide array of systemic abnormalities. Classic signs and symptoms of hypothyroidism in children include short stature resulting from a decline in growth rate, fatigue, cold intolerance, weight gain, dry skin, hair loss, constipation, hoarse voice, and coarse facial features. Myxedema coma is a severe manifestation of hypothyroidism that can occur in profoundly hypothyroid individuals exposed to an external stress, such as infection, surgery, hypnotics, or cold temperature. Myxedema coma can result in severe life-threatening heart failure or coma[132,133] and should be considered in any postoperative child with unexplained cardiovascular dysfunction, difficulty weaning from ventilator support, or delirium.[97] Other medical conditions associated with hypothyroidism include anemia, hyperlipidemia, and pubertal disorders.

#### Neonatal Hypothyroidism
Congenital hypothyroidism remains the most frequent cause of preventable mental developmental delay. Thyroid dysgenesis or agenesis accounts for the majority of cases, whereas a smaller percentage results from thyroid dyshormonogenesis and secondary or tertiary hypothyroidism.[134] Because neonates do not exhibit the classic signs or symptoms of hypothyroidism, testing for congenital hypothyroidism occurs with the neonatal screen. Newborn screening programs that employ a strategy based on TSH thresholds detect only primary thyroid deficiency and not the central hypothyroidism that accompanies hypopituitarism or CNS anomalies, such as septo-optic dysplasia. Early detection and implementation of thyroid replacement are essential to avoid permanent neurologic sequelae. The classic syndrome includes macroglossia, umbilical hernia, constipation, hypothermia, a low hoarse cry, and neonatal jaundice (Fig. 25-10). In general, affected children who receive adequate thyroid replacement starting early in the neonatal period lead normal lives.

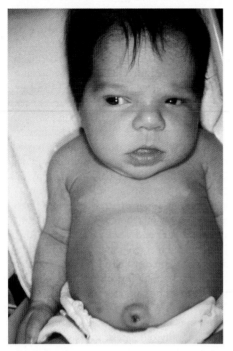

FIGURE 25-10 An infant with congenital hypothyroidism. ("Congenital hypothyroidism," Wikipedia: The Free Encyclopedia. Wikimedia Foundation, Inc. 24 Feb 2012, as of 31 Mar. 2012. http://en.wikipedia.org/wiki/Congenital_hypothyroidism.)

### Treatment

The goal of thyroid replacement is to normalize $T_4$ within 1-2 weeks and TSH within 4 weeks, and consequently reverse the metabolic derangements caused by hypothyroidism. In general, daily levothyroxine ($LT_4$) replacement leads to normalization in $T_4$ levels within a week but equilibration of TSH occurs more slowly, over 4 to 6 weeks.[135] The appropriate starting $LT_4$ dose varies with age and disease state. For neonates, the starting dose is 10 to 15 µg/kg/day, which is much greater than the conventional replacement dose of 2 to 4 µg/kg/day in older children and adolescents.[136] In healthy children with acute hypothyroidism (e.g., post thyroidectomy), full $LT_4$ replacement can be started immediately. However, symptomatic children with chronic hypothyroidism may develop pseudotumor cerebri or slipped capital femoral epiphysis if they are started on full $LT_4$ doses. Therefore treatment should begin at one-fourth of the expected dose, with slow titration every 4 to 6 weeks.[137,138] After dose stabilization, children and adolescents should continue to have regular clinical examinations and TSH monitoring owing to increased dose requirements during puberty and pregnancy.[139,140] Thyroid replacement can be given parenterally if needed. The IV dose of $LT_4$ is approximately half of the oral dose and should be given once daily.

### Preoperative Management

Because thyroid hormones play a critical role in regulating metabolism, children should be clinically and biochemically euthyroid before any type of elective surgery. Several case studies have shown decreased cardiac function, diminished breathing capacity, and increased sensitivity to anesthetic agents with moderate to severe hypothyroidism.[141-143] Children with known hypothyroidism should have documented normal thyroid function tests before surgery. For those with undiagnosed hypothyroidism,

a detailed history should be obtained regarding previous thyroid disorders, head and neck radiation, radioiodine therapy, thyroid surgery, and family history of thyroid disease.[144] In addition, children with autoimmune disorders, type 1 diabetes mellitus, celiac disease, and children with genetic syndromes such as trisomy 21 and Turner syndrome are at increased risk for developing autoimmune thyroiditis and should be screened if symptomatic.[145-147]

Children with subclinical or mild hypothyroidism often must undergo urgent surgery without delay. Thyroid replacement can be started and continued with the same regimen as described in the outpatient setting. For children with moderate to severe hypothyroidism, however, surgery should be postponed, if possible, until thyroid hormone levels normalize on replacement therapy. However, if urgent surgery is required, perioperative treatment with IV $LT_4$ with or without glucocorticoids should be given to prevent myxedema coma.[97,144] An exception to this strategy applies to the child who is scheduled for cardiovascular surgery or cardiac catheterization in which thyroid replacement could precipitate or worsen unstable coronary syndromes. Several studies in adults reported no adverse outcomes in cardiac patients undergoing surgery without thyroid replacement.[97,144,148] Therefore thyroid replacement could be initiated postoperatively in children with cardiovascular disease undergoing cardiac surgery or cardiac evaluation.

## HYPERTHYROIDISM

### Classification and Epidemiology

Hyperthyroidism is a condition caused by excess circulating thyroid hormones resulting in an increase in metabolic activity of various peripheral tissues in the body. Almost all children with hyperthyroidism have suppressed serum TSH concentrations resulting from negative feedback by increased concentrations of $T_4$ and $T_3$. Hyperthyroidism can be either overt or subclinical.[149] Overt hyperthyroidism is characterized by both clinical and biochemical manifestations of the disease. A child with subclinical hyperthyroidism typically is asymptomatic but with a suppressed TSH level.

Hyperthyroidism occurs less frequently than hypothyroidism in children and is nearly always caused by Graves disease. Other causes of childhood thyrotoxicosis include autoimmune thyroiditis (Hashimoto thyroiditis), infections of the thyroid gland, autonomously functioning thyroid nodules, iodine-induced hyperthyroidism, McCune-Albright syndrome, TSH-producing pituitary adenomas, and thyroid hormone ingestion.[150] A rare thyroid disorder that mimics hyperthyroidism is thyroid hormone resistance. However, unlike other causes of childhood thyrotoxicosis, thyroid hormone resistance should not be treated with antithyroid medications.[151,152]

### Graves Disease

Graves disease, an autoimmune disorder, is the most common cause of childhood hyperthyroidism. The pathophysiology of Graves disease involves thyroid-stimulating immunoglobulins that bind to the TSH receptor causing hyperstimulation of the thyroid gland. Most children with Graves disease have a diffuse goiter, and some develop autoimmune ophthalmopathy and myxedema. Because few children with Graves disease enter spontaneous remission, treatment of hyperthyroidism is required. Current treatment options include antithyroid medications (methimazole; propylthiouracil [PTU] is no longer recommended for treatment of Graves disease in children because of the risk of hepatotoxicity), surgical removal of the thyroid gland, or radioiodine.[153,154] Although virtually all children enter remission during therapy with antithyroid drugs, side effects are relatively common (see later discussion) and the majority of children treated for 2 to 3 years relapse shortly after discontinuation of therapy.[155,156] Radioactive ablation is usually definitive and carries less risk than surgery.[157]

## Thyroiditis

The term *thyroiditis* is used to describe a heterogeneous group of disorders that result in inflammation of the thyroid gland with subsequent release of preformed thyroid hormone. Transient hyperthyroidism can result from the initial inflammatory process, but symptoms generally last up to about 8 weeks, until preformed stored thyroid hormone is depleted. Some children will develop hypothyroidism after the recovery phase because of lymphocytic infiltration of the gland and destruction of thyroid tissue. Treatment with antithyroid drugs (thioamides) that block formation of thyroid hormone is not indicated for transient hyperthyroidism, but for symptomatic children, β-blockers should be used during the thyrotoxic phase to control symptoms.[158]

Thyroiditis can also manifest as painful inflammation of the gland and fever owing to bacterial or viral infection. *Haemophilus influenzae*, group A streptococci, and *Staphylococcus* are the most frequent causes of acute thyroiditis, which can be associated with thyroid gland cutaneous fistulas.[159] Viral infections of the thyroid gland are less severe and result in subacute thyroiditis.[160] Owing to the difficulty in distinguishing bacterial from viral infections, all cases of infectious thyroiditis are treated with antibiotics.

## Clinical Manifestations

Most of the symptoms that children experience are the same regardless of the cause of hyperthyroidism. Classic signs and symptoms of hyperthyroidism include goiter, tachycardia and/or palpitations, tremor, brisk reflexes, heat intolerance, dyspnea, insomnia, diarrhea, nervousness, and weight loss despite a normal or increased appetite. Many children with hyperthyroidism have inability to concentrate, resulting in poor school performance, and may be initially mistaken to have attention deficit hyperactivity disorder. Other medical conditions associated with long-standing hyperthyroidism include osteoporosis and irregular menses.[161]

Individuals with Graves disease may develop additional autoimmune manifestations, such as ophthalmopathy and pretibial myxedema. Eye involvement in Graves disease is characterized by inflammation of the extraocular muscles, connective tissue, and orbital fat, which results in proptosis, restricted eye movement, and periorbital edema.[162,163] Children with Graves ophthalmopathy may complain of eye irritation or dryness because of lid retraction (Fig. 25-11). If left untreated, corneal ulceration may develop and lead to irreversible eye damage, including blindness. Unfortunately, ophthalmopathy usually persists in spite of treatment of the hyperthyroidism.[153,164]

## Treatment

Antithyroid medications remain the first line of treatment for many physicians, because one-third of children enter remission after several years of drug therapy.[155,165] Long-term remission rates are greater in pubertal than prepubertal children. Other favorable prognostic indicators include a small thyroid gland and normal levels of TSH receptor antibodies at the time of diagnosis.[166,167] Methimazole (a thioamide) is the mainstay of antithyroid therapy. Minor adverse effects occur in 25% of children treated with

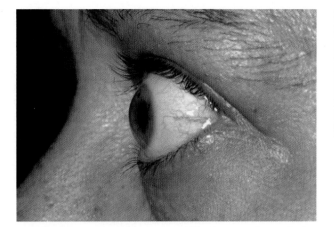

**FIGURE 25-11** Proptosis of the eyes in a child with Graves disease. (With permission of author and publisher, HealthInfoTimes, Symptoms of Graves disease, 14 Feb 2012, http://healthinfotimes.com/symptoms-of-graves-disease-in-children-14945.html.)

thioamides and include increases in liver enzymes, neutropenia, rash, and lymphadenopathy. Serious adverse effects, such as agranulocytosis and liver failure, are rare, occurring in up to 1% of individuals.[168]

## Perioperative Management

For children who relapse after antithyroid drug therapy or who require immediate definitive therapy, radioiodine is a safe and effective alternative to thyroidectomy. Treatment consists of iodine-131 uptake in the thyroid gland, which leads to cell destruction by internal radiation. Several longitudinal studies have shown that children are not at increased risk for developing thyroid cancer if appropriate ablative doses of radioiodine are used.[169,170] In cases in which radioiodine is contraindicated, surgical removal of the entire thyroid gland can also cure the hyperthyroid state. Children should be euthyroid or slightly hypothyroid before surgery to avoid precipitation of thyroid storm. In addition, because of potential serious complications from neck surgery, only surgeons with expertise in performing thyroidectomies in children should perform the surgery.[171]

In special circumstances, perioperative rapid control of hyperthyroidism can be achieved by using large doses of oral iodine (Lugol solution or saturated potassium iodine), which inhibit thyroid hormone synthesis. The effect is short-lived (several days) because of eventual escape from the Wolff-Chaikoff effect (iodine inhibition of thyroid hormone release); therefore, the addition of a thioamide is necessary for long-term treatment. Rarely, untreated or undertreated hyperthyroidism can lead to thyroid storm (approximately 1 in 1,000,000 young children), a potentially lethal complication.[172] Thyroid storm may be difficult to differentiate from an acute malignant hyperthermia (MH) reaction.[173,174] However, in contrast to MH, thyroid storm has a varied onset (usually an insidious onset 6 to 18 hours postoperatively, although it may develop precipitously during surgery), it induces a less severe acidosis than MH, and the serum creatine phosphokinase remains unchanged. Because the serum creatine phosphokinase peaks at 12 to 18 hours after an MH reaction, it is a late sign to differentiate from MH. Interestingly, IV dantrolene will ameliorate some of the clinical manifestations of thyroid storm, including rigidity and hyperthermia.[174,175] Thyroid storm usually responds to symptomatic treatment, including parenteral β-blockers, large doses of glucocorticoids (block conversion of

**TABLE 25-5** Management of Hyperthyroid Crisis

| Drug Class | Recommended Drug | Starting Dose | Mechanism of Action |
|---|---|---|---|
| Iodine | Potassium iodide (SSKI) | 3-5 drops by mouth q6h | Blocks release of thyroid hormone from gland |
| | Lugol solution | 4-8 drops by mouth q6-8h | Blocks release of thyroid hormone from gland |
| β Blockers | Propranolol | Infant: 2 mg/kg/day by mouth divided q8-12h<br>Child: 10-40 mg by mouth q6-8h | β-adrenergic blockade; decreased $T_4$ to $T_3$ conversion |
| | Esmolol | 100-200 µg/kg/min IV infusion | β-adrenergic blockade |
| Thioamide | Propylthiouracil | 5-10 mg/kg/day by mouth divided q8h | Inhibits new hormone synthesis; decreases $T_4$ to $T_3$ conversion |
| | Methimazole | 0.4 mg/kg/day by mouth divided q8-12h | Inhibits new hormone synthesis |
| Supportive treatment | Intravenous fluid | 20-40 mL/kg normal saline | Replacement of increased insensible losses resulting from fever, diaphoresis, vomiting, and diarrhea |
| | Cooling blankets, ice packs | | Reduce fever |
| | Acetaminophen | 15 mg/kg/dose by mouth q4-6h or 40 mg/kg per rectum loading dose then 20 mg/kg/dose q6h<br>Intravenous acetaminophen may be utilized in children with IV access. | |
| | Hydrocortisone | Adult: 100 mg IV q8h (no pediatric dose recommended) | Decreases $T_4$ to $T_3$ conversion; enhances vasomotor stability |

*SSKI*, Saturated solution of potassium iodide.

$T_4$ to $T_3$ and prevent relative adrenal insufficiency), and propylthiouracil, the last intervention administered with a nasogastric tube.[173] If left untreated, the mortality rate resulting from thyroid storm is 20% to 30%.[172] Several factors may precipitate thyroid storm, including surgery, infection, and stress. Because of the dramatically increased metabolic state, acute management of hyperthyroidism and targeted symptomatic treatment is essential to avoid death.[132,150,173] If the presentation proves difficult to distinguish from MH (both diseases may present with tachycardia, rigidity, and fever), it would be prudent to administer dantrolene 2.5 mg/kg IV in case the presumptive diagnosis of thyroid storm is incorrect.[175] However, if the hypermetabolic signs abate after dantrolene, one cannot conclude that the reaction was MH, as dantrolene does attenuate the hypermetabolic signs of thyroid storm.[174] The specific treatment for thyroid storm, however, remains a multidrug approach to (1) halt production and release of thyroid hormone, (2) prevent conversion of $T_4$ to $T_3$, (3) antagonize the peripheral (adrenergic) effects of thyroid hormone, and (4) control systemic disturbances with supportive therapy (Table 25-5).[133,153,168,176-179]

## Parathyroid and Calcium Disorders

### PHYSIOLOGY OF CALCIUM HOMEOSTASIS

The four parathyroid glands are usually present in pairs on the posterior aspect of the superior and inferior poles of the thyroid gland, with the inferior pair occasionally ectopic elsewhere in the neck or chest. Parathyroid hormone (PTH) is released from secretory granules in response to a decrease in serum ionized calcium; its secretion is inhibited by hyperphosphatemia, profound hypomagnesemia or hypermagnesemia, or increased 1,25-dihydroxyvitamin D (calcitriol). The calcium-sensing receptor in the parathyroid mediates PTH release and also directly regulates calcium reabsorption in the distal tubule. Inactivating mutations in the calcium-sensing receptor gene result in a greater

serum calcium set point in familial hypocalciuric hypercalcemia, now a relatively common and incidental diagnosis that is benign unless homozygotic, whereas activating mutations result in autosomal dominant hypocalcemia with hypercalciuria.[180,181] PTH has three primary modes of increasing serum calcium: (1) calcium reabsorption in the proximal convoluted tubule, and concomitant phosphaturia in the proximal tubule; (2) upregulation of osteoclast-mediated calcium and phosphate release from bone; and (3) renal conversion of 25-hydroxyvitamin D to the active metabolite, calcitriol. In turn, calcitriol increases absorption of calcium and phosphate from the gut and has direct calcium-releasing effects on bone. Calcitonin is secreted by the thyroid C cells and has calcium-reducing properties via its own G protein–coupled receptor. It has no known physiologic role at this time.

### HYPOCALCEMIA
#### Neonatal Hypocalcemia
Neonatal hypocalcemia owing to prematurity and maternal diabetes is common but is typically transient. Rare causes include maternal hyperparathyroidism, excessive diuretic use or phosphate load, and transient neonatal hypoparathyroidism.[182] Neonatal hypocalcemia requires exclusion of 22q11.2 deletion syndrome (which includes DiGeorge syndrome, velocardiofacial syndrome [VCF], and other clinical manifestations) by genetic testing.[183-185] The hypocalcemia of VCF results from an incomplete hypoparathyroidism that tends to normalize eventually but may recur. Reduced PTH or PTH resistance (pseudohypoparathyroidism) cause hyperphosphatemia beyond the already increased normal range in neonates, whereas vitamin D deficiency or resistance is associated with low to normal serum phosphate levels. Maternal 25-hydroxyvitamin D deficiency is another common cause of early or late infantile hypocalcemia in the United States, regardless of the infant's dietary intake.[186,187] Childhood hypocalcemia with reduced PTH may be the first

endocrine sign of polyglandular autoimmune disease type I, now called autoimmune polyendocrinopathy-candidiasis-ectodermal dystrophy (APECED).[188]

### Childhood Hypocalcemia

Persistent hypocalcemia in infants and children can have many manifestations, including poor feeding, tetany, seizures, laryngospasm, paresthesias, and muscle cramping. Initial evaluation of hypocalcemia, regardless of age, includes measurement of serum calcium, phosphate, magnesium, alkaline phosphatase, creatinine, PTH, 25-hydroxyvitamin D, and 1,25-dihydroxyvitamin D, plus urine calcium, phosphate, and creatinine. Therapy for acute hypocalcemia includes parenteral calcium, followed by oral calcium supplementation and 25-hydroxyvitamin D if reduced,[187] and calcitriol as a substitute for PTH, because PTH itself, an anabolic bone agent in adults,[189] is contraindicated in children owing to concerns about its possible role in osteosarcoma.

### Perioperative Management

Hypocalcemia is most frequently managed by IV infusion of calcium in the form of calcium chloride or calcium gluconate, with frequent measurement of serum ionized calcium levels to guide therapy (see Chapter 10). Calcium salts release free calcium ions and should be given via a central venous catheter because their hypertonicity and the increase concentration of ionized calcium causes intense local vasoconstriction that may lead to necrosis of the skin and subcutaneous tissues and possible gangrene of the affected limb if administered via a peripheral IV cannula that becomes interstitial. In the postoperative period after the child is tolerating oral intake, IV calcium supplementation may be converted to oral supplementation.

### HYPERCALCEMIA

Hyperparathyroidism (HPT) is much less common in children than in adults.[190] In most cases of HPT in children, an adenoma is present that is unresponsive to the increased serum calcium level. Other uncommon causes of HPT in children include generalized parathyroid hyperplasia and, rarely, parathyroid carcinoma.[191]

Parathyroid hyperplasia occurs in familial forms of HPT, including multiple endocrine neoplasia type 1 (MEN 1), in which HPT is a nearly universal manifestation of the mutation of the menin gene; the hyperparathyroid abnormality occurs more commonly and earlier in presentation than the associated pancreatic, pituitary, and gastrointestinal neuroendocrine tumors associated with MEN 1.[192,193] HPT is a less common manifestation of MEN 2A, in which medullary thyroid carcinoma and pheochromocytoma occur as a result of the proto-oncogene mutation.[194] Secondary HPT with relatively normal calcium levels is a common pediatric phenomenon that accompanies renal failure, renal tubular acidosis, and hypophosphatemic rickets.[195] When hypercalcemia is present, the differential diagnosis includes Williams syndrome, vitamin A intoxication, vitamin D excess and conversion to 1,25-dihydroxyvitamin D in granulomatous disorders, and infantile subcutaneous fat necrosis.[196] Solid tumors may secrete increased concentrations of parathyroid hormone–related protein (PTHrP). Tumors, such as leukemias, lymphomas, and others, may release excess cytokines and osteoclast-activating factors, with the hypercalcemia leading to the tumor diagnosis.[197,198]

Signs and symptoms of hypercalcemia are usually nonspecific, such as nausea and vomiting, polyuria, and fatigue. Initial laboratory evaluation of hypercalcemia matches the list for hypocalcemia given earlier.[199]

Evaluation of unexplained hypercalcemia includes measurement of PTHrP for malignancy, and of parental calcium levels for familial hypocalciuric hypercalcemia, additional hormones or genetic testing for MEN syndromes, tumor markers, bone marrow biopsy, and relevant imaging. When HPT is found, ultrasonography is helpful to assess the parathyroid glands, but MRI or technetium-sestamibi scan is more precise, and intraoperative measurement of PTH levels can be provided for tumor localization.

### Perioperative Management

Management of acute hypercalcemia begins with isotonic rehydration and administration of furosemide to induce calciuria. Treatment then proceeds to administration of calcitonin, to which tachyphylaxis may occur within 1 or 2 days, or to glucocorticoids. In the absence of a definitive therapy, such as surgical excision of the pathologic source of PTH, chronic hypercalcemia is responsive to bisphosphonates, such as pamidronate, which can be given by infusion every 3 months.[200,201] Acute management after parathyroidectomy requires careful monitoring and replacement of calcium and possibly the use of calcitriol for persistent hypocalcemia. In isolated parathyroid hyperplasia, MEN, or secondary HPT, surgeons may elect to leave a portion of one gland in the forearm to avoid permanent hypoparathyroidism, which is challenging to manage.

## Adrenal Endocrinopathies

### PHYSIOLOGY

Adrenal steroidogenesis begins with cholesterol as precursor and results in three types of steroids: mineralocorticoids, glucocorticoids, and sex steroids (androgen precursors).[202] Most of the enzymes involved in adrenal (or gonadal) steroidogenesis are cytochrome P450s. The adrenal cortex comprises three zones: the outer zona glomerulosa exclusively synthesizes mineralocorticoids owing to localized expression of CYP11B2, whereas the zona fasciculata and reticularis synthesize glucocorticoid and androgens owing to localized expression of CYP17.[203] Cortisol, the end-product of the glucocorticoid pathway, is the primary regulator of the hypothalamic-pituitary-adrenal (HPA) axis, in which hypothalamic corticotropin-releasing hormone regulates pituitary adrenocorticotropic hormone (ACTH) secretion and downstream adrenal production of all three categories of steroid. ACTH release follows a diurnal pattern with a peak at 0400 to 0800 hours and, most importantly, markedly increases in response to trauma, acute illness, high fever, and hypoglycemia.

Mineralocorticoid production is primarily controlled by the renin-angiotensin system, in which angiotensinogen secreted by the liver is cleaved by renin to angiotensin I, which is then converted to angiotensin II.[204] The mineralocorticoid pathway is also responsive to ACTH, as demonstrated by a rise in all mineralocorticoid precursors and the end-product aldosterone within minutes of exogenous ACTH stimulation. However, hypopituitarism does not lead to mineralocorticoid deficiency because an intact renin-angiotensin system independently stimulates aldosterone synthesis. Nevertheless, patients with ACTH deficiency may present with hyponatremia (glucocorticoids are required for free water excretion) and hypotension. The latter consequence of failure of the adrenal to release an adequate amount of glucocorticoid may be attributable to the role of cortisol in enhancing vascular responsiveness to catecholamines and inotropic activity.[205] This essential aspect of glucocorticoid activity is the most lethal potential consequence of both primary adrenal insufficiency and hypothalamic-pituitary deficiency and requires the utmost caution on the part of pediatrician, endocrinologist, surgeon, or anesthesiologist. When any question regarding adequacy of the HPA arises, it is prudent to provide exogenous glucocorticoid, particularly perioperatively.[206]

## CAUSES OF ADRENAL INSUFFICIENCY

Primary adrenal insufficiency is suspected from features such as weight loss, nausea and vomiting, poor appetite, and, specifically, the characteristic skin hyperpigmentation that is secondary to melanocyte-stimulating hormone receptor cross-stimulation by ACTH (which is present in extraordinarily large concentrations).[207] Primary adrenal insufficiency is uncommon in countries with advanced health care systems now that infectious diseases, such as tuberculosis, are less prevalent, but adrenal hemorrhage still causes adrenal failure.[208] Autoimmune adrenal insufficiency, sometimes as part of a polyendocrinopathy syndrome, is now the most common cause and includes both glucocorticoid and mineralocorticoid deficiency. Glucocorticoid deficiency with or without mineralocorticoid loss is characteristic of congenital adrenal hyperplasia.[209] Rare disorders causing adrenal insufficiency include adrenoleukodystrophy,[210] congenital adrenal hypoplasia, X-linked adrenal hypoplasia congenita, and ACTH receptor defects.[211]

Congenital or acquired lesions of the hypothalamus or pituitary may lead to ACTH deficiency. In general, these lesions cause other pituitary deficiencies, particularly growth hormone or TSH deficiency; isolated ACTH deficiency is rare. Both growth hormone and ACTH deficiency may cause hypoglycemia in infancy. CNS malformations leading to ACTH deficiency are usually detectable by MRI. A notable CNS anomaly with hypopituitarism is septo-optic dysplasia,[29,212-214] which may be associated with an assortment of midline defects, such as an absent or underdeveloped septum pellucidum and optic nerve hypoplasia, but isolated pituitary agenesis or hypoplasia is more common. Acquired lesions leading to hypopituitarism include hydrocephalus, meningitis, infiltrative disorders,[215] and tumors such as craniopharyngioma or histiocytosis X.[216] Tumor resection, especially craniopharyngioma, cranial irradiation, and chemotherapy, can lead to multiple pituitary deficiencies, often evolving over many years.[217]

## TESTING FOR ADRENAL INSUFFICIENCY

Cortisol levels follow a diurnal pattern, with peak levels resulting from an ACTH surge in the early morning and trough levels later in the day. Although a morning serum cortisol level of less than 5 μg/dL is less than normal and suggestive of adrenal insufficiency, it may be difficult to interpret the significance of a random cortisol concentration. A reduced concentration at any other time of day is uninformative and should not be used to test for adrenal function. In contrast, laboratory confirmation of primary mineralocorticoid deficiency by obtaining a random serum sample will show a low aldosterone concentration despite markedly increased plasma renin activity.

Primary adrenal insufficiency may be effectively assessed in two ways,[218] either by simultaneous measurement of serum cortisol and plasma ACTH concentrations or by stimulating the adrenal with exogenous ACTH (cosyntropin [Cortrosyn], the biologically active fragment of ACTH containing the first

24 amino acids). A markedly increased random plasma ACTH concentration is definitive evidence of primary adrenal insufficiency, but levels can be moderately increased by the stress of phlebotomy itself. Therefore blood for plasma ACTH levels should be obtained from an indwelling catheter to avoid false-positive values.

Hypothalamic-pituitary insufficiency is more difficult to assess. The complete absence of ACTH levels, as in the obvious case of pituitary ablation or destruction, leads eventually to adrenal atrophy and complete unresponsiveness to cosyntropin stimulation, a finding that necessitates maintenance glucocorticoid replacement. However, an "adequate" response to cosyntropin implies only tonic ACTH secretion and does not guarantee the ability to generate a normal surge of ACTH during stress. As a consequence, any patient with a CNS lesion that might cause HPA deficiency should receive stress doses of glucocorticoid (see later discussion). In practical terms, a post–cosyntropin-treatment cortisol value of 10 to 20 μg/dL in an at-risk child suggests the need for stress coverage, whereas a value less than 10 μg/dL indicates long-term replacement.[218,219]

## PERIOPERATIVE MANAGEMENT OF ADRENAL INSUFFICIENCY

### Glucocorticoid Dosing

Endogenous cortisol secretion is 6 to 8 mg/m$^2$/day. Because a fraction of oral cortisol is degraded by the liver, the typical oral replacement dose is 10 to 12 mg/m$^2$/day. A replacement dose of hydrocortisone depends on age and body size but might be 5.0 to 7.5 mg two to three times a day orally for an adolescent with chronic adrenal insufficiency. No dose monitoring is required, but the child's growth rate should be tracked according to age. With concomitant or isolated mineralocorticoid deficiency, replacement uses fludrocortisone (Florinef) at an approximate dose of 0.1 mg orally per day, independent of body size, with intermittent monitoring of blood pressure and plasma renin activity. When the primary goal of glucocorticoid therapy is not replacement but suppression of ACTH secretion, as in congenital adrenal hyperplasia, the daily hydrocortisone dose is generally 15 to 20 mg/m$^2$, guided by monitoring of serum levels of 17-hydroxyprogesterone, androstenedione, dehydroepiandrosterone sulfate, and testosterone. Alternatives to hydrocortisone include prednisone, which is four to five times more potent than hydrocortisone. Dexamethasone is 30 to 40 times more potent than hydrocortisone, but has no mineralocorticoid activity and carries much more significant risk of adverse effects, such as osteopenia and aseptic necrosis of the femoral head, and so should not be used for chronic routine replacement therapy. Single-dose use of dexamethasone has not been associated with aseptic necrosis of the femoral head.

Conventional stress glucocorticoid coverage is 3 to 10 times the patient's usual replacement dose, depending on the severity of illness or trauma, although this practice is not evidence based.[220] Therefore, with little risk associated with the transient use of excess glucocorticoid, for children who are on oral replacement therapy we recommend exogenous glucocorticoid replacement using three to five times the patient's usual oral maintenance dose for intercurrent illness or fever (greater than 101° F) and five to ten times the oral maintenance dose for major surgery, during critical illness, or in major emergencies. For children who require stress glucocorticoid coverage but who do not take outpatient steroids, or who are unable to take medications by mouth, we recommend using parenteral cortisol (Solu-Cortef) at a dose of 0.5 mg/kg/day every 12 hours for illness associated with nausea, vomiting, diarrhea, or fever (greater than 101° F) and 0.5 to 1 mg/kg every 6 hours for perioperative, intensive care, or emergency department indications for up to 72 hours.[221]

### Iatrogenic Adrenal Suppression and Tapering

Increased doses of exogenous glucocorticoids are used chronically for control of autoimmune disorders, suppression of transplant rejection, and control of inflammatory processes. Iatrogenic adrenal suppression depends on the duration and dose of glucocorticoid used. Periods of high-dose steroids up to 7 to 10 days do not suppress the HPA axis. Adrenal suppressive treatments lasting 3 to 6 weeks require a taper over 1 to 2 weeks to allow recovery of the HPA axis. Long-term high-dose treatment may require up to 6 to 9 months for complete return of HPA function and necessitates a taper during that period. At the termination of the taper, a repeat cosyntropin stimulation test should be performed to confirm recovery of function, and any repeat trauma or illness during the period of taper requires short-term stress coverage.

The glucocorticoid taper has two meanings. The tempo of therapeutic tapers of prednisone by gastroenterologists, rheumatologists, nephrologists, and oncologists, and of dexamethasone by surgeons, is entirely dependent on their assessment of the immune or inflammatory process. As long as the glucocorticoid dose is in excess of the replacement dose, and regardless of the dose, the HPA axis continues to be suppressed. It is only when the steroid dose is tapered down to the daily replacement dose (approximately 10 mg/m² hydrocortisone, 2 mg/m² prednisone, or less than 0.5 mg/m² dexamethasone) that the endocrine taper begins. At that point, the prednisone should be switched to hydrocortisone for ease of starting a gradual taper from replacement therapy to reduced doses while function of the HPA axis is reestablished. In the perioperative period, steroid coverage should be administered if there is any concern about the integrity of the HPA axis during a steroid taper (Table 25-6).

### HYPERCORTISOLISM (CUSHING SYNDROME)

Excess cortisol, whether exogenous or endogenous, results in muscle wasting, truncal obesity, moon facies, hypertension, hyperglycemia, osteopenia, and growth deceleration.[222,223] Iatrogenic hypercortisolism is common in pediatrics,[224] whereas Cushing disease or syndrome is rare.[225] Cushing disease refers to an ACTH-secreting pituitary adenoma. Cushing syndrome refers to other conditions of excess glucocorticoid, including ectopic ACTH-secreting tumors[226] and adrenal tumors that secrete cortisol.[227] An adrenal tumor (adenoma or carcinoma) is the most likely cause of hypercortisolism in a young child. These tumors can secrete any combination of steroids and commonly cosecrete

androgens, resulting in virilization.[228] A unilateral glucocorticoid-secreting tumor typically causes HPA axis suppression, requiring careful tapering of hydrocortisone replacement after resection to reestablish normal cortisol production in the contralateral adrenal gland.[229]

In a child with signs of hypercortisolism (and not simply obesity), screening tests include an overnight small dose dexamethasone suppression test, measurement of 24-hour urinary free cortisol and creatinine, and measurement of nocturnal salivary cortisol concentrations.[230] If screening tests suggest a diagnosis of hypercortisolism, additional adrenal steroids should be measured and an adrenal computed tomographic scan or magnetic resonance image obtained. In an adolescent with pure glucocorticoid effects and suspicious results of a corticotropin-releasing hormone stimulation test or longer dexamethasone suppression test[231] suggestive of a pituitary ACTH-secreting adenoma (Cushing disease), pituitary magnetic resonance imaging is warranted.[232] Because pituitary adenomas can be very small, bilateral inferior petrosal sinus sampling may be necessary to locate the adenoma.[233]

### PERIOPERATIVE MANAGEMENT OF HYPERCORTISOLISM

Therapy for Cushing disease and Cushing syndrome is surgical.[234,235] There are no specific anesthetic considerations except the supportive management of secondary manifestations, such as obesity and its attendant airway concerns, hypertension, and skin and bone fragility.

## ANNOTATED REFERENCES

[No authors listed]. Type 2 diabetes in children and adolescents. American Diabetes Association. Diabetes Care 2000;23:381-9.
*This consensus statement from the American Diabetes Association reviews the classification of diabetes in children, epidemiology of type 2 diabetes in U.S. children, along with recommendations for screening, treatment, and prevention of type 2 diabetes in children and adolescents.*

Andersen LJ, Andersen JL, Schutten HJ, et al. Antidiuretic effect of subnormal levels of arginine vasopressin in normal humans. Am J Physiol 1990;259:R53-60.
*The renal response to 120-minute infusions of arginine vasopressin (AVP) was investigated in healthy volunteers undergoing water diuresis induced by an oral water load. The human kidney is sensitive to changes in the rate of secretion of AVP of less than 1 pg/min/kg and maximal change occurs after 1 to 2 hours of constant infusion. It is estimated that the rate of infusion of AVP required to produce isosmolar urine during overhydration is approximately 3 pg/min/kg.*

Baylis PH. The syndrome of inappropriate antidiuretic hormone secretion. Int J Biochem Cell Biol 2003;35:1495-9.
*The author reviews the cardinal diagnostic criteria, clinical features, and pathophysiology of SIADH, which develops because of persistent detectable or elevated plasma arginine vasopressin concentrations in the presence of continued fluid intake. Inappropriate infusion of hypotonic fluids in the postoperative state is a common cause. For symptomatic patients with chronic SIADH, the mainstay of therapy is fluid restriction.*

LaFranchi S. Congenital hypothyroidism: etiologies, diagnosis, and management. Thyroid 1999;9:735-40.
*LaFranchi thoroughly reviews and discusses thyroid development and hypothyroidism in this article. He includes both embryologic and molecular defects of hypothyroidism.*

Rhodes ET, Ferrari LR, Wolfsdorf JI. Perioperative management of pediatric surgical patients with diabetes mellitus. Anesth Analg 2005;101: 986-99.
*The authors review the fundamental pathophysiology and perioperative management of type 1 and type 2 diabetes mellitus in children who are surgical patients.*

**TABLE 25-6** Steroid Equivalency Ratios and Doses

| Steroid | Relative Antiinflammatory Potency | Relative Mineralocorticoid Potency | Daily Replacement (mg/m²) |
|---|---|---|---|
| Hydrocortisone | 1 | 2 | 10 |
| Cortisone | 0.8 | 2 | 12 |
| Prednisone | 4 | 1 | 2.5 |
| Prednisolone | 5 | 1 | 2 |
| Dexamethasone | 20-30 | 0 | <0.5 |

Rivkees SA. The treatment of Graves' disease in children. J Pediatr Endocrinol Metab 2006;19:1095-111.

*This article reviews the pathophysiology of hyperthyroidism with particular focus on Graves disease. Rivkees outlines current treatment options for hyperthyroidism, including medical, surgical, and radioiodine ablation.*

Sarlis NJ, Gourgiotis L. Thyroid emergencies. Rev Endocr Metab Disord 2003;4:129-36.

*A concise review article on the presentation and management of extreme thyroid disorders, myxedema coma, and thyrotoxic storm.*

Seckl JR, Dunger DB, Lightman SL. Neurohypophyseal peptide function during early postoperative diabetes insipidus. Brain 1987;110: 737-46.

*Neurohypophyseal function, including serial measurements of plasma and urinary arginine vasopressin (AVP) and the AVP prohormone/carrier peptide neurophysin I concentrations, was investigated in 11 children undergoing pituitary or suprasellar surgery. The authors conclude that early postoperative diabetes insipidus is not a result of decreased levels of circulating AVP but may be related to the release of biologically inactive precursors from the damaged neurohypophysis. These may lead to renal refractoriness to AVP.*

Silverstein J, Klingensmith G, Copeland K, et al. Care of children and adolescents with type 1 diabetes: a statement of the American Diabetes Association. Diabetes Care 2005;28:186-212.

*This statement provides a comprehensive review of the diagnosis of diabetes, management of type 1 diabetes, and acute and chronic complications of type 1 diabetes.*

Sterns RH, Riggs JE, Schochet Jr SS. Osmotic demyelination syndrome following correction of hyponatremia. N Engl J Med 1986;314: 1535-42.

*This is a description of eight patients who developed a neurologic syndrome with clinical or pathologic findings typical of central pontine myelinolysis, which developed after they presented with severe hyponatremia. Each patient's condition worsened after relatively rapid correction of hyponatremia (greater than 12 mmol of sodium per liter per day). The data suggest that the neurologic sequelae were associated with correction of hyponatremia by more than 12 mmol/L/day. When correction proceeded more slowly, patients had uneventful recoveries. Osmotic demyelination syndrome is a preventable complication of overly rapid correction of chronic hyponatremia.*

Wolfsdorf J, Glaser N, Sperling MA. Diabetic ketoacidosis in infants, children, and adolescents: a consensus statement from the American Diabetes Association. Diabetes Care 2006;29:1150-9.

*The authors review the pathophysiology of diabetic ketoacidosis in childhood and discuss currently recommended treatment protocols. Current concepts regarding cerebral edema are presented, as are strategies for prediction and prevention of diabetic ketoacidosis.*

## REFERENCES

Please see www.expertconsult.com.

# Essentials of Nephrology

26

DELBERT R. WIGFALL, JOHN W. FOREMAN, AND ALLISON KINDER ROSS

THE ANESTHESIA PRACTITIONER IS OFTEN FACED with a patient who has acute kidney injury (AKI) or renal failure. Renal disease requires the practitioner to be vigilant about fluid homeostasis, acid-base balance, electrolyte management, choice of anesthetics, and potential complications. Maintaining a fine balance, particularly in the neonate and younger child, requires knowledge of the excretory and volume maintenance functions of the kidney. If not managed correctly, perioperative renal dysfunction can lead to multiorgan system compromise and significant morbidity or mortality. The anesthesia provider must understand renal physiology, appropriate preoperative preparation, intraoperative management, and postoperative care of the renal patient.

## Renal Physiology

The basic function of the kidney is to maintain fluid and electrolyte homeostasis. The first step in this tightly controlled process is the production of the glomerular filtrate from the renal plasma. The glomerular filtration rate (GFR) depends on renal plasma flow, which depends on blood pressure and circulating volume. The kidneys are the best perfused organs per gram of weight in the body. They receive 20% to 30% of the cardiac output maintained over a wide range of blood pressures through changes in renal vascular resistance. Numerous hormones play a role in this autoregulation, including vasodilators (i.e., prostaglandins E and $I_2$, dopamine, and nitric oxide) and vasoconstrictors (i.e., angiotensin II, thromboxane, adrenergic stimulation, and endothelin). Congestive heart failure and volume contraction severely limit the ability of the kidney to maintain autoregulation during changes in blood pressure.

When renal blood flow is adjusted for body surface area, it doubles during the first 2 weeks of postnatal life and continues to increase until it reaches adult values by the age of 2 years (see Figs. 6-10 and 6-11).[1,2] Increased blood flow results from an increase in cardiac output and a decrease in renal vascular resistance. Paralleling these changes, the GFR, when adjusted for body surface area, also doubles over the first 2 weeks of postnatal life and continues to increase until it reaches adult values by the age of 1 to 2 years. The initial GFR and the rate of increase correlate with gestational age at birth. For example, the GFR of an infant of 28 weeks gestation is half of that of a full-term infant (see Figs. 6-10 and 6-11).[3] An estimate of GFR can be made from the serum creatinine concentration and the height of the child according to the following formula[4,5]:

$$\text{GFR (mL/min/1.73 m}^2) = \text{height (cm)} \times \text{k/serum creatinine}$$

In the equation, k is 0.45 for infants, 0.55 for children, and 0.7 for adolescent boys. The serum creatinine concentration, especially in the first days of life, reflects the maternal serum creatinine concentration and therefore cannot be used to predict neonatal renal function until at least 2 days after birth.[6]

### FLUIDS AND ELECTROLYTES

The kidney regulates total body sodium balance and maintains normal extracellular and circulating volumes.[7] The adult kidney filters 25,000 mEq of sodium per day, but it excretes less than 1% through extremely efficient resorption mechanisms along the nephron. The proximal tubule resorbs 50% to 70%, the ascending limb of the loop of Henle resorbs about 25%, and the distal nephron accounts for 10% of the filtered load of sodium. Several hormones, including renin, angiotensin II, aldosterone, and atrial natriuretic peptide, and changes in circulating volume play roles in maintaining sodium balance.[8]

Serum osmolality is tightly regulated through changes in arginine vasopressin (AVP) release and the appreciation of thirst.[9-11] AVP, also called *antidiuretic hormone,* is synthesized in the hypothalamus and stored in the posterior pituitary, where it is released in response to an increasing plasma osmolality. AVP is also released in response to a decreased circulating volume or hypotension, including those responses to nausea, vomiting, and possibly opioids. AVP binds to receptors in the collecting duct, increasing the permeability of the tubules to water and leading to increased water resorption and concentrated urine. Neonates are much less able to conserve or excrete water compared with older children, rendering the fluid management and volume issues important tasks of the pediatric anesthesiologist in this young age-group.[12]

The regulation of serum potassium is managed by the kidney and depends on the concentration of plasma aldosterone. Aldosterone binds to receptors on cells in the distal nephron, increasing the secretion of potassium in the urine. Neonates are much less efficient at excreting potassium loads compared with adults, and the normal range of serum potassium concentrations is therefore greater in neonates; Table 26-1 provides the normal values.[13] Potassium regulation is affected by the acid-base status; excretion of potassium increases in the presence of alkalosis and decreases in the presence of acidosis. Causes of hyperkalemia and hypokalemia are presented in Tables 26-2 and 26-3, respectively.

### ACID-BASE BALANCE

The kidney is involved in the day-to-day regulation of acid-base balance and the response to the stress of illness. The kidney reclaims virtually all of the filtered bicarbonate in the proximal tubule. The kidney also regenerates the bicarbonate ($HCO_3^-$) lost in the neutralization of acid generated by the normal combustion of food, especially protein, and the formation of bone. New bicarbonate is generated by the cells of the distal nephron by decomposing the carbonic acid ($H_2CO_3$) formed from water ($H_2O$) and carbon dioxide ($CO_2$) by carbonic anhydrase. The protons ($H^+$) that are generated from this process are pumped into the lumen of the collecting duct, where they combine with hydrogen phosphate ($HPO_4^{2-}$) or ammonia ($NH_3$) generated by the catabolism of amino acids, mainly glutamine, in the tubule cells.

Infants, especially neonates, maintain a slightly acidotic pH (7.37) and decreased plasma bicarbonate concentration (22 mEq/L) compared with older children and adults (pH = 7.39; plasma bicarbonate = 24 to 28 mEq/L).[14] Neonates can maintain acid-base homeostasis but are limited in their ability to respond to an acid load.[15] This is especially true for preterm infants. This reduced plasma $HCO_3^-$ concentration in infants is the result of a reduced threshold, or the plasma concentration at which $HCO_3^-$ is no longer completely resorbed by the kidney.

**TABLE 26-1** Normal Values of Serum Potassium

| Age | Serum Potassium Range (mEq/L) |
| --- | --- |
| 0-1 month | 4.0-6.0 |
| 1 month-2 years | 4.0-5.5 |
| 2-17 years | 3.8-5.0 |
| >18 years | 3.2-4.8 |

**TABLE 26-2** Causes of Hyperkalemia

**Transcellular Shifts**

Acidosis

β-Adrenergic blockers

Insulin deficiency

Burns

Tumor lysis syndrome

Rhabdomyolysis

**Decreased Excretion**

Renal failure

Potassium-sparing diuretics

Cyclosporine

Nonsteroidal antiinflammatory drugs

Angiotensin-converting enzyme inhibitors

Mineralocorticoid deficiency
  Adrenal insufficiency
  Congenital adrenal hyperplasia
  Hyporeninemic hypoaldosteronism
  Primary mineralocorticoid deficiency

Mineralocorticoid resistance
  Prematurity
  Obstructive uropathy
  Pseudohypoaldosteronism

**Increased Intake**

Potassium supplements

Blood transfusions

Potassium-containing antibiotics

**TABLE 26-3** Causes of Hypokalemia

**Transcellular Shift**

Insulin

β-Adrenergic agonists

**Increased Excretion**

Vomiting

Diarrhea

Nasogastric suction

Laxatives

Diuretics

Cisplatin

Amphotericin B

Renal tubular acidosis

Bartter syndrome

Corticosteroids

**Decreased Intake**

Malnutrition

Anorexia nervosa

## Disease States

The causes of and differences in renal diseases between children and adults are substantive. Adult renal disease usually results from longstanding diabetes mellitus or hypertension with an associated compromise in cardiovascular function. Children may also have renal failure due to diseases such as sickle cell anemia or systemic lupus erythematosus, but cardiovascular function is far less commonly compromised. Depending on the cause of the renal disease, management may be different.

## ACUTE RENAL FAILURE AND ACUTE KIDNEY INJURY

Acute renal failure (ARF) or acute renal insufficiency can be defined as an abrupt deterioration in the kidney's ability to clear nitrogenous wastes, such as urea and creatinine. Concomitantly, there is a loss of ability to excrete other solutes and maintain a normal water balance. This leads to the clinical presentation of acute renal insufficiency: edema, hypertension, hyperkalemia, and uremia.

*Acute kidney injury* (AKI) has almost replaced the traditional term *acute renal failure,* which was used in reference to the subset of patients with an acute need for dialysis. With the recognition that even modest increases in serum creatinine are associated with a dramatic impact on the risk for mortality, the clinical spectrum of acute decline in GFR is broader. The minor deteriorations in GFR and kidney injury are captured in a working clinical definition of kidney damage that allows early detection and intervention and uses AKI as a replacement for the term ARF. The term ARF is preferably restricted to patients who have AKI and need renal replacement therapy.[16] The prognosis of AKI is assessed in part by the use of the RIFLE criteria, which include three severity categories (i.e., Risk, Injury, and Failure) and two clinical outcome categories (Loss and End-stage renal disease) (Table 26-4).

The term ARF has often been incorrectly used interchangeably with *acute tubular necrosis,* which usually refers to a rapid deterioration in renal function occurring minutes to days after an ischemic or nephrotoxic event. Although acute tubular necrosis is an important cause of ARF, it is not the sole cause, and the terms are not synonymous. For the purposes of this chapter, AKI refers to the disease formerly called ARF.

### Etiology and Pathophysiology

AKI is often multifactorial in origin or the result of several distinct insults. To treat AKI, it is important to understand its causes and pathophysiology. The causes of AKI are varied but in general can be classified as follows (Table 26-5):

- *Prerenal* implies poor renal perfusion.
- *Renal* implies intrinsic renal disease or damage.
- *Postrenal* implies an obstruction to urine excretion.

Prerenal insults are a common cause of AKI, accounting for up to 70% of all cases. Prerenal failure usually results from extracellular fluid loss, such as from gastroenteritis, burns, hemorrhage, or excessive diuresis. It also occurs in the setting of cardiac failure or sepsis. The common feature of this condition is diminished renal perfusion. In response to the reduction in flow, there is a compensatory increase in afferent tone, which decreases the GFR and increases the retention of salt and water. The net effect of these events is a drastic reduction in urine volume, often resulting in oliguria. If the underlying problem is recognized and treated aggressively, progressive renal insufficiency may be averted. Nonsteroidal antiinflammatory drugs, angiotensin-converting enzyme (ACE) inhibitors, and angiotensin receptor blockers can aggravate prerenal azotemia by further reducing glomerular capillary pressure and the GFR.[17]

AKI resulting from parenchymal disease or injury accounts for 20% to 30% of cases of abrupt renal insufficiency. Common causes in infants include birth asphyxia, sepsis, and cardiac surgery. Important causes of AKI in older children include trauma, sepsis, and the hemolytic uremic syndrome. Prolonged prerenal azotemia may result in overt renal injury. Similarly, intrarenal obstruction to blood flow from thrombi or vasculitis may cause renal failure. Drugs such as aminoglycosides or amphotericin B or other nephrotoxins, including radiocontrast agents, may induce AKI through tubular injury or cause interstitial injury as a result of allergic reactions, as can be seen with penicillins. Acute glomerulonephritis is another cause of AKI in children. Rarely, pyelonephritis can lead to AKI.

The remaining causes of AKI result from the obstruction to urine flow. In total, these conditions account for less than 10% of all cases of AKI and lead to obstruction of both kidneys. Complete cessation of urine may be a clue to a postrenal cause. The obstruction can occur within the collecting system of the kidney (intrarenal), in the ureter, or in the urethra (extrarenal). Intrarenal obstruction may occur with the tumor lysis syndrome with the deposition of uric acid crystals or from medications such as acyclovir and cidofovir. Extrarenal obstruction can be caused by the presence of stones in the ureters or from external compression due to lymph nodes or tumor. As with other forms of AKI, prompt recognition and appropriate intervention to relieve an obstruction may prevent a permanent reduction in renal function.

The exact pathophysiology of AKI remains unclear, but several factors have been identified.[18] There is a profound vasoconstriction in the initial phase of AKI that contributes to the reduced GFR (Fig. 26-1). Factors implicated in increased vasoconstriction include increased activity of the renin-angiotensin and the adrenergic systems and endothelial dysfunction with increased endothelin release and decreased nitric oxide synthesis. However, therapeutic interventions to increase vasodilatation, such as prostaglandin and dopamine infusions, ACE inhibitors, calcium channel blockers, and endothelin receptor antagonists, have not significantly improved established AKI.[19]

Another factor in the pathogenesis of AKI is renal tubule cell injury that is a direct result of a nephrotoxic agent or from an ischemic insult (Fig. 26-2). Cellular injury leads to sloughing of the brush border, swelling, mitochondrial condensation, disruption of cellular architecture, and loss of adhesion to the basement membrane with shedding of cells into the tubular lumen.[20] These changes, which occur within minutes of an ischemic event,

| **RIFLE Factors** | **GFR Criteria** | **Urine Output Criteria** | |
|---|---|---|---|
| Risk | Increased Cr × 1.5 or decreased GFR >25% | UOP <0.5 mL/kg/hr × 6 hours | High sensitivity |
| Injury | Increased Cr × 2 or GFR decrease >50% | UOP <0.5 mL/kg/hr × 12 hours | |
| Failure | Increased Cr × 3 or GFR decrease of 75% or Cr ≥4 mg/dL Acute rise ≥0.5 mg/dL | UOP <0.3 mL/kg/hr × 24 hours or anuria × 12 hours | |
| Loss | Persistent ARF: complete loss of kidney function >4 weeks | | High specificity |
| ESKD | End-stage kidney disease (>3 months) | | |

**TABLE 26-4** RIFLE Classification of Renal Failure and Kidney Injury

Modified from Bellomo R, Ronco C, Kellum JA, Mehta RL, Palevsky P; Acute Dialysis Quality Initiative Workgroup. Acute renal failure—definition, outcome measures, animal models, fluid therapy and information technology needs: the Second International Consensus Conference of the Acute Dialysis Quality Initiative (ADQI) Group. Crit Care 2004;8:R204-12.

*ARF,* Acute renal failure; *Cr,* creatinine; *ESKD,* end-stage kidney disease; *GFR,* glomerular filtration rate; *RIFLE,* Risk of renal dysfunction, Injury to the kidney, Failure of kidney function, Loss of kidney function, and End-stage kidney disease; *UOP,* urine output.

**TABLE 26-5** Causes of Acute Renal Failure

| Prerenal Failure | Renal Failure | Postrenal Failure |
|---|---|---|
| Hypovolemia<br>  Volume loss<br>  Gastrointestinal, renal losses<br>  Sequestration (burns, postoperative) | Acute glomerulonephritis<br>  Postinfectious<br>  Membranoproliferative glomerulonephritis<br>  Rapidly progressive glomerulonephritis<br>  Glomerulonephritis due to systemic<br>    disease (e.g., HUS, DIC, SLE) | Obstruction<br>  Intrinsic (papillary necrosis due to diabetes, sickle<br>    cell disease, or analgesic nephropathy)<br>  Intrarenal abnormalities, ureteral obstruction,<br>    obstruction of the bladder or urethra<br>  Extrinsic (tumor compression, lymphadenopathy) |
| Hypotension<br>  Shock<br>  Vasodilators | Acute interstitial nephritis<br>  Drug-induced hypersensitivity (penicillin)<br>  Infections | |
| Decreased effective blood flow<br>  Low cardiac output<br>  Cirrhosis<br>  Nephrotic syndrome | Tubular disease<br>  ATN (ischemic, nephrotoxic)<br>  Intratubular obstruction (uric acid, oxalate) | |
| Renal hypoperfusion<br>  Use of ACE inhibitors<br>  NSAIDs<br>  Hepatorenal syndrome | Cortical necrosis<br>  Gram-negative sepsis<br>  Hemorrhage<br>  Shock | |
| Vascular occlusion<br>  Thromboembolic phenomenon<br>  Aortic dissection<br>  Renal vein thrombosis (dehydration,<br>    hypercoagulable state, neoplasm) | Acute renal failure<br>  Toxins<br>  Organic solvents<br>  Heavy metals<br>  Insecticides<br>  Hemoglobin<br>  Myoglobin<br>Chronic renal failure<br>  Chronic interstitial nephritis<br>  Chronic glomerulonephritis<br>  Chronic glomerulosclerosis<br>  Nephrocalcinosis<br>  Obstructive uropathy<br>  Hypertension | |

*ACE*, Angiotensin-converting enzyme; *ATN*, acute tubular necrosis; *DIC*, disseminated intravascular coagulation; *HUS*, hemolytic uremic syndrome; *NSAIDs*, nonsteroidal antiinflammatory drugs; *SLE*, systemic lupus erythematosus.

contribute to the decreased GFR by obstructing the lumen of the tubule.[21] These cellular changes allow the filtrate to leak back into the peritubular blood, reducing the excretion of solutes and the effective GFR.

Some of these cell derangements in AKI, such as a decrease in ATP concentrations,[21] cell membrane injury by reactive oxygen molecules,[22] and increased intracellular calcium levels from changes in membrane phospholipid metabolism, lead to cell death. Reactive oxygen molecules also stimulate the production of cytokines and chemokines that play a role in cell injury and vasoconstriction.

Infiltrating neutrophils, recruited during reperfusion injury after renal ischemia, mediate parenchymal damage.[23] Reperfusion injury increases intracellular adhesion molecule 1 (ICAM-1) on endothelial cells promoting the adhesion of circulating neutrophils and their eventual infiltration into the parenchyma. Neutrophils then release reactive oxygen molecules, elastases, proteases, and other enzymes that lead to further tissue injury.

### Diagnostic Procedures

A thorough history and physical examination can yield important clues to the possible cause of renal failure. The initial laboratory assessment of a child with AKI should include the measurement of serum urea, creatinine, and electrolytes and a urinalysis. Prerenal azotemia is typically associated with a ratio of blood urea nitrogen (BUN) to creatinine that is usually greater than 20. In cases of renal parenchymal dysfunction, this ratio is approximately 10. Hematuria and proteinuria are seen in all causes of AKI, but the presence of cellular casts, especially red blood cell casts, in the urinary sediment suggests glomerulonephritis. Granular casts may be seen in prerenal azotemia.

One test to distinguish prerenal azotemia from established renal failure from ischemia or nephrotoxins is the fractional excretion of sodium ($FE_{Na}$). The $FE_{Na}$ is calculated using the following equation:

$$FE_{Na} = \frac{U_{Na} \times S_{Cr}}{S_{Na} \times U_{Cr}} \times 100\%$$

$U_{Na}$ and $S_{Na}$ are urine and serum sodium concentrations, and $U_{Cr}$ and $S_{Cr}$ are the urine and serum creatinine concentrations, respectively. In prerenal azotemia, the $FE_{Na}$ is usually less than 1% for adults and children and less than 2.5% for infants. In established AKI from ischemia and nephrotoxins, but not acute glomerulonephritis, the $FE_{Na}$ is usually increased above 1%. Diuretics confound the interpretation of this test.

The initial radiologic assessment of children with AKI is ultrasonography. Renal ultrasound does not depend on renal function and can define renal anatomy, changes in parenchymal density, and possible obstruction by demonstrating dilation of the urinary tract. Doppler interrogation of the renal vessels provides information on vascular flow. Further radiographic studies, such as voiding cystourethrography, nuclear renal flow scanning, and

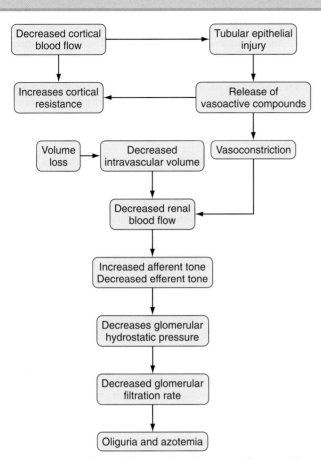

**FIGURE 26-1** Hemodynamic factors in the pathogenesis of acute renal failure.

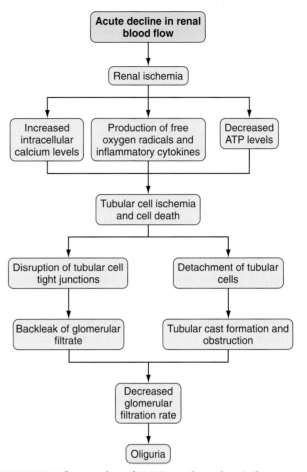

**FIGURE 26-2** Influences of specific injuries on the nephron in the pathogenesis of acute renal failure. *ATP,* Adenosine triphosphate.

abdominal computed tomography (CT) may be indicated in selected children.

### Therapeutic Interventions

Therapeutic interventions in children with AKI should be aimed at the underlying cause and at improving renal function and urine flow. Children with AKI due to hypovolemia should be fluid resuscitated with at least 20 mL/kg over 30 to 60 minutes of normal saline or a balanced salt solution. For children with significant hypotension, an alternative choice is a colloid-containing solution. Children with oliguria due to hypovolemia usually respond within 4 to 6 hours with increased urine output. Although there are anecdotal reports supporting low-dose dopamine in AKI, clinical trials have not shown a benefit from dopamine in preventing or improving AKI.[24]

Diuretics have been commonly used to treat oliguric AKI. There are several theoretical reasons why mannitol, furosemide, or other loop diuretics may ameliorate AKI. Diuretics may convert oliguric AKI to nonoliguric AKI. Loop diuretics decrease energy-driven transport in the loop of Henle, and this may protect cells in regions of hypoperfusion. However, neither mannitol nor loop diuretics can predictably convert an oliguric patient with AKI to a polyuric patient. Diuretics have not been shown in clinical studies to influence renal recovery, need for dialysis, or survival in patients with AKI.[25,26] Diuretics should be used only after the circulating volume has been adequately restored and should be stopped if there is no early response.

Dopamine has been widely used to prevent and manage AKI. In low doses (0.5 to 2.0 µg/kg/min), dopamine increases renal plasma flow, GFR, and renal sodium excretion by activating dopaminergic receptors. Infusion rates in excess of 3 µg/kg/min stimulate α-adrenergic receptors on systemic arterial resistance vasculature causing vasoconstriction; cardiac β₁-adrenergic receptors increasing cardiac contractility, heart rate, and cardiac index; and β₂-adrenergic receptors on systemic arterial resistance vasculature causing vasodilatation. In a meta-analysis of 24 studies and 854 patients, dopamine did not prevent renal failure, alter the need for dialysis, or change the mortality rate.[27] In a randomized clinical trial of low-dose dopamine in 328 critically ill patients, dopamine did not change the duration or severity of the renal failure, need for dialysis, or mortality.[28] From these data, the routine use of low-dose dopamine in patients with AKI cannot be supported.

Several other agents that were useful in experimental models of AKI have been investigated but not shown clinical success. Atrial natriuretic peptide increases GFR in animal models of AKI by increasing renal perfusion pressure and sodium excretion. Initial studies demonstrated some benefit in patients with AKI,[29] especially oliguric AKI,[30] but a subsequent study of 222 patients with oliguric AKI revealed no statistical difference between patients treated with atrial natriuretic peptide and placebo in terms of the need for dialysis or mortality.[31] Insulin-like growth factor 1 has been beneficial in animal models of AKI, presumably by potentiating cell regeneration. However, in a multicenter, placebo-controlled trial enrolling 72 patients with AKI, insulin-like growth factor 1 did not speed recovery, decrease the need for dialysis, or alter the mortality rate.[32] Thyroxine abbreviates the course of experimental acute renal failure but had no effect on the duration of renal failure in patients and increased mortality threefold (by suppression of thyroid-stimulating hormone).[33]

In patients with severe AKI, renal replacement therapy through dialysis is life sustaining. The indications for initiation of dialytic therapy are persistent hyperkalemia, volume overload refractory to diuretics, severe metabolic acidosis, and overt signs and symptoms of uremia such as pericarditis and encephalopathy. Many nephrologists advocate for initiation of dialysis if the BUN value approaches 100 mg/dL or even earlier, especially in the oliguric patient, although this has not proved to alter outcome. A retrospective study that compared early (BUN <60 mg/dL) versus late (BUN >60 mg/dL) initiation of dialysis in 100 adult patients suggested that early initiation improved survival.[34] However, the timing of the initiation of dialysis remains an unresolved question.

The three modalities of renal replacement for the support of critically ill children and adults are hemodialysis, peritoneal dialysis, and a variation of continuous replacement therapies, such as venovenous hemofiltration (CVVH), hemodialysis (CVVHD), and hemodiafiltration (CVVHDF). No form of replacement therapy has been clearly superior to the others. However, in the individual child, one form may be more practical than the others. Hemodialysis is technically more difficult than peritoneal dialysis in the infant and hemodynamically unstable child. Continuous replacement therapies appear to cause less hemodynamic instability compared with hemodialysis but offer more predictable solute and fluid removal than peritoneal dialysis. Hemodialysis and continuous replacement therapies require large-bore vascular access to achieve the high blood flow rates necessary for these modalities.

Although the modalities are technically different, they are based on the same principles (Fig. 26-3). The aim of all renal replacement therapies is to promote the removal of nitrogenous wastes (i.e., urea), excess fluid, and excess solute, especially potassium. This is achieved by exposing blood to a salt solution (i.e., dialysate), with the two separated by a semipermeable membrane. The movement of solute occurs by diffusion (i.e., solute moves across the membrane in response to a concentration gradient) and ultrafiltration (i.e., osmotic or hydrostatic pressures). The rate of removal of water and solute waste depends on membrane characteristics (i.e., pore size and selectivity), diffusion, and ultrafiltration.[35]

The permeability characteristics and surface areas are known for specific dialyzers used in hemodialysis and hemofiltration. The peritoneum serves as the dialysis membrane in peritoneal dialysis and remains physically unalterable, but changes in dialysate composition and length of time the dialysate is exposed to the peritoneal membrane changes the amount of solute and water removed. In all forms of renal replacement therapy, the therapeutic prescription is individualized for the child.

### Hemodialysis

Hemodialysis is useful for AKI and is the best modality for the rapid removal of toxins, such as drug overdoses or other ingestions. Hemodialysis is very efficient, with the ability to reduce the BUN by 60% to 70%, normalize the serum potassium concentration, and remove fluid equal to 5% to 10% of the body weight in 3 to 4 hours. To accomplish this, rapid blood flows are necessary (5 to 10 mL/kg/min), which requires large-vessel venous access, but this can usually be achieved even in infants by the insertion of a double-lumen catheter into the subclavian, internal jugular, or femoral vein. In small infants, two single-lumen catheters placed in different sites may be necessary for access and return of blood. Rarely, a single-lumen catheter is used for outflow and return of blood. Modern hemodialysis machines have microprocessors that can accurately measure fluid removal, allowing precise volumes of fluid to be removed.

Hemodialysis usually requires systemic anticoagulation with heparin, the effectiveness of which can be monitored by the activated clotting time. Hemodialysis can be done without the use of an anticoagulant in the child at significant risk for bleeding by using a rapid blood flow rate and frequent rinsing of the blood circuit with saline. However, clotting of the circuit with subsequent loss of the extracorporeal blood is common.

In addition to the risk of bleeding, hemodialysis is associated with several other complications. The most common side effect is hypotension, which is usually related to aggressive volume removal but can be caused by sepsis or the release of cytokines and autokines from blood passage over the hemodialysis filter surface. Muscle cramps, headache, nausea, and vomiting are also common complaints. A more serious complication of hemodialysis is the disequilibrium syndrome that is related to rapid removal of solute from the bloodstream with slow equilibration with the tissues, particularly in the brain. This can cause cerebral edema, manifested by headache, obtundation, seizures, or coma. The disequilibrium syndrome is usually reported in children undergoing dialysis for the first time. This can be avoided by short, frequent dialysis sessions initially, especially if the BUN concentration is increased substantially. Infection of the dialysis catheter is another common problem and can be minimized with sterile central line technique.

### Peritoneal Dialysis

Peritoneal dialysis has a long history as a renal replacement therapy in children.[36] It is relatively simple and easily performed

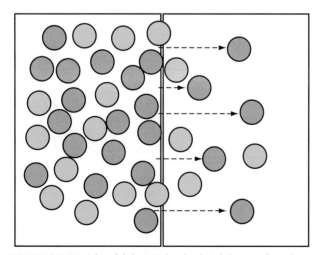

**FIGURE 26-3** Principles of dialysis. Solute (*pink circles*) moves from the blood to the dialysate (*broken arrows*) in response to a concentration gradient (i.e., diffusion). The obligate passive movement of water (*blue circles*) attempts to maintain appropriate osmolarity. This flux of solute and water (i.e., ultrafiltration) may be enhanced by increased osmotic pressure (i.e., glucose in peritoneal dialysis fluid) or by increased hydrostatic pressure, which is created mechanically as transmembrane pressure in hemodialysis.

even in small infants. Although not as efficient as hemodialysis, it is best done continuously to control solute and water balance. In contrast to hemodialysis, it is much less likely to cause hemodynamic instability. Peritoneal dialysis involves instilling dialysate fluid into the peritoneum for a set period and then draining the fluid and replacing it with fresh dialysate. This cycling removes waste products by diffusion and water by ultrafiltration as a consequence of a high glucose concentration in the dialysate. The efficacy of peritoneal dialysis depends on the volume instilled and the number of cycles per day. Most children with acute renal failure can be managed with 1- to 2-hour cycles of 5- to 30-mL/kg dwell volumes. Children with chronic renal failure are managed with greater cycle times and larger dwell volumes. The amount of fluid removed can be varied by changing the concentration of the glucose in the dialysate. Short-term peritoneal dialysis can be accomplished with a nontunneled catheter, but dialysis that should continue beyond 3 to 5 days is best achieved with a subcutaneously tunneled cuffed catheter to minimize the risk of peritonitis.

The principal complications of peritoneal dialysis are infection and mechanical problems related to the catheter. It is not uncommon to find poor drainage from the catheter, usually from fibrin occlusion of the catheter or from omentum or bowel covering the inlet holes. The catheter may leak at its point of insertion. Hernias, especially inguinal hernias in boys, may develop as a consequence of the increased abdominal pressure from the infused dialysate. Mild hyponatremia may develop in infants because of the relatively low sodium concentration (130 mEq/L) in commercial dialysate. Less common but serious complications include bowel injury and intraabdominal hemorrhage from catheter insertion and peritonitis.

## CHRONIC RENAL FAILURE

The loss of functioning renal mass results in a compensatory increase in filtration by the remaining renal tissue.[37] For example, after a unilateral nephrectomy, there is a demonstrable increase in the GFR and evidence of contralateral renal hypertrophy within the first 48 hours. By 2 to 4 weeks, the GFR has returned to 80% of normal, and there is no clinical evidence of renal dysfunction. With the loss of 50% to 75% of renal mass, there is an increase in the residual function to 50% to 80% of normal and often little evidence of clinical renal insufficiency. When the residual renal function decreases to 30% to 50% of normal, the term *chronic renal insufficiency* applies. At this point, acute illness and other stress states may result in acidosis, hyperkalemia, and dehydration. It is only when the residual function decreases to less than 30% of normal that the term *chronic renal failure* is used. At this point, electrolyte abnormalities begin to appear, and more importantly, there is limited ability of the kidney to adjust to variations in fluid and electrolyte homeostasis. The term *uremia* refers to the symptoms of anorexia, nausea, lethargy, and somnolence that develop as a result of chronic renal failure. Uremia ultimately results in death unless dialysis therapy or renal transplantation is performed. Initiating dialysis or transplanting a kidney is referred to as end-stage renal disease care.

Chronic renal insufficiency and chronic renal failure are both categories within the larger schema of chronic kidney disease (CKD). Although the stages are defined by categorizing continuous measures of function (i.e., GFR) and therefore are somewhat arbitrary, they do provide a context for the evaluation and management of kidney disease. There are six stages of CKD:

Stage I: The GFR is normal (>90 mL/min/1.73 m²), but there may be evidence of chronic renal disease, including an abnormal urinalysis, hypertension, or abnormal renal ultrasound results.

Stage II: The GFR of 60 to 89 mL/min/1.73 m² indicates mild kidney damage with a reduction in the GFR.

Stage III: The GFR of 30 to 59 mL/min/1.73 m² indicates a moderate reduction in the GFR.

Stage IV: The GFR of 15 to 29 mL/min/1.73 m² indicates a severe decline in the GFR, often accompanied by electrolyte or metabolic derangements.

Stage V: The GFR of less than 15 mL/min/1.73 m² indicates kidney failure requiring renal replacement therapy.

Stage VI: Patients are receiving dialysis or are transplant recipients.

Despite losses of up to 90% of renal function, sodium homeostasis usually is well maintained in chronic renal failure. With large decreases in the GFR, the kidney maintains normal serum sodium by increasing the $FE_{Na}$ from less than 1% up to 25% to 30%, largely through decreases in distal tubular resorption. Some of the hormonal factors involved in this adaptation include aldosterone, atrial natriuretic factor, and a poorly characterized natriuretic hormone that inhibits $Na^+/K^+$-ATPase. With chronic renal failure, the ability of the kidney to handle a wide range of sodium intake, from 1 to 250 mEq/m²/day, is lost. Instead, the kidney may be able to handle an intake of only 50 to 100 mEq/m²/day. It may be possible to decrease this obligatory excretion of sodium to 5 to 20 mEq/m²/day, although only after weeks of decreasing the sodium intake slowly. Certain children with renal disease, especially those with obstructive uropathy or tubulointerstitial disease, may be unable to adjust to a decreased sodium intake and display a salt-losing nephropathy. These children are prone to dehydration with salt restriction and may need salt supplementation for normal growth. In others, a regular diet may lead to sodium retention, volume overload, and hypertension; sodium intake must be individualized to fit the limitations of each child.

Water balance also is affected by chronic renal failure. There is an obligatory total osmolar excretion that limits the ability of the kidney to excrete free water. The concentrating ability of the kidney is affected, limiting its ability to make a maximally concentrated or dilute urine. These limitations may result in water retention and hyponatremia or dehydration if water is administered in amounts exceeding the kidney's capabilities. These limitations must be considered in the treatment of children with chronic renal failure, particularly before surgery when free access to water is restricted.

In patients with chronic renal failure, normal serum potassium concentrations usually are maintained until the GFR is less than 10% of normal. Potassium excretion in normal and uremic states is maintained by potassium secretion in the distal nephron. In response to an increase in potassium intake or loss of renal mass, there is an increase in $Na^+/K^+$-ATPase in the remaining collecting tubules that seems to be partly responsible for augmented excretion of potassium per nephron. In uremic animals, potassium is excreted from the renal tubules at a rate sixfold greater than in nonuremic animals and 1.5 times the filtered potassium load. Partial adaptation can occur in the absence of aldosterone, but aldosterone plays an important role in the maintenance of normal potassium homeostasis. This is demonstrated by the presence of hyperkalemia in children with hyporeninemic hypoaldosteronism or in those treated with the aldosterone antagonist spironolactone.

The colon normally is responsible for the excretion of less than 13% of dietary potassium. In patients with chronic renal failure, this can increase to 50% by the activation of colonic $Na^+/K^+$-ATPase. Aldosterone augments the activity of colonic $Na^+/K^+$-ATPase. An additional mechanism that plays an essential role in the adaptation to an acute potassium load is the redistribution of potassium from the extracellular to the intracellular compartment, which depends on insulin, β-adrenergic catecholamines, aldosterone, and pH. Despite the presence of total body potassium depletion in uremia, the uptake of potassium into the cells is impaired. This contributes to the intolerance to an acute potassium load in uremia despite the ability to excrete a potassium load.

Hyperkalemia is a major problem in chronic renal failure.[38] In contrast, significant hypokalemia is unusual in the absence of potassium restriction, alkalosis, or diuretic therapy. Hyperkalemia can result from an extrinsic potassium load, but it also can be caused by fasting or acidosis, in which case the source of the potassium is the intracellular compartment. This can be a particular problem when a child is fasted before surgery and can be ameliorated by an infusion of glucose and insulin. Drugs that can cause hyperkalemia in renal failure include spironolactone, β-adrenergic blockers, and ACE inhibitors. When clinically significant hyperkalemia develops in a child with chronic renal failure, the first-line therapy is to stabilize the myocardium with exogenous calcium and then to redistribute the potassium into the intracellular compartment with insulin and glucose. To deliver the same dose of ionized calcium, three times as much calcium gluconate (mg/kg) must be given than calcium chloride. All doses of calcium are optimally delivered through a central venous access line because calcium infusions are irritating to peripheral veins and can cause necrosis of the skin if extravasation occurs. More definitive correction of hyperkalemia is accomplished by removing potassium from the body using dialysis or Kayexalate. At eight times the usual asthma dose, nebulized albuterol has been effective in redistributing potassium intracellularly, whereas sodium bicarbonate ($NaHCO_3$) administration has not been effective (Table 26-6).

**TABLE 26-6** Treatment of Hyperkalemia

| Treatment | Dosage |
| --- | --- |
| **Stabilization of Myocardium** | |
| Calcium and bicarbonate | Calcium gluconate: 10% 30-100 mg/kg IV or Calcium chloride: 10% 10-33 mg/kg IV Sodium bicarbonate: 1 mEq/kg IV if acidotic |
| **Shifting of Potassium to Intracellular Space** | |
| Insulin and glucose | Insulin: 0.1-0.3 unit/kg or 0.1 unit/kg/hr infusion Glucose: $D_{50}$ 1-2 mL/kg or $D_{25}$ 2-4 mL/kg IV or $D_5$ 1-2 mL/kg/hr |
| Albuterol | Albuterol: 2.5-5 mg/mL nebulization |
| **Decreasing Total Body Potassium** | |
| Sodium polystyrene sulfonate (Kayexalate) | 1 g/kg up to 40 g every 4 hours PO or PR |
| Furosemide (diuretic) | 0.5 mg/kg up to 40 mg |

*D*, Dextrose; *IV*, intravenous; *PO*, per os (oral); *PR*, per rectum (suppository).

Metabolic acidosis is common in patients with chronic renal failure.[39] The metabolic acidosis is associated with a normal anion gap in moderate renal insufficiency, but with severe renal insufficiency, there is retention of phosphate, sulfate, and organic acids, resulting in an elevated anion gap. The primary cause of metabolic acidosis in chronic renal failure is the inability of the remaining proximal renal tubules to increase ammonium formation to keep pace with the loss of renal mass. The kidney becomes unable to generate the 1 to 3 mEq/kg/day of new bicarbonate that is necessary to compensate for that lost to buffer endogenous acid production. Previous studies have suggested a major role for decreased resorption of bicarbonate by the proximal renal tubule in chronic renal failure. Although this may occur in the presence of volume overload, severe secondary hyperparathyroidism, and disorders such as Fanconi syndrome, it is not a major mechanism causing acidosis in chronic renal failure. Except for severe phosphate depletion, decreased excretion of phosphate as a titratable acid normally does not contribute to metabolic acidosis.

One of the earliest manifestations of chronic renal failure is secondary hyperparathyroidism.[40] Secondary hyperparathyroidism, which results from inadequate formation of 1,25-(OH)$_2$ vitamin D (i.e., 1,25-dihydroxyvitamin $D_3$ or calcitriol), develops in moderate renal insufficiency in the presence of normal serum concentrations of calcium and phosphorus. With more severe renal insufficiency, overt hypocalcemia and hyperphosphatemia often develop. Hypocalcemia is caused by decreased calcium absorption from the gastrointestinal tract as a result of a true deficiency of 1,25-(OH)$_2$ vitamin D. Diminished release of calcium from bone occurs as a result of resistance to the action of parathyroid hormone, and calcium and phosphate are deposited in soft tissues as a consequence of hyperphosphatemia.

The kidney plays a key role in the maintenance of phosphate homeostasis by regulating its excretion. In the presence of a normal GFR, the kidney excretes 5% to 15% of the filtered load of phosphate, whereas in chronic renal failure, the kidney can increase its fractional excretion of phosphate to 60% to 80%. Through this adaptation, the kidneys are able to maintain a phosphate balance in chronic renal failure, but they do so at an increased serum phosphate concentration. At the same time, the kidneys have no reserve with which to increase phosphate excretion in response to a phosphate load. In children with chronic renal failure, a large phosphate load, such as can occur with the administration of a phosphate-containing enema, can lead to life-threatening hyperphosphatemia and hypocalcemia.

### Hematologic Problems

One of the most common manifestations of chronic renal failure is anemia. The anemia of chronic renal failure results from impaired erythropoiesis, hemolysis, and bleeding. Of these, impaired erythropoiesis is most important and usually the result of a deficiency of erythropoietin production. Erythropoietin is synthesized and secreted by peritubular cells in the renal cortex in response to decreased tissue oxygenation. It acts on receptors on the erythroid burst-forming units and erythroid colony-forming units. With loss of renal mass, erythropoietin secretion does not respond adequately to hypoxia, and anemia results. Children with chronic renal failure are now routinely treated with recombinant erythropoietin.[41,42] Current recommendations are to treat children with chronic renal failure in whom the hematocrit is less than 30%, starting at a dosage of 50 to 150 units/kg intravenously three times per week. When a target hematocrit of

36% is reached, a maintenance dosage of about 75 units/kg is instituted. Subcutaneous administration of erythropoietin is also effective, can be given only once each week, and obviates the need for intravenous injections. Doses greater than 150 units/kg increase the hematocrit faster than smaller doses, but both therapies take 4 to 8 weeks to reach target hematocrit values of 33% to 36%. The most common cause for failure of erythropoietin is concurrent iron deficiency. Children who are scheduled for erythropoietin therapy should begin oral iron, vitamin C, and folic acid 2 to 3 weeks in advance to ensure adequate iron and folic acid stores to facilitate erythropoiesis. Current recommendations are to maintain serum ferritin concentrations above 250 ng/mL and transferrin saturation above 25%. Other causes for failure of erythropoietin to increase or maintain the hematocrit are occult infections, hemolysis, aluminum overload, severe hyperparathyroidism, and occult bleeding. Complications of erythropoietin therapy include worsening of hypertension and a possible increased incidence of thrombosis of polytetrafluoroethylene vascular grafts.

The other major hematologic problem in chronic renal failure is bleeding. This is a classic and lethal complication in children with terminal uremia and results from platelet dysfunction in the presence of a normal coagulation profile and normal platelet counts. The best indicator of platelet dysfunction in children with chronic renal failure is a prolonged bleeding time. The platelet dysfunction is the result of poorly described abnormalities attributed to the uremic environment, and platelet transfusions are ineffective. Dialysis improves the platelet dysfunction, as does improvement in the hematocrit with transfusion or erythropoietin therapy. Preoperative intravenous desmopressin acetate (1-deamino-8-D-arginine vasopressin [DDAVP]) (0.3 µg/kg) has been shown to be effective in improving the bleeding time in children with uremia.

### Cardiovascular Complications

Hypertension is one of the most common complications of chronic renal failure and contributes significantly to the morbidity and mortality of these children. The cause is multifactorial and includes volume overload and hormonal abnormalities, such as increased secretion of renin, that result from the underlying renal disorder. In children who are being dialyzed, volume overload is the result of inadequate removal of volume by the process of ultrafiltration during dialysis. The goal of ultrafiltration is to remove sufficient salt and water to achieve the dry weight that is appropriate for each child. The *dry weight* is the weight at which the child has no signs of volume overload but below which the child has hypotension. The initial response to volume overload is to increase the cardiac output. Later, the cardiac output returns to normal, but the peripheral resistance increases because of peripheral vasoconstriction, resulting in hypertension. These children may have no other signs of volume overload, such as edema, but with a reduction in total body salt and water content, the blood pressure can be controlled with little or no antihypertensive medication.

In other children, intrinsic renal abnormalities play a primary role in hypertension. In these children, bilateral nephrectomy may be necessary to control severe refractory hypertension, although usually it can be controlled with oral antihypertensive agents. Of the mechanisms that cause hypertension in these children, increased renin secretion is the best understood. Renin activates the formation of angiotensin I, which is then converted to angiotensin II, a powerful vasoconstrictor. Children with renin-dependent hypertension respond poorly to control of blood pressure by salt and water removal alone but respond well to ACE inhibitors such as captopril.

Cardiovascular disease is the most common cause of death in patients receiving long-term dialysis, including children.[43] Patients with chronic renal failure can have abnormalities of the pericardium, myocardium, cardiac valves, and coronary arteries. Another cardiac manifestation, pericarditis, has long been recognized as a complication of uremia. Pericarditis was once considered a sign of the terminal phase of uremia, but it occurs in 15% of children receiving dialysis and can be symptomatic or clinically silent. In nondialyzed uremic patients with pericarditis, intensive dialysis often results in its resolution within about 2 weeks. Some children require surgical procedures such as pericardiocentesis, pericardial drainage with a catheter or through a pericardial window, or pericardiectomy.

Left ventricular failure is also a common complication of chronic renal failure. In older patients, coronary artery disease may lead to myocardial dysfunction, severely limiting cardiac output. Volume overload and hypertension, which increase preload and afterload, respectively, are important causes of heart failure. With proper fluid management and antihypertensive medication, these abnormalities can be controlled. Anemia is another contributing factor that can be controlled with the use of erythropoietin. An array of metabolic abnormalities associated with chronic renal failure, such as secondary hyperparathyroidism, electrolyte and acid-base imbalances, and the accumulation of nonspecific uremic toxins, contribute to abnormal myocardial function.

### Causes of Chronic Renal Failure

The causes of chronic renal insufficiency and failure can be correlated with age (Table 26-7). The chronic renal failure that is commonly encountered in early infancy results largely from congenital anomalies or perinatal asphyxia. Later in childhood, renal

**TABLE 26-7** Causes of Chronic Renal Failure

| Infancy (Congenital Anomalies) | Childhood | Adolescence |
|---|---|---|
| Prune-belly syndrome | Dysplasia | Focal segmental glomerulosclerosis |
| Congenital obstruction | Agenesis | Membranoproliferative glomerulonephritis |
| Posterior urethral valves | Autosomal dominant PKD | Secondary glomerulonephritis |
| Multicystic dysplasia | Reflux nephropathy | Systemic lupus erythematosus |
| Agenesis | Obstruction | Sickle cell disease |
| Autosomal recessive PKD | Focal segmental glomerulosclerosis | HIV-associated nephropathy |
| Reflux nephropathy | Membranoproliferative glomerulonephritis | Diabetes mellitus Vasculitis Hemolytic uremic syndrome Henoch-Schönlein purpura Interstitial nephritis Malignancy |

*HIV,* Human immunodeficiency virus; *PKD,* polycystic kidney disease.

failure may result from dysplasia, or acquired lesions, whereas those affected in adolescence may have deterioration of function related to acquired disease, manifestation of inherited disease, or secondary lesions resulting from other illnesses (e.g., systemic lupus erythematosus, sickle cell disease) or their treatments.

# Preoperative Preparation of the Child with Renal Dysfunction

The preoperative preparation of the renal patient depends on the type of renal disease and the presence of hypertension. Renal diseases that may affect the choice of anesthetic agents include renal failure, nephrotic syndrome, and tubular disorders. In children with known renal disease, careful delineation of the type of renal disease and a knowledge of the child's medications should be reviewed at the time of the preoperative visit to anticipate potential problems during the procedure. Identification of children with occult renal disease can be difficult. Clues to the presence of renal disease include edema, hypertension, failure to thrive, anemia, and rickets.

Children with tubular disorders, obstructive uropathy, or hypoplastic/dysplastic kidneys may have fixed polyuria and are at risk for dehydration if oral intake is restricted (NPO) for long periods. Following the American Society of Anesthesiologists (ASA) guidelines and allowing liberal amounts of clear fluids until 2 hours before the procedure may avoid potential dehydration and alleviate anxiety in a fasting child. Alternatively, for the in-house patient, maintenance intravenous fluids should be continued while the child is NPO.

Perioperative renal dysfunction may occur in children with normal renal function when subjected to perioperative insults such as hypoperfusion from hypotension or hypovolemia. Preexisting renal insufficiency compounds this risk, and precautions to preserve renal perfusion must be taken.[44] Associated risk factors include hypovolemia leading to vasoconstriction, nephrotoxic agents such as contrast media, embolic events in cases involving arterial vessel cross-clamping, renal ischemia, and inflammation. Perioperative renal failure is associated with mortality rates of 60% to 90%, and it is therefore important to avoid factors that may augment preexisting renal dysfunction.[45,46] A large national database has shown that 1% of all adult patients who underwent general surgical procedures developed postoperative AKI[47]; the patients at greatest risk were older men (≥56 years old). These data may not be applicable to children, but an increased incidence of AKI among children with congestive heart failure, hypertension, preoperative renal insufficiency, or ascites may help to identify children who are also at risk. Identification of those at risk is not a trivial exercise because postoperative AKI increased postoperative morbidity threefold and postoperative mortality fivefold.

## PREOPERATIVE LABORATORY EVALUATION

Several preoperative laboratory tests should be assessed before surgery in a child with renal insufficiency. This allows the practitioner to determine the severity of the presenting disease and provides a baseline that may be compared with intraoperative and postoperative laboratory values to ensure proper protective renal care.

Children with known renal failure, especially those with a significant reduction in renal function, require preoperative serum electrolyte and calcium concentrations and hemoglobin levels measured within 24 hours of the procedure and on the morning of the procedure if a known lability exists. Although the serum creatinine concentration is typically used as a marker for renal function, the value is not indicative of the degree of injury.

Abnormal potassium concentrations often occur in children with renal failure; acceptable limits depend on the status of the child and the trends in the potassium concentration over time. Chronic hypokalemic or hyperkalemic states are less likely to have cardiac effects than acute changes. Acute hypokalemia reduces arrhythmia threshold and increases cardiac excitability. Acute hyperkalemia may result in life-threatening arrhythmias from electrical conduction suppression. A child with chronic renal failure whose serum potassium concentrations are chronically 5.5 to 6.0 mEq/L does not need correction of the hyperkalemia, whereas a child with an acute increase to a potassium concentration greater than 5.5 mEq/L requires intervention before the surgical procedure and anesthesia. Existing acidosis must be taken into consideration in determining total body potassium concentrations, with the understanding that acute acidosis promotes extracellular hyperkalemia at a rate of 0.5 mEq/L for every decrease in pH of 0.1 unit. Treatment of hyperkalemia has several options (see Table 26-6).

Hypomagnesemia likewise predisposes a child to the risks of supraventricular and ventricular arrhythmias and should be corrected preoperatively. Hypermagnesemia or hypophosphatemia may cause muscle weakness and potentiate the action of muscle relaxants. Administration of calcium is helpful in treating hyperkalemia or hypermagnesemia.

Hemoglobin, hematocrit, and platelet counts should be part of the preoperative evaluation. Anemia is a common finding in children with renal disease, and morbidity and mortality are associated with hemoglobin concentrations less than 11 g/dL in adult patients with renal failure.[48,49] This relationship was based on the effect of anemia on the incidence of left ventricular hypertrophy and associated morbidity and may be less of a concern in children. Recombinant erythropoietin reduces the risks of cardiac compromise from left ventricular hypertrophy by increasing the hemoglobin to normal values.[50,51] Blood transfusion is generally not indicated if the hematocrit is more than 25%.

Platelet counts, although typically normal in children with renal failure, are not predictive of platelet dysfunction. The best indicator of platelet dysfunction in children with chronic renal failure is a prolonged bleeding time. Signs of coagulopathy such as petechiae should alert the practitioner of abnormal platelet function, which does not necessarily improve with platelet transfusion. Dialysis, red blood cell transfusion, and erythropoietin improve platelet dysfunction. Desmopressin (0.3 μg/kg given intravenously over 15 to 20 minutes) can improve the bleeding time in children with uremia and can minimize hypotension when given 1 hour before surgery. It releases endothelial von Willebrand factor/factor VIII complex and improves platelet function for 6 to 12 hours. Cryoprecipitate is an alternative that should be used in children who have received desmopressin and continue to have coagulopathy.

A preoperative urinalysis can be useful in identifying children with unknown renal disease, although a normal result does not always exclude the possibility that a child has significant renal disease. The use of an $FE_{Na}$ estimate assists differentiating prerenal azotemia from acute tubular necrosis.

Depending on the degree of renal failure and suspected cardiac involvement, additional testing, including an electrocardiogram, a chest radiograph, and an echocardiogram, should be considered. These tests can help the practitioner determine evidence of left ventricular hypertrophy, arrhythmias, and presence or absence of pericardial effusions.

Although not proved to be reliable markers of renal injury, concentrations of serum cystatin C, which reflects the GFR better than serum creatinine, and urinary neutrophil gelatinase-associated lipocalin, which is produced in response to injury by tubular cells, may be used more in the future to provide information preoperatively.[52,53]

## PERIOPERATIVE DIALYSIS

In the child with renal failure, dialysis is used to prevent hyperkalemia and remove excess water. However, excessive or overly aggressive dialysis may lead to electrolyte abnormalities and hypovolemia. Accordingly, the timing of this therapy or need for the therapy should be discussed with the child's nephrologist. Ideally, renal failure patients on *intermittent* hemodialysis should be dialyzed the day before surgery to optimize their fluid and electrolyte status and minimize problems with acute fluid shifts with hypotension, hypokalemia, and anticoagulation that may occur if hemodialysis occurs the day of surgery. Children being treated with peritoneal dialysis can be dialyzed up until the day of surgery. Peritoneal dialysis should be resumed with the consideration that the child's pulmonary function must be able to tolerate the increased abdominal distention. Consultation with the child's nephrologist is recommended to optimize the child's clinical status before the procedure and to arrange the appropriate timing of the peritoneal dialysis.

## MEDICATIONS

Children with renal failure may require that their medications be adjusted in the perioperative period. These medications typically include antihypertensives, and although proceeding with elective surgery with moderate hypertension may be acceptable, severe or labile hypertension should be controlled before surgery. Induction of anesthesia may cause hypotension in children with chronic hypertension, although preloading with balanced salt solution may offset this effect. There is a temporal relationship between adults who take ACE inhibitors for blood pressure control on the day of surgery and hypotension at induction of anesthesia and cardiac arrest.[54] Moderate hypotension was significantly more frequent in patients who discontinued their ACE inhibitor within 10 hours of their anesthetic induction compared with those who had not taken their medication for more than 10 hours before induction.[54] Additional studies and opinion leaders suggest that ACE inhibitors should be stopped the day before surgery to prevent hypotension after induction of anesthesia, although the hypotension can be easily managed, especially during total intravenous anesthesia in adults.[55-57] All other antihypertensives, immunosuppressives, and steroids should be continued. Most other medications can be safely held until they can be resumed postoperatively.

If acute hypertension is diagnosed before an urgent procedure, clonidine should be considered. Because of the risk of rebound hypertension when it is discontinued, oral therapy should be started as soon as the child can tolerate oral intake, or alternatively, a transdermal clonidine patch may be applied to avoid postoperative rebound hypertension.

# Intraoperative Management

## SPECIAL CONSIDERATIONS

Children with chronic renal failure frequently present with serious medical problems that complicate anesthesia when surgery is required.[58,59] These problems stem mainly from fluid and electrolyte abnormalities, complications of chronic renal failure such as anemia and hypertension, and differences in the pharmacokinetics of anesthetic agents in children with renal failure. Although several empirical measures have been advocated for renal protection in the perioperative period, a Cochrane review concluded that no interventions, whether pharmacologic or otherwise, protected the kidney in the perioperative period.[60]

In addition to routine monitoring, consideration should be given to the absolute need for arterial access because it may affect future shunt sites, careful positioning of children with renal osteodystrophy, and careful antiseptic techniques for vascular line placements due to the increased risk of infection. Strategies to maintain normothermia, including increasing the room temperature and application of a forced-air warming blanket, should be considered to avoid hypothermia. An arterial line may be useful to monitor blood pressure that may be labile during the perioperative period. An arterial or central line also facilitates checking laboratory values during prolonged procedures in children with large fluid shifts and in the severely compromised renal patient. Serum potassium concentrations must be monitored and corrected to avoid arrhythmias or conduction problems. Central venous monitoring may be valuable in this population for several reasons; peripheral venous access may be challenging due to their chronic disease, fluid management is more easily guided using central venous pressure monitoring when urine output cannot be used as an indicator of hydration status, and it ensures safe and reliable delivery of vasoactive medications and calcium.

## FLUIDS AND BLOOD PRODUCTS

In the child with renal insufficiency, fluid management requires a balanced approach. The child must receive adequate hydration to prevent further renal deterioration in an otherwise injured kidney. Children with renal failure and a history of hypertension are at risk for hypotension and hypertension and require some degree of fluid resuscitation for stability. However, they also may have hypoalbuminemia with low oncotic pressure that puts them at risk for pulmonary edema. Ideally, if the child is euvolemic, standard fluid therapy based on typical surgical fluid management may ensue. Fluid overload must be avoided in all anuric children and in outpatients. Although common sense and years of practice suggest that normal saline is preferable to lactated Ringer solution due to the potassium load in the latter, there is evidence to the contrary. In a series of adults who underwent kidney transplantation with normal saline or lactated Ringer solution, 19% of the patients in the saline group had a potassium concentration of 6 mEq/L and 31% had a metabolic acidosis that required treatment, compared with none for both metabolic disorders in the lactated Ringer group.[61] Consideration should be given to returning to lactated Ringer solution for renal failure patients.

In a child with AKI and low urine output, it is tempting to administer diuretics to increase renal blood flow and flush the renal tubules. However, the use of diuretics in a patient with renal disease may worsen renal failure by causing hypovolemia and decreased renal perfusion.

Because of the risk of bleeding in children with significant renal failure, hemoglobin concentrations should be followed closely. This is a classic and lethal complication in children with terminal uremia that results from platelet dysfunction in the presence of a normal coagulation profile and normal platelet counts. Blood and component therapy may be used in accordance with surgical losses and to keep the hemoglobin concentration greater than 11 g/dL. Other components that may be effective to alleviate surgical oozing or occult bleeding should be given based on clinical need because results of coagulation studies may not be true indicators of the coagulation status in children with platelet dysfunction.

## ANESTHETIC AGENTS

The pharmacokinetics and pharmacodynamics of anesthetic agents and perioperative medications may be altered in children with renal failure. The medications most likely to be affected are those that depend on renal excretion, such as the hydrophilic, highly ionized agents. Repeated doses of medications that depend primarily on renal excretion for elimination should be administered at longer intervals or in smaller doses than they are given otherwise. Examples of commonly used perioperative medications that primarily depend on renal elimination are penicillins, cephalosporins, aminoglycosides, vancomycin, and digoxin. Anesthetic agents should be tailored according to the circumstances and child. For example, the duration of action of medications that are delivered as a single bolus depends more on redistribution than on elimination. If the volume of distribution of the medication is unchanged, the single bolus dose should be unchanged. Medications that depend only in part on renal elimination have a normal duration of action when delivered as a bolus or short-term infusion. Many anesthetics depend in part on renal elimination, including pancuronium, vecuronium, atropine, glycopyrrolate, and neostigmine. The vasoactive agents milrinone and amrinone also belong to this group. Long-acting medications and infusions must be used with caution in renal failure patients due to the risk for drug accumulation.

Because uremic children are more susceptible to excessive sedation, premedication should be kept to a minimum in these children. However, a short-acting anxiolytic such as midazolam may be used with caution in the anxious child, but if the child is encephalopathic, no premedicant should be used.

Induction of anesthesia may be carried out safely as long as the child is euvolemic and the pharmacokinetics and pharmacodynamics of the induction agent are understood and accounted for. Anesthetic agents may be affected by the presence of anemia, acidosis, and altered drug binding due to hypoproteinemia in children with renal disease. Antihypertensives such as ACE inhibitors, particularly in combination with diuretics, may lead to profound hypotension.[62]

The dose of propofol to induce anesthesia using the bispectral index and clinical signs to indicate the state of hypnosis in adult patients with renal failure were significantly greater than in those without renal disease.[63] This was attributed to a larger volume of distribution in renal failure patients, consistent with previous studies of thiopental.[64] Anemia is another contributing factor. It may indirectly cause a greater plasma volume and greater cardiac output. When propofol is delivered as an infusion, no significant differences in pharmacokinetic or pharmacodynamic parameters have been observed.[65]

There are insufficient data on the use of inhalational anesthetics for induction in children with renal impairment. For maintenance of anesthesia in adults, desflurane and isoflurane do not further impair renal function in those with preexisting renal disease.[66] Sevoflurane at low flows is associated with increased circuit concentrations of compound A, which is nephrotoxic in rats.[67,68] In adult patients with normal renal function, low-flow sevoflurane anesthesia has been associated with mild, transient proteinuria but no changes in BUN, creatinine level, or creatinine clearance.[69] In adults with renal insufficiency, low-flow sevoflurane has been shown to be as safe as low-flow isoflurane in terms of kidney function.[68] Overall, sevoflurane is considered safe in patients with renal disease, but low flows should be avoided. Because desflurane is minimally metabolized (rate of 0.2%) in vivo, it may be preferred even at very low flows (1 L/min).

Neuromuscular blocking drugs (NMBDs) have evolved over the years to provide a choice of relaxants for use in children with renal disease. Children with chronic renal failure may have existing autonomic neuropathy and associated delayed gastric emptying that puts them at risk for aspiration. Along with renal implications, aspiration should be anticipated when choosing a NMBD for airway management. Succinylcholine is often avoided in children with renal failure because of its well-known propensity for increasing serum potassium. However, succinylcholine does not increase the plasma potassium concentration in patients with renal failure any more than in patients with normal renal function (0.5 to 0.8 mEq/L of potassium).[70,71] Plasma potassium concentration is chronically increased in renal failure, which means that the intracellular and extracellular potassium concentrations are in equilibrium. This contrasts with patients with acute hyperkalemia in whom the intracellular and extracellular potassium concentrations are not in equilibrium, which predisposes them to ventricular arrhythmias if succinylcholine is given. In the latter case, succinylcholine is relatively contraindicated, whereas in the former case, it is not contraindicated.

The pharmacodynamics of NMBDs in children with renal insufficiency merit consideration. The onset time of rocuronium in children with renal failure (139 seconds) was significantly greater than in the control children (87.3 seconds). This difference was attributed to a greater volume of distribution and decreased serum albumin concentrations and possibly to a reduced cardiac output in children with renal failure who were taking antihypertensives. The slower onset time of rocuronium in children with renal failure must be considered when a rapid-sequence intubation is required. The duration of action of rocuronium in children with end-stage renal disease and normal renal function is similar.[72] The time to recover a train-of-four ratio of 70% in children with renal failure was 28.9 minutes, and in those without renal failure, it was 29.4 minutes. The clearance of rocuronium is decreased in children with renal failure.[73] Vecuronium has an increased duration of action in adults with renal failure.[74]

NMBDs such as atracurium and cisatracurium are ideal choices for children with renal insufficiency because their elimination is independent of the kidney. Despite the fact that atracurium and cisatracurium undergo spontaneous degradation by plasma esterase and Hofmann elimination, neuromuscular blockade should be monitored.[75] With appropriate monitoring and dosing, atracurium, cisatracurium, vecuronium, and rocuronium are acceptable NMBDs in children with renal disease and provide reliable durations of action after a single bolus dose. However, depending on how rocuronium and vecuronium are administered during a case, their accumulation may ultimately affect their duration of action.[75]

If a prolonged neuromuscular blockade occurs, hypermagnesemia should be ruled out. In this case, calcium may be administered to help antagonize the blockade. The elimination of neostigmine may be delayed beyond elimination of atropine or glycopyrrolate, and muscarinic effects such as bradycardia, increased secretions, or bronchospasm may occur postoperatively after antagonism. Sugammadex, a selective relaxant binding agent, has reduced clearance in adults with severe renal failure.[76] The clearance of sugammadex was only 5.5 mL/min in renal failure patients but 95.2 mL/min in the control group. Despite this difference in pharmacokinetics, sugammadex can rapidly and effectively reverse the effects of rocuronium in patients with renal failure.[77]

Remifentanil may be a preferred choice for a maintenance opioid in the intraoperative period in children with renal insufficiency because of its rapid metabolism by nonspecific blood and tissue esterases. The pharmacokinetics and pharmacodynamics of remifentanil are not altered in patients with renal disease, but the principal metabolite of remifentanil has reduced elimination,[78,79] which is not expected to be clinically important. Doses of other opioids should be reduced by 30% to 50% to avoid unexpected respiratory depression in children with chronic renal failure. Active metabolites of morphine and meperidine can likewise accumulate in patients with renal failure, whereas those of fentanyl and sufentanil do not. The latter opioids are preferable on that basis alone.[80-84] Prolonged antagonism of opioid effects with naloxone can be expected in renal failure patients.

Esmolol or labetalol are useful to control tachycardia and hypertension, but large doses may exacerbate hyperkalemia by blocking intracellular potassium flux. Nicardipine is an effective, short-acting antihypertensive agent that does not affect serum potassium.

Delayed emergence, vomiting and aspiration, hypertension, respiratory depression, and pulmonary edema are potential problems that should be anticipated with anesthetic emergence. Hyperkalemia as a consequence of tissue injury, catabolism, blood transfusion, and acidosis is common. Children with chronic renal failure usually have chronic metabolic acidosis with limited buffer reserve. Modest hypercapnia with emergence may lead to significant acidosis and hyperkalemia. Careful attention should be given to the fluid needs of the child postoperatively to minimize volume overload and pulmonary edema.

Regional anesthesia is a viable alternative to general anesthesia or an adjunct in many cases. The anesthesia team must pay particular attention to coagulation studies and signs of coagulopathy before embarking on any central block because abnormal platelet function puts the renal failure patient at risk for epidural hematoma.

## Postoperative Concerns

The postoperative care of the child with renal disease must take into account the level of renal function, anemia, and preexistence of hypertension. In the child with limited ability to excrete a salt and water load, care must be given to the rate and amount of postoperative fluids administered, with consideration of the volume given during the procedure and operative losses. In children with renal insufficiency, nephrotic syndrome, or tubular disorders (especially those with concentration impairments), it is common to administer fluid volumes that approximate anticipated output and insensible needs. This volume needs to be

**TABLE 26-8** Management of Acute Malignant Hypertension

| Drug | Dose | Side Effects |
|---|---|---|
| Sodium nitroprusside | 1-10 µg/kg/min | Possible cyanide and thiocyanate toxicity, acute hypotension |
| Enalaprilat* | 0.01-0.06 mg/kg/day every 6 hours | Hypotension, angioedema, anaphylactoid reaction |
| Labetalol | 0.4-3 mg/kg/hr or 0.2-1 mg/kg every 10 minutes | Bradycardia |
| Nicardipine | 0.5-5 µg/kg/min | Acute hypotension |

*Intravenous angiotensin-converting enzyme inhibitor.

adjusted for third spacing, ongoing losses, and the administration of blood and blood products.

For children with known renal disease, care must be taken to identify medications that need to be resumed in the immediate postoperative period. Children who have been on chronic antihypertensive medications may be able to resume oral medications when awake. It may be necessary to treat isolated hypertensive episodes with intravenous medications during the postoperative period. It is important to assess the contribution of pain and anxiety to increased blood pressures to avoid overtreatment.

Because of ischemic tissue injury, it is possible that preexisting metabolic acidosis and hyperkalemia may worsen in the postoperative period. In children who have renal failure, careful monitoring of electrolytes during and after the procedure may prevent untoward emergencies. When clinically significant hyperkalemia develops in a child with chronic renal failure, treatment is imperative (see Table 26-6).

Acute hypertension can be treated with a variety of intravenous and oral medications (Table 26-8). Because the therapy for acute symptomatic hypertension should be directed toward rapid normalization of blood pressure, prompt and effective therapy must be initiated, often before the cause has been discerned. The rate of change of blood pressure can be just as important as its absolute level in the pathogenesis of hypertensive emergencies. Blood pressure itself may be a poor determinant of the severity of the clinical situation and the need for aggressive parenteral therapy. The decision to use aggressive parenteral therapy should be based on an absolute number and on clinical findings that define the situation as emergent. When it is determined that aggressive therapy is indicated, several antihypertensive agents can be used safely in children in the acute setting. The drugs most often chosen are potent vasodilators, such as hydralazine, diazoxide, or nitroprusside. There has been widespread use of nicardipine for acute hypertension in children, and they have the advantages of intravenous administration, safety, and rapid onset of action.

Hemodialysis or peritoneal dialysis can be safely resumed on the first postoperative day, with the exception of the occasional child who has operative placement of a dialysis access port for more emergent therapy. In these children, timing of renal replacement therapy must be individualized in consultation with the child's nephrologist.

Uremic encephalopathy may occur and should be considered in the child who exhibits confusion or prolonged sedation in the postanesthesia care unit. These children should be transferred to an intensive care setting for stabilization and airway management during further workup.

By careful preoperative assessment and review of preexisting disease, many postoperative complications can be anticipated and avoided. Hypervigilance during the entire perioperative period allows children with renal disease to be managed in a safe manner.

## ANNOTATED REFERENCES

Driessen JJ, Robertson EN, Van Egmond J, Booij LH. Time-course of action of rocuronium 0.3 mg/kg in children with and without end-stage renal failure. Paediatr Anaesth 2002;12:507-10.
*This study is one of the few that has specifically considered children with renal disease. It describes the differences in onset and issues related to recovery for agents that are used in children with renal disease.*

Kheterpal S, Trember KK, Heung M, et al. Development and validation of an acute kidney injury risk index for patients undergoing general surgery: results from a national data set. Anesthesiology 2009;110:505-15.
*This study is significant because it looks at patients with acute kidney injury undergoing surgery.*

Petroni KC, Cohen NH. Continuous renal replacement therapy: anesthetic implications. Anesth Analg 2002;94:1288-97.
*This article provides the anesthesiologist with a working knowledge of the various types of dialysis and how to manage the use of continuous renal replacement therapy in the perioperative period.*

Sear JW. Kidney dysfunction in the postoperative period. Br J Anaesth 2005;95:20-32.
*This article reviews the significance of renal dysfunction and the associated morbidity and mortality in the perioperative period. It discusses the causes of renal dysfunction and the prevention and treatment of postoperative renal impairment.*

Zaccharias M, Gilmore ICS, Herbison GP, Sivalingam P, Walker RJ. Interventions for protecting renal function in the perioperative period. Cochrane Database Syst Rev 2008;(4):CD003590.
*This work reports the evidence for interventions that are successful for protecting the kidney in the perioperative period.*

## REFERENCE

Please see www.expertconsult.com.

# General Abdominal and Urologic Surgery

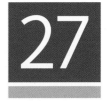

JERROLD LERMAN, YOICHI KONDO, YASUYUKI SUZUKI, RICHARD BANCHS, TAKAKO TAMURA, REIKO HAYASHI, AND KATSUYUKI MIYASAKA

ABDOMINAL SURGERY AND UROLOGIC interventions after infancy make up a large fraction of anesthetic practice for the pediatric anesthesiologist. The field is rapidly evolving, with increased use of laparoscopic surgery, including robot-assisted procedures.[1] This chapter focuses on the specific issues related to abdominal and urologic surgery, particularly in young children. The management of infants for pyloromyotomy and other neonatal abdominal procedures is discussed in Chapter 36.

## General Principles of Abdominal Surgery

### "THE FULL STOMACH": THE RISK FOR PULMONARY ASPIRATION OF GASTRIC CONTENTS

A large number of abdominal surgeries are emergency procedures that require a rapid induction of anesthesia and protection of the airway to prevent regurgitation and aspiration. Children who present with these emergencies should be considered to be at risk for vomiting and/or regurgitation and aspiration during induction of and emergence from anesthesia. Adhering to fasting guidelines for elective surgery[2] does not ensure that the stomachs of children with acute abdomens are empty of liquids and solids. The only metric that has been associated with gastric emptying after an acute emergency in children is the time interval between the last food ingested and the occurrence of the pathologic event or trauma.[2] However, there is no firm fasting interval after a trauma that predicts a zero risk of regurgitation and aspiration. In a postal survey, 83% of anesthesiologists use a rapid-sequence induction (RSI) for children with a forearm fracture within 2 hours of feeding and after opioid administration, whereas fewer than 20% use an RSI for this fracture if the child had not eaten for 6 hours since the injury.[3] The presence or absence of bowel sounds is also not predictive of gastric emptying or of the risk of regurgitation. Preoperatively, some children with acute abdomens are administered oral contrast agent before abdominal ultrasonography and/or computed tomography, in order to visualize the stomach contents and to estimate their volumes. However, these radiologic tools may not provide reliable estimates of the volume of the gastric contents.[4,5] Indeed, the absence of gastric contents in these scans does not eliminate the risk of vomiting and regurgitation. Consequently, there is no evidence that delaying the surgical procedure for the express purpose of emptying the stomach will reduce the risk of regurgitation; it cannot predict when the risk of regurgitation will be zero and may actually increase the risk of complications by delaying surgical attention to the acute abdomen.

## RAPID-SEQUENCE INDUCTION

RSI is recommended for children with a full stomach, to quickly secure the airway. This approach is intended to minimize the risk of aspiration, although it is not evidence based. The strategy is to predetermine the drug doses and have all the required airway equipment ready to use. Predetermined drug doses are administered in a rapid sequence and when muscle relaxation is present, the trachea is intubated and the cuff (if used) inflated. Many clinicians include cricoid pressure to occlude the esophageal lumen during RSI, although no randomized studies have demonstrated that this combination prevents regurgitation and aspiration compared with an inhalational or slow IV induction. This lack of evidence, combined with both theoretical and actual complications associated with RSI and cricoid pressure in children, has generated skepticism regarding their role in preventing vomiting in children who are at risk.[6] Only 74% of anesthesiologists in Northern Ireland perform RSI for children scheduled for appendectomy, 78% in the United States use it for pyloromyotomy and 83% in England use it for forearm fractures within 2 hours of eating and after recent opioid administration.[3,7,8] In two surveys, 16% and 28% of anesthesiologists in the United States and UK, respectively, reported that a number of children with full stomachs had experienced gastric regurgitation despite using RSI with cricoid pressure, and several of them had progressed to serious harm and even death.[7,9] Despite the lack of evidence that RSI is effective in children with full stomachs, we continue to recommend this approach for the majority of children at risk. Whether cricoid pressure contributes substantively to preventing regurgitation when RSI is performed remains unclear. Complications of RSI, for the most part, relate to improperly performed RSI (e.g., excessive cricoid pressure distorting the anatomy of the airway,[10] causing difficulty in securing the airway) or poor selection of patients (those with a known difficult airway, where a more measured approach must take precedence over concerns for possible aspiration).

RSI in infants and children requires more planning than it does in older children and adults for several reasons. First, the induction drugs should be flushed into the child's veins using a separate flush syringe, to ensure a rapid bolus administration of the drugs. Succinylcholine remains useful for rapid-sequence tracheal intubation for brief procedures. The introduction of intermediate-acting neuromuscular blocking drugs (NMBDs) with rapid onset, coupled with concerns about the risk of hyperkalemia after succinylcholine in children with undiagnosed neuromuscular diseases (especially males less than 8 years of age), have dramatically reduced the use of succinylcholine in elective surgery. With the shift from succinylcholine to nondepolarizing NMBDs for rapid paralysis in young children, inability to intubate and prolonged paralysis may present serious, possible life-threatening problems. Although sugammadex reverses some NMBDs, its effectiveness is limited to rocuronium and vecuronium and is not always available.[11-13] Second, preoxygenation is often difficult in infants and children because they commonly resist the tight application of the face mask needed to deliver high concentrations of oxygen. Failure to ventilate the lungs after induction and before tracheal intubation may result in desaturation more rapidly in young infants and children than older children, and in those with upper respiratory tract infections or other causes of a limited oxygen reserve.[14,15] During laryngoscopy and intubation, mask ventilation with 100% oxygen should begin when the saturation decreases to 95%, to attenuate the nadir in oxygen saturation that follows.[14] Third,

the force needed to occlude the esophagus when applying cricoid pressure to infants and children is poorly understood and poorly applied, can distort the view of the larynx during laryngoscopy, may not occlude the lumen of the esophagus, and may actually deform the lumen of the trachea if excessive force is applied.[6,10,16] Conversely, effective cricoid pressure that occludes the esophagus in children, may permit bag mask ventilation with up to 40 cm $H_2O$ peak inspiratory pressure without gastric insufflation.[17] This is known as a modified RSI. Thus, if the first attempt at tracheal intubation fails or the child desaturates during laryngoscopy, properly maintained cricoid pressure allows bag and mask ventilation of the lungs to restore oxygenation, without increasing the risk of regurgitation.

## INDICATIONS FOR PREOPERATIVE NASOGASTRIC TUBE PLACEMENT

Although there are no published guidelines on this subject, it is reasonable to insert a nasogastric tube preoperatively to allow drainage of gastrointestinal fluids in cases of documented bowel obstruction (e.g., ileus, strangulated bowel, pyloric obstruction) or in other situations in which aspiration is judged to be a substantial risk. The child may experience discomfort while a nasogastric tube is inserted, but this must be balanced against the need to decompress the stomach and reduce the risk of regurgitation during induction of anesthesia. In the remaining cases, the placement of a nasogastric tube can wait until after tracheal intubation. It should be noted that placement of a nasogastric tube may decrease lower esophageal sphincter tone, increase the risk for reflux, and reduce the ability to clear refluxed gastric contents from the distal esophagus.[18,19] Thus the anesthesiologist is faced with the dilemma of whether or not to remove the nasogastric tube before induction. It is reasonable to apply suction to the nasogastric tube, evacuate all of the gastric contents before induction, and to remove the nasogastric tube before induction, because it is unclear if even properly applied cricoid pressure can prevent wicking of gastric contents along the path created by the nasogastric tube. It should be further noted that placing a nasogastric tube, although comforting, does not ensure an empty stomach.

## FLUID BALANCE

Many acute abdominal emergencies are associated with pronounced shifts in fluid balance, mainly in the form of dehydration, electrolyte losses, third space fluid shifts, and hypovolemia. Adequate correction of these derangements is mandatory, in most instances, before proceeding with anesthesia and surgery. However, when a large fraction of the bowel becomes strangulated and ischemic, large volumes of fluid may be sequestered in the bowel. In these cases, hypovolemia should be suspected and resuscitation initiated as anesthesia is rapidly induced. In some elective cases (e.g., bowel resection because of inflammatory bowel disease), fluid and electrolyte resuscitation should routinely be a focus of special interest, because the child may not be fully compensated at the time of surgery.

To date, published studies indicate that resuscitation with crystalloid fluids yields similar results to that with colloids.[20] In most children, initial resuscitation is undertaken with balanced salt solutions. Although colloid therapy may result in less tissue edema and less volume infused, the added expense of colloids may not justify their routine use in children.

## POTENTIAL FOR STRANGULATED OR ISCHEMIC BOWEL

The need for anesthesia and surgery becomes more urgent when the bowel is suspected of being ischemic and/or necrotic. For example, if true volvulus is suspected, immediate action is necessary; otherwise the child is at risk for massive bowel resection with subsequent short bowel syndrome, a condition associated with serious lifelong medical problems. Even if the child is far from optimally resuscitated, anesthesia must be induced and maintained, preferably with anesthetics that do not depress the circulation excessively, while simultaneously correcting the dehydration (or hypovolemia) and electrolyte imbalance. The situation is somewhat less critical in the child with an incarcerated inguinal hernia, although delay of even this surgery should be minimized.

Translocation of bacteria from the intestinal tract and subsequent septicemia are possible with ischemic bowel. Ischemic bowel may release a host of mediators that can cause severe hemodynamic instability. Thus when a substantial segment of the bowel is becoming ischemic, the anesthesiologist must be prepared to maintain anesthesia without depressing the circulation excessively, acutely resuscitate the child with appropriate fluids, and administer inotropic and/or vasoactive medications as needed. It should be noted that hemodynamic instability might acutely worsen when reperfusion of the bowel is established or with simple opening of the abdomen. Close communication with the surgeon is paramount in these cases.

## PRESENCE OF CONCOMITANT SEPTICEMIA

Children with acute intraabdominal disease should always be regarded as being at risk for bacterial translocation with subsequent septicemia. Children with overt sepsis are usually easy to identify and may already be admitted to the pediatric intensive care unit. However, incipient or early sepsis may not exhibit overt signs, therefore signs of sepsis should be actively sought. If septicemia is present or suspected, appropriate intravenous (IV) antibiotics should be administered without delay, preferably before anesthesia and surgery. Septic or preseptic children can be extremely unstable; the possible need to administer inotropic and/or vasoactive drugs should be anticipated. Hemodynamic compromise may be dramatically revealed following anesthetic induction and loss of vascular sympathetic tone. Additionally, their lungs may be difficult to ventilate because of established or developing acute lung injury. Thus the anesthesiologist needs to be prepared to provide invasive monitoring (arterial and central venous pressures) and an anesthetic machine capable of providing positive end-expiratory pressure; in some situations an intensive care unit ventilator may be needed in the operating room.

## PRESENCE OF ABDOMINAL COMPARTMENT SYNDROME

Acute intraabdominal disease processes may lead to a critically increased intraabdominal pressure (IAP).[21] If the IAP increases above the capillary perfusion pressure of the intraabdominal organs, an abdominal compartment syndrome can develop. Organ perfusion will become compromised and ischemia and/or necrosis may develop. The most commonly affected organs in this situation are the bowels, kidneys, and liver. Abdominal compartment syndrome occurs less frequently in children than in adults.[22] Causes of abdominal compartment syndrome include burns, extracorporeal membrane oxygenation,[23] closure of gastroschisis or omphalocoele,[24] abdominal trauma,[25,26] abdominal surgery,[27] and a variety of other intraabdominal pathologies, including necrotizing enterocolitis, Hirschsprung enterocolitis,

perforated bowel, diaphragmatic hernia, and Wilms tumor.[23,28,29] Insufficient perfusion of the bowel may cause an ileus, translocation of bacteria, lactate accumulation, and production of mediators that cause hemodynamic instability. Increased IAP can reduce liver blood flow that will reduce hepatic function,[30] mainly manifested as an inability to metabolize lactate, a delay in drug metabolism,[30,31] and, in severe cases, impaired synthesis of coagulation factors. Because the pressure is also transmitted to the retroperitoneal space, renal function may become impaired, resulting in oliguria or anuria and reduced excretion of drugs.[28] In addition, cranial displacement of the abdominal contents and splinting of the diaphragm may seriously compromise ventilation.[32]

If acute intraabdominal compartment syndrome is suspected, then the IAP should be measured to determine if it exceeds the critical threshold of 20 to 25 mm Hg. Some suspect a compartment syndrome when the vesicular (bladder) pressure exceeds 10 to 12 mm Hg.[33,34] These pressures can be measured either via a nasogastric tube or bladder catheter.[35] The diagnosis of intraabdominal compartment syndrome should be suspected when the triad of (1) massive abdominal distention, (2) increased bladder pressures and increased peak inspiratory airway pressures, and (3) evidence of renal and/or cardiac dysfunction are present.[29,36,37]

Children with acute intraabdominal compartment syndrome can become extremely hemodynamically unstable. Although decompression of the abdomen by a laparotomy will immediately normalize the IAP, reperfusion of the ischemic tissues almost always releases a host of biologically active substances that cause serious hypotension. These substances may also precipitate acute renal failure and lead to a disseminated intravascular coagulopathy. As in the case of sepsis, the anesthesiologist must be fully prepared to address these challenges by having blood products in the operating room and vasopressors available before induction of anesthesia. Some children will require a patch abdominoplasty as a temporizing measure to protect abdominal organs with primary closure of the anterior abdominal wall at some time in the future.[29,36]

## PREOPERATIVE LABORATORY TESTING AND INVESTIGATIONS

Most minor elective cases (e.g., umbilical or inguinal hernia repair) do not require any further preoperative work-up beyond a basic history and physical examination. Many centers require a preoperative urine (or hemoglobin) screen for pregnancy in females who have reached menarche.[38] More complex elective cases may warrant additional laboratory testing, including basic hematology screening and electrolyte profile.

Preoperative laboratory testing is strongly advised in more critically ill children. Liver and renal function tests, coagulation profile, and serum albumin concentration should be assessed and blood typed and crossmatched. In children who are septic or who have an acute intraabdominal compartment syndrome, a preoperative chest radiograph may indicate the severity of pulmonary involvement. An echocardiogram may be needed to assess myocardial contractility and volume status if there is evidence of cardiac dysfunction.

## MONITORING REQUIREMENTS

Routine elective cases rarely require more than standard monitoring equipment. In children undergoing major intraabdominal procedures, invasive arterial and central venous blood pressure monitoring may be indicated. A multiple-lumen central venous line inserted at the beginning of the procedure will facilitate administration of inotropic and/or vasoactive drugs, in addition to measuring central venous pressure; ultrasound-guided insertion is strongly recommended.[39] These lines are of great value in the immediate postoperative period for blood sampling, drug administration, ongoing assessment of intravascular volume status, and parenteral nutrition. Transesophageal echocardiographic or transesophageal Doppler evaluation may provide valuable intraoperative and postoperative information regarding the child's volume status, as well as cardiac contractility.[40-50]

A urinary catheter with a pediatric urinometer (i.e., a graduated collection receptacle), which provides an accurate measure of urine output is a useful monitor for most intraabdominal procedures. The measurement of hourly urine output safeguards against the development of hypovolemia and possible prerenal azotemia (see the section on laparoscopy for discussion of changes in urine output with increased IAP).

Monitoring IAP is important during laparoscopic surgery, although it will be of minimal value in omphalocele and gastroschisis surgeries, as long as the abdomen remains open. Once the abdomen is closed however, IAP will provide useful prognostic information regarding intraabdominal organ blood flow, circulatory stability, and respiratory embarrassment (see Chapter 36).[32]

## CHOICE OF ANESTHETIC

The anesthesiologist may use his or her personal preference of anesthetic technique for the management of both elective and emergency intraabdominal surgery in children. However, airway management associated with intraabdominal surgery requires careful consideration. Even when the child is not at increased risk for regurgitation and aspiration, the risk of regurgitation can be increased if the surgeon manipulates the bowel, when the child is positioned head down, and if gas is insufflated into the peritoneal cavity (as occurs in laparoscopic procedures). A particular concern arises when the surgeon decides to decompress distended bowel. One method is to perform an enterotomy and directly drain the fluid, whereas the other is to massage (strip) the bowel in a retrograde direction until the contents can be vented with a nasogastric tube. The latter method has caused massive intestinal regurgitation that exceeded the capacity of the nasogastric tube, required clearance of the mouth with a Yankauer suction tip, and caused pulmonary aspiration.[51] The laryngeal mask airway should not be used during intraabdominal surgery in general, and instead we strongly recommend the use of tracheal intubation with a cuffed tracheal tube as the standard in the majority of these cases.

Regional anesthetic techniques may be useful adjuncts in children undergoing both minor and major abdominal surgery. However, in critically unstable or septic children, the use of epidural anesthesia is not recommended, because sympathetic blockade may further exacerbate the hemodynamic instability, and there is an increased risk of epidural abscess formation. Simple local infiltration of the port insertion sites contributes to adequate postoperative analgesia in most children who have had laparoscopic procedures,[52] whereas those who have had an open procedure will require IV opioids (see Chapter 43). Analgesia is commonly supplemented with NSAIDs and acetaminophen.

# General Principles of Urologic Surgery

With the exception of acute drainage of urinary obstruction (i.e., ultrasound-guided nephrostomy or cystostomy procedures) and torsion of the testis, most pediatric urologic surgeries are elective. In the vast majority of cases, these children are otherwise healthy or with stable medical conditions that do not require more than a careful history, physical examination, and review of the child's medical record. Children who undergo urologic procedures may be suffering from emotional disturbance because of repeated interventions and sensitivity of the surgical site. This mandates special psychological attention before and after anesthesia. The occurrence of anaphylaxis resulting from exposure to latex-related products is of special concern in children with chronic urologic disorders.[53-56] Children with spina bifida are at greater risk for latex allergy than those without spina bifida,[57-60] presumably because of early and repeated exposure to latex urethral catheters, although every child with congenital malformations of the urinary tract and repeat latex exposure to mucous membranes beginning in the neonatal period is at significant risk for developing latex hypersensitivity.[61,62] Thus latex-free management is highly recommended in this population.[63-65]

## REDUCED RENAL FUNCTION

Children with chronic renal disease have impaired renal function, which may affect drug dosing and disposition, as well as cause secondary effects on the cardiovascular system. In the most severe cases, the child may require dialysis to balance fluids and electrolytes. In children with renal disease, it is essential to determine the degree of renal impairment by consulting the child's nephrologist and reviewing the serum creatinine, blood urea nitrogen, sodium, and potassium concentrations (see also Chapter 26). Because renal impairment may also affect clotting, a coagulation profile, including platelet count, should be reviewed preoperatively if substantial blood loss is anticipated. These children are prone to fluid overload, particularly those who are anuric and dialysis dependent. Apart from clinical signs associated with fluid overload, measuring the child's weight and comparing it with their normal weight is a simple means to assess the child's current volume status. If cardiac function or volume status remains in doubt, an echocardiogram should be obtained. Children with chronic renal insufficiency often have impaired left ventricular function even before they require dialysis, so a preoperative echocardiogram may be indicated[66-70]; pericardial effusion is also a concern in these children.[67,71,72]

For children who are dialyzed, the most recent date of dialysis should be documented. Overhydration and/or hypervolemia should be corrected preoperatively with dialysis. Although dialysis corrects hyperkalemia and overhydration, and may transiently improve platelet function (peritoneal dialysis yielding more consistent improvement than hemodialysis), it is best to not perform dialysis within 12 hours of anesthesia, so as to avoid a relative hypovolemia and to allow sufficient time for body fluids to re-equilibrate (see Chapter 26).[73,74] Postdialysis laboratory indices of serum electrolytes (particularly potassium), hemoglobin or hematocrit, renal function (creatinine and blood urea nitrogen), and the child's weight loss should be recorded. For children who undergo hemodialysis, IV access should not be established in the extremity ipsilateral to the arteriovenous fistula.

## SYSTEMIC HYPERTENSION

Systemic hypertension is common in renal insufficiency in adults, but far less common in children. Nonetheless, some children with urologic disorders develop significant systemic hypertension associated with disturbances in the renin-angiotensin system.[75-78] As in adults, it is important to control systemic hypertension before induction to avoid wide swings in blood pressure. In contrast to adults, however, hypervolemia is an important cause of hypertension in children with renal insufficiency and should be considered and treated preoperatively. Children and adults are often treated with similar antihypertensive medications.[77,78] These medications should be continued up to and including the morning of surgery to maintain intraoperative and postoperative hemodynamic stability. However, angiotensin-converting enzyme inhibitors are exceptions to this rule[79]: consideration should be given to holding the medication at least 1 day before surgery to avoid intraoperative hypotension[80,81]; conversely, holding the medication may be associated with rebound hypertension postoperatively. If these medications are not withheld, vasopressors may be required during anesthesia to stabilize the blood pressure.[82] Because therapy-resistant renal hypertension is an indication for nephrectomy, one should anticipate and be prepared to treat wide fluctuations in blood pressure, including severe hypertension during the first stage of the operation and profound hypotension when the responsible kidney is removed. As a consequence, long-acting antihypertensive agents are best avoided during the early stages of a nephrectomy in a child.

### CORTICOSTEROID MEDICATIONS

Children with renal disease may be chronically treated with corticosteroids as part of their medical management (e.g., children with proteinuria or who have undergone previous renal transplant surgery). In such cases, a stress dose of parenteral corticosteroids during surgery is indicated, with continued supplementation until the child resumes his or her normal corticosteroid medication by the enteral route. In more complex situations, consultation with a pediatric nephrologist or endocrinologist is warranted to optimize corticosteroid supplementation, although in more straightforward cases, a dose of 2.5 mg/kg of IV hydrocortisone two to three times each day is usually adequate (see Chapter 25).

### INFECTION OR SEPSIS

Obstructive urinary tract disease or chronic renal insufficiency increases the risk for urinary tract infections. If treated properly, the infection is usually well controlled and should not interfere with anesthesia. However, in children who demonstrate overt signs of systemic illness or septicemia, the anesthetic and postoperative course may be difficult.

### MONITORING REQUIREMENTS

Standard noninvasive monitoring is adequate for the vast majority of urologic procedures in children, as they are of minor or moderate magnitude (e.g., circumcision, orchiopexy, pyeloplasty, and ureter neoimplantation). The anesthetic care that is required for infants and children undergoing penile surgery is routine, including a forced-air heating mattress to prevent hypothermia in surgeries lasting more than 1 hour. However, recognizing the minimal amount of skin that is exposed during this type of surgery, the child's temperature often increases steadily during the surgery necessitating close monitoring of the child's temperature to avoid iatrogenic overheating.

Invasive monitors (i.e., invasive blood pressure monitoring, central venous access for pressure measurements and administration of vasoactive drugs) are indicated for major surgical interventions, and in cases with concomitant problems (e.g., decreased renal function, significant hypertension, associated cardiac dysfunction, sepsis). If central venous access is deemed to be

necessary, the coagulation status of the child should be evaluated, because platelet function may be substantially compromised. Ultrasound guidance improves safety in securing central venous access in cases in which a coagulopathy is present or suspected on clinical grounds (see Chapter 48). In the unstable child, even more complex monitoring (e.g., esophageal Doppler monitoring or transesophageal echocardiography) should be considered.

It is important to monitor urine output, although the volume of urine may not reflect renal homeostasis. During surgery that involves the bladder or in children who are anuric, urine output will not be available for part or all of the surgery. Hence, other indices of fluid status and perfusion must be used. Heart rate and systolic blood pressure are reliable indices of volume status and perfusion in most children, although central venous pressure and invasive arterial pressure measurement may be indicated in special cases. Surgeons may be heartened to observe urine flowing into the bladder after reimplantation of ureters and kidney transplantation. Preloading with an IV balanced salt solution may be useful in such circumstances; occasionally a loop diuretic is requested.

## Laparoscopic Surgery

Although laparoscopic surgery was introduced more than 80 years ago, its role in pediatric surgery has only become notable in the past 10 to 15 years. To a large extent, this has been due to improved technology in optics and miniaturization of the instruments. An increasing number of general and urologic surgical procedures (including appendectomy, cholecystectomy, and splenectomy, as well as those to treat inguinal hernia and undescended testicles) are performed either laparoscopically or using robotic techniques in children of all ages, including neonates (Figs. 27-1 to 27-4).[83-91] More sophisticated laparoscopic techniques have enabled the performance of complex surgical procedures, including Nissen fundoplication, colectomy, pyeloplasty, bowel pull-through, and removal of large organs, including the kidney and spleen.[89,92-95] Technological advances now permit laparoscopic surgery in neonates and small infants, including those with hypoplastic left heart syndrome after stage 1 or 2 repair.[91,96-98]

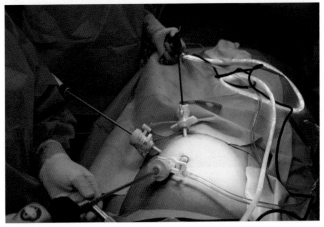

**FIGURE 27-1** A child undergoing laparoscopic appendectomy, presented as a paradigm for the surgical set-up for any multiple trocar laparoscopic surgery. Three incisions were made, two in the anterior abdominal wall and the third in the umbilicus. The first two trocars carry instruments to manipulate the appendix, while the third holds the camera for viewing by all personnel in the operating room. All cables swing widely off the surgical field.

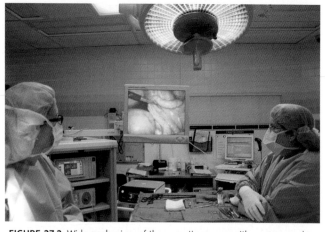

FIGURE 27-2 Wide-angle view of the operating room with surgeon and scrub nurse viewing the appendix being held by the grasper, shown on the overhead monitor.

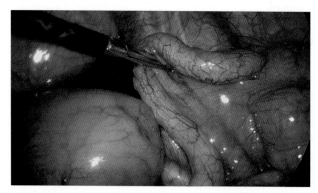

FIGURE 27-3 Inside the abdominal cavity with a view of the inflamed appendix that has been mobilized. The peritoneal attachments must be peeled off the appendix before it is ligated and removed.

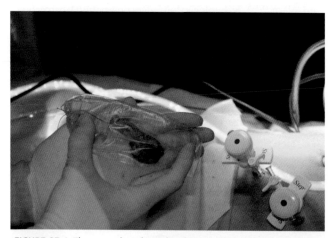

FIGURE 27-4 The appendix is ligated and inserted into a plastic container and withdrawn usually through the trocar or incision site without contaminating adjacent tissues. The appendix is shown in the surgeon's hand after removal.

It must be noted however that laparoscopic surgery in children with cyanotic heart disease carries with it a substantial risk that exceeds most other populations having this form of surgery. Although several reports suggest that infants and children of all ages, at all stages of palliative repair of their cyanotic heart

disease, tolerate laparoscopic surgery,[98-100] the risk for those with Fontan physiology undergoing laparoscopic surgery is substantial. It is essential to understand that in Fontan physiology, pulmonary blood flow is passive, and decreases in venous return (whether from increases in intrathoracic pressure or head-up positioning) or increases in pulmonary vascular resistance (because of carbon dioxide absorption or decreased minute ventilation) could severely reduce the cardiac output.[101] Creating a pneumoperitoneum, as in the case in laparoscopic surgery, and extreme positions increase IAP and arterial carbon dioxide tensions (increasing pulmonary artery pressure), reduce venous return, and increase the risk of reducing the cardiac output in children with Fontan physiology (see later discussion). Successful management of these children during laparoscopic surgery requires a multidisciplinary team that functions in concert to optimize the child's outcome (1) by optimizing the child's condition preoperatively and identifying any cardiac issues, (2) by recruiting surgeons who can complete the surgery quickly and efficiently, (3) by maintaining the children in the supine position throughout the surgery, (4) by maintaining normocapnia, (5) by monitoring the child with a transesophageal echo probe as needed, as well as with an arterial invasive pressure monitor for blood gas analysis, and (6) by insufflating the abdomen to the lowest (less than 8 mm Hg) IAP that is surgically feasible. Larger studies are required before children with cyanotic heart disease, particularly those with Fontan physiology, can routinely undergo laparoscopic surgery in any center except those with specialized teams to manage these children.

Laparoscopic surgery offers a number of advantages over open surgery, including more rapid emergence from anesthesia, faster ambulation, earlier discharge from the hospital, and reduced perioperative complications.[102-105] Robot-assisted surgical technology is discussed later.

Laparoscopic surgery involves the insufflation of gas into the abdominal cavity in order to visualize the intraabdominal organs. When preparing for laparoscopic surgery, if the surgery involves the upper abdomen, the stomach should be decompressed using a nasogastric or orogastric tube whereas if the surgery involves the lower abdomen, the bladder should be emptied using a urinary catheter. Surgical access to the peritoneal cavity is achieved with trocars introduced through three (or more) small (3 to 10 mm in diameter) incisions. Through the trocars, the laparoscopic instruments and a camera are then passed. Recently a laparo-endoscopic single site (LESS), single port, single incision laparoscopic surgery (SILS), single incision multiport laparoscopy (SIMPL), or "belly button" surgery has been developed, in which all instruments pass through a single incision and a single large trocar (often in the umbilicus).[106-109] Through the single trocar, the instruments and a camera are inserted.[109a] (E-Figs. 27-1 through 27-3). "Clashing" (or colliding of objects) is a common problem because of the close proximity of the cables exiting the single trocar, as well as the proximity of the multiple hands performing the procedure. The clashing of cables has been resolved by fusing them into a single cable as they exit the trocar.

Pneumoperitoneal pressure is a major concern for all laparoscopic approaches. Experimental evidence in adult and newborn pigs demonstrated that the risks of cardiorespiratory consequences and potentially fatal emboli were directly related to the peak pneumoperitoneal pressure.[110,111] In infants and children, the optimal pneumoperitoneal pressure is the least pressure that enables adequate surgical access. Carbon dioxide should be insufflated through one of the trocars until the IAP reaches 6 to

15 mm Hg; most surgeons currently limit the IAP in neonates and young infants to 6 to 8 mm Hg and in children to 10 to 12 mm Hg.[112] The IAP is maintained throughout the surgery by intermittently insufflating additional $CO_2$. Although carbon dioxide is most commonly used, a number of gases have been investigated (see later discussion).[113] Carbon dioxide is the preferred gas because it does not support combustion, is rapidly cleared from the peritoneal cavity at the end of surgery, and does not expand into bubbles or spaces.[93,114,115] However, the increased IAP may cause mechanical difficulties, such as circulatory or respiratory depression, hypothermia due to dry gas leakage, pneumothorax or subcutaneous emphysema, endobronchial intubation resulting from the upward shift of tracheal bifurcation, and injury due to paracentesis. The major disadvantage of $CO_2$ is that it is rapidly absorbed from the peritoneum, with the absorption and washout of $CO_2$ being more rapid and the peak end-tidal partial pressure of $CO_2$ ($PETCO_2$) less in infants than in older children.[116,117] The inverse relationship between age and rate of $CO_2$ absorption from the abdomen has been attributed to the thinner peritoneum and the reduced peritoneal fat deposits in the abdomen of infants compared with older children.[117] Evidence indicates that only 10% to 20% of the $PETCO_2$ originates from the insufflated $CO_2$ after 10 to 20 minutes of insufflation at an IAP of 10 to 15 mm Hg.[118] During $CO_2$ insufflation, both the $PETCO_2$ and $PaCO_2$ increase up to 20 mm Hg or 20% to 50% above baseline.[94,112,114,116,119] Hypercapnia may occur if surgery lasts more than 1 hour, particularly in neonates,[120] necessitating an increase in minute ventilation of 50% to 100% to maintain a physiologic pH.[93,121] Again, it must be emphasized that all of these adverse physiologic changes that occur with laparoscopic surgery could have catastrophic implications for children with Fontan physiology and that consideration to performing an open procedure may be the safest approach.

The difference between the partial pressures of arterial and end-tidal $CO_2$ ($Pa–PETCO_2$) often increases during insufflation of $CO_2$,[119,121] although a number of studies reported negative $Pa–PETCO_2$ gradients, particularly in infants. The explanation for these negative gradients has been elusive, but may be due to sampling or technical errors or ventilation-perfusion mismatch.[119,121] The $Pa–PETCO_2$ gradient before and after pneumoperitoneum increases from a mean of 5.7 mm Hg to 13.4 mm Hg.[122] In neonates and in children with cyanotic congenital heart disease, the $PETCO_2$ may not reliably track the $PaCO_2$ during $CO_2$ insufflation, leading some to recommend arterial blood gas monitoring to validate the $PETCO_2$ measurements.[119,122,123]

Increased $PaCO_2$ may also trigger spontaneous respiratory efforts that could interfere with surgery. Additionally it may also initiate a sympathetic response, including an increase in the heart rate, blood pressure, and cerebral blood flow, as well as ventricular arrhythmias, although this occurs rarely today because sevoflurane has replaced halothane in many countries. A sudden increase in $PETCO_2$ may also suggest a diagnosis of malignant hyperthermia. If this diagnosis proves to be difficult to confirm or reject (see Chapter 40), it may be necessary to desufflate the abdomen and determine if the clinical and laboratory findings suggestive of MH resolve. Insufflated $CO_2$ originating from the abdomen continues to be exhaled for the first 30 minutes after desufflation.[118]

Gas emboli have been reported in several laparoscopic studies, most of which were interesting curiosities of no clinical consequence, although in several, the result was profound cardiovascular collapse. Most consider the emboli to be intravascular

$CO_2$ bubbles. Intravascular embolization of $CO_2$ may occur when the insufflation pressure exceeds the venous pressure, forcing $CO_2$ bubbles into the venous circulation, resulting in sudden cardiovascular collapse.[124] Continuous precordial Doppler or $CO_2$ partial pressure are effective in detecting a gas embolus, although the Doppler may be overly sensitive, with numerous false-positives. It has been suggested that many episodes of subclinical gas embolisms are unrecognized because the symptoms are mild and nonspecific. However, children with right-to-left shunts or potential right-to-left shunts, such as a patent foramen ovale, are vulnerable to the systemic effects of these emboli. Although $CO_2$ is soluble in blood and rapidly buffered, $CO_2$ emboli dissolve slowly in blood, taking 2 to 3 minutes to disappear.[125] Hence, large emboli may block blood flow in the heart for several minutes or more, before they dissolve. The minimum rate of infusion of $CO_2$ into blood that triggers cardiovascular collapse in pigs is 1.2 mL/kg/min[125]; comparable data in humans are lacking. Anesthesiologists should be aware of the high-risk conditions that predispose to $CO_2$ emboli (e.g., increased abdominal insufflation pressure, hypovolemia and reduced venous pressure, spontaneous respirations, and resection of vessel-rich parenchymatous organs) and correct the condition or warn the surgeons.

Some investigators suggest that clinically important gas emboli are actually nitrogen, not carbon dioxide gas emboli.[124] Whereas transient emboli are thought to be composed of $CO_2$, emboli that persist may be nitrogen gas.[124] Nitrogen is insoluble in blood (blood/gas partition coefficient of 0.014), which explains its persistence as an embolus in blood. These emboli may arise from air either present in or entrained by the trocar during insufflation of the peritoneum, that is forced into a transected blood vessel while the carboperitoneum is pressurized.[124] This mechanism is a rare source for gas in the circulation, which may explain, in part, why the emboli that occur during laparoscopy very rarely result in cardiovascular instability and arrest.

In contrast to $CO_2$, insufflation with oxygen, air, and nitrous oxide for laparoscopic surgery has been eschewed because they all support combustion. However, repeat desufflations of the pneumoperitoneal gas during laparoscopy in pigs whose lungs were ventilated with 66% nitrous oxide in oxygen, has been shown to prevent concentrations of nitrous oxide from exceeding 10% in the pneumoperitoneal cavity.[126] Nitrous oxide is still not recommended for either insufflation or as an adjunctive anesthetic gas during laparoscopy, because it also expands into gas-filled cavities should gas emboli appear in the circulation.[114] Its use during laparoscopic surgery may distend the bowel in bowel obstruction and obscure the surgeon's view, as well as expand any $CO_2$ emboli that develop.

The inert gases argon and helium were also candidate gases for insufflation to create a pneumoperitoneum as they cannot be oxidized (and therefore ignited), although they are much more expensive than $CO_2$. When argon was used to create a pneumoperitoneum in pigs, embolization occurred more frequently than with $CO_2$.[127] In theory, both argon and helium can cause serious sequelae if embolized into the vascular system because they are insoluble in blood (blood/gas solubility of helium is 0.007 and argon is 0.029) and are likely to persist.[93,114,115,127]

## PULMONARY EFFECTS

As the pressure within the peritoneal cavity increases, so too do the possible adverse respiratory effects, particularly at IAP greater than 15 cm $H_2O$. The respiratory manifestations of increased IAP include cephalad displacement of the diaphragm, decreased excursion of the diaphragm, and decreases in pulmonary and thoracic compliance, vital capacity, functional residual capacity, and closing volume.[128] Cephalad displacement of the diaphragm shifts ventilation to the nondependent parts of the lungs, creating ventilation-perfusion mismatch which may require that minute ventilation is increased from 50% to 100% to offset these effects. With a small functional residual capacity in children, cephalad displacement of the diaphragm further compresses the lungs, causing collapse of the small airways, ventilation-perfusion mismatch, and possibly hypoxemia. Pulmonary mechanics after insufflation of a pneumoperitoneum increases peak inspiratory pressures by 27% and decreases compliance by about 39%.[129] These physiologic changes are compounded by the extreme body tilting (i.e., extreme head-up or head-down positions) often requested by surgeons.[114,130] Positioning the child head down (i.e., Trendelenburg position) decreases compliance by 17% and pneumoperitoneum decreases compliance by 27%, requiring increases in peak inflation pressures of 19% and 32%, respectively.[131] Pulmonary function appears to be restored more readily after laparoscopic than open surgery.[93] In some instances, the pneumoperitoneum and the extreme position shift the tracheal tube in a rostral direction, as far as 1.2 to 2.7 cm, possibly impacting on the carina or passing into a bronchus.[132] With these changes, inspired oxygen concentrations in excess of 30% may be required, along with positive end-expiratory pressure to restore adequate oxygenation. A persistent 5% decrease in oxygen saturation has been associated with partial or intermittent endobronchial intubation.[133]

Securing the airway for laparoscopic surgery requires particular attention. Cuffed tracheal tubes are preferred over uncuffed tubes to maintain an adequate minute ventilation.[123] If the child has a mature tracheotomy, the air leak around the tracheotomy must be assessed before surgery. If the leak is excessive, then the IAP may prevent adequate ventilation during surgery. In such a situation, the tracheotomy should be replaced with a cuffed tracheotomy or an armored (cuffed) tracheal tube. If the air leak around the tracheotomy is insignificant, then ventilation should be adequate in the presence of increased IAP during laparoscopic surgery.

Excessive IAP may cause gas to track across the diaphragm, causing a pneumomediastinum or pneumothorax.[115] This is more common in hiatus hernia surgery and Nissen fundoplication, during which dissection of the esophagus may create passages for gas to traverse the diaphragm. Pneumomediastinum should be suspected if subcutaneous emphysema appears. If surgery creates a transdiaphragmatic passage for $CO_2$ to accumulate in the pleural space, the resulting pneumothorax may produce cardiorespiratory manifestations. A chest radiograph should be obtained if subcutaneous emphysema appears during or after surgery, or if there is a high index of suspicion that a pneumothorax has formed. In laparoscopic surgeries that are brief (less than 30 minutes), both laryngeal mask airways and ProSeal supraglottic airways have been used without complications, although most clinicians prefer cuffed tracheal tubes.[115,134] Both pressure- and volume-controlled ventilation have been used during laparoscopic abdominal surgery in infants and children. In a single randomized study, both ventilation strategies with 5 mm Hg positive end-expiratory pressure maintained effective ventilation and gas exchange.[135]

Although pneumoperitoneum offers the surgeons excellent operating conditions, it is a source of cardiorespiratory compromise. An alternative to insufflating $CO_2$ to create a pneumoperitoneum is the gasless laparoscopic approach. This requires lifting the anterior abdominal wall to create an intra-abdominal tent.[115,136] Implementation of the gasless approach in pediatric medicine has been rather slow, presumably because of technical difficulties and the scarcity of instruments for infants and children.

## CARDIOVASCULAR EFFECTS

A pneumoperitoneum can adversely affect cardiovascular indices.[115,136] Three major factors contribute to cardiovascular changes: (1) IAP, (2) position (i.e., steep head-up or reverse Trendelenburg), and (3) release of neurohumoral vasoactive substances.[128] Increased IAP exerts a biphasic effect on venous return and cardiac output (CO). In neonatal pigs, the cardiac index (CI) decreased 55% when IAP exceeded 20 mm Hg.[115] The magnitude of the increase in IAP determines the degree to which the circulation is depressed.[123,137] For example, at IAP less than 15 mm Hg, blood is compressed out of the splanchnic circulation increasing venous return which either increases or results in no effect on CO. In contrast, at IAP greater than 15 mm Hg, the inferior vena cava is compressed, reducing venous return and therefore CO. Studies in children yielded similar results. When the IAP exceeded 12 mm Hg, myocardial contractility[138] and venous return[114] decreased mildly. In both infants and children, $CO_2$ insufflation to IAP 10 to 13 mm Hg decreased CI approximately 13%.[139-141] However, an IAP less than or equal to 5 mm Hg maintained the CI in infants during a $CO_2$ pneumoperitoneum.[142] In all of the studies in infants and children in which the CI decreased during increased IAP (10 to 12 mm Hg), the CI returned to preinsufflation values when the abdomen was desufflated.[138,139,141] Left ventricular systolic function was diminished and septal wall motion abnormalities have been reported with an IAP of 10 to 12 mm Hg in children with a $CO_2$ pneumoperitoneum.[138,139] No significant changes in echocardiographic indices of left ventricular work, preload or afterload, have been noted if the IAP was less than 10 mm Hg during the pneumoperitoneum.[112] When standard indices of hemodynamics were measured in infants and young children during laparoscopic Nissen fundoplication, IAP less than or equal to 10 mm Hg yielded no significant changes in heart rate and blood pressure but a slight increase in CI.[142,143] If IAP is maintained at less than or equal to 10 mm Hg, then the impact on hemodynamics (and in particular, CO) should be clinically insignificant, because venous return is enhanced as a result of displacement of blood from the splanchnic bed, and afterload is not increased.[114,123,142]

Body position during laparoscopic surgery may exaggerate cardiovascular changes. For Nissen fundoplication, a steep head-up position (greater than 20-degree incline) has been used, which reduces venous return.[130] In adult pigs, laparoscopic surgery for Nissen fundoplication increased pleural and mediastinal pressures that in turn, reduced CO episodically at an IAP of 15 mm Hg.[144] These decreases in CO were manifested by episodes of hypotension and hypoxia. When children were positioned in the steep head-up position, they developed transient hypotension and bradycardia that were reversed immediately with fluid loading and atropine.[145]

It is imperative to continuously monitor IAP to minimize the cardiorespiratory effects of laparoscopic surgery and to avoid excessive insufflation pressures. In adults, induction of anesthesia, IAP to 14 mm Hg, and 10-degree head-up tilt decreased the CI more than 50%.[146] Some clinicians recommend a maximum

IAP during laparoscopy in children of 6 to 8 mm Hg to limit the cardiorespiratory effects,[147] although the consensus appears to be closer to pressures of 10 to 12 mm Hg. In neonates and infants, 6 to 8 mm Hg appears to be the accepted peak IAP. Based on the current literature, the net cardiovascular effects of insufflating the abdomen to pressures less than or equal to 12 mm Hg, combined with the head-up position, are likely to be well-tolerated if adequate hydration is maintained and bradycardia is avoided.[145]

## CENTRAL NERVOUS SYSTEM EFFECTS

Laparoscopic surgery must be carefully evaluated if planned for a child with increased intracranial pressure, or in the presence of a ventriculoperitoneal (VP) shunt. The combination of increased IAP, increased systemic vascular resistance, increased $PaCO_2$ tension, and Trendelenburg position (as in lower abdominal surgery) may dramatically increase intracranial pressure. In adults during extreme head-down position (40 degrees) for prolonged periods, such as in robot-assisted surgery in the pelvis, cerebral tissue oxygen saturation is well-maintained, as evidenced by near-infrared spectroscopy.[148] Under similar surgical conditions, intraocular pressure increased 100%, and scleral edema and blurred vision may develop.[149]

Patency of a VP shunt should be evaluated before the procedure to prevent sudden increases in intracranial pressure during the procedure. Children with reduced brain compliance may sustain dramatic increases in intracranial pressure if the IAP is sufficient to attenuate the drainage of cerebrospinal fluid into the abdominal cavity. In these children, laparoscopic surgery may be relatively contraindicated.[130] The risks should be thoroughly explored and discussed with the neurosurgeon, general surgeon, anesthesiologist, and the family. Studies have reported a range of responses to laparoscopy in children with VP shunts, from dramatic increases in intracranial pressure to no change at all.[128,150,151] Accordingly, some advocate externalizing the shunt and clamping the distal (intraabdominal) end of the shunt before surgery to prevent carbon dioxide from passing retrograde up the shunt or from the laparoscopic pressure disrupting the shunt valve, although an IAP of 80 mm Hg is required for this to occur.[153] Others discourage externalizing the shunt as sequelae have been reported, and instead recommend monitoring the intracranial pressure to prevent and detect increases in intracranial pressure, and further recommend retraction of abdominal tissue during the laparoscopic surgery.[153] For the surgeon, using a SILS approach to laparoscopic surgery in these children reduces the risk of both traumatizing and infecting the VP shunt.[152] A recent review demonstrated that laparoscopy in children with VP shunts is safe and not associated with an increased risk of shunt infection.[153] No single strategy can provide the optimal management for every child with a VP shunt undergoing laparoscopic surgery.

## RENAL FUNCTION AND FLUID REQUIREMENTS

Increased IAP decreases renal blood flow, renal function (creatinine clearance and glomerular filtration rate), and urine output.[123,128,154] The effects on renal function and renal filtration are poorly understood. Decreases in urine output during laparoscopic surgery in children vary, in part, with the age of the child: oliguria occurs in older children and anuria in infants less than 1 year of age.[128,130,155] The etiology of the renal dysfunction and oliguria is multifactorial, but includes direct and indirect effects of IAP on renal perfusion, antidiuretic hormone (ADH), endothelin, and nitric oxide (NO).[128,156] ADH concentrations increase as a result of reduced renal blood flow, resorbing water, and decreasing urine output. IAP increases renal endothelin (endothelin-1), resulting in renal venoconstriction, which reduces renal blood flow and urine output.[128,156] Inhibiting endogenous NO exacerbates the renal dysfunction during pneumoperitoneum through several mechanisms, including reduced renal perfusion and increased salt and water resorption (e.g., oliguria).[156] Thus pretreating patients with an NO donor (such as L-arginine or nondepressor doses of nitroglycerine) may attenuate the detrimental effects of a pneumoperitoneum on renal dysfunction, a supposition that awaits human studies.[156] Renal tubular injury does not contribute to the renal dysfunction associated with increased IAP.[157] In adult donor nephrectomy patients, an overnight infusion of fluids followed by a colloid bolus immediately before the pneumoperitoneum attenuated the adverse hemodynamic effects and reduced the magnitude of changes in creatinine clearance associated with increased IAP.[158] Comparable data in children have not been forthcoming.

Fluid administration during laparoscopic surgery should be carefully monitored. Open abdominal surgeries may require 10 to 15 mL/kg/hr to account for "third space fluid" losses resulting from extensive bowel manipulation. Although the existence of and manipulation of a real "third space" are debated, the conceptual fluid shift is real. During laparoscopic surgery, however, these fluid requirements are reduced because little fluid is lost and the bowels are minimally manipulated. In fact, care must be taken to avoid fluid overload during these surgeries. Urine output is often used as an index of preload in children undergoing abdominal surgery, but 88% of infants (less than 1 year of age) and 33% of children develop anuria or oliguria during laparoscopic surgery. Because these completely resolve within several hours of desufflation, it is not necessary to fluid challenge these children, as fluid overload is a real possibility.[155] Transient oliguria in children after laparoscopic surgery should not be viewed as an early indicator of impending renal dysfunction.

## PAIN MANAGEMENT

Postoperative pain after open general and urologic surgery is primarily directed at the pain from the skin and muscle incisions. With the small incisions used during laparoscopic surgery, perioperative pain is less than with open surgery.[159-161] Pain after laparoscopic surgery arises from several sources, including the incision sites, residual gas in the abdomen, referred pain from the diaphragm, and stretch on nerves from peculiar patient positions. A long-acting local anesthetic should be infiltrated around the incision sites at the end of laparoscopic surgery to prevent postoperative incisional pain. Some children develop pain after laparoscopic surgery, including back and shoulder pain. In these instances, multimodal pain therapy, including acetaminophen, nonsteroidal antiinflammatory agents, and (less commonly) opioids, are effective.[94,95,115] Recent evidence suggests that SIMPL for appendectomy causes less pain than surgery with a multiport system.[162]

# Robot-Assisted Surgery

Robot-assisted surgery is relatively new to pediatric surgery and urology, with only limited experience reported, although it has been used extensively in adults since the late 1990s to facilitate minimally invasive endoscopic surgery. Enhanced with three-dimensional magnifying views and feedback-controlled enhanced motions of human hands, robot-assisted surgery enables very fine manipulation of surgical instruments without natural human tremor, in a way that was not possible in the past. It has great potential as the future direction for pediatric surgery and urology.[1,148,163,164]

Initially introduced as a tool for remote battlefield surgery, robotic surgery is now available to assist pediatric surgeons in performing complex surgery, with less tissue and organ damage on extremely small surgical targets. Most of the information that is currently available is limited to one product (da Vinci Surgical System, Intuitive Surgical, Sunnyvale, Calif.) and to adult urologic procedures. However, rapid innovation and miniaturization of equipment has resulted in several pediatric centers undertaking robot-assisted laparoscopic surgery, with excellent outcomes (Videos 27-1 and 27-2). Concerns from the anesthesiologist's perspective regarding this relatively new approach are summarized in Table 27-1. Most of the perceived problems relate to the steep Trendelenburg position used, although numerous surgeries have been performed without this position.[148,163]

---

**TABLE 27-1** Issues Regarding Current Robotic-Assisted Procedures from the Anesthetist's Perspective

**Dependence on Extreme Body Position, such as Extreme Trendelenburg Position (Because of Absence of Adequate Surgical Assistance for Surgical Field Exposure), May Lead to:**

Increased intracranial pressure, ocular pressure, and impairment of cerebral perfusion

Optic nerve or retinal morbidity

Cerebro-facial congestion, airway edema, vocal cord palsy, delayed awakening

Possible overstretching of nerves passing through the axilla and nerve plexus damage

Extended lithotomy leading to compartment syndrome in the lower legs

Tendency to apply greater intraabdominal pressure

Circulatory depression and respiratory depression

Carbon dioxide insufflation related complications

**Absence of Touch, Traction, and Compression Sensations of Holding Instruments or Tissues**

All the manipulations are dependent exclusively on the visual sense

Inability to know the events occurring in an invisible place, overt tissue damage

Possibility of overlooking overt bleeding or tissue damage

**Absence of Robot Legs and Easy Movability**

Once fixed, it is hard to change the position of the robot or body position

Difficulty to check intravenous access sites or the airway

**Unlimited and Unexpected Surgical Approaches**

Exploration of new surgical approaches and complex tasks at awkward angles

Longer surgical time and longer setting up time, hypothermia, pressure sores

Unpredictable movement of robot and camera arms,

Hitting or compressing the child's face

Organization of all tubing and cables, including intravenous tubing and breathing hoses.

**Need for Emergency Undocking of the Robot in Case of Mechanical Failure or Critical Events**

---

# Specific General Surgical and Urologic Conditions

## NISSEN FUNDOPLICATION

This surgery is indicated for children with documented gastric fluid reflux that failed medical management. It involves mobilizing the muscles around the esophagus and suturing them tightly around the esophagus at the level of the lower esophageal sphincter. This surgery requires general anesthesia and tracheal intubation, and is usually performed laparoscopically.

Children who require a Nissen fundoplication often have a cerebral neurologic injury (i.e., cerebral palsy) that causes esophageal dysmotility. This dysmotility heralds esophageal reflux that, if severe, may result in aspiration pneumonia. If medical and gastric tube therapies fail, a Nissen fundoplication may be considered. The anesthetic considerations are few because this surgery is not associated with postoperative pain, large fluid shifts, or large blood loss. Positioning a bougie within the esophagus during surgery allows the surgeons to gauge how tight to tie the muscles around the esophagus; without a bougie, the muscles around the esophagus may be overtightened, causing an esophageal obstruction. Care must be taken to avoid dislodging the tracheal tube in the perioperative period. At the end of the procedure, it is common for the surgeon to request that 50 to 60 mL of air be insufflated into the stomach via the gastric tube to ensure that there are no anastomotic leaks. In general, this surgery is completed in less than 1 hour in experienced hands, with a complication rate of about 10% and an average hospital stay of about 1.6 days. Postoperative pain is easily managed.[165,166]

## PECTUS EXCAVATUM

Although this is a deformity of the chest wall, pediatric surgeons most often carry out the corrective procedure. Correction of the pectus excavatum by the classic approach involves an open procedure with fracture of the sternum, removal of multiple costal cartilages, and lifting of the sternum anteriorly with fixation, using one or two stainless steel bars. The Nuss procedure, a less invasive technique,[167,168] was initially a technique whereby a U-shaped bar was blindly passed through the thorax hugging the undersurface of the sternum. Once across the chest, the bar was flipped, through which process the sternum was pushed anteriorly without fracturing it, thus avoiding the creation of a flail chest by the removal of the costal cartilages. This procedure has since been modified, whereby the bar is passed through the thorax under direct vision, using thoracoscopy to reduce possible perforation of major structures (e.g., the heart or lungs).[169-171] Although the risk of this complication is reduced when the Nuss procedure is performed under direct vision, it may still occur.[172-174] Both blind and thoracoscopic approaches cause significant postoperative pain, which may be treated with patient-controlled analgesia, a thoracic epidural catheter, or a lumbar epidural catheter and epidural morphine (see Chapters 41 to 44).[175] Because these procedures are generally performed in teenagers, the thoracic epidural is preferably placed with the teenager awake but sedated. Compliance with inserting the epidural catheter while awake may be difficult in less mature teenagers. It is unclear whether the thoracic epidural provides improved analgesia compared with standard patient-controlled analgesia for this procedure.[176] It should be noted that these children will return for removal of the pectus bar after several years. Occasionally, the bar has become adherent to the pericardium or lung, resulting in a severe, sudden, and catastrophic rupture of a major vessel or chamber in the heart when the pectus bar is removed.[177] It would be prudent to establish ample IV access to provide the means to rapidly transfuse fluids and blood should a catastrophic blood loss occur.

## PHEOCHROMOCYTOMA

*Pheochromocytoma* is a rare but potentially life-threatening neuroendocrine tumor that arises from the chromaffin cells of the adrenal medulla in 80% of cases, or extraadrenal paraganglionic tissue in 20% of cases.[178,179] Intraabdominal tumors are most commonly found around renal blood vessels or the corpora paraaortica (organs of Zu), which displays the largest collection of chromaffin tissue. Extraadrenal paragangliomas may occur anywhere in the body from the base of the skull to the pelvis.[180] Only cells that stain positive for chromaffin secrete catecholamines. These tumors derive their name from the dark grey-brown immunostaining of chromogranin A by chromium salts.[180] The Greek word "pheo," meaning twilight, refers to the dark grey or twilight-colored immunostaining.

The incidence of pheochromocytoma in the general population is approximately 0.3 to 1 per million per year.[180] In children, the incidence of benign pheochromocytoma is 1 per 10 million and of the malignant form, 1 per 50 million. Approximately 10% to 20% of all pheochromocytomas are diagnosed in childhood, with an average age at the time of onset of 11 years.[179,180] In childhood, there is a preponderance of males, whereas during the reproductive years, there is a preponderance of females. The net effect throughout childhood is an equal distribution in the sexes.[181] In contrast to adults, pheochromocytomas in children are more often benign, bilateral, multiple in number, and extraadrenal.[180] With adequate preparation preoperatively and close monitoring intraoperatively, the mortality associated with extirpation of the tumor is less than 3% in children.[178]

Most of these tumors are benign, with only 5% to 10% malignant (although some reports suggest a malignancy rate as great as 50%). Malignancies of pheochromocytomas have been found in the bones, lungs, lymph nodes, and liver.[178,179] A diagnosis of pheochromocytoma can be confirmed by positive staining for chromaffin cells. The paraganglioma tumors with mutations in succinate dehydrogenase subgroup B (see later discussion) are most likely to metastasize.[178] Malignant tumors are more likely to secrete dopamine than benign ones.[178] The 5-year survival of metastatic pheochromocytoma is 50%, with no effective treatment.[178] In adults, radical surgery and iobenguane I 123 therapy have been effective in 80% of adults, although only 5% go into remission.[182]

In children, 40% to 60% of pheochromocytomas are inherited[179,180] in an autosomal dominant pattern,[179,180] with the remainder occurring spontaneously. Four hereditary syndromes associated with pheochromocytomas have been identified in five genes' mutations[178,183-185]: von Hippel-Lindau type 2, multiglandular multiple endocrine neoplasia (MEN) type 2, neurofibromatosis 1, and paraganglionic syndromes (mitochondrial complex II succinate dehydrogenase type B and D). Two additional (nonhereditary) syndromes have also been associated with pheochromocytomas: Tuberous sclerosis and Carney triad. The gene defect responsible for the MEN syndromes is located on chromosome 10q11.2.[179] MEN type 2A (Sipple syndrome) includes medullary thyroid cancer, parathyroid adenoma, and pheochromocytoma. MEN type 2B includes medullary thyroid cancer, multiple neuromas, Marfan habitus, and pheochromocytoma. Pheochromocytomas associated with MEN secrete both epinephrine and norepinephrine.[178] These tumors are bilateral in 50% to 80% of cases, but rarely metastasize.[178] The

von Hippel-Lindau syndrome type 2 (type 1 does not involve pheochromocytomas) is the most common cause of familial pheochromocytoma.[180] The von Hippel-Lindau gene is located on 3p25-26.[178,179] Pheochromocytoma is present in 10% to 20% of children with the gene. Three subtypes of the gene are distinguished by their association with other organs: type 2A involves hemangioblastomas of the central nervous system, endolymphatic sac tumors, and ependymal cystadenomas; type 2B involves all the organs in type 2A, as well as renal cell and pancreatic cysts and tumors. The only tissues associated with type 2C are pheochromocytomas. When associated with the von Hippel-Lindau gene, pheochromocytomas secrete exclusively norepinephrine.[178] These tumors occur bilaterally in the adrenal glands, but rarely metastasize.[179] Neurofibromatosis type 1 involves neurofibromas and café au lait spots. The genetic mutation is found on chromosome 17q11.2.[178] Pheochromocytomas occur in less than 5% of children with neurofibromatosis.[179]

Paraganglioma syndromes arise from mutations in the gene that codes for succinate dehydrogenase on cytochrome oxidase II in the respiratory chain of mitochondria. Two genetic mutations involve pheochromocytomas: subgroup B, which is coded on chromosome 1p36 and subgroup D, which is coded on chromosome 11q23.[178,179] These mutations present with paragangliomas of the adrenal, extra-adrenal, and head and neck regions. Subgroup B occurs more commonly in children (approximately 20% of pheochromocytomas bear this mutation), with a 30% to 50% metastatic rate. Subgroup D is inherited strictly along paternal lines.[179]

Tuberous sclerosis presents with the clinical findings of epilepsy, neurocognitive dysfunction, polycystic renal disease, and retinal phakomas. Tuberous sclerosis arises from two gene mutations located on chromosomes 9q34 and 1613.3, which code for the production of hamartin and tuberin, respectively. The wild types of these proteins suppress tumor production.

Carney triad, which usually occurs in young women, comprises gastric leiomyosarcoma (currently recognized as gastrointestinal stromal tumors), pulmonary chondroma, and extra-adrenal pheochromocytoma.

Pheochromocytomas can secrete epinephrine, norepinephrine, and/or dopamine. Most pheochromocytomas secrete norepinephrine as the predominant hormone; only 10% to 20% secrete epinephrine and dopamine as the predominant hormones. Hypertension is the most common presenting sign of this tumor. It is often accompanied by regular, intermittent headaches that are associated with nausea and vomiting. In children, nausea is a common presenting finding. The classic triad of headaches, sweating and palpitations, along with hypertension constitute the presenting signs in greater than 90% of patients with pheochromocytomas. Sustained hypertension is present in 60% to 90% of children with the tumor, but is not a requirement for the diagnosis.[186] In fact, there is no relationship between circulating catecholamine concentrations and overt symptoms. Epinephrine-secreting tumors can present as circulatory shock due to decreased intravascular volume, as a result of sustained high concentrations of catecholamines and their effects on vascular resistance. Tumors that secrete predominantly dopamine do not usually present with hypertension.

Other presenting findings include weight loss, nausea and vomiting, polyuria, visual disturbances, and anxiety.[186] Presenting signs may include pallor, orthostatic hypotension, tremor, and syncope, as well as abdominal pain, diarrhea and other gastrointestinal manifestations, hyperglycemia, low-grade fever, and behavioral disturbances. On occasion, catecholamine release may be triggered by anesthesia, micturition (as in a urinary bladder pheochromocytoma), foods, and drugs, such as metoclopramide, tricyclic antidepressants, glucagon, and radiology contrast dye. Pheochromocytomas have been described as the great mimic, giving support to a differential diagnosis that includes acute coronary infarction, carcinoid tumor, thyroid storm, and cocaine (or other amphetamine-like drug) overdose. In other emergent circumstances, surgery undertaken for acute appendicitis with an undiagnosed pheochromocytoma has been terminated prematurely once the diagnosis of a pheochromocytoma was strongly suspected. The acute appendicitis resolved with conservative nonoperative management while the pheochromocytoma was investigated, the patient was treated with α-adrenergic blocking agents, and the pheochromocytoma removed electively.[187]

Surgical resection of pheochromocytoma is optimally managed on an elective basis, after the child's medical status has been properly investigated, medical conditions are stabilized, the location of the tumor(s) determined and the α-adrenergic receptors completely blocked. Preoperative α-adrenergic blockade is critical, as its routine use has reduced perioperative complications during pheochromocytoma resection from 60% to 3%.[188] It must be emphasized that β-adrenergic blockade should NEVER be introduced until α-adrenergic blockade has been well-established, because this could cause unopposed paroxysmal systemic hypertension, acute coronary or stroke signs, and death. Thus preoperative preparation of these children first requires the institution of a noncompetitive α-adrenergic blocker, such as phenoxybenzamine. Phenoxybenzamine irreversibly alkylates α-adrenergic receptors reducing the risk of an α-adrenergic medicated paroxysmal increase in blood pressure during surgery. Phenoxybenzamine may be administered either orally or IV.[183] Oral doses between 0.25 and 1.0 mg/kg/day in divided doses are most common, although doses as great as 2 mg/kg/day have been used.[180,183] Oral bioavailability of phenoxybenzamine is only 20% to 30% with a 24-hour onset of action.[183] Children are usually treated for 3 to 15 days with oral phenoxybenzamine before surgery, although there is no means to reliably assess the completeness of α-adrenergic blockade.[183] Some think that α-adrenergic blockade has been established when the systolic blood pressure returns to normal limits for the child's age.[179] Alternatively, IV phenoxybenzamine has been used to more rapidly and reliably block α₁ receptors, although aggressive monitoring for peripheral vasodilatation, decreases in blood pressure, and relative hypovolemia must be followed until the hemodynamics have equilibrated. The action of phenoxybenzamine is terminated only by synthesizing new α-adrenergic receptors. The disadvantage of irreversibly blocking α-adrenergic receptors, as conferred by phenoxybenzamine, is that reactive hypotension may follow removal of the tumor, with resistance to interventions that are intended to increase the peripheral vascular resistance. In contrast, phentolamine has also been used because it has a much shorter half-life than does phenoxybenzamine and it is reversible. Competitive α-adrenergic blockade with doxazosin, which also has a brief duration of action when compared with phenoxybenzamine, may be displaced from the α-adrenergic receptors by increased concentrations of circulating catecholamines.[178] It is important to reemphasize that β-adrenergic blockade should only be introduced once α-adrenergic receptor blockade has been established.

Perioperative fluid and electrolyte management in children as α-adrenergic blockade develops requires close monitoring. It is tempting to administer generous volumes of balanced salt solutions preoperatively to prevent hypotension, but this should be tempered with the understanding that children are at increased risk for catecholamine-induced pulmonary edema.[183] The plasma potassium concentration should be monitored closely as hypokalemia may develop as a result of increased renin concentrations.[179] Postoperative hypotension, a direct consequence of α-adrenergic receptor blockade, may be attenuated by augmenting the sodium intake in the diet preoperatively, and by the judicious use of IV balanced salt solutions in the perioperative period.[180]

### Perioperative Evaluation

The pretreatment blood pressure should be compared with their supine blood pressure after α-adrenergic blockade. The current blood pressure (and heart rate) should be within normal limits. If orthostatic hypotension is present, it should be treated with fluid boluses to render the child euvolemic. If the heart rate is not normal or within 20% of normal after α-adrenergic receptor blockade, boluses of balanced salt solutions (20 mL/kg, IV) should be administered until the tachycardia abates. A recent electrocardiogram and echocardiogram should be reviewed to rule out arrhythmias and myocardial dysfunction. Thyroid function tests and serum calcium and blood glucose concentrations should be evaluated, as indicated by the associated endocrinopathies present. The child should be examined for café au lait spots to rule out neurofibromatosis. If café au lait spots are present, a history and physical examination should focus on the presence of neurofibromas, particularly in the form of a pulmonic flow murmur (intracardiac tumor) or a change in the child's voice (suggesting a laryngeal neurofibroma).

Preparation should be made for general anesthesia with invasive arterial and central venous catheters, together with transesophageal echocardiogram, if deemed necessary. Infusions to manage hypertensive crises should be available, including sodium nitroprusside, magnesium sulfate, and esmolol. Magnesium causes vasodilation by inhibiting catecholamine receptors and catecholamine release as well as antagonizing endogenous calcium effects.[189] Vasopressors, including ephedrine and vasopressin, may be required to restore the blood pressure if hypotension occurs, especially postoperatively.[178,189,190]

### Laboratory Findings

Biochemical testing for pheochromocytoma should be performed in children who present with signs suggestive of pheochromocytoma, whether a primary tumor or a recurrence. The most accurate biochemical tests are those for free plasma metanephrine and normetanephrine concentrations, and 24-hour urine for fractionated metanephrines,[191] although even these tests are not without problems.[178,183,184] These tests have supplanted 24-hour urinary and plasma epinephrine, norepinephrine, and dopamine concentrations, and the degradation product, urinary vanillylmandelic acid. Reference standards for metanephrine must be adjusted for the child's age, because the concentrations may be up to 33% less than those in adults. The current tests are much more reliable than older methods (vanillylmandelic acid concentration) for establishing a diagnosis of a pheochromocytoma. Plasma catecholamine concentrations correlate well with the urine concentrations during sustained tumor catecholamine secretion, although they may be exaggerated during episodes of cardiovascular instability. In both sporadic and familial pheochromocytoma, the test with the greatest sensitivity for normetanephrine and metanephrine is the measurement of plasma free concentrations.[191] Plasma metanephrines are present in 99% of sporadic pheochromocytomas. However, this test may be difficult to perform in children because they must remain supine and relaxed for 30 minutes before sampling. The presence of increased urine and plasma catecholamine concentrations can be attributed to numerous physiologic and pathologic conditions, as well as to medications (e.g., acetaminophen, tricyclic antidepressants, β-adrenergic blockers, and calcium channel blockers). However, when the upper reference limits are adjusted, sensitivities of 100% and specificities of 80% to 94% can be obtained (sensitivities for familial forms are less than for sporadic forms, whereas specificities for familial forms are greater than for sporadic forms).[178,184] Concentrations of metanephrine and normetanephrine (as determined by high pressure liquid chromatography) that exceed the 99th percentile upper limit for normal levels, and thus suggest a "likely" diagnosis of a pheochromocytoma are: blood, free metanephrines greater than 0.42 nmol/L and normetanephrine greater than 1.4 nmol/L; urine, metanephrine greater than 2880 nmol per 24 hours and normetanephrine greater than 6550 nmol per 24 hours.[178] In some cases, results of the biochemical tests for diagnosing a pheochromocytoma are borderline. In such cases, oral clonidine may be administered as a suppression test, suppressing the release of norepinephrine. If clonidine suppresses the concentration of plasma normetanephrine greater than 40% below the upper reference limit, then a diagnosis of a pheochromocytoma may be excluded.[192] Caution should be exercised when administering clonidine, as $\alpha_2$-adrenoceptor agonists may cause substantial hypotension and bradycardia in children. Suppression tests are infrequently used today because of the sensitivity and specificity of the current catecholamine assays.

Preoperative hemoglobin and hematocrit should be determined, to gauge the adequacy of fluid replacement during α-adrenergic blockade. Careful examination of the biochemical profile preoperatively will confirm the involvement of other organs. Hypokalemia may be present if hyperaldosteronism is diagnosed. Excess catecholamines associated with pheochromocytomas may increase fasting glucose concentrations or cause an abnormal glucose-tolerance test. This may be exacerbated by hypoinsulinemia caused by α-adrenergic suppression of pancreatic insulin release. Testing should include total and ionized calcium concentrations to determine whether the parathyroid glands are involved, suggesting MEN syndrome.

Chronic exposure to increased circulating catecholamine concentrations may lead to a cardiomyopathy, congestive heart failure, and arrhythmias. Preoperatively, an electrocardiogram, chest radiograph, and echocardiogram should be performed.[183] The electrocardiogram may reveal arrhythmias, evidence of myocardial ischemia, or ventricular hypertrophy. The chest radiograph may show an increased cardiothoracic ratio suggestive of a cardiomyopathy or heart failure. Echocardiography will identify reduced cardiac function, heart failure, cardiomyopathy, or simply ventricular hypertrophy. Cardiac function should be optimized medically before embarking on general anesthesia. Transesophageal echocardiography and central venous pressure and arterial pressure monitoring may be indicated.

Once the biochemical diagnostic tests have been completed and the presence of a pheochromocytoma has been confirmed, the tumor(s) must be located. The most common location in children is in the abdomen, both within and without the adrenal gland; computed axial tomography (CAT) and magnetic resonance imaging (MRI) are used to locate these tumors in children.[183] CAT scans are very rapid, but they expose the children to radiation. MRI studies are slower and require general anesthesia, but they avoid radiation exposure. The accuracy of locating a pheochromocytoma with these two techniques is similar,[183] 96% to 100%, although both may, on occasion, have difficulty distinguishing a pheochromocytoma from other intraabdominal lesions, especially with small tumors (less than 1 cm in diameter). For small tumors or for extraadrenal tumors, a supplementary radiologic investigation known as the iobenguane I-123 test may be used. Studies with iobenguane yield positive responses with both pheochromocytomas and neuroblastomas, necessitating additional studies to distinguish between the two.[179] Iobenguane uptake by the tumor may be impaired in the presence of labetalol and tricyclic antidepressants. Although metastatic paragangliomas may lose their ability to take up iobenguane, the combination of a positive MRI and iobenguane uptake usually confirms the diagnosis. In cases where iobenguane cannot be used or yields negative results, or when the tumor remains elusive, positron emission tomography with fluorodeoxyglucose F-18 may be used. The latter test offers greater sensitivity and possibly specificity than does the iobenguane I-123 test, especially during investigation for a metastatic pheochromocytoma.

### Anesthetic Management

Anxiolytics (such as midazolam) are useful to maintain circulatory homeostasis before surgical resection of pheochromocytomas. General anesthesia and tracheal intubation is required whether the tumor is resected using an open laparotomy or a laparoscopy. Induction of anesthesia may be undertaken with IV anesthetics, while avoiding sympathomimetics (e.g., ketamine). Steroidal muscle relaxants (e.g., vecuronium), benzodiazepines, opioids, and inhalational anesthetics may be used. Some have suggested succinylcholine may trigger a sympathetic response via stimulation of the sympathetic ganglia or fasciculations, although the evidence for such a response is weak.[193] Surges in blood pressure may be managed with propofol, increasing the concentration of the inhalational anesthetic, or administering vasodilators (magnesium or sodium nitroprusside infusions). Most pheochromocytomas are resected using an open laparotomy approach, although more recently, laparoscopic surgery has found favor.[194] The latter approach reduces the duration of surgery and speeds recovery. However, insufflation of the abdomen with carbon dioxide may precipitate a sympathetic response and a decrease in venous return. If the child was not euvolemic before insufflating the abdomen, a rapid decrease in venous return and blood pressure may ensue. This should be treated aggressively, using balanced salt solutions while relieving the intraabdominal pressure until the blood pressure stabilizes. If abdominal insufflation triggers a sympathetic response, an IV bolus of propofol should be administered, the concentration of inhaled anesthetic increased, and/or antihypertensives administered as needed. Contraindications to laparoscopic surgery include large tumors (greater than 15 cm), coagulopathy, and invasive metastatic disease.

For those undergoing a laparotomy, an epidural catheter may be placed after induction of anesthesia and dosed only for perioperative analgesia after the tumor has been removed. This eliminates the contribution of the epidural analgesic and vasodilation to hypotension that may occur. If an epidural is not medically indicated or the parents refuse, then patient-controlled analgesia may be used.

Emergency surgery is a hotly debated subject; the vast majority of these tumors are scheduled for elective removal after α-adrenergic blockade has been pharmacologically established.

Rare instances of multiorgan failure from pheochromocytoma-associated "catecholamine crisis" have been reported. The crisis includes cardiomyopathy and congestive heart failure, hypertension, encephalopathy (with seizures), fever, and end-organ damage that required life-saving resection of the tumor to prevent a fatal outcome. In such situations, aggressive α-adrenergic blockade while concurrently supporting an adequate CO take precedence.

### Potential Perioperative Problems

Hypertension can occur during the surgery, before or during manipulation of the tumor, despite α-adrenergic blockade. Measures that may be used to control the blood pressure include increasing the inspired concentration of inhalational anesthetic, IV propofol (bolus or infusion), sodium nitroprusside infusion (0.5-8 μg/kg/min), IV magnesium sulfate (30 mg/kg loading dose over 30 minutes, followed by an infusion of 10 mg/kg/hr), α-adrenergic blockers (e.g., phentolamine) and calcium channel blockers (e.g., diltiazem or nicardipine).[189]

Tachycardia may occur in response to tumor manipulation, antihypertensive treatment or hypovolemia. β-adrenergic blockers should never be used without first blocking $α_1$ adrenoceptors. Cautious use of β-adrenergic blockers is advised particularly in the presence of myocardial dysfunction. The preferred β-adrenergic blocker is esmolol (100-300 μg/kg/min) because of its very brief duration of action.

Hypotension can occur once the tumor has been extirpated, as a result of the sudden removal of the source of catecholamines and/or irreversible α-adrenergic blockade by phenoxybenzamine. Hypotension may continue for several days postoperatively. Supportive treatment with fluids and vasopressors (including vasopressin) may be effective in restoring normal blood pressure.[189]

Fluid overload and left ventricular failure may present with the sudden onset of hemoglobin desaturation, increased airway pressures and pulmonary edema fluid in the tracheal tube. This should be prevented by the careful and judicious administration of balanced salt solution throughout the surgery and the avoidance of myocardial depressants. In the presence of a cardiomyopathy, it may be prudent to have a measure of central venous pressure or transesophageal echocardiography to assess for evidence of left ventricular decompensation during surgery.

Reactive hypoglycemia may occur upon removal of the source of catecholamines and relatively excess insulin levels. Blood glucose concentrations should be measured perioperatively until stabilized.

If bilateral adrenalectomy has been performed, steroid replacement may be required postoperatively. It is possible that after such surgery, the lack of an adequate concentration of steroids contributes to the development of hypotension, however, a much more likely cause for the hypotension is hypovolemia.

### CIRCUMCISION

Circumcision is performed in neonates, infants, children, and adults under local, regional, or general anesthesia. The indications for circumcision include phimosis, recurrent balanitis, religious beliefs, or parental preference. Inhalational anesthesia with additional regional analgesia is preferred. Classic circumcision involves cutting the foreskin and cauterizing and suturing the skin edges. The duration of surgery is usually less than 1 hour. The type of anesthetic and airway management do not significantly affect perioperative outcomes. The most common complication arising from circumcision is bleeding.

In infants and children, circumcision is performed under general anesthesia. Multimodal pain therapy includes acetaminophen 30 to 40 mg/kg rectally or 10 to 15 mg/kg IV, parenteral opioids (i.e., morphine 0.05-0.1 mg/kg), and/or local anesthetic without epinephrine (dorsal penile block, caudal block, subcutaneous ring block, and topical lidocaine–prilocaine [EMLA]) (see Chapter 41).[195] A comparison of a subcutaneous ring block of the penis with a suprapubic penile block, showed the latter provided better analgesia.[196] When a caudal block was compared with penile blocks and parenteral analgesics, a Cochrane review concluded that, with a caudal block, both rescue analgesia and nausea and vomiting were reduced compared with parenteral analgesics, although the analysis was limited because of a dearth of studies.[197]

### HYPOSPADIAS AND CHORDEE

This congenital malformation occurs in 1 of 250 liveborn males. It often occurs in isolation, without other congenital anomalies. *Hypospadias* refers to a malposition of the meatus of the urethra: rather than opening at the distal tip of the penis, the urethra opens along the undersurface of the penis anywhere from just proximal to the glans to the scrotum (Fig. 27-5). The majority of hypospadias defects are distal, occurring near or at the glans of the penis. Between 15% and 50% of hypospadii have an associated chordee, whereas 8% have an undescended testis. A small number of children with hypospadias have urethral openings remote from the glans of the penis, including the scrotum (Fig. 27-6, E-Figs. 27-4 and 27-5).

Surgery is undertaken with an expected duration of between 1 and 4 hours depending on the severity of the hypospadias. It is important to establish an understanding with the urologist

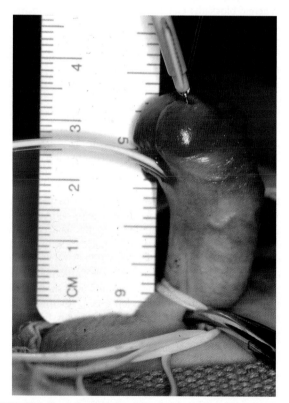

**FIGURE 27-5** Classic hypospadias. Saline is injected to perform an erection test before surgical correction of the hypospadias. (Courtesy Dr. P. Williot, Pediatric Urology, Women and Children's Hospital of Buffalo, Buffalo, N.Y.)

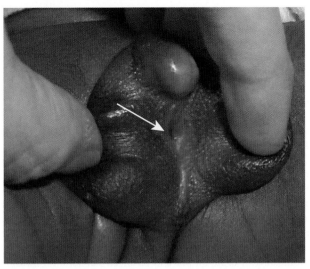

FIGURE 27-6 Scrotal hypospadias with the urethra opening in the midline of the scrotum. (Courtesy Dr. P. Williot, Pediatric Urology, Women and Children's Hospital of Buffalo, Buffalo, N.Y.)

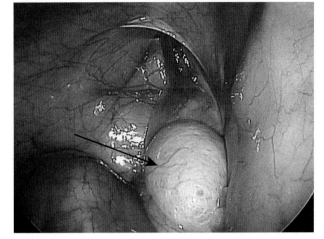

FIGURE 27-7 Intraabdominal testis in the hernia ring, discovered during laparoscopy for an undescended testicle. (Courtesy Dr. P. Williot, Pediatric Urology, Women and Children's Hospital of Buffalo, Buffalo, N.Y.)

of the type of regional block that will suit the extent of surgery: those requiring a minor hypospadias repair (single-stage procedure, i.e., MAGPI [meatal advancement and glanuloplasty technique] or Mathieu repair) may be managed with a facemask, laryngeal mask airway, or tracheal tube. The anesthetic is at the discretion of the anesthesiologist; the children are outpatients and receive either a penile block or a single-shot caudal block. Those with more extensive hypospadias who require longer surgery will require either a laryngeal mask airway or a tracheal tube. They will be admitted to a hospital for one to two nights and need a strategy for continuous postoperative analgesia. For the latter, either a caudal catheter or a lumbar epidural catheter can be used during surgery to reduce the anesthetic requirements and postoperatively for analgesia. If opioids are avoided, a caudal-epidural block consisting of only local anesthetic does not cause delayed micturition after the urinary catheter has been removed.[198]

## CRYPTORCHIDISM AND HERNIAS: INGUINAL AND UMBILICAL

These surgeries, together with hydrocele repair, are common outpatient procedures. *Orchiopexy* refers to mobilizing the undescended testis that is either in the inguinal canal or, less commonly, within the abdominal cavity (Fig. 27-7), and securing it firmly in the scrotum. Approximately 33% of preterm infant males are born with one undescended testis, whereas only 3% of full-term males are similarly afflicted. Although the incidence of undescended testis decreases to 1% by 3 months of age, the incidence remains at 1% thereafter. Cryptorchidism usually occurs in isolation, although it is associated with a number of conditions, including Prader-Willi syndrome, Noonan syndrome, and cloacal exstrophy.

Undescended testes are categorized, based on physical examination, to include testes that are truly undescended, those that are ectopic, and those that are retracted. The retracted ones are not true undescended testis because they can be massaged into the scrotum and require no further treatment. In the case of true undescended testes, the testes must be located, mobilized, and then fixed within the scrotal sac to ensure viability. Failure to

mobilize the testes out of the inguinal canal or abdomen may result in atrophy, torsion, testicular cancer, or hernias.

An *inguinal hernia* in a child is a congenital failure of the processus vaginalis to obliterate. In this case, a loop of bowel protrudes beyond the internal ring, causing a bulge in the inguinal region or scrotum. These protuberances may appear periodically, with complete resolution in the interim. On occasion, a small sac of fluid is present in the scrotum, known as a *hydrocele*, and is confused for a loop of bowel in the scrotum (E-Fig. 27-6). Hydroceles are removed electively with the same approach as for an inguinal hernia. On occasion, the loop of bowel does not reduce spontaneously from the hernia and remains trapped in the canal, necessitating a visit to the emergency department. A surgeon is often required to manually reduce the trapped bowel. In these cases, the hernia repair is then scheduled as an urgent or elective surgery, depending on whether there is suspicion of persistent or potential recurrent ischemia to the bowel. In some cases, the entrapped bowel cannot be reduced and an incarcerated hernia or obstructed bowel is diagnosed. Incarcerated hernias and bowel obstructions are surgical emergencies that require general anesthesia, and muscle relaxation to reduce the strangulated bowel. The emergency nature of the surgery requires careful questioning regarding the time interval between the last meal and the onset of abdominal pain and strangulated bowel. It is usually assumed that these children have a full stomach. At the time of open reduction, if the bowel does not appear to have adequate perfusion, a segment of the ischemic or necrotic bowel may have to be resected.

Management of cryptorchidism and inguinal hernia requires general anesthesia (facemask, laryngeal mask airway, or tracheal tube) and an adequate pain management strategy. Multimodal pain therapy, as described earlier, may be used together with a regional block. When the surgeon pulls on the foreskin, hernia sac, or testis during surgery, laryngospasm may occur if the depth of anesthesia is inadequate. Anesthesia can be deepened most rapidly by an IV bolus of propofol, although some increase the inspired concentration of inhalational anesthetic. Regional blocks (ilioinguinal, iliohypogastric, scrotal block; caudal-epidural block; or transversus abdominis plane block) are used for both orchiopexy and inguinal hernia surgery, using either a landmark-based or ultrasound-guided method[199] (see Chapter 41).

An *umbilical hernia* is a 1- to 5-cm defect in the anterior abdominal wall (usually halfway between the umbilicus and the xiphisternal junction), with intermittent protuberance of bowel through the defect. This defect occurs in 15% of children, more commonly in children of African rather than European descent, and equally in males and females. Many resolve spontaneously in the first year of life. It also occurs frequently in preterm and low birth weight infants. If the defect is small, then a laryngeal mask airway may be sufficient to manage the airway, provided a deep level of anesthesia is maintained when the suture needles pass through each side of the rectus muscle. If the defect is large, tracheal intubation and, depending on the surgeon, muscle relaxation may be required. Deepening anesthesia while the defect is being closed by increasing the inspired concentration of inhalational anesthetic or administering an IV bolus of propofol (1 to 2 mg/kg) provides adequate relaxation to reduce the defect in most cases.

## TORSION OF THE TESTIS

Presentation of a male with sudden onset of acute scrotal pain in the absence of trauma requires immediate investigation and possible surgery to preserve a potentially viable testis. The differential diagnosis of acute onset of torsion of the testis (Fig. 27-8) includes torsion of the testicular appendix, torsion of the spermatic cord, epididymitis, and incarcerated hernia. The majority of testes can be saved if surgery is performed within 6 hours of the onset of pain if the diagnosis is confirmed by Doppler ultrasonography or suspected on clinical grounds.[200] The salvage rate for the testis decreases to 50% if surgery is undertaken 6 to 12 hours after the onset of pain. Children with suspected acute testicular torsion are assumed to have a full stomach and require RSI and tracheal intubation. Although pain at the time of induction of anesthesia may be intense, when the torsion is relieved, the pain abates. Hence, at the conclusion of surgery many of these children no longer have substantive pain that warrants aggressive treatment.

## POSTERIOR URETHRAL VALVES

Posterior urethral valves (PUV) is a spectrum of urethral obstruction that varies from mild to severe. The diagnosis is often made

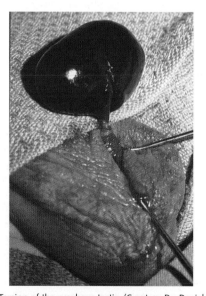

**FIGURE 27-8** Torsion of the newborn testis. (Courtesy Dr. Daniel P. Doody, MD, Pediatric Surgery, MassGeneral Hospital for Children, Boston.)

antenatally (preferably by 24 weeks gestation) by ultrasound identification of bladder distention, megaureters, and hydronephrosis. When PUV is diagnosed antenatally, the severity of the disease tends to be greater.[201] Decompression of the urogenital system may be achieved by a vesicoamniotic shunt in utero. Although some recommend that an intervention should be undertaken as quickly as possible to minimize the impact on renal function, evidence suggests that early intervention does not substantively affect the outcome, because renal damage may have already occurred in utero.[202,203]

Postnatally, a lack of or decrease in urine output, urinary retention, or a poor urine stream may be the only indications of the presence of these valves.[204] Affected children can have associated renal insufficiency resulting from congenital renal dysplasia and urethral valve obstruction. Because the renal concentrating mechanism is often impaired, these infants commonly present with greater than normal urine output. Consequently, careful monitoring of urine output and balanced salt solution infusion rate is necessary. Primary valve ablation is required to decompress the urogenital system.

Several indices have been postulated as predictors of poor long-term renal function in infants with PUV, including a creatinine 0.8 mg/dL or greater at birth, antenatal diagnosis, proteinuria, moderate or severe hydronephrosis, and renal dysplasia.[201,205] A recent analysis indicated that a nadir creatinine greater than 1 mg/dL and bladder dysfunction were the only independent predictors of long-term renal dysfunction.[206]

Children with PUV are scheduled for elective surgery. A general anesthetic is required, with the specific management left to the discretion of the anesthesiologist. There are few special considerations needed.

## PRUNE-BELLY SYNDROME

Prune-belly syndrome is a disorder that occurs predominantly (97% of the time) in males, with an incidence of 1 in 40,000 births. Affected infants present with a range of findings, from stillborn to a full-term neonate, with a host of possible organ and chromosomal abnormalities.[205] Affected organs may involve orthopedic in 50% (congenital hip dislocation and scoliosis), gastrointestinal in 30% (malrotation and volvulus), congenital heart disease in 10% (tetralogy of Fallot and ventricular septal defect), and chromosomal defects (trisomy 18 and trisomy 21).[205]

In utero, the child's abdomen often swells with fluid (in the presence of oligohydramnios) that is resorbed by birth, leaving the characteristic wrinkled redundant abdominal wall (Fig. 27-9 and E-Fig. 27-7). The pathophysiology of this syndrome is unclear, but it has been suggested that a urethral obstruction in utero leads to dilatation of the urethra (megaurethra is a common finding), which, combined with bladder distention and ascites, causes distention of the abdomen in utero. This ultimately leads to vesicoureteral reflux and ureteral dilatation in 80% of affected children.

Abdominal overdistention in utero causes weak rectus abdominis muscles that undermine the child's ability to exhale forcefully, and to generate a strong cough to clear secretions. As a result, chronic aspiration pneumonia may contribute to an early demise. Some have suggested that aggressive intervention to correct the weak rectus muscles by plication and muscle transfer may improve respiratory function,[207,208] reduce back strain and pain, decreased bladder volume, and arrest scoliosis.[209] However, this view is not shared by others who prefer to observe the child for signs of regurgitation and aspiration before intervening.[210]

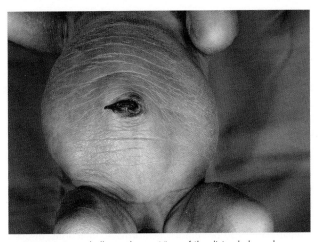

**FIGURE 27-9** Prune-belly syndrome. View of the distended, weak muscled abdomen in a child with prune-belly syndrome. The muscle wall is so thin that the abdominal surface is bulging in front of the bowels. (Courtesy Dr. P. Williot, Pediatric Urology, Women and Children's Hospital of Buffalo, Buffalo, N.Y.)

Controlling the type of feeds, preventing gastrointestinal reflux disease, and using antibiotics to treat pneumonia permit the child to grow. Constipation is a frequent problem that may be exacerbated by their inability to increase their IAP during defecation. Stool softeners are often prescribed to prevent constipation and abdominal distention. Pneumonia must be aggressively treated and completely resolved before entertaining surgery. Percutaneous endoscopic gastroscopy tubes are generally eschewed in these children when feeding is a problem, as abdominal wall surgery is difficult. These children often require urologic surgery to correct vesicoureteral reflux and orchiopexy. Urethral obstruction may be due to the angulation of the urethra within the prostate.

Trisomy 18, the second most common autosomal trisomy, occurs in 1 in approximately 7,000 live births, and is associated with prune-belly syndrome. In contrast to the simple prune-belly syndrome, 60% to 80% of these infants are female. Trisomy 18 is characterized by severe neurologic developmental problems (including microcephaly), micrognathia and/or retrognathia, microstomia, auricular abnormalities, and others. In fact, 95% die in utero, with only 5% to 10% surviving 1 year and only 1% reaching 10 years of age. Mortality results from cardiac anomalies (90% of affected children have a ventricular septal defect, valvular heart defect, atrial septal defect, hypoplastic left heart syndrome, tetralogy of Fallot, or other cardiac defect), renal anomalies, failure to thrive, and apnea.[211,212] Additional findings include pulmonary hypoplasia and gastrointestinal anomalies (including prune-belly syndrome, omphalocele, ileal atresia, and esophageal atresia).

General anesthesia with tracheal intubation is required for most surgeries in these children. Controlled ventilation is recommended, because of the variability in the strength of the abdominal muscles. It is prudent to suction the lungs once the trachea has been intubated, in order to assess the severity of secretions. As little muscle relaxant as possible should be used during the surgery, with preferably no muscle relaxant administered during the last hour, to ensure the child's strength has had time to recover to have a successful extubation. Although opioids should be used cautiously, regional anesthesia may be preferred, in view of their difficulty with clearing secretions from the tracheobronchial tree.[213]

## URETERAL REIMPLANTATION

Vesicoureteral reflux, in which urine passes retrograde up the ureter, is a congenital disorder affecting 0.5% to 2% of children. Recurrent episodes of pyelonephritis may occur, leading to renal scarring and reduced renal function, depending on the severity of the reflux. The pathology is thought to be an anatomically abnormal insertion of the ureter into the bladder that fails to close tight when the bladder fills and contracts. A voiding cystourethrogram is the test required to diagnose the reflux and assess its severity. Mild forms of vesicoureteral reflux are managed with daily antibiotics until the child outgrows the reflux. However, more severe forms or those who develop kidney infections despite antibiotic therapy, require surgical correction. The classic surgical approach for vesicoureteral reflux is an open procedure in which the affected ureters are reimplanted into the bladder wall, re-creating a normal muscle flap valve.[214] This involves a lower abdominal incision and 3 to 4 hours of surgery. Postoperatively, the pain is often intense, necessitating 2 to 3 days of continuous infusion of local anesthetic via an indwelling caudal or epidural catheter.

More recently, laparoscopic techniques have been developed, with and without robotic control, for reimplantation of the ureters.[214] Preliminary evidence suggests an excellent success rate (greater than 90%) for this approach,[215] although the time for the surgery is more than twice the open technique and more complications were identified in children with small bladders.

Surgical alternatives in the past 20 years have spawned a number of compounds for injection into the terminal submucosal tract of the ureter, by passing a needle through a specially designed cystoscope. Initially, polytetrafluoroethylene (Teflon) was injected endoscopically, but a safer, more durable polymer has been developed over the past 20 years that is a mixture of dextranomer and hyaluronic acid (Deflux). In this way, surgeons create a swelling just inferior to the opening of the ureter into the bladder that prevents urine from refluxing (Fig. 27-10, before and after injection of polymer). The technique is successful in 80% of cases after one injection and in greater than 90% after two injections. Although this procedure still requires general anesthesia, its advantages far outweigh any disadvantages, in that the duration of the procedure is very brief (usually 15 to 30 minutes), the procedure avoids an abdominal incision, causes no postoperative pain, and its greatest advantage is that the child can be an outpatient. However, the results of this injection

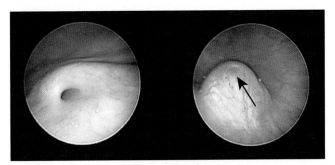

**FIGURE 27-10** A female with ureteral reflux. Preinjection (*at left*) with the bladder orifice wide open. There is no valve to prevent the backwash of urine up the ureter. Polymer was injected into the submucosa of the bladder, raising a mound to seal off the orifice of that ureter. Postinjection (*at right*) with the orifice now appearing as a dimple on the peak of the mound (*arrow*). (Courtesy Dr. P. Williot, Pediatric Urology, Women and Children's Hospital of Buffalo, Buffalo, N.Y.)

technique continue to be monitored because long-term outcomes and sequelae have not been determined.

## PYELOPLASTY

Pyeloplasty is performed to decompress the renal pelvis either because of intrinsic (congenital) or extrinsic (major vessel) compression of the ureter. A distended renal pelvis is often diagnosed antenatally and, in some instances, decompressed in utero by percutaneous nephrostomy. The ureteric narrowing often occurs at the ureteropelvic junction, where the ureter exits the renal pelvis. Surgery involves disconnecting the ureter at the renal pelvis, reshaping it, and then reinserting it into the kidney. Such surgery is often performed in the lateral or prone position, with the table jackknifed. The duration of this surgery is approximately 2 hours, with a success rate of approximately 95%. Dissection is often retroperitoneal, but the incision is placed immediately below the rib cage. This procedure has been performed laparoscopically and with the use of robotics.[105,215b]

Anesthetic considerations include the prone or lateral decubitus position (complicated by placing the table in the "jackknife position"), postoperative pain, and adequate fluid resuscitation. IV access should be established in an upper extremity to maintain adequate atrial filling pressures. If the table is placed in the jackknife position, it is very important to measure the child's blood pressure before and after the table is jackknifed, because venous return may become severely compromised, necessitating reducing the extent of the jackknife and resuscitating the child with fluid. The laparoscopic approach to pyeloplasty in children is new. In renal surgery, $CO_2$ is insufflated in the retroperitoneal space to provide surgical access.[216] Because of the anatomic differences between the retroperitoneal and intraperitoneal spaces, greater pressures may be required to provide adequate surgical visibility. A mean retroperitoneal pressure of 12 mm Hg increases $PETCO_2$ and peak inspiratory pressures, and decreases blood pressure.[217] Early evidence indicates that laparoscopic surgery yields similar outcomes to the open approach, although the duration of surgery is approximately one-third greater.[218,219] In part, this has been attributed to the learning curve of this technique. Evidence suggests that the laparoscopic approach decreases the length of hospital stay and may decrease postoperative pain[105,219] (see previous discussion of pain management after laparoscopic surgery).

## NEPHRECTOMY

Indications for nephrectomy and partial nephrectomy in children include nonfunctioning kidney, dysplastic kidney, urolithiasis, Wilms or other tumor, end-stage renal failure (pretransplantation or to control hypertension), hemolytic uremic syndrome, and polycystic disease. Children who require a nephrectomy will require a thorough preoperative assessment in terms of history, physical examination, and laboratory testing, depending on their underlying pathology. These children are often anemic because of chronic disease and possibly decreased erythropoietin concentrations. If the child is being staged for kidney transplant, the nephrologists may prefer to avoid blood transfusions at this time. If time is available and the patient is anemic, oral $FeSO_4$ and vitamin C should be commenced 3 to 6 weeks before surgery (vitamin C increases gut absorption of $FeSO_4$) to increase the hemoglobin concentration, particularly if erythropoietin supplementation is planned.[220,221] These children are often small in size and this should be considered when preparing the anesthetic equipment.

Nephrectomies are commonly performed using a retroperitoneal approach with the child in the lateral decubitus position and the table jackknifed. The incision is usually large and located just subcostal to the twelfth rib. If an open approach is planned, a low thoracic epidural catheter may be placed before positioning the child. If, however, a laparoscopic or robotic-assisted approach is planned,[89] then no neuraxial block is necessary but the same surgical approach occurs. Outcomes after laparoscopic nephrectomy in children are similar to those after an open procedure, according to the experience from one center,[222] although recent evidence points to less pain and earlier discharge from the hospital.[89]

## NEUROBLASTOMA

The adrenal glands are located in the retroperitoneal space, adjacent to the superior pole of the kidneys. Masses that arise in the adrenal gland may be tumors, hemorrhage, infections, or cysts. The tumors in the adrenal glands may arise from the cortex (as in adenoma) or medulla (including the sympathetic chain, as in neuroblastoma or ganglioneuroma), and may be either hyperfunctioning or nonfunctioning.

Neuroblastoma is the most common extracranial solid tumor that presents in childhood, comprising 10% of all tumors and 15% of all deaths from tumors.[223] It is the second most common abdominal tumor, after Wilms tumor. Its incidence is approximately 1 in 100,000 children in the United States.[224,225] Neuroblastomas arise in the abdomen in 75% of cases and along the sympathetic chain anywhere from the neck to the pelvis in 25%. Only one-third of those that arise in the abdomen arise in the adrenal glands. The median age at presentation is 2 years, with up to 90% occurring in children under 5 years of age. In some series, up to 50% of the cases appear in the first month of life, with some diagnosed antenatally. This tumor occurs equally in boys and girls. Reports of familial neuroblastoma are rare. However, these tumors may be associated with other disorders, including Beckwith-Wiedemann syndrome, neurofibromatosis, Hirschsprung disease, and central hypoventilation syndrome.[223]

Most neuroblastomas are first detected as palpable masses in the abdomen. Symptomatic presentation may present as local pressure on adjacent organs or structures (liver, kidney, or spine), as metastases (lymph nodes, bone marrow, liver, and skin), or with manifestations of excess neurohumoral production (i.e., from catecholamine [e.g., systemic hypertension] or vasoactive intestine polypeptides [e.g., diarrhea]).[223] Urinary catecholamines are increased in greater than 90% of children (more than 1 year of age) with neuroblastoma. In a minority of instances, the diagnosis is made through incidental examination, either by radiography or ultrasonography.

Staging of these tumors follows two protocols.[224] The International Neuroblastoma Staging System depends on tumor resectability, lymph node involvement, and metastases. However, if patients are not surgical candidates, the staging score holds little relevance. To further stage these tumors, a second scoring system was developed, the International Neuroblastoma Risk Group classification system, which is based on the preoperative radiologic findings only. Survival likelihood depends on a low score, extraabdominal (as opposed to intraabdominal) primary tumor, and younger age. Therapeutic intervention is tailored to the staging of the tumor at presentation and the size of the tumor. Those with favorable tumor biology, no distant metastases, and younger than 18 months of age, are often curable with surgical resection alone. Those with less favorable tumor biology, metastases, and a large tumor size that may present a challenge surgically, are ideally treated with a combination of chemotherapy, radiation, and/or bone marrow transplantation to reduce the tumor size first, and then with surgical resection. Patients with less favorable biology present a challenge for surgical resection because of local infiltration, large tumor size, and vascular extension. Debulking the tumor with incomplete resection has been met with mixed reviews. The most promising treatments for neuroblastomas with poor prognoses include molecular profiling of the tumor.[224] The long-term survival after treating these tumors is 88% for infants and children less than 18 months of age, 49% for children 18 months to 12 years of age, and 10% for those 12 years old or older.[226] Preoperative assessment requires a general systems review, with particular focus on the organ systems involved with the tumor. These tumors may present as a large intra-abdominal mass that compromises respiration, most commonly manifested as tachypnea. Those with catecholamine-secreting tumors may also present with chronic hypertension. This is mitigated to a large extent if the tumor is shrunk preoperatively, but intraoperative hypertensive episodes still occur in 25% of the children (with urinary catecholamines) during surgery. Children with catecholamine-secreting neuroblastomas should have both α-adrenergic and β-adrenergic blockades established preoperatively (see previous discussion of pheochromocytoma) to avoid swings in blood pressure during manipulation of the tumor.[227] Less frequently, chronic diarrhea from vasoactive intestine polypeptides may cause chronic dehydration and electrolyte derangements that require correction.

The anesthetic plan depends on the nature and extent of the surgery. A general anesthetic with tracheal intubation and controlled respiration, as well as standard anesthetic monitors, is required. These should be supplemented with invasive monitoring, including arterial and central venous access for catecholamine secreting tumors, large tumors, and those that are expected to bleed excessively. Anticipation of massive blood loss will necessitate using large bore upper extremity IV access, blood warmers, and possibly a rapid transfusion device. No specific anesthetic regimen has been recommended for these surgeries.

Although the blood pressure may be controlled with established α-adrenergic blockade, manipulation and squeezing of the tumor during its removal may cause a surge in catecholamine release, necessitating the use of antihypertensive medications intraoperatively (see previous discussion of pheochromocytoma).[227] Labetalol may be effective in children with hypertension during resection of neuroblastomas[227]; however, it may cause paroxysmal hypertension and heart failure in children who have only β-adrenergic blockade established, because of the predominant β-adrenergic blocking action of labetalol.

## WILMS TUMOR

Renal tumors comprise 2.5% to 7% of tumors in children. Wilms tumor is the most common abdominal tumor in children, with an incidence of 8 in 1,000,000 children less than 15 years old, and the most common solid renal tumor beyond the first year of life.[225,228] These tumors arise from persistent immature parenchymal renal tissue (referred to as Wilms tumorlet cells) often in the periphery of the kidney (as opposed to the collecting ducts), enclosed by a pseudocapsule (Fig. 27-11). They may achieve a large size before detection, often compressing adjacent renal parenchyma. Histologically, the tumor often includes up to three distinct tissue cell lines: epithelial, blastemal, and stromal cells.[228] The presence of anaplastic cells (in 4% of Wilms tumors) and, more specifically, whether the cells are focal or diffuse in the

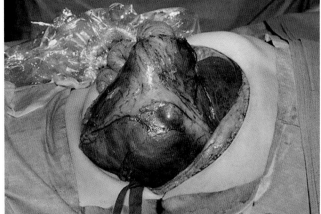

**FIGURE 27-11** A Wilms tumor was mobilized and exteriorized from the abdomen. Note that it is encapsulated and contiguous with the left kidney. (Courtesy Daniel P. Doody, MD, Pediatric Surgery, MassGeneral Hospital for Children, Boston.)

tumor, and older age at the time of presentation suggests a less favorable response to chemotherapy and less favorable long-term prognosis.[228] With tailored multimodal therapy, the survival from Wilms tumor in the past several decades has increased dramatically, from 30% to 90%.

Eighty percent of the children with of Wilms tumor present between 1 and 5 years of age (peaking at 3 to 4 years of age), with no gender or racial bias.[225,228] Presentation of Wilms tumor is similar to that of other intraabdominal tumors in the form of an incidental mass on physical examination; approximately 6% are bilateral. Congenital anomalies coexist with Wilms tumors in 12% of children, notably in genitourinary anomalies (5%), hemihypertrophy (2.5%), and aniridia (1%).[228] A number of genetic syndromes predispose to Wilms tumors, including Beckwith Wiedemann syndrome.[225] Wilms tumors occur twice as frequently in children with horseshoe kidneys than in those with normal kidneys, and is also more frequent in those with multicystic dysplastic kidneys.

Preoperatively, most children with Wilms tumors appear well, presenting with constitutional findings, including weight loss, loss of appetite, and malaise. Occasionally, they have an associated syndrome that should be detailed. Physical examination includes a palpable abdominal mass in 75% to 90% of children. Laboratory investigations before nephrectomy include routine complete blood count, electrolytes, renal function, as well as coagulation indices. Polycythemia may be present from tumor-induced excess erythropoietin production. Acquired Von Willebrand disease is present in less than 10% of these children.[225] Blood should be cross-matched for the surgery. Microscopic hematuria occurs in 25% of children whereas gross hematuria is rare,[228] suggesting tumor invasion of the collecting ducts. Systemic hypertension is present in 25% of children, presumably as a result of hyperreninemia. Preoperative investigations should include radiography and ultrasonography, the latter highlighting hyperechogenic structures within the kidney. Tumor extension into the ipsilateral renal vein and inferior vena cava must be examined before embarking on surgery, as chemotherapy may lead to involution of these tumors (Fig. 27-12).[225] Magnetic resonance imaging and computed tomography are valuable tools for delimiting the tumor borders within the kidney, as well as metastases in the lungs or other organs.[225] Most recent summaries of

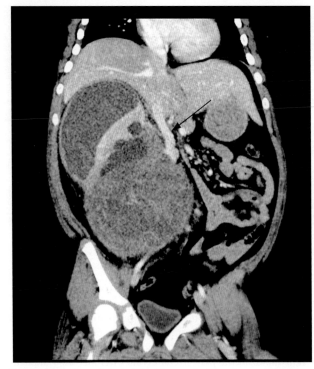

FIGURE 27-12 Coronal view of the CT scan of a Wilms tumor. Note the massive tumor enveloping the inferior vena cava, as the vena cava is only visible where it enters the liver in the upper midportion of the radiograph (*arrow*). (Radiograph courtesy Daniel P. Doody, MD, Pediatric Surgery, MassGeneral Hospital for Children, Boston.)

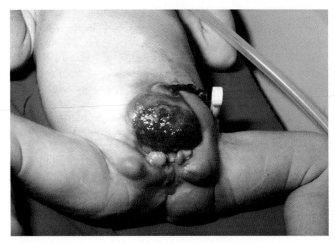

FIGURE 27-13 Bladder exstrophy in a neonate. Note the open anterior abdominal wall, protuberant bladder, distorted genitalia, and splayed hips.

the radiologic investigations may determine the need for additional interventions, including echocardiogram and lung scan to determine the presence of tumor in the heart and lungs, respectively. An echocardiogram may be specifically required to evaluate myocardial function if doxorubicin and other anthracycline chemotherapeutic agents had been administered.[225]

Anesthetic management of children with Wilms tumor is similar to that with neuroblastoma. No specific anesthetic regimen is preferred. Invasive monitoring and large bore IV access (upper extremities to avoid interference from tumor extension into the inferior vena cava) with adequate blood warming capability is mandatory. Anesthesia may be further complicated by hypertension (precipitated by tumor handling), coagulopathy (acquired von Willebrand disease), extension of the tumor into the proximal inferior vena cava or right atrium, pulmonary tumor emboli, acute right heart failure, and considerations concerning preoperative or previous treatment with chemotherapeutic drugs.[225] These drugs may impair hepatic or hematopoietic function (actinomycin D), cause inappropriate antidiuretic hormone release (vincristine), or myocardial damage (doxorubicin).[225] Pain may be controlled using either IV or regional anesthesia, though the risk of a coagulopathy must be ruled out before administering an epidural block.

## BLADDER AND CLOACAL EXSTROPHY

Bladder exstrophy is a rare congenital anomaly of the genitourinary tract occurring in 1 in 50,000 births with a 2:1 male to female ratio.[229] It occurs as a failure of the abdominal wall to close during fetal development and results in defects of the anterior wall of the bladder and overlying midline abdominal wall. Bladder exstrophy may present with a spectrum of anomalies,

including widening of the symphysis pubis, and genital anomalies, such as epispadias, bifid clitoris, and undescended testes (Fig. 27-13). Some regard bladder and cloacal exstrophies as distinct entities, whereas others consider them both extremes in a continuum of antenatal defects. Cloacal exstrophy includes features of bladder exstrophy plus an omphalocele and spinal defects, and always includes imperforate anus. Because the antenatal diagnosis of bladder exstrophy using ultrasound may be technically difficult, and thus dependent on indirect signs (absence of bladder filling, a low-set umbilicus, widening of the pubic ramus, small external genitalia, or a lower abdominal mass), the diagnosis is confirmed at birth when the anterior abdominal wall defect with the exposed bladder mucosa are evident.

Therapy is aimed at the surgical reconstruction of the bladder with preservation of renal function while achieving urinary continence and satisfactory appearance of the external genitalia. Surgical repair is usually achieved via a planned surgical approach.[230,231] In a very carefully selected group of infants, surgical management may be carried out as a single-stage procedure.[232] Alternatively, a planned staged surgical repair may be chosen with management directed at closure of the bladder, posterior urethra, and abdominal wall. In addition, a bilateral iliac osteotomy is often performed to facilitate surgical closure, decrease the stress on the midline soft tissues, and reduce the risk of postoperative wound dehiscence.

Wound dehiscence, bladder prolapse, and multiple attempts at bladder closure are among the risk factors for decreased bladder growth and the inability for the later development of continence.[233] In addition to the immediate postoperative complications, children who have undergone surgical repair of bladder exstrophy carry an increased risk for the development of renal, bladder, and colon adenocarcinoma.[234] Children who require frequent bladder catheterizations or repeat surgeries are at risk for developing latex allergy if latex products are used.[56] Today, most bladder catheters exclude latex.

Surgical management of the epispadias is usually performed at 6 to 12 months of age, and reconstruction of the bladder neck by 5 years, the latter to allow for bladder training. After the initial surgical repair, children are immobilized for 4 to 6 weeks,[235] with a successful outcome likely when a modified Buck traction with an external fixator or a modified Bryant traction[236] and adequate postoperative analgesia are used.[237]

The preoperative assessment should evaluate the presence and severity of all congenital anomalies, particularly cardiac abnormalities. Signs or symptoms of renal insufficiency and electrolyte balance may be present. If the child has renal insufficiency, the dose and frequency of administration of potentially nephrotoxic drugs, as well as the commonly used anesthetic drugs, must be carefully evaluated. Typically, surgery is performed with the child in the supine and lithotomy positions. The duration of surgery is often prolonged, requiring alternating urologic and orthopedic teams for their respective segment of the surgery, and repositioning the child depending on the stage of the surgery. These neonates require judicious management of fluids, blood loss, and temperature control, as is typical for surgical procedures in the neonatal period. In formulating the anesthetic plan, the anesthesiologist must partner with the surgical teams to ensure an optimal strategy for balanced salt solutions, colloids, and blood products. This allows for optimal intraoperative management, as well as planning for a multimodal perioperative pain management strategy and postoperative ventilatory support, if needed. After applying the standard monitors, anesthesia may be induced either by inhalation or IV; after induction, at least one large bore peripheral IV should be placed. A second IV may be placed, or a central venous catheter and possibly an arterial catheter. In general, if blood loss occurs, it is slow and steady, but if posterior iliac osteotomies are performed, the blood loss may become brisk, requiring aggressive fluid resuscitation and administration of blood products. Beat-to-beat variability of arterial blood pressure and serial laboratory evaluations are valuable during goal directed resuscitation. Appropriate padding, a fluid warmer, and a forced-air heating system should be standard. The anesthetic plan varies according to the age of the child and whether the surgery is completed in a single or staged repair. Postoperatively, children are transferred directly to the pediatric intensive care unit for recovery. Careful attention must be paid to maintain fluid and electrolyte homeostasis, to prevent reduced oxygen carrying capacity, and to assure adequate analgesia.

A general anesthetic in combination with an epidural or caudal continuous infusion technique is often used if there are no associated spine abnormalities.[238] Opioids (other than remifentanil) have had a limited role in neonates because of their potential to cause postoperative respiratory depression, although pediatric anesthesiologists today are much more aggressive in anticipating pain and administering opioids to neonates and infants, even if it delays extubation.

Maintenance of anesthesia may be achieved using an inhalation anesthetic, small doses of opioids, and intermittent boluses (0.5 to 1 mL/kg) or continuous infusions of bupivacaine (0.125% to 0.25%) or ropivacaine (0.2%) with or without epinephrine through a lumbar or caudal epidural catheter. Caudal or epidural analgesia may be provided by advancing the catheter to the appropriate surgical dermatomal level after induction of anesthesia. The catheter is either secured directly to the skin or tunneled using the epidural insertion needle.[239] A continuous infusion of a local anesthetic may be used and maintained for up to 3 days to provide analgesia and a mild motor blockade that favors immobility. However, care must be taken to avoid systemic toxicity. Neonates are at increased risk for developing local anesthetic toxicity because of their low serum protein concentration and metabolism. Albumin and $\alpha$1-acid glycoprotein are reduced in this age group,[240] which reduces protein binding and increases the free-fraction of bupivacaine. This free form is metabolized to a lesser extent in the neonate because of immature metabolic pathways, and contributes to an increased risk of cardiac and systemic toxicity.[241,242] This is especially true of the amide local anesthetics. If the epidural infusion is maintained beyond 48 to 72 hours, serum concentrations of local anesthetic should be sampled once or twice a day to guide therapy and minimize the risk of complications. Because serum concentrations of bupivacaine increase after only 48 hours of a continuous epidural infusion,[241] and serum concentrations are difficult to assay, lidocaine 0.1% (0.8 mg/kg/hr) may be preferable. Ropivacaine is also currently being used for infusions that last less than 72 hours.[243]

The outcome of this complex surgery is determined primarily by the surgical expertise. Urologic incontinence, bladder prolapse, and epispadias revisions will require additional urologic surgery, as well as possible osteotomies, for satisfactory closure and surgical outcomes. Renal function is usually well-maintained throughout. Complications of complete repair are reported to be similar to those of the staged repair, but usually involve additional soft tissue defects.[244]

## Acknowledgment

The authors thank P.A. Lonnqvist for his contributions to this chapter in the previous edition.

Videos 27-1 and 27-2 on page 27-10. Video 27-1: Robotic-assisted laparoscopic ureteral reimplantation. Video 27-2: Robotic-assisted laparoscopic pyeloplasty. Courtesy Dr. C. Koh et al, Institute of Urology, Children's Hospital of Los Angeles, University of Southern California.

## ANNOTATED REFERENCES

Kim PH, Patil MB, Kim SS, et al. Early comparison of nephrectomy options in children (open, transperitoneal laparoscopic, laparo-endoscopic single site (LESS), and robotic surgery). BJU Int 2012;109:910-5.
*This up-to-date review provides us with comparative results of both laparoscopic techniques and robotic surgery in children.*

Lasersohn L. Anaesthetic considerations for paediatric laparoscopy. S Afr J Surg 2011;49:22-6.
*In this very detailed review, the author provides a comprehensive review of the physiology and anesthetic considerations of laparoscopic surgery in children.*

Lenders JW, Eisenhofer G, Mannelli M, Pacak K. Phaeochromocytoma. Lancet 2005;366:665-75.
*Pheochromocytoma is a rare and dangerous disorder that has many hidden problems that may complicate anesthesia. This review provides a single but most thorough analysis of the basic science and practical clinical issues needed to safely anesthetize children with this disorder and to anticipate and minimize complications and risks.*

Ure BM, Suempelmann R, Metzelder MM, Kuebler J. Physiological responses to endoscopic surgery in children. Semin Pediatr Surg 2007;16:217-23.
*Understanding the physiology of laparoscopic surgery is key to preventing complications and minimizing their impact when they occur. These authors detail the physiology in this type of surgery in a logical and understandable manner, tying many loose ends together to present a comprehensive understanding of the effects of $CO_2$ pneumoperitoneum.*

Walker RW, Ravi R, Haylett K. Effect of cricoid force on airway calibre in children: a bronchoscopic assessment. Br J Anaesth 2010;104:71-4.
*This investigation documents the magnitude of the external force required to distort the cricoid ring from infants until adolescents. In infants, force as little as 5 N distorts the cricoid rings. The force required to distort the ring increases with age, reaching 15 to 25 N in adolescents.*

## REFERENCES

Please see www.expertconsult.com.

# Essentials of Hepatology

MARCUS RIVERA, ROBERT H. SQUIRES, AND PETER J. DAVIS

## Anatomy

THE LIVER AND BILIARY TREE are derived from the endoderm of the dorsal foregut during the late third to the early fourth week of gestation. By the sixth week, the fetal liver primarily serves as a hematopoietic organ, while critical biologic functions such as glycolysis, bile acid synthesis, and metabolic waste processing are managed by the maternal liver through the fetoplacental circulation. Oxygenated blood is shunted from the placenta to the right atrium through the ductus venosus. Functional closure of the ductus begins immediately after birth, with complete functional closure occurring in up to 95% of infants by 2 weeks of age and anatomic closure taking place shortly thereafter.

Hepatic developmental changes occur throughout gestation. Hepatic hematopoiesis develops in utero at 5 to 6 weeks gestation, followed closely by protein synthesis.[1] The ability to metabolize carbohydrates and lipids begins by 10 weeks gestation, followed closely by the development of drug metabolizing systems.

At the time of delivery, the liver weighs between 120 and 160 g but remains structurally and physiologically immature. Peripheral branches of the intrahepatic biliary system require an additional 4 to 8 weeks before portal bile ducts can be identified histologically. The liver is composed of eight structurally independent segments, and each contains a feeding hepatic artery, portal vein, draining hepatic vein, and bile duct. Segment 1 is the caudate lobe. Segments 2 and 3 form the left lateral segment, and with segment 4, the left lobe of the liver is defined. Segments 5, 6, 7, and 8 constitute the right lobe of the liver.

The liver receives blood from two sources: the portal vein, which drains the spleen and intestine, and the hepatic artery, which provides systemic oxygenated blood directly to biliary epithelium and to the hepatic sinusoids. The portal vein accounts for approximately 70% of the blood flow to the liver. In the sinusoids, the hepatic arterial and portal venous blood mix and intercalate among the hepatocytes, fenestrated sinusoidal cells, and a host of resident immune cells (e.g., Kupffer cells). Sinusoids drain into terminal hepatic venules, which eventually coalesce to form the left and right hepatic veins. The veins merge into the inferior vena cava immediately before entering the right atrium. At any time, the liver contains approximately 13% of the circulating blood volume.

During the neonatal period, liver function is immature in its ability to metabolize and clear xenobiotics. Factors believed to affect the clearance of medications include hepatic blood flow and the developmental status of hepatic transport and enzyme systems. Size alone does not account for this observed degree of immaturity, because the fetal and neonatal liver account for a greater percentage of body weight than the adult counterpart (3.6% of body weight versus 2.4% in adults).[2] The neonatal liver contains approximately 20% fewer hepatocytes than the adult liver, and the cells are almost one half of the size of adult hepatocytes. These structural features may play some role in the functional deficiencies exhibited by infant livers. Cellular growth and hypertrophy of the liver continue at a rapid pace into young adulthood.

The structural unit of the liver parenchyma is the lobule, a hub-and-spoke structure with the central vein serving as the hub that is bordered by portal tracts, which contain a bile duct and tributaries of the portal vein and hepatic artery. While the mixed venous and arterial blood flows from the portal tract to the central vein, bile flows in the opposite direction through a canalicular matrix that then enters the bile ductule in the portal tract. The functional unit of the liver is the hepatic acinus, which is centered on the portal track and extends in three concentric zones (i.e., zones of Rappaport) outward to the central vein (Fig. 28-1). The more central zones (zones 1 and 2) are most active in oxidative processes, whereas the distal zone 3, which is closer to the central vein, is more dependent on glycolysis and more susceptible to ischemic and toxic injury.

## Principles of Hepatic Drug Metabolism

Lipid solubility, an important and desired feature of most administered drugs, allows passive diffusion across cellular membranes. Lipophilic drugs are also difficult to excrete. They have a propensity to accumulate in the body's fat stores and are bound to proteins in plasma, thereby limiting renal excretion. Renal and

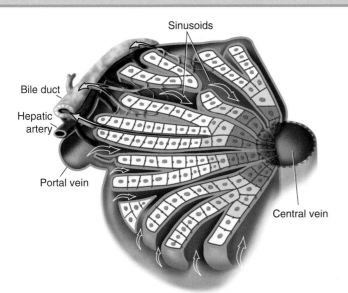

**FIGURE 28-1** Blood flows from the hepatic arteries and portal vein along the sinusoids toward the central vein. The hepatic triad consists of the bile duct, a branch of the portal vein, and the hepatic artery, with zone 1 (*white*) surrounding the triad, followed by zone 2 (*pink*), and zone 3 (*red*). Cytochrome P-450 expression is higher in zone 3, which has more extensive drug metabolism. (From Oinonen T, Lindros KO. Zonation of hepatic cytochrome P-450 expression and regulation. Biochem J 1998;329:17-35.)

biliary excretion of lipid-soluble compounds can result in their resorption across their respective membranes. A major role of the liver is to transform lipid-soluble drugs into water-soluble compounds that become easily excreted metabolites. An interesting example of the need for this biotransformation is the anesthetic compound thiopental, which if not transformed into its less lipophilic counterpart would have a plasma half-life of approximately 25 years.[1]

The primary family of liver enzymes assigned the task of metabolizing these exogenous substances is the cytochrome P-450 (CYP) family. *P* designates a red *pigment*, which is related to a heme molecule and absorbs light at a wavelength of 450 nm.[3] The primary reactions involved in the drug biotransformation and metabolism are hydroxylation and conjugation. Hydroxylation prepares the metabolite for conjugation (i.e., phase II reaction). The CYP family of enzymes is responsible for most phase I reactions, and the members were first thought to be chemically similar to mitochondrial cytochromes.

## PHASE I REACTIONS

The CYP enzymes likely evolved as a mechanism by which the host was able to protect itself from toxins ingested from the environment. Most enzymes involved in hepatic drug metabolism are categorized in three distinct families: CYP1, CYP2, and CYP3. Each family is further divided into subfamilies that are designated with capital letters and numbered in the order in which they were discovered. The CYP enzymes are generally conserved across species, but their regulation and catalytic activity vary among species, which highlights the challenges associated with laboratory analysis of drug metabolism.[3]

Genetic and nongenetic factors contribute to the variability in the enzymatic activity seen across all CYP enzymes.[4] Approximately 5% of Caucasian populations lack CYP2D6 activity, which is associated with altered metabolism of some drugs.[5] For

example, a lack of CYP2D6 activity enhances the effect of drugs such as haloperidol and metoprolol that require the enzyme for efficient metabolism, whereas codeine, which is metabolized to morphine by CYP2D6, provides little analgesia in a child with CYP2D6 deficiency.[6]

Nongenetic factors that influence CYP activity include concomitant disease states, malnutrition,[7] and exposure to a host of pharmacologic and naturally occurring compounds. Many drugs can inhibit or stimulate the enzyme system (Table 28-1). Inhibition of the CYPs occurs when drugs compete for the same enzyme. The degree to which this competition becomes clinically significant depends on five factors: the relative amount of the specific CYP, the concentrations of each drug, the degree of pharmacologically active metabolite generated through this system, the importance of the enzyme in elimination of the drugs, and the therapeutic index of the drug.[3]

Enhanced CYP expression occurs after amplified transcription of the specific gene that is induced by a variety of compounds. For example, rifampin and phenytoin induce CYP3A4 by binding the cytosolic human pregnenolone-X receptor (hPXR) or the steroid xenobiotic receptor (SXR).[8] The activated receptor translocates into the nucleus, where it binds the regulator elements of the *CYP3A4* gene and promotes increased transcription of CYP3A4, which can lead to toxic levels of intermediate

**TABLE 28-1** Major Human Liver Forms of Cytochrome P-450

| P-450 | Substrate | Inhibitors | Inducers |
|---|---|---|---|
| CYP1A2 | Caffeine Clozapine Estradiol Theophylline | Fluvoxamine Furafylline | Omeprazole Tobacco smoke |
| CYP2A6 | Halothane Nicotine | Methoxsalen | |
| CYP2C8 | Rosiglitazone Taxol | | Phenytoin Rifampin |
| CYP2C9 | Diclofenac Ibuprofen Tolbutamide Warfarin | Sulfaphenazole | Rifampin Secobarbital |
| CYP2C19 | Omeprazole | Fluvoxamine Ketoconazole | |
| CYP2D6 | Codeine Chlorpromazine Desipramine Dextromethorphan Encainide Haloperidol Metoprolol | Fluoxetine Quinidine | |
| CYP2E1 | Acetaminophen Halothane | Disulfiram | Ethanol Isoniazid |
| CYP3A4 | Cyclosporine Estradiol Indinavir Lovastatin Midazolam Nifedipine Quinidine Docetaxel | Delavirdine Erythromycin Grapefruit juice Ketoconazole Ritonavir Troleandomycin | Carbamazepine Phenobarbital Phenytoin Rifampin St. John's wort Troglitazone |

Modified from Watkins PB. The role of cytochrome P450s in drug-induced liver disease. In: Kaplowitz N, Deleve LD, editors. Drug-induced liver disease. New York: Marcel Dekker; 2003, p. 15-33.

compounds, as is the case with erythromycin, or to subtherapeutic levels of cyclosporine in transplant recipients.[9]

## CYTOCHROME P-450 ACTIVITY

The superfamily of CYP enzymes is divided into subfamilies based on sequence homology and on demonstration of broad substrate specificities. An important example is the CYP3A subfamily, which is the most abundant group of cytochromes involved in the metabolism of xenobiotics. The three identified isoforms are CYP3A4, CYP3A5, and CYP3A7. CYP3A4 is the most abundant single enzyme in the human liver, accounting for the metabolism of approximately 50% of clinically used pharmaceuticals.[10] CYP3A5 is more commonly found in the kidneys and lungs and to a lesser degree in the liver. CYP3A7 is the predominant isoform in the neonatal liver but is replaced after birth by CYP3A4. Given its critical involvement in hepatic biotransformation of xenobiotics, the CYP3A family of enzymes is used to study and estimate hepatic drug clearance in various age and gender groups.

Changes in the distribution and activity of the CYP enzyme systems occur with hepatic growth and maturation (Fig. 28-2). The CYP3A family is homogeneously distributed across the liver parenchyma in the fetal liver and shortly after birth. However, during postnatal growth, expression of the CYP3A protein shifts toward the centrilobular region of the acinus (i.e., Rappaport zone 1). By adulthood, expression of CYP2A becomes increasingly limited to the zone 1 and zone 2 hepatocytes, with sparse expression occurring in zone 3.[11] Other examples of developmental changes in the CYP system include the CYP2C and CYP3A3/4 subfamilies, which have negligible expression in the fetus but have increased expression in the first few weeks of life.[12,13] CYP2D6 reaches adult activity levels within 1 month chronological age; variability thereafter is determined primarily by genetic polymorphisms.[13a]

Changes in activity of CYP enzyme families and subfamilies have correlated with drug clearance. For example, midazolam clearance correlates with changes in CYP3A4 activity, with decreased clearance in fetal and neonatal livers and with adult clearance rates achieved by 3 months of age.[14,15] In contrast, CYP3A7 activity peaks at about 1 week postpartum and steadily diminishes during the first year of life, reaching approximately 10% of fetal liver activity by adulthood.

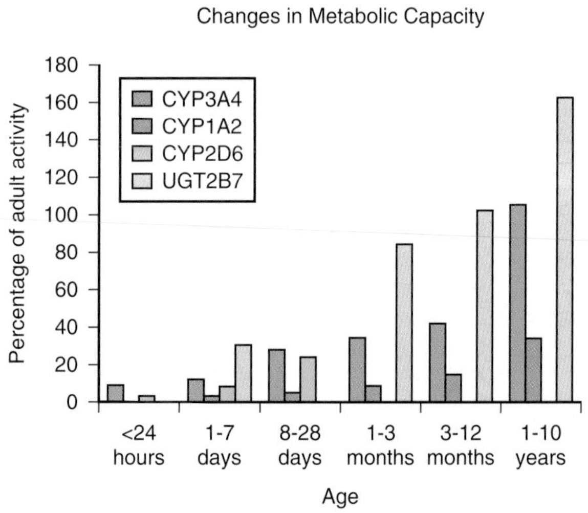

## PHASE II REACTIONS

Conjugation of lipophilic compounds decreases their lipid solubility and facilitates renal excretion.[16,17] Conjugation reactions (i.e., glucuronidation, sulfation, glutathione conjugation, acetylation, and methylation) are decreased in infants compared with adults.[18]

Glucuronidation is catalyzed by uridine 5'-diphosphate (UDP)–glucuronosyltransferase (UGT) family of enzymes, which are derived from assimilation of proteins from separate genes or alternate splicing from single-gene transcripts.[19] UGT enzymes are responsible for the metabolism of several drugs, including phenols, estrogens, and opioids (see Chapter 6). As with the CYP enzymes, individual UGT enzymes demonstrate substrate specificity and can act in concert to metabolize single compounds. Glucuronidation is not fully active in infants and can place this population at risk for toxic drug accumulation.[20] Hepatic UGT enzyme concentrations are reduced during fetal and early postnatal development. At 3 months of age, the levels of many UGTs are 25% of those in adults.[21]

UGT1A enzyme activity, which is involved in the conjugation of bilirubin and ethinylestradiol, is decreased in the fetus, but it increases to adult levels within 3 to 6 months after a term delivery.[22] UGT1A6, which conjugates acetaminophen and naproxen, has 10% of adult activity in the fetus and neonate, and it achieves only 50% of adult activity by 6 months of age.[18] UGT2B7 is active in the metabolism of the nonsteroidal antiinflammatory drugs naloxone, codeine, and lorazepam. Fetal activity of this enzyme approaches 10% to 20% of adult levels, with a rapid increase to adult levels by 2 months of age.[23]

Sulfation is accomplished by sulfotransferases, a family of cytosolic enzymes that are divided into two categories: catechol and phenol sulfotransferase. These enzymes conjugate inorganic sulfate from 3'-phosphoadenosine-5'-sulfophosphate (PAPS) with compounds containing functional hydroxyl groups.[16] The catechol transferases develop earlier in fetal life than the phenol counterparts and appear to exhibit decreased activity in the developing neonate. Although specific sulfotransferase substrates require identification, the activity of these enzymes is increased in fetuses and neonates and theorized to be an efficient conjugation pathway in this age group.

Glutathione S-transferases (GSTs) conjugate glutathione with a broad spectrum of lipophilic and electrophilic compounds. The family of GSTs is composed of up to five different groups in various classes designated μ, α, θ, and π, which are derived from at least three genetic loci.[24] Tissue-specific expression of these enzymes has been demonstrated, with the liver expressing the greatest amount of protein. Variable time-dependent expression has also been shown, with α- and π-class GSTs having enhanced expression between 16 and 24 weeks gestation, whereas only the α-class enzymes predominate in the neonate and adult liver.[25] The hepatic π-class enzymes disappear from their hepatocellular location by 6 months of age and can be found only in the epithelial cells of the biliary canaliculi. Variations in the developmental expression of this class of enzymes have made it challenging to fully appreciate what is likely a multitude of clinical interactions.[25]

Acetylation reactions are catalyzed by N-acetyltransferases, which transfer an acetyl group from acetyl coenzyme A to a

**Changes in Metabolic Capacity**

FIGURE 28-2 Changes in metabolic capacity versus percentage of adult activity. (Modified from Kearns G, Abdel-Rahman SM, Alander SW, et al. Developmental pharmacology—drug disposition, action, and therapy in infants and children. N Engl J Med 2003;349:1157-67.)

variety of substrates (e.g., *p*-aminobenzoic acid, *p*-aminosalicylic acid, procainamide). Two genes, *NAT1* and *NAT2*, are responsible for yielding two specific enzymes with different allelic forms. Despite having 87% sequence homology, these enzymes exhibit different substrate specificities.[26] Both are cytosolic enzymes involved in the biotransformation of several drugs and the bioactivation of several human carcinogens. NAT1 is present in multiple fetal and postnatal tissues and accounts for the most *N*-acetyltransferase substrate metabolism in children younger than 1 year of age. NAT2 is located primarily in the liver and becomes the dominant acetylator after 1 year of age. NAT2 has polymorphisms with enzyme kinetics that differentiate patients with slow or rapid acetylation capabilities. Infants younger than 1 year of age usually are slow acetylators; subsequent age-dependent alterations lead an individual's targeted acetylator status.[27] Individuals who are genetically destined for rapid acetylation manifest this feature by 2 to 4 years of age.

## Anesthetic Agents

### INHALATIONAL ANESTHETIC METABOLISM
Inhalational anesthetics are poorly metabolized, with 15% to 20% of halothane undergoing biotransformation. Although both oxidative and reductive pathways are involved, the primary pathway of metabolism of halothane is through oxidation to a reactive intermediate, trifluoroacetyl chloride,[28] which then undergoes glutathione conjugation.[29]

Isoflurane is metabolized by CYP2E1 to a limited extent (0.2%).[30] Isoflurane is excreted as inorganic fluoride and trifluoroacetic acid after oxidative metabolism in the liver.[31] Desflurane is the least metabolized (0.02%) of the volatile anesthetics, which is approximately 10% of the rate of isoflurane.[32] Both are metabolized in the liver along similar paths because the urinary metabolite for desflurane, trifluoroacetic acid, is the same as for isoflurane.

Only 2% to 5% of inhaled sevoflurane is metabolized in humans by means of the hepatic CYP2E1 enzyme, as occurs for the other ether anesthetics.[33] Oxidation of sevoflurane generates the intermediate formyl fluoride, a highly reactive species thought to generate liver protein adducts. Carbon dioxide and inorganic fluoride are released through this oxidative mechanism, and the final product is hexafluoroisopropanol, which undergoes glucuronide conjugation and is further excreted in the urine (see Chapter 6).[34]

### NEUROMUSCULAR BLOCKING DRUGS
Neuromuscular blockade is achieved by depolarizing or nondepolarizing neuromuscular blocking agents (see Chapter 6). The only depolarizing agent still in use is short-acting suxamethonium (i.e., succinylcholine).[35] Succinylcholine is hydrolyzed completely by plasma cholinesterases, which are synthesized by the liver.[36] Enzyme activity varies with age, but it is decreased in liver disease and has been used as a metric of liver prognosis.[37]

Nondepolarizing muscle relaxants are divided into aminosteroids (i.e., pipecuronium, pancuronium, vecuronium, and rocuronium) and benzylisoquinolinium diesters (i.e., doxacurium, atracurium, and cisatracurium besylate). Renal and hepatic diseases affect their safety and efficacy.[38] Hepatic elimination depends on protein binding, hepatic blood flow, and drug extraction. The volume of drug distribution is increased in hepatic disease, leading to a slower onset and prolonged effect. In children with cholestatic liver disease, such as biliary atresia, uptake of these compounds by the liver is decreased, which decreases plasma clearance and prolongs their effects.[39,40] Approximately 75% of the administered dose is bound to plasma proteins, with most bound to albumin. Despite these problems, children with liver disease and a correspondingly low albumin concentration are at minimal risk for the adverse effects from this group of drugs.[41]

Rocuronium is an analogue of vecuronium with a more rapid onset of action. Unlike other aminosteroids, which largely undergo renal excretion, only 12% to 22% of rocuronium is cleared through the kidney.[42] In patients with hepatic disease, the volume of distribution of rocuronium increased by 33% compared with healthy controls.[43] In patients undergoing liver transplantation, the clearance of rocuronium was only slightly reduced by the diseased native liver compared with the functioning allograft and healthy individuals.[44] Reduced infusion requirements of rocuronium during liver transplantation may indicate graft dysfunction.[45]

Hepatic elimination of the benzyl isoquinolinium agents is poorly understood, but hepatic dysfunction has been observed to affect their efficacy. Despite increased concentrations in biliary secretions, the pharmacokinetics of doxacurium are unchanged in the presence of hepatocellular injury, but recovery indices are prolonged.[46] Although no longer available in the United States, mivacurium is a mixture of three stereoisomers. Clearance of the *trans-trans* and *cis-trans* isomers is reduced in patients with liver disease,[47] whereas clearance of the *cis-cis* isomer is unchanged. Prolonged recovery occurs as a result of a decrease in plasma cholinesterases in significant liver disease.[47] Clearance of cisatracurium is decreased, although patients with liver disease experience no delay in recovery and minimal delay in onset of action. Children with liver disease, regardless of cause, usually tolerate this class of compounds, and there is no observed toxicity.[48]

### SEDATIVES, OPIOIDS, AND LIVER DISEASE
The commonly used sedatives midazolam, propofol, and ketamine undergo hepatic metabolism through oxidation and conjugation. These compounds are all lipid soluble, and their effects are altered by liver disease.[49] Midazolam has an increased clearance rate that depends in part on hepatic blood flow. In children with cirrhosis, the clearance of midazolam is halved with a corresponding doubling of the half-life compared with healthy controls.[50] With 95% to 97% bound to albumin, diseases that decrease the concentration of albumin dramatically increase the free fraction of drug, which leads to a greater effect.[51,52] Propofol is eliminated primarily (>88%) in the urine, and hepatocellular injury does not alter its pharmacokinetics.[53] Ketamine is also highly lipophilic and undergoes metabolism in the liver. However, unlike the other drugs described, it does so through methylation, and its clearance is minimally affected by liver dysfunction.[54]

Clinical effects from opioids result from their binding to opioid receptors. A greater serum concentration of opioid binds a greater number of receptors, resulting in a correspondingly greater opioid effect. Hepatic clearance and protein binding govern the serum concentration of an opioid.[55] Most opioids are oxidized in the liver. However, morphine and buprenorphine undergo glucuronidation, and remifentanil is metabolized by plasma and tissue esterases, enzymes that are mature in term neonates. The ability of the diseased liver to oxidize opioids is diminished, leading to increased oral bioavailability due to decreased first-pass metabolism and decreased drug clearance. The clearance of morphine, despite being metabolized by glucuronidation, is also negatively affected by the presence of cirrhosis.[56]

Clearance of drugs that are highly extracted by the liver, such as meperidine and morphine, depend on hepatic blood flow.[57,58] Clearance (CL) is a function of hepatic blood flow ($Q_H$) and the extraction ratio ($E_H$), describing the ability of the liver to efficiently remove the drug from the circulation:

$$CL_H = Q_H \times E_H$$

When $E_H$ is greater than 0.7, as with meperidine, lidocaine, and pentazocine, $CL_H$ approaches $Q_H$. Conditions that alter hepatic blood flow, such as cirrhosis, portal vein thrombosis, and portacaval shunting, significantly alter opioid clearance. Drugs with a low $E_H$, such as methadone and naproxen, do not depend on hepatic blood flow. The metabolic activity of the liver and the plasma protein-binding fraction affect the clearance to a greater degree. The hepatic clearance of these drugs is described by the following equation:

$$CL_H = CL_{INT} \times f_u$$

In the formula, $f_u$ is the fraction of unbound drug and $CL_{INT}$ describes the metabolic activity. When $f_u$ is small as with methadone (<0.1), clearance is mainly affected by reduced enzyme capacity.[55]

The pharmacology of the opioids is variably affected by liver disease. The analgesic effect of codeine, obtained after its demethylation to morphine, is reduced in the presence of liver disease. Liver disease can affect glucuronidation and thereby decrease clearance and prolong the half-life of morphine.[59] The protein binding and clearance of alfentanil are reduced in the presence of hepatic dysfunction,[60,61] whereas the half-life and volume of distribution of methadone are increased.[62] The pharmacokinetics of fentanyl, remifentanil, and sufentanil are unchanged in the presence of significant hepatic dysfunction.[63-65] Because the degree of hepatic dysfunction exhibits interindividual variability, the level of adverse events of these medications also varies. Careful monitoring of children with liver disease is required when administering opioids.

## Anesthetic Effects on Hepatic Cellular Functions

### CARBOHYDRATES

Glucose metabolism is influenced by the availability of the substrate, the rate of entry into cells, and the ability of the target organ to convert glucose into energy or to use it to synthesize fats. In healthy individuals, hepatic glucose production accounts for most whole-body glucose production and is narrowly regulated directly and indirectly by insulin.[66] Insulin directly inhibits gluconeogenesis and glycogenolysis by binding to insulin receptors in the liver, thereby diminishing hepatic glucose production.[67] Of the glucose available to the liver, about 50% undergoes glycolysis and is converted to energy. Between 30% and 40% is converted to fat for storage, and 10% to 20% is shunted to glycogen.[68] Anesthetics inhibit glucose uptake by hepatocytes, an action referred to as the *anti-insulin effect of anesthesia.*[69] Although all inhalational anesthetics exhibit this tendency, halothane has the greatest impact on serum glucose, with isoflurane and sevoflurane having lesser effects.[70] Inhalational anesthetics at 1 to 2 minimal alveolar concentrations (MACs) inhibit glucose uptake by up to 50%. The combined effects of anesthetics and stress from surgery or trauma increase the serum glucose concentration,

which is one reason why glucose-containing intravenous fluids are no longer recommended for most healthy children undergoing elective surgery.

### PROTEIN SYNTHESIS

The impact of anesthesia and surgery on protein synthesis and metabolism is poorly understood. Albumin, a large, soluble, single polypeptide protein with a molecular weight of 66 kD, is an important protein synthesized by the liver. Between 6 and 12 g of albumin are produced each day, and production can increase twofold to threefold according to the individual's needs. Albumin functions as a binding and transport protein and maintains colloid oncotic pressure. Hepatic dysfunction may result in decreased synthesis of albumin and other proteins. Anesthetics may also inhibit protein synthesis. Diethyl ether causes reversible inhibition of protein synthesis in rat hepatocytes,[71] whereas halothane and enflurane block protein synthesis in a dose-dependent manner.[72] Halothane, sevoflurane, and enflurane inhibit protein synthesis and secretion, which may be an early indicator of hepatic cytotoxic injury.

### BILIRUBIN METABOLISM

Bilirubin, the end product of heme metabolism, is converted to unconjugated bilirubin by macrophages in the spleen and bone marrow and transported to the liver bound to plasma albumin. Unconjugated bilirubin is transported into the hepatocyte by bile acids and bacterial endotoxins. In the hepatocyte, bilirubin is conjugated with glucuronate, taurine, and to a lesser extent, glucose by glucuronyl transferase. Deficiencies of glucuronyl transferase manifest clinically in Gilbert syndrome, with more severe forms seen in Crigler-Najjar syndrome types I and II. Gilbert syndrome affects 2% to 13% of individuals, who have increases in bilirubin associated with stress or fasting. Although postoperative jaundice has been described, Gilbert syndrome has not been associated with serious adverse effects in the perioperative anesthesia period.[73] Patients with Crigler-Najjar syndrome can be managed safely by minimizing their exposure to drugs that may displace bilirubin from albumin and by using anesthetics that undergo minimal hepatic metabolism.[74]

### HEPATOTOXICITY

Increases in serum aminotransferase concentrations and bilirubin up to two times the upper limit of normal occur commonly in the postoperative period.[75,76] These increases are typically self-limited and inconsequential. However, serious liver injury can be caused by anesthetics.[77] The Drug-Induced Liver Injury Network, established by the National Institutes of Health in 2003, has and continues to standardize the nomenclature and causality assessment of drug-induced liver injury (DILI).[78] Diagnosis of DILI is entertained when increases in alanine aminotransferase (ALT), aspartate aminotransferase (AST), alkaline phosphatase, γ-glutamyl transferase (GGT), and bilirubin occur coincident with xenobiotic exposure. Patterns of injury are classified as hepatocellular, with predominantly increased ALT and AST levels; cholestatic, with increases in alkaline phosphatase, GGT, and bilirubin; and mixed pattern, with features of both hepatocellular and cholestatic injury. Differences between predictable and unpredictable DILI and the associated clinical and histologic variability led to the clinical pearl known as the *Hy rule*, named after Hyman Zimmerman: If increased serum aminotransferase levels (greater than three times the upper limit of normal) and cholestasis (bilirubin greater than two times the upper limit of normal) without evidence of biliary obstruction occur at the same time in the setting of DILI, a mortality rate of at least 10% can be expected.[79]

In the absence of a unique test to assess liver function, surrogate markers for liver dysfunction include a prolonged prothrombin time (PT) greater than 15 seconds or an international normalized ratio (INR) greater than 1.5, or both. Other clinical and biochemical markers, such as hypoalbuminemia, hypoglycemia, and an altered mental status, should be included in the assessment of hepatic dysfunction, but they can also result from conditions not related to liver function, such as malnutrition, protein-losing enteropathy or nephropathy, or medications for sedation or pain management.

Halothane hepatitis is well described and used as a model for hepatotoxicity of all inhalational anesthetics.[80-85] Patients who develop halothane hepatitis typically have no history of preexisting liver disease, alcohol use, or concurrent exposure to other hepatotoxic drugs. The incidence is small, with 1 case reported for every 10,000 to 30,000 patients, making it difficult to clinically establish a causal link between exposure to halothane and the development of liver injury. Although halothane hepatitis can occur in all age-groups, the most common demographic is the obese, middle-aged woman. Although liver injury can occur after a single exposure, recurrent exposure to halothane, particularly when the interval between exposures is brief, increases the risk of liver injury and, in some cases, of liver failure. Health care workers exposed to halothane are also at increased risk through occupational exposure.[86]

The clinical symptoms observed in patients with halothane-induced liver injury are nonspecific and include malaise, fatigue, and anorexia. Patients may have subtle gastrointestinal symptoms such as nausea and abdominal pain. Some patients develop fever (albeit delayed), nonspecific rash, and arthralgias. Increases in serum transaminases are observed after exposure, with some patients becoming jaundiced. Jaundice can occur as late as 28 days after exposure. Many who develop halothane hepatitis do not progress to liver failure, and the inflammation usually resolves.[87] If continued exposure to halothane does not occur, chronic liver disease usually does not develop. However, in a few selected patients, fulminant hepatic failure does occur, and the mortality rate associated with developing halothane-induced hepatic necrosis is 20% to 50%.[88] A mild form of DILI occurs in up to 30% of patients after exposure. They tend to be asymptomatic and have increased transaminase levels, but they lack the serologic markers for immune activation, a feature common among those who develop significant liver disease.[84-86,89-90]

Histologic findings associated with halothane hepatitis include primarily centrilobular necrosis, although a range of findings from multifocal necrosis to massive fulminant necrosis is described. Ballooning degeneration, steatosis, and fibrosis have also been documented; in a small subset of patients, there are electron microscopic findings of mitochondrial injury. The histology of halothane hepatitis has a significant overlap with features of acute viral hepatitis and toxic hepatitis from other pharmaceutical exposures.[91]

Patient-specific metabolic and immunologic factors combine to account for this unpredictable hepatotoxicity. Variable expression and activation of CYP2E1 and the GSTs likely account for the different degrees of liver injury. Immunologic factors probably play a role in this process and may account for the individual variability in effects. The halothane-induced liver injury is associated with circulating antibodies to tissue antigens, peripheral eosinophilia, and the finding of halothane-induced liver neoantigens.[92-94]

Evidence suggests that molecular mimicry exists between the trifluoroacetylated proteins and the lipoyl-lysine regions of the E2 subunits (i.e., dihydrolipoyl transacetylase) of the mitochondrial pyruvate dehydrogenase complex because they are epitopes recognized by the antibodies in patients with halothane hepatitis.[95,96] Molecular mimicry may account for immunologic tolerance to the trifluoroacetylated proteins resulting from anesthetic metabolism, providing an explanation for the lack of tissue-specific injury observed in most patients exposed to these compounds.[97] Various levels of expression of the E2 component of the pyruvate dehydrogenase complex have been observed, with abnormally low levels seen in tissue specimens from patients with halothane hepatitis. It is postulated that individuals with low levels of the E2 subunit of the pyruvate dehydrogenase complex are more likely to develop injury because of a decrease in immune tolerance of triacetylated proteins.[97] However, many thousands of children have been safely anesthetized with halothane, and its use has proved to be very safe for most children. Concern about the rare occurrence of halothane hepatitis should not discourage the use of this anesthetic agent in children.

The obesity epidemic and associated nonalcoholic fatty liver disease and nonalcoholic steatohepatitis have raised concerns that these patients may be at increased risk for DILI.[98] Obesity and hypercholesterolemia can induce CYP2E1, which may facilitate development of liver injury.[99] Few data are available to inform the best practice of anesthesia management for the obese child, and adequately powered prospective studies are needed.[100]

Enflurane, isoflurane, desflurane, and sevoflurane have also been associated with liver injury. Agents such as enflurane, isoflurane, and desflurane are associated with a lesser degree of toxic hepatitis, possibly because they are metabolized to a lesser extent than halothane.[101] Case reports have documented that each is capable of producing liver injury. Enflurane, for example, was associated with the development of severe liver disease, with an estimated incidence of 1 case per 800,000 exposed patients. The clinicopathologic features are similar when compared with halothane-induced disease, including histologic findings, delayed onset of jaundice, and a history of previous exposure to the anesthetic. There is also a correspondingly high mortality rate.[102] It is thought that previous exposure to halothane leads to an increased risk of disease, occurring through previous cross-sensitization among chemicals.

Isoflurane has been associated with development of liver disease, although significantly less frequently than other agents. Features of isoflurane hepatic injury mimic those found with halothane. Detection of hepatic metabolite–modified neoantigens that occur in a small percentage of patients demonstrates an immune-mediated pathogenesis similar to that of halothane.[103] Desflurane-associated liver injury has been described, and the finding of modified liver neoantigens supports an immune-mediated mechanism of injury similar to that of the other inhalation anesthetics.[104,105] Hepatic disease after exposure to sevoflurane has been reported, but an immunologic correlation, as seen with the other inhalational drugs, has not been established.[106]

## Perioperative Considerations in Liver Disease

Patients with known or suspected liver disease should be assessed for hepatocellular and bile duct injury, coagulopathy, ascites, and encephalopathy. Hepatopulmonary syndrome and portopulmonary hypertension are rare but important complications in children with known chronic liver disease, and they may serve as relative or absolute contraindications to elective surgery.[107] Perioperative mortality is greatest among those who have acute hepatitis compared with those with chronic liver disease.[108-110] The physiologic stress associated with surgical procedures decreases portal blood flow. Liver disease may decrease the degree to which hepatic artery blood flow can compensate for reduced portal blood flow,[111] which can increase the risk of developing ischemic injury.

Parenteral nutrition–associated liver disease (PNALD) occurs in children requiring parenteral nutrition for longer than 60 days. Children with short bowel syndrome are at greatest risk for PNALD. Aside from the disturbances to hepatic and portal blood flows seen in children with liver disease, those exposed to total parenteral nutrition (TPN) are at increased risk for perioperative glucose derangements.[112-114] Frequent perioperative glucose monitoring with adjustment of dextrose infusion appears to be the standard of care, which is associated with various rates of TPN discontinuation. A survey administered to members of the Study Group of Pediatric Anesthesia found that approximately 50% of respondents checked glucose levels as often as every 1 to 2 hours.[115] They also found that 19% discontinued TPN and administered a glucose-containing solution, whereas 35% decreased the fluids to one half of maintenance rates and 33% continued maintenance rates unchanged.[115]

## Summary

Understanding the basics of hepatic biotransformation is crucial in providing effective and safe care to children with or without evidence of liver disease. Hepatic injuries and hepatic dysfunction can alter baseline processes and increase the risk of toxicity and complications from sedatives and anesthetics. Drugs directly metabolized by the liver should be used with caution in the setting of hepatic injury. However, a multitude of drugs that undergo extrahepatic metabolism or are bound to plasma proteins may also be affected by hepatic injury. Assessing hepatic function before sedation or anesthesia and monitoring those parameters throughout treatment can diminish the risk of injury and increase the targeted effect of the medication.

## ANNOTATED REFERENCES

Bjorkman S. Prediction of drug disposition in infants and children by means of physiologically based pharmacokinetic (PBPK) modeling: theophylline and midazolam as model drugs. Br J Clin Pharmacol 2004;59:691-704.

*This paper attempts to generate data for an age-group that provides significant challenges to study and examines two very different drugs. The predicted pharmacokinetics are then thoroughly compared with the adult literature, with very reassuring results.*

Kharasch ED, Hankins D, Mautz D, Thummel KE. Identification of the enzyme responsible for oxidative halothane metabolism: implication for prevention of halothane hepatitis. Lancet 1996;347:1367-71.

*This paper outlines a rare but serious complication of the inhaled anesthetic and provides a mechanism for its toxicity. These researchers also tested the hypothesis that the involved cytochrome enzyme was cytochrome P-450 2E1 (CYP2E1).*

Watkins PB. The role of cytochrome P450s in drug induced liver disease. In: Kaplowitz N, Deleve LD, editors. Drug-induced liver disease. New York: Marcel Dekker; 2003. p. 15-33.

*This summary of cytochrome P-450 enzymes provides a thorough review of this complex enzyme system and demonstrates their role in toxin-mediated liver disease.*

## REFERENCE

Please see www.expertconsult.com.

# Organ Transplantation

## FRANKLYN CLADIS, MIRIAM ANIXTER, STEVEN LICHTENSTEIN, JAMES CAIN, AND PETER J. DAVIS

## Liver Transplantation

The first successful liver transplant was performed by Dr. Tom Starzl in a child in 1967, but the history of liver transplantation begins in 1955, with Stuart Welch in Albany, and Jack Cannon at UCLA. Welch was the first to describe auxiliary liver transplantation in the dog and Cannon was the first to attempt orthotopic liver transplantation in dogs. Unfortunately, none of the dogs survived the operation.[1] Francis Moore and Tom Starzl continued the research in the dog model. From 1958 to 1959, they each were able to successfully transplant the liver in the dog but the animals all died from rejection within 4 to 20 days. These deaths highlighted the barriers that prevented the first application in humans.

In the early stages of animal experimentation with liver transplantation, the main barriers to success involved surgical technique, organ preservation, and immunosuppression. Regarding organ preservation, the liver used to be preserved with chilled electrolyte solutions like lactated ringers and normal saline. Preservation time with these solutions was only 5 to 6 hours. In 1987, the University of Wisconsin developed a solution which increased the preservation time of livers to 18 to 24 hours. The third barrier, immunosuppression, was the most significant and likely explained most of the canine deaths. Medawar discovered the role of the immune system in organ rejection in 1944. Since that time, several unsuccessful attempts to deliberately weaken the immune system and control rejection failed. It was not until an animal

model demonstrated that the combination of azathioprine and prednisone were synergistic and ameliorated rejection. This combination was first used in human kidney transplants, and then expanded to liver transplantation. Later, in 1967, antilymphocyte globulin was introduced, providing lymphoid depletion, and supplemented azathioprine and prednisone, providing better immunosuppression.[2]

The first human liver transplantation was performed in 1963 on a 3-year-old boy with biliary atresia. This attempt ended in failure secondary to fatal intraoperative hemorrhage from venous collaterals. Six more attempts at three different institutions (Denver, Boston, and Paris) produced the same results. Attempts to control the intraoperative hemorrhage with coagulation factor replacement and ε-aminocaproic acid resulted in clots and fatal pulmonary emboli in the venovenous bypass system. Inadequate immunosuppression played a significant role in these fatalities as well. At this time a self-imposed moratorium was established. Thymoglobulin, a lymphoid depleting agent was introduced into the immunosuppression regimen in 1967 and Starzl successfully transplanted a liver in a 1 year old with hepatoblastoma; this child survived 13 months.

Despite the initial success of the first pediatric liver transplant, the 1-year survival rate in subsequent transplant patients remained no greater than 50%. In 1979, with the introduction of cyclosporine, the 1-year patient survival increased to 70%.[3,4] FK-506 (tacrolimus) was introduced in 1989, replacing cyclosporine,[5] and the 1-year survival further increased to approximately 80%.

## DEMOGRAPHICS AND EPIDEMIOLOGY

There has been a steady increase in the number liver transplants performed yearly in the United States since 1988 (1713 that year, increasing to 6291 in 2010). The vast majority of this increase is attributed to adult transplants. The total number of pediatric liver transplants in 1990 was 513. This increased to 589 in 2000 and has essentially remained unchanged 10 years later, with 560 in 2010. The increase from 1990 to 2000 is only a 10% to 11% increase, compared with the 169% increase in adult liver transplants (2177 in 1990 to 5875 in 2005, according to the United Network for Organ Sharing [UNOS] Scientific Registry 2011). However, the total number of adult liver transplants has plateaued since 2005, with 5731 transplants performed in 2010.

Indications for liver transplantation in children include the presence of an underlying primary liver pathology with acute or chronic liver failure caused by cholestatic liver disease, acute hepatic failure, metabolic disorders, cirrhosis, tumors, toxins, and other derangements (i.e., Budd-Chiari syndrome) (E-Table 29-1). The most common cause for liver transplantation in children is cholestatic liver disease secondary to biliary atresia, particularly in children less than 1 year of age, where it accounts for 50% or more of transplants.[6] Biliary atresia continues to be the most common overall cause for liver transplantation, and the most common cholestatic cause, but cholestatic liver disease secondary to total parenteral nutrition has become more prominent over the past 10 years and accounts for just over 4% of all pediatric liver transplants. After cholestatic liver disease, acute hepatic failure and metabolic disorders are the next most common causes for pediatric liver transplantation. In the past, the most common metabolic disorders, in decreasing frequency, were $\alpha_1$-antitrypsin deficiency, tyrosinemia, Wilson disease, oxalosis, and glycogen storage diseases. The three most common disorders that lead to liver transplantation have changed, with cystic fibrosis now the second most common metabolic indication for pediatric liver transplantation, according to the United Network for Organ Sharing/Organ Procurement and Transplantation Network (UNOS/OPTN.org).

The cause for acute or fulminant hepatic failure is not known in the majority of patients. Neonatal hepatitis is the primary cause for acute hepatic failure in children. Drugs and toxins are the second leading cause of acute hepatic failure and viral hepatitis is third. Acetaminophen is the most common cause of drug- or toxin-induced liver failure.[7]

There are not many absolute contraindications to pediatric liver transplantation. Children with neoplastic processes, such as hepatocellular carcinoma, and infectious processes, such as infection with human immunodeficiency virus (HIV), are transplanted. However, patients with acute infections from bacterial or fungal agents, metastatic neoplasm, or disease processes that are considered an immediate threat to life (severe cardiopulmonary disease, sepsis, or septic shock) are generally not transplanted.

Allocation of the available livers to the appropriate recipients has been a challenge. Initially liver transplant candidates were prioritized based on geographic location and medical condition, as defined by Child-Turcotte-Pugh (CTP) score. Patients were ranked as status 1, 2a, 2b, or 3. Status 1 patients received the highest priority and were defined by the presence of acute liver failure of less than 6 weeks or a failed liver transplant within 1 week. Status 2a, 2b, and 3 were defined by their CTP score and time on the wait list.[8] Efforts by the UNOS/OPTN Liver Disease Severity Scale (LDSS) committee to identify predictors of mortality in patients with chronic liver disease resulted in the implementation of the model for end-stage liver disease (MELD) and the pediatric end-stage liver disease (PELD) severity score in 2002.[9] The PELD score incorporates variables for age, growth failure, serum albumin, bilirubin, and international normalized ratio (INR) (E-Table 29-2). In 2005, the cutoff for using the PELD score was revised to include only children 12 years of age or younger; the MELD score was extended downwards to include those as young as 12 years of age.[10] Serum creatinine is incorporated in the MELD score because it predicts mortality for adult patients waiting for liver transplantation. Although this value may predict mortality after liver transplantation in adults, it is not predictive in children.[11]

The allocation of deceased liver donors has changed with the new MELD/PELD policy. Before this policy, organs from donors younger than 18 years old were distributed only to those younger than 18 years old. With the new policy, the donor graft is first allocated to a status 1 child (less than 12 years of age) in the local region. If none is available, it is offered to the first status 1 adult in the region. If no status 1 adult is available, the liver is made available to children with more than 50% risk of mortality. Adults with mortality risk above 50% are next, and then all children are offered the graft over all other adult candidates. If there are no appropriate pediatric recipients in the region, the donor organ is offered to the national pool.[12] The introduction of the MELD/PELD score appears to have decreased the wait time for deceased donor liver grafts. Analysis of prescore and postscore MELD/PELD data indicates that the median time to transplant, defined as the number of days for half of the new registrants to receive organs, has significantly decreased from 981 days in 2002 to 361 days in 2007.[10]

Survival of deceased-donor organs is age dependent. Infants less than 1 year old have the lowest 3-month and 1-year survival, at 88% and 83%, respectively, when compared with other pediatric groups. If the infant recipient of a transplanted liver survives the first year, the survival for this age group increases. In fact the *5-year* survival is the greatest for infants less than 1 year old, at 84%. The 10-year survival for infants less than 1 year old is 77%, for children 1 to 5 years old, 79%, and for children 6 to 11 years old, 81%.[10] However, outcomes other than survival, such as growth and cognitive function, should also be taken into consideration.[13]

## PATHOPHYSIOLOGY OF LIVER DISEASE

The liver is the only organ that can regenerate itself when damaged. The stigmata and multiorgan involvement from end-stage liver disease occurs because of loss of hepatocytes and the resulting fibrosis. The hepatic injury and loss of hepatocytes leads to decreased synthetic function. This cellular dysfunction results in coagulopathy, hypocholesterolemia, hypoalbuminemia, and encephalopathy. Attempts at regeneration result in fibrosis and destruction of the portal triad, with increased resistance to blood flow through the liver. Portal hypertension is the final consequence of this increased resistance. Much of the characteristic features of liver disease occur because of portal hypertension, specifically varices (esophageal, bowel), hemorrhoids, ascites, spontaneous bacterial peritonitis, splenomegaly with thrombocytopenia, and hepatic encephalopathy.

### Cardiac Manifestations

Cardiac disturbances occur in children with liver disease because of altered physiology, congenital heart defects, and toxic side effects. A hyperdynamic circulation secondary to vasodilation characterizes the altered cardiac physiology from liver disease, with a compensatory increase in cardiac output (CO). Vasodilation is central to the hyperdynamic circulation that accompanies portal hypertension. It likely occurs because of the presence of vasoactive mediators. These mediators or gut-derived "humoral factors" (e.g., nitric oxide [NO], tumor necrosis factor α, endocannabinoids) enter the systemic circulation through portosystemic collaterals and bypass hepatic detoxification.[14] Shunting also occurs at the level of the skin and the lungs. Mixed venous saturation increases in children with liver disease because of poor tissue oxygen extraction. Arterial-venous oxygen difference is reduced because of the combination of decreased oxygen consumption and hypoxia from arterial-venous shunting.

Cardiomyopathy associated with portal hypertension is well described in adults but is not well characterized in children with liver disease. However, children with liver disease can develop a cardiomyopathy for other reasons. Inborn errors of metabolism and other syndromes are associated with cardiomyopathies and cardiac anomalies. Some of the inborn errors include Wilson disease, oxalosis, glycogen storage disease type III, and Gaucher disease.[15] Tacrolimus and cyclosporine A have also been associated with hypertrophic cardiomyopathy in animal studies and in pediatric liver transplant recipients.[16,17,18] Echocardiographic assessment of cardiac function is generally well preserved in children receiving tacrolimus, but there may be evidence of subtle cardiovascular changes, which predispose a small percentage of children to develop hypertrophic cardiomyopathy.[19]

Other diseases that may lead to liver failure are associated with congenital heart disease. For example, children with Alagille disease may have pulmonary stenosis, coarctation, tetralogy of Fallot, atrial and ventricular septal defect.

QT prolongation has also been described in adults with alcoholic liver disease and may be associated with sudden cardiac death.[20] A decrease in $K^+$ currents observed in rat cardiomyocytes with cirrhosis may provide a possible mechanism for the QT prolongation. Children with liver failure have also been shown to have an increase in QT interval (QTc greater than 450 msec in 18% of children with liver disease), possibly increasing the risk of ventricular arrhythmias, however, there is no evidence of an increased dispersion of repolarization (see Chapter 14). These changes appear to be transient and reversible after liver transplantation.[21] Nonselective β-adrenergic blockade has also been shown to reduce the QT prolongation, but it is unclear if this reduces the risk of arrhythmias or improves survival.[22] Although previous data suggested that prolonged QT did not predict decreased survival,[23] more recent evidence suggests that the presence of a prolonged QT was associated with an increased PELD score and portal hypertension. Children with chronic liver disease and prolonged QT may be at increased risk of mortality while waiting for a transplant.[24]

## Pulmonary Manifestations

The hallmarks of the pulmonary manifestations of liver disease are hypoxia and pulmonary hypertension. Hypoxia is secondary to hepatopulmonary syndrome (HPS) and ventilation/perfusion ($\dot{V}/\dot{Q}$) mismatch from atelectasis caused by tense ascites, hepatosplenomegaly, and/or pleural effusions. HPS is characterized by hypoxia from intrapulmonary arteriovenous shunting and intrapulmonary vascular dilatation.[25] The diagnosis is predicated on either arterial hypoxia ($PaO_2$ less than 70 mm Hg in room air) or an increased alveolar-arterial gradient of more than 20 mm Hg

in the setting of pulmonary vascular dilatation. Intrapulmonary vascular dilatation can best be demonstrated on echocardiography or lung perfusion scan with macroaggregated albumin.[26] HPS occurs in 15% to 20% of adults and in 0.5% to 20% of infants and children with cirrhosis[27] as young as 6 months of age. It appears to be more prevalent in children with biliary atresia and polysplenia syndrome.[28,29]

Treatment for hypoxia is long-term supplemental oxygen; definitive treatment is liver transplantation. In a case series of seven children with HPS who were successfully transplanted, all recovered postoperatively with their hypoxia resolving within an average of 24 weeks.[30]

Portopulmonary hypertension (PPH) is defined by the World Health Organization as pulmonary artery hypertension (pulmonary systolic pressure of 25 mm Hg or greater) in the setting of a normal pulmonary capillary wedge pressure and portal hypertension.[31] The incidence of PPH is 0.2% to 0.7% in adults with cirrhosis but increase to 3% to 9% in adults presenting for liver transplantation.[32] The incidence in children is unknown, with accounts limited to case reports and one case series. Signs and symptoms on presentation are new heart murmurs, dyspnea, and syncope. Echocardiography can successfully identify pulmonary hypertension in pediatric and adult patients with PPH[33]; the severity of PPH predicts mortality. In a retrospective review, mild PPH did not increase mortality; however, those children who underwent liver transplantation with moderate PPH (pulmonary artery pressure [PAP] is 35 to 45 mm Hg) had a 50% mortality rate and those with severe PPH (PAP greater than 50 mm Hg) had a 100% mortality rate.[34]

There are no definitive guidelines for the management of children with PPH. Early identification is essential, and this may be accomplished with echocardiography. If PPH appears likely, cardiac catheterization should be performed to confirm the diagnosis, measure pulmonary artery pressures, and assess the response to NO and epoprostenol. Children who respond to medical management may be candidates for liver transplantation.[35] Otherwise, severe PPH is generally a contraindication for liver transplantation because of the increased risk of mortality.

## Neurologic Manifestations

Hepatic encephalopathy (HE) is a significant neurologic complication that is classified as either acute (seen in fulminant hepatic failure) or chronic (seen in chronic cirrhosis or chronic portal hypertension). The classification of the severity of acute and chronic HE is similar and is shown in Table 29-1. The pathophysiology is not entirely known, but cerebral edema appears to

**TABLE 29-1** West Haven Staging Classification of the Severity of Acute and Chronic Hepatic Encephalopathy

| Grade | Description |
|-------|-------------|
| 0 | Detectable only by neuropsychological testing |
| 1 | Lack of awareness, euphoria, or anxiety; shortened attention span; impaired addition and subtraction |
| 2 | Lethargy, minimal disorientation to time, personality change, inappropriate behavior |
| 3 | Somnolence but responsive to verbal stimuli, confusion, gross disorientation, bizarre behavior |
| 4 | Comatose |

be a feature of both acute and chronic HE. Cerebral edema is more severe in acute HE and can result in increased intracranial pressure. Ammonia is repeatedly implicated in the pathogenesis of HE and may participate in the process by causing astrocyte swelling and low-grade cerebral edema.[36,37] The two major sources of ammonia in humans are catabolism of endogenous protein and gastrointestinal absorption. Bacterial breakdown of nitrogen-containing products in the gut results in ammonia formation, which is then absorbed in the portal circulation. Factors that increase blood ammonia concentrations can exacerbate the signs and symptoms of HE. These typically include increased catabolism from infection, increased gut absorption from high-protein diets, constipation, and gastrointestinal bleeding. Other neurotoxins that have been implicated in the exacerbation of HE include endogenous production of benzodiazepines, hyponatremia, and inflammatory cytokines; these may all share the final common pathway of increasing cerebral edema.

Management of HE should begin with assessing the child's ability to manage their airway. Children with grade 3 (somnolence to semi-stupor, responsive to verbal stimuli but confused) and 4 (coma, unresponsive to verbal or noxious stimuli) HE may require tracheal intubation to protect the airway and to provide adequate oxygenation and ventilation. Otherwise, management typically focuses on reducing gastrointestinal production and absorption of ammonia. Lactulose is often prescribed to create an osmotic gastrointestinal diuresis and to acidify the lumen of the gut to trap ammonia and minimize absorption. Antibiotics (e.g., neomycin and metronidazole) kill the gastrointestinal bacteria that are involved in metabolizing nitrogen products to ammonia. Other medications include sodium benzoate, which combines in the liver with ammoniagenic amino acids, like glycine, to facilitate their excretion.[38] Ornithine aspartate may also provide a substrate to the liver for enhancing urea cycle and glutamine synthesis, and reduce ammonia levels. Flumazenil may reduce the symptoms of HE by inhibiting endogenous benzodiazepines and γ-aminobutyric acid, although 0.01 mg/kg in children with fulminant hepatic failure failed to correct the HE.[38]

Children with fulminant hepatic failure can have increased intracranial pressure (ICP), which is the major cause of mortality and may be a contraindication for liver transplantation. Intracranial hypertension occurs in 38% to 81% of adult patients with fulminant hepatic failure[39] and is often monitored in those with fulminant hepatic failure (grade 3 to 4 HE). The risk of intracranial hemorrhage secondary to coagulopathy can be reduced by replacing clotting factors and platelets, and by placing an epidural rather than a subdural monitor.[40] Management strategies for children with increased ICP should focus on maintaining cerebral perfusion pressure above 60 mm Hg, and ICP at less than 20 mm Hg. Management strategies often include tracheal intubation and ventilation with the head in midline position and slightly elevated to 30 degrees to facilitate venous drainage. Ventilation is adjusted to achieve a $PaCO_2$ of 30 to 35 mm Hg with minimal positive end-expiratory pressure (PEEP). Medical management to reduce ICP includes administering barbiturates or propofol to minimize stimulation and to directly reduce ICP.[41] Mannitol can be administered if ICP remains increased. Hypothermia has also been described, and in a small trial with 14 patients with fulminant hepatic failure, ICP was reduced by maintaining core body temperature at 32° C to 33° C.[42] Orthotopic liver transplantation is the definitive treatment for children with acute or chronic HE.

## Hematologic Manifestations

There are several hematologic alterations associated with liver disease. Anemia is common because of a combination of gastrointestinal bleeding, poor nutrition, and decreased erythropoietin production from renal failure. Portal hypertension can result in splenomegaly, which causes platelet sequestration and thrombocytopenia. All of the coagulation factors (except factor VIII) are synthesized in the liver. As synthetic functions decline, coagulation factor production diminishes. The reduction in bile salt also decreases the absorption of fat-soluble vitamins (A, D, E, K) and contributes to the deficiency of factors II, VII, IX, and X. The result is an increase in prothrombin time (PT) and partial thromboplastin time (PTT). Children with acute or fulminant hepatic failure can present with a hematologic profile similar to disseminated intravascular coagulation.

## Renal Manifestations

Renal failure is common in children with acute and chronic liver disease and its cause is multifactorial. Renal failure can be classified as prerenal azotemia, acute tubular necrosis (ATN), or hepatorenal syndrome (HRS). Prerenal azotemia from hypovolemia is a common cause for renal failure and occurs secondary to diuretic therapy, gastrointestinal bleeding, splanchnic pooling, and sepsis. ATN occurs because of decreased central blood volume secondary to central splanchnic pooling, and decreased prostaglandin synthesis. HRS is characterized by renal failure in the setting of liver failure and portal hypertension. The incidence in adults with chronic liver disease is approximately 10% to 15%; in children the incidence is even less, at approximately 5%. The reduced incidence in children may reflect the lack of definitive criteria for diagnosis of HRS in children.[43] HRS occurs secondary to intense renal vasoconstriction from activation of the renin-angiotensin, arginine vasopressin, and sympathetic nervous systems. This activation is a homeostatic response to the profound splanchnic vasodilation that occurs with portal hypertension.[44] HRS presents similarly to prerenal azotemia (increased creatinine, decreased urine sodium [$U_{Na}$ less than 10 mM, $Fe_{Na}$ less than 1%]), but is differentiated from azotemia by its lack of response to a fluid challenge. HRS has been classified based on the rate of progression of renal failure into types 1 and 2: type 1, which has a worse prognosis, is characterized by a rapid progression of renal failure with a 100% increase in creatinine in less than 2 weeks. It usually occurs in patients with acute liver failure. In type 2, renal failure progresses over weeks to months, and usually occurs in patients with chronic liver disease. Regardless of the type, prognosis is poor in children with HRS, with a mortality of 80% to 95%.[45] The definitive treatment for HRS is liver transplantation, because the renal failure is reversible if the liver is replaced.[46]

The primary goal in the management of patients with liver disease and renal failure is to exclude treatable and reversible causes, such as nephrotoxins (NSAIDs), hypovolemia (diuretics, gastrointestinal bleeding), and sepsis. All nephrotoxins should be stopped and children should be given a fluid challenge, ideally with a colloid solution. If sepsis is suspected patients should be extensively cultured and antibiotics that are not nephrotoxic administered.

Pretransplant renal function predicts mortality in adult patients undergoing transjugular intrahepatic shunt and liver transplantation, and serum creatinine is used in the MELD score. Preexisting renal failure is also a major determinant of survival after liver transplantation in adults. Efforts to improve renal function pretransplant may improve posttransplantation outcome.[47] At this time it is not clear that serum creatinine is a predictor of mortality in children with liver disease.[48] Before transplantation, type 1 HRS can be managed with vasoconstrictors (vasopressin analogs, norepinephrine), although there are limited data on their use in children. Critically ill children may require continuous renal replacement therapy (continuous venovenous hemofiltration or hemodiafiltration) as a bridge to transplantation.

### Metabolic Manifestations

The metabolic derangements seen in liver disease include glucose, ammonia, electrolyte, and acid-base disturbances. Electrolyte abnormalities include hyponatremia, hypo- and hyperkalemia, hypocalcemia, and hypomagnesemia. Hypoglycemia may occur in children with fulminant hepatic failure or abrupt discontinuation of total parenteral nutrition, but hyperglycemia is more common in the perioperative period. During the dissection and anhepatic phase there are several causes of hyperglycemia. Typically glucose concentrations will increase immediately after reperfusion. Serum glucose increases if there is an exogenous source of glucose or if there is altered glucose metabolism. Exogenous sources include glucose from blood products,[49] dextrose containing intravenous (IV) fluids, and damaged hepatocytes from the liver graft.[50] Glucose uptake is altered by methylprednisolone steroid-induced insulin resistance. Hepatic denervation likely results in alterations in insulin and glucose clearance during the postoperative period, and may explain the frequent occurrence of impaired glucose tolerance and diabetes in liver transplant recipients.[51]

Acid-base disturbances commonly occur during liver transplantation. Children with renal disease may have a preexisting metabolic acidosis from bicarbonate elimination. A metabolic acidosis is typically present during the dissection and anhepatic phase, but it is usually most pronounced immediately after reperfusion. Lactic acid and citrate (from blood products) are not metabolized during the anhepatic phase and contribute to the acidosis. Cross clamping of the inferior vena cava (IVC) and aorta alters blood flow to gut and lower extremity tissue beds and may also contribute to the lactic acidosis. Once the liver graft begins to function, the metabolism of lactate and citrate may lead to a metabolic alkalosis.[49]

### PREOPERATIVE EVALUATION

The preoperative evaluation begins with a history and physical examination to identify the primary cause of liver failure and to identify liver- and non–liver-related alterations in physiology that may affect the anesthetic and surgical plan. A complete review of the systems will identify most of the perioperative concerns (Table 29-2).

The primary cardiovascular concerns include acquired cardiomyopathies from liver disease and inborn errors of metabolism, congenital cardiac defects, and QT prolongation. Aside from a cardiovascular physical examination, the preoperative cardiac evaluation should include an echocardiogram and a 12-lead electrocardiogram.

The pulmonary concerns include hypoxia and PPH. Hypoxia can occur from V/Q mismatch caused by pleural effusions and ascites, and HPS. Oxygen saturation on room air and with oxygen will identify those who are hypoxic and whether they respond to oxygen. Children with significant intrapulmonary shunts from HPS will not increase their oxygen saturation significantly while

**TABLE 29-2** Preoperative Evaluation of Liver Transplant Candidates

**History and Physical Examination**

Cause for liver failure

Identifiable syndrome or metabolic disorder

Past medical history: medical problems not related to liver (e.g., asthma)

Past surgical history: portoenterostomy (Kasai), previous anesthetic concerns

Medications: diuretics, lactulose

Allergies

Family history of anesthesia-related problems

Immediate eating and drinking history

**Cardiovascular**

Echocardiography: to identify cardiomyopathy, pulmonary hypertension, and congenital cardiac defects

Electrocardiogram: to identify arrhythmias and QT prolongation

**Pulmonary**

Oxygen saturation (possible arterial blood gas): to assess hypoxia (HPS)

Radiography: to identify pleural effusions and central line position

**Hematology**

Complete blood count: to assess anemia, leukocytosis, and leukopenia (sepsis)

Prothrombin time and partial thromboplastin times

Platelet count

**Renal**

Blood urea nitrogen (BUN)

Creatinine (Cr)

**Neurologic**

Assessment of increased intracranial pressure in acute and/or fulminant hepatic failure

**Electrolytes**

$Na^+$ and $K^+$: hyponatremia and hypokalemia secondary to diuretics

Calcium

Albumin

Magnesium

Glucose

*HPS*, Hepatopulmonary syndrome.

receiving oxygen. HPS can be diagnosed by demonstrating intrapulmonary vascular dilatation on echocardiography or lung perfusion scan with macroaggregated albumin.[52]

PPH can usually be identified on echocardiography (tricuspid regurgitation). Children suspected of having PPH may undergo a cardiac catheterization to define the severity of pulmonary hypertension and to assess the response to therapeutic agents (NO, epoprostenol). Children with severe pulmonary hypertension (PAP greater than 50 mm Hg) are at increased risk of perioperative mortality and liver transplantation is contraindicated.[34]

Anemia, deficiency of hepatic coagulation factors (decreased vitamin K absorption, smaller concentrations of clotting factors II, VII, IX, X), and thrombocytopenia are common and should also be evaluated preoperatively. A PT and PTT should also be obtained before commencing surgery.

Renal failure is common and in adults predicts decreased survival in the period after transplantation.[53] Both a blood urea nitrogen and creatinine measurement should be obtained preoperatively.

Children should be evaluated for evidence of HE, particularly those with acute hepatic failure. Increased intracranial pressure is common and it is the most common cause of mortality. Children with advanced HE (grade 3 and 4) may already have had their airways intubated to protect them from regurgitation and control their PaCO$_2$.

Baseline laboratory values should be obtained for liver function tests, sodium, potassium, calcium, magnesium, glucose, and albumin. Hyponatremia and hypokalemia are common with diuretic therapy. Children who have already received citrate-containing blood products may be hypocalcemic secondary to citrate induced chelation. Hypoglycemia occurs secondary to depleted glycogen stores in the failed liver and/or removal of chronic total parenteral nutrition.

An important issue that is rarely communicated to the ward team when the child is admitted for surgery, is that all preoperative IV access should be placed in the lower extremities. This ensures that none of the veins that the anesthesiologist will require intraoperatively (i.e., those originating in the upper extremities or neck) will be compromised preoperatively.

A key portion of the preoperative evaluation is the preparation of the child and family for the anticipated risks, benefits, and clinical course. Specifically, the child's airway will likely remain intubated and the child sedated to facilitate mechanical ventilation of the lungs in the immediate postoperative period. After surgery, the child may have significant facial and extremity edema. Likewise informing the family about the potential number and location of the intravascular catheters and their associated risks can be helpful in preparing them to see the child after surgery. Informed consent should also include a discussion about the use of blood products and risks associated with prolonged positioning (peripheral nerve injury, occipital alopecia).

## INTRAOPERATIVE CARE

Appropriate intraoperative care requires an understanding of the surgical and anesthetic issues. Several factors affect the child's physiology, including the underlying pathophysiology of liver disease, surgery, and response to anesthetics. A sound understanding of both surgical and anesthetic issues is needed to safely manage these children. In general, the surgical approach for liver transplantation in children is similar to that in adults. The most significant difference is the reduced size of the recipient. The obstacles imposed by the size of the child include a smaller blood volume, more challenging vascular access, size restriction of donor graft, venovenous bypass, and the incidence of surgical complications, such as hepatic artery thrombosis.

The initial anesthetic management begins with a thorough preoperative evaluation, as discussed previously. Children over the age of 1 year old will likely be anxious and may benefit from an anxiolytic like midazolam. Midazolam can be administered IV, orally, nasally, or rectally; children with HE should not receive midazolam because of the theoretic possibility of exacerbating the encephalopathy (see previous discussion).

Most children are considered to have a full stomach because of delayed gastric emptying from ascites, gastrointestinal bleeding, HE, and the nonelective nature of most transplants (i.e., a rapid-sequence induction is required). The exception may be the child presenting for an "elective" transplant without any stigmata of portal hypertension (e.g., Crigler-Najjar syndrome). Induction agents should be tailored to meet the needs of the patient but etomidate (0.2 to 0.3 mg/kg), sodium thiopental (4 to 6 mg/kg), propofol (2 to 4 mg/kg), and ketamine (2 mg/kg) are suitable options. Appropriate neuromuscular blocking drugs for rapid-sequence induction include succinylcholine and high-dose rocuronium (1.2 mg/kg), because of their rapid onset. Children who are not at risk for aspiration can have an inhalation induction with sevoflurane and nitrous oxide. The use of nitrous oxide is not recommended after induction because it may increase the risk of bowel distension and expansion of gas emboli.

The trachea should be secured with a cuffed or uncuffed tracheal tube. If the tracheal tube is uncuffed there should not be a leak at less than 15 to 20 cm H$_2$O. High inspiratory pressures may be required to achieve adequate ventilation in the intraoperative and postoperative periods because of atelectasis from pleural effusions and ascites, surgical retractors placed on the abdominal and chest wall, and a tight abdominal closure. Positive end-expiratory pressure should be used in all patients.

Anesthesia is typically maintained with an inhalational agent, an opioid, and a neuromuscular blocking drug. Isoflurane, sevoflurane or desflurane may be used because they are readily available, undergo minimal hepatic metabolism, and appear to have minimal adverse effects on the liver, although all three have been associated with isolated case reports of hepatotoxicity.[54,55,56] Propofol is also an option to maintain anesthesia during liver transplantation. It is relatively short-acting and even though the primary metabolic pathway is hepatic, there appears to be extrahepatic metabolism in the lung, kidney, and intestine.[57,58] However, when used for a prolonged period, the pharmacokinetics of propofol switch from those of a short-acting to those of a long-acting anesthetic, and the risk of propofol infusion syndrome becomes a substantive concern (see Chapter 6). Neuromuscular blockade can be maintained with a variety of agents. Rocuronium, vecuronium, pancuronium, atracurium, and cisatracurium have all been described. Pancuronium may have the added advantages of increased heart rate, long duration, and reduced cost. The disadvantage of pancuronium, rocuronium, and vecuronium is their partial hepatic metabolism, but this can be overcome with appropriate monitoring and dose adjustments. Dose requirements of continuous infusions of rocuronium, vecuronium, and pancuronium are reduced during the anhepatic phase of liver transplantation, but return to initial values after reperfusion.[59] There is no change in the dose requirements of atracurium during the anhepatic phase.[60] Atracurium or cisatracurium may be ideal in patients with combined hepatic and renal insufficiency, because they are cleared by nonspecific esterases in tissues, and erythrocytes and do not rely on hepatic or renal function.

The liver metabolizes all opioids, with the exception of remifentanil, which is metabolized by plasma and tissue esterases. The metabolic pathway for most opioids is oxidation, although morphine undergoes glucuronidation.[61] There is evidence that the elimination half-life and clearance of alfentanil and fentanyl are not dramatically altered in patients with cholestatic and cirrhotic liver disease.[62,63] Fentanyl, sufentanil, alfentanil, and morphine have all been used during liver transplantation. Fentanyl is commonly selected and is usually administered as a bolus during induction (2 to 10 µg/kg) and maintained as an infusion throughout the anesthetic and the immediate postoperative period (2 to 5 µg/kg/hr).

Vascular access is important for resuscitation and monitoring. At least two peripheral upper extremity IV catheters should be placed, along with a central venous line. The central venous line is used to monitor trends in central venous pressure and measure superior vena cava oxygen saturation (a surrogate marker for venous oxygen saturation). Larger children tolerate rapid infusion catheters placed in the upper extremities. Blood loss can be significant, with estimates between 0.5 to 25 blood volumes (mean is approximately four blood volumes).[49] Fluid warmers and rapid infusion devices (e.g., Level 1 Rapid Infuser, SIMS Level One INC, Rockland, Mass.) need to be available to facilitate resuscitation if significant hemorrhage occurs (see Chapters 10 and 51). The Level 1 Rapid Infuser has been associated with massive air emboli, and all air must be removed from the infusion bags before using the device, or the device should be used with air-detection add-on modifications.[64] The Rapid Infusion System (RIS, Haemonetics, Braintree, Mass.) is no longer manufactured and has been replaced by the Belmont FMS (Belmont Instrument Corp., Billerica, Mass.). This device is not routinely used in small children (less than 30 kg) but may be indicated in larger children and adolescents (see Chapter 51). Choice of resuscitation fluids should be limited to 0.9% normal saline and Plasmalyte. Lactated ringers is not recommended because the lactate will accumulate unmetabolized during the anhepatic stage. Many children with liver disease are hypoalbuminemic, and the use of 5% albumin is appropriate.

Standard monitoring should include electrocardiogram, pulse oximetry (×2), noninvasive blood pressure, invasive arterial blood pressure, central venous pressure, and temperature. Other high-technology monitoring that is commonly employed in adult liver transplantation includes transesophageal echocardiography (TEE), continuous cardiac output (CCO) catheter, bispectral index (BIS), venovenous bypass (VVBP), and more than one arterial catheter. In children, there are limitations to the use of these monitors because of patient size. A United States–based utilization survey found that TEE, CCO, BIS, and VVBP are used in 0%, 7.7%, 15.4%, and 7.7% of pediatric transplant centers, respectively.[65]

Hematologic and electrolyte changes are common and measurements of arterial blood gases, sodium, potassium, calcium, magnesium, glucose, hemoglobin, platelets, and coagulation parameters (PT, PTT, fibrinogen, and D-dimers) need to be performed frequently throughout the procedure. Most centers use either portable devices or an operating room (OR) laboratory to obtain these data. Assessment of coagulation variables can be obtained with thromboelastography. However, only 28% of pediatric transplant centers used TEG routinely[65] (E-Fig. 29-1). Positioning is critical to prevent soft tissue and peripheral nerve injuries. All extremities should be padded and all cables and wires need to be wrapped to protect the skin. The head should be rotated and repositioned periodically to prevent pressure sores and alopecia. To minimize the risk of peripheral neuropathy, the upper extremities should not be abducted more than 90 degrees and the wrists should not be hyperextended for the arterial catheter.

## SURGICAL TECHNIQUE

The surgical approach can divided into four stages; hepatectomy, anhepatic, reperfusion, and biliary reconstruction.

### Hepatectomy (Stage 1)

The initial description of orthotopic liver transplantation is referred to as the "classic" technique. In the "classic" approach

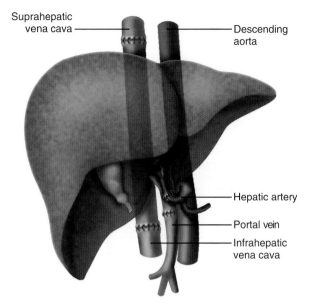

**FIGURE 29-1** The classic approach for orthotopic liver transplantation. The suture lines are visible at the suprahepatic and infrahepatic anastomoses. (From Starzl TE, Iwatsuki S, VanTheil DH, et al. Evolution of liver transplantation. Hepatology 1982;2:614-36.)

the liver is dissected to its vascular supply and the supra- and infrahepatic IVC are clamped, along with the portal vein and hepatic artery. The liver is removed enbloc (Fig. 29-1). The disadvantage of this approach is that the IVC is cross clamped, thus reducing preload. The piggyback technique was described 1989 and is the preferred approach for pediatric transplants, because there is more flexibility with the organ size and it only requires partial clamping of the IVC.[66] The liver is dissected away from the IVC, the short hepatic veins, portal vein, and left, right, middle hepatic vein. The infrahepatic vena cava of the donor is oversewn and the suprahepatic vena cava is anastomosed to the native hepatic veins (Figs. 29-2 and 29-3). This only requires partial clamping of the IVC. A portacaval shunt can be established for children who do not tolerate clamping of the portal vein (see Fig. 29-3). Typically these are recipients who have not developed collateral flow secondary to portal hypertension (e.g., maple syrup urine disease).

There are several physiologic considerations that take place during the hepatic dissection that affect the anesthetic management. Hypotension is common and can occur for a variety of reasons. These include changes to the cardiovascular, hematologic, and metabolic systems. The most common cause of hypotension includes hypovolemia secondary to hemorrhage and third space volume losses. Resuscitation with citrated blood products can result in hypocalcemia and surgical manipulation can cause mechanical compression of the IVC or right ventricle. Bleeding occurs from fragile collaterals, adhesions from prior surgery (Kasai procedure), and coagulopathy.[67] Blood conservation during this portion of the surgery by maintaining low central venous pressure (decrease of 30% from baseline) has been described in adults. The reported benefit of a low central venous pressure is less bleeding, with subsequent decrease in allogeneic blood requirements and decreased morbidity. Some studies have suggested an overall reduction in 1-year mortality.[68,69] The technique is controversial and the potential risks include end-organ

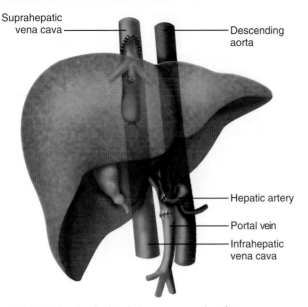

Suprahepatic vena cava

Descending aorta

Hepatic artery

Portal vein

Infrahepatic vena cava

**FIGURE 29-2** The piggyback technique preserves the inferior vena cava (IVC). This is the view of the liver graft after the recipient's hepatic confluence is anastomosed to the donor's IVC (the infrahepatic IVC of the donor is ligated). (From Tzakis A, Todo S, Starzl TE. Orthotopic liver transplantation with preservation of the inferior vena cava. Ann Surg 1989;210:649-52.)

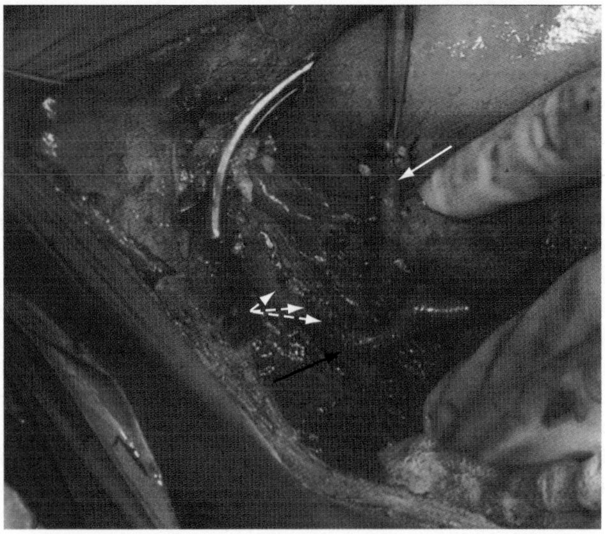

**FIGURE 29-3** The native liver has been removed. There is a clamp across the right, middle, and left hepatic veins. The *black arrow* shows the portacaval shunt. The *white arrow* shows the hepatic artery. The *dashed white arrows* show the short hepatic veins. (From Kuo PC, Davis RD. Comprehensive atlas of transplantation. Philadelphia: Lippincott Williams & Wilkins; 2005, p. 132.)

injury, such as renal or graft failure.[70] This technique has not been described in the pediatric liver transplant population.

Hematologic abnormalities include anemia, thrombocytopenia, coagulation factor deficiency, and low fibrinogen. A progressive coagulopathy can develop during this stage. Metabolic derangements include hyperkalemia, hypocalcemia, hypomagnesemia, and acidosis from resuscitation with blood products.

### Anhepatic Stage (Stage 2)

The anhepatic phase begins once the hepatic veins, hepatic artery, and portal vein are cross clamped. The dissection of the recipient's liver is completed and the organ is removed. This phase ends when the hepatic and portal vein cross clamps are removed and the graft is reperfused.

Cardiovascular changes that occur during this stage can result in hypotension. This occurs from the IVC cross-clamp, which causes a decrease in preload. Hemodynamically, there is a decrease in cardiac output, central venous pressure, and pulmonary artery pressure, with an increase in systemic vascular resistance.[67] Preload should be gently augmented to maintain mean arterial pressure (MAP) with the lowest filling pressures possible. Hypervolemia may cause hepatic congestion during reperfusion. Inotropic agents like dopamine or epinephrine may need to be used to maintain MAP. A portacaval shunt, if performed, may moderate some of these hemodynamic changes by preserving preload from the portal vein (if venovenous bypass is going to be used, it is initiated during this period). Unmetabolized citrate causes hypocalcemia and hypomagnesemia because it chelates both. Acidosis occurs from the unmetabolized citrate, lactate, and other acids. Bicarbonate may be administered if there is a significant metabolic acidosis (base deficit less than 5 mEq/L). Once the liver is on the surgical field warm ischemia time begins. The time to reperfusion should be brief, and steps should be in place for reperfusion. Before reperfusion, potassium should be in

the low-normal range and calcium and bicarbonate should be in the high-normal range. Hemoglobin should be maintained between 9 and 10 g/dL. If the potassium is greater than 5 mEq/L, steps need to be taken to reduce it. This may be achieved by increasing the serum pH with hyperventilation, and the administration of sodium bicarbonate (1 to 3 mEq/kg). Glucose and insulin can be administered to acutely reduce potassium (see Chapter 8). Potassium-wasting diuretics like furosemide (0.5 to 1 mg/kg) can also be used. Administering fresh blood or washed red blood cells will minimize the increase in potassium during transfusion therapy. $\beta_2$-Adrenoceptor agonists may decrease potassium and can be used. Calcium and epinephrine should be immediately available for reperfusion.

### Reperfusion (Stage 3)

The liver graft can be reperfused once the hepatic and portal vein anastomosis are complete. Before reestablishing hepatic blood flow, the graft is flushed to remove the preservation solution to minimize the reperfusion syndrome. Many changes can occur acutely during the reperfusion period secondary to cardiovascular, hematologic, and metabolic derangements. Postreperfusion syndrome is characterized by a decrease in MAP of greater than 30%.[71] Several factors participate in this event, including myocardial dysfunction, arrhythmias, and bleeding. The myocardial dysfunction is thought to occur from release of NO and tumor necrosis factor $\alpha$.[72] Cardiovascular collapse can occur and the child may require epinephrine to correct the hemodynamic effects of reperfusion.[71] Hyperkalemia is a common event immediately after reperfusion and may cause ventricular arrhythmias. It should be treated with calcium chloride (10 to 30 mg/kg) initially to stabilize the cardiac membrane and then insulin and dextrose, hyperventilation, furosemide, $\beta_2$-adrenoceptor agonists, and sodium bicarbonate to decrease the serum potassium concentration (see previous section). The high potassium content of the preservation solution is the cause of the hyperkalemia. University of Wisconsin (UW) solution, a very commonly used preservation solution contains large amounts of potassium (120 mmol/L). Histidine-tryptophan-ketoglutarate (HTK) solution was introduced in 1980 as a cardioplegic solution, and contains substantially less potassium (10 mmol/L) than the UW solution.[73] A recent study comparing the two found equal 1-month and 1-year graft survival with HTK and UW solutions. The viscosity is reduced with HTK and may introduce itself more easily into the vascular spaces in the donor liver.[74] Although hyperkalemia is the hallmark electrolyte disturbance in the immediate reperfusion period, hypokalemia is more common in children throughout the intraoperative period and may require correction.[75]

Fibrinolysis can occur after reperfusion, and in one study it occurred in 60% of children and 80% of adults.[76] This results from increased tissue plasminogen activator activity and decreased synthesis of fibrinolysis inhibitors. Heparin effect is produced by endogenous heparinoids from the graft, residual heparin from the preservation, and release of tissue plasminogen activator from endothelial cells of the revascularized graft. Aprotinin blunts this response by inhibiting kallikrein and plasmin, which led to the wide spread use of aprotinin. The beneficial effects of aprotinin to reduce blood loss in orthotopic liver transplant in adults and children had been considered inconclusive until the European Multicenter Study on the Use of Aprotinin in Liver Transplantation (EMSALT) study in 2000.[77] However, the benefits of aprotinin in pediatric patients are not as clear. A retrospective study in 18 pediatric transplant patients receiving a high or regular dose of aprotinin demonstrated a reduction of red cell and fresh frozen plasma transfusion by half, but it was not found to be statistically significant. There is concern that there may be an association between aprotinin and intraoperative thrombotic events (hepatic artery and portal vein thrombosis) in pediatric recipients of liver transplants. Children may be at increased risk for developing intraoperative thrombi or emboli. Children are hypercoagulable after liver transplantation because of a decrease in protein C and antithrombin III,[78] and they may be more likely to develop hepatic artery thrombosis.[79,80,81] Aprotinin has been removed from the market because of the increased risk of death in adult cardiac patients. Tranexamic acid, an alternative antifibrinolytic is being used in adults for liver transplants; a nonrandomized prospective study did not find a difference in transfusion requirements or thromboembolic events after changing from aprotinin to tranexamic acid.[82] Currently there are no pediatric data to support or refute the use of tranexamic acid or ε-aminocaproic acid.

### Biliary and Hepatic Artery Reconstruction (Stage 4)

The final step is reestablishing hepatic artery blood flow and reconstructing the biliary system. In smaller children, the hepatic artery may require an anastomosis via a conduit to the infrarenal aorta. This requires temporary cross clamping of the aorta. Biliary reconstruction is established by directly connecting the graft and the recipient's common bile ducts or by connecting the common duct of the graft to a Roux-en-Y limb of the recipient's jejunum.

During biliary reconstruction, metabolic and hematologic alterations are addressed. As the liver graft begins to function, the citrate administered during the previous three phases is metabolized, and metabolic alkalosis may develop. The hemodynamic goals include maintaining a normal central venous pressure. If the central venous pressure is high (greater than 8 mm Hg), there is a concern that the liver graft can become congested and may not function normally. The risk of hepatic artery thrombosis

ranges from 0% to 25% and is greater in infants and children.[80,81] This risk increases if the PT and PPT are corrected. Also, the viscosity from a greater hematocrit may increase the risk of hepatic artery or portal vein thrombosis. The hematocrit does not need to be corrected to normal values. In fact, maintaining the hematocrit at 8 to 9 g/dL is safe and reasonable. Anticoagulation strategies with heparin, dextran, aspirin, and alprostadil may reduce the risk of hepatic artery thrombosis.

### Split Liver Techniques and Living Donor Liver Transplants

Advances in surgical technique, tissue preservation, and immunosuppression have resulted in improved survival in children undergoing liver transplantation. The result is more children are awaiting liver transplantation, but the number of available organs has not increased significantly. Children are at a particular disadvantage because of size limitations. Two techniques have attempted to address these issues. The reduced liver technique does not increase the number of available grafts, and efforts were made to perform split liver techniques to make two grafts from one adult donor. The initial results were poor, with an increase in complications and mortality.[83,84] The technique has evolved, and today the graft is split while still in vivo (in the heart-still-beating donor), as compared to ex vivo (splitting performed after the graft is removed from the donor). This decreases cold ischemia time and facilitates hemostasis of the liver edge. The result is improved child and graft survival,[85] which has increased from 60% to 70% in the 1990's to 80% to 90% in 2003. In one series, 218 split-liver grafts were transplanted between 1995 and 2002. Overall child survival at 1 year was 81.7%, and overall graft survival was 75.8%. Surgical complications that caused a return to the OR were bleeding (9.2%), bowel perforation (8.3%), and biliary problems (7.5%); hepatic artery complications occurred in 6.7%.[85]

Living-donor liver transplantation was first described in 1989.[86] This approach has reduced mortality among children awaiting liver transplantation. The benefit of a living donor (especially if related), is improved posttransplant results because of better graft quality, smaller ischemic times, and better immune compatibility. In fact, these improved results have been observed in several institutions that perform this procedure.[87] In a recent study, the 1- and 5-year patient survivals were 94% and 92% respectively.[88] The left hepatic segment is removed for pediatric recipients, whereas the right hepatic lobe is removed for adult recipients. The regenerative capacity of the liver allows the donor to regenerate the liver without hepatic insufficiency. Despite the success of this technique for the recipients, there is considerable risk to the donor. Complications include exposure to blood products, peripheral nerve injuries, biliary leakage, abdominal wall defects, pleural effusions, pneumonia, pulmonary emboli, and death.[88,89,90] Other than death, these complications were without long-term sequelae, except for a peripheral nerve injury.[88]

### Outcomes

The Studies of Pediatric Liver Transplantation (SPLIT) registry was initiated in 1995 and consists of 38 centers in the United States and Canada. These centers contributed 85% of the pediatric liver transplants in 2002. Transplants performed more recently had greater survival rates. In the past, age less than 1 year was considered an increased risk factor for mortality, but over the past 20 years there is little mortality difference between children less than 2 years of age and those greater than 2 years of age at transplant.[91]

Survival also depends on the preoperative MELD/PELD score. Patients stratified to status 1 had a significantly smaller 1-year survival rate when compared to other transplant recipients (76% vs. 87%). Adults with MELD scores greater than 35 demonstrated decreased 1-year patient and graft survival. There is a suggestion that pediatric patients with greater PELD scores have decreased 1-year patient and graft survival, but that association was not statistically significant. The overall 1-year survival remained excellent, at more than 85%[92] (E-Fig. 29-2).

## IMMEDIATE POSTOPERATIVE CARE

At the completion of surgery, the child is transported to the intensive care unit (ICU). All of the preoperative pathologies will continue into the postoperative period. Children with underlying cardiac, pulmonary, and renal dysfunction will be more difficult to manage.

Hemodynamically, patients after liver transplantation will continue to lose intravascular volume because of bleeding and third-space losses. These losses need to be replaced to maintain a normal central venous pressure and adequate urine output (0.5 to 1 mL/kg/hr). Replacement with a lactate free isotonic solution (0.9% normal saline or Plasmalyte) and albumin is appropriate. Particular attention should be focused on children with underlying ventricular dysfunction or PPH because they tolerate fluid overload poorly. In adults, evidence suggests that fluid overload was responsible for ICU readmission,[93] whereas hypovolemia could lead to renal insufficiency and increase the risk of hepatic artery thrombosis. Preexisting pulmonary hypertension will not dissipate immediately, and children that were previously on prostaglandins will need to continue these infusions in the OR and in the postoperative period. Systemic hypertension is common after liver transplantation and has been described in as many as one-third of children[94]; this is typically attributed to cyclosporine therapy.

Most children require tracheal intubation, mechanical ventilation, and sedation in the immediate postoperative period. This is particularly true for smaller pediatric patients who may have received a relatively large graft and in children with underlying lung disease (HPS). Ascites, pulmonary edema, and pleural effusions may prolong the period of mechanical ventilation.[95] Efforts to minimize atelectasis include positive-pressure ventilation with PEEP. Diuretics may be required on the second or third postoperative day to treat edema and effusions. There is speculation that prolonged mechanical ventilation may have a negative effect on the hemodynamics of transplant patients and may contribute to overall morbidity and mortality.[96] High levels of PEEP may play a role in this morbidity. Some have advocated for early extubation to decrease the incidence of pulmonary complications and to facilitate discharge from the ICU.[97]

Renal failure secondary to HRS usually resolves after successful liver transplantation. The goal in the immediate postoperative period is to maintain normovolemia and to avoid nephrotoxic agents. These include aminoglycoside antibiotics and immunosuppressant agents like cyclosporine and tacrolimus. The immunosuppressant agents may need to be delayed until renal function improves.

Neurologic complications after liver transplantation are common. In adults, 10% to 40% develop these complications.[98] Comparable pediatric data are lacking. In adults, neurologic complications manifest as encephalopathy, seizures, or coma. The causes of encephalopathy and coma include drugs (immunosuppressive agents like tacrolimus and OKT3), infection (meningitis and brain abscess), strokes (bleeding), and hyponatremia with central pontine myelinolysis (CPM). The most common cause of seizures is an adverse drug reaction associated with immunosuppressant agents.[99] Hyponatremia, which can contribute to neurologic complications, should be corrected slowly to prevent CPM. Correcting the hyponatremia no faster than 0.5 mEq/L/hr is considered safe. If the correction proceeds faster than recommended, then evidence from animal models indicates that dexamethasone administered within 6 hours of the correction may minimize the risk of CPM.[100]

Surgical complications after transplantation include vascular complications, acute rejection, and infections; frequent monitoring for their occurrence is important to ensure prompt treatment. Vascular complications include hepatic artery and portal vein thrombosis, bleeding, and bowel perforation.[94] Hepatic artery thrombosis is identified with frequent hepatic Doppler flow imaging. Children may be anticoagulated with aspirin, heparin, dextran, and alprostadil to reduce the risk of thrombosis.[101] Infections are common and contribute to significant morbidity. The primary source for infections appears to be central lines, percutaneous catheter drainage, and mechanical ventilation. Acute rejection should be suspected in children with fever and elevated liver enzymes. The diagnosis is made by histologic examination.[94]

Rejection is an immune response, and efforts to understand and control this immune response lie at the heart of transplant medicine. Initial efforts to control the response involved suppressing the recipient's immune system. There has been a move from immunosuppression to immunotolerance. Immunotolerance describes the concept of immune cells from both the recipient and the donor coexisting without attacking each other.[102] The goal of managing immunosuppression medication is to get to this state of tolerance. In this state of immunotolerance, minimal immunosuppression can be used. The benefits of decreasing immunosuppression include the reduced risk of infection, hypercholesterolemia, malignancy, hypertension, and diabetes mellitus. Protocols to induce tolerance include exposing patients to lymphoid-depleting agents (antilymphoid antibodies), like antithymocyte globulin, before liver engraftment, to reduce the antidonor response to a more controllable or "deletable" range and allow maintenance therapy (e.g., tacrolimus) to begin with one agent. Other agents are added only when there is evidence of rejection.[103] The immunosuppressant agents currently used include calcineurin inhibitors (CNIs) like tacrolimus and cyclosporine, and they provide the mainstay of therapy. Other options include azathioprine or mycophenolate mofetil, for children who cannot tolerate the CNIs because of toxicity. Adverse effects of the CNIs include hypertension, tremor, and renal failure. Other agents being used include monoclonal antibodies against interleukin-2 (IL-2).[104]

## LONG-TERM ISSUES

Recipients of liver transplants require repeated anesthetics for a variety of reasons (central line placement, wound irrigation, dental rehabilitation, bowel obstruction, cholangiogram, biliary dilation, esophagogastroduodenoscopy). A primary concern in the posttransplant child is the adverse effects of immunosuppressant agents. Most organ systems become involved, and a thorough review of systems is important.

The cardiovascular effects of immunosuppressant agents includes hypertension from cyclosporine and cardiomyopathy (rare) from tacrolimus.[105,106] Renal insufficiency can occur secondary to cyclosporine, diuretics, or hypertension. Baseline blood urea nitrogen and creatinine should be obtained preoperatively in children with a history of renal insufficiency, and medications that are renally cleared (morphine, rocuronium, vecuronium) should be adjusted or avoided. Hyperkalemia may accompany renal failure and should be evaluated before induction of anesthesia.

Pediatric recipients of a liver transplant can have multiple hematologic abnormalities. Azathioprine can cause anemia, leucopenia, and thrombocytopenia. Gastrointestinal bleeding from corticosteroid-induced ulcers may also cause occult anemia. Children receiving azathioprine should have a complete blood count before surgery, particularly if the procedure may involve blood loss.

The endocrine effects of chronic steroid exposure include diabetes, growth retardation, and adrenal insufficiency. Children receiving insulin for diabetes need intraoperative blood glucose monitoring and dextrose-containing IV fluids if they are hypoglycemic or are at risk of developing hypoglycemia. Children receiving chronic steroids need stress-dose steroids during the perioperative period (see Chapter 25).

Most recipients of a liver transplant have been exposed to multiple procedures and may benefit from an anxiolytic preoperatively.[107] Midazolam is safe, provided there is no evidence of residual HE. Anesthesia can be induced with an inhalational technique, provided the liver graft is functioning normally and nothing-by-mouth (NPO) guidelines have been followed. Children who are hospitalized, septic, bleeding, encephalopathic, or rejecting the graft should have an IV induction and their airways should be secured with an endotracheal tube. Isoflurane, sevoflurane, and desflurane are suitable for maintenance of anesthesia.

## Kidney Transplantation

### DEMOGRAPHICS AND EPIDEMIOLOGY

Renal transplantation improves development, quality of life, and survival[108,109] in children with chronic renal failure. The OPTN maintains the national transplant registry in the United States; the OPTN data as of 2011 shows 826 children under the age of 18 on the active waiting list; this represents fewer than 1% of the 89,169 patients in the US waiting for a kidney.[110] Characterization of such a small patient population is challenging. The North American Pediatric Renal Trials and Collaborative Studies (NAPRTCS) group has obtained the voluntary participation of all centers in the United States and Canada performing renal transplants on more than four children per year. Since the advent of the NAPRTCS in 1987, it has registered 11,603 pediatric renal transplants in 10,632 recipients.[111] This represents a capture rate of approximately 68% of the 16,000 kidney transplants that have been performed in the United States in children younger than 18 years of age[110] (E-Table 29-3). The inclusion into the NAPRTCS of pediatric patients requiring dialysis began in 1992, and the inclusion of children in chronic renal failure (creatinine clearance of 75 mL/min/1.73 m² or less) began in 1994. Currently, there are 16,874 children in the NAPRTCS registry based on the above indications (E-Table 29-4).

### PATHOPHYSIOLOGY: IMPLICATIONS OF THE PATIENT IN RENAL FAILURE

The kidneys perform a number of vital functions; both their dysfunction and the current methods of mechanical renal-replacement therapy have systemic implications. Because renal

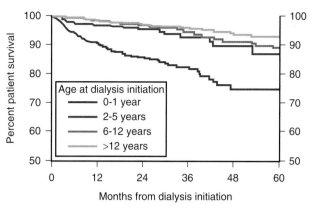

**FIGURE 29-4** Patient survival while on dialysis. (Exhibit 1.9 from The North American Pediatric Renal Trials and Collaborative Studies 2011 Annual Dialysis Report. Available at https://web.emmes.com/study/ped/annlrept/annlrept.html [accessed June 17, 2011].)

dysfunction creates profound disturbances in normal homeostasis, morbidity and mortality is increased in children with renal failure, especially the very young (Fig. 29-4).

Disturbances in growth and development occur with renal failure, and depend on both the age of onset and the severity of the disease.[112] Infants, in particular, are vulnerable to growth retardation caused by renal failure. Appropriate management of nutrition, with[113] or without[114] the provision of renal replacement therapy, is necessary to ameliorate this effect. Renal transplantation may provide for some "catch-up" growth, although this is limited to younger children; the child's final height is a function of the height at the time of transplant, graft function, and the immunosuppression regimen.[111,114,115] Growth hormone therapy can be used for children, both pretransplant and posttransplant, to manage height deficits. However, when therapy is initiated before severe growth retardation has occurred, growth hormone therapy is more effective.[114,116,117,118] A possible complication of growth hormone replacement in transplant recipients has been scoliosis.[119]

In addition to the effects on growth, renal failure also effects intellectual and behavioral development. Children requiring renal-replacement therapy from infancy are particularly vulnerable. Nutritional invasive enteral support and renal replacement therapy, along with early transplantation, can lead to near-normal cognitive function.[120] However, these children may have more problems with hyperactivity and conduct disorder. In addition, if these children are suffering from other comorbid conditions, they are very likely to have diminished IQ.[121] In older children and adults with end-stage renal disease since childhood, age at diagnosis and increased duration of dialysis are risks for decreased mental capacity. Renal transplantation status did not appear to be protective from the risks of decreased mental capacity.[122,123]

Chronic renal failure is associated with cardiovascular changes. Between 20% and 33%[116,124] of deaths in children on dialysis are cardiac in nature. Approximately 25% to 33%[125,108] of deaths in children and young adults with end-stage renal disease whose disease began in childhood are from cardiac causes. The incidence of coronary artery calcifications and carotid intimal-medial thickening, two surrogate measures of coronary artery disease, are increased in dialysis-dependent children[126] and in young adults with childhood-onset chronic renal failure.[127] Hyperhomocysteinemia, associated with cardiovascular disease in adults, is common in children with chronic renal failure,[128] as is dyslipidemia.[129] Hypertension is frequent, and is a risk factor for deterioration of renal function.[130,131] Left ventricular hypertrophy (LVH) is prevalent, both in children with chronic renal failure and in children on dialysis.[132-134] LVH may be associated with diastolic dysfunction.[135] Both LVH[134] and diastolic dysfunction[135] were noted to be more severe in children requiring dialysis.

In transplanted children, cardiac deaths constitute 15% of the causes of death.[104] Renal transplantation does decrease the risk of cardiac death, compared to that of children in chronic renal failure or dialysis-dependent children.[108,125] However, transplanted children have a persistence of pretransplant risk factors. LVH is still found in 50% to 75% of transplant recipients.[136,137] Risk factors for LVH in the posttransplant patient include a history of dialysis, anemia, and hypertension.[136] LVH can occur in renal transplant patients with normal 24-hour ambulatory blood pressure measurements.[137] In addition to LVH, 10 of 73 posttransplant patients in one study[136] demonstrated left ventricular dilation with systolic dysfunction. The incidence of coronary artery calcification in young adults who were transplanted as children is greater than in control patients,[127,138] and may be associated with carotid intimal-medial thickening.[127] Hyperhomocysteinemia is present in 63% to 77%[138,139] of transplanted children, and its presence is associated with poor graft function.[139] Folate supplementation may normalize homocysteine levels.[140] Even with good graft function following transplantation, dyslipidemia persists and is generally related to immunosuppression medications.[129] The incidence of diabetes requiring insulin treatment is 2.6%. Tacrolimus use and African American race are the two major risk factors for insulin requiring diabetes.[141]

Anemia is common both before and after transplantation. Anemia is caused by a decrease in erythropoietin production and iron deficiency. In posttransplant patients, CNIs, especially tacrolimus, are additional risk factors for anemia.[142] In pediatric patients requiring dialysis for the first time, anemia was associated with a greater risk of death and prolonged hospitalization.[109] Treatment of anemia has been shown to retard the progression of renal disease in adults.[143] In children with chronic renal failure, a hematocrit less than 33% is a risk factor for progression to end-stage renal disease.[112] Anemia may be associated with LVH in children[132-136] and in adult patients with chronic renal disease; erythropoietin has been shown to improve LVH.[144]

## PREOPERATIVE EVALUATION

Immediately before transplantation, the child should be stable, and fluid or electrolyte imbalances should be corrected. It is important to assess the urine output (anuric, polyuric) so that appropriate intraoperative fluid replacement can be administered before unclamping the blood vessels of the donor organ. Active infection is a contraindication for transplantation. Any concurrent systemic disorders should be optimized. Finally, the NPO status of the child should be ascertained; many who present for cadaveric transplantation will have a full stomach.

## SURGICAL TECHNIQUE

The surgical techniques used in the pediatric recipient differ from those used in the adult and depend on the child's size and underlying preexisting abnormalities, as well as the approach to the transplant (intraperitoneal or extraperitoneal). The extraperitoneal approach may be more technically difficult in smaller children. Removal of native tissue, either concurrently or (ideally)

previously, occurred in approximately 22% of children registered in the NAPRTCS database.[111] Preservation of urine-producing native kidneys may be desirable to prevent fluid overload during dialysis, especially for small children.[145]

Native nephrectomy may be required for polycystic kidney disease, uncontrollable hypertension, urinary tract infection, or nephrotic syndrome.[145-148] Removal of polycystic kidneys may be necessary for space reasons, especially in small children. Children with severe vesicoureteral reflux and intractable urinary tract infections may also require native nephrectomy. Nephrectomy for severe nephrosis may be necessary to resolve associated hypoalbuminemia, malnutrition, and hypercoagulability. Ideally, native nephrectomy is performed before transplant.[147-149] Native nephrectomy performed at the time of transplant increases operative time and cadaveric graft ischemic time,[140] and has been shown to be a risk factor for ATN in the grafted organ.[111]

### Children Weighing More Than 20 kg

In larger children (more than 20 kg), the surgical approach is similar to that in the adult transplant patient; the kidney is placed in the iliac fossa, and the vascular anastomoses are to the common iliac vein and artery.[146,147] In larger children, the external iliac vessels may be used.[147] An extraperitoneal approach has the advantage of increased ease of future graft biopsy and ability to resume peritoneal dialysis in case of delayed graft failure.[145]

### Children Weighing Less Than 20 kg

If renal transplantation in smaller children were restricted to size-compatible organs, then the surgical approach would be similar to that of the larger patient. However, a 1992 NAPRTCS report noted an increased loss of cadaveric grafts from pediatric donors. These pediatric donor organs had a greater rate of graft thrombosis and primary nonfunction, as well as a greater risk for acute rejection.[150,151] Consequently, the use of pediatric donors has declined and living donors increased (Fig. 29-5). More importantly, the improvement in graft survival (Figs. 29-6 and 29-7) and patient survival (Fig. 29-8) with a living donor, although present across age-groups, is markedly greater in these young children.[111]

For these reasons, the surgical technique for renal transplantation in the infant and small child has been modified to accommodate the adult-sized kidney. The use of a size-discrepant organ precludes the traditional approach. As Starzl et al[152] describe: "the adult organ almost completely fills a child's right paravertebral gutter, extending from the undersurface of the liver to the pelvis." Typically, a midline incision from pubis to xiphoid is used and the cecum and right colon are mobilized.[146,149,152,153] An alternate approach used by some centers, is a right lower quadrant incision, dissecting extraperitoneally;[147,154] this may have the advantage of quicker return of bowel function. Depending on the size of the recipient's vessels, the donor organ anastomoses may be made to the common iliac artery and vein, or directly to the aorta and vena cava.[146,147,149,153]

In addition to difficulties in surgical technique, adult organs in pediatric recipients present physiologic challenges. The adult-sized organ sequesters a disproportionate amount of the infant's blood volume and cardiac output.[145,146,155] In one study[156] that involved nine infant recipients of adult-sized kidneys, pretransplant, early posttransplant, and late posttransplant blood flows were determined in both the infant's aorta and the adult graft. Pretransplant graft flow was approximately 618 mL/min, whereas 8 to 12 days posttransplant, graft flow had decreased to

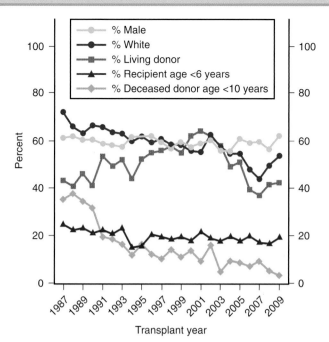

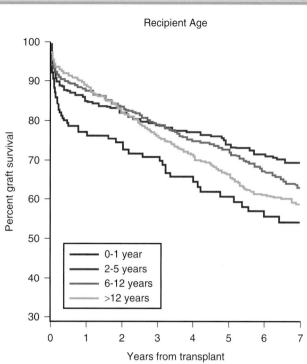

**FIGURE 29-5** Patient registrations, transplants, and selected characteristics. (Exhibit 1.1 from The North American Pediatric Renal Trials and Collaborative Studies 2010 Annual Transplant Report. Available at https://web.emmes.com/study/ped/annlrept/annlrept.html [accessed June 17, 2011].)

**FIGURE 29-7** Deceased-donor graft survival by recipient age. (Exhibit 5.5 from The North American Pediatric Renal Trials and Collaborative Studies 2010 Annual Transplant Report. Available at https://web.emmes.com/study/ped/annlrept/annlrept.html [accessed June 17, 2011].)

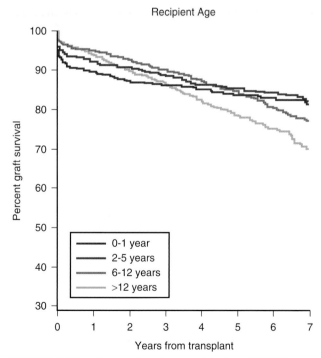

**FIGURE 29-6** Living-donor graft survival by recipient age. (Exhibit 5.4 from The North American Pediatric Renal Trials and Collaborative Studies 2010 Annual Transplant Report. Available at https://web.emmes.com/study/ped/annlrept/annlrept.html [accessed June 17, 2011].)

385 mL/min, despite aortic blood flow increasing from 331 mL/min to 761 mL/min. A further decrease was observed at 4 to 6 months, with aortic blood flow at 665 mL/min and graft flow at 296 mL/min. At 4 months the graft size had decreased by 26%. Even with excellent conditions, optimal hydration, and a doubling of aortic blood-flow, these adult grafts are still underperfused, both during transplant and in the late posttransplant period. In addition, the transplanted kidney is vulnerable to further reductions of flow resulting from gastrointestinal illness, poor oral intake, or hypotension during nontransplantation surgery.[151] This may explain why early graft loss in these smaller children is either primary nonfunction or thrombosis (E-Fig. 29-3).[157]

## ANESTHETIC APPROACH

### Periinduction

A living-donor renal transplantation is an elective procedure, whose only time constraints involve coordination with the donor harvest team, whereas in a cadaveric transplant, any delay could potentially increase donor organ cold-ischemic time. As such, most recipients of living-donor kidneys will arrive in the OR with an IV, empty stomach, completed blood work, and any immunosuppressant induction treatment underway. Conversely, recipients of cadaveric kidneys likely have a full stomach, have pending blood work, and may have immunosuppressant induction medications ordered but not yet given. An acceptable electrolyte panel, assurance that any cross-matching is under way, and confirmation with the treatment team regarding the type of immunosuppressant induction (and premedicant) planned is necessary. In particular, it is important to confirm that any

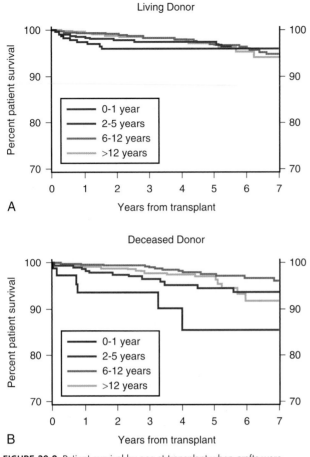

A

**FIGURE 29-8** Patient survival by age at transplant when grafts were received from living (**A**) and deceased (**B**) donors; transplant era 1996 to 2006. (Exhibit 7.6 from The North American Pediatric Renal Trials and Collaborative Studies 2010 Annual Transplant Report. Available at https://web.emmes.com/study/ped/annlrept/annlrept.html [accessed June 17, 2011].)

immunosuppressant induction drug and its premedicant (if any) is ordered and will be immediately available when the child arrives in the OR.

### Immunosuppressant Induction Therapy

Children may receive immunotherapy perioperatively (Fig. 29-9) to assist the development of immunotolerance[158] of the implanted graft, and potentially to delay the administration of the nephrotoxic CNIs.[145,146] Antilymphocyte antibodies include alemtuzumab (Campath), equine antilymphocyte globulin (Atgam), and polyclonal rabbit antithymocyte globulin (Thymo-globulin), and the infusion of these agents cause a cytokine response. This cytokine response can include fever, chills, rigors, and malaise that should be pretreated with acetaminophen, cor-ticosteroids, and diphenhydramine.[158,159] Anti–IL-2 antibodies include basiliximab (Simulect) and daclizumab (Zenapax), and these drugs do not cause a cytokine response. Adverse effects from anti–IL-2 antibodies are comparable to those from a placebo, save for an acute hypersensitivity reaction that can occur with basiliximab.[158]

Depending on the child, premedication may be adminis-tered to facilitate separation from the family. The cytokine effects of the antilymphocyte induction drugs can be unpleas-ant, and can erode the coping mechanisms of any age child. In children with a suspected full stomach, a rapid-sequence induc-tion should be performed. Succinylcholine may be used in the absence of contraindications, such as hyperkalemia. In children with an empty stomach, an inhalational, IV, or combination technique may be used. Drug choices should avoid those drugs primarily metabolized or excreted by the kidney. One should not assume immediate resumption of renal function by the new graft. Because renal failure affects both protein-binding and volume of distribution, anesthetic agents and adjuncts should be titrated to effect. Preferential use should be made of drugs that undergo organ-independent elimination (cisatra-curium, remifentanil), or do not rely exclusively on the

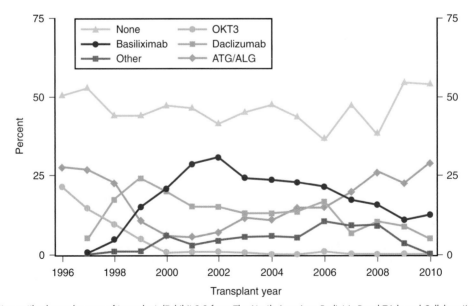

**FIGURE 29-9** Induction antibody use by year of transplant. (Exhibit 3.2 from The North American Pediatric Renal Trials and Collaborative Studies 2010 Annual Transplant Report. Available at https://web.emmes.com/study/ped/annlrept/annlrept.html [accessed June 17, 2011].) *ATG/ALG,* Polyclonal antibodies antithymocyte globulins and antilymphocyte globulins.

kidney for metabolism (propofol), or whose renally excreted metabolites are inactive (midazolam, fentanyl). Regarding drugs with renally excreted metabolites that are active (morphine), these agents should be used cautiously and titrated to effect. Drugs with renally excreted metabolites that are toxic (i.e., meperidine) should be avoided.

## Monitors and Vascular Access

Standard monitors, including core temperature, should be used. The need for vascular access should reflect third-spacing requirements, and the potential for brisk blood loss inherent in a long intraabdominal procedure in which the surgeon will be directly accessing large vessels. Urine output may not reflect intravascular volume status secondary to native renal dysfunction, the ureter not yet anastomosed with the bladder, or polyuria in the reperfused graft.[145,146] Smaller children will have the most severe fluid shifts and will be the most vulnerable to graft hypoperfusion. Therefore central venous and arterial catheters to monitor intraoperative and postoperative pressures are extremely useful.[145,145,155,160] In the larger child, for whom assessment and maintenance of intravascular volume is more reliable, a central venous catheter may not be necessary in the presence of adequate peripheral access.[153]

## Maintenance and Reperfusion

The anesthetic management plan should take into account hemodynamic conditions necessary for adequate perfusion of the donor organ. Combined general-regional techniques have been used, but have been associated with larger intraoperative fluid requirements and the need for IV opioid supplementation in half the children.[160] A hypnotic agent supplemented with an opioid to minimize negative inotropy is appropriate, and avoiding nitrous oxide in a long intraabdominal case is prudent. Sevoflurane has been associated with the production of inorganic fluoride and compound A (see Chapter 6). Although no negative outcome data exist for the use of this agent in renal transplant recipients, case numbers are not sufficient to demonstrate its safety in this population.

Optimal hemodynamic conditions for reperfusion are more important when a large size discrepancy exists between the native organ and the graft. The extreme of this situation would be in the infant receiving an adult graft. In children, recommendations for central venous pressure range from 8 to 12 mm Hg to 16 to 20 mm Hg,[146,154,155] with most centers in the middle.[145,147,149] Some authors suggest a systolic blood pressure above 120 mm Hg,[146] and MAP above 65 to 70 mm Hg.[145,146] In the smaller child, blood sequestration in the graft will constitute a significant portion of the patient's total blood volume,[145,146,155] and the anastomosis will likely require the clamping, and subsequent unclamping, of the aorta. Both preload supplementation with blood, crystalloid, and colloid, and possible dopamine infusion to optimize cardiac output may be necessary.[145,146] Furosemide and/or mannitol may be given at the completion of the anastomoses to promote diuresis, and sodium bicarbonate may be given after aortic unclamping to attenuate subsequent acidosis.[145-148] Avoidance of blood products is desirable, as children with more than five lifetime transfusions are at increased risk of ATN.[111] Although there are data regarding prevention of anemia in the chronic management of the renal transplant patient, there does not appear to be an optimal hematocrit in the immediate postoperative period. Blood therapy must therefore be specific for each child.

## IMMEDIATE POSTOPERATIVE MANAGEMENT

In the immediate postoperative period, maintenance of the child's blood volume remains important. In small children, the volume resuscitation required to adequately perfuse the graft may preclude early extubation.[147,154,155,160] Maintenance of an adequate blood volume continues into the postoperative period, where usually copious urine output is replaced mL for mL.[145-148,154,155] Prevention of graft hypoperfusion and subsequent ATN potentially prevents acute rejection,[151] as ATN in the early postoperative period is a major risk factor for graft loss.[111,130] Maintenance of the circulating blood volume continues to be important even in the late postoperative period. One study[161] noted improved glomerular filtration rates at 6 months in their transplant recipients after starting an aggressive 2500 mL/m$^2$/day fluid regimen (via nasogastric or gastrostomy tube) for 6 months; this difference persisted into the 12-month period.

## LONG-TERM ISSUES

Much has been accomplished in preservation of graft function for kidney transplant children. Unfortunately, cardiovascular morbidity, infection, and malignancy are the major long-term concerns. Almost half of renal transplant recipients die with a functioning graft.[111]

### Infection

Increased success in immunotolerance for transplant recipients, unfortunately, can result in an increase in opportunistic infections from exogenous pathogens. After the first 5 months posttransplantation, infection surpasses acute rejection as the cause of hospitalization.[111] In particular, fungal infection is a significant risk for graft loss.[162] Deaths from infection eclipse cardiovascular causes of death for transplant recipients. Infection accounts for 28.4% of deaths in the NAPRTCS database.[111] Epstein-Barr virus (EBV) related adenotonsillar hypertrophy is common in the transplant population, occurring in 11 of 16 children in one series.[163] Risk factors for EBV-related adenotonsillar hypertrophy include young age and seronegativity at time of transplant.[164] Posttransplant lymphoproliferative disorder (PTLD), a result of EBV infection, is common and occurs earlier in the renal transplant population.[165]

### Malignancy

Malignancy accounts for between 11.3% and 14% of the deaths after transplant in children.[111,108] A case report[166] describes the graft loss of two living-donor related kidney grafts to renal cell carcinoma 9 and 11 years posttransplant; neither donor developed cancer in their remaining kidney. In one series of 282 pediatric kidney recipients with cancer, PTLD and skin cancer were the most common cancers, 31% each, followed by cancers of the perineum, 7%, and Kaposi sarcoma, 5%; PTLD and Kaposi sarcoma were more likely to manifest in childhood.[167]

## SUMMARY

Anesthetic management of the child for renal transplant may be complicated by a number of factors. Impaired renal function may be present pre- and posttransplant. Comorbidities as a result of impaired renal function are numerous, and may require altered anesthetic management. Although the renal transplant patient is not normal, the continued function of the transplanted kidney allows for near normal function, growth, and development. Therefore the ultimate goal of management is preservation of both patient and graft.

# Cardiac Transplantation

Cardiac transplantation, as a viable treatment strategy in infants and children with congenital and acquired heart disease, has matured considerably since Kantrowitz performed the first heart transplant in a 16-day-old infant in 1967.[168] As the indications for pediatric cardiac transplantation continue to evolve and expand, donor organ availability is the major limiting factor.[169] The advances in immunosuppression, coupled with a better understanding of rejection, have resulted in improved graft and child survival, fewer adverse effects, and an improved quality of life.

However, rejection, infection, and posttransplant neoplasia continue to remain the major causes of death.

## DEMOGRAPHICS AND EPIDEMIOLOGY

Cardiac transplantation has become a valuable therapeutic option for a broad range of pediatric cardiac abnormalities. Approximately 20% of the pediatric recipients are younger than 1 year of age (Fig. 29-10).[169] The primary indication for cardiac transplantation in infants younger than 1 year of age is a severe structural congenital cardiac defect (Fig. 29-11).[169] Dilated, hypertrophic, or restrictive cardiomyopathies are less frequent

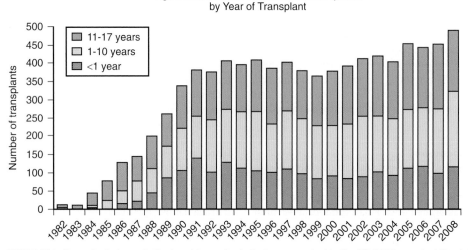

NOTE: This figure includes only the heart transplants that are reported to the ISHLT Transplant Registry. As such, this should not be construed as evidence that the number of hearts transplanted worldwide has increased and/or decreased in recent years.

**FIGURE 29-10** Age distribution of pediatric heart recipients by year of transplant. (From Kirk R, Edwards LB, Kucheryavaya AY, et al. Registry of the International Society for Heart and Lung Transplantation: thirteenth official pediatric heart transplantation report—2010. J Heart Lung Transplant 2010;29:1119-28.)

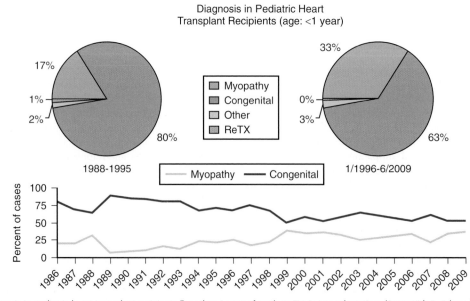

**FIGURE 29-11** Diagnosis in pediatric heart transplant recipients (less than 1 year of age). *ReTX*, Retransplantation. (From Kirk R, Edwards LB, Kucheryavaya AY, et al. Registry of the International Society for Heart and Lung Transplantation: thirteenth official pediatric heart transplantation report—2010. J Heart Lung Transplant 2010;29:1119-28.)

indications in infants. However, in children 1 to 17 years of age, cardiomyopathies account for at least half of all indications for transplantation.[169] Unresectable cardiac tumors, severe life-threatening arrhythmias, and other diseases, such as Kawasaki syndrome, are uncommon indications in all age-groups (Figs. 29-12 and 29-13).[170]

## PATHOPHYSIOLOGY OF THE DISEASE

An understanding of the basic cardiac anatomy and pathophysiology in recipients presenting for cardiac transplantation is the key to safe perioperative management. Many recipients have underlying lesions that allow alterations in the balance between systemic and pulmonary blood flow. Changes that accompany normal anesthetic management can radically alter this balance and thereby result in the recipient's deterioration. Other recipients have marginal cardiac output secondary to their underlying myopathies, or structural defects that hinder normal myocardial function.

### Congenital Heart Disease

This group of children includes those with complex lesions for which no option for palliation exists, children with end-stage

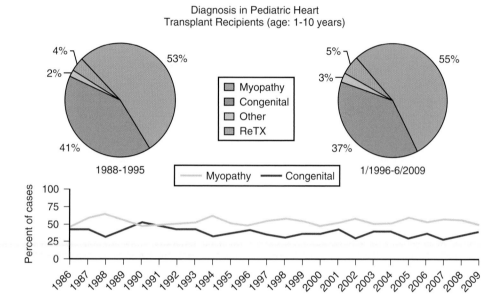

**FIGURE 29-12** Diagnosis in pediatric heart transplant recipients (1 to 10 years of age). *ReTX,* Retransplantation. (From Kirk R, Edwards LB, Kucheryavaya AY, et al. Registry of the International Society for Heart and Lung Transplantation: thirteenth official pediatric heart transplantation report—2010. J Heart Lung Transplant 2010;29:1119-28.)

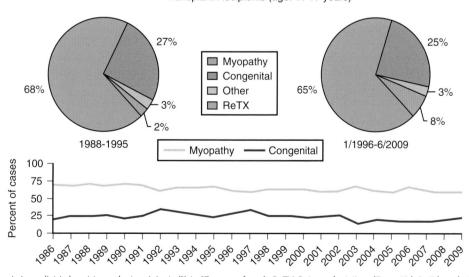

**FIGURE 29-13** Diagnosis in pediatric heart transplant recipients (11 to 17 years of age). *ReTX,* Retransplantation. (From Kirk R, Edwards LB, Kucheryavaya AY, et al. Registry of the International Society for Heart and Lung Transplantation: thirteenth official pediatric heart transplantation report—2010. J Heart Lung Transplant 2010;29:1119-28.)

heart failure after surgical repair of congenital heart defects, children with failed palliation for single-ventricle physiology (Fontan type), and neonates with hypoplastic left heart syndrome (HLHS). There are children who have undergone surgical palliation with successful early results who later in life present with dilated cardiomyopathies secondary to long-standing valvular regurgitation, ventricular outflow tract obstruction, or dysrhythmias. Although the right ventricle has been shown to be capable of adapting to work as the "systemic" ventricle in cases of HLHS or in children who have undergone an "atrial type" switch operation for transposition of the great vessels, with time, these systemic right ventricles fail and develop both systolic and diastolic dysfunction. Thus in these children, the only therapeutic option left is transplantation.

### Dilated Cardiomyopathy

The etiology of dilated cardiomyopathy is often unknown or complex but includes viral myocarditis and drug-induced, ischemic, metabolic (disorders of fatty acid, amino acid, glycogen and mucopolysaccharide metabolism), genetic, or mitochondrial disorders.[171] The primary disorder in dilated cardiomyopathy is an abnormality of systolic function. Congestive heart failure is the most common presentation. Predictors of poor outcome include a family history of cardiomyopathy, syncope, ventricular arrhythmia, left ventricular end-diastolic pressure greater than 25 mm Hg, and left ventricular ejection fraction less than 30%.

### Restrictive Cardiomyopathy

Restrictive cardiomyopathies are uncommon disorders, with generally poor prognoses, that are associated with infiltration of the myocardium, such as glycogen storage disease, amyloidosis, mucopolysaccharidosis, hemochromatosis, and sarcoidosis. The infiltration results in diastolic dysfunction and diminished stroke output. Endocardial fibroelastosis also causes a restrictive cardiomyopathy and an increased pulmonary vascular resistance (PVR).[172,173] The increased PVR is secondary to an increased left ventricular end-diastolic pressure with associated increases in PAP.

### Hypertrophic Cardiomyopathy

Hypertrophic cardiomyopathy is a concentric thickening of the left ventricular wall that can lead to both a fixed and a dynamic obstruction to left ventricular outflow (see Chapter 14). A number of sarcomeric genotypes have been described for this lesion. Many children with hypertrophic cardiomyopathy first present as infants. Their clinical course depends on the presence or absence of outflow tract obstruction. If obstruction is present, more than 25% of infants will present with failure to thrive and feeding intolerance as manifestations of congestive heart failure. A large septal muscular prominence can lead to mitral regurgitation secondary to abnormal systolic anterior motion of the mitral valve leaflets. The major consequence of this diagnosis is sudden death. Risk factors for sudden death include a family history of sudden death, marked concentric left ventricular wall thickness, age at presentation, and a reduced fractional shortening Z score.[174]

### Other Conditions

Although rare, some children require cardiac transplantation for unresectable cardiac tumors or sequelae of other diseases, such as Kawasaki disease. The pathophysiology of these lesions varies with the disease, but the end result is similar: systolic dysfunction, diastolic dysfunction, or both.

Contraindications to pediatric cardiac transplantation include multiple severe congenital anomalies, marked prematurity (before 36 weeks), low birth weight (less than 2 kg), ectopia cordis, diffuse pulmonary artery hypoplasia, pulmonary venous hypoplasia, active malignancy, active infection, severe metabolic disease, irreversible noncardiac end-organ damage, and a fixed pulmonary vascular resistance index (PVRI) greater than or equal to 6 Wood units, or a fixed transpulmonary pressure gradient greater than or equal to 15 mm Hg (1.9 kPa).[175,176] The increase in PVR is usually assessed during cardiac catheterization. These contraindications are considered by some to be relative, rather than absolute contraindications to cardiac transplantation. Additional potential contraindications include severe psychosocial problems that may impede proper postoperative care, the lack of reliable caretakers, and an unstable family structure; these are critical factors in the decision to offer transplantation as a treatment option.

## DONOR SELECTION

Donor selection for pediatric heart transplantation is often complicated by difficult social settings associated with the death of the donor. In addition, the usual criteria for selection of adult donors may not correlate well with myocardial pathologic findings in infants and children, thereby potentially limiting the availability of donor organs for infants and children.[177] There have been reports of neonatal transplants crossing the ABO barrier.[178,179,180] Donor-to-recipient weight ratios up to 3.0 have been used successfully. In a comparison with more equally matched donor-to-recipient weight ratios, children who received hearts from oversized donors had no differences in ICU ventilator days, fractional shortening as assessed by echocardiography, ability to close the chest, or duration of inotropic support.[181] In contrast to the use of oversized donor organs, undersized donor organs were associated with an increased rate of donor organ failure. Recipient PVR is a major determinant for appropriate donor selection, and larger donor hearts should be considered for those with increased PVR to permit the right ventricle to compensate for the increased afterload.[182] Myocardial preservation of the donor organ is aimed at minimizing the ischemia time. Ischemic times of 6 hours were thought to be ideal, but pediatric allograft ischemic times may be extended to 8 hours with little adverse consequence.[183,184]

## PREOPERATIVE EVALUATION

A comprehensive, multidisciplinary evaluation of a potential cardiac allograft recipient is required to determine the recipient's suitability for transplantation. This evaluation includes an assessment of the child's underlying cardiopulmonary, hepatic, renal, neurologic, infectious disease, and immune system status, as well as socioeconomic and psychosocial function (Table 29-3).

Assessment of cardiopulmonary function usually begins with a thorough history, with attention to exercise tolerance, oxygen requirements, and need for diuretics and inotropic support. Examination of the electrocardiogram, chest radiographs, echocardiograms, and Holter monitors may be helpful in the discovery of pleural or pericardial effusions, conduction disturbances, cardiac function, and arrhythmias. Radionuclide angiography may be useful in defining systemic ventricular dysfunction in children with complex cardiac morphology. The pretransplant assessment ultimately includes cardiac catheterization with angiography. The anatomy and hemodynamics of the recipient must be carefully delineated, because this influences anesthetic

**29**

## TABLE 29-3 Routine Pre–Cardiac Transplant Evaluation

**History and Physical Examination**

Age, height, weight, body surface area
Diagnoses
Medical history
Medications
Allergies
Immunization record

**Laboratory Data**

Liver and kidney function studies
Urinalysis
Glomerular filtration rate
Prothrombin time, partial thromboplastin time, INR, platelet count
Complete blood cell count with differential
PPD skin test
Serologies for HIV, hepatitis, cytomegalovirus, Epstein-Barr virus, toxoplasmosis, syphilis
ABO type
Panel-reactive antibody

**Cardiomyopathy Work-Up**

Thyroid function studies
Blood lactate, pyruvate, ammonia, acyl carnitine
Urine organic acids, acyl carnitine
Skeletal muscle biopsy
Karyotype

**Cardiopulmonary Data**

Electrocardiogram
Chest radiograph
Echocardiogram
Radionuclide angiography
Cardiac catheterization
Endomyocardial biopsy
Pulmonary function studies
Oxygen consumption

**Psychosocial Evaluation**

History of abuse or neglect
Parental substance abuse
Long-term supportive care and reliability of caregivers
Possible relocation

**Other Consultations as Needed**

Dental services
Social services
Other

Modified from Boucek MM, Shaddy RE. Pediatric heart transplantation. In: Allen HD, Gutgesell HP, Clark EB, et al., editors. Moss and Adams' heart disease in infants, children, and adolescents including the fetus and young adult 6th ed. Philadelphia: Lippincott Williams & Wilkins; 2001, p. 295-407.
*INR*, International normalized ratio; *PPD*, purified protein derivative.

$$\text{PVRI (units/m}^2) = (\text{PAP [mm Hg]} - \text{PAWP [mm Hg]})/\text{CI (L/min/m}^2)$$

$$\text{TPG (mm Hg)} = \text{PAP (mm Hg)} - \text{PAWP (mm Hg)}$$

where PAP is the mean pulmonary artery pressure, PAWP is the mean pulmonary artery wedge pressure, and CI is the cardiac index.

A PVRI greater than 6 Wood units/m$^2$ or a TPG in excess of 15 mm Hg can lead to acute right ventricular graft failure, although the upper limit of PVR associated with successful cardiac transplantation has not been established in children. An endomyocardial biopsy can identify acute myocarditis and myocardial infiltrates. Pulmonary function studies may be useful in older children with chronic lung disease.

Laboratory evaluation should include serum electrolytes, complete blood cell count with differential, coagulation profile, viral titers for possible latent viral infections, such as cytomegalovirus (CMV) and EBV, and metabolic or genetic work-ups. Donor matching is based on ABO typing, although successful transplantation of ABO-incompatible hearts in infants has increased the potential donor pool for infants in critical need.[185,186] ABO-incompatible hearts are possible because of the immaturity of the infant immune system and the lack of production of ABO antibodies during the first 3 to 6 months of life. The use of triple-volume exchange transfusions also minimizes the potential reaction to maternally transmitted, preformed ABO antibodies. The recipient's blood is also screened for antibodies against sera of random blood donors and, if reactive, a serum crossmatch with the donor may be performed. Panel reactive antibodies are preformed circulating human leukocyte antigen (HLA) alloantibodies that, in high titers, are associated with diminished graft survival.[187,188,189] These antibodies arise from the use of homologous blood products, and blood products should be avoided if at all possible in the pretransplant period. Treatments to reduce panel-reactive antibodies may include IV immunoglobulin, cyclophosphamide, and plasmapheresis.[190] Although HLA compatibility may improve graft survival, HLA matching is not routinely performed, owing to time constraints and limited availability of donor organs.

The mean time from listing for transplant to the actual surgery is about 3 months, but varies with the child's age, blood group, and list status. UNOS has developed allocation procedures that give priority to the most urgently ill children. Status 1 children have a projected life expectancy of less than 6 months, and status 2 children have a projected life expectancy of more than 6 months. Status 1 children generally require mechanical or pharmacologic support to sustain life, and most require support in ICUs. These children are further subdivided into 1A and 1B, where 1A is reserved for those with a projected life expectancy of less than 1 month. Physicians of status 1A children must recertify every 7 to 14 days if their patients do not require mechanical support for acute hemodynamic decompensation, and even those who require mechanical support are only guaranteed 30 days until physician recertification becomes necessary. Approximately 20% of children with cardiomyopathy and 30% of those with end-stage congenital heart disease die while waiting for a donor heart.[191-193] Medical stabilization frequently includes the use of diuretics, inotropic agents, arrhythmia therapy, oxygen or subatmospheric oxygen, and mechanical ventilation, if warranted. Studies of β-adrenergic blockade therapy (carvedilol) have shown promise in children with dilated cardiomyopathy and chronic heart failure.[194,195] Those with severe chamber

management, surgical donor harvesting, and recipient transplant technique. For instance, in children with unrepaired HLHS, the donor harvest team has to conserve a large segment of donor aorta to facilitate reconstruction of the recipient aorta. The anesthetic management of this child before bypass must account for the possibility of pulmonary overcirculation. Determination of the PVRI, transpulmonary gradient (TPG), and reactivity of the pulmonary vascular bed to pharmacologic manipulation is crucial to the assessment of suitability for cardiac transplant.

enlargement, arrhythmias, and low cardiac output may require systemic anticoagulation to prevent thrombus formation and systemic embolization. Implantable defibrillators have been effective in children large enough for these devices, and biventricular pacing has shown promise as well.[196,197]

Children with end-stage myocardial failure will require mechanical circulatory support as a bridge to transplantation (see Chapter 19). Extracorporeal membrane oxygenation (ECMO) has been used for up to 1200 hours as a bridge to cardiac transplantation.[198]

Newer ventricular assist devices show more promise and applicability to a broad range of children for a much more prolonged period of support.[199-202] Renal failure that requires dialysis reduces survival.[203] Sepsis, neurologic injury, and bleeding are also serious complications of mechanical circulatory support.

Congenital heart disease is the primary indication for cardiac transplantation in infants younger than 1 year of age, and many of these recipients will have HLHS. The patency of the ductus arteriosus must be maintained with prostaglandin $E_1$, initially as a continuous infusion, and perhaps by stenting the ductus in the catheterization laboratory later, if a suitable donor organ is not found. Alteration of flow across the atrial septal defect can be addressed as well by the interventional cardiologist (see Chapter 20). If the balance between systemic and pulmonary blood flow cannot be managed medically, pulmonary artery banding may be necessary to reduce pulmonary overcirculation while waiting for a donor organ.

### SURGICAL TECHNIQUE

The original orthotopic technique devised by Lower and Shumway in adults was popular for many years in children in whom the anatomy was straightforward.[204] This technique avoided individual systemic and pulmonary venous anastomoses by leaving a large cuff of right and left atrial recipient tissue behind and anastomosing the donor right and left atria to these cuffs. The resulting atrial chambers were a combination of donor and recipient atria that contracted asynchronously. Because the atrial contribution to cardiac output may be augmented with total cardiac transplantation, most centers have converted to the "bicaval" technique with a modification to use the standard left atrial anastomosis.[205-208] This technique improves sinus node function, causes less tricuspid regurgitation, and improves exercise tolerance.[209,210]

Cardiac transplantation in children with congenital heart disease may require surgery of greater complexity, involving reconstruction of the great vessels or alterations in venous anastomoses. It is important that the donor harvesting team understand the recipient's anatomy and the potential harvest needs that may require large portions of aorta, pulmonary arteries, and venae cavae. In children with HLHS who require aortic arch reconstruction, deep hypothermic circulatory arrest may be necessary.[211-213]

The recipient is placed on cardiopulmonary bypass (CPB) after median sternotomy with aortic and bicaval cannulation. Cannulation may be modified, depending on the cardiac anatomy encountered. The aorta is cross clamped, and both the aorta and the pulmonary artery are divided at the level of their semilunar valves. The superior and inferior vena cavae are transected, preserving a cuff of atrial tissue on each to facilitate the anastomoses. The interatrial groove is prepared, an encircling left atriotomy is performed, and the recipient heart is removed from the field. The donor organ is prepared and brought to the field.

The left atrial anastomosis is completed first; and while iced saline is bathing the interior and exterior of the heart, the aortic anastomosis is completed. A vent is left in the left ventricular cavity for decompression and evacuation of air as the caval anastomoses are completed while the child is rewarming. The cross clamp is removed, and the donor heart is reperfused while the pulmonary arterial anastomosis is completed. Ventilation is resumed, and the child is liberated from CPB after return of cardiac function is documented by transesophageal echocardiography. Epicardial pacing wires are placed, mediastinal drainage tubes are positioned, and the chest is closed.

### INTRAOPERATIVE PROBLEMS AND MANAGEMENT

Some children listed for cardiac transplantation may be hemodynamically stable and living at home. Preoperative fasting may be an issue in these children. The anesthesiologist must carefully assess the relative risks of a full stomach compared with the potential complications associated with an unexpected difficult airway in a child undergoing a rapid-sequence induction. Several hours may lapse between the call to mobilize the team and the actual surgery, but therapy to modify gastric pH and volume, and the application of cricoid pressure may be warranted. It is equally likely that the pediatric recipient is hospitalized and requires a host of treatments designed to promote hemodynamic stability while a donor organ is sought. These children have minimal cardiovascular reserve. Anesthetic agents, positive-pressure ventilation, and surgical stress frequently result in hemodynamic instability. Anesthetic preparation should include the immediate availability of a variety of medications for the perioperative manipulation of myocardial function and hemodynamics. Vasoactive drugs and inotropic agents, such as epinephrine, phenylephrine, dopamine, dobutamine, isoproterenol, milrinone, nitroprusside, and nitroglycerin, should be readily available. For children with underlying congenital heart disease, the anesthesiologist needs to understand the child's underlying pathophysiology. The anesthetic management before CPB is similar to that for nontransplant cardiac surgery. For children with end-stage myocardial dysfunction, the sympathetic nervous system is chronically activated, with downregulation of the cardiac $\beta_1$-adrenoceptors and an impaired response to $\beta$-adrenoceptor agonists.[214] Reduced renal perfusion stimulates the renin-angiotensin system, leading to increases in vasoconstriction, venoconstriction, and increased intravascular volume. These compensatory changes further aggravate the congestive heart failure by increasing preload and afterload. A dysfunctional, dilated myocardium is very sensitive to changes in preload, afterload, heart rate, and contractility. Both systolic and diastolic myocardial function is impaired, and an increased mean atrial pressure is needed to ensure adequate ventricular filling volume. Increasing heart rate results in a decreased diastolic filling time and, therefore, a diminution in stroke volume as a result of the poor systolic and diastolic ventricular function, atrial pressure increase, and atrial enlargement. There is a loss of preload reserve. Cardiac output then becomes more heart rate dependent, and a decrease in heart rate results in a decreased cardiac output. Furthermore, small increases in afterload result in an increased end-systolic volume, decreased stroke output, and a further decrease in cardiac output. Dysrhythmias are poorly tolerated in these children.

Coordination of the arrival of the child to the OR with the donor team ensures the briefest possible ischemic time for the donor organ. Premedication is best administered under monitored conditions. If the child was receiving supplemental oxygen, it should be continued during the preinduction period. Before induction, monitoring devices, such as a precordial stethoscope, electrocardiogram, noninvasive blood pressure cuff, and pulse oximeter, are applied. Meticulous airway management is critical, because hypoxemia and hypercarbia may alter PVR and further depress cardiac output. A wide variety of anesthetic agents have been used, depending on the nature of the cardiac disease and the risk of pulmonary aspiration. After induction, invasive monitoring does not differ from that used during routine pediatric cardiac open-heart surgery. Some centers avoid right internal jugular vein cannulation because that vessel may be repeatedly accessed for posttransplant endomyocardial biopsy. TEE is useful to assess graft function, mechanical issues, and pulmonary hypertension. In children, TEE has been shown to be a more sensitive monitor for changes in cardiac function than hemodynamic changes.[215,216] Many experienced centers do not use pulmonary artery catheters routinely because the value of the information gained does not warrant the additional risk. In children who have undergone multiple cardiac operations, the potential risks of reoperation should be addressed and should include the need for adequate-sized vascular catheters, the availability of blood products in the OR, the preparation for alternate cannulation sites, and the use of antifibrinolytics. The use of ultrafiltration during CPB may be beneficial by removing free water, hemoconcentrating the red blood cells and coagulation factors, and modulating the inflammatory response.[217-221]

Anesthesia is generally maintained with opioids, benzodiazepines, isoflurane, and a nondepolarizing muscle relaxant. In children with congenital heart disease, this anesthetic technique preserves cardiac output better than some inhalational agents, provided the heart rate is maintained.[222] In preparation for termination of CPB, it is critical that the hemodynamics are optimized. A stable cardiac rhythm and acceptable heart rate are desirable. Chronotropic support, using IV therapy with β-adrenergic agents, such as isoproterenol and epinephrine, or the use of epicardial pacing, may be needed to maintain an appropriate heart rate between 120 and 150 beats per minute. The denervated transplanted heart does not respond in the normal fashion to hypotension. Medications with indirect cardiac effects, such as atropine, glycopyrrolate, or ephedrine, will likewise be ineffective. Direct-acting medications, such as dopamine, dobutamine, epinephrine, or isoproterenol, are required if inotropic or chronotropic support is needed. Some children benefit from vasodilator infusions to improve left ventricular stroke volume and cardiac output.[223] The use of inotropic agents to separate from CPB and provide early postoperative stability is common. The choice of agents is based largely on the perceived balances between pulmonary and systemic vascular resistance, the patient's underlying myocardial function, blood pressure, and cardiac output. Ventilation should be managed to ensure mild respiratory alkalosis and adequate oxygenation. Factors that potentially increase PVR, such as hypothermia, acidosis, hypercarbia, hypoxemia, increased adrenergic tone secondary to light anesthesia, and polycythemia, should be eliminated. Children with increased PAP before bypass show a greater response to ventilatory changes than those without increased PAP. In addition, children with congenital heart disease and associated pulmonary hypertension may develop severe pulmonary hypertension in response to hypoxemia.[224-226] The narrow range of afterload that the donor right ventricle is capable of handling is critical; if managing the pulmonary hypertension with conservative methods is unsuccessful, more aggressive pharmacotherapy is

warranted. The use of prostaglandin, prostacyclin, nitroglycerin, high-dose milrinone, calcium-channel blockers, sildenafil, and inhaled NO have all been effective in treating pulmonary hypertension in children (see Chapter 16).[227-239] In extreme cases, mechanical assist devices or ECMO have been used (see Chapter 19).[240,241]

Dysrhythmias may be common in the postbypass period, and, depending on the technique of implantation, there may be two independent P waves on the electrocardiogram, one from the recipient sinoatrial node and the other from the donor sinoatrial node. It is only the donor sinoatrial node that transmits impulses to the atrioventricular node and thus to the ventricle. The most common dysrhythmias are junctional rhythms, underscoring the utility of direct-acting β-adrenoceptor agonists and epicardial atrioventricular sequential pacing. This denervated state results in the loss of the baroreceptor reflex, forcing cardiac output to become primarily dependent on venous return and circulating catecholamines, and thus unable to respond acutely to changes in the circulating blood volume and blood pressure.[242-243]

After separation from CPB, hemodynamic stabilization, and control of surgical bleeding, protamine sulfate is administered slowly to reverse anticoagulation. Risk factors for hypotension in children after protamine administration following bypass include female sex, greater protamine doses, and smaller heparin doses.[244] Transfusion of blood products is determined by a balance of the need against the associated risks of administration. There may be significant acid-base and electrolyte disturbances associated with large-volume transfusions. These disturbances may be decreased by washing the cells before transfusion.[245,246] Donor blood should be screened for CMV and, ideally, CMV-negative recipients should receive blood that has screened negative for CMV.[247] Leukocyte reduction by filtration may be associated with a diminished risk of exposure to CMV through transfusion.[248,249] Another concern associated with transfusion in cardiac transplant recipients is the risk of transfusion-associated graft-versus-host disease (TAGVHD). This results from active T lymphocytes in the transfused blood of a recipient who is unable to reject them, such as a neonate, those undergoing chemotherapy, and the otherwise immunocompromised child.[250,251] To limit the risk of TAGVHD in cardiac transplant recipients, some centers routinely irradiate cellular blood products with γ-radiation before administration. At recommended doses, γ-radiation has an insignificant effect on platelet, red cell, or granulocyte function, but it may increase the free potassium concentrations (see Chapter 10).[252,247]

Transport of the child from the OR proceeds as in any other open-heart procedure. In selected recipients with excellent allograft function and hemodynamics, extubation of the trachea is possible in the OR or within a few hours of arrival in the ICU. It is important that these children are comfortable, but otherwise ventilating adequately to prevent atelectasis, hypoxemia, or hypercarbia that may increase PAP and thus strain the donor right ventricle. Newer agents, such as dexmedetomidine, may facilitate early extubation in these children.[253] Other children may require sedation and mechanical ventilation as a result of hemodynamic instability or because of delayed sternal closure, particularly if a large donor-to-recipient size mismatch is present.

## IMMEDIATE POSTOPERATIVE MANAGEMENT
Early postoperative management consists primarily in maintaining hemodynamic stability. Infusions and volume needs are adjusted to maintain an optimal balance of preload, afterload, cardiac output, and peripheral perfusion. Attention should be

directed toward maintaining normal acid-base and electrolyte balance. In some children, pulmonary hypertension remains a serious concern, and management of sedation, ventilation, inotrope infusions, and pulmonary vasodilator administration is required to optimize right ventricular function. Ventilation modes may need to be adjusted to reduce the mean intrathoracic (airway) pressure. Renal dysfunction continues to be a major source of morbidity and mortality after cardiac transplantation. Decreased perioperative renal function can occur in as many as 20% of children after cardiac transplantation.[254,255] A peritoneal dialysis catheter, placed at the time of cardiac transplant, can be used to reduce ascites and improve ventilatory mechanics in those with right-sided heart dysfunction, and in the treatment of renal insufficiency. Arrhythmias in the postoperative period may herald rejection.

Immunosuppression begins with corticosteroids administered before removal of the aortic cross clamp, and continues into the postoperative period. Immunosuppression induction continues postoperatively, with infusions of antibodies to reduce early rejection and to diminish dose requirements of corticosteroids and calcineurins. T-cell–depleting antibodies include polyclonal rabbit antithymocyte globulin (Thymoglobulin), equine antithymocyte globulin (Atgam), and monoclonal muromonab-CD3 (OKT3). IL-2 blockers (basiliximab and daclizumab) may also be used for induction. Maintenance therapy is guided largely by institutional experience and the recipient's clinical profile. The goal of maintenance therapy is to prevent acute and chronic rejection, while minimizing the adverse effects of immunosuppression. All maintenance regimens involve a CNI along with antiproliferative agents, or sirolimus. Corticosteroids may also be used, although most centers limit or avoid their long-term use. CNIs include cyclosporine and tacrolimus. Antiproliferative agents include azathioprine and mycophenolate mofetil (CellCept). Sirolimus (rapamycin) is a macrolide antibiotic that acts synergistically with the CNIs and can be used to reduce the dose of cyclosporine or tacrolimus. Sirolimus may also inhibit the process of coronary arteriopathy.[256]

First-line therapy for acute rejection is high-dose corticosteroids. Other agents, including monoclonal and polyclonal anti–T-lymphocyte antibodies, are reserved for refractory or recurrent severe acute rejection, or rejection with severe hemodynamic compromise. Recurrent moderate rejection is usually controlled with modulation of the maintenance-therapy dosing.[257]

In spite of the remarkable improvements in immunosuppression and patient selection, acute and chronic rejection remain the major cause of death after pediatric cardiac transplantation (E-Tables 29-5 and 29-6).[258,259] Monitoring and diagnosis of allograft rejection remain a challenge. Some studies suggest that transplant before 1 year of age offers protection from episodes of acute rejection, and significantly greater freedom from rejection and time to first rejection.[260] Rejection surveillance in children includes three levels of detection. The clinical assessment includes nursing and parental accounts of changes in the child's activity and appetite, nausea, emesis, malaise, resting heart rate 15 to 20 beats per minute above normal, and presence of ectopia. Echocardiography has become very important in the postoperative follow-up, especially in neonates. These studies are performed frequently, especially in the first months after the transplant. Acute changes in left ventricular end-diastolic dimension, posterior wall thickness, and shortening fraction are potential signs of acute rejection.[261] Endomyocardial biopsy remains the standard in the diagnosis

of acute cardiac allograft rejection. It provides tissue for both precise documentation of the presence or absence of rejection, and allows more accurate titration of immunosuppression, to avoid the adverse effects of increased use of immunosuppression based on clinical and noninvasive examinations only. Biopsy specimens are also analyzed for signs of humoral and vascular rejection. The biopsy specimen is examined for evidence of lymphocytic accumulations in the graft interstitium and perivascular tissue, and in severe forms of cellular rejection, myocardial necrosis and polymorphonuclear cell infiltrates. Over time, it is also possible to develop chronic rejection, which is primarily a vasculopathy that involves vascular inflammation, with binding of IgG and/or IgM and complement. This produces a diffuse and concentric stenosis affecting the mid and distal coronary arteries and is often asymptomatic. Although annual coronary angiography is recommended, accelerated graft arteriosclerosis is underestimated angiographically.

New techniques are being developed to identify early evidence of rejection. Serum vascular endothelial growth factor may be a marker for cellular rejection.[262] Vascular endothelial growth factor is an established angiogenesis factor and is expressed in allografts undergoing rejection, but its function in the rejection process has not been defined. The possibility also exists for the detection of graft rejection by the examination of the characteristic gene expression patterns in peripheral blood mononuclear cells of heart transplant recipients.[263]

## LONG-TERM OUTCOME AND QUALITY OF LIFE
Over 500 pediatric heart transplants are performed annually, giving a total of more than 6000 worldwide since 1982. Approximately 50% of the recipients do not require hospitalization in the first year after transplantation and, by 3 years, more than 70% are free from hospitalization. One year after transplant, 93% of survivors are without functional limitations. This increases to 95% by 5 years after transplant (E-Figs. 29-4 and 29-5; Table 29-4). The prevalence of posttransplant morbidities for 5-year transplant survivors is as follows: hypertension (61%), hyperlipidemia (21%), coronary vasculopathy (11%), renal dysfunction (9%), and diabetes mellitus (5%) (Table 29-5). At one center, 13% of pediatric cardiac recipients returned to the ORs for noncardiac procedures.[264] Preoperative evaluation requires an understanding of the unique features associated with the transplanted heart, such as its denervation, risk of vasculopathy (coronary artery disease), and arrhythmias. The interaction of the immunosuppressive regimens with anesthetic agents and their association with hypertension and renal dysfunction are additional considerations. Medication and monitoring choice should be tailored to the individual needs of the child to minimize anesthetic morbidity. Most medically stable cardiac transplant patients can undergo routine noncardiac surgical procedures in a similar fashion to children who haven't received transplants (see Chapter 21). It is important to remember that reflex mechanisms are impaired in the denervated heart, and changes as a result of light anesthesia, hypovolemia, or contractility will be delayed until circulating catecholamines can influence the cardiac β-adrenoceptors directly.[265,266] As cardiac-transplant children live longer, the risks of coronary vasculopathy increase, with coronary ischemia becoming a major concern. Therefore attention to the maintenance of coronary perfusion is paramount. As in all immunocompromised patients, these children are vulnerable to infection, and strict adherence to aseptic and sterile technique is mandatory.

**TABLE 29-4** Post–Heart Transplant Morbidity for Pediatric Patients: Cumulative Prevalence in Survivors within 1 Year Posttransplant (Follow-ups: April 1994 to June 2004)

| Outcome | Morbidity within 1 Year (%) | Total with Known Response |
|---|---|---|
| Hypertension | 46.7 | 2184 |
| Renal dysfunction | 5.8 | 21 |
| Abnormal creatinine <2.5 mg/dL | 3.8 | 83 |
| Creatinine >2.5 mg/dL | 1.3 | |
| Chronic dialysis | 0.6 | |
| Renal transplant | 0.0 | |
| Hyperlipidemia | 10.1 | 2285 |
| Diabetes | 3.2 | 2188 |
| Coronary artery vasculopathy | 2.5 | 1996 |

Data from Boucek MM, Edwards LB, Keck BM, et al. Registry of the International Society for Heart and Lung Transplantation: eighth official pediatric report—2005. J Heart Lung Transplant 2005;24:968-82.

**TABLE 29-5** Post–Heart Transplant Morbidity for Pediatric Patients: Cumulative Prevalence in Survivors within 5 Years Posttransplant (Follow-Ups: April 1994 to June 2004)

| Outcome | Morbidity within 5 Years (%) | Total with Known Response |
|---|---|---|
| Hypertension | 61.4 | 696 |
| Renal dysfunction | 9.4 | 715 |
| Abnormal creatinine <2.5 mg/dL | 8.0 | |
| Creatinine >2.5 mg/dL | 0.8 | |
| Chronic dialysis | 0.4 | |
| Renal transplant | 0.1 | |
| Hyperlipidemia | 21.4 | 746 |
| Diabetes | 4.6 | 694 |
| Coronary artery vasculopathy | 11.0 | 480 |

Data from Boucek MM, Edwards LB, Keck BM, et al. Registry of the International Society for Heart and Lung Transplantation: eighth official pediatric report—2005. J Heart Lung Transplant 2005;24:968-82.

# Pediatric Heart-Lung and Lung Transplantation

## DEMOGRAPHICS AND EPIDEMIOLOGY

Pediatric heart-lung and lung transplants, unavailable just a generation ago, are now relatively commonplace at a number of pediatric specialty hospitals. There are 35 to 40 centers that perform pediatric lung transplants, and roughly 10 centers perform heart-lung transplants. The first successful pediatric heart-lung transplant was performed at the Children's Hospital of Pittsburgh in 1985. Pediatric lung transplantation followed in Toronto in 1986, recalling the success of adult lung transplantation in the early 1980's.

In 1962 the first adult lung transplant recipient survived for eighteen days after transplantation. It was not until the early 1980s that advances in surgical technique and immunosuppressive therapy ushered in the modern era of lung transplantation. Subsequently, heart-lung and lung transplantation have become a well-accepted treatment for both adults and children with end-stage cardiopulmonary and pulmonary disease. There have been over 1500 pediatric lung transplants since the first pediatric lung transplantation in 1986, with an additional 550 heart-lung transplants.[267] The management of the heart-lung transplant patient enjoys many similarities with that of the lung transplant patient, including a sharing of many of the underlying disease processes. Nonetheless, the number of heart-lung transplants continues to decrease yearly, from a high of seventeen in the late 1990's. Only 4 centers reported performing a pediatric heart-lung transplant in 2008.[268] Although this decrease in transplants may be related to a decrease in suitable donor availability, it is more likely a result of an increasing awareness that even longstanding right ventricular dysfunction in the face of significant pulmonary hypertension exhibits reversibility post–lung transplant. Therefore heart-lung transplants are less necessary than previously thought.

Children with end-stage pulmonary and cardiopulmonary disease who receive heart-lung transplant or lung transplants, frequently undergo a variety of interventions both pre- and post-transplant. These ill children require special considerations in all phases of their anesthetic care.

The number of children listed on all transplant waiting lists continually outstrips the donor supply. Donor identification and management are more selective for heart-lung and lung transplant candidates than isolated heart transplants. One example of this increased selectivity is that the thoracic capacity of the donor should not be greater than that of the recipients. If it is larger the transplanted lungs will be at an increased risk of postoperative atelectasis and infections.[269] Donor supply remains the largest obstacle in transplantation. As many as one-third of all children listed on the waiting list die before receiving lung transplantation.[270-271] The average waiting time for cadaveric lungs is 20 months for adolescents and 6 to 12 months for children less than 2 years old. As experience in pediatric lung transplantation increases, it is likely that accepted indications for transplantation will increase as well. In that eventuality, time spent on the waiting list is likely to grow, given that there is no indication the donor pool is increasing.

A variety of strategies have been undertaken to increase the size of the donor pool. Television, radio, and print advertisements have been provided to the public. Everyone has the opportunity to declare themselves a potential donor when obtaining a drivers license in the United States. Some states go further. Pennsylvania has laws requiring nurses to ask the patient's family members whether they will consent for donation in the event of the patient's death.

Some countries have a longstanding reluctance to donate organs. These barriers to transplantation can come down by increasing education. More often it takes a dramatic event to engender change. Nicholas Green, a 7-year-old American boy, was vacationing in Italy in 1999 when he was shot in the head by a random act of violence and subsequently declared brain dead. His parents elected to donate his organs. Seven Italian citizens received his organs. In the wake of the publicity of the shooting and subsequent organ donation, signed organ donation cards in Italy quadrupled, and actual donations tripled. Donors' families may also gain some solace from donation. Green's father stated: "There is some consolation with the process. It puts something on the other side of the balance. It will never bring my son back, but it can help somewhat with the grief."[272] However, in other countries, such as Japan, organ donation rate is much less than in North America. In part, this is because of cultural concerns and fears that patients might be declared brain-dead just for their organs and, in part, because Japanese culture expects reciprocal gift giving rather than selfless altruism of organ donation, as is more common in Western cultures. Despite the 1997 inculcation of "brain-death" criteria in Japan, it was not until July 17, 2010, that the revised Organ Transplant Act permitted children less than 15 years of age to donate organs.

## PATHOPHYSIOLOGY OF THE DISEASE

The indication for heart-lung and lung transplantation is severe end-stage pulmonary disease, for which there is no other medical treatment, and a life expectancy less than 18 months. The listing criteria for the prospective transplant patient additionally includes consideration of the functional status of the child, the child's hemodynamic parameters, and the natural history of the underlying disease. For example, children with pulmonary hypertension may progress to end-stage pulmonary disease rapidly. Most pediatric lung transplant patients are 11 to 17 years old, with a smaller subset of children less than 2 years old.[273] The most common underlying disease in elder pediatric lung transplantation patients is cystic fibrosis, accounting for nearly half of all pediatric lung transplants. Of children with cystic fibrosis who do not receive transplants, 95% will eventually succumb because of pulmonary issues. Factors associated with why less than 50% of cystic fibrosis patients survive include an $FEV_1$ (forced expiratory volume in 1 second) of less than 30%, a predicted $PaO_2$ less than 55 mm Hg or a $PaCO_2$ greater than 50 mm Hg.[274] Pulmonary vascular disease accounts for nearly one-fourth of the remaining transplantations. Infants who require transplantation, most often have a variety of relatively rare diseases, such as surfactant B deficiency, primary alveolar proteinosis, or pulmonary vascular disease.[275] These infants are often severely ill at the time of their transplantation. Their tracheas are frequently intubated and they receive mechanical assistance for oxygenation and ventilation, or even require ECMO. Independent risks for mortality after lung transplant include repeat transplant, mechanical ventilation at time of transplant,[276] and congenital heart disease.[277,278] Although at one time it was thought that prior thoracic surgery was a contraindication for lung transplantation, as experience has grown, this is no longer considered a contraindication.[279] In fact, a significant number of children who receive lung transplant have had prior thoracic surgery for congenital heart disease. Furthermore, prior lung transplantation is not a contraindication for subsequent lung transplantation.[280] Today the primary contraindications for lung transplantation are (1) active malignant disease within the prior 2 years, which may be unmasked by the immunosuppressive therapy required in transplantation, (2) significant active infectious processes (including HIV and hepatitis B and C), (3) significant coexisting cardiac disease, (4) hepatic or renal disease (although these children may be candidates for multiple organ transplants), (5) collagen vascular disease, (6) major irreversible neurologic injury, and (7) patient or family history of poor medical compliance or severe psychiatric illness that would preclude the child from effective posttransplant care. Relative contraindications include (1) significant musculoskeletal disease, (2) invasive ventilation, (3) colonization with atypical mycobacterium or fungi, (4) poor nutritional status (body mass index at either extreme), and (5) inability to reduce dependency on corticosteroids. A lung allocation score is calculated for each patient on the waiting list aged twelve years or older.[281] Variables

considered in calculating the individual child's score include age, underlying illness, forced vital capacity, functional status, and need for supplemental oxygen.[282] The UNOS also includes ABO compatibility and distance between the donor and the recipient in its considerations for organ allocation.

UNOS adopted a new allocation system for children younger than 12 years old in 2010. There are now two distinct priority levels, with the most ill children given a priority 1 ranking. Priority 1 candidates will have respiratory failure with the need or presence of continuous mechanical ventilation, fraction of inspired oxygen ($FIO_2$) greater than 0.5 to maintain arterial oxygen saturation levels of more than 90%, an arterial or capillary $PCO_2$ of more than 50 mm Hg or a venous $PCO_2$ of more than 56 mm Hg and/or significant pulmonary hypertension despite medical therapy. Children not meeting the above conditions are listed as priority 2. Donor lungs are first allocated to the priority 1 candidate longest on the waiting list who matches the donor's size and blood type. If there is no suitable priority 1 candidate, the lungs are then offered to the priority 2 candidate with the most waiting time.

The care of the donor is critical. The donor must first meet criteria for brain death. Additionally, the donor should have been intubated less than 5 days to decrease the risk of lung injury, particularly ventilator-associated pneumonia. The donor should have no active infection. In particular, tracheal secretions must be void of infection. The donor should have either a $PaO_2$ greater than 300 mm Hg at an $FIO_2$ 1.0, or greater than 100 mm Hg at an $FIO_2$ of 0.4, with an inflation pressure less than 30 cm $H_2O$, with tidal volumes of 15 mL/kg, and a PEEP of 4 cm $H_2O$. For lung donation, the donor is kept euvolemic to slightly hypovolemic, with central venous pressures in the range of 8 to 10 mm Hg. On occasion this places the physicians desiring to use the donor kidneys at odds with those desiring to use the heart and lungs. In such situations, the goal is to meet the desires of all, within reason, so that as many of the potential organs may be used as possible. When lungs are harvested, they are perfused with a preservative solution and prostaglandins, which reduces the incidence of graft failures. The lungs are inflated and the trachea is stapled closed to maintain an inflated position. The organs are then transported to the recipient at a temperature of 4° C. Ischemic times of less than 8 hours are desired; less than 3 to 4 hours is ideal.

Another avenue being explored to increase the availability of organs suitable for lung transplantation is the nonheartbeating donor (NHBD).[283] Kidneys,[284] livers,[285] and other tissues have been used successfully from NHBDs. NHBDs may prove to be an as yet untapped resource and facilitate an expansion of pediatric lung transplantation. A system has been developed in Madrid that allows out-of-hospital emergency services personnel and transplant teams to initiate a protocol to harvest organs from NHBDs. They reported success in two children who were discharged to home after receiving lung transplants from NHBDs.[286] NHBDs are typically younger than traditional donors.

An additional resource of lung donation is the living related-donor with transplantation of adult lobes into the child.[287,288] Living related transplants overcome some of the difficulties inherent in attempting to predict the clinical course of the underlying disease, by being able to electively schedule the transplant. However, the inherent size mismatch limits the use of this technique to children 5 years and older. Typically, the left lower lobe is harvested from one donor while the right lower lobe is harvested from another donor. The harvest technique is similar to that of a lobectomy; however, the technique requires an appropriate length of bronchus and adequate vascular pedicles. Morbidity in the donor is significant.[289]

## PREOPERATIVE EVALUATION

Children listed for lung transplantation undergo an extensive work up. Commonly included are chest radiographs, pulmonary function tests, arterial blood gas, complete metabolic panel, electrocardiogram, and echocardiogram. If the child has pulmonary hypertension and/or associated cardiac defects, they also require a cardiac catheterization. The catheterization will define the patient's anatomy and allow measurement of pulmonary vascular resistance.

When the decision is made to proceed with transplantation, the donor is notified. A short ischemic time (the time from when the donor lungs are explanted to when they are implanted into the recipient) is desired. Prolonged ischemic times have been implicated in increasing the risk of bronchiolitis obliterans (BO), a major source of morbidity in the posttransplant period. In light of this desire to proceed expeditiously, the anesthesiologist commonly has limited time to collate all the data and perform their preoperative evaluation. The cautious use of premedication may be beneficial. Commonly used anxiolytics include midazolam and ketamine, with consideration of a relatively new agent, dexmedetomidine, an $\alpha_1$-adrenoceptor agonist sedative with minimal depression of respiratory drive.

## SURGICAL TECHNIQUE

Children most commonly receive bilateral lung transplants with CPB.[290,291] To facilitate this, most pediatric lung transplantations are performed via a bilateral anterolateral transsternal "clamshell" incision. Before institution of CPB, as much dissection as possible is carried out. The anastomosis itself is made with two bronchial anastomoses rather than one tracheal anastomosis. Tracheal anastomoses have been found to produce less satisfactory results than bilateral bronchial reanastomosis and have largely fallen out of favor. Bilateral bronchial anastomosis has been found to produce better results, without the concern of tracheal stenosis. Traditionally each bronchus is anastomosed with an end-to-end anastomosis. The most popular technique now is the telescoping anastomosis, in which the larger bronchus is telescoped several centimeters over the smaller bronchus portion, with peribronchial tissue being wrapped around the anastomosis to ensure blood supply, because bronchial blood supply is not reestablished. If the end-to-end anastomosis technique is used, this traditional method may include an omental wrap around the suture line. Once the bronchus is anastomosed, the pulmonary artery is anastomosed. The donor lung includes an atrial cuff, which is sutured directly to the left atrium of the recipient. Use of the donor atrial cuff avoids the complication of pulmonary vein stenosis. Although donor lungs are selected to be a size match, occasionally the lungs are too large for the recipient and can not be used en toto without predisposing to significant areas of atelectasis. If deemed too large, volume reduction may be undertaken to remove areas prone to atelectasis.[292,293]

Single lung transplants are infrequently performed in children and are specifically avoided in cystic fibrosis patients, to avoid damage from the remaining diseased lung. If single lung transplantation is performed for the non–cystic fibrosis patient, the side chosen to transplant is the most diseased side, preserving the best lung to remain in situ. Additionally, if emphysema changes

are present, the most emphysematous lung is removed to decrease the risk of compression of the donor lung. Single lung transplants are most often performed without CPB. Single lung ventilation is procured and a thoracotomy is performed, exposing the bronchus and vessels. A test occlusion by the surgeon of the pulmonary artery to the proposed explant lung is then performed to evaluate the ability of the child to withstand the procedure without CPB. Presuming the child tolerates the test clamp, the surgery proceeds with the removal of the native diseased lung. The donor lung is anastomosed by first connecting the pulmonary vein atrial flap to the native left atrium, followed by anastomosing the pulmonary artery. As in the technique for sequential bilateral lung transplants previously described, the smaller of the two bronchial ends is telescoped into the other, with an overlap of one cartilage ring. The lung is then gently inflated. Air within the lung vasculature is vented via the pulmonary artery or the atrial cuff, with the left atrium partially occluded. Once de-airing is accomplished, ventilation and perfusion of the donor lung are both established.

## INTRAOPERATIVE PROBLEMS AND MANAGEMENT

Children arriving for lung and heart-lung transplant are often critically ill. Cystic fibrosis patients are often quite compromised when they arrive for transplant, frequently unable to comfortably lie down because of excess secretions. Children with pulmonary fibrosis or end-stage chronic obstructive pulmonary disease may be marginally hypoxic and hypercarbic at baseline, with elevated pulmonary artery pressures and right heart dysfunction. If premedication is necessary, caution must be exercised to not decrease respiratory drive to any significant degree, which would possibly precipitate worsening hypoxemia, hypercarbia, and right heart failure.

Pretransplant, children commonly have a "full stomach" because of the often short interval between their notification of impending transplant and the timing of the transplant itself. In such circumstances, a rapid sequence or modified rapid sequence induction may be considered. However, if possible, the best route is likely one of a more gentle induction. The choice of induction agents is broad and must take into account comorbid illnesses, such as significant right heart dysfunction or other congenital anomalies, in addition to the end-stage pulmonary disease. A one-size-fits-all anesthetic technique is not appropriate for heart-lung and lung transplantations. Once standard monitors have been applied, propofol, sodium thiopental, etomidate, or even volatile anesthetics may be considered as primary induction agents, either alone or in combination with narcotics or benzodiazepines. Much of the peritransplant anesthetic considerations focus on the optimization of pulmonary vascular resistance. Elevations in pulmonary vascular resistance may cause acute right ventricular failure, with reduced cardiac output. Right sided pressures can increase enough to cause significant right-to-left shunting through intracardiac lesions, and result in desaturation. Heart-lung transplants are generally reserved for those children with the worst pulmonary hypertension and right heart dysfunction. Ketamine does not appear to significantly alter pulmonary vascular resistance in infants[294] and may be considered as a first-choice drug.[295,296,297] Given the desire to rapidly intubate and control the airway, a relatively rapid-onset neuromuscular blocking agent, such as rocuronium, is most commonly used. Initial ventilator settings must take into account the underlying disease process. For example, fibrotic lungs may be better served by smaller tidal volumes with a faster rate, allowing a decreased peak inspiratory pressure while preserving minute ventilation. On the other hand, severe obstructive disease may best be served by a slower pattern, with an expiratory time long enough that it does not induce dynamic hyperinflation (auto-PEEP). PEEP may be beneficial to improve oxygenation and ventilation, and decrease atelectasis. Nonetheless, both dynamic hyperinflation and PEEP, by increasing intrathoracic pressure, may decrease venous return and cause hemodynamic compromise, particularly in relatively hypovolemic children. Should hemodynamic collapse occur with the institution of ventilation in a child with severe obstructive lung disease, dynamic hyperinflation should be immediately considered among the possible etiologies. Rapid treatment is provided by just disconnecting the child from the ventilator circuit and allowing the child to exhale. When ventilation is reinstituted, care must be taken to allow for adequate expiratory time.

Anesthetic maintenance is most commonly with a balanced anesthetic, typically opioid-based and supplemented with volatile anesthesia to ensure amnesia. Volatile anesthetic based techniques are less common because of their cardiovascular depression and vasodilation. Furthermore, volatile anesthetics blunt hypoxic pulmonary vasoconstriction, and may make it more difficult to maintain adequate oxygenation should off CPB lung transplantation be desired. Nitrous oxide is avoided because of its propensity to increase pulmonary vascular resistance[298,299,300] and its property of expanding small air bubbles, which may be present in the microcirculation of the transplanted lung on reimplantation. Consideration may also be given to regional anesthesia techniques. Because of concerns regarding the use of CPB for these procedures and its attendant need for systemic heparinization, epidural thoracic catheters used for postoperative pain control are generally placed postoperatively, when the child's coagulation profile has normalized.

The anesthesiologist is also likely responsible for the administration of the preoperative antibiotics and immunosuppressive medications required for lung transplantation. Many transplant centers include the use of immunosuppressive induction therapy. More than half of all recipients are now receiving either IL-2 receptor antagonists or cytolytic medications. There is no clear-cut consensus on this point; however, some centers believe it best to avoid this treatment because of the profound immunosuppression and the risk for perioperative infections.

The vast majority of pediatric lung transplants are performed with the assistance of CPB. This contrasts to the non-CPB technique most commonly employed in adults. There are several reasons for the evolution of this distinction. Cystic fibrosis patients have a significant risk of cross contamination of the donor lung during a bilateral sequential lung transplant. This risk of damage is minimized by the simultaneous removal of both lungs. Furthermore, children with pulmonary hypertension are frequently too unstable to tolerate single-lung ventilation. An additional difficulty is that many children are too small to accommodate a double-lumen tube and single-lung ventilation may be difficult. CPB alleviates these issues and allows the surgeon a quiet field with good exposure and predictable hemodynamics, thus speeding the time for anastomosis and decreasing the overall ischemic time.

If the child does undergo either single-lung transplant or sequential bilateral lung transplant without CPB, continual vigilance and reassessment of the patient's condition is required. These are extremely ill children undergoing dramatic perturbations to their homeostasis. Single-lung ventilation often precipitates hypoxemia and hypercarbia. The combination of the increased afterload on the right heart by the clamping of the pulmonary artery, along with hypercarbia and hypoxemia-induced pulmonary hypertension on the other lung, may precipitate right heart failure. Attempts to diminish pulmonary hypertension may be undertaken with pulmonary vascular dilators and inotropes, such as milrinone, prostaglandins, or NO, along with maintaining an adequate right-sided filling pressure. Nonetheless, continued right heart failure may necessitate CPB. If the child can tolerate clamping of the pulmonary artery, it is typical that the gas exchange improves as the shunting through the nonventilated lung is stopped and the perfusion-ventilation mismatch is diminished.

Bilateral sequential lung transplants performed on CPB do not offer these problems. Nonetheless, CPB does not come without cost. Gas exchange may worsen as a result of reperfusion injury and pulmonary edema, with the concomitant decrease in lung compliance. Inflammatory mediators are liberated and the complement cascade is initiated, perhaps contributing to reperfusion injury in the transplanted lungs. The systemic heparinization required for CPB further increases the risk for perioperative bleeding and the need for transfusion of blood products. Packed red blood cells, platelets, and clotting factors are typically required. Some of these needs may be mitigated with the addition of fibrinolytics.

When the procedure is performed with CPB, there is no need to perform single-lung ventilation, so airway management of the child is accomplished with a single lumen endotracheal tube after the patient has been anesthetized. Cuffed endotracheal tubes are typically chosen for the ability to provide a better tracheal fit and allow for the potential ventilation of the lungs with relatively high pressures, both pretransplant and posttransplant, with less concern about excessive air leak. In the rare circumstances that the operation of pediatric lung transplantation is performed without CPB, single-lung ventilation will be required. Double-lumen tubes may be used in older children. If a double-lumen tube is used, it is exchanged for a single lumen endotracheal tube at the conclusion of the operation, unless there is a desire to continue with differential lung ventilation or there is a concern about contralateral lung contamination. In small children either a bronchial blocker or selective intubation of a single bronchus may be considered. These options, however, preclude the ability to suction the nonventilated lung. Once the child has been intubated, additional invasive monitoring is placed, typically an arterial catheter and a central venous catheter, along with two large-bore IV catheters. Some centers will place a pulmonary artery catheter, in addition to or in place of the percutaneous central venous line. Occasionally, the surgeon will place a right atrial catheter. If a pulmonary artery catheter is placed, it must be withdrawn into the main pulmonary artery before pneumonectomy. A transesophageal echocardiography (TEE) probe is then placed to assist in evaluation of residual cardiac abnormalities and cardiac performance, particularly right ventricular performance, both pretransplant and posttransplant, while weaning from CPB.[301]

Perioperative bleeding is common, both in the OR after coming off CPB and in the immediate postoperative period. Extensive pulmonary-to-systemic collaterals, coagulopathies resulting from hepatic dysfunction, and significant adhesions from prior surgeries or cystic fibrosis may make the surgical dissection difficult and precipitate blood loss. Fibrinolytics have been demonstrated to reduce bleeding in children with prior thoracic surgery.[302]

During CPB the patient is typically cooled to 32° C. Cystic fibrosis patients are uniformly colonized with bacteria, and after the native lungs are removed, their tracheal stump is irrigated with antibiotic solution to reduce contamination of the transplanted lungs. Despite best efforts, occasionally these children develop sepsis or a syndrome similar to septic shock caused by liberation of bacteria and toxic mediators during the removal of the native lungs. Such children require intensive therapy and often do poorly.

Following the first lung being implanted, a small amount of blood is allowed to eject into the pulmonary artery while the second lung is being anastomosed, reducing ischemic time for the first lung. After the second lung is implanted, the lungs are ventilated to remove all areas of atelectasis. Posttransplant ventilation strategy limits tidal volumes to maintain peak inspiratory pressures less than 35 cm $H_2O$ and PEEP in the range of 5 to 10 cm $H_2O$. It is typical to augment myocardial performance with inotropic support before termination of CPB. Occasionally, a combination of inotropes, dilators, or pressors may be required. Some centers routinely use NO and/or prostaglandin $E_1$ ($PGE_1$) to reduce pulmonary vascular resistance, whereas others reserve their use only to treat problematic pulmonary hypertension. Fiberoptic bronchoscopy may be performed to assess the bronchial anastomotic sites, either in the OR, or within the first 24 hours postoperatively, along with a lung perfusion scan.

In the heart-lung transplant patient, weaning from CPB is analogous to that for the cardiac transplant patient, described elsewhere in this chapter. There remains the need to support the denervated heart with adequate fluids and inotropy. Maintaining adequate fluid status in these children may require a bit more effort because of increased bleeding when compared to heart transplant patients. Bleeding is further exacerbated in these children as a result of bronchial circulation and extensive collaterals, which have often developed. Blood products are uniformly required in these children.

The onset of acute graft dysfunction may present with persistent hypoxemia after weaning from CPB. Although this may be attributable to relatively reversible causes, such as inadequate ventilation, atelectasis, or right ventricular dysfunction with right-to-left shunting, a more ominous problem may be reperfusion injury. Free radicals and inflammatory mediators are readily produced by the lung during both the ischemic time and during reperfusion. Reperfusion injury is correlated with greater ischemic times. Reperfusion injury presents as hypoxemia in the face of adequate ventilation and no other clear etiology of the hypoxemia. Pink frothy secretions noted in the endotracheal tube often indicate reperfusion injury. $PGE_1$ may reduce reperfusion injury risk and symptoms. Although some routinely start $PGE_1$ infusion at 0.025 µg/kg/min, even before returning circulation to the first anastomosed lung, and continue this treatment for the first 24 to 48 postoperative hours, prevention of prolonged ischemic times is the best treatment. Ventilation strategy aims at maintaining adequate oxygenation and ventilation with adequate PEEP and the lowest peak inspiratory pressures possible. $FIO_2$ is aimed to keep $PaO_2$ less than 120 mm Hg to avoid oxygen toxicity. NO, a potent smooth muscle relaxant, is gaining favor for use in this setting as well. Although it has not been shown that prophylactic NO prevents reperfusion injury, NO in the dose range of 20 to 60 parts per million has been demonstrated to be effective in children with elevated pulmonary artery and right heart pressures coupled with hypoxemia.[303,304] Another option may be inhaled prostacyclin, which

had been demonstrated to be safe and useful in the treatment of pulmonary hypertension and reperfusion injury.[305] Nonetheless, on occasion, all these measures remain inadequate. In this event, ECMO should be instituted to allow the donor lungs to recover.[306]

## IMMEDIATE POSTOPERATIVE MANAGEMENT

The immediate postoperative care of the patient is individualized based on the child's age, pretransplantation diagnosis and pretransplantation comorbidities. Older children with cystic fibrosis usually require mechanical ventilation for several days. Their time-to-discharge from the critical care unit averages less than 1 week.[307] After extubation, these children may still require some supplemental oxygen for exercise therapy. Infants and children without cystic fibrosis, typically more acutely ill pretransplant, require an average of more than 3 weeks of mechanical ventilation and average nearly 2 months of critical care stay.[308] These younger transplantation patients are smaller in size, have an increased incidence of airway complications, and may suffer from associated congenital cardiac defects. Children with significant pretransplantation pulmonary hypertension often manifest significant hemodynamic instability postoperatively. In anticipation of this, these children are kept intubated, sedated, and frequently paralyzed for the first 2 postoperative days.

Posttransplantation patients require aggressive chest physiotherapy to avoid lung congestion that could lead to infection and respiratory failure. The child's cough reflex is absent and mucociliary transport is disrupted across the bronchial suture line. Frequent endotracheal suctioning is mandatory. Therapeutic bronchoscopy for pulmonary toilet may also be required. In addition to the risk for infections resulting from pulmonary considerations, the surgical sites, catheters, and drains also add to the risk of infection. Prophylactic antibiotics are given perioperatively, including antivirals and antifungals, particularly if underlying fungal infection or viral infection (such as cytomegalovirus)[309] are present in either the donor or recipient.

Postoperative pain control is critical to ensure effective pulmonary toilet. It is most readily obtained with judicious use of opioids. Patient-controlled analgesia may be considered in those children deemed able to use such a device. Regional anesthesia may also be used, but because of the systemic heparinization on CPB, many are reluctant to place a catheter prebypass. If regional anesthesia is desired, a thoracic epidural or paravertebral catheters may be placed postoperatively when the coagulation status of the child has normalized. Dexmedetomidine may also be used as adjunct pain management. Dexmedetomidine is an $α_2$-adrenoceptor agonist, offering an arousable sedation with minimal effect on respiratory drive. Dexmedetomidine has been demonstrated to decrease opioid use by one-half in postoperative children, and may additionally decrease the incidence of opioid tolerance.

## LONG-TERM ISSUES

Because of the large endothelial surface in the lungs and the resulting large number of immunologically active cells that predispose to major histocompatibility class antigens, and an extreme lymphocyte-directed host response, immunosuppressive drugs are used in greater doses in lung transplant and heart-lung transplant patients than in other organ transplant patients. Induction immunosuppression is used in more than half of the heart-lung and lung transplant centers.[310] Most transplant centers use a continuing multiple-drug immunosuppressive regimen.[311]

Bearing in mind the adverse effect profiles and efficacy of immunosuppression, the International Pediatric Lung Transplant Collaborative has recommended that tacrolimus, mycophenolate mofetil, and prednisone form the mainstay of immunosuppressive therapy. The most widely used regimens rely on a CNI, coupled with a cell cycle inhibitor, and a corticosteroid. The most commonly used CNIs are cyclosporine and tacrolimus. Both work similarly, and both have clinically important side-effect profiles. Neither one appears to offer a significant benefit over the other in preventing BO from occurring. The major adverse effects of tacrolimus include hyperglycemia, alopecia, possibly worsening renal function, and possibly increased risk of PTLD. Cyclosporine's major adverse effects include hypercholesterolemia, hirsutism, gingival hyperplasia, and hypertension. Cyclosporine may prolong the neuromuscular blockade of atracurium and vecuronium.[312] Cyclosporine blood concentrations must be monitored closely, particularly in patients with cystic fibrosis who are prone to variable absorption. Elevated concentrations of cyclosporine have been implicated in central nervous system adverse effects, such as seizures, headaches, and even strokes.[313,314] Steroids are included in nearly all lung transplant programs. Over time the steroid dose is weaned to prevent complications, such as hyperglycemia and osteoporosis, yet at 1 year and 5 years posttransplant, nearly all lung transplant patients remain on a dose of prednisone. Cell cycle inhibitors are used in addition to the CNIs and corticosteroids. Mycophenolate use is increasing, but there has not been a clearly demonstrated benefit over azathioprine. Azathioprine may prolong neuromuscular blockade of succinylcholine.[315] Sirolimus acts by blocking IL-2–induced T-cell proliferation. Its role as a primary medication is limited by its hindrance of wound healing, potentially contributing to a dehiscence. It may be used as rescue therapy for children with BO who have mature suture lines.

More than one-third of children on chronic immunosuppression develop hypertension during the first posttransplant year. By 5 years that number is nearly three-quarters of all survivors. Additionally, a significant number of these children, particularly those receiving tacrolimus, develop chronic renal insufficiency with decreasing creatinine clearance. Occasionally, renal insufficiency progresses such that the child requires dialysis and renal transplantation.

A variety of perioperative complications may occur.[316] Posttransplant airway complications may be devastating. Although life-threatening bronchial dehiscence is uncommon, bronchial stenosis and tracheomalacia remain problematic.[317,318] Bronchial stenosis is thought to be related to relative ischemia at the anastomotic site, recurrent infections, and possibly high-dose corticosteroids. Initial treatment of stenosis is balloon dilation; however, up to half of the children with bronchial stenosis will require placement of bronchial stents. In younger children, dynamic obstruction may be a complication that makes extubation difficult. This dynamic airway obstruction usually is self limited, improves over time, and does not require intervention.

Posttransplantation, patients are followed closely for signs of rejection, infection, and/or BO. Pulmonary function tests are followed and the results examined for change. The choice of anesthetic agents and techniques for these patients after transplantation must be individualized, accounting for comorbidities, such as right heart dysfunction, decreased ability to handle secretions, and airway involvement affecting bronchial suture lines. Flexible fiberoptic bronchoscopies with bronchoalveolar lavage and transbronchial biopsies are the most common indications

for anesthesia in children after transplantation.[319] Bronchoscopies are performed at regular intervals, typically every 3 months, to evaluate even very early pathologic changes. Flexible fiberoptic bronchoscopies are most frequently performed under general anesthesia in children. A supraglottic airway (SGA) is the preferred manner of airway management. The SGA lumen is significantly larger than that of an endotracheal tube and allows the bronchoscopist to use a larger fiberoptic bronchoscope, facilitating improved view, improved suctioning, easier bronchoalveolar lavage, along with enhancing the ability to obtain adequate transbronchial biopsies.[320] Acute rejection is common in the first several weeks to months posttransplantation. Although acute rejection is often asymptomatic, fever and dyspnea may be present. Radiographic findings may include infiltrates and pleural effusions. Pulmonary function tests may demonstrate a decreased $FEV_1$ and decreased forced vital capacity. Diagnosis is confirmed by bronchoscopy, bronchoalveolar lavage and transtracheal biopsy. Acute rejection is graded on a scale of A0 to A4. Grade A2 and above are treated with increased immunosuppression. The major manifestation of chronic rejection, BO,[321] remains the bane of the lung transplantologists, occurring in nearly 50% of all post–lung transplant patients within 5 years of transplant. BO is the leading cause of death after the first posttransplant year. BO presents as progressive deterioration of exercise tolerance, and deterioration in airflow. BO is characterized by fibrosis of small airways and thickening of blood vessels. BO is diagnosed by a decrease in $FEV_1$, compared to the immediately previous $FEV_1$. Known risk factors for BO include prolonged ischemic time of the donor lung, more than two rejection episodes, and age greater than 3 years.[322] Unfortunately, there is no consistently reliable treatment for BO. A variety of immunosuppressive medications have been used with variable results. The primary treatment for BO is immunosuppressive prevention of acute rejection and prompt CMV treatment. In severe instances of BO, retransplantation is the only treatment option.

Posttransplant vascular complications are uncommon, but when they do occur are most commonly a result of mechanical obstruction of blood flow secondary to redundant tissue in either the pulmonary artery or at the cuff of the atrial tissue, impeding venous return. Vascular complications may be difficult to distinguish from reperfusion injury, presenting with elevated right sided and pulmonary artery pressures, with pink frothy secretions in the endotracheal tube. Pulmonary arterial or venous stenosis may be diagnosed in the OR, or at bedside in the critical care unit, with a TEE. If there are still questions regarding the diagnosis, cardiac catheterization may be required. Depending on the findings, the children may be treated with a stent placed during cardiac catheterization, or they may require reoperation to alleviate the stenosis. Furthermore, transplanted lungs do not have lymphatics anastomosed. Therefore there is a loss of lymphatic drainage in the transplanted lungs. This loss of lymphatic drainage increases the risk for pulmonary edema in the postoperative period. Increased parenchymal water and increased vascular filling further serve to decrease the compliance of the posttransplant lungs.[323]

Posttransplantation donor lungs are denervated. Although this produces minimal effect on airway reflexes, mucociliary transport, and bronchial reactivity,[324] the larger effect is the loss of stimuli to the respiratory drive center, with a loss of coordination of the respiratory accessory muscles. This lack of coordination may be visually apparent. Additionally, in the early posttransplantation period, children often demonstrate episodes of bradycardia. A later effect is a tendency toward an elevated sympathetic tone and an increased heart rate.[325]

Phrenic, recurrent laryngeal, and vagus nerve injuries are common after lung transplant.[326] Although phrenic nerve injury is typically transient, the resulting diaphragmatic paralysis may result in prolonged need for mechanical ventilation or even consideration of placement of a diaphragmatic pacer. Recurrent laryngeal nerve injury may occur in up to 10% of pediatric lung transplants. The left recurrent laryngeal nerve is most often involved, resulting in a left vocal cord paralysis, from which most patients will recover.[326]

Gastroesophageal reflux disease (GERD) is a considerable problem for post–lung transplant patients. A significant number of children with GERD require a Nissen fundoplication. Laparoscopic Nissen fundoplication may be the preferred technique.[327] GERD and gastroparesis may be precipitated by vagal nerve injury. Not only do recurrent-aspiration pneumonias contribute to the transplanted lung's failure, but the delayed gastric emptying results in unreliable absorption of the child's immunosuppressive drugs.

Children with cystic fibrosis, in particular, have a high incidence of intestinal obstruction after lung transplantation. These children may require gastrostomy, jejunostomy, or other procedures for ileus. As many as one in ten children with cystic fibrosis also have intestinal obstruction after lung transplantation.[328]

Post–lung transplant graft rejections are common. Older children average 10 times more episodes of rejection than infants,[329,330] likely because of the infants more immature immune system. The signs and symptoms of rejection are nonspecific. Any diminished clinical measure is generally aggressively investigated to rule out rejection. If rejection is confirmed, aggressive treatment with immunosuppressive therapy is instituted.

CMV is one of the most common infections in children, posttransplantation. CMV infections may present with mild symptoms, but they may progress to pneumonitis, gastrointestinal symptoms, or even a sepsis syndrome with multiorgan failure. CMV has been associated with both acute cellular rejection and chronic rejection.[331] Antiviral medications have decreased the severity of this infection. Prophylactic treatment is often considered if either the donor or the recipient are CMV positive.

Patients with cystic fibrosis remain at a greater risk for infection postoperatively. *Pseudomonas aeruginosa* or fungal organisms may be noted. Aggressive antibiotic therapy is warranted. Additionally, a number of malignancies have been reported in post–lung transplant patients at greater rates than their age-matched counterparts, and may be attributed to immunosuppressive therapy. PTLD has a greater incidence in lung and heart lung transplant patients than in other solid organ transplants, perhaps owing to the greater level of immunosuppression required in these children. Even in this group of children, the cystic fibrosis subgroup of transplant patients has an even greater incidence of PTLD. PTLD includes a group of tumors, ranging from B-cell hyperplasia to immunoblastic lymphoma. Mortality has been reported to be as much or greater than 60% for those afflicted, with a number of the deaths attributed to graft failure resulting from the treatment of PTLD (by the need to decrease immunosuppressive therapy). As many as 25% of cystic fibrosis patients may suffer from PTLD. PTLD is, in most cases, associated with EBV infection, either as a reactivation of the virus with immunosuppression, or with new infection acquired from the donor lung. EBV occurs uncommonly in children who are seropositive

for EBV pretransplantation. In those seronegative, EBV-associated disease occurs in one in five children. The diagnosis of PTLD is made by the symptoms, evidence of lymphoproliferation on biopsy, and EBV DNA or RNA in the biopsied tissue. PTLD presents with a variety of nonspecific symptoms, including a mononucleosis-type syndrome. The most common symptoms include elevated temperature, lymphadenopathy, and gastrointestinal symptoms. Most PTLD occurs in the first year posttransplantation. EBV infection results in both a humoral and cellular immune reaction in children. In immunodeficient children, the normal immune responses are blunted at best. The natural regulation by T cells and natural killer cells is impaired. Natural killer cells' function is impaired for several months posttransplantation. The immunosuppression required to prevent graft rejection impairs T-cell immunity and allows for unchecked proliferation of EBV-infected B cells.

The treatment of PTLD is reduction or withdrawal of immunosuppressive therapy,[332] which may double survival rates.[333] Unfortunately, reduction or withdrawal of immunosuppressive therapy places these children at risk for graft failure. Additional treatments that have been demonstrated to be effective include localized excision of the lesion, antiviral therapy,[334] monoclonal antibodies,[335] interferon,[336,337] immunoglobulin, and cytotoxic T lymphocytes.[338] Chemotherapy does not appear to offer an advantage and may worsen survival.[339] One method to follow the efficacy of treatment is to measure EBV titers weekly. Declining viral load is indicative of response to treatment, whereas persistently high or increasing titers indicate continuing or progressing disease. Continuing surveillance includes serial physical examinations and radiographic studies. Reintroduction of immunosuppression may precipitate recurrence. Recurrence rates for PTLD average 10%.

Dysrhythmias may also occur post–lung transplant, but are relatively uncommon and typically do not require treatment. Atrial dysrhythmias associated with extensive left atrial suture lines were among the first dysrhythmias to be described.[340,341] However, the types of dysrhythmias after lung transplant surgery include junctional escape rhythm, nonsustained ventricular tachycardia, accelerated junctional rhythm, sinus bradycardia, nonsustained supraventricular tachycardia, ectopic atrial tachycardia, and second degree heart block. The incidence of the dysrhythmias is low, less than 5%, without apparent sustained supraventricular tachycardia, atrial flutter, atrial fibrillation, or complete heart block. Treatment is not commonly required in these children.[342]

Chronic kidney disease is a major comorbidity in pediatric lung transplant recipients.[343,344] More than one-third of children have a degree of renal dysfunction within 7 years posttransplantation. Renal dysfunction is associated with increased mortality.

Children who have received a lung transplant fall behind their contemporaries in height and weight (typically between the fifth and tenth percentile for age) with the overall growth rate only two-thirds of the predicted value. It appears, based on pulmonary function tests, radiographic studies, and histologic examination, that the transplanted lung's grow in the recipient is appropriate for the recipient's height and weight. Functional reserve capacity,[345] airway size,[346] and absolute number of alveoli increase as height and weight grow, in a manner comparable to their normal counterparts. Furthermore, recipients of mature lobar lungs from living related-donors are also noted to grow. Transplanted mature lung lobes expand and fill the entire chest. In these mature lung lobes, however, although the airways appear to grow in size, the alveoli appear to become distended rather than increasing in absolute number. Pediatric post–lung transplant survival after the first year has remained the same for the past 20 years.[347] Just over half of the transplant patients will survive 5 years. This follows overall 1-year and 3-year survival rates of three-quarters and two-thirds of the children, respectively.[310] Children with idiopathic pulmonary hypertension do slightly better, with 1- and 5-year survival rates of 95% and 61%, respectively, but still have a median survival posttransplantation of 5.8 years.[348]

The early death rate in infants is substantive, at 25%. Children with significant pretransplantation pulmonary hypertension and those who undergo retransplantation also have a greater than average death rate. More than half of the early (first month) deaths in all ages are a result of primary graft failure. The main culprits in later deaths are infections, BO, and malignancies. The leading cause of death from 1 month through 1 year of age is non-CMV infections. The leading cause of death in 1- to 3-year-olds is BO, followed by non-CMV infections. After 3 years of age, BO is the leading cause of death, accounting for nearly half of all deaths. The majority of malignancies are from posttransplant lymphoproliferative disease. In those children who do survive, more than 75% have minimal limitation on activity at 1, 3, and 5 years posttransplantation.

## ANNOTATED REFERENCES

Aggarwal S, Kang Y, Freeman JA, et al. Postreperfusion syndrome: cardiovascular collapse following hepatic reperfusion during liver transplantation. Transplant Proc 1987;19(Suppl 3):54-5.
*This is a classic paper describing the hemodynamic instability following reperfusion of the liver during transplantation.*

Bailey LL. Heart transplantation techniques in complex congenital heart disease. J Heart Lung Transplant 1993;12:S168-75.
*The author provides an excellent discussion of transplantation techniques in children with complex congenital heart defects.*

Beebe DS, Belani KG, Mergens P, et al. Anesthetic management of infants receiving an adult kidney transplant. Anesth and Analg 1991;73:725-30.
*The authors present a good description of intraoperative management of renal transplantation in infants.*

Boucek MM, Edwards LB, Keck BM, et al. Registry of the International Society for Heart and Lung Transplantation: eighth official pediatric report–2005. J Heart Lung Transplant 2005;24:968-82.
*The Registry of the International Society's eighth official pediatric report examines and reports the current cumulative international experience of pediatric thoracic transplantation regarding survival rates and trends in therapeutic care.*

Boucek MM, Mathis CM, Boucek Jr RJ, et al. Prospective evaluation of echocardiography for primary rejection surveillance after infant heart transplantation: comparison with endomyocardial biopsy. J Heart Lung Transplant 1994;13:66-73.
*The authors compare techniques used in rejection surveillance after cardiac transplantation.*

Coupe N, O'Brien M, Gibson P, de Lima J. Anesthesia for pediatric renal transplantation with and without epidural analgesia–a review of 7 years experience. Pediatr Anesth 2005;15:220-8.
*This is a description of intraoperative management of renal transplantation in patients of a mix of ages.*

Egan TM, Murray S, Bustami RT, et al. Development of the new lung allocation system in the United States. Am J Transplant 2006;6:1212-27.
*The development of the new lung allocation system in the United States is described, including the change in the in donor lung allocation in the United States from one based primarily on waiting time to a system based on a newly defined lung allocation score (LAS), taking into account pretransplant and posttransplant survivability.*

Haddow GR. Anaesthesia for patients after lung transplantation. Can J Anaesth, 1997;44:189-97.
*The author discusses the unique consideration in the perioperative care of the postlung transplant patient.*

Huddleston CB, Bloch J, Sweet S, et al. Lung transplantation in children. Ann Surg 2002;236:270-6.
*This article describes one center's experience in lung transplantation of 190 patients, from 1990 to 2002, providing an overview of the patients selected, their therapeutic interventions, and outcomes.*

Jacobs JP, Quintessenza JA, Boucek RJ, et al. Pediatric cardiac transplantation in children with high panel reactive antibody. Ann Thorac Surg 2004;78:1703-9.
*The authors discuss techniques to improve outcomes in cardiac transplantation in children with high panel reactive antibody titers.*

Magee JC, Campell DA. Renal Transplantation. In: Fonkalsrud EW, Coran AD, editors. Pediatric Surgery. 6th ed. Philadelphia: Mosby; 2006. p. 699-716.
*This is an overview, from a surgical perspective, of renal transplantation in the pediatric patient.*

NAPRTCS Annual Reports. Available at www.naprtcs.org
*The NAPRTCS follows trends in pediatric patients with renal disease, on dialysis, and with renal transplants. Morbidity, mortality, and treatment characteristics are available, as well as a list of publications using the database.*

Otte JB, de Ville de Goyet J, Alberti D, Balladur P, de Hemptinne B. The concept and technique of the split liver in clinical transplantation. Surgery 1990;107:605-12.
*This classic paper describes the surgical technique involving split livers, a technique where one donor can potentially create a liver for two recipients.*

Silverstein DM. Risk factors for cardiovascular disease in pediatric renal transplant patients. Pediatr Transplant 2004;8:386-93.
*This is a comprehensive review article regarding multifactorial etiologies for the development of cardiovascular disease in the patient with a renal transplant.*

Spray TL. Use of aprotinin in pediatric organ transplantation. Ann Thorac Surg 1998;65:S71-3.
*The author describes the clinical benefits of aprotinin in both high- and low-risk thoracic organ transplant patients.*

Starzl TE, Klintmalm GB, Porter KA, et al. Liver transplantation with the use of cyclosporine a and prednisone. N Engl J Med 1981;305:266-9.
*This is one of the earliest papers to report on the successful use of cyclosporine to enhance survival in liver transplantation.*

Sweet SC. Pediatric lung transplantation update 2003. Pediatr Clin North Am 2003;50:1393-417.
*The author discusses the current status of pediatric lung transplantation, including indications, outcomes, and complications.*

Tzakis A, Todo S, Starzl TE. Orthotopic liver transplantation with preservation of the inferior vena cava. Ann Surg 1989;210:649-52.
*This is a classic paper describing the surgical techniques and modifications to liver transplantation.*

Van Doorn C, Karimova A, Burch M, Goldman A. Sequential use of extracorporeal membrane oxygenation and the Berlin Heart Left Ventricular Assist Device for 106-day bridge to transplant in a two-year-old child. ASAIO J 2005;51:668-9.
*The authors discuss the use of mechanical assist devices as a bridge to transplantation.*

West LJ, Pollock-Barziv SM, Dipchand AI, et al ABO-Incompatible heart transplantation in infants. N Engl J Med 2001;344:793-800.
*The authors present a discussion of ABO-incompatible heart transplantation in infants.*

## REFERENCES

Please see www.expertconsult.com.

# Orthopedic and Spinal Surgery

## 30

NIALL C. WILTON AND BRIAN J. ANDERSON

ANESTHESIA FOR ORTHOPEDIC AND SPINAL SURGERY provides a multitude of challenges. Children often present with concomitant diseases that affect cardiovascular and respiratory function. The ability to maintain a clear airway during anesthesia is not straightforward for some children, such as those with arthrogryposis multiplex congenita.[1] Operating times can be protracted. Significant blood loss can occur that requires strategies for blood product management and transfusion reduction (see Chapter 10). Major trauma causing orthopedic injuries invariably involves other organ systems that may adversely interact with or compromise anesthesia management (see Chapter 38). The risks of aspiration of gastric contents into the lungs and the requisite fasting times,

after even minor trauma involving an isolated forearm fracture, continue to be debated. Fat embolus is uncommon in children with long-bone fractures but should be considered in any child with hypoxia and altered consciousness in the perioperative period.[2] Tumor surgery may be complicated by chemotherapy, altered drug disposition, or bone grafting considerations akin to those for plastic and reconstructive surgery (see Chapter 33) and complex postoperative pain management may be required (e.g., phantom pain, reflex sympathetic dystrophy) (see Chapter 44).

Children with chronic illnesses present repeatedly for surgical or diagnostic procedures. A single bad experience can blight attitudes about anesthesia for a long time. Positioning children on the operating table involves care, especially for those with limb deformities and contractures (Video 30-1). Padding, pillows, and special frames are required to protect against damage from inadvertent pressure ischemia while achieving the best posture for surgery. Plaster application, particularly around the hip, should allow for bowel and bladder function, avoid skin breakdown due to pressure or friction, and allow access to epidural catheters. Postoperative management of casts on peripheral limbs must account for the possibility of compartment syndromes attributable to restrictive casts or compartment pathology. Major plexus blocks may mask pressure effects under plaster casts or compartment syndrome, but epidural blocks using low-dose amide anesthetics are ineffective against the discomfort of pressure.[3,4] Intraoperative temperature regulation may be affected by tourniquet application or disease (e.g., osteogenesis imperfecta, arthrogryposis multiplex congenita). The use of radiology is common during orthopedic surgery, and precautions against excessive radiation exposure should not be neglected by the anesthesiologist.

Regional anesthesia (see Chapter 41) reduces anesthesia requirements intraoperatively and provides analgesia postoperatively. The use of ultrasound techniques to locate neural tissue improves success and reduces local anesthetic doses (see Chapter 42).[5,6] This has heralded increasing use of peripheral nerve blockade rather than central blockade for unilateral lower limb surgery. Acetaminophen (paracetamol) and nonsteroidal antiinflammatory drugs (NSAIDs) are the most common analgesics prescribed for moderate pain. Regular administration of acetaminophen and NSAIDs decreases the amount of systemic opioids administered,[7] but NSAIDs decrease osteogenic activity and may increase the incidence of nonunion after spinal fusion.[8,9] Intravenous acetaminophen improves the early effectiveness of this drug before the child is able to tolerate oral intake, but this formulation is not available in all countries.[10] Long-term pain associated with limb-lengthening techniques (e.g., Ilizarov frame) may require oral opioids after hospital discharge.

## Scoliosis Surgery

Children presenting for scoliosis surgery represent a spectrum, ranging from uncomplicated adolescents to severely compromised patients with neuromuscular disease, respiratory failure, and cardiac problems. The age range at presentation varies from infancy to young adulthood. Anesthesia techniques for scoliosis surgery vary with individual patient requirements.[11,12] Approaches aimed at minimizing blood loss and transfusion requirements have progressed from extremes of hypotension and hemodilution to a more balanced approach involving moderate degrees of both, use of antifibrinolytic agents, predonation programs, and intraoperative cell salvage. The impact of anesthetic agents on complex physiologic signals has become increasingly important as more sophisticated measurements of neural transmission using somatosensory evoked potentials (SSEPs) and motor evoked potentials (MEPs) have become the standard of care.

### TERMINOLOGY, HISTORY, AND SURGICAL DEVELOPMENT

Early Hindu literature (3500 to 1800 BC) describes Lord Krishna curing a woman whose back was "deformed in three places."[13] The terms scoliosis (i.e., crooked), kyphosis (i.e., humpbacked), and lordosis (i.e., bent backward) originated with the Greek physician Galen. *Scoliosis* is a lateral deviation of the normal vertical line of the spine, which is greater than 10 degrees when measured by radiographs. Scoliosis consists of a lateral curvature of the spine with rotation of the vertebrae within the curve. *Lordosis* refers to an anterior angulation of the spine in the sagittal plane, and *kyphosis* refers to a posterior angulation of the spine as evaluated on a side view of the spine. Curves may be simple or complex, flexible or rigid, and structural or nonstructural. Primary curves are the earliest to appear and occur most frequently in the thoracic and lumbar regions. Secondary (or compensatory) curves can develop above or below the primary curve and evolve to maintain normal body alignment. Various combinations of curve types have different pathophysiologic consequences.

The magnitude of the scoliosis curve is most commonly measured using the Cobb method.[14] Measurement is made from an anteroposterior radiograph and requires accurate identification of the upper and lower end vertebrae involved with the curve. These vertebrae tilt most severely toward the concavity of the curve. The Cobb method of angle measurement is shown in Figure 30-1.

Hippocrates (circa 400 BC) developed treatments that relied primarily on manipulation and traction, using an elaborate traction table called a *scamnum*.[15] Nonsurgical treatments for spinal deformities persisted until 1839, when a surgical treatment in the form of a subcutaneous tenotomy and myotomy was described by a French surgeon, Jules Guerin.[16]

Posterior spinal fusion was first described by Russell Hibbs for tuberculous spinal deformity in 1911.[17] The original spinal instrumentation system was the Harrington rod system.[18] Modification of this technique that allowed segmental fixation of the rods and early mobilization followed.[19] These systems treated the lateral curve but did not allow for correction of the axial rotation. Subsequent developments allowed both corrections by cantilever maneuvers using Cotrel-Dubousset instrumentation.[20]

Pedicle screws rather than hooks were the next advance. They were initially used as a distal anchor for lumber curves and were found to enhance correction and stabilization, even when used with hooks for the more proximal curves (i.e., hybrid constructs).[21] Pedicle screw instrumentation techniques for total curve correction are a recent development that offer better curve

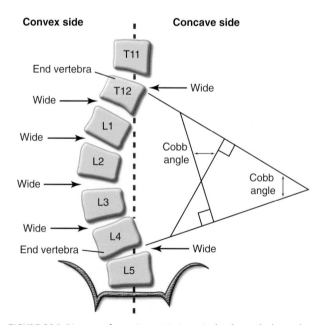

**FIGURE 30-1** Diagram of an anteroposterior spinal radiograph shows the Cobb method of scoliosis curve measurement.

correction than hook techniques [22] and the hybrid pedicle screw and hook technique.[23]

## CLASSIFICATION

Classification of scoliosis deformities is imperfect because the systems used are clinically rather than etiologically based. Most classifications are surgically based and used for surgical decision making. Curves can be described on the basis of age at onset, associated pathology, and anatomic configurations of the curve, such as single, double, or triple curves; amount of pelvic tilt;

curve flexibility; and three-dimensional analysis of the curve.[24] A classification that could indicate the risk of an adverse outcome of anesthesia, particularly respiratory failure, would be of clinical benefit. Children younger than 5 years of age with early-onset scoliosis or with independent cardiac or pulmonary disease appear to be at increased risk for respiratory failure, whereas those with idiopathic scoliosis in whom the curve develops at adolescence appear to have minimal risk.[25] A classification adapted from that proposed by the Scoliosis Research Society in 1973 remains relevant for anesthesiologists (Table 30-1).[26]

**TABLE 30-1** Classification of Scoliosis with Associated Key Anesthetic Risk Factors

| Classification | Issues Associated with Scoliosis Surgery | Increased K⁺ with Succinylcholine | Expected High Blood Loss | Respiratory Complications and Ventilatory Support |
|---|---|---|---|---|
| **Idiopathic** | | | | |
| Infantile <3 years | Repeat operations, small size | | ✓ | ✓ |
| Juvenile 3-9 years | | | | |
| Adolescent 9-18 years | Regarded as cosmetic by patient; perfect result expected | | | |
| **Congenital** | | | | |
| Bony abnormalities | Acute angle deformity; high risk of spinal cord injury, genitourinary malformations | | | |
| Neural tube defects | | | | |
| Meningomyelocele, spina bifida, syringomyelia | Latex allergy, pressure sores, hydrocephalus, Arnold-Chiari and Chiari malformations (avoid neck extension) | | | |
| **Neuromuscular** | | | | |
| *Neuropathic* | | | | |
| Upper motor neuron | | | | |
| Cerebral palsy, cerebral hypoxia | Upper airway obstruction, recurrent pneumonia, postoperative pain management | | ✓✓ | ✓✓ |
| Lower motor neuron | | | | |
| Poliomyelitis | | | | |
| *Myopathic* | | | | |
| Progressive | | | | |
| Duchenne muscular dystrophy | Cardiomyopathy, mitral valve prolapse, conduction abnormalities | ✓ | ✓✓ | ✓✓ |
| Spinal muscular atrophy | Electrocardiographic abnormalities | ✓ | ✓ | ✓ |
| Facioscapulohumeral muscular dystrophy | Hypertrophic cardiomyopathy, cardiac failure | ✓ | | |
| Other | | | | |
| Freidrich ataxia | | ✓ | | |
| **Neurofibromatosis** | Hypertension, other neurofibromas | | | |
| **Mesenchymal** | | | | |
| Marfan syndrome | Mitral and aortic regurgitation | | | |
| Mucopolysaccharidoses (e.g., Morquio syndrome) | Atlantoaxial subluxation, difficult intubation | | | |
| Arthrogryposis | Difficult intubation, severe contractures | | ✓ | |
| Osteogenesis imperfecta | Small size | | | |
| **Trauma** | | | | |
| **Tumor** | | | | |

Modified from Goldstein LA, Waugh TR. Classification and terminology of scoliosis. Clin Orthop Relat Res 1973;93:10-22.
✓, Anesthetic risk is likely; ✓✓, anesthetic risk is very likely.

The Lenke classification system, developed in 2001 for idiopathic scoliosis, provides a means to categorize curves and guide surgical treatment.[27] It is increasingly used by the surgeons as an integral part of their decision making.[28] Major and structural minor curves included in the instrumentation and fusion are used for the classification, and the nonstructural minor curves are excluded. The system has three components: curve type, a lumbar spine modifier, and a sagittal thoracic modifier. The resulting six curve types have specific radiographic characteristics that differentiate structural and nonstructural curves as proximal thoracic, main thoracic, and thoracolumbar/lumbar regions such that the number, curve type, and main structural curves are related as follows:

Type 1, main thoracic: single; main thoracic structural curve

Type 2, double thoracic: double; proximal, and main thoracic structural curves

Type 3, double major: double; main thoracic (major curve) and thoracolumbar/lumbar structural curves

Type 4, triple major: triple; all three structural curves

Type 5, thoracolumbar/lumbar: single; thoracolumbar/lumbar structural curve

Type 6, thoracolumbar/lumbar main thoracic: double; thoracolumbar/lumbar (major curve) and main thoracic structural curves

In types 1 through 4, the main thoracic curve is the major curve, and in types 5 and 6, the thoracolumbar/lumbar curve is the major curve.

### PATHOPHYSIOLOGY AND NATURAL HISTORY

Vertebral rotation and rib cage deformity usually accompany any lateral curvature. With progression of the curve, the vertebral bodies in the area of the primary curve rotate the convex aspect of the curve and the spinous process to the concave side. This vertebral rotation can be determined by measurement of the position of the pedicles from the midline (i.e., Moe method).[29] The vertebral bodies and the discs develop a wedge-shaped appearance, with the apex of the wedge toward the concave side. On the convex side of the curve, the ribs are pushed posteriorly, which narrows the thoracic cavity and causes the characteristic hump. On the concave side, the same rotation forces the ribs laterally, with consequent crowding toward their lateral margins (Fig. 30-2). These changes result in an increasingly restrictive lung defect. Exactly when this becomes a problem depends on the child's accompanying pathology. The thoracic and lumbar regions are the most common sites of the primary curve. In children in whom the primary curve is in the lumbar region, the rotation of the vertebral bodies and spinous processes should be taken into consideration when spinal or epidural insertion is attempted because the spinal canal is relatively displaced toward the convex aspect of the curve.

The physical distortion in the thorax results in restriction of lung volumes and function. Ventilation depends on the mobility of the thoracic cage, the volume of each hemithorax, and the muscle power and elastic forces required to move the thorax. Children with idiopathic scoliosis with a mild decrease in vital capacity also have reduced forced expired volume at 1 second ($FEV_1$), gas transfer factor, and maximal static expiratory airway pressures (PEmax) (see Fig. 11-4). The predominant deformity of lateral flexion and vertebral rotation results in the lung on the concave side being able to achieve a near-normal end-expiratory position but not end-inspiratory position, whereas the lung on the convex side achieves a normal end-inspiratory position but

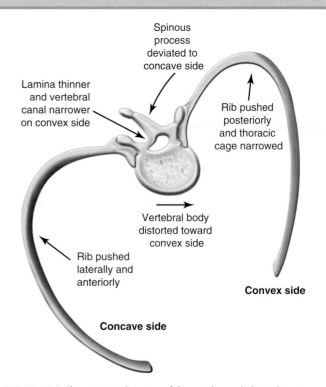

**FIGURE 30-2** Characteristic distortion of the vertebra and ribs in thoracic scoliosis. (Modified from Kleim HA. Scoliosis. Ciba foundation symposium, Vol. 1. Summit, N.J.: Ciba; 1978, p. 609; Gregory GA, editor. Anesthesia for orthopaedic surgery. In: Paediatric anesthesia. 3rd ed. Edinburgh: Churchill Livingstone; 1994.)

cannot reach a normal end-expiratory position. The concave side contributes less than normal at total lung capacity, resulting in a decrease in PEmax. Similarly, because the convex side does not reach a normal end-expiratory position, the intercostal muscles and hemidiaphragm will be less efficient, resulting in a reduced maximum static inspiratory airway pressure (PImax), although this reduction may not be quite so marked.[30] The main effect of scoliosis on respiratory function is mechanical, and the anatomic changes in the chest wall cause impaired movement and reduced compliance. Potential long-term respiratory problems when these defects are left untreated include hypoxemia, hypercarbia, recurrent lung infections, and pulmonary hypertension.

### Congenital, Infantile, and Juvenile Scoliosis

Congenital spinal anomalies are caused by failures of formation and segmentation that result in scoliosis and kyphosis. The hemivertebra, caused by failure of formation, is the most common anomaly. Fully segmented hemivertebrae contribute to progressive deformity during periods of rapid spinal growth (e.g., first 5 years of life). The most severe deformities are seen in the thoracolumbar spine. Congenital spinal anomalies may be associated with malformations of the ribs, chest wall, and hemifacial microsomia.[31] Children with congenital scoliosis have a 25% chance of urologic abnormalities and 10% chance of a cardiac abnormality. Bracing or casting techniques are not effective for this form of scoliosis. Surgical options for these patients include fusion in situ, convex hemiepiphysiodesis, hemivertebra excision, growing rods, and vertical expandable prosthetic titanium rib (VEPTR) treatment.[32] Although short-term correction is easily achievable, a short thoracic or even thoracic insufficiency syndrome can result.[33] Approximately one half of the children who have extensive thoracic fusions and those whose fusions involve the proximal thoracic spine develop restrictive pulmonary disease (FEV$_1$ <50%).[34] Expansion thoracoplasty and stabilization using a VEPTR may be used.[35]

Infantile and juvenile scoliosis are part of the spectrum of idiopathic scoliosis but are considered here because they manifest and require treatment at an early age. Infantile scoliosis accounts for less than 1% of idiopathic scoliosis and is defined as scoliosis appearing between birth and 3 years of age.[32] It usually occurs in the thoracic spine, and the curve is convex to the left. Bracing and serial casting techniques are used for infantile scoliosis. Improvement and resolution in some cases have been achieved at 9-year follow-up.[36]

Treatment of infantile scoliosis may begin as early as 4 to 5 months of age or as soon as the diagnosis of scoliosis has been made. Body casting appears useful in selected children, such as those with smaller, flexible spinal curves, but curve progression and the need for secondary treatments affect a significant proportion of these children.[37] Bracing is considered when the curve reaches 30 degrees.[32] Success has also been reported for more severe curves (60 degrees) when casting was started before 20 months.[38] After induction of anesthesia, the child is positioned on the frame (first described by Cottrell and Morel), securing the pelvis to the caudal end of the frame and tethering the head by a chin strap to the rostral end. The spine is mildly distracted, but the main maneuver derotates the spine through the ribs (Fig. 30-3, *A*). General anesthesia with tracheal intubation is required to facilitate positioning the child, stretching the spine, and molding the body cast. Hemoglobin desaturation frequently occurs when the cast is molded to correct the spinal deformity. An oral airway is also needed to prevent compression of the tracheal tube after the chin strap is applied and tightened. After the cast has hardened, it is cut back and trimmed to maintain the correction to the spine while facilitating breathing, gastrointestinal function, and day-to-day living (see Fig. 30-3, *B*). Halo traction may be used to stretch and improve the curves. Pin infections occur in almost half of the children.[39]

Juvenile idiopathic scoliosis comprises 10% to 15% of idiopathic scoliosis and is defined as scoliosis that is first diagnosed between the ages of 4 and 10 years. Approximately 20% of these children and those with infantile scoliosis with a curve greater than 20% have an underlying spinal condition, particularly Arnold-Chiari malformation and syringomyelia.[40] Although bracing is used to manage these curves, almost all children in this group with curves greater than 30% require surgical intervention.[41]

Growing rods may be used for congenital, infantile, or juvenile scoliosis to maintain the correction obtained at initial surgery while allowing spinal growth to continue. Several procedures are required before a definitive fusion.[42] All the systems (i.e., growing rods and VEPTR) have a moderate complication rate (i.e., rod breakage and hook displacement). VEPTR systems are being used to correct large-magnitude curves in this group of children when conservative treatment is inadequate.[43]

## Idiopathic Scoliosis

Although adolescent idiopathic scoliosis is relatively common, severe morbidity is seen only in children with early-onset (infantile or juvenile) idiopathic scoliosis.[44] Respiratory deterioration alone is seldom the reason for surgery in those who develop

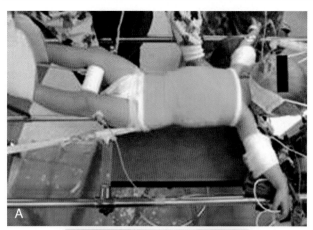

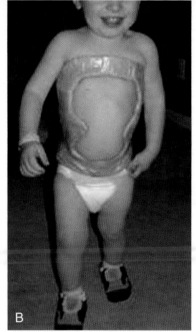

FIGURE 30-3 **A,** Nonoperative correction of scoliosis in infants and toddlers may be achieved with repeated casting. **B,** Cutting and trimming of the cast allows correction of the spine while facilitating daily living.

scoliosis after the age of 5 years.[25] This is explained by the fact that the respiratory alveoli are mature by this age.[45,46]

Scoliosis evolves during growth spurts. The earlier the age of onset and the more immature the bone growth at the time the process begins, the more severe the outcome. The relentless progression of infantile-onset idiopathic scoliosis with rapidly deteriorating curves and lung function is often not amenable to surgery. Treatment involving spinal instrumentation and anterior epiphysiodesis does not prevent the reappearance of the deformity or the decrease in pulmonary function.[47]

Pulmonary impairment correlates directly with the magnitude of the thoracic curve. Severity of the scoliosis is the most accurate predictor of impaired lung function.[48] The morphology of the thoracic curve, the number of vertebrae in the major curve, and the rigidity of the curve also are associated with deteriorating pulmonary function.[49] Conventional wisdom has held that there is minimal impact on the vital capacity until the curve exceeds 60 degrees, with clinically relevant decreases in respiratory function occurring only after the thoracic scoliosis has progressed

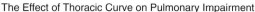

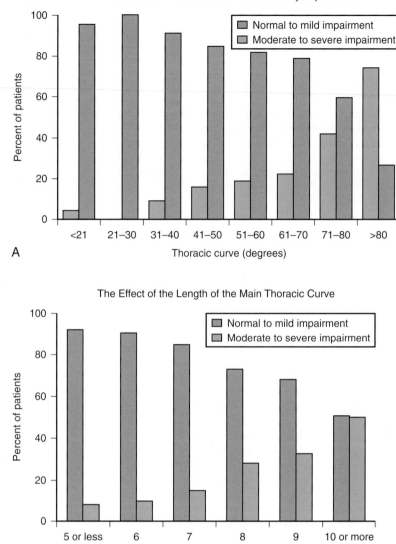

**FIGURE 30-4 A,** The bar graph demonstrates increasing pulmonary impairment with increasing curve severity as measured by degrees. **B,** Pulmonary impairment increases with increasing length of the thoracic curve. (From Newton PO, Faro FD, Gollogly S, et al. Results of preoperative pulmonary function testing of adolescents with idiopathic scoliosis. A study of six hundred and thirty-one patients. J Bone Joint Surg Am 2005;87:1937-46.)

beyond 100 degrees.[34] However, it has been shown that children with adolescent idiopathic scoliosis may have pulmonary impairment that is disproportionate to the severity of the scoliosis and that it occurs well before the curve reaches 100 degrees. Forced vital capacity (FVC) may decrease below the normal threshold (<80% of predicted) after the magnitude of the thoracic curve exceeds 70 degrees; $FEV_1$ decreases to less than the normal threshold after the main thoracic curve exceeds 60 degrees.[35] Twenty percent of children with a thoracic curve of 50 to 70 degrees have moderate or severe pulmonary impairment (i.e., less than 65% of predicted) (Fig. 30-4, *A*).[50] Those with thoracic hypokyphosis are more likely to have moderate or severe pulmonary impairment; complex curves have a greater prevalence of moderate or severe pulmonary impairment, and the number of vertebrae in the thoracic curve is the most significant predictor of impaired respiratory function (see Fig. 30-4, *B*).[51] These data indicate that children with a structural cephalad thoracic curve, a major thoracic curve spanning eight or more vertebral levels, or thoracic hypokyphosis are at increased risk for moderate to severe pulmonary impairment.

**Neuromuscular Scoliosis**

Children with neuromuscular scoliosis have the burden of deteriorating muscle function in addition to mechanical distortion. Crowding of the ribs on the concave side of the curve limits chest wall expansion, and the sitting posture restricts diaphragmatic excursion. This inevitably leads to more rapid deterioration in the curve and respiratory function. These children also have the potential for rapid and unpredictable deterioration of the curve.[36] It is important to consider the natural history of the specific neuromuscular disease when trying to balance the risks of surgery against conservative management.

Children with Duchenne muscular dystrophy (DMD) suffer from progressive muscular weakness and increasing disability until death occurs, usually by the beginning of the third decade.[52] These children tend to become wheelchair bound by 8 to 10 years of age because of increasing motor muscle weakness. Scoliosis then progresses with an acute deterioration during the growth spurt between the ages of 13 and 15 years, such that it becomes difficult or impossible to sit unaided. After the lumbar curve exceeds 35 degrees, further progression becomes inevitable.[53] A normal cough requires an inspiratory effort of more than 60% of total lung capacity and effective glottic closure to produce an effective peak flow (more than 160 L/min in adults). Forced expiratory flows are typically reduced proportionally to the decrease in lung volume. As muscle weakness progresses, patients hypoventilate, initially at night. If nocturnal ventilatory support is not provided at this stage, diurnal hypercapnia will result.[54]

There have been two significant changes in the overall management of children with DMD: the use of steroids and the earlier use of nocturnal noninvasive positive-pressure ventilation (NPPV). Steroid treatment in the early phase of the disease appears to slow disease progression for a few years; treatment with prednisone can stabilize strength and function for 6 months to 2 years.[55,56] This may delay the presentation of children for corrective surgery. Earlier adoption of nocturnal NPPV for nocturnal hypoventilation improves survival and quality of life. Clinically unsuspected nocturnal hypoventilation occurs in about 15% of patients with DMD and can be predicted by moderate impairment according to pulmonary function tests (FVC <70% and $FEV_1$ <65% of predicted) and scoliosis. Those with nocturnal hypoventilation have increased gas trapping, decline of muscle strength, and worse perception of health status despite NPPV.[57]

A 2007 multidisciplinary consensus statement on the "Respiratory and Related Management of Patients with Duchenne Muscular Dystrophy undergoing Anesthesia or Sedation" provided recommendations to standardize the approach to these patients[58] and others with flaccid neuromuscular diseases undergoing anesthesia; the most important of these are as follows: An FVC less than 50% of predicted indicates an increase in postoperative respiratory complications, and an FVC less than 30% suggests a further increase in that risk. Respiratory function tests should be part of the preoperative evaluation whenever possible and should include FVC, maximal inspiratory pressure, maximal expiratory pressure, peak cough flow, $SpO_2$ on room air, and $PaCO_2$ if the $SpO_2$ value is less than 95%. Consider preoperative training and postoperative use of NPPV if FVC is less than 50% of predicted, and strongly consider NPPV if FVC is less than 30%. Consider preoperative training and postoperative use of manual and mechanically assisted cough in those with impaired cough. In older children, this can be predicted by a peak cough flow less than 270 L/min or maximal expiratory pressure less than 60 cm $H_2O$. Strongly consider planning to extubate the trachea directly to NPPV when the FVC is less than 30%.

Dilated cardiomyopathy occurs in up to 90% of DMD individuals older than 18 years of age. The severity of the physical disability in boys with DMD in their late teens often masks the clinical symptoms of cardiac failure. Cardiomyopathy has been considered responsible for death of up to 20% of individuals with DMD, but this proportion may increase in the future for individuals in whom NPPV prevents respiratory-related mortality.[56] (See also Chapter 22.)

# Risk Minimization and Improving Outcome from Surgical Intervention

## RESPIRATORY FUNCTION AND COMPLICATIONS IN THE EARLY POSTOPERATIVE PERIOD

Decreases in lung volumes and flow rates similar to thoracic and upper abdominal surgery occur after scoliosis surgery. The FVC and $FEV_1$ decrease with a nadir at 3 days and are about 60% of

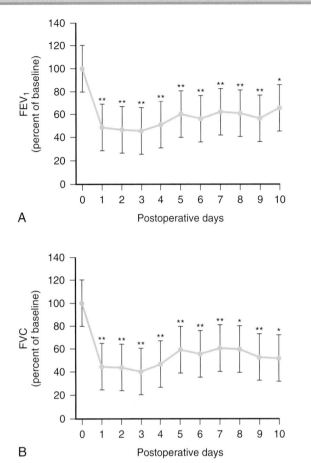

**FIGURE 30-5 A,** Changes in forced expiratory volume in 1 second ($FEV_1$) during the 10 days after scoliosis surgery. **B,** Changes in forced vital capacity (FVC) during the 10 days after scoliosis surgery. (From Yuan N, Fraire JA, Margetis MM, et al. The effect of scoliosis surgery on lung function in the immediate postoperative period. Spine 2005;30:2182-5.)

preoperative values 7 to 10 days after surgery (Fig. 30-5). It is not until 1 to 2 months after surgery that pulmonary function test results again approach baseline values. The magnitude of this decrease is not affected by the type of surgery performed or whether the scoliosis has an idiopathic or neuromuscular cause.[59]

Children with neuromuscular disease are more likely to require prolonged mechanical ventilation after spinal surgery because of more severe preoperative respiratory impairment.[60] The marked decrease in vital capacity and peak flows is undoubtedly related to the risk of postoperative complications, but determining when it is no longer safe to anesthetize those with a restrictive lung defect remains an imperfect science.

Equipment is available to assist the postoperative management of children with impaired respiratory function. The routine use of NPPV and cough augmentation therapy should be planned if the preoperative FVC is less than 30%. Cough augmentation can be provided manually by hyperinflation and forced expiration, alone or together, and by mechanical insufflation-exsufflation (MIE) therapy.[61] The effectiveness of MIE may be limited in children with a weak or enlarged tongue if it blocks exsufflation flow.

Less extensive surgery with the newer pedicles screw systems decreases the need for pelvic fixation to correct pelvic obliquity.

The procedures require less extensive surgery and shorter operating times, which may benefit children with impaired respiratory function.[62-65]

Respiratory complications after surgery for idiopathic scoliosis are relatively uncommon. In contrast, respiratory complications after surgery in children with nonidiopathic scoliosis is reported to be fivefold greater.[66] The risk increases as the degree of curvature increases and the respiratory function decreases.[67] Anterior spinal procedures are associated with a greater incidence of complications than posterior spinal fusion, such that some consider this to be the main risk factor for postoperative respiratory complications.[67] Modern pedicle screw systems may decrease the need for anterior procedures, thereby decreasing the complication rate.[68]

Atelectasis, infiltrates, hemothoraces, pneumothoraces, pleural effusions, and prolonged intubation have the greatest incidence, whereas pneumonia, pulmonary edema, and upper airway obstruction occur less frequently. These problems are more common when the scoliosis is associated with mental retardation and developmental delay. The greatest complication rate occurs for those with cerebral palsy and flaccid neuromuscular scoliosis.[66-69] Although respiratory complications increase as the severity of scoliosis and the degree of respiratory impairment increase, reported complication rates vary considerably. Studies of children with neuromuscular scoliosis suggest an overall respiratory complication rate of 15% to 30%[69-73] and minimal mortality. In one of these studies, which identified three groups by respiratory impairment (FVC <30%, FVC = 30% to 50%, FVC >50%), an overall complication rate of 31% occurred independent of the degree of respiratory impairment,[69] perhaps reflecting improvement with modern management techniques (Table 30-2).

Children with cerebral palsy have additional problems associated with their lack of muscular control (e.g., swallowing incoordination, excessive salivation, gastroesophageal reflux) and sometimes have developmental delay that contribute to a postoperative complication rate of 30%.[70,71,74] Nonambulatory patients and those with curves greater than 60 degrees are at increased risk for major complications, with nonambulatory patients almost four times more likely to have a major complication.[74] Gastrointestinal dysmotility in cerebral palsy patients can be exacerbated after scoliosis surgery and cause persistent vomiting and bloating.[75] Pancreatitis may occur in up to 30% of cerebral palsy patients after surgery, with a greater incidence among those with documented gastroesophageal reflux and reactive airway disease.[76]

## LONG-TERM CHANGES
### Idiopathic Scoliosis
Improvements in pulmonary function are not impressive after correction of idiopathic scoliosis. Early studies suggested that spinal fusion stabilized the respiratory dysfunction that existed preoperatively, but failed to offer any improvement.[77]

Improvements may be possible in certain subgroups of patients with some surgical techniques, but it takes months to years for pulmonary function to improve. Children with a preoperative curve less than 90 degrees undergoing a posterior procedure only had a greater than 10% increase in vital capacity, maximum voluntary ventilation, and maximum respiratory mid-flow rate after 2 years; this improvement did not occur in those who underwent anterior surgery.[78] Harrington rod instrumentation in children with idiopathic scoliosis resulted in only a small improvement in vital capacity.[79]

The newer instrumentation systems, such as the Cotrel-Dubousset instrumentation that allows segmental realignment and approximation, result in further improvements in pulmonary volumes.[80] Pulmonary function returns to preoperative values within 3 months after the posterior approach using the newer instrumentation systems, with additional improvements occurring and being sustained for 2 years.[81] Pedicle screws provide greater curve correction in adolescent idiopathic scoliosis, with a trend toward improved pulmonary function after 2 years compared with other instrumentation techniques.[23] A 10-year follow-up analysis demonstrated an absolute increase in the FVC (3.25 versus 3.66 L) and $FEV_1$ (2.77 versus 3.10 L) but no changes in percent of predicted values in children who underwent a posterior fusion and instrumentation only. In the same analysis, those with chest wall disruption experienced no change in FVC and $FEV_1$ over 10 years, but the assessment demonstrated a significant decrease in percent of predicted FVC (85% versus 79%,) and $FEV_1$ values (80% versus 76%).[82]

Chest cage disruption (i.e., thoracoplasty or anterior thoracotomy) is associated with reduced pulmonary function at 3 months and a 10% to 20% decrease in total lung capacity and FVC. These values do not return to baseline until 1 to 2 years after surgery. Improvements in lung function with this approach are seldom seen.[44,45] Video-assisted thoracoscopic surgery (VATS) for anterior release and instrumentation appears to result in less pulmonary morbidity and a smaller decrease in pulmonary function at 3 months. One year after surgery, values for children treated thoracoscopically had returned to baseline, but this did not occur for those undergoing open thoracotomy (Fig. 30-6).[83,84] Two- and 5-year follow-up evaluations of those undergoing VATS showed no significant changes with regard to the correction of the major Cobb angle (56% ± 11% and 52% ± 14%, respectively) or average total lung capacity as a percent of the predicted value (95% ± 14% and 91% ± 10%) over the study period.[85]

Changing surgical techniques may challenge these findings in the future because some surgeons think that anterior fusions with modern systems offer short-term benefits of reduced blood loss and transfusion and long-term benefits due to shorter fusions, better maintenance of thoracic kyphosis, and improved spontaneous lumbar curve correction. A 2-year postoperative study concluded that VATS for thoracic curves and open procedures

| **TABLE 30-2** Incidence of Pulmonary Complications | | | | | | |
|---|---|---|---|---|---|---|
| Forced Vital Capacity | Total Number of Patients | Patients with Pulmonary Complications | Pneumonia | Atelectasis | Pneumothorax | Ventilator Care (>3 days) |
| <30% | 18 | 6 | 3 | 0 | 1 | 2 |
| 30-50% | 18 | 7 | 3 | 1 | 0 | 4 |
| >50% | 38 | 10 | 2 | 1 | 0 | 7 |

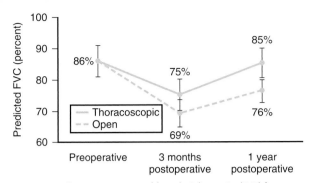

**FIGURE 30-6** Changes in percent of forced vital capacity (FVC) for thoracoscopic versus open anterior instrumentation during the first year after surgery. (From Faro FD, Marks MC, Newton PO, Blanke K, Lenke LG. Perioperative changes in pulmonary function after anterior scoliosis instrumentation: thoracoscopic versus open approaches. Spine 2005;30:1058-63.)

for thoracolumbar curves resulted in minimal to no permanent pulmonary impairment 6 months after the procedure compared with posterior spinal fusion, despite a short-term decrease observed after VATS.[86]

**Neuromuscular Scoliosis**

Improvements in the scoliosis angle and the degree of pelvic obliquity are achieved after spinal instrumentation in children with neuromuscular disease. Significant improvement can usually be shown in the ability to sit unaided, particularly if children are unable to do so beforehand.[87-91] Some investigators have reported an increase in the quality of life perceived by the child or caregiver.[89,91]

There is little evidence for any improvement in respiratory function in this group of children. There may be a period of delay or even stabilization of the inevitable deterioration of respiratory function.[52,88,92] Other investigators have shown no difference in respiratory function after 5 years compared with patients managed conservatively[90,93] or an early loss in vital capacity after surgery with a progressive decrease of 25% over 4 years, with 66% of patients requiring mechanical respiratory assistance by that time.[89] A Cochrane review was unable to find any data evaluating the effectiveness of scoliosis surgery in patients with DMD and even suggested, "Patients should also be informed about the uncertainty of benefits on long-term survival and respiratory function after scoliosis surgery."[94]

Some retrospective analyses, however, deserve consideration. A review of the long-term survival of children with DMD after spinal surgery and nocturnal ventilation demonstrated that those having spinal surgery and ventilation had a median survival of 30 years, whereas those receiving nocturnal ventilation only survived to 22.2 years. This result occurred despite a decrease in mean vital capacity from 1.4 to 1.13 L in the first postoperative year.[95] Posterior spinal fusion for scoliosis in DMD was associated with a significant slowing in the rate of decrease in respiratory function; the rate of 4% per year before surgery decreased to 1.75% per year (over 8 years) after surgery.[96] In a study of 14 children with DMD and an FVC of less than 30%, the mean rate of decrease in percent of FVC after surgery was 3.6% per year. Most children and parents thought scoliosis surgery improved their function, sitting balance, and quality of life and gave it high satisfaction scores.[97]

Less outcome information is available for children with cerebral palsy. Surgery is perceived as having a positive impact on patients' quality of life, overall function, and ease of care by parents and other caregivers,[98] despite the high complication rates described earlier. A 3-year follow-up after a pedicle screw construct for scoliosis, which reduced the mean Cobb angle to 31%, demonstrated improved functional ability in 42% of children. Most children had improved sitting balance and nursing care requirements. A 32% complication rate occurred; most were pulmonary in origin but ultimately reversible. There were two perioperative deaths and one transient neurologic deficit due to screw impingement among 56 patients.[68]

Less morbidity has been claimed for the same-day (one-stage) surgery compared with the two-staged approach in children with neuromuscular disease requiring anterior and posterior spinal surgery.[99,100] However, it seems reasonable to avoid anterior thoracotomy in neuromuscular patients in view of the poor respiratory function after chest cage disruption.[81,83] Currently, pedicle screw systems in children with neuromuscular scoliosis produce outcomes similar to those of earlier systems but with quicker operating times and less blood loss.[63]

# Spinal Cord Injury during Surgery

## ETIOLOGY

Spinal cord injury can occur by four main mechanisms: direct contusion of the cord during surgical exposure; contusion by hooks, wires, or pedicle screws; distraction by rods or halo traction; and reduction in spinal cord blood flow.[101] Epidural hematoma should be included in the differential diagnosis of deficits occurring postoperatively. The areas of the spinal cord most vulnerable to ischemic injury are the motor pathways, which are supplied by a single anterior spinal artery. This is fed in a segmental manner by the radicular arteries that arise from the vertebral, cervical, intercostals, lumbar, and iliolumbar arteries. The largest radicular artery is the artery of Adamkiewicz, which arises between T8 and L4. A watershed area between T4 and T9 is prone to ischemia because the blood supply in this region of the cord is poorest.[102] Paraplegia is the most feared neurologic complication, but partial spinal cord injury resulting in areas of localized weakness and numbness as well as bladder and bowel disturbances also have been reported.

The increasing use of pedicle screws in spinal surgery raises the possibility of increased risk to individual nerve roots. A systematic review of pedicle screw complications that involved a total of 4570 pedicle screws in 1666 patients reported an overall 4% malposition rate that increased to 16% in studies that systematically examined their patients postoperatively.[103] Eleven patients required revision surgery for the malpositioned screws, and there was one temporary neurologic complication (i.e., epidural hematoma). No vascular injuries were reported, although six cases of aortic abutment were described.

## RISK OF SPINAL CORD INJURY AND SPINAL CORD MONITORING

Combined surveys undertaken by the Scoliosis Research Society and the European Society for Deformities of the Spine investigating idiopathic scoliosis suggested an incidence of neurologic impairment of 0.72% in 1975.[104] At the end of the last millennium, that incidence had decreased to less than half (0.3%), and all were partial cord lesions.[101] Patients with curves greater than 100 degrees, congenital scoliosis, kyphosis, and postirradiation deformity appear to be at greatest risk for complications. The use of pedicle screws may have increased the immediate neurologic complication rate. Nine neural complications were reported among 1301 patients, for an incidence of 0.69% in 2007. Three thecal penetrations occurred, two as a result of pedicle screws, all without sequelae. There were two nerve root injuries and four spinal cord injuries, all of which resolved within 3 months.[105]

A retrospective review of 19,360 cases of pediatric scoliosis showed significantly different overall complication rates among idiopathic (6.3%), congenital (10.6%), and neuromuscular (17.9%) scoliosis. Neurologic deficits had a different distribution, with the greatest rate among congenital cases (2%), and lower rates with neuromuscular (1.1%) and idiopathic scoliosis (0.8%).[106] Mortality rates of 0.3% were observed for neuromuscular and congenital scoliosis, with an idiopathic scoliosis rate of 0.02%. Rates of new neurologic deficits were greater with anterior screw–only constructs (2%) or wire constructs (1.7%) than with pedicle screw constructs (0.7%).

Spinal cord function is monitored to ensure that the complication rate is as small as possible. The Scoliosis Research Society issued a position statement concluding that neurophysiologic monitoring can assist in the early detection of complications and can possibly prevent postoperative morbidity in patients undergoing operations on the spine. For any monitoring technique to be effective, it needs to have a sensitivity and specificity that allows true changes to be recognized with a very low occurrence of false-negative and false-positive results. The test or technique must also produce its results in a time frame that allows the problem to be reversed or prevented. Recognition of the limitation of individual techniques has seen the development of increasingly sophisticated monitoring systems to identify and minimize this risk. Older tests, such as the wake-up test and ankle clonus test, have largely been superceded by monitoring of SSEPs, MEPs, and triggered electromyographic techniques (EMGs). The importance of using a multimodal approach is increasingly recognized and is well addressed in the literature.[107-110] The capabilities and limitations of the various techniques are summarized in E-Table 30-1.

## METHODS OF MONITORING SPINAL CORD FUNCTION
### Wake-up Test
The wake-up test measures gross motor function of the upper and lower extremities. It has been used widely since it was first described.[111] The test consists of decreasing the depth of anesthesia almost to the point of wakefulness and asking the patient to respond to verbal commands. Failure to move the feet and toes while being able to squeeze a hand suggests a problem with the spinal cord. The test requires limiting or reversing muscle relaxation and reducing the depth of anesthesia sufficiently to enable the patient to follow commands. When the test was initially described, 3 of 124 patients had a positive result (i.e., no movement) and were saved from paraplegia.[111] A major concern is that the test is conducted after maximal spinal correction, which may occur after any neurologic insult has occurred; however, removal or modification of the spinal instrumentation within 3 hours of the onset of the neurologic deficit has been reported to prevent the risk of permanent neurologic sequelae.[112] The wake-up test is unlikely to detect isolated nerve root injury or sensory changes. It is limited to neurologically normal patients with an appropriate developmental age who can follow instructions.

With the clinical application of SSEP and MEP monitoring (Fig. 30-7) well established and in the absence of intraoperative changes, there is no justification to perform the wake-up test.[113] Nonetheless, some surgeons still regard the wake-up test to be the gold standard, and it may be used to confirm changes demonstrated by SSEP or MEP monitoring.[114] Risks include lack of nerve root and sensory information, accidental extubation, dislodgement of the instrumentation, intraoperative recall with subsequent psychological trauma, air embolism, and cardiac ischemia. If a wake-up test is planned, it is prudent to fill the wound with saline to reduce the risk of an air embolism.

### Ankle Clonus Test
The ankle clonus test uses the clonus that occurs just before consciousness is regained during wakening from anesthesia. Rhythmic muscle contractions are thought to result from spinal reflexes returning while the higher neurologic centers remain inhibited by anesthesia, and the oscillations demonstrate an intact spinal cord. Inability to demonstrate clonus suggests spinal cord injury.[115] Like the wake-up test, it is a post hoc test rather than real-time monitoring. However, in a review of more than 1000 patients undergoing spinal procedures in which six postoperative neurologic deficits occurred, this test identified all the deficits but produced three false-positive findings, giving a sensitivity of 100% and a specificity of 99.7%. In comparison, the wake-up test produced false-negative results for four of the five patients who developed deficits.[115]

### Somatosensory Evoked Potentials
SSEPs involve stimulating a peripheral nerve and measuring the response to that stimulation using scalp electrodes (i.e., cortical SSEPs).[116,117] Alternatively, the response can be measured subcortically near the spinal cord by electrodes placed in the epidural space, interspinous ligament, or spinous processes of the vertebrae.[118] An intranasally placed pharyngeal electrode can act as a surrogate for these. The advantage of the subcortical evoked potential is that the responses are more stable, reproducible, and resistant to the effects of anesthesia.

The signal produced with SSEP monitoring travels from the peripheral nerve through the nerve root and up the ipsilateral dorsal column. The impulses then cross over at the level of the brainstem and progress rostrally through the thalamus to the primary sensory cortex. The rationale for using SSEP to monitor motor deficits is based on the fact that the sensory tracts are in proximity to the motor tracts of the spinal cord. Injury to the motor tracts indirectly affects the sensory tracts and causes changes in the SSEP. When spinal cord function is significantly impaired, there is usually an increase in latency and a decrease in amplitude in the SSEP, with eventual loss of signal. A 10% increase in latency of the first cortical peak (P1) or 50% decreases in the peak-to-peak amplitude (P1N1) constitute an indication for intervention.[119,120] Although SSEP signals primarily monitor transmission through the sensory dorsal columns, they are effective,[120] and SSEP monitoring is associated with a 50% decrease in the incidence of neurologic deficits.

It is unusual for motor tract injury to occur when SSEPs remain unchanged, but false-positive and false-negative results have been reported.[120,121] Seventy percent of the postoperative complications were detected by the monitor, but 30% (false negatives) were not detected. Pedicle screw misplacement leading to radiculopathy may not be detected by SSEP monitoring.[122] Several case reports of paraparesis also attest to the limitations of

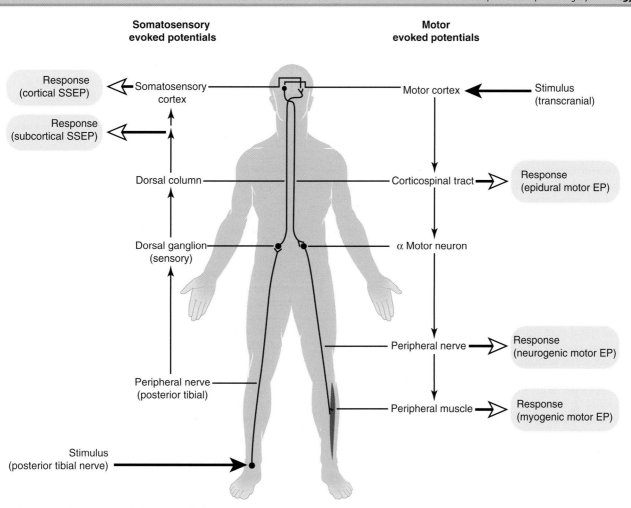

**Somatosensory evoked potentials**

Response (cortical SSEP) ← Somatosensory cortex

Response (subcortical SSEP) ←

Dorsal column

Dorsal ganglion (sensory)

Peripheral nerve (posterior tibial)

Stimulus (posterior tibial nerve)

**Motor evoked potentials**

Motor cortex ← Stimulus (transcranial)

Corticospinal tract → Response (epidural motor EP)

α Motor neuron

Peripheral nerve → Response (neurogenic motor EP)

Peripheral muscle → Response (myogenic motor EP)

**FIGURE 30-7** Comparison of pathways involved in somatosensory evoked potential (SSEP) and motor evoked potential (MEP) monitoring. (Modified from de Haan P, Kalkman CJ. Spinal cord monitoring: somatosensory- and motor-evoked potentials. Anesthesiol Clin North Am 2001;19:923-45.)

SSEP monitoring. These problems are caused by injury occurring outside the monitored domain of SSEP rather than a failure of this modality. These concerns encouraged development of methods to monitor the motor tracts of the spinal cord. SSEP monitoring is possible in patients with cerebral palsy, whereas MEPs may not be.[123]

### Motor Evoked Potentials

The motor pathways can be activated by transcranial stimulation of the motor cortex or by spinal cord stimulation. Transcranial stimulation is achieved using electrical or magnetic stimulation applied to the scalp. Electrical stimulators are most commonly used in spinal surgery and operate by applying high-voltage pulses to the scalp using corkscrew, needle, or surface electrodes. The stimulation pulses can be applied as single stimuli or brief pulse trains with intervals between the pulse trains. Multiple stimuli result in a stronger signal with less variability due to temporal summation of the excitatory postsynaptic potential.[124] Epilepsy and proconvulsant medicines are considered relative contraindications to MEP monitoring because of concerns about brain injury from prolonged seizure activity due to the electrical current required for stimulation.[125,126] Not surprisingly, MEPs may be difficult to record and interpret in patients with cerebral palsy and should not be attempted if the child has seizures.

MEP monitoring may be a problem in younger children, particularly those younger than 6 or 7 years of age.[125,127] Use of a spatial summation technique in addition to temporal summation increased the success rate from 78% to 98% over all ages. Using this technique along with ketamine anesthesia in children younger than 6 years of age, reliable MEPs were documented in 98% (111 of 113) of children older than 6 years of age and in 86% (18 of 21) in children younger than 6 years of age.[127] There is also evidence that younger children require a greater stimulating voltage and pulse train frequency for MEP monitoring, probably because of immaturity of the central nervous system, specifically the descending corticospinal tracts.[128]

Spinal cord stimulation is achieved electrically and can be applied using electrodes placed outside or inside the spinal cord rostral to the area of interest. Single stimuli rather than brief pulse trains typically are used for spinal cord stimulation.[129] This approach is not commonly used in scoliosis surgery.

Responses can be recorded anywhere distal to the area of interest. They have included the lower lumbar epidural space (i.e., epidural MEP), peripheral nerve (i.e., neurogenic MEP), and peripheral muscles using compound muscle action potential (CMAP) (see Fig. 30-7).[130] Each recording site has its limitations regarding the accuracy of the information displayed and the susceptibility to anesthetic drug interference. Epidural MEPs are the least affected by neuromuscular blocking drugs (NMBDs), but they only monitor conduction in the corticospinal tract and provide no information about the anterior horn gray matter.[131] They have a much slower response to acute spinal cord ischemia when compared with myogenic responses (i.e., CMAPs).[132] Neurogenic MEPs are also resistant to anesthetic interference but appear not to accurately measure motor conduction. Most of the spinally elicited peripheral nerve responses seen with neurogenic MEPs occur through the dorsal columns in a retrograde fashion and are sensory rather than motor.[133] Anterior spinal cord injury has been demonstrated with normal neurogenic MEPs.[134] CMAPs after transcranial stimulation are thought to be exclusively generated by motor tract conduction, and unlike epidural MEPs, they include the ischemia-sensitive anterior horn alpha motor neurons.[130] These responses are very sensitive to anesthetic agents. The responses obtained with CMAPs after spinal cord stimulation also appear to contain signals that include transmission through the dorsal columns and may represent a mixed response.[135]

One outstanding problem with MEP monitoring is deciding when and how much change in the signal is significant and indicative of spinal cord ischemia. Some centers use the same criteria they have adopted for SSEP monitoring, whereas others require a greater degree of change, such as a 75% decrease in amplitude.[136] An amplitude decrease of 80% at one of six sites using transcranial myogenic MEP monitoring was demonstrated to have a sensitivity of 1.0 and a specificity of 0.91 when used as the sole monitor during spinal surgery.[137] A 65% decrease in amplitude identified all postoperative motor deficits (SSEP changes identified only 43%) in children with idiopathic scoliosis.[138] An alternative technique of measuring MEP has been described in which a minimum threshold for producing a response is established, and a significant increase in that threshold is used to signal a problem.[139] Supportive data for this technique are lacking.

The dorsal columns may be injured without involvement of the motor tract.[140] Occasionally, adverse changes in SSEPs occur without changes in MEPs.[129,141] Because of these reports, MEP monitoring should be used in addition to SSEP monitoring rather than as a replacement.[107-110,142]

### Triggered Electromyographic Techniques

The increasing use of pedicle screws allows greater curve and rotational correction than earlier techniques but has an additional risk of direct nerve root trauma. Triggered EMGs using a monopolar needle or bipolar handheld stimulator have been described, with a threshold stimulation level of more than 8 mA considered to be normal, 5 to 8 mA to be critical, and less than 5 mA to be pathologic, indicating that there was not enough distance between the screws and the neural tissue.[142] This technique requires monitoring rectus abdominis or intercostal muscles when used for thoracic curves.[143,144]

## Preoperative Assessment and Postoperative Planning

### RESPIRATORY ASSESSMENT AND PLANNING FOR POSTOPERATIVE VENTILATORY SUPPORT

The preoperative pulmonary assessment should identify patients at increased risk for postoperative respiratory compromise. Patients with idiopathic scoliosis tend to have less decrease in pulmonary function with correspondingly reduced complication rates, so most studies have focused on nonidiopathic patients.[66] The rate of postoperative pulmonary complications correlates broadly with the decrease in vital capacity.[60,145,146] Vital capacity less than 30% to 35% of predicted values indicates marginal respiratory reserve and a level at which complications and a need for postoperative respiratory support are likely. Many patients with these low vital capacities are unable to cough effectively, rendering them prone to postoperative atelectasis, pneumonia, and respiratory failure.

Studies involving a mixed population with a vital capacity less than 40% (but few with neuromuscular disorders) suggest that although short-term and middle-term pulmonary complications occur, these patients can be successfully managed to achieve discharge to home, although some require prolonged postoperative ventilation.[147,148] Modest numbers of patients with a vital capacity of less than 25% of the predicted value are described in these studies and do not appear to have greater complication rates than those with greater vital capacity values. Anterior or combined approaches increase the likelihood of respiratory complications, particularly due to pleural effusion.[147,148]

Children with neuromuscular scoliosis are likely to need postoperative ventilation that is often prolonged.[60,146] These patients may also have abnormalities in the central control of breathing and impaired airway defense mechanisms. Impaired coordination of laryngeal and pharyngeal muscles may result in impaired swallowing and inadequate cough with increased risk of aspiration. Initial work suggested that as the vital capacity decreased to less than 35% of predicted, most patients would need a short period of postoperative ventilation.[84] The earlier use of nocturnal NPPV and use of NPPV in the postoperative period may alter our perception of risk by decreasing the impact or severity of postoperative respiratory complications while allowing children with increasingly severe respiratory impairment to be considered for surgery. Scoliosis surgery can be successfully undertaken in patients with a vital capacity of less than 35% of predicted, often with no more than 24 hours of planned ventilation followed by a period of noninvasive ventilation (e.g., bi-level positive airway pressure [BiPAP]).[60,69,149,150] In one study ($n = 30$), the overall complication rate was similar whether the FVC was more than or less than 30%, and the average hospital stay was approximately 3 weeks (see Table 30-2). Tracheostomy was required in two children, and the overall pulmonary complication rate was 30%.[150] Similar results are reported by others.[69] It seems reasonable to anticipate using noninvasive ventilator support for several days after spine stabilization surgery in children with a vital capacity of less than 25% of predicted values. Children with a mean FVC of 20% of predicted have been successfully managed with a brief period of postoperative ventilation and transitioned to BiPAP within 48 hours.[151]

Whether a child should be denied surgery requires consideration of individual patient factors. The successful management of children with a vital capacity of 15% to 20% of predicted has been described, although the numbers were small.[147-150] Although the risk of an unsuccessful outcome can increase at this level, individual circumstances may justify the risk.

### CARDIOVASCULAR ASSESSMENT

Muscle disorders may affect the myocardium and the skeletal system. Children with DMD develop a cardiomyopathy that may be difficult to evaluate because the child is wheelchair bound. Sinus tachycardia is an early manifestation, and in terms of frequency and severity, cardiac function declines from early adolescence.[152] More than 90% of adolescents with DMD have subclinical or clinical cardiac involvement.[153] Echocardiography is an essential part of the preoperative evaluation of any wheelchair-bound patient presenting for scoliosis surgery. (See also Chapter 14.)

## POSTOPERATIVE PAIN MANAGEMENT

Scoliosis surgery is associated with severe pain that lasts for at least 3 days.[154] Effective analgesia minimizes postoperative respiratory complications by allowing deep breathing, chest physiotherapy, early ambulation, and rehabilitation. Postoperative pain may be managed with systemic or epidural analgesics. A multimodal approach is likely to be most effective.

### Intraoperative Intrathecal and Intravenous Opioids

Intraoperative intrathecal morphine (2 to 5 µg/kg) has provided potent analgesia during the first 24 hours after spinal fusion in children.[155,156] Intrathecal morphine also decreases the amount of remifentanil required intraoperatively, contributing to less pain on cessation of remifentanil.[157,158] However, perioperative administration of intravenous morphine, when using remifentanil as part of the anesthesia technique, does not result in any measurable benefit.[159]

Methadone (0.2 mg/kg) decreases pain scores and opioid requirements for 36 hours in children undergoing surgery, but it seems to have been ignored in modern practice.[160] This drug is used in adult spinal surgery, but reports of its use in children are few.[161]

### Nonsteroidal Antiinflammatory Drugs

NSAIDs, but not acetaminophen, impair fracture healing in animal models.[162] Cyclooxygenase-2 (COX-2) activity plays an important role in bone healing, and the use of NSAIDs decreases osteogenic activity that may increase the incidence of nonunion after spinal fusion.[8,9] The effect on osteogenic activity is dose dependent and reversible.[163] Similar effects have not been demonstrated in humans. Nonetheless, based on animal evidence, NSAIDs should be used with caution and in consultation with the surgeon during the first 3 to 5 days after scoliosis surgery.[164]

### Systemic Analgesics

Morphine remains the mainstay of systemic analgesic regimens. Morphine infusions of 20 to 40 µg/kg/hr are required during the first 48 hours after surgery. Achieving a balance of effective analgesia while avoiding sedation can be difficult in children with neurodevelopmental delay. Regular evaluation of these children is important if complications are to be avoided. Patient-controlled analgesia (PCA) is appropriate for children older than 6 to 7 years of age. It can be used with a typical bolus dose of 20 µg/kg and a lockout interval of 5 to 10 minutes. The use of a background morphine infusion may be effective in some patients, although its inclusion is controversial.[165,166] Our preference is to use a nighttime background infusion at 5 to 10 µg/kg/hr but to use PCA alone during the day (see Chapter 43). Nurse- and parent-controlled analgesia are effective if the child is too young or unable to use PCA.[167] Intrathecal morphine plus PCA appears to offer the optimal combination of effective analgesia and minimal adverse effects in idiopathic scoliosis patients compared with PCA morphine alone or epidural morphine.[168]

Low-dose ketamine infusion (0.05 to 0.2 mg/kg/hr) has been used as an adjunct to morphine infusions or PCA, although its role is debated.[169-174] Ketamine may be initiated intraoperatively

(initial infusion of 5 µg/kg/min, decreasing to 2 µg/kg/min at the end of surgery) as part of the anesthetic technique to minimize the hyperalgesia reported after high-dose remifentanil infusions.[175,176] The literature continues to be confused with conflicting reports showing no effect[177] or a modest decrease in pain scores and morphine consumption.[178] Ketamine added to morphine PCA has produced mixed results, with no clear beneficial effect in orthopedic surgery, despite such evidence being apparent for thoracic surgery.[179] If added to PCA, the optimal combination of morphine: ketamine is a 1:1 ratio.[172] Despite scoliosis causing severe pain, it is probably best to reserve the use of ketamine for those with significant preoperative pain or morphine-resistant pain.

Gabapentin and pregabalin provide some benefit with an opioid-sparing effect,[180] although postoperative nausea and vomiting benefits are limited.[181] Gabapentin (15 mg/kg followed by 5 mg/kg three times daily for 3 days) reduced morphine consumption by about 30% over the study period but without any improvement in morphine's adverse effects. Improved pain relief was observed only until the morning after surgery.[182]

### Epidural Analgesia

Continuous epidural analgesia using single- and double-catheter techniques may provide effective analgesia after spinal surgery. The single-catheter technique using bupivacaine-fentanyl and sited at T6-7 for patients undergoing a mean 12-level scoliosis surgery resulted in analgesia similar to that of PCA but with more postoperative nausea and vomiting and pruritus. Bowel sounds returned earlier in the epidural group, but liquid intake and hospitalization were similar.[183] Similar results were reported with a bupivacaine-morphine combination in patients undergoing 10-level spinal fusions. Full diet and discharge from hospital were achieved one-half day earlier with the epidural technique than with PCA.[184] A retrospective review of more than 600 patients treated with an epidural or PCA for analgesia after scoliosis surgery, in which the average number of segments fused was 8.5, confirmed the effectiveness of epidural analgesia.[185] In that study, a bupivacaine-hydromorphone epidural combination was used, and although pain management was effective, more complications occurred in the epidural group. Respiratory depression and transient neurologic changes were the most common complications observed. Thirteen percent of patients with an epidural catheter required discontinuation of the epidural, most commonly for inadequate pain relief.[185] Effective analgesia and a large incidence of postoperative nausea and vomiting and pruritus have been features of studies that combined bupivacaine and morphine.[186,187]

Patient-controlled epidural analgesia (PCEA) has been successfully used in children older than 5 years of age for orthopedic surgery and thoracotomies.[188] In scoliosis surgery, PCEA with bupivacaine and hydromorphone compared with PCA resulted in a slightly improved pain score but a 37% failure rate.[189] PCEA with a single- or double-catheter technique, depending on the number of spinal segments involved, and using a bupivacaine, fentanyl, and clonidine solution has been successful and is associated with a relatively small incidence of complications.[190]

Improved pain control and bowel function with decreased adverse effects may be possible by using a double-epidural technique using moderate amounts of fentanyl and clonidine with local anaesthetics.[191] Double-epidural techniques comprise an upper catheter positioned in the upper to middle thoracic segments and a lower catheter at the upper to middle lumbar level.[192,193] This modality resulted in improved pain control compared with morphine infusion and had fewer gastrointestinal adverse effects.

## Anesthetic and Intraoperative Management

### POSITIONING AND RELATED ISSUES

The patient must be positioned so that extreme pressure points are avoided, the limb positions are adjusted to prevent nerve injury, and the abdomen is free to minimize venous congestion. This is usually achieved by the use of the Relton-Hall frame or a variant.[194] The frame comprises four well-padded supports arranged into V-shaped pairs, with the upper pads supporting the thoracic cage and the lower pair supporting the anterolateral aspects of the pelvic girdle at the anterior iliac crests. The arms must not be abducted or extended greater than 90 degrees from their natural position. The weight of the arms is evenly distributed across the forearm to avoid pressure on the ulnar nerve at the elbow. The range of motion of the shoulders should be assessed preoperatively for optimal positioning during anesthesia. This can present quite a challenge in children with severe deformities, and creative positioning may be required. In some centers, the nipples are covered with Tegaderm (3M, St. Paul, Minn.) and positioned free of direct pressure. It is also essential that the head is maintained in a neutral position and that pressure is evenly distributed between the forehead and face, avoiding direct pressure on the eyeballs. Care must be taken to avoid any direct pressure on the knees, and the patient's weight should be distributed throughout the lower limb (Fig. 30-8). Reston self-adhering foam (3M, St. Paul, Minn.) may be used to pad the pelvic brim and knees.

Not all spinal tables and frames affect cardiac function in the same way. There is some evidence that the Jackson spine table or longitudinal bolsters have minimal effects on cardiac function, whereas Wilson, Siemens, and Andrews frames may negatively impact cardiac function.[195]

Postoperative visual loss is an uncommon, unpredictable, and devastating complication associated with spinal surgery in the prone position. It may occur in up to 0.2% of cases, and although most of the reports involve adult patients, older children are not immune.[196,197] The most common cause is ischemic optic neuropathy, but the cause remains obscure. Prolonged operating time (>6 hours) and increased or uncontrolled blood loss are features of most of the reports.[198-201] The phenomenon is unrelated to pressure on the globe and usually occurs without evidence of any other ischemia-related complications.[201] There is nothing to support controlled hypotension or hemodilution as contributory factors despite occasional expert opinion to the contrary.[198,201,202]

### TEMPERATURE REGULATION

The long preparation time and exposure of an undraped patient on the spinal frame render them susceptible to hypothermia. Hypothermia is associated with hemodynamic instability and increased blood loss.[203] A threefold increase in surgical wound infection occurs with a 2° C decrease in core temperature.[204] Efforts should be made to increase the ambient temperature in the operating room while the patient is prepared for surgery. Subsequent hypothermia can be minimized if the room temperature is maintained at 24° C during this period rather than at 18° to 21° C, as is often encountered during surgery.[205] After the patient has cooled during preparation and positioning, it may take several hours before the core temperature begins to return toward normal. Even with forced air warming systems, it is often difficult to restore normothermia because only a small amount of the patient's body is exposed to these devices. It may be possible to position a warming blanket underneath the frame so that warming from below and above occurs (see Fig. 30-8 and Video 30-1).

### PATIENT MONITORING

Patient monitoring needs to be tailored to the individual case, but at a minimum, arterial oxygen saturation, end-tidal carbon dioxide ($CO_2$), electrocardiographic (ECG) patterns, core temperature, and urine output should be recorded. In most cases, invasive arterial and central venous pressures are monitored because of large blood losses, fluid shifts, and the risk of cardiovascular instability. Direct pressure by the surgeon during dissection or curve correction may compromise cardiac function or filling. Central venous pressure is an accurate and valid measurement in the prone position, providing the zero is adjusted for the patient's position on the spinal frame. Patients with a significant kyphotic component are at increased risk for venous air embolism and should be monitored for this possibility. Depth of anesthesia monitoring should be considered, particularly when MEP monitoring limits the concentrations of anesthetic drugs. Care should be taken when positioning the head because pressure on the forehead by the sensor while the patient is in the prone position for many hours may cause erythema, localized swelling, and tissue necrosis. Contact dermatitis from the adhesive has also been reported.[206] Mixed venous oxygen tension trends may be helpful for children with myocardial compromise. Transesophageal echocardiography can be useful for determining ventricular filling and function when hemodynamic compromise is identified or suspected preoperatively.

### MINIMIZING BLOOD LOSS AND DECREASING TRANSFUSION REQUIREMENTS

Scoliosis surgery involves exposure of a large wound over a considerable period. Positioning the patient with the abdomen free to avoid venous compression is important to control and minimize blood loss. Increased intraabdominal pressure attributable to positioning can double intraoperative blood loss.[207]

Posterior spinal fusion procedures tend to lose more blood than anterior procedures. This loss probably corresponds to the

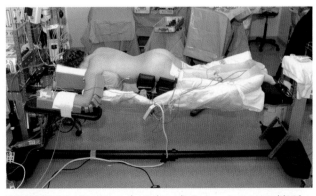

**FIGURE 30-8** Positioning on the Orthopedic Systems Incorporated (OSI) Jackson frame, showing protected pressure points and an underframe forced-air warming blanket.

greater number of vertebral levels fused with the posterior approach. Blood loss increases as the number of vertebrae included in the fusion increases. The estimated blood loss (EBL) is approximately 750 to 1500 mL in patients with idiopathic scoliosis, or 60 to 150 mL per vertebral segment fused. The blood loss of 1300 to 2200 mL (100 to 190 mL per vertebral segment) is significantly greater in patients with cerebral palsy. Children with DMD experience the largest EBL–2500 to 4000 mL (200 to 280 mL per vertebral level).[208]

Children with neuromuscular scoliosis demonstrate a prolonged prothrombin time and a decrease in factor VII activity intraoperatively, suggesting that consumption of clotting factors and dilution of clotting factors enhance the blood loss.[209] It has been postulated that children with DMD lack dystrophin in all muscle types and that the poor vascular smooth muscle vasoconstrictor response may be a factor in the increased blood loss.[210] Hypothermia exacerbates blood loss by decreasing platelet function, decreasing coagulation factor activity, and slowing vasoconstriction.[203]

Adverse reactions to blood appear to be more common in children than adults, with human error as the most common cause.[211] Several techniques have been used to decrease blood loss and minimize exposure to blood products.

### Hypotensive Techniques

Controlled hypotension has been used to minimize blood loss during scoliosis surgery since it was first described more than 30 years ago. A greater than 50% decrease in blood loss with a decreased need for blood replacement and a reduced operating time was demonstrated in early studies. Ganglion-blocking agents (i.e., pentolinium and trimethaphan) have been superseded by β-blockers, direct arterial vasodilators, calcium channel blockers, and α$_2$-agonists. It remains uncertain whether reduced blood loss results from lowered blood pressure[212] or lower cardiac output.[213] A target mean arterial pressure (MAP) of 50 to 65 mm Hg has been recommended. Although this appears to be safe, concerns that the margin of safety for cerebral and spinal cord ischemia is reduced by controlled hypotension apply to operations of prolonged duration, and there is the potential for periods of hypovolemic hypotension in addition to drug-induced (controlled) hypotension.[214,215] The incidence of these feared complications is fortunately very small with or without hypotension. Renal function appears well preserved even when hypotensive anesthesia is used during scoliosis surgery.[216,217] Because of these concerns and the concomitant use of hemodilution, less extreme degrees of hypotension are usually employed. Robust data supporting the beneficial effects of controlled hypotension in scoliosis surgery is minimal, although clear benefits have been demonstrated for orthognathic and orthopedic surgery.[218,219]

In modern practice, moderate hypotension with good control of the heart rate can often be achieved without the use of specific vasoactive drugs by using a remifentanil infusion titrated to the desired blood pressure.[220] Although not considered a hypotensive agent, intrathecal morphine decreases blood loss and may facilitate blood pressure control, particularly with a remifentanil infusion. At an analgesic dose of 5 μg/kg, a decrease in EBL from 41 to 14 mL/kg occurred.[156] Using this technique, blood pressure control can frequently be achieved without any additional agents. We have found that using an anesthetic combination of less than 1 minimal alveolar concentration (MAC) of inhalational agent plus remifentanil with clonidine (2 μg/kg)[221] provides controlled hypotension in most patients without the need for additional

agents. Dexmedetomidine may be used as part of a technique for controlling blood pressure.[222,223]

Short-acting calcium channel blockers have been used for controlled hypotension for scoliosis surgery, and although they are effective, experience is limited. Nicardipine is associated with less blood loss at the same MAP compared with sodium nitroprusside, although a slower return to baseline blood pressure (27 versus 7 minutes) is seen.[224,225] Clevidipine has been used without evidence of clear benefit, but it may be associated with an increase in heart rate.[226] If a hypotensive technique is to be used, invasive arterial monitoring is essential, and central venous pressure catheters are useful for the safe conduct of anesthesia (see Chapter 10).

### Hemodilution

Decreasing the hemoglobin concentration by removing red cells and replacing the volume with a combination of crystalloid and colloid means that for a given volume loss, there is less red cell loss (see Chapter 10). The decreased metabolic rate during anesthesia suggests that oxygen delivery can be maintained with a reduced hemoglobin concentration if normovolemia is maintained.

It has been estimated that more than 2 to 3 units of blood must removed during hemodilution to significantly reduce transfusion requirements. Hemodilution modeling in adult patients has suggested that as many as 5 units of blood must be removed before there is a decrease in transfusion requirements.[227] Deciding on the degree of hemodilution and establishing a threshold for transfusion may be difficult. In scoliosis surgery, reduction to an initial hematocrit of 30% has been effective for reducing and minimizing transfusion requirements.[228] Some posit that only modest benefits are gained from the technique.[229] Hypotensive anesthesia, hemodilution, and a cell saver used as part of a "bloodless surgery" program with erythropoietin and supplemental iron resulted in an average EBL of 855 mL (blood returned by the cell saver averaged 341 mL), with an average drop in hemoglobin after surgery of 3.1 g/dL.[230]

Tachycardia and hemodynamic instability are common at hemoglobin concentrations less than 7 g/dL. Myocardial ischemia becomes a risk as the hemoglobin concentration decreases below 5 g/dL.[231] At this level of anemia, cyanosis cannot develop because 5 g/dL of desaturated hemoglobin are required for cyanosis to be detected. Extreme hemodilution techniques such as these are reserved for patients who oppose blood transfusion. One report detailed patients who had hemodilution during scoliosis surgery that produced a hemoglobin concentration of 3 g/dL in the absence of preexisting cardiac disease.[232] Cardiac output increased by more than 30%, with only a modest increase in heart rate and decrease in blood pressure.[232] Although no cerebral sequelae were reported, *this degree of extreme hemodilution is not recommended.*

### Autologous Predonation

Preoperative strategies, including predonation of blood and preoperative red cell augmentation, may be used alone or in addition to intraoperative techniques to minimize exposure to blood (see Chapter 10). In idiopathic scoliosis surgery, preautologous blood donation plus intraoperative red cell salvage and controlled hypotension resulted in an average EBL of 1055 mL, avoided transfusion, and the hematocrit only decreased by 10% (35.6 to 32.4) at discharge.[233] The advantages of preoperative erythropoietin in addition to preautologous blood donation include a greater preoperative hemoglobin concentration and fewer donated units. Its effect on blood use depends on the total blood loss.[234,235] In children with neuromuscular scoliosis, erythropoietin alone did not affect the amount of blood transfused, although the preoperative and discharge hematocrits were greater in treated patients.[236]

### Antifibrinolytic Agents

The use of synthetic antifibrinolytic agents to decrease perioperative blood loss after scoliosis surgery has produced mixed results. To be most effective, an effective plasma concentration of the antifibrinolytics should be established before skin incision. ε-Aminocaproic acid (Amicar) decreases the EBL by 25% during the perioperative period,[237] mainly attributable to decreasing the postoperative suction drainage.[238] In contrast, an initial dose of tranexamic acid (10 mg/kg) followed by an infusion of 1 mg/kg/hr failed to significantly decrease blood loss in a small sample.[239] High-dose tranexamic acid (100 mg/kg loading dose, followed by an infusion of 10 mg/kg/hr) did decrease blood loss by 40% but did not affect transfusion requirements. Post hoc analysis in patients with secondary (neuromuscular) scoliosis showed significant reduction in blood loss and transfusion requirements.[240] The correct dose of tranexamic acid remains elusive, but it may be one half of the high dose reported previously.[241]

A meta-analysis of aprotinin, tranexamic acid, and ε-aminocaproic acid on blood loss and use of blood products in children undergoing scoliosis surgery showed that all antifibrinolytic drugs decreased the amount of blood transfused and that aprotinin, tranexamic acid, and ε-aminocaproic acid were equally effective.[242] A similar meta-analysis of major pediatric surgery showed that in the scoliosis studies, aprotinin and tranexamic acid reduced blood loss compared with placebo (385 mL, 95% confidence interval [CI] 42 to 727 mL, versus 682 mL, 95% CI 214 to 1149 mL).[243] In all operations, both drugs also decreased red cell transfusion. Demonstration that tranexamic acid is as effective as aprotinin is fortunate, because aprotinin has been withdrawn in many countries after reports of increased morbidity and mortality in adults after cardiac surgery.[244] However, after a review of the evidence, aprotinin has been reintroduced in Canada, citing off-label use of the drug as the cause of complications. Studies are being conducted in the United States. Use of ε-aminocaproic acid reduces mean intraoperative blood loss (1125 mL versus 2194 mL), total perioperative blood loss (1805 mL versus 3055 mL), and transfusion requirements (660 mL versus 1548 mL) compared with placebo.[245] Reduced blood loss has significant cost savings from decreased operating room time and blood products use.[246] Desmopressin is ineffective in decreasing blood loss associated with spinal surgery. Initial beneficial results with desmopressin[247] have not been reproduced in patients with idiopathic scoliosis[248,249] or in those with neuromuscular scoliosis.[250,251]

### Intraoperative Salvage of Shed Blood

Decisions concerning the use of intraoperative salvage of shed blood (e.g., cell saver) depend on the anticipated blood loss, size of the patient, and use of other methods to minimize blood transfusion, such as predonation and hemodilution (see Chapter 10). It is important to have some idea of the blood loss associated with idiopathic scoliosis in your institution when deciding to use cell saver techniques. For example, the cell saver was found to be beneficial in less than 5% of adolescents with idiopathic scoliosis involved with an autologous predonation program or

modest intraoperative hemodilution in one institution.[228] At another institution, however, allogeneic transfusion rates were reduced from 55% to 18% when the cell saver was used. The allogeneic transfusion relative risk was 2.04 for patients undergoing surgery lasting more than 6 hours and 5.87 for patients not receiving cell saver blood.[252]

Pediatric systems are available with small spinning bowls (55 to 75 mL). These systems benefit children with smaller body weights and greater than anticipated blood loss such as patients with neuromuscular scoliosis undergoing extensive spinal fusion.[253,254] Among children undergoing anterior instrumentation for thoracolumbar curves, cell saver use decreased the number requiring allogenic blood transfusion from 39.4% to 6.7% and with similar mean postoperative hemoglobin values (10.2 versus 9.6 g/dL).[255]

## MANAGING BLOOD LOSS

Autologous blood before donation requires an organized schedule of donation with or without the administration of erythropoietin.[256,257] This may be the safest and most effective method of avoiding or minimizing the use of allogenic blood products in this group of patients.[258] A predonation program was effective in minimizing blood exposure in idiopathic adolescents undergoing surgical correction for their scoliosis. A mean of 3.7 units of blood was donated by each patient before surgery, and 97% of adolescents avoided the use of allogeneic blood during and after surgery.[256]

Measurement of blood loss during scoliosis surgery is difficult. Accuracy is lost as measurements embrace blood suctioned from the operative field that includes irrigation fluid, weighing or estimating blood collected on swabs and sponges, approximations of blood on drapes and gowns, and estimations of evaporation from the wound.

The decision about when to administer blood component therapy (i.e., non–red cell blood components) is often based on clinical judgment. Dilutional thrombocytopenia is expected only after several blood volumes have been lost and depends on the preoperative platelet count (see Chapter 10). Platelet concentrations should be measured after loss of one blood volume and at periodic intervals after this. Dilution of coagulation factors may also lead to surgical bleeding when only packed red blood cells are used to replace blood loss. Prolongation of prothrombin time and activated partial thromboplastin time may occur when the blood loss exceeds one blood volume, and they should be checked for at this time. These coagulation tests are not usually associated with increased bleeding until values are greater than 1.5 times mean control values, at which time increased surgical bleeding can be effectively treated with fresh frozen plasma.[259] Platelet counts after one blood volume loss, whether associated with normal or abnormal clotting, were within the normal range.[259] Blood component therapy should probably be based on abnormal clotting test results, uncontrolled bleeding, or the absence of normal clotting in the surgical field. It is preferable to intervene with blood component therapy before uncontrolled bleeding develops. If pooled blood in a dependent part of the operative field fails to show evidence of clotting, it is time to transfuse with blood components starting with fresh frozen plasma and administering platelets only if this approach is not effective.[259]

Massive transfusion protocols, in which predefined ratios of red blood cells, plasma factors, and platelets (usually in a 1:1:1 ratio) are administered early in the resuscitation phase of massive trauma, are being increasingly used in all situations of uncontrolled blood loss.[260,261] Evidence that these protocols decrease morbidity and mortality in the trauma setting has resulted in their implementation in surgery, in which significant and uncontrolled bleeding may be expected.[262,263] This approach results in proportionally greater administration of factors and platelets than with conventional approaches to severe hemorrhage, but it is associated with increased survival.[264]

The thromboelastogram is also useful in refining blood product administration if multiple blood volumes are required for resuscitation.[262,264] Scoliosis surgery in patients with neuromuscular scoliosis or cerebral palsy, particularly in those with severe complex curves in whom pelvic stabilization and iliac crest grafts are considered, fulfill these criteria. In this group of patients, early administration of blood and factors using a massive transfusion protocol may be beneficial.[265]

Recombinant factor VIIa may be a useful therapy for patients with a dilutional coagulopathy who are unresponsive to blood component replacement therapy. Successful use with doses as small as 20 μg/kg, has been described in spinal surgery.[266-269]

## EFFECTS OF ANESTHETICS ON SOMATOSENSORY EVOKED AND MOTOR EVOKED POTENTIALS

Anesthetic agents act by directly inhibiting synaptic pathways or by indirectly changing the balance of inhibitory and excitatory influences.[270,271] The greater the number of synapses and the more complex the neuronal pathway being monitored, the greater the potential impact of anesthetic agents on the evoked potentials. Most anesthetic agents depress the amplitude and increase the latency of SSEPs and MEPs. For this reason, cortical SSEPs are more sensitive than spinal cord or brainstem measured SSEPs. MEPs are susceptible to anesthetic agents at three sites: the motor cortex, the anterior horn cell, and the neuromuscular junction. Consequently, transcranial stimulation with peripheral muscle detection (using CMAPs) is most susceptible to anesthetic interference. Although inhalational anesthetics and most intravenous anesthetics markedly depress SSEPs and MEPs, ketamine and etomidate appear to enhance the amplitudes of both, possibly by attenuating inhibition.[271]

### Inhalational Anesthetics

Inhalational anesthetics cause dose-dependant depression of the SSEP and myogenic MEP. At equipotent concentrations, the MEP is affected to a greater degree than the SSEP. This means that while inhalation agents can be used during SSEP monitoring, they often need to be administered in subanesthetic doses during MEP monitoring. Adequate cortical SSEPs and subcortical SSEPs can be measured with up to 1 MAC of isoflurane, sevoflurane, and desflurane, although some increase in latency and decrease in amplitude may be detected.[272,273] It is important to maintain constant end-tidal concentrations throughout anesthesia after baseline measurements have been established. Concentrations of these anesthetics that allow adequate monitoring are significantly less than was possible with halothane.[274]

Myogenic MEPs (i.e., CMAPs) are recordable only at low concentrations of inhalational anesthetics. The exact concentration depends on the system being used and is greatly influenced by the number of pulses in the stimulus. Single-pulse transcranial stimuli may be inhibited by end-tidal concentrations as small as 0.2 MAC and abolished by end-tidal concentrations as small as 0.5 MAC.[275-277] This suppression can be partially overcome by using greater intensity stimuli with multipulse stimulation of up to 6 pulses per stimulus. An increasing number of patients lose recordable myogenic MEPs, even when multipulse stimuli are used, as the concentration of inhalational anesthetic exceeds 0.5 MAC. At end-tidal concentrations in excess of 0.75% isoflurane, monitoring conditions become unacceptable.[278-282] Stimulus intensity and pulse train frequency probably are factors in determining successful myogenic MEPs with inhalational anesthetics. Using direct stimulation of the cortex during craniotomy, CMAP was easily recordable at 1 MAC of isoflurane and sevoflurane.[283] Similar results have been demonstrated with sevoflurane using transcranial stimulation.[284] Information regarding desflurane is limited, and although it causes a dose-dependent depression, myogenic MEPs have been successfully recorded at 0.5 MAC.[282,285] Using a multipulse stimulation technique, intraoperative recording of MEPs was equally successful during desflurane or propofol anesthesia.[286] In contrast to its effects on SSEPs, halothane depresses myogenic MEPs to a lesser extent than the newer inhalational anesthetics.[284]

### Nitrous Oxide

Nitrous oxide reduces the amplitude of the cortical SSEP, but comparisons with other inhalational anesthetics are limited. Nitrous oxide (0.5 MAC) depresses SSEPs to a greater extent than isoflurane at a similar MAC.[287] Similarly, 66% nitrous oxide depressed SSEPs to a greater extent than propofol (6 mg/kg/hr; 100 μg/kg/min).[288] Nitrous oxide depresses myogenic MEPs.[273] The effect relative to other inhalational anesthetics is difficult to determine. Nitrous oxide appears to affect CMAP amplitude to a lesser extent than isoflurane.[289] Multipulse stimulus techniques can partially reverse nitrous oxide–induced depression of amplitude. Compared with a propofol infusion designed to maintain a target concentration of 3 μg/mL, 50% nitrous oxide decreases CMAPs with single or paired stimuli to a lesser extent.[290] When 60% nitrous was added to low-dose propofol infusion at a target concentration of 1 μg/mL, adequate CMAPs were obtained using multipulse transcranial stimulation.[291] Conversely, the addition of nitrous oxide to a variety of different total intravenous techniques significantly depressed the CMAP such that some were not recordable.[292] With the widespread availability of remifentanil and the variable but mostly negative effects of nitrous oxide on SSEP and MEP signals, it seems that nitrous oxide is best avoided when spinal cord monitoring is used.

### Propofol

Propofol decreases the amplitude of the cortical SSEP, but adequate signals can be recorded, even in the presence of nitrous oxide, at doses used for anesthesia (6 mg/kg/hr; 100 μg/kg/min).[293] Propofol better preserves cortical SSEP amplitude and provides a deeper level of hypnosis as measured by processed electroencephalographic values than combinations of low-dose isoflurane and nitrous oxide or low-dose isoflurane or sevoflurane alone.[294-296]

Propofol depresses the amplitude of myogenic MEPs. In addition to its cortical effect, it suppresses activation of the alpha motor neuron at the level of the spinal gray matter.[297,298] Low-dose propofol infusions have become popular as part of the anesthetic technique used with MEP monitoring due to the rapid improvement of signals when the drug is terminated and because multipulse stimulation techniques can improve the response amplitude.[279,299] Propofol, even in combination with nitrous oxide, depresses multipulse transcranial CMAPs less than isoflurane.[279] Propofol (5 mg/kg/hr; 83 μg/kg/min) combined with 66% nitrous oxide produced satisfactory CMAP recordings in 75% of patients when a four-pulse stimulation sequence was used. In contrast, no recordings were possible with 1 MAC of isoflurane.[280] The infusion rates or target concentrations that allow acceptable myogenic MEP recordings vary considerably and reflect different adjuvants (e.g., opioids, ketamine, nitrous oxide), degrees of neuromuscular blockade, and transcranial pulse rates. Propofol at a target of 4 μg/mL or at an infusion rate of 6 mg/kg/hr (100 μg/kg/min) produces acceptable signals with multipulse stimuli.[299-301]

### α₂-Adrenoreceptor Agonists: Clonidine and Dexmedetomidine

The cerebral effects of the α₂-agonists appear to act mainly at the locus ceruleus, rather than by the more generalized inhibition of synaptic pathways, as in the case of general anesthetics.[302] Clonidine at doses of 2 to 5 μg/kg given intravenously had minimal effects on cortical SSEPs when added to isoflurane.[303-305] In view of its lack of effect on SSEPs and its anesthetic-sparing properties with inhalational agents and propofol,[305-307] it seems reasonable to consider clonidine at a dose of 2 to 4 μg/kg as part of an anesthetic technique. Dexmedetomidine has similar beneficial properties on SSEPs.[308,309]

There are no published studies on the effects of clonidine on MEPs, but a few publications have examined dexmedetomidine and MEPs with variable results.[310-313] The effects of dexmedetomidine, like other anesthetic agents, produce a dose-dependent depression of MEPs, and the ability to interpret these signals may depend on the depth of anesthesia, which suggests that depth of anesthesia monitoring should be used when recording MEPs to maintain a plane of anesthesia that is adequate to prevent recall but still enable good MEP signals to be recorded.

We have observed similar effects with clonidine as an adjunct to desflurane anesthesia. A temporary decrease in MEPs sometimes occurs if clonidine is administered too rapidly, but signals are improved if the bispectral index (BIS) is maintained at 50 to 60.

### Opioids

Alfentanil, fentanyl, sufentanil, and remifentanil minimally depress SSEP and MEP signals.[314,315] Dose-dependent depression of the CMAP does occur at doses of opioids that far exceed those used in clinical anesthesia.[316,317] Comparison of alfentanil, fentanyl, and sufentanil at doses sufficient to suppress noxious stimuli suggested that sufentanil exerted the least effect.[316] A similar study that included remifentanil showed that this drug had the least depressive effects, with CMAPs measurable at infusion rates of 0.6 μg/kg/min.[317] It is likely that greater doses can be used if clinically indicated.

### Ketamine and Etomidate

Ketamine enhances the cortical SSEP amplitude and has a minimal effect on subcortical and peripheral SSEP responses.[318] It also produces minimal effects on the myogenic MEP responses as a bolus of 0.5 mg/kg[319] or when used in moderate doses (1 to 4 mg/kg/hr; 17 to 83 μg/kg/min) as a supplement to a nitrous oxide–opioid anesthesia.[319,320] Experimental evidence suggests S(+)-ketamine modulates the CMAP by a peripheral mechanism at or distal to the spinal alpha motor neuron.[321] Ketamine (4 μg/kg/min) has been successfully used with MEP monitoring during propofol-remifentanil anesthesia for scoliosis correction.[127,322]

Etomidate, although capable of inducing general anesthesia, behaves more like ketamine in its effect on evoked potentials. It improves the quality of SSEPs and enhances the amplitude of MEPs.[323] It produces minimal changes in MEPs compared with barbiturates or propofol.[297] Etomidate infusions (10 to 35 μg/kg/min) produce adequate MEP monitoring signals.[319,324] Concerns regarding adrenocortical depression with etomidate infusions remain and limit its widespread use.[325] Bolus doses of etomidate, however, can transiently depress MEPs.[319]

### Midazolam

Intravenous midazolam (0.2 mg/kg) decreases the SSEP amplitude by 60%.[326] This does not occur with subcortical SSEPs, for which a slight increase in latency but no change in amplitude has been demonstrated.[327] Although midazolam (0.5 mg/kg) caused marked depression of MEPs in monkeys that persisted during awakening,[328] this finding does not hold true in human studies. MEP amplitude was unaffected by a midazolam-ketamine infusion technique compared with propofol-ketamine or propofol-alfentanil techniques.[292] Midazolam did not suppress myogenic MEPs, even at doses sufficient to produce anesthesia.[317] Effects were similar to those with etomidate.[317]

### Neuromuscular Blockade

NMBDs exert little or no effect on the SSEP. They prevent or limit recording of CMAPs during myogenic MEP recording because of their effects on the neuromuscular junction. Partial neuromuscular blockade, however, is commonly used during MEP monitoring because it improves conditions for surgery by providing adequate muscle relaxation when retraction of the tissues is required and limits any patient movement during the stimulus generation. Partial muscle relaxation may also reduce noise caused by spontaneous muscle movement. Constant neuromuscular blockade must be maintained during the procedure. Many centers avoid neuromuscular blockade after intubation, the initial incision, and muscle dissection.

Two methods have been used to assess the degree of neuromuscular blockade for MEP monitoring. One is measurement of the amplitude of the CMAP produced by single supramaximal stimulation (T1) before an NMBD is administered. When T1 is maintained between 20% and 50% of the baseline level, reproducible CMAP responses can be obtained with a degree of muscular blockade that allows surgery.[324,329] The other technique is adjustment of the neuromuscular blockade based on the train-of-four responses. Comparison of the fourth twitch (T4) with that of first twitch (T1) suggests acceptable CMAP monitoring is possible when two of the four twitches remain.[329-331] Neuromuscular blockade should be evaluated in the specific muscle groups that are used for electrophysiologic monitoring because different muscle groups have different sensitivities to the NMBDs. Patients with preoperative neuromuscular dysfunction tend to demonstrate greater effect after partial neuromuscular blockade than those with normal preoperative motor function. It is appropriate to avoid neuromuscular blockade in most of these patients.[324]

## CHOOSING ANESTHETIC DRUGS AND TECHNIQUES

The choice of anesthesia depends on the patient's pathology and the type of electrophysiologic monitoring for the operation. A marked increase in the use of MEPs and advances in MEP techniques have occurred since the previous edition of this text. CMAPs appear to provide the most useful data for minimizing the risk of spinal cord injury.

The key to success is to use a technique that allows a stable concentration of the hypnotic component of anesthesia. There is probably no difference between the inhalational anesthetics (<1 MAC) and propofol (<6 mg/kg/hr; 100 μg/kg/min). Concentrations of the inhalational anesthetics approaching 1 MAC are now compatible with multipulse MEP monitoring systems that did not appear possible several years ago. Short-acting medications offer greater flexibility if the monitored signals deteriorate. The use of a remifentanil infusion allows a rapidly titratable analgesic component with minimal effect on spinal cord monitoring. Clonidine or dexmedetomidine may be used to decrease the concentration of hypnotic drugs during SSEP monitoring and MEP monitoring, but the depth of anesthesia should be also be monitored.

Ketamine as the main component of anesthesia may improve MEP monitoring because it better preserves the MEP signals and allows reduced doses of other hypnotic agents to be used, but low-dose ketamine used as an adjunct to a conventional anesthetic does not. If processed electroencephalographic monitoring is used to determine anesthetic depth, the addition of ketamine may confound the reading by increasing it.[332,333] This occurs despite a deepening level of hypnosis.[332] An NMBD improves the SSEP monitoring and may be used in conjunction with MEP monitoring within the confines described earlier. However, even in patients with idiopathic scoliosis, adequate operating conditions after the initial muscle dissection can be produced in the absence of neuromuscular blockade. In the absence of muscle relaxation, muscle contractions, including those of the masseter muscles, occur during stimulation. In this situation, it is prudent to insert a bite block to prevent obstructing the tracheal tube or to intubate the patient nasally.

## Tourniquets

### INDICATIONS AND DESIGN
The tourniquet was used by the Romans to control bleeding during amputation.[334] The arterial tourniquet is used during orthopedic procedures to reduce blood loss and provide good operating conditions, for intravenous regional blockade and sympathectomy, and for isolated limb perfusion in the management of localized malignancy.[335]

The word *tourniquet* is derived from the French verb *tourner,* meaning "to turn," referring to the twisting or screwing action applied to the constricting bandage to tighten it. In 1873, von Esmarch introduced the use of a flat rubber bandage wrapped repeatedly around a limb.[334] Although this rubber bandage is still used to render a limb bloodless, the pneumatic tourniquet, introduced by Cushing in 1904, has replaced the rubber bandage to maintain ischemia. Compressed nitrogen or air is used for inflation. The target pressure is preset, and compensatory feedback mechanisms maintain that pressure during inflation. Curved and wider tourniquet cuffs, which are designed to fit conical limbs, are associated with lower arterial occlusion pressures than standard cuffs.[336] A soft dressing applied to the limb before tourniquet application helps to prevent wrinkles and blisters that may occur when the skin is pinched.[337] Adequate exsanguination can also be achieved by elevation of the arm at 90 degrees or the leg at 45 degrees for 5 minutes.[338,339]

### PHYSIOLOGY
#### Ischemia
Ischemia leads to tissue hypoxia and acidosis. The severity and consequences of the associated changes (e.g., increased capillary permeability, coagulation alteration, cell membrane sodium pump activity) depend on the tissue type, duration of ischemia, and collateral circulation. Muscle is more susceptible to ischemic damage than nerves. Histologic changes are more pronounced in muscle beneath the tourniquet compared with muscle distal to the tourniquet.

### Reperfusion
Reperfusion removes toxic metabolites and restores energy supplies. There is a sudden release of lactic acid, creatinine phosphokinase (i.e., creatine kinase), potassium (peak increase of 0.32 mEq/L), and $CO_2$ (peak increase of 0.8 to 18 mm Hg) when the cuff is deflated suddenly. Metabolic changes increase after longer periods of ischemia but return to baseline within 30 minutes. Muscle damage may release myoglobin, which can collect in the collecting tubules of the kidney, precipitating renal failure.

Systemic effects after deflation of the tourniquet include a shift of blood volume back into the limb with a transient decrease in blood pressure that is exacerbated by a postischemic reactive hyperemia in the limb. $CO_2$ release transiently increases the minute volume. The rapid increase in $CO_2$ is also associated with a transient (8 to 10 minutes) increase in cerebral blood volume that may affect patients with raised intracranial pressure.[335]

Increased microvascular permeability of muscle and nerve tissue occurs with tourniquet release after 2 to 4 hours of ischemia. Interstitial and intracellular edema and capillary occlusion due to endothelial edema and leukocyte aggregation may take months to resolve.

### Ischemic Conditioning
Short periods of ischemia followed by reperfusion render muscle more resistant to subsequent ischemia. Ischemic preconditioning improves skeletal muscle force, contractility, and performance and decreases fatigue of skeletal muscle. This preconditioning may enable prolongation of orthopedic and reconstructive procedures.[340]

### COMPLICATIONS
#### Local Complications
##### Muscle Damage
Histologic changes in the muscle beneath the tourniquet occur after 2 hours of tourniquet time (at 200 mm Hg [26.7 kPa]), but similar changes can occur in the distal ischemic muscle after 4 hours of tourniquet use. Direct pressure and mechanical deformation contribute to increased severity of muscle damage under the cuff.[335] These changes include an increase in the number of inflammatory cells in the perivascular space, focal fiber necrosis, and signs of hyaline degeneration.

The combination of muscle ischemia, edema, and microvascular congestion contributes to posttourniquet syndrome: edema, stiffness, pallor, weakness without paralysis, and subjective numbness of the extremity without objective anesthesia. The common use of postoperative casts may conceal the true incidence of this syndrome. Recovery usually occurs over 7 days.[341]

##### Nerve Damage
The cause of nerve injuries after tourniquet use probably is direct compression under the cuff rather than ischemia. Sheer forces that are maximal at the upper and lower edges of the tourniquet cause the most damage. These forces are greater with the Esmarch bandage than with the pneumatic tourniquet. The incidence of

nerve injuries is greater in the upper limb (1 case per 11,000 patients) than in the lower limb (1 case per 250,000 patients); the radial nerve is the most vulnerable nerve in the upper extremity, and the sciatic nerve is the most vulnerable in the lower extremity.[342]

### Vascular Damage

Arterial injury is uncommon in children. It is an injury of adults with atheromatous vessels, and the tourniquet should be avoided in patients with absent distal pulses, poor capillary return, a calcified femoropopliteal system, or a history of vascular surgery on the involved limb.[343]

### Skin Safety

Pressure necrosis and friction burns may occur with poorly applied tourniquets, and some form of skin protection should be used routinely.[344] Chemical burns may result from antiseptic skin preparations that seep beneath the tourniquet and are then retained and compressed against the skin.

### Tourniquet Pain

The tourniquet causes a vague, dull ache that becomes intolerable after approximately 30 minutes.[345] This pain is associated with an increase in heart rate and blood pressure that is not ameliorated by general anesthesia and neuraxial blockade.[345] The pain is transmitted by unmyelinated C fibers, which are normally inhibited by fast pain impulses transmitted by myelinated A-delta fibers, but in this case, mechanical compression reduces transmission through the larger A-delta fibers.[346]

### Systemic Complications
#### Temperature Regulation

The combination of decreased heat loss from the ischemic limb and reduced heat transfer from the central to ischemic peripheral compartment increases core body temperature.[347,348] Bilateral tourniquets increase the temperature more than use of a unilateral tourniquet.[348] Children who require intraoperative tourniquets should not be aggressively warmed during surgery.[348] Redistribution of body heat and the efflux of hypothermic venous blood from the ischemic area into the systemic circulation after deflation of the tourniquet decreases the core body temperature, which may switch off thermoregulatory vasodilation and decrease the skin-surface temperature.[349]

### Deep Vein Thrombosis and Emboli

The incidence of emboli after release of the tourniquet in children is unclear. The tourniquet appears to have no influence on deep vein thrombosis, but release of the tourniquet may be associated with an increased risk of embolism in adults. Some clinicians have suggested that heparin be used during total joint arthroplasty in adults to prevent emboli formation,[350] although this practice is not routine in children. Some surgeons use such therapy in adolescents.

### Sickle Cell Disease

Hypoxia, acidosis, and circulatory stasis contribute to the sickling of sickle cells in susceptible individuals. However, several institutions routinely use tourniquets in children with sickle cell disease while maintaining acid-base status and oxygenation throughout the procedure.[351,352] Each case must be assessed individually for the balance between the advantages of a bloodless field and the risks of precipitating sickling crises (see Chapter 9).

### Drug Effects

Antibiotics given after the tourniquet is inflated do not produce effective concentrations in the blood and tissue of the ischemic limb. Inflation of the tourniquet should be delayed at least 5 minutes after administration of the antibiotics.[353,354] Medications administered before inflation of the tourniquet may be sequestered in the ischemic limb and then re-released into the systemic circulation when the tourniquet is deflated. The antibiotic effect depends on the amount of antibiotic sequestered, the tissue binding, and the concentration-response relationship for the antibiotic, although the impact is minimal for most medications used in anesthesia. Volume of distribution may be reduced if the drug is administered after tourniquet inflation, but the plasma clearance remains unaffected.

## RECOMMENDED CUFF PRESSURES

Tourniquets usually should remain inflated for less than 2 hours, and most clinicians suggest a maximal time of 1.5 to 2 hours. Techniques such as hourly release of the tourniquet for 10 minutes, cooling of the affected limb, and alternating dual cuffs may reduce the risk of injury.[355] Nerve and muscle injuries that occur beneath the tourniquet cuff are related to the pneumatic pressure. Consequently, the lowest possible pressure that maintains ischemic conditions should be sought. Hypotensive anesthetic techniques have been used in adults to reduce the need for high cuff inflation pressures,[356] but there seems to be little need for this in children. Lieberman and colleagues suggested that pediatric occlusion pressures should be measured by Doppler and the tourniquet pressure set at 50 mm Hg above this value.[357] Maximum mean pressures recommended for the upper and lower extremities are 173.4 ± 11.6 mm Hg (range, 155 to 190 mm Hg) and 176.7 ± 28.7 mm Hg (range, 140 to 250 mm Hg), respectively.[357] Wider cuffs exert less force per unit area and reduce the risk of local sequelae. Recommendations for adults suggest that the cuff should exceed the circumference of the extremity by 7 to 15 cm. This is difficult to achieve in infants, in whom the proximal limb length is proportionally shorter than in adults and the wide cuffs impinge on the surgical field.

## Acute Bone and Joint Infections

The mainstay of management for osteomyelitis and septic arthritis are antibiotics and surgical drainage. The incidence of these infections is increasing, particularly in immunocompromised children with human immunodeficiency virus (HIV) infection. Tuberculosis remains a scourge in many developing countries. Mortality rates for hospital-acquired staphylococcal disease in compromised children[358] and community-acquired disease in healthy children[359,360] range from 8% to 47% for those presenting with severe sepsis.[361] *Mycobacterium* and *Staphylococcus* species resistant to conventional antibiotics increase morbidity and mortality rates.

## PATHOPHYSIOLOGY

*Staphylococcus aureus* is the most common pathogen. Osteomyelitis develops after bacteremia and occurs mostly in prepubertal children. Normal bone is highly resistant to infection, but *S. aureus* adheres to bone by expressing receptors for components of bone matrix, and the expression of collagen-binding adhesin permits the attachment to cartilage.[362] After the microorganisms adhere to bone, they express phenotypic resistance to antimicrobial treatment.[362]

The metaphyseal region around the growth plate is the predominant area of infection. Sluggish blood flow in the metaphysis predisposes children to bacterial infection, and endothelial gaps in developing vessels allow bacteria to escape into the metaphysis. Subsequent abscesses may decompress into the joint or subperiosteally. Infection may involve adjacent tissue planes, and hematogenous spread causes multiple pathologic processes beyond the primary site of infection.

Septic arthritis is more common in neonates because transphyseal vessels link the metaphysis and epiphysis. Growth plate and epiphyseal destruction may occur in this age group. Articular cartilage damage is attributable to the release of proteolytic enzymes by the pathogen and activated neutrophils.

## CLINICAL PRESENTATION

Most children with staphylococcal disease present with musculoskeletal symptoms and fever, but those with disseminated disease may be critically ill (4% to 10%) with severe sepsis and lung disease.[359,360] There is often a history of trauma.[359,360] It can be difficult to diagnose extracutaneous foci. One report found that 50% of extracutaneous foci of staphylococcal infection were not detected on hospital admission, and one third of these lesions were observed for the first time at autopsy.[358] An absolute polymorphonuclear cell count of greater than 10,000/mm$^3$ or an absolute band-form count of greater than 500/mm$^3$, or both, correlates with the presence of one or more inadequately treated sites of staphylococcal infection.[358] Tuberculosis is the great mimic and must always be suspected in endemic areas.

Diagnosis is confirmed by blood, bone, or joint aspirate culture. Radiologic procedures (e.g., plain radiographs, computed tomography, magnetic resonance imaging, radionuclide scans) are often required to identify foci, and the anesthesiologist is often requested to provide sedation.

## TREATMENT OPTIONS

Antibiotic therapy is the mainstay of treatment. Initial antibiotic choice is dictated by age and by local pathogen and sensitivity profiles. Antibiotic treatment should be extended to cover gram-negative enterococci in neonates and *Streptococcus* in older children. *Haemophilus influenzae* remains a pathogen in unvaccinated regions. Surgical decompression of acute osteomyelitis that is responding poorly to antimicrobial therapy may release intramedullary or subperiosteal pus and lead to clinical improvement. Pus within fascial planes also requires release. Venous thrombosis attributable to pus in soft tissue planes around major joints was associated with a high mortality rate in one series.[359] Determining and eradicating the primary focus improves the mortality and reduces recurrence rates.[363] An aggressive search for foci and surgical drainage of infective foci is required.

Highly active antiretroviral therapy (HAART) has positively altered the mortality rates for HIV-infected children. However, acute bone and joint infections still occur,[364] and these drugs can cause significant morbidity due to changes in fat distribution, lipid profiles, glucose concentrations, homeostasis, and bone turnover.[365] Infarction may replace infection as the major cause of morbidity and mortality from HIV.[365] It is uncertain whether HAART should be continued during acute osteomyelitis. Worsening cell-mediated immune function may occur during tuberculosis treatment if HAART is continued.[366] The combination of HIV infection and tuberculosis can be lethal in children, and antituberculosis treatment is continued for 12 to 18 months.

## ANESTHESIA CONSIDERATIONS

Anesthesiology services are commonly required for sedation during diagnostic investigation, anesthesia for surgical exploration and release of pus or fixation of pathologic fractures, management of pulmonary complications (e.g., intercostal chest drain insertion, pleurodesis), central venous cannulation for long-term antibiotic treatment, and analgesic modalities.

Children with disseminated staphylococcal disease may be critically ill with multisystem disease and require fluid volume augmentation, inotrope support, positive-pressure ventilation, extracorporeal renal support, and coagulation factor replacement. Others may appear clinically stable before induction of anesthesia; the assessment of hypovolemia in children is subject to moderate to poor interrater agreement.[367] Intravenous access and rehydration are required before beginning anesthesia to avoid a precipitous blood pressure drop immediately after induction. Bacteremic showering during manipulation and drainage of pus causes further decompensation. Excessive bleeding due to altered coagulation status should also be anticipated.

The presence of a septic arthritis in the shoulder or neck may cause cervical ligamentous laxity predisposing to C1-2 subluxation during intubation.[368] Pneumatoceles from staphylococcal pneumonia can rupture during positive-pressure ventilation. A spontaneous breathing mode, however, may be difficult to achieve because of laryngospasm, breath holding, increased secretions, and bronchospasm. The use of NMBDs and positive-pressure ventilation in these patients with a low threshold for introducing inotropes to support the cardiovascular system is an easier option. Vigilance is required for acute pneumothorax.

Myocarditis, pericarditis, and pericardial effusions compromise myocardial function. A 12% prevalence of infective endocarditis among children with hospital-acquired *Staphylococcus aureus* bacteremia has been reported.[369] This prevalence of infective endocarditis was frequently associated with congenital heart disease and the necessity for multiple blood cultures.[369] The incidence of infective endocarditis among children with community-acquired disease without preexisting cardiac abnormalities was low,[359] suggesting that echocardiography could be reserved for children with preexisting cardiac disease, those with suspicious clinical findings, those whose temperature fails to stabilize, or those who have prolonged bacteremia without an obvious source of infection.

## PAIN MANAGEMENT

Morphine and acetaminophen are the analgesics commonly used for postoperative pain management. The use of tramadol in children is increasing as our understanding of the pharmacokinetics of this medication increases.[370,371] The low incidence of respiratory depression and constipation, fewer controls on use, and similar frequency of nausea and vomiting (10% to 40%) compared with opioids make tramadol an attractive alternative.[372-374] NSAIDs are relatively contraindicated in the presence of coagulation disorders, altered renal function, and COX-2–mediated osteogenesis.

The performance of regional blockade in children with acute bone or joint infection is controversial. There are no studies addressing the risk/benefit ratios of regional techniques in this population. It seems reasonable to use these techniques only after 24 hours of appropriate antibiotic therapy in apyrexial children who show no signs of a coagulopathy.

# Common Syndromes

Children with some specific conditions present repeatedly for orthopedic procedures. It is worthwhile maintaining a database that details their anesthetic management. There should be 24-hour access to standard texts or electronic information concerning anesthesia and uncommon pediatric diseases.

## CEREBRAL PALSY
### Clinical Features
*Cerebral palsy* is an umbrella term that describes a group of non-progressive, but often changing motor impairment syndromes caused by lesions or anomalies in the brain that occur during the early stages of its development.[375] It is the leading cause of motor disability during childhood, with a prevalence of approximately 2 cases per 1000 live births in developed countries.[376]

Disorders include cognitive impairment, sensory loss (i.e., vision and hearing), seizures, and communication and behavioral disturbances. Systemic disorders resulting from cerebral palsy affect the gastrointestinal, respiratory, urinary tract, and orthopedic systems. Cerebral palsy is divided into three broad categories: spastic (70%), dyskinetic (10%), and ataxic (10%). Children with spastic cerebral palsy commonly present for orthopedic procedures because of contractures at major peripheral joints.[377,378] Functional improvement after surgery in children with spastic diplegia and spastic hemiplegia is better than in those suffering spastic quadriplegia.[377]

### Orthopedic Considerations
Orthopedic manipulations form only part of the treatments designed to improve performance or improve the ease of care. Management, including orthopedic surgery, physical and occupational therapy, recreational therapy, orthotics, and assistive devices, improve functional outcomes. Medical modalities such as intramuscular injections of botulinum toxin and intrathecal administration of baclofen by means of an implanted pump may also be of benefit.[379] Selective dorsal rhizotomy has been used to control spasticity.[380,381]

The indications for and timing of surgical interventions vary. Gait analysis increases the age of the patient at the first orthopedic surgical procedure, and botulinum toxin type A treatment delays and reduces the frequency of surgical procedures on the lower extremities.[382,383] Bone and soft tissue surgical procedures are designed to lengthen or weaken spastic muscles to give opposing muscles a chance to attain muscle balance.

### Anesthetic Considerations
Children with cerebral palsy who present for orthopedic surgery often have previous experience of operating rooms. They should be handled with sensitivity because communication disorders and sensory deficits may mask mildly impaired or normal intellect. They may be accompanied by a parent or caregiver or be premedicated for induction of anesthesia or in the recovery room. If there is a communication problem, the parent or caregiver should be present before and after anesthesia.[377,384]

Medical conditions (e.g., seizure control, respiratory function, gastroesophageal reflux) should be optimized preoperatively. Contracture deformities, spinal deformities, decubitus ulceration, and skin infection must be considered when positioning the child for anesthesia and surgery. Poor nutritional status affects postoperative wound healing and the risk of infection. Concurrent medications may influence anesthesia; cisapride for gastroesophageal reflux is associated with prolonged QT interval, sodium valproate can cause platelet dysfunction and affect drug metabolism, and anticonvulsant use increases resistance to NMBDs.[385] A history of latex allergy should be sought because of exposure to latex allergens from an early age.[386]

Intravenous access may be difficult. Drooling, a decreased ability to swallow secretions, and gastroesophageal reflux may dissuade some against an inhalational induction, but there is no evidence that rapid-sequence induction is safer. Succinylcholine may be used because it does not cause hyperkalemia in these children, whose muscles have never become denervated. Non-communicative or nonverbal children with cerebral palsy require less propofol to obtain the same BIS values (i.e., 35 to 45) than do otherwise healthy children.[387] The minimum alveolar concentration of halothane is 20% less in children with cerebral palsy, whether they took anticonvulsant drugs or not (MAC of 0.62 and 0.71, respectively).[388]

Intraoperative hypothermia is common in children with disordered temperature regulation due to hypothalamic dysfunction, reduced muscle bulk, and fat deposits. Thermal homeostasis should be managed aggressively from the moment the child enters the operating room.

Extensive plaster casting is an important component of bone and soft tissue surgical procedures. These casts may conceal blood loss, and limb swelling within the cast may contribute to compartment syndromes. Plaster jackets and hip spicas have been associated with mesenteric occlusion and acute gastric dilatation.

Pain and spasm are regular features postoperatively. Epidural analgesia is particularly valuable when major orthopedic procedures are performed. Occasionally, two epidurals at different spinal sites may be required for multilevel surgery. Systemic benzodiazepines, baclofen, dantrolene, and clonidine have been used to reduce muscle spasms. Selective dorsal rhizotomy is associated with severe pain, muscle spasms, and dysesthesia. Epidural and intrathecal forms of morphine have been used to control this pain. Intravenous morphine and midazolam also have been successfully used.[389] Oral benzodiazepines may be required to reduce the incidence and severity of muscle spasms but should be used with caution if combined with opioid analgesia.

Pain assessment is difficult in these children, but several scoring systems are available.[390,391] (See also Chapter 43.) The opinions of parents and caregivers are extremely valuable in the assessment of pain and discrimination from other factors such as irritability on anesthetic emergence, poor positioning, a full bladder, or nausea.

## SPINA BIFIDA
Spina bifida is characterized by developmental abnormalities of the vertebrae and spinal cord that may be associated with changes in the cerebrum, brainstem, and peripheral nerves. The failure of fusion of the vertebral arches is commonly known as *spina bifida*. *Spina bifida occulta* refers to spina bifida that occurs when skin and soft tissues cover the defect. *Spina bifida aperta* is used to describe lesions that communicate with the outside as a meningocele or a myelomeningocele (incidence of 1 case per 1000 live births). The myelomeningocele sac contains nerve roots that do not function below the level of the lesion.

### Clinical Features
Nerve root dysfunction results in muscle paralysis and a neurogenic bowel and bladder. Eighty percent of children develop

hydrocephalus because of aqueductal stenosis (Arnold-Chiari [type II] malformation). Skeletal abnormalities such as clubfoot and congenital dislocation of the hip are common. Scoliosis may result from congenital vertebral abnormalities or, more commonly, abnormal neuromuscular control. Epilepsy and learning disorders can also occur, but most children have normal intelligence.

## Orthopedic Considerations

Denervation causes muscle imbalance that results in abnormalities at the hip, knee, and foot. The aims of surgery are to reduce flexor posture at the hip and knee and plantigrade feet. Children with clubfeet, hip subluxation, or scoliosis commonly present for orthopedic correction.

## Anesthetic Considerations

The potential for infection of the central nervous system dictates closure of the sac within the first few days of life. Subsequent surgical procedures and urinary catheterizations set the stage for a sensitivity to latex.[392] Primary prophylaxis (i.e., avoiding all latex materials and using a latex-free operating room) is recommended for prevention of latex allergy and anaphylaxis.[393]

Preoperative assessment should include motor and sensory deficits, respiratory and renal function, and functioning of a ventriculoperitoneal shunt. Positioning on the operating table may require additional pillows for support of limbs with contractures. As a result of hypesthesia in the lower extremities, intravenous cannulae can be inserted painlessly. However, venous access is usually poor in the lower extremities because of limited use. The risk of endobronchial intubation is increased because of a short trachea (36% of patients).[394] Kyphoscoliosis may distort tracheal anatomy. Renal dysfunction may dictate NMBD choice and avoidance of NSAIDs. Succinylcholine may be used because it does not cause hyperkalemia in these children.[395] A reduced hypercapnic ventilation response means that these children should be closely observed in the recovery period.

## OSTEOGENESIS IMPERFECTA

Osteogenesis imperfecta (OI) is thought to have afflicted Ivar the Boneless (Ivar Ragnarsson), a Viking chieftain who led a successful invasion of the East Anglia region of England in 865 AD. Because he "had legs as soft as cartilage," he was unable to walk and had to be carried on a shield. Ivar's name is also associated with an early form of thoracoplasty. When King Ælla of Northumbria was captured, Ivar subjected him to the horrific "Blood Eagle" ordeal. His ribs were torn out and folded back to form the shape of an eagle's wings, and his lungs were removed.

## Clinical Features

OI is a genetically determined disorder of connective tissue that is characterized by bone fragility. The disease state encompasses a phenotypically and genotypically heterogeneous group of inherited disorders that result from mutations in the genes that code for type I collagen.[396] The disorder manifests in tissues in which the principal matrix protein is type I collagen—mainly bone, dentin, sclerae, and ligaments. Musculoskeletal manifestations vary in severity along a continuum ranging from perinatal lethal forms with crumpled bones to moderate forms with deformity and propensity for fracture to clinically silent forms with subtle osteopenia and no deformity.[396]

Classification (types I through IV) is based on the timing of fractures or on multiple clinical, genetic, and radiologic

features. Type I is the most common (1 case per 30,000 live births), and type I and type IV have autosomal dominant inheritance patterns. These children have the classic triad of blue sclera, multiple fractures, and conductive hearing loss in adolescence. Bowing of the lower limbs, genu valgum, flat feet, and scoliosis develop with age. Type IV is characterized by osteoporosis, leading to bone fragility without many of the other features of type I. Types II and III are more severe forms of OI and have autosomal recessive inheritance patterns. Molecular genetic studies have identified more than 150 mutations of the *COL1A1* and *COL1A2* genes, which encode for type I procollagen.[396]

## Orthopedic Considerations

The goals of treatment of OI are to maximize function, minimize deformity and disability, maintain comfort, achieve relative independence in activities of daily living, and enhance social integration. Physiotherapy, rehabilitation, and orthopedic surgery are the mainstays of treatment for moderate and severe forms of OI. Medical treatment with the antiresorptive bisphosphonates (e.g., pamidronate) can decrease pain, lower the fracture incidence, and improve mobility. Initial investigations have demonstrated an acceptable safety profile for pamidronate. Long-term follow-up data are lacking and will be necessary for the development of responsible therapeutic guidelines.[397] Medical therapies other than bisphosphonates, such as growth hormone and parathyroid hormone, have only minor roles. Gene-based therapy remains in the early stages of preclinical research.[398,399]

Operative intervention is indicated for recurrent fractures or deformity that impairs function.[396] Fractures in mild to moderately severe cases of OI type I are treated using the same methods as for patients without OI. Deformed bones that are fracturing are realigned, frequently followed by providing external or internal support. In selecting various modes of treatment, it is important to consider the natural history of the particular type of OI and to set realistic goals.[400-404]

## Anesthetic Considerations

In common with other children suffering chronic disabilities, children with OI are veterans of the operating room. Chronic pain from frequent fractures complicates handling. Deafness may hinder communication. Preoperative assessment centers on the chest wall deformity because it determines the severity of restrictive lung disease and subsequent cardiovascular compromise. Neck mobility, mouth opening, and dentition should also be assessed.

There is a risk of further fractures with positioning, tourniquet application, airway handing, and use of a blood pressure cuff. Invasive pressure monitoring may be less traumatic than a blood pressure cuff for some patients. If noninvasive blood pressure monitoring is used, less frequent monitoring of the blood pressure is recommended if possible. A laryngeal mask airway may avoid pressure from facemasks. An individual history may help determine the risk/benefit ratio for each child. Succinylcholine has the potential to cause fasciculation-induced fractures.

Abnormal temperature homeostasis may result in intraoperative hyperthermia that may be severe and accompanied by tachycardia and metabolic acidosis. This response is different from that of malignant hyperthermia in that there is an absence of respiratory acidosis and muscle rigidity.[405] Surface cooling is usually effective in restoring thermal homeostasis.

## DUCHENNE MUSCULAR DYSTROPHY

### Clinical Features

DMD is the most common of the progressive muscular dystrophies. It is an X-linked recessive disorder with an incidence of 3 cases per 10,000 births (see Chapter 22). The *DMD* gene (located at Xp21.2) codes for a large sarcolemmal membrane protein, dystrophin, which is associated muscle cell membrane integrity and signal transduction. Dystrophin is missing or nonfunctional in DMD patients. Both sexes can carry the *DMD* mutation, but girls rarely exhibit signs of the disease.

Children usually present before school age with a waddling gait and later develop a lumbar lordosis and difficulty climbing stairs. Children use their arms to assist standing up (i.e., Growers sign) due to proximal weakness of the hip girdle. Distal muscles, such as the calves, appear hypertrophied. The disease process is progressive, with increasing muscle weakness occurring with age. These boys often become wheelchair bound by 10 to 11 years of age. Respiratory weakness, often exacerbated by scoliosis and by difficulty swallowing secretions due to pharyngeal involvement, can progress to a terminal pneumonia in late teenage years.[406] By late adolescence, most children with DMD have cardiac disease, whether it is an abnormal electrocardiogram, arrhythmias, or a cardiomyopathy. Death from cardiorespiratory failure usually occurs before age 30, although respiratory support is extending life expectancy.

DMD is not a static disease. In early childhood, skeletal muscle is constantly catabolized and becomes unstable. The use of membrane-destabilizing medications such as succinylcholine and potent inhalational anesthetics (halothane in particular) in these young children can result in hyperkalemia, rhabdomyolysis, and cardiac arrest. However, after the children reach adolescence, the bulk of the skeletal muscle catabolism has arrested, and membrane-destabilizing medications are left with no substrate. Succinylcholine and potent inhalational anesthetics may be used without sequelae in adolescents with DMD who were undergoing scoliosis surgery and instrumentation. In contrast, the cardiac and smooth muscle consequences of DMD are minor and insignificant in childhood but become life-threatening during adolescence and adulthood. The anesthesiologist must appreciate the developmental nature of DMD and recognize the risks that may be associated with the use of succinylcholine and inhalational anesthetics in this group of children.

DMD can affect cardiac, smooth, and skeletal muscle. Right ventricular function may be compromised by nocturnal oxygen desaturation and sleep apnea contributing to pulmonary hypertension. Sinus tachycardia and arrhythmias may occur at an early age, but clinically apparent cardiomyopathy usually does not develop before 10 years of age. One third of children have some degree of intellectual impairment.

DMD should be suspected in male preschool children with delayed walking ability, and measurement of high serum creatinine phosphokinase concentrations provides a screening tool. Steroids are increasingly used for the management of DMD because they appear to increase muscle mass by decreasing protein breakdown.[407]

Becker muscular dystrophy (BMD) is a milder form of DMD with an onset at puberty or later in adolescence. Clinical expression varies, but even adolescents presenting with mild or subclinical weakness can develop cardiomyopathy with age progression. Death from cardiac or respiratory failure does not usually occur until the fourth or fifth decade. Because of improvements in respiratory care, dilated cardiomyopathy has become the major cause of death.[408]

BMD is an autosomal recessive myopathy that also results from mutations of dystrophin caused by a deletion of the exons 11 to 13 in the *DMD* gene (located at Xp21.2).[409] Dystrophin exerts its effect at the voltage-gated chloride channel 1 (CLCN1). Genetic analysis is an essential step in confirming the diagnosis. Additional EMG procedures may be of diagnostic value even when muscle biopsy may reveal no evidence of dystrophy.

Of importance to anesthesiologists, two thirds of patients with mild or subclinical BMD have evidence of right ventricular dilation, and one third have evidence of left ventricular dysfunction.[410] A thorough cardiac evaluation (similar to that for DMD) is recommended before scoliosis surgery.[408] Hyperthermia and heart failure, mimicking malignant hyperthermia and hyperkalemia with rhabdomyolysis after inhalational agents, have been reported in patients with BMD.[411,412] Despite these reports, the relationship between BMD and malignant hyperthermia remains unclear.

### Orthopedic Considerations

Orthopedic surgery is indicated to improve or maintain ambulation and standing. Early treatment of contractures of the hips and the lower limbs prevents severe contractures and delays the progression of scoliosis.[413] Techniques designed to improve deformities and permit early postoperative mobilization include subcutaneous release of contracted tendons and percutaneous removal of cancellous bone with corrective manipulation of the feet. Maintenance of upright posture extends the ability of patients to attend to the tasks of daily living.[414] Spinal deformities attributable to muscle imbalance or a collapsing spine are corrected to improve or maintain sitting posture. Spinal fusion may also decrease the rate of deterioration of respiratory function, although this has been questioned.[415]

### Anesthetic Considerations

Respiratory and cardiovascular compromise dominates preoperative assessment. Deformities and contractures of limb joints hinder vascular access, regional anesthetic techniques, and positioning on the operating table. Hypertrophy of the tongue may cause difficulty during intubation. Gastric motility is delayed, and gastric emptying times are prolonged.[416] Tracheobronchial tree compression has been described in a child positioned prone for spinal instrumentation.[417] These children tend to have greater blood loss during surgery. The precise cause remains unclear, but it may be because fat and connective tissue have replaced muscle or because of abnormalities in the blood vessels.[210]

Nondepolarizing NMBDs have a slow onset and prolonged duration of action.[418-420] All NMBDs should be monitored with a peripheral nerve stimulator.[421] *Succinylcholine is contraindicated in these children because of the risk of hyperkalemia, muscle rigidity, rhabdomyolysis, myoglobinuria, arrhythmias, and cardiac arrest.* There is no clear link between DMD and malignant hyperthermia.[422,423] The predominant candidate gene (*RYR1*) for malignant hyperthermia is located on the long arm of chromosome 19, whereas the *DMD* gene is located on the short arm of the X chromosome.[424] Although volatile anesthetic agents continue to be used in young children with DMD, rhabdomyolysis and hyperkalemia have been reported in the recovery room after halothane, isoflurane, desflurane, and sevoflurane anesthesia.[425-429] Potent inhalational anesthetics are best avoided in young children with DMD;

instead, alternative anesthetics that do not trigger rhabdomyolysis and hyperkalemia, such as propofol, ketamine, opioids, and benzodiazepines, are preferred.[430]

Regional techniques such as epidurals may be technically more difficult due to kyphoscoliosis and obesity. The use of ultrasound-guided peripheral nerve blockade can improve the quality and reduce complications of neuronal blockade.[6] Opioids are not contraindicated in the postoperative period but should be used with caution in children with respiratory compromise. Tramadol is an effective alternative. Noninvasive ventilation support using BiPAP or continuous positive airway pressure is sometimes required after major surgery or in those already receiving this treatment overnight.

## ARTHROGRYPOSIS MULTIPLEX CONGENITA
### Clinical Features
Arthrogryposis multiplex congenita is a spectrum syndrome of multiple, persistent limb contractures often accompanied by associated anomalies, including cleft palate, genitourinary defects, gastroschisis, and cardiac defects.[431] The incidence is 1 case per 3000 births. Joint contractures are present at birth and are a result of immobility in utero, commonly related to a neurogenic abnormality or myopathy.[432] These children have been likened to a "thin, wooden doll," because muscles connected to affected joints are atrophic and replaced by fibrous tissue and fat.[433] The temporomandibular joint may also be involved, causing restricted jaw opening and micrognathia. Scoliosis commonly develops. Restrictive lung disease, rib cage deformities, and pulmonary hypoplasia predispose to recurrent chest infections.

### Orthopedic Considerations
The aim of surgery is to improve function. Most operations involve the soft tissues, tendons, and osteotomies of the lower limbs and hips.[434] Upper limb surgery is less common. Extension contracture of the elbow joint makes it impossible to reach the mouth or to perform hygienic necessities. Improvement in passive elbow flexion by capsulotomy or in active flexion by triceps transfer can increase independence and personal hygiene. When both arms are involved, consideration may be given to maintaining one arm in flexion for reaching the head and mouth passively or even actively and one arm in extension for basic hygiene cares.[435]

### Anesthetic Considerations
Arthrogryposis multiplex congenita is commonly associated with other syndromes that may complicate anesthesia.[431,436] Venous cannulation is difficult because veins tend to be small and fragile. The concavity of joints is difficult to access. Care must be taken in positioning the patient on the operating table and protecting skin overlying bony joints to prevent pathologic fractures.

These children should be evaluated for a difficult airway because of temporomandibular joint limitation and micrognathia.[437-439] Fusion or underdevelopment of the first and second cervical vertebrae may further complicate laryngoscopy and tracheal intubation with a severe reduction in neck mobility. Tracheal intubation may become progressively more difficult with age. During infancy, however, evaluating mouth opening may be difficult; it may be necessary to insert a tongue blade into the mouth to determine whether the mandible can be distracted from the maxilla.

Succinylcholine has been used without incident in these children, although teleologically, the use of a depolarizing muscle relaxant in the presence of anterior horn cell disease is contentious. The response to nondepolarizing NMBDs should be monitored.

Hyperthermia and persistent tachycardia have been reported during general anesthesia.[431,440-442] These signs occur irrespective of the anesthetic agent and are not associated with malignant hyperthermia. In this case, hyperthermia responds to simple cooling techniques.

Pulmonary dysfunction and an increased sensitivity to opioids dictate suitable monitoring postoperatively. Regional techniques may be difficult in the presence of contractures, but if successful, they offer intraoperative and postoperative analgesia.[433] Success can be improved by using ultrasound-guided techniques.

## ANNOTATED REFERENCES

Harper CM, Ambler G, Edge G. The prognostic value of preoperative predicted forced vital capacity in corrective spinal surgery for Duchenne's muscular dystrophy. Anaesthesia 2004;59:1160-2.

*Performing scoliosis surgery on children with Duchenne muscular dystrophy who have a forced vital capacity (FVC) of 30% has been questioned because of the high incidence of postoperative pulmonary complications. This clinical paper demonstrated that with careful attention to detail, children with an FVC less than 30% can undergo scoliosis surgery with results similar to those with an FVC greater than 30%. Early extubation followed by the use of noninvasive ventilation was identified as key to reducing respiratory complications.*

Malhotra NR, Shaffrey CI. Intraoperative electrophysiological monitoring in spine surgery. Spine 2010;35:2167-79.

*The authors undertook a pooled data analysis to review intraoperative neuromonitoring changes that occur during the course of spine surgery, and they describe the appropriate application of this monitoring.*

Nolan J, Chalkiadis GA, Low J, et al. Anaesthesia and pain management in cerebral palsy. Anaesthesia 2000;55:32-41.

*Children with cerebral palsy frequently present for a variety of orthopedic procedures. This well-written review from a large children's hospital details the many issues and concerns involved with anesthetizing and caring for these patients postoperatively.*

Reinacher PC, Priebe HJ, Blumrich W, et al. The effects of stimulation pattern and sevoflurane concentration on intraoperative motor evoked potentials. Anesth Analg 2006;102:888-95.

Scheufler KM, Reinacher PC, Blumrich W, et al. The modifying effects of stimulation pattern and propofol plasma concentration on motor-evoked potentials. Anesth Analg 2005;100:440-7.

*The authors of this pair of complicated but interesting articles investigated the influence of anesthetic agent concentration (i.e., sevoflurane and propofol) and stimulation pattern on intraoperative motor evoked potentials (MEPs). Although conducted in children undergoing craniotomy, the finding that the MEP characteristics depended more on stimulation pattern than anesthetic agent concentration is important for spine surgery. Their finding that using a train of three or more stimuli (MEP recording was possible at 1 minimal alveolar concentration (MAC) of sevoflurane or with propofol target-controlled infusion at 6 μg/mL) demonstrates that with modern monitoring systems, anesthetic concentrations of these agents can be used for spine surgery while preserving MEPs.*

Yemen TA, McClain C. Muscular dystrophy, anesthesia and the safety of inhalational agents revisited again. Paediatr Anaesth 2006;16:105-8.

*In this thought-provoking editorial, the authors discuss the risk of rhabdomyolysis in patients with Duchenne muscular dystrophy. The paper challenges us to reevaluate our approach to patient safety based on an increasing number of case reports (but in the absence of scientific evidence), linking rhabdomyolysis to inhalational agents in this group of patients.*

Yuan N, Fraire JA, Margetis MM, et al. The effect of scoliosis surgery on lung function in the immediate postoperative period. Spine 2005;30:2182-5.

*This study clearly demonstrated the dramatic decrease in pulmonary function in the days after scoliosis surgery, readily explaining why children are at risk for pulmonary complications during this period. Pulmonary function tests (FEV$_1$, FVC, FEV$_1$/FVC, and FEF$_{25-75\%}$) were measured daily for 10 days after scoliosis repair. Results of pulmonary function tests decreased by up to 60% after surgery, with a nadir at 3 days. The FEV$_1$ and FVC values were still only at 60% of the preoperative values on the 10th postoperative day.*

## REFERENCES

Please see www.expertconsult.com.

# Otorhinolaryngologic Procedures

RAAFAT S. HANNALLAH, KAREN A. BROWN, AND SUSAN T. VERGHESE

OTORHINOLARYNGOLOGIC PROCEDURES REPRESENT A large segment of elective pediatric surgery. Anesthetic management of these children is provided by both pediatric and general anesthesiologists, frequently working in anesthesia care teams, most commonly in ambulatory surgery centers and office practices.[1] Additionally, anesthesiologists are often consulted to help manage potentially life-threatening pediatric otolaryngologic emergencies. These include airway obstruction suffering from croup, foreign body aspiration, airway trauma and acute epiglottitis.[2] In both the elective and emergent scenarios, it is essential to understand the pathophysiology, and to discuss the anesthetic plan in advance of the procedure with the surgeon, who will frequently be sharing the airway with the anesthesiologist. This ensures safe anesthetic management and ideal conditions for both children and surgeons.

## Anesthesia for Otologic Procedures

### MYRINGOTOMY AND VENTILATING TUBE INSERTION

Chronic serous otitis media is common in young children. If untreated or poorly managed, it can lead to hearing loss and formation of cholesteatoma. When conservative medical management fails, surgical drainage of accumulated fluid in the middle ear is indicated. Myringotomy creates an opening in the tympanic membrane through which fluid can drain. If performed alone, when the incision heals, the drainage path is occluded. Therefore myringotomy is frequently accompanied by placement of a ventilation tube. A small plastic tube (a variation of the grommet or the T-tube) inserted in the tympanic membrane serves as a stent for the ostium, facilitating continuous drainage from the middle ear until the tubes are naturally extruded in 6 months to a year, or surgically removed at an appropriate time.

Children with cleft palate have a high frequency of middle ear disease compared with the noncleft population, because of associated abnormalities of the cartilage and muscles surrounding the eustachian tubes. Surgical drainage and ventilation tube insertion is a standard treatment for chronic otitis media in these children. This is usually performed at the time of the surgical repair of the cleft.

Most young children require general anesthesia for tympanotomy tube placement, although an occasional older child may tolerate topical anesthesia. This may be accomplished by iontophoresis or instillation of lidocaine–prilocaine cream (EMLA cream), which remains in the ear canal for an hour and is then suctioned out before the procedure.

Myringotomy with tube insertion is a very brief operation, usually performed as ambulatory surgery using a potent inhalational agent (e.g., sevoflurane), oxygen, and nitrous oxide administered by facemask with spontaneous respirations. An oropharyngeal airway may assist in maintaining a patent airway when the head is laterally rotated and reduces head movement (which is amplified through the microscope). Gentle manual assistance of ventilation can also help reduce head movement. Occasionally, a laryngeal mask airway (LMA) may be used in children in whom the procedure is expected to be prolonged (e.g., children with narrow ear canals) or those with a difficult airway. Most children can be managed safely without intravenous (IV) access,[3] but it is reasonable to have an IV setup ready. Some children with severe underlying medical or surgical conditions will require IV access, despite the anticipated brief duration of the minor procedure. Although premedication is often omitted because their duration of action exceeds that of the procedure, an anxious child may still benefit from a sedative premedication.

In some instances, it is desirable to remove a retained tympanostomy tube. This can be easily accomplished in the surgeon's office without anesthesia. Some stiff-flanged grommet tubes require general anesthesia for removal. If the incision does not heal spontaneously, a paper patch or fat graft may have to be placed to stimulate healing of the tympanic membrane. The anesthetic would be the same as that for the tube placement, except that nitrous oxide is best avoided to minimize the chance of graft dislodgment (see later discussion).

Discomfort after myringotomy and tube insertion is usually managed by the administration of acetaminophen, either via the oral route preoperatively or the rectal route intraoperatively. The recommended dose of acetaminophen to achieve therapeutic blood levels is 10 to 20 mg/kg when administered via the oral route, and 30 to 40 mg/kg when administered via the rectal route.[4-7] Oral acetaminophen is very rapidly absorbed, achieving therapeutic blood levels in minutes, whereas rectal acetaminophen is slowly absorbed, with a time to onset of action of 60 to 90 minutes, and a time to peak effect of 1 to 3 hours.[8-11] Consequently, the oral route is preferred for this procedure.

Preschool-aged children who receive sevoflurane without an analgesic for myringotomy and tube insertion may exhibit emergence delirium and postoperative agitation (see Chapter 4). Although pain may be partially responsible for these responses, their etiologies are not completely understood. Because the procedure is so brief and IV access is not usually established, intranasal fentanyl, 1 to 2 µg/kg, has been shown to provide analgesia and to reduce the frequency of emergence agitation.[12,13] The only significant side effect is a 12% incidence of vomiting when oral fluids are administered in the early postoperative period.[5] Other medications, including IV ketorolac (1 mg/kg), or intranasal butorphanol (25 µg/kg), and intranasal dexmedetomidine (1 to 2 µg/kg), have been shown to reduce the pain after myringotomy and tube insertion.[14-16] However larger doses of dexmedetomidine (2 µg/kg) significantly prolong the duration of stay in the postanesthesia care unit (PACU). Some practitioners prefer to use more soluble anesthetics, such as isoflurane, for anesthesia maintenance to reduce the incidence of agitation after myringotomy and tube insertion, although there is limited evidence to support this practice.

Children with chronic otitis frequently have persistent rhinorrhea and suffer recurrent upper respiratory tract infection (URI) (see Chapter 11). Eradication of middle ear congestion and improved fluid drainage often resolves the concomitant symptoms. The frequency of perioperative complications in children with mild URIs is similar to that in children who are asymptomatic. In general, morbidity is not increased in children who present for minor surgery with acute uncomplicated mild URIs, provided tracheal intubation can be avoided.[17,18] Canceling this surgery because of rhinorrhea or recurrent mild respiratory symptoms is not usually justifiable. It is, however, recommended that children with respiratory symptoms have their oxygen saturation measured before induction of general anesthesia, and that supplemental oxygen is administered postoperatively to those whose oxygen-saturation readings are less than 93%.[19]

## MIDDLE EAR AND MASTOID SURGERY

Tympanoplasty and mastoidectomy are two of the most common major ear operations performed in children. General anesthesia usually consists of an inhalational anesthetic and IV opioids. Surgical identification and preservation of the facial nerve are necessary because of its proximity to the surgical field. To ensure the facial nerve can be identified using electrical stimulation, neuromuscular blockade is usually avoided. If a muscle relaxant must be used, a small dose should be given to facilitate tracheal intubation; if a muscle relaxant is used for maintenance, suppression of the twitch response should not exceed 70%.

To gain access to the surgical site, the child's head is placed on a headrest, which may be positioned below the operating

table. In addition, extreme degrees of lateral rotation may be required to visualize the middle ear anatomy. The anesthesiologist and surgeon must be especially vigilant to ensure that nerves, muscles, and bony structures are not injured as a result of this unusual positioning; the sternocleidomastoid muscles generally limit the safe degree of lateral head rotation. Left or right tilting (airplaning) of the operating room (OR) table minimizes the need for extreme lateral head rotation as in the case of children with Down syndrome. The laxity of the ligaments of the cervical spine, as well as immaturity of the odontoid process in these children predisposes them to C1-C2 subluxation. Of children with Down syndrome or achondroplasia, 15% to 31% have atlantoaxial instability.[20-23] Anteroposterior positioning requires the utmost care to avoid injury. Positioning of the OR table to allow access to the respective middle ear and accommodate all the extra surgical equipment can also pose a challenge. Depending on the room configuration, the table may be rotated 90 degrees or even 180 degrees away from the anesthesia machine, necessitating the use of extra-long breathing circuits (Fig. 31-1). As a result of the limited access to the airway, very careful attention must be paid to securing the tracheal tube. Draping must allow immediate access to the airway should that be required.

Bleeding must be kept to a minimum during surgery on the small structures of the middle ear. Relative hypotension (i.e., mean arterial pressure 10% to 25% less than baseline) may help to reduce bleeding. Concentrated epinephrine solution, 1:8000, is frequently applied to the tympanic membrane to induce vasoconstriction of the blood vessels. Close attention should be paid to the dose of epinephrine used to avoid arrhythmias and wide swings in blood pressure. The maximum dosage of topical epinephrine is 10 µg/kg, which may be repeated after 30 minutes.

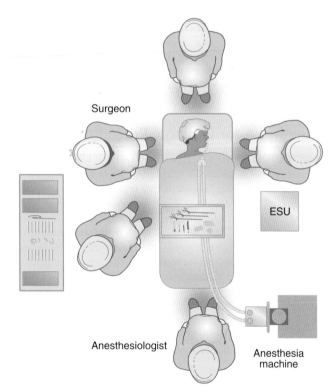

**FIGURE 31-1** An operating room table turned 180 degrees may limit access to the child during ear surgery. *ESU* is the electrosurgical unit.

The middle ear and sinuses are air-filled, nondistensible cavities. An increase in the volume of gas within these cavities increases the pressure within the cavities. Nitrous oxide diffuses along a concentration gradient into air-filled middle ear spaces more rapidly than nitrogen moves out because nitrous oxide is 34 times more soluble in blood than nitrogen. The middle ear is vented through the opening of the eustachian tube. Normal passive venting of the eustachian tube occurs at 20 to 30 cm $H_2O$ pressure. Nitrous oxide increases the pressures within the middle ear such that they exceed the ability of the eustachian tube to vent the middle ear within 5 minutes, leading to pressure buildup.[24] If the function of the eustachian tube is compromised during the surgical procedure, then pressure in the middle ear can increase further. Venting the middle ear occurs intermittently, and leads to constant fluctuations in middle ear pressure that cause movement of the tympanic membrane.[25] During procedures in which the tympanic membrane is replaced or a perforation is patched, nitrous oxide should be discontinued or, if this is not possible, limited to a maximum of 50% of the concentration before the application of the tympanic membrane graft to reduce the potential for pressure-related displacement.[26] The omission of nitrous oxide does not significantly increase the requirements (minimal alveolar concentration) for the less-soluble inhaled anesthetics, desflurane, or sevoflurane in children.[27] After nitrous oxide is discontinued, it is quickly reabsorbed, creating a void in the middle ear, with resulting negative pressure. This negative pressure may result in serous otitis, disarticulation of the ossicles in the middle ear (especially the stapes), and hearing impairment, which may last up to 6 weeks postoperatively. The use of nitrous oxide may increase the incidence of postoperative nausea and vomiting (PONV), as a direct result of negative middle ear pressure during recovery. The negative pressure created by the reabsorption of nitrous oxide stimulates the vestibular system by producing traction on the round window. Although all children are at risk for PONV, older children and adolescents, in particular, seem to be at greatest risk.[28] Prophylactic administration of antiemetics (e.g., dexamethasone and ondansetron) is usually warranted. Local infiltration of the great auricular nerve can provide pain relief equivalent to that of opioids and may reduce the incidence of opioid-induced vomiting (see Chapter 41).[29]

A smooth, quiet emergence is desirable. Deep tracheal extubation can be accomplished if the child breathes spontaneously during the last 15 to 20 minutes of surgery, the concentration of inhalational anesthetic is greater than 1.3 times the minimal alveolar concentration, and opioids are titrated to produce regular slow respirations. Gentle suctioning of the oropharynx and possibly the use of IV lidocaine (1 to 1.5 mg/kg) in children older than 1 year of age can minimize or even prevent coughing after the tracheal tube is removed.

## COCHLEAR IMPLANTS

In recent years, the indications for cochlear implants have broadened and continue to evolve. With the application of universal neonatal hearing screening programs, a large pool of hearing-impaired infants has been identified. The benefits of early intervention with cochlear implants are being explored. Younger children with severe to profound hearing loss markedly improve their auditory, speech, and language skills after cochlear implants, and more of these children can be mainstreamed with their age-appropriate hearing peers when they receive an implant early in life. Experience has shown that cochlear implant surgery is safe

in infants older than 6 months of age, provided that special attention is paid to the physiologic and anatomic differences present in this age-group. Surgery requires meticulous care with hemostasis, soft tissue dissection, and bone drilling because bleeding from bone can be difficult to control and can complicate the surgical outcome. Availability of skilled postoperative nursing and a pediatric intensive care unit (ICU) is also essential.[30] Postoperative fitting of the externally worn speech processor is very important for successful use of the cochlear implant. However, this fitting process can be difficult, particularly in infants and young children, because of limited communication capabilities. Stapedius reflex thresholds obtained intraoperatively have been used for postoperative speech processor fitting, although the influence of anesthetics on the threshold values must be taken into account. More reliable threshold values can be obtained by adjusting the dosage of hypnotics to achieve a lighter level of hypnosis during stapedius reflex measurement.[31] In most children, increasing the concentration of inhalational anesthetics increases the stapedius reflex threshold. As always, appropriate communication with the surgeon will help ensure a successful outcome.

## Anesthesia for Rhinologic Procedures

Chronic sinusitis in children can be caused by antibiotic-resistant bacteria and is usually treated with broad-spectrum antibiotics. In some children with obstructive adenoid pads, adenoidectomy will improve the signs and symptoms of sinusitis. Functional endoscopic sinus surgery using sharp biting instruments and/or a microdebrider has become the primary method of surgical therapy for chronic sinusitis.[32] Current techniques aim to leave the mucosa intact to prevent scarring in the frontal recess. Although sometimes controversial, there is no evidence at present that functional endoscopic sinus surgery affects facial growth in children. Of interest to the anesthesiologist is that many children who require functional endoscopic sinus surgery have coexisting medical problems, such as asthma and cystic fibrosis. These conditions must be optimized before surgery (see Chapter 11).

Anesthetic management usually requires tracheal intubation to secure the airway; the use of an oral preformed tracheal tube (e.g., the Ring-Adair-Elwyn [RAE] tube) allows secure fixation to the mandible and unobstructed access to the maxilla and sinuses. The use of a cuffed tracheal tube is particularly advantageous to eliminate a gas leak that could fog up the endoscopic instruments. A throat pack is frequently inserted to absorb blood in the oropharynx and limit the gas escaping around an uncuffed endotracheal tube (ETT). It is critically important that the pack is removed before tracheal extubation. Occasionally, an LMA may be used to facilitate a quick "second look."

Because bleeding is inevitable with this surgery and can interfere with the surgical exposure, packing the nasal cavity with a vasoconstricting solution is frequently done before surgery commences. The most commonly used topical vasoconstrictors include oxymetazoline 0.025% to 0.05%, phenylephrine 0.25% to 1%, and cocaine 4% to 10%. It is important for the anesthesiologist to be aware of the type and dose of the vasoconstrictor used and that no more than the maximum effective dose is applied. Application of topical phenylephrine or other potent vasoconstrictors to mucous membranes or open surgical sites can cause severe hypertension, reflex bradycardia, and even cardiac arrest.[33] Hypertension that is induced by topically applied vasoconstrictors often resolves spontaneously and may not require aggressive treatment. The use of β-adrenergic blockers or calcium-channel blockers to control blood pressure in these circumstances can depress cardiac output, leading to pulmonary edema and cardiac arrest.[33] It is recommended that the initial topical dose of phenylephrine should not exceed 20 μg/kg in children.[33]

Corticosteroids, such as IV dexamethasone (0.25 to 0.5 mg/kg), are usually administered to reduce swelling and scarring. Frequently, the surgeon will want to leave an absorbable stenting material, such as MeroGel (Medtronic ENT, Jacksonville, Fla.), at the end of surgery. Unfortunately, this will interfere with nasal breathing and may increase the incidence of emergence agitation. An anesthetic technique that ensures adequate analgesia and rapid return of consciousness at the end of surgery is therefore desirable. One of us (RSH) has found that a combination of desflurane, fentanyl, and low-dose propofol works well in this regard. A unilateral or bilateral infraorbital nerve block can also be performed via the intraoral or extraoral route to provide analgesia (see Chapter 41).[34] One further concern is the need to avoid nonsteroidal antiinflammatory drugs (NSAIDs) in children with asthma and sinusitis secondary to nasal polyps (Samter triad).[35]

## Adenotonsillectomy

Adenotonsillectomy is one of the oldest and most commonly performed pediatric surgical procedures worldwide. More selective indications, however, have reduced the annual caseload.[36,37] Chronic or recurrent tonsillitis and obstructive adenotonsillar hyperplasia are the major indications for surgical removal, although other indications do exist (Table 31-1).[38,39] Surgical treatment is required when tonsillitis recurs despite adequate medical therapy, or when it is associated with peritonsillar abscess or acute airway obstruction. Halitosis, persistent pharyngitis, and cervical adenitis may accompany chronic tonsillitis. Tonsillar hyperplasia may lead to chronic airway obstruction, resulting in sleep apnea, $CO_2$ retention, intermittent nocturnal hypoxemia, cor pulmonale, failure to thrive, swallowing disorders, and speech abnormalities (Fig. 31-2). Many of these adverse effects are reversible with surgical excision of the tonsils. Certain children with cardiac lesions may be at risk for endocarditis caused by recurrent streptococcal bacteremia secondary to infected tonsils and will require prophylactic antibiotics (see Chapter 14).

Adenoidectomy is usually performed in conjunction with tonsillectomy although, in some situations it is performed as the sole surgical procedure. Indications for adenoidectomy alone include chronic or recurrent purulent adenoiditis (despite adequate medical therapy), recurrent otitis media with effusion secondary to adenoidal hyperplasia, and chronic sinusitis. Advanced degrees of adenoidal hyperplasia may lead to nasopharyngeal obstruction, obligate mouth breathing, poor feeding resulting in failure to thrive, speech disorders, and sleep disturbances. Longstanding nasal obstruction can result in orofacial abnormalities with a narrowing of the upper airway and dental abnormalities, which may be avoided by removal of hypertrophied adenoid tissue.

Surgical techniques for adenotonsillectomy include guillotine and snare techniques, cold and hot knife dissection, suction, radiofrequency ablation, and unipolar and bipolar electrocautery techniques. A major advantage of the electrocautery dissection technique is a reduction in the incidence of intraoperative blood loss, as well as postoperative hemorrhage; a major disadvantage is greater pain and poor oral intake postoperatively.[40-44]

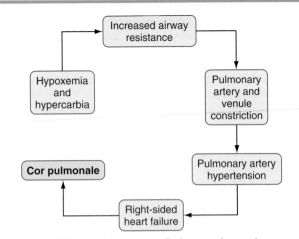

**FIGURE 31-2** Children with chronic tonsillar hypertrophy may have long-standing hypoxemia and hypercarbia, which can lead to cor pulmonale.

| TABLE 31-1 Indications for Adenotonsillectomy |
| --- |
| **Infection** |
| Acute tonsillitis or adenoiditis |
| Recurrent tonsillitis or adenoiditis |
| Chronic tonsillitis or adenoiditis |
| Peritonsillar abscess |
| Halitosis |
| **Obstruction** |
| Nasal airway (adenoids) |
| Pharyngeal airway (tonsils) |
| Sleep apnea |
| Cyanosis |
| Failure to thrive |
| Cor pulmonale due to airway obstruction |
| **Mass Lesion** |
| Tonsillar/adenoidal |
| Benign |
| Malignant |

The mortality associated with adenotonsillectomy is estimated at 1 per 16,000 to 1 per 35,000 procedures.[45,46] Hospital-based reviews of anesthetic mortality continue to list adenotonsillectomy as a surgical procedure associated with perioperative cardiac arrest and death.[47,48] Bleeding, burns, and airway fires account for over one third of malpractice claims associated with this procedure.[49]

Surgical complications after adenotonsillectomy are rare but include uvular amputation, uvular edema, velopharyngeal insufficiency, and nasopharyngeal stenosis. Atlantoaxial subluxation manifesting as neck pain and torticollis, mandibular subluxation and condylar fracture, cervical adenitis, and cervical osteomyelitis have also been reported.[46,50]

Throat pain, otalgia, emesis, poor oral intake, and dehydration are common morbidities. Respiratory morbidity after adenotonsillectomy in the otherwise healthy child affects less than 1%,[51-53] but has assumed a greater importance since obstructive breathing has replaced infection and halitosis as the most common indication for adenotonsillectomy.

Age has a major influence on postadenotonsillectomy complications. Secondary postadenotonsillectomy hemorrhage is more common in children older than the age of 10 years.[54,55] Young age is a risk factor for both poor oral intake and respiratory complications. The majority of children younger than age 3 years experience airway problems after adenotonsillectomy for obstructive breathing.[56,57]

## PREOPERATIVE EVALUATION

The general health of the child and the indications for surgery must be reviewed. URIs are frequent in these children and can interfere with the timing of adenotonsillectomy because the risk of respiratory morbidity and hemorrhage is increased.[46,51,58,59] A history of bleeding tendencies requires investigation. Medications that interfere with coagulation include aspirin, NSAIDs, and valproic acid. Discontinuation of these drugs preoperatively is sometimes problematic, and preoperative consultation with neurology, cardiology, and hematology specialists may be indicated.

A careful cardiorespiratory history and physical examination is essential. Children with chronic tonsillar hypertrophy may have long-standing hypoxemia and hypercarbia, which can lead to cor pulmonale (see Fig. 31-2). The oropharynx should be evaluated and the tonsillar size classified (Fig. 31-3).[60] In some centers, a complete blood cell count is required before adenotonsillectomy. There is no evidence that routinely performed preoperative coagulation studies are beneficial unless they are indicated by history.[61,62] The indications for the procedure should be clearly delineated. If the indication is for obstructed breathing, then further evaluation for symptoms of possible obstructive sleep apnea (OSA) is indicated. Parents should be asked if the child

### A Standardized System for
### Evaluation of Tonsillar Size

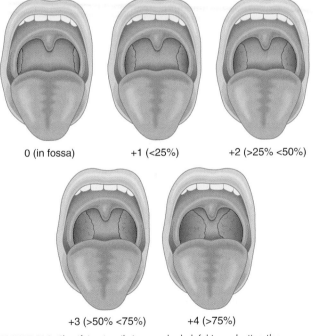

0 (in fossa)        +1 (<25%)        +2 (>25% <50%)

+3 (>50% <75%)        +4 (>75%)

**FIGURE 31-3** Classifying tonsil size may be helpful in evaluating the degree of airway obstruction. Children classified as +3 or greater (i.e., having more than 50% of the pharyngeal area occupied by hypertrophied tonsils) are at an increased risk of developing airway obstruction during anesthetic induction. (Modified from Brodsky L. Modern assessment of tonsils and adenoids. Pediatr Clin North Am 1989;36:1551-69; illustration by Jon S. Krasner.)

snores loudly, if the snoring can be heard through a closed door, if there are gasps or pauses in respirations, if there is daytime somnolence, night terrors, nocturnal enuresis, attention deficit disorder, or poor school performance. A positive response to any of these questions is suggestive of OSA, in particular when combined with obesity (weight greater than the 95th percentile).[63-67]

### Special Considerations for the Child with OSA

*The single most important task during the preoperative evaluation of the child for adenotonsillectomy is to distinguish the child with OSA from the child with obstructive breathing, because the former is at greater risk for developing severe perioperative respiratory complications, possibly including death, after adenotonsillectomy.*[68-71b]

OSA is the most severe form of sleep-disordered breathing. Sleep-disordered breathing ranges from normal respirations to primary snoring, upper airway resistance syndrome (UARS), obstructive hypopnea, and OSA. At the most extreme form of sleep-disordered breathing, OSA, clinical signs of partial or complete upper airway obstruction (UAO) must be present during sleep, as well as some degree of hypercarbia and/or hypoxemia.[72] Although it is important to recognize the significance of OSA in children who are scheduled for adenotonsillectomy, children who do not meet the criteria for OSA but who have less severe forms of sleep-disordered breathing, such as UARS or obstructive hypopnea, may also be at increased risk for morbidity after surgery. Guidelines for the perioperative management of these children continue to be developed.[71a,73,74]

A high index of suspicion is required to identify the child with OSA on clinical criteria, although clinical criteria do not distinguish primary snoring from OSA in children.[75] There is a greater incidence of OSA in Asian and African American populations.[76,77] In addition, African American children desaturate more profoundly during sleep-related obstructive airway events than do Caucasian and Hispanic children[78]; the reason for this difference is unclear.

Anatomic features, including increased nasal resistance, may underlie the pathogenesis of OSA; common medical conditions and syndromes that predispose to the development of OSA are listed in Table 31-2. Infants suffering acute life-threatening events have a greater incidence of OSA in childhood and adolescence.[79-81]

The obstructive events that characterize OSA result in recurrent episodes of hypoxia, hypercarbia, and sleep disruption, a trilogy that has been linked to the development of medical sequelae that accompany severe OSA. Because adenotonsillectomy is very often the initial treatment for the majority of children, these children may present with a spectrum of disease affecting multiple organ systems. Failure to thrive is common. Cardiovascular abnormalities, including ventricular dysfunction, a depressed ventricular ejection fraction, right ventricular hypertrophy, and pulmonary hypertension, may be present.[82-85] Repeat infections affecting the lower respiratory tract have been linked to chronic aspiration.[86]

The severity of OSA is assessed by the frequency and severity of the obstructive respiratory events during sleep; both vary with sleep stage and occur most often during rapid eye movement (REM) sleep. The frequency and severity of obstructive events worsen after midnight, a finding that may reflect the greater proportion of REM sleep in the latter part of the night and fatigue of the upper airway musculature.[87-89]

Apneas are classified as central, obstructive, and mixed. Central apnea occurs when there is no apparent respiratory effort. Obstructive apnea is associated with apparent, often vigorous,

**TABLE 31-2**  Medical Conditions in Children That Predispose to Development of Obstructive Sleep Apnea

**Craniofacial Syndromes**

Crouzon syndrome
Apert syndrome
Pfeiffer syndrome
Treacher Collins syndrome
Pierre Robin sequence
Goldenhar syndrome
Larsen syndrome

**Disorders of Cranial Base**

Arnold-Chiari malformation
Achondroplasia
Syringobulbia

**Neuromuscular Disorders**

Cerebral palsy

**Trisomy 21**

**Infiltrative Disorders**

Mucopolysaccharidoses
Acromegaly
Obesity
Prader-Willi syndrome

**Temporomandibular Joint Ankylosis**

**TABLE 31-3**  Clinical Diagnostic Criteria for Pediatric Obstructive Sleep Apnea Syndrome

1. Predisposing physical characteristics
   a. Body mass index greater than 95th percentile for age and gender
   b. Craniofacial abnormalities affecting the airway
   c. Anatomic nasal obstruction
   d. Tonsils nearly touching or touching in the midline
2. History of apparent airway obstruction during sleep (*two or more of the following*)
   a. Loud snoring (loud enough to be heard through a closed door)
   b. Frequent snoring
   c. Observed pauses in breathing during sleep
   d. Frequent arousals from sleep
   e. Intermittent vocalization during sleep
   f. Parental report of restless sleep, difficulty breathing, or struggling respiratory efforts during sleep
   g. Nocturnal enuresis
3. Somnolence (*one or more of the following*)
   a. Parent or teacher comments that the child appears sleepy during the day, is easily distracted, is overly aggressive, or has difficulty concentrating
   b. Child often is difficult to arouse at the usual awakening time

*Note:* If signs and symptoms in at least two categories are present, there is a significant probability of moderate obstructive sleep apnea (OSA). If severe abnormalities are present, children should be treated as having severe OSA.
Modified from Table 1 in Gross JB, Bachenberg KL, Benumof JL, et al. Practice guidelines for the perioperative management of patients with obstructive sleep apnea: a report by the American Society of Anesthesiologists Task Force on Perioperative Management of patients with obstructive sleep apnea. Anesthesiology 2006;104:1081-93.

inspiratory efforts that are ineffective because lack of upper airway patency. A mixed obstructive apnea is diagnosed when both central and obstructive apnea occur without interruption by effective respirations. The presence of sleep-disordered breathing is documented by polysomnography and is quantitated by the frequency of obstructive events and by oxygen-desaturation indices. The polysomnogram simultaneously records the electroencephalogram, electromyogram, electrocardiogram, pulse oximetry, airflow, and thoracic and abdominal movement during sleep. A recent consensus paper on the criteria for diagnosing OSA in children has been developed.[71a,84] A common definition of obstructive apnea in children is an obstructive effort that includes more than two obstructive breaths, regardless of the duration of the apnea.[87] An obstructive apnea index of 1 is the cutoff for normality in children.[90] *Hypopnea* is defined as a reduction in airflow of more than 50%.[87] The apnea hypopnea index (AHI) is the summation of the number of obstructive apnea and hypopnea events and is analogous to the respiratory disturbance index (RDI). A common definition of desaturation is a 4% decrease in oxygen saturation from baseline. The saturation nadir is the minimum oxygen saturation recorded during the sleep study. A saturation nadir of 92% is the minimum normal saturation in children.[90,91]

The severity of OSA predicts the nature of perioperative respiratory complications (Table 31-3). An RDI of greater than 20 events per hour is associated with breath holding during induction, whereas an RDI greater than 30 is associated with laryngospasm and desaturation during emergence.[92] Ten obstructive events per hour during a screening polysomnogram is the threshold for severe postoperative respiratory complications.[69] An oxygen-saturation nadir less than 80% is associated with a greater incidence of respiratory morbidity after adenotonsillectomy, compared with a saturation nadir greater than 80%.[68,71]

The RDI and AHI correlate inversely with the oxygen-saturation nadir,[93,94] making simplified testing with continuous pulse oximetry a meaningful metric. The McGill oximetry score has been shown to correlate with the risk of respiratory complications after adenotonsillectomy in children (Fig. 31-4). Of children with a McGill oximetry score of 4, 24% experienced major postoperative respiratory complications.[94]

Children with severe OSA may require additional preoperative testing before adenotonsillectomy. A capillary blood gas sample drawn in the morning can be evaluated for an increased concentration of bicarbonate, suggestive of $CO_2$ retention during sleep. When indicated, a preoperative electrocardiogram or echocardiogram may provide evidence of right ventricular hypertrophy and/or pulmonary hypertension. A chest radiograph may suggest lower airway disease or cardiomegaly.

Consultations to plan the perioperative care of children with severe OSA are important. Young children with profound oxygen desaturation during sleep and $CO_2$ retention may require admission to the pediatric ICU for optimization before and/or after adenotonsillectomy.[36,94] Urgent adenotonsillectomy for severe OSA is associated with significant respiratory morbidity after surgery.[70,95] On occasion, adenotonsillar hypertrophy may progress to compromise the upper airway during wakefulness. In some instances the anesthetic considerations for the obstructed and difficult airways may overlap.

## ANESTHETIC MANAGEMENT AND POSTOPERATIVE CONSIDERATIONS

The anesthetic goals for adenotonsillectomy are (1) to provide a smooth, atraumatic induction; (2) to provide the surgeon with optimal operating conditions; (3) to establish IV access for

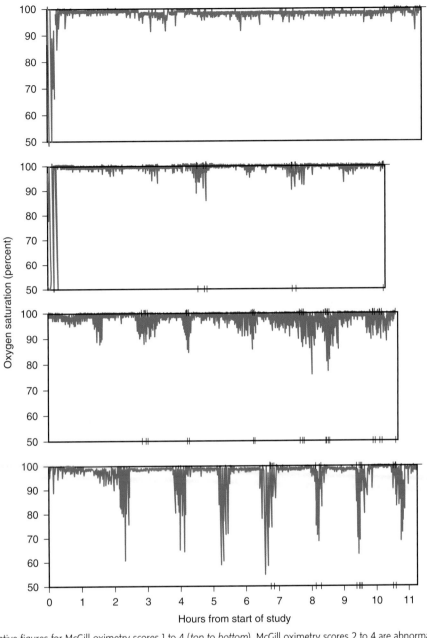

**FIGURE 31-4** Representative figures for McGill oximetry scores 1 to 4 (*top to bottom*). McGill oximetry scores 2 to 4 are abnormal in that they all show at least three clusters of desaturation. The severity of the saturation nadir determines the score such that McGill oximetry scores 2, 3, and 4 correspond to saturation nadirs of less than 90%, less than 85%, and less than 80%, respectively. (From Nixon GM, Kermack AS, Davis GM, et al. Planning adenotonsillectomy in children with obstructive sleep apnea: the role of overnight oximetry. Pediatrics 2004;113:e19-25.)

volume expansion and medications as indicated; and (4) to provide rapid emergence so that the child is awake and able to protect the recently instrumented airway. The need for a premedication is determined during the preanesthetic evaluation. *Children with symptoms of sleep-disordered breathing who require premedication should be closely observed*, although the desaturation is transient and infrequent (1.5% of cases) after oral midazolam premedication.[96] *Monitoring with pulse oximetry after premedication may be indicated for select children with severe OSA and confounding variables.[96] Premedication with short-acting drugs and/or those that can be antagonized is advised (see further).*

The anesthetic techniques for adenotonsillectomy are varied and include the choice of an inhalational or IV technique, the choice of an ETT or LMA, and the choice of spontaneous or controlled ventilation. Of the currently available inhalational agents, sevoflurane provides a smooth induction of anesthesia, and desflurane (for those whose airway is secured with an ETT) used for maintenance provides a rapid emergence and recovery.[97,98] The rapid return of airway reflexes is particularly important when the dose of opioids must be titrated after extubation.

Children who are scheduled for adenotonsillectomy have a high incidence of airway reactivity and laryngospasm. This will influence the choice of airway management. Placement of an oral RAE or standard uncuffed ETT with a leak at 20 cm $H_2O$ (the leak increases with neck extension and insertion of the mouth gag) is generally sufficient to prevent soiling of the trachea during the surgery, yet reduces the incidence of postextubation croup. Cuffed ETTs have become increasingly used in children of all age-groups.[99] A cuffed tube prevents an air leak and the consequent bubbling of gases through the oropharyngeal secretions and blood that can interfere with surgery. It also minimizes pollution by anesthetic gases and decreases the risk of an airway fire when electrocautery is used.

Blood and secretions may be present in the oropharynx at the conclusion of surgery and should be carefully suctioned before emergence from anesthesia. Emptying the stomach with an orogastric tube, a maneuver frequently performed by the surgeon under direct vision after completion of surgery, does not reduce the incidence of PONV, although the study was underpowered to detect a difference.[100]

It is preferable to wait until the child is fully awake and able to clear blood and secretions from the oropharynx before removing the ETT. A common practice is to position the child in the lateral position (known as the "tonsil" or "recovery" position) with the head slightly down at the time of extubation to permit blood and secretions to pool in the dependent cheek and drain out of the mouth rather than accumulate at the laryngeal inlet. Intact airway and pharyngeal reflexes are of utmost importance in preventing aspiration, laryngospasm, and airway obstruction.[101] The child should remain in the tonsil position postoperatively, while being carefully observed and monitored during transport to the recovery room.

The use of the LMA for adenotonsillectomy was described in 1990, but it was not until the widespread availability of a model with a flexible spiral, metallic reinforced shaft that it was widely used (E-Fig. 31-1).[102,103] The wide, rigid tube of the original model did not fit under the mouth gag and was easily compressed or dislodged during full mouth opening. The newer, flexible model has a soft, reinforced shaft, which easily fits under the mouth gag without becoming dislodged or compressed. Adequate surgical access can be achieved and the airway is reasonably well protected from exposure to blood during the surgery.[104,105] Early advantages cited for the LMA over the ETT include a decrease in the incidence of postoperative stridor and laryngospasm, and an increase in immediate postoperative oxygen saturation,[106] although recent evidence disputes any difference in the frequency of laryngospasm.[107] Insertion of the LMA, however, may be difficult in the presence of tonsillar enlargement, and careful placement to avoid kinking of the LMA is essential.[108] Although it has been recommended that the LMA be used only in spontaneously breathing children and that positive-pressure ventilation be avoided, gentle assisted ventilation is both safe and effective if peak inspiratory pressure is limited to 20 cm $H_2O$ or less. If there is any leak of gases around the LMA then the potential for an airway fire must be considered and appropriate precautions taken if electrocautery is used.

### Analgesic Management

Surgical technique has a major impact on the analgesic requirements after adenotonsillectomy because electrocautery techniques are generally associated with greater pain, presumably owing to increased thermal injury,[40,41,109] although this is debated.[110] Opioids have been the mainstay of perioperative analgesia. However, because opioids increase the incidence of emesis[111] and respiratory morbidity, the use of opioid-sparing adjuncts has been advocated, including dexamethasone, acetaminophen, NSAIDs, and ketamine.

A single intraoperative dose of dexamethasone reduces postadenotonsillectomy pain and edema when electrocautery has been used. Large doses are traditionally used, especially in children with OSA. Dexamethasone (1 mg/kg) administration is associated with reduced parental- and physician-rated pain scores after adenotonsillectomy (Table 31-4).[41] The minimum morphine-sparing dose for dexamethasone is reported to be 0.5 mg/kg.[112] For dexamethasone doses between 0.0625 mg/kg and 1.0 mg/kg, the frequency of postoperative vomiting, pain scores, and times to first liquid and first analgesics were similar.[113] A similar absence of a dose response for dexamethasone between 0.050 and 0.15 mg/kg for vomiting after tonsillectomy was reported in another study.[114] Single doses of dexamethasone have not been associated with aseptic necrosis of the hip or infections, but have been responsible for several cases of acute tumor lysis syndrome, including one death.[115-117] One study suggested an increased risk of bleeding after tonsillectomy in children who received dexamethasone up to 0.5 mg/kg (maximum 20 mg).[118] These findings have been refuted by a recent meta-analysis and several studies.[119-122a]

The routine use of NSAIDs for adenotonsillectomy remains controversial because of the potential for postadenotonsillectomy hemorrhage. A meta-analysis of seven randomized controlled trials (505 children) on the effects of NSAIDs on bleeding risk after tonsillectomy reported the number needed to harm, in terms of reoperation for hemostasis, to be 29.[123] NSAIDs were associated with a greater risk of both postoperative bleeding that required treatment and reoperation for hemostasis. The Cochrane Collaboration assessed the effect of NSAIDs on bleeding after pediatric tonsillectomy in 13 trials (955 children) and found no increase in bleeding that required reoperation for hemostasis.[124] An audit of more than 4800 pediatric tonsillectomies in which the NSAIDs diclofenac and ibuprofen were routinely used, reported a primary hemorrhage rate of 0.9%.[55] Because the effects of ketorolac on platelet function are reversible, the effect is dependent on the presence of ketorolac within the body.[125] Thus, unlike the effect of aspirin, this effect is short-lived. However, we recommend administering NSAIDs only after consulting with

**TABLE 31-4** Effect of Single Intraoperative Dose of Dexamethasone on Postoperative Pain in Pediatric Tonsillectomy or Adenotonsillectomy: A Comparison of Randomized, Double-Blind Studies

| Source | No. of Children | Dexamethasone Dose | Electrocautery Technique | Effect on Pain |
|---|---|---|---|---|
| Catlin and Grimes[292] | 25 | 8 mg/m² | No | No difference |
| Ohlms et al.[293] | 69 | 0.5 mg/kg | No | No difference |
| Tom et al.[294] | 58 | 1.0 mg/kg | Yes | Reduced |
| April et al.[295] | 80 | 1.0 mg/kg | Yes | No difference |
| Hanasono et al.[41] | 219 | 1.0 mg/kg | Yes | Reduced |

Modified from Hanasono MM, Lalakea ML, Mikulec AA, et al. Perioperative steroids in tonsillectomy using electrocautery and sharp dissection techniques. Arch Otolaryngol Head Neck Surg 2004;130:917-21.

the surgeon and, if in agreement, administering them after hemostasis is achieved.[126] Acetaminophen is commonly used as a component of multimodal analgesic approach in these children.[127] IV formulations of acetaminophen are now available in many countries, offering the theoretical advantage of greater predictability than the oral and rectal routes. However, recent studies suggest that the duration of analgesia after 15 mg/kg of acetaminophen given IV is less than that after 40 mg/kg given rectally.[128] Furthermore, although introduced only 7 years ago, two reports of 10-fold overdoses of IV acetaminophen with near-catastrophic outcomes in infants should alert clinicians to the very serious risk of dosage errors with this medication.[129]

An IV infusion of dexmedetomidine 2 μg/kg over 10 minutes followed by 0.7 μg/kg/hr combined with an inhalation agent can provide satisfactory intraoperative conditions for adenotonsillectomy without adverse hemodynamic effects. In children with OSA syndrome, postoperative opioid requirements are significantly reduced and the incidence and severity of severe emergence agitation is reduced, with few children desaturating.[130] After larger doses of dexmedetomidine (2 and 4 μg/kg), the opioid-free interval increases and the postoperative opioid requirements decrease. However, duration of stay in the PACU is prolonged.[131]

Infiltration of local anesthetics into the tonsillar fossa during tonsillectomy is sometimes reported to decrease postoperative pain, but the pain relief is transient (E-Fig. 31-2).[132] In addition, life-threatening complications have been reported after local anesthetic infiltration in the tonsillar fossa, including intracranial hemorrhage, bulbar paralysis, deep cervical abscess, cervical osteomyelitis, medullopontine infarct, and cardiac arrest. The risks associated with injection of local anesthesia in the tonsillar fossa may outweigh its potential benefits, particularly in inexperienced hands.[133,134]

## Postoperative Nausea and Vomiting

Emesis and poor oral intake are common comorbid conditions after adenotonsillectomy. Opioids increase the incidence of PONV, with two thirds of treated children experiencing PONV.[37,55,135] The incidence of PONV increases with morphine dose.[111,136] Propofol infusions,[136a,136b] ondansetron and dexamethasone are widely used to reduce the incidence of emesis after adenotonsillectomy. Postdischarge vomiting continues for days in some children. One study has shown that at-home use of oral ondansetron disintegrating tablets may prevent emesis during the first 3 days after adenotonsillectomy.[137] A single intraoperative dose of dexamethasone reduces the incidence of emesis during the first 24 hours after adenotonsillectomy.[138] The number of children needed to treat was only four, which means that the use of dexamethasone in four children undergoing adenotonsillectomy results in one less child experiencing PONV. In addition, children who received dexamethasone were more likely than those receiving placebo to advance to a soft diet on postoperative day 1, with a number needed to treat of five. Given the antiemetic and possible morphine-sparing advantages of a single dose of dexamethasone, and its low cost and safety profile, the evidence suggests that routine use of dexamethasone reduces morbidity after adenotonsillectomy in children.[41,138] Although the literature supports the effectiveness of a single dose of dexamethasone, the smallest effective dose remains somewhat unclear. One study suggested an IV dose of 0.15 mg/kg,[139] whereas another reported no difference in postoperative vomiting, pain scores, time to first liquid, and time to first analgesics between doses of 0.0625 and 1.0 mg/kg (Fig. 31-5).[113] Acupuncture, acupressure, as well as therapeutic suggestion, have also been used with variable results.[140-142]

### Special Considerations for Children with OSA

Children with OSA who require premedication should be closely observed, because transient oxygen desaturation has been reported in 1.5% of children with OSA who received 0.5 mg/kg oral midazolam.[96]

#### Induction of Anesthesia

Compared with children undergoing adenotonsillectomy for chronic tonsillitis, those whose indication was OSA experienced more respiratory complications during induction of anesthesia.[92] The vulnerability of the upper airway musculature described for halothane[143] has subsequently been reported for most anesthetic agents, resulting in a graded reduction in airway caliber with increasing anesthetic concentration.[144-148] Airway obstruction occurs in the upper two thirds of the pharyngeal airway, and the smallest pharyngeal dimension is in the area of overlap between the adenoids and tonsils.[147] During induction of anesthesia, early pharyngeal airway obstruction may require a jaw thrust maneuver, insertion of an oral or nasopharyngeal airway, and the application of continuous positive airway pressure (CPAP). Propofol-associated loss in airway caliber is reversed with the application of CPAP.[148] CPAP acts as a pneumatic splint to increase the caliber of the pharyngeal airway (Fig. 31-6).[149] Of equal importance, CPAP increases longitudinal tension on the pharyngeal airway, thereby decreasing the collapsibility of the upper airway (see Fig. 12-10), and increases lung volumes.[150,151] Small increments in CPAP between 5 and 10 cm $H_2O$ increase the dimension of the pharyngeal airway dramatically (Fig. 31-7).[152,153] The closing pressure of the pharynx increases with OSA severity, such that greater levels of CPAP are required in children with severe OSA compared with those with mild OSA. It is prudent to consider securing IV access before induction of anesthesia in children with severe OSA, to expedite administration of muscle relaxants or IV agents should pharyngeal obstruction or laryngospasm occur during induction. The small oropharynx and adenotonsillar hypertrophy associated with severe OSA may increase the difficulty in properly inserting an LMA.

#### Analgesic Management in Children with OSA

Severe OSA is characterized by recurrent episodes of transient hypoxia and hypercarbia during sleep. In animal models, exposure to intermittent hypoxia during development affects the opioid system, increasing the density of μ-opioid receptors in the respiratory-related areas of the brainstem. The cellular mechanism whereby this increased density is achieved has yet to be elucidated, but it may represent an adaptive response to the effects of recurrent intermittent hypoxia that allows μ-receptor–mediated opioid respiratory effects to predominate.[154-157]

For children with severe OSA, the severity of the nocturnal oxygen desaturation correlates with the sensitivity to exogenously administered opioids (Fig. 31-8).[158-160] The morphine dose required to achieve a uniform analgesic endpoint in children with OSA who exhibited a low preoperative oxygen-saturation nadir during sleep (less than 85%) (Fig. 31-9) was less than in those whose preoperative saturation nadir was greater.[159] Young age was also associated with an increased sensitivity to opioids. *An unforeseen risk of perioperative opioid use in children with severe OSA is that smaller-than-expected doses of opioids may produce exaggerated*

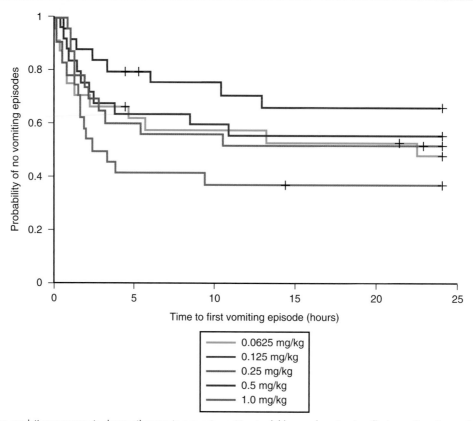

| | 0.0625 mg/kg |
|---|---|
| | 0.125 mg/kg |
| | 0.25 mg/kg |
| | 0.5 mg/kg |
| | 1.0 mg/kg |

**FIGURE 31-5** No dose-escalation response to dexamethasone to prevent vomiting in children undergoing tonsillectomy. Time-to-event analysis for first vomiting episode was performed; tick marks indicate time of censoring for patients who did not have complete follow-up (N = 13). No significant difference was found between dose levels, P = 0.28 (Cox Proportional Hazard Likelihood Ratio Test). (Redrawn with permission from Kim MS, Coté CJ, Cristoloveanu C, et al. There is no dose-escalation response to dexamethasone (0.0625-1.0 mg/kg) in pediatric tonsillectomy or adenotonsillectomy patients for preventing vomiting, reducing pain, shortening time to first liquid intake, or the incidence of voice change. Anesth Analg 2007;104:1052-8.)

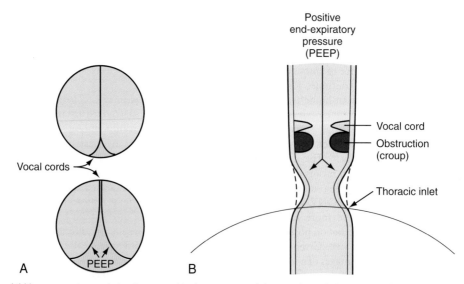

**FIGURE 31-6** When a child has upper airway obstruction caused by laryngospasm (**A**) or mechanical obstruction (**B**), application of approximately 10 cm H₂O of positive end-expiratory pressure (PEEP) during spontaneous breathing often relieves obstruction. PEEP helps to hold the vocal cords apart (**A**) and the airway open (*broken lines* in **B**). (From Coté CJ. Pediatric anesthesia. In Miller RD, editor. Miller's anesthesia. 8th ed. New York: Churchill Livingstone; 2012. In press.)

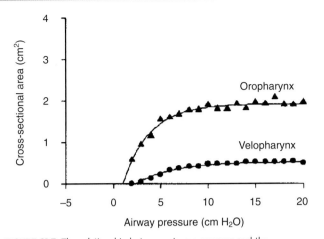

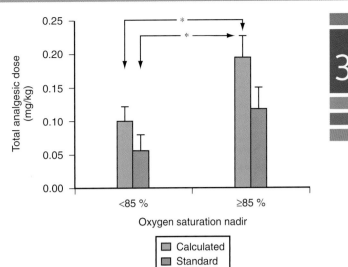

**FIGURE 31-7** The relationship between airway pressure and the cross-sectional area of the pharynx. Maximal airway dimension is achieved between 15 and 20 cm $H_2O$. At reduced airway pressures, around 5 cm $H_2O$, small increments in airway pressure make a large difference in airway caliber. (From Isono S, Tanaka A, Nishino T. Dynamic interaction between the tongue and soft palate during obstructive apnea in anesthetized patients with sleep-disordered breathing. J Appl Physiol 2003;95:2257-64.)

**FIGURE 31-9** The total analgesic dose of morphine required to achieve a uniform analgesic endpoint in children with obstructive sleep apnea (OSA). Children were grouped by severity of OSA into those who had a preoperative oxygen saturation nadir of <85% or ≥85%. The asterisks indicate post hoc differences between groups, $p < 0.05$. (From Brown KA, Laferrière A, Lakheeram I, Moss IR. Recurrent hypoxemia in children is associated with increased analgesic sensitivity to opiates. Anesthesiology 2006;105:665-9.)

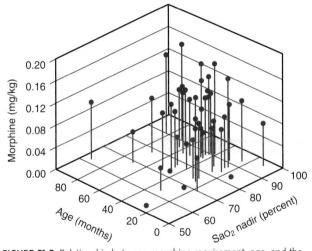

**FIGURE 31-8** Relationship between morphine requirement, age, and the preoperative arterial oxygen-saturation nadir in 46 children who were otherwise well. The lengths of the stems supporting the 46 dots are proportional to the morphine dose. The stems in the foreground are shorter than those in the background, indicating a significant correlation between the three variables. $Sao_2$, Arterial oxygen saturation. (From Brown KA, Laferrière A, Moss IR. Recurrent hypoxemia in young children with obstructive sleep apnea is associated with reduced opioid requirements for analgesia. Anesthesiology 2004;100:806-10.)

*respiratory depression.* Of children with severe OSA who were anesthetized with halothane, 46% experienced apnea after a uniform dose of fentanyl, compared with 4% of controls.[161] This increased sensitivity to the respiratory depressant effects of fentanyl in children with OSA is supported by the exaggerated respiratory depression to subsequent administration of a uniform dose of fentanyl in rat pups exposed to intermittent hypoxia.[162] Hence, allowing spontaneous respirations during maintenance of anesthesia enables an assessment of the response to small challenges of opioid analgesics. In this manner, the anesthesiologist can assess the sensitivity of the child with OSA to opioids.

Controlling respiration precludes such an evaluation. Sleep fragmentation blunts the arousal response to acute airway occlusion during sleep.[163,164] In addition, exposure to intermittent hypoxia during development is associated with an increase in the arousal latency to hypoxia.[165-167] Morphine acting at the level of the basal forebrain blunts arousal.[168] If the increased sensitivity to both the analgesic and respiratory effects of exogenously administered opioids reported in children with OSA extends to arousal mechanisms, the use of opioids in children with severe OSA may further impair arousal mechanisms. Guidelines for the perioperative management of OSA assign a greater risk score if opioids are used for postoperative analgesic regimens in children with OSA.[91] Although these guidelines suggest that the use of low-potency oral opioid analgesia carries a reduced perioperative risk, the use of codeine, a "low-risk" oral opioid commonly used in the ambulatory setting, may also be problematic in children with OSA. Codeine is metabolized by the cytochrome P450 debrisoquine 4-hydroxylase (CYP2D6) to its active analgesic metabolites. The CYP2D6 gene displays polymorphism, including gene duplication (ultra-rapid metabolizers) and inactive genes. Gene duplication may lead to ultra-rapid metabolism, which for prodrugs, such as codeine, might yield a 50% greater fraction of morphine and its glucuronides compared with extensive metabolizers.[169] Respiratory arrest after codeine has been reported in both adults and children who demonstrate ultra-rapid metabolism of codeine.[170-171a] Whereas the ultra-rapid metabolizing genotype is present in 3% of Caucasians, it is present in 10% to 30% of Arabian and Northeast African populations. In contrast, almost 10% of children lack CYP2D6, rendering codeine an ineffective analgesic. Given the broad variability in codeine metabolism and our lack of knowledge of which polymorphism is carried by each child, the use of codeine and the dose prescribed for children with OSA must be very carefully considered or an alternate opioid selected.

### Neural Blockade

Blockade of neural input to the upper airway dilator musculature in children with OSA is also problematic. Serious life-threatening complications, including severe UAO and pulmonary edema, have been reported after local anesthetics have been infiltrated in the tonsillar fossa to prevent pain after adenotonsillectomy. The pharynx in children with OSA is not only smaller in size,[147,172] but also more collapsible, even during wakefulness, compared with those children who do not have OSA.[173-175] Topical anesthesia applied to the mucosa of the pharynx of children with OSA reduces the caliber of the pharynx compared with control subjects.[176]

### Extubation Strategy and Management of the Postoperative Period in Children with OSA

Extubation of the trachea is usually performed when the child is fully awake. Techniques that involve minimal stimulation of the airway have been suggested.[101] Although a minority of children receive muscle relaxants for adenotonsillectomy, residual neuromuscular blockade in the recovery room will selectively depress the function of the upper airway dilators relative to the diaphragm, promoting collapse of the pharyngeal airway.[177] Full antagonism of neuromuscular blockade is strongly recommended before extubating the tracheas of children with OSA.[91] Antagonism of neuromuscular blockade with atropine and neostigmine after tonsillectomy has been associated with less PONV than antagonism with glycopyrrolate and neostigmine.[178]

Several other factors may increase the risk of respiratory difficulties after adenotonsillectomy in children with OSA. Otherwise healthy children with severe OSA, whose adenotonsillectomy is performed in the morning, are less likely than those whose surgery is performed in the afternoon to desaturate when managed in a PACU setting.[179] In addition, meticulous attention to the position of the head and neck is required during recovery from anesthesia, because hypercarbia and a loss of lung volume (functional lung capacity) both promote collapse of the pharyngeal airway.[151,180,181] Extension of the cervical spine, the sniffing position, the lateral recovery position, and mouth opening with anterior advancement of the mandible all increase the dimension of the pharynx[182-186] and reduce the risk of UAO.

Two drugs, atropine and naloxone, have the potential to augment the function of the upper airway. Atropine administered after induction of anesthesia decreased the risk of postadenotonsillectomy respiratory complications.[70] Of possible relevance is the report that muscarinic blockade of the hypoglossal nucleus in the rat model enhances activity of the genioglossus muscle.[181] Agonists of opioid μ-receptors have been shown to depresses activity in the pharyngeal dilator muscles, including the genioglossus muscle.[155,187-189] Given the increased sensitivity to both analgesic and respiratory effects of exogenously administered opioids in children with severe OSA, a similar sensitivity may also apply to the respiratory-related activity of the pharyngeal musculature. Small doses of naloxone may alleviate UAO after adenotonsillectomy if exogenous opioids have been administered.

The severity of OSA is a predictor of the outcome after adenotonsillectomy.[190] A preoperative RDI above 19 may predict an RDI in excess of 5 in long-term follow-up.[75,93] Children with OSA continue to demonstrate obstructive apnea and desaturation during sleep on the first night after adenotonsillectomy, with the frequency of the obstructive events and the severity of desaturation usually greater in those children with severe OSA (Fig. 31-10).[191,192] Thus despite removal of the hypertrophied

tonsils and adenoids, children with OSA continue to experience symptoms on the first postoperative night. This underscores the need to admit these children to a hospital for continuous overnight monitoring postoperatively, rather than discharge them home. Long-term follow-up studies more than 6 months after tonsillectomy in children with OSA show that symptoms completely resolve in those with mild OSA (AHI less than 10) but are persistent in 35% of those with severe OSA (AHI greater than 20).[190] Furthermore, recent epidemiologic evidence suggests that residual sleep-disordered breathing is more likely to be present after adenotonsillectomy in older children (more than 7 years of age) and obese children. It has also been suggested that obese children with large tonsils and OSA also show evidence of systemic inflammatory disease that persists after the tonsillectomy.[190,193]

Measures to support airway patency in the postoperative period have included insertion of nasal airways, administration of noninvasive ventilatory support (e.g., CPAP), reintubation, ventilation, and the administration of bronchodilators, racemic epinephrine, and heliox. Bilevel positive airway pressure and/or CPAP may be useful in children with preexisting neurologic disorders.[194] However, nasal secretions may be copious after adenotonsillectomy, limiting the efficacy of noninvasive ventilatory support. Children with complex medical diseases, who are critically dependent on the function of upper airway musculature, may benefit from delayed extubation. Acute relief of chronic UAO favors the exudation of intravascular fluid into the pulmonary interstitium and noncardiogenic pulmonary edema, which may present preoperatively, intraoperatively, and postoperatively. Supportive measures include the administration of oxygen, endotracheal intubation, mechanical ventilation with positive end-expiratory pressure, and administration of furosemide.[195-197]

## DISCHARGE POLICY FOR AMBULATORY ADENOTONSILLECTOMY

Children younger than 3 years of age and those with complex medical disorders are not candidates for adenotonsillectomy as outpatients.[38,198] *Although children undergoing adenotonsillectomy for obstructive breathing without apnea may undergo ambulatory surgery, those with OSA should not.* A diagnosis of OSA increases the likelihood of respiratory complications after adenotonsillectomy from 1% in otherwise healthy children to 20% in those with OSA.[37]

The majority of children who are scheduled for adenotonsillectomy have symptoms of obstructive breathing,[42,199,200] yet only 55% with clinical criteria suggestive of OSA subsequently meet sleep laboratory criteria for OSA.[201] Sleep screening of children undergoing routine adenotonsillectomy for chronic tonsillitis revealed unexpectedly that 20% had severe obstructive episodes associated with desaturation.[202] Because only a minority of children undergoing adenotonsillectomy undergo diagnostic testing for sleep-disordered breathing, the recently published guidelines on management of OSA have empowered clinical diagnostic criteria, such that a child with severe symptoms must be assumed to have moderate to severe OSA until proven otherwise by sleep laboratory testing (see Fig. 31-4). Ambulatory programs may now find it cost effective to screen children with a positive clinical history.

In otherwise healthy children, conversion from ambulatory to inpatient status was most frequently prompted by respiratory events in children whose indication for surgery was obstructive breathing.[42] A systematic reduction in postoperative morphine use was associated with a reduced rate of hospital admission from 8% to 2.4%.[55] Same-day discharge, which abbreviates the

Perioperative Overnight Oximetry in a Child with Severe OSA

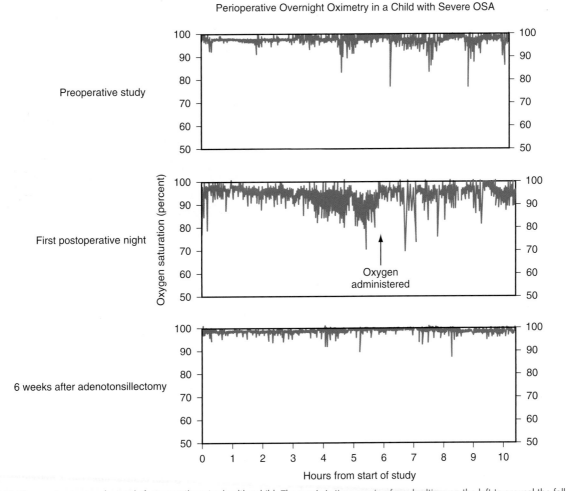

FIGURE 31-10 Three oximetry trend records from an otherwise healthy child. The x-axis is time ranging from bedtime on the left to arousal the following morning on the right. The *top* panel is the preoperative record showing clusters of desaturation. The *middle* panel is the record from the first night after adenotonsillectomy. With sleep onset, a decrease in saturation is evident that worsens after midnight. Oxygen therapy is administered after midnight. The *bottom* panel is the recording 6 weeks after adenotonsillectomy, which is within normal limits. (From Nixon GM, Kermack AS, McGregor CD, et al. Sleep and breathing on the first night after adenotonsillectomy for obstructive sleep apnea. Pediatr Pulmonol 2005;39:332-8.)

postoperative stay in hospital and the minimum period of observation before discharge from hospital, has been the subject of much debate. Because the onset of respiratory complications in these children may be delayed,[69,179,191] a 6- to 8-hour period of observation for respiratory complications after adenotonsillectomy for OSA has been suggested. However, this extended period of observation does not preclude the delayed onset of sleep-related respiratory compromise after adenotonsillectomy. Table 31-5 presents common admission criteria for children undergoing elective tonsillectomy.

## POST-TONSILLECTOMY BLEEDING

Post-tonsillectomy bleeding is a surgical emergency. This can occur either within the first 24 hours (primary) or 5 to 10 days after surgery when the eschar covering the tonsillar bed retracts (secondary). Approximately 75% of postoperative tonsillar bleeding occurs within 6 hours of surgery. Sixty-seven percent of cases of postoperative bleeding originate in the tonsillar fossa, 27% in the nasopharynx, and 7% in both.[203] Primary bleeding is typically more serious than secondary bleeding because it is usually more brisk and profuse. It is considered a surgical complication that is responsible for converting tonsillectomy from ambulatory surgery to a hospital admission in 1.6% of cases.[42]

| **TABLE 31-5** Criteria for Overnight Admission after Tonsillectomy and Adenoidectomy |
| --- |
| • Obstructive sleep apnea |
| • Sleep disturbance |
| • <3 years of age |
| • Craniofacial abnormalities (e.g., Down syndrome, Treacher Collins syndrome) |
| • Lives >1 hour away |
| • Lives in an unstable home environment that precludes adequate supervision |
| • Postoperative problems (e.g., fever, failure to take oral fluids, or continued vomiting) |
| • Possible or documented coagulopathy |
| • Extreme obesity |

From Zalzal G: Personal communications, survey of major pediatric hospitals, 2006.

In a review of more than 9000 adenotonsillectomies in children performed with blunt and sharp (cold) dissection, the incidence of postoperative bleeding was 2.15%, with 76% of the hemorrhages occurring in the first 6 hours postoperatively.[204] The authors of an audit of 4800 pediatric tonsillectomies for which hemostasis was secured with electrocautery (hot) techniques, reported a primary postoperative hemorrhage rate of 0.9%, with 83% presenting within 4 hours of surgery.[55] The consensus is that the period of observation for primary hemorrhage depends on the surgical technique: 6 hours and 4 hours, for cold and hot dissection, respectively,[55,203,204] although abbreviated periods of observation have been advocated by some.[42]

The management of anesthesia in this situation can be challenging even in the hands of an experienced pediatric anesthesiologist.[205] It often requires dealing with anxious parents, an upset surgeon, and a frightened anemic, hypovolemic child with a stomach full of blood. A thorough review of the anesthetic record of the original surgery will provide pertinent information about any existing medical condition, use of medications (such as aspirin), difficulty with airway management, and a rough estimate of intraoperative blood loss and fluid replacement, as well as the duration of known bleeding and the volume of blood vomited since the bleeding began. A quick history and examination of the child will provide vital information about the child's current volume status. A history of dizziness and the presence of orthostatic hypotension may suggest a loss of more than 20% of the circulating blood volume and the need for aggressive fluid resuscitation and crossmatch of blood before induction.[206] Even when severe hypotension is not present, the child with the bleeding tonsil is hypovolemic and has a decrease in cardiac output secondary to ongoing blood loss. If blood loss is severe, and/or fluid resuscitation is not vigorous, lactic acidosis and an eventual state of shock will develop. The compensatory response to acute blood loss is an outpouring of catecholamines. This causes peripheral vasoconstriction, which delays the clinical onset of hypotension in the awake child. When anesthesia-induced vasodilation occurs, profound hypotension may develop. Vigorous fluid resuscitation with crystalloids (repeated boluses of 20 mL/kg of balanced salt solution) and/or colloids is therefore the key to improve the cardiac output and achieve hemodynamic stability before induction of anesthesia. Hemoglobin or hematocrit determination should be interpreted in light of the child's volume status and the type of fluid resuscitation administered. If the hemoglobin concentration is low, blood may be required; however, blood is rarely the primary solution for volume replacement in these children. If severe hypovolemia is suspected or if there may be a delay in obtaining blood, blood should be crossmatched for two or more units of packed red blood cells before the child reaches the OR. If a child bleeds after the tonsillectomy, and a bleeding blood vessel is not identified, it may be necessary to measure the prothrombin time, partial thromboplastin time, platelet count, and a bleeding time to rule out a bleeding diathesis. It cannot be overemphasized that the child must be adequately volume resuscitated before proceeding to the OR.

A child who presents with a bleeding tonsil has a full stomach (filled with swallowed blood) and may still be hypovolemic. A child who is spitting bright red blood may quickly exsanguinate, but the bleeding may be temporarily controlled by compression of the carotid artery ipsilateral to the bleeding source. The anesthesiologist may have difficulty visualizing the larynx because of the bleeding tonsillar bed and clots in the pharynx. A styletted ETT, two sets of well-illuminated laryngoscope blades and handles, and two large-bore Yankauer-type suction tubes must be available before induction of anesthesia (see also Chapter 4 and Fig. 38-5). On arrival in the OR and application of routine monitors, the child should be preoxygenated while positioned in the left lateral position and head down to drain blood out of

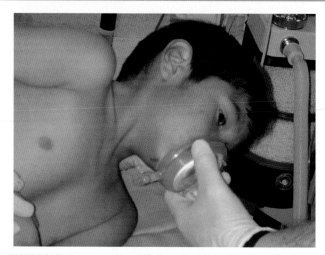

**FIGURE 31-11** Preoxygenation with the patient in the lateral position to control post-tonsillectomy bleeding before induction of anesthesia.

the mouth (Fig. 31-11). The child is then turned supine, and a rapid-sequence induction is carried out with cricoid pressure (Sellick maneuver) applied by an assistant, to minimize the risk of aspirating blood into the lungs.[207] There is no evidence that a rapid-sequence induction with cricoid pressure decreases the risk of aspiration in children with full stomachs, although this practice is commonplace. It should also be recognized that aspiration of blood into the lungs is not synonymous with acid particulate aspiration, unless the volume of blood aspirated compromises pulmonary oxygenation. The use of a full induction dose of propofol in a hypovolemic child could result in significant hypotension. A reduced dose of these induction agents (e.g., propofol, 1 to 2 mg/kg), or ketamine (1 to 2 mg/kg) or etomidate (0.2 mg/kg) for induction followed by atropine (0.02 mg/kg) combined with succinylcholine (1.5 to 2 mg/kg) or rocuronium (1.2 mg/kg) for tracheal intubation should facilitate a rapid control of the airway without hypotension. However, the systolic blood pressure after induction of anesthesia will provide a direction indication of the volume status of the child.

When possible, a cuffed ETT (one-half size smaller than usual for age or weight) should be used to minimize the chance of aspirating blood. The use of a stylet is strongly recommended in spite of a previous history of easy intubation. Titration of an inhalational anesthetic, such as sevoflurane or desflurane with nitrous oxide and oxygen,[97] supplemented with an opioid, such as fentanyl, 1 to 2 μg/kg, will facilitate rapid recovery at the end of surgery.[208] Often these surgeries are not excessively painful because surgery is limited to the area of bleeding. Controlling the bleeding vessel in the tonsillar bed can be accomplished rapidly if the blood pressure is maintained in the normal range. Hence, these surgeries are often quite brief and the anesthetic should be planned accordingly. Suctioning the stomach with a large-bore catheter under direct vision after the procedure does not guarantee an empty stomach, because much of the blood may be clotted and the clots are often too large to be suctioned. The use of prophylactic antiemetic therapy (e.g., ondansetron 0.1 mg/kg) is indicated.

The most important postoperative consideration is to extubate these children when they are fully awake and able to control their airway reflexes. Extubating the trachea while the child is in the lateral position may be the safest practice to minimize the risk of aspiration. If there is a medical indication to substitute high-dose rocuronium (1.2 mg/kg) for succinyl-choline, then a prolonged period of relaxation may be anticipated. Sugammadex may allow early reversal of residual deep neuromuscular blockade with high-dose rocuronium, although at the time of this writing, sugammadex is neither approved for use in children nor available in the United States or Canada. Postoperatively, a repeat determination of the hemoglobin level may be indicated.

## PERITONSILLAR ABSCESS

Peritonsillar abscess (quinsy tonsil) occurs in older children and young adults. It is the most common deep neck-space infection treated by otolaryngologists. Infection originates in the tonsil and spreads to the peritonsillar space between the tonsillar capsule and the superior constrictor muscle, and usually into the soft palate in the region of the superior pole of the tonsil. Commonly cultured organisms include aerobes, such as *Streptococcus pyogenes, S. milleri, S. viridans,* β-hemolytic streptococci, *Haemophilus influenzae,* as well as anaerobes, such as *Fusobacterium* and *Prevotella* species.[209]

Clinically, these children present with fever, pharyngeal swelling, sore throat, dysphagia, odynophagia, and often trismus. Trismus is caused by compression of nerves by the tense peritonsillar mass, spasm of the pterygoid muscles, and inflammation of the muscles of the face and neck. Dehydration can ensue because of fever and the persistent difficulty with swallowing.

Preoperative evaluation includes careful assessment of the airway, with special emphasis on the degree of trismus. Blood specimens should be analyzed for total and differential white blood cell count to ascertain the response to the infection, and for cultures for appropriate antibiotic therapy. Computed tomography of the tonsillar area will identify airway deviation or compromise and the extent of spread of the abscess (Fig. 31-12).

While awaiting the results of the cultures, treatment should begin with establishing IV access, hydration, and appropriate antibiotic coverage. The majority of organisms, including anaerobes, are penicillin sensitive. Consequently, penicillin is usually the antibiotic of choice.[209] The three different procedures currently used to drain a peritonsillar abscess are needle aspiration, incision and drainage, and abscess tonsillectomy.[210] Most children undergo general anesthesia for treatment of peritonsillar abscess by incision and drainage, although in some centers, moderate to deep sedation has been successfully used.[211] If the abscess is small and well confined, immediate tonsillectomy is performed.

The anesthetic management of these children can be challenging. Rupture of the abscess and possible aspiration of purulent material during laryngoscopy and intubation should be avoided during induction of anesthesia. Although the airway may appear to be compromised, most peritonsillar abscesses are in a fixed location in the lateral pharynx and do not interfere with mask ventilation. Visualization of the vocal cords is usually not impaired, because the pathology is supraglottic and well above the laryngeal inlet, although a right-sided abscess may interfere with the usual sweeping of the tongue to the left during laryngoscopy. Laryngoscopy must be carefully approached to avoid excessive manipulation of the larynx and surrounding structures. Occasionally, the pharyngeal swelling and the distortion of normal anatomy, along with excessive secretions, may create difficulty for laryngoscopy and intubation. The OR should be prepared as for any difficult airway case, with different sizes of ETTs, stylets, two sets of well-illuminated laryngoscopes, a Glidescope or other device to facilitate difficult intubation, and a

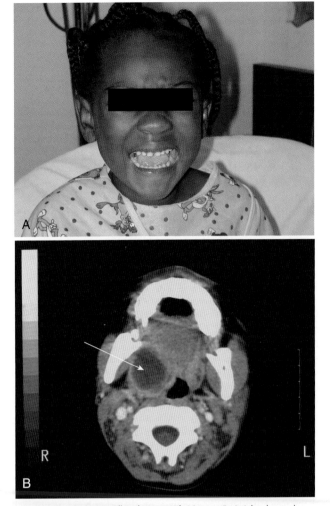

**FIGURE 31-12 A,** Peritonsillar abscess with trismus. **B,** Axial enhanced computed tomography scan through the oropharynx showing a 3-cm ring-shaped, enhancing, low-density mass (*arrow*) replacing the left tonsil, typical of a tonsillar abscess.

tonsil-tip suction catheter attached to a powerful suction device. The surgeon must be present in the OR during induction of anesthesia, should airway obstruction occur. Equipment for cricothyrotomy or tracheotomy must be readily available.

These children are often older and do not require preoperative sedation. If trismus is present, an inhalational induction should be performed, using sevoflurane and oxygen while the anesthesiologist assesses mobility of the temporomandibular joint under anesthesia. An oropharyngeal airway is best avoided, lest the abscess is traumatized. Usually, awake trismus resolves once an adequate depth of anesthesia has been achieved. When this is confirmed, or if there was minimal trismus to begin with, then a short-acting muscle relaxant (or propofol) should be given to facilitate tracheal intubation. Alternatively, if there is minimal trismus and the preoperative airway assessment indicates minimal distortion, a rapid-sequence IV induction after adequate preoxygenation may be the best way to avoid trauma to the pharyngeal structures while struggling with a mask induction, needing to insert an oropharyngeal airway, and possibly rupturing the abscess.[2]

To avoid aspiration of purulent material during intubation and drainage, a cuffed ETT is recommended and the child is placed in Trendelenburg position. At the end of surgery, the child should be extubated awake, preferably in the lateral decubitus position.[2]

# Anesthesia for Endoscopy

Anesthesia for rigid bronchoscopy in young children presents a significant challenge. Not only does the child have a compromised airway, but we also must share it with the surgeon. The importance of constant communication between the endoscopist and the anesthesiologist cannot be overstated. In general, the goals of anesthesia for endoscopy are analgesia, an unconscious child, and a quiet surgical field.[212] Coughing, bucking, or straining during instrumentation with a rigid bronchoscope may cause difficulty for the surgeon and damage the child's airway. At the conclusion of the procedure, children should be returned to consciousness quickly with airway reflexes intact to protect the recently instrumented airway. General principles for the anesthetic management will be outlined first. Disease-specific requirements will be discussed under appropriate subheadings.

For most children, a pulse oximeter, blood pressure cuff, electrocardiogram, and precordial stethoscope are applied before induction. Continuous monitoring of ventilation by capnography is not always possible during bronchoscopy, particularly when the Hopkins optical telescope is in place for optimal viewing. Clinical observation of the chest wall movement and the use of a precordial stethoscope are useful. In many cases, intermittent capnography is possible when the bronchoscope is withdrawn by the surgeon. Although greater than normal $CO_2$ tensions are inevitable with intermittent ventilation, they are generally well tolerated in the presence of sevoflurane. In contrast, if halothane is used, ventricular arrhythmias may occur and should be treated by hyperventilation and deepening halothane anesthesia, or by substituting isoflurane or sevoflurane for halothane (see Chapter 6).[213] Hypoxia, on the other hand, is not well tolerated, and the procedure should be stopped while the child is oxygenated.

In many instances, endoscopists prefer that the child breathes spontaneously throughout the procedure. Inhalation induction by mask is accomplished with oxygen and an inhalational agent, usually sevoflurane. Nitrous oxide can be used initially, if tolerated, to speed the induction and then discontinued before the examination. Once a sufficient depth of anesthesia has been achieved, IV access is established and the depth of anesthesia is increased. Alternatively, in those children in whom IV access was established before anesthesia, anesthesia may be induced IV with a sleep-dose of propofol, followed by mask ventilation with a volatile agent.

An antisialagogue (atropine or glycopyrrolate) may be administered IV to decrease secretions that may impair the view through the bronchoscope. Topically treating the vocal cords and subglottic airway with local anesthetic decreases the incidence of coughing or bucking during instrumentation, and allows the child to tolerate a lighter level of anesthesia. Lidocaine, either 2% or 4%, is the most frequently used topical anesthetic. It may be applied to the vocal cords either by atomizer or sprayed with a 3-mL Luer-Lok syringe fitted with a 24-gauge IV catheter (without the needle). With constant pressure applied on the plunger, a fine stream of lidocaine is directed to the supraglottic structures and through the vocal cords to the tracheal mucosa. The dose of lidocaine should be limited to 3 to 4 mg/kg divided between the laryngeal and tracheal surfaces because rapid absorption via the

mucosa occurs. It is important to confirm whether the surgeon intends to observe for movement of the vocal cords or evaluate tracheal or bronchial dynamics so that the anesthetic may be planned accordingly (i.e., spontaneous respirations preserved during light levels of anesthesia versus no respiratory efforts and the use of short-acting muscle relaxants).

## DIAGNOSTIC LARYNGOSCOPY AND BRONCHOSCOPY

Although diagnostic laryngoscopy and bronchoscopy procedures are usually of brief duration, the anesthetic management can be challenging in small infants with an already compromised airway. Stridor, or noisy breathing due to obstructed airflow, is a common indication for a diagnostic laryngoscopy and bronchoscopy in infants and children. Inspiratory stridor results from UAO, expiratory stridor results from lower airway obstruction, and biphasic stridor is present with mid-tracheal lesions (see Chapters 11 and 12). Subglottic stenosis may follow prolonged tracheal intubation in an infant that was born preterm.

The evaluation of a child with stridor begins with taking a thorough history. The age at symptom onset helps suggest a cause; for instance, laryngotracheomalacia and vocal cord paralysis are usually present at or shortly after birth, whereas cysts or mass lesions develop later in life (Table 31-6). Information indicating positions that make the stridor better or worse should be obtained, because placing a child in a position that allows gravity to aid in reducing obstruction can be of benefit during induction.

Physical examination reveals the general condition of a child or infant, as well as the degree of the airway compromise. Laboratory examination may include a chest radiograph and barium swallow, which can aid in identifying lesions that may be compressing the trachea. Computed tomography, magnetic resonance imaging, and tomograms may be helpful in isolated instances but are not routinely indicated.

| TABLE 31-6 Causes of Stridor |
| --- |
| **Supraglottic Airway** |
| Choanal atresia |
| Cyst |
| Mass |
| Large tonsils |
| Large adenoids |
| Craniofacial abnormalities |
| Foreign body |
| **Larynx** |
| Laryngomalacia |
| Vocal cord paralysis |
| Hemangiomas |
| Cysts |
| Laryngocele |
| Infection (tonsillitis, peritonsillar abscess) |
| Foreign body |
| **Subglottic Airway** |
| Subglottic stenosis |
| Tracheomalacia |
| Vascular ring |
| Foreign body |
| Infection (croup, epiglottitis) |
| Hemangiomas |

Laryngomalacia is the most common cause of stridor in infants and most often results from a long epiglottis that prolapses posteriorly and prominent arytenoid cartilages with redundant aryepiglottic folds that prolapse into the glottic opening during inspiration.[214] The definitive diagnosis is obtained by direct laryngoscopy and by rigid or flexible bronchoscopy.

Preliminary examination is usually carried out in the surgeon's office. A small flexible fiberoptic bronchoscope is inserted through the nares into the oropharynx. Nasal insertion provides an excellent view of the movement of the vocal cords and pharyngeal structures. Topically treating the nasopharynx with lidocaine facilitates passage of the nasal pharyngoscope or bronchoscope. Alternatively, the examination can be accomplished in the OR in a lightly anesthetized child during spontaneous respirations. Children must be spontaneously breathing so that the vocal cords move freely. After movement of the vocal cords is observed and recorded, the anesthetic level can be increased as appropriate, a rigid bronchoscope (or just the telescope in small infants) is inserted through the vocal cords, and the subglottic area, the lower trachea, and bronchi are evaluated.

The use of premedication in these children should be individualized. Small infants may be brought into the OR unpremedicated; older children may experience respiratory depression and worsening of airway obstruction if heavily premedicated.

Usually an inhalational induction with sevoflurane is performed. Nitrous oxide can be used initially, if tolerated, to speed the induction and then discontinued before the examination. Because sevoflurane is relatively insoluble and is rapidly eliminated, ventilation will be intermittently interrupted during the examination, and the Hopkins optical telescope prevents adequate ventilation through the smallest diameter bronchoscopes, supplementation with IV agents, such as propofol (1 mg/kg boluses or a 50- to 100-μg/kg/min infusion), is necessary to maintain an appropriate depth of anesthesia. If an inhaled technique is used by insufflation, scavenging may be attempted by positioning a suction device near the child's mouth.

A propofol-based total intravenous anesthesia (TIVA) technique has the advantage that it can be given continuously during the procedure, resulting in a more stable level of anesthesia than can be achieved with inhalational agents and intermittent ventilation. Propofol can be supplemented with small (0.5 mg/kg) doses of ketamine to enhance analgesia. Opioids can also be used but will frequently induce apnea.

The key to a stress-free bronchoscopy is properly placed topical anesthesia. Although topically treating the laryngeal structures with local anesthetic helps the child tolerate the procedure, it may interfere with assessment of normal vocal cord movement. For that reason, a local anesthetic is often topically applied after initial evaluation of the upper airway and just before insertion of the bronchoscope for evaluation of the distal airway structures.

After completion of pharyngoscopy and/or laryngoscopy, the surgeon generally proceeds to rigid bronchoscopy. The size of a rigid bronchoscope refers to the internal diameter (ID). Because the external diameter may be significantly greater than that of an ETT of similar size, care must be taken to select a bronchoscope of proper external diameter, to avoid damage to the laryngeal structures (Table 31-7). The rigid bronchoscope can be used for ventilation through the side port attached to the anesthesia circuit with a flexible extension. It is often most useful to paralyze the child with a fixed lesion, which diminishes the risk of vocal

**TABLE 31-7** External Diameter of Standard Endotracheal Tube versus Rigid Bronchoscope

| Internal Diameter (mm) | EXTERNAL DIAMETER (mm) | |
| --- | --- | --- |
| | Endotracheal Tube* | Rigid Bronchoscope† |
| 2.0 | 2.9 | |
| 2.5 | 3.6 | 4.2 |
| 3.0 | 4.3 | 5.0 |
| 3.5 | 4.9 | 5.7 |
| 3.7 (bronchoscope) | | 6.3 |
| 4.0 | 5.6 | 6.7 |
| 5.0 | 6.9 | 7.8 |
| 6.0 | 8.2 | 8.2 |

*Mallinckrodt Medical, Inc., St Louis.
†Karl Storz Endoscopy-America, Inc., El Segundo, Calif.

cord injury secondary to movement. For nonfixed lesions, such as an aspirated foreign body, and for assessment for bronchomalacia or tracheomalacia, it is preferable to proceed with spontaneous ventilation, a deep level of anesthesia, and good topical anesthesia of the vocal cords and carina. Adequate oxygenation should be maintained in these infants throughout the procedure. Because ventilation may be intermittent and at times suboptimal, it is recommended that 100% oxygen be used as the carrier gas during the bronchoscopic examination. During ventilation of the infant with the optical telescope in place, high resistance may be encountered as a result of partial occlusion of the lumen. This is especially likely when the 2.5-, 3.0-, and 3.5-mm ID scopes are used. Large fresh-gas flow rates, large tidal volumes with high inflation pressures, and large concentrations of inspired inhalational anesthetic (or TIVA) are often necessary to compensate for leaks around the ventilating bronchoscope and the high resistance encountered when the optical telescope is in place. Hand ventilation at greater than normal rates is most effective in achieving adequate ventilation. Sufficient time for exhalation must be provided for passive recoil of the chest. In small infants, there may be room for only the optical telescopic light source, which does not have a ventilation channel. In these cases, insufflation of oxygen via a small tube placed in the hypopharynx via the nose or mouth will delay the onset of desaturation in a spontaneously breathing child. If (when) desaturation occurs, the surgeon must stop and allow the child to be oxygenated before continuing with the examination.

At the conclusion of bronchoscopy, the surgeon may wish to determine the size of the larynx and determine the degree of airway narrowing. An uncuffed ETT is inserted beyond the narrowest portion of the obstructed airway, and the airway is assessed by applying positive pressure between 10 and 25 cm $H_2O$ to the airway and listening with a stethoscope for an air leak around the ETT at the level of the suprasternal notch. The outer diameter of the appropriate ETT is compared with the inner diameter of the child's larynx and trachea, and the percentage of obstruction is calculated. Grade I obstruction involves up to 50% of the airway, grade II is from 51% to 70%, and grade III is greater than 70% (Fig. 31-13, B).[215]

An alternative method of ventilation during bronchoscopy is the Sanders jet ventilation technique. The principle of jet ventilation involves intermittent bursts of oxygen delivered at a maximum pressure of 50 psi from a hand-regulated

Percent Subglottic Stenosis by Endotracheal Tube Size (mm ID)

| Age | ETT | 2 | 2.5 | 3 | 3.5 | 4 | 4.5 | 5 | 5.5 | 6 |
|---|---|---|---|---|---|---|---|---|---|---|
| Preterm (<1500 gm) | | 40 | | | | | | | | |
| Preterm (>1500 gm) | | | 30 | | | | | | | |
| 0-3 months | | | 48 | 26 | | No obstruction | | | | |
| 3-9 months | No detectable lumen | 75 | | 41 | 22 | | | | | |
| 9 months to 2 years | | 80 | | | 38 | 20 | | | | |
| 2 years | | 84 | 74 | | 50 | 35 | 19 | | | |
| 4 years | | 86 | 78 | | | 45 | 32 | 17 | | |
| 6 years | | 89 | 81 | 73 | | | 43 | 30 | 16 | |
| | Grade IV | Grade III | | | Grade II | | Grade I | | | |

A

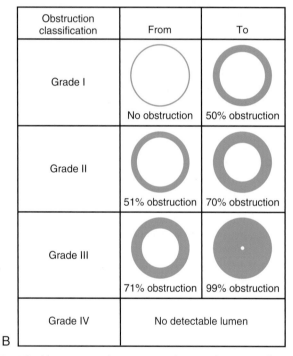

| Obstruction classification | From | To |
|---|---|---|
| Grade I | No obstruction | 50% obstruction |
| Grade II | 51% obstruction | 70% obstruction |
| Grade III | 71% obstruction | 99% obstruction |
| Grade IV | No detectable lumen | |

B

FIGURE 31-13 **A,** Method for estimating the percentage of airway obstruction. After easy passage of an uncuffed endotracheal tube (*ETT*), a manometer is placed at the connection of the elbow of the anesthesia circuit and the ETT. A stethoscope is placed over the larynx and the circuit is slowly pressurized. The pressure at which a leak is auscultated (10 to 25 cm H₂O) is matched with the age of the child and the size of the ETT to estimate the percent of laryngeal narrowing shown in numbers in teal boxes. Clear boxes indicate the usual size ETT for child's age. Grade I, *light teal*, Grade II, *medium teal*, and Grade III, *dark teal*. **B,** Schematic representation of subglottic stenosis classification system. This chart is based on one institution's experience, and the manufacturer of the ETTs was not described, thus the actual external diameter of the ETTs used is unknown. *ID,* Internal diameter. (Reproduced and modified with permission from Myer CM III, O'Connor DM, Cotton RT. Proposed grading system for subglottic stenosis based on endotracheal tube sizes. Ann Otol Laryngol 1994;103:319-23.)

pressure-reducing valve to the lungs, through a 16-gauge catheter attached to a rigid bronchoscope.[216] Current jet ventilators include adjustable pressure-control valves that permit attenuation of the peak pressure, a desirable feature if this device is to be used in a child. Intermittent flow is accomplished by depressing the lever of an on-off valve. A jet of oxygen is released at the tip of the 16-gauge catheter, creating a Venturi effect that entrains room air into the bronchoscope. This jet of oxygen and room air mixture allows inflation of the lungs to occur. Exhalation is passive and depends on the recoil of the chest wall. Although this technique is usually effective for both oxygenation and ventilation in experienced hands, a number of potential problems exist. Because of potentially high inflation pressure, pneumothorax, pneumomediastinum, and death can occur.[217] Blood or infectious or particulate matter in the airway may be forced distally by high-pressure bursts. There is also the possibility of hypoxemia in some children, because the high-pressure oxygen entrains room air, diluting the oxygen.

High-frequency jet ventilation is also possible for upper airway endoscopy and laryngotracheal surgery. Obstruction to expiratory flow is a major concern and is dependent on good positioning of the rigid laryngoscope. Complications, such as barotrauma, pneumopericardium, $CO_2$ retention, necrotizing tracheobronchitis, and gastric rupture, dictate a fastidious technique.[218]

Dexamethasone in a dose of 0.5 mg/kg IV (maximum dose, 10 to 20 mg) is frequently administered during the procedure to decrease postoperative laryngeal swelling and the possibility of croup. At the conclusion of rigid bronchoscopy, an ETT can be placed in the trachea to control the airway during recovery from anesthesia or, if ventilation is adequate and the anesthetic depth is not excessive, the child can be allowed to emerge breathing 100% oxygen by a facemask.

# Upper Airway Obstruction

### LARYNGOTRACHEOBRONCHITIS (CROUP)

Croup is a symptom complex of inspiratory stridor; suprasternal, intercostal, and substernal retractions; barking cough; and hoarseness that results from swelling of the mucosa in the subglottic area of the larynx.[2] There are two common entities that account for most cases of croup: spasmodic croup, and laryngotracheobronchitis. Spasmodic croup has been diagnosed in about 3% of children with stridor.[219] The child is otherwise healthy and afebrile, presenting with nocturnal episodes of spasmodic cough, which is described as barking and high pitched. The disease is self-limiting. Besides viruses, allergic and psychological factors are blamed for this acute phenomenon. It differs from acute laryngotracheitis in that it is considered an allergic reaction to viral antigens rather than a true infection with the viruses.[220] Besides lack of fever, spasmodic croup is usually remarkable for lack of severe laryngeal inflammation, and, in general, supportive therapy on an outpatient basis is all that is required.

Viral laryngotracheitis is by far the most common form of infectious croup. The disease has a gradual onset, usually after a URI in a young child. Low-grade fever is common. Children who have more than two episodes of croup requiring hospitalization should be evaluated for subglottic narrowing from stenosis or cysts. Clinical scoring systems based on objective criteria are helpful in following the progress of the disease and in judging the effectiveness of therapy (Table 31-8).[221]

Anteroposterior radiographs of the neck will confirm the diagnosis and rule out acute epiglottitis or the possibility of a foreign body in the airway (Table 31-9).[222] The viral infection affects the subglottic region of the larynx, causing edema. The characteristic radiograph of croup, therefore, includes blurring of the tracheal air shadow on lateral neck films, and symmetrical narrowing of the subglottic air shadow, described as "church steeple" or "sharpened pencil" sign on anteroposterior films (Fig. 31-14 and E-Fig 31-3). The lateral neck radiographs show normal supraglottic structures and normal epiglottic shadow.

The majority of cases will resolve quickly with simple conservative measures, such as breathing humidified air or oxygen. Less than 10% of cases require hospitalization because of significant respiratory difficulty, and fewer still require an artificial airway.[214] Humidification of inspired gases is usually effective in improving respiratory distress, and it prevents drying of secretions, although despite the popularity of cool mist therapy, it is

**TABLE 31-8** Clinical Croup Score

|  | 0 | 1 | 2 |
|---|---|---|---|
| Inspiratory Breath Sounds | Normal | Harsh with rhonchi | Delayed |
| Stridor | None | Inspiratory | Inspiratory/expiratory |
| Cough | None | Hoarse cry | Barking |
| Retractions | None | Flaring and suprasternal retractions | Flaring, suprasternal and intercostal retractions |
| Cyanosis | None | In air | In 40% $O_2$ |

Modified from Downes JJ, Raphaely RC. Pediatric intensive care. Anesthesiology 1975;43:238-50.

**TABLE 31-9** Differential Diagnosis of Croup and Epiglottitis

|  | Croup* | Epiglottitis |
|---|---|---|
| Incidence | More common | Less common |
| Obstruction | Subglottic | Supraglottic |
| Age | Younger (<3 years) | Older (3-6 years) |
| Etiology | Viral | Bacterial |
| Recurrence | Possible (5%) | Rare |
| **Clinical Features** | | |
| Onset | Gradual (days) | Sudden (hours) |
| Fever | Low grade | High |
| Dysphagia | None | Marked |
| Drooling | None | Present |
| Posture | Recumbent | Sitting |
| Toxemia | None | Present |
| Cough | Barking | Usually none |
| Voice | Hoarse | Clear to muffled |
| Respiratory rate | Rapid | Normal/slow |
| Larynx palpation | Not tender | Tender |
| Leukocytosis | + (Lymphocytic) | +++ (Polymorphonuclear cells) |
| Neck radiographs | Anteroposterior: steeple sign | Lateral: thumb-like mass |
| Clinical course | Longer | Shorter |
| **Treatment** | | |
| Primary therapy | Medical and supportive | Secure airway first |
| $O_2$ and humidity | Essential | Usually desirable |
| Hydration | Oral or IV | Intravenous |
| Racemic epinephrine | Usually effective | No value |
| Corticosteroids | Controversial | Not indicated |
| Antibiotics | Not indicated | Effective |
| Airway support | Occasionally needed (<3%) | Always indicated (100%) |
| Preferred airway | Nasotracheal Tracheostomy (rarely) | Nasotracheal |
| Extubation | 4-7 days | 1-3 days |

From Hannallah R. Epiglottitis. In: Stehling L, editor. Common problems in pediatric anesthesia. 2nd ed. St Louis: Mosby-Year Book; 1992, p. 277-81.
*Foreign bodies in the airway should also be considered.

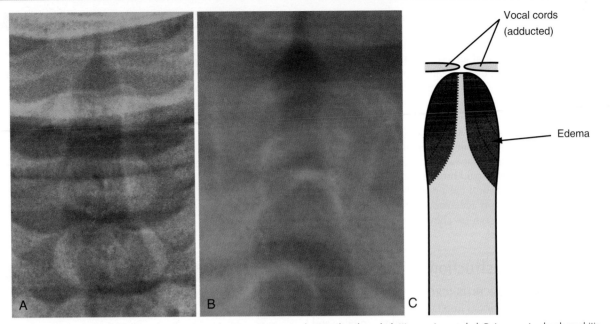

**FIGURE 31-14 A,** Radiograph of the normal upper airway (anteroposterior view). Note that the subglottic area is rounded. **B,** Laryngotracheobronchitis (croup) produces swelling (edema and inflammation), which obliterates the normal rounded subglottic area, producing the so-called sharpened pencil or steeple sign. **C,** Schematic representation showing progressive swelling of the subglottic area. For an additional view, see E-Figure 31-3.

not evidence-based practice.[223] Oxygen is obviously essential to prevent or to treat hypoxemia, which may result from ventilation-perfusion mismatching caused by accumulation of secretions. Hydration prevents thickening of tracheal secretions.

Racemic epinephrine is the most effective drug therapy for these children, although L-epinephrine has also been effective. Racemic epinephrine is available as a 2.25% solution, which is diluted in water or saline, and administered either by intermittent positive-pressure ventilation via a face-mask or nebulization.[224] Nebulized racemic epinephrine is administered in cases of mild-to-moderate obstruction. The solution is prepared by diluting a volume of 2.25% racemic epinephrine in 2 mL of saline or sterile water according to the child's weight in kilograms (i.e., 0.25 mL of racemic epinephrine for 0 to 20 kg, 0.5 mL for 20 to 40 kg and 0.75 mL for greater than 40 kg).[225] Because the duration of action of racemic epinephrine is brief, rebound edema may occur. Treatments are required every 1 to 2 hours, and the child should be observed for at least 2 hours after treatment. For L-epinephrine, the volume of a 1% solution is the same as that for racemic epinephrine.

If treatment with racemic epinephrine is unsuccessful, in addition to edema, the underlying problem may be obstruction caused by thick, inspissated secretions possibly related to bacterial superinfection, such as bacterial tracheitis.[226,227] In this situation, or if the child appears exhausted from the increased work of breathing, relief of the obstruction must be obtained through endotracheal intubation, followed by pulmonary suctioning. The clinical assessment of "exhaustion" in children with croup may be difficult. An alternative approach is to consider intubating the tracheas of those children who have arterial oxygen saturation less than 90% when breathing air, despite nebulized epinephrine and steroid treatment. Laryngotracheobronchitis is also a disease of the lower airways. An inability to clear secretions contributes to atelectasis and arterial oxygen desaturation. Intubation is often required to allow suctioning of the copious yellow secretions.

One large series (512 consecutive admissions in a single year) reported that approximately 6% of children who had sternal and chest retractions on admission and failed to respond to conventional medical therapy required endotracheal intubation.[228] Intubation should be performed in the OR under controlled anesthetic conditions, as for a child with severe epiglottitis. The tracheal tube selected should be at least one-half size smaller (0.5 mm ID) than would normally be chosen, to avoid aggravating the subglottic edema and possibly causing subglottic stenosis.[229-231] Children whose airways have been intubated are admitted to the ICU, and special care is provided for suctioning of inspissated secretions. The tracheal tube usually remains in place for 3 to 5 days.

Corticosteroid therapy for laryngotracheobronchitis has become the standard of care.[232] Single-dose corticosteroid therapy appears safe and effective,[233] although large studies of the risk of progression of viral infection or the development of secondary bacterial infections in moderate to severe laryngotracheobronchitis are lacking; reports suggest that IV dexamethasone (0.5 to 1 mg/kg) may be effective.[234] There is evidence that there is rapid clinical improvement 12 and 24 hours after steroid treatment, which significantly reduces the incidence of endotracheal intubation.[235-237] Antibiotics are generally not indicated in the treatment of uncomplicated viral croup.

The child is usually ready for extubation within 2 to 4 days. Criteria to consider include abatement of fever, diminished tracheal secretions, change in the character of secretions to a thin and watery type, and an audible air leak that develops around the nasotracheal tube as the edema subsides.

## ACUTE EPIGLOTTITIS

Although rarely seen today, acute epiglottitis can be fatal because it can produce seemingly unprovoked sudden and complete airway obstruction. It is a clinical and pathologic entity that should more correctly be termed supraglottitis, because the arytenoids and aryepiglottic folds, as well as the epiglottis itself, are usually affected. All supraglottic structures become swollen and stiffened by inflammatory edema. Although the main focus of infection is the oropharynx, the disease produces a generalized toxemia. Epiglottitis is most common between the ages of 3 and 5 years, but it can occur in any age; historically, the causative organism was typically *Haemophilus influenzae* type B.[2,238-240] However, with the widespread use of *H. influenzae* vaccination, the incidence of epiglottitis in children has all but disappeared in medically advantaged countries.[241,242] *Streptococcus*,[243] *Staphylococcus*,[244] *Candida*,[245] and other fungal pathogens[246] have become more frequent causes of this now rare disorder in children, although the incidence in adults has not diminished substantially.[247] It should be noted that vaccine failures may occur or parents may refuse proper immunizations of their child, resulting in susceptibility to *H. influenzae* type B infection.[248,249] Epiglottitis has become more of a disease of adults.[250]

The onset is usually abrupt, with a brief history of high fever, severe sore throat, and difficulty in swallowing. Stridor, if present, is usually inspiratory, and because the subglottic structures are usually unaffected, there is little or no hoarseness. An expiratory snore, rather than inspiratory stridor can often be heard. The child appears toxic, and, in an attempt to improve airflow past the swollen epiglottis, assumes the sitting position, leaning forward in the sniffing position (E-Fig. 31-4). The mouth is open, with the tongue protruding. The child frequently drools because of difficulty and pain on swallowing. The mnemonic *SNORED* is often useful for diagnosis: *Septic, NO cough, Rapid onset, Expiratory snore, Drool.*

In addition to high fever, other signs of generalized toxemia may include tachycardia, a flushed face, and prostration. The respiratory pattern is usually slow and quiet to allow more comfortable breathing.

Acute epiglottitis is a clinical diagnosis. It must remain prominent in the differential diagnosis of a child presenting with signs and symptoms of UAO. However, in some early cases, the clinical presentation alone may be inconclusive. If so, a lateral radiograph of the neck will usually demonstrate a swollen epiglottis and aryepiglottic folds (Fig. 31-15 and E-Fig 31-5). The vallecula may be obliterated, but subglottic structures are usually clear. A physician capable of establishing an airway should always be in the child's attendance (especially if in a remote area of the hospital, such as Radiology), because total airway obstruction can develop during the radiologic examination, especially if the child is forced to lie supine. This is one reason why the use of lateral neck radiographs in the differential diagnosis of UAO is avoided. Examination of the pharynx and larynx should only be attempted in an area with adequate equipment and staff prepared to intervene should UAO develop; ideally, the OR. The safest, most conservative approach to the management of acute epiglottitis is to establish an artificial airway as soon as the diagnosis is made, and then, with the airway secured, to proceed with appropriate antibiotic and supportive therapy. The child should remain in the sitting position at all times and never forced into the supine position. No attempts to examine the larynx should be made in the emergency room.[2]

These children should not be premedicated. Instead they should be brought to the OR calm and undisturbed. If it takes the presence of a parent to achieve this, then that is what should be done. In the OR, with equipment and personnel who can insert a surgical airway immediately present, a precordial stethoscope, pulse oximeter, and other standard monitors are applied. General anesthesia is induced with oxygen and sevoflurane with the child still sitting up. Spontaneous respiration is continued as the child is gently allowed to recline. If the child is moribund, then an awake intubation should be considered.

When a surgical stage of anesthesia is achieved, IV access is established and secured. A large fluid bolus of balanced salt solution is infused (20 to 30 mL/kg) because these children are often dehydrated and will require a deep plane of anesthesia to permit tracheal intubation while spontaneous respirations are preserved. Some anesthesiologists would also administer an antisialagogue to reduce secretions. Epiglottitis is marked by progressive swelling of the lingual surface of the epiglottis with resultant obliteration of the vallecula (see Fig. 31-15). Viewing the glottic opening without traumatizing the epiglottis may usually be accomplished by forcing the tip of the laryngoscope blade along the center of the base of the tongue into the vallecula, where the vallecula has been obliterated by the swollen lingual surface of the epiglottis (see Fig. 31-15, *C*). Lifting the base of the tongue, without directly touching the epiglottis, can then expose the glottis. A stylet within the ETT may be helpful because it provides increased rigidity to facilitate introduction through a partially obstructed glottic aperture. The size of the ETT should be one-half size smaller (0.5 mm ID) than otherwise selected for the same age child. By choosing an ETT with a smaller ID than usual, one also lessens the risks of pressure necrosis on the mucosa. Figure 31-16 illustrates a case of severe epiglottitis (before [*A*] and after [*B*] the airway was secured). A styletted orotracheal tube is inserted first, and may be replaced by a nasotracheal tube of appropriate size. However, if the glottic opening was difficult to visualize, then no attempt should be made to replace the oral tube with a nasal one. The orotracheal tube may displace supraglottic edema, improving the view of the glottic opening and facilitating placement of the nasotracheal tube. An air leak at 20 to 25 cm of $H_2O$, when present, confirms the selection of an appropriate size tube. Because the airway obstruction in epiglottitis is supraglottic, not subglottic, the nasotracheal tube size is often the usual size or one-half size smaller for the child's age. A larger tube is not necessary and may contribute to the possible development of serious laryngeal complications, such as subglottic stenosis. The child should be able to breathe around the tube, as well as through it. If the anesthesiologist is unable to intubate the trachea, then a rigid bronchoscope should be used. If both of those maneuvers fail, then a tracheostomy or cricothyrotomy should be performed (see Fig. 12-25).[251,252]

Once the airway is secured, a culture of the pharynx and blood cultures are obtained, and aggressive medical therapy beginning with antibiotics should be commenced. It is recommended that cephalosporins (such as ceftriaxone 50 mg/kg/day)[253-255] be used initially for antibiotic therapy, with the first dose immediately after the diagnosis is made and appropriate cultures taken.[2] The duration of the treatment is controversial, but at least 3 to 5 days of IV antibiotics followed by oral therapy is usually the minimum. Steroids are not indicated. Supportive measures include IV hydration, airway care, sedation as necessary, and acetaminophen for fever. Negative-pressure pulmonary edema can develop after tracheal intubation in children with severe epiglottitis.[195] When the child resumes swallowing and the fever abates, usually 24 to 48 hours after initiation of therapy, the acute supraglottic edema should be resolving and the child may be prepared for tracheal extubation.

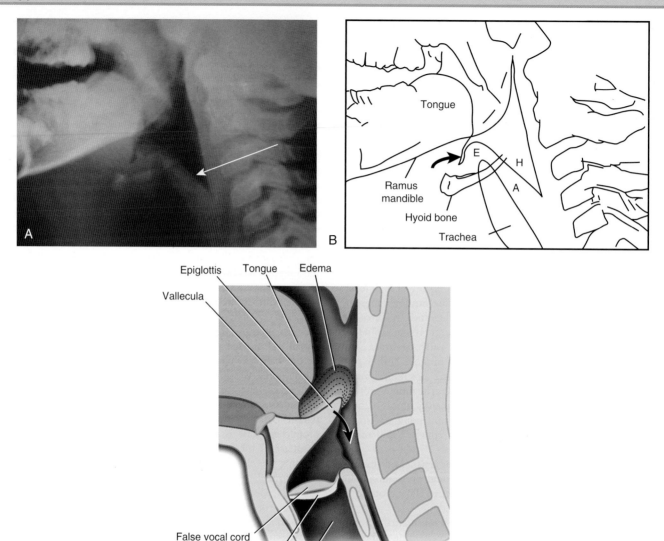

FIGURE 31-15 **A,** Lateral neck radiograph of child with epiglottitis. Note the marked thickening of the aryepiglottic folds (*arrow*). **B,** Schematic representation of **A.** Note the marked thickening of the aryepiglottic folds (*A*), loss ("amputation") of the vallecula (*curved arrow*), swelling of the epiglottis (*E*), and distention of the hypopharynx (*H*). **C,** Schematic representation of epiglottitis demonstrating progressive swelling of the lingual surface of the epiglottis, resulting in "amputation" of the vallecula. Progressive swelling leads to trapdoor-like occlusion of the glottic opening (*curved arrow*). For additional views, see E-Figure 31-5.

## OBSTRUCTIVE LARYNGEAL PAPILLOMATOSIS

Recurrent respiratory papillomatosis, also known as juvenile laryngeal papillomatosis, is the most commonly found tumor in the larynx and upper airway in children. Recurrent respiratory papillomatosis is caused by the human papilloma virus (HPV). The incidence is only 1 in 400 births, even though active or latent viral infection is present in 10% to 25% of pregnant women.[256] This disease is caused by HPV 6 and 11; the incidence may markedly decrease in the future, with the introduction of a maternal vaccine to prevent HPV infection for types 6, 11, 16, and 18.[257-260] The papillomas are usually found in the larynx on the vocal cord margins, epiglottis, pharynx, or trachea (Fig. 31-17). If left untreated, symptoms of aphonia, respiratory distress, hoarseness, stridor, right ventricular hypertrophy, and cor pulmonale may occur.

The current treatment is primarily surgical removal of the papillomatous tissue using the $CO_2$ laser under microscopic visualization. Alternatively, papillomas can be surgically debulked using an ultrasonic microdebrider or cup forceps before laser treatment. Topical application of mitomycin C (usually in combination with debulking procedures) has also been shown to be effective in suppressing these tumors. Nonsurgical treatment using interferon alfa-n1 has been beneficial in some children.[261] The main goal of the treatments is to reduce the bulk of the lesion without scarring and permanent damage to the underlying mucosa.

Because of the recurrent nature of this condition, most children will return frequently for treatment. Many may require monthly scheduled visits to the OR to prevent recurring

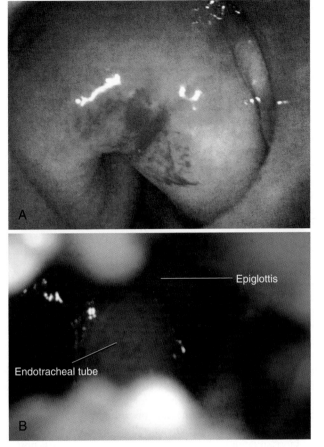

FIGURE 31-16 Acute epiglottitis. **A,** The entire upper airway is inflamed and there is marked swelling of the epiglottis. **B,** Photograph taken after securing the airway with an endotracheal tube.

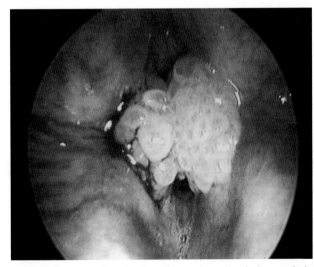

FIGURE 31-17 Large pedunculated papillomas obstructing the laryngeal inlet.

obstruction. If some of these scheduled sessions are missed, or if the progress of the disease is accelerated, the child will present with an acute exacerbation of obstructive symptoms requiring emergent endoscopic resection. In all cases, it is important to obtain a careful history, including inquiry about changes in voice or increased difficulty breathing during daily activities, that may indicate progressive airway obstruction.

Because of frequent hospitalizations, these children become psychologically sensitized to the perioperative experience. Premedication is usually avoided if the degree of airway obstruction is significant and there are concerns about compromising spontaneous ventilation. In selected cases, when the children are extremely anxious and/or upset, the parents (or a child-life surrogate) may accompany the child to the OR for induction, to provide emotional support.

The perioperative care can be very challenging and often depends on the degree of obstruction to airflow and the type and location of the papillomas.[262] Pedunculated papillomas can produce complete ball-valve obstruction of the upper airway in certain positions. It is therefore prudent to avoid paralysis and to maintain spontaneous respirations until the airway is examined and the anesthesiologist is certain that assisted or controlled ventilation is possible. These children must be approached and monitored in the same manner as any child with anticipated severe airway obstruction (e.g., acute epiglottitis). The surgeon must be present in the OR when anesthesia is induced, with equipment immediately available to deal with complete airway obstruction, including rigid bronchoscopes and a tracheostomy–cricothyrotomy set. The problem of sharing the already compromised airway with the surgeon is worsened by the need to use a laser to excise these lesions. A laser (an acronym for *l*ight *a*mplified by *s*timulated *e*mission of *r*adiation) consists of a tube with reflective mirrors at either end with an amplifying medium between them to generate electron activity in the form of light. The $CO_2$ laser is the most widely used in medical practice, having particular application in the treatment of laryngeal or vocal cord papillomas, laryngeal webs, and resection of subglottic tissue and hemangiomas. A laser is useful for endoscopic procedures because the beam may be directed down open-tube endoscopes and is invisible, thereby affording the surgeon an unobstructed view of the lesion during resection. Laser energy is absorbed by tissue water, rapidly increasing its temperature, denaturing protein, and causing vaporization of the target tissue. The thermal energy produced by the laser beam cauterizes capillaries as it vaporizes tissues; therefore, bleeding is minimal and very little postoperative edema occurs.

These properties give the laser a high degree of specificity; however, they also provide the route by which a misdirected laser beam may cause injury to a child or to unprotected OR personnel.[263] Laser radiation increases the temperature of absorbent material; therefore, flammable objects, such as surgical drapes, must be kept away from the path of the laser beam. Unprotected surfaces, such as skin, can be burned and must be shielded. Wet towels should be applied to cover the skin of the face and neck when the laser is being used to avoid burns from deflected beams.

The anesthetic management of these children depends on the approach the surgeon will use to remove the lesions. The basic choice is between intubation and nonintubation techniques. For the latter approach, the choice is between intermittent apnea versus jet ventilation.[217] The ETT used during laser surgery can affect the safety of the technique. All standard polyvinylchloride ETTs are flammable and can be ignited and vaporized by a laser beam. Although red rubber ETTs do not vaporize, they deflect the laser beam when wrapped with metallic tape. The metallic tape can only be applied along the stem of the tube down to the cuff. As a result, the laser may damage the tube below the vocal cords. Alternatively, nonlatex ETTs are manufactured specifically for use during laser surgery. Some have a double cuff to protect the airway in the event the outer cuff is damaged by the laser beam. Others have a special matte finish that is effective in deflecting the laser beam along its entire length. Nonreflective flexible metal ETTs and specifically wrapped ETTs are also specifically manufactured for use during laser surgery (Fig. 31-18). The outer diameters of these special tubes are considerably larger than the polyvinylchloride counterpart, especially in the small sizes. Thus they may not be appropriate for use in very small infants or children with a severely narrowed airway. Table 31-10

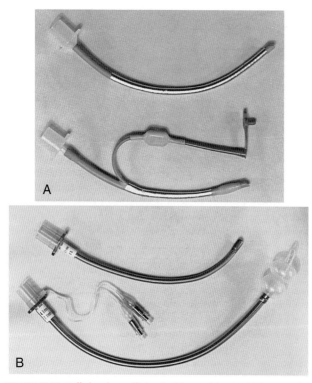

**FIGURE 31-18** Cuffed and uncuffed red rubber endotracheal tubes may be wrapped with reflective metallic tape for use during laser airway surgery. Note that this metallic tape is not approved by the Food and Drug Administration for this application. **A,** Cuffed and uncuffed commercially available foil-wrapped laser tubes are available (Laser-Shield II, Medtronic Xomed, Jacksonville, Fla.). **B,** An example of several commercially available stainless steel laser endotracheal tubes (V. Mueller Stainless Co., Chicago). Note that the external diameters of these devices are greater than those of standard endotracheal tubes.

presents a variety of such specialized tubes compared with standard ETTs. Although these ETTs offer some advantage, they are considerably more expensive than metallic-tape–wrapped red rubber ETTs. A syringe or a bag (500 or 1000 mL) of normal saline should be immediately available to douse ignited tissues in the event of an airway fire.

Once the airway is secured, one anesthetic approach is to use intermittent apnea with paralysis, TIVA, and topical lidocaine. An antisialagogue, such as glycopyrrolate, is often given at the beginning of the anesthesia, together with dexamethasone (0.5 mg/kg [maximum dose 10 to 20 mg]) to reduce mucosal swelling resulting from repeated intubations; this dose of dexamethasone however is empiric and not evidence based. Anesthesia is typically induced with oxygen and sevoflurane while the anesthesiologist gradually assists respiration as the depth of anesthesia increases. Once IV access is established, the anesthesia is deepened further and the larynx is anesthetized with topical lidocaine (3 to 4 mg/kg). The airway is then evaluated and tracheal intubation is performed. The ETT chosen is usually several sizes smaller than what is normally appropriate for the child's age, because most of these children have some degree of laryngeal scarring from repeated resections, and there is the need to prevent the ETT from obscuring the surgeon's view and interfering with access to the lesions.

Although the goal is to achieve the desired depth of anesthesia to secure the airway with the child still spontaneously breathing, partial obstruction is frequently encountered before an adequate depth of anesthesia for laryngoscopy is achieved. In these cases, thrusting the jaw forward and applying positive pressure in the anesthetic circuit will maintain an open airway in most situations (see Chapter 4). If complete obstruction is encountered, then a single IV bolus of propofol (2 to 3 mg/kg) or a short-acting muscle relaxant may be necessary for immediate laryngoscopy and intubation, or to allow the surgeon to perform rigid bronchoscopy.

Once the correct position of the ETT is confirmed, a neuromuscular blocking agent (e.g., rocuronium) can be administered and the TIVA technique with propofol (200 to 300 μg/kg/min) and fentanyl (2 to 3 μg/kg) or remifentanil infusion (0.1 to 0.25 μg/kg/min or more, as needed) is started. Muscle relaxation is desirable to produce an immobile surgical field. A neuromuscular blockade monitor should be used to assess the degree of relaxation.

**TABLE 31-10** External Diameter of Standard Plastic versus Endotracheal Tubes Used for Laser Surgery

| ID (mm) | EXTERNAL DIAMETER (mm) | | | | | | |
|---|---|---|---|---|---|---|---|
| | Standard ETT (uncuffed)* | Standard ETT (cuffed)* | Laser-Shield (cuffed)† | Laser-Flex (uncuffed)* | Laser-Flex (cuffed)* | Lasertubus (double cuffed)‡ | Red Rubber (cuffed without copper wrap) |
| 3.0 | 4.2 | 4.2 | | 5.2 | | | 4.7 |
| 3.5 | 4.9 | 4.9 | | 5.7 | | | 5.3 |
| 4.0 | 5.5 | 5.5 | 6.6 | 6.1 | | 6.0 | 6.0 |
| 4.5 | 6.2 | 6.2 | 7.3 | | 7.0 | | 6.7 |
| 5.0 | 6.8 | 6.8 | 8.0 | | 7.5 | 7.3 | 7.3 |
| 5.5 | 7.5 | 7.5 | 8.6 | | 7.9 | | 8.0 |
| 6.0 | 8.2 | 8.2 | 9.0 | | 8.5 | 8.7 | 8.7 |

*ETT,* Endotracheal tube; *ID,* internal diameter.
*Mallinckrodt, Inc., St Louis.
†Medtronic, Inc., Minneapolis.
‡Rüsch GmbH, Kernen, Germany.

An apneic anesthetic technique without an ETT offers the best unobstructed view of the larynx and avoids the presence of flammable material (e.g., the ETT) in the path of the laser beam. The child is positioned for suspension laryngoscopy with eyes protected with moist eye pads, and the otomicroscope and $CO_2$ laser equipment are aligned. The ETT is then removed and surgical resection is carried out during repeated periods of apnea. The need for reintubation is guided by the adequacy of oxygenation as reflected by the pulse oximeter. Reintubation can be readily performed by the surgeon by introducing the tracheal tube through the suspension laryngoscope under direct vision. After each reintubation, the lungs are ventilated manually to restore both the oxygen saturation and end-tidal $CO_2$ to baseline. When those baselines are reached and surgery can resume, the trachea is extubated. This process is repeated until the surgery is complete.[2]

A modification of the apneic technique that avoids tracheal intubation is the jet ventilator. The operating laryngoscope may be fitted with a catheter through which $O_2$ flows, entraining ambient air. In this manner, the lungs are intermittently inflated by the pressure delivered by the jet. The advantage of this technique is twofold. The surgical field is extremely quiet because large excursions of the diaphragm are eliminated and ventilation is uninterrupted. However, transtracheal jet ventilation carries a greater risk of pneumothorax in children than the transglottic approach.[217] In the past, tension pneumothorax and pneumomediastinum occurred because of excessive peak inspiratory pressures during jetting. Maximum peak inspiratory jet pressures of approximately 15 mm Hg have reduced this risk dramatically. In morbidly obese children and those with severe disease of the small airways, effective ventilation may be difficult with this technique, and an alternate approach should be used.[264] In addition, jet ventilation may theoretically distribute papilloma virus throughout the tracheobronchial tree, although this technique continues to be used.

When surgery is completed, the ETT is reinserted and secured until the child is completely awakened. Postoperative measures to prevent laryngeal edema, such as racemic epinephrine inhalation and/or the use of dexamethasone, are usually indicated.

### ASPIRATED FOREIGN BODIES

Curious young children can push many loose objects into almost any orifice in their body. Objects inserted in the nose or ear are usually benign in nature and simple to remove once the child is anesthetized. Small button-sized battery foreign bodies require urgent removal because of their potential for extensive local damage.[265] Impacted, or displaced objects present greater challenges for the anesthesiologist and endoscopist, and the danger of misplacement into the respiratory tract must always be considered.[266]

Tracheobronchial foreign-body aspiration is most common in toddlers 1 to 3 years of age. The majority (95%) of foreign bodies lodge in the right main-stem bronchus.[267] A history of choking while eating or playing, persistent cough, or wheezing that does not respond to medical treatment may be the only manifestations. If the foreign body completely obstructs a bronchus, or creates a ball-valve phenomenon, distal hyperinflation from air trapping may occur; a hyperinflated lung during the expiratory phase may be the only indication of an aspirated foreign body on chest radiography (Fig. 31-19). The more distal the object is lodged in the airway, the more atelectatic changes are noted.

Foreign bodies lodge in the trachea (less than 5% of airway foreign bodies) if they are too large to pass the carina.[268] The signs of a tracheal foreign body may include a brassy cough with or without abnormal voice, bidirectional stridor, or complete airway obstruction in the case of laryngeal foreign bodies. Any sharp object, or any object that causes acute UAO with cyanosis and an inability to maintain ventilation, requires emergent removal. Unroasted peanuts (with unsaturated double bonds in the oils) should be removed promptly, because the oil can cause an inflammatory response and subsequent pneumonitis (Fig. 31-20).[269] In contrast, roasted peanuts (with saturated double bonds in the oils) may be present in the lungs for greater periods without inducing as severe an inflammatory response. In addition, peanuts tend to swell, fragment, and crumble over time, making removal "en bloc" extremely difficult. The child who presents with a history of cyanosis after aspiration of a nut, very likely has aspirated material into the trachea or into the lungs bilaterally (as in the case of a broken nut or multiple nuts) and should be assessed emergently. It should be noted that esophageal foreign bodies may compress the trachea as well (Fig. 31-21).

The anesthetic management of these children depends on the level, degree, and duration of obstruction. A child who aspirates a foreign body while eating, or soon thereafter, presents with the additional risk of a full stomach. Waiting for the stomach to empty may not be appropriate or even effective in the acute situation. IV metoclopramide (0.15 mg/kg) may be used to hasten stomach emptying but does not guarantee that the stomach empties.[270] If time permits, the administration of an anticholinergic agent may be useful to reduce secretions. In the debate of how best to anesthetize a child with a full stomach and a compromised airway from an aspirated foreign body, concern for the airway takes precedence over the full stomach and an inhalational induction is recommended.

One of the major controversies in the anesthetic management of foreign body aspiration is whether to control ventilation or allow spontaneous respirations during bronchoscopy. Some endoscopists prefer a spontaneously breathing child, to prevent movement of the foreign body as it is being retrieved out of the airway. Sevoflurane is the preferred inhalational anesthetic in these children because it maintains spontaneous respirations, does not trigger upper airway reflex responses, and maintains hemodynamic stability.[271] Anesthesia is usually maintained with 100% oxygen and sevoflurane, or a propofol-based TIVA technique.[2] Halothane has some advantages over sevoflurane during maintenance because it is more soluble and more slowly eliminated, which allows more time to manipulate the airway without the child recovering from the anesthetic and reacting to the procedure. Alternatively, a propofol TIVA technique allows a steady level of anesthesia that is independent of ventilation and does not expose the OR personnel to waste anesthetic agents that inevitably egress from the airway around the bronchoscope. In some cases, a combined approach of sevoflurane in oxygen, as well as IV propofol, may be used. Often these children have very irritable airways because of the presence of the foreign body. The use of topical lidocaine (3 to 4 mg/kg) divided between the laryngeal structures and tracheal mucosa may be used to suppress airway reflexes and prevent coughing and bronchospasm.

## Tracheostomy

Tracheostomy in infants and children is usually performed electively, as a planned procedure after an airway has already been

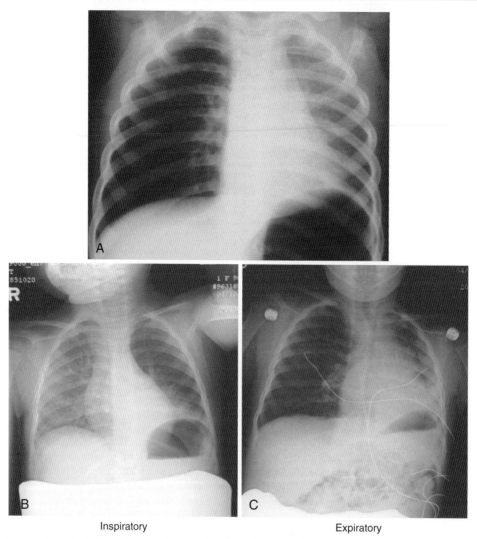

FIGURE 31-19 **A,** Expiratory radiograph of the chest demonstrates marked right-sided hyperinflation because of air trapping by the ball-valve effect of the foreign body. Chest radiograph may appear normal during inspiration after foreign body aspiration. A hyperinflated right lung (**B**) and a leftward mediastinal shift during expiration (**C**) suggest a foreign body in the right main-stem bronchus. (Radiographs courtesy Sjirk J. Westra, MD, Division of Pediatric Radiology, Massachusetts General Hospital.)

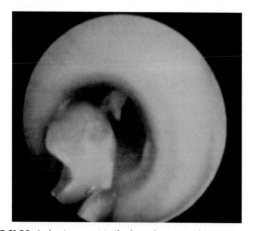

FIGURE 31-20 A classic peanut in the bronchus. Note the irritation caused by the oil of the peanut.

established with an ETT. Indications for a planned tracheostomy include lesions, such as congenital or acquired vocal cord paralysis, central hypoventilation syndrome (Ondine curse), craniofacial abnormalities (e.g., Pierre Robin malformation), persistent laryngotracheomalacia, and congenital or acquired subglottic stenosis (see Fig. 36-3). Usually these children have had a period of watchful waiting, with the hope of avoiding tracheostomy. However, persistent hypoxemia, hypercarbia, or intermittent obstruction that cannot be eliminated with the natural airway, or failed extubation will force the need to secure the airway via a tracheostomy. Children from intensive care sometimes require tracheostomy for long-term ventilation or secretion management. Still other children have acute deteriorations of the airway and require tracheostomy on an emergent basis.

In either case, the surgeon will frequently want to perform a thorough examination of the airway (i.e., diagnostic laryngoscopy and bronchoscopy) before proceeding with the tracheostomy. This requires that the tracheal tube be removed, the airway examined with a rigid bronchoscope, and then the child reintubated for the procedure. After the diagnostic laryngoscopy

Children whose airways cannot be intubated may undergo an "awake" tracheostomy with sedation and local anesthesia. Ketamine is an attractive alternative, but promotes secretions, which may further compromise an already marginal airway; an antisialagogue may reduce the secretions. Children who can be anesthetized with an inhalational agent administered by mask, but who cannot be intubated because of severe subglottic stenosis or inability to visualize the vocal cords by direct laryngoscopy, may have the airway maintained with spontaneous ventilation and a face mask or an LMA until a surgical airway is obtained.

Once the trachea has been entered, a portion of the delivered tidal volume is lost through the incision, and ventilation may become inadequate. This is less of a problem if spontaneous respirations are maintained at this point. It is prudent to leave the ETT within the lumen of the trachea but withdrawn just proximal to the tracheal incision, so that it can be readily advanced should difficulty be encountered with passing the tracheotomy tube. Once the tracheotomy tube is in place and ventilation is confirmed, the ETT is removed, the sterile distal end of the clean anesthesia circuit is attached to the tracheotomy tube (and the proximal end to the anesthesia machine), and the wound is closed. In the event of the tracheostomy tube becoming dislodged or removed, the tracheal incision will close and attempts at reinsertion may cause bleeding, the creation of a false passage, or trauma to the tracheal wall. The tracheal lumen is identified by internal traction sutures, which are placed by the surgeon at the end of the surgical procedure (E-Fig. 31-6). With the surgeon pulling up on the external ends of these sutures, the tracheal incision is identified and the tracheotomy is opened so that an artificial airway can be inserted. The child should not leave the OR without the potentially lifesaving sutures in place and their laterality (right vs. left) properly identified. Flexible fiberoptic bronchoscopy through the new tracheostomy tube can be performed to confirm appropriate location of the tip of the tracheostomy tube above the carina.

## Laryngotracheal Reconstruction

Glottic and subglottic stenosis, although rare, can be life threatening and difficult to manage, from both the surgeon's and anesthesiologist's points of view. Congenital laryngeal atresia and congenital laryngeal webs can be incompatible with life unless an emergent tracheostomy is performed at birth. When diagnosed antenatally, such an intervention can be undertaken before placental separation, described as an operation on placental support, or the ex-utero intrapartum treatment (EXIT) procedure (see Chapter 37). Treatment depends on the severity of laryngeal obstruction. In some instances, the defects are sufficiently severe to require immediate intubation or tracheostomy (see Fig. 36-2). Others may be discovered as an incidental finding while attempting to intubate the trachea for an unrelated surgical problem.[272,201] Most membranous defects can be broken down by passing a bronchoscope through the lumen or incised using a surgical knife or scissors. Thin anterior webs can be managed by microendoscopic incision with a microsurgical knife or CO$_2$ laser, staging the procedure for each side separately to avoid recurrence. The anesthetic management is similar to that for children undergoing laser excision of laryngeal papillomatosis.

Acquired subglottic stenosis is usually the result of prolonged tracheal intubation for respiratory support of infants born prematurely. In older children, it is often the result of laryngeal trauma. Symptoms usually relate to airway, voice, and feeding

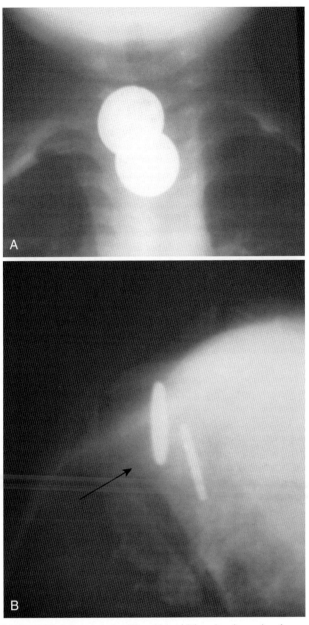

**FIGURE 31-21** Anteroposterior (**A**) and lateral (**B**) neck radiographs of a child who swallowed two coins. Note tracheal compression caused by these foreign bodies in the esophagus (*arrow*).

and bronchoscopy and reintubation, the child is positioned supine, with the head maximally extended over a shoulder roll, and the head taped to the end of the bed. It is a good practice to have a separate clean anesthesia circuit, or an extension, to hand to the surgeon to connect to the freshly inserted tracheostomy cannula.

Anesthesia is maintained with spontaneous respirations of inhalational agents so that, if there is airway compromise at any point, the child may still be able to maintain oxygenation. One hundred percent oxygen should be administered throughout the procedure, because the airway may be lost at any time. If, however, electrocautery is required, then fire prevention precautions should be taken. IV opioids or local anesthetic infiltration, or both, should be used to manage postoperative pain. A thrashing, crying child who is in pain will compromise the integrity of the newly established surgical airway.

and, in the case of a laryngeal insult, often occur 2 to 4 weeks later. Progressive respiratory difficulty with biphasic stridor, dyspnea, air hunger, and retractions are typical. These children usually have a tendency toward prolonged courses of URIs. Soft tissue radiographs of the neck and computed axial tomography will locate the exact site and length of the stenotic segment. Because both gastroesophageal and gastrolaryngopharyngeal reflux disease are thought to contribute to the development and exacerbation of subglottic stenosis, these conditions must be excluded, usually by a 24-hour esophageal pH probe placement. However, direct endoscopic visualization of the larynx is ultimately required to fully evaluate the stenosis. Rigid and flexible endoscopy of the airway and esophagus is performed in the OR. Because of the small diameter of the airway, the rigid rod-lens telescope and/or a flexible bronchoscope are used to visualize the larynx and trachea beyond the obstruction. The trachea is then intubated, and the degree of air leak around the tube helps establish the degree of stenosis (see Fig. 31-13; see also Fig. 36-3, *A*).

The surgical management of these infants must be individualized according to the degree of obstruction and the general condition of the child.[273] Most cases of moderate or severe subglottic stenosis require a tracheostomy at or below the third tracheal ring to establish a safe airway. The presence of a tracheostomy also helps to facilitate the airway management during subsequent procedures. For less severe cases, endoscopic dilation or $CO_2$-laser endoscopic scar excision may be sufficient.

The more severe cases of laryngeal stenosis require external reconstruction. Of the many available options, an anterior cricoid split operation and laryngotracheal reconstructions are more frequently used. The cricoid split operation is performed with the use of general endotracheal anesthesia. The largest possible tracheal tube is inserted through the nose. An incision is made through the cricoid, and the cartilage springs open. The ETT will be readily visible in the lumen. Frequently, the incision will be extended to include the upper two tracheal rings and even the lower third of the thyroid cartilage (Fig. 31-22). Stay sutures are placed on each side of the incised cricoid, and the skin is loosely approximated. The ETT is left in place for about 7 days to act as a splint while the mucosal swelling subsides and the split cricoid heals. Endoscopy is not usually required, but corticosteroids are administered before extubation.

Open reconstructive surgical techniques are done at the youngest age possible to help the development of speech and language skills. They basically combine the use of laryngeal and cricoid splits, cartilage grafts, and stenting.

For laryngotracheal reconstruction procedures, the infant is positioned with a roll under the shoulders and the head is extended. The tracheostomy cannula is replaced with an ETT that is introduced through the stoma to allow easy and secure access to the airway. A sterile, shortened, preformed oral RAE tube is ideal to allow secure fixation. The distal end is cut to an appropriate length to avoid bronchial intubation and then sutured to the skin of the neck. A costal cartilage graft is harvested and fashioned to fit the intended site of transplantation (anterior or posterior splits). Repair of laryngotracheal stenosis in almost all cases, except anterior subglottic stenosis, requires brief stenting to keep the graft in place and lend support to the reconstructed area. Stents will counteract scar contracture and provide a scaffold for epithelium to cover the lumen of the airway. Many types of stents have been used. T-tubes are popular in adults, but are associated with more complications and blockage in children. The lower end of the stent is sutured in place during surgery. The stent is eventually removed endoscopically, after cutting the sutures and retrieving the tube.

Single-stage laryngotracheal reconstruction is sometimes used in children without significant obstruction. A full-length nasotracheal tube is used to support the graft for 3 to 7 days, depending on the type of graft. The advantages of immediate decannulation, and possible avoidance of a tracheostomy altogether, make this approach appealing in appropriate candidates (Fig. 31-23).

The anesthetic challenges in these cases are many. The general condition of the child may not be perfect. Residual stigmata of prematurity are often present. The airway will be shared with the surgeon, and the tracheal tube that is placed in the stoma will need to be intermittently removed for surgical access and stent placement. A quiet surgical field is essential. The possibility of a pneumothorax during the cartilage graft harvesting should be kept in mind. The need to ensure that the stent, or the tracheal tube in case of a single-stage laryngotracheal reconstruction, is not dislodged in the ICU cannot be overstated. Accidental extubation cannot be allowed. A combination of sedation techniques and/or pharmacologic relaxation is necessary. The choice is often dictated by the individual policy in each ICU. Dexmedetomidine sedation may offer advantages as an alternative to propofol by providing a relatively rapid recovery from short-term sedation.[274]

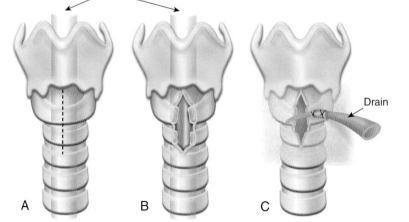

**FIGURE 31-22** Anterior cricoid split. After a midline laryngeal incision through cartilage and mucosa (**A**), the cricoid cartilage is decompressed and the endotracheal tube (*ETT*) is pictured in (**B**). The skin is loosely closed with a *drain* (**C**). (From Zalzal GH, Cotton RT. Glottic and subglottic stenosis. In Cummings CE, editor. Otolaryngology head & neck surgery. 4th ed. St Louis: Mosby; 2005.)

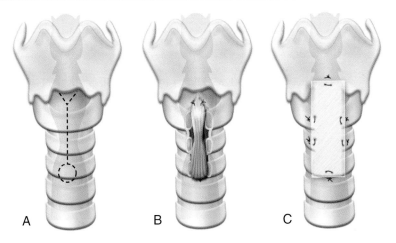

A                    B                    C

**FIGURE 31-23 A,** Laryngotracheal resection with anterior cartilage graft. **B,** After a midline incision into the thyroid cartilage, the intraluminal scar and lining mucosa are incised along the length of the stenotic segment (**C**). Costal cartilage is shaped into a modified boat and placed in position with the lining of the perichondrium facing internally. (From Zalzal GH, Cotton RT. Glottic and subglottic stenosis. In Cummings CE, editor. Otolaryngology head & neck surgery. 4th ed. St Louis: Mosby; 2005.)

## TRACHEOCUTANEOUS FISTULA

Approximately 12% of children who have had their tracheostomy removed will retain a tracheocutaneous fistula.[275] Surgical repair is generally required to remove the fistula track, followed by a primary closure of the defect.[276-278] In some, this may be accomplished with simple endoscopic cauterization.[279] Usually there is a preliminary endoscopic assessment of the stoma site, removal of residual granuloma, and then a determination of the best approach to closure.[280] A multilayered closure is commonly used to close the fistula,[281,282] whereas others recommend direct primary closure of the defect.[283] The anesthesia approach generally includes maintenance of spontaneous respirations, and methods to avoid coughing or straining at the time of extubation. The main concern is the potential for the development of subcutaneous emphysema caused by residual air leak if the child coughs or strains.[279,284-287] This complication may result in life-threatening pneumothorax or pneumomediastinum, which may occur up to 7 days following closure[280]; these complications require emergent removal of sutures, reestablishment of a tracheostomy, and thoracostomy and/or pericardial drainage.[288] Some children may require postoperative ventilation, but most are extubated and admitted for observation after extubation and conclusion of the surgery. The vast majority have an uneventful recovery.

## Airway Trauma

Nasal fractures are frequently seen in older children and adolescents. They may result from a direct hit (fight) or an accident.[289] Because the nasal mucosa is very vascular, a lot of blood is usually swallowed. A stomach full of blood is to be assumed for the first 24 to 48 hours after the injury. A rapid-sequence intubation is the safest approach during that period. However, closed reduction of a nasal fracture is often delayed for a few days to allow swelling to subside. At that time, gastroparesis has resolved and an LMA may be considered. These operations can be very brief. Frequently, the surgeon will leave a nasal pack in situ and apply an external splint over the nose. If a throat pack was not inserted, then the stomach should be suctioned to remove blood that may have accumulated during the surgery. At the conclusion of the surgery, the stomach and pharynx should be suctioned. The tracheal tube or LMA should be removed only when the child is awake, cooperative, and understands the need for mouth breathing; a combative,

semi-awake adolescent who is unable to breathe through the nose, can hurt himself or herself and others.

Closed or open injuries to the larynx and trachea in children can result from bicycle accidents, falls, direct trauma from sharp objects, and, rarely, a "clothesline" injury. The more cephalad cervical position of the pediatric larynx behind the mandibular arch and the pliability of the cricothyroid structures usually limit the extent of injury and prevent severe fractures.[289] However, the small size of the laryngotracheal airway and the potential for massive soft tissue swelling because of the loose attachment of the submucosal tissue to the perichondrium make early diagnosis and treatment critical. The injury can range from minor laryngeal hematoma to a severe form of laryngotracheal separation. This extreme and often fatal condition can occur after a clothesline mechanism of injury and is often associated with bilateral vocal cord paralysis resulting from recurrent laryngeal nerve damage.[290] Hoarseness, cough, dyspnea, hemoptysis, and voice changes suggest laryngeal damage. Clinical subcutaneous emphysema, pneumothorax, and pneumomediastinum signify definite disruption of the laryngotracheal complex. Computed tomography is the most appropriate imaging modality to identify the extent of laryngeal injury.[291]

Positive-pressure ventilation by mask, excessive coughing, or struggling can worsen the subcutaneous emphysema and cause the airway to further deteriorate. Administration of nitrous oxide, application of cricoid pressure, multiple vigorous attempts at laryngoscopy and intubation, and passage of blind nasotracheal tubes or nasogastric tubes should be avoided to prevent further trauma by creating a false passage through a mucosal tear. A good approach to this type of injury, if the child is stable, is to use the fiberoptic bronchoscope to visualize the airway before tracheal intubation. Ideally, the airway should be secured in the OR after induction of general anesthesia with an inhalational agent, and with the child breathing spontaneously. However, tracheostomy below the level of the injury, under local anesthesia or over a bronchoscope, may be necessary if there is extensive injury to the mouth and larynx that requires major reconstruction.

Postoperatively, these children require management in a monitored setting, usually the ICU. The resolution of other complications, such as subcutaneous emphysema, pneumothorax, or pneumomediastinum, will dictate the duration of the child's stay. Postoperative analgesia must be carefully titrated to balance the need for pain relief with the adequacy of ventilation.

**ACKNOWLEDGMENT**

The authors wish to acknowledge the prior contributions to this chapter by Lynne R. Ferrari, MD, Susan A. Vassallo, MD, Lucinda L Everett, Gennadiy Fuzaylov, and I. David Todres.

## ANNOTATED REFERENCES

Brown KA, Laferrière A, Lakheeram I, Moss IR. Recurrent hypoxemia in children is associated with increased analgesic sensitivity to opiates. Anesthesiology 2006;105:665-9.

*This study makes a clear case that younger children with OSA syndrome are at increased risk from opioid-induced respiratory depression; equal analgesia can be achieved with one half the usual opioid dose.*

Gross JB, Bachenberg KL, Benumof JL, et al. Practice guidelines for the perioperative management of patients with obstructive sleep apnea: a report by the American Society of Anesthesiologists Task Force on Perioperative Management of patients with obstructive sleep apnea. Anesthesiology 2006;104:1081-93.

*A practice guideline by a panel of experts discussing different levels of evidence for said guidelines.*

Marcus CL, Brooks LJ, Draper KA, et al. Diagnosis and management of childhood obstructive sleep apnea syndrome. Pediatrics 2012;130: 576-84.

*A comprehensive review from the American Academy of Pediatrics regarding assessment and management of children with OSA.*

Nixon GM, Kermack AS, Davis GM, et al. Planning adenotonsillectomy in children with obstructive sleep apnea: the role of overnight oximetry. Pediatrics 2004;113:e19-25.

*When a full sleep study in a sleep pathology laboratory is not possible, overnight oximetry can be a more practical approach.*

Nixon GM, Kermack AS, McGregor CD, et al. Sleep and breathing on the first night after adenotonsillectomy for obstructive sleep apnea. Pediatr Pulmonol 2005;39:332-8.

*At-risk children become more hypoxemic on the first night after tonsillectomy than they were preoperatively. This study makes a compelling case for in-hospital monitoring postoperatively.*

Schwengel DA, Sterni LM, Tunkel DE, Heitmilller ES. Perioperative management of children with obstructive sleep apnea. Anesth Analg 2009;109:60-75.

*A recent review of the pathophysiology, current treatment options, and recognized approaches to perioperative management of pediatric OSA patients.*

Verghese ST, Hannallah RS. Otolaryngological emergencies. Anesthesiol Clin North Am 2001;19:237-56.

*A comprehensive review of pediatric airway emergencies is presented.*

## REFERENCES

Please see www.expertconsult.com.

# Ophthalmology

R. GREY WEAVER, JR. AND JOSEPH R. TOBIN

THE INFANT OR CHILD presenting for elective ophthalmic surgery requires careful preanesthesia assessment. In addition to ophthalmologic issues, the infant or child may have associated or unassociated systemic disorders. In this chapter, we review some of the more important issues that should be addressed preoperatively and some of the difficulties that may be anticipated in the perioperative period for ophthalmologic procedures.

Many ophthalmologic diagnoses can be confirmed only by the ophthalmologist examining a cooperative infant or child. An examination under anesthesia (EUA) often is essential for an accurate diagnosis and evaluation of many processes, including trauma, tumors, infiltrative diseases, coloboma, glaucoma and other vascular diseases of the retina, Coats disease, and incontinentia pigmenti. Inpatient preterm infants often require serial EUAs to monitor the development and progress of retinopathy of prematurity (ROP) and the response of the disease to surgery. These examinations may be performed in the neonatal intensive care unit or operating room and may require sedation or general anesthesia.[1] Other inpatient trauma victims may require serial EUAs to monitor the development of glaucoma or retinal injury. Serial EUAs are also necessary to monitor progress during outpatient retinoblastoma radiation treatments. The anesthesiologist is essential to the provision of pediatric ophthalmologic diagnostic and therapeutic techniques.

Ophthalmologic procedures that require an absolutely immobile child for maximal safety include surgery in which the globe is open (e.g., cataract removal), vitrectomy, laser or cryotherapy for retinopathy, retinal detachment repair, anterior chamber paracentesis, and repair of an open globe injury. Other procedures may require a child to be cooperative only for a nonpainful examination, but because the target organs (orbits) are close to the airway, a strategy must be devised to ensure safe management of the airway.

The child in need of ophthalmologic surgery typically requires general anesthesia or deep sedation rather than exclusive use of local or regional anesthesia. Many infants and children cannot cooperate for anything beyond a brief eye examination. Although the ophthalmologist may be able to tolerate small movements by the child during an EUA, unnecessary head or eye globe movement during an ophthalmologic procedure should be prevented. Retrobulbar block is sometimes performed for postoperative analgesia in children before emergence from general anesthesia[2]; all complications associated with a retrobulbar block identified in adults may also occur in children.[3,4]

## Preoperative Evaluation

The perioperative environment should be welcoming to the child and family.[5,6] All team members should be comfortable with the anesthesia considerations for infants and children for ophthalmologic procedures.[6] Anticipation and prevention of postoperative nausea and vomiting (PONV) and understanding of anesthesia emergence and postoperative analgesia are essential.

Before an elective ophthalmologic procedure, the patient undergoes a thorough physical examination, including a review of all systems, and a complete medical history is obtained, including a surgical and anesthesia history, list of current medications, known allergies, and family history.[7] Because many ophthalmologic diagnoses are commonly associated with systemic conditions, all implications of the systemic illness are a concern for the anesthesiologist.

The physical examination should evaluate whether the ophthalmologic condition demands an alteration in airway management or affects the ability to obtain an appropriate mask fit. The airway should be carefully assessed for issues arising from other systemic conditions. Assessments of cardiorespiratory

**TABLE 32-1** Common Ophthalmologic Procedures in Children

Examination under anesthesia
Strabismus repair
Retinopathy of prematurity: laser or cryotherapy
Ptosis repair
Cataract excision with or without intraocular lens placement
Corneal transplantation
Evaluation of penetrating eye injuries
Dacryocystorhinotomy and dacryocystocele repair
Enucleation
Retro-orbital cellulitis decompression
Vitrectomy

**TABLE 32-2** Ophthalmologic Conditions Associated with Systemic Syndromes and Illnesses

| Syndrome or Illness | Ophthalmologic Conditions |
| --- | --- |
| Fetal alcohol syndrome | Strabismus, optic nerve hypoplasia |
| Galactosemia | Neonatal cataracts |
| Mucopolysaccharidoses | Corneal involvement; may require transplantation |
| Retinitis pigmentosa | Heart block |
| Sturge-Weber syndrome | Glaucoma |
| Prematurity | Retinopathy of prematurity, strabismus |
| Fabry disease | Whorled corneal opacities |
| Tay-Sachs disease | Cherry-red macular spot |
| Osteogenesis imperfecta | Blue sclerae |
| Craniofacial syndromes (e.g., Crouzon, Apert, Pfeiffer) | Proptosis, strabismus, glaucoma |

and neurologic systems are important in formulating the anesthesia plan.

## Common Ophthalmologic Diagnoses Requiring Surgery

Common pediatric diagnoses and surgical procedures are listed in Table 32-1. A diagnosis may exist in isolation or be one aspect of a more complex group of diagnoses. Many involve systemic illnesses, and the anesthesiologist should be familiar with the implications of ophthalmologic disease in these settings.

Some procedures and examinations can be performed without insertion of an artificial airway; however, communication with the ophthalmologist about requirements is essential in planning anesthesia. Other procedures may be performed very quickly and require only induction of anesthesia (often by mask in children) and then removal of the facemask from the nasal bridge to give the ophthalmologist full access to both orbits, eyelids, and nasolacrimal ducts. With experience and use of soft, inflatable-cushion facemasks, a close fit can be obtained to reduce environmental contamination with anesthetic gases and to maintain a suitable plane of anesthesia. The EUA may be brief or intermediate in length, and as information is generated, surgical correction may be contemplated during the same episode of anesthesia.

Communication and flexibility are mandatory in anesthesia planning. Anesthesia may start with a plan for a brief EUA using an inhalational anesthetic with a facemask and no intravenous catheter. However, if corrective surgery becomes necessary, airway control may require placement of a laryngeal mask airway (LMA) or tracheal tube. Intravenous access is required if the airway is instrumented to administer medications, including those to prevent or treat the oculocardiac reflex (OCR), postoperative pain, and nausea and vomiting.[8]

For procedures of brief or intermediate duration, the use of an LMA allows excellent access to all periorbital structures and provides good airway control in most circumstances. Compared with mask anesthesia, the LMA has the advantage of decreasing environmental contamination by inhalational anesthetics. It is relatively easy to insert and remains secure while avoiding the need for the anesthesiologist to hold a facemask near the surgical site. Compared with the tracheal tube, the LMA does not increase the heart rate, blood pressure, and intraocular pressure (IOP) to the same degree.[9]

Some of the more common ophthalmologic presentations and associated systemic illnesses or syndromes are listed in Table 32-2. Some systemic conditions have significant cardiorespiratory or central nervous system implications for perioperative management, and they should be fully evaluated before anesthesia (see Chapter 4). Many procedures are performed on preterm infants or formerly preterm infants, and prematurity and its complications have some of the most clinically important implications for anesthesia management.

## Ophthalmologic Conditions Associated with Systemic Disorders

### PREMATURITY

The preterm infant may present for many surgical procedures early in life. ROP, congenital cataracts, and glaucoma may require surgery even when the infant weighs less than 1000 g. The preterm infant may have significant systemic illnesses. Common complications of prematurity include acute and chronic pulmonary disease,[10] respiratory failure and pulmonary hypertension, congenital heart disease (unrepaired or with a limited palliative repair), and intraventricular hemorrhage,[11] with or without obstructive hydrocephalus.

Acutely ill preterm infants and those younger than 1 year of age are at greater risk than older children and adults for perioperative complications.[12] Careful attention to airway management, assisted ventilation, and titration of oxygen therapy with specified goals are essential for success.[13] In preterm infants whose airways are already intubated and whose lungs are ventilated mechanically, the anesthesiologist should confirm the position of the tube, transport the infant safely to the operating room, and limit the exposure to high concentrations of oxygen. Although institutional goals are not uniform regarding supplemental oxygen therapy,[14] communication with the neonatal team is often helpful in gauging the infant's previous oxygen requirement and current targeted goals (e.g., hemoglobin-oxygen saturation levels of 90% to 95%). Because most inhalational anesthetics impair hypoxic pulmonary vasoconstriction, a greater fraction of inspired oxygen ($FIO_2$) may be necessary to maintain the targeted hemoglobin saturation.

Hypercarbia and hypoxia may increase choroidal blood volume and increase IOP. Partial pressures of carbon dioxide ($PCO_2$) and oxygen ($PO_2$) should be controlled. Infants may be at greater risk for the OCR than older children and adults, and intravenous access should be obtained before the surgical procedure or any examination that may involve traction on the extraocular muscles or pressure on the globe.

Infants with extremely low birth weight require many weeks to grow and develop to a weight of approximately 1800 g and to maintain normothermia without special environmental control. These infants commonly have a history of short-term or intermediate-term assisted ventilation and may not require supplemental oxygen before an EUA or planned operative procedure for ROP.[15] Many of these infants undergo ophthalmologic examinations while their lungs are ventilated in the neonatal intensive care unit.[16] During surgical therapy (i.e., laser or cryosurgical stabilization) for ROP, these infants require anesthesia to provide optimal conditions (Fig. 32-1). Perioperative apnea may preclude

tracheal extubation or require close postoperative monitoring after anesthesia.

Perioperative apnea in the preterm infant is widely described.[17,18] Whether the child is still hospitalized or presenting for elective surgery as an outpatient, the preoperative assessment should determine the pattern and frequency of apnea before the planned surgical procedure and anesthesia. If the child has been discharged, the current use of respiratory stimulants (i.e., caffeine or theophylline) and oxygen should be determined. Is an apnea monitor being used, or has it been discontinued? Guidelines have not been developed to manage some of the scenarios, but infants who continue to require supplemental oxygen, who are younger than 60 weeks postconceptional age, or who are monitored for apnea or bradycardia should have continuous cardiorespiratory and oxygen saturation monitoring postoperatively for at least

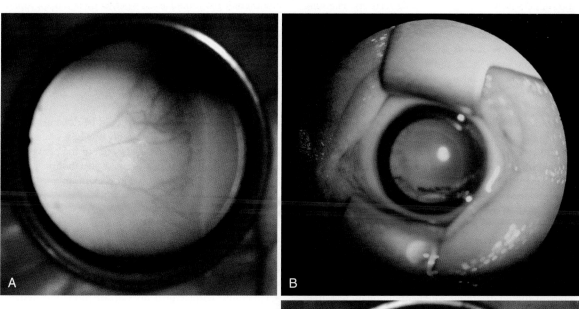

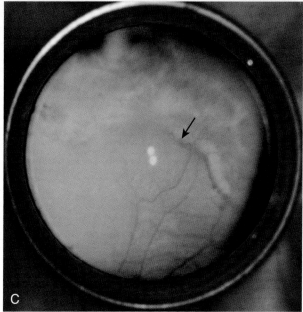

**FIGURE 32-1 A,** Grade III retinopathy of prematurity with neovascularization of the retina requires surgical therapy to halt the growth of vessels. **B,** Retinal detachment caused by retinopathy of prematurity. This degree of damage results in permanent visual impairment. **C,** Appearance after cryotherapy. Cryotherapy causes a well-demarcated ridge of tissue scarring (*arrow*) that prevents further growth of the neovasculature (*left to right in the middle*).

12 hours or until they are apnea free (see Chapter 4). The risk of apnea after general anesthesia and sedation decreases with advancing gestational age at birth and with advancing postnatal-postconceptual age. The risk of apnea is independent of opioid use; its multifactorial origins include the presence of general and neuraxial anesthetics and the immature central nervous system and respiratory center in the preterm infant. Flexible planning for possible postoperative ventilatory support is essential, and families should be informed of this possibility preoperatively.

The airway of the preterm infant who is younger than 52 to 60 weeks postconceptual age is usually intubated for ophthalmologic surgery (except for a very brief EUA) due to the immature respiratory drive, unpredictable respiratory response to anesthetic agents, and possible lag before recovery of respiratory drive after completion of the procedure and discontinuation of anesthetic agents. If the infant does not appear to have a stable respiratory drive and strength after anesthesia, assisted ventilation should be provided postoperatively and weaned during recovery. Planning for this contingency is vital. *Ophthalmologic procedures may be brief and have a low risk of blood loss, but the risks of general anesthesia mandate full postoperative support.* Intensive care resources for assisted ventilation in preterm and formerly preterm infants should be available before embarking on anesthesia.

Although chronic lung disease due to prematurity is prevalent, its intensity has been significantly reduced with the routine use of surfactant and advances in ventilator management strategies. Long-lasting respiratory effects from prematurity may include reactive airway disease, subglottic stenosis from prolonged intubation, and alveolar or interstitial disease with an oxygen requirement lasting weeks to years.[10] Because many anesthetics impair hypoxic pulmonary vasoconstriction, an increased oxygen requirement in the perioperative period should be anticipated. Tracheal intubation, a light level of anesthesia, or topical use of β-adrenergic antagonists may exacerbate reactive airway disease, requiring further treatment to reduce air trapping and hypercarbia.

Along with assessing for airway and alveolar diseases, the anesthesiologist should determine whether pulmonary hypertension or right ventricular dysfunction is or was present.[19] Some infants may be receiving continuing oxygen therapy as treatment for pulmonary hypertension and to reduce intermittent episodes of hypoxemia due to crying or while sleeping. If pulmonary hypertension was diagnosed previously, an updated evaluation is warranted. Because pulmonary hypertension is exacerbated by hypoxia and hypercarbia, tracheal intubation should be considered to ensure control of ventilation and oxygenation. At emergence, pulmonary hypertension may be exacerbated as hypercapnia develops, causing physiologic or anatomic shunting with systemic hemoglobin-oxygen desaturation. Immediate and continued evaluation of the airway is imperative to rule out an independent respiratory contribution to the systemic hypoxia.

Congenital cardiac disease may be diagnosed in the preterm neonate, infant, or child who presents for ophthalmologic procedures. A patent ductus arteriosus may not close spontaneously or after administration of cyclooxygenase inhibitors. This may lead to persistent congestive failure, reduced pulmonary compliance, and complications of fluid management. Congenital cardiac anomalies require assessment before elective surgery. The various complex congenital cardiac lesions have a wide spectrum of interactions with multiple anesthetic agents.[20] Many cardiac conditions require surgery or palliation (e.g., systemic-to-pulmonary shunts) before elective ophthalmologic procedures.

Correction of congenital heart disease is limited by the difficulty of using cardiopulmonary bypass in infants weighing less than 2 kg. There may be an urgent need for ophthalmologic evaluation (e.g., congenital tumor, cataract, glaucoma) before repair of the congenital cardiac condition. Preoperative consultation with the infant's pediatric cardiologist can provide useful information on the infant's current ventricular function and the risk of dysrhythmias associated with cardiac defects. Medical management must be optimized before undertaking anesthesia and surgery.

Intraventricular hemorrhage is a major source of morbidity and mortality for preterm infants.[11] Obstructed hydrocephalus may occur and require cerebrospinal fluid diversion procedures to decompress the obstructed ventricular system and treat the associated increased intracranial pressure. Many of these infants require ophthalmologic surgery for repair of strabismus due to a neurologic insult. If a ventriculoperitoneal shunt is in place, its proper function should be determined by direct evaluation. The anesthesiologist should assess whether there is inappropriate macrocephaly or a bulging or tense fontanelle. Obstructed hydrocephalus may occur after the infant's discharge from hospital, even though a ventriculoperitoneal shunt was not required previously. The preoperative assessment should include the child's developmental and neurologic status at the time of surgery. Because intraventricular hemorrhage is associated with long-term morbidity, any history of seizures should be elicited, and the antiepileptic drugs being used should be documented.

Preterm and small infants rapidly lose heat when anesthetized. Prevention of hypothermia is essential in the perioperative environment. Hypothermia can decrease metabolism of most drugs and depresses respiratory drive in preterm infants (see Chapters 35 and 36).

## DOWN SYNDROME

Children with Down syndrome (i.e., trisomy 21) frequently present for ophthalmologic surgery because of associated pathologic processes such as neonatal cataracts, significant refractive errors (e.g., hypermetropia, astigmatism), strabismus, glaucoma, keratoconus, nasolacrimal duct obstruction, and nystagmus.[21-23] Infants with trisomy 21 should have an ophthalmologic evaluation in the neonatal period. If this requires an EUA, the anesthesiologist should be prepared for the extensive medical implications associated with trisomy 21.[24,25] Almost half of these infants are born with congenital heart disease, including septal defects, complete or partial atrioventricular canal, tetralogy of Fallot, transposition of the great arteries, and valvular insufficiency or stenosis. Any child with a left-to-right shunt may develop pulmonary hypertension, and children with trisomy 21 develop irreversible pulmonary hypertension at an earlier age. Bradycardia (25% to 60%) and hypotension (12% to 73%) have been reported during sevoflurane anesthesia in these children.[26,27] Complete understanding of the child's cardiac defects is essential to planning anesthesia (see Chapters 14, 16, and 21).

Airway abnormalities such as narrowed nasopharyngeal passages, macroglossia, pharyngeal hypotonia, and subglottic stenosis are frequently observed in children with trisomy 21. These abnormalities may contribute to development of chronic intermittent hypoxia, further exacerbating pulmonary hypertension, and these children should be expected to demonstrate exacerbations of airway obstruction and hypoxia after general anesthesia.[28]

Children with trisomy 21 have a wide spectrum of developmental delays. Cervical spine instability occurs, and occiput-C1 and C1-2 instabilities have been described.[29,30] Subluxation of the cervical spine has rarely been reported in these children during anesthesia. Nonetheless, the anesthesiologist and the surgeon should avoid extremes of neck flexion and extension and lateral rotation during head positioning for laryngoscopy and surgery. While the child is awake, the range of motion of the neck in flexion and extension should be assessed, along with complaints of numbness or tingling in the hands or feet in a particular position. Previous spine and neck investigations or operations should be reviewed. These infants and children may have ligamentous laxity of the cervical spine and other locations. No consensus exists for the radiologic workup of children who are asymptomatic for cervical disease, although many children have been evaluated radiologically before about 5 years of age.

Children with trisomy 21 may be born with congenital hypothyroidism, or it may develop at any time during their life span. They may develop junctional bradycardia during sevoflurane anesthesia.[31] The bradycardia may be associated with or result from occult hypothyroidism. If the child is found to have a goiter on examination or has symptoms consistent with hypothyroidism (i.e., prolonged jaundice, hypothermia, constipation, dry skin, macroglossia, or relative bradycardia), thyroid function studies should be obtained before anesthesia for an elective procedure.

## ALPORT SYNDROME

Alport syndrome (i.e., progressive hereditary nephritis) is one of the disorders in a group of familial oculorenal syndromes. This classification includes Lowe (oculocerebral) syndrome and familial renal-retinal dystrophy. Alport syndrome involves sensorineural hearing loss, progressive renal disease, and multiple ophthalmologic disorders, including cataracts, retinal detachment, and keratoconus.[32,33] Development of myopathy and renal failure constitutes the major anesthesia concern. If the patient has myopathy, it is prudent to avoid succinylcholine and the risk of a hyperkalemic response. Renal insufficiency may alter the choice of pharmacologic agents to very-short-acting agents or agents that are not renally excreted.

## MARFAN SYNDROME, EHLERS-DANLOS SYNDROME, AND HOMOCYSTINURIA

Marfan syndrome, Ehlers-Danlos syndrome, and homocystinuria are considered together only from the perspective of a general body phenotype. The metabolic and molecular causes of these syndromes are well described. They share problems with connective tissue development, possible joint laxity, and cardiovascular disorders.

Marfan syndrome is caused by a defect in the fibrillin 1 gene (*FBN1*), which affects elastic and nonelastic connective tissues. These children have an increased risk of retinal detachment, lens dislocation, glaucoma, and cataract formation (E-Fig. 32-1).[34] They may have significant pulmonary (scoliosis) and cardiovascular problems,[35] which may include aortic, mitral, or pulmonic valve insufficiency. Preoperative cardiovascular evaluation is indicated to determine the progression of cardiovascular abnormalities that inevitably occur. Blood pressure control is essential to prevent aortic dissection.

Homocystinuria has at least three forms and different inborn errors. Enzymatic deficiency of the metabolism of sulfur-containing amino acids causes the intermediate metabolite, homocysteine, to accumulate. These children suffer from cataracts, retinal degeneration, optic atrophy, glaucoma, and lens dislocation. The cardiovascular pathology includes coronary artery disease at a young age. Thromboembolic phenomena occur more frequently because the children may be hypercoagulable.[36] Nitrous oxide should be avoided because it inhibits methionine synthase, further limiting the conversion of homocysteine to methionine.

At least 10 forms of Ehlers-Danlos syndrome have been described. Not all forms express significant ocular pathology. From the anesthesiologist's perspective, positioning is important to avoid trauma to the skin because these children develop hemorrhages with minor trauma and experience delayed wound healing. A thorough preoperative assessment should be performed for cardiac lesions. Hypertension should be avoided to reduce the risk of rupturing an aneurysm. The duration of effect of local anesthetics in patients with class III Ehlers-Danlos syndrome may be less than that in normal patients, and contingency plans should be in place to address these possibilities, including retrobulbar block or general anesthesia.[37]

## MUCOPOLYSACCHARIDOSES

The mucopolysaccharidoses are a group of disorders with enzyme defects that result in incomplete degradation of glycosaminoglycans. These children have various degrees of cognitive dysfunction, macroglossia, airway obstruction, cervical spine instability, and systemic involvement with deposition of mucopolysaccharide material. This leads to cardiac and respiratory dysfunction, airway obstruction, corneal opacities, and glaucoma.

The systemic complications of these disorders are sufficiently severe that even well-planned anesthesia management for ophthalmologic procedures may cause death.[38] Airway management can be extremely difficult with poor mask fit, dynamic airway obstruction with narrowed passages, a floppy epiglottis, and difficulty visualizing the larynx.[39] Infiltrative material may be deposited in the laryngeal inlet and pretracheal tissues; an LMA is particularly useful in maintaining a patent airway. Tracheal intubation may require the use of advanced airway management techniques, and the anesthesiologist should have several plans for airway management (see Chapter 12). Cardiac evaluation should be considered before an elective procedure to assess ventricular function and arrhythmias. Intravenous access may be difficult due to subcutaneous deposition of mucopolysaccharides.

## CRANIOFACIAL SYNDROMES

Craniofacial syndromes may manifest as craniosynostosis or have only middle and lower facial structure involvement.[40] Apert and Crouzon syndromes are both disorders of craniofacial development, but syndactyly occurs only in the former (E-Fig. 32-2). They share the potential for many ocular disorders, including severe proptosis, and mask airway management may be difficult.[41] Other mutations of the fibroblast growth factor receptor 2 gene (*FGFR2*) cause Antley-Bixler and Pfeiffer syndromes. These children may develop chronic airway obstruction, and some have complete tracheal rings. Tracheal narrowing should be anticipated, and smaller tracheal tube sizes should be used.

Children with asymmetry of facial and mandibular bone growth may present with limited mouth opening. Children with Goldenhar syndrome (i.e., hemifacial microsomia), Treacher Collins syndrome, and Pierre Robin sequence can be expected to present a challenge to airway management (see Chapters 12 and 33).[42] Children with craniosynostosis have an increased risk of congenital heart disease, and a cardiac evaluation should be performed before anesthesia.[43] Neurologic morbidity and seizure disorders occur more frequently in this group of patients.

### PHAKOMATOSES

The phakomatoses are neurocutaneous syndromes with multiple ocular pathologic processes. These syndromes include neurofibromatosis,[44,45] encephalotrigeminal angiomatosis (i.e., Sturge-Weber syndrome),[46] tuberous sclerosis,[47,48] incontinentia pigmenti, and ataxia telangiectasia. Central nervous system involvement varies with each of these diseases. Patients may have developmental delay, seizures, and significant neurologic morbidity. Anticonvulsant drugs should be continued in the perioperative period. Electrolyte and hepatic function studies should be done, and plasma levels of antiepileptic agents should be evaluated preoperatively.

## Ophthalmologic Physiology

Two major considerations of ophthalmologic physiology are of great interest to the anesthesiologist. The first is the dynamics of aqueous humor production and transport and the effects on IOP. The second is the OCR that may occur during any surgical procedure around the orbit. Anesthetic agents affect the IOP. In a patient with a penetrating eye injury, any increase of IOP may be associated with extravasation of elements of the globe and irretrievable loss of vision.

### INTRAOCULAR PRESSURE

IOP is the pressure exerted by the internal components of the globe on the covering (i.e., sclera and conjunctiva). The normal IOP is 12 to 15 mm Hg. An IOP greater than 20 mm Hg is considered abnormal. Aqueous humor is a clear fluid that is secreted by the ciliary body and released into the anterior chamber of the globe. It traverses the anterior chamber and bathes the iris. It flows through the canal of Schlemm into the pores of Fontana and then drains into the episcleral veins (Fig. 32-2). The posterior chamber, which is larger than the anterior chamber, is composed of a gelatinous mix known as vitreous humor. The sclera and globe that encase the intraocular constituents are relatively noncompliant and are protected by the bony orbit. However, intraorbital masses may impinge on the globe and increase the relative IOP or alter the flow of aqueous humor, resulting in increased IOP. Any obstruction to the drainage of aqueous humor causes fluid to build up within the anterior chamber and increases IOP.[49] Increased central venous pressure (e.g., Trendelenburg position, coughing, Valsalva maneuver, straining, increased intrathoracic pressure) attenuates the drainage of aqueous humor from the eye. Arterial pressure does not directly effect changes in IOP. However, as arterial blood pressure increases beyond the normal range, approximately 30% of the increase in systolic blood pressure is reflected in IOP increases. Aqueous humor formation is described in the following equation:

$$IOP = K\left[(OP_{aq} - OP_{pl}) + P_c\right]$$

$K$ is the coefficient of outflow, $OP_{aq}$ is the osmotic pressure of aqueous humor, $OP_{pl}$ is the osmotic pressure of plasma, and $P_c$ is the capillary pressure. These variables allow calculation to intervene by increasing the plasma osmolality acutely with mannitol to lower the IOP. This increases the gradient of osmolality and draws water out of the aqueous humor, thereby reducing the IOP.

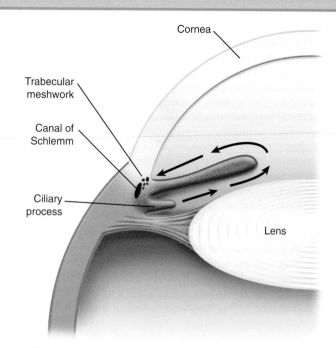

**FIGURE 32-2** Aqueous humor is synthesized in the ciliary process and then circulates around the iris, past the lens, and into the anterior chamber. After flowing through the trabecular meshwork, aqueous humor enters the canal of Schlemm (*arrows*), which drains into the episcleral venous system. Pathologic conditions that increase venous pressure, obstruct the canal of Schlemm, or increase aqueous humor production may increase intraocular pressure.

In the relatively noncompliant globe, any pharmacologic or metabolic process that increases choroidal blood volume (e.g., hypercapnia, coughing, increased central venous pressure) produces choroidal congestion and an increased IOP. Although well tolerated in the healthy eye, this congestion may lead to extrusion of contents if the globe is ruptured. The anesthesiologist should carefully control the child's physiology during the induction and maintenance of anesthesia to minimize increases in IOP, regardless of whether there is a preoperative concern about increased IOP.

Congenital or trauma-induced glaucoma requires therapy to reduce the IOP. If the IOP remains elevated, blood flow in the retina will be impaired, possibly leading to loss of vision. Unfortunately, there are many causes of glaucoma in childhood. Hypercarbia, hypoxia, and drugs known or suspected to increase IOP (e.g., succinylcholine, ketamine) should be avoided or used with care. Reducing a child's apprehension and crying and avoiding increases in central venous pressure are also important considerations.

The effect of succinylcholine on IOP is well documented.[50,51] Succinylcholine increases IOP 6 to 10 mm Hg, an effect that begins within 1 minute after administration and continues for up to 10 minutes, at which time the IOP returns to normal. This effect has been attributed to four possible mechanisms:

- Cycloplegia induced by succinylcholine, which obstructs the outflow of aqueous humor
- Tonic contraction of extraocular muscles
- Increased choroidal blood volume
- Relaxation of orbital muscles, which increases external pressure on the globe

Specific muscles develop a sustained tonic tension after succinylcholine that may in the presence of a ruptured globe cause extrusion of intraocular contents.[52] Extrusion in response to increased IOP depends on the diameter of the orifice; a smaller laceration (<2 mm) is less likely to facilitate extrusion of intraocular contents than a larger laceration (>4 mm). Pretreatment with a nondepolarizing agent (one-tenth the usual intubating dose) and paralysis with succinylcholine are still advocated by some anesthesiologists to minimize the risk of aspiration when dealing with an open globe injury. Alternatively, rocuronium (1.2 mg/kg given intravenously) can provide optimal intubating conditions in 30 seconds for the child with an open globe injury while minimizing the risk for aspiration or succinylcholine-associated increases in IOP.

Most general anesthetics decrease IOP,[53] although ketamine has been shown to increase IOP in some studies and decrease it in others.[54-56] When intravenous access is unavailable or the cardiovascular status of the patient warrants the use of ketamine,

the child's overall safety takes precedence over the possible ramifications of ketamine on IOP.

Measurement of IOP is performed by applanation tonometry on the external surface of the globe. Tonometry is often performed along with the EUA during general anesthesia to avoid an overestimation of IOP in struggling, uncooperative infants or children. Borderline measurements must take into account the possibility of anesthetic agents temporarily reducing or increasing the IOP.

## OCULOCARDIAC REFLEX

First described in 1908, the OCR is as a consequence of ophthalmologic surgery and other conditions.[49] Traction on the extraocular muscles and levator (eyelid elevator) or external pressure applied to the globe triggers an afferent signal through the trigeminal nerve that activates parasympathetic output through the vagus nerve, resulting in many types of dysrhythmias (Fig. 32-3, *A*), which include sinus or junctional bradycardia,

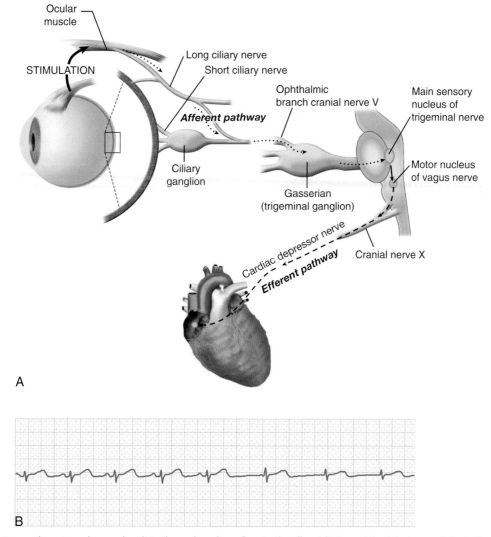

**FIGURE 32-3** Traction on the extraocular muscles elicits the oculocardiac reflex. **A,** The afferent limb consists of the long and short ciliary nerves, which synapse in the ciliary ganglion (*dotted arrows*). The ophthalmic division of the trigeminal nerve (cranial nerve V) carries the impulse to the gasserian ganglion, and the arc continues to the sensory nucleus of cranial nerve V in the brainstem. Fibers in the reticular formation synapse with the nucleus of the vagus nerve (cranial nerve X). Efferent fibers from the vagus nerve terminate in the heart (*dashed arrow*). The neurotransmitter from the vagus nerve to the sinoatrial node is acetylcholine, and the reflex is blocked by antimuscarinic pharmacologic agents (i.e., atropine and glycopyrrolate). **B,** Electrocardiogram shows conversion from normal sinus rhythm to a nodal rhythm.

atrioventricular block, ventricular ectopy, and asystole (see Fig. 32-3, *B*). Retrobulbar block with local anesthetic may precipitate the trigeminovagal (oculocardiac) reflex due to external pressure sensed on the globe, and the local anesthetic may not completely prevent the OCR response to further surgical stimulation or manipulation. For this reason, an anticholinergic medication, such as atropine (20 µg/kg) or glycopyrrolate (10 to 20 µg/kg), is routinely given intravenously at induction of anesthesia or early thereafter. Although these medications do not preclude the occurrence of bradycardia, both decrease its intensity and duration. Because anticholinergics cause pupillary dilatation, they do not present a problem for the ophthalmologist, but they may slightly increase the IOP.

If significant bradycardia occurs, the anesthesia team should have the surgeon release the extraocular muscle or stimulation in the surgical field. An additional intravenous dose of atropine (5 to 10 µg/kg) usually interrupts the reflex and corrects the situation, but it may recur. Intravenous epinephrine (1 to 10 µg/kg) is rarely necessary but should always be available. The anesthesiologist should ensure adequate oxygenation and ventilation because hypercarbia or hypoxia may compound or intensify the reflex activity.

Other strategies to attenuate the OCR include topically applied lidocaine[57] or intravenous ketamine.[58] In a four-armed study, a ketamine-based anesthetic (10 to 12 mg/kg/hr) was associated with a decreased incidence of OCR compared with the three other anesthetic regimens: propofol/alfentanil, sevoflurane/nitrous oxide, or halothane/nitrous oxide.[59] The prevalence of the OCR during sevoflurane and desflurane anesthesia was similar.[60]

## Ophthalmologic Pharmacotherapeutics and Systemic Implications

Topical ophthalmologic medications are usually placed directly on the cornea or in the inferior cul-de-sac. Most of these agents need many minutes to 1 hour for maximal effectiveness. Medications delivered topically to the eye are absorbed through the conjunctiva and nasal mucosa into the systemic circulation. When systemically absorbed, their pharmacologic mechanisms of action predict the systemic consequences. Some medications are diluted for use in children to reduce possible systemic toxicity. Anticholinergics, sympathomimetics, and antihistamines can cause pupillary dilation and decrease the movement of aqueous humor, increasing the IOP. Table 32-3 lists the more commonly used topical agents in pediatric ophthalmology.

Topical mydriatic agents are used to induce pupillary dilatation. The most common agent used is phenylephrine, an $\alpha_1$-adrenergic agonist. Phenylephrine (2.5% solution) is easily absorbed, and in small infants, it may cause significant hypertension. If hypertension is severe, reflex bradycardia may occur.

Topical cycloplegic agents dilate the pupil, and these drugs eliminate lens accommodation by paralyzing the ciliary muscle. This effect aids in retinal evaluation with the indirect ophthalmoscope and scleral depression and in evaluating refractive errors for which the child is using accommodation for compensation. These agents are muscarinic cholinergic antagonists (i.e., antimuscarinic agents). Cyclopentolate hydrochloride (0.5%) can cause central nervous system toxicity with disorientation, seizures, and blurred vision. Atropine (0.5% to 2.0%) and scopolamine (0.25%) solutions are used for cycloplegia and pupil

dilatation. Tropicamide (0.5% and 1.0%) is less commonly used in children. When systemically absorbed, these agents may result in antimuscarinic, anticholinergic toxicity, including tachycardia, dry mouth, pupillary dilation, flushing of the skin, heat intolerance or fever, and disorientation (E-Fig. 32-3).

β-Adrenergic blockers (e.g., timolol, betaxolol) are used to reduce IOP in the treatment of glaucoma. Systemic absorption causes symptoms of sympathetic nervous system blockade. β-Adrenergic antagonists induce bradycardia and cardiovascular collapse and may precipitate bronchospasm. If β-adrenergic intoxication is suspected, direct-acting cardiovascular stimulants (epinephrine) should be used to antagonize the β-adrenergic blockade rather than indirect-acting stimulants such as ephedrine.

Topical local anesthetics are infrequently used in children except for the very cooperative child for tonometry or removal of sutures. Proparacaine and tetracaine are available for topical use, and lidocaine and bupivacaine are used for retrobulbar blocks. Absorption of the esters (i.e., proparacaine and tetracaine) has little potential for systemic toxicity due to the extensive metabolism by cholinesterases. Ophthalmic amide agents, however, do have the potential for systemic toxicity (i.e., cardiac dysrhythmias and seizures) but are not frequently used in children. Topical cocaine is rarely used in pediatric ophthalmology except to test for Horner syndrome and as a vasoconstrictor to reduce nasal bleeding during nasal and nasolacrimal duct surgery.

Nonsteroidal antiinflammatory drugs (NSAIDs) are used for certain inflammatory conditions of the eye, but perioperative use in a child is uncommon. Some NSAIDs (i.e., ketorolac and ibuprofen) pose a concern for ophthalmology because their anticoagulant profiles may increase local perioperative bleeding. However, five NSAIDs are approved for ocular use: diclofenac, bromfenac, flurbiprofen, ketorolac, and nepafenac. Diclofenac, bromfenac, and nepafenac are used postoperatively for their antiinflammatory effects. Ketorolac has been used to treat macular edema after cataract extraction.

Echothiophate (i.e., phospholine iodide) is a cholinesterase inhibitor used to induce miosis in the treatment of glaucoma. When absorbed systemically, it impairs plasma cholinesterase, reducing the metabolism of some drugs (e.g., succinylcholine) and prolonging their duration of action. Decreased metabolism of acetylcholine may result in increased relative cholinergic tone, inducing bradycardia and bronchiolar muscle activity and resulting in bronchospasm. Toxicity from echothiophate may be antagonized by administration of pralidoxime (2-PAM) (25 mg/kg given intravenously). Otherwise, its action to reduce effective systemic cholinesterases lasts 4 to 6 weeks.

Pilocarpine, a direct-acting cholinergic agonist that is commonly used to treat glaucoma, has replaced echothiophate iodide. Through multiple actions, it improves the flow of aqueous humor. If absorbed, it may acutely cause bradycardia.

Many vitreal substitutes are used in ophthalmologic procedures. They include nonexpansile and expansile gases (e.g., sulfur hexafluoride), perfluorocarbon liquids, and silicone oils. The anesthesia team should be informed when the ophthalmologist plans intraocular use of one of these substances. If a gas pocket is anticipated, nitrous oxide should be discontinued or not used at all. When a perforated globe is closed, any residual environmental air pocket can be expanded by nitrous oxide. Increased ocular pressure and reduced retinal blood flow may result.

A novel agent being studied in the treatment of retinal angiogenic diseases is bevacizumab (Avastin), which inhibits the

**TABLE 32-3** Commonly Used Ophthalmologic Agents

| Drug | Indication | Side Effect Profile |
| --- | --- | --- |
| **Cholinergic Agonists** | | |
| Carbachol | Induce miosis | Corneal edema, retinal detachment |
| Pilocarpine | Glaucoma | Corneal edema, retinal detachment |
| **Cholinesterase Inhibitors** | | |
| Physostigmine | Glaucoma | Retinal detachment, miosis |
| Echothiophate | Glaucoma | Retinal detachment, miosis |
| **Muscarinic Antagonists** | | |
| Atropine | Cycloplegic retinoscopy | Photosensitivity, blurred vision, increased heart rate, dry mouth |
| Scopolamine | Cycloplegic retinoscopy | Photosensitivity, blurred vision, increased heart rate, dry mouth |
| Homatropine | Cycloplegic retinoscopy | Photosensitivity, blurred vision, increased heart rate, dry mouth |
| Cyclopentolate | Cycloplegic retinoscopy | Photosensitivity, blurred vision, increased heart rate, dry mouth |
| Tropicamide | Cycloplegic retinoscopy | Photosensitivity, blurred vision, increased heart rate, dry mouth |
| **Sympathomimetic Agents** | | |
| Dipivefrin | Glaucoma | Photosensitivity, hypersensitivity |
| Epinephrine | Glaucoma | Photosensitivity, hypersensitivity |
| Phenylephrine | Mydriasis | Photosensitivity, hypersensitivity |
| Apraclonidine | Glaucoma | Photosensitivity, hypersensitivity |
| Brimonidine | Glaucoma | Photosensitivity, hypersensitivity |
| Cocaine | Local anesthetic | Anisocoria, corneal injury, photosensitivity, hypersensitivity |
| Hydroxyamphetamine | Glaucoma | Anisocoria, photosensitivity, hypersensitivity |
| Naphazoline | Decongestant | Photosensitivity, hypersensitivity |
| Tetrahydrozoline | Decongestant | Photosensitivity, hypersensitivity |
| **α- and β-Adrenergic Antagonists** | | |
| Dapiprazole (α) | Reverse mydriasis | Conjunctival hyperemia |
| Betaxolol (β$_1$-selective) | Glaucoma | Bradycardia, hypotension |
| Carteolol (β) | Glaucoma | Decreased heart rate, blood pressure, bronchospasm |
| Levobunolol (β) | Glaucoma | Decreased heart rate, blood pressure, bronchospasm |
| Metipranolol (β) | Glaucoma | Decreased heart rate, blood pressure, bronchospasm |
| Timolol (β) | Glaucoma | Decreased heart rate, blood pressure, bronchospasm |

Modified from Brunton LL, Lazo, JS, Parker KL, editors. Goodman and Gilman's the pharmacological basis of therapeutics. 11th ed. New York: McGraw-Hill; 2006.

formation of new blood vessels.[61] In the doses prescribed, it should not be an anesthesia concern, but the visual outcome of any infant must be monitored for all perioperative care provided.

## EMERGENT, URGENT, AND ELECTIVE PROCEDURES

One of the greatest controversies in pediatric anesthesia is defining the optimal technique to induce anesthesia in a child with an open globe injury and a full stomach.[52] The issue of aspiration while securing the airway versus the possible extravasation of intraocular contents due to an increase in IOP is a difficult risk–benefit assessment. The debate is likely to continue because the risks are real and the incidence of either phenomenon is rare, difficult to study, and probably underreported.

Among adults, aspiration is an uncommon event with a small mortality rate. The incidence is less than 1 case of aspiration per 200,000 children, precluding an estimate of the mortality rate.[62-65] The rapid-acting, depolarizing muscle relaxant succinylcholine, when used for a rapid-sequence induction in the treatment of a perforated globe, has been challenged because of its known propensity to increase IOP. Development of rapid-acting,

nondepolarizing agents such as rocuronium has provided the anesthesiologist with alternatives to succinylcholine. High-dose rocuronium provides excellent intubating conditions[66] and has the advantage of reducing IOP by blocking the neuromuscular junction of extraocular muscles. However, if the child is not adequately anesthetized and fully paralyzed during instrumentation of the airway, any episode of coughing, retching, or increased systolic blood pressure may increase IOP. Lidocaine (1 to 2 mg/kg given intravenously) usually attenuates the hemodynamic responses to laryngoscopy and tracheal intubation, but this is not a consistent experience.[67,68] Pretreatment with opioids (0.05 to 0.15 µg/kg of sufentanil, 0.03 mg/kg of morphine, and 0.1 µg/kg of remifentanil) has been proposed to achieve a similar effect, although they are not consistently recommended. Although reported to blunt the IOP response to intubation, opioids may also induce vomiting, increasing the IOP.

Intravenous access is essential for a rapid induction of anesthesia. In most instances, children with ruptured globes present with intravenous access because intravenous antibiotics must be started as soon as possible (i.e., within 6 hours of the rupture) to prevent endophthalmitis, which untreated may result in complete loss of vision in that eye. In some instances, however, intravenous access has not been established. When intravenous access is not available, other options may be used to induce anesthesia:

- Placement of a central line
- Intramuscular ketamine (and succinylcholine or rocuronium)
- Mask induction with sevoflurane or halothane
- Placement of an intraosseous needle
- Rectal methohexital or ketamine

None of these alternatives is easy or ideal, and all have significant drawbacks and risks. Placement of a central line may be very challenging in a nonsedated or noncooperative child. Absorption of agents given intramuscularly varies greatly. Although succinylcholine can dependably induce paralysis in a few minutes, the child may cry from pain, develop hypertension, vomit, or experience direct succinylcholine-induced increases in IOP. The latency to action (possibly 2 to 8 minutes) and the gradually paralyzed airway reflexes in a child with a full stomach are clinically important risks.

An argument can be made for placement of an intraosseous needle for induction when intravenous access has not already been established. Even with local anesthesia, placement of an intraosseous needle is poorly tolerated by a conscious child. Mask induction with sevoflurane may facilitate induction of anesthesia, but if only a light plane of anesthesia is reached, coughing and vomiting may occur. The overpressure technique should be used to achieve a rapid and deep plane of anesthesia. Intravenous access should then be established. If this is unsuccessful, an intramuscular dose of muscle relaxant may be administered.[69-71] In this circumstance, IOP may increase, and regurgitation remains a possibility. Rectal methohexital (30 mg/kg) is used only in infants; and if the child evacuates part of the dose, induction is incomplete.[72] Because there is no reliable absorption of neuromuscular relaxant rectally, intramuscular or intravenous administration is necessary.

A moderate approach to the child who needs emergent or urgent ophthalmologic surgery is to secure intravenous access as quickly and painlessly as possible. An attempt is made to preoxygenate the child without causing distress. If a tight mask fit is not easily achieved, forcing the tight fit to the child's face is not desirable because of the likelihood of increasing the IOP as the child resists. Anesthesia should be induced intravenously with propofol and rocuronium. After 30 to 60 seconds by the clock or with train-of-four monitoring, tracheal intubation is performed as expeditiously as possible and the gastric contents evacuated as soon as feasible. The ophthalmologist should be intimately involved in the induction. He or she can physically protect the injured eye with a metal or plastic shield to prevent further injury and assist the anesthesiologist by holding the tracheal tube and suction apparatus immediately within reach of the field of view of the airway.

Other urgent procedures may include treatment of retinopathy or decompression of orbital cellulitis. These procedures may be urgent but still allow several hours of *nil per os* (NPO) status. Concern about aspiration may not be as great. Nonetheless, the surgeon will wish to proceed as expeditiously as is safe. Options for induction and maintenance may or may not include succinylcholine.

Most ophthalmologic procedures are performed on a scheduled basis, allowing routine preoperative evaluation and planning. This includes establishing all relevant medical information about the child, implementing NPO status, and placing an intravenous catheter if desired.

## INDUCTION AND MAINTENANCE OF ANESTHESIA

Intravenous or inhalational induction of anesthesia may be performed in infants and children for most elective ophthalmologic procedures. Most infants do not require a premedicant for anxiolysis, and the use of premedication after the first year of life is usually discussed between the anesthesiologist and the parents and child. Separation anxiety or struggling during induction usually does not affect most ophthalmologic diagnoses, except for a penetrating eye injury, which may become worse if the child struggles.

Intravenous propofol, etomidate, or ketamine produce a smooth induction, and the anesthesiologist can then support and secure the airway as planned. Inhalational induction with oxygen, nitrous oxide, and sevoflurane or halothane also produces smooth induction states. If laryngospasm develops during induction, an intravenous or intramuscular neuromuscular relaxant or intravenous propofol (1 to 2 mg/kg given intravenously) should be administered promptly. Atropine (20 μg/kg) should be given intravenously or intramuscularly before bradycardia occurs. For planned tracheal intubation, an intravenous nondepolarizing muscle relaxant is preferred because succinylcholine may raise the IOP. Intramuscular administration of succinylcholine or rocuronium may also break laryngospasm if an intravenous catheter has not been placed.[64-71,73-75]

Alternative induction methods include intramuscular administration of ketamine (4 to 10 mg/kg) and, in infants, rectal methohexital (25 to 30 mg/kg). Ketamine may increase IOP, but it has been successfully used in ophthalmologic procedures in children.[58] Rectal methohexital has a dependable latency to induction of general anesthesia of 7 to 8 minutes, but its elimination can vary widely, and its respiratory depressant effects may linger. Currently, rectal methohexital is infrequently used.

Tracheal intubation is our preference for most pediatric ophthalmologic procedures, except for a rapid EUA or nasolacrimal duct probing. With the tracheal tube secured, the child and operating table may be safely turned 90 or 180 degrees for optimal positioning of the table and child for surgery.

An immobile child may be essential to ensure the optimal surgical outcome. If the surgeon requires immobility, a tracheal tube should be placed and neuromuscular relaxants administered for as long as is required to complete the procedure. A cuffed or uncuffed tracheal tube may be used. If the uncuffed tube has too large a leak, we do not hesitate to change to a larger uncuffed tube or replace the first tube with a cuffed tube to seal the airway. The tracheal tube is secured so that the sterile surgical field is maintained during the procedure. Access to the tracheal tube and anesthesia circuit by the anesthesia care team without trespass of the surgical field is imperative. Extensions to the anesthetic circuit have no bearing on the dead space of the breathing circuit, whereas extensions between the Y connector in the circuit and the patient (i.e., adjacent to the tracheal tube) adds dead space that may increase $PCO_2$.

Anesthesia can be maintained with a variety of techniques. Inhalational sevoflurane, isoflurane, or desflurane may provide excellent conditions for maintenance of anesthesia[60] and rapid emergence. Emergence from halothane anesthesia is slower. We communicate with the ophthalmologist and reinforce the need for an absolutely immobile field. When neuromuscular blockade is necessary, we routinely use nondepolarizing neuromuscular relaxants and train-of-four monitoring to ensure the adequacy of surgical conditions. Carefully titrated doses of opioids are used as an anesthetic adjunct if postoperative pain is anticipated.

The anesthetic and type of surgery affect the incidence of PONV. Strabismus surgery in children is associated with the greatest incidence (45% to 85%) of PONV.[76] The type of ventilation does not attenuate the incidence of PONV.[77] Fluid replacement has a significant effect on the risk of PONV. Avoiding opioids during strabismus surgery may also be effective.[78,79] Nonopioid analgesics such as acetaminophen,[80] diclofenac,[81] and ketorolac[78,79] may be used. If opioids are needed, short-acting medications are preferred: remifentanil, alfentanil, or fentanyl. Some evidence suggests that the more extraocular muscles that require surgery and specific muscles that require more traction (e.g., inferior oblique), the greater the incidence of PONV, although these data have not been firmly established.

A host of medications can significantly affect the risk of PONV.[82] Preoperative use of benzodiazepines,[83] avoidance of nitrous oxide,[84] and superhydration with balanced salt solutions[85]; using of propofol,[84,86] clonidine,[87] 5-HT$_3$ receptor antagonists,[88-92] dimenhydrinate,[93,94] metoclopramide,[92,95] or dexamethasone[96-100]; and delaying oral fluid ingestions after surgery[101] attenuate the incidence of PONV. With clonidine and 5-HT$_3$ receptor blockers, but not dexamethasone, there is a dose-response relationship with PONV.[87,88,96] Older antiemetics such as droperidol that have been very effective in attenuating the incidence of PONV[80,102-105] have fallen into disfavor because of their sedative side effects and concerns associated with prolonged QT intervals,[106] although the latter has not been a common problem in children.[107]

Anesthesiologists have adopted a multimodal approach to PONV in the case of strabismus surgery. A commonly used regimen includes premedication with oral midazolam, choice of anesthesia, superhydration with intravenous fluid, and the combination of 5-HT$_3$ receptor antagonists and dexamethasone. There is no evidence in children undergoing strabismus surgery that dosing 5-HT$_3$ receptor antagonists at the end of surgery provides better protection against PONV than earlier in the surgery.[108] However, dosing 5-HT$_3$ receptor antagonists during emergence in children with congenital prolonged QT interval increases the risk of adverse events.[109] There is a dichotomy of practice with respect to maintenance of anesthesia. Some avoid nitrous oxide, maintaining anesthesia by propofol infusion and including the previously mentioned supplementary medications. Others use nitrous oxide and an inhalational anesthetic for maintenance but also include the remainder of the preoperative and intraoperative supplementary medications.

Intravenous fluid replacement can reduce PONV.[110] Children who present for elective surgery drink clear fluids up to 2 hours before surgery, reducing the fasting period. However, it is important to identify those who have fasted for a prolonged period and to administer sufficient intravenous fluids to reestablish euvolemia, avoiding the activation of antidiuretic hormone and aldosterone that may cause fluid retention. When using balanced salt solutions, children should receive 10 mL/kg/hr of the solution intravenously during the first 4 hours of surgery and recovery to reestablish euvolemia and to avoid activation of the antidiuretic hormone and aldosterone pathways. This should be followed postoperatively by a maintenance intravenous fluid infusion rate

at one half of the previously considered rate, using 2 mL/kg/hr for the first 10 kg, 1 mL/kg/hr for the next 10 kg, and 0.5 mL/kg/hr for every kilogram greater than 20 kg until the child takes fluids by mouth.[111-113] The incidence of PONV is reduced when large volumes of balanced salt solution (20 to 30 mL/kg) are administered compared with smaller volumes (10 mL/kg).[85] When the surgical procedure is not likely to involve an increased IOP, we routinely replace almost 100% of the calculated deficit. We have not observed children to experience urinary retention or hypertension from this strategy. However, if the duration of surgery exceeds 3 hours, then we catheterize the bladder to reduce the risk of urinary retention and overdistention of the bladder.

At the completion of surgery, neuromuscular relaxation is antagonized, maintenance agents are discontinued, and the child is allowed to awaken. Deep extubation is preferred by some to reduce coughing and increases in IOP at the time of extubation.[114] Others prefer extubating the trachea when the child is fully awake with intact airway reflexes, although coughing and increases in IOP may occur. For most procedures in children, a short interval of increased IOP does not damage a surgical correction, such as strabismus, ptosis, or ROP treatment. Appropriate postoperative analgesics may include local anesthetics, acetaminophen, and opioids. Nonsteroidal agents usually are not given to these children due to concerns about perioperative bleeding at the surgical site because of their mild anticoagulant profile, but ketorolac has been useful.[78] Lorazepam may also have some utility.[83] Postoperatively, withholding oral fluids until the child expresses a desire to drink reduces the incidence of PONV.[101]

## Specific Ophthalmologic Procedures

Strabismus repair is common in children.[91] Corrective surgery realigns the divergent visual axes of the eyes by detaching and reattaching extraocular muscles to the globes (Fig. 32-4). The procedures may be brief if only one or two muscles are involved. In infants, inhalational or intravenous induction is performed, and neuromuscular blockade is provided with nondepolarizing neuromuscular relaxants. Strabismus may be an isolated finding in a child or a manifestation of other systemic diseases or syndromes.[115] The anesthesiologist should carefully review the birth history, history of prematurity, central nervous system disorders, syndrome identification, possible coexistent myopathy, and cardiovascular and respiratory history. He or she should also anticipate the OCR and pretreat with atropine or glycopyrrolate. PONV is common and may be reduced by multiple strategies (Table 32-4).

We avoid succinylcholine for routine use in children in general, and in this circumstance, if succinylcholine is used, the

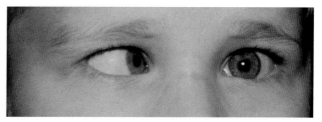

**FIGURE 32-4** Strabismus repair is a common pediatric ophthalmologic procedure. The child demonstrates significant right esotropia that requires surgical correction.

**TABLE 32-4** Antiemetic Strategies for Prophylaxis and Treatment of Postoperative Nausea and Vomiting

| Strategy | Drug and Dose |
| --- | --- |
| Butyrophenone (dopamine antagonist) | Droperidol (10-70 µg/kg) |
| Serotonin (5HT$_3$ receptor antagonists) | Ondansetron (0.1 mg/kg)<br>Granisetron (10-40 µg/kg)<br>Dolasetron (0.35 mg/kg) |
| Propofol-based total intravenous anesthesia | Propofol (100-175 µg/kg/min) |
| Local anesthetic | Lidocaine local-topical and systemic (1-1.5 mg/kg) |
| Opioid-sparing analgesics or anesthetics | Retrobulbar block with bupivacaine |
| Other pharmacology | Dexamethasone (10-500 µg/kg); maximum, 8 mg<br>Dimenhydrinate (0.5-1 mg/kg)<br>Metoclopramide (0.15-0.25 mg/kg)<br>Benzodiazepines (e.g., lorazepam, midazolam) (10-100 µg/kg)<br>Avoid nitrous oxide (N$_2$O)<br>Avoid opioids<br>Use ketorolac (Toradol) (0.5 mg/kg PO, IV, IM), acetaminophen (30-40 mg/kg PR or 15 mg/kg IV), or diclofenac (1 mg/kg PR), or short-acting opioids (e.g., remifentanil, alfentanil, fentanyl) |
| Nonpharmacologic adjuvants | Intravenous hydration<br>Gastric decompression |

*IV,* Intravenous; *IM,* intramuscular; *PO,* per os (oral); *PR,* per rectum (suppository).

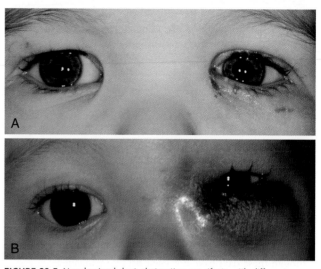

**FIGURE 32-5** Nasolacrimal duct obstruction manifests with different degrees of infraorbital inflammation, from mild obstruction with minor infection and mucoid material accumulation (**A**) to severe obstruction with periorbital or preseptal cellulitis (**B**). Both may require dacryocystorhinostomies.

surgeon should be informed because it may alter the forced duction testing and affect the planned repair.[116] After induction of anesthesia and tracheal intubation, the operating room table is rotated to permit complete access to the orbits. It is common to use a preformed tube that lies flat against the mandible.[117] The tracheal tube is positioned away from the surgical field. Ventilation may be spontaneous or controlled if the surgery is extraocular. If the surgery is intraocular or medical conditions dictate, controlled ventilation should be considered. Some anesthesiologists are willing to perform strabismus repair using an LMA with spontaneous ventilation.[118] Although regional block is performed in some adults, strabismus surgery in children is routinely performed with general anesthesia.

## ANTERIOR CHAMBER PARACENTESIS

An anterior chamber paracentesis may be performed in children for evaluation of uveitis, infection,[119] or leukemia[120] or for removal of fluid to decrease IOP. Because the field needs to be sterilized and the needle must enter a small target area of the anterior chamber, the child should be placed under general anesthesia to make the field immobile for the surgeon.

## DACRYOCYSTORHINOSTOMY

Infants may be born with nasolacrimal duct stenosis (i.e., congenital dacryostenosis) (Fig. 32-5 and E-Fig 32-4). If conservative measures do not demonstrate improvement, the ophthalmologist may need to dilate the duct or pierce a hole in the intact

membrane using a metal probe.[121,122] These infants are induced with general anesthesia, and when the level of anesthesia is sufficient, the ophthalmologist completes the procedure in a few minutes. To confirm that the duct is patent, the ophthalmologist can touch the metal probe within the duct with a second probe that is inserted into the nostril. Alternatively, the ophthalmologist may inject fluorescein into the nasolacrimal duct and detect the fluorescein on a pipe cleaner in the nasal airway. In both instances, fluorescein or blood may reach the larynx and trigger breath holding or laryngospasm. To avoid this, it is prudent to tilt the operating table to a 5- to 10-degree Trendelenburg position and place a small roll under the child's shoulders to pool the fluids away from the larynx. These secretions are suctioned out of the oropharynx and nasopharynx before emergence. Anesthesia may be maintained by facemask inhalation or with intravenous agents. The airway and respirations are carefully monitored visually and by capnography. The infant is awakened, and postoperative analgesia may be offered with acetaminophen or opioids, or both, as necessary.

Alternatively, an endonasal endoscopic approach may be used for complicated or recurrent dacryorhinocystotomy.[123,124] This makes the procedure significantly longer, and it requires airway control to facilitate the surgeon's approach and to protect the child from aspirating blood during the procedure.

## PTOSIS REPAIR

*Ptosis* (i.e., blepharoptosis) means "drooping of the eyelid." This condition can be congenital or acquired, and it may be associated with amblyopia or astigmatism. If eyelid closure is complete in infancy, occlusion amblyopia will occur, and this may require urgent attention. Otherwise, surgery for ptosis is often performed in later childhood. The surgical approaches require a quiet surgical field, and the surgeon makes a great effort to produce a symmetric repair.

## CATARACT SURGERY

Cataracts are opacifications of the lens of the eye (Fig. 32-6). Cataracts in children may be congenital, posttraumatic, or

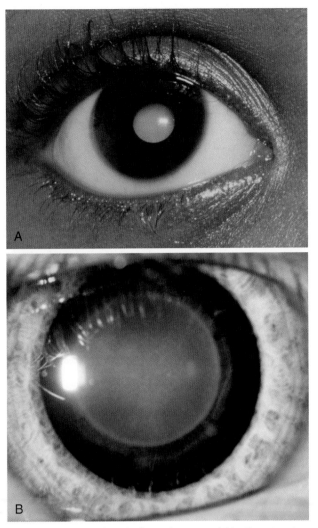

**FIGURE 32-6 A,** The right red reflex is absent in a child with a cataract that requires removal. **B,** The close-up photograph shows a nuclear cataract, which is associated with many inborn errors of metabolism in childhood. Cataracts that are not central or spherical may be caused by trauma or abuse.

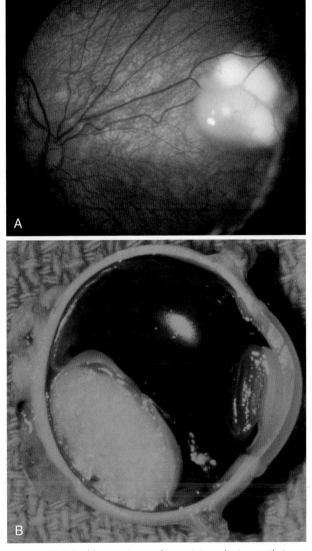

**FIGURE 32-7** Retinoblastoma is one of many intraocular tumors that may require enucleation. **A,** Retinoblastoma seen by direct ophthalmoscopy. **B,** Pathologic specimen of a retinoblastoma in the globe after enucleation.

metabolic in origin.[125] Congenital cataracts require surgery very early in life to permit photostimulation of the retina.[126] Although the surgery can be performed as an outpatient, the formerly premature and young infant may require monitoring for postoperative anesthetic-induced respiratory depression or apnea. Cataracts are associated with some systemic diseases, and intraocular lens implants are often offered to improve the long-term visual prognosis.[127] The child should be examined carefully for dysmorphology, with close attention to issues of airway management and the cardiorespiratory system.

### ENUCLEATION

Enucleation of the eye may be necessary when a child has an intraocular tumor (e.g., retinoblastoma) (Fig. 32-7),[128] a ruptured globe or ocular trauma,[129] recurrent or chronic infections, or a blind, painful eye. *Leukocoria* is the term meaning "white pupil." The differential diagnosis is extensive and includes many intraocular tumors. Other disorders causing leukocoria include Coats disease, cataract, coloboma, and *Toxocara canis* infection.

When necessary, the entire globe must be removed, and all bleeding points are coagulated. The OCR may occur during this procedure and may be attenuated by infiltration with a local anesthetic. Prophylactic antiemetics are often administered after enucleation surgery because PONV is common.

### VITRECTOMY

Vitrectomy may be necessary for retinal injury or detachment induced in circumstances of nonaccidental trauma or ROP.[130] Any infant or child presenting acutely with a closed head injury from suspected abuse should have an ophthalmologic consultation to completely evaluate all orbital structures.[131] These delicate tissues may demonstrate pathology that requires long-term follow-up or urgent medical or surgical therapy. Glaucoma may occur with hyphema or lens subluxation or dislocation with tearing of the support tissue. Early diagnosis is paramount if surgical intervention is to have the greatest benefit.

## RETINOPATHY OF PREMATURITY TREATMENT

Preterm infants may present with multiple ocular pathologic conditions, but none is more common than ROP. It has been extensively studied,[15] and multiple collaborative trials have reported their results and recommendations for medical and surgical intervention.[132-136] The cause is unknown, but oxygen-related theories have been described for more than 40 years. Because of this concern, oxygen range targeting has become common[137-139] to reduce the oxidative stress[140] on the infant in general and to reduce the effect of oxygen on neovascularization in the eye.

Laser and cryotherapy are common treatments for this condition.[132,133] Because of the delicacy and exacting accuracy required in laser procedures, we routinely intubate the trachea and use neuromuscular relaxants. This facilitates the immobile field necessary for the surgeon, and it provides better perioperative physiologic stability for the infant.[141] The complications of prematurity determine whether extubation is possible, and many infants require postoperative ventilation, if only for a brief period or overnight. The operative environment should be kept warm to reduce thermal stress on the infant.

## ACKNOWLEDGMENT

We wish to acknowledge the prior contributions to this chapter of Susan A. Vassallo, MD, and Lynne R. Ferrari, MD.

## ANNOTATED REFERENCES

Borland LM, Colligan J, Brandom BW. Frequency of anesthesia-related complications in children with Down syndrome under general anesthesia for noncardiac procedures. Pediatr Anaesth 2004;14:733-8.

*Children with Down syndrome have multiple systemic conditions of importance to the anesthesiologist. They are not exclusively of interest due to congenital heart disease. Anesthesia-related complications occur more frequently in children with Down syndrome than other children presenting for noncardiac surgery, and prevention of complications is essential by means of thorough evaluation and planning.*

Cunningham AJ, Barry P. Intraocular pressure–physiology and implications for anaesthetic management. Can Anaesth Soc J 1986;33: 195-208.

*This review elegantly details the physiology of intraocular pressure and conditions that may increase it. Structural, physiologic, and pharmacologic considerations are reviewed in detail.*

Donahue SP. Clinical practice. Pediatric strabismus. N Engl J Med 2007;356:1040-7.

*Strabismus is a common presenting condition requiring surgical therapy in children. Significant improvements in the detection and treatment of strabismus are reviewed. Surgical approaches and recent advances are presented.*

Saugstad OD, Aune D. In search of the optimal oxygen saturation for extremely low birthweight infants: a systematic review and metaanalysis. Neonatology 2011;100:1-8.

*Advances in neonatology continue to reduce morbidity and mortality for these fragile children. Oxygen-saturation targeting is becoming a mainstream technique. This has implications for the management and oxygen support strategies for infants coming to the operating room for ocular and other surgical procedures. Because volatile anesthetics impair hypoxic pulmonary vasoconstriction, a supplemental oxygen requirement should be anticipated, but oxygen-saturation targets should be considered for optimal care.*

Stephen E, Dickson J, Kindley AD, et al. Surveillance of vision and ocular disorders in children with Down syndrome. Dev Med Child Neurol 2007;49:513-5.

*Children with Down syndrome have many different ocular disorders. Along with the multiple systemic issues of concern for the anesthesiologist described in the chapter, this reference provides insight into the ocular diseases that may require surgical therapy.*

## REFERENCES

Please see www.expertconsult.com.

# Plastic and Reconstructive Surgery

## 33

THOMAS ENGELHARDT, MARK W. CRAWFORD, RAJEEV SUBRAMANYAM,
AND JERROLD LERMAN

PEDIATRIC PLASTIC SURGERY is performed in children of all ages, even in utero.[1] However, the majority of children who undergo plastic surgical and reconstructive procedures are between 2 and 9 years of age, with a median age of 5 years.[2] A wide spectrum of associated craniofacial abnormalities, underlying medical conditions, and surgical procedures characterize this pediatric population. Consequently, a thorough preoperative assessment, consultation with medical and surgical teams, and anticipation and preparation for potential complications are of paramount importance to ensure a successful perioperative outcome. The incidence of major morbidity and mortality has been reduced over the last 30 years from 16.5% and 1.6% to less than 0.1% and 0.1%, respectively, in children undergoing major craniofacial surgeries.[3]

## Cleft Lip and Palate

Cleft lip and palate are among the more common congenital malformations, occurring with an estimated incidence of approximately 1 in 700 births worldwide.[4] More common in males than in females, this malformation likely results from both environmental and genetic causes. Parental occupation, in particular paternal farming, increases the risk of cleft lip or palate in the offspring, whereas the maternal occupation presents no additional risk.[5] Folate metabolism disturbances and increased maternal homocysteine levels also may be contributory.[6] Cleft lip with or without cleft palate has been linked to several loci on chromosomes 1, 2, 4, 6, 14, 17, and 19, suggesting a genetic basis for some of these anomalies.[7-9]

These disorders are associated with more than 400 syndromes; the more common syndromes are presented in Table 33-1. Cleft lip and palate begin as a defect in palatal growth in the first trimester of pregnancy. Fetal magnetic resonance imaging (MRI) provides a greater degree of resolution of defects in the posterior palate and lateral extent of cleft with greater diagnostic accuracy than ultrasound. MRI also enables early detection of potential syndromic conditions by providing a complete study of the fetal head and biometric development of the facial bones.[10]

Primary cleft lip repair is usually undertaken at approximately 3 months of age, whereas primary cleft palate repair occurs at 6 months. Surgery for lip or nose revision usually takes place in early childhood, and palatal revision and alveolar bone grafts occur at approximately 10 years of age. Rhinoplasty and maxillary osteotomy to complete the repair may take place at 17 to 20 years of age. Pharyngoplasty may be required for velopharyngeal incompetence secondary to anatomic or neurologic dysfunction to improve speech development and prevent nasal regurgitation during eating.

### ANESTHETIC CONSIDERATIONS

Surgical correction of cleft lip defect is usually performed at 3 months of age to allow sufficient time for maturation and associated abnormalities to become apparent. Preoperative assessment may reveal abnormalities such as mandibular hypoplasia in Pierre Robin sequence (Fig. 33-1 and E-Fig. 33-1) or restricted neck movement as in Klippel-Feil syndrome (E-Fig. 33-2).[4] *Pierre Robin sequence* is defined as the triad of micrognathia, glossoptosis (caudally displaced insertion of the tongue), and respiratory distress in the first 24 to 48 hours after birth. The presence of other anomalies might warrant additional clinical or laboratory investigations. Cleft lip repair usually involves minimal blood loss, so for children with hematocrit values greater than 30%, homologous blood donation is unnecessary. Type and screen of donated blood is usually sufficient for a hematocrit value less than 30%.[11]

The frequency of difficult airways in children with cleft lip and palate varies from 4.7% to 8.4%.[12-14] The incidence of difficult intubation in children with bilateral cleft is greater than that with unilateral cleft.[14] Furthermore, micrognathia is an independent predictor of a difficult airway. The incidence of difficult laryngoscopy is approximately 50% in children with micrognathia but only about 4% in those without. In infants and young children, micrognathia may be subtle and not always easily detected. However, the presence of microtia, particularly bilateral microtia, which has a 42% incidence of difficult intubation with bilateral compared with 2% with unilateral microtia, should

| **TABLE 33-1** Syndromes Commonly Associated with Cleft Lip and Palate |
| --- |
| Pierre Robin sequence |
| Down syndrome |
| Klippel-Feil syndrome |
| Treacher Collins syndrome |
| Velocardiofacial syndrome |
| Fetal alcohol syndrome |
| Nager syndrome |
| Goldenhar syndrome |

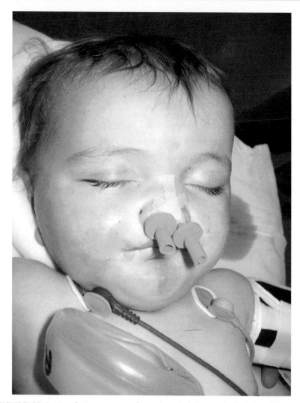

**FIGURE 33-2** Nasal airways are often placed at the end of cleft palate or pharyngoplasty surgery to ensure that a patent airway is maintained.

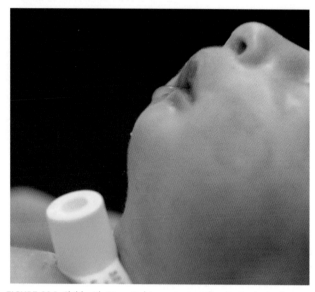

**FIGURE 33-1** Child with Pierre Robin sequence who required a tracheostomy because of respiratory distress in the first 24 hours postnatally. The retrognathia is often associated with glossoptosis, which makes visualization of the glottic aperture more difficult.

prompt a closer examination of the mandible for hypoplastic growth and raise the possibility of a hemifacial microsomia or Treacher Collins syndrome.[15] Intubation difficulty with isolated micrognathia decreases with increasing age, with the greatest difficulty presenting in infants younger than 6 months. Tracheal intubation becomes easier with age in isolated micrognathia. This has been attributed to rapid growth of the mandible, which catches up to the maxilla, thereby aligning the two bones, by 2 years of age in most cases. A careful review of previous anesthetic records may forewarn of a difficult airway. In our experience, tracheal intubation is not particularly difficult in most infants and children with cleft lip or palate, unless concomitant defects such as micrognathia are present.

Induction of anesthesia via facemask is usually uncomplicated in infants with cleft lip and palate. Laryngoscopy should be performed using a straight blade via a right paraglossal approach (blade inserted into the pharyngeal gutter with tongue displaced to the opposite side)[16] (or a left approach if a left-handed blade is available), taking care to avoid inserting the blade into the cleft (see also Fig. 12-28, *A-C*). If the mandible is hypoplastic, external laryngeal manipulation may be required to visualize the larynx. In some centers, the tongue is sutured to either the mandible or lower lip to preclude airway obstruction in infants with Pierre Robin sequence in the postnatal period. In such instances, the tongue cannot be displaced to the left to expose the larynx. To

facilitate laryngoscopy in such cases, the tongue is first released from the lower lip using ketamine sedation. Direct laryngoscopy follows. If direct laryngoscopy fails to expose the larynx, then alternative airway maneuvers such as fiberoptic intubation through a laryngeal mask airway (LMA) may be used after an inhalational induction of anesthesia and release of the tongue (see Chapter 12 and Fig. 12-22, *A-C*).

A variety of tracheal tubes can be used to secure the airway for cleft lip and palate surgery, although the ideal tracheal tube is perhaps the oral Ring-Adair-Elwyn (RAE) tube, which can be fixed centrally to the chin to facilitate optimal surgical access. Reinforced tracheal tubes are suitable alternatives, but in both cases care must be taken to fix the tube at the correct depth to avoid endobronchial intubation. Throat packs usually impinge on the surgical field and are not normally required for cleft palate repair. The lungs are ventilated for the duration of the procedure, usually 1 to 2 hours. Inhalational or intravenous anesthetics combined with a short-acting opioid such as fentanyl (1 to 2 μg/kg) can be used for maintenance of anesthesia. Bilateral infraorbital nerve blocks may be used to provide postoperative analgesia for cleft lip repairs (see Fig. 41-11, *A-C,* and Chapter 41 videos). Such blocks reduce the need for opioids and antiemetics, improve the ability to feed,[17] and increase parental satisfaction.[18] A combination of infraorbital and external nasal nerve blocks for pain control after cleft lip repair is an alternative.[19]

During cleft palate surgery, the pharyngeal space is reduced dramatically (Fig. 33-2 and E-Fig. 33-3). The trachea is extubated after the upper airway reflexes have returned and the child is completely awake. These children are at particular risk for acute upper airway obstruction in the immediate postextubation period as a result of upper airway narrowing, edema, blood, and residual anesthetic effects.[20-25] Accordingly, it is very important to extubate the trachea only when the child is completely awake. Late postoperative edema[26] and severe subcutaneous emphysema are additional complications. Upper respiratory tract infections are common in this age group, and if these infections are present, they should weigh heavily in favor of delaying surgery until they are resolved. Antibiotics may reduce the incidence of postoperative respiratory complications.[27]

A nasopharyngeal airway may be inserted by the surgeon before extubation to ensure a patent airway after extubation and permit suctioning the airway without damaging the palatal repair (see Fig. 33-2). Arm restraints are used in many centers to prevent suture disruption. These children are monitored for signs of upper airway obstruction during the recovery period for approximately 48 hours.[20] As soon as the child is awake, feeding with clear fluids is allowed. Postoperative pain is managed with a combination of opioids and acetaminophen. Sphenopalatine and infraorbital nerve blocks with a long-acting local anesthetic can be placed at the end of the procedure to prevent pain after cleft lip and palate repair.[17] Palatal nerve block (nasopalatine, greater and lesser palatine)[28] or a bilateral suprazygomatic maxillary nerve block reduce postoperative pain and favor early feeding.[29]

Children who are scheduled for elective pharyngoplasty are usually school age, having undergone cleft palate repair at an earlier age. The primary objective of this procedure is to restore velopharyngeal competence for speech development, which can be achieved by a pharyngeal flap, sphincter pharyngoplasty, or palatal lengthening (Furlow double-opposing Z-plasty palatoplasty). The anesthetic goals and management are similar to those discussed for cleft palate repair.

## Craniosynostosis

Craniosynostosis, a congenital anomaly in which one or more cranial sutures closes prematurely, occurs in approximately 1 in 2000 births, and affects males more frequently than females. Embryologically, the cranial vault starts to ossify at 8 weeks after conception. Fusion of the parietal and frontal bones is usually completed by 7 months after conception. Postnatally, the anterolateral fontanelle closes by 3 months, the posterior fontanelle by 3 to 6 months, the anterior fontanelle by 9 to 18 months, and the posterolateral fontanelle by 2 years. Premature osseous obliteration of a bony suture might result from the absence of osteoinhibitory signals from the suture. Craniosynostosis may be categorized as simple (or nonsyndromic) (65% to 80% of cases), involving closure of one suture, or complex (or syndromic) (20% to 30%), involving closure of two or more sutures and often associated with a variety of clinical features and metabolic diseases (Table 33-2).[30,31]

In the child with craniosynostosis, the head may assume various shapes depending on the sutures involved (Fig. 33-3 and E-Fig. 33-4). The frequency of single suture closures varies with the specific suture: sagittal (50%), coronal (20%), and metopic (10%).[30] The coronal suture is more commonly associated with syndromic craniosynostoses.

Although approximately 80% of premature suture closures are isolated defects, the remaining 20% involve multiple suture closures associated with more than 150 syndromes that present with a myriad of clinical features (see Table 33-2).[30] Apert syndrome occurs in approximately 1 in 100,000 live births, usually as a sporadic mutation, although autosomal dominant inheritance patterns can occur. This syndrome phenotypically manifests as cloverleaf skull (craniosynostosis), hypertelorism, proptosis,

| TABLE 33-2 Classification of Craniosynostosis |
| --- |
| **Nonsyndromic (primary) ~80%: Single suture closed, isolated finding** |
| **Syndromic ~20%: Two or more sutures closed, often with associated clinical findings. More than 150 syndromes have been described; the more common syndromes are as follows:** |
| Crouzon |
| Apert |
| Pfeiffer |
| Saethre-Chotzen |
| Carpenter (acrocephalopolysyndactyly type II) |
| Muenke |
| Crouzonodermoskeletal |
| Shprintzen-Goldberg |
| Loeys-Dietz |
| Jackson-Weiss |
| Beare-Stevenson |
| Cole-Carpenter |
| Kleeblattschädel |
| Fibroblast growth factor receptor mutations 1 and 2 |
| Metabolic and Other Causes |
| Rickets |
| Bone metabolic disorders (hypophosphatasia) |
| Achondroplasia |
| Prematurity |

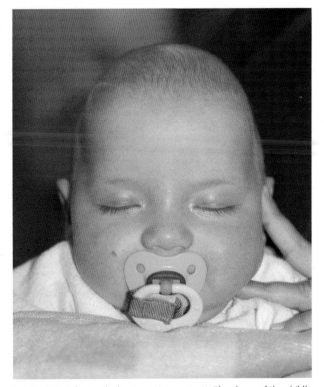

**FIGURE 33-3** Infant with classic craniosynostosis. The shape of the child's head may not reflect the severity of the defect. The defect is best appreciated by three-dimensional magnetic resonance imaging reconstruction.

midface hypoplasia, and syndactyly (upper or lower extremity). Development is often complicated by increased intracranial pressure (ICP) and obstructive sleep apnea (OSA).[32,33] Whether children with Apert syndrome develop normal intelligence quotients (IQs) is unclear. One study reported that 32% of children with Apert syndrome had IQs greater than 70.[34] Timing of cranial surgery may affect the child's IQ; surgery in the first year of life was associated with an IQ greater than 70 in more than 50% of children in one study, whereas surgery after the first year of life was associated with an IQ greater than 70 in only 7%. Two other factors predicted improved IQ indices: absence of a defect in the septum pellucidum and noninstitutional residence (i.e., family home residence). Crouzon syndrome is phenotypically similar to Apert syndrome but has different ophthalmologic defects, specifically, optic atrophy occurring in up to 20%, and the absence of digital involvement.[35] Fifty percent of Crouzon syndrome defects are sporadic mutations, and the remainder are familial. Pfeiffer syndrome occurs in approximately 1 in 25,000 live births. Most cases are familial with an autosomal dominant inheritance pattern, although many remain sporadic. The phenotype of Pfeiffer syndrome is similar to that of Apert syndrome but includes broad thumb, large first toe, and polydactyly. Children with Pfeiffer syndrome have normal intelligence. Carpenter syndrome is associated with craniosynostosis, syndactyly, cardiac defects, and obesity.[36] Cognitive impairment is common.[36] A relatively new but rare syndrome, Shprintzen-Goldberg, is characterized by craniosynostosis and a phenotype that resembles that of Marfan syndrome.

Indications for cranial vault reconstruction include increased ICP, severe exophthalmos, OSA, craniofacial deformity, and psychosocial reasons. If uncorrected, the deformed cranium may cause severe neurologic sequelae, including visual loss and developmental delay (see Chapter 23).[37-49] Because rapid brain growth during infancy determines skull shape, surgical correction is undertaken within the first months of life to achieve the best cosmetic results.

Cranial vault reconstruction may involve the anterior or posterior aspect of the skull or both (total cranial vault reconstruction). Less invasive approaches to correct craniosynostosis are available and may be associated with reduced morbidity. Surgical correction may employ an extended strip craniectomy in which the cranial vault is split in multiple segments, allowing the skull to grow with the brain (Fig. 33-4 and E-Fig. 33-5). This technique is used in children younger than 6 months of age and is believed to be less invasive than total cranial vault reconstruction, although children are required to wear a protective helmet after surgery.[50,51] Endoscopic strip craniectomy is increasingly being used in early infancy and has various benefits compared with the open procedures. Spring-assisted cranioplasty, a technique preferentially used in infants, involves performing a midline osteotomy along the fused sagittal suture and placing springs across the osteotomy to increase the biparietal dimension. Spring-assisted cranioplasty may be associated with reduced intraoperative blood loss, reduced transfusion requirement, and shorter duration of hospital stay.[52] In a single-center study of 100 children with spring-assisted craniosynostosis, no child was transfused and none was admitted to the intensive care unit.[53]

Preoperative assessment of children with craniosynostosis should focus on airway management, eye protection, and ICP. An important consideration in children with midfacial hypoplasia and large tonsils is the presence of OSA. OSA may be present in 50% to 70% of children with syndromic craniosynostosis.[33,54,55] Although some recommend preoperative adenotonsillectomy to treat OSA in children with craniosynostosis, neither airway dimensions nor airway collapse is improved. Midfacial advancement may be required to resolve OSA, and even then, residual airway obstruction may persist.[33,54] Preoperative endoscopy has been recommended to assess the severity of midfacial hypoplasia and whether OSA is likely to persist after midface advancement. Careful titration of opioids in the perioperative period is indicated if the child exhibits severe nocturnal desaturation (i.e., if the $SaO_2$ nadir is less than 85%) (see Chapter 31). Upper airway obstruction may also occur postoperatively in children who received opioids as a direct effect of opioids on the hypoglossal nucleus.[56]

Postoperative pain is generally not severe and is managed effectively with a combination of acetaminophen, nonsteroidal antiinflammatory drugs (NSAIDs), and intravenous opioids. Opioids remain the mainstay of pain management, but careful titration of reduced doses (approximately 50% less) must be considered if OSA is present. Given the small incidence of craniosynostosis and the large variability in the management of these patients, multicenter trials are required to determine the optimal management strategy for these children.[57]

## AIRWAY MANAGEMENT

Meticulous preoperative planning and evaluation of the airway is essential, particularly for OSA.[54] A facemask may prove to be a challenge to seal on their flat faces and the nasal passages may be obstructed, together creating a difficult mask ventilation.[58] External fixator devices on the face may also present challenges in managing the airway (E-Fig. 33-6).

Upper airway obstruction may readily occur during mask induction because of the narrowed nares, midfacial hypoplasia, pharyngeal collapse, and large tonsils. Subluxing the temporomandibular joint or inserting an oropharyngeal airway should resolve the obstruction and permit the inhalational induction to continue. In the majority of these children, the anatomy of the mandible and the temporomandibular joint is normal, as are upper airway dimensions, resulting in an easy laryngoscopy and tracheal intubation. Rarely, mandibular hypoplasia may complicate an otherwise straightforward laryngoscopy and tracheal intubation. Abnormal neck mobility also may pose additional challenges for laryngoscopy and tracheal intubation.

## BLOOD LOSS, COAGULOPATHY, AND HYPONATREMIA

Crystalloid solutions are commonly administered for minimal to moderate surgical blood loss and fluid shifts during craniosynostosis surgeries. Although lactated Ringer's solution is most commonly used in North America, some advocate using normal saline because it may be less likely to induce hyponatremia and an acid-base disturbance than lactated Ringer's solution. However, a recent study comparing the two solutions suggests that normal

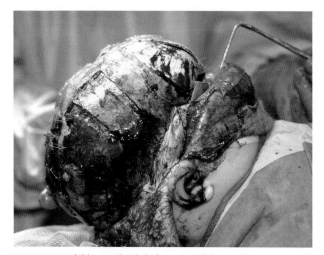

**FIGURE 33-4** Child immediately before surgical closure after total cranial vault reshaping using strip craniectomy for sagittal craniosynostosis.

saline is more likely to induce (metabolic) acidosis than lactated Ringer's solution in infants undergoing craniosynostosis.[59] The explanation for this finding has been elusive, but it has been attributed to hyperchloremia, a dilutional acidosis, or both.

Surgery for craniosynostosis is associated with an increased incidence of cardiac arrest as a result of sudden massive blood loss.[3,30,60,61] Although these procedures are extradural, significant blood loss from the scalp and cranium can occur. The blood loss can be so rapid during the surgery that the expression "trauma in progress" is applicable. The risk of massive blood loss and the need for invasive monitoring are determined in part by the specific suture involved, number of sutures scheduled for repair, type of surgery, and expertise of the surgeon.[61] In children undergoing endoscopic strip craniectomy, weight less than 5 kg, those undergoing sagittal endoscopic craniectomy, those with syndromic craniosynostosis, and earlier date of surgery in the series were associated with blood transfusion.[62] Some centers advocate commencing blood transfusions at the time of skin incision (particularly in infants) to prevent hemodynamic instability and the need for a rapid transfusion, but this must be tempered by whether the surgery is open or endoscopic (see later discussion).

To manage the large volume and rapidity of the blood loss, it is essential to establish large-bore peripheral venous access. Central venous access (see also Fig. 48-2), usually via the femoral route, can provide a useful estimate of the cardiac filling pressures but should not be used for rapid transfusion in small infants, because hyperkalemic cardiac arrests may occur with old blood infused rapidly into the right atrium and the lumens may limit the rate of blood infusion. Estimation of ongoing blood loss can be difficult because of the use of large volumes of irrigation fluid and blood loss onto surgical drapes and gowns.[63] Invasive arterial blood pressure (BP) monitoring and serial blood gas sampling are indicated in this type of surgery (see Fig. 48-10, *A-D*). A urinary catheter should be inserted to monitor urine output.

Several blood conservation strategies have been proposed for this type of surgery, including preoperative recombinant human erythropoietin, directed blood donation (from the parents or siblings), acute normovolemic hemodilution, antifibrinolytics, and induced hypotension (see Chapter 10 for a more detailed discussion). These strategies should be combined with meticulous surgical technique and attention to hemostasis. Furthermore, bleeding from the scalp incision may be reduced by infiltration with a dilute (1:400,000) epinephrine-containing solution. The use of the reverse Trendelenburg position may help to decrease venous pressure and blood loss from osteotomy sites but also increases the risk of venous air embolism (which has been reported to be 5% to 80%; see later discussion). For this reason, the horizontal position is preferred.

Blood-conserving dual therapy with recombinant human erythropoietin (to optimize preoperative hematocrit) and use of a cell saver reduces transfusion in children undergoing craniosynostosis repair.[64] Administration of preoperative recombinant human erythropoietin, in combination with elemental iron (6 mg/kg/day to a maximum of 200 mg/day for 6 weeks) increases the preoperative hematocrit value and decreases the need for autologous blood transfusion.[65,66] If iron stores are at all compromised, iron therapy combined with oral vitamin C (to increase gastrointestinal absorption) should begin 3 weeks before erythropoietin therapy.[67]

Little evidence exists to suggest that autologous or directed blood donation decreases perioperative morbidity in craniosynostosis surgery, although it will decrease the number of blood unit exposures.[68,69] Infants as young as 3 months have predonated, although the limited volume of predonated blood is unlikely to preclude all blood transfusions during craniosynostosis or repeat craniosynostosis surgery.[68,69]

Acute normovolemic hemodilution is a labor-intensive technique in which blood is collected from the child after induction of anesthesia but immediately before surgery and replaced with an equal volume of crystalloid or colloid, such as 5% albumin. Although acute normovolemic hemodilution may be beneficial in children with rare blood types, no evidence exists that it reduces either the incidence of homologous transfusion or the amount of homologous blood transfused in children undergoing craniosynostosis repair.[70]

The coagulation profile and clotting factors after fresh frozen plasma (FFP) or 5% albumin during craniofacial surgery have been compared in a nonrandomized study in infants younger than 12 months of age.[71] The increases in activated partial thromboplastin time (aPTT) and decreases in the plasma concentration of factors XI and XIII and antithrombin 3 were less after intraoperative FFP than after 5% albumin. Fibrinogen concentrations remained stable in the FFP-treated group but decreased in the albumin-treated group. However, it should be emphasized that no clinical indication exists to administer FFP when the blood loss is less than 1 blood volume (Chapter 10). Recombinant factor VIIa has been used successfully for intractable hemorrhage during cranial vault reconstruction in an infant, although this is an isolated report.[72]

Antifibrinolytic therapy may decrease blood loss during craniosynostosis repair in children. Tranexamic acid (TXA) is a widely used agent, and several dosing regimens have been described: (1) A loading dose of 15 mg/kg TXA after induction of anesthesia, followed by an infusion of 10 mg/kg/hr until skin closure[73]; (2) 50 mg/kg TXA loading dose, followed by an infusion of 5 mg/kg/hr[74] until skin closure; and (3) 15 mg/kg at induction of anesthesia, every 4 hours during surgery, and every 8 hours after surgery for 24 hours after surgery. Although dose-response data from a single study are lacking, two studies[73,74] report that TXA reduces intraoperative and postoperative bleeding and transfusion requirements.[75] Another antifibrinolytic, ε-aminocaproic acid (EACA), is effective in reducing bleeding in cardiac and spinal procedures, although its effectiveness in reducing blood loss during craniosynostosis has not been established. The dose that has been used for spinal surgery is 75 to 100 mg/kg loading dose intravenously over 15 to 20 minutes before skin incision, followed by 10 to 15 mg/kg/hr until skin closure.[76]

Induced hypotension defined as a 10% to 20% reduction in the mean arterial BP decreases intraoperative surgical blood loss and operating time,[77] although studies demonstrating its efficacy during craniosynostosis surgery are lacking. A variety of pharmacologic agents have been used to induce hypotension, including inhalational agents, vasodilators, β-blockers, and remifentanil.[77,78] Invasive arterial pressure monitoring is essential whenever hypotensive anesthesia is used. Induced hypotension should be used with caution in the presence of increased ICP because of the risk of compromising cerebral perfusion pressure (i.e., the difference between mean arterial pressure [MAP] and either ICP or central venous pressure, whichever is greater). Increases in ICP mandate invasive monitoring of MAP to ensure an adequate cerebral perfusion pressure. It is considered prudent to maintain normovolemia and normocapnia when induced hypotension is used (see Chapter 10 for a more detailed description of these techniques).

Whether used alone or in combination,[79-81] the preceding techniques seldom obviate the need for all blood transfusions during craniofacial surgery. Therefore intravenous access with large-bore catheters remains essential and at least 2 units of packed red blood cells (PRBCs) should be crossmatched and available in the operating room at all times. All intravenous fluids should be administered via a fluid warmer to prevent hypothermia. Maintaining normothermia preserves normal coagulation indices and theoretically reduces bleeding and transfusion-related complications.[82] A coagulopathy should always be anticipated once the blood loss exceeds 1 blood volume. Serial determinations of the international normalized ratio, partial thromboplastin time, platelet count, and fibrinogen concentration will identify an evolving coagulopathy and indicate which blood products, FFP, platelets, or cryoprecipitate, will best correct the abnormalities (see Chapter 10).

Endoscopic repair of craniosynostosis has become a rapidly growing surgical approach to reduce bleeding and decrease morbidity.[83,84] Independent risk factors for bleeding during endoscopic strip craniectomy include low body weight (<5 kg), sagittal suture surgery (related to proximity to the sagittal vein), syndromic craniosynostosis, and earlier date of surgery.[62]

Hyponatremia and cerebral salt wasting syndrome are associated with craniosynostosis repair.[85-89] Both intraoperative and postoperative hyponatremia have been described, with the latter occurring in approximately 30% of children. In a retrospective review of a cleft palate and craniofacial database, postoperative hyponatremia was significantly associated with preoperative increased ICP, blood loss, and female gender with normal preoperative ICP.[89] The average reduction in sodium concentration was more pronounced in children who received hyponatremic (hypotonic) (5% dextrose and 0.2% or 0.5% NaCl) compared with normonatremic (isotonic) postoperative intravenous fluids.[89] The perioperative use of balanced salt solutions is recommended to prevent hyponatremia (see Chapter 8 for a more in-depth discussion of new perioperative fluid management recommendations). In infants, the addition of 5% dextrose to the balanced salt solution may be required to avoid intraoperative or postoperative hypoglycemia.

### Increased Intracranial Pressure

Early surgery for craniosynostosis is often indicated to prevent increases in ICP.[31,32] One third of children with craniofacial dysostosis syndrome and 15% to 20% of children with single-suture craniosynostosis have increased ICP (>15 mm Hg).[90] Approximately 40% to 50% of children with syndromic craniosynostosis have associated hydrocephalus, although differentiation from nonprogressive ventriculomegaly may be difficult.[90-92] Timing of surgery may affect neurocognitive development and intelligence because these are adversely affected by sustained increased ICP. Associated OSA resulting in hypoxemia and hypercapnia may lead to an increase in cerebral blood volume and thereby exacerbate intracranial hypertension.[93] Untreated intracranial hypertension may lead to optic atrophy and visual impairment.[35,94] As a consequence, when increased ICP has been identified either preoperatively or postoperatively, placement of a ventriculoperitoneal shunt should be considered.[92] This is more common an occurrence in Crouzon and Pfeiffer syndromes.[92]

For children who present with signs of intracranial hypertension, it is important to follow basic principles of neuroanesthesia to prevent further increases in ICP and decreases in cerebral perfusion pressure (see Chapter 24 for a more in-depth discussion). It may be prudent to use protective measures to attenuate the hypertensive response to laryngoscopy and intubation,

including the administration of a short-acting opioid, a β-blocker, or topical local anesthesia to the upper airway. Intraoperatively, the anesthesiologist faces numerous challenges to control ICP. Mild to moderate hyperventilation (to an end-tidal carbon dioxide of 30 to 35 mm Hg), especially when signs of herniation are evident, avoidance of hypervolemia, and, where indicated, appropriate use of mannitol, furosemide, and dexamethasone may be employed to reduce ICP, reduce brain volume, and facilitate brain retraction. Although cranial vault reconstruction increases intracranial volume and reduces ICP,[95] children remain at risk of increased ICP after surgery and require close ophthalmologic and clinical follow-up, even after a cosmetically successful cranial expansion.[96,97]

### Venous Air Embolism

Venous air embolism (VAE) may occur during any operative procedure in which the operative site is above the level of the heart and noncollapsible veins are exposed to atmospheric pressure.[98-105] The incidence of VAE in children undergoing craniectomy for craniosynostosis repair has been reported to be as great as 83%,[105] although hemodynamically significant VAE is rare. The incidence associated with endoscopic craniectomy may be as small as 2%.[62] Significant hypovolemia resulting from surgical blood loss can lead to a decrease in both systemic and central venous pressures and the development of a pressure gradient between the right atrium and the surgical site. This gradient increases the potential to entrain air via open dural sinuses or bony venous sinusoids.[105,106] If the entrained volume of air is sufficiently large, right ventricular outflow obstruction may ensue, causing acute right-sided heart failure and cardiovascular collapse. Smaller volumes of air may cause a reduction in cardiac output, hypotension, and myocardial or cerebral ischemia.[103] Transesophageal echocardiography (documenting the presence of air in the right ventricular outflow tract), precordial Doppler ultrasonography (continuous machinery mill murmur), end-tidal carbon dioxide (precipitous decrease in carbon dioxide tension), and nitrogen monitoring (sudden increase in nitrogen concentration in the exhaled breath) have been used to identify VAE with different sensitivities, well before cardiovascular collapse occurs (see Figure 24-6).[103,107-110] Applying bone wax to the open edges of cut bone, reducing the degree of or avoiding the reverse Trendelenburg position, introducing positive-pressure ventilation with 5 cm of positive end-expiratory pressure, and maintaining normovolemia help to prevent VAE. Fluid resuscitation, vasopressors, and aspiration of air from the right side of the heart may prevent episodes of VAE from progressing to cardiovascular collapse.[99,105,110]

### Prolonged Surgery

As with all surgeries that last several hours, preventing the complications associated with prolonged anesthesia is paramount.[111] Nerve palsies, pressure necrosis of the skin, ophthalmic complications, hypothermia, and acidosis may occur. Careful positioning of the extremities, use of an egg-crate type mattress, and avoiding pressure to the eyes, particularly when the surgical procedure requires the prone position, will prevent the majority of these adverse outcomes. In children with proptosis, such as Crouzon syndrome, it is particularly essential to suture the eyelids closed after applying lubrication to prevent corneal abrasions. Anterior ischemic optic neuropathy that can cause transient or permanent postoperative blindness is a rare complication that occurs in the absence of external pressure to the eyes.[112]

Hypothermia is another major concern. Factors that predispose to hypothermia include the relatively large surface area exposed during surgery and the transfusion of large volumes of relatively cold intravenous fluids. Effective measures to prevent hypothermia include warming the operating room, insulating the child, and the use of forced air warmers and warming devices for blood and intravenous fluids. Preventing hypothermia and limiting blood loss and transfusion requirements are key factors in preventing the development of perioperative metabolic disturbance.[113]

## Orbital Hypertelorism

The term *orbital hypertelorism* describes abnormally separated orbits. This deformity may occur in isolation or in association with other congenital abnormalities, such as facial clefts and Apert syndrome (Fig. 33-5). Surgical repair involves mobilization and repositioning of the orbit through either a subcranial approach, which leaves the roof of the orbit intact, or an intracranial approach via a frontal craniectomy. This procedure is performed in children older than 5 years who may have already undergone extensive surgical reconstruction. Surgical manipulation of the globe may elicit the oculocardiac reflex, resulting in bradyarrhythmias or asystole. Oculocardiac reflex may also occur during midface and orthognathic procedures (see also Fig. 32-3, *A* and *B*).[114] These arrhythmias are prevented by administering a prophylactic anticholinergic such as atropine (10-20 µg/kg) or glycopyrrolate (5-10 µg/kg). Discontinuing the surgical stimulus almost always increases the heart rate.

The presence of a difficult airway influences the anesthetic technique, although in most instances, an inhalational induction is performed while spontaneous ventilation is maintained until the trachea is intubated. After establishing intravenous access, the

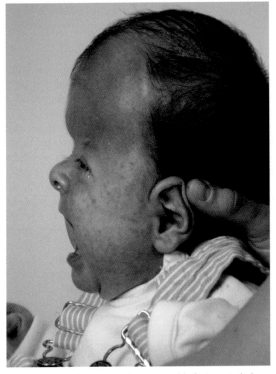

**FIGURE 33-5** Child with Apert syndrome. Notable features include proptosis, cloverleaf skull, maxillary hypoplasia, and syndactyly (syndactyly is present in Apert syndrome but not in Crouzon syndrome).

airway should be secured using a preformed orotracheal tube. Blood loss from multiple osteotomies may be significant, and, as in the case of craniosynostosis surgery, methods to reduce the use of homologous blood should be considered. Intraoperative management follows the principles outlined for craniosynostosis surgery. At the conclusion of surgery, the trachea is extubated and the child is monitored overnight in a high-dependency setting with the capability of managing acute airway obstruction.

## Midface Procedures

Midface advancement to improve facial appearance is commonly required for children with maxillary hypoplasia, such as those with Crouzon, Apert (see Fig. 33-5), and Pfeiffer syndromes (E-Fig. 33-7).[115-117] This procedure is typically performed in preschool children, although complications such as proptosis, corneal ulceration, ocular dislocations, and airway obstruction may necessitate earlier intervention.[117-120] A LeFort II procedure is similar to a LeFort III, with the difference that the osteotomy is oriented vertically through the infraorbital rim. Thus the nasal pyramid and the maxilla move forward as a single unit. Le Fort III osteotomy and monobloc procedures (Fig. 33-6) have the potential for significant complications, including massive blood loss, airway difficulties, cerebrospinal fluid leak, and infection.[111,121-123]

Anesthetic concerns are similar to those for orbital hypertelorism and craniosynostosis. Children with Apert and Crouzon syndromes often present with incomplete or complete nasal obstruction that results from choanal atresia or midface hypoplasia. As a consequence, mask anesthesia can be difficult, even with an oral airway in situ. However, laryngoscopy and tracheal intubation in these children is usually uncomplicated. The diameter of the tracheal tube requires careful consideration because these children may require prolonged postoperative ventilation until postoperative facial and laryngeal edema has resolved. The decision to intubate the trachea via the oral or nasal route must be discussed with the surgeon before induction of anesthesia. A nasotracheal tube can be used throughout the procedure, or the surgeon may request an intraoperative change from the oral to the nasal tracheal position after completing the midfacial osteotomies.[124] To perform the latter maneuver, the anesthesiologist wears a sterile surgical gown and gloves and uses sterile equipment, including laryngoscope, Magill forceps, and tube exchange catheter (see E-Fig. 12-3). Visualizing the glottis during surgery may be difficult because of the presence of airway edema and blood in the hypopharynx. A tube exchange catheter is passed through a naris and into the trachea alongside the orotracheal tube. The nasal tube is then passed over the exchange catheter, and its tip is positioned at the glottic opening. The oral tube is then removed, and the nasal tube is advanced (rotating the bevel 90 degrees clockwise or counterclockwise as needed to pass the vocal cords and arytenoids)[125,126] and visualized as it passes through the glottic aperture. Once the tube position is confirmed, the catheter is removed and the nasal tube is sutured securely to the nasal septum. Given the proximity of the tracheal tube to the surgical site, damage to the tracheal tube can occur during surgery.[127,128] Vigilance is required at all times to detect an accidental disconnection or damage to the tracheal tube. The anesthesiologist must be prepared to respond immediately to an unexpected interruption in ventilation and replace the tracheal tube. A nasogastric tube is placed after surgery to prevent gastric distention and reduce the likelihood of postoperative nausea and vomiting. A wire cutter must be available at the bedside at all

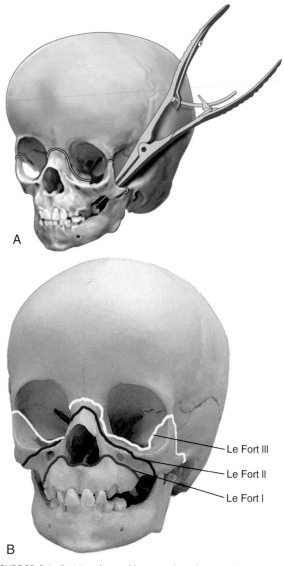

FIGURE 33-6 Le Fort III and monobloc procedures for correction of midface hypoplasia. **A,** The osteotomies in the Le Fort III procedure pass through the nasofrontal junction, across the medial orbital wall and floor, and into the inferior orbital fissure. A cut through the frontozygomatic suture, pterygomaxillary junction, and zygomatic arch allows separation of the midface. **B,** The monobloc procedures are similar, but the nasofrontal junction and frontozygomatic suture are not mobilized. This technique allows simultaneous correction of supraorbital and midface deformities at the expense of an increased incidence of postoperative complications.

times if intermaxillary fixation is used to stabilize the facial bones and mandible. In the intensive care unit, the presence of an audible leak around the tracheal tube is an important criterion to determine absence of laryngeal or periglottic edema and therefore readiness for tracheal extubation.[127] Intraoperative blood loss is not typically as great as for craniosynostosis surgery. Hypotensive anesthesia may reduce or prevent the need for blood transfusions during maxillary orthognathic surgery.[129]

## Hemifacial Microsomia, Treacher Collins Syndrome, and Goldenhar Syndrome

Hemifacial microsomias, also known as otomandibular dysostosis (Fig. 33-7), result from a malformation of the first and second branchial (or pharyngeal) arches. This is the second most common facial defect after clefts. These disorders are classified according to the classification *o*rbital distortion, *m*andibular hypoplasia, *e*ar anomaly, *n*erve involvement, and *s*oft tissue deficiency (OMENS).[4,130-133] Piezosurgery is a relatively new technique used to perform osteotomies using ultrasonic frequencies during mandibular distraction in children with hemifacial microsomia.[134] Airway difficulty increases with the complexity of the defect from unilateral to bilateral mandibular or temporomandibular involvement. The disorder may include mandibular hypoplasia, temporomandibular joint dysostosis, cleft palate, and auricular, ophthalmologic, and facial nerve defects. Goldenhar syndrome (Fig. 33-8 and E-Fig. 33-8) is the most common form of this disorder. Vertebral anomalies are present in 40% and congenital heart defects occur in 35% of children with this syndrome. Airway management is complicated by midfacial hypoplasia, asymmetry of mouth opening, and mandibular retrognathia. Overall, tracheal intubation in children with unilateral hemifacial microsomia is easy in 70% and very difficult in 9%.[130] In contrast, tracheal intubation in children with bilateral mandibular hypoplasia is evenly distributed among easy, difficult, and very difficult.[130] The airway anomalies associated with this syndrome predispose to OSA.

The craniofacial abnormalities of mandibular hypoplasia, macrostomia, and cleft palate in Treacher Collins syndrome (Fig. 33-9 and E-Fig. 33-9) often present difficulties for airway management that increase with increasing age.[4,130] Other clinical features of the syndrome include hypoplastic zygomatic arches, ophthalmic features (including sloping palpebral fissures, coloboma of the eyes, and notched lower eyelids) and microtia, choanal atresia, cardiovascular defects, and renal anomalies. Mandibular distraction osteogenesis is a surgical option considered when upper airway obstruction is due to mandibular deficiency. This avoids tracheostomy or other surgical intervention and allows for future growth of the mandible. Children with hemifacial microsomia have a poor psychosocial outcome.[135]

### AIRWAY MANAGEMENT

Airway management of children with hemifacial dysostoses is traditionally known to be difficult. It is essential that all equipment for management of the difficult airway be present in the operating room before induction of anesthesia (see Table 12-10). For infants and children with difficult airways, an inhalational induction is the most commonly used technique. In contrast, in older children and adolescents, either an inhalational induction or intravenous sedation (using dexmedetomidine or propofol) with topical local anesthesia applied to the upper airway may be used to facilitate tracheal intubation. In all cases, it is essential to maintain spontaneous respirations until the airway is secured so that oxygenation and ventilation will be maintained if the airway cannot be secured.

A variety of techniques may be used to control the difficult airway, including a flexible fiberoptic bronchoscope, Glidescope (Verathon Inc., Bothell, Wash.), the Airtraq (Prodol Meditec S.A., Vizcaya, Spain) disposable optical laryngoscope, Truview Infant laryngoscope (Truphatek International Truview Infant laryngoscope Limited, Netanya, Israel), LMA,[136] and others (see Chapter 12). We have used the two-person intubation technique, in which the first anesthesiologist applies external posterior laryngeal pressure while performing laryngoscopy to optimize the view of the glottis, while the second anesthesiologist inserts the tracheal tube into the trachea when the view is adequate (see Fig. 33-9).[137] The

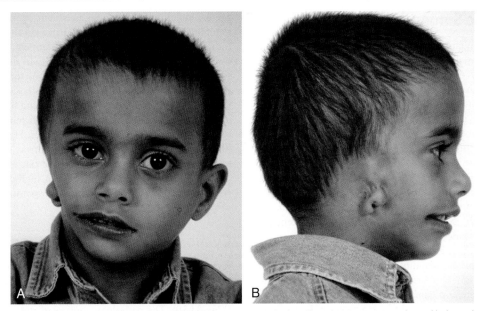

FIGURE 33-7 Frontal (**A**) and lateral (**B**) views of unilateral hemifacial microsomia. In the lateral view, microstomia and mandibular and ocular deformities are evident. These children may present with either unilateral or bilateral hemifacial microsomia, a hypoplastic mandible and maxilla, and ear deformities.

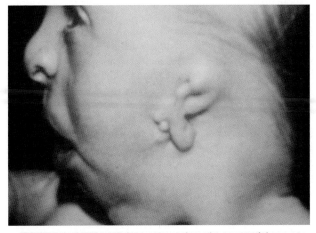

FIGURE 33-8 Goldenhar syndrome in an infant. This is one of the most common forms of hemifacial microsomia. With unilateral hemifacial microsomia, the airway is usually managed and instrumented without difficulty, but with bilateral mandibular hypoplasia, the airway may be very difficult to manage in one third of afflicted children.

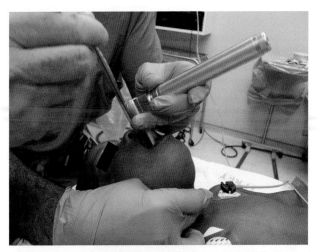

FIGURE 33-9 Two-person intubation technique. The intubator (first person) performs laryngoscopy and manipulates the larynx with external laryngeal manipulation (gloved hands). With the larynx in view, the intubator cocks his or her head to the left while holding position and the assistant (second person, nongloved hand) who is standing on the intubator's right, then passes the tracheal tube through the larynx.[137]

second anesthesiologist also may assist with more advanced airway management both in terms of helping to observe the child and assisting with the use of advanced airway devices.

Preformed tracheal tubes are generally used via the oral or nasal route, depending on the site of surgery. The use of an LMA can be very helpful to maintain airway patency or as a guide to facilitate fiberoptic bronchoscopy. When a nasotracheal tube is used, it can be secured by suturing it to the membranous nasal septum or taping it after the skin has been prepared with benzoin. An oral tube may be wired to the mandible.

For children with a history of upper airway obstruction or midfacial hypoplasia who present with a tracheostomy, the tracheostomy tube can be replaced with a cuffed tracheostomy tube or an armored tube that is sutured in place for the duration of the surgery. Changes in the position of the head and neck can

cause displacement of the tracheal tube, so care should be taken to confirm tracheal tube position after the child is positioned for surgery.[138] This is especially important for cranial vault procedures that involve extremes of neck extension, such as might occur during reconstruction of the supraorbital bar. Airway equipment and additional tracheal tubes must be available in the operating room at all times. It is essential to document an audible leak around the tracheal tube at the time of tracheal intubation (with the cuff on the tracheal tube deflated), because the presence of a leak is often used postoperatively to determine suitability for extubation when significant airway edema has developed. OSA associated with midfacial anomalies may result in supraglottic obstruction during induction and emergence.[54,58]

## Orthognathic Surgery

Malocclusion secondary to maxillary or mandibular hypoplasia (such as occurs in hemifacial microsomia and Treacher Collins syndrome), tumors, trauma, as well as temporomandibular joint dysfunction are generally accepted indications for orthognathic surgery. LeFort I procedures for maxillary hypoplasia involve a transverse incision through the maxilla to advance the upper teeth into normal occlusion with the mandible. Children who are candidates for this surgery are typically adolescents, because these procedures are performed once maxillary and mandibular growth is complete. Because this age group usually exhibits increased perioperative anxiety, preoperative assurance and education as well as premedication with oral midazolam (0.3 to 0.4 mg/kg, up to 20 mg for older children and adolescents) or intravenous midazolam (2 to 4 mg) are often necessary.

Airway management is a major concern, particularly in children with a hypoplastic mandible or temporomandibular dysfunction.[4] A high index of suspicion for atlantoaxial instability is required if juvenile rheumatoid arthritis is the underlying disease process. The anticipated difficult airway can be managed using fiberoptic intubation, with sedation or topical local anesthesia or an inhalation induction and maintenance of spontaneous ventilation until the trachea is intubated, as discussed earlier. Nasotracheal intubation using a preformed tracheal tube is the preferred method of tracheal intubation. Careful stabilization and fixation of the tube using transseptal suturing to prevent unintended extubation is often employed. Excessive pressure on the ala nasi (causing ischemia) can be avoided by fixing the nasal RAE tube to the forehead with the nasal curve positioned away from the ala. LeFort I advancements require close communication between the surgery and anesthesia teams because the nasotracheal tube has been dislodged once the maxilla is fully mobilized. If intermaxillary fixation is used postoperatively, wire cutters must be immediately available at all times while the child is monitored in an intensive care setting.

To reduce intraoperative blood loss, controlled hypotension is commonly employed using any of a range of pharmacologic agents, including inhalational anesthetic agents, β-blockers, and remifentanil. The literature is extensive on the salutary effect of induced hypotension in reducing intraoperative blood loss and improving the quality of the surgical field during orthognathic surgery.[129,139-148] Invasive BP monitoring is indicated to monitor BP continuously during controlled hypotension and to facilitate intraoperative evaluation of blood gases and hematocrit. In some cases, a mild degree of hypotension is sufficient for optimal surgical conditions (systolic BP 85 to 90 mm Hg). Dexamethasone (0.2 mg/kg) may reduce postoperative airway edema.[149] After the return of protective airway reflexes, the trachea is extubated and the child is monitored overnight in a high-dependency setting with the ability to establish an airway should acute airway obstruction develop.

## Cystic Hygromas and Hemangiomas

Cystic hygroma is a rare congenital malformation of the lymphatic system occurring with an incidence of 1 in 16,000 births, most frequently involving the axilla and neck (Fig. 33-10 and E-Fig 33-10). The pathology consists of multiple loculated cysts that contain lymph fluid or blood (see Fig. 33-10, B). In most cases, cystic hygromas are present at birth, although 80% to 90% are diagnosed within the first 2 years of life. The natural history is spontaneous resolution, although most require repeated aspirations, sclerotherapy, or surgical excision to debulk the mass (see E-Fig. 33-10, B).[150-152] Cystic hygroma can be associated with other chromosomal abnormalities such as Noonan and Turner syndromes, in which case the anesthetic management is guided by the underlying syndrome. Some children require an urgent tracheostomy in the first hours of life to relieve an obstructed airway (Chapter 37). During the preoperative assessment, the airway should be examined and evaluated by radiographs for involvement of supraglottic and infraglottic structures. Acute airway obstruction can occur during induction if cystic lesions are present in the upper airway. Fiberoptic intubation may be required if the larynx is distorted by the lesions, in which case spontaneous ventilation should be maintained until the airway

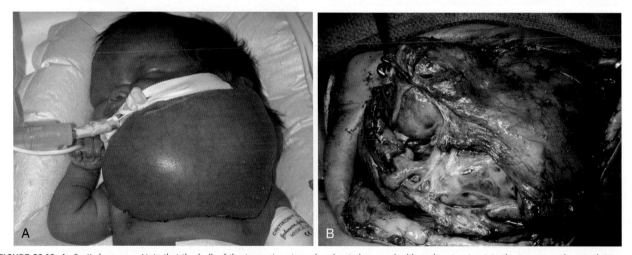

**FIGURE 33-10 A,** Cystic hygroma. Note that the bulk of the tumor is extraoral and extralaryngeal, although extension into the tongue and supraglottic region may complicate direct laryngoscopy. The tumor on the surface of the neck may rapidly expand owing to bleeding into the cysts or accumulation of fluid in the lymphatics. Such large tumors may put the overlying skin under great tension. They may also be situated such that they preclude tracheostomy. **B,** Gross pathologic condition in cystic hygromas consists of a combination of multiloculated cysts that may contain a combination of lymph fluid and blood. Debulking may result in substantial blood loss. Sequential debulking of the hygroma may be required as the residual cysts expand with fluid and blood and reexpand the hygroma.

is secured.[153] Postoperative complications of surgical excision include laryngeal edema, airway obstruction, pneumonia, facial palsy, and infection.[150,151,154]

Hemangiomas, also known as juvenile or infantile hemangiomas, are the most common benign tumors in infancy, affecting up to 10% of infants.[155] The majority of hemangiomas are uncomplicated and require no treatment. The natural course begins with a proliferation phase that starts within the first few months of life, followed by an involution phase of variable length. It is estimated that involution occurs at a rate of 10% per year. Hemangiomas can affect all organs, and intervention is required when the lesion affects the function of vital organs such as the eyes, airway, or liver.[156] Hemangiomas that occur in the subglottic region must be considered in the differential diagnosis of a noninfectious cause of croup in infants younger than 3 months of age. When present around the eyes and on the face (Fig. 33-11), hemangiomas are often associated with lesions in the airway.[157,158] They can occur in any part of the airway and can cause airway and feeding difficulties. Airway procedures to resect or remove hemangiomas are generally undertaken between 1 and 11 months of age.[159] Limb hemangiomas generally present with cosmetic concerns and bleeding. Rarely, children with large hemangiomas develop high-output heart failure.

Treatment options for hemangiomas include nonintervention, systemic corticosteroid treatment, corticosteroid injection, surgical excision, and laser ablation. Propranolol is an emerging treatment option for hemangiomas.[160] It may be used in children without contraindications either as an oral monotherapy at a dose of 2 mg/kg/day divided into three doses or in combination with oral prednisone 3 mg/kg/day tapered after 4 to 6 weeks of therapy. Propranolol reduces the need for surgical intervention but requires 6 months to 1 year of therapy.[161] Surgical treatment is reserved for superficial hemangiomas in locations that are surgically accessible.[156] Laser treatment for superficial lesions is commonly performed as an outpatient procedure,[162] and routine anesthetic precautions should be taken. Children with hemangiomas who had airway procedures received more steroids and had increased admissions and mortality compared with those without airway procedures.[159]

Arteriovenous malformations are present at birth but can go unrecognized for years, especially when they are intracranial. Large arteriovenous malformations may cause high-output cardiac failure, necessitating therapeutic intervention. Treatment options may include chemotherapy, corticosteroid therapy, embolization, and surgical excision. Children who undergo excision of the hemangiomas often require blood products during surgery, but platelets should be transfused with care because an accumulation within the malformation may increase its size.[163] NSAIDs should be avoided because of their effects on platelet function.

## Möbius Syndrome

Möbius sequence is a rare neurologic disorder (2 to 20 in 1,000,000 births) characterized by congenital palsy of the facial (VII) and abducens (VI) cranial nerves, resulting in unilateral or bilateral facial weakness and defective extraocular eye movement (E-Fig. 33-11). These classic features may be associated with other cranial nerves palsies, ophthalmic abnormalities, developmental delay, and various craniofacial, limb, and musculoskeletal malformations, resulting in a variable pattern of clinical expression.[164-168] Involvement of cranial nerves IX and X is associated with pharyngeal dysfunction, dysphagia, feeding difficulties, retention of oral secretions, and recurrent aspiration pneumonia. Associated micrognathia, microstomia, limited mouth opening, and other orofacial abnormalities may make tracheal intubation difficult.[169] Other associations include gastroesophageal reflux, hypotonia of skeletal muscles, congenital cardiac abnormalities, spinal abnormalities, and peripheral neuropathies. Central alveolar hypoventilation has been described in association with Möbius sequence and may be secondary to hypoplasia of midbrain respiratory centers.[170] Central alveolar hypoventilation, compounded by upper airway hypotonia and the effects of sedatives, opioids, and anesthetic agents, can predispose to postoperative respiratory compromise. The absence of facial expression secondary to paresis of the facial nerve can make it difficult to assess and evaluate postoperative pain.[171] The anesthetic plan for the child with Möbius sequence must be tailored to the individual based on the clinical expression of the syndrome.

The most common surgical procedure performed in children with Möbius sequence is a segmental gracilis muscle transplantation, in which the muscle is transplanted to the face and revascularized to the facial artery and vein.[172] Motor innervation of the gracilis requires a functioning cranial nerve such as the masseter branch of the trigeminal nerve. The aim of this facial reanimation is to facilitate facial expression and provide lower lip support to reduce drooling and improve speech.[172] Anesthetic considerations include those for prolonged surgery, avoidance of neuromuscular block to facilitate intraoperative nerve stimulation, and avoidance of hypocapnia, hypothermia, and hypotension to ensure graft perfusion. The latter considerations are also applicable to the postoperative period. Other surgical procedures commonly performed in children with Möbius sequence include

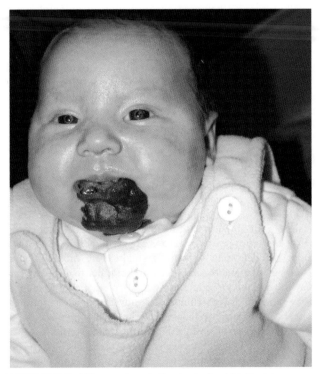

**FIGURE 33-11** Facial hemangioma in the cheek of a child. The hemangioma involves the skin overlying the mandible centrally from the lower lip to the tip of the mandible. Hemangiomas vary widely in size but can enlarge precipitously as a result of bleeding into the tumor.

strabismus surgery and orthopedic procedures to improve limb function.

## Congenital Intraoral Fibrous Bands

Congenital intraoral fibrous bands (e.g., pterygium syndrome and syngnathia) can present an almost impossible airway to secure even with advanced pediatric fiberoptic skills (E-Fig. 33-12). Syngnathia reduces mouth opening as a result of fusion of maxilla and mandible and often presents as a part of Van der Woude and popliteal pterygium syndromes.[173] These children often present with airway and feeding difficulties. Depending on the severity of the bands, these children may present formidable anesthetic challenges. Intravenous ketamine anesthesia in the spontaneously breathing neonate may allow division of the adhesions in the first few days of life, precluding the need for a surgical airway or facilitating tracheal intubation if other surgery is required.[173]

## Intraoral Tumors

Intraoral tumors are rare in children (E-Fig. 33-13) but, if massive, may present great challenges in securing the airway. Those that present the greatest difficulties preclude visualizing the larynx (E-Fig. 33-14) and present an increased risk of intraoperative bleeding. Preoperative radiographic studies are required to delineate the extent of involvement of the upper airway and whether the supraglottic region or the nasopharynx is clear for passage of a bronchoscope. If the tumors are sufficiently large that laryngoscopy is precluded, fiberoptic nasal intubation must be considered. If the tumor is resectable, a tracheostomy could be a back-up plan. The risk of bleeding depends on the vascularity of the tumor and whether the tongue is involved. If the vascular supply of the tumor can be isolated, bleeding should be easily controlled. If, however, the tumor cannot be separated from the tongue, bleeding can be controlled only by clamping the tongue before resecting the tumor. This should prevent excessive blood loss and permit a hemostatic closure of the resection surface. The trachea should remain intubated postoperatively until both airway and lingual edema have abated.

## Brachial Plexus Surgery

Brachial plexus injury occurs in 0.5 to 5 infants per 1000 live births as a result of birth trauma.[174,175] Erb palsy involves damage to nerve roots C5, C6, and C7, whereas Klumpke palsy involves roots C8 and T1.[175] Complete plexus palsies are the most devastating injuries, resulting in a flail and insensate arm.[175,176] Although 75% of brachial plexus injuries resolve spontaneously and completely within the first month after birth, 25% result in permanent disability and impairment.[175,177,178] Surgical intervention is indicated if the motor function does not improve after 3 months of age.[177,178] Clinically significant diaphragmatic palsy is associated with 2.4% of neonates with brachial plexus injury. In the very young, diaphragmatic palsy requires aggressive intervention before brachial plexus repair. For brachial plexus surgery to be successful, the nerve root cannot be completely avulsed from the spinal cord. Therefore detailed imaging is required to characterize the nature of the injury: avulsion of the nerve root from the spinal cord, disruption of the nerve within the nerve sheath, or disruption of the nerve and the nerve sheath. Because irreversible loss of the neuromotor end plate may occur, surgery is often undertaken before 12 months of age.[174,177-181] Microsurgical intervention is performed in infants with global lesions and Horner syndrome by 3 months of age. The aim is to improve function with no expectation of complete recovery; without intervention these children have severe functional deficits. Conversely, if recovery of biceps occurs by 3 months, treatment is performed without microsurgical intervention.[182] The treatment of choice includes resection of neuromas with interpositional nerve grafting.[183] Nerve grafting is being increasingly performed for treating neonatal brachial plexus injury. Donor nerves include motor branches of C4, intercostal nerves, inferior branches of the 11th cranial nerve, pectoral nerves, and sural nerves.[184] Synthetic collagen nerve conduits have been approved as nerve guidance channels in microsurgery and may be an option for the future.

Preoperative MRI for assessing bone and joint deformities may require administration of general anesthesia. Repair of brachial plexus may be challenging because the only extremity for intravenous access and monitoring (BP and pulse oximetry) is the contralateral upper extremity. Both lower extremities are usually prepped and draped for harvesting the sural nerves or other donor nerves for the repair. Because these infants are usually 9 to 12 months of age, they are chubby, making intravenous access more difficult. This surgery often takes up to 12 hours, so the considerations for prolonged anesthesia must be invoked, such as protecting pressure points during positioning. Muscle relaxants are avoided to facilitate intraoperative electrophysiologic testing.[185] An indwelling urinary catheter is essential to decompress the bladder. Analgesic requirement is minimal except during brief periods of surgical stimulation. Remifentanil provides excellent intraoperative analgesia and permits rapid adjustment of the depth of anesthesia. Maintenance of normothermia and prevention of fluid overload are important during this prolonged surgery. Blood loss is minimal, and maintenance fluids usually suffice.[174] Prolonged administration of propofol is not recommended because of the risk of propofol infusion syndrome and delayed emergence. In its stead, remifentanil combined with inhalation agent may be a more appropriate regimen. Postoperative analgesia requirements are minimal, and acetaminophen and NSAIDs usually provide adequate pain relief. Shoulder spica casts may be applied to avoid sudden neck movements postoperatively if the lower branches of the accessory nerve are used for reconstruction.[185]

## Otoplasty

Protruding ears (commonly known as "bat ears") are common in the Caucasian population, occurring with an incidence of up to 5% (E-Fig. 33-15).[186] Children with protruding ears are generally healthy, with about two thirds undergoing surgical correction before the age of 8 years or as soon as the child expresses concern about the deformity.[187] Younger children are more likely to require general anesthesia, whereas those older than age 8 years may tolerate the procedure using local anesthetic infiltration or nerve blocks.[188] Laser techniques are now employed increasingly to perform cartilage reshaping.[189] The main complication of general anesthesia is postoperative nausea and vomiting, which can last up to 2 days after surgery in approximately 80% of children.[190] However, postoperative nausea and vomiting may be reduced by surgical and anesthetic techniques, including the use of propofol and avoidance of packing of the external auditory meatus and concha.[190,191] To provide optimal surgical access and positioning of the child, a preformed, low-profile tracheal tube, such as the RAE tube, may be required, but flexible LMAs provide equally satisfactory conditions in the ventilated or spontaneously breathing child.[192] Infiltration with local anesthetic (usually less than 10 mL of 1% lidocaine with 1:100,000 epinephrine) attenuates the surgical stimulus and reduces the intraoperative opioid requirements. The use of a long-acting local anesthetic combined with a nerve block, acetaminophen, and NSAIDs provides adequate postoperative analgesia in most children. This multimodal approach may obviate the need for opioids and thereby reduce the incidence of postoperative nausea and vomiting.[193] Multimodal therapy (ondansetron and dexamethasone) provides specific antiemetic prophylaxis or therapy.

## Congenital Hand Anomalies

Congenital limb malformations exhibit a wide spectrum of phenotypic manifestations. Syndactyly may occur as an isolated malformation (Fig. 33-12 and E-Fig. 33-16) or part of a syndrome, the most common being Apert syndrome but also with Poland syndrome, in association with skeletal abnormalities and gastrointestinal and cardiac malformations. Limb malformations are more frequent in males than females, and they affect both upper and lower limbs in approximately 50% of children with a deformity. Early separation of digits is favored if the ring and little fingers or index finger and thumb are involved, because the differing longitudinal growth rates will lead to greater deformities.[194] Surgery is usually performed between 6 and 18 months of age.[195,196] An association has been reported between syndactyly and prolonged QT interval, with life-threatening arrhythmias reported in one child during anesthesia.[197] Timothy syndrome is

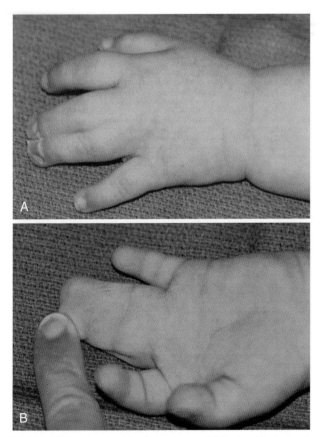

**FIGURE 33-12** Syndactyly of the first and second digit of an infant: dorsal aspect (**A**) and volar aspect (**B**).

a multisystem disorder with cardiac, facial, limb, and neurodevelopmental features.[198]

Duplicated thumb can be present as an isolated anomaly and is present in approximately 1 in 3000 births. Hypoplastic thumbs are associated with systemic syndromes such as Holt-Oram syndrome; **v**ertebral, **a**nal, **c**ardiac, **t**racheal, **e**sophageal, **r**enal, **l**imb (VACTERL) anomalies; Fanconi anemia; Nager syndrome; and thrombocytopenia-absent radius.[199] A complete evaluation of the child is generally warranted because abnormalities can occur in the cardiovascular, neurologic, and hematopoietic systems.[199] Genetic testing is not generally needed in isolated thumb duplications.

## Tissue Expanders

Tissue expansion has become a major treatment modality in the management of giant congenital hairy pigmented nevi (see E-Fig. 33-17), hemangiomas, meningomyelocele, abdominal wall defects, and secondary reconstruction of extensive burn scars.[200-208] Tissue expanders effectively allow removal of the affected area and preserve sensation in a durable flap with minimal donor site morbidity.[209] These devices consist of a silicone shell that stretches to accommodate serial injections of saline when placed subcutaneously or, in the case of the scalp, under the galea, through an incision made in normal tissue adjacent to the lesion or defect (Fig. 33-13).[204,210] Osmotic tissue expanders have been used in burn scars, congenital nevi, alopecia, or foot deformities with reduced infection rates and low cost. Tissue expansion requires at least two surgical procedures, one to insert the expander and a second to remove it when expansion is complete; some children may require serial insertions or multiple expanders.[204] Reconstruction of areas of the head and neck constitute a particular challenge because expansion without oral, visual, or airway compromise is required.[211] Complications of tissue expansion include infection, skin erosion, leakage, migration, and flap necrosis.[207,212-215] Perioperative antibiotics are given at insertion and removal, although their effectiveness in preventing infection has not been established.[202,207,209,213,214]

## Hairy Pigmented Nevi

Congenital melanocytic nevi characteristically vary in size, shape, surface texture, and hairiness. They are frequently excised because

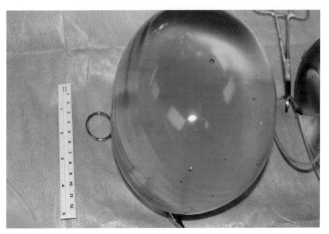

**FIGURE 33-13** Tissue expander that is approximately 18 cm long. These expanders are inserted in a partially deflated state and then expanded by sequentially injecting saline over a period of weeks.

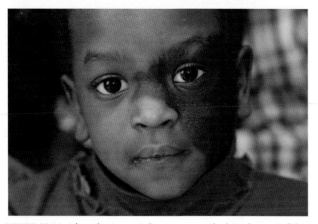

**FIGURE 33-14** A heavily pigmented nevus covers the lateral aspect of the face from the eyebrow, over the bridge of the nose, and down to the skin covering the mandible. These large and disfiguring pigmented nevi must be resected in staged events.

they are disfiguring and have the potential to become malignant. Serial surgical excision is common, but skin grafting and tissue expanders are also used (E-Fig. 33-17).[209] The position and size determine the frequency of excision and anesthetic technique. If the face, head, or neck is involved, airway management should be discussed with the surgeon to allow optimal surgical access (Fig. 33-14).

In general, these children are healthy. In the cooperative and motivated child, subcutaneous infusion of a very dilute local anesthetic (e.g., ropivacaine 0.08% to 0.3%) mixed with epinephrine 1:1,000,000 can be used to provide painless tumescent anesthesia.[216] The local anesthetic is infused through a 30-gauge needle at an initial rate of 120 mL/hr. Blanching of skin identifies the area that is anesthetized. This method has been used successfully in children 7 years of age and older.[217] To avoid toxicity, local anesthetic volume and dosing guidelines should be followed (see Chapter 41). The addition of longer-acting local anesthetics to the infiltrate will enhance postoperative analgesia. Repeated reconstructive procedures are often required, and attention should be paid to providing appropriate premedication where necessary (see Chapter 4).

## Cosmetic Procedures

According to American Society of Plastic Surgeons, the most common cosmetic surgeries performed in adolescents are nose reshaping, male breast reduction, ear surgery, laser hair removal, laser treatment of leg veins, and laser skin resurfacing.[218] Breast implants and liposuction are the most controversial cosmetic procedures performed in this age group, although combined they only comprise 5% of cosmetic surgery in this age group. In 2011, 73% of male breast reduction and 28% of otoplasty occurred in this age group.[218] The breast augmentation procedures were performed on an outpatient basis.[219] These patients are generally healthy. Routine anesthetic induction with endotracheal intubation with no additional invasive monitoring is generally all that is required. This group of patients may be at increased risk of postoperative nausea and vomiting and will benefit from multimodal prophylaxis. Postoperative discomfort is common, requiring administration of systemic opioids or nerve blocks.

Liposuction is usually scheduled as outpatient surgery, although extensive liposuction may require an overnight admission to the hospital. This latter procedure is associated with acute complications, including itching, bruising, and swelling, damage to nerves or vital organs, blood loss, and embolization of fat or blood. Lidocaine toxicity and fluid accumulation at the surgical site are directly proportional to the volume of aspirated fat and number of treated sites.[220]

## Trauma

A considerable proportion of plastic surgical procedures in children are performed for trauma and emergency surgery. Procedures include treatment of simple lacerations, animal bites, tendon, nerve and vascular repair, reimplantation of digits and limbs, and treatment of burns (see Chapter 34). The cooperative and fasted child with minor trauma can often undergo minor surgical procedures using local anesthesia, commonly administered by the plastic surgeon in the emergency department. This can be supplemented with inhalation of a 50:50 mixture of nitrous oxide and oxygen (Entonox),[221] intravenous administration of small doses of a benzodiazepine and opioid (e.g., midazolam 50 μg/kg, and fentanyl 0.5 μg/kg) or ketamine according to locally established sedation protocols (see Chapters 45 and 47). Alternatively, a single-injection digital nerve block is safe and effective for minor surgical procedures in children.[222]

Surgery for extensive injuries to digits and limbs usually requires general anesthesia because children do not tolerate prolonged application of a tourniquet. The severity and urgency of the injury dictate the timing of the surgery. The general principles of care for the child with trauma should be followed (see Chapter 38), with particular attention directed to identifying more life-threatening injuries. For urgent surgery in the presence of a full stomach, precautions against aspiration of gastric contents should be considered. For postoperative pain control, a combination of regional anesthesia or systemic analgesia is usually adequate. Continuous brachial plexus or other nerve blocks may improve tissue perfusion[223] and facilitate cooperation during postoperative physiotherapy for procedures such as digital reimplantation. Continuous nerve block may attenuate the signs associated with compartment syndrome, and frequent and meticulous attention must be paid to perfusion of the extremity.

**ACKNOWLEDGMENTS**
The authors thank R. Zuker, MD, FRCS, Professor of Surgery, Division of Plastic Surgery; C. Forrest, MD, FRCS, Associate Professor of Surgery, Head of the Division of Plastic Surgery, The Hospital for Sick Children, University of Toronto, Toronto, Ontario; and J. Girotto, MD, Assistant Professor of Pediatrics, Neurosurgery and Plastic Reconstructive Surgery, Director of the Cleft and Craniofacial Center, Golisano Children's Hospital at Strong Memorial Hospital, University of Rochester, Rochester, N.Y., for providing photographs to illustrate this chapter.

## ANNOTATED REFERENCES

Antony AK, Sloan GM. Airway obstruction following palatoplasty: analysis of 247 consecutive operations. Cleft Palate Craniofac J 2002; 39:145-8.
*Two hundred forty-seven children underwent palatoplasty, yielding a 6% incidence of perioperative airway obstruction. The airway obstruction occurred as late*

as 48 hours postoperatively. Of the 14 children with severe airway compromise, 12 required continued tracheal intubation, reintubation, and tracheostomy. Of these 14 children (93%), 13 had coexisting craniofacial abnormalities, with 7 having Pierre Robin sequence.

Faberowski LW, Black S, Mickle JP. Incidence of venous air embolism during craniectomy for craniosynostosis repair. Anesthesiology 2000; 92:20-3.

*This case series of 23 children undergoing craniosynostosis reported an 83% incidence of venous air embolism using precordial Doppler monitoring. Although cardiovascular collapse did not occur, 32% developed hypotension. Detection and early intervention are important strategies to prevent cardiovascular collapse associated with this type of surgery.*

Goobie SM, Meier PM, Pereira LM, et al. Efficacy of tranexamic acid in pediatric craniosynostosis surgery: a double-blind, placebo-controlled trial. Anesthesiology 2011;114:862-71.

*This randomized, placebo-controlled trial examined the effects of tranexamic acid on blood loss during reconstructive craniosynostosis surgery. Both blood loss and blood transfusion requirements were significantly reduced, by almost 50%.*

Lavoie J. Blood transfusion risks and alternative strategies in pediatric patients. Pediatr Anesth 2011;21:14-24.

*This review summarizes blood conservation modalities such as acute normovolemic hemodilution, hypervolemic hemodilution, deliberate hypotension, antifibrinolytics, intraoperative blood salvage, and autologous blood donation. The* transfusion triggers and algorithms and the current literature in blood transfusion alternatives are discussed.

Meier PM, Goobie SM, DiNardo JA, et al. Endoscopic strip craniectomy in early infancy: the initial five years of anesthesia experience. Anesth Analg 2011;112:407-14.

*This retrospective chart review studied 100 infants ranging from 4 to 34 weeks of age (weight: 3.2 to 10.1 kg) who underwent single and multiple endoscopic strip craniectomy. Four infants had craniofacial syndrome; 87 infants underwent single and 13 multiple craniectomy. The risk factors for bleeding are identified, along with an emphasis on venous air embolism, intensive care unit admissions and reoperation.*

Nargozian C. The airway in patients with craniofacial abnormalities. Pediatr Anesth 2004;14:53-9.

*This review summarizes the salient features and airway implications of the major craniofacial disorders that afflict children, including Pierre Robin sequence, Treacher Collins syndrome, Goldenhar syndrome, and Klippel-Feil syndrome. The anatomic pathology is very well described, and the clinical implications of the pathologic condition are thoroughly discussed.*

## REFERENCES

Please see www.expertconsult.com.

# Burn Injuries

# 34

ERIK S. SHANK, CHARLES J. COTÉ, AND J.A. JEEVENDRA MARTYN

EVERY YEAR IN THE UNITED STATES millions of people are treated for burns; of these, hundreds of thousands are hospitalized, with a significant mortality rate.[1-3] The National Burn Repository Report for 2006 reviewed their 10-year experience; overall mortality for 140,318 records was 5.3%. Inhalation injury was reported in 5.7% of cases; approximately 30% of burns were in children or adolescents age 20 years or younger, and the majority were scald burns or contacts with hot objects. Unfortunately, approximately 1166 cases were suspected child abuse. It is estimated that around 120,000 pediatric burn injuries are treated in the emergency department each year in the United States and the majority of patients are younger than 6 years of age.[4] Children with burn injuries are well managed only when their care providers thoroughly understand the pathophysiologic and pharmacologic abnormalities associated with burn injury.[5,6] These abnormalities include metabolic derangements, neurohumoral responses, massive fluid shifts, sepsis, and the systemic effects of massive tissue destruction. In this chapter we address the pathophysiology, the initial evaluation and resuscitation, and the anesthetic and pain management of children with burn injury. Some of the principles presented are the result of more than 30 years of experience in caring for children with burn injuries, and others are derived from experiences with adults and applied to children.

Each year, in the United States, approximately 15,000 children are hospitalized with burn injuries.[1] The mortality rate has declined steadily over the past decades, owing to the advent of dedicated hospital burn centers,[7,8] improved surgical techniques, and safer anesthetic management. However, almost 1100 children still die each year from fire and burn injuries. Safety prevention efforts such as smoke detectors do not seem to have reduced pediatric flame injuries because many flame injuries are related to children playing with matches,[9,10] although there has been a small overall decrease in total burn injuries to children.[11]

## Pathophysiology

Thermal injury to the skin disrupts the vital surface barrier that is responsible for thermal regulation, bacterial defenses, and fluid and electrolyte balance.[12] It is essential to appreciate, however, that even minor, localized burn injuries may be associated with diffuse and dramatic systemic responses. These injuries may have an impact on all of the systems of the body.[5] Several mediators released from the burned areas activate the inflammatory response and cause local and remote edema. Complement, arachidonic acid metabolites, and oxygen radicals are involved in this response.[6] Cytokines are the key mediators of the systemic effects.[13] Abnormal cytokine values reflect the severity of injury, and these abnormalities may persist for years after injury.[14-18] Endotoxins are frequently detected in the period immediately after the burn, usually correlate with the burn size, and are predictive of the development of multiple organ failure and the subsequent demise of the patient.[19] The clinical symptoms and pathologic changes are relatively more severe in children, and, unfortunately, the gravity of the injury is often underestimated because of their greater ratio of body surface area to weight (Fig. 34-1).

Soon after the injury, massive volumes of fluid shift from the vascular compartment to the burned tissue, resulting in sequestration of fluid, even in nonburned areas of the body, resulting in significant hemoconcentration.[5] Despite the massive fluid loss, systemic blood pressure is usually maintained through an outpouring of catecholamines and antidiuretic hormone, both of which are potent vasoconstrictors.[20] In the first 4 days after a burn of moderate size or larger (approximately 40% of the body surface area), an amount of albumin equal to about twice the total body plasma content is lost through the wound. In addition to the direct effects of the burn (thrombosis, increased capillary permeability), changes in vascular integrity occur in areas remote

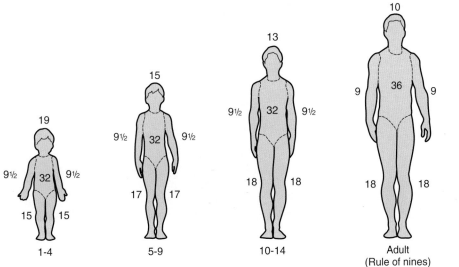

**FIGURE 34-1** The different proportions of body surface area are illustrated for calculation of percentage of burn according to a patient's age. Note the large proportion of body surface area that the head and face account for in an infant. (From Carvajal HF, Goldman AS. Burns. In: Vaughan VC III, McKay RJ, Nelson WE, editors. Nelson's textbook of pediatrics. Philadelphia: WB Saunders; 1975, p. 281.)

from the injury, resulting in tissue edema.[21] In the pulmonary capillary network, these changes may be life-threatening; severe pulmonary edema and vascular congestion may result.

## CARDIAC

Immediately after an injury, cardiac output is dramatically reduced.[22,23] This decrease is often related to the rapid reduction in circulating blood volume and the severe compressive effects of circumferential burns on the abdomen and chest that impair venous return.[24] Despite adequate cardiac filling pressures, cardiac output often remains reduced. This may result from other factors, such as direct myocardial depression from the burn injury. Some investigators have described circulating myocardial depressant factors such as interleukins, tumor necrosis factors, or oxygen free radicals existing in subjects with extensive third-degree burns.[25-28] Transesophageal echocardiography may be helpful in guiding supportive care in the early phase.[29] At our institution, acutely burned children frequently require inotropic support during the acute period of depressed cardiac function. Carefully titrated inotropic support improves cardiac output, without the need for volume overload–mediated improvement in cardiac function.

Children develop a hypermetabolic state 3 to 5 days after a burn injury. This state is associated with a twofold to threefold increase in cardiac output, which persists for weeks to months, depending on the extent of the injury and the time needed for wound closure; heart rate, cardiac output, cardiac index, and rate-pressure-product are increased for at least 2 years after burns that involve 40% or greater of body surface area.[30] Some children develop a reversible cardiomyopathy.[31] Hypertension has been reported to occur during this hypermetabolic period. The most common cause of the hypertension in this period is inadequate pain control, and this should be ruled out. However, other circulating mediators such as increased catecholamines, atrial natriuretic factor, renin-angiotensin, endothelin-1, and vasopressin and other circulating vasoactive mediators can cause intermittent or persistent hypertension in patients with burn injuries.[32-36] If decreased cardiac output is observed during this hypermetabolic state, gram-negative sepsis or hypovolemia should be suspected.

Closure of the burn wound usually decreases metabolic demand, resulting in a concomitant reduction in cardiac output.[37,38] Some children may benefit from treatment with propranolol, which reduces cardiac work and decreases the systemic inflammatory response.[39,40]

## PULMONARY

Pulmonary function may be adversely affected from the upper airway to terminal alveoli. The upper airway is an excellent heat exchanger; just as it warms cold air, it cools hot air. The cooling of hot inspired air may cause a thermal injury to the tissues of the larynx; the air in a closed space (e.g., house or automobile fire) may reach 538° C (1000° F) 2 feet above floor level. Inspiration of superheated air damages the upper airway. Airway obstruction occurs as a result of massive edema formation involving laryngeal and tracheal structures above the carina (see later). The thermal insult also may injure the ciliated epithelium and mucosa in the proximal bronchi. The inhalation of toxic fumes, such as nitrogen dioxide and sulfur dioxide released from burning plastic, which combine with water in the tracheobronchial tree to form nitric and sulfuric acids, may damage the distal bronchi and alveoli. Thus upper airway injury is usually a thermal insult, whereas lower airway injury is a chemical or toxic insult. Acid gases such as hydrochloric acid, sulfuric acid, and phosgene form small aerosolized particles that penetrate deep into the tracheobronchial tree, damaging the alveolar membranes and surfactants.[41] Wool and cotton combustion forms aldehydes, which may cause pulmonary edema in concentrations as small as 10 ppm.[42] Combustion of synthetic materials (insulation, wall paneling) releases hydrogen cyanide. Although cyanide is a rare toxin in fires,[43] cyanide poisoning can lead to histotoxic hypoxia and death,[44] mimicking carbon monoxide (CO) poisoning. Inhalation of hydrogen cyanide is an often unrecognized cause of immediate death.

The overall effect of a pulmonary inhalation injury is necrotizing bronchitis, bronchial swelling, alveolar destruction, exudation of protein, loss of surfactant, loss of the protective bronchial lining, and bronchospasm, all of which contribute to

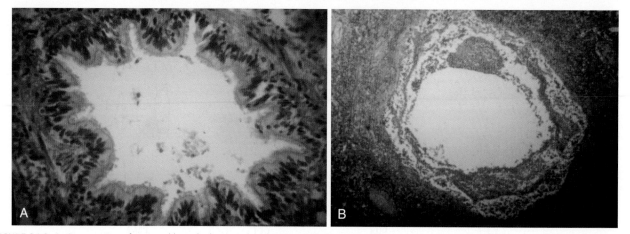

**FIGURE 34-2 A,** Cross section of a normal bronchiole. Note the ciliated epithelial layer. **B,** Compare with a cross section of a distal bronchiole from a child who died of an inhalation injury. Note the marked thickening of the bronchial wall, the massive inflammatory cell infiltrate, the sloughing of the mucosa, and the total destruction of the ciliated columnar epithelium.

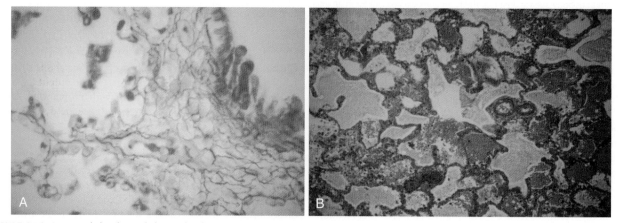

**FIGURE 34-3 A,** Normal alveoli. **B,** Inhalation alveolar injury is generally related to noxious fumes such as nitrogen dioxide and sulfur dioxide that are carried far down the tracheobronchial tree, combine with exhaled water, and form nitric acid and sulfuric acid, resulting in pulmonary congestion, alveolar injury, and hyaline membrane formation.

the development of bronchopneumonia (Figs. 34-2 and 34-3). Inhalation of particulate matter (smoke, soot) and lower airway edema also obstruct the airway mechanically. Edema of the bronchi, combined with loss of integrity of the pulmonary capillary endothelium, decrease pulmonary compliance. Circumferential chest burns may have a tourniquet-like effect that decreases chest wall compliance.[24] All of these injuries lead to clinically important ventilation-perfusion abnormalities and right-to-left intrapulmonary shunting, with hypoxemia and hypercarbia. In adults, the $PaO_2/FIO_2$ ratio and baseline carboxyhemoglobin concentrations are predictive of mortality.[45] One pediatric trial of inhaled heparin and acetylcysteine suggested a benefit with decreased airway cast formation and mucus plugging.[46] However, subsequent studies have yielded contradictory results.[47,48] CO inhalation can further compromise both hemoglobin's oxygen ($O_2$)-carrying capacity and its ability to deliver $O_2$ to tissues. CO also impairs $O_2$ usage at the cellular level (cellular respiration). Severe smoke inhalation alone may occur without externally visible injuries.[49] One clue that smoke inhalation has occurred is the presence of singed nasal hairs or nasal passages. Extrapulmonary factors such as changes in cardiac output also can contribute to hypoxemia. Blood gas analysis alone may not

indicate these factors. Rational therapy of arterial $O_2$ desaturation requires evaluation of both extrapulmonary and intrapulmonary factors,[21,50] including cardiac output, mixed venous $O_2$ content or saturation, and shunt fraction.[22] In general, the prognosis of cutaneous burn is compounded by the presence of an inhalation injury; the presence of an inhalational injury doubles the mortality rate from cutaneous burns,[41] with pediatric mortality reported to be approximately 16%.[51]

### RENAL

Renal function may be adversely affected soon after injury, primarily as a result of myoglobinuria and hemoglobinuria.[52] The former is most common after electrical injury,[53,54] whereas the latter is common after severe cutaneous burns of 40% or greater of body surface area. Hypovolemia, hypotension, and hypoxemia may further aggravate renal dysfunction, leading to acute tubular necrosis. Catecholamines, angiotensin, and vasopressin production increase, leading to systemic vasoconstriction, compounding the renal insufficiency.[55,56] Release of vasoactive peptides such as endothelin-1 may cause acute vasoconstriction, which also may adversely affect renal function.[57,58] Fluid retention is common during the first 3 to 5 days after injury and is followed by diuresis thereafter. Thus renal function may be impaired soon after the injury, delaying the excretion of some drugs or their active metabolites. At 3 to 7 days after the burn injury, glomerular filtration rate increases pari passu with an increased cardiac output and metabolic rate.[59] The serum half-life of many antibiotics and other medications that depend on renal excretion may be altered as a result of changes (increased or decreased) in the glomerular filtration rate.[60-64] Children who sustain a burn that covers greater than 40% of their body surface area demonstrate renal tubular dysfunction, in the form of an inability to concentrate the urine.[20] Even during hyperosmolar states, antidiuresis is not observed, suggesting an inadequate renal response to antidiuretic hormone and aldosterone. Thus an adequate urine output may be observed even in the presence of hypovolemia.[65] Episodic or persistent hypertension is frequent in children, in part mediated by an increase in renin and catecholamine production.[66,67] If hypertension persists, treatment that decreases stress on the cardiovascular system or reduces the potential for hypertensive encephalopathy should be instituted.

## HEPATIC

The liver may be damaged by hypoxemia or hypoperfusion during the early postburn phase as a result of inhaled or absorbed chemical toxins, hypovolemia, or hypotension.[68,69] Reperfusion injury may harm the liver when adequate circulation is reestablished. Delayed hepatic dysfunction may result from drug toxicity, sepsis, the hypermetabolic response to burns, or blood transfusions.[70] Studies in adults have found increased hepatic blood flow, increased protein synthesis and breakdown, and increased hepatic gluconeogenesis during the hypermetabolic phase of burn injury. With the onset of sepsis, hepatic glucose output and alanine uptake may decrease sharply but hepatic blood flow and $O_2$ usage can remain increased.[68,71] Fatty infiltration of the liver also has been reported.[72] Sustained increases in hepatic blood flow deliver more drug to the liver; this effect, combined with drug-induced enzyme induction, may decrease the half-life of drugs that are perfusion limited.[73] Although all studies of animals suggest decreased clearance of drugs after burn injury, clinical studies of the capacity of the liver to metabolize drugs are conflicting, even for the same class of drugs.[74-79] The magnitude of the burn, the time after injury, and the effects of co-administered drugs, alone or in combination, as well as alterations in protein binding and volume of distribution, may have a role in these conflicting reports.

## CENTRAL NERVOUS SYSTEM

The central nervous system (CNS) may be adversely affected by inhalation of neurotoxic chemicals or by hypoxic encephalopathy; other contributing factors include sepsis, hyponatremia, and hypovolemia.[80] CNS dysfunction includes hallucinations, personality changes, delirium, seizures, abnormal neurologic symptoms, and coma.[81] These effects may be due to the burn injury or to the administration of drugs necessary for sedation, anxiolysis, and analgesia.[82] Such effects usually clear after several weeks. Abnormalities of CNS neurotransmitters have been postulated to mediate the anorexia associated with extensive burn injury.[83] The possibility of cerebral edema and increased intracranial pressure also must be considered during the initial phases of burn injury. Under such circumstances, the usual measures for treating increased intracranial pressure would be instituted (see Chapter 24). Data suggest that rapid overcorrection of hyponatremia also may be associated with cerebral injury.[84]

## HEMATOLOGIC

Blood viscosity may increase as a result of hemoconcentration secondary to fluid shifts and because of alterations in plasma protein content.[85] The hematopoietic system is also adversely affected. Ongoing microangiopathic hemolytic anemia secondary to the burn injury is common.[86] An inhibitor of erythroid stem cells has been found in the sera of burn patients, which may in part contribute to the anemia of burn injury. Another study has demonstrated a normal erythropoietin response to anemia in patients with burn injury.[87] The half-life of red blood cells is diminished in burn patients, and multiple blood draws may contribute to the development of anemia.[88,89] The possible role of recombinant erythropoietin in the care of children with burns has yet to be defined.[90,91] One study in adults reported no reduction in either mortality or blood transfusion requirements in patients who received recombinant erythropoietin compared with controls.[92]

In the early stage, thrombocytopenia secondary to increased platelet aggregation and trapping of platelets in the lungs is followed by an increase in platelet count 10 to 14 days after the burn injury. A prolonged period of thrombocytopenia and reduced nadir in platelet count compared to survivors are both associated with increased mortality.[93] This thrombocytopenia may persist for several months.[89,93] An increase in fibrin split products (disseminated intravascular coagulopathy), which lasts for 3 to 5 days, may occur.[62] Factors V, VII, and VIII and fibrinogen are also increased several-fold over baseline for the first 3 months after severe injury uncomplicated by sepsis.[94,95] Children with increased platelet counts (>1 million/mm$^3$) who then developed sepsis in our unit experienced a marked decrease in the platelet count. The sudden onset of thrombocytopenia should prompt an evaluation of the child for sepsis.[96] Likewise, large swings in the fibrinogen concentration can occur (up to 2 g/dL),[97] although these do not appear to herald an increase in the incidence of thrombotic events.

## GASTROINTESTINAL

Gastrointestinal function is diminished immediately after thermal injury secondary to the onset of gastric stasis and intestinal ileus.[98] Because of the risk of pulmonary aspiration of gastric contents during this time, the stomach should be adequately vented and appropriate gastric acid ulcer prophylaxis instituted. At 48 to 72 hours after a burn injury, when generalized edema is resolving, gastrointestinal function usually resumes. Enteral feeding should be established at this time to provide calories, to blunt the hypermetabolic response, and to attenuate gluconeogenesis and stress ulceration.[85,99,100] Early enteral feeding has the added advantages of diminishing muscle catabolism, reducing bacterial translocation through the intestinal mucosa and is associated with reduced mortality.[101-104]

In children who do not tolerate enteral feeding, parenteral nutrition must be initiated.[99,105-107] Stress ulcers (Curling ulcers) are associated with any burn injury and may be life-threatening, although the incidence has decreased in critically ill patients, in part because of improved pharmacologic control of gastric acidity.[108] Prospective studies of pediatric and adult burn patients and patients in intensive care indicate that cimetidine or ranitidine in the usual doses does not adequately protect critically ill patients from increases in gastric acidity.[60,61] The increased requirement for drugs is due to differences in their pharmacokinetics.[60] Therefore frequent feedings when tolerated and the liberal use of antacids, combined with larger or more frequent doses of $H_2$-receptor antagonists (or proton pump inhibitors), may be required to prevent development of stress ulcers.[60,85,98]

### ENDOCRINE

The endocrinologic response to acute thermal injury is complex, involving most organ systems. Stimuli that trigger endocrine responses include the thermal injury itself and subsequent fluid shifts, as well as the stress responses that are associated with critical illness.[109] These may include decreased circulating hormone concentrations (e.g., triiodothyronine, dehydroepiandrosterone, and testosterone), as well as increased concentrations of other hormones (antidiuretic hormone, catecholamines, renin, angiotensin II, and cortisol).[110] Replacement therapy with synthetic androgenic steroids (e.g., oxandrolone) shortens acute hospital stay and improves body composition (lean body mass) and hepatic protein synthesis.[111,112] Glucose control may be poor, owing to the increased levels of cortisol and insulin resistance.[113] Tight control of hyperglycemia may improve mitochondrial oxidative capacity,[114] decrease the incidence of urinary tract infection, and improves the survival of critically ill burn patients, although the last finding resulted from a single study.[115,116] Avoiding hyperglycemia may attenuate the risk of cerebral injury from hypoperfusion states (see Chapters 24 and 39); one group recommends a target blood glucose level of 130 mg/dL.[116] Blocking the renin-angiotensin system may improve the insulin response after burn injury.[117] It should be noted that insulin resistance might persist for 6 to 9 months after discharge.[114]

### SKIN

Extensive skin destruction results in the inability to regulate body heat, conserve fluids and electrolytes, and protect against bacterial invasion. Permeability of burned tissues is markedly increased and proportional to the number of layers of tissue damaged.[118] Because children have a much greater ratio of body surface area to weight compared with adults, they are even more likely to become hypothermic (see Fig. 34-1). Thus it is important to keep these children covered as much as possible, to increase the environmental temperature, and to use radiant warmers, plastic wrap around extremities, reflective insulated blankets, artificial "noses" (in-line moisture and heat exchangers), and hot-air heating blankets. Late complications affecting the skin include progressive scar formation, which results in movement-restricting contractures.[24,119] Topical antibiotic and antibacterial therapy is necessary to prevent burn wound sepsis.[120-125]

### METABOLIC

Many metabolic alterations follow extensive burn injury. Increased usage of glucose, fat, and protein results in greater $O_2$ demand and increased carbon dioxide ($CO_2$) production.* Mediators that have been implicated in these metabolic changes include interleukin-1, tumor necrosis factor, catecholamines, prostanoids, and other stress hormones.[2,133] Centrally mediated or sepsis-induced hyperthermia also increases $O_2$ consumption and $CO_2$ production. Some of these abnormalities may persist even after complete closure of the burn wounds, when metabolic demand is already reduced.† Intravenous alimentation, particularly with increased glucose concentrations, may also increase $CO_2$ production and therefore increase ventilatory requirements.[105] Increase in $O_2$ demand[135] and $CO_2$ production must be compensated for during controlled mechanical ventilation. Treatment of fever reduces metabolic demand.[136]

### CALCIUM HOMEOSTASIS

The ionized calcium concentrations in many acutely burned patients are dramatically decreased. Marked abnormalities in the indices of calcium and magnesium metabolism, including hypoparathyroidism in both acute and recovery phases, may persist for weeks after injury (E-Fig. 34-1).[137,138] One study suggested that short-term therapy with pamidronate, a drug that inhibits bone resorption, conserves bone mass after burn injury in children.[139] Hypophosphatemia and hypermagnesemia revert toward normal during the latter phase of recovery from the acute injury. The usual reciprocal relationship between calcium and inorganic phosphate is not evident in those with major burns. Therefore supplemental calcium therapy is extremely important, particularly when rapid colloid infusions are required intraoperatively during burn surgeries, because ionized hypocalcemia dramatically impairs cardiovascular homeostasis. In general, frequent small boluses of calcium are safer and more effective than intermittent large boluses (see also Figs. 10-8 and 10-9).[140] Doses of 2.5 mg/kg calcium chloride or 7.5 mg/kg calcium gluconate ionize at equivalent rates and produce equivalent increases in calcium concentration. After recovery from burn injury, vitamin D supplements are strongly recommended to offset the decreased conversion of 7-dehydrocholesterol to previtamin $D_3$.[141]

### PSYCHIATRIC

It is imperative to recognize that physical trauma is not the only trauma sustained by the pediatric burn patient; psychological trauma and its associated long-term sequelae is also common.[142,143] A large percentage of acutely burned children present with acute stress or develop posttraumatic stress disorders.[142-145] Risk factors for developing acute stress disorders include the size of burn, the degree of pain, the pulse rate, and parental issues.[146] Treatment with fluoxetine or imipramine may ameliorate these stress disorders,[147-149] although one randomized controlled study found no difference from placebo.[150] Another study found risperidone to be of value in reducing stress symptoms.[151] There is an increased incidence of attention-deficit disorders in pediatric burn patients, likely owing to impulsivity.[152,153] Finally, the normal psychosocial support network may be impaired in the families of the burn patient, even before the burn injury.[154-156]

## Pharmacology

Subsequent to any major thermal injury, many physiologic changes occur that have an impact on the disposition of drugs in the body. During the hypovolemic period, uptake and clearance of drugs may decrease because of impaired organ perfusion.[2,73-76,157] During the hypermetabolic phase, the activity of organs that clear drugs from the circulation (e.g., the liver and kidneys) may be enhanced because of enzyme induction and increased blood flow to those organs.* The massive volume of edema present and the loss of drug through burn wounds can increase the central or total volume of drug distribution.[162]

Many drugs are highly bound by plasma proteins. The activity of such drugs depends primarily on the unbound rather than

---

*References 2, 68, 85, 105, 121, 126-132.
†References 14, 17, 18, 38, 40, 134.

*References 59, 60, 63, 68, 73, 79, 157-161.

total drug concentrations, and small changes in the unbound fraction may have a dramatic effect on the response to the drug. The two major binding proteins, $\alpha_1$-acid glycoprotein and albumin, increase and decrease, respectively, after burn injury, resulting in either decreased or increased free fractions of those drugs to which they bind.[73,161] For example, the clearance of morphine and meperidine is enhanced or impaired, depending on the size of the burn, with a trend to reduced morphine or meperidine clearance after large burns compared with moderate burns. In general, burned children clear drugs more readily than those without burn injuries.[75-77,162-164] Similarly, pharmacokinetic studies of lorazepam and diazepam indicate that the clearance of the former is increased whereas that of the latter decreases.[78,79] In the case of oral ketamine, the pharmacokinetics were unaffected in children with small burns.[165]

Evidence indicates that burn injury, with its complications and hormonal responses, may affect the number of receptors in tissues.[78,83,157,161,166-173] Therefore reports of aberrant responses to drugs acting on adrenergic and cholinergic receptors are not surprising. These include altered sensitivity to succinylcholine at the neuromuscular junction, increased sensitivity to dopamine in the pulmonary circulation, and decreased sensitivity to non-depolarizing neuromuscular blocking drugs.[73,166,168-170,174-176] Other examples of drugs affected by burn-induced kinetic and dynamic changes include aminoglycoside antibiotics, diazepam, and cimetidine. Burn-induced alterations in kinetics and dynamics make the clinical response to any medication unpredictable. Therefore clinical effects should always be closely monitored and plasma concentrations, protein binding, and clearance evaluated whenever possible.[60,63,73,177-181] Dexmedetomidine (see later) also may have altered pharmacodynamics in the burned child. Because of the known hypotensive effects of the $\alpha_{2a}$-adrenoceptor

agonists, particular attention to limit the dose and to ensure euvolemia may minimize the hemodynamic consequences.

## Resuscitation and Initial Evaluation

Resuscitation of children with a burn injury requires a clear and secure airway, as well as maintenance of adequate oxygenation, perfusion, and circulating blood volume. The diagnosis and evaluation of associated injuries also must be considered.

### AIRWAY AND OXYGENATION

Every burn patient, especially those with inhalation injuries, must be considered hypoxemic and exposed to carbon monoxide (CO). Therefore during transport to the hospital and on admission, administration of high inspired concentrations of $O_2$ is mandatory, pending evaluation of the severity of CO poisoning and pulmonary injury (see later).[181] Direct injury to the airway and alveoli occurs in children who have sustained pulmonary injury from the inhalation of smoke, flames, noxious gases, heated air, or steam.[42,51,133,182-211] When a child is burned in an enclosed space (house, automobile) or if thermal burns or carbonaceous materials are evident about the mouth and nose, inhalational injury is probable.[192,212] Upper airway obstruction caused by edema of the lips, nose, tongue, pharynx, glottis, and subglottis is very common. The resultant airway obstruction can be compared with the combined effects of acute macroglossia, epiglottitis, macro uvula, and laryngotracheobronchitis. The decreasing patency of the airway resulting from rapidly increasing edema, beginning in the first hours after the injury and lasting several days, makes delayed intubation hazardous if not impossible (Fig. 34-4). Prophylactic intubation should be performed in any case of severe facial burns or when pulmonary burn and upper

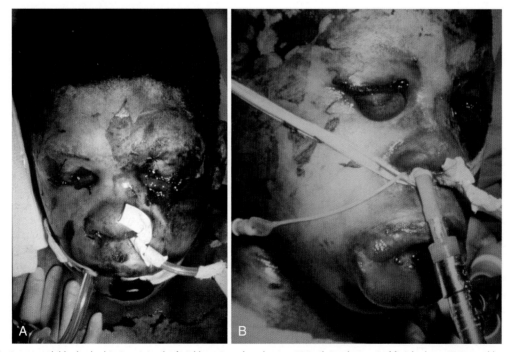

**FIGURE 34-4 A,** A young child who had just sustained a facial burn in a closed space. Note the early onset of facial edema. **B,** Several hours later there is massive edema that extends into the oropharynx, larynx, and trachea (similar to the combined effects of macroglossia, epiglottitis, and laryngotracheobronchitis). Early prophylactic intubation is mandatory in any facial burn or in any child when there is potential for inhalation injury. Note that the cuffed endotracheal tube was changed from an oral to a nasal position and that it is secured with cloth tape rather than adhesive tape.

airway inhalation injury are suspected. The severity of adverse outcomes is related to the presence or absence of inhalation injury.[51,200-211,213]

Control of the airway in children is usually accomplished under general anesthesia. In the case of pure inhalational injury without facial or upper airway burns, the need for intubation should be considered on a case-by-case basis. Early clinical experience at our hospital showed that tracheal tubes could be left in place in these children for weeks with fewer risks than the alternative, tracheostomy.[214,215] Tracheostomy in thermally injured children was associated with high mortality rates; in one pediatric series the death rate approached 100%.[216] However, in recent years there has been a move back to performing tracheostomy for children who are expected to require long-term ventilatory management. Although one review of burn centers in North America found that the practice of performing a tracheostomy in burned children was variable, there has been increasing tendency to perform a tracheostomy in children over age 7.[217] Some report that an early tracheostomy secures the airway and reduces the risk of subglottic stenosis.[218,219] When early airway instrumentation is indicated, a cuffed tracheal tube is preferred to reduce the need for changing the tube to deliver high peak inspiratory pressures should they be required.[220] Traditionally, cuffed tracheal tubes have not been used in children younger than 8 years. This practice may not be necessary with proper attention to leak pressures (pressure at which gas can be heard "leaking" around the tracheal cuff by auscultating over the trachea while administering positive pressure) or the use of the MICROCUFF (Kimberly-Clark, Roswell, Ga.) tube (see later), although long-term studies with these tubes are needed (see Chapter 12).[221,222] We routinely use cuffed tracheal tubes, appreciating the added flexibility they offer in not requiring replacement because of decreasing edema (with associated increased leak if uncuffed tubes were used). Another important means of minimizing barotrauma is the use of permissive hypercarbia.[223] New tracheal tubes that are designed to have the cuff located more distally and made of thinner material (MICROCUFF) may also reduce the potential for airway injury (see also Figs. 12-15 and 12-17), although in the hot environment of a burn unit they may have a greater tendency toward kinking.[224-228]

## CARBON MONOXIDE POISONING AND CYANIDE POISONING

The majority of smoke inhalation victims have CO poisoning. Direct measurement of carboxyhemoglobin (COHb) is an important guide to the adequacy of treatment. Estimates of the COHb concentration may be derived by measuring (not calculating) $O_2$ saturation or arterial $O_2$ content. The half-life of COHb is approximately 5 hours when the patient is breathing room air but decreases to 90 minutes when 100% $O_2$ is administered.[229,230] Immediate administration of $O_2$ is therefore essential to achieve the maximum possible level of $O_2$ in the blood; positive-pressure ventilation may be indicated in severe cases.[231-233] Hyperbaric oxygen may be a useful adjunct for this purpose (see later).

Standard pulse oximeters do not differentiate between oxyhemoglobin and COHb; in contrast, transcutaneous $O_2$ analyzers and cooximeters are useful.[234] Thus pulse oximetry cannot be used to accurately monitor the oxygenation of patients with CO poisoning because COHb produces an overestimation of $O_2$ saturation; the photo detector is "fooled" into interpreting

COHb as oxyhemoglobin.[234-236] A more recent eight-wavelength pulse oximeter capable of measuring COHb and methemoglobin may prove useful in the management of burn patients[237,238]; however, the sensors are quite expensive and likely should be reserved for use in those with an established diagnosis, unless arterial blood gas analysis is not immediately available.[239]

COHb is produced by the combination of CO with the iron of the heme radical at the $O_2$-binding site. CO combines more slowly with hemoglobin than $O_2$ but is bound 200 times more firmly.[240,241] Inhalation of 1% CO for 2 minutes can result in COHb values of 30% (E-Fig. 34-2).[242] The toxic effects of CO poisoning are due to tissue, organ, and cellular hypoxia from decreased $O_2$ delivery. Decreased delivery occurs because CO reduces $O_2$ binding capacity both to the hemoglobin molecule at the tissue level and to cytochromes in the respiratory chain at the cellular level; even in small amounts, COHb shifts the $O_2$-dissociation curve to the left (E-Fig. 34-3), thus reducing release of $O_2$ from hemoglobin.[42,181,231,241-245] For example, if an individual had 40% carboxyhemoglobin, this would reduce $O_2$ carrying capacity from 20 mL/100 g of hemoglobin to 12 mL/100 g and with the leftward shift further compromise $O_2$ delivery.

The evidence supporting the use of hyperbaric oxygenation (HBO) therapy as an adjunct therapy for burns remains controversial.[85,246-250] A Cochrane review of six randomized controlled trials with 1361 patients concluded that at present insufficient data exist to demonstrate reduced adverse neurologic outcomes with HBO therapy and that additional research is needed to "better define the role, if any, of HBO in the treatment of patients with CO poisoning."[251] The most common indication for hyperbaric therapy in burned children is concomitant CO poisoning.[42,252,253] As previously mentioned, CO binds avidly to hemoglobin[254] and other iron-containing enzymes, such as intramitochondrial cytochromes, interfering with the delivery and usage of $O_2$, respectively.[255,256] Children suffering significant CO exposure are at risk of developing both acute and delayed neurologic sequelae. The pathophysiology of neurologic sequelae is not known, although imaging studies suggest a potentially reversible demyelinating process.[257,258] Data supporting the use of hyperbaric $O_2$ to prevent and treat these complications may be weak[259-266] but cannot be discounted, given the seriousness of these sequelae.[248,249,267,268]

The important practical question is whether hyperbaric treatment will decrease the frequency and severity of delayed neurologic sequelae in burned children with concomitant CO poisoning. This is a difficult question because the incidence of delayed sequelae is unknown and determining the severity of an individual exposure is often not possible. Delayed sequelae include headaches, irritability, personality changes, confusion, memory loss, and gross motor deficits. The frequency with which those exposed develop symptoms is unknown, although they are reported to occur in approximately 10% of patients with serious exposures.[243] A symptom-free interval of several days is commonly reported. Delayed hyperbaric treatment may relieve symptoms, and spontaneous resolution of delayed sequelae may be expected in up to 75% of patients within 1 year.[269-275] The severity of the CO poisoning is often difficult to pinpoint because there is a poor correlation between serum COHb and degree of CO exposure.[276,277] Neuropsychiatric testing has been proposed as a more accurate way to determine this,[229] but such detailed examinations are difficult in burned children secondary to pain medications and hemodynamic instability. Some clinicians believe that a history of unconsciousness indicates that an exposure has been severe enough to warrant treatment.[271,278-280] However, the relatively few randomized prospective studies evaluating this have returned conflicting results.[262,266] Hyperbaric $O_2$ treatment is not without expense, inconvenience, and risk, and the indications for treatment of burned children with concomitant CO poisoning are debated.[256,281] One study described complications during treatment of a heterogeneous groups of patients: emesis (6%), seizures (5%), agitation requiring restraints or sedation (2%), cardiac dysrhythmias or cardiac arrests (2%), arterial hypotension (2%), and tension pneumothorax (1%).[256] Complications may be expected more frequently in the critically ill.[282]

Hyperbaric $O_2$ treatment is probably appropriate in burned children with documented or strongly suspected serious CO poisoning who are hemodynamically stable, not requiring ongoing burn resuscitation, and not wheezing or air trapping and in whom such treatment does not require interfacility transport, which is inconsistent with good general burn treatment.

Cyanide toxicity may occur in inhalational burn injuries as well.[283] If cyanide poisoning is confirmed in the child's blood, administration of hydroxycobalamin or sodium thiosulfate, alone or in combination, is warranted (see Chapter 10).[284] HBO therapy has been shown to facilitate movement of cyanide out of tissues and into blood, thereby potentially facilitating treatment,[283] although the use of HBO for treatment remains investigational.

## ADEQUACY OF CIRCULATION

The various formulas for determining fluid replacement are estimates and often need modification, depending on clinical and laboratory findings.* The most widely accepted fluid protocols in current use are the Parkland (Baxter) and Brooke formulas. All formulas and guidelines for fluid therapy require modification according to the individual child, depending on the child's response (Table 34-1).[6] The most important metric of fluid homeostasis remains a good urine output (0.5 to 1 mL/kg/hr).

Both formulas provide estimates of the fluid volume required for resuscitation, in addition to the calculated normal maintenance fluid requirement for each day. *These formulas are of great value in guiding the fluid resuscitation of older children; however, serious underestimation of the fluid volume may occur if applied to infants weighing less than 10 kg.* In such infants, it is reasonable to estimate the normal hourly maintenance fluid requirements and then add to this the fluid volume of the Parkland or Brooke formula.[2] Alternatively, the crystalloid fluid regimen for resuscitation can be increased to 6 mL/kg × the percent surface area burn per 24 hours.[297,298]

The degree of edema depends on the volume and composition of the resuscitation fluid administered. Consequently, colloids or hypertonic saline (with or without albumin) are used in some burn centers during early burn wound resuscitation.[299] These modified regimens have been shown to be particularly effective in the very young and the elderly.† The purported advantage is less tissue edema. It is of interest that a Cochrane review of 15 studies using hypertonic saline in 614 patients found that less intravenous fluid was needed for resuscitation and higher sodium values occurred, although the overall morbidity and mortality was unchanged.[301]

A growing practice in burn programs has been to begin the fluid resuscitation with colloid, usually 5% albumin, early during

---

*References 2, 5, 19, 85, 130, 133, 285-296.
†References 2, 85, 133, 290, 291, 296-298, 300.

**TABLE 34-1** Parkland and Brooke Formulas

| Formula | FLUID THERAPY | | |
|---|---|---|---|
| | Crystalloid (mL/kg) | Colloid (mL/kg) | |
| Parkland | 4.0 | +0 | × Percent burn × wt (kg) |
| Brooke | 0.45 | +1.5 | × Percent burn × wt (kg) |

NOTE: Half this volume is administered during the first 8 hours and the remainder during the next 16 hours. Infants who weigh less than 10 kg may have even greater fluid requirements (see text).

resuscitation of seriously burned children.[302] No consensus has been reached on such a colloid protocol.[303] In seriously burned children in our unit, we begin with a 5% albumin solution at a maintenance rate immediately on admission. We administer an amount equal to that of their calculated crystalloid requirements, tapering the crystalloid first, and continuing albumin fusion for 48 hours. Further work is required before advocating hypertonic fluid regimens in burned children routinely.[304]

The syndrome of hyperosmolar hyperglycemic nonketotic coma (severe dehydration, marked hyperglycemia, serum hyperosmolality, and coma in the absence of ketoacidosis) may be associated with burns. Avoiding this syndrome is critically important because it carries a high mortality.[285] Glucose-containing solutions should be restricted at all times, particularly during the initial volume resuscitation. Serum glucose concentrations should be measured frequently during this period. Blood glucose concentrations should be managed with insulin with a target blood glucose of 130 mg/dL.[116]

The general appearance of the child and his or her sensorium provide important guides to the effectiveness of the resuscitative therapy. In addition, urine output is a useful metric to determine the need for additional fluid administration, recognizing that antidiuretic hormone secretion may be increased and renal tubular dysfunction may be present.[20,158] Every effort must be made to protect kidney function by providing adequate fluid replacement.[2,304] Renal failure in the presence of a major burn is usually lethal. However, overly aggressive fluid administration may induce pulmonary and tissue edema. Therefore, when a burned child is being volume resuscitated, all fluids to replace the circulating blood volume must be carefully titrated. Commonly used end points of satisfactory fluid resuscitation include heart rate, systemic arterial blood pressure, urinary output, central venous pressure, arterial oxygenation, and pH. Cardiovascular function estimated by transthoracic or transesophageal echocardiography[29] and technetium-99m ventriculography may be of value in critically ill patients.[305,306] These advanced cardiac evaluations are not required in most children; they are mostly useful in the presence of cardiovascular compromise and a need to consider the use of a vasopressor or additional volume loading.

In a child, the evaporative fluid losses exceed 4000 mL/m² of burn surface each day, compared with only 2500 mL/m² in an adult.[290] Concomitantly, for each square meter of burn surface, 2500 to 4000 kcal of heat is lost each day. Minimizing caloric expenditure and providing caloric supplementation simultaneously are the only ways to minimize catabolism of body tissues. The tendency for children to be poikilothermic, particularly in the absence of protective skin as a result of the burn injury, causes profound temperature derangements. Efforts to maintain

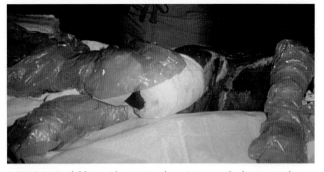

**FIGURE 34-5** Children with extensive burn injury can be kept warm by having the extremities wrapped with sterile plastic bags. Covering the head is also an important method of heat preservation.

a normal body temperature are essential in both the operating room and the intensive care unit. These measures are especially important during the initial volume resuscitation and in the operating room when dressings are removed for examination and excision (Fig. 34-5).

## ASSOCIATED INJURY

Associated injuries such as a tension pneumothorax, a ruptured spleen or liver, long-bone fractures, or head injury may be missed, especially during the initial assessment and early phase of burn wound fluid resuscitation. Taking a detailed history, especially from the emergency medical personnel and family, combined with a careful physical examination, is mandatory during the initial resuscitation because such injuries may compound or be hidden by the need for an increased volume of resuscitation fluids. The type of burn injury (e.g., explosion, electrical) may trigger concerns for associated injuries (e.g., shrapnel wounds).

## CIRCUMFERENTIAL BURNS

Adverse cardiovascular and respiratory responses are immediate to circumferential burns of the chest, abdomen, and extremities.[2,24,196,197] Circumferential burns of the thorax can restrict respiratory effort, resulting in respiratory failure as a result of decreased chest wall compliance. Functional residual capacity is reduced with airway closure and atelectasis, resulting in profound hypoxemia.[42,183-187,190-198,307] Deep circumferential burns of the chest and abdomen may generate excessive intrathoracic and intraabdominal pressure, which, in addition to restricting diaphragmatic movement, may further reduce the already decreased cardiac output by impairing venous return (Fig. 34-6).[24,196,197] When this occurs, both extrapulmonary and intrapulmonary factors can contribute to arterial desaturation.[50]

The edema of damaged tissues also can generate severe compressive forces, restricting or occluding the blood flow to burned extremities. The net result may be ischemia of the limb, which if left untreated, may lead to partial or total amputation. Escharotomies of circumferential burns of the chest, abdomen, and extremities must be performed urgently because impaired hemodynamics and respiratory mechanics can cause irreversible damage within hours of the burn injury. Escharotomy is often undertaken without the need for general anesthesia because a full-thickness burn usually destroys skin innervation. Abdominal compartment syndrome may develop in children who require large volume resuscitation. To detect any evolving compartment syndrome, some burn centers advocate routine monitoring of bladder pressure.[307,308]

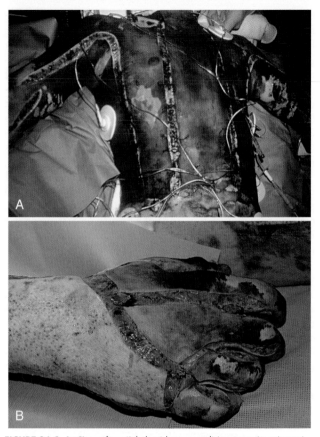

**FIGURE 34-6 A,** Circumferential chest burns result in severe impairment of respirations secondary to the tourniquet effect of the shrinking eschar and subcutaneous edema. The widely separated escharotomy lines indicate the severity of the constriction. **B,** Similar effects occur in circumferentially burned extremities. Early escharotomy may help to preserve blood flow and obviate amputation.

## ELECTRICAL BURNS

Electrical burns occur with household voltage (electric cords and sockets) and nonhousehold high-voltage current (power line or lightning). Children often disconnect extension cords by stabilizing one end in their mouths and pulling the other end with a hand, resulting in circumoral and lingual burns.[4,53,309,310] High-voltage injuries are often associated with loss of limbs and other injuries that are not immediately obvious.[311-314] The extent of this injury is unpredictable. The surface injury is often small, but the extent of underlying tissue damage and necrosis is massive. Such an injury is a combination of electrical and thermal damage.[314,315] Victims often have concurrent injuries such as fractures of vertebrae or long bones, ruptured organs, myocardial injury, or numerous contusions. Even children with low-voltage injuries may have abnormalities of cardiac conduction.[312] Children with electrical burns may be comatose or have sustained seizures at the time of admission to the hospital. Muscle tissue adjacent to bone is usually more damaged than superficial muscles because bone is a poor conductor of electrical current, and therefore heats up when high currents are passed through it, resulting in damage to the muscles surrounding bone. Early fasciotomy may be needed to preserve the blood flow to extremities (Fig. 34-7). Myonecrosis necessitates general anesthesia during the first day of injury at the time when fluid shifts, hyperkalemia, and myoglobinuria are maximal. Massive myonecrosis and hemolysis may result in hyperkalemia, as well as myoglobinuria and hemoglobinuria. In the presence of hemoglobinuria or myoglobinuria, increased fluids and mannitol will ensure a continuous urine output (>1 mL/kg/hr).[316,317] Alkalization of the urine may prevent these proteins from precipitating in the renal tubules. Follow-up of patients with electrical injuries often reveals

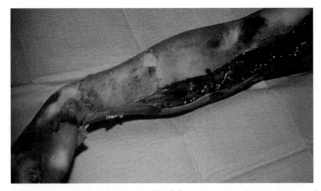

**FIGURE 34-7** Electrical injuries tend to follow neurovascular structures and have an entry as well as an exit wound. The skin might appear normal but the underlying structures may have had extensive injury. These children require a fasciotomy rather than just a simple escharotomy to preserve blood flow to the deep structures. In general, this is required on the first day of injury for best results in tissue preservation.

unpredictable sequelae, which may manifest months to years later. These injuries may occur in organs or areas that do not appear abnormal during the acute course of illness. These late complications most frequently include neurologic dysfunction, ocular damage, damage to the gastrointestinal tract, circumoral strictures, changes in the electrocardiogram, and delayed hemorrhage from large vessels.[315,317]

## Guidelines to Anesthetic Management

Anesthetic management of children with severe thermal injury begins with the initial resuscitation and continues for many years through reconstructive surgery. Knowledge and understanding of the pathophysiology of burn injury enable anesthesiologists to plan appropriate anesthetic management and recognize and treat complications arising as a result of burn injury or its therapy (Table 34-2).[2,12,318]

Children who require surgery for burn wound excision and grafting must be properly prepared physiologically and psychologically, and specific equipment must be available in the operating room. Children who have not had surgical debridement and have had the burn for a week or longer must be considered septic. Such children often demonstrate severe cardiovascular instability during burn wound excision likely because of acute bacteremia.

**TABLE 34-2** Systemic Effects of Burn Injury

| System | Early Effects | Late Effects |
|---|---|---|
| Cardiovascular | ↓ CO as a result of decreased circulating blood volume, myocardial depressant factor | ↑ CO as a result of sepsis<br>↑ CO 2 to 3 times > baseline for months (hypermetabolism)<br>Hypertension secondary to vasoactive substances such as renin |
| Pulmonary | Upper airway obstruction as a result of edema<br>Lower airway obstruction as a result of edema, bronchospasm, particulate matter, sloughing of airway mucosa<br>↓ FRC<br>↓ Pulmonary compliance<br>↓ Chest wall compliance | Bronchopneumonia<br>Tracheal stenosis, vocal cord granuloma<br>↓ Chest wall compliance |
| Renal | ↓ GFR secondary to<br>  ↓ circulating blood volume<br>  Myoglobinuria<br>  Hemoglobinuria<br>  Tubular dysfunction | ↑ GFR secondary to ↑ CO<br><br>Tubular dysfunction |
| Hepatic | ↓ Function as a result of ↓ circulating blood volume, hypoxia, hepatotoxins | Hepatitis<br><br>↑ Function as a result of hypermetabolism, enzyme induction, ↑ CO<br>↓ Function as a result of sepsis, drug interactions |
| Hematopoietic | ↓ Platelets<br>↑ Fibrin split products, consumptive coagulopathy, anemia | ↑ Platelets<br>↑ Clotting factors |
| Neurologic | Encephalopathy<br>Seizures<br>↑ ICP | Encephalopathy<br>Seizures<br>ICU psychosis |
| Skin | ↑ Heat, fluid, electrolyte loss | Contractures, scar formation, difficult IV access, difficult intubation |
| Metabolic | ↓ Ionized calcium | ↑ Oxygen consumption<br>↑ Carbon dioxide production<br>↓ Ionized calcium |
| Pharmacokinetics | Altered volume of distribution<br>Altered protein binding<br>Altered pharmacokinetics<br>Altered pharmacodynamics | Tolerance to opioids, sedatives<br>Enzyme induction, altered receptors<br>Drug interaction |

↓, Decrease in; ↑, increase in; *AIDS,* acquired immunodeficiency syndrome; *CO,* cardiac output; *FRC,* functional residual capacity; *GFR,* glomerular filtration rate; *ICP,* intracranial pressure; *ICU,* intensive care unit.

In such cases, it is advantageous to have infusions of dopamine, epinephrine, or norepinephrine prepared for administration before induction of anesthesia.

Psychological support must be provided by parents, nurses, physicians, and trained psychologists. It is important for anesthesiologists to understand that the families of children who have sustained a severe burn injury feel a great deal of psychological stress and guilt. This stress may be transferred to anger at the physicians, nurses, and other members of the burn care team. The parents are angry that their child has sustained a devastating injury and occasionally vent this anger and frustration. It is therefore vital that the entire burn care team understand this response, that they spend as much time as possible listening to the parents' concerns, and that they emphasize all that is being done to ensure the very best care for their child. Specific nurses and physicians should be designated to communicate with the family to avoid misunderstandings and confusion about issues of patient care. The anesthesia care team, while explaining the risks of anesthesia, must emphasize the extensive monitoring and the central role that anesthesiologists have in ensuring the well-being of their child. Special emphasis must be placed on methods for minimizing physical and psychological pain during transport to the operating room, in the operating room, and postoperatively.

Keeping children with severe burn injuries on nothing by mouth (NPO) status for 8 hours or longer before sedation for a dressing change or anesthesia for a surgical procedure severely compromises caloric intake; therefore we advocate the use of continuous orojejunal or nasojejunal alimentation. Generally children can receive calories up to about 4 hours before sedation or induction without fear of significant gastric residual volumes. Feeding can be resumed almost immediately after the procedure. In children with large injuries who will quickly develop a negative nitrogen balance with cessation of enteral feedings, short-term use of parenteral protein-sparing support is justified and safe.[319]

Adequate sedation and pain control are necessary before moving children to the operating room. This move is painful, both physically and emotionally, for the child. Intravenous opioids, such as fentanyl, which has minimal histamine release, are particularly helpful. Intravenous midazolam is also helpful for its sedative and amnestic properties. Drug doses should not be based on standard doses used in children without thermal injury. Burned children develop tolerance to most opioids and sedatives, thus requiring increasing doses over time to achieve a satisfactory clinical response.[320,321] The dose of sedative or opioid should be titrated to effect while the child is carefully observed and monitored. Children with burn injuries rapidly develop tolerance. It is not unusual for children with burns over greater than 25% of the body surface to require 1 mg/kg/hr of both morphine and midazolam to provide adequate analgesia and sedation.

Correction of intravascular volume before induction of anesthesia may require fluid boluses during and after sedation and before transport. Establishing adequate intravenous access preoperatively may be especially difficult in children with large burns. We use both topical anesthetic creams and needle-free subcutaneous local anesthetics to help make this process painless and stress free.

It is critically important to minimize heat loss and maintain normothermia. This is may be difficult to achieve because of the massive evaporative heat loss that occurs through open wounds. Operating room temperatures during extensive excisions are commonly maintained near 98.6° (37° C).[133] Attention must be paid to minimize heat loss both during transport and in the operating room. Multiple blankets or thermal reflective covers are helpful. Special equipment is used to maintain body temperature, including a warming blanket, radiant warmer, blood warmer, and heat/moisture exchangers and forced hot air warmers. Simply wrapping the extremities in sterile plastic bags and covering the head with plastic or thermal insulation material markedly reduces heat and fluid losses (see Fig. 34-5). Although a hot operating room is uncomfortable for staff, maintaining the child's temperature may be helpful in maintaining normal blood clotting. Each calorie that does not have to be spent to maintain body temperature is one more that can be used in the healing process.

Adequate monitoring for major blood loss and fluid shifts includes arterial and central venous cannulas, a urinary catheter, an electrocardiograph, a pulse oximeter, a capnograph, and an esophageal stethoscope. A secure intravenous route for volume infusion is essential. If the potential for rapid blood loss exists, multilumen catheters may not be adequate because of their high-flow resistance. Rapid infusion devices may be particularly helpful (see Chapter 51).[322-324] The femoral vein is an alternative cannulation site, in addition to the internal jugular and subclavian veins (see Chapter 48).

Specific anesthetic equipment is used, including various sterilized laryngoscope blades, tracheal tubes, airways, and blood pressure cuffs.

Invasive arterial and central venous pressure monitoring may be established after induction of anesthesia in most children. Propofol, thiopental (if available), or ketamine in incremental doses is usually well tolerated, provided the children are not hypovolemic (onset of effect is noted by lateral nystagmus. (See Video 6-1: Nystagmus after Ketamine Administration.) Studies in children long recovered from acute burn injury found a 40% increase in the thiopental dose needed to ablate the lid reflex, compared with children without burn injury (Fig. 34-8).[325] Our experience suggests that the clinical response to propofol appears to be equally shifted to the right; however, clinical studies are lacking. Ketamine may, on occasion, be preferred if the adequacy of intravascular volume is in question or if invasive monitoring lines must be inserted before anesthetic induction; tolerance to ketamine with repeated administration has been reported.[326] High-dose fentanyl or morphine combined with nitrous oxide ($N_2O$) for those children who will undergo ventilation postoperatively is also an acceptable anesthetic technique. In general, an inhalation agent is titrated to clinical effect to supplement the opioid-based anesthetic. When using large bolus doses of fentanyl, chest wall rigidity is a possibility. A slow inhalation induction is preferable for children with a compromised airway, bearing in mind the potential for cardiovascular depression.[327]

Succinylcholine is contraindicated in burned children because of a potentially lethal efflux of potassium ions from muscle.[166,169,172] However, within the first 24 hours after a burn, succinylcholine can be used without apparent risk of triggering a hyperkalemic response. This abnormal response first appears 24 to 48 hours after the burn and continues for an indeterminate, but prolonged, period. Some have suggested that the hyperkalemic response continues until all areas of burn have been covered by scar tissue, although this is not evidence-based. Because the end point for succinylcholine-induced hyperkalemia is unknown, we advise avoiding succinylcholine in children with large burns (≥40%) for at least 1.5 years after the burn. The smallest burn reported to trigger a hyperkalemic response was a 9% burn. This

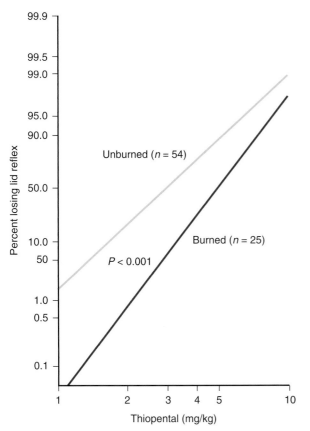

**FIGURE 34-8** The percentage of children (burned and unburned) who lost the lid reflex is compared with the intravenous bolus dose of thiopental. Note the marked shift in the dose-response curve. (From Coté CJ, Petkau AJ. Thiopental requirements may be increased in children reanesthetized at least one year after recovery from extensive thermal injury. Anesthesiology 1981;55:S338.)

abnormal response occurs because the entire muscle membrane, rather than just the myoneural junction, is occupied by acetylcholine receptors. The muscle tissue of burn victims also demonstrates resistance to nondepolarizing muscle relaxants.[169,328] We observed a child who demonstrated marked resistance to nondepolarizing neuromuscular blocking drugs (NMBDs) 463 days after burn injury. This response indirectly suggests that the hyperkalemic response may persist long after the acute injury phase of the burn.[329] The nondepolarizing NMBDs are therefore the relaxants of choice in children with a burn injury. It has been found that after burns over greater than 25% of body surface area, both the total dose of *d*-tubocurarine administered and the serum concentration necessary to attain a given degree of muscle twitch depression are three to five times greater than in children without burn injury.* Although *d*-tubocurarine is no longer used, similar observations have been made with the more modern nondepolarizing NMBDs (Fig. 34-9). If rapid intubation is needed and it is clear that the child's lungs can be ventilated, high doses of rocuronium (1.2 mg/kg) can be used. However, even 1.2 mg/kg of rocuronium may not provide adequate conditions for rapid intubation and larger doses may be indicated (Fig. 34-10).[330] Recovery from neuromuscular blockade has been observed at serum concentrations that would cause 100% twitch depression

---

*References 73, 157, 160, 169, 179, 180.

in children without burn injury. Studies with nondepolarizing NMBDs indicate that the hyposensitivity correlates well with the magnitude of burn ($r = 0.88$).[180,331-333] Protein binding and pharmacokinetic studies with *d*-tubocurarine indicate that these two factors contribute little to the enhanced requirements.[73,157,160,169] An increase in the number of acetylcholine receptors at junctional and extrajunctional areas and an altered affinity for the NMBD by those receptors have a major role in the elevated demand for nondepolarizing NMBDs.[168,174,328] Even with high doses of rocuronium, the onset time is prolonged compared with that in nonburned children.[334] Pharmacologic reversal of neuromuscular blockade, however, poses no special problem in burned children. Studies with intermediate- and short-acting nondepolarizing relaxants have shown resistance, but it is not as pronounced as has been observed with the long-acting relaxants.

Maintenance of anesthesia is usually accomplished with $N_2O$, $O_2$, an NMBD, and an opioid or inhalation agent. All of the commonly used anesthetic agents can be administered to burned children. Sevoflurane offers an advantage of smooth inhalation induction; isoflurane, desflurane, or halothane can be used for maintenance. No data show that repeated halothane anesthetics in burned children cause hepatotoxicity. All anesthetics cause concentration-dependent depression of cardiac output. In very ill children, anesthetic doses, but not NMBD requirements, are drastically reduced. In this injury, high-dose fentanyl-$O_2$ anesthesia is well tolerated. Ketamine may be the anesthetic agent of choice in specific circumstances, including those in which we wish to avoid airway manipulation after application of fresh facial grafts, for very brief procedures, or children who are unable to open their mouth for a standard laryngoscopy. Ketamine sedation may also be used along with midazolam for sedation before a trial of extubation. E-Figure 34-4 illustrates extubation of a child with a severe facial burn with the use of an airway exchange catheter to provide a ready means for possible reintubation should the trial fail. Some burn centers use ketamine as the sole anesthetic and find it quite satisfactory.[335] Ketamine can be used to potentiate the analgesic effects of opioids.[336] The postoperative analgesia and somnolence for prolonged periods produced by high-dose ketamine may be considered an advantage in some instances in which postoperative agitation might dislodge fresh skin grafts; one report describes long-term ketamine for sedation and analgesia.[337] Conversely, prolonged somnolence will delay reinstitution of critical enteral nutrition. Low-dose ketamine may be used postoperatively for its opioid-sparing effects.[338] Ketamine either alone or with propofol is commonly used for burn dressing changes.[339,340] An emerging experience with dexmedetomidine in children appears to demonstrate safety and efficacy in reducing otherwise common opioid tolerance and dose escalation.[341]

The inspired $O_2$ concentration is regulated according to the arterial blood gases and $O_2$ saturation. A pulse oximeter may not function properly on tissue discolored with silver nitrate; scraping the fingernail and cleaning the skin allow proper transmission and reception of the pulse oximeter light.[342] Pulse oximetry has a vital role in identifying evolving hypoxemia before the desaturation becomes life-threatening.[343] A pulse oximeter probe generally can function even on burned digits. If a child's digits are swollen or vasoconstriction prevents normal pulse oximeter function, alternative sites must be sought, such as the earlobe, nasal septum, or tongue. We have found the tongue to be particularly valuable. An additional benefit of using the tongue is that the tissues of the mouth apparently direct the interfering electrons

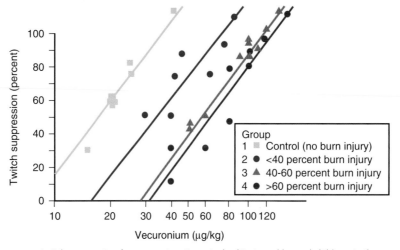

FIGURE 34-9 Logarithm of dose versus twitch suppression for vecuronium in control subjects and burned children. In the presence of acute injury, the vecuronium effective dose values increased with increasing burn size. The slopes of the curves were not different, but the intercepts were significantly different ($P < 0.01$). *Solid squares,* Children without burn injury; *purple circles,* children with less than 40% burn injury; *triangles,* children with 40% to 60% burn injury; *pink circles,* children with greater than 60% burn injury. (From Mills AK, Martyn JA. Neuromuscular blockade with vecuronium in paediatric patients with burn injury. Br J Clin Pharm 1989;28:155-159.)

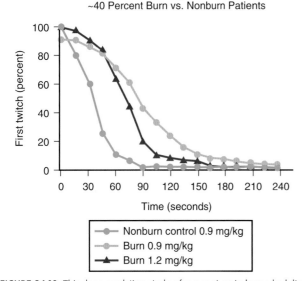

FIGURE 34-10 This dose escalation study of rocuronium in burned adults (approximately 40% body surface area) demonstrated severe resistance to the onset of neuromuscular blockade (percent of train-of-four first twitch). The time of onset could be reduced with higher doses; however, a dose of 1.2 mg/kg did not achieve complete paralysis until longer than 2 minutes had elapsed. These data suggest that if a rapid sequence induction were needed in patients with severe burns, an even higher as yet undefined dose would be required to shorten the time to complete relaxation. (Modified from Han TH, Kim HS, Bae JY, et al. Neuromuscular pharmacodynamics of rocuronium in patients with major burns. Anesth Analg 2004;99:386-392.)

of the electrocautery unit away from the pulse oximeter probe placed on the tongue (i.e., minimal electrocautery artifact occurs even when multiple electrocautery devices are used simultaneously).[243] A sealed oximeter probe that prevents electrical current leakage and leaching of adhesive can be easily modified (E-Fig. 34-5).[344,345] Newer reflectance oximeters may also have a role in the care of burned children.[346]

Because of increased metabolic rate, increased $CO_2$ production, and inhalation injury, an increase in alveolar ventilation compared with healthy children is often required. Blood gas analysis must therefore be assessed early and frequently throughout the anesthetic procedure. Constant monitoring of expired $CO_2$ is vital during intraoperative management. It is also necessary to be cognizant of the possibility of significant differences between arterial and expired $CO_2$ values as a result of shunting and dead space ventilation in children with severe pulmonary injury. *For these reasons, an expired $CO_2$ monitor may be used for trending and as a disconnect alarm but should not be relied on to adjust and assess the adequacy of ventilation.* The tracheal tube must be secured with tracheostomy tape because standard adhesive tape does not stick to burned tissue and wet dressings. Electrocardiographic leads also do not adhere and for this reason are placed under dependent portions of the body or sutured or stapled onto the skin after the patient is anesthetized. The standard measures for protecting the cornea from drying (including ophthalmic ointment and closing the eyelids when possible) and for positioning the limbs to prevent nerve compression must be observed.

The most important consideration of the intraoperative course is monitoring and correcting a child's blood losses. For this reason, invasive intravascular monitoring is essential. Children may lose as much as 1 to 3 blood volumes during each burn excision. It is therefore necessary to be familiar with the surgical approach to burn excision. During a tangential excision (Fig. 34-11 and Video 34-1), a child might lose 3 to 5 times more blood than during excisions down to fascia (Video 34-2). The liberal use of very dilute concentrations of epinephrine (500 μg/L in normal saline) injected subcutaneously in both donor and excision sites markedly reduces surgical blood loss (Fig. 34-12 and Video 34-3)[347]; our institution uses a 1:2,000,000 epinephrine-containing solution (0.5 μg/mL). As much as, or even more than, 10 μg/kg epinephrine may be injected every 20 minutes because of the desensitization to catecholamines.[173] It should be noted that significant fluid overload may occur several hours after surgery if excessive clysis or tumescent fluid is injected by the surgeons to facilitate harvesting of skin (Video 34-4). We have observed a number of infants (~≤10 kg) who developed pulmonary edema several hours after their surgical procedure. Blood loss also depends on the expertise of the surgical team,[348] and relatively "blood-free" excision and grafting has been described. It is difficult to estimate blood and fluid loss despite accurate weighing of surgical sponges because of significant losses hidden by the surgical drapes and evaporation. Other indicators of circulating blood volume, such as urine output, central venous pressure, arterial pressure, and shape of the arterial waveform (see Fig. 10-10), must be closely monitored.

Early excision of full-thickness burns has improved survival and shortened hospital stays.[349-351] In the past, we routinely observed that 5% of the blood volume was lost for every 1% of the body surface excised and grafted.[352,353] This extensive blood loss was a major source of morbidity and expense.[354,355] During the last several years, effective blood-conserving techniques for excision have been developed that have drastically reduced intraoperative blood loss. These techniques include (1) clearly planning the excision to be performed before its initiation; (2) performing all extremity excisions under pneumatic tourniquet, exsanguinating the extremity before tourniquet inflation, and wrapping the extremity in a hemostatic dressing before tourniquet deflation; (3) conducting all fascial excisions with coagulating electrocautery; (4) performing major layered excisions as soon as possible after injury, before significant wound hyperemia develops; (5) executing all layered torso excisions after subeschar

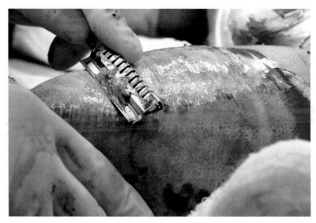

**FIGURE 34-11** Tangential skin excision in which multiple thin areas of burn tissue are excised until a viable vascular bed is achieved. This is indicated by brisk bleeding. This type of excision results in less scarring because the majority of fat tissue remains intact. However, this also results in significantly greater blood loss.

epinephrine clysis; (6) maintaining normothermia, primarily through maintaining a hot operating room (near 98.6° F [37° C]); and (7) subcutaneous injection of diluted epinephrine (with and without dilute bupivacaine) in donor areas.[356]

Large doses of epinephrine are well tolerated and markedly diminish bleeding. In a series of 25 consecutive children undergoing extensive layered excision, we used a total dose of epinephrine averaging 25 ± 3 μg/kg without complication.[347] Based on preoperative and postoperative hematocrit and known volume of transfusion, the percent of the total blood volume lost per percent of total wound excised generated an average 0.98 ± 0.19% of the blood volume per percent of the body surface excised. This was about one fifth of our earlier experience with this type of excision.[357,358] Operating with epinephrine clysis or tourniquets requires the surgeon to accurately determine wound bed viability in the absence of free bleeding. This is an important acquired skill that may be difficult to develop if the surgeon is not performing these procedures frequently.

Chronic ionized hypocalcemia is commonly observed with major thermal injury.[137] Prophylactic intermittent administration of calcium chloride or calcium gluconate is strongly recommended during the rapid infusion of citrated blood products.[359-362] We observed children experience electromechanical dissociation or cardiac arrest during the rapid administration of fresh frozen plasma (FFP). This observation prompted a controlled prospective study in which highly significant reductions in calcium were found when FFP was administered at a rate of 1 mL/kg/min or greater (see Fig. 10-9).[362] Of interest, no relation was seen between adverse cardiovascular responses, rate of FFP infusion, or calcium concentration. A careful review of the previous cases of cardiac arrest revealed that all children were anesthetized with halothane, whereas in our prospective study most were anesthetized with "balanced" techniques. Because all inhalation agents depress cardiac function in part through their calcium channel–blocking activity, a sudden citrate-induced decrease in ionized calcium would be expected to cause additional cardiac dysfunction. Studies in our laboratory have, in fact, documented this interaction.[21,362,363] Additional exogenous calcium is administered during rapid infusion of FFP or citrated whole blood, especially in infants (see Chapter 10).[362] It is our clinical impression that the rapid administration of (cold) FFP or citrated whole blood through a central line, without additional exogenous calcium, may be more likely to induce severe hypotension, bradycardia, and electrical mechanical dissociation. Our experience has been that rapid administration of citrated blood products is safer through peripheral lines. Rapid administration of washed packed

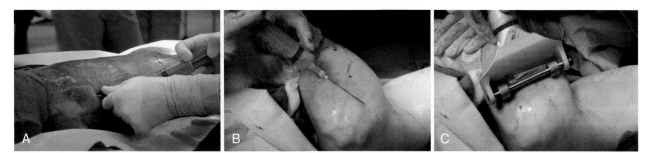

**FIGURE 34-12 A,** Subcutaneous injection of normal saline with a dilute concentration of epinephrine (0.5 μg/mL) from an area to be excised. **B,** Note the blanching of the donor skin secondary to the epinephrine. This helps greatly reduce the amount of blood loss observed from both the donor sites and burn wound excision. It should be noted, however, that in the case of a large quantity administered to a small patient, late absorption can result in fluid overload. **C,** Skin is now harvested with minimal blood loss owing to the vasoconstriction of the tumescence solution with low dose epinephrine.

or citrated packed red blood cells does not cause ionized hypocalcemia. It would also seem advantageous to administer exogenous calcium through a peripheral line to avoid excessive concentrations in coronary vessels. However, calcium administered simultaneously in the same intravenous line with FFP or citrated blood products may cause clot formation unless the calcium is rapidly flushed through the intravenous system.

## SPECIAL CONSIDERATIONS
### Pharmacologic Responses
As a general rule, children with burn injuries require larger than normal doses of all medications, including antibiotics, NMBDs, opioids, and benzodiazepines.* Cardiovascular response to catecholamines may be attenuated because of a reduced affinity of β-adrenergic receptors for ligands and diminished second messenger production,[173] thus the need for greater than standard doses to achieve the desired clinical response. Pharmacokinetic studies in acutely burned children indicate that the increased requirement for antibiotics is due in part to leakage through the burn wound, rapid urinary excretion, and altered volume of distribution.[43] Thermal injuries of more than 30% of body surface area cause an upregulation of acetylcholine receptors and consequent resistance to NMBDs.[167-169,171-174,364] In addition, there appears to be increased tolerance to sedatives and opioids. In adult burn patients, the free fraction (pharmacologically active component) of diazepam was greater than in nonburned patients, whereas the clearance of free diazepam was reduced. An increased tolerance to diazepam despite a greater fraction of the pharmacologically active compounds combined with a decreased clearance suggests resistance at tissue receptors similar to that observed for NMBDs at the neuromuscular junction.[78] A similar tolerance has been observed with opioids. The persistence of such pharmacodynamic changes for both NMBDs and anesthetic drugs long after recovery from burn injury must be kept in mind and doses titrated according to patient responses.[73,177,325,329]

The pharmacology of many medications commonly used in burned children remains to be investigated.[177] In general, it is necessary to be aware of both pharmacokinetic and pharmacodynamic changes. Furthermore, these children are frequently taking multiple medications, and therefore drug interactions, potentiations, and incompatibilities must be considered. Of particular importance in this context are the $H_2$-receptor antagonists, which are commonly used in burned children and are known to inhibit the clearance of many other medications (see Chapter 6).

### Methemoglobinemia
A less common, but important source of intraoperative cyanosis and hypoxemia is the development of methemoglobinemia. When silver nitrate dressings are used on the burn sites, there are some strains of gram-negative bacteria capable of reducing nitrates to nitrites, which diffuse into the bloodstream and convert hemoglobin into methemoglobin.[120,121,285] The methemoglobin decreases the available $O_2$-carrying capacity and increases the affinity of the unaltered hemoglobin for $O_2$, thereby further impairing the delivery of $O_2$. As a consequence, the $O_2$-hemoglobin P50 curve is shifted to the left. Therefore methemoglobinemia should be considered in the differential diagnosis of cyanosis. Approximately 5 g of deoxyhemoglobin for each deciliter of blood is necessary to produce visible cyanosis, but a

comparable skin color is produced by 1.5 to 2 g of methemoglobin for each deciliter of blood. Blood that contains more than approximately 10% methemoglobin usually appears dark red or even brown, despite a high measured $PaO_2$, and does not change color even with vigorous agitation in room air. Measured $O_2$ saturation or content is low. However, pulse oximetry, although demonstrating a decrease in saturation, provides a falsely increased value.[235,236] Treatment consists of removing the toxic agent and administering methylene blue (2 mg/kg) and high inspired $O_2$ concentrations.

### Tracheal Tube Size
Because burned children frequently undergo multiple anesthetic procedures, special considerations must be given to the tracheal tube type and size. As mentioned previously, cuffed tracheal tubes are preferable. The size of the tracheal tube, the volume of air inflated into the cuff, and the pressure at which leakage occurs around the cuff should be recorded at each anesthetic. It is common to note that the requirement for a smaller diameter tracheal tube as weeks go by suggests the development of a subglottic lesion (stenosis, granuloma, polyps), which should be investigated with bronchoscopy. When $N_2O$ is used, the intraoperative cuff pressure should be checked to avoid excessive pressure on the tracheal mucosa, although MICROCUFF tubes provide a greater margin of safety than conventional tracheal tubes (see Chapter 12). We generally inflate the cuff to the minimum pressure that allows controlled ventilation and check the cuff pressure regularly.

### Airway Control
The pediatric burn patient may present an especially difficult airway challenge to the anesthesiologist. This may be due to external airway factors such as temporomandibular joint limitation, macroglossia from thermal injury, and neck contractures.[12,327] It also may be due to direct thermal or inhalational injuries to the glottis and respiratory tree. A detailed history and physical examination focusing on airway injury is vital. History details such as victim of fire in a closed space (e.g., house or automobile fire [very commonly associated with inhalational injuries]), vocal changes, stridor, and hoarseness may be important predictors of difficulty in establishing an airway.

Fiberoptic intubation is a very useful method of securing the airway. We use this technique frequently after induction when we are confident we can maintain a mask airway as well for "awake" but sedated children who are breathing spontaneously. Recently, we have used dexmedetomidine as our sole sedative while performing fiberoptic intubations on spontaneously breathing children. Dexmedetomidine, an $\alpha_2$-adrenoceptor agonist, may provide a relatively stable hemodynamic environment, without respiratory depression, making it an ideal sedative when loss of respiratory drive could be catastrophic.

Fiberoptic intubation is often aided in these children with manual distraction of the tongue (especially if macroglossia is present) and a jaw lift (Fig. 34-13). If the tongue is difficult to grasp, moderately high suction applied to the tip of the tongue or a gauze wrapped around the tongue and then gently pulling the tongue forward facilitates visualization of glottic structures (see Fig. 12-29).[365] Fiberoptic intubation sometimes is more easily performed if the bronchoscope is guided through a laryngeal mask airway (LMA) that has already been seated and used to ventilate the lungs. This can be especially advantageous if there is a lot of perioral edema from inhalational burn injury.

---

*References 2, 59-61, 73, 77-79, 160-164, 169, 177-180, 331-333, 356.

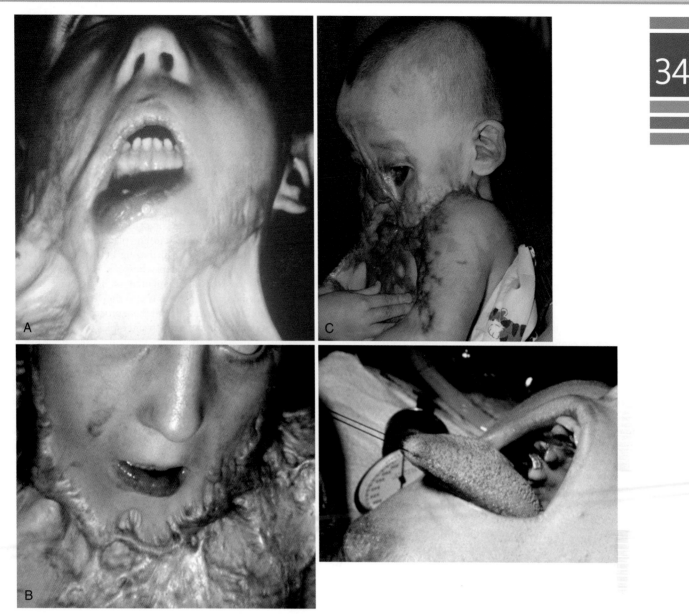

**FIGURE 34-13 A,** Child with inadequately treated facial burn. Note that skin contracture has resulted in complete distortion of the face with inability to close the right eye. **B,** Child with another example of an inadequately treated neck burn; note that her chin is fused with the sternum, resulting in very difficult airway management. **C,** An acute burn injury with an even more extreme example of inability to access the airway. To manage this child safely for the initial neck release, extracorporeal membrane oxygenation was used. This child is also unable to close her eyes. **D,** Some children with severe neck burns may have their airway visualized only by pulling back on the tongue (zero silk suture, suction applied to the tip of the tongue, or grasping forceps may be used [see also Fig. 12-29]) so as to pull the tongue and larynx cephalad.

In addition to direct laryngoscopy, fiberoptic intubations, and LMA-assisted intubations, other techniques have been described, including retrograde wires and light-wand intubations. These techniques may be difficult to use in a child with a severely burned neck and contractures. In children with severe neck or oral contractures, the surgeon may release the contracture during ketamine sedation and spontaneous ventilation to facilitate access to the airway (Video 34-5). The airway may then be instrumented either directly or indirectly (see Chapter 12).

### Hyperalimentation
Hyperalimentation fluids are frequently administered to burned children.[99,366] These fluids should be continued intraoperatively; however, we generally reduce the rate of infusion to half to two thirds of the initial infusion rate because metabolic rate is usually decreased during anesthesia. These fluids should be administered with a constant-infusion pump to avoid accidental overinfusion or underinfusion. If the hyperalimentation fluids must be terminated (e.g., to permit blood transfusion), monitoring of blood glucose levels is recommended. Dangerous rebound hypoglycemia may occur if infusion of these solutions is abruptly interrupted and no compensation is made with other glucose-containing solutions. It should be noted that most blood products, particularly whole blood and FFP, provide a significant glucose load. Compatibility of hyperalimentation solutions with drugs, blood, and other infusions must be addressed.

### Ultrasound-Guided Vascular Access, Regional Analgesia, and Cardiovascular Assessment

The use of high-resolution portable ultrasound continues to increase among anesthesiologists. The perioperative care of the pediatric burn patient is arguably one of the areas with the greatest use of this new and advancing technology. At Shriners Hospital for Children in Boston we employ ultrasound as an adjunct for vascular access, regional anesthesia, and cardiopulmonary diagnosis.

Vascular access for the pediatric burn patient can be extremely challenging. However, placing central venous and arterial catheters in the operating room under carefully controlled conditions is associated with a rate of acute mechanical complications and deep vein thrombosis of less than 1%.[367] This applies to both central and peripheral access as a result of thermal damage from the burn, surgical grafting over peripheral vessels, and increased clotting and thrombi from multiple factors such as multiple prior cannulations, hypercoagulable state from the burn, and long periods of being bedbound. Ultrasound is useful not only to more rapidly and safely access arteries and veins but also to diagnose clotted vessels, saving the child many futile attempts at obtaining vascular access.[368] Ultrasound also helps establish the location of cannulae. For peripherally inserted central catheters (PICCs), we first use ultrasound to assist in cannulating a vein, then place the probe over the internal jugular to verify that the PICC is not traveling cephalad, and scan the subclavian vein to verify placement.

Ultrasound-guided regional anesthesia is also a valuable tool in the care of the burned child undergoing reconstructive surgery. Typically, the complaints children have after reconstructive procedures involve the pain of the graft donor site. For the past 5 years we have improved the postoperative experience by placing ultrasound-guided blocks of donor sites, sometimes with catheters for further postoperative analgesia. Specific blocks we have found very useful include the lateral femoral cutaneous nerve and fascia iliaca to cover the most common donor site— the lateral thigh. Using ultrasound, reliability of these blocks is significantly improved over typical blind techniques.[369,370] We find that block of the lateral femoral cutaneous nerve provides better pain control for the donor site than infiltrating the donor site with local anesthetics. Longer analgesia can be provided by leaving a catheter in place. Usually we place fascia iliaca catheters; lateral femoral cutaneous nerve catheters also work, but we have found the learning curve for successful placement to be a bit steeper.[371]

Ultrasound is one of several strategies to rapidly assess intraoperative cardiac function during burn surgery. We have used real-time ultrasound while decompressing a spontaneous pneumothorax in a burn patient as a rapid and reliable indicator of when the lung has reexpanded as indicated by return of the pleural "sliding" sign.[372-374] Hemodynamic measurements also can be estimated intraoperatively; we use the Bedside Assessment for Trauma/Critical Care (BEAT) examination as a quick assessment of volume status.[375,376]

### Awakening

In the immediate postoperative period, $O_2$ consumption increases even in the absence of shivering.[37] If $O_2$ debt develops (metabolic acidosis), appropriate measures must be taken to correct it. Special consideration also must be given to the likelihood of severe pain. Analgesic drugs should be administered in increasingly liberal doses because of increased drug tolerance. Adequacy

of air exchange and patency of the airway, however, must be given first priority. It is important to assess the leak pressure at the end of the surgical procedure. The airway patency of the burned child is highly dynamic, and the child whose airway had minimal edema at the beginning of a procedure may have a very edematous airway at the end and be a poor candidate for extubation.

## PAIN MANAGEMENT AND POSTOPERATIVE CARE

Treatment of the child with a burn who has pain, both perioperatively and in the intensive care unit, remains a major challenge for anesthesiologists and intensivists. Our experience is that the pain is proportional to the size of the thermal injury. Nearly every maneuver involving the care of the child with a burn is associated with pain. This includes dressing changes, excision and grafting, physical therapy, weighing, and line placements.

Part of the challenge in managing burn pain is due to the overlay of physiologic and psychosocial responses to thermal injury. Besides physical stimulation of nociceptors and other direct pain mechanisms, there is also the very real anticipation, anxiety, and fear associated with these procedures. Evidence suggests that skillful communication and explanations of why certain treatments are necessary, despite the pain caused, decreases analgesic requirements.[320,377-379]

Opioid administration for pain control has been an evolving science for the child with a burn. Twenty years ago there was significant fear that treatment of pain with opioids would create addictions. However, no reports of children developing opioid addiction after therapeutic uses of opioids have been published and studies in adults revealed a very low addiction rate.[380-384] This has led to liberalization of opioid dosing. It is not unusual for children to receive more than 1 mg/kg/hr of morphine intravenously while recovering from burn injuries in our intensive care unit. Once the thermal wounds are closed, opioid requirements rapidly decrease (Fig. 34-14).

Although the fear of post–burn care addiction to opioids has not been realized, there are other reasons why this class of drugs may be detrimental to the child with a burn. Recent evidence from rats suggests that thermal injury itself may lead to a hyperalgesic state with both reduced efficacy of morphine (presumably from downregulation of spinal μ receptors) and increases in N-methyl-D-aspartate (NMDA) receptors. The increases in NMDA receptors induced by burns provide the rationale for the widespread use of ketamine to treat pain in these children. Opioids may also increase sensitivity to pain. Morphine has been shown in a mouse model to downregulate μ-opioid receptors within the spinal cord and cause injury to spinal inhibitory interneurons.[383,384] Opioids in mice have also been shown to cause postburn immunosuppression in the mouse model.[385]

The fact that opioids may have disadvantages when used for pain management has led to a search for alternative analgesics. Among these are potentially dexmedetomidine,[386-392] gabapentin,[393] and, until their recent withdrawal from the market, cyclooxygenase-2 inhibitors.[394-396]

Dexmedetomidine is a parenterally administered $\alpha_2$-adrenoceptor agonist with good sedative and anxiolytic properties. In adults, it has been demonstrated to decrease opioid requirements postoperatively.[387-391,397] In children with burns, it has been used successfully for sedation,[386] although larger dexmedetomidine doses may be needed than those required in nonburned adults or nonburned children.[386] Dexmedetomidine does not appear to be a remarkable analgesic for children with

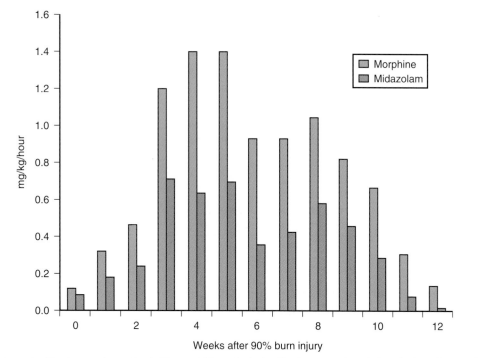

**FIGURE 34-14** Morphine and midazolam requirements of a 16-year-old boy who had suffered an approximately 90% body surface area burn injury. Note the marked rapid rise in analgesia and sedation requirements during the first 4 to 5 weeks after injury and then the rapid decline in requirements as his wounds were successfully grafted.

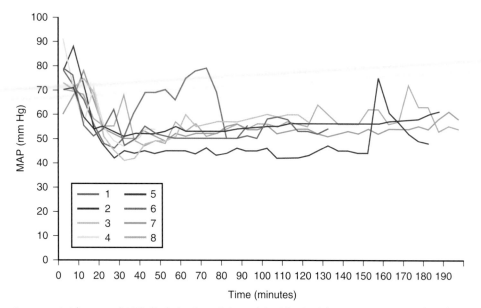

**FIGURE 34-15** Change in mean arterial pressure (MAP) after bolus dose of dexmedetomidine in eight consecutive acute pediatric burn patients. *NOTE:* Given these observations, we now avoid a bolus dose; however, should a bolus dose be considered necessary, we suggest that the need for volume resuscitation (10 mL/kg or greater of balanced salt solution) or mild pressor support must be anticipated. (From Shank ES, Sheridan RL, Ryan CM, Keaney TJ, Martyn JA. Hemodynamic responses to dexmedetomidine in critically injured intubated pediatric burned patients: a preliminary study. J Burn Care Res 2012 Aug 27 [Epub ahead of print].)

burns. In a prospective study of dexmedetomidine in acutely burned children,[398] a bolus dose of intravenous dexmedetomidine (1 µg/kg over 10 minutes) was followed by an ascending infusion protocol (0.7 µg/kg/hr to 2.2 µg/kg/hr).[399] We found no instances of heart block or other arrhythmias, but noted a consistent and significant decrease in mean arterial blood pressure (MAP) after the bolus (approaching 30% change in mean pressure) (Fig. 34-15). This occurred in all ages studied (2 to 18 years), although the decrease in the MAP did not correlate with size of burn, time out from burn, or central venous pressure, before the study. Given these observations, we avoid a bolus dose of dexmedetomidine. However, should a bolus dose be indicated, we recommend 10 mL/kg or more of balanced salt solution or mild pressor support before commencing dexmedetomidine.

**TABLE 34-3** Pain Treatment Plan

| Clinical State | Background Anxiety | Background Pain | Procedural Anxiety | Procedural Pain | Transition to Next Clinical State |
|---|---|---|---|---|---|
| Mechanically ventilated acute burn | Midazolam infusion | Morphine infusion | Midazolam intravenous titration | Morphine intravenous titration | Wean infusions 10%-20% per day and substitute nonmechanically ventilated acute guideline |
| Nonmechanically ventilated acute burn | Scheduled enteral lorazepam | Scheduled enteral morphine | Lorazepam intravenous titration or enteral dose | Morphine enteral or intravenous titration | Wean scheduled drugs 10%-20% per day and substitute chronic acute guideline |
| Chronic acute burn | Scheduled enteral lorazepam | Scheduled enteral morphine | Lorazepam enteral dose | Morphine enteral dose | Wean scheduled and bolus drugs 10%-20% per day to outpatient requirements and pruritus medications |
| Reconstructive surgical patient | Scheduled enteral lorazepam | Scheduled enteral morphine sulfate | Lorazepam enteral dose | Morphine enteral dose | Wean scheduled drugs and bolus drugs to outpatient requirement |

Other investigators have retrospectively examined cardiovascular stability of pediatric burn patients sedated with dexmedetomidine and concluded that in the absence of a loading dose, blood pressure was maintained in the dexmedetomidine treatment group.[400] Dexmedetomidine pharmacokinetics in nonburned children appear similar to those in adults, but they have not been reported in pediatric burn patients.[401-403] When dexmedetomidine was compared with midazolam as an adjunct to ketamine in sedation and analgesia for burn dressing changes, the authors determined that both were effective adjuncts but that the dexmedetomidine ketamine group had better sedation with less hemodynamic instability.[404] Dexmedetomidine has also been used in anxious children with burns as an intranasal premedication.[405] The authors concluded that dexmedetomidine (2 μg/kg) intranasally as a premedication compared with oral midazolam (0.5 mg/kg), induced preoperative sleep faster and was equally effective for induction conditions and rapidity of emergence. In our experience, the majority of our children prefer oral midazolam despite its bitter aftertaste, to intranasal dexmedetomidine. A substantial detractor from dexmedetomidine use is its cost (more than $44 for a 100-μg vial at our institutions). One study in adult volunteers compared intravenous with intranasal dexmedetomidine; pharmacodynamic responses were similar, but the peak blood concentration occurred sooner in the intravenous group.[406] Bioavailability after nasal administration was 65% (range 35% to 93%).

Dressing changes sometimes present one of the greatest analgesic challenges. This is because they are very painful, cause a rapid rise above baseline pain, and are associated by the child with anticipation of impending pain. Various methods to manage this pain have been used, including additional opioids and benzodiazepines, ketamine,[335] intranasal fentanyl,[407] immersive virtual reality,[408,409] and music therapy.[410] Management of the child's pain depends on physiologic and pharmacologic factors, as well as the psychological state of the child. Unfortunately, some children become so tolerant that one author observed that doses of intravenous fentanyl as large as 100 μg/kg administered as a bolus did not cause respiratory depression nor did it control the pain (CJC).

When poorly controlled, pain and anxiety have adverse psychologic[146,411,412] and physiologic effects.[19] Posttraumatic stress disorder has been reported to occur in up to 30% of those with serious burns[413,414] and may be related to both the accident and the treatment, particularly in the setting of inadequate control of pain and anxiety. An inconsistent approach to pain and anxiety will be associated with inappropriate degrees of child discomfort, nonuniform drug selection with inconsistent dosing of unfamiliar drugs, varying tolerance of child discomfort among staff members, and bedside disagreements over management of the child's distress.

To address this issue, a pain and anxiety guideline should be developed by all facilities routinely treating burned children.[415-418] We developed one such guideline that we have followed for several years, which is briefly described in Table 34-3.[321] The ideal characteristics of such a guideline include (1) safety and efficacy over the broad range of ages and injury acuities seen in the particular unit; (2) explicit recommendations for drug selection, dosing, and escalation of dosing; (3) a limited formulary that generates staff familiarity with agents used; and (4) regular assessment of pain and anxiety levels and guidance for intervention as needed through dose ranging. We have found this structured approach to manage this predictable problem to be very effective over the broad range of injury severity and child ages seen in our unit. Substantial escalation of drug doses, particularly in children with large injuries, is commonly required; doses should be titrated to the child's needs. When the child is being weaned toward extubation, background medications should be tapered toward a sensorium consistent with airway protection; many children's tracheas are safely extubated while they are still receiving opioid and benzodiazepine infusions. Finally, it is essential to emphasize that the most effective of all analgesics and anxiolytics is prompt, definitive wound closure.

Tolerance to opioids occurs over time and must be considered so that adequate analgesia is provided throughout the recovery period. It is common to observe children who receive 1 mg/kg of morphine at the beginning of a 2-hour operative procedure not only to be ready for extubation but also to require additional opioids for continued pain relief postoperatively. Similar trends have been observed for fentanyl.[162] Thus an increased rate of excretion and degradation may influence the effect of some opioids. As the child recovers, the painful stimuli diminish and the opioid requirements are gradually reduced. This is generally such a prolonged process that withdrawal is not an issue. Anesthesiologists can have a central role in the treatment of thermal injury pain and, with an understanding of pharmacology, pharmacokinetics, and pharmacodynamics, are a vital resource for the care of these children (see Chapters 43 and 44).

## Summary

The care of burned children involves detailed knowledge of the early and late effects of burn injury on the respiratory, cardiac, renal, central nervous, hepatic, gastrointestinal, hematopoietic, and metabolic systems. An awareness of the pharmacokinetics and pharmacodynamics of anesthetic agents, combined with an understanding of the problems of massive blood transfusion, also contribute to the safe conduct of anesthesia. Finally, the importance of adequate analgesia, sedation, and concern for the psychological well-being of these devastatingly injured children cannot be overemphasized. Knowledge of all of these factors combines to produce a successful outcome.

### ACKNOWLEDGMENT

We wish to thank S.K. Szyfelbein for his previous contributions to this chapter.

## ANNOTATED REFERENCES

Han T, Kim H, Bae J, et al. Neuromuscular pharmacodynamics of rocuronium in patients with major burns. Anesth Analg 2004;99: 386-92.

*Currently, rocuronium is the fastest acting nondepolarizing muscle relaxant available. This paper discusses its pharmacodynamics in burn patients and in particular describes both delayed onset and resistance in burned adults with doses as great as 1.2 mg/kg.*

Scheinkestel CD, Bailey M, Myles PS, et al. Hyperbaric or normobaric oxygen for acute carbon monoxide poisoning: a randomised controlled clinical trial. Med J Aust 1999;170:203-10.

*This study is the first large-scale randomized prospective study of hyperbaric oxygen versus normobaric oxygen for the treatment of carbon monoxide poisoning. It raised important questions about hyperbaric oxygenation's role in the treatment of acute carbon monoxide poisoning.*

Sheridan RL, Szyfelbein SK. Staged high-dose epinephrine clysis is safe and effective in extensive tangential burn excisions in children. Burns 1999;25:745-8.

*The use of epinephrine clysis of both donor and recipient sites is one of the important techniques in minimizing blood loss during burn excisions.*

Weaver LK, Hopkins RO, Chan KJ, et al. Hyperbaric oxygen for acute carbon monoxide poisoning. N Engl J Med 2002;347:1057-67.

*This is an important follow-up randomized prospective study suggesting that there is a benefit to hyperbaric oxygen therapy for avoiding delayed neurologic sequelae.*

## REFERENCES

Please see www.expertconsult.com.

# The Extremely Premature Infant (Micropremie)

35

JAMES P. SPAETH AND C. DEAN KURTH

THE PRETERM INFANT IS defined by birth before 37 weeks gestation. Preterm infants can be classified as low–birth-weight infants (less than 2500 g), very low–birth-weight infants (less than 1500 g), and extremely low–birth-weight (ELBW) infants (less than 1000 g). Morbidity and mortality in this population has decreased over the past 25 years, especially in the ELBW infant group, in which the mortality in 2011 is less than 30% in Level 3 hospitals, compared with 80% in 1980.[1-3] This decrease in mortality is the result of many factors, including the use of surfactant shortly after birth, antenatal glucocorticoid administration, specialization of neonatal care units, and changes in mechanical ventilator therapy. However, many of these surviving infants develop coexisting diseases that require care by an anesthesiologist. For the purpose of this chapter, we will focus on the very low and extremely low–birth-weight infant, or "micropremie," and discuss developmental physiology and its impact on anesthetic care; neonatal emergencies are discussed in Chapter 36.

## Physiology of Prematurity Related to Anesthesia

### RESPIRATORY SYSTEM

The small airways predispose the micropremie to obstruction and difficulty with ventilation. Resistance to airflow is inversely proportional to the fifth power of the radius in the upper airway and to the fourth power of the radius beyond the fifth bronchial division (see also Fig. 12-7). As a result, insertion of an endotracheal tube (ETT) increases resistance and work of breathing far greater for the micropremie (2.5 or 3 mm inside diameter [ID]) than for a larger infant (4 mm ID), child (5 mm ID), and adult (7 mm ID) (Fig. 35-1). Similarly, partial occlusion of the ETT by secretions, blood, or kinking increases the work of breathing to a much greater extent in the micropremie. Partial occlusion of the natural airway from loss of muscle tone during anesthesia and sedation also increases the work of breathing more in the micropremie. Consequently, general anesthesia often requires placement of an ETT to ensure airway patency, and assisted ventilation to overcome the increased work of breathing.

Diseases that narrow the airway, such as subglottic stenosis, tracheal stenosis, and tracheobronchomalacia, occur commonly in the micropremie, and the associated reduction in airway diameter further increases both resistance to airflow and work of breathing. Subglottic stenosis necessitates the placement of a smaller ETT than would otherwise be placed, further increasing airflow resistance. Tracheal stenosis often occurs near the carina and, although not necessitating a smaller ETT, it increases airway resistance from the stenosis distal to the ETT. With tracheobronchomalacia, the intrathoracic airways collapse during exhalation, again increasing resistance and the work of breathing (see also Fig. 12-10). Positive end-expiratory pressure (PEEP) or continuous positive airway pressure (CPAP) helps stent open the airway.

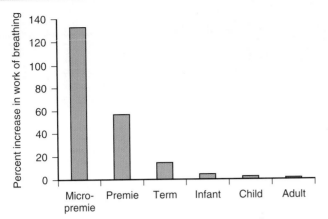

**FIGURE 35-1** Change in work of breathing after placement of an appropriate size endotracheal tube in extremely low–birth-weight infants (less than 1000 g), premature infants (1500 g), full-term infants, children, and adults (see text for details). (Redrawn with permission from Spaeth JP, O'Hara IB, Kurth CD. Anesthesia for the micropremie. Semin Perinatol 1998;22:390-401.)

| TABLE 35-1 | Severity-Based Diagnostic Criteria for Bronchopulmonary Dysplasia (BPD) |
|---|---|
| Gestational age | <32 weeks |
| Time point of assessment | 36 weeks postmenstrual age or discharge home, whichever comes first |
|  | Therapy with oxygen >21% for at least 28 days *plus:* |
| Mild BPD | Breathing room air |
| Moderate BPD | Need for <30% oxygen |
| Severe BPD | Need for ≥30% oxygen and/or positive-pressure ventilation or nasal continuous airway pressure |

From Ehrenkranz RA, Walsh MC, Vohr BR, et al. Validation of the National Institutes of Health consensus definition of bronchopulmonary dysplasia. Pediatrics 2005; 116:1353-60.

Mechanical ventilation, rather than spontaneous ventilation during anesthesia, prevents fatigue from increased work of breathing, and maintains ventilation and oxygenation. During anesthesia the use of *smaller inspiratory-to-expiratory ratios* prevent air trapping and hyperinflation of lung segments.

The structure and function of the immature lung predisposes to alveolar collapse and hypoxia. The alveoli are primarily composed of thick-walled, fluid-filled saccular spaces that are surfactant deficient and require greater pressures to initially expand. Production of surfactant begins at between 23 to 24 weeks gestation, although surfactant concentrations often remain inadequate until 36 weeks gestation. These factors lead to reduced lung volumes and lung compliance, increased intrapulmonary shunting, and ventilation-perfusion mismatch. Decreased lung volumes and ventilation-perfusion mismatch may also occur as a consequence of anesthesia. The effects of immature structure, disease, and anesthesia on lung function all increase the risk of hypoxia during surgery and anesthesia.

Micropremie lungs are particularly susceptible to oxygen toxicity, volutrauma, and the development of bronchopulmonary dysplasia (BPD). Mechanical lung injury is no longer thought to be caused by the use of high peak-inspiratory pressures, but rather related to increased end-inspiratory lung volumes and frequent collapse and reopening of alveoli. A ventilation strategy using small tidal volumes (4 to 6 mL/kg), greater respiratory rates, PEEP sufficient to avoid alveolar collapse, and permissive hypercapnia reduces lung injury in the premature lung.[4] Randomized controlled trials of permissive hypercapnia (PaCO$_2$ 45 to 55 mm Hg) showed smaller periods of assisted ventilation, reduced incidence of BPD, and no increase in adverse neurodevelopmental effects.[5] The use of high inspired oxygen concentrations leads to the development of free radical species, which contribute to pulmonary epithelial cell injury.

A severity index for BPD based on the need for supplemental oxygen and/or positive-pressure ventilation or nasal CPAP has been developed and shown to identify a spectrum of risk for adverse pulmonary and neurodevelopmental outcomes in preterm infants (Table 35-1).[6] Although this severity index has not been studied in the context of anesthetic risk, experience suggests that such infants requiring supplemental oxygen, positive pressure, or medications for reactive airways are at greater risk for perioperative pulmonary complications. Anesthetic goals include minimizing the inspired oxygen concentration and tidal volumes while maintaining oxygen saturation (SaO$_2$ 90% to 94%) and ventilation (PaCO$_2$ 50 to 55 mm Hg). The use of smaller tidal volumes decreases the risk of pneumothoraces and interstitial emphysema.

## RESPIRATORY CONTROL

Micropremies possess a biphasic ventilatory response to hypoxia. Initially, ventilation increases in response to hypoxia, but after several minutes, ventilation decreases and apnea may ensue.[7] The ventilatory response to carbon dioxide is decreased in the micropremie, and hypoxia further blunts this response.[8,9] Anesthetic drugs depress the ventilatory responses to both hypoxia and hypercapnia. Hypoxia and hypercapnia occur commonly as a result of apnea and hypoventilation during emergence and recovery from anesthesia. Thus the combination of anesthetic effects and an immature respiratory control system, as well as immature intercostal and diaphragmatic muscles,[10,11] increase the risk of hypoxia, hypercapnia, and apnea in the postoperative period.

Apneic episodes occur commonly in the micropremie but decrease with advancing postconceptional age.[12] These apneic episodes usually involve both a failure to breathe (central apnea) and a failure to maintain a patent airway (obstructive apnea). Central apnea results from decreased respiratory center output, although it may be precipitated by abrupt changes in oxygenation, pulmonary mechanics, brain hemorrhage, hypothermia, or airway stimulation. Apnea may also occur without a precipitating event (i.e., idiopathic). Preterm infants with apnea do not increase ventilation in response to hypercapnia, compared with those without apnea, thereby delaying resumption of breathing and prolonging the apneic episode.[13] During obstructive apnea, the airway becomes obstructed in the hypopharynx and larynx as a result of pharyngeal muscle incoordination. Anesthetic drugs may further decrease pharyngeal muscle tone, precipitating airway obstruction during recovery from anesthesia. The combination of anesthetic effects and immature respiratory control place the micropremie at risk for central and obstructive apnea for a prolonged period of time during recovery from anesthesia.

Not surprisingly, apnea occurs commonly after anesthesia and surgery in preterm infants.[14,15] Like apnea of prematurity, postoperative apnea may be central, obstructive, or mixed in origin.[16] The term *postoperative apnea* usually means prolonged apnea (greater than 15 seconds) or brief apnea accompanied by

bradycardia (heart rate 80 beats per minute or less). Postoperative apnea typically occurs as a cluster of episodes over several minutes, with minutes of normal breathing in between the clusters. Bradycardia may occur with apnea, usually beginning at the onset of apnea and not in response to hypoxia. Arterial oxygen desaturation usually follows the apnea, although many apneic episodes may not have any associated desaturation. Arterial desaturation is worse with obstructive apnea than with central apnea.[16]

Several different terms have been used to describe the age of the fetus, leading to some confusion in the literature. Gestational age, menstrual age, conceptional age, and postnatal age are all used with somewhat different meanings, even in this book, so we present here the definitions of these terms according to the American Academy of Pediatrics, Committee on the Fetus and Newborn from 2004.[17] The gestational or menstrual age of the neonate is the interval from the first day of the mother's last menstrual cycle until birth of the fetus. The postmenstrual age is the sum of the menstrual age and the postnatal age. The conceptional age is defined as the interval between conception and birth, although the former is generally unknown. The postconceptional age (PCA) is the sum of the conceptional age and the postnatal age. Postconceptual age actually refers to a concept, not conception, but this term has been used interchangeably with postconceptional age in the apnea literature in anesthesia. The postnatal (or chronological) age is the age of the infant since birth. Controversy over this terminology continues, as some argue that the menstrual age overestimates the "in utero" age of the fetus because 10 to 14 days may lapse between the onset of menses and conception. On the other hand, terms such as conceptional (and postconceptional) age are imprecise because the date of conception is usually unknown, and thus these terms are not recommended.[17]

The incidence of postoperative apnea depends on PCA, hematocrit, and the type of surgical procedure (Fig. 35-2; see also Fig. 4-7 and E-Fig. 4-5).[14-16,18] The most significant risk factor is the PCA; the lesser the PCA, the greater the risk, with the incidence of postoperative apnea in the micropremie greater than 50%.[14,15] Postoperative apnea can occur in the micropremie even without a history of apnea of prematurity.[14] Anemia (hematocrit less than 30%) and younger gestation increase the risk of apnea for a given PCA.[15,18]

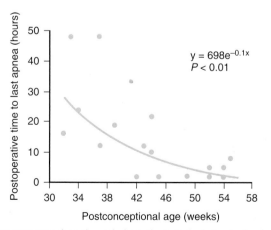

**FIGURE 35-2** Time from the end of anesthesia to the last episode of postoperative apnea in prematurely born infants. ($r^2 = 0.49$.) (Redrawn with permission from Kurth CD, Spitzer AR, Broennle AM, et al. Postoperative apnea in preterm infants. Anesthesiology 1987;66:483-8.)

Postoperative apnea usually begins within an hour of emergence from anesthesia.[14] In the micropremie, it can continue to occur up to 48 hours postoperatively, despite the elimination of anesthetic agents (see Fig. 35-2). In fact, postoperative apnea can occur after surgery with desflurane- or sevoflurane-based anesthetics, or even after surgery for which a regional anesthetic was administered and no general anesthetic drugs were used.[19,20] Postoperative apnea is more common after major procedures, such as a laparotomy, compared with peripheral surgical procedures, such as inguinal hernia repair. These observations indicate that the neurohormonal response to surgery and postoperative pain may play an important role in the origins of postoperative apnea. Management of postoperative apnea includes close observation with a cardiorespiratory monitor and pulse oximeter, administration of intravenous (IV) methylxanthines (e.g., caffeine, theophylline),[21] and prevention of anemia or hypovolemia. Nasal CPAP or tracheal intubation and mechanical ventilation may be required for several days postoperatively if these measures fail.

N7-methylation of theophylline (or aminophylline) to produce caffeine is well-developed in the neonate, whereas oxidative demethylation (CYP1A2) responsible for caffeine metabolism is deficient. Theophylline is effective for the management of postoperative apnea in the preterm neonate, in part because it is a prodrug of caffeine, which is effective in controlling apnea in this age group and can only be cleared slowly by the immature kidney. Consequently, the half-life of caffeine is ~72 hours in the extreme premature neonate, which decreases to 4 to 6 hours by 6 months of age. Clearance increases from 0.004 L/kg/hr in the premature neonate to 0.119 L/kg/hr by 6 months.[22-26] Although therapeutic drug monitoring is not required, target concentrations 5 to 20 mg/L are considered therapeutic.[27] One study suggests a loading IV or oral dose of 10 mg/kg followed by 2.5 mg/kg by mouth, once daily.[26]

## CARDIOVASCULAR SYSTEM

The micropremie remains at greater risk of cardiovascular collapse during anesthesia and surgery than does the full-term infant for several reasons. The fetal heart differs from the infant heart in that it has more connective tissue, less organized contractile elements, and increased dependence on extracellular calcium concentration. In addition, the less compliant fetal heart has a flatter Frank-Starling curve and is less sensitive to catecholamines because of near-maximal baseline β-adrenergic stimulation (see Chapter 16).[28,29] Consequently, cardiac output depends more on heart rate in the micropremie than it does in the term neonate. The increased resting heart rate in the micropremie also does not permit cardiac output to increase to the same extent as in an infant or child. The micropremie has a small absolute blood volume (Table 35-2). Therefore, relatively little blood loss during surgery can cause hypovolemia, hypotension, and shock. Because autoregulation is not well developed in the micropremie, the heart rate may not increase with hypovolemia, and blood flow and oxygen delivery to the brain and heart may decrease with relatively little blood loss.[30] Anesthesia blunts baroreceptor reflexes in the micropremie, further limiting the ability to compensate for hypovolemia.[31] The combination of limited ventricular stroke volume reserve, an increased heart rate, small blood volume, and limited autoregulation predispose the micropremie to cardiovascular collapse during major surgery.

Failure of the ductus arteriosus to close in the micropremie further increases this risk. A patent ductus arteriosus (PDA) promotes pulmonary hypertension and congestive heart failure.

**TABLE 35-2** Circulating Blood Volume in Micropremies, Premies, Full-Term Neonates, Infants, and Children

| | Blood Volume (mL/kg) | Weight (kg) | Total Blood Volume (mL) | 25-mL Blood Loss Proportion of Total Blood Volume (%) |
|---|---|---|---|---|
| Micropremie | 110 | 1 | 110 | 23 |
| Premie | 100 | 1.75 | 175 | 14 |
| Full-term neonate | 90 | 3 | 270 | 9 |
| Infant | 80 | 10 | 800 | 3 |
| Child | 70 | 20 | 1400 | 2 |

Changes in systemic or pulmonary vascular resistance alter the direction of flow through the PDA or the foramen ovale.[32] Increased pulmonary vascular resistance predisposes to right-to-left shunting that worsens with hypoxia, hypercarbia, acidosis, and hypothermia. Paradoxical embolism is another concern.[33] Fluid restriction and diuretic therapy, often used to treat congestive heart failure from left-to-right shunting through a PDA, further increase the risk of hypotension during surgery. In contrast to full-term neonates, the success of inhaled nitric oxide in the micropremie with hypoxic respiratory failure and pulmonary hypertension remains unclear.[34-36]

## NEUROLOGIC DEVELOPMENT

Although mortality in extremely preterm infants has improved over the years, many survivors experience cognitive impairment and long-term disability.[37,38] Regions of the central nervous system develop at different times during gestation; consequently, the impact of premature birth on the central nervous system (CNS) depends on gestational age at birth and the severity of cardiovascular, respiratory, and other postnatal stressors. The area of the brain most susceptible to injury in the micropremie is the periventricular white matter.[38] The white matter consists of preoligodendrocytes, astrocytes, and neuronal axons. Late in the second trimester (24 to 27 weeks gestation), preoligodendrocytes and astrocytes multiply tremendously and most cortical and subcortical structures begin to develop.[38] During this period, the periventricular white matter is particularly susceptible to neurologic injury. The periventricular white matter is perfused by arteries penetrating from the cortical surface and by lenticulostriate arteries from the circle of Willis. As a result, the periventricular white matter is a "watershed region" and susceptible to poor perfusion and hypoxic-ischemic injury during conditions of hypotension, reduced cardiac output, hypoxemia, and hypocarbia.

Neural pathways allowing for perception of pain develop during the first, second, and third trimesters (see Chapter 43).[39] During the first trimester, peripheral sensory receptors and spinal reflex arcs develop that lead to the presence of a "withdrawal reflex" to non-noxious stimuli. Neurons that transmit nociception appear in the dorsal root ganglia at 19 weeks gestation, and afferent neurons from the thalamus reach the cortical subplate and cortical plate between 20 and 24 weeks gestation. However, it is not until early in the third trimester (29 weeks) that pathways between the thalamus and somatosensory cortex are functional. Significant controversy exists regarding the exact gestational age at which perception and memory of pain occur. Nevertheless, our approach in the micropremie is to administer anesthesia during surgery and provide pain management postoperatively.

## LONG-TERM NEUROLOGIC COMPLICATIONS OF PREMATURITY

Long-term neurologic and developmental disabilities remain common in the micropremie and include cerebral palsy, cognitive deficits, behavioral abnormalities, as well as hearing and visual impairment. In one cohort of ELBW infants, only 25% were classified as normally developed at 5 years of age, whereas 20% exhibited major disabilities.[37] Brain magnetic resonance imaging (MRI) identifies a spectrum of abnormalities. The most common abnormality is diffuse high signal intensity on T2-weighted imaging in the periventricular cerebral white matter. Diffusion-weighted imaging shows increased apparent diffusion coefficient values, indicative of increased water content and delayed white matter maturation, suggesting ischemia-reperfusion injury in periventricular white matter, which has activated microglia and damaged preoligodendrocytes.[38,40] Damage to preoligodendrocytes impairs myelination of cerebral white matter axons and accounts for many of the fine motor, speech, and cognitive deficits. On MRI, tissue volumes in the basal ganglia, corpus callosum, amygdala, and hippocampus are reduced and correlate with smaller full-scale, verbal, and performance IQ scores.[41] Collectively, these MRI findings indicate that different regions of the brain vary in their susceptibility to injury during development and that such injuries lead to specific long-term disturbances in neurocognitive function.

## INTRAVENTRICULAR HEMORRHAGE

Intraventricular hemorrhage (IVH) occurs in as many as one-third of micropremie infants. The severity of IVH, as defined by head ultrasound, is graded as follows:

- Grade 1: hemorrhage limited to the germinal matrix
- Grade 2: hemorrhage extending into the ventricular system
- Grade 3: hemorrhage into the ventricular system and with ventricular dilatation
- Grade 4: hemorrhage extending into brain parenchyma.

Although micropremie infants with grade 3 or 4 IVH are more likely to exhibit severe long-term neurocognitive sequelae, even micropremie infants with grade 1 and 2 IVH display poorer neurodevelopmental outcomes compared with those without IVH.[42] Early onset of IVH appears during the first day of life. Risk factors include fetal distress, vaginal delivery, reduced Apgar scores, metabolic acidosis, severe hypercapnia, and the need for mechanical ventilation.[43,44] Late onset of IVH appears days to weeks after birth. Risk factors include respiratory distress syndrome, seizures, pneumothoraces, hypoxemia, acidosis, severe hypocarbia, and the use of vasopressor infusions.[43] Rapid fluctuations in cerebral blood flow, cerebral blood volume, and cerebral venous pressure appear to play a role in the development of IVH.[45] Factors that may decrease the incidence and severity of IVH include administration of antenatal glucocorticoids, or indomethacin.

## RETINOPATHY OF PREMATURITY

Retinopathy of prematurity (ROP) occurs in approximately 50% of ELBW infants, with the incidence being inversely proportional to birth weight and gestational age (see Chapter 32).[46] Although the pathogenesis of ROP is not completely understood, extremes in arterial oxygenation (hypoxia or hyperoxia)[47] and exposure to bright light appear to play a role.[48] One theory holds that the combination of hyperoxic vasoconstriction of retinal vessels (also known as vaso-obliteration), induction of vascular endothelial growth factor, and free oxygen radicals damage the spindle cells in the retina.[49] A Cochrane review concluded that liberal oxygen delivery to a preterm infant is more harmful to the retina than restrictive oxygen delivery, although the data reviewed failed to specify the optimum blood oxygen concentrations that should be delivered.[50] Evidence points to additional factors in the pathogenesis of ROP, including genetic polymorphisms[51] and antenatal and neonatal exposure to inflammation.[52]

ROP appears to be multifactorial in origin and oxygen tension is just one of many contributory factors. During anesthesia, our goal is to deliver the minimum inspired oxygen concentration that provides oxygen saturations between 90% and 94% and to avoid significant fluctuations in oxygen saturations. It should be noted however that ROP has occurred in children with cyanotic congenital heart disease[53] and that no anesthesia-associated cases have been reported over the past 25 years. Nevertheless it is reasonable to aim for saturation values in the ranges described here.

## TEMPERATURE REGULATION

The micropremie is susceptible to hypothermia. Heat loss in children occurs by four possible routes: radiation (39%), convection (34%), evaporation (24%) and conduction (3%). In the micropremie, evaporative heat loss and insensible fluid loss are increased because the epidermis has less keratin.[54] Conductive and convective heat losses are also increased because the micropremie has little subcutaneous fat for insulation and a large surface area to mass ratio. Thermal regulation is not well developed in the micropremie. Nonshivering thermogenesis, which depends on brown fat stores, is decreased and regulation of skin blood flow is less efficient.[55] During anesthesia, measures should be undertaken to minimize radiation and convective heat loss by warming the operating room (OR) to 78° F to 80° F (25.5° C to 26.6° C) before the neonate arrives, and minimize convective heat loss during transport (i.e., use a thermoneutral incubator). Using a warming pad on the operating table reduces conductive heat loss; use of overhead heat lamps reduces radiant heat loss; and keeping the skin dry reduces evaporative heat loss. The most effective means for warming is a forced-air warmer. Temperature should be carefully monitored as overheating the infant may readily occur.

## RENAL AND METABOLIC FUNCTION

In the micropremie, kidney function is decreased as a result of fewer nephrons and smaller glomerular size.[56] Glomeruli continue to form postnatally until approximately 40 days.[57] During this period, reduced cardiac output, hypotension, and nephrotoxic drugs may inhibit glomerular growth and development. Creatinine concentrations depend on production that is reduced in micropremies with limited muscle mass, and on excretion that is reduced because of immature renal function. Baseline plasma creatinine concentrations increase with increasing prematurity and remain increased until 3 weeks of age.[58] In addition, the normal increase in creatine clearance in term infants occurs more slowly in the micropremie. Creatinine concentrations in the first few days after birth are increased and reflect maternal transplacental transfer.[59] It is for this reason that antibiotic dosing must be adjusted to take renal immaturity into consideration, so as not to administer excessive doses that might result in ototoxicity.[60]

Very preterm infants easily become hyponatremic because of reduced proximal tubular reabsorption of sodium and water, and reduced receptors for hormones that influence tubular sodium transport. As many as one-third of ELBW neonates develop hyponatremia.[61] Frequent assessment of sodium and free water requirements is important during critical illness. Increased plasma potassium concentrations occur in preterm infants during the first few days after birth. The increase results from a shift in potassium from the intracellular to extracellular space.[62] These increases are greater as gestational age and birth weight decrease.[63] Reduced cardiac output and urine output may further increase serum potassium concentrations and predispose to cardiac arrhythmias.[64]

## GLUCOSE REGULATION

The micropremie is at risk for both hypoglycemia and hyperglycemia. Decreased glycogen and body fat predispose to fasting hypoglycemia, whereas decreased insulin production with infusion of dextrose predisposes to hyperglycemia.[65,66] Glucose production is poorly regulated within a large range of glucose and insulin concentrations. The micropremie is also relatively insulin resistant and requires a greater infusion rate of insulin to achieve normoglycemia.[67] The use of total parenteral nutrition and glucocorticoids places the micropremies at increased risk for hyperglycemia.

## GLUCOSE AND THE BRAIN

Multiple animal models and clinical studies implicate hyperglycemia as detrimental to the adult brain during global and focal ischemia.[68] In contrast, hyperglycemia in neonates appears to protect the brain from ischemic damage.[69-71] Studies in both neonatal rat and pig hypoxia-ischemia models observed less brain damage with greater glucose concentrations. Many mechanisms exist for this strikingly different outcome between neonates and adults.[72] Relatively mild hypoglycemia is known to cause brain damage in preterm infants.[73] Micropremies with critical illness are especially prone to hypoglycemia because they contain limited stores of glucose and consume glucose anaerobically. Thus the administration of dextrose-containing fluids (carefully controlled with an infusion pump so as to minimize wide fluctuations in glucose values) and close monitoring of blood glucose concentrations is vital during anesthesia. Mild or moderate hyperglycemia during surgery is best managed by reducing the rate of infusion of dextrose-containing solutions and not administering insulin, with its attendant risk of hypoglycemia.

## HEPATIC AND HEMATOLOGIC FUNCTION

Immature hepatic function leads to a reduction in many hepatic proteins important for drug metabolism. In addition, reduced albumin synthesis decreases albumin concentrations compared with term neonates (see Fig. 6-6), thus enhancing the "free" (unbound) concentration of anesthetic drugs that are highly bound to albumin (see Chapter 6). The micropremie is at particular risk for spontaneous liver hemorrhage.[74,75] This occurs most commonly during laparotomy for necrotizing enterocolitis (NEC), is associated with large IV fluid resuscitation, and is difficult to control surgically. Recombinant factor VIIa has been used to stop liver hemorrhage when administration of other blood products has been unsuccessful.[76]

The ideal hematocrit level for the micropremie remains controversial. In the micropremie with reduced oxygen saturations and cardiac output, tissue oxygen delivery will be maximized by maintaining the hematocrit between 44% and 48%. In a randomized study of liberal versus restrictive transfusion in neonates between 500 and 1300 grams, intraparenchymal brain hemorrhage, periventricular leukomalacia, and episodes of apnea occurred more frequently in the restrictive transfusion group.[77] The risks of blood transfusion in the micropremie must be balanced against the benefits of improved oxygen delivery and fewer medical complications.

Thrombocytopenia (platelet count less than 150,000/mm³) occurs in as many as 70% of micropremies.[78] Although the etiology of thrombocytopenia is often unknown, pathophysiologic processes such as sepsis, disseminated intravascular coagulation, and NEC are common causes. Preoperative evaluation should include a recent platelet count and the availability of platelets for major procedures.

## Anesthetic Agents and the Micropremie

Anesthesia provides insensibility to pain during surgical procedures. Although anesthesia may be provided by regional or general techniques, general anesthesia is the most commonly used technique in the micropremie. During the past 25 years, general anesthesia has been delivered using both inhaled and IV drugs in very premature infants for a variety of surgical procedures.

### ANESTHETICS AND THE IMMATURE BRAIN
Research in immature animals indicates that anesthetics are both neuroprotective and neurotoxic. Inhalational anesthetics protect against hypoxic-ischemic injury in neonatal pigs and rats.[79-81] The anesthetic must be administered before and during the ischemic event at a concentration of 1 MAC (minimal alveolar concentration) to be effective. Thus for surgery in which there is a risk of brain ischemia, use of an inhalational anesthetic may afford some advantage over IV agents. Cardiac surgery, ventricular shunt insertion, and vein of Galen embolization represent examples of procedures that are performed in preterm infants and that carry a risk of brain ischemia. The MAC for sevoflurane has not been established in preterm infants and many sick preterm infants cannot tolerate even relatively modest concentrations of potent anesthetic agents.

Of particular concern are the reports in immature rats and other animals, including primates, that prolonged exposure to commonly used anesthetics, such as isoflurane, ketamine, and midazolam, induces apoptosis in many regions of the brain (see Chapter 23).[82,83] In rodents, exposure for at least 2 hours at 1 MAC of isoflurane produces apoptosis. A combination of isoflurane, midazolam, and nitrous oxide produces more neuronal degeneration than isoflurane or midazolam alone; nitrous oxide alone is not neurotoxic. When affected rats matured to adulthood, neurocognitive impairment was detected.[82] The neurotoxicity is brain-region specific and very dependent on the developmental age of the rodent. Rats are most sensitive to the neurotoxic effects of anesthetics on postnatal day 7, more so than on postnatal day 4 or beyond postnatal day 10.[84] The most susceptible age in rats, 7 days, corresponds to human brain development around mid-gestation. This suggests that if this phenomenon applies to humans, the preterm infant could potentially be more susceptible to anesthetic neurotoxicity than is the full-term infant.

The mechanism for the neurotoxicity appears to be attributable to the neurotransmitters glutamate and γ-aminobutyric acid, which act as trophic factors in the developing brain.[85] In the immature brain, these trophic factors promote synaptic growth

and plasticity and are obligate for neuronal survival. The inhaled anesthetics, ketamine, and midazolam exert their anesthetic effects by altering synaptic transmission through blockade of glutamate and γ-aminobutyric acid receptors. In the immature brain, this blockade also precipitates neuronal cell death by apoptosis.[86] In contrast, several anesthetics and medications may protect against apoptosis (see Chapter 23). A confounding factor is that neurodegeneration and apoptosis is a normal developmental phenomenon in the maturing fetal brain. Furthermore, anesthesia-induced neuronal cell death in neonatal animals may not directly translate into long-term neurologic abnormalities. Indeed, evidence suggests that sevoflurane-induced cognitive impairment, in the form of short-term memory deficiency in neonatal rodents, is offset by delayed exercise.[87] Moreover, immature animals that undergo painful procedures without anesthesia experience neuronal degeneration.[88,89] Preterm infants who receive anesthesia and sedation for painful procedures experience less morbidity and mortality than those who do not.[90] Curiously, the combination of surgery and anesthesia in neonatal rats produces more apoptosis than either intervention alone suggesting that in this model, anesthetics are neither neuroprotective themselves nor do they offset the apoptotic effects of surgery.[91] In summary, the neurodegeneration precipitated by inhaled anesthetics, ketamine, and benzodiazepines depends on developmental age, brain region, and duration of exposure. Based on the animal models, the micropremie exposed to several hours of large concentrations of inhaled agents with nitrous oxide and midazolam is potentially at risk, as is the micropremie exposed to surgery with insufficient anesthesia. Thus our approach at the present time for emergency surgery is to use small concentrations of inhaled agent with opioids and regional anesthesia whenever possible.

Of even greater concern may be the sedatives that are administered for prolonged periods of time in the intensive care unit (ICU), although one study found "no evidence of an association between dose and duration of sedation and/or analgesia drugs given during the preoperative, intraoperative, and postoperative period and major adverse developmental outcomes" in children undergoing repair of congenital heart disease in the first 6 weeks of life.[92]

### INHALATION ANESTHETIC AGENTS
The MAC defines the anesthetic depth for inhaled agents at which 50% of patients respond to a painful stimulus with movement; this measure allows comparison of the effects of inhaled anesthetics at equipotent doses. The MAC of isoflurane in the micropremie (less than 32 weeks PCA) is approximately 20% less than that in full-term neonates (E-Fig. 35-1; see also Fig. 6-16), and that at equipotent doses of isoflurane (1 MAC), systolic arterial pressure decreased similarly in all age-groups, 20% to 30%.[93] Sevoflurane affords a rapid induction and emergence from general anesthesia. Desflurane is contraindicated for induction of anesthesia but is widely used for maintenance of anesthesia administered through an ETT. However, desflurane causes more airway irritability than isoflurane or sevoflurane, and as a result, it is not recommended for infants with severe BPD. Desflurane, sevoflurane, and isoflurane decrease arterial blood pressure in a dose-dependent manner, possibly through decreasing the systemic vascular resistance or by myocardial depression. One possible mechanism to explain the myocardial depression is that the baseline ionized calcium concentrations in preterm infants, especially critically ill neonates are reduced.[94,95] Because inhalational

anesthetics block the calcium channels,[96] and because the neonatal heart depends on the plasma ionized calcium for contractility to a greater extent than do the hearts of older children,[97] preterm infants may be more susceptible to the cardio-depressant effects of inhalational anesthetics.

Nitrous oxide is not routinely used in the micropremie for several reasons. First, nitrous oxide must be delivered in inspired concentrations ranging from 50% to 75% to reduce the MAC of other agents; therefore, its role in micropremies, a group often requiring supplemental oxygen, is limited. Second, because of its blood gas solubility, nitrous oxide rapidly enters air-filled cavities; therefore it is not recommended for use in infants with bowel obstruction, NEC, pulmonary interstitial emphysema, or pneumothoraces, which are common disorders in micropremies.[98] Third, in neonatal and young rats, nitrous oxide demonstrates no antinociceptive effects, which contrasts its antinociceptive effect in adolescent and adult rats.[99] This observation requires validation in humans.

## INTRAVENOUS AGENTS

IV agents include opioids, benzodiazepines, barbiturates, propofol, ketamine, and dexmedetomidine. Fentanyl possesses analgesic and sedative properties, however, it does not reliably produce unconsciousness or amnesia and, by itself, is not considered an anesthetic in children or adults. Nevertheless, the use of fentanyl as an anesthetic has been justified in preterm infants because they were deemed to be inherently amnestic by virtue of their age, even though the age at which "consciousness" and memory occurs is unknown. Preterm infants (less than 1500 g) who receive IV fentanyl (30 to 50 µg/kg) and pancuronium for ligation of a PDA exhibit remarkable hemodynamic stability, with only a 5% decrease in blood pressure.[100] Another study examined the dose response of 25 neonates undergoing a variety of thoracic and abdominal procedures. A dose of 10 to 12.5 µg/kg administered together with a muscle relaxant produced hemodynamic stability for 75 minutes.[101] Hypertension and tachycardia did not occur with skin incision, suggesting that analgesic concentrations necessary for surgery are achieved with this dose of fentanyl.

The pharmacokinetics of fentanyl (30 µg/kg) in preterm infants yielded plasma concentrations that remained constant for up to 120 minutes, indicating a reduced clearance.[102] The elimination half-life of fentanyl ranged from 6 to 32 hours in preterm infants, significantly greater than the 2- to 3-hour half-life observed in children and adults.[102] The clearance of fentanyl is 7 mL/min/kg at 25 weeks, 10 mL/min/kg at 30 weeks, and 12 mL/min/kg at 35 weeks postmenstrual age.[103] These studies demonstrated that the half-life and volume of distribution of fentanyl are increased, whereas the clearance is reduced in preterm infants compared with adults.[104] These changes may be explained by immature CPY450 3A4, reduced proteins, immature kidneys, and a patent ductus venosus. In a subset of infants with increased intra-abdominal pressure (after repair of a gastroschisis or omphalocele), the elimination half-life of fentanyl is 1.5- to 3-fold greater than that in other infants of the same age.[104] This likely results because increased intraabdominal pressure decreases hepatic blood flow, the rate limiting step in the metabolism of drugs with a large hepatic extraction ratio, such as fentanyl.[104] The increased volume of distribution decreases the initial plasma concentration of fentanyl compared with that in adults. These pharmacokinetic differences, combined with an increased propensity to apnea, serve to prolong analgesia, as well as prolong

respiratory depression, increase the risk of postoperative apnea, and slow recovery of consciousness. In the micropremie, mechanical ventilation may be required for several days after large doses of fentanyl.

Similarly, the elimination half-life of morphine is markedly prolonged in preterm infants compared with that in children and adults.[105-108] The elimination half-life of morphine ranges from 6 to 16 hours in the micropremie, compared with 2 to 4 hours in the adult. We prefer fentanyl instead of large-dose morphine (2 to 3 mg/kg) for anesthesia because it has fewer hemodynamic adverse effects.

Remifentanil, a relatively new synthetic, short-acting opioid, is rapidly inactivated by plasma and tissue esterases and, because of its short half-life, is administered by continuous infusion. The half-life of remifentanil in adults is 3 to 4 minutes, independent of the duration of infusion, and similar to that in infants or children.[109] A multicenter study that compared halothane and remifentanil for maintenance of anesthesia in infants undergoing pyloromyotomy showed similar intraoperative hemodynamic stability intraoperatively with the two techniques, but significantly fewer "new onset apneas" with remifentanil compared with halothane.[110,111] Interestingly, the most rapid clearance of remifentanil was in infants and children younger than 2 years of age, thus allowing an intense opioid effect intraoperatively that rapidly dissipates on terminating the infusion.[112] Remifentanil has been used to provide anesthesia in infants weighing 400 to 580 grams with apparent good hemodynamic stability.[113,114] A study examining cord blood from preterm infants found high nonspecific esterase activity, comparable to that of term infants, thus suggesting that preterm infants should be able to rapidly metabolize remifentanil.[115]

Ketamine, a phencyclidine derivative, affords several advantages compared with inhaled and other IV agents. It provides analgesia, amnesia, and unconsciousness yet minimally depresses cardiovascular function (Fig. 35-3).[116] However, ketamine anesthesia depresses ventilation and airway reflexes, which predisposes to airway obstruction, apnea, and gastric aspiration. Thus we recommend the use of an ETT when ketamine is used for surgical procedures in the micropremie. In the setting of brief painful procedures, IV ketamine can be used as an anesthetic without an ETT.[117]

Other IV agents include thiopental, propofol, and benzodiazepines. These agents induce loss of consciousness but possess less analgesia than ketamine. Thiopental is a short-acting barbiturate primarily used for the induction of anesthesia. The micropremie requires less thiopental for induction than does the infant (2 to 3 mg/kg vs. 5 to 6 mg/kg, respectively), a relationship similar to the MAC of isoflurane.[118] In the micropremie, we only use thiopental for neurosurgical procedures involving increased intracranial pressure. However, thiopental is no longer available in the USA. Propofol is primarily used to induce anesthesia and has largely replaced thiopental for this purpose. A word of caution is needed regarding the use of propofol for induction of anesthesia in neonates. Several reports highlight episodes in otherwise stable infants of protracted hypotension and low cardiac output state that were associated with hypoxia after propofol boluses (1 to 3 mg/kg IV). The mechanism underlying these responses remains unclear although acute pulmonary hypertension with reversion to persistent fetal circulation remains a strong possibility.[119,120] In our experience, the micropremie can be anesthetized with a propofol infusion (50 to 200 µg/kg/min) supplemented with fentanyl as needed for analgesia. The selection of

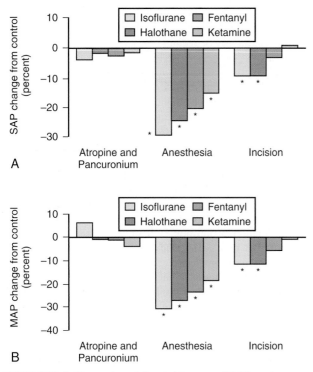

**FIGURE 35-3 A,** Changes in systolic arterial pressure (*SAP*) in preterm infants after anesthesia with either isoflurane, halothane, fentanyl, or ketamine, and after surgical incision. **B,** Changes in mean arterial pressure (*MAP*) in premature infants after anesthesia with either isoflurane, halothane, fentanyl, or ketamine, and after surgical incision. (Reprinted with permission from Friesen RH, Henry DB. Cardiovascular changes in preterm neonates receiving isoflurane, halothane, fentanyl, and ketamine. Anesthesiology 1986;64:238-42.)

infusion pumps that allow for delivery of small volumes accurately is vital. The infusion rate of propofol in these small infants must be carefully and meticulously checked, as a 10-fold overdose of propofol has been reported, with a successful recovery.[121] Recovery from propofol anesthesia is delayed in micropremies compared with term infants, because micropremies have both less fat and muscle tissue to redistribute the drug, and reduced clearance. In pediatric ICUs, propofol infusions have been implicated in unexpected deaths (propofol infusion syndrome).[122] Until the safety of long-term administration of propofol has been examined in preterm infants, other alternatives for prolonged sedation should be considered.

Benzodiazepines, such as midazolam and diazepam, have been used in the neonatal intensive care unit (NICU) for sedation. As with thiopental and propofol, these drugs do not provide analgesia and are not recommended as the sole anesthetic for surgery. However, the combination of a benzodiazepine and opioid provides complete anesthesia for surgery. Midazolam clearance is markedly decreased in the micropremie when compared with the term neonate or infant, and will be further prolonged in the setting of decreased liver function.[123] Midazolam can cause systemic hypotension, depress ventilation, and impair airway reflexes in preterm infants. The hypotension caused by midazolam is greater in the presence of fentanyl; thus both drugs must be titrated in small doses when administered concomitantly.[124] One study noted an 8% to 23% decrease in arterial pressure after a bolus of 0.1 mg/kg of midazolam in preterm infants.[125]

## Anesthetic Considerations for Surgical Procedures

The extremely preterm infant rarely requires surgical intervention unless the condition is life-threatening or incurs long-term disability if not treated promptly. Preoperative preparation focuses on optimization of cardiac and respiratory status and on treatment of anemia, electrolyte abnormalities, metabolic acidosis, and coagulopathy. In conditions such as NEC, surgical intervention may be necessary before these can be corrected. For non-emergency procedures, such as inguinal hernia repair, preoperative evaluation occurs well in advance of surgery, to optimize the medical status before administration of anesthesia. Communication between the anesthesiologist, surgeon, and neonatologist before and after surgery is vital for safe care.

To ensure the safe delivery of care in these micropremies, particular attention must be paid to ensuring the accurate delivery of medications and fluids. These infants require only small fractions of the medications in most vials and ampoules. As a result, either tuberculin syringes should be used to carefully measure the very small aliquots of medications or the medication in the vial should be diluted so that a measurable and accurate fraction of the content of the vial can be given. Tuberculin syringes present several challenges, including difficulty in removing air bubbles from the syringe, and the very small volume that will be administered. The volume of medication may be so small that it is no larger than the volume of the stem of the clave or stopcock, resulting in less drug than intended being administered to the infant. To prevent this problem, a saline flush should follow each medication administration. Diluting every medication introduces the risk of a drug dosing error that could lead to an overdose or underdose. In all instances, it is prudent to verify the dose and dilution of the medication with a colleague. To ensure drug is not lost in the dead space of the IV set, each clave or stopcock should be flushed with saline after the medication has been given. All medications should be administered into the IV set as close to the skin insertion as possible, to minimize the volume of fluids needed to flush the medication into the child (see Figure 51-3).

Fluid overload is always a concern in these small infants. To minimize the fluids administered, all IV infusions should be delivered through a pump. Free-flowing IVs are dangerous sources for fluid overload, which may open a ductus arteriosus and cause congestive heart failure. Finally, meticulous care must be taken to remove air bubbles from all IV administration systems, solutions, and medications that are administered. See Chapter 51 for further discussion on infusion pumps and the implications of IV administration dead space on drug delivery.[126,127]

In the past, some surgeons chose to perform surgery at the bedside in the NICU without an anesthesiologist because it was deemed unsafe to transport the infant, there was lack of an OR or anesthesiologist to perform the surgery in a timely manner, or it was thought that the micropremie did not need anesthesia. The neonatologist often administered sedation and/or muscle relaxants during surgery. We believe that this approach does not provide optimal patient care; there is ample evidence that the micropremie requires anesthesia for surgery. As far as operating at the bedside is concerned, there is reduced access to the child, suboptimal lighting, reduced sterility, limited monitors (usually capnography is absent), and an inability to control room temperature, although NICU incubators use built-in overhead radiant heaters. In our institution we addressed the issue of transporting an unstable infant to the OR by building a surgical suite in the NICU, thus minimizing the period of transport and providing optimal surgical conditions. In most institutions, anesthesiologists attend to preterm neonates in the NICU when the infants are too small or unstable (because of hemodynamic instability) to transport, the transport requires inter-hospital travel, or they are ventilated with an oscillator or high-frequency jet ventilator. Adapting to the working environment requires planning and organization in concert with communication with the surgeons, neonatologists, and nurses in the NICU. If bedside anesthesia is to be provided, then appropriate IV equipment for transfusion, pumps, and monitors compatible with electrocautery and expired carbon dioxide monitoring should be available, just as in the OR.

## EXPLORATORY LAPAROTOMY FOR NECROTIZING ENTEROCOLITIS

Necrotizing enterocolitis, a life-threatening condition mainly afflicting preterm neonates, occurs in about 5% of ELBW infants (see Chapter 36).[128] Although NEC may be treated medically, the micropremie with NEC is more likely to require surgery; mortality ranges from 10% to 50%.[129-131] The pathogenesis of NEC is incompletely understood; intestinal mucosal ischemia is thought to play a key role. Other key contributing factors include inflammation of bowel mucosa, alterations in normal intestinal flora by antibiotic therapy, gastric alkalinity, low systemic cardiac output, and red blood cell transfusion in the preceding 48 hours.[132-135] Early signs of NEC include feeding intolerance, increased work of breathing, lethargy, and temperature instability; later signs include hypotension, abdominal distention, apnea, thrombocytopenia, coagulopathy, and multisystem organ failure. Classic radiographic findings include gas in the intestinal wall (pneumatosis intestinalis) and biliary tract, and free air within the abdomen. Indications for surgical exploration include the presence of perforation or continued clinical deterioration despite medical management (Fig. 35-4).

Surgical management of the micropremie with NEC involves either initial primary peritoneal drainage or a laparotomy with resection of necrotic bowel. Primary peritoneal drainage requires a small surgical incision and fewer anesthetic requirements and

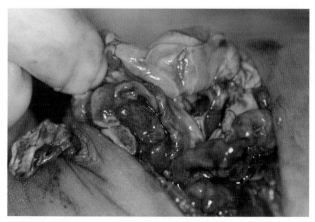

**FIGURE 35-4** Early necrotizing enterocolitis with bowel perforation. Note that the perforation was diagnosed early and that there is soiling of the peritoneum but there does not appear to be any dead bowel. This type of perforation is generally associated with a positive outcome.

can be performed at the bedside. Some infants who undergo initial peritoneal drainage will subsequently require laparotomy if their condition worsens. Peritoneal drainage has generally been favored in the smaller and more unstable preterm infants for logistical reasons; thus the ability to compare the two management strategies has been difficult because of multiple confounding variables.[128,136] A prospective randomized, multicenter trial comparing laparotomy and peritoneal drainage in infants weighing less than 1500 g with perforated NEC found no difference in survival, development of short-gut syndrome, or length of hospital stay between the two approaches.[137]

NEC is a surgical emergency, and preoperative preparation in a timely fashion is vital. NEC predisposes to hypovolemia, cardiovascular and respiratory failure, capillary leak syndrome, disseminated intravascular coagulation, and hypoglycemia. It is important to prepare for all these sequelae. We have albumin, fresh frozen plasma, platelets, and packed red blood cells available; calcium gluconate, dopamine, and epinephrine are prepared for treatment of hypotension and reduced cardiac output. Because pulmonary function may deteriorate, we ensure the availability of sophisticated ventilators for increased mechanical ventilatory support. Newer anesthesia machines provide modes of ventilation similar to the ventilators used in the ICU. Coagulopathy and thrombocytopenia increase bleeding and necessitate blood product administration during surgery. Before transporting the micropremie to the OR, a transfer note is written to include the current medications, size and location of IV catheters, and dextrose infusion rate. We also obtain a current plasma glucose concentration and assess the ETT for size, equality of breath sounds, how well it is secured, and when it was last changed.

Vascular access remains critical for this surgery. At least two venous cannulas and an arterial catheter should be considered for optimal care. Usually the venous cannulas are 24-gauge catheters. In-line filters designed to prevent air within tubing, easily become blocked when one attempts to transfuse blood through them. Packed cells, even if they are reconstituted with plasma, do not flow rapidly through 24-gauge catheters; therefore it is important to avoid falling behind in fluid administration in these infants, so that there is no need to force a catch-up to stave off hypotension. A central venous catheter facilitates the delivery of infusions, such as dopamine or epinephrine. In our institution, many preterm infants have peripherally inserted central catheters (PICCs), allowing for delivery of vasopressors. These catheters are not well-suited for rapid delivery of anesthetic drugs or blood, or for measurement of central venous pressure. An arterial catheter provides continuous blood pressure monitoring and the ability to sample blood gases, electrolytes, complete blood cell count (CBC), platelet count, and prothrombin time/partial thromboplastin times (PT/PTT). In recent years, automated blood pressure cuffs have improved enormously in their ability to measure blood pressure non-invasively in young infants, although cases still occur in which they fail to measure arterial pressure during this surgery. A Foley catheter allows for the assessment of urine flow. A nasogastric tube should be present. Time spent by the anesthesia and surgical team to place these lines must be weighed against the need for urgent laparotomy.

General endotracheal anesthesia with neuromuscular blockade remains the anesthesia technique for NEC surgery. NEC increases the risk for aspiration. Tracheal intubation may be achieved by "awake intubation" or by rapid-sequence anesthetic induction. We prefer an awake intubation in the micropremie because effective cricoid pressure is difficult to apply, a very small force may distort the airway in the infant rendering intubation difficult,[138] and arterial desaturation occurs rapidly during apnea. After the administration of IV atropine, awake intubation is performed using an *oxyscope*, a laryngoscope with an oxygen port to allow for oxygen delivery during direct laryngoscopy (see E-Fig. 12-12, *A* and *B*). Awake intubation should be completed efficiently and rapidly in less than 15 seconds. To accomplish this, all equipment and monitors should be prepared, including an ETT with a "hockey stick" bend using a stylet. After preoxygenating the infant and administering 10 to 20 μg/kg IV atropine, the infant's arms are brought up by an assistant and held against the head (hands pointing to the anesthesiologist) with the elbows adjacent to the ears. This secures the child's arms and shoulders, preventing the infant from laterally rotating the neck, raising the shoulders, or moving the arms during laryngoscopy. Once the infant is positioned, a #1 straight blade is inserted into the mouth at the right commissure and the tip is advanced toward the glottic opening in one smooth motion. When the infant gags, the ETT, which is being held in the other hand, is poised to pass through the cords. Once the position of the tube is confirmed with the presence of carbon dioxide on the capnogram, the assistant immediately administers a predetermined dose of IV propofol to rapidly induce anesthesia. Inhalational anesthesia and muscle relaxant, as indicated, should be administered while the ETT is taped in place. Chest auscultation in the axillae will confirm a properly placed ETT.

The anesthetic regimens that we prefer for maintenance include (1) IV fentanyl (5 to 10 μg/kg), an inhaled anesthetic (such as isoflurane, sevoflurane, or desflurane), and neuromuscular blocking drug (balanced technique), or (2) IV fentanyl (20 to 50 μg/kg), IV midazolam (0.1 mg/kg), and a neuromuscular blocking drug (high-dose opioid technique). We select the high-dose opioid technique for hemodynamically unstable infants. Pancuronium is an ideal neuromuscular blocking drug when combined with large doses of fentanyl because of its anticholinergic properties, but should be avoided in infants with renal dysfunction. If hypotension persists despite a trial of 10 to 20 mL/kg of IV fluid, we begin an infusion of epinephrine (0.02 to 0.1 μg/kg/min) or dopamine (5 to 20 μg/kg/min). Hypocalcemia during administration of citrated blood products may contribute to hypotension, and requires replacement with either calcium chloride or calcium gluconate (see Chapter 10). When severe shock persists despite IV fluid resuscitation, calcium, and inotropic support, rescue treatment with "stress dose" glucocorticoids may be beneficial. Treatment with hydrocortisone and dexamethasone has been effective in improving arterial pressure in low–birth-weight infants with refractory hypotension.[139,140]

Intraoperative fluid management in micropremies should begin with continuing the solution that arrives with the infant from the NICU; usually this is a calcium- and/or glucose-containing solution. Alternately, some infants may arrive with a hyperosmolar glucose or dextrose (10%) parenteral nutrition solution. In both cases, these solutions should not be discontinued, but rather continued at the same rate (by infusion pump) or slightly less throughout the surgery to avoid reactive hypoglycemia from increased circulating insulin concentrations. There is no evidence regarding the optimal infusion rates for these solutions during anesthesia. If no solution is being infused, a balanced salt solution (e.g., lactated Ringer's solution) could be initiated at 4 mL/kg/hr, supplemented with the same solution for third space loss (at least 10 mL/kg/hr), and replacement of blood loss. If no glucose solution is being administered, then a balanced salt solution containing glucose may be administered through a pump. Serum glucose concentrations should be monitored regularly to avoid hypoglycemia. Third space losses include evaporation and vascular leak and are replaced with an isotonic salt solution. Blood losses are replaced with packed red blood cells and fresh frozen plasma to maintain the hemoglobin greater than 10 g/dL and the PT/PTT within normal range. Platelets are administered to keep the platelet count greater than 100,000/mm³. Continuous measurement of arterial pressure and serial measurement of urine output, blood gases, CBC, platelet counts, and PT/PTT aid in the fluid replacement process. Arterial blood gas analysis helps guide ventilation and inspired oxygen concentration. Warming of the operating suite to 80° F (26.7° C), a forced air warmer underneath the infant, and warmed fluids help maintain normothermia during surgery. In preterm infants with NEC, postoperative mechanical ventilation remains the rule. Postoperative analgesia can be provided with a continuous infusion of fentanyl (1 to 3 μg/kg/hr) or intermittent doses of morphine (0.1 mg/kg every 4 to 6 hours). The time it takes for the micropremie to emerge from anesthesia depends on the anesthetic technique (balanced vs. high-dose opioid) and the need for postoperative analgesics. After a high-dose opioid technique, the micropremie may take 12 to 24 hours to emerge, as compared with several hours for a balanced technique. Remifentanil may provide an alternative, which allows an intense opioid effect that rapidly dissipates on discontinuation of the infusion[113,114,141-143]; an alternate form of analgesia is required for postoperative pain management.

## LIGATION OF PATENT DUCTUS ARTERIOSUS

Failure of the ductus arteriosus to close after birth is common in the micropremie.[144] A PDA may incur significant left-to-right shunting of blood, causing excess pulmonary blood flow, congestive heart failure, and respiratory failure. In fact, the diameter of the PDA may be greater than the aorta. In the micropremie with respiratory distress syndrome or persistent pulmonary hypertension, right-to-left shunting across the PDA may occur, producing cyanosis. Significant controversy exists regarding whether a PDA should be aggressively treated, the timing of therapy, and merits of medical versus surgical therapy.[145] Medical therapy involves the administration of a cyclooxygenase inhibitor, such as indomethacin or ibuprofen. Indomethacin therapy is less likely to close the PDA in micropremies compared with preterm infants, and more likely to produce complications, including thrombocytopenia, renal failure, hyponatremia, and intestinal perforation.[146] Ibuprofen is equally effective for PDA closure in the micropremie, with a reduced frequency of renal failure.[147] When surgery is performed by experienced teams, the incidence of major intraoperative complications is small.[148] However, as many as one-third of preterm infants develop severe cardiovascular instability following PDA ligation, as evidenced by systemic hypotension, pulmonary hypertension, and myocardial dysfunction.[149]

During preoperative preparation, arterial pressure, heart rate, arterial blood gases, ventilator settings, and inspired oxygen concentration should be noted. The PDA is ligated through a left thoracotomy and requires retraction of the left lung, which decreases lung compliance, ventilation, and oxygenation. Preoperative difficulty with ventilation and oxygenation forecasts trouble in the OR. Because the aorta and pulmonary artery lie in proximity to the PDA, severe bleeding may occur abruptly and unexpectedly during the procedure. Packed red blood cells

should be immediately available for transfusion. Intraoperative monitoring includes a blood pressure cuff (right arm reflects cerebral perfusion of preductal blood), continuous end-tidal carbon dioxide monitoring, and a pulse oximeter placed on digits on the right arm and a lower extremity. This will help the surgeon to confirm that the vessel about to be ligated (clipped) is in fact the ductus and not the aorta. It should be noted that with a left-sided arch, the pulse oximeter may need to be applied to the left hand instead of the right to ensure monitoring of a preductal blood vessel. Invasive monitoring of arterial pressure and blood gases is helpful in the micropremie with significant heart failure and/or lung disease, although we do not consider it a requirement for surgery. An IV catheter through which blood can be rapidly administered should be available.

The anesthetic technique of choice for PDA ligation remains fentanyl (20 to 50 μg/kg) and pancuronium (0.2 mg/kg).[100] Although this technique usually does not cause hypotension or bradycardia, reduction in arterial pressure after anesthetic induction may occur because of loss of sympathetic tone, especially in the setting of hypovolemia from diuretic therapy. Thus we commonly administer 5% albumin or balanced salt solution (10 mL/kg) before induction. During mechanical ventilation, mild hypoventilation and a reduced inspired oxygen concentration help to reduce pulmonary over-circulation from the PDA. However, during surgical retraction of the lung it is usually necessary to increase the ventilator inspiratory pressure setting as well as the inspired oxygen concentration. Surgical complications of PDA ligation include inadvertent ligation or laceration of the aorta or pulmonary artery. The lower extremity oxygen saturation provides a monitor of perfusion to the legs, and loss of this signal immediately after PDA ligation may indicate aortic ligation. With ligation of the pulmonary artery, oxygen saturation in both extremities and end-tidal $CO_2$ decrease. With successful PDA ligation, arterial diastolic and mean pressure increase, and the PDA murmur disappears.

The time until emergence from anesthesia depends on the fentanyl dose. In the micropremie with normal renal function, pancuronium will disappear in 2 to 3 hours, whereas the fentanyl (20 to 50 μg/kg) will last for at least 6 hours. Thus a trial of spontaneous ventilation and extubation is generally not planned until the following day.

## INGUINAL HERNIA REPAIR

Inguinal hernias are common in preterm infants. In ELBW infants, an inguinal hernia occurs in approximately one-third of patients, whereas in full-term neonates, it occurs in 1%.[150] Complications related to inguinal hernias and their surgical repair include incarcerated bowel, intestinal obstruction, gonadal infarction, infection, hematoma, and recurrent hernias.[151] Because of the risk of incarceration and bowel infarction, the hernia should be repaired as soon as the infant is medically stable.

General and/or regional anesthesia may be used for inguinal hernia repair. Induction of general anesthesia can be achieved with IV propofol or inhalation of sevoflurane. We prefer IV induction for the infant with an IV catheter in place. Indications for emergency surgery include incarceration of the bowel or gonads. When the micropremie with intestinal obstruction or incarceration requires emergency surgery, we secure the airway by awake tracheal intubation (see previous section on Exploratory Laparotomy for Necrotizing Enterocolitis). When hernia repair is performed electively, we induce anesthesia with propofol if IV access is present, or by mask with sevoflurane.

A non-depolarizing muscle relaxant may be administered as needed. Cisatracurium or atracurium are preferred because their action is terminated by Hofmann elimination in plasma, whereas the action of rocuronium and vecuronium is terminated primarily by hepatic metabolism. After induction of anesthesia, the trachea is intubated and the lungs ventilated mechanically.

General anesthesia is maintained with an inhalational anesthetic agent. We avoid nitrous oxide when intestinal obstruction is present, or when the infant has complex hernias that may take several hours to repair. Preterm infants with BPD often exhibit a compensated respiratory acidosis and will have increased end-tidal $CO_2$ during anesthesia. In these infants the ventilation parameters are set to allow permissive hypercapnia. Mechanical ventilation with small tidal volumes (4 to 6 mL/kg), increased respiratory rates, and PEEP minimizes atelectasis and reduces the risk for lung injury. If extubation is planned after surgery, caffeine (10 mg/kg) is administered IV to reduce the risk of postoperative apnea.[21,152] IV fluids consist of lactated Ringer's solution (4 mL/kg/hr) with dextrose (5 mg/kg/min administered by infusion pump) to maintain normoglycemia. A warm OR and forced-air warming blanket should be used to prevent hypothermia during the procedure.

Postoperative analgesia may be provided by regional analgesia or systemic analgesics; the choice depends on whether extubation of the trachea occurs immediately after surgery. Ilioinguinal and iliohypogastric nerve blocks or caudal epidural blocks may be used (see Chapter 41). We do not advocate percutaneous blockade because the local anesthetic injectate may distort the local tissues, making an already difficult surgery more difficult. Ilioinguinal and iliohypogastric nerve blocks consist of injecting 0.25% bupivacaine with epinephrine (1 : 200,000) (1 mg/kg/side) around the nerve by the surgeon under direct vision. This block provides 6 to 8 hours of analgesia. Caudal epidural blockade consists of injecting 0.125% bupivacaine with epinephrine (1 : 200,000) (1 mL/kg) through the sacral hiatus, providing several hours of analgesia. Orally administered acetaminophen (10 to 15 mg/kg) can also be given, providing analgesia for several hours. We do not administer opioids to the micropremie whose trachea will be extubated immediately after surgery because of the risk of postoperative apnea.

The micropremie with BPD who requires supplemental oxygen, but who is not intubated, is an excellent candidate for regional anesthesia.[153-156] Regional anesthesia circumvents the need to intubate the trachea and administer a general anesthetic, which may exacerbate the BPD and create a situation in which extubation after surgery may be difficult to achieve. Either a spinal or epidural anesthetic may be used to provide surgical conditions with a regional block. For spinal anesthesia, an intrathecal injection of a hyperbaric solution of tetracaine (1 mg/kg) or isobaric bupivacaine (1 mg/kg) provides 1 to 2 hours of surgical anesthesia (see Chapter 41) The addition of epinephrine (10 μg) to the tetracaine solution increases the duration of anesthesia by 30 to 60 minutes.[154] Hypotension rarely occurs after spinal anesthesia in an infant.[157] For epidural anesthesia, 0.75 mL/kg of 0.375% bupivacaine with epinephrine is injected into the epidural space through the sacral hiatus.[155,156] Ultrasound can be used to map out the anatomy of the spinal cord and cauda equina, dura mater, and intrathecal space. During injection one can visualize the local anesthetic tracking up the epidural space to confirm its proper location (see also Chapters 41 and 42). Preterm infants are more sensitive to local anesthetic blockade than are children and adults; therefore surgical anesthesia may

be achieved with reduced concentrations of local anesthetic. Another route to the epidural space is by the lumbar approach (L3-4 interspace).[19] The use of the lumbar route allows a smaller dose of local anesthetic compared with the caudal route, thus decreasing the risk of toxicity, however, this route is technically more challenging.

Epidural anesthesia offers several advantages over spinal anesthesia in the awake infant, in that it is often easier to perform, and a catheter can be placed to repeatedly administer local anesthetic to extend the duration of the block (see Chapter 41). General anesthesia offers several advantages over regional anesthesia, including better operating conditions and greater ease in titrating anesthetic duration. An often cited advantage of regional anesthesia is the decreased incidence of postoperative apnea. However, the evidence in support of this notion is conflicting. When the incidence of postoperative apnea after spinal anesthesia, spinal anesthesia with IV ketamine, and general endotracheal inhalational anesthesia was compared,[158] no postoperative apnea was reported in the spinal anesthesia group, whereas an 89% incidence was noted in the spinal/ketamine group and a 31% incidence was noted in the general anesthesia group. Thus, if there is a benefit to regional anesthesia over general anesthesia, spinal anesthesia must be administered without supplemental sedatives, such as ketamine.

In contrast, Krane and colleagues compared general endotracheal inhalational anesthesia with spinal anesthesia and found no difference in the incidence of postoperative apnea.[159] In a study of more than 250 preterm infants receiving spinal anesthesia for inguinal hernia repair at a single institution experienced with this technique, spinal block was successfully placed on the first attempt in more than 90% of infants.[160] Despite a high rate of successful block placement, more than 20% of the infants required supplemental anesthesia at some time during the surgery. Postoperative apnea occurred in 4.9% of infants, and all infants who developed this complication had a preoperative history of apnea. Given the technical challenges of spinal block placement for practitioners who do not perform it routinely, failure rate even with successful block placement, and persistent risk of postoperative apnea, we commonly administer general anesthesia for hernia repair in the micropremie, except for those with severe BPD, in whom we use spinal anesthesia.

## EYE SURGERY FOR RETINOPATHY OF PREMATURITY

ROP may be treated with cryotherapy, laser photocoagulation, or scleral buckling surgery and/or vitrectomy. Diode laser photocoagulation is typically performed at the bedside in the NICU for moderate ROP, whereas cryotherapy and scleral buckling surgery are performed in the OR. Cryotherapy involves applying a freezing probe under direct visualization to the avascular retina anterior to the fibrovascular ridge. Scleral buckling surgery and vitrectomy, performed for severe ROP with retinal detachment, are less frequently employed because early detection and treatment with laser photocoagulation prevents ROP progression to severe disease. Laser surgery has been shown to be as effective as cryotherapy for moderate ROP, and is most commonly used because the systemic side effects are significantly less, the ocular tissues are less traumatized, and this technique has a smaller incidence of late complications (see Chapter 32).

Laser photocoagulation may be performed under topical anesthesia alone, with IV sedation, or under general anesthesia. Cryotherapy and scleral buckling surgery require general anesthesia. For laser photocoagulation, the incidence of cardiorespiratory

complications is greater with topical anesthesia alone than with topical anesthesia with sedation or general anesthesia.[161] Factors that influence the selection of anesthetic technique include the infant's medical condition, gestational age, and availability of pediatric anesthesia services. The vast majority (95%) of preterm infants who require laser photocoagulation or cryotherapy develop threshold disease between 32 and 42 weeks PCA. The usual age for scleral buckling or vitrectomy is much older, between 6 months and 1 year.

Laser photocoagulation takes 10 to 30 minutes to perform and often involves a series of treatments every few weeks. For laser photocoagulation, the anesthetic goals are to provide optic analgesia and to prevent eye and head movement. Many preterm infants younger than 32 weeks PCA are naturally inactive. With topical anesthesia alone they will remain motionless and do not require sedation or general anesthesia. As the infants mature beyond 32 weeks PCA, their activity naturally increases, along with the need for sedation and general anesthesia. Given the brevity and frequency of the procedure, we prefer a combination of topical anesthesia with an infusion of propofol and spontaneous ventilation through a natural airway. After applying the local anesthetic, we administer a series of IV propofol boluses (1 mg/kg) until there is no movement to tactile stimulation, and then begin a propofol infusion (150 µg/kg/min). We use an oral airway as necessary. We administer supplemental oxygen and monitor end-tidal $CO_2$ through a nasal cannula. Alternative sedative agents include IV midazolam (0.1 to 0.2 mg/kg), pentobarbital (2 mg/kg), or oral chloral hydrate (75 mg/kg). We employ standard monitors and conduct the procedure with the ophthalmologist, in a treatment room in the NICU; size-appropriate airway equipment should be immediately available should airway obstruction or apnea occur. Cryotherapy and scleral buckling surgery take more time to complete and require surgical preparation in the OR. As a result, our preferred technique is inhalational anesthesia with tracheal intubation and neuromuscular relaxant, along with topical anesthesia. After an inhalational induction with sevoflurane using standard monitors, we paralyze the child, intubate the trachea orally, and mechanically ventilate the lungs. Administration of caffeine reduces the incidence of postoperative apnea. At the end of surgery, we discontinue the inhaled agent, antagonize the neuromuscular blockade as appropriate, and extubate the trachea after the return of appropriate breathing and airway reflexes.

## ANESTHESIA OR SEDATION FOR RADIOLOGIC IMAGING

Very preterm infants frequently experience neurocognitive complications. With advances in the capabilities of MRI, and new therapies to improve neurologic outcome based on MRI findings, preterm infants are increasingly undergoing MRI evaluation. At many centers, virtually all preterm infants less than 30 weeks gestational age at birth undergo brain MRI during their hospitalization. In past years, head ultrasound and computed tomography were the modalities of choice to diagnose IVH and hydrocephalus. MRI is gradually replacing these modalities for this purpose because there is no exposure to radiation. Moreover, MRI is able to identify congenital lesions, vascular malformations, and ischemic injury, which the older modalities were less effective in detecting.

Although not painful, MRI requires absolute immobility for the duration of the scan, typically 45 to 60 minutes. Immobility may be achieved through simulated feeding, sedation, or anesthesia. In very preterm infants (less than 30 weeks PCA) and

in good-tempered older preterm infants, swaddling the infant in warm blankets and applying sugar water ("sweet-ez") to a pacifier often promotes natural sleep, enabling the scan to be obtained. In healthy preterm infants ("premie growers") aged 30 to 70 weeks PCA, orally administered chloral hydrate (75 mg/kg) 30 to 60 minutes before the procedure provides sedation lasting 2 hours. We perform a history and physical examination and prescribe the sedation regimen, and specially trained sedation nurses in our department administer the regimen and monitor the infant during the scan, under our supervision. It should be noted that chloral hydrate has an extremely long half-life in this population, placing the infants at risk for late re-sedation and/or apnea.[162-164]

In preterm infants with medical problems, we administer propofol anesthesia for the scan, titrated to effect similarly to that with laser photocoagulation for ROP. We monitor expired $CO_2$ through a nasal cannula, sometimes insert an oral airway, and less often use a laryngeal mask airway or an ETT. In critically ill preterm infants with an ETT and mechanical ventilation, we administer IV midazolam and fentanyl or inhaled sevoflurane for the scan. In anesthesia cases, monitors include electrocardiogram, blood pressure, pulse oximetry, and expired $CO_2$. IV pumps being used for administration of fluids or drugs must remain outside the MRI room, thus requiring extra-long tubing. All anesthesia equipment, the infant, and personnel must not contain ferrous materials. As with general anesthesia, monitoring for postoperative apnea for 24 hours after sedation is recommended (see Chapters 45 and 47).

## ANNOTATED REFERENCES

Baum VC, Palmisano BW. The immature heart and anesthesia. Anesthesiology 1997;87:1529-48.

*This article examines developmental aspects of cardiac function and, in particular, how anesthetic agents affect the immature heart.*

Coté CJ, Zaslavsky A, Downes JJ, et al. Postoperative apnea in former preterm infants after inguinal herniorrhaphy. Anesthesiology 1995;82:809-22.

*This is a combined analysis of eight papers that studied postoperative apnea after general anesthesia for inguinal herniorrhaphy.*

Friesen RH, Henry DB. Cardiovascular changes in preterm neonates receiving isoflurane, halothane, fentanyl, and ketamine. Anesthesiology 1986;64:238-42.

*This is one of the few studies that compares the cardiovascular effects of different anesthetic agents on the preterm infant.*

Mikkola K, Ritari N, Tommiska V, et al. Neurodevelopmental outcome at 5 years of age of a national cohort of extremely low birth weight infants who were born in 1996-1997. Pediatrics 2005;116:1391-400.

*This study assesses neurodevelopmental outcome at 5 years of age in a cohort of extremely low–birth-weight infants. The authors found that only 25% of these children were classified as developmentally normal.*

Thome UH, Ambalavanan N. Permissive hypercapnia to decrease lung injury in ventilated preterm neonates. Semin Fetal Neonatal Med 2009;14:21-7.

*This review article discusses the use of permissive hypercapnia in the extremely premature infant. It also discusses the mechanism of lung injury and ventilation strategies that are believed to decrease the subsequent development of BPD in this population.*

## REFERENCES

Please see www.expertconsult.com

# Neonatal Emergencies

PATRICIA R. BACHILLER, JOSEPH H. CHOU, THOMAS M. ROMANELLI,
AND JESSE D. ROBERTS, JR.

**36**

| Neonatal Physiology Related to Anesthesia | Preparation for Surgery |
|---|---|
| Cardiopulmonary | The Operating Room |
| Temperature Regulation | The Family |
| Renal and Metabolic Function | **Emergency Surgery** |
| Gastrointestinal and Hepatic Function | Respiratory Problems |
| Neurologic Development | Gastrointestinal Problems |

ADVANCES IN PERINATAL CARE have greatly reduced the morbidity and mortality of critically ill neonates. Anesthesiologists have contributed to the improvement in neonatal outcome by applying advanced principles of developmental biology and pharmacology to the care of critically ill neonates undergoing surgical procedures. The goal of this chapter is to describe developmental processes in neonates and how they affect the anesthetic management of neonatal emergencies.

## Neonatal Physiology Related to Anesthesia

### CARDIOPULMONARY

#### Oxygen Consumption

The cardiopulmonary system of the neonate is driven by the need to deliver sufficient oxygen ($O_2$) to maintain a high metabolic rate. The $O_2$ consumption of an average neonate is 5 to 8 mL/kg/min, whereas that of an adult is 2 to 3 mL/kg/min (Table 36-1). It is this high rate of $O_2$ consumption that primarily leads to the rapid decrease in blood $O_2$ partial pressures in the neonate during periods of hypoventilation. Although ventilatory gas exchange volume is nearly 10-fold greater in adults than in neonates, the tidal volume relative to body weight for both is approximately equal (6 mL/kg). In neonates, increasing the respiratory rate facilitates the elimination of carbon dioxide ($CO_2$) generated by their relatively high metabolic processes; alveolar ventilation is approximately 130 mL/kg/min in the perinatal period, compared with 60 mL/kg/min in adulthood. In neonates, the thoracic gas volume on a weight basis is similar to that in adults. These metabolic and volume changes are consistent with those predicted by allometric scaling (see Chapter 6).[1]

#### Pulmonary Gas Exchange

Preterm neonates may have abnormalities in lung surfactant activity. Surfactant production by type II alveolar pneumocytes occurs predominantly after 32 weeks of gestation. Infants born prematurely may develop respiratory distress syndrome (RDS) because of surfactant deficiency. However, infants of mothers with gestational diabetes may develop RDS even when born near term. RDS is characterized by grunting respirations, nasal flaring, and chest retractions, developing soon after birth. Radiographic examination demonstrates decreased lung volume resulting from widespread atelectasis. The resultant intrapulmonary shunting of blood through atelectatic lung units causes intrapulmonary shunt and systemic hypoxemia and reduces $O_2$ delivery to the tissues. Judicious application of positive end-expiratory pressure (PEEP) and treatment with exogenous surfactant may reduce intrapulmonary shunting in RDS and decrease hypoxemia.[2-6] In addition, the incidence and severity of RDS has been decreased by the now routine treatment of mothers who are in preterm labor with glucocorticoids.

Atelectasis in neonates also might be caused by anatomic forces that decrease lung volume. For example, the relatively large abdomen in a neonate displaces the diaphragm cephalad, placing the lungs' closing capacity within the expiratory reserve volume. Moreover, increases in intraabdominal pressure from gastric distention associated with overzealous assisted ventilation with a facemask, replacement of bowel in the abdomen during repair of gastroschisis or omphalocele, or surgical retraction or manipulation of the abdominal contents also might shift the closing capacity to within the infant's expiratory reserve volume. The resulting atelectasis and intrapulmonary shunting may require controlled ventilation with PEEP to recruit closed lung units and improve oxygenation, emptying of the stomach, or changes in surgical maneuvers.

In the neonate, apnea decreases pulmonary gas exchange and can lead to hypoxemia and bradycardia. Conceptually, apnea is differentiated in terms of its cause: (1) *central apnea*, resulting from immaturity or depression of the respiratory drive; (2) *obstructive apnea*, caused by an infant's inability to maintain a patent airway; and (3) *mixed apnea*, a combination of both central and obstructive apnea.[7]

Apnea of central origin may be secondary to the poor organization and integration of input from proprioceptive receptors, which are located in the diaphragm and intercostal muscles, and from medullary and peripheral chemoreceptors. Preterm infants are at greater risk for central apnea because chemoreceptor signaling is incompletely developed. Exaggerated responses to chemoreceptor signaling during periods of mild hypercarbia and hypoxia can cause apnea in preterm infants, in whom it might stimulate the respiratory rate in those born at term. Susceptibility to central apnea is also exacerbated by metabolic disturbances such as hypothermia, hypoglycemia, and hypocalcemia, even in

**TABLE 36-1** Lung Function in Infants and Adults

| Parameter | Infants | Adults | Infant-to-Adult Ratio |
|---|---|---|---|
| Oxygen consumption (mL/kg/min) | 5-8 | 2-3 | 2 |
| Respiratory rate (breaths/min) | 40-60 | 12 | 3-5 |
| Tidal volume (mL/kg/min) | 6-8 | 7 | 1.0 |
| Total lung capacity (mL/kg) | 53 | 85 | 0.6 |
| Airway diameter (mm) Trachea | 5 | 14-16 | 0.3 |
| Bronchus | 4 | 11-14 | 0.3 |
| Bronchiole | 0.1 | 0.2 | 0.5 |

Data from Polgar G, Weng TR. The functional development of the respiratory system: from the period of gestation to adulthood. Am Rev Respir Dis 1979; 120:625-95.

**TABLE 36-2** Primary Categories of Apnea in Infants

| Cause | Treatment |
|---|---|
| Central | Increase $O_2$ delivery |
| |    Increase fraction of inspired $O_2$ |
| |    Increase hematocrit (?) |
| | Xanthine derivatives |
| |    Theophylline |
| |    Caffeine |
| Obstructive | Neck extension |
| | Prone or lateral position |
| | Oral airway |
| | Nasal continuous positive-airway pressure |

full-term neonates. For these reasons, central apnea may be associated with anemia and sepsis in babies. Blood transfusions may decrease the incidence of apnea in preterm infants with a hematocrit less than 27%[8,9]; however, data suggest a poor correlation between anemia and the incidence of apnea or bradycardia episodes.[10] Central apnea resulting from immaturity of the respiratory drive center is often treated with xanthine derivatives, such as caffeine and theophylline (Table 36-2).[11-14] Of particular importance to the anesthesiologist is that central apnea in neonates can be exacerbated by opioids. In some cases, apnea in neonates exposed to opioids may be alleviated by treatment with naloxone. Because of these reasons, all neonates require careful continuous monitoring of blood $O_2$ saturations and heart rate in the postoperative period.

Apnea of an obstructive or mixed origin is responsible for the majority of apneic episodes in preterm infants.[15-17] Obstructive apnea may be due to incomplete maturation and poor coordination of upper airway musculature. These forms of apnea often respond to changes in head position, insertion of an oral or nasal airway, or placing the infant in a prone position. Application of continuous positive airway pressure (CPAP) also may reduce obstructive apnea.[18]

Postoperative apnea is a common morbidity associated with anesthesia in neonates with a history of prematurity, apnea, or chronic lung disease.[19] Nearly 20% of such infants have apnea exacerbated by anesthesia or surgery in the postoperative period. Apnea may result from prolonged action of anesthetic agents, a shift of $CO_2$ response curve, immaturity of respiratory control, or fatigue of respiratory muscles.[20] Early studies suggested that preterm infants who were younger than 46 weeks

postconceptional age (PCA*) at the time of general anesthesia require continuous cardiopulmonary monitoring in the hospital afterward until they are apnea-free.[15] Kurth and colleagues[21] extended these recommendations to include monitoring for premature infants younger than 60 weeks PCA for at least 12 apnea-free hours after surgery. Although several studies suggest that regional anesthesia techniques reduce the incidence of postoperative apnea, others reported that apnea may still occur if the regional technique is supplemented with a sedative (e.g., ketamine).[22-25] An analysis of several hundred former preterm infants studied prospectively from four centers over 6 years revealed the following[26]:

- The incidence of postoperative apnea is inversely and independently related to PCA and gestational age; for example, the younger a preterm infant was born and the earlier after birth that the preterm infant undergoes surgery, the greater the incidence of apnea.
- Preterm infants younger than 56 weeks PCA are at greatest risk for apnea; the risk of postoperative apnea does not fall to less than 1% until approximately 55 weeks PCA (see Chapter 4).
- Even infants who were born at full term can experience postoperative apneas, although this is extremely rare.[27-30]
- Preterm infants without a history of apnea are still susceptible to the development of postoperative apnea.
- Preterm infants with anemia (hematocrit less than 30%) are particularly vulnerable even up to and possibly beyond 60 weeks PCA.[31]

Apnea also might be associated with nasal obstruction in infants. Although most neonates prefer to breathe through their nose, a few are *obligate* nasal breathers and do not overcome nasal airway obstruction by changing to mouth breathing.[32,33] In such neonates, nasal obstruction caused by choanal stenosis or atresia or a nasogastric tube may lead to apnea and cyanosis. Obstruction resulting from nasal edema may be relieved by instillation of saline or phenylephrine nose drops.

The work of breathing comprises compliance and resistive components. Although the work of breathing from compliance is 20- to 40-fold greater in the adult than in the neonate, the compliance work relative to tidal volume is nearly the same. However, the resistive work of breathing in the neonate is nearly 6 times greater than in the adult because of the relatively small airways in the neonate. Breathing through a tracheal tube especially increases resistive work in neonates because the airway resistance is inversely proportional to the fifth power of the radius of the tube and directly proportional to the length of the tracheal tube. The relatively narrow and long tracheal tubes through which neonates breathe can greatly increase their work of breathing (see Fig. 12-7). The work is also increased when a neonate breathes spontaneously through a circle system because of the inspiratory force required to open the one-way valves in the system. Although valveless ventilatory circuits, such as the Mapleson D systems, are recommended for spontaneously breathing neonates, studies suggest that a circle system may be used in these patients provided compensation is arranged for the problems associated with this circuit; that is, a neonate requires assisted ventilation and adequate inflation pressures to reduce the work of breathing and ensure adequate ventilation (see Chapter 51).[34-36]

---

*When evaluating the age of a newborn, be aware that by convention postconceptional age is 2 weeks shorter than postmenstrual age.

Bronchopulmonary dysplasia (BPD) is an important chronic lung disease of neonates born prematurely.[37] Although the use of antenatal steroids, exogenous surfactant treatment, and advanced ventilator therapies has decreased the incidence of BPD, it still afflicts nearly 10,000 premature infants in the United States every year and is a significant contributor to infant morbidity and mortality. BPD is identified in preterm infants with abnormal chest radiographs that require supplemental $O_2$ at 36 weeks postmenstrual age (PMA). Other factors that increase the risk for developing BPD include chorioamnionitis and the persistence of a patent ductus arteriosus (PDA).[38] Lung injury in the preterm infant decreases pulmonary maturation; infants who have died from BPD have impaired pulmonary alveolar and disrupted microvascular development.[39] BPD is most often seen in preterm infants who are subjected to high levels of $O_2$ and ventilation therapy and may be caused by lung injury–induced increase in cytokine activation.[40] Decreased lung development in infants with BPD diminishes the surface area for pulmonary gas exchange that increases $O_2$ requirements. Moreover, some infants with BPD have reduced lung compliance and increased airway resistance and hence have prolonged pulmonary time constants. Some infants with severe BPD have abnormal muscularization of the vessels in the periphery of their lungs, pulmonary hypertension, and right ventricular hypertrophy.

Pulmonary disease in infants with BPD is associated with abnormal pulmonary function tests and chest radiograph findings (small radiolucent cysts and hyperexpanded lungs), hypercarbia, chronic hypoxemia, and reactive airway disease.[41-46] Nitric oxide (NO) is a free radical gas formed in endothelial cells and diffuses into subjacent smooth muscle cells, where it stimulates cyclic guanosine monophosphate (cGMP) production and mediates vasorelaxation (Fig. 36-1). Inhaled NO decreases abnormal cell proliferation in the injured developing lung[47,48] and improves alveolar development in preterm animal models of BPD.[49,50] Given the biologic plausibility and the results from animal studies, clinical trials have examined whether preterm neonates would benefit from NO. However, 14 randomized controlled trials of inhaled NO in preterm infants 34 weeks gestational age or younger failed to demonstrate benefit in survival or pulmonary or neurodevelopmental outcomes.[51] It is likely that decreased NO signaling enzyme activity in the injured newborn lung reduces the effectiveness of inhaled NO in protecting pulmonary development. Emerging laboratory studies suggest that modulating cytokine signaling might improve the development of the injured lung and decrease BPD. For example, investigations in newborn animal models suggest that lung injury increases cytokine signaling. Moreover, in a mouse pup model of BPD, antibody-mediated inhibition of excess transforming growth factor-beta (TGF-β) activity was observed to improve NO signaling and pulmonary alveolar and microvascular development.[52] Studies are under way to examine the mechanisms through which TGF-β modulates injured lung development.

The treatment of BPD in neonates often requires ventilatory and medical therapies.[53] Early and aggressive CPAP may eliminate the need for positive-pressure ventilation. Air trapping during assisted ventilation is associated with the long lung time constants in babies with BPD and may be reduced by using a prolonged expiratory time. Respiratory infection (e.g., *Ureaplasma urealyticum*) may contribute to the inflammatory response. Bronchodilators such as aminophylline, albuterol, or ipratropium may be beneficial in reducing airway resistance in some infants with BPD.

Infants with BPD are often treated with diuretics. As a result of chronic furosemide treatment, metabolic abnormalities may exist. Hypercalciuria may occur from the action of furosemide on the ascending loop of Henle, leading to secondary hyperparathyroidism and nephrocalcinosis in some infants. Hydrochlorothiazide and spironolactone produce less severe metabolic abnormalities. Finally, large doses of steroids, especially dexamethasone, have been shown to provide relief for some infants with severe BPD that is refractory to other medical and ventilator therapies.[54,55] However, dexamethasone treatment may result in systemic hypertension, hyperglycemia, hypertrophic cardiomyopathy, and alteration of neurologic and pulmonary development in some children.[56,57] Preoperative evaluation of infants with BPD requires a very careful history and physical examination, particularly focused on the pulmonary and cardiovascular systems.

### Oxygen Uptake and Circulation

Uptake of $O_2$ in the pulmonary microvasculature of neonates is facilitated by the greater hemoglobin concentration in the neonate and the increased amount of fetal hemoglobin. Fetal hemoglobin has a reduced affinity for 2,3-diphosphoglycerate and hence a greater affinity for $O_2$. Although this affinity facilitates fetal hemoglobin $O_2$ uptake in the placenta, it can reduce $O_2$ release from hemoglobin to the tissues. Red blood cells containing fetal hemoglobin have an average life span of 100 days, compared with 120 days for those containing adult hemoglobin. The higher hematocrit in neonates causes an increased bilirubin load for an immature hepatic clearance pathway. However, preterm infants frequently experience anemia of prematurity, a normocytic, normochromic hypoproliferative anemia with the hallmark of inadequate production of erythropoietin.[58]

The $O_2$ delivery to systemic tissues in neonates is facilitated by a cardiac output greater than in adults on a per–kilogram body-weight basis. The relationships among myocardial preload, contractility, afterload, and heart rate determine cardiac output. Passive myocardial fiber tension is reflective of myocardial compliance, which is significantly reduced in the perinatal period.[59] Active myocardial tension, reflecting contractility, is

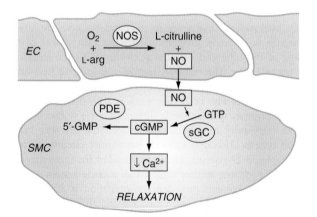

**FIGURE 36-1** Nitric oxide (*NO*) produced by nitric oxide synthase (*NOS*) in endothelial cells (*EC*) diffuses into subjacent smooth muscle cells (*SMC*), interacts with soluble guanylate cyclase (*sGC*), and increases the concentration of cyclic guanosine monophosphate (*cGMP*) to cause vascular relaxation. The effect of NO is decreased by metabolism of cGMP by specific phosphodiesterases (*PDE*). *L-arg*, L-Arginine.

also significantly reduced in the neonate.[59] At smaller end-diastolic volumes, mild increases in preload in the neonate are associated with increased cardiac output. At greater end-diastolic volumes, as a result of poor ventricular compliance in the neonatal heart, this positive effect is soon overcome and cardiac output becomes more dependent on heart rate (see Chapters 14 and 16).[60-62] The heart rate of a term neonate is approximately 120 beats/min; it increases to 160 beats/min by 1 month of age.[63] Parasympathetic control of heart rate in lambs, and probably in developing humans, matures earlier in gestation and to a greater extent than β-adrenergic control.[64,65] For this reason, neonates tend not to respond to adrenergic signaling associated with hypovolemia or an inadequate depth of anesthesia with tachycardia. Additionally, the vagotonic response caused by succinylcholine or its metabolites (succinylmonocholine) and synthetic opioids may lead to bradycardia. These cardiac reflexes can be offset by the vagolytic effects of pancuronium or atropine.[66,67]

Preterm infants may have pulmonary hypertension. In utero, the lungs are not required for gas exchange; the placenta performs this function. Thus the fetal circulatory pattern consists of atria and ventricles working as units in parallel (see Fig. 16-1). As little as 10% of the fetal right ventricular output may circulate through the lungs.[68] Most of the blood returned from the lower extremities and a portion of the umbilical venous blood supply passes into the pulmonary arteries and subsequently through the PDA into the systemic circulation (see Chapters 14 and 16). The superior vena caval blood supply circulates through the patent foramen ovale (PFO) into the left atria and subsequently into the systemic circulation. With expansion of the lungs during the first breath, pulmonary vascular resistance decreases and blood flow to the lungs increases, matching perfusion with new ventilation.[68,69] Any factor that increases pulmonary vascular resistance, (e.g., hypoxia, hypercarbia, or acidosis) may cause the circulation to revert to a fetal circulatory pattern with shunting of deoxygenated blood from the right to the left side of the heart via the PFO or PDA. This right-to-left shunting of blood explains in part why some infants remain hypoxemic despite ventilation with 100% $O_2$ after severe desaturation.

The ductus arteriosus may remain patent in neonates, especially in those born prematurely.[70] Bounding peripheral pulses, a harsh systolic ejection murmur at the left sternal border, and widened pulse–pressure difference, suggest the presence of a PDA. The presence of a PDA and of right-to-left shunting of blood may contribute to ventilation-perfusion ($\dot{V}$-$\dot{Q}$) mismatch as deoxygenated blood is shunted from the pulmonary arteries to the systemic circulation through the PDA and differential upper and lower extremity $O_2$ saturations result. Later, as the pulmonary vascular resistance decreases, left-to-right shunting of blood from the systemic to pulmonary circulation across the PDA may cause flow-mediated endothelial cell injury and abnormal pulmonary artery remodeling and hypertension. Infants with a PDA often require increased ventilatory support.

A PDA in the neonate may be treated with indomethacin or ibuprofen. If the PDA persists despite medical treatment, surgical ligation may be required.[71-73] Treatment with indomethacin is associated with renal and platelet dysfunction. Although experience suggests that infants who have received large volumes of intravascular fluid have a greater incidence of PDA,[74] the mechanism behind this is unknown, and the relationship may not be causal. In fact, if the PDA is associated with ventricular dysfunction and poor organ perfusion, it is *imperative* to provide adequate intravascular volume and to improve cardiac output rather

than expose the infant to hypotension mediated by left-to-right shunting across the PDA. Occasionally, systemic perfusion in infants with PDA may be improved with a dopamine infusion and judicious intravenous fluid administration.

In neonates, increased pulmonary vascular resistance causes shunting of desaturated blood through the PFO and PDA and thereby causes severe systemic hypoxemia. Although the cause of persistent pulmonary hypertension of the newborn (PPHN) is incompletely understood, it is associated with increased muscularization of pulmonary arterial vessels[75] and sepsis and aspiration syndromes.[76] PPHN is suspected in severely hypoxic neonates who do not have a significant increase in postductal $O_2$ saturation when they breathe 100% $O_2$. A difference in preductal and postductal $O_2$ saturations supports the diagnosis because it reflects the extrapulmonary right-to-left shunting of deoxygenated blood via the PDA. PPHN is diagnosed when pulmonary hypertension and no other structural heart lesions are observed by cardiac ultrasound.

Treatment of PPHN is directed at decreasing pulmonary vascular resistance and the extrapulmonary shunting of deoxygenated blood. In cases of pneumonia and aspiration syndromes, in which airway disease can lead to atelectasis and intrapulmonary shunt, PEEP and exogenous surfactant are sometimes used to recruit alveoli. To treat the pulmonary vasoconstriction that is pathognomonic of PPHN, hyperoxia and alkalosis therapies have been used. Although inspired $O_2$ is a potent vasodilator, maximum dilation of the pulmonary vasculature is achieved by relatively low levels of $O_2$. For this reason, increasing the $FIO_2$ often does not improve gas exchange in PPHN. Through a mechanism that is incompletely understood, alkalosis causes pulmonary vasodilation. In many infants with PPHN, alkalosis induced by hyperventilation or the infusion of base decreases pulmonary vascular resistance and increases systemic $O_2$ partial pressures. In general, the vasodilation induced by alkalosis occurs when the arterial pH is 7.55 or greater. With the advent of inhaled NO, alkalosis has been largely replaced with avoiding acidemia, but not inducing marked alkalosis. Intravenous vasodilator drugs cause inconsistent vasodilation in infants with pulmonary hypertension.[77] Unfortunately, because these agents dilate the systemic as well as the pulmonary vasculature, they often cause severe systemic hypotension.

Inhaled NO selectively decreases pulmonary vascular resistance and increases systemic $O_2$ partial pressures in infants with PPHN.[78-80] NO is a gas that is synthesized by NO synthase from L-arginine and $O_2$ in endothelial cells and diffuses into subjacent smooth muscle cells, where it stimulates soluble guanylate cyclase to increase cGMP levels. It is probably through cGMP's stimulation of cGMP-dependent protein kinase I and the phosphorylation of several cytoplasmic targets that regulate intracellular calcium levels and vasomotor protein function that NO causes vascular relaxation (see Fig. 36-1). Inhaling small concentrations of NO caused selective pulmonary vasodilation, decreased right-to-left shunting of blood, and increased systemic $O_2$ partial pressures in neonate animals and infants with pulmonary hypertension.[81-83] Acutely breathing up to 80 parts per million (ppm) by volume of NO rapidly and selectively decreases pulmonary vascular resistance and increases systemic $O_2$ partial pressures by decreasing extrapulmonary shunting of deoxygenated blood. Although methemoglobin is produced during the metabolism of NO, no important increases in methemoglobin were observed in infants breathing low concentrations of NO. Large multicenter studies suggest that breathing 20 ppm NO decreases the requirement for extracorporeal membrane oxygenation (ECMO). Although ECMO can be lifesaving for severely hypoxemic neonates,[84-86] it is expensive and invasive, sometimes causes important complications, and is not available at most hospitals. For these reasons, inhaled NO is used in most intensive care nurseries to treat the severe hypoxemia associated with PPHN.

Studies also suggest that chronic NO inhalation protects the neonatal lung from injury.[47] In cell cultures, NO has been observed to decrease pulmonary smooth muscle cell proliferation and increase programmed cell death (apoptosis). Inhaled NO has been observed to decrease pulmonary artery neomuscularization in animals with lungs injured by breathing gases with low concentrations of inspired $O_2$. Although inhaled NO may decrease lung artery remodeling by preventing hypoxic pulmonary vasoconstriction, studies suggest that it prevents abnormal pulmonary artery remodeling in injured lungs without hypertension.[78] Although the protective mechanism of inhaled NO is unknown, it does decrease smooth muscle cell proliferation in vitro,[87] possibly by altering the expression of transcriptional regulators and the progression of the cell cycle.[88-90] It is likely that studies that identify the protective mechanisms of NO/cGMP signaling will guide the development of novel therapies to prevent pulmonary disease in the injured lung.

Appreciation has been increasing of the potential harmful effects of even brief periods of hyperoxia.[91] Six randomized controlled clinical studies have shown no apparent advantage of initiating resuscitation of neonates with 100% supplemental $O_2$ instead of 21% $O_2$. In fact, some studies suggest slightly greater mortality rates with 100% $O_2$. In light of these findings, the 2010 Neonatal Resuscitation Program has been updated to recommend initiating resuscitation of full-term neonates with 21% $O_2$ and that pulse oximetry be used if supplemental $O_2$ is needed.[92]

## TEMPERATURE REGULATION

The neonatal body habitus favors heat loss. The large surface area of the head relative to that of the body of neonates increases heat dissipation. A head cover may significantly reduce temperature loss.[93,94] Neonates do not shiver or sweat effectively to maintain body temperature and rely primarily on brown fat metabolism to maintain body heat. Brown fat cells begin to differentiate at 26 to 30 weeks of gestation and hence are not available in extremely preterm infants to provide fat for metabolism and heat generation.[95] Warming the operating room to 85° F (30° C), using radiant warming units, forced-air heating pads, and adding humidity to the inspired gases in the ventilator circuits help maintain the neonate's temperature in the neutral thermal range.[96-98] The sources of heat loss in infants is 39% radiation, 37% convection, 21% evaporation, and 3% conduction. Warming intravenous and irrigation fluids before they are used may also be beneficial.

## RENAL AND METABOLIC FUNCTION
### Renal Function

The placenta acts as an excretory organ for the fetus. A neonate's kidneys are not fully developed at birth, and development is closely related to PCA.[98,99] At full-term birth, the glomerular filtration rate (GFR) is only 30% of normal adult rates (see Chapter 6).[100] The GFR reaches adult values at approximately 1 year of age (see Figs. 6-10 and 6-11). The kidneys' tubular function, and hence sodium-retaining ability, does not develop until about 32 weeks of gestation.[101,102] The immaturity of the

kidney at birth also affects the metabolism of many drugs in the neonate The renal excretion of medications such as penicillin, gentamicin, and some neuromuscular blocking drugs (NMBDs), such as pancuronium, may be prolonged, resulting in increased duration of action or the development of excessive blood concentrations. This effect is particularly important when administering medications to an extremely preterm infant. Thus the use of NMBDs that do not require renal function are most advantageous (e.g., cisatracurium).

The total body water content in neonates is greater than it is in infants, children, or adults. In the preterm infant 75% to 85% of body weight is water; in general, the less the PCA of the neonate, the greater the percentage of water. In a term infant, 70% of body weight is water.[103] By 6 to 12 months of age, 50% to 60% of body weight is water (see also Figs. 6-7 and 6-8). Differences between the total body water, renal maturity, and serum protein concentrations (see also Fig. 6-6) in a neonate affect the volume of distribution of many medications. Because of the increase in the volume of distribution of drugs confined to the extracellular fluid, the initial doses of some medications (e.g., NMBDs, aminoglycosides) may be greater on a weight basis in neonates than for adults to achieve the desired blood concentration. In contrast, because of immaturity of renal function, the interval between doses of these drugs may be increased (see also E-Fig. 6-4).

## Fluid Management

The basic principles of fluid maintenance in neonates are similar to those in older children and adults. The highly variable body fluid composition, degree of renal maturity,[104] neuroendocrine control of intravascular fluid status, and insensible fluid loss with age[105] make precise estimates of fluid requirements in neonates very difficult (see Chapter 8). Urine volume and concentration may be difficult to determine intraoperatively and may not always correlate with volume status. Moreover, blood pressure and heart rate may not correlate with intravascular volume status in preterm infants, and anesthetics may mask subtle cardiovascular changes that occur with changes in intravascular volume. Increased insensible fluid loss, which often occurs in the operating room environment, requires judicious titration of intravenous fluids. Congenital abnormalities (e.g., gastroschisis, omphalocele) may markedly increase insensible fluid loss through exposure of large mucosal surfaces. The use of humidified gas mixtures reduces insensible fluid loss through the respiratory tract. However, overzealous intraoperative administration of fluids can result in pulmonary complications and worsened third-spacing of fluids.

## Methods of Intravenous Access and Monitoring

Infants who are dehydrated after a prolonged period of fasting or vomiting or because of increased insensible fluid losses may require special procedures for intravenous access. With severe hypovolemia, scalp and peripheral veins may be difficult to cannulate. Many of the superficial veins may be thrombosed from prior use. Fiberoptic light sources or ultrasound may help visualize deeper veins and peripheral arteries. Femoral and axillary veins may be accessed percutaneously or via a surgical approach for the delivery of fluids and medications.[106-108] Knowledge of femoral artery and vein anatomy decreases the incidence of accidental injury of the femoral head joint and possible septic arthritis (see Fig. 48-5).[109] The external or internal jugular veins can also provide alternative sites for venous access.

36

In neonates, fluids and many medications may be infused through the umbilical vessels. The tip of umbilical arterial lines should be placed either in a "low" position, at the level of the bifurcation of the femoral arteries (L3-4), or in a "high" position, in the descending aorta above the diaphragm (T6-9). The catheter tip of the umbilical artery catheter should not be left in the descending aorta in the area of the renal or mesenteric arteries (L1-2) because renal or mesenteric artery thrombosis might result (see Figs. 48-8 and 48-9). Aortic thrombosis occurs in approximately 1% of umbilical artery catheterizations, although thrombi can be detected with radiologic techniques in 20% to 95% of infants.[110-112] Infants with renal artery thrombosis may present with hypertension, oliguria, hematuria, and elevated blood creatinine concentrations. The tip of an umbilical venous catheter should rest in the inferior vena cava above the level of the ductus venosus and hepatic veins so that solutions are not directly infused into the liver parenchyma. The delivery of hypertonic solutions into the liver might result in liver damage and portal cirrhosis. Aspiration of arterial oxygenated blood suggests that the venous catheter has entered the left atrium through the foramen ovale. Catheters in the left atrium should be pulled back to the level described earlier.

Some drugs may be delivered through the tracheal tube. Rapid uptake and minimal effects on gas exchange or the pulmonary parenchyma occur with epinephrine, atropine, and lidocaine (see Chapter 39). The doses of some drugs administered through the tracheal tube are increased in comparison with that delivered intravenously (e.g., epinephrine 0.05 to 0.1 mg/kg via the tracheal tube versus 0.01 to 0.03 mg/kg intravenously).[92] It is important to understand that administration of solutions via the endotracheal tube can cause adverse effects. For example, complications associated with the tracheal administration of exogenous surfactant include occasional transient hypoxia and bradycardia and are likely due to the relatively large volume of fluid (2.5 to 6 mL/kg) associated with the proper dose of surfactant.

Intraosseous cannulation of the tibia with a special intraosseous infusion needle (e.g., Easy-IO, Vidacare, San Antonio, Tex.) or a styleted spinal needle provides a rapid route for emergency fluid and drug administration and can be lifesaving (see Fig. 48-6 and E-Fig. 48-1, *A* through *E*).

## Glucose Homeostasis

Although the placenta allows the delivery of glucose from the maternal circulation to the fetus, the development of significant glycogen stores does not occur until late in gestation. Various conditions may lead to hypoglycemia in a neonate. Preterm and small-for-gestational-age (SGA) infants have very high glucose requirements; they require glucose infusion rates of 8 to 10 mg/kg/min. In full-term infants, a glucose infusion rate of 5 to 8 mg/kg/min prevents hypoglycemia. Full-term infants who have been excessively fasted, SGA infants, and infants of diabetic mothers are all prone to develop hypoglycemia. Although hypoglycemia may result in respiratory distress, apnea, cyanosis, seizures, tremors, high-pitched cry, irritability, limpness, lethargy, eye-rolling, poor feeding, temperature instability, and sweating, the signs and symptoms in infants are often blunted and nonspecific.[113,114] In infants younger than 24 hours old, a plasma glucose concentration of less than 40 mg/dL is a cause for concern and should be treated.[115] After 24 hours of life, plasma glucose values less than 45 mg/dL should be considered abnormally low. Although hypertonic glucose administration has been used to treat hypoglycemia in neonates, studies reveal that

administration of hypertonic sodium bicarbonate solutions increases the incidence of intraventricular hemorrhage in preterm infants.[116] For this reason, it is prudent to avoid bolus administration of hypertonic glucose to treat hypoglycemia to prevent sudden changes in blood tonicity and hyperglycemia. A bolus of 2 to 4 mL/kg of $D_{10}W$ (0.2 to 0.4 g/kg of glucose) and an increase in the basal glucose infusion are prudent measures to treat hypoglycemia. It is extremely important to reassess the blood glucose concentration after these treatments to determine the effectiveness of the therapy.

Infants undergoing surgical procedures often require less glucose supplementation.[117] This reduced need may be attributed to hormonal responses that decrease glucose uptake as a result of catecholamine release in excess of insulin activity, as well as a decrease in metabolic demand from the effects of the anesthetic agents.[118-120] Nevertheless, it is important to administer glucose-containing solutions using a constant-infusion device to avoid large fluctuations in blood glucose values and monitor blood glucose values in critically ill neonates. All other fluids (e.g., to replace third-space losses, blood loss, and fluid deficits) should be glucose-free to avoid hyperglycemia.[117] Infants treated with high levels of glucose via total parental nutrition (TPN) may develop severe hypoglycemia if the infusion rate is abruptly lowered; thus it is important to continue these infusions (possibly at a slightly reduced rate) during surgery and to check the serum glucose concentrations.

## Calcium Homeostasis

Calcium exists in the serum in three fractions: (1) protein bound; (2) chelated to bicarbonate, phosphate, and citrate; and (3) free or ionized calcium ($iCa^{2+}$). The ionized fraction is the physiologically active component. The serum calcium concentration is mainly regulated by the action of parathyroid hormone (PTH) and vitamin D metabolites. PTH acts directly in the bone and kidneys and indirectly through calciferol in the gut.[121]

Hypocalcemia has been observed in nearly 40% of critically ill neonates.[122] Causes of hypocalcemia include (1) PTH insufficiency and peripheral resistance to PTH, (2) inadequate calcium supplementation, and (3) altered calcium metabolism caused by transfusion with citrated blood products (see also Fig. 10-9), bicarbonate administration, or diuretics (furosemide). Hypocalcemia may be asymptomatic or accompanied by nonspecific symptoms (e.g., seizures and tremors). Thus the diagnosis rests on the determination of total and $iCa^{2+}$ levels. In critically ill children, total calcium concentrations do not accurately reflect the $iCa^{2+}$ concentrations; therefore the diagnosis of hypocalcemia in these infants should be determined by direct measurement of $iCa^{2+}$ with an ion-specific electrode.[123] Neonatal hypocalcemia may be defined as a serum $iCa^{2+}$ less than 1 mmol/L in full-term infants and less than 0.75 mmol/L in preterm infants. Persistent hypocalcemia necessitates determination of magnesium, phosphorus, PTH, and vitamin D concentrations.

Treatment of hypocalcemia is not effective in the presence of hypomagnesemia. In this situation, administration of supplemental magnesium and calcium and treatment of the underlying cause of hypocalcemia are necessary.[122] Symptomatic hypocalcemia is treated with 100 mg/kg calcium gluconate (10%) by slow intravenous infusion (5 minutes) in a patent intravenous line. Thereafter, maintenance calcium is administered at 100 to 200 mg/kg/day elemental calcium and the clinical response and serum $iCa^{2+}$ levels are carefully monitored.

## GASTROINTESTINAL AND HEPATIC FUNCTION

The fetal gut is not functionally developed until late in gestation. In full-term neonates, the maturation of esophageal function occurs soon after birth. However, in comparison with adults, gastric emptying in neonates is prolonged and lower esophageal sphincters are incompetent, making reflux of stomach contents common. Early feeding of hypertonic formulas in preterm infants increases intestinal energy demands and is associated with bowel ischemia and necrotizing enterocolitis.[124] On the other hand, the use of hypocaloric or trophic feeds in preterm infants is associated with subsequent feeding intolerance, indirect hyperbilirubinemia, cholestatic jaundice, and metabolic bone disease.[125,126]

After birth, increased concentrations of unbound serum bilirubin introduce the risk of kernicterus, particularly in infants who are preterm, hypoxemic, and acidotic and have low serum protein concentrations.[127] Highly protein-bound agents such as furosemide, sulfonamides, ceftriaxone, and benzyl alcohol (found as a preservative in many drugs such as diazepam) may displace bilirubin and increase the possibility of kernicterus.[128] Hepatic metabolism is immature in neonates and particularly in preterm infants. Drug metabolism may be prolonged as a result of both immaturity of enzymatic processes and a relatively low hepatic perfusion (less drug delivered to the liver). Any factor that further compromises hepatic blood flow (e.g., increased intraabdominal pressure) may have profound adverse effects on drugs with perfusion-limited hepatic clearance.[129] Therefore careful titration of these drugs (e.g., opioids, propofol) is required to optimize therapeutic effects and prevent toxicity. Just as consideration is given to immature renal function, the use of NMBDs that do not require hepatic metabolism can be advantageous, (e.g., cisatracurium). The use of remifentanil during the procedure followed by a low dose of longer-acting opioid or regional block at the end of the procedure might facilitate early extubation.

## NEUROLOGIC DEVELOPMENT

The central nervous system is incompletely developed at birth. However, early in gestation, the pain pathways are integrated with the somatic, neuroendocrine, and autonomic systems. The hormonal responses to pain and stress may be exaggerated in neonates,[118,119] although the clinical significance of this has not been defined. The potential lack of autoregulation of cerebral blood flow and an infant's fragile cerebral blood vessels may be important factors in the development of intraventricular hemorrhage.[130,131] Although an association has been noted between the incidence of intraventricular hemorrhage and fluctuations in blood pressure,[130,132] it is difficult to confirm any causal relationship. This association has been a concern during "awake" or nonanesthetized laryngoscopy and intubation of neonates; however, one study reported no significant change in blood pressure or heart rate in neonates even after awake intubation.[133] In addition, another study questioned the lack of autoregulation of cerebral blood flow in preterm infants. Using near infrared spectroscopy, investigators found that preterm infants could maintain adequate cerebral perfusion at a mean arterial blood pressure in the range of 23 to 39 mm Hg.[134]

In neonates, the spinal cord extends to a lower segment of the spine than in older children and adults (see E-Fig. 41-3). The volume of cerebrospinal fluid and the spinal surface area are proportionally larger in neonates (see also E-Fig. 41-4), whereas the amount of myelination is less than in older children and

adults.[135,136] These factors may account in part for the increased amount of local anesthetics (milligram per kilogram) required for successful spinal anesthesia in infants.

Hyperoxia has been associated with retinopathy of prematurity (ROP).[137-139] Although two case reports of ROP associated with anesthesia in preterm infants implicated hyperoxia as a primary etiologic factor, the cause of ROP appears to be multifactorial[140-149]; the association between arterial $O_2$ tension and ROP is unclear (see also Chapter 32). ROP begins as retinal vascular narrowing and obliteration followed by increased vascularity (neovascularization), hemorrhage, and, in the most severe cases, retinal detachment and blindness (see also Fig. 32-1). In two clinical trials (the SUPPORT[150] and BOOST II[151] trials) infants born at less than 28 weeks gestation were randomized to saturation ranges of either 85% to 89% or 91% to 95%. In the SUPPORT trial, for every 11 infants treated in the lower saturation range, one case of severe ROP was prevented (results for the BOOST II trial are not yet available). However, in both the SUPPORT and BOOST II trials, the latter of which was terminated early, the mortality was greater in infants who were randomized to the 85% to 89% range than those in the 91% to 95% range. Although the optimal saturation range has not been defined in preterm infants, it seems prudent to target the $O_2$ saturation in the range of 91% to 95% and avoid a saturation less than 89%.

# Preparation for Surgery

## THE OPERATING ROOM

Conditions that require emergency surgery in neonates are often accompanied by medical problems, and, as a consequence, management and monitoring considerations can be complex. Routine standard monitoring equipment includes an electrocardiograph, chest or esophageal stethoscope, blood pressure monitor, temperature probe, pulse oximeter and a $CO_2$ analyzer. Rapid decreases in arterial $O_2$ content in neonates after brief periods of ventilatory compromise, coupled with the possible risk of ROP as a result of hyperoxia, dictate the need for continuous $O_2$ saturation monitoring. A pulse oximeter probe placed in a preductal position (right hand) can be compared with one placed in a postductal position (foot or left hand ) to determine the severity of extrapulmonary shunting of deoxygenated blood via the PDA. Pulse oximetry may prove to be particularly useful for infants in whom the risk of intraarterial monitoring cannot be justified.[152] This device can diagnose hypoxemia but not hyperoxia; however, maintaining the $O_2$ saturation at 91% to 95% (preductal) places most infants on the steep portion of the $O_2$ hemoglobin dissociation curve and avoids severe hyperoxia.[153]

Expired $CO_2$ can be measured using capnography. However, dilution of the exhaled gases with those of the dead space of the tracheal tube or by the fresh gas may underestimate the true alveolar $CO_2$ partial pressure. If desired, a more accurate estimate of expired $CO_2$ concentration may be obtained by using a special tracheal tube with a sample port located at its tip, by inserting a narrow catheter through the $CO_2$ sampling port in the elbow and into the lumen of the tracheal tube or by using a needle introduced through the side wall of the tracheal tube 2 to 3 cm distal to the 15-mm tube connector (see Chapter 51).[154,155] Using a circle system provides a reasonably accurate measurement of expired $CO_2$ concentrations because the fresh gas flows are small and less mixing of exhaled and inhaled gases occurs. However, regardless of the circuit configuration, the value obtained by the capnograph may not accurately reflect PaCO$_2$ in the presence of congenital heart disease (e.g., cyanotic heart disease or a mixing shunt) or significant intrapulmonary shunting.[156]

In neonates, changes in blood pressure, heart rate, and the intensity of heart sounds are excellent indicators of cardiac function, intravascular volume status, and depth of anesthesia. Under most circumstances, a urinary catheter permits adequate determination of urine output and aids in the monitoring of fluid balance during prolonged operations. In cases in which major blood or fluid losses are expected, or the physiology is complicated by the presence of cardiac disease, a central venous catheter is warranted. Any neonate with significant underlying cardiovascular instability should have an arterial catheter placed for continuous monitoring of blood pressure and to provide the means to obtain arterial blood samples for determination of blood pH and gas levels and serum glucose and electrolyte concentrations. Many neonates arrive in the operating room from the intensive care unit (ICU) with an umbilical artery line in place. Because of the risk of renal artery thrombosis with these lines, it is important to verify the location of the tip of the umbilical artery catheter. Infrahepatic umbilical venous lines may not be reliable under operative conditions because they may become wedged in the liver. In this position, infusion of hypertonic solutions may lead to parenchymal necrosis and ultimately fibrosis.[157,158]

Nonrebreathing (open) circuits are simple and effective for delivering anesthetic agents to infants weighing less than 10 kg. The system must have provisions for a humidifier to warm and hydrate the cold, dry anesthetic gases. However, a trend exists away from the use of nonrebreathing circuits to save money and reduce air pollution.[34-36,59] With the increasing need for cost savings there appears to be no significant disadvantage to using circle systems, which allow the use of small fresh gas flows. This substitution should only be made if the provider has a clear understanding of the marked increase in compression volume/compliance volume losses (see also Fig. 51-7) compared with nonrebreathing circuits.[159] The anesthesia machine should also provide compressed air in addition to O$_2$ and NO. The use of air allows regulation of inspired O$_2$ concentrations during cases in which NO treatment is contraindicated and a high PaO$_2$ is not desired. Table 36-3 lists basic equipment for conducting emergency anesthesia on a neonate.

### THE FAMILY

Close interaction between the parents and the anesthesia, medical, surgical, and nursing staff promotes effective communication of medical concerns and continued emotional support for parents. The birth of a preterm neonate or illness in a full-term infant often does not allow time for emotional preparation for or acceptance of the situation by the family. With the institution of aggressive medical and surgical interventions, parents sometimes feel excluded from the care of their infant and develop feelings of isolation and lack of control. The development of rapport between the parents of critically ill infants and hospital staff is essential to ensure adequate psychological support during this intensely anxiety-provoking event.

## Emergency Surgery

### RESPIRATORY PROBLEMS

Lesions of the respiratory system can be categorized into those that involve the large airways or the small airways and lung parenchyma.

**TABLE 36-3** Suggested Equipment for Emergency Neonatal Anesthesia

| Airway Equipment | Environment | Agents | Intravenous Fluids |
|---|---|---|---|
| Suction catheters | Room temperature (80°-85° F) | Gases Air/O$_2$/NO | Lactated Ringer solution |
| Oral airways | Forced warm air delivery device | Volatile anesthetics | D$_{10}$W |
| Facemasks | | Drugs | Normal saline |
| Breathing circuit | Underbody warming blanket | IV anesthetics Propofol | 5% albumin |
| Miller 0, 1, blades and handle | Circuit humidifier | Ketamine | |
| Uncuffed endotracheal tubes (2.5, 3.0, 3.5, 4.0 mm) | IV fluid warmer Infusion pumps for both maintenance fluid and for opioid or vasoactive drugs | Muscle relaxants Succinylcholine Cisatracurium Vecuronium Pancuronium | |
| Stylet | | Opioids Fentanyl Morphine Remifentanil | |
| | | Local anesthetics Tetracaine 1.0% Bupivacaine 0.25% | |
| | | Emergency drugs Atropine Epinephrine (1:10,000) Dopamine Calcium Bicarbonate Isoproterenol | |

### Abnormalities of the Airway

#### Choanal Atresia and Stenosis

Not all neonates are able to change to oral breathing when nasal obstruction occurs.[32,33] Choanal atresia can present as cyanosis at rest that resolves with crying or placement of an oral airway. Choanal atresia and stenosis result from the failure of the bone or membranous portion of the nasopharynx to undergo regression during development. The incidence is approximately 1 in 8000 births. Unilateral lesions are seldom symptomatic and may escape early detection. Although bilateral lesions may be asymptomatic, occasionally they may lead to respiratory distress.[160] Choanal atresia and stenosis are generally not associated with other craniofacial anomalies. Choanal atresia may be found as part of a constellation of congenital anomalies, the CHARGE association: **c**oloboma, **h**eart disease (tetralogy of Fallot, PDA, double-outlet right ventricle with atrioventricular canal, ventricular septal defect, atrial septal defect, right-sided aortic arch), **a**tresia choanae, **r**etarded growth (including other central nervous system anomalies), **g**enital anomalies (hypogonadism), and **e**ar anomalies.[161,162] These neonates may develop airway obstruction during anesthetic induction. Early placement of an oral airway, facilitated by preinduction topical application of viscous lidocaine to the tongue, aids in airway management.

Functional choanal obstruction may result from traumatic nasal suctioning. Obstructive symptoms are often ameliorated by treatment with cool mist therapy or vasoconstrictors such as phenylephrine. The upper airway may also be stented open by nasal placement of a shortened endotracheal tube. Such treatment, however, is only temporary; prolonged use of a nasal airway may increase edema and obstruction.

### Laryngeal and Upper Tracheal Obstruction

Obstruction at the level of the larynx or upper trachea may be due to laryngeal and tracheal webs or subglottic lesions. Subglottic lesions may be due to congenital stenosis, hemangioma, web, or vascular ring (Figs. 36-2 and 36-3; see also Videos 12-1, 12-2, and 12-5). Anesthetic management of obstructive lesions in older children and adults usually includes an inhalation anesthetic induction while maintaining spontaneous respirations. This method may be difficult in neonates for the following reasons: (1) the combined effects of inhalation anesthetic agents and immature ventilatory drive regulation may predispose to hypoventilation; (2) hypoventilation leads to an increased alveolar $CO_2$, which displaces alveolar $O_2$; and (3) anesthetic agents decrease intercostal muscle function, resulting in decreased

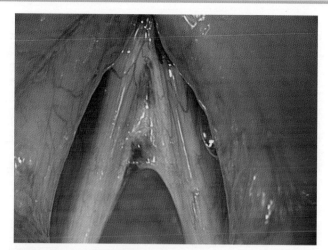

**FIGURE 36-2** Laryngeal web in a neonate. (Courtesy Dr. Christopher Hartnick.)

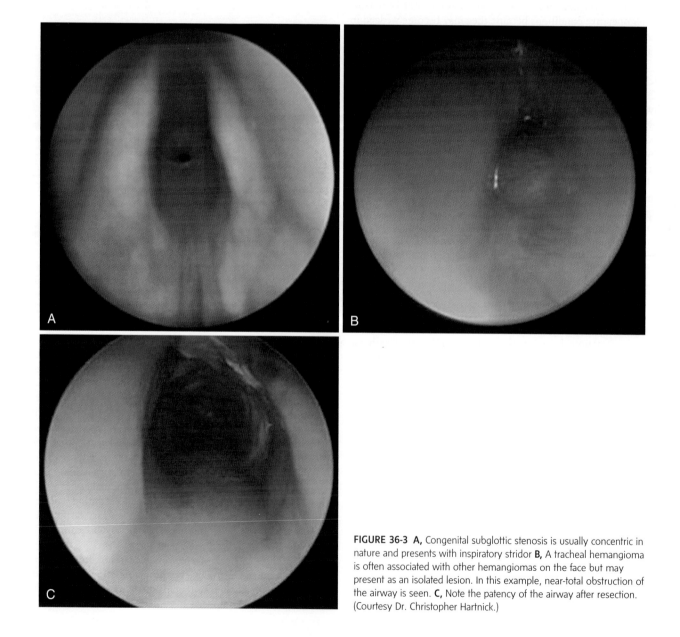

**FIGURE 36-3 A,** Congenital subglottic stenosis is usually concentric in nature and presents with inspiratory stridor **B,** A tracheal hemangioma is often associated with other hemangiomas on the face but may present as an isolated lesion. In this example, near-total obstruction of the airway is seen. **C,** Note the patency of the airway after resection. (Courtesy Dr. Christopher Hartnick.)

functional residual capacity (FRC).[163,164] The hypoventilation and reduced FRC combined with high $O_2$ consumption predispose infants to desaturation during anesthetic induction while the infant maintains spontaneous ventilation.

WEBS. Laryngeal or tracheal webs generally produce incomplete fibrous membranes that lead to obstruction of the airway with acute respiratory distress or stridor shortly after birth (Fig. 36-2).[165] Complete airway obstruction occasionally results in an emergency in the delivery room. A tracheal tube may be used as a stent to open an incomplete lesion. If tracheal intubation is not possible, an intravenous catheter passed through the cricothyroid membrane may allow oxygenation and be lifesaving (see Figs. 12-25 through 12-27).[166] A tracheostomy is then established.

CONGENITAL SUBGLOTTIC STENOSIS. The severity of the symptoms resulting from congenital subglottic stenosis depends on the degree of airway occlusion (see Fig. 36-3, *A*). Treatment depends on the location and length of stenosis. For severe narrowing, a tracheostomy is placed and a series of dilations attempted.[167] Tracheal dilations may cause airway disruption, pneumomediastinum, and pneumothorax. Anesthesia may be induced using an inhalation technique with a facemask and appropriate ventilatory assistance. If a tracheostomy is considered, a small-diameter tracheal tube may be placed to facilitate ventilation until a tracheostomy is performed. This tracheal tube should be of smaller diameter so that it passes beyond the level of obstruction. As resistance increases inversely with the airway radius to the fifth power, ventilatory assistance is required to overcome this substantial increase in the work of breathing. The greater time constants that result from the increased airway resistance require a greater time for expiration to avoid gas trapping.

SUBGLOTTIC HEMANGIOMA. Subglottic hemangioma may produce respiratory distress during the first few weeks of life as it rapidly increases in size (see Fig. 36-3, *B* and *C*). The presence of other hemangiomas on an infant's body, especially on the face, is a clue that a subglottic hemangioma may be the source of the respiratory distress.[168] These infants often present with symptoms of upper airway obstruction, which may be life-threatening when additional exacerbating factors such as upper respiratory tract infections or other causes of inspissated mucus result in further airway compromise.[169] Any infant who is younger than 3 months of age and presents with symptoms of "croup" must be considered to have causes other than infection as a source of the airway obstruction. If tracheal intubation is required, it should be carried out as gently as possible because bleeding may occur secondary to trauma from the intubation procedure.

ESOPHAGEAL ATRESIA AND TRACHEOESOPHAGEAL FISTULA. Esophageal atresia and tracheoesophageal fistula (TEF) are often associated with other congenital abnormalities, in particular the VACTERL association (**v**ertebral abnormalities, imperforate **a**nus, **c**ongenital heart disease, **t**rache**o**esophageal fistula, and **r**enal abnormalities and **l**imb abnormalities (typically radial atresia).[170,171] The specific cause of these associations is unknown. Although esophageal atresia may be an isolated occurrence, in 90% of cases it is associated with TEF.

Affected neonates usually present with excessive oral secretions, regurgitation of feedings, and occasionally respiratory distress exacerbated by feedings; recurrent pneumonia is associated with an H-type TEF (~2% to 6% of cases) and is usually diagnosed later in life. The diagnosis of esophageal atresia is confirmed by the inability to pass a moderately rigid orogastric tube into the stomach or the demonstration of a blind esophageal pouch by air contrast or radiopaque dye and radiographic studies.

The presence of bowel gas suggests a TEF; on occasion, the abdominal distention may be severe enough to cause atelectasis and impede ventilation. In the most common form of TEF, the esophagus ends in a blind proximal pouch with the distal end of the esophagus connected to the trachea (usually posteriorly) just above the carina. In the less common form of isolated TEF without esophageal atresia, radiologic studies may be inconclusive (Fig. 36-4 and E-Fig. 36-1).

Neonates with TEF should be nursed prone or in a lateral position on an incline of 30 degrees head up to decrease the risk of pulmonary aspiration. A sump suction catheter placed in the upper esophageal pouch preoperatively and connected to constant suction decreases the accumulation of saliva and reduces the potential for aspiration. Neonates with esophageal atresia and TEF may have a staged repair of their lesions. A gastrostomy tube to vent the stomach and a central line for parenteral nutrition may be placed with the patient under sedation with local anesthesia or general anesthesia. The procedures will permit the infant to receive long-term nutrition so that growth may occur and an esophageal anastomosis can be performed when the infant is older and the distance between the esophageal pouch and stomach decreases.

Several approaches may be used to secure the airway in these infants. Awake intubation may be conducted with topical anesthesia of the airway or with intravenous suction if the neonate is medically stable. Alternatively, inhalational induction and spontaneous ventilation may be used until the trachea is secured, particularly if rigid bronchoscopy is used to define the anatomy of the airway before ligation of the fistula. To properly position the tracheal tube, an intentional right main-stem bronchial intubation is sometimes performed; subsequently, the tracheal tube is slowly withdrawn while auscultating the left thorax until breath sounds are heard. During this maneuver, it is key to ensure the bevel of the tube is on the left side (particularly if a Murphy eye is not present on the tube) to facilitate detection of air exchange with the left lung as soon as the tube is withdrawn above the level of the carina. At this position, the tip of the tracheal tube is just above the carina and usually below the level of the fistula. When the tracheal tube is secured in this location, less gastric insufflation will occur through the fistula. The use of fiberoptic bronchoscopy after tracheal intubation has simplified positioning and verifying the position of the tracheal tube and has reduced the need for rigid bronchoscopy. *The tracheal tube should be carefully secured; if the tracheal tube is withdrawn to the position of the fistula opening, adequate pulmonary ventilation cannot be guaranteed.* A stethoscope placed over the left chest (usually best in the axilla) may be helpful in detecting accidental advancement of the tracheal tube into the right main-stem bronchus. An arterial line allows monitoring of blood gas values during the procedure. Pulse oximetry is particularly helpful in detecting partial displacement of the tracheal tube. Preterm infants with poorly compliant lungs occasionally require positive-pressure ventilation.[172,173]

Preferential ventilation through the fistula (the path of least resistance) may result in inadequate pulmonary gas exchange because the air leak through the fistula and into the stomach might increase the intraabdominal pressure, causing the diaphragm to press on the lungs and thereby lead to atelectasis. A staged preoperative gastrostomy was commonly used in the past to avoid this complication. However, although gastrostomy may avert life-threatening gastric rupture, it also may contribute to ineffective ventilation as a result of a bronchocutaneous fistula. A spontaneous breathing technique often results in little gastric

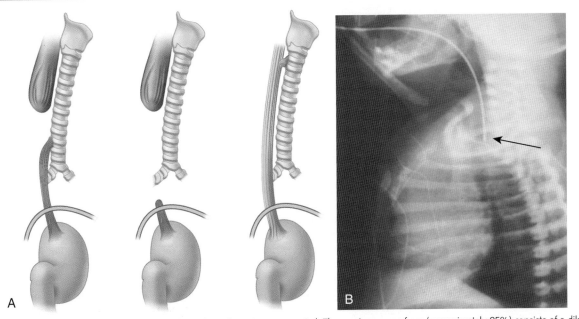

**FIGURE 36-4 A,** The three most common forms of esophageal atresia are presented. The most common form (approximately 85%) consists of a dilated proximal esophageal pouch and a fistula between the distal trachea and distal esophagus (*left*). The second most common form consists of esophageal atresia alone (*middle*). Neonates with tracheoesophageal fistula alone (*right*) often present with pneumonia as the initial manifestation. **B,** The classic presentation is of a newborn with excessive secretions who spits up during the initial feeding; inability to pass a nasogastric tube (*arrow*) is pathognomonic. (**A,** From Coran AG, Behrendt DM, Weintraub WH, Lee DC: Surgery of the neonate. Boston: Little, Brown; 1978, p. 46. **B,** Courtesy Dr. Daniel P. Doody.)

insufflation. Although positive-pressure ventilation may cause gastric dilation, ventilation is usually successful because the compliance of the lungs is greater than that of the distended stomach. Pneumoperitoneum can be managed by emergent needle decompression of the left upper abdominal quadrant. Strategies to ensure adequate ventilation include one-lung ventilation, tracheal intubation distal to the fistula, or Fogarty catheter occlusion of the fistula. If a staged gastrostomy has been performed, a Fogarty catheter passed retrograde through the gastrostomy can be used to occlude the esophagus from below. This approach offers the advantage of avoiding bronchoscopy to pass a Fogarty catheter into the fistula through the trachea in an infant with pulmonary compromise.[174] An epidural catheter threaded from the caudal to the thoracic space may provide a means to give postoperative analgesia in patients who have had TEF repairs (E-Fig. 36-2).

Following correction of the defect, absorptive atelectasis in pulmonary segments may require ventilation with long inspiratory times to reexpand alveoli. This measure is generally a transient necessity. Early extubation is desirable because it prevents prolonged pressure of the endotracheal tube on the suture line. However, a substantial proportion of these infants will require reintubation because of secretions or tracheobronchomalacia. Therefore, at the end of the procedure, a joint decision is made with the surgeon regarding whether to extubate, balancing the child's cardiopulmonary stability with the desire to remove the tracheal tube as soon as possible. Recurrent laryngeal injury, overlooked additional fistulas, and recurrent fistulas may also complicate recovery.

### Diseases of the Lung Parenchyma

Parenchymal lesions may be congenital or acquired. Lesions may include lung hypoplasia if interruption of parenchymal growth occurs early in gestation. Pulmonary cysts may be clinically insignificant until inflation with NO or excessive positive-pressure ventilation leads to gas trapping followed by atelectasis of adjacent areas as a result of compression. Shift of mediastinal contents from marked cyst distention may compromise cardiovascular function.

The small diameter of a neonate's airway makes double-lumen tracheal tubes impractical. Nevertheless, selective bronchial intubations may be successful, especially on the right. Fiberoptic bronchoscopes and guidewires aid in the placement of left-sided tracheal tubes. Bronchial blocking with 5F embolectomy catheters or the intrathoracic use of a clamp by the surgeons may allow selective ventilation of the lung.[175-177]

Avoiding increases in pulmonary artery pressure by preventing hypoxemia, hypercarbia, acidosis, hypothermia, and surgical stress is an essential aspect of managing neonates with compromised pulmonary systems.

#### Specific Lesions

CONGENITAL DIAPHRAGMATIC HERNIA. As the diaphragm completes its formation during weeks 7 to 10 of gestation, anatomic defects that occur will permit the intrusion of abdominal contents into the thoracic cavity, resulting in congenital diaphragmatic hernia (CDH). Although infrequent, this defect in the diaphragm has profound consequences for the further development of the fetus's cardiopulmonary structure, necessitating extensive tertiary care center interventions.

Failure of the diaphragm tissues to fuse appropriately most often appears as the posterolateral Bochdalek type of hernia (90%). Approximately 9% are the anterior, Morgagni type of defects. Less than 1% are bilateral hernias, which are often fatal. The incidence of CDH ranges from 1 in 2000 to 1 in 5000 live births, the variation being attributable to underdiagnosed postdelivery

36

deaths among those neonates severely affected. Equal representation occurs among the genders, although some larger, population-based studies have demonstrated a male preponderance.[178]

Environmental and genetic variables (some poorly understood) contribute to the frequency and presentation of CDH. In neonates in whom the hernia is the only health issue, the risk of recurrence for future pregnancies is small (2%). Neonates with the Bochdalek type of hernia are more likely to have concurrent birth defects, including a 20% to 40% chance of congenital heart defects and a 5% to 15% chance of chromosomal abnormalities.[179] CDH is associated with genitourinary and gastrointestinal malformations, as well as chromosomal anomalies, including trisomy 13, trisomy 18, tetrasomy, and 12p mosaicism.

Prenatal diagnosis of CDH has become an effective tool in furthering the treatment modalities of affected neonates and counseling expectant parents. Level 2 ultrasonography is required for antenatal diagnosis of CDH.[180] Ultrasound examination findings suggestive of the presence of CDH include polyhydramnios, an intrathoracic gastric bubble, and mediastinal shift away from the herniation site. Additional diagnostic testing may include amniocentesis and karyotyping for the delineation of any coexisting chromosomal abnormalities. Abnormally low levels of maternal serum α-fetoprotein are also associated with CDH. The importance of prenatal diagnosis cannot be overemphasized because prior knowledge of the defect will permit the arrangement for delivery at a tertiary care center equipped to provide support. In addition, a handful of research centers offer advanced treatment options such as fetal-based corrective surgical procedures.[181,182] Antenatal diagnosis has allowed the development of risk stratification for fetuses with CDH. The constellation of CDH with liver herniation and a small lung-to-head ratio is often indicative of high postnatal mortality. However, newer surgical techniques performed in utero have attempted to address this issue. Temporary fetoscopic tracheal plugging, performed between 25 and 28 weeks gestation, prevents the normal outflow of surfactant-rich fetal lung fluid.[183] The retained volume subsequently enlarges the fetal lungs, accelerates growth, and reduces the mass effect of herniated viscera. This is coupled with another advanced technique (the ex utero intrapartum tracheoplasty [EXIT] procedure) used to unplug the trachea at the time of birth. During the EXIT procedure, placental support of the fetus continues until the airway has been secured (see Chapter 37). Only a small number of centers offer this treatment option, so only a few randomized, controlled studies have been performed to determine long-term outcomes for fetuses with CDH.[183-185] Further clinical experience is needed before the comparative long-term efficacy of such fetal therapies can be determined.

Emergent surgical closure of the defect was the standard of care in the 1980s, because of the prevalent belief that reduction of the herniated viscera would facilitate lung growth and a return toward normal lung size and function. A thorough understanding of the specific pathophysiology of the defect prompted the application of new medical therapies and changed the timing of open surgical repair.[186] Although the mere presence of abdominal viscera (which may include intestine, liver, spleen and stomach) in the thoracic cavity is not in itself life-threatening, the compressive effects of these viscera on the developing pulmonary structures presents a significant obstacle to the smooth transition from a fetal to neonatal circulatory pattern. The abnormal compression of pulmonary structures is the hallmark of CDH and its cardiopulmonary sequelae.[187-190] Lung growth is severely restricted, especially during the pseudoglandular phase,

when multiplication of proximal airway divisions and the formation of supporting pulmonary arterial vasculature usually occur. Subsequently, fewer functional alveolar units and a grossly diminished surface area for effective gas exchange in the hypoplastic lungs develop. Lung hypoplasia is also associated with a decreased number of alveolar type II cells that results in a deficiency of surfactant apoprotein A (SP-A), which can be associated with alveolar instability, atelectasis, intrapulmonary shunting of deoxygenated blood, and inadequate gas exchange. These biochemical deficiencies are only partially ameliorated with exogenous surfactant treatment. A unilateral CDH may still restrict the normal growth of both lungs depending on the degree of mass effect. The severity of the lung hypoplasia, and its associated morbidity and mortality, were negatively correlated with the gestational age at the time the hernia occurred. The abdominal mass effect, which hinders normal lung growth, also reduces the total cross-sectional area and may alter the reactivity of the arterioles, resulting in pulmonary hypertension. Decreased pulmonary blood flow prevents the normal transition from an intrauterine to extrauterine circulatory pattern. Right-to-left shunting via the PFO and PDA, with associated severe hypoxemia, poses an immediate threat to the neonate. The increased volume of intrathoracic contents may also cause caval compression, with subsequent reductions of preload and cardiac output.

CDH most often presents as severe respiratory distress in the neonate, a direct consequence of lung hypoplasia and inadequate pulmonary gas exchange. Tachycardia, tachypnea, and cyanosis can be observed shortly after delivery. The abdomen may appear concave because of the displacement of viscera into the thorax (the classically described scaphoid abdomen). The mediastinum may be shifted as a result of the herniated viscera (E-Fig. 36-3). Neonates with the Morgagni type of hernia may present with less severe respiratory compromise but with symptoms of bowel obstruction.

The initial management of neonatal respiratory failure associated with CDH is directed at refining oxygenation and ventilation. Definitive airway control is a priority and should be achieved soon after delivery. Mask ventilation is generally avoided in an attempt to limit gastric insufflation that can cause visceral distention and increase the mass effect within the thorax. Once the airway has been secured, mechanical ventilation should be instituted at the lowest peak airway pressures to achieve clearance of $CO_2$ and adequate oxygenation at an acceptable inspired $O_2$ concentration. A nasogastric tube should be passed to decompress the intestinal contents. Serial arterial blood gas analysis and chest radiographs are essential in establishing the prognosis. Studies suggest that alveolar-arterial $O_2$ differentials (A-a$O_2$) and serial $PaCO_2$ measurements are useful predictors for survival.[191,192] If the blood gas values are unacceptable, further strategies, including high-frequency ventilation, oscillation, and ECMO may be considered (see later). An echocardiogram will identify the cardiac anatomy and specific flow characteristics, permitting assessment of pulmonary hypertension and right heart dysfunction, as well as major vessels that may be used for ECMO. Concurrent congenital heart defects also may be diagnosed at this time. Cranial ultrasonography is useful to diagnose intraventricular bleeding, an important consideration for potential institution of ECMO. Appropriate intravenous access and invasive blood pressure monitoring should be established as soon as feasible.

Several ventilator strategies have been successfully used and include conventional mechanical ventilation, high-frequency

oscillatory ventilation, gentle ventilation with permissive hypercapnia, and intratracheal pulmonary ventilation. All of these methods seek to avoid the harmful effects of volutrauma and conditions known to increase pulmonary vascular resistance (hypoxemia, acidosis, hypotension, and significant hypercarbia).[190,193-195] CDH may have variable presentations and degrees of severity; thus no single technique may address all ventilation requirements. Settings that allow for rapid low tidal volumes and limit peak inspiratory pressures will reduce the degree of volutrauma and the potential for pneumothorax. Deliberate alkalosis may increase pulmonary blood flow and decrease $\dot{V}$-$\dot{Q}$ mismatch, but possibly worsening the risk of volutrauma. In neonates in whom oxygenation remains compromised, global tissue hypoxemia will result in significant metabolic acidosis, which may be treated with intravenous bicarbonate infusions, if adequate ventilation is ensured.

Sedation with opioids and benzodiazepines is important to ensure the neonate tolerates the instrumented airway and limit catecholamine responses, which may increase pulmonary vascular resistance. The benefit of vasodilator therapies (prostaglandin $E_1$ [$PGE_1$] and nitrates) remains controversial. Although these agents may reduce pulmonary vascular resistance, they often do so at the expense of systemic hypotension, because they are not specific pulmonary vasodilators. Severe cardiovascular compromise should be treated with volume replacement and inotropic support, although the physician must be aware of the risk of volume overload and pulmonary edema.

Inhaled NO has been used for infants with CDH complicated by refractory pulmonary hypertension because it is a specific pulmonary vasodilator. Reducing pulmonary vascular resistance in the neonate with CDH will decrease right-to-left shunting and improve oxygenation. Despite the decrease in pulmonary resistance, $PGE_1$ infusion may be required to keep the PDA open and avoid right ventricular failure. A significant advantage of inhaled NO therapy is the avoidance of systemic hypotension. The agent is short acting and must be delivered through a specially metered flow apparatus. Although several studies suggest that inhaled NO is not effective in treating hypoxemia associated with CDH, it has been an effective rescue therapy in some cases, particularly when ECMO is not readily available. Animal studies suggest that exogenous surfactant enhances the effectiveness of inhaled NO in CDH, perhaps by recruiting pulmonary tissue. However, these observations have not yet been conclusively confirmed.

ECMO has been used in several centers to treat infants with CDH in whom other medical and ventilator therapies have not been effective. Although the mechanism whereby ECMO improves the outcome of infants with CDH is not fully understood, ECMO can act as a temporizing measure, permitting the lungs to rest and mature while providing appropriate gas exchange through membrane oxygenators.[196] ECMO has also been used as a rescue technique in postoperative infants who decompensate following surgical closure (most often from the incompletely understood phenomenon of rebound pulmonary hypertension). There are multiple inclusion and exclusion criteria (e.g., the presence of high-grade intraventricular hemorrhage is a contraindication because of systemic heparinization).[197] Venovenous (VV) and venoarterial (VA) are two variations of the extracorporeal circuit, and refer to the location of the inflow and outflow catheters. In VV circuits, a double-lumen catheter resides in the internal jugular vein. VA circuits require the placement of two catheters (internal jugular vein and carotid artery) and the ligation of the carotid ipsilateral artery to prevent backflow. In general, VA ECMO is used for neonates who require additional hemodynamic support and greater delivered $O_2$ concentrations. The widespread institution of ECMO has promoted the early stabilization of infants with CDH. The procedure is invasive, however, and complications may arise as a result of systemic anticoagulation and intracranial bleeding. Emboli, infection, vascular damage, and circuit failure are additional concerns.

Currently, surgical repair is delayed until the neonate has been optimized using applicable treatment modalities. Timing of the procedure is variable, based on individual infant condition and institutional experience. A transabdominal approach will replace the herniated viscera and conclude with primary closure of the defect, or if the defect is large, a synthetic patch will be needed to augment the repair. Anesthetic management focuses on supportive care during transport and surgery. Adequate central access should be established, and ventilator settings should mimic those used in the ICU. Serial blood gas sampling will guide changes in respiratory management during closure of the diaphragm. It should be noted that the compliance of the chest actually decreases after surgical correction of the hernia and return of the displaced abdominal organs to the abdomen.[198] This paradoxical effect is the result of distending the abdomen and increasing tension on the diaphragm without relief above the diaphragm (i.e., the hypoplastic lung remains unchanged and nondistensible). If the compliance decreases substantively, the outcome may be fatal.

High-dose opioid techniques decrease catecholamine and other stress hormonal responses to surgical manipulation. Inhalational anesthetics may be tolerated in small concentrations, depending upon the hemodynamic status. Nitrous oxide ($N_2O$) should be avoided because it will expand any air-filled cavities (e.g., the bowels) and limit the inspired $O_2$ concentration.

The use of current multimodal therapies presents a special challenge to the anesthesiologist. Transporting a neonate on ECMO and other agents such as inhaled NO remains a dangerous part of the anesthetic care. Machine malfunctions and disconnects can be sudden and catastrophic. In addition, standard anesthesia machines may not be able to deliver special ventilation modes such as high-frequency oscillatory ventilation. Some tertiary care centers possess facilities for the surgical repair to be conducted within the ICU.[199] Neonates receiving ECMO may require higher doses of opioids delivered via the extracorporeal circuits because of the increased volume of distribution within the circuit, altered plasma clearance rates, and variable degrees of drug adhesion to the synthetic tubing.[200-203]

Despite many years of clinical investigation and the introduction of multiple new approaches, the overall survival for neonates with CDH has remained essentially unchanged, with widely varying mortality rates among institutions.[204] The optimal therapy for the neonate with CDH is unclear. Survivors often have medical issues that require further treatment after hospital discharge, including gastroesophageal reflux, growth impairment, developmental delay, and sensorineural hearing loss. Additional research and multicenter trials are needed to improve clinical outcomes and advance our understanding of long-term issues associated with survival.[205]

### Congenital Bronchogenic and Pulmonary Cysts

Congenital bronchogenic and pulmonary cysts represent arrests of embryologic pulmonary tissue during early fetal lung development.[206] These cysts may be centrally located within the mediastinum and produce obstruction by a mass effect.[207] They may

also be located at the carina and cause obstruction or distal gas trapping by a ball-valve effect. Those located in the hilum, in the paratracheal region, or in the lung parenchyma may lead to chronic respiratory illness from infection and abscess formation.[208,209] Congenital cysts are occasionally diagnosed only after rupture of the cyst produces hemorrhage or bronchopulmonary fistula formation.[206,209]

Anesthetic management is directed at minimizing further enlargement of the cyst because a communication may exist with the airway. Awake (sedated) intubation or intubation with an inhalation induction, followed by maintenance of spontaneous ventilation, if possible, until the thorax is opened, may reduce the potential for sudden enlargement of the cyst. If assisted ventilation is required, low peak inspiratory pressures should be used. Should the cyst be fluid filled or infected, selective bronchial blocking may be helpful in protecting the unaffected lung.[175,176] Nitrous oxide and positive-pressure ventilation without adequate expiratory time should be avoided to decrease the possibility of enlarging the cyst. If these attempts are not successful and the cyst enlarges to the point of occluding the airway or compromising the circulation, needle aspiration to reduce the size of the cyst and facilitate oxygenation and ventilation should be considered. If this method is unsuccessful, emergency thoracostomy may be lifesaving.

### Congenital Lobar Emphysema

Congenital lobar emphysema most commonly affects the left upper lobe but may involve the entire lung (Fig. 36-5).[210,211] Congenital heart disease coexists in approximately 15% of infants.[212] Patients usually have with progressive respiratory failure, unilateral thoracic hyperexpansion, atelectasis of the contralateral lung, and possibly mediastinal shift with cardiovascular compromise.[213] The anesthetic care is focused on minimizing expansion of the emphysema and is similar to that for patients with pulmonary cysts.

## GASTROINTESTINAL PROBLEMS

The types of emergency surgical conditions can be categorized as (1) lesions that are obstructive, (2) those that represent a compromise in intestinal blood supply, and (3) a combination of these two.

Obstructive lesions may be congenital or acquired. Congenital obstruction of the gastrointestinal tract may be suggested by an abnormal increase in maternal weight, polyhydramnios, fetal size greater than normal for gestational age, and fetal abdominal distention detected by ultrasonography. Neonates with acquired lesions may soon after birth have vomiting, abdominal distention, and late passage of meconium (Fig. 36-6). Associated findings may include aspiration pneumonia, dehydration, hypovolemia, and metabolic abnormalities. Unless lifethreatening compromise of organ blood flow occurs, these lesions do not require emergent care. Instead, a priority is to reestablish euvolemia and a metabolically stable state before surgery. Neonates with obstructive lesions usually undergo general anesthesia with tracheal intubation. Induction of general anesthesia may follow an awake intubation if a difficult intubation is anticipated or if active vomiting occurs; a rapid-sequence induction may be used if no airway anomaly is apparent. A rapid-sequence intubation may proceed in a manner similar to that for children and adults. Desaturation after apnea is more rapid, however, because the $O_2$ consumption of a neonate is twice that of an adult and the alveolar stores are reduced. If

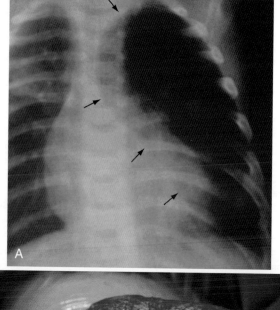

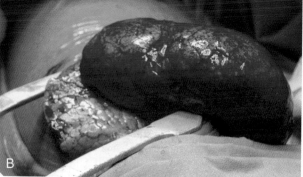

**FIGURE 36-5  A,** Radiograph from an infant with congenital lobar emphysema demonstrates hyperinflation of the left lung with herniation across the midline (*arrows*) and mediastinal shift.
**B,** Intraoperative photograph shows the emphysematous lobe bulging through the thoracotomy incision. (From Coté CJ: The anesthetic management of congenital lobar emphysema. Anesthesiology 1978;49:296.)

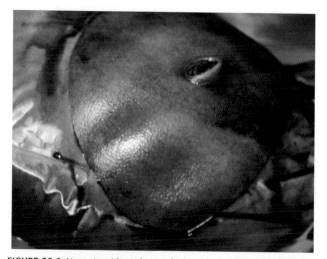

**FIGURE 36-6** Neonate with evidence of a bowel obstruction. Note the distended loops of bowel. This infant will require either an awake intubation or a rapid sequence induction to secure the airway.

surgery is an emergency and the intravascular volume status of the neonate is tenuous, ketamine may be used for induction in place of propofol. A stylet within the tracheal tube should be used to facilitate placement during awake intubations but is infrequently needed in neonates with normal airways. If a stylet is used, it may cause injury to the airway if it extends beyond the bevel of the tube. After tracheal intubation, general anesthesia with either an inhalation (without $N_2O$) or opioid technique and neuromuscular blockade is generally used. Air should be blended with $O_2$ to decrease the inspired $O_2$ concentration to a safe concentration. As described earlier, these neonates may have poor renal perfusion; therefore pancuronium and many antibiotics may have prolonged action. In addition, if hepatic blood flow is compromised, metabolism of opioids and muscle relaxants may be delayed.[214,215]

Infants with lesions that compromise bowel blood flow and cause ischemia are extremely ill. These infants may have a tender and distended abdomen, bloody stools, vomiting, hypotension, metabolic abnormalities, anemia, leukopenia, and thrombocytopenia. Abdominal radiographic examination may reveal distended intestinal loops, decreased bowel gas, and perforation.

Emergency surgery is required and directed at removing necrotic tissue, closing perforations, and reestablishing normal perfusion to the intestine. Blood and blood products should be immediately available, including uncrossmatched blood if crossmatched blood is not available, fresh frozen plasma, and platelets. These infants are not appropriate candidates for regional anesthesia. Before anesthetic induction, adequate venous access should be ensured because they require increased intraoperative fluids and may require rapid transfusion of blood products (which is in general not possible through 24-gauge intravenous catheters or peripherally inserted central catheter [PICC] lines). It may be prudent to replace the umbilical arterial line with a peripheral arterial line if it is possible that the line may obstruct mesenteric blood flow. The volume status should be optimized and dopamine 5 μg/kg/min) infused to increase blood flow to the gut. If poor peripheral perfusion occurs secondary to shunting of blood through a PDA, carefully titrated intravenous fluids and sympathomimetics may improve cardiac output and organ perfusion.

### Specific Lesions

#### Hypertrophic Pyloric Stenosis

Pyloric stenosis usually manifests within weeks 2 to 6 of life with nonbilious vomiting. This lesion occurs more frequently in first-born males; the incidence is approximately 1 in 500 live births (Fig. 36-7).[216] Pyloric stenosis represents hypertrophy of the muscularis layer of the pylorus and can often be palpated as an olive-shaped mass between the midline and right upper quadrant. The lesion is most commonly delineated by ultrasonography[217] or rarely with a barium swallow and radiographic examination.

With protracted vomiting, these infants may become hypokalemic, hypochloremic, and alkalotic.[218] The renal response to vomiting is twofold. Initially, serum pH is defended by excretion of alkaline urine with sodium and potassium loss; later, with depletion of these electrolytes, the kidneys secrete acidic urine (paradoxical aciduria), further increasing the metabolic alkalosis. Hypocalcemia may be associated with the hyponatremia. With further fluid loss prerenal azotemia may portend hypovolemic shock and metabolic acidosis. Hemoconcentration may result in polycythemia. This lesion does not mandate an emergency surgical procedure; therefore intravascular volume and metabolic stabilization and correction are a priority.

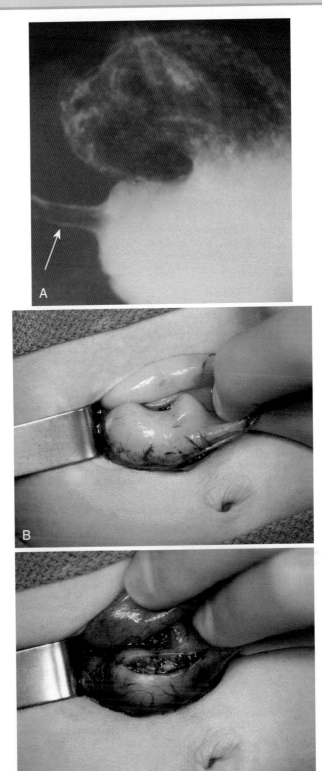

**FIGURE 36-7 A,** Barium swallow and abdominal radiograph of an infant with pyloric stenosis demonstrates a high degree of obstruction of the gastric outflow tract with a "wisp" of barium escaping through the pylorus (*arrow*). **B,** The hypertrophied pylorus. **C,** Surgical myotomy relieved the obstruction. (Courtesy Dr. Daniel P. Doody.)

Suctioning an in situ orogastric or nasogastric tube seldom empties the stomach. A freshly inserted wide-bore orogastric tube almost always removes additional residual gastric contents; this step is especially important for infants who have had a barium contrast radiographic study. One study found nearly complete emptying of the gastric contents if the infant's stomach is suctioned in the right and left lateral as well as the supine positions with a vented catheter (e.g., Salem sump).[219] Therefore the stomach is aspirated immediately before induction using a large-bore orogastric tube as described. These infants are most commonly managed with an intravenous induction (although some centers have performed inhalational inductions for more than 30 years for this abdominal defect) because vomiting during induction might result in serious pulmonary aspiration. A rapid-sequence induction is preferred. Intermediate acting NMBDs are infrequently required. However, if the intubation is anticipated to be difficult, a sedated "awake" intubation is carried out before the induction of anesthesia. Inhalation or balanced anesthesia may then be used for maintenance. These surgeries are brief and thus the concentration of inhalational anesthetic must be carefully titrated because these infants are notoriously slow to recover from anesthesia. Infants should be extubated once fully awake and vigorous. Feedings are usually begun soon after surgery, and the postoperative course is generally uncomplicated. Local infiltration of the incision site with a long-acting local anesthetic generally provides complete analgesia.

Some surgeons will perform this procedure laparoscopically or through a periumbilical incision. Laparoscopic techniques may have profound hemodynamic and respiratory effects (see Chapter 27).[220,221] One further consideration is the number of case reports describing apnea in this population[222]; some centers advocate postoperative apnea monitoring.

### Duodenal and Ileal Obstruction

Congenital duodenal and ileal obstructions (atresia, stenosis, annular pancreas, meconium ileus) are often associated with other anomalies. For example, 20% to 30% of neonates with duodenal atresia have trisomy 21, with a high likelihood of associated cardiac lesions such as atrial septal defect, ventricular septal defect, or atrioventricular canal. Neonates with intestinal atresia are frequently preterm or may have other associated anomalies, such as malrotation of the gut, volvulus, and abdominal wall defects.[223] Meconium ileus occurs in 10% to 15% of neonates with cystic fibrosis. It may present either as terminal ileal obstruction by viscid meconium or as bowel atresia. Hyperosmolar enemas are frequently administered to these infants in an effort to clear the viscid meconium plugs. These enemas may result in serious shifts in intravascular volume, leading to hypovolemia requiring aggressive treatment before anesthetic induction.

Duodenal atresia is associated with bilious vomiting beginning within the first 24 to 48 hours after birth. Radiographs of the abdomen demonstrate the pathognomonic double-bubble sign formed by air contrast of the dilated stomach and proximal duodenum; the remaining bowel is devoid of air (Fig. 36-8). With jejunoileal atresia, air–fluid levels are observed throughout the abdomen. With distal ileal obstruction, a barium enema may demonstrate a microcolon. The typical radiographic presentation of meconium ileus is a soap-bubble mass in the right lower abdomen and absence of air–fluid levels. Initial stabilization of neonates with these lesions is directed at fluid and metabolic resuscitation. Anesthetic management proceeds after suctioning of contrast agent and other stomach contents. Awake intubation

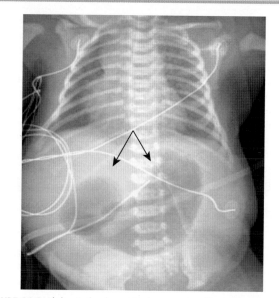

**FIGURE 36-8** Abdominal radiograph of a neonate with congenital duodenal atresia demonstrating a classic double-bubble sign (*arrows*). Note that the remainder of the bowel is devoid of air, indicating complete obstruction.

may be indicated in volume-depleted or actively vomiting infants; rapid-sequence induction is used in hemodynamically stable infants with normal airway anatomy. $N_2O$ should be avoided to minimize intestinal distention. Neuromuscular blockade is generally necessary to facilitate abdominal exploration; use of a neuromuscular blocking agent also decreases or avoids the need for high concentrations of potent inhalation agents, which are poorly tolerated by hypovolemic neonates.

### Infantile Hernia

Infantile hernia usually presents within the first 6 months after birth. Although the potential for incarceration through the inguinal canal is present in greater than 90% of neonates, it occurs in only 3% to 5% of full-term infants and 30% of preterm infants.[224] With incarceration or strangulation of bowel or gonads, emergency correction is indicated. Incarcerated hernias with or without strangulation should be treated similarly to bowel obstruction. A rapid-sequence or awake intubation should be used at the induction of general anesthesia. An inhalation technique without $N_2O$ or an opioid technique may be used after intubation.

Elective repair of a nonincarcerated hernia can be carried out with either general or regional anesthesia when there is no acute bowel obstruction (e.g., a reduced inguinal hernia).[225-228] An intravenous line should be placed before anesthetic induction if there is any concern about the volume status. Because blood pressure instability is unusual in infants undergoing spinal anesthesia,[229] placement of an intravenous line in the lower extremity may follow the onset of sensory block. Similarly, blood pressure monitoring may be accomplished by using a blood pressure cuff placed on the lower (anesthetized) extremity. Swaddling and a pacifier often are all that is required for sedation.

Spinal anesthesia may be administered through a 1½-inch, 22-gauge spinal needle (see also Fig. 41-8). Once the block is placed, the infant should be maintained in the supine position. Leg lifting, especially during placement of the electrocautery grounding pad, should be avoided because it has been associated

with a high spinal blockade (see also Fig. 41-9).[230] Rather, log-roll or lift the entire infant to apply the cautery pad. Apnea or sudden cessation of crying may be the presenting sign of a high spinal blockade in a neonate.

Because hernia repair is a common operation in former preterm infants, this population is at greatest risk for postoperative life-threatening apnea.[19-21,231,232] Outpatient repair of inguinal hernia in former preterm infants is contraindicated in those infants 55 weeks or younger postconceptional age (see also Fig. 4-7 and E-Fig. 4-6). Because apnea may occur even after regional anesthesia, provision for postoperative monitoring must be available.[233]

### Imperforate Anus

Imperforate anus is generally recognized at the initial physical examination or by failure to pass meconium within the first 48 hours of life. Neonates with imperforate anus are likely to have associated anomalies of the urogenital sinus, as well as those associated with the entire spectrum of the VACTERL association.[171] Some infants require a decompressive colostomy before definitive surgery. It may be prudent to perform echocardiography to rule out associated congenital heart disease before anesthetic induction. Preductal and postductal $O_2$ saturation determinations may be of value. If these infants exhibit signs of bowel obstruction, they should undergo anesthesia in a manner similar to that in others with obstructive lesions.

### Necrotizing Enterocolitis

Necrotizing enterocolitis is not an anomaly but an illness found predominantly in preterm infants.[234] The incidence is 5% to 15% in infants less than 1500 grams birth weight, and the mortality rate is 10% to 30%.[235] Morbidity associated with necrotizing enterocolitis includes short-bowel syndrome, sepsis, and adhesions associated with bowel obstruction. Necrotizing enterocolitis is associated with birth asphyxia, hypotension, RDS, PDA, recurrent apnea, intestinal ischemia, umbilical vessel cannulation, systemic infections, and early feedings.[110,236-238]

Initial signs of necrotizing enterocolitis include temperature instability, poor feeding with gastric residuals or vomiting, malabsorption of feedings (positive stool-reducing substances), lethargy, hyperglycemia, and heme-positive or overtly bloody stools. Affected infants may appear very ill and have a distended and tender abdomen. Radiographic examination may initially suggest an ileus with edematous bowel and later demonstrate gas in the intestinal wall (pneumatosis intestinalis) and in the hepatobiliary tract or portal venous system (Fig. 36-9). When perforation has occurred, free air within the abdominal cavity can be appreciated by radiologic examination of the abdomen.

Infants generally have metabolic and hematologic abnormalities, including hyperglycemia, thrombocytopenia, coagulopathy, and anemia. Hypotension, metabolic acidosis, and prerenal azotemia are other significant findings in severe cases. Initial treatment includes discontinuation of enteral feedings and decompression of the abdomen by means of low-pressure continuous nasogastric or orogastric suctioning. Wide-spectrum antibiotics are administered, although no specific bacteria are associated with necrotizing enterocolitis. Dopamine infusions may be required to increase the cardiac output and improve intestinal perfusion. Umbilical arterial lines are replaced with a peripheral arterial line so that mesenteric blood flow is not compromised. Indications for surgery can vary from surgeon to surgeon but may include abdominal viscus perforation resulting

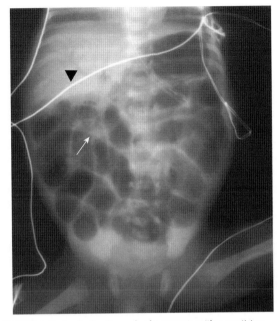

**FIGURE 36-9** Abdominal radiograph of a neonate with necrotizing enterocolitis demonstrates generalized bowel distention (ileus), small amount of pneumotosis intestinalis in left upper quadrant (*arrow*), and gas outlining the intrahepatic portal vein (*arrowhead*). (Courtesy Dr. Sjirk J. Westra.)

in free air, persistence of a bowel loop on serial abdominal radiographs, or persistent metabolic acidosis with clinically important hyperkalemia, indicating the presence of necrotic tissue.[239]

Adequate preparation before surgery is important. Blood, fresh frozen plasma, and platelets likely will be required. Dopamine infusions may be necessary to improve renal and intestinal perfusion and cardiac output. Patients often are already intubated; otherwise, rapid-sequence or awake intubation is indicated. Because these infants are septic and volume depleted, potent inhalation agents are poorly tolerated and generally avoided. An opioid and muscle relaxant technique, avoiding $N_2O$, is preferred. These infants usually have very large volume requirements; it is common for 1 or more blood volumes of fluid infusion to be required as a result of massive third-space losses. In addition, severe coagulopathy may result in sudden, catastrophic generalized hemorrhage (Fig. 36-10). Platelet transfusion is often needed before surgical incision.

### Omphalocele and Gastroschisis

Neonates with omphalocele and gastroschisis have defects in the abdominal wall and may present with impaired blood supply to the herniated organs, intestinal obstruction, and major intravascular fluid deficits. The differences between omphalocele and gastroschisis are summarized in Table 36-4.

Omphalocele represents a failure of the gut to migrate from the yolk sac into the abdomen during gestation (Fig. 36-11, *A*).[240,241] It occurs in 1 in 6000 births.[242] Infants with omphalocele may have associated genetic, cardiac, urologic (exstrophy of the bladder; see Fig. 36-11, *B*), and metabolic abnormalities (Beckwith-Wiedemann syndrome with visceromegaly, hypoglycemia, polycythemia).[243] The herniated viscera emerge from the umbilicus and are covered with a membranous sac; the bowel is morphologically and usually functionally normal.

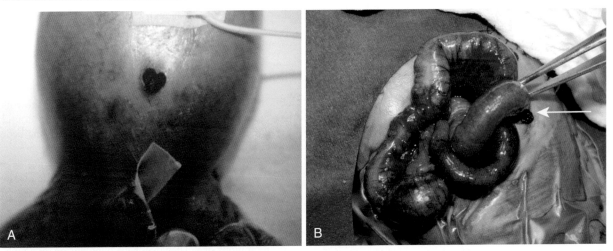

**FIGURE 36-10** A preterm neonate with severe necrotizing enterocolitis and intestinal necrosis. **A,** Abdominal discoloration consistent with dead bowel. **B,** Necrotizing enterocolitis with segment of dead bowel (*top*) and evidence of free stool in the abdomen (*arrow*). These infants often have bowel perforation and hemorrhage from bowel or liver. They can have severe hypotension requiring vasopressor support and enormous volume requirements. Moreover, because of hemorrhage and disseminated intravscular coagulopathy, these infants will generally require transfusions of blood, platelets, and fresh frozen plasma. Some practitioners also advocate administration of vitamin K. (Courtesy Dr. Daniel P. Doody.)

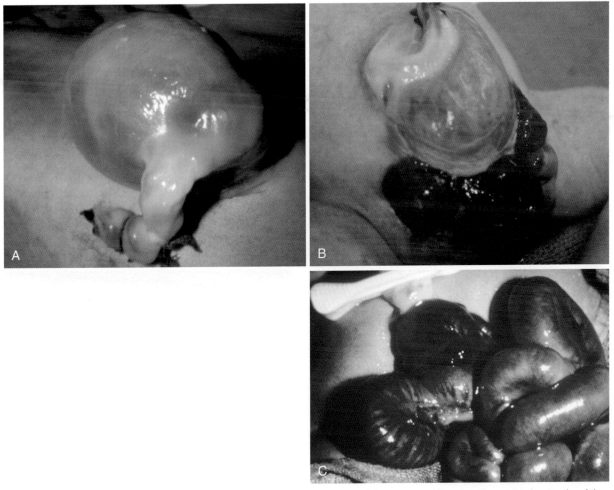

**FIGURE 36-11 A,** Omphalocele covered with a membranous sac; the defect arises at the umbilicus. **B,** Ompahlocoele with associated exstrophy of the bladder. **C,** Gastroschisis; note the absence of a membranous sac. In contrast to omphalocele, the gastroschisis anomaly is periumbilical.

**TABLE 36-4** Comparison of Omphalocele and Gastroschisis

| Comparison Factors | Omphalocele | Gastroschisis |
|---|---|---|
| Cause | Failure of gut migration from yolk sac into abdomen | Occlusion of omphalomesenteric artery |
| Location | Within umbilical cord | Periumbilical |
| Associated lesions | Beckwith-Wiedemann syndrome (macroglossia, gigantism, hypoglycemia, hyperviscosity)<br>Congenital heart disease<br>Exstrophy of bladder | Exposed gut inflammation, edema, dilation, and foreshortened |

Gastroschisis develops as a result of occlusion of the omphalomesenteric artery during gestation.[241,244] It occurs in 1 in 15,000 births and is usually not associated with other congenital anomalies. The herniated viscera and intestines are periumbilical, usually on the right, and are exposed to air after delivery, resulting in inflammation, edema, and dilated, foreshortened, and functionally abnormal bowel (see Fig. 36-11, *C*).[245, 246]

Management of these lesions from birth until surgery is directed at maintaining perfusion to the herniated viscera and reduction of fluid loss from exposed visceral surfaces by covering the mucosal surfaces with sterile, saline-soaked dressings. A plastic wrap further decreases evaporative volume losses and the tendency to develop hypothermia. These anomalies represent a wide spectrum of pathology and require individualized assessment of intravascular volume status and fluid replacement. When these infants arrive in the ICU, fluid resuscitation is instituted; neonates with gastroschisis lose more fluid than those with omphalocoeles and thus require repeat boluses of 20 mL/kg isotonic fluids to replace evaporative and third-space losses.[247]

Anesthetic management is directed at continued volume resuscitation and measures to prevent hypothermia. Aspiration of stomach contents should be performed. Rapid-sequence induction or awake intubation is carried out. Neuromuscular blockade facilitates reduction of the eviscerated organs and bowel; however, abdominal closure may be associated with markedly increased intraabdominal pressure (E-Fig. 36-4). The effects of increased intraabdominal pressure are twofold: (1) decreased organ perfusion and (2) decreased ventilatory reserve. The increase in intraabdominal pressure may lead to decreased intestinal, renal, and hepatic perfusion and secondarily impaired organ function. This may lead to markedly altered drug metabolism and prolonged drug effect. The bowel may become edematous, and urine output may be reduced as a result of renal congestion. Venous return from the lower body also may be reduced, resulting in lower extremity congestion and cyanosis. Blood pressure and pulse oximetry determinations from a lower extremity may be different from those in the upper extremity. Significantly decreased diaphragmatic function and bilateral lower lobe atelectasis may occur, leading to respiratory failure.[248] Transduction of intragastric or bladder pressures may be a diagnostic adjunct.[249]

If complete reduction is not possible, a staged reduction is carried out. The intestine is covered with a silastic pouch, and the size of the pouch is subsequently reduced in stages either in the operating room or intensive care unit, thus allowing the abdominal cavity gradually to accommodate the increased mass without severely compromising ventilation or organ perfusion.[250,251]

### Malrotation and Midgut Volvulus

Malrotation and midgut volvulus result from abnormal migration or incomplete rotation of the intestines from the yolk sac back into the abdomen.[252] Rotation of the intestine around the mesentery may produce the abnormal location of the ileocecal valve in the right upper quadrant and kinking or compression of its vascular supply. If the malrotation occurs during development, atretic segments of bowel are formed. If the kinking or compression occurs after the bowel is normally developed, bowel necrosis may result.

These infants present with bilious emesis, a tender and distended abdomen, and increasing abdominal girth; bloody stools are an ominous sign. They may have hypotension, hypovolemia, and electrolyte abnormalities. Because delay in surgery may result in necrosis of the entire small intestine, fluid and electrolyte resuscitation begins preoperatively and continues during surgery. This is a true neonatal emergency, and surgery should proceed as expeditiously as possible. Blood and blood products should be available in the operating room. Note that the hematocrit may be falsely increased secondary to marked intravascular volume depletion. The indications for intraarterial monitoring depend on the severity of the infant's illness. Central venous pressure monitoring may improve assessment of intravascular volume status and assist in directing replacement and postoperative fluid management. However, if peripheral venous access is adequate, the operation should not be delayed to insert the central venous pressure line.

### Hirschsprung Disease and Large-Bowel Obstruction

Hirschsprung disease is the most common cause of neonatal colon obstruction and consists of the absence of parasympathetic ganglion cells (Auerbach and Meissner plexus) in the large intestine.[253,254] This deficiency creates a nonperistaltic segment of variable length, a tonically contracted anorectal sphincter, and delayed passage of meconium. Functional obstruction occurs at the level of the affected segment. The bowel may occasionally become distended to the point at which its blood supply is

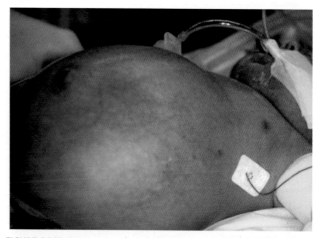

**FIGURE 36-12** Toxic megacolon results in massive abdominal distention, fluid requirements, and sepsis. These infants require special consideration in airway management because of the high risk for aspiration and increased abdominal pressure.

36

compromised; perforation may occur, with resultant peritonitis. If the condition is not recognized and is left untreated, enteric bacteria may invade the bowel wall and subsequently enter the bloodstream, producing the toxic megacolon syndrome. Infants thus affected present with a distended, tender abdomen and hypotension and require massive volume replacement and vasopressor support (Fig. 36-12).

The majority of these neonates are diagnosed early because of bowel distention and failure to pass meconium. Bowel obstruction may be intermittent. Initial management is directed at stabilizing the infant's fluid status. Infants with lower intestinal obstruction may require rapid-sequence induction or awake intubation. If the infant is volume depleted, potent inhalation agents are poorly tolerated. $N_2O$ should be avoided to prevent increasing bowel distention.

## REFERENCES

Please see www.expertconsult.com.

# Fetal Intervention and the EXIT Procedure

ROLAND BRUSSEAU

THE ADVENT OF FETAL intervention introduced the concept of surgically correcting a known congenital defect in utero to avoid certain fetal demise. With improvements in prenatal imaging and surgical techniques, fetal interventions have grown to include diagnoses associated with intrauterine demise, as well as diseases associated with significant postnatal morbidity. The goal of fetal intervention is to improve the chances of normal fetal development and minimize postnatal morbidity.[1] Advances have changed some procedures from open in-utero interventions, which are associated with significant maternal risk, to percutaneous or fetoscopic techniques, thus improving the maternal risk-to-benefit ratio while diminishing postoperative uterine contractions associated with open procedures.

Fetal surgery differs from any other subspecialty of anesthesia because the anesthesiologist must care for two or possibly three patients at once, all with distinctive and, at times, conflicting requirements. The first is the mother who can express her level of discomfort, who can be monitored directly, and to whom drugs can be administered easily. The second (and possibly third) is the fetus. For the latter, detecting pain depends solely on indirect evidence, monitoring is limited at best, administering drugs is more complicated, and there is the possibility of long-term effects from procedures and drugs administered during early development. The anesthesiologist is required to provide both maternal and fetal anesthesia and analgesia while ensuring both maternal and fetal hemodynamic stability; a plan must be prepared to resuscitate the fetus if problems occur during the intervention.

# A Range of Anesthetic Options for Mother and Fetus

## MOTHER

Fetal interventions have been successfully performed with various anesthetic techniques; both maternal and fetal anesthetic requirements must be considered and may, in fact, be quite different. With some endoscopic interventions, the site of surgical intervention is not innervated; thus the fetus may not sense a noxious stimulus, and its anesthetic requirements are presumably minimal. Nevertheless, fetal immobility remains essential to procedural safety and success. Other interventions may require that a needle be inserted into the fetus, which may elicit a noxious stimulus and possibly even cause pain. Open procedures can produce significant noxious stimuli. In addition to surgical demands, each mother and fetus exhibit a unique physiologic, pharmacologic, and pathophysiologic profile; the anesthesiologist must evaluate the advantages and disadvantages of each anesthetic technique and select the safest anesthetic.[2]

### Local Anesthesia

Local anesthesia is almost exclusively used for trocar insertion sites with percutaneous procedures. The most obvious advantage is maternal safety, because the mother receives no intravenous (IV) medications. The disadvantages of this technique include increased risk of injury to the nonanesthetized, nonparalyzed fetus, no fetal analgesia, and no uterine relaxation. Patients on tocolytic therapy or those with polyhydramnios and uterine contractions may be at further risk of worsening contractions with this approach.

### Monitored Anesthesia Care

IV sedation involves the maternal administration of benzodiazepines, opioids, and occasionally low-dose induction agents. Advantages include possible provision of anesthesia and analgesia to the fetus via transplacental transfer of agents, as well as decreased maternal anxiety and pain. Depending on the amount and effect of the drugs administered, this sedation may increase the mother's risk of aspiration because of an unprotected airway. This technique also provides no uterine relaxation.

### Regional Neuraxial Blockade

Neuraxial techniques (spinal, epidural, or combined spinal and epidural anesthesia) have been used with fetoscopic techniques and, rarely, without an adjunct general anesthetic, for open techniques. A T4 sensory-level blockade is required for most surgical uterine manipulations. Neuraxial techniques provide no uterine relaxation, nor do they provide fetal analgesia or anesthesia. Neuraxial anesthesia is associated with an increased maternal risk (e.g., failed block, high spinal, total spinal, or intravascular injection of local anesthetic).

### Regional Neuraxial Blockade with Sedation

The addition of IV sedation to regional anesthesia may provide the fetus with analgesia/anesthesia via placental drug transfer. Although IV fentanyl, propofol, and benzodiazepines can be administered to patients receiving regional anesthesia, they may place the mother at increased risk of bradyarrhythmias, respiratory depression, and pulmonary aspiration; the need for a T4 sensory block may produce alterations in respiratory mechanics additive to those caused by pregnancy. In addition, the level of sympathetic blockade is often two to six levels greater than the sensory level.[3] Hence, a T4 sensory block may completely block cardiac accelerator fibers (T1 to T4); severe bradyarrhythmias and cardiac arrest have been reported.[4-6] When IV agents with vagotonic properties are administered in this clinical setting, the risk of significant bradyarrhythmias may be increased.[7]

### General Anesthesia

General anesthesia with inhalational anesthetics provides both maternal and fetal anesthesia and dose-dependent uterine relaxation even in patients who have received tocolytic therapy for preoperative premature uterine contractions.[8-11]

### Combined Regional and General Anesthesia

A combined regional and general anesthesia technique is often used for open procedures, as well as for patients with anterior placentas, in whom externalization of the uterus for safe trocar insertion is anticipated. In addition to providing the advantages of both the regional and the general anesthetic techniques listed previously, this method allows for planned postoperative pain control.[12] The physical window for trocar insertion is often smaller in this patient cohort, necessitating either externalization of the uterus or extreme lateral decubitus position. Externalization of the uterus requires a larger surgical incision than for standard cesarean sections.

## FETUS

Maternal anesthetic techniques that do not include inhalational anesthetics may not provide adequate analgesia and/or anesthesia for the fetus. However, fetal analgesia and anesthesia may also be accomplished by delivery of anesthetics and analgesics directly to the fetus. Potential methods include transplacental, direct intramuscular, direct intravascular, and intraamniotic administration; each route of administration has advantages and disadvantages that can have a direct impact on overall outcome.

### Transplacental Access

Many fetal interventions (open or endoscopic) employ transplacental drug administration to provide anesthesia and analgesia for both mother and fetus. Many, but not all, drugs cross the placenta via Fick's law of passive diffusion (Fig. 37-1). Lipid solubility, the pH of both maternal and fetal blood, the degree of ionization, protein binding, perfusion, placental area and thickness, and drug concentration are factors that influence the extent of transplacental drug diffusion.[13] The most obvious disadvantage with this approach is that the mother must be exposed to every drug that the fetus is intended to receive, often at large concentrations, to achieve adequate drug concentrations in the fetus. In addition, the uptake of drugs may be impaired if there is reduced placental blood flow. This has implications for successful anesthesia and analgesia both in terms of the delivered fetal dose and the time interval that must be allowed from maternal administration to the start of the fetal intervention. All inhaled anesthetics cross the placental barrier, but uptake in the fetus is slower than in the mother.[13] However, this is offset by the reduced minimal alveolar concentration (MAC) for anesthesia in the fetus, resulting in a similar onset of anesthesia as in the mother.[2] Fetal anesthesia is also important to reduce the fetal stress response, which, through catecholamine release, can reduce placental blood flow and exacerbate any asphyxia.[14-17]

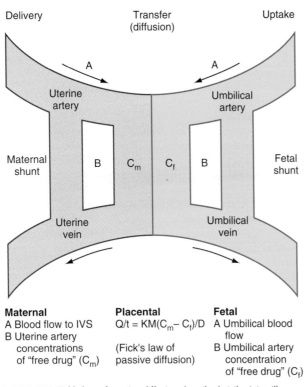

**Maternal**
A Blood flow to IVS
B Uterine artery
concentrations
of "free drug" ($C_m$)

**Placental**
$Q/t = KM(C_m - C_f)/D$

(Fick's law of
passive diffusion)

**Fetal**
A Umbilical blood
flow
B Umbilical artery
concentration
of "free drug" ($C_f$)

**FIGURE 37-1** Fick's law of passive diffusion described at the intervillous space (*IVS*). *D,* Membrane thickness; *K,* diffusion constant of the drug; *M,* membrane surface area; *Q/t,* rate of diffusion.

### Intramuscular Access

Intramuscular (IM) injection involves inserting a needle under ultrasound guidance into a fetal extremity or buttocks. Unlike umbilical cord injection, the noxious stimulus to the fetus by the IM injection stimulates the fetal stress response. Although the bleeding risk from IM injection is less than that with intravascular injections, there remains a risk of bleeding and injury from the needle itself. Furthermore, if the fetus is already stressed, blood will be diverted away from muscle (the site of drug administration) and toward the fetal heart and brain. In this case, it may be impossible to estimate the time course for the drug to be absorbed from the IM site.

### Intravascular Access

Intravascular fetal drug administration ensures immediate drug levels, and no additional dosing calculations are necessary because placental perfusion does not significantly alter dosing. Intravascular access can be obtained via the umbilical cord (which is not innervated), larger fetal veins (e.g., hepatic vein), or intracardiac, as the specific intervention dictates.[18] One advantage of administering drugs via the umbilical vein is the ability to provide analgesia before the surgical insult. Muscle relaxants, analgesics, and vagolytic agents, as well as resuscitation drugs, can be given with assurance of immediate access to the fetal circulation. This method is also useful when alterations in peripheral blood flow occur (i.e., a "central sparing response"), which significantly diminishes the blood distribution to sites of potential IM access.

Establishing intravascular access in the fetus requires inserting a needle in a fetus that is often not sedated from maternally administered agents. The needle may injure the moving fetus, and there is a risk of bleeding from the fetus, umbilical cord, and

placenta. Uncontrolled bleeding could impair the surgical view and it places the fetus and mother in jeopardy, because an open hysterotomy may be necessary to control the bleeding. Establishing access via the umbilical cord vessels may also produce vascular spasm, potentially compromising fetal perfusion.

### Intraamniotic Access

Intraamniotic fentanyl, sufentanil, thyroxine, vasopressin, and digoxin have been safely administered in pregnant large-animal models, with only minimal drug detected in the mother.[19,20] If the safety and efficacy of this method of drug delivery hold true in human trials, intraamniotic drug administration may become the preferred method for fetal drug delivery.

## Fetal Development

### PATHOLOGIC LUNG DEVELOPMENT

In the context of fetal interventions, there are two important causes of respiratory morbidity to consider: insufficient amniotic fluid and prematurity. With both, the timing of the insult in terms of the stage of lung development is critical to estimating the degree of likely morbidity. Deficiency of amniotic fluid may result from prelabor premature rupture of the amniotic membranes (PPROM), which may be spontaneous or iatrogenically induced either directly through trauma or by introducing infection into the uterus. Small amniotic fluid volume may also be secondary to reduced fetal urine output, from either poor renal function (e.g., with renal agenesis or urinary tract obstruction) or growth restriction secondary to placental insufficiency. Amniotic fluid deficiency contributes to pulmonary hypoplasia. In general, the likelihood of pulmonary insufficiency is inversely related to gestation at membrane rupture, a long latency to delivery, and the amount of residual amniotic fluid.[21-23] The risk is relatively small if PPROM occurs after 24 weeks gestation,[24] as demonstrated by one series of fetuses with PPROM before 26 weeks reporting pulmonary hypoplasia in 27% of fetuses.[25] In contrast, with severe oligohydramnios of more than 2 weeks duration after PPROM arising before 25 weeks gestation, the predicted neonatal mortality exceeds 90%.[26]

Studies in sheep show that oligohydramnios causes spinal flexion, which compresses the abdominal contents, displacing the diaphragm upward and thus compressing the developing lungs.[27] This increase in the pressure gradient between the lungs and the amniotic cavity causes a net loss of lung fluid through the trachea, preventing lung expansion.[27] Lung fluid produced in the airways is thought to act as a stent for the developing lungs.[28] Normally, it passes out through the trachea and is either swallowed or passes into the amniotic cavity. Ligation of the trachea causes lung hyperplasia[29] or ipsilateral lung hyperplasia if a main bronchus is ligated.[30] Experimental drainage of amniotic fluid in animals has been shown to result in pulmonary hypoplasia.[31] Later restoration of amniotic fluid prevents the onset of pulmonary hypoplasia.[32] There is evidence to support amnioinfusion in humans to maintain fluid volumes around the fetus after PPROM, in an effort to improve lung development.[26,33]

Surfactant is a complex of phospholipids secreted by type II alveolar cells, which reduces lung surface air tension, thereby preventing the lungs from collapsing at low volumes. Glucocorticoids, thyroid hormone, and β-adrenergic agonists stimulate surfactant synthesis. It is first detected in the lungs around 23 weeks gestation, but mature levels necessary for unassisted ventilation are not present until about 34 weeks. The degree of

**FETAL CIRCULATION**

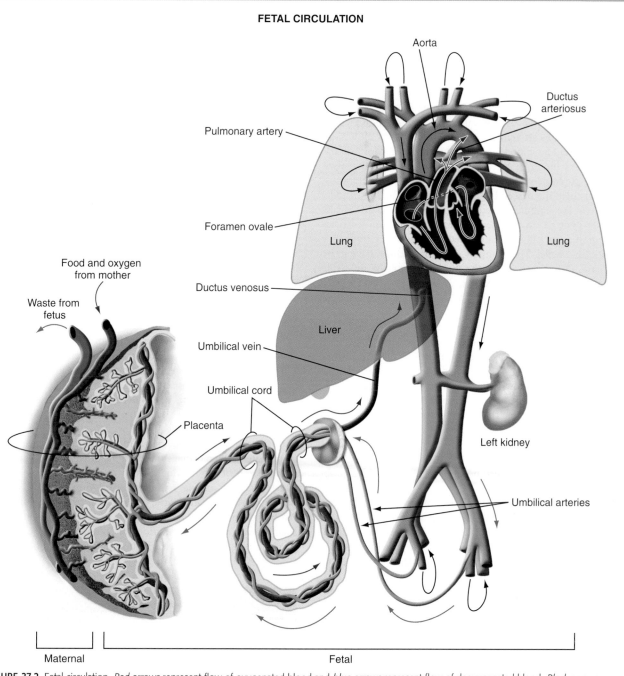

**FIGURE 37-2** Fetal circulation. *Red arrows* represent flow of oxygenated blood and *blue arrows* represent flow of deoxygenated blood. *Black arrows* indicate direction of blood flow and represent travel of blood from the central circulation through capillary membranes and return to central circulation. Shading (from red to purple to blue) represents the corresponding relative oxygenation of the blood at that site, from oxygenated to deoxygenated. Note the mixing of blood as the ductus venosus delivers oxygenated blood from the placenta to the central fetal circulation and the progressive desaturation of blood in the fetal aorta secondary to shunts, consumption, and the return of deoxygenated blood from the fetal pulmonary circulation.

lung maturity can be evaluated by amniocentesis using the lecithin to sphingomyelin ratio or, more recently, by the lamellar body count.[34] Acceleration of surfactant synthesis may be achieved with corticosteroids administered to the mother.[35]

## FETAL CARDIOVASCULAR DEVELOPMENT

The differences between the fetal and postnatal circulations are complex (Fig. 37-2). In the fetal circulation, oxygenated blood returns from the placenta via the umbilical veins and ductus venosus (bypassing the liver) into the right atrium. At 20 weeks, 30% of the umbilical venous return (40 to 60 mL/kg/min) is

shunted through the ductus venosus.[36] This flow decreases over the second half of gestation as hepatic blood flow increases so that, by term only 20% of umbilical venous return (less than 20 mL/kg/min) is shunted through the ductus venosus.[36] Hypoxia and hemorrhage increase the resistance in the liver, shunting a greater proportion of blood toward the brain and heart via the ductus venosus.[37] The proportion of blood that perfuses the liver, which exits 15% less saturated in oxygen, rejoins the ductus venosus blood in the inferior vena cava. However, this deoxygenated blood has less kinetic energy and flows more slowly into the right atrium toward the right ventricle.[37] The greater-velocity oxygenated blood from the ductus venosus is preferentially directed through the foramen ovale into the left side of the heart and out via the aortic arch to the developing head and upper body. The integrity of the foramen ovale is thus imperative. Blood returning from the placenta along the umbilical vein is 80% to 85% saturated. Despite this streaming within the right atrium, some mixing does occur, resulting in blood that is 65% saturated in the ascending aorta. The blood in the left ventricle, however, is 15% to 20% more saturated than the blood in the right ventricle. Most of the deoxygenated blood in the right ventricle bypasses the high-resistance pulmonary vasculature to enter the ductus arteriosus, and from there the descending aorta to supply the lower body, or pass via the umbilical arteries for reoxygenation in the placenta. In contrast to extrauterine life, when the two ventricles function in series and thus have equal outputs, before birth they function in parallel. Their outputs, therefore, do not have to be equal and, in fact, are not. In the third trimester, the right side of the heart has a greater output, as determined by Doppler ultrasonography studies, showing a 28% greater stroke volume than the left side.[36]

Fetal heart rate (FHR) is maintained above the intrinsic rate of the sinoatrial node by a combination of vagal and sympathetic inputs, as well as circulating catecholamines.[38-40] FHR decreases throughout gestation,[41,42] accompanied by an increase in stroke volume as the heart grows. Hypoxic stress in late gestation produces a reflex bradycardia, with a normal heart rate or tachycardia developing a few minutes later. The chemoreceptor reflex nature of the bradycardia is demonstrated by its abolition after section of the carotid sinus nerves.[43] The later tachycardia is a result of an increase in plasma catecholamines causing β-adrenergic stimulation.[44] Hemorrhage can also produce increases in FHR, probably via a baroreceptor reflex.

Cardiac output in the fetus is determined largely by heart rate.[45] The combined ventricular output of the left and right ventricles in the human fetus is 450 mL/kg/min.[46] During development, the ability of the fetus to increase stroke volume is limited by a reduced proportion of functioning contractile tissue and a limited ability to increase the heart rate because of a relatively reduced β-adrenergic receptor density and immature sympathetic drive. Thus if blood volume is reduced by hemorrhage, the heart cannot compensate by increasing stroke volume, or, conversely, if volume is increased, the walls are less able to distend and cardiac efficiency is reduced (although this second effect is reduced substantially by the huge, relatively compliant placental circulation). Thus the only way for the fetus to increase cardiac output is to increase heart rate. Despite this homeostatic limitation, the fetus is able to withstand significant hemorrhage. Sheep studies have shown that the fetal lamb can restore arterial blood pressure and heart rate very quickly, without any measurable disturbance in acid-base balance after acute loss of 20% of their blood volume.[47] Even after a 40% reduction in blood volume, the ovine fetal blood pressure recovers to normal within 2 minutes and the heart rate within 35 minutes.[48] Oxygen delivery to the brain and heart is maintained secondary to vascular redistribution (*central sparing effect*) and blood volume replacement from the placenta and extravascular space, with 40% of the hemorrhaged loss being corrected within 30 minutes.[48] The development of acidemia indicates that the fetus is not able to compensate; acidosis shifts the oxygen dissociation curve to the right, thereby decreasing fetal hemoglobin oxygen saturation but improving release of oxygen from hemoglobin. Blood flow

during periods of asphyxia increases more than 100% to the brainstem, but only 60% to the cerebral hemispheres.[49]

## FETAL OXYGENATION

The fetus exists in an environment of low oxygen tension, with arterial oxygen partial pressure ($PO_2$) being approximately one-fourth that of the adult. The maximum $PO_2$ of umbilical venous blood is approximately 30 mm Hg. The affinity of fetal hemoglobin for oxygen is modulated in utero by two principal factors: fetal hemoglobin and 2,3-diphosphoglycerate (2,3-DPG). The hemoglobin oxygen dissociation curve is shifted to the left because of fetal hemoglobin (hemoglobin F), thereby increasing the affinity for oxygen. 2,3-DPG is also present and might be expected to shift the oxyhemoglobin dissociation curve to the right, decreasing the affinity of the fetal hemoglobin for oxygen and favoring oxygen unloading. However, 2,3-DPG only appears to exert approximately 40% of the effect on fetal hemoglobin as it does on adult hemoglobin, thereby preserving a net leftward shift on the oxyhemoglobin dissociation curve. Thus for any given $PO_2$, the fetus has a greater affinity for oxygen than does the mother. The P50 (the $PO_2$ at which hemoglobin is 50% desaturated) is approximately 27 mm Hg for the adult and 20 mm Hg for the fetus. The concentration of 2,3-DPG increases with gestation, as does the concentration of hemoglobin A[50]; the greater hemoglobin concentration (18 g/dL) results in a greater total oxygen carrying capacity.

Oxygen supply to fetal tissues depends on a number of factors (Table 37-1). First, the mother must be adequately oxygenated. Second, there must be adequate flow of well-oxygenated blood to the uteroplacental circulation. This blood flow may be reduced from maternal hemorrhage (reduced maternal blood volume) or compression of the inferior vena cava (reduced venous return), which increases uterine venous pressure, thus reducing uterine perfusion. Additionally, aortic compression reduces uterine arterial blood flow.[51] Care must be taken to position the mother in such a way as to prevent aortocaval compression. The surgical incision of hysterotomy itself reduces uteroplacental blood flow

| TABLE 37-1 | Causes of Impaired Blood Flow and Oxygenation to Fetal Tissues | |
|---|---|
| **Causes of Impaired Uteroplacental Blood Flow/Oxygenation** | **Causes of Impaired Umbilical Blood Flow/Fetal Circulatory Redistribution** |
| Reduced maternal oxygenation/hemoglobin concentration | Umbilical vessel spasm |
| Maternal hemorrhage | Reduced fetal cardiac output |
| Aortocaval compression | Fetal hemorrhage/reduced hemoglobin concentration |
| Drugs reducing uterine blood flow | Fetal hypothermia |
| Uterine trauma | Impaired uteroplacental blood flow/oxygenation |
| Uterine contractions | Umbilical cord kinking |
| Placental insufficiency (PET, IUGR) | |
| Polyhydramnios: pressure effect | |
| Maternal catecholamine production increasing uteroplacental vascular resistance | Fetal catecholamine production increasing fetoplacental vascular resistance |

*IUGR,* Intrauterine growth restriction; *PET,* preeclamptic toxemia.

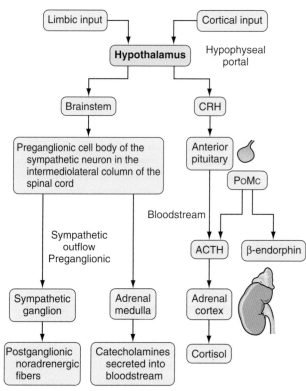

**FIGURE 37-3** Human fetal endocrine responses to stress. *ACTH,* Adrenocorticotropic hormone; *CRH,* corticotropin-releasing hormone; *PoMc,* proopiomelanocortin.

by as much as 73% in sheep, whereas fetoscopic procedures with uterine entry have no effect.[52]

Even if the uterine circulation is adequate, the fetus still depends on uteroplacental blood flow and umbilical venous blood flow for tissue oxygenation. Care must be taken not to interrupt umbilical vessel blood flow by manipulation or kinking the cord, which can cause vasospasm. Umbilical vasoconstriction can also occur as part of a fetal stress reaction resulting from a release of fetal stress hormones (Fig. 37-3). Increases in amniotic fluid volume increase amniotic pressure and impair uteroplacental perfusion.[53,54] Placental vascular resistance can be increased, raising fetal cardiac afterload, by the surge in fetal catecholamine production stimulated by surgical stress.[55] Fortunately, animal studies suggest that adverse effects on the arterial blood gas in the fetus do not occur until uteroplacental perfusion has been reduced by 50% or more.[56]

Inhalational anesthetics may cause maternal vasodilatation and, thus, in theory, could cause or exacerbate preexisting fetal hypoxia. Studies of anesthetics in hypoxic ovine fetuses have shown that isoflurane exacerbates preexisting acidosis.[57] It also causes blunting of the usual vascular redistribution response to fetal hypoxia, but, owing to a reduction in cerebral oxygen demand, the balance of cerebral oxygen supply and demand is unaffected. β-Adrenergic blockade renders a fetus less able to cope with asphyxia. Compared with controls, these fetuses have a smaller increase in heart rate, cerebral blood flow, and cardiac output, and recover from acidosis more slowly.[58]

## CENTRAL AND PERIPHERAL NERVOUS SYSTEM DEVELOPMENT

By the beginning of the second trimester, the spinal cord is largely formed; development of the brain and spinal cord begins

as early as postconception week 3. Neural crest cells migrate laterally to form peripheral nerves from about 4 weeks, with the first synapses between them forming a week later.[59] Synapses within the spinal cord develop from about 8 weeks gestation, suggesting the first spinal reflexes may be present at this time. Between 8 and 18 weeks gestation is the time of maximal neuronal development. The first neurons and glial cells develop in the ventricular zone (an epithelial layer) along which the newly formed neurons migrate out in waves to form the neocortex. Synaptogenesis occurs after neural proliferation, first in peripheral structures and then more centrally from around 20 weeks; this process is at least partly dependent on sensory stimulation.[60]

The development of the nociceptive apparatus proceeds in parallel with basic central nervous system development. The first essential requirement for nociception is the presence of sensory receptors, which develop first in the perioral area at around 7 weeks gestation. From here, they develop in the rest of the face and in the palmar surfaces of the hands and soles of the feet from about 11 weeks gestation. By 20 weeks, they are present throughout all of the skin and mucosal surfaces.[61] The nociceptive apparatus is initially involved in local reflex movements at the spinal cord level without higher cortical integration. As these reflex responses become more complex, they, in turn, involve the brainstem, through which other responses, such as increases in heart rate and blood pressure, are mediated. However, such reflexes to noxious stimuli have not been shown to involve the cortex and, thus, are not thought to be available to conscious perception. The nature of fetal consciousness itself is complicated, both physiologically and philosophically, and a discussion of such is beyond the scope of this chapter. However, there is a working consensus that for consciousness to be present there must be electrical activity in the cerebral cortex.[62] It appears that, far from being "switched on" at any one moment, consciousness evolves in a gradual process that has been likened to a "dimmer switch," making attribution of fetal consciousness to any particular developmental moment a difficult undertaking.

## PROGRAMMING EFFECTS

When considering the effects of noxious stimuli on the developing fetus and the rationale for fetal anesthesia and analgesia, we must consider not just the humanitarian need to alleviate the possible distress of pain sensation, but also whether being subjected to surgical stress during early development might cause permanent alterations in physiology. This concept is known as *programming,* defined as "the process whereby a stimulus or insult at a critical, sensitive period of development has permanent effects on structure, physiology, and metabolism."[63] Studies in rats and nonhuman primates have shown permanent reductions in the numbers of hippocampal and hypothalamic glucocorticoid receptors in the offspring of antenatally stressed animals. This attenuates the negative feedback response, resulting in increased basal and stress-induced cortisol levels in the offspring, which last into adulthood. Behavioral changes, such as poor coping behaviors, have also been observed.[63]

## Fetal Monitoring

The goal during any fetal intervention is to optimize fetal well-being by avoiding fetal hypoxia and hypothermia while optimizing stable fetal hemodynamics. It is essential that the physiologic response of the fetus to anesthetic and surgical stresses be understood and addressed, to avoid the known detrimental effects of stress on an already compromised fetus. However, access to the fetus is limited at best and the technologies for continuous intraoperative and postoperative fetal vital sign monitoring are still in development.

A hysterotomy is not needed for many surgical interventions; thus the fetus remains within the uterus, often making access for direct monitoring impossible. Even for those fetuses that are partially delivered for an invasive procedure, monitoring is obtainable only intermittently and is frequently unreliable, because the fetus must remain within a fluid environment during the procedure, making the direct placement of available monitors difficult. Current methods for monitoring fetal well-being include FHR monitoring, direct measurement of fetal blood gases, fetal electrocardiography (ECG), fetal pulse oximetry (FPO), fetal echocardiography, and Doppler ultrasonography of fetal cerebral blood flow.

## USE OF FETAL HEART RATE MONITORING FOR FETAL INTERVENTIONS

Currently, FHR monitoring with Doppler ultrasonography is the standard for the intrapartum assessment of fetal well-being. FHR monitoring is also used perioperatively during fetal interventions. The FHR is documented before maternal induction of anesthesia, to serve as a baseline for comparison and to reassure the perinatologist, surgeon, and anesthesiologist that the fetus is stable. The FHR may be continuously monitored intraoperatively by fetal echocardiography and with intermittent palpation of the umbilical cord in open cases. It is known that the most commonly used anesthetic induction agents at appropriate doses (propofol and thiopental) rapidly cross the placenta and thus also rapidly reach the fetus.[64,65] The inhalation anesthetics also cross the placenta,[66] but the uptake of the anesthetic occurs more slowly in the fetus than in the mother.[67,68] These anesthetics decrease FHR and FHR variability. Although it is reassuring if the FHR is within the normal range for the gestational age, fetal bradycardia is a reliable indicator of fetal distress that needs to be immediately addressed.

With the advent of minimally invasive fetal endoscopic surgery, new problems in monitoring have surfaced. The fetus is no longer physically accessible to the surgical team, and the trocars used for fetoscopic surgery currently prohibit the placement of radiotelemetric probes. At present, fetoscopic or cardiac intervention use direct visualization of the heart with fetal echocardiography, which gives an accurate estimation of the FHR. Although very beneficial, the continuous use of fetal echocardiography requires the presence of a skilled ultrasonographer working in the operative field.

## USE OF FETAL BLOOD SAMPLING DURING FETAL INTERVENTIONS

In suspected cases of fetal compromise during an open intervention, fetal blood can be obtained from capillary vessels, a peripheral vein, a central vein, or a puncture of the umbilical vessels. The fetus' small size and friable tissue make vascular access difficult. Puncture of the umbilical vessels can lead to cord spasm, hematoma, and even fetal death, and thus should be reserved for circumstances when no other options are available. During an endoscopic intervention, access to the fetal circulation is possible through puncture of the umbilical vessels. With most fetal cardiac interventions, a needle and/or catheter is placed directly through the fetal myocardium, allowing access for blood samples; only a very small sample should be withdrawn because of the small circulating fetal blood volume.

## FETAL ELECTROCARDIOGRAPHY

Several groups have used fetal ECG analysis to determine whether changes in time interval (PR and RR interval) and signal morphology (T to QRS ratio) correlate with fetal or neonatal outcome. Studies in animals and humans have shown that under normal conditions, there is a negative correlation between the PR interval and the FHR: as the FHR slows, the PR interval lengthens, and as the FHR increases, the PR interval shortens. *The opposite relationship occurs in acidemic infants.*[69-75] During periods of fetal compromise, it is hypothesized that the sinoatrial node and the atrioventricular node respond differently.[73] Periods of mild hypoxemia will induce increases in epinephrine levels, which will increase the FHR and shorten the PR interval. However, with periods of prolonged hypoxemia, the oxygen-dependent calcium channels of the sinoatrial node will demonstrate reduced sensitivity to epinephrine, resulting in a decrease in FHR. The fast sodium channels of the atrioventricular node are not affected by the reduction in the oxygen supply, and the increased levels of epinephrine will shorten the PR interval. As a result, the relationship between the PR interval and FHR changes from negative to positive.[73] Measurements of this relationship have been divided into short-term and long-term measures.[73,74] The short-term measure or the conduction index can be intermittently positive over short periods of time without an adverse outcome. However, a prolonged positive conduction index (greater than 20 minutes) has been associated with an increased risk of fetal acidemia.[75]

## FETAL PULSE OXIMETRY

Standard pulse oximeters use the transmission and absorption of light through a vascular bed to a photodetector on the opposite side of the tissue. However, the development of reflectance oximetry allowed measurement of oxygen saturation from light-emitting diodes that are positioned next to each other on the same skin surface and absorption is determined from the light that scatters back to the tissue surface[76,77]; any fetal condition that decreases vascular pulsations (e.g., hypotension, vasoconstriction, shock, or strong uterine contractions) can produce inaccurate oximetry readings.[78] Because direct contact of the oximeter must be made with the fetal skin surface, anything that interferes with light transmission or skin adhesion (e.g., fetal or maternal movement, vernix caseosa, caput succedaneum) can influence the quality and accuracy of the oximeter.[79-83] Oximetry readings also vary in relation to the site of sensor application; several studies have found reduced baseline oxygen saturation values with the use of the oxygen sensor on the fetal buttock compared with the fetal head.[84-87]

The development of a 735/890-nm wavelength system (compared with the older 660/890-nm system) has improved the accuracy in monitoring arterial oxygen saturation ($FSaO_2$) in the fetus[88]; because the normal range of $FSaO_2$ of 30% to 70% lies in the middle of the oxygen-hemoglobin dissociation curve, small changes in pH or oxygen partial pressure cause large changes in $FSaO_2$.[89] FPO can also identify an acidotic fetus. Increased concentrations of both the hydrogen ion and 2,3-DPG cause a rightward shift of the oxygen dissociation curve (Bohr effect) such that a chronically acidemic or hypoxemic fetus will have a low $FSaO_2$ even though the $PO_2$ is within normal limits.[89]

## FETAL ECHOCARDIOGRAPHY

When technically feasible, fetal echocardiography should be available to assess fetal myocardial contractility and function, heart rate, intravascular volume status, and amniotic fluid volume. We have also used echocardiography to correctly identify proper endotracheal tube placement during an EXIT procedure[90]; a sterile sleeve is placed over the ultrasonographic probe that is then placed over the fetal chest.

## DOPPLER ULTRASONOGRAPHY OF FETAL CEREBRAL BLOOD FLOW

Antepartum Doppler ultrasonography studies of the fetal circulation in cases of intrauterine growth restriction with presumed hypoxia have shown a compensatory redistribution, with an increase in peripheral vascular resistance in the fetal body and placenta and a compensatory reduction in peripheral vascular resistance in the fetal brain, producing a brain-sparing effect.[91] Intrapartum Doppler ultrasonography and FPO have verified the brain-sparing response in the presence of intrapartum arterial hypoxemia ($FSaO_2$ less than 30% for 5 minutes or more), as reflected by increased mean flow velocity in the fetal middle cerebral artery.[92] Preliminary studies of the middle cerebral artery pulsatility index in minimally invasive procedures, such as fetal blood sampling, transfusion, shunt insertion, tissue biopsy, and ovarian cyst aspiration, have demonstrated significant cerebral hemodynamic responses (decreases in the middle cerebral artery pulsatility index) in fetuses that underwent procedures involving transgression of the fetal body. This response was not noted in the fetuses undergoing procedures at the noninnervated placental cord insertion.[93]

Although not yet advocated for routine intrapartum management, it has been suggested that the combination of reduced arterial oxygen saturation and increased cerebral blood flow may indicate an ominous phase during labor. The redistribution of the fetal circulation is not an unlimited protective mechanism, and with persistent cerebral hypoxia, the active vasodilation of the cerebral vessels may fail, leading to disastrous consequences for the fetus.[94]

# Physiologic Consequences of Pregnancy

## RESPIRATORY AND AIRWAY CONSIDERATIONS

There is an increase in metabolic demand of both the mother and the fetus, and this, along with anatomic and hormonal influences, accounts for the changes in maternal pulmonary physiology (Table 37-2). Pregnancy results in progressive increases in oxygen consumption and minute ventilation, along with a decreased residual volume and functional residual capacity.[95] The

increased metabolic demands and anatomic changes can make adequate oxygenation and perfusion of the parturient and the fetoplacental unit a constant challenge during maternal general anesthesia. During periods of apnea or hypoventilation, the parturient is prone to rapid development of hypoxia and hypercapnia. Even after adequate preoxygenation, the $PaO_2$ in an apneic anesthetized parturient decreases by about 8 mm Hg more per minute than in nonpregnant women.[96] Acidosis rapidly develops from hypoxia during difficult airway situations because of a decreased buffering capacity during pregnancy. The decreased pulmonary oxygen stores and increased oxygen consumption make parturients more susceptible than nonpregnant women to the consequences of airway mismanagement.

Not all physiologic changes of pregnancy are deleterious to the performance of anesthesia. For example, both the induction of and emergence from anesthesia with inhalational anesthetics occur faster in parturients than in nonpregnant women because the combination of increased alveolar ventilation and decreased functional residual capacity speeds the rate at which denitrogenation occurs and at which inspired and alveolar concentrations of inhalational agents reach equilibrium[97]; a faster induction, coupled with a decreased MAC, make parturients susceptible to relative anesthetic overdose and severe hypotension.[98]

## CARDIOVASCULAR CONSIDERATIONS

Cardiovascular function is appropriately increased during pregnancy to meet the increased metabolic demands and oxygen requirements of the mother (Table 37-3). Cardiac output increases by 35% to 40% by the end of the first trimester and continues to increase throughout the second trimester until it reaches a level 50% greater than that in nonpregnant women.[99] Heart rate increases 15% to 25% above prepregnancy rates and remains stable after the second trimester, and stroke volume progressively increases 25% to 30% by the end of the second trimester and remains stable until term.[100,101] Aortocaval compression by the gravid uterus can cause a 30% to 50% decrease in cardiac output; lesser decreases occur in the sitting or semirecumbent positions. Maternal position is a major factor contributing to hypotension and fetal well-being.[102]

Maternal blood flow and pressure are directly linked to fetal perfusion via the placenta, and uterine blood flow represents about 10% of maternal cardiac output. The avoidance of aortocaval compression by left or right uterine displacement is imperative to prevent a decrease in the maternal blood pressure. Because large doses of inhalational agent are often necessary for uterine relaxation during fetal intervention, prompt treatment of hypotension is vital. Because uteroplacental blood flow is not autoregulated, a decrease in maternal blood pressure will eventually

---

**TABLE 37-2** Anesthetic Considerations of Respiratory Changes of Pregnancy

Decreased functional residual capacity
  Faster denitrogenation
  Rapidly prone to hypoxia during apnea
  Faster induction and emergence of anesthesia with inhaled agents

Increased oxygen consumption
  Rapidly prone to hypoxia during apnea

Capillary engorgement of the respiratory mucosa
  Predisposes upper airway to trauma, bleeding, and obstruction
  Laryngeal edema increases the frequency of difficult intubation

Decreased $PaCO_2$ and no $PETCO_2$-$PaCO_2$ gradient
  Capnograph reading similar to $PaCO_2$
  Hyperventilation may lead to a reduction in uterine blood flow

$PETCO_2$, End-tidal carbon dioxide pressure.

---

**TABLE 37-3** Anesthetic Considerations of Cardiovascular Changes of Pregnancy

Aortocaval compression
  Supine position leads to a decline in cardiac output
  May lead to supine hypotensive syndrome
  Mostly prevented by left or right uterine displacement

Decreased colloid oncotic pressure
  Parturient is at greater risk for developing pulmonary edema

Increased maternal blood volume
  Parturient tolerates more blood loss than nonparturients
  Hypotension and acidosis may develop with significant blood loss

decrease placental blood flow and, therefore, blood flow to the fetus. IV ephedrine (5 to 10 mg) or phenylephrine (50 to 100 μg) per dose should be used to treat maternal hypotension unless contraindicated.[103]

Careful attention to the volume status of the parturient is imperative; aggressive volume hydration, the normal decrease in colloid oncotic pressure that occurs during pregnancy, the decrease in colloid oncotic pressure post partum, and the use of tocolytic agents (e.g., magnesium or β-adrenoceptor agonists) may all predispose the parturient to pulmonary edema.

## CENTRAL AND PERIPHERAL NERVOUS SYSTEMS

Pregnancy-mediated analgesia is affected by changes in spinal opioid antinociceptive pathways and peripheral processes, including the effect of ovarian sex steroids (estrogen and progesterone) and uterine afferent neurotransmission. It is thought that pregnancy-mediated analgesia increases the woman's threshold for pain during the latter stages of pregnancy before labor.[104,105] Pregnant women are more sensitive to the action of many anesthetic agents and require less local anesthetic for spinal and epidural anesthesia and less inhalational anesthetics than their nonpregnant counterparts. The MAC of inhalational anesthetics in pregnancy is approximately 30% less than in nonpregnant females; and for this reason the concentration of inhalational anesthetic needs to be carefully titrated.[106]

## PHARMACOLOGIC CONSEQUENCES OF PREGNANCY

Physiologic changes of pregnancy alter the pharmacokinetics and pharmacodynamics of many anesthetic drugs. An increase in total body water and adipose tissue, and a decrease in plasma protein concentrations alter the volume of distribution. An increased renal blood flow and glomerular filtration rate can enhance the elimination of renally excreted drugs; hepatic metabolism of some drugs may be inhibited by competition with steroid hormones during pregnancy, whereas others may have a greater clearance associated with the increased basal metabolic rate. Therefore drug administration must consider the pharmacokinetics within the maternal-placental-fetal unit. Most drugs cross the placenta to some extent and the proportion transferred increases with the duration of gestation. The fetus has reduced plasma protein binding, producing relatively greater concentrations of free drug (i.e., unbound and available to cross biologic membranes).[107] Despite detection of oxidation and reduction reactions in the fetal liver from as early as 16 weeks, enzyme concentrations and reaction rates are minimal, exposing the fetus to more prolonged drug effects than occur in the mother.[108] Early in gestation, the primary mode of drug excretion is via blood flow to the placenta, but later, as the fetal kidneys mature, they become a route of drug excretion into the amniotic fluid for water-soluble drugs and metabolites. Amniotic fluid, however, can act as a reservoir for drugs, from which they can be reabsorbed.[107]

### Induction

Pregnancy increases the parturient's sensitivity to induction agents.[109] Propofol has been safely used for induction of anesthesia for cesarean delivery, in doses of 2 mg/kg, with minimal effects on the neonate.[110] Ketamine has also been used as the sole induction agent for parturients undergoing elective cesarean section; ketamine (1.5 mg/kg) has not been associated with maternal awareness or neonatal depression at delivery and parturients required fewer analgesics in the first 24 hours after delivery.[111] It is speculated that ketamine's analgesic properties may reduce the sensitization of pain pathways and subsequently confer extended benefit into the postoperative period. Induction agents decrease spontaneous uterine contractions of isolated pregnant rat myometrium, but only in concentrations greater than those seen in clinical obstetric practice.[112]

### Neuromuscular Blocking Drugs

Although serum cholinesterase activity decreases 30% during pregnancy, recovery from a dose of 1 mg/kg of succinylcholine is not prolonged.[113] Succinylcholine has a very low placental transfer, owing to its low lipid solubility and high degree of ionization.[114] Similarly, cisatracurium has been safely used for cesarean section without routine neostigmine antagonism, despite decreased plasma cholinesterase activity.[115] Pregnant women may be more sensitive to the action of nondepolarizing muscle relaxants, with the administration of vecuronium resulting in a more rapid onset and delayed recovery of neuromuscular block when compared with nonpregnant control patients. The prolonged action of vecuronium persists into the postpartum period for at least 4 days[116]; the clinical duration of vecuronium in term and postpartum women is twice that of nonpregnant women.[117] However, in a study comparing cisatracurium 0.2 mg/kg for intubation in immediate postpartum and nonpregnant women, both the mean onset and recovery times in the postpartum period were significantly smaller.[118] Nondepolarizing muscle relaxants have no effect on uterine relaxation and, as quaternary amines, do not cross the placenta.

### Inhalational Anesthetics

Pregnant women are more sensitive to the anesthetic action of the inhalational anesthetics (MAC is reduced approximately 30% from nonpregnant females).[119] This may lead to a deeper level of anesthesia than predicted during fetal surgery, and a relative overdose associated with maternal cardiac depression and hypotension. All inhalational anesthetics rapidly cross the placenta, but their uptake occurs more slowly in the fetus than in the mother.[120,121] At light (1.0 MAC) isoflurane or halothane anesthesia, neither maternal pulse rate, cardiac output, and acid-base status, nor fetal pulse rate, acid-base status, and oxygen saturation changed significantly.[122] During moderately deep (1.5 MAC) isoflurane or halothane anesthesia, maternal arterial pressure and cardiac output decreased. Uterine vasodilation occurred, but uteroplacental perfusion was maintained; fetal oxygenation and base excess were also maintained. However, at concentrations of inhalational anesthetics that exceeded 2.0 MAC, maternal hypotension decreased uteroplacental perfusion despite uterine vasodilation, leading to fetal hypoxia and acidosis. Inhalational anesthetics produced a dose-related uterine relaxation.[123] At 0.5 MAC of enflurane, isoflurane, or halothane, uterine contractility decreases 20% whereas at 1.5 MAC, contractility decreases 60%.[124] Sevoflurane produces a dose-dependent depression in uterine muscle contractility, with complete abolition of uterine activity at greater than 3.5 MAC.[125] The large concentrations of inhalation anesthetic needed for profound uterine relaxation generally requires tracheal intubation and aggressive use of vasopressors.

# Fetal Preoperative Evaluation

Prenatal imaging of all fetal anomalies, including anatomic areas of involvement, the relationship to normal structures, and tracheal location, is needed to plan the most appropriate surgical and anesthetic interventions. The accuracy and quality of preoperative fetal ultrasonography and magnetic resonance imaging (MRI) are of the utmost importance because some lesions, especially pulmonary lesions, may spontaneously regress in utero; an inaccurate diagnosis could lead to suboptimal or inappropriate intervention. In addition, extremely valuable information can be obtained that would aid in the decision-making process for a given treatment, namely, the presence of ascites, hydrops, mediastinal shift, degree of lung hypoplasia and lesion involvement, airway involvement and potential tracheal distortion, or compression from intrathoracic masses. Preoperative imaging can also determine other anticipated alterations in anatomy that may acutely alter fetal cardiopulmonary physiology (e.g., mediastinal shift and the known associated potential alterations in fetal preload). Serial radiologic examinations can also monitor the growth of certain masses, the development of hydrops, and the response to treatment medications (e.g., transplacental digoxin). Significant fetal ventricular dysfunction or heart failure should alert the anesthesiologist to the possibility of fetal cardiac arrest during a fetal intervention. Other congenital abnormalities may be detected that may render a potential fetal intervention useless.

In addition, a fetal karyotype must be obtained to rule out the presence of any genetic disorders that are associated with significant fetal morbidity or mortality, making further intervention pointless. An estimated fetal weight, obtained by ultrasonography immediately before surgical intervention, allows for preparation of unit doses of fetal medications. Any previous attempts at fetal intervention should be evaluated, including the number of interventions, fetal tolerance of the procedures, transient reversal in fetal symptoms, the presence of fetal cardiac dysfunction, and the reason or reasons for failed intervention. Assuming that fetal hydrops is present, any attempts to treat this condition should also be documented, including the effectiveness of digoxin therapy, total dose administered, method of administration, and response to treatment.

## Maternal Evaluation

A complete medical history and physical examination, especially a focused airway evaluation, are of the utmost importance. Details regarding fetal pathophysiology and its effects on secondary maternal morbidity should be addressed. Any patient with significant polyhydramnios and associated preterm contractions is at great risk for preterm labor and rupture of membranes with uterine manipulation. Patients with significant polyhydramnios despite multiple amnioreductions have required greater amounts of intraoperative tocolysis and greater inhalational anesthetic concentrations to obtain uterine relaxation and acceptable surgical conditions.

The presence of fetal hydrops should alert the practitioner to the possibility of maternal mirror syndrome. *Mirror syndrome* refers to characteristic maternal pathophysiologic changes associated with a variety of fetal disorders, including nonimmune hydrops, molar pregnancies, congenital cystic adenomatoid malformation of the lung, and sacrococcygeal teratoma. Polyhydramnios and placentomegaly are usually present. Although the etiology of this condition is unclear, the end result is a maternal hyperdynamic state with associated hypertension and total body edema.[126] Respiratory insufficiency or pulmonary edema may develop, requiring prompt and aggressive treatment. If preterm uterine contractions develop, treatment options may be limited because tocolytic agents can greatly exacerbate respiratory decompensation.

Treatment is aimed at maternal supportive care; even correction of the underlying fetal pathology will not completely resolve the maternal abnormalities. Delivery of the fetus is the only sure method to completely reverse this maternal pathologic process.

The anesthesiologist should specifically investigate for the presence of placentomegaly; increased placental blood flow may alter pharmacologic treatment in both the mother and the fetus because increased drug metabolism may occur. The presence of placentomegaly may also increase risk for acute intraoperative bleeding, and preparation must be made to rapidly transfuse the mother. Several reports describe inadvertent inclusion of the placental edge during the hysterotomy incision, causing a sudden, massive loss of blood with a completely relaxed uterus[127,128]; immediate surgical control, resuscitation with blood products, and vasopressors that do not increase placental vascular resistance must be administered.

## Tocolysis and Tocolytic Agents

The occurrence of contractions and preterm labor is an expectation for the first few postoperative days. Fortunately, in many cases, delivery can be postponed until after 32 weeks, giving the fetus time to heal from the procedure and allowing the lungs to mature. However, for many women, the onset of surgically induced preterm contractions heralds premature labor and delivery that, at best, eliminates the positive results of the procedure, and, at worst, ends in the loss of the pregnancy. Although most women who require fetal surgery can be successfully prevented from delivering immediately after surgery, the current generation of medications used for tocolysis have been ineffective in preventing premature labor and delivery. Preterm labor remains the single most common complication that limits the success of fetal surgery.

### HORMONAL RECEPTORS IN LABOR
The adrenergic hormonal system plays a very influential part in the activity of the myometrium; several types of adrenergic receptors are found in the uterus (Fig. 37-4). Stimulation of the α-adrenergic receptor causes an increase in the rate and intensity of uterine contractions, whereas activation of the $\beta_2$-adrenergic receptors produce myometrial relaxation.[129] In addition, the term uterus is heavily populated with receptors for endogenously released oxytocin responsible for initiating uterine contractions. Prostaglandins also play a significant role in modulating myometrial tone. In general, prostaglandins are produced in or near the local environment where they exert their effect; both uterotonic and tocolytic prostaglandins have been identified. The balance of intrauterine and maternal uterotonic prostaglandins is thought to play an essential part in the preparation for both term and preterm labor. Prostaglandins, especially prostaglandin $E_2$, are an essential component of every aspect of natural labor.[130]

### TREATMENT OF ACUTE PRETERM LABOR
#### Nonsteroidal Antiinflammatory Drugs
Nonsteroidal antiinflammatory drugs (NSAIDs) block the action of cyclooxygenase, preventing the formation of prostaglandins. In-vitro studies of indomethacin have found consistent inhibition or complete arrest of overall myometrial activity.

#### β-Adrenergic–Mimetic Agents
Currently, only $\beta_2$-adrenoceptor–selective medications are routinely used for acute preterm labor. Most adverse effects result

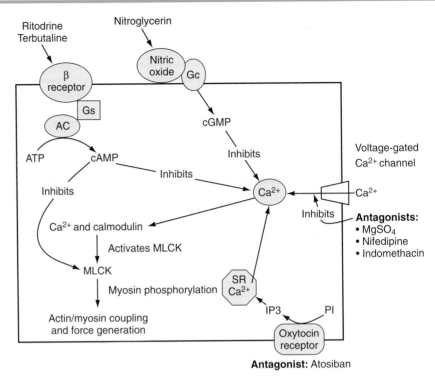

**FIGURE 37-4** Biochemistry of uterine contraction and its inhibition. *AC,* Adenylate cyclase; *ATP,* adenosine triphosphate; *cAMP,* cyclic adenosine monophosphate; *cGMP,* cyclic guanosine monophosphate; *Gc,* G-protein c; *Gs,* G-protein s; *IP3,* inositol triphosphate; *MLCK,* myosin light-chain kinase; *PI,* phosphatidylinositol; *SR,* sarcoplasmic reticulum.

from their lack of pure specificity, that is, simultaneous stimulation of $\beta_1$- and $\beta_2$-adrenergic receptors. Adverse effects include fetal tachycardia, maternal tremors, palpitations, tachycardia, a decreased or increased blood pressure, lethargy, sleepiness, ketoacidosis, and pulmonary edema. Pulmonary edema occurs in up to 5% of patients, especially when used with other tocolytics (e.g., magnesium).[131] Because the $\beta$-adrenergic–mimetic agents are nonspecific receptor agonists, in large concentrations these agents can stimulate $\alpha$-adrenergic receptors, which promotes uterine contractions, leading to treatment failure.

### Magnesium

Magnesium competes with calcium for transmembrane channel entry into cells.[132] Because the myometrium depends on stores of calcium for adequate contraction, a decrease in intracellular transport prevents the activation of the actin and myosin complex, resulting in uterine relaxation.

### Nitric Oxide Donors

Nitroglycerin is an effective uterine relaxant used in select situations to produce rapid uterine relaxation (e.g., extraction of a retained placenta and uterine inversion). In pregnant sheep, nitroglycerin causes a decrease in mean maternal arterial pressure and increase in heart rate, without compromising uterine blood flow.[133] During fetal surgery, nitroglycerin has been used to relax the myometrium and halt breakthrough contractions. Adverse effects include maternal hypotension, tachycardia, headache, development of tachyphylaxis, and a high incidence of maternal pulmonary edema.[134]

### Calcium-Channel Blockers

Calcium-channel blockers are better tolerated than $\beta$-adrenergic–mimetic agents. Nifedipine may be more effective than $\beta_2$-adrenergic agonists in postponing delivery, especially in those women with intact membranes.[135] Neonates born to women

treated with calcium-channel blockers have a reduced frequency of respiratory distress, necrotizing enterocolitis, and intraventricular hemorrhage.[136] The most serious adverse effect is maternal hypotension; the combination of calcium-channel blockers and magnesium sulfate should generally be avoided.

### PAIN CONTROL

Pain control after fetal surgery is an essential component of tocolytic therapy, because it is thought that adequate pain control prevents the stress-induced hormonal impetus for preterm labor. Surgical stress elicits the release of adrenocorticotropic hormone that increases production of cortisol; cortisol production, in turn, leads to the deleterious changes in the placenta that increase fetal estrogen and prostaglandin production, promoting increased uterine activity.

### FETAL COMPLICATIONS OF TOCOLYTIC THERAPY

The adverse effects of tocolytics in the fetus present a number of problems, albeit usually less so than in the mother. Sympathomimetics that act through $\beta$-adrenoceptors cause fetal tachycardia.[137] Whereas cyclooxygenase inhibitors have been shown to be more effective than other tocolytics in delaying labor,[138] the adverse effects of fetal oliguria and ductus arteriosus constriction have limited their long-term use.[139] However, after short-term use, these adverse effects are fully reversible within 72 hours from cessation of treatment.[139] Longer-term use of indomethacin has been associated with renal dysfunction and increased rates of necrotizing enterocolitis, intracranial hemorrhage, and patent ductus arteriosus in infants delivered at less than 30 weeks gestation.[140] Magnesium sulfate reduces FHR variability[141] and depresses fetal right ventricular function.[142] Because this drug rapidly crosses the placenta but is excreted more slowly by the fetal kidneys than by the maternal kidneys, there are concerns about fetal toxicity, resulting in respiratory and central nervous

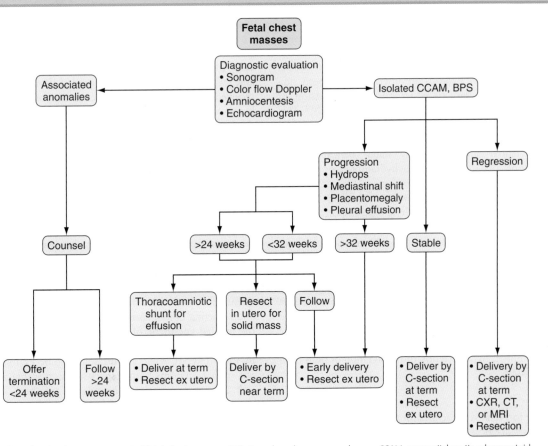

**FIGURE 37-5** Algorithm for the management of fetal chest masses. *BPS,* Bronchopulmonary syndrome; *CCAM,* congenital cystic adenomatoid malformation; *CT,* computed tomography; *CXR,* chest radiography; *MRI,* magnetic resonance imaging. (Reprinted with permission from Myers LB, Bulich LA, editors. Anesthesia for fetal intervention and surgery. Philadelphia: BC Decker; 2005.)

system depression.[143] Nitric oxide donors, such as nitroglycerin, appear to have minimal fetal side effects.[144]

### POSTOPERATIVE PULMONARY EDEMA

Noncardiogenic pulmonary edema is a known complication of tocolysis. Most often, obstetric pulmonary edema is a result of increased hydrostatic pressures and resolves rapidly with diuretics, cessation of tocolytics, and fluid restriction. One study observed a prevalence of pulmonary edema of 0.5%, but that rate increased to 23% in fetal surgical patients; 93% of those with pulmonary edema required intensive care and 20% required tracheal intubation.[134] It has been hypothesized that extensive uterine manipulation during surgery may result in release of mediators that increase the permeability of lung vasculature. The class of medications most strongly associated with pulmonary edema is β-adrenergic–mimetic agents. An additional important observation is that patients receiving nitroglycerin for tocolysis have demonstrated more pronounced pulmonary edema (more severe hypoxemia, greater time to resolution, worse chest radiograph, and a greater composite lung injury scores) than those who received other tocolytics.[134]

## Congenital Cystic Adenomatoid Malformation: The Open Procedure

Congenital cystic adenomatoid malformation (CCAM) serves as a prime example of a fetal condition requiring open intervention.

Fetuses with lung masses presenting before extrauterine viability represent a complex group of congenital disorders. Before the advent of preterm fetal intervention, management of fetal lung masses consisted of limited options, which included (1) delivery with hydrops once fetal viability was determined with regard to lung maturity while acknowledging the potential need for emergent postpartum resuscitation, (2) transplacental digoxin therapy in an effort to treat severe forms of cardiac dysfunction,[145,146] and (3) termination of the pregnancy if the fetus was considered nonviable (Fig. 37-5). Fetuses demonstrating in-utero tumor regressions as documented by serial sonograms are allowed to progress to term gestation. Most infants with smaller lung masses or those with masses demonstrating in-utero regression do well with standard delivery and neonatal resection.[147] However, a subset of fetuses experience significant fetal lung mass growth, ultimately compromising normal lung development. Treatment options for these fetuses have expanded to include cyst aspiration, thoracocentesis, double-J stents for permanent thoracic drainage, and in-utero resection of the lung mass.[147-149] All treatment options aim to reduce the size of the lung mass to allow the remaining fetal lung to develop.

### CONGENITAL CYSTIC ADENOMATOID MALFORMATION OF THE LUNG

CCAM of the lung consists of cystic masses of pulmonary tissue and bronchial structures, neither of which participate in gas exchange,[150,151] that may represent a form of pulmonary hypoplasia.[152] CCAMs can compress surrounding lung tissue and impede normal lung development, resulting in pulmonary hypoplasia.[153] Of all the fetal lung masses, CCAM is the lesion most frequently associated with hydrops fetalis that often indicates a premorbid fetal state. Although the exact mechanisms for the development of hydrops are unclear, it has been suggested that it is secondary to either cardiac compression or vena caval obstruction from the intrathoracic mass.[154,155] This condition is associated with a significant imbalance of fetal fluid, resulting in accumulation of fetal fluid causing increases in fetal interstitial and total body water, pericardial and pleural effusions, ascites, anasarca, polyhydramnios, or placental thickening.[156,157]

Fetal lung abnormalities themselves may lead to excessive fluid accumulation because the fetal lung is an important organ for amniotic fluid balance. The average fetal lung fluid production is estimated to be approximately 300 mL/day or about 4 mL/kg/hr.[158] Fetal urine output is approximately 700 mL/day, and fetal swallowing is about 700 mL/day. The remaining 300 mL/day is postulated to exit the amnion through the chorioamnionic membrane. CCAMs may impair fetal swallowing via esophageal obstruction and therefore disrupt normal fluid balance; fetal swallowing is the major method by which amniotic fluid water is returned to the fetal vascular compartment. A second possibility is hypersecretion or transudation of fluid from the CCAM itself.

## Management

Experts have formulated guidelines for the fetal surgical management of fetuses diagnosed with CCAM lesions; overall prognosis depends on the size of the lung mass and the presence of secondary physiologic derangements.[147] Special consideration is given to fetuses exhibiting signs of hydrops fetalis, especially those who are less than 32 weeks gestation.[159] Although these conclusions were based primarily on the experience with CCAM infants, it might be appropriate to extend this experience to the management of fetuses with other lung lesions. The primary goal of treatment is to reduce lesion size so that the fetal lung has an improved chance of normal development.

## Operating Room Preparation

Like all other types of fetal intervention, ultrasonography should be performed before the induction of anesthesia to assess fetal well-being and to obtain an estimated fetal weight. In addition to the normal preanesthesia preparation checklist, additional maternal airway equipment, resuscitation drugs, and tocolytic agents should be prepared and immediately available. The availability of type-specific packed red blood cells for the mother and O-negative irradiated packed red blood cells, divided into 50 mL aliquots for the fetus must be confirmed. The operating room (OR) temperature should be warmed to at least 80° F (26.7° C) to prevent hypothermia of the partially exposed fetus during thoracotomy. Resuscitation drugs for the fetus (atropine 10 to 20 µg/kg, epinephrine 1 to 10 µg/kg), as well as a neuromuscular blocking drug (NMBD; e.g., vecuronium 0.2 mg/kg or pancuronium 0.1 mg/kg), and fentanyl (10 µg/kg) are prepared under sterile conditions, thus making them available during the procedure.[160] A rapid infusion system with warmed isotonic saline is used to replace amniotic fluid loss during fetal lung resection, and is ready to administer onto the surgical field via a sterile tubing system. A pulse oximeter with a sterile extension cord should be available for application to the upper extremity of the fetus.

## Induction

The preferred method of maternal anesthesia for these cases is general anesthesia with endotracheal intubation and neuromuscular blockade. Before entering the OR, an IV line is started and sedation is administered as needed. If the mother has not received indomethacin (50 mg rectal suppository) for tocolysis before arrival, it is administered after induction of general anesthesia. Indomethacin is used in conjunction with magnesium in the postoperative period for tocolysis but does not play a significant tocolytic role in the intraoperative period. After placement of standard monitors, a lumbar epidural catheter may be inserted for postoperative pain management. With the exception of a test dose, most practitioners avoid local anesthetic administration through the epidural catheter until the fetal intervention is completed. This is done to avoid possible decreases in maternal mean arterial pressure from an epidural-associated sympathectomy. The mother is then positioned in a uterine displacement position, preoxygenated, and a rapid-sequence induction is performed with an induction agent, succinylcholine (and subsequently followed with a short-acting nondepolarizing agent), and a rapid-acting opioid. Anesthesia is maintained with 1 MAC of the inhaled anesthetic of choice (usually sevoflurane or desflurane, should a rapid reinstatement of uterine tone be required) in 100% oxygen, while an ultrasonographic examination maps out surface anatomy with respect to the placenta and fetus, as well as reassuring fetal well-being after anesthetic induction. A second large-bore peripheral IV catheter, radial arterial catheter, urinary catheter, and nasogastric tube are then inserted. Because the maternal anesthesia induction is the same as a standard cesarean section, invasive blood pressure monitoring is not necessary until the inhalational anesthetic is increased to 2 to 3 MAC. Fetal hemodynamics (heart rate, right ventricular contractility) are monitored intraoperatively by continuous fetal echocardiography.[160]

Alternatively, in cases where a long period of time is expected to transpire between maternal induction and hysterotomy, a substitution or combination with an IV anesthetic (typically propofol and remifentanil) may reduce fetal cardiac acidosis seen with greater concentrations of inhalational anesthetics (most notably desflurane).[161] In such cases, large concentrations of inhalational anesthetics should be reinstituted before uterine incision to assure adequate uterine relaxation. Alternatively, recent reports have described total IV anesthesia techniques employing remifentanil, nitrous oxide, midazolam as general anesthetic agents with IV nitroglycerin used for uterine relaxion.[162] Remifentanil, which moves across the placenta freely, has also been described as an agent for fetal immobilization under combined spinal epidural anesthesia.[163]

## Maintenance

Before hysterotomy the concentration of inhalational anesthetic is increased to 2 MAC to ensure myometrial relaxation and tocolysis.[160,164] Satisfactory uterine relaxation can be achieved, but these concentrations may decrease maternal arterial pressure, uteroplacental perfusion, and fetal oxygenation, and may require pressor support.[160,165] Although only small increases in fetal $PaO_2$ occur with maternal inspired oxygen concentrations of 100%, this small increase may be advantageous. Additionally, the increased concentration of inhalational anesthetic needed for uterine relaxation dictates that only medications that augment uterine relaxation be administered.[166] Given that nitrous oxide does not affect the uterine tone to any measurable degree and thus provides no direct surgical benefit, it is best omitted and 100% oxygen is used. Maternal eucapnia (PaCO$_2$ of 31-33 mm Hg) is the physiologic goal,[156] because maternal hyperventilation may lead to decreases in fetal PaO$_2$.[167,168] Some have suggested that maternal hypercarbia can, in fact, increase fetal PO$_2$.[169] At this time, however, extrapolation of these conclusions to fetal intervention cases should be done with caution.

When recovery from the short-acting nondepolarizing agent has been achieved, additional doses of muscle relaxant should be titrated as needed. If preoperative tocolytic agents were administered, combined with the anticipated administration of magnesium sulfate during the abdominal closure, long-acting NMBDs are best avoided, to ensure that neuromuscular blockade can be antagonized at the end of the surgery.

Meticulous attention to maternal blood pressure is essential to ensure adequate uterine blood flow and uterine perfusion; maternal systolic pressure is maintained at 110% of mean awake values with IV ephedrine or phenylephrine. Total IV fluids are limited unless blood loss is excessive, so as to minimize the risk of postoperative maternal pulmonary edema.[170]

Once the uterus has been completely exposed, the surgeons assess uterine tone. Because there is no objective method to assess the degree of uterine relaxation, surgical palpation remains the standard. The concentration of inhalational anesthetic is adjusted as needed, with bolus doses of nitroglycerin administered, followed by an infusion to diminish uterine tone. Any attempted surgical manipulation before complete uterine relaxation may increase uterine vascular resistance, reduce uterine perfusion, and place the fetus at risk for hypoxia.

After adequate uterine relaxation, the hysterotomy site is prepared by placement of two sutures parallel to the proposed incision site and through the full thickness of the uterine wall. A hemostatic uterine stapling device is inserted. Once the stapler is deployed, the amniotic membranes are secured to the uterine wall, effectively minimizing excessive maternal bleeding. However, if the stapling device misfires or if the placental edge is mistakenly incorporated into the hysterotomy, significant hemorrhage may occur.

### Intervention

The fetal hemithorax and upper extremity are delivered through the hysterotomy. Warm fluids are continuously infused into the uterine cavity from a high-volume fluid warmer to replace amniotic fluid losses, provide a thermoneutral environment for the fetus, and prevent umbilical cord kinking or stretching. Limiting the size of the uterine incision helps prevent fetal evaporative fluid loss, uterine hemorrhage, and postoperative uterine contractions. Once the fetal hemithorax and upper extremity have been delivered into the operative field, fentanyl (5 to 20 µg/kg), atropine (20 µg/kg), and an NMBD (usually vecuronium 0.2 mg/kg or pancuronium 0.1 mg/kg) are given IM as a single injection into the exposed shoulder of the fetus.[160] Fentanyl is administered for intraoperative and postoperative fetal analgesia and to suppress the fetal stress response, atropine ablates the expected bradycardic response with fetal surgical manipulation, and an NMBD will ensure an immobile fetus during surgery. Although the fetus receives anesthesia from transplacental transfer of maternal inhaled anesthetic, these additional IM medications augment fetal anesthesia and ensure fetal analgesia before thoracotomy.

A pulse oximetry probe can be applied to the exposed fetal extremity. Fetal echocardiography provides information about

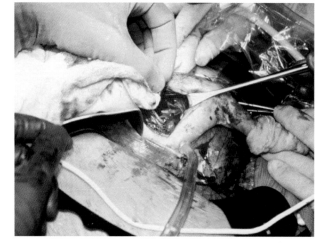

**FIGURE 37-6** In-utero thoracotomy in a 22-week fetus after excision of congenital cystic adenomatoid malformation. (Courtesy N. Scott Adzick, MD, Children's Hospital of Philadelphia.)

FHR and ventricular filling, which is particularly useful in those procedures in which fetal blood loss is anticipated (Fig. 37-6). Fetal lung lesions, especially if composed of multiple tissue types, may have a very irregular vascular supply, and significant fetal hemorrhage is possible. Direct vascular access in the exposed upper extremity allows immediate resuscitation and blood administration as needed. Even surgical manipulations alone can lead to hemodynamic instability, requiring urgent resuscitation. This may be secondary to mediastinal torsion, resulting in a sudden loss of cardiac preload.

### Intraoperative Fetal Resuscitation

Fetal bradycardia (FHR less than 100 beats per minute) usually results from hypoperfusion with low cardiac output, umbilical cord kinking, or surgical manipulation, but it may also be a result of increased uterine vascular resistance or unrecognized bleeding from the tumor site. Other expected surgery-related complications include blood loss from the tumor, hypothermia, dehydration, and unintended delivery of the fetus. Despite identification and correction of precipitating factors, the fetus may remain severely bradycardic and require resuscitation. Efforts should be made to maximize fetal perfusion and ensure adequate fetal intravascular volume. Maneuvers include confirming maternal FIO$_2$ of 100%, increasing maternal mean arterial pressure to 15% to 25% above awake values, increasing the concentration of the inhalational anesthetic to minimize the resistance of the uterine vessels, confirming adequate intrauterine volume with warmed replacement Ringer's lactate solution, and identifying the umbilical cord via ultrasonography to verify that twisting or kinking has not occurred are essential to avoiding untoward events. Pharmacologic support may also be needed. In cases with no fetal intravascular access, IM epinephrine (1 to 2 µg/kg) and atropine (20 µg/kg) can be administered and repeated if necessary. If intravascular access is available, pharmacologic resuscitation should be administered via this route to guarantee immediate effect. In addition, blood transfusions (5 to 10 mL/kg O-negative irradiated packed red blood cells [PRBCs]) can be administered in cases of severe fetal hypovolemia, by either an upper extremity intravascular route or by percutaneous access to the umbilical vein with ultrasound guidance.

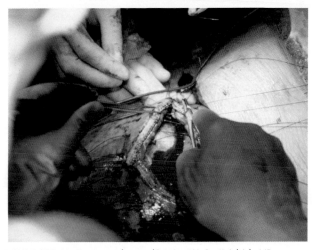

**FIGURE 37-7** Hysterotomy closure. (Courtesy N. Scott Adzick, MD, Children's Hospital of Philadelphia.)

### Closure

Once the lung lesion has been resected and fetal well-being is confirmed, the fetus is returned to the intrauterine environment and the hysterotomy incision closed. Closure consists of two separate layers, thus minimizing the risk for postoperative amniotic fluid leak and uterine wall dehiscence (Fig. 37-7). It is important to maintain complete uterine relaxation during closure, because uterine manipulation can alter blood flow and place the fetus at risk of hypoperfusion. Before the last uterine stitches, intraamniotic volume is assessed via ultrasonography and any deficit is replaced with warmed Ringer's lactate solution.

Once the uterine incision is closed, the surgeon begins to close the maternal abdominal wall. At this time, a loading dose of magnesium sulfate (6 g) is administered IV over 20 minutes, followed by a 3-g/hr infusion that is continued postoperatively. The epidural catheter can be dosed with local anesthetic (15 to 20 mL of 0.25% bupivacaine) and an opioid (e.g., fentanyl 1 to 2 μg/kg) as the inhalational anesthetic is decreased or discontinued. Careful attention to the degree of neuromuscular blockade is needed, as magnesium sulfate potentiates the action of the muscle relaxants. Extubation occurs as soon as the usual criteria for extubation are met.

### Postoperative Management

As soon as the procedure is completed, the mother should be monitored by experienced staff with necessary equipment to immediately address any complications that might occur. Ultrasonography is performed in the immediate postoperative setting and frequently over the subsequent week to monitor fetal hemodynamic stability. Tocodynamometers to assess the degree of uterine activity and irritability are used to guide tocolytic therapy.

Serious postoperative complications include premature labor, pulmonary edema, amniotic fluid leak, wound seroma, infection, and fetal demise.[156,160,171-175] Virtually all patients experience premature uterine contractions in the immediate postoperative period, thereby necessitating a continuous magnesium sulfate infusion until premature labor is significantly diminished. In some instances, additional tocolytic agents may be necessary. Despite maximal tocolytic therapies, continued uterine irritability may result in premature delivery. Amniotic fluid leak can lead to oligohydramnios and significant reductions in amniotic fluid volume that may necessitate replacement. In refractory cases, the mother may return to the OR for reclosure of the hysterotomy incision.

The etiology of fetal demise after open fetal surgery is usually secondary to a primary complication (see earlier discussion). As such, every effort is made to minimize and promptly treat potential postoperative complications to ensure a positive fetal intervention and to provide an environment for a successful term gestation. Surgical stress and pain can lead to release of cortisol and inflammatory cytokines in both the mother and the fetus, which, in turn, may lead to premature uterine maturation and contractions.[176] Maternal pain control can be provided by patient-controlled analgesia and epidural or spinal analgesia. One disadvantage of epidural analgesia is that the systemic opioid concentrations are reduced; therefore less is transferred to the fetus for postoperative analgesia. The benefit from a greater concentration of systemic opioids produced by IV analgesia is the possibility of improved fetal analgesia. However, IV analgesia does not reliably prevent a maternal stress response. To address this, the optimal choice for epidural analgesia may be a reduced concentration of the local anesthetic with a large concentration of a fat-soluble opioid, such as fentanyl (e.g., bupivacaine [0.05%] and fentanyl [10 μg/mL]).[171]

## Other Diseases Eligible for Open Procedures

### PULMONARY SEQUESTRATION

Pulmonary sequestration, also known as bronchopulmonary sequestration, accessory lung, or bronchopulmonary foregut malformation, represents 0.5% to 6% of congenital lung disease (0.15% and 1.7% of live births).[30-32] Pulmonary sequestrations consist of nonfunctional lung tissue that does not communicate with the normal tracheobronchial tree and hence does not participate in gas exchange.[31] Pulmonary sequestration may be differentiated from CCAM by investigation of its blood supply. Unlike pulmonary sequestrations, CCAMs derive their blood supply and venous drainage from the pulmonary circulation. A multitude of somatic anomalies have been associated with sequestration, most commonly diaphragmatic hernia. If not treated in utero, these lesions often present as respiratory distress in the neonatal period or as chronic respiratory infections in older children.

### BRONCHOGENIC CYSTS AND MIXED OR HYBRID PULMONARY LESIONS

Bronchogenic cysts are embryonic abnormalities considered to be a type of bronchopulmonary foregut malformation.[177] These cysts are thought to result from an abnormal budding of the primitive bronchial tree between weeks 4 and 8 of gestation, thus representing abnormal lung development at an early stage of ontogeny.[178] In most cases, bronchogenic cysts are asymptomatic in the first months of life. A notable exception is a mediastinal cyst that usually manifests as stridor.

Although in-utero complications are less likely than with the other fetal lung lesions previously described, the propensity of these lesions to cause life-threatening postnatal complications warrants close attention throughout the prenatal period. Fetal intervention with intermittent or continuous drainage of cysts can prevent the secondary morbidity; definitive fetal surgery with thoracotomy has also been successful.[179]

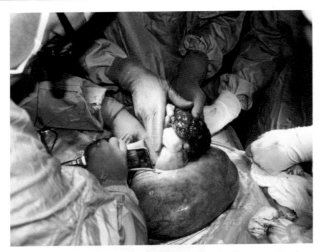

**FIGURE 37-8** Fetal sacrococcygeal teratoma before in-utero resection in a 22-week fetus. (Courtesy N. Scott Adzick, MD, Children's Hospital of Philadelphia.)

## SACROCOCCYGEAL TERATOMA

Sacrococcygeal teratomas (SCTs, Fig. 37-8) are one of the most common congenital neonatal tumors (1 per 40,000 live births).[180-182] A variety of tissues from the three primary germ layers are usually found, and the size of the tumor is quite variable.[183,184] Most SCTs are external, usually protruding from the perineal region. The majority include both solid and cystic components, with only 15% being entirely cystic.[185,186] Although usually benign, SCTs can cause significant secondary morbidity in selected cases because of the tumor's mass effect and vast blood supply.[187] With smaller tumors, complete surgical resection usually occurs after delivery under elective, controlled conditions. In extreme cases, the tumor can cause fetal congestive heart failure (usually high output failure), and even fetal demise if no treatment is performed.[188] Death is usually secondary to an enlarged tumor mass and associated polyhydramnios, resulting in preterm labor and delivery, with ultimate survival dependent on fetal lung maturity. Massive hemorrhage into the tumor with fetal exsanguination may occur spontaneously in utero or be precipitated by labor and delivery. Prenatal intervention may be necessary, including intrauterine transfusion or fetal surgery for those fetuses that develop significant secondary morbidity (e.g., hydrops).

# Hypoplastic Left Heart Syndrome: Percutaneous and Fetoscopic Procedures

A variety of congenital heart defects (CHDs) may be considered for fetal intervention. To date, the most studied defects include severe aortic stenosis with evolving hypoplastic left heart syndrome (HLHS) and pulmonary valve atresia with an intact ventricular septum with evolving hypoplastic right heart syndrome.[189-193]

## RATIONALE FOR FETAL CARDIAC INTERVENTION

Most CHDs can be safely repaired in infancy, with excellent surgical survival and long-term prognosis. For these defects, there would be no need for in-utero intervention; and for many defects, in-utero intervention would not be technically possible (e.g., arterial switch procedure for transposition of the great arteries). For other defects, surgical correction itself may not be possible and the only option is staged surgical palliation, which is often associated with significant surgical morbidity and mortality.[189,194,195] As such, the risk of performing any fetal intervention must be balanced against the potential benefits of improving the anticipated outcome of surgery performed in the neonatal period to correct the specific cardiac defect. It is the intention of prenatal intervention for certain types of CHD to reverse the pathologic process in an attempt to preserve cardiac structure and function and, thus, it is hoped, prevent serious postnatal disease. A secondary aim of prenatal intervention is to modify the severity of the disease and improve postnatal surgical outcomes.

## DEFECTS AMENABLE TO IN-UTERO REPAIR

Certain congenital heart defects cause aberrations in blood flow, which are usually secondary to valvular stenosis or regurgitation. Regardless of the etiology, the end result is often an abnormally developed ventricle.[196] Several case reports have characterized the progression of valvular stenosis to ventricular hypoplasia from reduced flow through the chamber during gestation.[197-199] It has been hypothesized that relief of valvular stenosis in utero could reverse the progression toward ventricular hypoplasia. In these cases, there may be a window of opportunity in which ventricular growth can be salvaged. Because most routine prenatal ultrasonographic screening is performed between 16 and 24 weeks gestation, the window of opportunity for prenatal intervention is likely between 20 and 26 weeks gestation.

To date, the defect most amenable to correction is severe aortic stenosis with evolving HLHS.[197-200] Without prenatal intervention, severe aortic stenosis can lead to marked left ventricular dysfunction, diminished flow through the left heart, arrest of left ventricular growth, ventricular fibroelastosis, and, consequently, HLHS. Aortic valve dilation may be performed percutaneously with ultrasound guidance. Optimal fetal positioning, placental location, or maternal habitus may require exposure of the uterus through an abdominal incision to obtain ideal access to the fetal thorax. These procedures have been performed under both maternal regional and general anesthesia, although general anesthesia is often preferred to obtain optimal uterine relaxation and an anesthetized fetus. Preliminary results are promising, but larger prospective investigations are warranted to determine long-term outcomes.[201]

## TECHNICAL ASPECTS OF FETAL CARDIAC INTERVENTIONS

Open cardiac surgery on the fetus is not presently technically possible.[202-206] In humans, all of the reported procedures to date have been attempted using the transcutaneous or transuterine approach with ultrasound-guided access into the fetal heart.[191-193] Although hysterotomy would provide means for more direct fetal access (e.g., femoral artery, transumbilical or carotid artery access), maternal morbidity would be significantly increased and postoperative premature labor certain. After valvuloplasty, the fetus requires time for the ventricle to recover. Therefore, any procedure that substantially increases the likelihood of early delivery would likely be counterproductive.

Although initial percutaneous techniques for fetal cardiac valvuloplasty were performed with only the mother receiving sedation,[191,192] recent advances in surgical techniques have led to provision of maternal and fetal analgesia and anesthesia.[207] The mother usually receives general anesthesia. After ultrasonographic confirmation of placental location, the maternal abdomen and uterus are punctured with a 22-gauge spinal needle. An IM

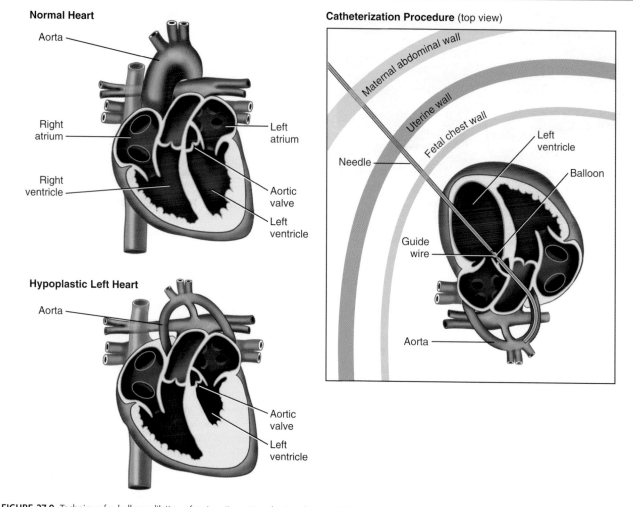

**Normal Heart**

Aorta

Right atrium

Right ventricle

Left atrium

Aortic valve

Left ventricle

**Hypoplastic Left Heart**

Aorta

Aortic valve

Left ventricle

**Catheterization Procedure** (top view)

Maternal abdominal wall

Uterine wall

Fetal chest wall

Needle

Left ventricle

Balloon

Guide wire

Aorta

**FIGURE 37-9** Technique for balloon dilation of a stenotic aortic valve in a fetus with hypoplastic left heart syndrome. (Reproduced with permission from Dream Magazine, Spring/Summer 2002, Boston: Children's Hospital Boston; 2002. p. 20.)

injection of fentanyl, atropine, and a muscle relaxant is delivered to the fetus. A 19-gauge needle is subsequently directed into the fetal thorax, and access to the fetal heart is obtained. A small coronary balloon-tipped catheter is threaded over a guidewire through the needle, and passed through the stenotic valve or closed septum. The catheter balloon is then dilated, and blood flow is confirmed using Doppler ultrasonography (Fig. 37-9). The technique has been modified in certain cases, such that a laparotomy to expose the uterus is performed. Using this technique, better ultrasonography and ideal fetal positioning are possible to achieve optimal access to the fetal thorax.

## ANESTHETIC MANAGEMENT FOR THE MOTHER

Most cases of fetal cardiac intervention are performed using a percutaneous technique or through a laparotomy incision with direct uterine exposure. The surgical approach will vary according to patient habitus, placental position (anterior vs. posterior), and fetal position. For the less invasive percutaneous approach, the choice of a regional anesthetic accompanied by IV sedation for the mother may be acceptable. However, it must be remembered that although the placental transfer of sedative drugs administered to the mother may sedate the fetus, an anesthetized or immobile fetus is not guaranteed. Excessive fetal movement makes most cardiac interventions impossible and even dangerous to both the fetus and mother.

Patients who received an epidural anesthetic technique required significantly more IV fluids but less IV opioid. The administration of large amounts of crystalloid and tocolytics during fetal surgery increases the risk of maternal pulmonary edema.[208,209] Neuraxial techniques (e.g., spinal, epidural, and combined spinal-epidural anesthesia) have been used in other percutaneous and fetoscopic procedures; a T4 sensory level blockade is required. It should be noted that neuraxial anesthesia provides no uterine relaxation and no analgesia or anesthesia to the fetus unless supplemented with IV maternal analgesics and sedatives (e.g., fentanyl, benzodiazepines, propofol). Because of these issues, it is generally recommended, even in anticipated percutaneous procedures, to deliver a general anesthetic to the mother. If there is a high suspicion of a laparotomy being performed, a dose of spinal Duramorph (morphine sulfate) may be delivered to the mother before the anesthetic induction for postoperative pain relief and resultant suppression of myometrial contractility after laparotomy.[197,198]

## ANESTHETIC MANAGEMENT FOR THE FETUS

Anesthesia for percutaneous and fetoscopic interventions, of which fetal cardiac interventions are a significant subset, pose several unique challenges for the anesthesiologist. The combination of immature organ systems and the underlying cardiac anomaly places the fetus at considerable anesthetic risk. Unlike adults and older children, fetal cardiac output depends more on heart rate than on stroke volume. Because fetal myocardial contractility is likely maximally stimulated, the fetus has a limited ability to increase stroke volume. Therefore, it is plausible that fetal patients with congenital heart disease and evidence of failure (i.e., hydrops) will exhibit more pronounced physiologic limitations. Notably, anesthetic-induced decreases in contractility, combined with intracardiac catheter manipulation in a structurally compromised heart, can result in fetal hypotension, bradycardia, and eventual cardiac collapse and death. It is generally accepted that neonates manifest a greater degree of hypotension in response to isoflurane and halothane at equipotent anesthetic concentrations when compared with older children.[210,211]

Because direct exposure of the fetus is not warranted during most cardiac interventions, intraoperative monitoring is limited to echocardiography. An ultrasonographer continually monitors the fetal heart during placement of the intracardiac needle and during catheter balloon inflation. A continuous echocardiogram is also useful for measuring FHR, contractility, and volume status.

### INTRAOPERATIVE FETAL RESUSCITATION DURING PERCUTANEOUS INTERVENTIONS

If fetal bradycardia (heart rate less than 100 beats per minute) or significantly reduced ventricular function develops, resuscitation proceeds immediately. Because direct vascular access to the fetus may not be immediately available, several other treatments can be employed. Intracardiac and IM administration of epinephrine (1 to 2 µg/kg) may be used to treat severe sustained bradycardia. Other maneuvers improve uterine perfusion and hence fetal oxygenation and include increasing maternal mean arterial pressure to 15% to 25% above awake values with volume loading and ephedrine or phenylephrine, and decreasing uterine vascular resistance by ensuring adequate uterine relaxation. Occasionally, pericardial tamponade may cause impaired cardiac function; needle drainage of the effusion may be necessary for fetal survival. If fetal echocardiography indicates a decreased ventricular volume, an intracardiac blood transfusion with O-negative irradiated blood (5 to 10 mL/kg) may be indicated.

### POSTOPERATIVE CONSIDERATIONS

The fetus is monitored postoperatively with intermittent ultrasonographic examinations. The incidence of premature contractions and labor is less after fetoscopic surgery than after open hysterotomy.[212,213] Fetoscopic intervention also appears to have reduced requirements for tocolysis and a reduced rate of premature delivery.[213] If early delivery should occur, many of these fetuses are considered nonviable owing to their young gestational age (usually less than 24 weeks gestation) and serious cardiac disease.

## Other Diseases Eligible for Fetoscopic Procedures

### TWIN–TWIN TRANSFUSION SYNDROME

Twin–twin transfusion syndrome (TTTS) is a serious complication occurring in 10% to 15% of monozygotic monochorionic twin pregnancies.[214] Although all monochorionic twin pregnancies demonstrate one or more placental vascular anastomoses, TTTS represents a pathologic form of circulatory imbalance between the monochorionic twin fetuses.[215] As a result of this

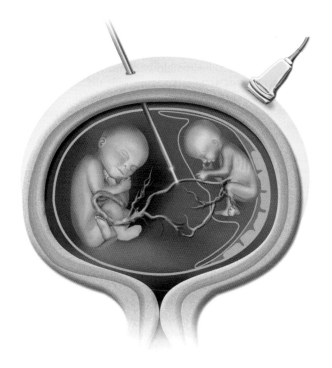

**FIGURE 37-10** Schematic representation of umbilical cord ligation in twin reversed arterial perfusion sequence. (Courtesy T.M. Crombleholme, MD.)

imbalance, a net fetofetal transfusion occurs, from one twin (the donor) to the other (the recipient) (Fig. 37-10). Symptoms develop rapidly and, in the donor twin, include hypovolemia, oliguria, oligohydramnios, and growth retardation. In turn, the recipient twin develops hypervolemia, polyuria, polyhydramnios, and signs of circulatory volume overload, resulting in congestive heart failure.[214-218] In severe cases, if untreated, TTTS may result in intrauterine fetal death and miscarriage. Even if twins with TTTS survive, there remains a high incidence of secondary neurologic and pulmonary morbidities.

Fetoscopic laser photocoagulation of the communicating vessels associated with TTTS is based on three fundamental assumptions: (1) the syndrome occurs in the presence of vascular communications between fetuses in a monochorionic gestation, (2) obliteration of these vessels can halt the pathophysiologic process, and (3) both deep and superficial communications can be interrupted at the surface of the placenta.[219] Fetoscopic laser surgical occlusion of superficial communicating vessels is associated with a reported survival rate of 55% to 83% and a reduced neurologic complication rate (5%) among survivors.[214,216]

There are few data on the reported anesthetic techniques used for fetoscopic laser ablation. The procedure has been performed with local, general, epidural, and combined general and epidural anesthesia.[220-223] Factors that may influence the anesthetic technique include (1) the planned surgical approach and probability of converting to open fetal surgery; (2) the likelihood of surgical perturbation of innervated fetal tissues; (3) maternal preference; and (4) a history of prior uterine activity. The surgical approach for fetoscopic laser photocoagulation is determined by (1) the location of the placenta (anterior vs. posterior), (2) the position of the fetuses, and (3) the potential window(s) for trocar insertion.[224]

## TWIN REVERSED ARTERIAL PERFUSION SEQUENCE

Twin reversed arterial perfusion (TRAP) sequence denotes a common pathophysiology of several different conditions, all of which describe a twin pregnancy in which one twin is normal and the second twin exhibits multisystem malformations, including anencephaly or acardia. The twin with the hemodynamic advantage is denoted as the "pump" twin, perfusing deoxygenated blood in a retrograde direction to the other twin, "the recipient twin." The term *reversed perfusion* is used to describe this scenario because blood enters the acardiac or anencephalic twin through its umbilical artery and exits through the umbilical vein. This eventually places the normal or "pump" twin at a hemodynamic disadvantage because this normal twin provides cardiac output to both itself and the nonviable sibling. This anomaly places the pump twin at risk of cardiac overload and congestive heart failure, often with associated hepatosplenomegaly.

Perinatal complications with TRAP sequence range in severity, with reported death rates for the pump twin ranging from 39% to 59% in untreated pregnancies.[225] Treatment options include observation, medical therapy with digoxin and indomethacin, selective delivery, umbilical cord blockade with a coil, and fetoscopic cord ligation. Although all endoscopic procedures have the primary aim of interrupting umbilical cord blood flow to the nonviable twin, this invasive technique is generally employed after failed medical therapy or after signs of cardiac failure in the viable twin.[226,227]

## NEEDLE ASPIRATION AND PLACEMENT OF SHUNTS

A variety of fetal disorders may benefit from in-utero needle aspiration or shunt placement. These disorders include posterior urethral valves, aqueductal stenosis, fetal hydrothorax, ovarian cyst, and fetal ascites. Various shunts have been attempted to provide long-term decompression, with variable results.[221]

# The EXIT Procedure

Ex utero intrapartum treatment, or the EXIT procedure, was initially described as a method for reversal of tracheal occlusion in fetuses with prenatally diagnosed severe congenital diaphragmatic hernia that had undergone in-utero tracheal clip application.[228] Although these infants demonstrated no reduced morbidity compared with those who underwent conventional treatment, this novel technique provided a new therapeutic option for fetuses with a variety of potentially fatal diseases. Improvements in prenatal imaging and widespread use of prenatal ultrasonography have increased the identification of potentially lethal fetal structural malformations, which has had a direct impact on perinatal management and outcomes.

Also referred to as the OOPS procedure (operation on placental support),[229] the EXIT procedure allows for a controlled delivery and intrapartum assessment strategy to treat fetuses with certain life-threatening diseases. By maintaining uteroplacental circulation with only partial delivery of the infant, crucial time is provided to perform procedures critical to infant survival. These procedures include direct laryngoscopy, bronchoscopy, intubation, tracheostomy, tumor decompression and resection, and extracorporeal membrane oxygenation (ECMO) cannulation before clamping the umbilical cord (Fig. 37-11). In this way, continuous oxygenation is maintained at all times to the threatened infant, thereby improving the chances of overall survival. The EXIT procedure is now used for infants in whom prenatal imaging suggests a very low probability of survival

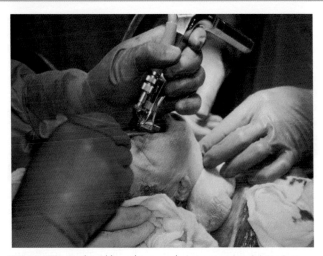

**FIGURE 37-11** Fetal rigid bronchoscopy during an ex-utero intrapartum treatment procedure. (Courtesy N. Scott Adzick, MD, Children's Hospital of Philadelphia.)

with conventional treatment methods. This group includes fetuses with known tracheal obstruction and other life-threatening airway abnormalities, as well as those who will likely require ECMO support (i.e., congenital cardiac disease and diaphragmatic hernia).

Unlike many other fetal interventions, however, a planned delivery of the infant is the end result of these interventions. This unique difference creates significant increases in maternal morbidity because these procedures require complete uterine relaxation and serious maternal hemorrhage could result.[230] An intimate understanding of the EXIT procedure, the fetal pathophysiology involved, and pregnancy-induced alterations directly affecting anesthesia care is required to minimize maternal and fetal morbidity and mortality.

## FETAL DISEASES ELIGIBLE FOR THE EXIT PROCEDURE
### Cervical Teratoma

Cervical teratomas are rare (1 per 20,000 to 40,000 live births) and can extend from the mastoid process to the sternal notch inferiorly and to the trapezius muscle posteriorly. They can also invade the oral floor and extend into the anterior mediastinum. Many of the larger teratomas diagnosed prenatally cause maternal polyhydramnios, which is secondary to esophageal compression by the tumor and impaired fetal swallowing. Most of these tumors are benign but are associated with substantial mortality rates caused by airway compression and difficulty in establishing an adequate airway after delivery (Fig. 37-12).[231] Of neonates with cervical teratomas, 30% die of airway obstruction shortly after delivery[232]; for infants not diagnosed prenatally, mortality rates are even greater.[233,234] In addition, some larger tumors may interfere with normal delivery methods and necessitate emergent alterations in maternal care, placing the mother at increased risk.[231,235]

Until recently, treatment options for infants with cervical teratomas who survived the intrauterine period were limited. The standard of care incorporated scheduled cesarean section followed by various airway maneuvers, including the establishment of a surgical airway. Even with skilled help immediately available, dismal outcomes were common.[231-233] Despite securing the airway,

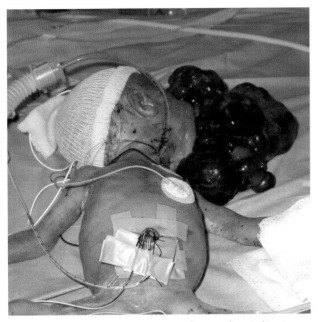

**FIGURE 37-12** Newborn with a massive oropharyngeal cervical teratoma immediately after ex utero intrapartum treatment was performed to secure the airway. Immediate resection of the teratoma followed in an adjacent operating room.

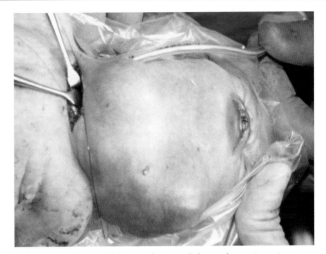

**FIGURE 37-13** Fetus (with a cystic hygroma) that underwent ex utero intrapartum treatment to establish a surgical airway before delivery. (Courtesy N. Scott Adzick, MD, Children's Hospital of Philadelphia.)

critical time is needed to perform this task, often at the expense of neonatal oxygenation. With the introduction of the EXIT procedure, precious time is provided to locate the trachea and provide a definitive airway before clamping the umbilical cord, thereby maintaining continuous fetal oxygenation and decreasing morbidity and mortality.

### Cystic Hygroma

Cystic hygromas arise from the failure of the jugular lymph sacs to join the lymphatic system early in fetal development, resulting in the development of endothelium-lined cystic spaces that eventually compress normal surrounding structures. This compression may result in fetal hydrops, including skin edema, ascites, and pleural or pericardial effusions (Fig. 37-13).[233,234] In infants with isolated cervical cystic hygroma and no evidence of hydrops, airway compromise at birth or shortly thereafter is the main therapeutic concern. These infants are considered candidates for EXIT procedures.

### Congenital High Airway Obstruction Syndrome

Congenital high airway obstruction syndrome (CHAOS) is a clinical syndrome consisting of extremely large echogenic lungs, flattened or inverted diaphragms, a dilated tracheobronchial tree, ascites, and evidence of nonimmune hydrops, including fetal ascites, placentomegaly, and pleural or pericardial effusions.[236-238] Airway obstruction may be because of laryngeal atresia, laryngeal cyst, or tracheal atresia. Diagnosis of prenatal CHAOS is confirmed by ultrasonographic evidence of complete or near-complete upper airway obstruction. Most diagnostic findings result from increased intratracheal pressure and distention of the tracheobronchial tree secondary to the accumulation of fluid in the lungs. Cardiac changes include the appearance of an elongated heart, septal shift, and small, compressed heart chambers.[233]

Management guidelines for fetuses with CHAOS are not definitive. In third trimester fetuses with a diagnosis of CHAOS and no evidence of hydrops, there is most probably incomplete airway obstruction, and management is aimed at establishing an airway before complete delivery. This subset of fetuses would likely benefit from an EXIT procedure.[233,239] Those fetuses with a diagnosis of CHAOS made in the second trimester and those with evidence of complete airway obstruction and/or nonimmune hydrops present a dilemma, because insufficient data exist to determine their best treatment options.

### Congenital Goiter

Congenital goiter is associated with fetal hypothyroidism, euthyroidism, or hyperthyroidism. Goiter associated with fetal hypothyroidism is almost always associated with the transplacental passage of a thyroid-stimulating immunoglobulin G antibody from the mother. Such antibodies are present in 90% of women with Graves disease. These antibody levels may not reflect maternal thyroid status, making the fetus of any woman with Graves disease at increased risk for fetal goiter. Less common causes include iodine deficiency, iodine intoxication, congenital metabolic disorders of thyroid hormone synthesis, or hypothalamic-pituitary hypothyroidism. Ultrasonographic findings of fetal hyperthyroidism include cardiac hypertrophy, tachycardia, or nonimmune hydrops fetalis. Fetal hypothyroidism may be associated with fetal cardiomegaly and heart block. Fetal blood sampling is required to determine the fetal thyroid status.[233,240,241]

The possibility of significant airway compression immediately after delivery is similar for all fetuses with goiter. In severe cases, even the presence of experienced personnel in the delivery room may not ensure prompt ability to secure the airway. These infants may benefit from the EXIT procedure; it can provide the time that may be necessary to identify and secure the compromised fetal airway.

### EXIT TO ECMO

In addition to airway management, the EXIT procedure may be considered for other instances in which separation from uteroplacental support is expected to cause critical cardiac or pulmonary compromise. Fetuses with congenital heart disease who are expected to need emergent ECMO at birth and fetuses with poor-prognosis congenital diaphragmatic hernias may benefit from the "EXIT to ECMO" strategy.[230,242] Neonates undergoing this procedure are partially delivered via the EXIT procedure, and arterial and venous cannulas are inserted while uteroplacental perfusion is maintained. Although CHD remains the most common disease entity considered for potential EXIT to ECMO therapy, this technique has been used for neonates with other disease processes associated with almost certain chance of immediate cardiorespiratory collapse after conventional delivery.

### Intraoperative Considerations

A multidisciplinary team consisting of an obstetrician, pediatric surgeon, ultrasonographer, anesthesiologist, neonatologist, scrub nurses, and technicians provides the expertise in each respective field to aid in the overall success of the procedure. In cases in which immediate surgical intervention is planned (e.g., resection of a neck mass), a prepared adjacent OR with separate personnel should be available. A meeting of the entire team is held before the start of the case to clearly identify individual roles and to discuss any concerns or questions. This is also a good opportunity to address any clinical changes, either in radiographic findings or in fetal position, or other factors that may alter the surgical plan.

### Uterine Relaxation and Perfusion

To preserve maternal-fetal gas exchange at the placental interface, ensure fetal oxygenation, and avoid life-threatening hypoxemia, it is of primary importance to ensure complete uterine relaxation throughout the duration of fetal uteroplacental support. Factors affecting uterine blood flow include, but are not limited to, anesthetic induction agents, maternal hyperventilation, maternal hypotension, maternal catecholamine release, and other causes of increased noradrenergic activity and uterine tone. Any increase in uterine vascular resistance will decrease uterine perfusion, as is seen with uterine contractions. Of all factors ensuring the overall success of the EXIT procedure, minimal uterine vascular resistance is the most important, because decreases in uterine blood flow will cause fetal hypoxemia, acidosis, and, potentially, fetal demise.[243]

### Surgical Procedure

After the hysterotomy site has been created and hemostasis achieved, the fetal head, neck, and shoulders are delivered. Because many of these procedures involve large neck masses, a generous hysterotomy incision is needed to partially deliver the fetus without injury to the mass or fetus. Furthermore, if a uterine contraction occurs at this time, inadvertent expulsion of the fetus could occur, interrupting the fetoplacental unit and thus critically jeopardizing the viability of the fetus. In some cases, a fetal extremity may be delivered to apply a pulse oximetry probe and to obtain IV access.[244,245] Although the fetus is anesthetized via placental transfer of maternally administered inhaled anesthetics in most cases, additional analgesia and paralytics are administered (e.g., fentanyl, atropine, muscle relaxant). The additional medications may be given as a single IM dose in an upper extremity, or can alternatively be delivered under ultrasound guidance before hysterotomy. An advantage to earlier administration is increased time for fetal absorption via the IM route. If peripheral IV access is obtained, additional medications can be given through this route.

### ACCESS TO THE FETAL AIRWAY

Most EXIT procedures are currently performed to access a compromised fetal airway before delivery; successful access depends on meticulous preoperative evaluation and careful preparation.[246,247] Portions of the trachea can be completely compressed and distorted such that even successful intubation may result in an inability to achieve adequate ventilation. For this reason, most surgeons perform a direct laryngoscopy and rigid bronchoscopy to examine the status of the fetal airway. In one series, successful endotracheal intubation by conventional means was reported in 77% of cases.[230] In those cases in which tracheal intubation is impossible, a surgical tracheostomy can be performed as soon as the trachea is identified. The trachea can be located with the aid of preoperative radiographic studies, often identifying the tracheal location relative to fixed external anatomic landmarks. Gentle surgical palpation may also aid in the identification of cartilaginous tracheal rings. In cases in which the former options have failed, ultrasonography with the sterile probe inserted directly into the surgical incision may help to locate the trachea.[248] When tracheal rings are identified, the trachea may be accessed directly with an endotracheal tube by tunneling through the fetal soft tissue, or with the aid of a retrograde wire inserted by the Seldinger technique. The trachea, exposed through a neck incision, may be incised via a temporary tracheotomy to allow passage of a feeding tube or wire from the trachea to the mouth or nose. The guidewire is then attached to the endotracheal tube, which is then pulled down into the proper position. After suturing the endotracheal tube securely to the mouth, the tracheotomy can then be closed.

Regardless of the method used to secure the trachea, the anesthesiologist must be prepared to control ventilation in the fetus. In some institutions, an anesthesiologist may be scrubbed at the operative field to assume this responsibility. In other institutions, one of the surgeons or neonatologists assumes this role. Adequate ventilation may be difficult to achieve for several reasons. Certain types of tumors, specifically cervical teratomas, may secrete thick mucus into the trachea, and this must be aggressively removed before ventilation. As soon as the airway is satisfactorily cleared, surfactant should be administered via the tracheal tube to diminish expected airway resistance. Surfactant is provided for two principal reasons. First, the majority of infants treated for such lesions are delivered at some point before term and their pulmonary development (considered both by gestational age and underlying pathophysiology) cannot be assumed to be normal. Second, the thick mucoid secretions and the aggressive lavage necessary to clear them may interrupt the normal surfactant layering and functionality, suggesting that surfactant therapy may provide a benefit if administered before lung ventilation. These steps should result in increases in fetal oxygen saturation to levels greater than 90%. If this does not occur, the position of the tracheal tube should be rechecked and the lungs should be auscultated with the aid of a sterile stethoscope. In addition, ultrasound examination for the presence of air bronchograms may be used to confirm tracheal intubation. Ventilation occurs most commonly with the aid of a sterile Jackson-Rees circuit. When adequate ventilation has been established, the fetus can be delivered.

### Delivery of the Infant and Maternal Management

Before umbilical cord clamping and delivery, coordination between the surgery and anesthesia teams is crucial to prevent uterine atony and excessive maternal hemorrhage. Because a decrease in the tocolytic agent, whether an inhalational or an IV agent, would result in increased uterine vascular resistance and decreased fetal oxygenation, reversal of the tocolysis must not occur before the umbilical cord is clamped. However, at clamping, a near-total reversal of tocolysis is required to limit uterine bleeding. This is best achieved with a low-solubility inhalational anesthetic (e.g., desflurane). As the cord is clamped, the anesthetic is immediately discontinued and oxytocin is administered as a bolus followed by a continuous infusion and titrated to uterine response (e.g., 40 units oxytocin in 500 mL of normal saline over 30 minutes, followed by 20 units over 8 hours). Additional uterotonic medications may be necessary and must be immediately available should uncontrolled maternal hemorrhage occur.[249] These medications include methylergonovine, carboprost, and calcium carbonate. Anticipation of massive and rapid maternal hemorrhage is essential. Appropriate IV access (e.g., rapid infusion catheters, introducer sheaths) with a rapid infusion device in place for blood product administration may be life saving, should uncontrolled and persistent bleeding occur. In cases of uncontrolled hemorrhage despite maximal drug therapy, a hysterectomy may be necessary. When maternal hemostasis has been achieved, uterine tone restored, and the placenta delivered, then a low-dose inhalational anesthetic and nitrous oxide can be administered, provided that the mother is hemodynamically stable.

A separate team of neonatologists, anesthesiologists, and nurses should be available for the neonate because additional medications, blood products, and vascular access may be needed. A brief physical examination, confirmation of bilateral breath sounds, and hemodynamic stability must be ensured soon after delivery. In some instances, immediate surgical intervention is planned, necessitating entirely separate anesthetic, surgical, and nursing teams in an adjacent OR as the maternal abdomen is closed.

### Postoperative Considerations

Mothers recovering from an EXIT procedure differ from those who undergo standard cesarean deliveries. Potential postoperative complications include wound dehiscence, infection, bleeding, and urinary retention.[230] Although every attempt is made to place the hysterotomy incision in the lower uterine segment during EXIT procedures, those patients with anterior placentas may require incisions in different areas of the uterus. As a result, these patients are at increased risk of uterine rupture in any subsequent pregnancy. Practitioners should also consider the fact that, unlike with a standard cesarean section, the parents cannot immediately interact with or even view their neonates after delivery. Because many of these neonates undergo immediate surgical intervention, the parents' first glimpse of their child will be of an intubated, sedated child with monitors, invasive catheters, and swollen, distorted facies. Continued emotional support, social services, and education will help ease this transition.

## Movement toward Intervention for Non–Life-Threatening Diseases: Myelomeningocele

At present, nearly all human fetal interventions are performed to prevent almost certain fetal demise secondary to a known congenital defect or pathophysiologic process. Myelomeningocele (MMC) is the first nonfatal birth defect to be treated in utero. MMC affects 0.5 to 1 per 1000 live births annually, with variations in both population and geography.[250-252] At least 75% of affected individuals reach early adulthood; most deaths occur

during infancy and the preschool years secondary to respiratory and neurologic complications.[253] There is significant risk associated with this early fetal intervention. Many infants with MMC may be delivered prematurely as a direct result of intrauterine intervention, further adding to the risks of an already compromised infant.[252] Some have argued that because MMC is a nonlethal defect, intrauterine intervention for potential reduced secondary morbidity may not justify the significant maternal morbidity or fetal mortality associated with this procedure. However, the severe morbidity associated with MMC, combined with the promising results of animal research, have led to consideration of prenatal intervention for this disorder. Initial human outcomes have demonstrated some improvement in secondary morbidity.[252,254,255] Recent publication of the results of the Management of Myelomeningocele Study (or the MOMS trial) demonstrated a reduced need for placement of cerebrospinal fluid shunts and improved motor outcomes (e.g., earlier ambulation) at 30 months in the fetal intervention group, compared to infants whose repairs were deferred until after delivery. Nevertheless, significant maternal and fetal morbidities were reported.[256]

## Future Considerations

With the advances in surgical and anesthetic techniques and technologies, significant progress may be made in mid-gestation fetal intervention, and in moving from treatment of only life-threatening fetal pathologic processes toward preemptive management of fetal disorders that are not necessarily life-threatening but have significant, disabling postpartum morbidities. However, these benefits may have to be balanced against the possibility of long-term neurocognitive disorders in anesthetized fetuses, particularly in those fetuses undergoing prenatal repair of anomalies that are not life threatening.[257-259]

The particular challenges for anesthesiologists are to develop methods to provide selective fetal anesthesia and analgesia, and techniques of targeted uterine relaxation such that safer, specifically tailored anesthesia may be provided to all patients involved in the fetal intervention. Furthermore, techniques and technologies that will enhance tocolysis and retard PPROM and preterm labor will allow increased time for fetuses to heal and mature in utero, while reducing the incidence of postoperative pulmonary edema in mothers. Finally, enhanced fetal monitoring will help the anesthesiologist provide better care for the fetus both in utero and in the postoperative period. With such advances, the provision of fetal anesthesia may become a more routine part of pediatric surgical and anesthetic practice, bringing with it new opportunities for practice and research, and new problems to be solved.

## ANNOTATED REFERENCES

Boat A, Mahmoud M, Michelfelder EC, et al. Supplementing desflurane with intravenous anesthesia reduces fetal cardiac dysfunction during open fetal surgery. Paediatr Anaesth 2010;20:748-56.

*In a retrospective study, Boat and colleagues found that early institution of high concentrations of volatile agents for extended periods before hysterotomy resulted in the development of intraoperative fetal bradycardia, most notably when desflurane was used as the maintenance agent. Based on their findings, they suggest alternative utilization of supplemental IV anesthesia with propofol and remifentanil until just before the hysterotomy incision is made, at which point high volatile-anesthetic concentrations may be used to achieve the desired uterine relaxation.*

Courtier J, Poder L, Wang ZJ, et al. Fetal tracheolaryngeal airway obstruction: prenatal evaluation by sonography and MRI. Pediatr Radiol 2010;40:1800-5.

*The authors reviewed the sonographic and MRI findings of tracheolaryngeal obstruction in the fetus, including extrinsic causes, such as lymphatic malformation, cervical teratoma, and vascular rings, and intrinsic causes, such as congenital high airway obstruction syndrome (CHAOS). The authors found that accurate radiologic distinction of these conditions by sonography or MRI may facilitate optimizing patient selection for ex utero intrapartum treatment (EXIT) procedure, as well as identifying associated procedural risks for surgeons, anesthesiologists, and neonatologists.*

Fink RJ, Allen TK, Habib AS. Remifentanil for fetal immobilization and analgesia during the ex utero intrapartum treatment procedure under combined spinal-epidural anaesthesia. Br J Anaesth 2011;106:851-5.

*The authors report three cases of ex utero intrapartum treatment performed under neuraxial anesthesia, with maternal administration of remifentanil used to provide fetal immobilization and analgesia via placental transfer. No clinically significant maternal sedation or respiratory depression were observed. In all cases, the authors argue, remifentanil provided adequate fetal immobilization and obviated the need to administer other analgesics or NMBDs.*

Ngan Kee WD, Khaw KS, Tan PE, Ng FF, Karmakar MK. Placental transfer and fetal metabolic effects of phenylephrine and ephedrine during spinal anesthesia for cesarean delivery. Anesthesiology 2009; 111:506-12.

*The authors randomized 104 healthy parturients having elective Cesarean section under spinal anesthesia, to receive infusions of either phenylephrine or ephedrine, titrated to maintain approximate baseline systolic blood pressure. The authors found that, although ephedrine crosses the placenta to a greater extent and undergoes less early metabolism (or redistribution) in the fetus compared with phenylephrine, its associated increased fetal concentrations of lactate, glucose, and catecholamines may favor phenylephrine as the preferred vasopressor for such indications, despite historical evidence suggesting uteroplacental blood flow may be better maintained with ephedrine.*

Tran KM, Maxwell LG, Cohen DE, et al. Quantification of serum fentanyl concentrations from umbilical cord blood during ex utero intrapartum therapy. Anesth Analg 2012;114:1265-7.

*The authors quantified the concentration of fentanyl in umbilical vein blood drawn following IM injection from 13 human fetal subjects undergoing EXIT procedures. The median dose of fentanyl was 60 μg (range, 45 to 65 μg) for fetuses with a mean weight at delivery of 3000 g. The median time between IM administration of fentanyl and collection of the sample was 37 minutes (range, 5 to 86 minutes). Fentanyl was detected in all of the samples, with a median serum concentration of 14.0 ng/mL (range, 4.3 to 64.0 ng/mL).*

## REFERENCES

Please see www.expertconsult.com.

# Trauma

## DAVID A. YOUNG AND DAVID E. WESSON

ANESTHESIOLOGISTS COMMONLY PROVIDE CARE TO CHILDREN who have suffered traumatic injuries. These injuries vary in complexity, and patients range from the healthy older child with an isolated elbow fracture to the infant with a life-threatening epidural hematoma. The anesthesiologist should view the management of children with traumatic injuries as a continuum of care that may originate in the prehospital setting with emergency medical services (EMS), progress to the emergency department (ED), and continue through the operating room, the postanesthesia care unit, and the intensive care unit. Anesthesiologists may become involved in all phases of care of the traumatically injured child, with the possible exception of the prehospital setting. The care required is often complex but can be effectively accomplished in a collaborative environment incorporating a standardized process for initial evaluation and management.[1] Anesthesiologists should be familiar with these processes to effectively continue this care in the perioperative setting.

Anesthesiologists are essential participants in many capacities during the care of injured children. Operative interventions demand full involvement of the anesthesiologist. In many institutions, anesthesiologists also provide emergency airway and critical care management. From the perspectives of airway control, ventilation, hemodynamic resuscitation, metabolic management, and effective control of pain, anesthesiologists can play a central role in the care of the injured child. Common diseases of childhood are now better understood and more effectively treated, which has resulted in more cures, better outcomes, and an improved quality of life. Despite major reductions in the overall mortality rate for pediatric trauma in recent years, unintentional injuries remain the leading cause of death and disability in the pediatric population of the United States.[2] Injury has also emerged as the most common public health threat to children around the world.[3]

This chapter reviews the key principles of anesthesia management of traumatic injuries to children. This discussion is intended to augment the principles established in the widely accepted Advanced Trauma Life Support (ATLS) program, which is produced by the American College of Surgeons Committee on Trauma.[4] Additional resources for the management of the pediatric trauma patient include the Advanced Pediatric Life Support (APLS) course administered by the American Academy of Pediatrics and the American College of Emergency Physicians.[5] Many of the topics discussed in this chapter are being investigated to determine the most effective strategy, including volume resuscitation, evaluation of the cervical spine, and prehospital tracheal intubation.

## Epidemiology of Pediatric Trauma

Traumatic injuries are the most common cause of death within the United States for children older than 1 year of age.[6] Approximately 20,000 deaths of children occur annually as a result of trauma. Most traumatic injuries in children are a result of motor vehicle accidents (the leading cause of death), falls, nonaccidental trauma (Fig. 38-1), drowning, or extremes of temperature.

The epidemiology of trauma reflects its continued growth as a significant health risk for children of the world. Table 38-1 illustrates the recent incidence of injury types per 100,000 U.S. children.[2] Motor vehicle trauma is a major threat to the health of children in the United States, which has spurred research to identify methods to improve their protection.[7-9]

Pediatric and adult injury patterns and treatment protocols are different.[10] Head injuries are the leading cause of death in children. One explanation for this is the proportionately large head of children compared with adults. Thoracic injuries are the second leading cause of death for pediatric trauma patients. Due to increased rib cage pliability from a lack of bony calcification and the flexible cartilaginous component, severe internal injury can occur in children without obvious external signs such as rib fractures. Blunt abdominal trauma frequently can be treated with close observation, avoiding operative intervention. Penetrating abdominal trauma usually requires surgical exploration. However, diagnostic laparoscopy is being used in lieu of exploratory

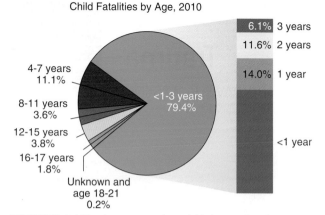

Child Fatalities by Age, 2010

**FIGURE 38-1** Fatalities by age group from child abuse and neglect in 2010. Most of these children are 3 years of age or younger. (Data from the U.S. Department of Health and Human Services, Administration for Children and Families, Administration on Children, Youth, and Families, Children's Bureau; Child Maltreatment 2010. Available at http://www.acf.hhs.gov/programs/cb/pubs/cm10/cm10.pdf#page=70 [accessed September 2012]).

| TABLE 38-1 Incidence of Injury Type per 100,000 U.S. Children by Age in 2008 | | | | | |
|---|---|---|---|---|---|
| | AGE (years) | | | | |
| Cause of Injury | 1-4 | 5-9 | 10-14 | 15-19 | Overall (1-19) |
| Unintentional | 8.8 | 4.1 | 5.1 | 25.7 | 11.3 |
| Assault | 2.5 | 0.6 | 1.0 | 9.8 | 3.6 |
| Self-harm or suicide | | | 1.1 | 7.5 | 2.3 |

Data from Mathews TJ, Miniño AM, Osterman MJ, et al. Annual summary of vital statistics: 2008. Pediatrics 2011;127:146-57.

laparotomy in hemodynamically stable children to evaluate and repair many types of abdominal injuries.[11]

## Nonaccidental Trauma

Nonaccidental trauma, also referred to as shaken baby syndrome or child abuse, is an epidemic that continues to grow in virtually all parts of the world. Although 3 million reports of nonaccidental trauma are filed every year in the United States, most experts believe that this represents less than one third of the actual cases.[12,13] Every state has stringent laws for reporting nonaccidental trauma. These laws are designed to assist the health care provider who suspects mistreatment and to punish health care providers who do not appropriately report potential neglect. It is the responsibility of every physician involved, including the anesthesiologist, to be aware of the potential for nonaccidental trauma in all infants and children and to report all suspicious observations accurately to the appropriate authorities.

Characteristics of nonaccidental trauma include a history inconsistent with the character and extent of the injuries and a delay in seeking medical assistance.[14,15] Nonaccidental trauma should be considered when the history appears improbable. Funduscopic examination may disclose retinal hemorrhages or papilledema, which may suggest forceful shaking of the head or increased intracranial pressure (ICP), respectively. Examination of the skin may show bruises, burns, or other injuries in several stages of healing (Fig. 38-2). A skeletal survey may reveal multiple fractures of various ages occurring typically at the metaphyses of long bones. Occasionally, a child who has

previously been silent in the company of the parents or caregiver tells operating room or recovery room personnel about the events surrounding his or her injuries. These reports should be carefully documented and relayed to the appropriate personnel. Maltreated children are often terrified of painful procedures, and the need for sensitivity and reassurance in these settings cannot be overemphasized.

The anesthesiologist encountering a potential victim of nonaccidental trauma may provide the first impartial assessment of the child's status.[16] Physicians, nurses, and other professionals who provide initial resuscitation may be preoccupied with the small child's acute and potentially life-threatening injuries. Historical data associated with the event may be inaccurate or fictitious at the time of initial presentation. An objective evaluation by the anesthesiologist in preparation for operative intervention may reveal the first objective evidence of nonaccidental trauma. Indications of mistreatment may be subtle, ranging from lack of parental availability for perioperative counseling and consent to irrational refusal of permission for a necessary operative intervention.[17,18]

## Prehospital Care of the Pediatric Trauma Patient

### TRAUMA SYSTEMS

The evolution of pediatric trauma systems has significantly improved outcomes and quality of life for trauma victims.[19,20] Countries such as the United States have a trauma system philosophy more in line with the military approach. in which prehospital personnel such as paramedics are the initial team to make rapid assessments, initiate efforts at stabilization, obtain radio contact with the medical facility, and transport the child to the trauma center as rapidly as possible.[21] This philosophy of minimizing the time on the scene and emphasizing prompt transport to the closest trauma center is called *scoop and run*.

In parts of Canada and several European countries, initial resuscitation of injured children is commonly performed by physicians who are charged with evaluating the child at the scene, securing the airway, initiating resuscitative measures to maintain hemodynamic stability, and transporting the child to an appropriate trauma center (Fig. 38-3). Instituting these management procedures may result in additional time on the scene. This approach has been called *stay and play*. Many aspects of this system are being integrated into existing American trauma systems as part of mass casualty disaster management plans.[22,23]

Developing a systematic approach to the care of the pediatric trauma patient is crucial. This includes acquiring age- and size-appropriate equipment. Luten and Broselow developed a system that provides immediate guidance for the identification of appropriate equipment and drug doses based on the child's length.[24-27] This system assigns a specific color based on the child's body length. A corresponding color-coded, length-based wristband can then be placed onto the child, which designates drug doses and devices that match the assigned color. The system is designed to minimize delays, medication miscalculations, and equipment errors.

Over the past 2 decades, there have been dramatic advances in the capability of prehospital providers to recognize the need for and initiate resuscitation of pediatric trauma patients. Part of this progression has been attributed to the development of trauma systems and the commitment of trauma centers to provide more effective medical direction to prehospital providers. Effective management of the continuum of care for trauma patients is optimized if the prehospital personnel communicate the details regarding the child's injuries directly to the hospital personnel. This information may include details about the mechanism of injury, forces involved, time elapsed from the event, loss of consciousness, estimated blood loss, treatment given, and a summary of suspected injuries.

As trauma systems have evolved and EDs have become overwhelmed by larger patient volumes, effective triage for the pediatric trauma patient has become increasingly important. Care of

traumatically injured children requires the use of significant personnel and resources from many services, including the operating room and ancillary services such as diagnostic imaging and transfusion services.[28] Inappropriate triage may waste precious resources and potentially limit access to patients most in need if every patient with traumatic injuries, regardless of their severity, is sent to a trauma center. Conversely, not recognizing that a child must be brought to a trauma center may increase morbidity and result in preventable deaths.[29,30]

The Glasgow Coma Scale (GCS) (E-Table 38-1) and the modified GCS for children (Table 38-2) are the most common scales used to estimate the severity of neurologic injury. The GCS

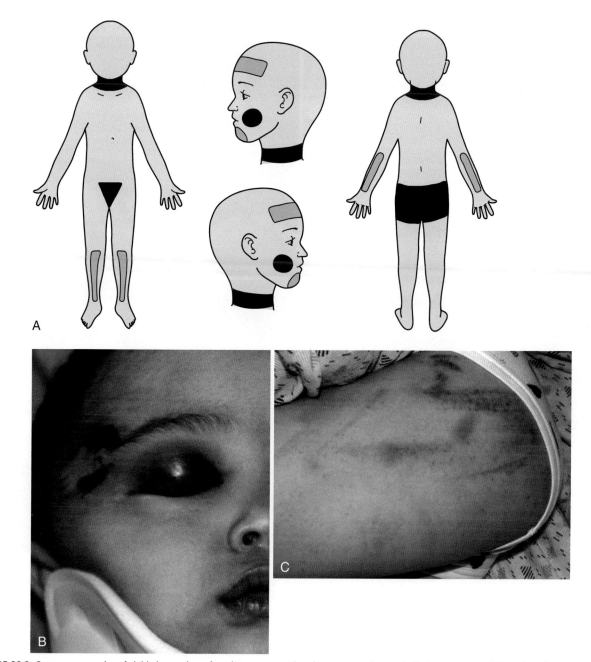

**FIGURE 38-2** Common examples of child abuse, also referred to as nonaccidental trauma, are shown. **A,** Typical areas on children where bruising can be caused by daily living activities. The *blue areas* indicate regions where normal bruising may occur. The *black areas* are regions of unusual bruising. Any bruise in the black areas must be considered for possible child abuse. Cutaneous manifestations of child abuse vary. **B,** A child with obvious facial trauma. **C,** A whipping injury from a belt plus additional bruises.                                                              *Continued*

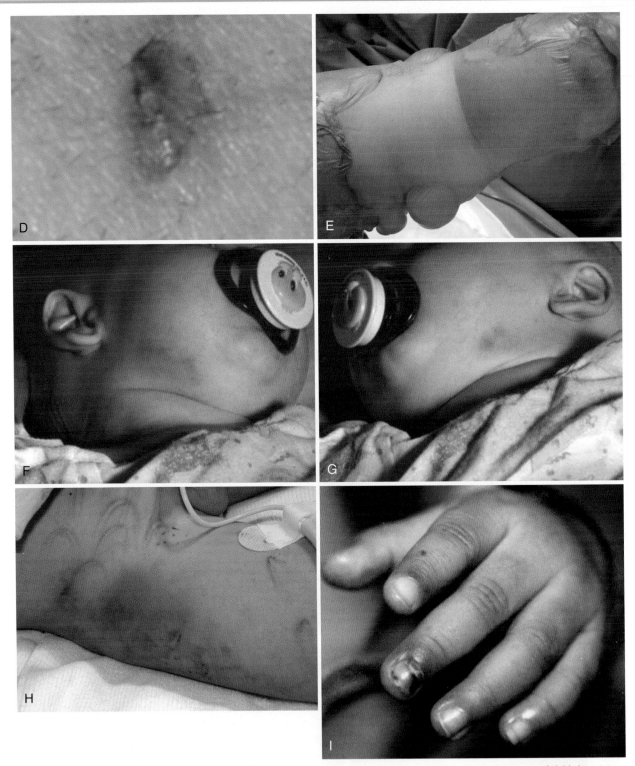

**FIGURE 38-2, cont'd D,** A cigarette burn. **E,** An immersion burn; notice sparing of the popliteal fossa, which is typical of this type of child abuse injury. **F** and **G,** Facial bruises. **H,** Whipping injury from an electrical cord. **I,** Unusual finger injuries in an infant. (Photographs courtesy of several child advocates from several institutions who asked to remain anonymous.)

assigns a total score with a range of 3 to 15 that quantifies eye opening, verbal, and motor functions. The Pediatric Trauma Score (PTS) was developed to facilitate the initial assessment and triage of injured children (Table 38-3). As trauma systems have matured and prehospital providers have become more experienced with assessment and field management, the GCS and PTS have emerged as effective tools for determination of appropriate direct transfer to a trauma center.[31,32]

## PREHOSPITAL AIRWAY MANAGEMENT

Effective airway management in the prehospital environment has many challenges, including poor access to the child, lack of use

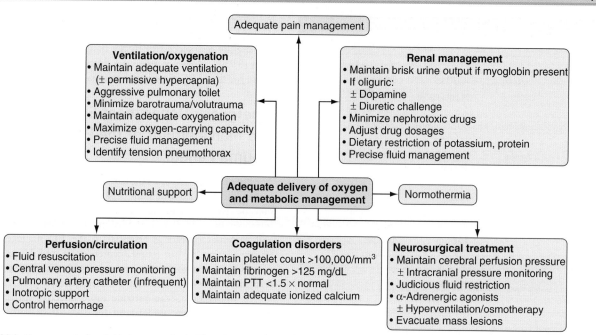

**FIGURE 38-3** Management of pediatric trauma patients. The primary goals are delivery of oxygen, appropriate ventilation, perfusion to vital organs, maintenance of normothermia to mild hypothermia, stability of renal and neurologic function, correction of coagulopathies, avoidance of overhydration, and meticulous management of metabolic demands. (Modified from Todres ID, Fugate JH, editors. Critical care of infants and children. Boston: Little, Brown; 1996, p. 17.)

**TABLE 38-2** Modification of the Glasgow Coma Scale for Pediatric Patients

| Type of Response | Score* | AGE-RELATED RESPONSES | | |
|---|---|---|---|---|
| | | *>1 Year* | *<1 Year* | |
| Eye-opening response | 4 | Spontaneous | Spontaneous | |
| | 3 | To verbal command | To shout | |
| | 2 | To pain | To pain | |
| | 1 | None | None | |
| | | *>1 Year* | *<1 Year* | |
| Motor response | 6 | Obeys commands | Spontaneous | |
| | 5 | Localizes pain | Localizes pain | |
| | 4 | Withdraws to pain | Withdraws to pain | |
| | 3 | Abnormal flexion to pain (decorticate) | Abnormal flexion to pain (decorticate) | |
| | 2 | Abnormal extension to pain (decorticate) | Abnormal extension to pain (decorticate) | |
| | 1 | None | None | |
| | | *>5 Years* | *2-5 Years* | *0-2 Years* |
| Verbal response | 5 | Oriented and converses | Appropriate words, phrases | Babbles, coos appropriately |
| | 4 | Confused conversation | Inappropriate words | Cries but is consolable |
| | 3 | Inappropriate words | Persistent crying or screaming to pain | Persistent crying or screaming to pain |
| | 2 | Incomprehensive sounds | Grunts or moans to pain | Grunts or moans to pain |
| | 1 | None | None | None |

Modified from James HE, Trauner DA. The Glasgow Coma Scale. In: James HE, Anas NG, Perkin RM, editors. Brain insults in infants and children. Orlando: Grune & Stratton; 1985, p. 179-82.
*Scoring: severe, <9; moderate, 9-12; mild, 13-15.

of pharmacologic agents, inclement weather conditions, trauma to the face, and providing care in challenging environments such as an ambulance. Several studies of adult patients undergoing tracheal intubation in the prehospital setting have reported an increased incidence of difficult tracheal intubation,[33] need for multiple attempts,[34] and undiagnosed esophageal intubation.

These events have been reported by all levels of providers, including anesthesiologists.[35] However, anesthesiologists have increased success rates and lower complication rates during tracheal intubation compared with other providers.[36-38]

Unsuccessful prehospital airway management in children may be due to a combination of training, experience, equipment, and

**TABLE 38-3** Pediatric Trauma Score

| | SCORE | | | |
|---|---|---|---|---|
| Factor | +2 | +1 | −1 | Totals* |
| Size (weight) | >20 kg | 10-20 kg | <10 kg | |
| Airway | Normal | Maintainable | Not maintainable | |
| Systolic blood pressure | >90 mm Hg | 90-50 mm Hg | <50 mm Hg | |
| Central nervous system | Awake | Obtunded or loss of consciousness | Comatose | |
| Open wound | None | Minor | Major or penetrating | |
| Skeletal trauma | None | Closed fracture | Open or multiple fractures | |

*The Pediatric Trauma Score is the sum of all rows. Scoring: minor injury, 12 (maximum); severe injury, <7; uniformly fatal, −6 (minimum).

environmental issues. A significant proportion of the unsuccessful prehospital tracheal intubations result from ineffective operator training and lack of professional experience. Most prehospital providers, such as paramedics, receive minimal dedicated training in pediatric airway management, including tracheal intubation.[39] These providers may not have an opportunity to use their skills on a routine basis. Over time, the psychomotor skills required for pediatric tracheal intubation decay, which likely contributes to the increased complication and failure rates associated with tracheal intubation in children.

Guidelines have proposed that avoidance of airway instrumentation in the prehospital setting may be just as effective as tracheal intubation for pediatric trauma patients. For example, the American Heart Association Pediatric Advanced Life Support (PALS) guidelines state, "Bag-mask ventilation can be as effective as ventilation through an endotracheal tube for short periods and may be safer."[40] The 2010 PALS guidelines state, "In the prehospital setting, ventilate and oxygenate infants and children with a bag-mask device, especially if transport time is short."[40] As a result, many EMS personnel have developed policies containing a scoop and run philosophy for pediatric trauma patients that avoid definitive airway management if the transport time is brief and bag-mask ventilation is effective. Several investigators have also questioned whether prehospital tracheal intubation is the best approach in children who require positive-pressure ventilation. The infrequent need for tracheal intubation in pediatric trauma patients has created obstacles for members of the emergency medical teams to maintain their skills. Multiple studies have demonstrated an increased mortality rate or worsening neurologic outcomes for adult patients who received prehospital tracheal intubation compared with those who received standard bag-mask ventilation.[41,42] Several studies that focused on children also reported increased complication rates associated with prehospital tracheal intubation.[43-46]

There is a trend for using alternative airway devices in the field in adult and pediatric trauma patients. Among the devices that have found favor, supraglottic airway devices have proved easy to use and reliable in the field. Although these devices do not protect the airway from regurgitation and aspiration, they may prevent airway obstruction during transport. One meta-analysis of prehospital alternative airway devices in adults and children

indicated that LMAs were very successful in the hands of anesthesiologists and nonphysician flight crews (success rate of 96%) and slightly less successful in the hands of nonphysician clinicians (83%).[47] However, there is a dearth of evidence to support a role for the LMA in pediatric trauma.

## Emergency Department Evaluation and Management of the Pediatric Trauma Patient

Anesthesiologists should familiarize themselves with the initial management of pediatric trauma patients in the ED because they may be asked to assist in emergency airway management and intraoperative care. Rapid establishment of provisional diagnoses and priorities of care is essential in the ED management of trauma victims.[48] Most trauma centers use a multilayered assessment system consisting of a primary survey with resuscitation, a secondary survey, and definitive management.[1]

Anesthesiologists can provide more effective intraoperative management if they understand the care of pediatric trauma patients commonly used in the ED. During initial resuscitation, a team member should attempt to obtain a history from the parents, the prehospital personnel, and perhaps the child. It should include the usual questions about drug allergies, medications, and past illnesses and inquiries about loss of consciousness, estimated blood loss, and treatment rendered before arrival at the ED.

Based on the ATLS course, evaluation of the trauma patient occurs in three progressive steps: primary survey, secondary survey, and definitive care.[4] The initial evaluation of all trauma patients is the primary survey. The sequence of the primary survey can be remembered as "ABCDE": airway (A), breathing (B), circulation (C), disability (D), and exposure or environment (E). Many trauma centers have the personnel and resources to simultaneously perform several activities and have prepared trauma rooms, usually in the ED. A trauma cart should be maintained daily in the trauma room and be prepared with all necessary equipment to resuscitate a child (E-Fig. 38-1 and E-Table 38-2). In this circumstance, it would be acceptable for the primary and secondary surveys to occur simultaneously—that is, the primary survey (e.g., volume resuscitation) can occur as a part of the secondary survey (e.g., drawing blood samples).

The airway (A) should be evaluated for patency and opened using a jaw-thrust technique if obstruction is encountered. Immobilization of the cervical spine should be maintained. The child's breathing (B) and ventilation should be evaluated, and immediate intervention should take place if they are inadequate. Circulation (C) is evaluated by palpation of peripheral pulses, blood pressure, sensorium, and skin turgor. Control of external hemorrhage by the application of direct pressure is also part of the circulation phase. Disability (D) is evaluated by examining the child for neurologic injuries. A GCS score of 8 or less implies severe neurologic injury (see Table 38-2), and immediate intubation (with in-line neck stabilization if indicated) is strongly recommended. Exposure (E) of the whole child is essential for a complete examination. The environment (E) should consist of a heated treatment area that is ideally prepared in advance of the child's arrival.

The importance of an adequate and secure airway cannot be overemphasized. All trauma patients should initially receive 100% supplemental oxygen. Tracheal intubation of most children

with major trauma occurs by using a rapid-sequence induction (RSI) with appropriate medications or, in some situations, while the child remains awake. When increased ICP is suspected, measures to prevent further increases during tracheal intubation should be undertaken. Regardless of site or mode of tracheal intubation, proper position and patency of the tracheal tube must be confirmed as soon as the child arrives in the ED.[49] Techniques to verify correct tracheal tube position may initially include auscultation, direct laryngoscopy, and determination of the tracheal tube length from the lips and the detection of end-tidal carbon dioxide (E-Fig. 38-2). All children should be monitored with frequent blood pressure measurements and continuous electrocardiography and pulse oximetry.

In trauma patients, shock is most commonly the result of hypovolemia. Cardiogenic shock, although rare in children, may be associated with chest trauma or preexisting cardiovascular disease. Attempts should be made to place two large-bore intravenous lines that are appropriate for age. One strategy for a child who has hypotension is to administer an initial bolus of 20 mL/kg of an isotonic crystalloid solution such as lactated Ringer's solution or normal saline. Fluid administration may be repeated with additional boluses of isotonic crystalloid as required to stabilize the blood pressure into the normal range. Blood products should be considered when the volume of isotonic crystalloid surpasses 40 to 60 mL/kg and the blood pressure remains unstable. Glucose-containing solutions usually should not be administered because they may produce unacceptable hyperglycemia and worsen the neurologic outcome.

For traumatic injuries that are primarily located in the abdomen, attempts should be made to place intravenous access in the upper extremities. Traumatic injuries that are located in the chest should have vascular access placed in the upper and lower extremities to account for disruption of a major vessel above or below the right atrium. If vascular access cannot be obtained promptly, femoral venous or intraosseous access should be strongly considered (see Fig. 48-6, *A-D*, and E-Fig. 48-1, *A-E*).[50]

When the primary survey and initial resuscitation have been completed, a secondary survey is initiated. The secondary survey is a complete head-to-toe examination designed to identify additional injuries not recognized during the primary survey. Frequent reassessment of the vital signs is critical during this phase. If clinical deterioration occurs, the primary survey and initial resuscitation should be repeated. Head examination should include visual inspection, palpation, assessment of pupillary size and reactivity, and a funduscopic examination. The cervical spine, chest, and abdomen should be evaluated in detail. Chest examination should involve inspection for wounds, palpation for tenderness and crepitance, and auscultation for bilateral breath sounds. The abdomen should also be examined carefully. In children, the physical signs of intraabdominal injuries can be subtle, especially in sedated or neurologically depressed children. The extremities should be inspected for tenderness, bruising, deformities, and vascular insufficiency.

Diagnostic testing is completed during the secondary survey.[51,52] Imaging studies, including computed tomography (CT) scans of the brain, neck, chest, abdomen, and pelvis, may be obtained, along with a bedside focused abdominal sonography for trauma (FAST) examination, which is used to detect intraperitoneal free fluid. Standard radiographs of the chest and extremities may also be obtained during the secondary survey. Laboratory studies, including blood count, electrolytes, and blood product crossmatching, are completed during the secondary survey. If the child remains unstable despite aggressive resuscitation, the patient should be considered for emergent transfer to the operating room for surgical intervention. After the child has been stabilized and all injuries have been identified, plans for definitive care can be made. This may include admission to the intensive care unit, an acute care bed, or an observation unit; discharge home with outpatient follow-up and consultation with specialists; or transfer to the operating room.

## Anesthesia Management of the Pediatric Trauma Patient

Anesthesiologists, surgeons, and other personnel should work as a coordinated team when managing children with trauma. This collaborative approach can optimize the prompt and reliable identification of suspected injuries so that the anesthesiologist can more effectively anticipate the magnitude of bleeding, physiologic effects, and nature of the surgical procedures. By understanding the appropriate evaluation and initial management of the pediatric trauma patient, the anesthesiologist can recognize injuries that might have been undiagnosed and anticipate the resultant effects intraoperatively.[53]

The approach to diagnosis and treatment for the pediatric trauma patient is dictated by the degree of urgency (see Fig. 38-3). For critically ill and hypotensive children who need immediate surgical intervention, resuscitation and the administration of anesthesia may need to be provided simultaneously. Basic principles are applied in this circumstance, including establishment and protection of the airway, maintenance of adequate ventilation, and support of hemodynamics with fluids, blood products, and vasoactive medications. Establishment of generous vascular access is recommended in the critically injured child; this may necessitate a vascular cutdown or placement of an intraosseous needle for volume resuscitation. Anesthetic medications should be cautiously administered in this situation by carefully titrating the dose of the medication to the child's hemodynamic status.

For the child who requires emergent transfer to the operating room, does not have a secure airway in place, and is not anticipated to have a difficult airway, induction of anesthesia should begin with preoxygenation and be followed by intravenous RSI. If the child is thought to be hypovolemic, a preoperative fluid bolus of balanced salt solution (20 mL/kg) should be administered before induction of anesthesia and drugs selected that maintain circulatory homeostasis. If concern exists regarding a possible cervical spine injury, which applies to most trauma patients, the practitioner should also incorporate in-line immobilization of the cervical spine during airway management and all transfers (Fig. 38-4).[54] Arterial and central venous line placements should be selected on a case-by-case basis. The anesthesiologist should be vigilant for the development of undiagnosed traumatic injuries that may manifest in the operating room. For a child who is critically ill, surgery should proceed without delay, and monitoring may initially include only a blood pressure cuff, pulse oximeter, and electrocardiogram.

As conditions permit, hemodynamic monitoring with arterial and central venous catheters may be established. Arterial catheters for trauma patients may be helpful in some situations, including concern about the adequacy of ventilation and need to frequently sample arterial blood gases, the need for frequent and repeated blood sampling (i.e., severe hemorrhage or

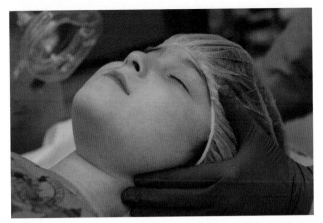

**FIGURE 38-4** Cervical spine control must be maintained during intubation. The child with a cervical spine injury requiring a definitive airway should be intubated under controlled circumstances. A neurosurgeon or the primary trauma physician should stabilize the head and neck during intubation. Oral intubation is the preferred route. In-line stabilization before attempts at laryngoscopy should be made so that the head is stabilized and prevented from rotating from side to side and from flexion and extension. No traction should be placed on the cervical spine because it is associated with increased neurologic deficits in patients with proven cervical fractures.

metabolic derangements), hemodynamic instability; and the need to alter the blood pressure rapidly. In a setting with significant actual or anticipated blood loss, establishment of large-bore venous access is of much greater priority than obtaining arterial access. Establishment of central venous access may be delayed until hemodynamic stability is established, because peripheral venous lines typically can be obtained quickly and provide effective volume resuscitation. Rotating the neck to place an internal jugular central line in a trauma patient with a possible cervical spine injury should be avoided.

After oxygenation, ventilation, and circulation have been stabilized, the anesthesiologist may need to address other concerns. If it has not been possible to administer acceptable doses of anesthetic medications, they are administered in stepwise increments after hemodynamic stability has been achieved. Evidence from adult victims of major trauma indicates that recall is more common in these cases. It is reasonable to assume that a similar risk holds true in children.[55-57] An intravenous dose of midazolam is strongly recommended,[58] although a single agent may be insufficient to guarantee amnesia. If inhalational anesthetics cannot be tolerated, the anesthesiologist may include a ketamine infusion (1 to 5 mg/kg/hr, titrated to the child's hemodynamic responses; infants may require up to 15 mg/kg/hr).

An important principle is maintenance of body temperature. Hypothermia occurs commonly in victims of major trauma. Hypothermia may potentiate neuromuscular blockade, exacerbate coagulopathy, and contribute to delayed emergence, although moderate hypothermia (34.5° C) may be protective in children with traumatic brain injury.[59] Measures to warm the child should be instituted as early as possible. They include warming the blood products and intravenous fluids, using forced-air warming devices and heat lamps, wrapping the head and extremities in plastic bags, and increasing the temperature of the operating room. Ideally, the operating room should be warmed in advance of the child's arrival to minimize radiant heat loss.

The features and mechanisms of trauma are different in children and adults. In children, abdominal trauma is more common than thoracic trauma, and blunt traumatic injuries are more common than penetrating traumatic injuries. In thoracic trauma, hemothorax and pneumothorax are common; needle decompression followed by chest tube placement may be lifesaving for a tension pneumothorax. Strong consideration should be given to needle decompression or the placement of a chest tube before instituting positive-pressure ventilation in a child with a tension pneumothorax. The greater mobility of the mediastinum in children makes it more likely for tension pneumothorax to occur and to produce hemodynamic instability. Chest injuries in children may be overlooked because rib fractures are less common than in adults.[60]

Head injury is the most common cause of traumatic death in children.[61] Although the principles of managing head injuries in polytrauma patients are mostly similar in adults and children, there are some differences. In neonates and infants, unlike adults, intracranial bleeding can lead to hypovolemic shock because the head is a significantly larger fraction of the body. The open fontanelles in children may provide greater compliance and a potential space for a proportionately larger amount of blood to accumulate. However, the open fontanelles may also provide additional protection against initial increases in ICP. A key goal for children with neurosurgical emergencies is maintenance of hemodynamic stability to preserve cerebral perfusion pressure. A child with suspected intracranial hemorrhage is at risk for increased ICP. Acute treatment for increased ICP due to intracranial hemorrhage includes hyperventilation, intravenous administration of hyperosmolar medications such as hypertonic saline, administration of medications such as opioids, cerebrospinal fluid drainage, and surgical removal of an intracranial hematoma.

## PREOPERATIVE EVALUATION

Advances in health care have produced an increased patient population with significant preinjury comorbid conditions. For example, children with repaired congenital heart disease may become victims of a traumatic injury. It is common for an acutely injured child to have a preexisting diagnosis of a medical condition such as asthma, developmental delay, seizure disorder, and significant psychosocial issues exacerbated by an unstable home environment. Each of these issues must be carefully considered when planning appropriate anesthesia management.

Emergency surgery is a great source of fear and anxiety for children and their parents.[62] The unexpectedness of the event provides little time for the child and family to adjust to the crisis and often limits the time the anesthesiologist has to develop rapport with the child and parents. The anesthesiologist who appears calm and reassuring is of great benefit to all parties.

If the child's condition permits, the preoperative evaluation should include a complete assessment. Vital signs should be stable and appropriate for age. Sensorium, urine output, skin turgor, and vital signs can be used to evaluate and estimate the child's preoperative volume status. A comprehensive airway evaluation should be done, including assessing the cervical spine. The medical and surgical history is obtained when possible. A list of previous injuries and interventions should be acquired before entering the operating room. Special attention to fluid management helps to estimate preoperative volume status and assist with intraoperative fluid administration. Assessment should include review of available laboratory reports, such as

hemoglobin, electrolyte, and coagulation studies and arterial blood gas determinations, including CO-oximetry results. Diagnostic imaging studies, including plain radiographs and CT scans, should be obtained.

Evidence suggests that the gastric residual volume in children undergoing emergency surgery is greater than in those undergoing elective surgery.[63,64] There is evidence to suggest that in emergency cases, the size of the gastric residual volume (measured in milliliters per kilograms) depends in part on the time interval between the last food ingestion and the injury.[64] There is some reassurance in these numbers, but the anesthesiologist should consider these children to have a full stomach and take appropriate measures to reduce the risk of aspiration.[65-68] The possible value of $H_2$-blocking agents, metoclopramide, and clear antacids may be considered but their use in these circumstances is not evidence based.

Premedication for emergency procedures, if indicated, usually is administered by the intravenous route. Benzodiazepines, such as midazolam, may help to reduce preoperative anxiety. If pain is present, opioids may be beneficial for children who are hemodynamically stable and have no airway compromise. Other than ketamine, anesthetics rarely cause profuse secretions, and the use of antisialagogues before induction should be reserved for specific indications. The administration of premedications to alleviate pain or control anxiety must be balanced against their disadvantages, including the potential for respiratory compromise, increased sedation, or hemodynamic instability.

## CERVICAL SPINE EVALUATION

Cervical spine injuries occur less often in children than in adults and typically occur in different locations.[69] Cervical spine injuries in children tend to be located at a more cephalad spinal level than in adults, usually at or above C3. In contrast to actual injuries, pseudosubluxation of the cervical spine is a common and benign finding in children. Pseudosubluxation of the cervical spine usually occurs as the anterior displacement of C2 on C3. In the pediatric trauma patient, the examiner may need to differentiate benign pseudosubluxation from a true cervical spine injury.[70] After consultation with the surgeon, pseudosubluxation can be excluded by placing the child's head in the sniffing position and repeating the radiograph; pseudosubluxation is reduced with this maneuver. In older children, an odontoid or open mouth view can also be considered to evaluate the superior cervical vertebrae. The physician must assume a cervical spine injury exists if the child complains of tenderness in response to palpating the spinous processes of the cervical spine, if the sensorium is decreased, or if neurologic deficits are found. Any of these findings demand a neurosurgical consultation and cervical spine immobilization.

Injury to the cervical spine is less common in children than in adults because the child's spine is more elastic and mobile, and their incompletely calcified vertebrae are less likely to fracture with minor trauma. Nevertheless, the risk of spine injury is increased when the child is subjected to a substantial force from a fall or the substantial forces associated with motor vehicle crashes.[71] Any child with a suspected neck injury should have cervical spine precautions implemented (e.g., placement of a cervical collar, backboard to provide immobilization). Cervical spine immobilization (see Fig. 38-4) should always be maintained when airway management is attempted (Fig. 38-5).

Challenges in obtaining plain radiographs of the cervical spine include difficulty in obtaining a complete view of the spine

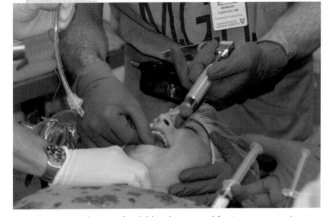

**FIGURE 38-5** Intubation of a child with a cervical fracture may require up to four individuals: one person to provide in-line stabilization, a second person to perform the intubation, a third person to perform cricoid pressure and hold the endotracheal tube or retract the cheek for the individual performing the intubation, and a fourth person to administer the medications.

below C6 and the odontoid process. As CT technology has advanced to more rapid and precise imaging, many centers have replaced standard radiographic examinations with CT scans for evaluation of the cervical spine in the trauma patient. The American College of Surgeons updated the ATLS guidelines, stating that a CT scan of the neck can be substituted for a cervical spine radiograph.[4] Replacing plain films with CT scans resulted in a doubling of the rate of cervical spine fractures identified in one study.[72]

It is challenging to rule out spinal cord injuries in children by standard radiography alone because up to 50% of spinal cord injuries may exist without positive radiographic findings. However, spinal cord injury without radiographic abnormality (SCIWORA) has been estimated in as many as 25% to 50% of children with spinal cord injuries.[73,74] These occult cases may reflect ligamentous damage that cannot be detected with standard radiographic examinations or CT scans but can be visualized with magnetic resonance imaging (MRI).

Imaging must be used in conjunction with the physical examination to evaluate the cervical spine, but the cervical spine cannot be considered cleared of pathology only on the basis of diagnostic imaging studies.[75,76] Appropriate spine immobilization should continue during the intraoperative and postoperative periods if the cervical spine of the child cannot be confirmed to be uninjured by a negative imaging study and by unremarkable results of the physical examination. The cervical spine cannot be considered undamaged if the child is not alert, is nonconversant, has positive neurologic deficits, has midline cervical tenderness, or has a painful, distracting injury. If the cervical spine cannot be clinically cleared in the postoperative period, MRI should be considered after the child is stable.

## AIRWAY MANAGEMENT

Children undergoing emergency surgery are assumed to have a full stomach. They often have considerable gastric contents because of a recent meal,[65] increased acid secretion, and delayed gastric emptying caused by pain, trauma, and the administration of opioids. Many experts recommend using an RSI to secure the airway to protect against pulmonary aspiration of gastric contents

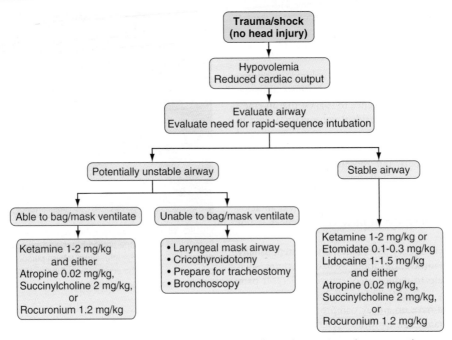

**FIGURE 38-6** Algorithm for the airway management of children with multiple trauma but without traumatic brain injury. These are commonly used doses and combinations of medications. The selection of sedatives, anxiolytics, opioids, and neuromuscular blocking agents depend on each child's condition and should be modified accordingly. (Modified from Todres ID, Fugate JH, editors. Critical care of infants and children. Boston: Little, Brown; 1996, p. 36.)

in the pediatric trauma patient. However, evidence-based data supporting this approach are lacking.[77] The anesthesiologist must balance the risks of an RSI with the risks of other airway management techniques. RSI is associated with an inability to intubate the trachea and rapid desaturation during periods of apnea. The risks of using this approach must be weighed against the benefit of reducing the risk for aspiration. The decision to use an RSI assumes that the anesthesiologist has completed an airway evaluation and predicts that the intubation will be uncomplicated and that mask ventilation while maintaining cricoid pressure will be possible as a backup temporizing measure.

In the operating room, induction of anesthesia depends on the child's injuries, condition at the time of presentation, whether the airway has been secured, and anticipated airway difficulty. The most common approach to the initial airway management is to follow a protocol for RSI.[78,79] Awake intubation is another approach for airway management and usually is reserved for those with severely depressed consciousness, cardiac arrest, or suspected difficult airway. The selection of medications depends on individual circumstances (e.g., head injury, hypovolemia, contraindication to succinylcholine) and preferences of the anesthesiologist. Table 38-4 lists dosages, advantages, and disadvantages of selected anesthetic medications for RSI. Figure 38-6 presents an algorithm for management of children with multiple traumatic injuries but without a suspected traumatic brain injury. Specific considerations for children with multiple trauma that include a traumatic brain injury are outlined in Figure 38-7.

Before an RSI is performed, the anesthesiologist must ensure that the proper equipment is present and functioning, including laryngoscope blades and handles, suction, a leak-free anesthesia circuit, an anesthesia machine, monitors, tracheal tubes of appropriate sizes, and a tracheal tube stylet. All monitors should be properly functioning, and at a minimum, the pulse oximeter and blood pressure cuff should be applied before induction, even though these monitors may not function properly in a crying,

uncooperative child until after induction of anesthesia. After intravenous access is confirmed, the child's lungs are denitrogenated with 100% oxygen for several breaths (as tolerated). Studies of adult patients demonstrate that oxygen saturation remains greater than 95% for 6 minutes after only four vital capacity breaths of 100% oxygen by mask.[80] Similar studies have not been performed in children, although the rates at which the $PaO_2$ decreases[81] and the $SaO_2$ decreases to 95%[82] in infants and younger children after breathing 100% oxygen through a tracheal tube and then performing an apnea maneuver was more rapid than in older children and adults. Even with an uncooperative child, it is possible to increase the $PaO_2$ by enriching the immediate environment with high flows of oxygen. Preoxygenation should not involve forcefully holding the facemask on the awake child; this will likely result in increased anxiety, increased oxygen consumption, and decreased effectiveness of denitrogenation. Premedication (e.g., 0.05 to 0.1 mg/kg of intravenous midazolam) in divided doses may be considered to alleviate fear and anxiety before induction. All drugs intended for use during the RSI should be prepared and labeled along with the doses predetermined for the child's weight and hemodynamic status.

RSI consists of preoxygenation with 100% oxygen and application of cricoid pressure, followed by the bolus administration of an induction agent such as ketamine (2 mg/kg), etomidate (0.2 to 0.3 mg/kg), or propofol (2 to 3 mg/kg), as well as atropine (20 µg/kg) if succinylcholine is selected and along with a neuromuscular blocking agent such as succinylcholine (2 mg/kg) or high-dose rocuronium (1.2 mg/kg), depending on the age of the child. This is followed immediately by laryngoscopy and tracheal intubation (see Chapters 4 and 12). We recommend using a modified Bier block technique with 1 mg/kg of lidocaine applied using an occlusive tourniquet for 30 to 60 seconds to prevent pain from injection before the administration of propofol or etomidate through a small peripheral vein. Positive-pressure ventilation before tracheal intubation is avoided during an RSI.

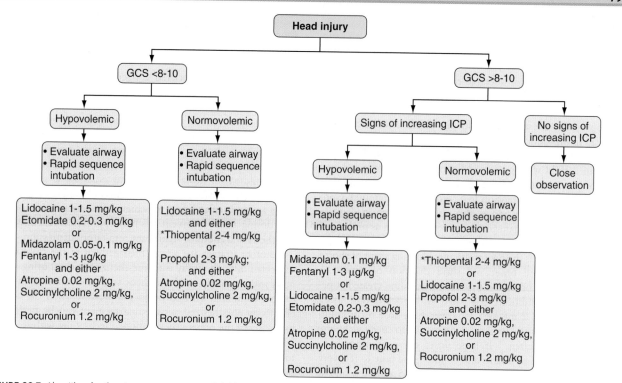

**FIGURE 38-7** Algorithm for the airway management of children with multiple trauma, including traumatic brain injury. Specific considerations to avoid increased intracranial pressure in traumatized children are outlined. *GCS,* Glasgow Coma Scale score; *ICP,* intracranial pressure. (Modified from Todres ID, Fugate JH, editors. Critical care of infants and children. Boston: Little, Brown; 1996, p. 36.) *Thiopental is no longer available in the United States.

**TABLE 38-4** Medications Used in Pediatric Trauma Patients for Rapid-Sequence Induction

| Medication | Intravenous Dose (mg/kg) | Advantages | Disadvantages |
|---|---|---|---|
| Atropine | 0.01-0.02 | Attenuates vagal response | Flushed skin, tachycardia, mild hyperpyrexia; possible sedation/agitation |
| Glycopyrrolate | 0.01 | Attenuates vagal response and antisialogogue; lacks sedation/agitation | Longer acting |
| Lidocaine | 1-1.5 | Attenuates hemodynamic and intracranial responses to intubation | Can cause toxicity in large doses (e.g., >5 mg/kg) |
| Fentanyl | 0.001-0.003 | Analgesic and attenuates hemodynamic and intracranial responses to intubation | Can cause bradycardia, chest wall and glottic rigidity |
| Midazolam | 0.05-0.2 | Sedation, amnesia, anxiolysis | May cause hypotension when combined with opioids in hypovolemic patients |
| Thiopental* | 3-5 | Sedative-hypnotic, some neuroprotective properties | May decrease blood pressure, increase heart rate, decrease cardiac output; usually avoided in hypovolemic patients |
| Ketamine | 1-2 | Sympathomimetic, used when hypovolemia is suspected | Increases oral secretions (administer with atropine or glycopyrrolate to reduce secretions), may increase intracranial pressure |
| Propofol | 1-3 | Sedative-hypnotic, some neuroprotective properties | May cause hypotension |
| Etomidate | 0.2-0.3 | Hemodynamic stability with no cardiac depression, some neuroprotective properties, used in patients with hypovolemia and cardiac instability | Possible adrenal suppression |
| Rocuronium | 0.6-1.2 | Rapid onset (with high doses), vagolytic properties; is a substitute for succinylcholine; sugammadex rapidly reverses neuromuscular blockade if "cannot intubate, cannot ventilate" occurs | Intermediate to long duration depending on dose; in the absence of sugammadex, neuromuscular blockade cannot be quickly antagonized if the airway is lost |
| Succinylcholine | 2 (precede with atropine or glycopyrrolate) | Rapid onset and ultra-short duration | May cause bradycardia if not preceded by an anticholinergic; may cause hyperkalemia in children with muscular dystrophy, crush injury, prolonged immobilization, burns, intraabdominal sepsis and upper and lower motor neuron lesions; may increase intracranial pressure and gastric pressures |

*Thiopental is no longer available in the United States.

Cervical spine immobilization is typically indicated for most trauma patients during RSI (see Fig. 38-4) and requires an assistant to perform manual in-line stabilization during laryngoscopy (see Fig. 38-5).

An RSI can be a considerable risk for children with cardiovascular problems such as hypovolemia or congenital heart disease. When performing an RSI, it may be difficult to select the appropriate anesthetic dose for the child's needs because it may lead to profound hypotension due to myocardial depression and vasodilation. Strategies for dosing intravenous induction agents in a child with presumed hypovolemia include reduced doses of propofol (e.g., 1 mg/kg) or using agents that are less likely to produce hypotension (e.g., etomidate, ketamine). Conversely, severe hypertension is also possible due to inadequate dosing during airway management procedures such as prolonged direct laryngoscopy.

Succinylcholine is the neuromuscular blocking agent of choice because of its rapid onset and short duration of action. A Cochrane Review concluded that succinylcholine created superior intubating conditions compared with rocuronium using doses of less than 1.2 mg/kg.[83] However, high-dose rocuronium may also be effectively used as an alternative to succinylcholine for an RSI in children.[84] If large doses of rocuronium (e.g., 1.2 mg/kg) are used in infants and children, the time to recovery of the train-of-four to 25% averages about 45 minutes, and it may take as long as 75 minutes.[84] It is possible that the duration of action may be longer than the planned procedure. Moreover, if the child's lungs are impossible to ventilate and the trachea cannot be intubated, the situation may become life-threatening. The use of high-dose sugammadex if available (see Chapter 6) can abbreviate the duration of the neuromuscular block in these situations. If rocuronium (or any nondepolarizing muscle relaxant) is combined with thiopental, the thiopental must be cleared from the intravenous tubing before administering the relaxant to prevent the former from precipitating.[85] The routine use of succinylcholine for elective tracheal intubation in children has lost popularity among pediatric anesthesiologists due to reports of hyperkalemia-induced cardiac dysrhythmias and cardiac arrest, which led the U.S. Food and Drug Administration to issue a black box warning about the use of succinylcholine in children undergoing elective surgery.[86] Many of the male children who developed hyperkalemic cardiac arrest were subsequently diagnosed with various forms of muscular dystrophy (mostly Duchenne's muscular dystrophy, which may manifest with few clinical signs in boys 8 years of age or younger).

Establishing a definitive airway may be required for children with a suspected difficult airway due to facial, laryngeal, or thoracic trauma. Alternative approaches for airway management should be considered when difficult intubation is anticipated.[87,88] In these situations, the urgency of securing the airway takes priority over the increased risk of tracheal aspiration of gastric contents. These cases can be managed by using an awake intubation approach, which commonly includes topical anesthesia and sedation combined with one of the following airway techniques:

- Awake intubation under direct laryngoscopy or rigid bronchoscopy
- A lighted stylet
- Indirect laryngoscopy using a fiberoptic bronchoscope (FOB) or video laryngoscope
- Supraglottic airway device–assisted tracheal intubation with or without an FOB
- Awake tracheostomy

In a nonemergent situation, the FOB is the gold standard approach to manage a difficult airway. An FOB can be very effective, especially in children with limited mouth opening, restricted neck movement (common in the trauma patient with a cervical collar in place), or associated congenital syndromes that make direct laryngoscopy difficult or impossible.[89,90] The alternative approaches are advantageous because their main goals are to maintain spontaneous ventilation, to maintain oropharyngeal reflexes to prevent aspiration if regurgitation occurs, and to allow the option of aborting the procedure if the airway cannot be secured. However, these airway techniques can be challenging in small children, in those whose airway anatomy is severely distorted, and those with copious secretions or blood in the pharynx. Large amounts of sedation to achieve effective patient cooperation during airway interventions may approach levels of general anesthesia and produce significant respiratory depression.

Another strategy for airway management in the child with a suspected difficult airway is to anesthetize the child using a facemask with an inhalational anesthetic such as sevoflurane in 100% oxygen combined with gentle cricoid pressure. After the child is effectively anesthetized, airway management can be performed using any of the previously mentioned techniques with the child breathing spontaneously. In addition to or instead of using an inhalational anesthetic, total intravenous anesthesia (TIVA) can be used with medications such as propofol or dexmedetomidine while maintaining spontaneous respirations during instrumentation of the airway. An infusion of ketamine can provide sedation and analgesia while maintaining spontaneous respirations, although glycopyrrolate may be required to attenuate increased production of oral secretions.

In emergency situations, blind placement of a supraglottic airway device such as an LMA is recommended as part of the American Society of Anesthesiologists' difficult airway algorithm.[91] The LMA does not protect the airway from tracheal aspiration of gastric contents, but it may be used as a conduit to facilitate blind or fiberoptic intubation of the trachea.[92] The development of an LMA (LMA North America, San Diego, Calif.) with a modified cuff and drainage tube (ProSeal) and that is available in sizes 1 to 5 may make this process even safer by allowing evacuation of gastric contents and providing a better airway seal than earlier LMA devices.[93,94] The Fastrach LMA (LMA North America) provides an additional supraglottic device that is useful when direct visualization of the laryngeal inlet is not possible. This device has been designed to blindly place a tracheal tube into the trachea from within the supraglottic airway.[95] However, this is only of benefit in children larger than 30 kg because pediatric sizes (1 to 2) are not available.

## CRICOID PRESSURE

Cricoid pressure was popularized for RSI by Sellick in his seminal report in 1961,[96] which carefully described the position of the head and neck during the maneuver. The patient assumes the supine position with the neck fully extended in a slight head-down tilt, and the nasogastric tube, if present, is removed. The concavity of the cervical neck is maintained during cricoid pressure using a firm support placed under the cervical spine. Cricoid pressure is applied by an assistant using the thumb and second finger; the first finger stabilizes the thumb and finger on the cricoid ring. Pressure is applied firmly as consciousness is lost and released only after the tracheal tube cuff has been inflated.

In current practice, the head and neck are often not positioned as described by Sellick. Although Sellick's preliminary

38

evidence suggested that his technique was very effective for occluding the esophagus, there have been no randomized, controlled trials that document its effectiveness or its superiority over other techniques in preventing aspiration during RSI.[97,98] Radiologic evidence suggests that cricoid pressure may not completely occlude the lumen of the esophagus because the contours of the vertebral bodies are asymmetric and the esophagus is not aligned directly over the vertebral bodies.[99] The application of cricoid pressure in children may result in even further lateral displacement of the esophagus than it does in adults.[100] Sellick never described the amount of force required to occlude the lumen of the esophagus, although in adults, a force of 30 to 40 N (equivalent to a 3- to 4-kg mass) is considered sufficient to occlude the esophagus. In a study of the force required to occlude the esophagus in infants, investigators determined that a force of only 5 N distorts the airway in infants weighing less than 5 kg and that a force of only 12 N produces the same distortion in 15-year-old adolescents.[101] This begs the question of how much force is required to reliably occlude the esophagus without distorting the airway in infants and children. The answer is unknown.

Many assistants who perform cricoid pressure apply insufficient force,[102] apply force at an incorrect location[103] or use excessive force that may distort the larynx and make tracheal intubation more difficult. One study found that correctly applied cricoid pressure in children 2 weeks to 8 years of age with or without paralysis resulted in no leak of air into the stomach with up to 40 cm $H_2O$ of peak inflation pressure.[104]

In children, the application of cricoid pressure has been viewed with some skepticism because the force required has been considered excessive in younger children. However, in the current medicolegal climate, many have perceived an obligation on their part to apply it to prevent regurgitation. In support of this perception, the results of a survey documented that even though 71% do not believe cricoid pressure occludes the esophagus, 90% use it when there is an increased risk for aspiration.[105]

## VOLUME ADMINISTRATION

Better understanding of the mechanisms of the stress response and particularly of the factors that contribute to sepsis and ongoing proliferation of proinflammatory cytokines has helped redefine the immediate and long-term goals of acute resuscitation and definitive management of the unstable trauma patient.[106] The original concept of resuscitation was restoration of adequate circulating volume with appropriate red cell mass and adequate oxygenation, but this has evolved to become a continuum of critical care focused on restoration of total body homeostasis. The initial priority is focused on hemodynamic stabilization and should progress seamlessly to the aggressive management of metabolic derangements. The anesthesiologist who is involved in immediate resuscitation of the severely injured child should focus on these initial hemodynamic goals.

The preservation of intravascular volume is a primary priority during resuscitation of the severely injured child. When immediate surgical intervention in the operating room is not necessary, it is advisable to replace fluid deficits before induction of anesthesia. Mild to moderate deficits can be replaced with isotonic crystalloid solutions. In severe hypovolemia with ongoing blood loss, colloids such as 5% albumin can be considered for use as an intravascular volume expander along with packed red blood cells. If time permits and if clinically indicated, crossmatched blood products should be administered, starting with an initial dose of 10 mL/kg. Type-specific uncrossmatched blood has a

very low incidence of transfusion reactions and is typically available before crossmatched blood.[107] In an emergency situation requiring the immediate transfusion of blood products, type O negative packed red blood cells should be administered if the ABO blood type of the child has not been determined.

Life-threatening exsanguination is most commonly caused by a massive disruption of the solid viscera or major vascular structures within the abdomen and chest. The most important part of this resuscitation process is restoration of adequate red cell mass and circulating volume to promote effective tissue perfusion and oxygenation. Evaluation of 103,434 cases in phases II and III of the National Pediatric Trauma Registry (NPTR) study suggests that massive exsanguination is relatively uncommon.[108] Children who sustain massive exsanguinating injuries typically die at the scene.

If volume resuscitation is vigorous and large volumes of crystalloid solutions are administered, hemorrhage-induced red blood cell loss may be further exacerbated by dilution with crystalloids. Overzealous fluid resuscitation may worsen bleeding by abrupt elevation of the systolic blood pressure from circulatory expansion that disrupts clots from injured vessels. Clinical evidence of this has been limited to assessment of penetrating injury in adults and elective cardiac surgery, emphasizing the necessity of a proper balance between restoration of adequate peripheral perfusion and avoidance of gross fluid overload.[109-110] Effective circulatory resuscitation of the injured child requires a combination of clinical data, anticipation of pending physiologic challenges, and coordination of planned operative interventions by all specialists involved in the child's acute care. Large-volume transfusions without consideration of coagulation status, electrolyte shifts, or critical serum protein depletion may produce coagulopathy. Injudicious or inadequate crystalloid infusions may worsen capillary leak locally in injured organs and remotely in the interstitium of lung and brain. It is postulated that the concentrations of systemic inflammatory mediators increase after traumatic injuries. Increased serum secretory phospholipase $A_2$ levels have been associated with increased injury magnitudes in patients after traumatic injuries,[111] and increased plasma high-mobility group box 1 (HMGB1) levels have been identified after traumatic injuries, although clear correlations with patient outcomes were not established.[112]

Injured children tend to be reasonably free of the acquired cardiovascular diseases that complicate the care of injured adults. However, transient myocardial ischemia can quickly undermine contractility of even the healthiest heart. In the presence of cardiovascular collapse from massive or ongoing hemorrhage, this can rapidly lead to cardiac failure and peripheral hypoperfusion. Children who are being resuscitated from major hemorrhage and who have been exposed to prolonged low flow states may require inotropic support to maintain adequate peripheral perfusion. Because an accurate definition for what was previously referred to as myocardial contusion is not easily quantifiable, a high index of suspicion based on an understanding of the child's mechanism of injury is the best guide to preemptive management, especially if rhythm disturbances are observed.[113,114]

Studies are being conducted to determine the ideal products and dosing schedules for fluid resuscitation of injured children. Several studies have evaluated hypertonic saline for use as a resuscitation solution and for the management of traumatic brain injury.[115-117] Investigators from several studies suggest that no definitive recommendations can be made because no fluid product is superior.[118-120] However, children with evidence of

significant hypovolemia who are bleeding significantly and receiving isotonic crystalloids probably should be initially resuscitated with lactated Ringer's solution due to its pH of 6.6, compared with a pH of 5.5 for normal saline, although Plasmalyte has a more normal physiologic pH. The critical objectives are immediate control of the sources of hemorrhage, restoration of red cell mass to ensure adequate oxygen delivery, and appropriate rheology to enhance tissue microperfusion.

## VASCULAR ACCESS

Vascular access can be overlooked as one of the more important priorities in the initial care of injured children. In some circumstances, placement of two large-bore intravenous lines may be very challenging in the hypovolemic child. In some cases, the child arrives in the ED with no vascular access. In the setting of the ED or operating room, adequate vascular access can usually be readily obtained by a standard percutaneous approach through a peripheral vein or by direct percutaneous cannulation of the femoral vein. These two methods are consistently successful in achieving immediate vascular access without resorting to invasive cutdown techniques. The success rate for percutaneous femoral catheterizations using a Seldinger technique is so high that using a cutdown approach is rarely required (see also Fig. 48-2). If the child is severely exsanguinated and percutaneous femoral vascular access is unsuccessful, surgical exposure through an incision 1 cm below the inguinal ligament can expose the saphenous vein at the saphenofemoral junction. This provides immediate access to a large-caliber vessel and facilitates the placement of a femoral arterial line for ongoing management. Ultrasound-guided vascular access techniques may also be used to place peripheral and central lines in the venous and arterial systems.[121,122] Many trauma centers do not routinely use subclavian or internal jugular veins for vascular access during acute resuscitation. Personnel responsible for airway management usually obstruct access to the neck, as does the cervical collar that should be in place as part of standard prehospital management protocols. In an orchestrated approach, one individual or group of individuals should concentrate fully on management and support of the airway while a second group addresses access to the vascular system.

Intraosseous infusion devices are being increasingly used in adults and children for whom percutaneous vascular access is unavailable or unsuccessful.[123] In the pediatric population, intraosseous needles are usually placed in the tibial plateau medial to the tibial tuberosity approximately 3 to 5 cm below the knee. These devices can be lifesaving and usually are inserted after several attempts at venous access have failed. If appropriately placed, they are useful conduits for infusion of all medications, crystalloids, and dilute blood products.[124] Intraosseous needles should be replaced by effective and reliable venous access as soon as possible (see also Fig 48-6, A-D). Pneumatic-driven devices for placement of intraosseous needles have also been described. Some of these devices have been extraordinarily difficult to remove and require specific training from the product manufacturer; their overall usefulness remains to be evaluated. One type of intraosseous infusion device, the EZ-IO (Vidacare Corporation; San Antonio, Tex.) operates like a battery-powered drill and is relatively simple to train providers in its use (see E-Fig. 48-1, A-E).[125]

## DAMAGE CONTROL SURGERY

Children with massive anatomic derangements associated with uncontrollable hemorrhage usually require emergent operative intervention. In many trauma centers, these hemodynamically unstable children are treated by *damage control surgery*,[126] which is based on the premise that rapid control of abdominal bleeding by placing abdominal packing and immediate coverage of the open abdomen enables more effective resuscitation before exposing the child to a more prolonged definitive repair.

Over the past decade, the use of damage control surgery for the initial stabilization rather than definitive repair has moved the focus of resuscitation away from simple circulatory volume management to a need for immediate correction of whole-body metabolic derangements associated with the stress response.[127] Acute abdominal packing and coverage avoids development of abdominal compartment syndrome, allows reevaluation of the injured tissue, and provides access for repeated lavage of contaminated spaces. Although there have been concerns that this approach may be used more often than necessary, the risks of leaving an abdomen open are minimal compared with the ventilatory and circulatory consequences that may develop from an abdominal compartment syndrome. Damage control surgery has proved to be a lifesaving technique in isolated circumstances by allowing an unstable child to receive comprehensive resuscitation in a more controlled environment.

## PAIN MANAGEMENT

Acute pain occurring as a result of traumatic injuries is one of the most common adverse stimuli experienced by children.[128] There has been fear that treating pain due to trauma may mask the symptoms of progressive injury. Historically, adults have received significantly more analgesia after injuries than children.[129] As a result, many physicians withhold significant pain relief, especially opioids, because they fear serious side effects such as respiratory depression or hypotension may develop. All medications used for analgesia and sedation in children can have significant side effects; however, careful titration to the desired effect along with appropriate monitoring should ensure safe administration.

The management of acute pain in the injured child can be accomplished by using nonpharmacologic interventions and pharmacologic therapies. Nonpharmacologic interventions include positive reinforcement, distraction, hypnotherapy, acupuncture, massage and touch relaxation, and guided imagery.[130] Pharmacologic therapies include oral and intravenous acetaminophen and nonsteroidal antiinflammatory drugs (NSAIDs) for mild to moderate pain and oral and intravenous opioids for moderate to severe pain.[131] Regional anesthesia can be very useful in the acutely injured child, especially for orthopedic injuries.

Injured children are often in pain at the time of arrival in the ED. For unstable children and those with evolving neurologic dysfunction, opioids must be used with caution. In many circumstances, injured children are sufficiently stable to allow judicious administration of opioids. Opioids free of histamine release (e.g., fentanyl) are preferable to those that release histamine (e.g., morphine), especially for children who are potentially hypovolemic. Fentanyl should be titrated in small increments (e.g., 0.5 to 1.0 µg/kg) to reduce the risk for respiratory depression and side effects such as chest wall or glottic rigidity.

In certain cases, regional nerve blocks can be used to provide analgesia in the ED; as primary anesthesia in a cooperative or older child to avoid some of the risks associated with general anesthesia, including aspiration; and as a supplement to general anesthesia for postoperative analgesia.[132,133] For example, analgesia for children with midshaft fractures of the femur can be

38

provided by a traditional femoral nerve block or fascia iliaca compartment block, diminishing pain from the femur and quadriceps muscle spasm. Similarly, an axillary or supraclavicular nerve block may be used in children with forearm fractures. Central neuraxial techniques, such as epidural analgesia, can be useful for children with major thoracoabdominal trauma, including rib fractures. Close communication with orthopedic and general surgical colleagues is advised so that there are no misunderstandings about the ability to perform sensory and motor examinations and about coordination of additional analgesic medications.

## Future Directions in Pediatric Trauma

As traumatic injuries have become recognized as a significant public health threat, numerous initiatives have emerged to improve prevention of this hazard, management of its victims, and measurement of system performance and outcomes. Exciting areas of investigation continue to emerge in aspects of clinical management, systems development, patient safety, and injury prevention.[134-136]

Prevention and public education are important areas of ongoing research in pediatric trauma. There has been great progress in educating the public that many injuries are avoidable, but there are still many factors that undermine the best intentions to produce a safe and nurturing environment for children. A significant advance in effective prevention and public education has occurred through the Injury Free Coalition for Children sponsored by the Robert Wood Johnson Foundation.[137-139] This coalition has evolved into a network of 40 institutions throughout the country, and each focuses on specific areas of enhanced public education to define opportunities for improvement within the environment of children. Although there is no such thing as a completely risk-free environment, ongoing and effective public awareness campaigns can enhance the likelihood that risks to children throughout the world will diminish.

As the transition from fluid resuscitation to metabolic management has evolved, there has been increasing interest in identifying tissue-specific biomarkers that reflect the severity and prognosis of injury.[140,141] The efficacy of resuscitation could be enhanced by routine assay of biomarkers that accurately reflect levels of physiologic derangements or effective restoration of homeostasis. Numerous studies are focusing on identification of various components of neuronal tissue markers that reflect the presence and severity of brain injury.

The combination of hypovolemia, coagulopathy, hypothermia, and acidosis is associated with increased morbidity and mortality. There have been many efforts to control these issues, and most significant has been the evolution of damage control surgery. There is growing laboratory animal evidence that hypothermia, if induced in a rapid and controlled fashion, is cytoprotective.[59,142-144] In the near future, the use of hypothermia in the minutes after traumatic injury may widen the margin of safety for injured children, especially those with significant cerebral injury. This is an area that must make the transition from animal observations in the basic science laboratory to well-designed, randomized, controlled trials involving prehospital providers and established trauma programs. Emerging evidence suggests that premature death in bleeding patients with severe trauma may be attenuated by administering antifibrinolytics, such as tranexamic acid.[145-147] Institution of tranexamic acid within 3 hours of the insult, particularly in countries with low to middle incomes, is likely to have the greatest impact on outcome. However, there is insufficient evidence to recommend antifibrinolytics in patients with traumatic brain injury.[148] Randomized, controlled trials enrolling traumatized children are warranted to identify a possible role for antifibrinolytics to prevent premature death.

## Summary

Trauma remains the most common cause of death for children older than 1 year of age. Pediatric patients develop unique traumatic injuries compared with adults, resulting in the need for specific knowledge and specialized anesthesia management. Anesthesiologists may function in several essential roles in the perioperative management of the pediatric trauma patient. They may provide urgent airway management in the ED, intraoperative care in the operating room, and anesthesia and pain control in the intensive care unit. The transition from acute resuscitation to definitive care should be a seamless continuum focusing on immediate recognition of threats to life, rapid restoration of homeostasis, definitive treatment of injuries, and effective rehabilitation and convalescence.

Care of the trauma patient is a perfect example of a team-driven approach that requires thoughtful coordination and adherence to established protocols. The investment of time necessary to prepare for this level of multidisciplinary, comprehensive care produces returns in diminished mortality and enhanced quality of life for all children.

**ACKNOWLEDGMENT**
We thank J. Tepas, MD, and H. DeSoto, MD, for their prior contributions to this chapter.

## ANNOTATED REFERENCES

Bhananker SM, Ramamoorthy C, Geiduschek JM, et al. Anesthesia-related cardiac arrest in children: update from the Pediatric Perioperative Cardiac Arrest registry. Anesth Analg 2007;105:344-50.

*The update from the POCA registry compares the causes of cardiac arrest during 1998 to 2004 data to the previous data 1994 to 1997. Cardiovascular and respiratory causes continue to dominate the causes of cardiac arrest in children.*

De Ross AL, Vane DW. Early evaluation and resuscitation of the pediatric trauma patient. Semin Pediatr Surg 2004;13:74-9.

*This review article focuses on the initial treatment of the pediatric trauma patient.*

Hubble MW, Wilfong DA, Brown LH, et al. A meta-analysis of prehospital airway control techniques. Part II: alternative airway devices and cricothyrotomy success rates. Prehosp Emerg Care 2010;14:515-30.

*This review discusses airway devices that are reliable, easy to use, and easy to maintain and describes the expertise needed to use it. The laryngeal mask airway has emerged as a suitable airway for initial resuscitation of children in the field.*

Peterson K, Carson S, Carney N. Hypothermia treatment for traumatic brain injury: a systematic review and meta-analysis. J Neurotrauma 2008;25:62-71.

*This review of the evidence supports the benefit of mild to moderate hypothermia in managing traumatic brain injury for more than 48 hours. It reduces mortality and improves neurologic outcomes, although at the risk of promoting pneumonia.*

Ross AK. Pediatric trauma. Anesthesia management. Anesthesiol Clin North Am 2001;19:309-37.

*This article reviews the implications of anesthesia in managing pediatric trauma.*

## REFERENCES

Please see www.expertconsult.com.

# Cardiopulmonary Resuscitation

## 39

POOJA KULKARNI, MARILYN C. MORRIS, AND CHARLES L. SCHLEIEN

THE PEDIATRIC ANESTHESIOLOGIST must be prepared to resuscitate a child who suffers a cardiac arrest in the course of a routine elective anesthetic, during a high-risk surgery, or outside the operating room (OR) during the delivery of an anesthetic or as a vital part of the "code team." The goal of this chapter is to provide pediatric anesthesiologists with an in-depth understanding of cardiopulmonary-cerebral resuscitation physiology and recommended resuscitative techniques.

## Historical Background

In 1814, a description in poetical form of the Rules of the Humane Society for recovering drowned persons included the following description of mouth-to-mouth resuscitation[1]:

> Let one the mouth, and either nostril close
> While through the other the bellows gently blows.
> Thus the pure air with steady force convey,
> To put the flaccid lungs again in play.
> Should bellows not be found, or found too late,
> Let some kind soul with willing mouth inflate;
> Then downward, though but lightly, press the chest.
> And let the inflated air be upward prest.

External cardiac massage was successfully conducted more than 100 years ago in two children (ages 8 and 13 years) after circulatory arrest precipitated by chloroform anesthesia during a surgical procedure.[2] In 1904, Crile described the effectiveness of external cardiac compressions in maintaining the circulation of dogs.[3]

After multiple reports that attested to the effectiveness of mouth-to-mouth resuscitation,[4-6] in 1958 the National Academy of Sciences National Research Council recommended mouth-to-mouth resuscitation with maximum backward tilt of the head as the preferred technique for all individuals requiring emergency artificial ventilation. In 1960, external cardiac compression was revived as a resuscitation technique when Kouwenhoven, Jude, and Knickerbocker[7] demonstrated its effectiveness when combined with artificial respirations. Many of their patients, including the first, were in cardiac arrest as a result of anesthesia. Before this study, internal cardiac compression was the accepted technique, with its effectiveness demonstrated by experience in cardiac bypass surgery. In 1947, Beck and associates[8] successfully internally defibrillated the human heart; and in 1956, Zoll and colleagues[9] performed the first successful external defibrillation of a human heart.

## Epidemiology and Outcome of In-Hospital Cardiopulmonary Arrest

A 2009 review of cardiac arrest events submitted to the National Registry of Cardiopulmonary Circulation included 3342 pediatric events, excluding events in a delivery room or neonatal intensive care unit (NICU).[10] Seventy-three percent of the inpatient cardiac arrests reported occurred in an ICU, 7% in a general inpatient area, 11% in an emergency department, and 3% in an operating room or postanesthesia care unit. Return of spontaneous circulation (ROSC) was achieved in 65%, 24-hour survival occurred in 47%, and 30% of children survived until hospital discharge. Other large series of in-hospital pediatric cardiac arrest report survival until hospital discharge ranging from 14% to 44%,[11-14] with the 44% survival representing cardiac arrests that occurred in a pediatric cardiac ICU. In another multicenter cohort study of in-hospital pediatric cardiac arrest,[15] 48.7% of the 353 children survived until hospital discharge. Survivors had greater body temperatures, greater pH values, and reduced serum lactate concentrations compared with nonsurvivors. Nonsurvivors were more likely to have a tracheal tube before the arrest, and to receive sodium bicarbonate, calcium, and vasopressin during the arrest. In this study, postoperative cardiopulmonary resuscitation (CPR) was associated with decreased mortality.

## Diagnosis of Cardiac Arrest

For the child who suffers a cardiac arrest in the OR, electronic monitoring will generally alert the anesthesiologist to an actual or impending cardiac arrest. The electrocardiogram (ECG) may indicate nonperfusing rhythms such as ventricular fibrillation and asystole, end-tidal carbon dioxide (ETCO$_2$) may decrease precipitously reflecting a decrease in cardiac output as a result of a decreased delivery of carbon dioxide (CO$_2$) to the lungs, and a pulse oximeter may lose its regular waveform in the absence of pulsatile blood flow. Granting the importance of these monitors, the diagnosis of cardiopulmonary arrest still rests on the absence of a pulse in a major artery (e.g., carotid, femoral, or brachial artery) as determined by palpation in the presence of unconsciousness and apnea.

Attention must be paid in the early minutes of resuscitation to determining the cause of the arrest. Many children will not be successfully resuscitated without correction of the underlying cause. A focused physical examination should be conducted and a brief history elicited if it is not already known. If not present, a cardiorespiratory monitor should be placed and the ECG examined. In an intraoperative arrest, the surgeon may be able to provide clues to the diagnosis, such as excessive blood loss, compression of major blood vessels, decreasing venous return to the heart, or manipulation of anatomic structures (e.g., manipulation of the peritoneum resulting in a severe vagal bradycardia or asystole). Equipment malfunction must always be considered as a potential cause of arrest. Early in the course of an attempted resuscitation, a blood gas analysis should be performed and key electrolytes measured (ideally as point-of-care testing).

## Mechanics of Cardiopulmonary Resuscitation

Management proceeds along the well-known airway, breathing, circulation (ABC) algorithm with the exception that the child with ventricular fibrillation or pulseless ventricular tachycardia should receive electrical defibrillation without delay. Airway access in children with ventricular fibrillation or pulseless ventricular tachycardia should be performed secondarily. CPR should be continued without interruption until a shock can be delivered.

### AIRWAY

Before tracheal intubation, the child's airway can usually be managed effectively with bag-valve-mask (BVM) ventilation with proper head positioning and jaw thrust. Although tracheal intubation ensures optimal control of the airway for effective ventilation, multiple attempts at tracheal intubation by an inexperienced operator may seriously compromise the airway and increases the cumulative duration of "no flow" (i.e., no CPR) time.

In the child without an artificial airway, the use of BVM devices may result in a significant risk of gastric inflation, followed by pulmonary aspiration of gastric contents. Abdominal distention (gastric and bowel) can significantly compromise oxygenation; therefore the stomach should be vented when excessive gastric inflation occurs. One study found a 28% incidence of pulmonary aspiration in a series of failed resuscitations.[16] For this reason as well as for the risk of barotrauma and volutrauma, excessive inflation pressures should be avoided. However, effective bilateral ventilation is best judged by visualizing bilateral chest excursions and listening to the quality of the breath sounds rather than setting a preset maximal inflation pressure.

Tracheal intubation should be performed as soon as appropriate personnel and equipment are available. The ETCO$_2$ is a valuable method of confirming correct placement of the tracheal tube. In the absence of capnography, a disposable colorimetric ETCO$_2$ device serves the same purpose. However, it is important to appreciate that ETCO$_2$ measurements are meaningful only in the presence of effective pulmonary circulation, such that a lack of color change may reflect either improper placement of the tube or a lack of pulmonary blood flow resulting from ineffective chest compressions or a massive pulmonary embolism. It is also essential to use the proper size colorimetric device for the child's weight because the adult size may not detect the presence of CO$_2$ and may lead the user to misdiagnose a successful intubation.

### BREATHING

In the inpatient environment, equipment necessary to ventilate the lungs emergently should be readily available. Because the equipment provided for emergency ventilatory support may differ from standard equipment, depending on the location within a hospital, the anesthesiologist needs to be familiar with all of the equipment in the hospital in which he or she practices. Anesthesiologists are skilled providers of ventilatory support, but in the context of a cardiac arrest, must return to the basics and remember that *if there is no chest movement, there is no ventilation.* If no chest movement occurs during BVM ventilation despite an apparently good seal between the mask and the child's face, the underlying cause, be it upper airway obstruction, whether anatomic or presence of a foreign body, bilateral tension pneumothoraces, or severe bronchospasm must be considered.

Overventilation is common during CPR, resulting in greater mean intrathoracic pressures than required, which decreases venous return and reduces cardiac output.[17] In cardiopulmonary arrest, a less than normal minute ventilation may be appropriate, because cardiac output and delivery of CO$_2$ to the lungs are diminished. If an artificial airway is not in place for single person rescue, two breaths should be given for each 30 chest compressions. If an artificial airway is not in place for two person rescue, two breaths should be given after each 15 chest compressions. Once an artificial airway is in place, a ventilator rate of 8 to 10 per minute *without* pausing during rapid chest compressions should be used (Table 39-1).

**TABLE 39-1** Ventilation and Chest Compressions during Pediatric Cardiopulmonary Pulmonary Resuscitation (all ages)

|  | Respirations | Chest Compressions | Notes |
|---|---|---|---|
| Bag-mask ventilation | 2 respirations after each 15 chest compressions (if one rescuer only, 2 respirations after each 30 compressions) | 100/minute | Aspirate (vent) the stomach if gastric inflation interferes with ventilation. |
| Endotracheal intubation | 8 to 10/minute | 100/minute | Do not pause compressions during ventilation. |

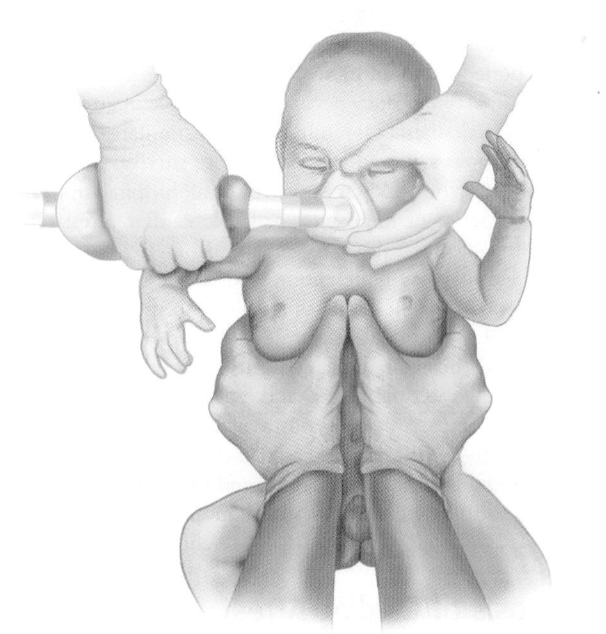

## CIRCULATION

During cardiac arrest, chest compressions provide the sole perfusion to a child's vital organs; therefore optimal performance of CPR is critical. Key elements to providing quality chest compressions include (1) ensuring an adequate rate (100 compressions per minute), (2) ensuring adequate chest wall depression (one third to half of the anteroposterior chest diameter), (3) releasing completely between compressions to allow full chest wall recoil, (4) minimizing interruptions in chest compressions, and (5) ensuring that the child is on a sufficiently hard surface to allow effective chest compressions.[18] In short, push hard and push fast, release completely, and do not interrupt compressions unnecessarily. Incomplete recoil during CPR is associated with higher intrathoracic pressures and significantly decreased venous return, and coronary and cerebral perfusion.[19]

If a child is small enough (e.g., younger than 6 months) that the person providing chest compressions can comfortably encircle the chest with his or her hands, chest compressions should be performed using the circumferential technique, with thumbs depressing the sternum and the fingers supporting the infant's back and circumferentially squeezing the thorax (Fig. 39-1). In larger infants, the sternum can be compressed using two fingers; and in the child, either one or two hands can be used, depending on the size of the child and of the rescuer.[19] Whichever method is used, focused attention must remain on delivering effective compressions with *minimal interruptions*.[20] In all cases other than circumferential CPR, a backboard must be used. Properly delivered chest compressions are tiring to the provider, and providers should rotate approximately every 2 minutes to prevent compressor fatigue and deterioration in the quality and rate of chest compressions.[19]

### Mechanisms of Blood Flow

External chest compressions provide cardiac output through two mechanisms: the cardiac pump mechanism and the thoracic pump mechanism. By the cardiac pump mechanism of blood flow, blood is squeezed from the heart by compression of the heart between the sternum and the vertebral column, exiting the heart only anterograde because of closure of the atrioventricular valves. Between compressions, ventricular pressure decreases below atrial pressure, allowing the atrioventricular valves to open and the ventricles to fill. This sequence of events resembles the normal cardiac cycle. Although the cardiac pump is likely not the dominant blood flow mechanism during most closed-chest

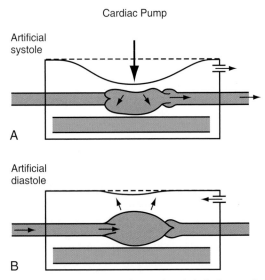

**FIGURE 39-1** Chest-encircling method for cardiac compressions in a neonate: thumbs are placed one finger's breadth below the nipple line. (Modified from Todres ID, Rogers MC. Methods of external cardiac massage in the newborn infant. J Pediatr 1975;86:781-2.)

Cardiac Pump

Artificial systole

A

Artificial diastole

B

**FIGURE 39-2 A,** Cardiac pump mechanism by which the heart is directly squeezed between the sternum and vertebral column, representing artificial systole. **B,** Artificial diastole occurs with relaxation of the compressions. (From Babbs CF. New versus old theories of blood flow during CPR. Crit Care Med 1980;8:191-5, © by Williams & Wilkins.)

CPR, specific clinical situations have been identified in which the cardiac pump mechanism is more prominent. For example, a smaller, more compliant chest may allow for more direct cardiac compression (Fig. 39-2). Increasing the applied force during chest compressions also increases the likelihood of direct cardiac compression.

Several observations do not support the cardiac pump as the primary mechanism of blood flow during CPR. Angiographic studies show that blood passes from the vena cava through the

39

right heart into the pulmonary artery and from the pulmonary veins through the left heart into the aorta during a single chest compression.[21,22] Echocardiographic studies show that the atrioventricular valves are open during blood ejection.[21,23,24] Without closure of atrioventricular valves during chest compression, the cardiac pump mechanisms cannot account for forward movement of blood during CPR.

In 1976, Criley and colleagues[25] made the dramatic observation that several patients who developed ventricular fibrillation during cardiac catheterization produced enough blood flow to maintain consciousness by repetitive coughing.[25] The production of blood flow by increasing thoracic pressure without direct cardiac compression describes the thoracic pump mechanism, in which the heart is a passive conduit for blood flow. The intrathoracic pressure is greater than the extrathoracic pressure during the compression phase of CPR, at which time blood flows out of the thorax, with venous valves preventing excessive retrograde blood flow (Fig. 39-3). Experimental and clinical data support both mechanisms of blood flow during CPR in human infants.

### Rate and Duty Cycle

The recommended rate of chest compressions for all patients is 100 per minute, with great care taken to minimize interruptions in chest compressions and to ensure adequate compression depth.[20] This rate represents a compromise that attempts to maximize contributions from both the thoracic pump and cardiac pump mechanism of blood flow.

Duty cycle is defined as the percent of the compression–relaxation cycle that is devoted to compression. If blood flow is generated by direct cardiac compression, then primarily the force of compression determines the stroke volume. Prolonging the compression (increasing the duty cycle) beyond the time necessary for full ventricular ejection should have no additional effect on stroke volume. Increasing the rate of compressions should increase cardiac output, because a fixed volume of blood is

ejected with each cardiac compression. In contrast, if blood flow is produced by the thoracic pump mechanism, the volume of blood that is ejected comes from a large reservoir of blood contained within the capacitance vessels in the chest. With the thoracic pump mechanism, flow is enhanced by increasing either the force of compression or the duty cycle but is not affected by changes in compression rate over a wide range of rates, given a set duty cycle.[26]

Different animal models yield conflicting results as to the optimal compression rate and duty cycle. However, a rate of compression during conventional CPR of 100 per minute satisfies both those who prefer the faster rates and those who support a longer duty cycle. This is true because it is easier to produce a longer duty cycle when compressions are administered at a faster rate.[27,28]

## Defibrillation and Cardioversion

In children with ventricular fibrillation or pulseless ventricular tachycardia, the immediate management should be defibrillation, without delay to secure an airway.

### ELECTRIC COUNTERSHOCK

Electric countershock, or defibrillation, is the treatment of choice for ventricular fibrillation and pulseless ventricular tachycardia. Defibrillation should not be delayed to secure an airway, because the likelihood of restoring an organized rhythm decreases with increased duration of fibrillation. Ventricular fibrillation is terminated by simultaneous depolarization and sustained contraction of a critical mass of myocardium,[29] allowing return of spontaneous, coordinated cardiac contractions, assuming the myocardium is well oxygenated and the acid-base status is relatively normal. Drug treatment may be required as an adjunct to defibrillation, but by itself cannot be relied on to terminate ventricular fibrillation.

An older generation of defibrillators that is still present in many hospitals delivers energy in a monophasic damped sinusoidal waveform (Fig. 39-4, *A*). This type of instrument delivers a single, unidirectional current with a gradual decrease to zero current. By contrast, the newer generation of biphasic defibrillators delivers a current in a positive direction for a set period, followed by a reversal in current (see Fig. 39-4, *B*). Biphasic defibrillators are more effective than monophasic defibrillators in terminating ventricular fibrillation in adults; therefore their use is recommended where possible.

In the majority of adult cases, energy levels of 100 to 200 joules are successful when shocks are delivered with minimal delay.[30,31] The goal of defibrillation is to deliver a minimum of electrical energy to a critical mass of ventricular muscle while avoiding excessive current that could further damage the heart. The most reliable predictor of success of defibrillation is the duration of fibrillation before the first countershock.[32] Acidosis and hypoxemia also decrease the success of defibrillation.[32]

### PRACTICAL ASPECTS OF DEFIBRILLATION IN CHILDREN

Correct paddle size and position are critical to the success of defibrillation. The largest paddle size appropriate for the child should be used because a larger size reduces the density of current flow, which in turn reduces myocardial damage. In general, adult paddles should be used in children weighing more than 10 kg and infant paddles should be used in infants weighing less than 10 kg. Paddle force is important as well. If the entire paddle does

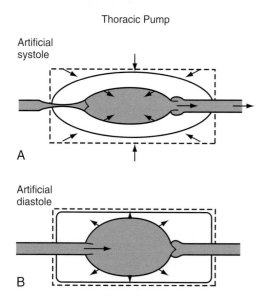

**FIGURE 39-3 A,** Thoracic pump mechanism by which blood flow occurs through a general increase in intrathoracic pressure with external compressions (i.e., the heart is a passive conduit). **B,** Artificial diastole occurs with release of external compressions. (From Babbs CF, New versus old theories of blood flow during CPR. Crit Care Med 1980;8:191-5, © by Williams & Wilkins.)

## Conventional Monophasic (dampened sine wave)

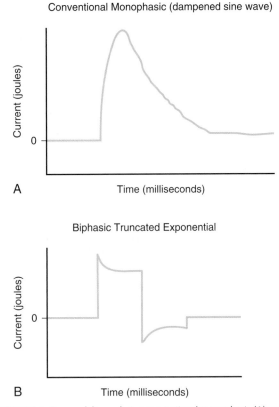

A

## Biphasic Truncated Exponential

B

**FIGURE 39-4** Energy delivery during conventional monophasic (**A**) and biphasic truncated exponential (**B**) defibrillation.

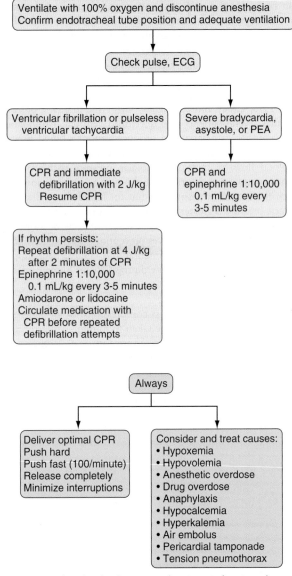

**FIGURE 39-5** Algorithm for diagnosis and treatment of acute cardiac dysfunction in the operating room. *CPR*, Cardiopulmonary resuscitation; *ECG*, electrocardiogram; *PEA*, pulseless electrical activity.

not rest *firmly* on the chest wall, a current of increased density will be delivered to a small contact point. Paddles should be positioned on the chest wall so that the bulk of myocardium lies directly between them. One paddle is placed to the right of the upper sternum below the clavicle; the other is positioned just caudad and to the left of the left nipple. For children with dextrocardia, the position of the paddles should be a mirror image. An alternative approach is to place one paddle anteriorly over the left precordium and the other paddle posteriorly between the scapulae.

The interface between the paddle and chest wall can be gel pads, electrode cream, or electrode paste. The electrode cream produces less impedance than the paste. *Electric current follows the path of least resistance, so care should be taken that the interface material from one paddle does not touch that of the other paddle. This is especially important in infants, in whom the distance between paddles is small.* If the gel is continuous between paddles, a short circuit is created and an insufficient amount of current will traverse the heart. Use of bare metal paddles increases the risk of arcing and worsens cutaneous burns from defibrillation. The use of self-adhesive pads is preferable when feasible.

In an oxygen ($O_2$)-enriched atmosphere, sparking from poorly applied defibrillator paddles can cause a fire. Therefore any sources of free-flowing $O_2$ should be removed to a distance of at least 1 meter from the child. These potentially hazardous $O_2$ sources include nasal cannula $O_2$, "blow-by" $O_2$, and nebulizers powered by $O_2$. By contrast, $O_2$ in a closed circuit may remain on the child. For example, it is not necessary to disconnect the ventilator from the child's tracheal tube (if a ventilator is disconnected, the fresh gas flow should be turned off because large volumes of $O_2$ flow through disconnected ventilators).

For children with in-hospital ventricular fibrillation or pulseless ventricular tachycardia, defibrillation should be attempted as soon as possible, with optimal CPR until the defibrillator is ready to deliver a shock. For the first defibrillation attempt, 2 joules/kg of delivered energy should be administered (Fig. 39-5). After shock delivery, CPR should resume immediately with chest compressions for five duty cycles (2 minutes). If one shock fails to eliminate ventricular fibrillation, the incremental benefit of another immediate shock is small. Resumption of CPR is likely to confer a greater benefit than another shock. CPR may provide coronary perfusion, increasing the likelihood of defibrillation with a subsequent shock. It is important to minimize the time between chest compressions and shock delivery and between shock delivery and resumption of postshock compressions.[20] Approximately 2 minutes of CPR should be delivered before a second attempt at defibrillation at twice the original energy level (4 joules/kg).[20]

If ventricular fibrillation or pulseless ventricular tachycardia persists beyond the second defibrillation attempt, standard doses of epinephrine should be administered (with subsequent doses every 3 to 5 minutes during persistent cardiac arrest). After 2 minutes of chest compressions, defibrillation should be attempted again, followed by administration of amiodarone (5 mg/kg) or lidocaine (1 mg/kg) with subsequent defibrillation attempts. It is not necessary to increase the energy level on each successive shock during defibrillation after the second dose. However, successful defibrillation has been reported with currents in excess of 4 joules/kg without adverse sequelae, up to a maximum dose not exceeding 10 joules/kg or the adult level, whichever is less.[20] This sometimes occurs when a fixed energy level, adult automated external defibrillator (AED) is used in a small child.

## OPEN-CHEST DEFIBRILLATION

If the chest is already open in the OR or easily opened as in a fresh postoperative cardiac patient, ventricular fibrillation should be treated with open-chest defibrillation, using internal paddles applied directly to the heart. These should have a diameter of 6 cm for adults, 4 cm for children, and 2 cm for infants. Handles should be insulated. Saline-soaked pads or gauzes should be placed between the paddles and the heart. One electrode is placed behind the left ventricle and the other over the right ventricle on the anterior surface of the heart. The energy level used should begin at 5 joules in infants and 20 joules in adults.

## AUTOMATED EXTERNAL DEFIBRILLATION

Use of AEDs is now standard therapy in out-of-hospital resuscitation of adults.[19,30] AEDs are now deemed appropriate for use in children older than 1 year. If available, use of pediatric attenuator pads or a pediatric mode on the AED should be used in children 1 to 8 years of age, but if unavailable (and a standard defibrillator is similarly unavailable), an unmodified AED should be used.

## TRANSCUTANEOUS CARDIAC PACING

In the absence of in situ pacing wires or an indwelling transvenous or esophageal pacing catheter, transcutaneous cardiac pacing (TCP) is the preferred method for temporary electrical cardiac pacing in children with asystole or severe bradycardia. TCP is indicated for children whose primary problem is impulse formation or conduction, with preserved myocardial function. It is most effective in those with sinus bradycardia or high-grade atrioventricular block, with slow ventricular response but adequate stroke volume. TCP is not indicated for children during prolonged arrest, because in this situation it usually results in electrical but not mechanical cardiac capture and its use may delay or interfere with other resuscitative efforts.

To set up pacing, one electrode is placed anteriorly at the left sternal border and the other posteriorly just below the left scapula. Smaller electrodes are available for infants and children, but adult-sized electrodes can be used in children weighing more than 15 kg. ECG leads should be connected to the pacemaker, the demand or asynchronous mode selected, and an age-appropriate heart rate used. The stimulus output should be set at zero when the pacemaker is turned on and then increased gradually until electrical capture is identified on the monitor. After electrical capture is achieved, whether an effective arterial pulse is generated must be determined. If not, additional resuscitative efforts should be initiated.

The most serious complication of TCP is the induction of a ventricular arrhythmia. Fortunately, this is rare and may be prevented by pacing only in the demand mode. Mild transient erythema beneath the electrodes is common. Skeletal muscle contraction can be minimized by using large electrodes, a 40-msec pulse duration, and the smallest stimulus required for capture. If defibrillation or cardioversion is necessary, a distance of 2 to 3 cm must be allowed between the electrode and paddles to prevent arcing of the current.

# Vascular Access and Monitoring during Cardiopulmonary Resuscitation

## VASCULAR ACCESS AND FLUID ADMINISTRATION

One of the key aspects of successful CPR is early establishment of a route for administration of fluids and medications. If intravenous access cannot be established rapidly, the intraosseous or endotracheal route should be used (see Chapter 48).

### Intravenous Access

Many children who suffer an in-hospital cardiac arrest will already have established vascular access. For children with impending cardiac arrest and no vascular access, a brief attempt should be made to establish peripheral intravenous access. If access is not achieved quickly, an intraosseous needle should be placed. For young children in cardiac arrest without vascular access, an intraosseous needle should be placed immediately, to avoid any delay from repeated attempts at establishing intravenous access.

### Intraosseous Access

The intraosseous route can be used to administer all medications and fluids used during CPR, including whole blood. An intraosseous needle also may be used to obtain initial blood samples, although acid-base analysis will be inaccurate after administration of sodium bicarbonate via the intraosseous needle. Intraosseous access should be considered a temporary measure during emergencies when other access is not available. The placement of an intraosseous needle in the older child (older than 10 years) and adult, although possible, is difficult owing to the thick bony cortex; however, a 50% success rate has been reported in these age-groups.[33]

The technique of placing an intraosseous line is straightforward. A specialized intraosseous needle or, if not available, a standard 16- or 18-gauge needle, a spinal needle with stylet, or bone marrow needle is inserted into the anterior surface of the tibia 1 to 2 cm below and 1 cm medial to the tibial tuberosity (avoiding the epiphyseal plate). The needle is directed at 90 degrees to the anteromedial surface of the tibia, just distal to the tuberosity (see Fig. 48-6 and E-Fig. 48-1). When the needle passes through the cortex into the marrow, a sudden loss of resistance is sensed. Successful placement has been achieved if the needle is in the marrow cavity, as evidenced by the needle standing upright without support. If the needle has slipped into the subcutaneous tissue, its upright position cannot be maintained without support. Free flow of the infusate without significant subcutaneous infiltration should also be demonstrated. The technique has a small complication rate,[34] although possible complications include osteomyelitis, fat and bone marrow embolisms, and compartment syndrome. To avoid these potential complications, intravenous access should replace intraosseous access as soon as possible. The onset of action and concentration of most drugs after intraosseous administration are comparable with venous administration.[35] A relatively new device, the EZ-IO

(Vidacare, Shavano Park, Tex.) provides the most rapid means for intraosseous access (see E-Fig. 48-1).

### ENDOTRACHEAL MEDICATION ADMINISTRATION

In the absence of other vascular access, medications including lidocaine, atropine, naloxone, and epinephrine (mnemonic LANE) can be administered via the endotracheal tube.[36,37] The use of ionized medications such as sodium bicarbonate or calcium chloride is not recommended by this route. The peak concentration of epinephrine or lidocaine administered via the endotracheal route may be less compared with the intraosseous route. For example, the peak drug concentration of epinephrine after endotracheal administration was only 10% of that after intravenous administration in anesthetized dogs. The recommended dose for epinephrine via the endotracheal tube is 10 times the intravenous or intraosseous dose or 0.1 mg/kg for bradycardia or pulseless arrest.

The volume and the diluent in which the medications are administered through an endotracheal tube may be important. When large volumes of fluid are used, pulmonary surfactant may be altered or destroyed, resulting in atelectasis. The total volume of fluid delivered into the trachea with each drug administered should not exceed 10 mL in children and 5 mL in infants and neonates.[38] However, administering an adequate volume of a drug is important to reach a large area of mucosal surface beyond the tip of the endotracheal tube for absorption. Absorption into the systemic circulation may be further enhanced by deep intrapulmonary administration by passing a catheter beyond the tip of the tracheal tube deep into the bronchial tree. The risk associated with the endotracheal route of drug administration is the formation of an intrapulmonary depot of drug, which may prolong the drugs' effect. This could theoretically result in postresuscitation hypertension and tachycardia or the recurrence of fibrillation after normal circulation is restored.

### MONITORING DURING CARDIOPULMONARY RESUSCITATION

A basic clinical examination is vital during cardiac arrest. The chest is carefully observed for adequacy of bilateral chest expansion with artificial ventilation and for equal and normal breath sounds. In addition, the depth of compression and the position of the rescuer's hands should be constantly reevaluated in performing chest compressions by palpation of a major artery. Palpation is essential in establishing absence of a pulse and in assessing the adequacy of blood flow during chest compressions. Palpating the peripheral pulses may be inaccurate, especially during intense vasoconstriction associated with the use of epinephrine.

An indwelling arterial catheter, when available, is a valuable monitor in assessing the arterial blood pressure. Specific attention should be paid to diastolic blood pressure as it relates directly to adequacy of coronary perfusion during CPR. In addition, arterial access allows for frequent blood sampling, particularly for measurement of arterial pH and blood gases. Pulse oximetry can be used during CPR to determine the $O_2$ saturation and may be of value in assessing the adequacy of cardiac output, as reflected in the plethysmograph. The ECG can suggest metabolic imbalances and diagnose electrical disturbances.

The ETCO$_2$ monitor provides important information during the course of resuscitation. Because the generation of exhaled $CO_2$ depends on pulmonary blood flow, it can provide a useful indicator of the adequacy of cardiac output generated by chest compressions. As the cardiac output increases, the ETCO$_2$

increases and the difference between end-tidal and arterial $CO_2$ becomes smaller.[39] In animal models, ETCO$_2$ during CPR correlates with coronary perfusion pressure and with ROSC.[40,41] In adults during cardiac arrest, an ETCO$_2$ greater than 10 mm Hg is positively associated with ROSC and hospital survival.[42,43] When the ETCO$_2$ is less than 10 mm Hg, efforts should be taken to enhance the quality of chest compressions (push hard, push fast, release completely, minimize interruptions, and optimize hand position). A reduced ETCO$_2$ may occur transiently in the presence of adequate chest compressions after administration of epinephrine owing to an increase in intrapulmonary shunting.

Temperature should be monitored during and after CPR. The resuscitation of the child with hypothermia as the cause of cardiac arrest must be continued until the child's core temperature exceeds 95° F (35° C). A glass bulb thermometer measures the temperature to very low values. Repeated measurements of core body temperature should be made at several sites (rectal, bladder, esophageal, axillary, or tympanic membrane) where possible, to avoid misleading temperature readings from a single site, because local body temperature may vary with changes in regional blood flow during CPR. Hyperthermia should be aggressively treated in the periarrest period, because postarrest hyperthermia is associated with worse outcomes in children.[44] Evidence suggests a benefit to induced hypothermia after resuscitation from cardiac arrest in adults[45,46] and after perinatal hypoxic or ischemic injury.[47] The data available to support the use of hypothermia in infants and children after cardiac arrest is from case series and retrospective studies. Pending results of a randomized controlled trial (Therapeutic Hypothermia After Pediatric Cardiac Arrest), clinicians may choose to control a child's temperature in the range of 91.4° to 95° F (33° to 35° C) for 12 to 48 hours after resuscitation with slow subsequent rewarming (see section on Postresuscitation Stabilization).

# Medications Used during Cardiopulmonary Resuscitation

## α- AND β-ADRENERGIC AGONISTS

In 1963, only 3 years after the original description of closed-chest CPR, Redding and Pearson[48] demonstrated that early administration of epinephrine in a canine model of cardiac arrest improved the success rate of CPR. They also demonstrated that the increase in aortic diastolic pressure with the administration of α-adrenergic agonists was responsible for the improved success of resuscitation. They theorized that vasopressors such as epinephrine were of value because the drug increased peripheral vascular tone and, hence, coronary perfusion pressure. The relative importance of α- and β-adrenergic agonist actions during resuscitation has been widely investigated. In a canine model of cardiac arrest, only 27% of dogs that received a pure β-adrenergic receptor agonist along with an α-adrenergic antagonist were resuscitated successfully, compared with 100% of dogs that received a pure α-adrenergic agonist and a β-adrenergic antagonist. Other investigators have demonstrated that the α-adrenergic effects of epinephrine resulted in intense vasoconstriction of the resistance vessels of all organs of the body, except those supplying the heart and brain.[49] Because of the widespread vasoconstriction in nonvital organs, adequate perfusion pressure and thus blood flow to the heart and brain can be achieved despite the fact that cardiac output is very low during CPR.[49-51]

The increase in aortic diastolic pressure associated with epinephrine administration during CPR is critical for maintaining coronary blood flow and enhancing the success of resuscitation.[52,53] Even though the contractile state of the myocardium is increased by the use of β-adrenergic agonists in the spontaneously beating heart, β-adrenergic agonists may actually decrease myocardial blood flow by increasing intramyocardial wall pressure and vascular resistance during CPR.[54] By its inotropic and chronotropic effects, β-adrenergic stimulation increases myocardial $O_2$ demand, which, when superimposed on low coronary blood flow, increases the risk of ischemic injury.

Any medication that causes systemic arterial vasoconstriction can be used to increase aortic diastolic pressure and resuscitate the heart. For example, pure α-adrenergic agonists can be used in place of epinephrine during CPR. Phenylephrine and methoxamine, two α-adrenergic agonists, have been used in animal models of CPR with success equal to that of epinephrine. Their use results in a greater $O_2$ supply to demand ratio in the ischemic heart and at least a theoretical advantage over the combined α- and β-adrenergic agonist effects of epinephrine. These agonists, as well as other classes of vasopressors such as vasopressin, have been used successfully for resuscitation.

The merits of using a pure α-adrenergic agonist during CPR have been questioned by some investigators. Although the inotropic and chronotropic effects of β-adrenergic agonists may have deleterious hemodynamic effects during CPR for ventricular fibrillation, increases in both heart rate and contractility will increase cardiac output when spontaneous coordinated ventricular contractions are achieved.

## EPINEPHRINE

Epinephrine (adrenaline) is an endogenous catecholamine with potent α- and β-adrenergic stimulating properties. The α-adrenergic action increases systemic and pulmonary vascular resistance, increasing both systolic and diastolic blood pressure. The increase in diastolic blood pressure directly increases coronary perfusion pressure, thereby increasing coronary blood flow and increasing the likelihood of ROSC.[52,53] The β-adrenergic effect increases myocardial contractility and heart rate and relaxes smooth muscle in the skeletal muscle vascular bed and bronchi. Epinephrine also increases the vigor and intensity of ventricular fibrillation, increasing the likelihood of successful defibrillation.[55]

Larger than necessary doses of epinephrine may be deleterious. Epinephrine may worsen myocardial ischemic injury secondary to increased $O_2$ demand and may result in postresuscitative tachyarrhythmias, hypertension, and pulmonary edema. Epinephrine causes hypoxemia and an increase in alveolar dead space ventilation by redistributing pulmonary blood flow.[39,56] Prolonged peripheral vasoconstriction by excessive doses of epinephrine may delay or impair reperfusion of systemic organs, particularly the kidneys and gastrointestinal tract.

Routine use of large-dose epinephrine in in-hospital pediatric cardiac arrest should be *avoided*. A randomized, controlled trial in 2003 compared high-dose with standard-dose epinephrine for children with in-hospital cardiac arrest refractory to initial standard-dose epinephrine. Survival was reduced at 24 hours, with a trend toward decreased survival to hospital discharge in the children who received large doses of epinephrine.[57] Despite these data, large doses of epinephrine may be considered in special cases (e.g., β-blocker overdose), particularly when diastolic blood pressure remains low despite excellent chest compression and several standard doses of epinephrine.

## VASOPRESSIN

Vasopressin is a long-acting endogenous hormone that causes vasoconstriction (V1 receptor) and reabsorption of water in the renal tubule (V2 receptor). In experimental models of cardiac arrest, vasopressin increases blood flow to the heart and brain and improves long-term survival compared with epinephrine.[58,59] In a randomized trial comparing the efficacy of epinephrine to vasopressin in shock-resistant out-of-hospital ventricular fibrillation in adults, vasopressin produced a greater rate of ROSC.[60] In a study of in-hospital adult cardiac arrest, vasopressin produced a rate of survival to hospital discharge similar to that of epinephrine.[61]

In a pediatric porcine model of prolonged ventricular fibrillation, the use of vasopressin and epinephrine in combination resulted in greater left ventricular blood flow than either vasopressor alone, and both vasopressin alone and vasopressin plus epinephrine resulted in superior cerebral blood flow than epinephrine alone.[62] By contrast, in a pediatric porcine model of *asphyxial* cardiac arrest, ROSC was more likely in piglets treated with epinephrine than in those treated with vasopressin.[63] Pediatric[64-66] case series and reports suggested that vasopressin[64] or its long-acting analog, terlipressin,[65,66] may be effective in refractory cardiac arrest. In a 2009 National Registry of Cardiopulmonary Resuscitation (NRCPR) review, vasopressin was associated with reduced ROSC and a trend toward reduced 24-hour and discharge survival. There is insufficient evidence to make a recommendation for its routine use during cardiac arrest.[20]

## ATROPINE

Atropine, a parasympatholytic agent, blocks cholinergic stimulation of the muscarinic receptors in the heart, increasing the sinus rate and shortening atrioventricular node conduction time. Atropine may activate latent ectopic pacemakers. Atropine has little effect on systemic vascular resistance, myocardial perfusion pressure, or contractility.[67]

Atropine is indicated for the treatment of asystole, pulseless electrical activity, bradycardia associated with hypotension, second- and third-degree heart block, and slow idioventricular rhythms. Atropine is particularly effective in clinical conditions associated with excessive parasympathetic tone. *However, for children with asystole or symptomatic bradycardia associated with severe hypotension, epinephrine is the medication of choice and atropine should be regarded as a second-line drug.*

The recommended pediatric dose of atropine is 0.02 mg/kg, with a maximum dose of 2 mg. The increase in heart rate after intravenous atropine (20 μg/kg) in infants and children may be attenuated compared with that in adults.[68] Although a minimum dose of 0.1 mg has been entrenched in the literature, it is not evidence-based.[68,69] Atropine may be given by any route, including intravenous, intraosseous, endotracheal, intramuscular, and subcutaneous. After intravenous administration, its onset of action is within 30 seconds and its peak effect occurs in 1 to 2 minutes. The recommended adult dose is 0.5 mg every 3 to 5 minutes until the desired heart rate is obtained, up to a maximum of 3 mg.

## SODIUM BICARBONATE

The routine use of sodium bicarbonate during CPR remains controversial, and it remains American Heart Association Class Indeterminate. Acidosis may depress myocardial function, prolong diastolic depolarization, depress spontaneous cardiac activity, decrease the electrical threshold for ventricular fibrillation, and reduce the cardiac response to catecholamines.[70-72] Acidosis also vasodilates systemic vessels and attenuates the vasoconstrictive response of peripheral vessels to catecholamines,[73] which is the opposite of the desired vascular effect during CPR. In children with a reactive pulmonary vascular bed, acidosis causes pulmonary hypertension. Therefore correction of even mild acidosis may be helpful in resuscitating children with increased pulmonary vascular resistance. Additionally, the presence of severe acidosis may increase the threshold for myocardial stimulation in a child with an artificial cardiac pacemaker.[74] Other situations in which administration of bicarbonate is indicated include tricyclic antidepressant overdose, hyperkalemia, hypermagnesemia, or sodium channel blocker poisoning.

Potentially deleterious effects of bicarbonate administration include metabolic alkalosis, hypercapnia, hypernatremia, and hyperosmolality. In a 2004 multicenter cohort study of in-hospital pediatric cardiac arrest, the use of sodium bicarbonate was associated with increased mortality.[15] Alkalosis causes a leftward shift of the oxyhemoglobin dissociation curve and thus impairs release of $O_2$ from hemoglobin to tissues at a time when $O_2$ delivery may already be reduced.[75] Alkalosis also can result in hypokalemia by enhancing potassium influx into cells and in ionic hypocalcemia by increasing protein binding of ionized calcium. The marked hypercapnic acidosis that occurs during CPR in the venous circulation, including the coronary sinus, may be exacerbated by the administration of bicarbonate.[76] Myocardial acidosis during cardiac arrest is associated with decreased myocardial contractility.[72] Hypernatremia and hyperosmolality may decrease tissue perfusion by increasing interstitial edema in microvascular beds.

Paradoxical intracellular acidosis after bicarbonate administration can occur with the rapid entry of $CO_2$ into cells with a slow egress of hydrogen ions out of cells; however, in neonatal rabbits recovering from hypoxic acidosis, bicarbonate administration increased both arterial pH and intracellular brain pH as measured by nuclear magnetic resonance spectroscopy.[77,78] Likewise, in rats, intracellular brain adenosine triphosphate concentration did not change during severe intracellular acidosis in the brain produced by extreme hypercapnia.[78] In a separate animal study, bicarbonate slowed the rate of decrease of both arterial and cerebral pH during prolonged CPR, suggesting that the blood-brain pH gradient is maintained during CPR.[79] Given the potentially deleterious effects of bicarbonate administration, its use should be *limited to cases in which there is a specific indication*, as discussed earlier.

## CALCIUM

Calcium administration during CPR should be restricted to cases with a specific indication for calcium (e.g., hypocalcemia, hyperkalemia, hypermagnesemia, and calcium channel blocker overdose). These restrictions are based on the possibility that exogenously administered calcium may worsen ischemia-reperfusion injury. Intracellular calcium overload occurs during cerebral ischemia by the influx of calcium through voltage-dependent and agonist-dependent (e.g., N-methyl-D-aspartate [NMDA]) calcium channels. Calcium plays an important role in the process of cell death in many organs, possibly by activation of intracellular enzymes such as nitric oxide synthase, phospholipase A and C, and others.[80]

The calcium ion is essential in myocardial excitation-contraction coupling, in increasing ventricular contractility, and in enhancing ventricular automaticity during asystole. Ionized hypocalcemia is associated with decreased ventricular performance and the peripheral blunting of the hemodynamic response to catecholamines.[81,82] Severe ionized hypocalcemia has been documented in adults suffering from out-of-hospital cardiac arrest[82] and in animals during prolonged CPR.[83] Thus children at risk for ionized hypocalcemia should be identified and treated as expeditiously as possible. Both total and ionized hypocalcemia may occur in children with either chronic or acute disease. Ionized hypocalcemia also occurs during massive or rapid transfusion of blood products (particularly whole blood and fresh frozen plasma) because citrate and other preservatives in stored blood products rapidly bind calcium. Because of this effect, ionized hypocalcemia is a known cause of cardiac arrest in the OR and should be treated immediately with calcium chloride or calcium gluconate (see Chapter 10). The magnitude of hypocalcemia in this setting depends on the rate and volume of blood products administered and the hepatic and renal function of the child. Administration of fresh frozen plasma at a rate in excess of 1 mL/kg/min significantly decreases the ionized calcium concentration in anesthetized children.[84]

The pediatric dose of calcium chloride for resuscitation is 20 mg/kg with a maximum dose of 2 g. Calcium gluconate is as effective as calcium chloride in increasing the ionized calcium concentration.[85,86] The dose of calcium gluconate should be three times that of calcium chloride (milligram per kilogram,) (i.e., 20 mg/kg calcium chloride is equivalent to 60 mg/kg calcium gluconate), with a maximum dose of 2 g in children. Calcium should be given slowly through a large-bore, free-flowing intravenous cannula, or preferably a central venous line. When administered too rapidly, calcium may cause bradycardia, heart block, or ventricular standstill. Severe tissue necrosis occurs when calcium infiltrates into subcutaneous tissue. Calcium administration is not recommended for pediatric cardiopulmonary arrest in the absence of documented hypocalcemia, calcium channel blocker overdose, hypermagnesemia, or hyperkalemia (Class III, level of evidence [LOE] B). Routine calcium administration in cardiac arrest provides no benefit and may be harmful.[74,87]

## GLUCOSE

The administration of glucose during CPR should be restricted to children with documented hypoglycemia because of the possible detrimental effects of hyperglycemia on the brain during or after ischemia. The mechanism by which hyperglycemia exacerbates ischemic neurologic injury may be due to an increased production of lactic acid in the brain by anaerobic metabolism. During ischemia under normoglycemic conditions, brain lactate concentration reaches a plateau. In a hyperglycemic milieu, however, brain lactate concentration continues to increase for the duration of the ischemic period.[88]

Clinical studies have shown a direct correlation between the initial post–cardiac arrest serum glucose concentration and poor neurologic outcome,[89-92] although the greater glucose concentration may be a marker rather than a cause of more severe brain injury.[90] However, given the likelihood of additional ischemic and hypoxic events in the postresuscitation period, it seems prudent to maintain serum glucose concentrations within the normal range. Additional studies are needed to determine if the benefit from tight control of serum glucose after cardiac arrest outweighs the risk of iatrogenic hypoglycemia. Some groups of children, including preterm infants and debilitated children with small endogenous glycogen stores, are more prone to

developing hypoglycemia during and after a physiologic stress such as surgery. Bedside monitoring of the serum glucose concentration is critical during and after a cardiac arrest and allows for the opportunity to administer glucose before the critical point of small substrate delivery has been reached. The dose of glucose generally needed to correct hypoglycemia is 0.5 g/kg given as 5 mL/kg of 10% dextrose in infants or 1 mL/kg of 50% dextrose in an older child. The osmolarity of 50% dextrose is approximately 2700 mOsm/L and has been associated with intraventricular hemorrhage in neonates and infants; therefore the more dilute concentration is recommended in infants.

## AMIODARONE

Amiodarone has now supplanted lidocaine as the first drug of choice for medical management of shock-resistant ventricular tachycardia and fibrillation. The role of amiodarone was established for cardiac arrest after a series of studies showed it to be more effective than lidocaine in the management of refractory tachyarrhythmias in adults. Compared with lidocaine, amiodarone results in an increased rate of survival to hospital admission in patients with shock-resistant out-of-hospital ventricular fibrillation.[93]

Early reports on the use of oral amiodarone in children were favorable.[94-96] Recent data on amiodarone use in children are limited to case reports and descriptive case series. Nevertheless, it is now used widely for serious pediatric arrhythmias in the nonresuscitation environment and appears to be effective and have an acceptable short-term safety profile.

The pharmacology of amiodarone is complex and may explain the wide range of its usefulness. It is primarily classified as a Vaughn-Williams class III agent that blocks the adenosine triphosphate–sensitive outward potassium channels causing prolongation of the action potential and refractory period; however, this effect requires intracellular accumulation. On intravenous loading, the antiarrhythmic effects are primarily due to noncompetitive α- and β-adrenergic receptor blockade, calcium channel blockade, and effects on inward sodium current causing a decrease in anterograde conduction across the atrioventricular node and an increase in the effective atrioventricular refractory period. The α-adrenergic blockade leads to vasodilation, which may increase coronary blood flow. It is poorly absorbed orally, requiring intravenous loading in urgent situations. The full antiarrhythmic impact requires a loading period of up to 1 to 3 weeks to achieve intracellular levels and full potassium channel–blocking effects.

Hypotension is commonly reported with intravenous administration and may limit the rate at which the drug can be given; however, the development of hypotension is less common with the newer, aqueous formulation.[97] The overall hemodynamic impact of intravenous administration will depend on the balance of its effect on rate control, myocardial performance, and vasodilation. Dosage recommendations for children are based on limited clinical studies. The dose is extrapolated from data on adults; 5 mg/kg intravenously for life-threatening arrhythmias. This dose can be repeated if necessary to control the arrhythmia. Intravenous loading doses are followed by a continuous infusion of 10 to 20 mg/kg/day if there is a risk of arrhythmia recurrence. The ideal rate of bolus administration is unclear; in adults, once diluted, it is given as an intravenous push. It is best administered over 20 to 60 minutes to avoid profound vasodilation. We recommend slow intravenous push (2 to 3 minutes) for pulseless

ventricular tachycardia or ventricular fibrillation until the arrhythmia is controlled and then a slower bolus (up to 10 minutes) for the remainder of the dose. An alternative dosing regimen for children is 1 mg/kg intravenous push every 5 minutes up to 5 mg/kg. The use of the small aliquot bolus technique may be particularly appropriate for infants younger than 12 months of age.

Amiodarone-induced torsades de pointes has been described.[98] The use of amiodarone should be avoided in combination with other drugs that prolong the QT interval, as well as in the setting of hypomagnesemia and other electrolyte abnormalities that predispose to torsades de pointes. Severe bradycardia and heart block have also been described, especially in the postoperative period, and ventricular pacing wires are recommended in this setting. Both amiodarone and inhalation anesthetic agents prolong the QT interval; however, no specific data exist to evaluate the use of amiodarone for ventricular arrhythmias in children receiving inhalation anesthetics. It would seem prudent to be especially vigilant for this adverse effect in this circumstance.

Noncardiac adverse effects are often seen, especially with chronic dosing.[99] The most serious of these has been the development of interstitial pneumonitis seen most commonly in patients with preexisting lung disease.[100] The incidence in children is unknown. Rarely, an acute illness similar to acute respiratory distress syndrome illness has been reported in both infants and adults at the initiation of treatment.[101] The lung disease may remit with early discontinuation of the drug. Hypothyroidism, hepatotoxicity, photosensitivity, and corneal opacities are also common side effects with chronic use.[99]

## LIDOCAINE

Lidocaine is a class IB antiarrhythmic that decreases automaticity of pacemaker tissue that prevents or terminates ventricular arrhythmias as a result of accelerated ectopic foci. Lidocaine abolishes reentrant ventricular arrhythmias by decreasing the action potential duration and the conduction time of Purkinje fibers and increases the effective refractory period of Purkinje fibers, reducing the nonuniformity of contraction. Lidocaine has no effect on atrioventricular nodal conduction time, so it is ineffective in the treatment of atrial or atrioventricular junctional arrhythmias. In healthy adults, no change in heart rate or blood pressure occurs with lidocaine administration. In patients with cardiac disease there may be a slight decrease in ventricular function when a lidocaine bolus is administered intravenously.

In children with normal cardiac and hepatic function, an initial intravenous bolus of 1 mg/kg of lidocaine is given, followed by a continuous intravenous infusion at a rate of 20 to 50 μg/kg/min. If the arrhythmia recurs, a second intravenous bolus at the same dose can be given. In children with severely decreased cardiac output, a bolus of no greater than 0.75 mg/kg is administered, followed by an infusion at the rate of 10 to 20 μg/kg/min. In children with hepatic disease, dosages should be decreased by 50%. Children with renal insufficiency have normal lidocaine pharmacokinetics; however, toxic metabolites may accumulate in children receiving infusions over a long period. In children with hypoproteinemia, the dose of lidocaine also should be lowered, because of the increase in free fraction of the drug.

Toxic effects of lidocaine occur when the serum concentration exceeds 7 to 8 μg/mL and include seizures, psychosis, drowsiness, paresthesias, disorientation, agitation, tinnitus, muscle spasms,

and respiratory arrest. The treatment of choice for lidocaine-induced seizures is a benzodiazepine (midazolam or lorazepam) or a barbiturate (e.g., phenobarbital; chronic therapy also increases the hepatic metabolism of lidocaine).[102] Conversion of second-degree heart block to complete heart block has been described,[103] as has severe sinus bradycardia. Lidocaine is not as effective as amiodarone for improving ROSC or survival to hospital admission among adults with ventricular fibrillation refractory to ventricular fibrillation and shock.[104]

## Special Cardiac Arrest Situations

### PERIOPERATIVE CARDIAC ARREST

The incidence, causes, and risk factors associated with anesthesia- and operative-related cardiac arrest have been evaluated by the Pediatric Perioperative Cardiac Arrest registry.[105,106] Cardiovascular causes of cardiac arrest were the most common (41% of all arrests), with hypovolemia from blood loss and hyperkalemia from transfusion of stored blood the most common identifiable cardiovascular causes. Among respiratory causes of arrest (27%), airway obstruction from laryngospasm was the most common cause. Vascular injury incurred during placement of central venous catheters was the most common equipment-related cause of arrest. The cause of arrest varied by phase of anesthesia care.

Cardiac arrest in the OR should have the greatest potential for a successful outcome, because it is a witnessed arrest with virtually instantaneous availability of skilled personnel, monitoring equipment, resuscitative equipment, and drugs. Whenever a cardiac arrest occurs in the OR, the circumstances causing the arrest should be rapidly determined. The circumstances of the arrest may provide a clue as to the cause, such as hyperkalemia after succinylcholine administration or rapid blood transfusion, hypocalcemia during a rapid infusion of fresh frozen plasma or large blood transfusion, or a sudden fall in $ETCO_2$ indicating air, blood clot, or tumor embolism. A bradyarrhythmia always must be assumed to be first resulting from hypoxemia; second, caused by anesthetic overdose (real or relative); and third, possibly related to a vagal reflex caused by surgical or airway manipulation. Administering 100% $O_2$ and ensuring adequate ventilation is always the first maneuver, regardless of the cause of the bradycardia. In reflex-induced bradycardia, atropine may be the first drug of choice, but in extreme cases of bradycardia, whatever the mechanism, epinephrine should be used. Hypotension and a low cardiac output state must be rapidly corrected by appropriate administration of intravenous fluids, vasopressors, and adequate chest compressions to circulate drugs to have the needed clinical effect. Once chest compressions are required, the standard American Heart Association recommendations for CPR generally apply and this includes the frequent administration of epinephrine. Figure 39-5 presents an algorithm for the differential diagnosis and treatment of the more common causes of acute OR-associated cardiac dysfunction.

### HYPERKALEMIA

A child with a hyperkalemic cardiac arrest may be identified by history, by the progression of ECG changes leading up to the arrest, or by initial laboratory results. A high index of suspicion must be maintained for hyperkalemia as a cause of cardiac arrest because it requires specific therapy. Along with the usual resuscitation algorithms, immediate therapy to antagonize the effects of an increased serum potassium level is necessary. Calcium gluconate or calcium chloride will antagonize the effects of hyperkalemia at the myocardial cell membrane, increasing the threshold for fibrillation. Sodium bicarbonate and hyperventilation will increase the serum pH and shift potassium from the extracellular to the intracellular compartment; insulin (with concomitant dextrose) will also cause potassium to shift intracellularly (0.1 unit/kg of insulin with 0.5 g/kg of dextrose; 2 mL/kg of dextrose 25%). The serum potassium concentration must be monitored frequently during this treatment, preferably by point-of-care testing modalities. Because these therapies shift potassium intracellularly, therapy to remove potassium from the body (furosemide, hemodialysis, sodium polystyrene sulfonate) also may be indicated.

### ANAPHYLAXIS

Anaphylaxis is an unusual, but usually reversible, cause of cardiac arrest. Manifestations of anaphylaxis include skin reaction (usually flushing, pallor, or urticaria), airway edema and possible obstruction, bronchospasm, and cardiovascular collapse. Anaphylaxis may be particularly severe in situations of decreased endogenous catecholamines, such as in a child taking β-blockers or in children receiving spinal or epidural anesthesia.

Resuscitation of the child with anaphylaxis rests on reversing airway obstruction and restoring intravascular volume and vascular tone. In the child with cardiac arrest, standard-dose epinephrine should be administered intravenously. In the child with impending cardiac arrest, 0.01 mL/kg of subcutaneous epinephrine (1 : 1000 concentration) may be preferred. Children with anaphylactic shock have profound intravascular depletion requiring rapidly administered, large-volume fluid resuscitation (20 mL/kg boluses). In addition to the usual resuscitation medications, treatment should include an antihistamine and corticosteroid, such as diphenhydramine (Benadryl), 1 mg/kg, and methylprednisolone (Solu-Medrol) 2 mg/kg. Inhaled bronchodilators such as albuterol may help reverse bronchospasm. If severe airway obstruction occurs, endotracheal intubation or even cricothyroidotomy may become difficult or impossible. Therefore the airway should be secured early on by a skilled practitioner.

### SUPRAVENTRICULAR TACHYCARDIA

Supraventricular tachycardia (SVT), a common arrhythmia in infants and children, may be associated with severe circulatory compromise or even cardiac arrest. Therapy for this arrhythmia should be based on the child's hemodynamic status. SVT associated with inadequate circulation should be treated immediately with synchronized cardioversion beginning at a dose of 0.5 J/kg. If intravenous access is available, adenosine can be administered while cardioversion is being prepared; however, cardioversion should not be delayed while intravenous access is being obtained.

Adenosine is the medical treatment of choice for SVT. The underlying mechanism in children is usually a reentry circuit involving the atrioventricular node. Adenosine causes a temporary block in the atrioventricular node and interrupts this reentry circuit. The initial dose is 0.1 mg/kg given as a rapid intravenous bolus. Central venous administration is preferable because the drug is rapidly metabolized by red blood cell adenosine deaminase and therefore has a half-life of only 10 seconds. When the drug is given peripherally, the intravenous line should be immediately and rapidly flushed with 10 mL of saline. If there is no interruption in the reentry circuit, successive doses of 0.2 and 0.4 mg/kg should be given. In neonates, a smaller initial dose of 0.05 mg/kg is given and increased by 0.05 mg/kg/dose until termination of the arrhythmia up to a maximum dose of

0.3 mg/kg.[107] When SVT appears without any circulatory compromise, conversion of the arrhythmia may first be attempted with a vagal maneuver such as ice to the face. If this is ineffective, then adenosine should be utilized.

Other medications used to treat SVT have a greater incidence of adverse effects than adenosine. Digoxin is often ineffective and causes frequent arrhythmias. Verapamil should be avoided in infants because of its association with congestive heart failure and cardiac arrest because of its negative inotropic effects.[108] Flecainide is effective in treating SVT but has many cardiac and noncardiac adverse effects[109]; its role for hemodynamically unstable SVT remains to be established. Other therapies include β-adrenergic blockers, edrophonium, and α-agonists. If SVT persists despite medical therapy and the child progresses to circulatory instability, electrical cardioversion should proceed immediately.

## PULSELESS ELECTRICAL ACTIVITY

Pulseless electrical activity (PEA) is defined as organized ECG activity, excluding ventricular tachycardia and fibrillation, without clinical evidence of a palpable pulse or myocardial contractions. It may occur spontaneously after cardiac arrest or as an intervening rhythm associated with treatment for cardiac arrest. The causes of PEA is divided into primary (cardiac) and secondary (noncardiac) causes. Primary PEA, associated with cardiac arrest, is due to depletion of myocardial energy stores and thus responds poorly to therapy. Drugs used to treat primary PEA include epinephrine, atropine, calcium, and sodium bicarbonate.

The causes of secondary PEA are often remembered using the 4 Hs and 4 Ts mnemonic: *h*ypovolemia, *h*ypoxia, *h*ypothermia, and *h*ypo- or *h*yper-electrolytemia (hyperkalemia, hypocalcemia), *t*ension pneumothorax, pericardial *t*amponade, *t*hromboembolism, and *t*oxins (anesthetic overdose). In secondary PEA, intervention is directed at the underlying disorder and usually results in a successful resuscitation. When the cause of PEA is unknown and the child does not respond to medications, giving a fluid bolus and inserting needles into the pleural space to rule out pneumothorax and into the pericardial space to rule out cardiac tamponade should considered.

# Adjunctive Cardiopulmonary Resuscitation Techniques

## OPEN-CHEST CARDIOPULMONARY RESUSCITATION

The use of open-chest cardiac massage, although generally replaced by closed-chest CPR, still has an active role in the OR and ICU especially during and after thoracic surgery. Compared with closed-chest CPR, open-chest CPR generates greater cardiac output and vital organ blood flow. During open-chest CPR, less elevation occurs in intrathoracic, right atrial, and intracranial pressure, resulting in greater coronary and cerebral perfusion pressure and greater myocardial and cerebral blood flow.[110-112]

Typically, in the OR and ICU, open-chest CPR is preferable to closed-chest CPR in the child who has had a recent sternotomy. Open-chest CPR is also indicated for selected children when closed-chest CPR has failed, although exactly which children should receive this method of resuscitation under this condition is controversial. When initiated early after failure of closed-chest CPR, open-chest CPR may improve outcome.[113-115] When performed after 15 minutes of closed-chest CPR, open-chest CPR significantly improves coronary perfusion pressure and the rate of successful resuscitation.[116]

## EXTRACORPOREAL MEMBRANE OXYGENATION

In institutions with the ability to rapidly mobilize an extracorporeal circuit, extracorporeal cardiopulmonary bypass (CPB) should be considered for refractory pediatric cardiac arrest when the condition leading to arrest is reversible and when the period of no flow (cardiac arrest without CPR) was brief. Survival with a good neurologic outcome is possible after more than 50 minutes of CPR in selected children who were resuscitated via extracorporeal CPB.[117,118] CPB requires major technical support and sophistication but can be rapidly implemented in hospitals set up to do so. However, absence of a formal rapid deployment extracorporeal membrane oxygenation (ECMO) team does not preclude resuscitation ECMO in pediatric cardiac patients with good results.[119] Extracorporeal CPB should be reserved for children who have effective CPR initiated immediately after cardiac arrest.

## ACTIVE COMPRESSION-DECOMPRESSION

Active compression-decompression CPR uses a negative-pressure "pull" on the thorax during the release phase of chest compression using a handheld suction device. This technique has been shown to improve vascular pressures and minute ventilation during CPR in animals and humans.[120-124] The hemodynamic benefit of this technique is attributed to enhancement of venous return by the negative intrathoracic pressure generated during the decompression phase. Thus, when this technique was used with a device adding impedance to inspiration, vascular pressures and flow increased further.[125] Its effectiveness in adults shows promise, with increased survival and a trend toward neurologic improvement in prehospital victims.[126-128] However, two recent, larger trials did not demonstrate improved survival in in-hospital or prehospital victims of cardiac arrest, nor did any subgroup demonstrate benefit from active compression-decompression CPR.[129-131] The complication rate, including fatal rib and sternal fractures, may be greater with this technique.[132]

# Postresuscitation Stabilization (Post–Cardiac Arrest Care)

The goals of postresuscitation care are to prevent secondary organ injury, preserve neurologic function, diagnose and treat the cause of illness, and prevent recurrent arrest. Respiratory support should be tailored to minimize the risk of oxidative damage while maintaining adequate $O_2$ delivery. $FIO_2$ should be limited to the lowest necessary amount. Ventilation should be closely monitored, because both hypercarbia and hypocarbia have the potential for deleterious effects.

Mitigation of neurologic injury after cardiac arrest has been a goal of many investigator groups. In adult patients with out-of-hospital ventricular fibrillation and in asphyxiated newborns,[47] therapeutic hypothermia has been shown to be of benefit. In a retrospective study involving five hospitals, the effectiveness of hypothermia therapy was neither supported nor refuted.[133] Fink and colleagues[134] studied the feasibility of achieving mild hypothermia after pediatric cardiac arrest and found that they were reliably able to achieve a target temperature of 89.6° to 93.2° F (32° to 34° C) in less than 3 hours. A multicenter, randomized, controlled trial of systemic hypothermia for 48 hours after nontraumatic cardiac arrest (Therapeutic Hypothermia After Pediatric Cardiac Arrest [THAPCA]) is currently ongoing.

## ANNOTATED REFERENCES

American Heart Association. American Heart Association guidelines for cardiopulmonary resuscitation and emergency cardiovascular care. Circulation 2010;122:S640-933.

*This publication provides comprehensive guidelines for pediatric and adult advanced life support, with comprehensive references.*

Nadkarni VM, Larkin GL, Peberdy MA, et al. First documented rhythm and clinical outcome from in-hospital cardiac arrest among children and adults. JAMA 2006;295:50-7.

*In this multicenter registry of in-hospital cardiac arrest, the first documented pulseless arrest rhythm was typically asystole or pulseless electrical activity in both children and adults. Because of improved survival after asystole and pulseless electrical activity, children had better outcomes than adults despite fewer cardiac arrests resulting from ventricular fibrillation or pulseless ventricular tachycardia.*

Perondi M, Reis A, Paiva E, et al. A comparison of high-dose and standard-dose epinephrine in children with cardiac arrest. N Engl J Med 2004;350:1722-30.

*This blinded, randomized controlled trial compared high-dose to standard-dose epinephrine as rescue therapy in children with in-hospital cardiac arrest. No benefit of high-dose epinephrine was detected. The data suggest that high-dose therapy may be more deleterious than standard-dose therapy.*

## REFERENCES

Please see www.expertconsult.com.

# Malignant Hyperthermia

JEROME PARNESS AND JERROLD LERMAN

MALIGNANT HYPERTHERMIA (MH) is a pharmacogenetic disease of skeletal muscle that may precipitate a potentially fatal sequence of metabolic responses in the presence of triggering anesthetics. The primary triggers for MH–inhalational anesthetics and succinylcholine–induce an uncontrollable release of intramyoplasmic calcium ($Ca^{2+}$) that results in sustained muscle contractures, which produce a hypermetabolic response. The hypermetabolic response manifests with hypercarbia, hyperpnea, tachycardia, and if not treated early, a mixed metabolic and respiratory acidosis. It is usually accompanied by some form of muscle rigidity: isolated muscle rigidity (e.g., masseter muscle tetany in the temporomandibular joint) or total body muscle rigidity (e.g., sustained contraction of major peripheral muscle groups).

MH was first described by Denborough and Lovell in 1960, who reported a 21-year-old man with compound fractures of his right tibia, who, with great trepidation, underwent general anesthesia with halothane.[1] After 10 minutes of anesthesia, he became hemodynamically unstable with hypotension, tachycardia, and mottled skin that was hot to the touch. The soda lime canister was found to be hot and was changed because it appeared to be exhausted. The anesthetic was discontinued, the patient was packed in ice, and he recovered without sequelae. Postprocedural examination did not reveal any known medical abnormalities. A careful family history disclosed that 10 blood relatives had previously died after ether anesthesia, suggesting an autosomal dominant pattern of inheritance for the disorder. This patient required a subsequent operation and was administered a spinal anesthetic without incident, demonstrating the effectiveness of nontriggering anesthetics.[2] Subsequent reports from around the world established this disorder as a familial entity that was potentially fatal.[3,4] The term *malignant hyperpyrexia* (later changed to *malignant hyperthermia*) was coined in 1967 at the first international meeting on this disorder.

The incidence of MH based on occurrences of MH reactions has been reported to be 1 case per 50,000 to 100,000 adults and 1 case per 3000 to 15,000 children.[5,6] Subsequent surveys of suspected MH reactions revealed even greater incidences; the incidence of suspected MH was 1 case per 16,000 anesthetics in adults in Denmark, an incidence that increased to 1 case per 4200 adults when an inhaled anesthetic and succinylcholine were combined.[7] However, a survey of anesthesia in a pediatric hospital in the United States during the halothane era revealed an MH incidence of 1 case per 20,000 to 40,000 children, almost one half of that reported previously.[8] The incidence of fulminant MH (i.e., rapid increase in temperature accompanied by life-threatening metabolic changes, arrhythmias, and increased serum creatine kinase level) was 1 case per 250,000 general anesthetics in Denmark.[7] A similar incidence of 1 case of fulminant MH per 200,000 general anesthetics was reported from the United Kingdom.[9] The Danish survey found an incidence of 1 case of masseter muscle spasm per 12,000 anesthetics among children who received succinylcholine, whether in combination with inhalational or intravenous anesthetics.[7] Clinically, the demographic data suggested that the incidence or suspicion of MH was greater among children than adults and that the incidence was even greater among children in whom succinylcholine was used.

The frequency of MH reactions is greatest in childhood, with a peak age of 3 years, although recent data suggest that only about 18% of MH reactions occur in childhood.[10,11] Reactions have also been reported in neonates and infants, although they have been infrequent.[12] Many have perceived a decrease in the incidence of MH reactions in the past 2 decades, although some have challenged this perception.[11] Two reasons for the perception that the incidence of MH reactions have decreased are that many families with a genetic predisposition to MH have been identified and bring it to the attention of their surgical and anesthetic care providers preoperatively, and that the routine use of succinylcholine has decreased dramatically as a result of concerns regarding rare complications, such as hyperkalemic cardiac arrest. The latter has resulted in a black box warning admonishing against the routine use of succinylcholine in children, particularly male children younger than 8 years of age who may have unrecognized muscular dystrophy or other myopathy.[13,14]

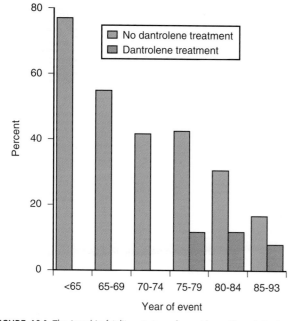

FIGURE 40-1 The trend in fatality rate in malignant hyperthermia is shown over time. The *blue bars* represent data from 361 patients, and the *magenta bars* represent data from 142 patients. Notice the marked decrease in mortality with dantrolene treatment. (Modified from Strazis KP, Fox AW. Malignant hyperthermia: a review of published cases. Anesth Analg 1993;77:297-304.)

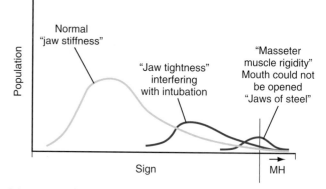

FIGURE 40-2 The spectrum of masseter muscle responses to succinylcholine varies from a slight jaw stiffness that does not interfere with endotracheal intubation to the extreme "jaws of steel," which is masseter muscle tetany that does not allow the mouth to be opened. The latter response is likely highly associated with malignant hyperthermia (MH). Even with the inability to open the mouth, the child's lungs should still be able to be ventilated by bag and mask because all other muscles are relaxed. (From Kaplan RF. Malignant hyperthermia. Annual refresher course lectures. Washington, DC: American Society of Anesthesiologists; 1993.)

It remains certain that all inhalational anesthetics and succinylcholine are potent triggers of MH reactions in susceptible patients,[15-19] with the possible exception of xenon based on evidence from MH-sensitive pigs[20] and caffeine-halothane contracture tests (CHCTs) from MH-susceptible and normal humans.[21] No other drugs used for intravenous or regional anesthesia trigger MH reactions. A comprehensive list of triggering and nontriggering drugs is available from the Malignant Hyperthermia Association of the United States (MHAUS) (http://www.mhaus.org/ [accessed July 2012]).

The mortality rate for MH has decreased dramatically from more than 80% in the 1960s to 1.5% to 5% in recent years (Fig. 40-1).[11,22-24] For children, the MH mortality rate (0.7%) is 15-fold less than the rate (14%) for adults.[11] The overall decrease in mortality may be attributable to several factors: better identification of MH-susceptible individuals; the routine use of capnography and pulse oximetry, facilitating early identification of the signs and symptoms of an acute MH reaction[25,26]; a better understanding of the pathogenesis of MH; and the widespread availability of dantrolene.[10]

## Clinical Presentation

The most common presentation of MH is a hypermetabolic response to the inhalational anesthetics, with or without succinylcholine (Table 40-1). Among the earliest clinical signs is a marked increase in the end-tidal $CO_2$ that resists control by either mechanical ventilation or an increase in minute ventilation when the patient is breathing spontaneously.[23,27] Other nonspecific early signs include tachycardia and hemodynamic instability with a trend toward hypertension. Severe masseter muscle spasm (i.e., masseter tetany) refers to the inability to insert a laryngoscope blade into the mouth, the so-called "jaws of steel," even with no

### TABLE 40-1 Clinical and Laboratory Findings Associated with Malignant Hyperthermia

| Clinical Findings | Laboratory Findings |
|---|---|
| Tachycardia, tachypnea and hypertension | Increased $PaCO_2$ |
| Hypercarbia (ETCO$_2$) | Acidosis (mixed respiratory and metabolic) |
| Greatly increased minute ventilation | Relative hypoxia, increased alveolar to arterial partial pressure gradient for oxygen |
| Generalized muscle rigidity (unresponsive to nondepolarizing muscle relaxants) | Hyperkalemia |
| Skin mottling | Elevated plasma lactate concentration |
| Hyperthermia (late sign) | Abnormal coagulation studies (late sign) |
| Cardiac arrhythmias (hyperkalemia-induced: PVC, VT, VF) | Myoglobinuria, myoglobinemia |
| Cola-colored urine (late sign) | Increased CPK level (usually a late sign) |
| Disseminated intravascular coagulation (late) | |

Data from Malignant Hyperthermia Association of the United States. Available at http://www.mhaus.org (accessed July 2012).
*CPK*, Creatinine phosphokinase; *ETCO₂*, end-tidal carbon dioxide; *PaCO₂*, arterial partial pressure of carbon dioxide; *PVC*, premature ventricular contraction; *VF*, ventricular fibrillation; *VT*, ventricular tachycardia.

twitches evident on a blockade monitor after administration of succinylcholine, and it strongly indicates MH susceptibility (Fig. 40-2). In vitro live muscle biopsy testing revealed a 28% to 50% incidence of MH susceptibility among children with jaws of steel (Table 40-2).[28-30] Generalized muscle rigidity develops as a result of the excessive accumulation of myoplasmic $Ca^{2+}$ concentrations in MH-susceptible skeletal muscle, causing sustained muscle contractures.[27] This occurs even in the presence of

**TABLE 40-2** Limited Excursion of the Mandible: Differential Diagnosis

Temporomandibular joint dysfunction: congenital, inflammatory/infectious, trauma, neoplasm, collagen vascular disease (rheumatoid arthritis)

Muscle disease: malignant hyperthermia, Duchenne or Becker muscular dystrophy, myotonia congenita

Integumentary disease: inflammatory or infectious disease, neoplasm, radiation effects, collagen vascular disease (scleroderma)

Neurologic injury

Ultra-rapid metabolizer of succinylcholine (Nietlich or Cynthiana [C5 enzyme] variant of pseudocholinesterase) (see Chapter 6)

Ineffective succinylcholine

**TABLE 40-3** Arterial Blood Gas Data from a Child in Early Malignant Hyperthermia

| Data | TIME AT MEASUREMENT | | | |
|---|---|---|---|---|
| | 08:52 | 08:59 | 09:05 | 09:27 |
| pH* | 7.34 | 7.03 | 7.29 | 7.39 |
| $Pco_2$ (mm Hg) | 46.3 | 109.4 | 47.9 | 42.7 |
| $Po_2$ (mm Hg) | 236 | 159 | 589 | 635 |
| Base excess | −1 | −2 | −3 | 1 |
| $HCO_3^-$ (mmol/L) | 25.1 | 29 | 23.1 | 25.6 |

*Notice the pure respiratory acidosis in this patient from Figure 41-3 and the rapid decrease in $Paco_2$ after dantrolene administration between 08:59 and 09:05.

**TABLE 40-4** Differential Diagnosis of Malignant Hyperthermia

| Diagnosis | Distinguishing Traits |
|---|---|
| Hyperthyroidism | Patients often present with similar symptoms and physical findings; blood gas abnormalities gradually evolve; creatine phosphokinase value does not increase substantively. |
| Sepsis | Usually, blood gases are normal early, and metabolic acidosis occurs late; creatine phosphokinase remains normal. |
| Pheochromocytoma | Similar to MH, except for marked blood pressure swings |
| Metastatic carcinoid | Flushing, diarrhea, hypotension |
| Cocaine intoxication | Fever, rigidity, rhabdomyolysis similar to NMS |
| Heat stroke | Similar to MH, except that the patient is outside the operating room |
| Masseter muscle rigidity (MMR) | May progress to MH; total body spasm more likely than isolated MMR |
| Neuroleptic malignant syndrome (NMS) | Similar to MH but evolves over weeks; usually associated with the use of antipsychotics |
| Serotonergic toxicity | Similar to MH and NMS; associated with the administration of mood-elevating drugs (e.g., selective serotonin reuptake inhibitors) |
| Nonmalignant hyperthermia syndrome | Reported only once; severe hyperthermia seemingly associated with fentanyl |

neuromuscular blockade with nondepolarizing neuromuscular blocking drugs (NMBDs).

Hyperthermia, often a late sign, results from the greatly increased aerobic and anaerobic metabolic activity of triggered skeletal muscle; the overlying skin soon becomes hot to the touch. In many instances, the large muscle groups such as calf or thigh muscles feel tight or knotted. This is accompanied by exaggerated carbon dioxide ($CO_2$) production, which usually is the first sign of an evolving MH reaction, and the accumulation of lactate fueled by markedly increased glycogenolysis and glycolysis (i.e., mixed respiratory and metabolic acidosis).[31,32] If an acute MH reaction is diagnosed and treated early in its evolution, before the body becomes unable to maintain this exaggerated aerobic metabolism, arterial blood gases may show an almost pure respiratory acidosis, which can make the diagnosis of MH difficult (Table 40-3). A mixed venous or peripheral venous blood gas analysis can be helpful in establishing the presence of hypermetabolism because it is more likely to demonstrate an increased $CO_2$ level, significant oxygen desaturation consistent with increased oxygen consumption ($\dot{V}o_2$ less than 40 mm Hg, despite administering supplemental oxygen for which the expected $\dot{V}o_2$ is greater than 60 mm Hg), and a possible increased lactate concentration.

In fulminant cases, untreated MH may increase the temperature as rapidly as 1° C every 10 minutes.[27] In one case, the temperature reached 43.8° C (110.8° F) within 18 minutes.[33] In addition to the profound hypercarbia and tachycardia, severe hypoxia, skin mottling, exuberant metabolic acidosis, rhabdomyolysis, coagulopathy, and hyperkalemia may follow. Unstable hemodynamics and ventricular arrhythmias inevitably follow. Intractable ventricular arrhythmias, pulmonary edema, disseminated intravascular coagulation, cerebral hypoxia or edema, and

renal failure due to myoglobin deposition in the renal tubules are often associated with fatal outcomes.

In the early years of treating acute MH reactions, before dantrolene was identified as the specific antidote, symptomatic treatment was the mainstay of therapy. This included treatment of the acidosis and hyperkalemia with bicarbonate, and insulin with glucose, respectively; active cooling with iced saline gastric lavage; infusion of cold intravenous saline; and infusions of procainamide (a drug that was later shown to be ineffective). These interventions helped to reduce the mortality rate to about 50%, but with the availability of dantrolene, the mortality rate has decreased dramatically.

The presenting signs of MH vary (see Table 40-1). The syndrome may be fulminant or indolent, not all features of a classic MH reaction may be immediately evident, and it may occur intraoperatively or postoperatively, although the frequency of MH reactions occurring postoperatively is only 2%.[27,34] The latest that an MH reaction has reportedly occurred postoperatively is 11 hours, although a recent review of reports of postoperative MH in the North American Malignant Hyperthermia Registry has not found any case occurring beyond 40 minutes after the end of the anesthetic.[34,35] The likelihood that an MH-susceptible patient will develop MH in the presence of inhalational anesthetics is exasperatingly unpredictable. In one study, 50% of susceptible individuals reported two or more uneventful general anesthesias before an MH reaction was triggered.[23,36] Only 6.5% of probands in a retrospective review reported a family or personal history of MH.[36] A negative personal or family history is insufficient to conclude that a child is not susceptible to MH. Other disease states may be confused with MH (Table 40-4) and must be distinguished from it to provide correct therapy.

Given the variability of the clinical presentation of MH and the dearth of pathognomonic signs for this syndrome,

**TABLE 40-5** Clinical Indicators for Determining the Malignant Hyperthermia Raw Score

| Process | Indicator | Points |
|---|---|---|
| Rigidity | Generalized muscular rigidity | 15 |
| | Masseter spasm | 15 |
| Muscle breakdown | Creatine kinase >20,000 IU after succinylcholine | 15 |
| | Creatine kinase >10,000 IU with no succinylcholine | 15 |
| | Cola-colored urine in perioperative period | 10 |
| | Myoglobin in urine >60 μg/L | 5 |
| | Myoglobin in serum >170 μg/L | 5 |
| | Blood, plasma, or serum $K^+$ >6 mEq/L, no renal illness | 3 |
| Respiratory acidosis | $PETCO_2$ >55 mm Hg with controlled ventilation | 15 |
| | Arterial $PaCO_2$ >60 mm Hg with controlled ventilation | 15 |
| | $PETCO_2$ >60 mm Hg with spontaneous ventilation | 15 |
| | Arterial $PaCO_2$ >65 mm Hg with spontaneous ventilation | 15 |
| | Inappropriate hypercarbia, anesthesiologist's call | 15 |
| | Inappropriate tachypnea | 10 |
| Temperature increase | Inappropriately rapid increase | 15 |
| | Inappropriately increased temperature >38.8° C (101.8° F) | 10 |
| Cardiac involvement | Inappropriate sinus tachycardia | 3 |
| | Ventricular tachycardia or fibrillation | 3 |
| Family history | Positive family history for first-degree relative | 15 |
| | Positive family history for more distant relative | 5 |
| Others | Arterial base excess more negative than −8 mEq/L | 10 |
| | Arterial pH <7.25 | 10 |
| | Rapid reversal of malignant hyperthermia (MH) signs after intravenous administration of dantrolene | 5 |
| | Positive MH family history with another indicator from the patient's anesthesia experience other than increased creatine kinase level | 10 |
| | Elevated creatine kinase level and a family history of MH | 10 |

From Larach MG, Localio AR, Allen GC, et al. A clinical grading scale to predict malignant hyperthermia susceptibility. Anesthesiology 1994;80:771-9.

**TABLE 40-6** Malignant Hyperthermia Clinical Grading Scale

| Raw Score Range | Rank | Likelihood |
|---|---|---|
| 0 | 1 | Almost never |
| 3-9 | 2 | Unlikely |
| 10-19 | 3 | Somewhat less than likely |
| 20-34 | 4 | Somewhat greater than likely |
| 35-49 | 5 | Very likely |
| ≥50 | 6 | Almost certain |

Modified from Larach MG, Localio AR, Allen GC, et al. A clinical grading scale to predict malignant hyperthermia susceptibility. Anesthesiology 1994;80:771-9.

## Patient Evaluation and Preparation

Optimal treatment begins with prevention and preparation. Obtaining an accurate family history of suspicious or unusual reactions to general anesthesia in blood relatives, unexpected admissions to intensive care after surgery, or unexplained sudden death during anesthesia should signal the surgeon and anesthesiologist to consider MH or another problem related to anesthesia. These questions assume the patient is part of a classic nuclear family, but with increasing levels of adoption, artificial insemination, surrogate motherhood, and egg donations, standard probing may not elicit clear family histories. The anesthesiologist must be sensitive but decisive in determining the true genetic relationship between the guardians and the child. Despite attempts to obtain an accurate history, misinterpretation of the questions may occur. In one case, an adopted child died of succinylcholine-induced hyperkalemic cardiac arrest, even though the parents denied that anyone in the family had anesthesia problems or muscle disease during the preoperative assessment. Only immediately after the event did the parent reveal that the child had been adopted and that the child's birth uncle had muscular dystrophy.

If the anesthesiologist is informed that the child has a blood relative who had an MH reaction or who has a myopathy with high concordance with MH, the most prudent course of action is to plan using a nontriggering anesthetic for total intravenous or regional anesthesia, or both. In the rare circumstance in which such prudence cannot be followed, extreme vigilance and preparation to treat MH are of the utmost importance.

Ambulatory surgery has rapidly expanded to include most pediatric surgery. Consequently, the safety of discharging children with a personal or family history of MH after an uneventful, trigger-free anesthesia on the day of surgery has raised concerns. Two retrospective studies concluded that the risk of a child developing an MH reaction after an uneventful, trigger-free anesthesia was exceedingly small.[38] Postoperative monitoring for an MH reaction while in the hospital was gradually reduced from 6 hours to 2 hours before discharge.[39,40] For MH-susceptible children, parents should be provided with a written description of the signs and symptoms of an MH reaction and a phone number for the on-call anesthesiologist for further advice. Families should contact an anesthesiologist rather than return to the emergency department, because the emergency physician may be unfamiliar with MH, particularly in children. Additional advice for the parents should include the use of an oral antipyretic drug (e.g., acetaminophen) to treat a mild fever. If the fever abates after a dose or two of acetaminophen, the fever was not caused by

establishing the diagnosis can be difficult. In response to the need for an objective measure to verify a clinical episode of MH, a retrospective, multivariable clinical grading scale was developed.[37] This grading scale was devised to clarify the cutoff value for a positive muscle CHCT result. It was not intended to be a clinical guide in the operating room. Despite recommendations not to use this scale to guide treatment and to be more conservative in its application, Tables 40-5 and 40-6 are provided to help clinicians identify true MH reactions. Although this clinical grading scale is somewhat cumbersome and has not been prospectively validated in clinical settings for use by nonexperts, it is a useful guide for the clinician.

MH. If the fever persists despite acetaminophen and sponge baths, and is accompanied by tachycardia and tachypnea, the parents should notify the on-call anesthesiologist and return the child to the hospital.

When a child with a known susceptibility to MH is scheduled for general anesthesia, the anesthesia machine (i.e., anesthetic workstation [AWS]) must be prepared to preclude the delivery of triggering agents. First, succinylcholine should be removed from the local vicinity to avoid inadvertent administration. Second, all vaporizers should be physically disengaged from the AWS, which is preferable because they can leak trace concentrations of inhalational anesthetics even in the off state, or if they cannot be removed from the AWS, tape should be placed across them in the off position to avoid accidentally turning them on.[41] Third, to accelerate the washout of anesthetics, the $CO_2$ absorbent should be replaced, a new anesthetic breathing circuit installed, and the ventilator bellows flushed and left operating.[41-43] Fourth, to eliminate inhalational anesthetics from the AWS, many clinicians follow a standardized protocol of flushing the workstation with 10 L/min of oxygen for 10 to 20 minutes, depending on the manufacturer and age of the machine.[44] However, the assumption that one protocol fits all to reduce the anesthetic concentration to less than 10 ppm, which is assumed to be the threshold below which an MH reaction cannot be triggered,[45] may not hold true for every AWS, particularly the newer ones, which are more complex in construction and more likely to contain internal working parts made of plastic, which act as sumps for inhalational anesthetics. To address the various types of AWS, the duration of flushing with large fresh gas flows (Table 40-7) and the need to exchange contaminated internal components with clean versions must be determined for each AWS. For some types of AWS, more than 60 minutes may be required to reach anesthetic concentrations less than 10 ppm.[44,46,47] To achieve an anesthetic concentration of 10 ppm or less in the Drager Primus, Fabius, and Zeus machines in a timely manner, the ventilator diaphragm and integrated breathing system should be replaced with autoclaved components and then flushed for 20 minutes at a fresh gas flow of 10 L/min.[46,47] Table 40-7 lists the published times required to reach an anesthetic concentration of less than 10 ppm without replacing any AWS components.[44,47,48] These data support the notion that the previously held protocols

**TABLE 40-7** Time to Wash Out Inhalational Anesthetics to Less than 10 ppm from Anesthetic Workstations

| Ohmeda Machines | Time (minutes) | Non-Ohmeda Machines | Time (minutes) |
|---|---|---|---|
| Modulus 1 | 5-15 | Narkomed | 20 |
| Excel 210 | 7 | Drager Primus | 70 |
| AS/3 | 30 | Drager Fabius GS | 104 |
| Aestiva (sevoflurane)* | 22 | Drager Zeus† | 85 |
| Aisys (sevoflurane)* | 25 | Kion | >25 |

Data from Kim TW, Nemergut ME. Preparation of modern anesthesia workstations for malignant hyperthermia-susceptible patients; a review of past and present practice. Anesthesiology 2011;114:205-12; Lerman J. Pediatric anesthesia. In: Barash P, Cullen B, Stoelting R, editors. Clinical anesthesia. St Louis: Lippincott Williams & Wilkins, 2012; *Sabouri AS, Lerman J, Heard C. Residual sevoflurane may be present after flushing the GE anesthesia workstation for MH susceptible patients. Anesthesiology 2011;115:A1276; †Shanahan H, O'Donoghue R, O'Kelly P, Synnott A, O'Rourke J. Preparation of the Drager Fabius CE and Drager Zeus anaesthetic machines for patients susceptible to malignant hyperthermia. Eur J Anaesthesiol 2012;29:229-34.

to wash out inhalational anesthetics from older AWSs do not hold true for the newer AWSs. The need for a single protocol or intervention that consistently achieves an anesthetic concentration of less than 10 ppm in all AWSs is of even greater importance because none of the available anesthetic agent analyzers is capable of measuring anesthetic concentrations in the 10 ppm range to confirm adequate removal of inhalational anesthetics.

After the AWS has been flushed with 10 L/min of an air and oxygen mixture, most anesthesiologists reduce the fresh gas flow during anesthesia. However, evidence has shown that the concentration of inhalational anesthetic surges (≥50 ppm) when the fresh gas flow is reduced, and the magnitude of the rebound directly depends on the fresh gas flow rate.[48,49] Those who reduce the fresh gas flow after purging the AWS may be exposing their patients to concentrations of inhalational anesthetics that may trigger an MH reaction, although no MH reactions have been reported in patients in whom a reduced fresh gas flow was used in an AWS that had been purged using a large (>10 lpm) fresh gas flow. To avoid confusion, a single, consistent, effective, and reliable intervention is required to prevent MH reactions in patients exposed to trace gases from a previously contaminated AWS.

A commercially available charcoal filter (Vapor-Clean, Dynasthetics, LLC, Salt Lake City) fitted to the expiratory and inspiratory limbs of the AWS reduces the concentration of inhalational anesthetics to less than 5 ppm within several minutes.[50] These filters are sold in pairs. The manufacturer recommends that a filter should be inserted into both limbs of the anesthesia breathing circuit just distal to the valves, which is reasonable during an acute MH reaction. However, when only the machine is contaminated with inhalational anesthetic (e.g., after flushing the AWS for elective MH cases), we apply a single filter in the inspiratory limb and keep the second of the pair to replace the first after 60 to 90 minutes, since it may become expended by that time.[50]

## Monitoring

Capnography and pulse oximetry, key monitors for early signs of an MH reaction, are required for all children who receive general anesthesia, irrespective of the duration of the procedure. Measurement of the body temperature is recommended for all children who undergo general anesthesia when fluctuations may be anticipated, according to the American Society of Anesthesiologists 2011 standards for basic anesthesia monitoring (www.asahq.org/For-Members/Standards-Guidelines-and-Statements.aspx). Monitoring the axillary temperature site (opposite the extremity with the intravenous line) is recommended rather than a core site for early detection of an MH reaction because the axillary region is surrounded by large muscle bulk in the pectoral shoulder girdle. Although most consider an increasing temperature a late sign of an MH reaction, a retrospective review suggested that an increasing body temperature may occur early in an evolving MH reaction.[36,51] Evidence also suggests that crystalline skin temperature tapes may not reliably track temperature changes during MH reactions.[36]

## Diagnosis

Because the underlying disorder in MH is a hypermetabolic reaction (i.e., increased $CO_2$ production and oxygen consumption), massive volumes of $CO_2$ are released into the circulation, which rapidly increase the partial pressure of $CO_2$ ($PCO_2$) and respiratory rate in the unparalyzed child. The cardiovascular response is an increased cardiac output, heart rate, and in some cases, blood pressure (E-Fig. 40-1). The first clinical signs and symptoms of this hypermetabolic reaction in a spontaneously breathing patient are hypercapnia, tachypnea, and tachycardia (see Table 40-1).[36] A steady and relentless increase in the end-tidal $CO_2$ pressure (PETCO$_2$) is the earliest sign of a reaction and is usually evident whether respirations are spontaneous or controlled. In some instances, the increase in PETCO$_2$ and heart rate occur contemporaneously, alerting the clinician to consider an evolving MH reaction (Fig. 40-3). Sudden unexpected cardiac arrest is a very rare presentation of MH and suggests a disease process other than MH, such as acute rhabdomyolysis and hyperkalemia after succinylcholine in a (male) child with an undiagnosed myopathy.

The presenting signs of an MH reaction are nonspecific and may suggest several possible disease states or equipment problems. The earliest sign of an MH reaction, an increase in end-tidal pCO$_2$, may result from one or more of three factors from the $CO_2$ mass balance equation:

$$PCO_2 = (\dot{V}CO_2 / \dot{V}A) + FICO_2$$

The circulating PCO$_2$ depends on the production of $CO_2$ ($\dot{V}CO_2$), the elimination of $CO_2$ (i.e., alveolar ventilation ($[\dot{V}A]$), and the inspired concentration of $CO_2$ (FICO$_2$). The differential diagnosis of an increased PCO$_2$ can be analyzed by considering the causes for each of these three factors. Causes of an increased $\dot{V}CO_2$ include fever, MH, thyroid storm, and sepsis. Causes of a decreased $\dot{V}A$ include a deep level of anesthesia, endobronchial intubation, bronchospasm, and a kinked tracheal tube or airway breathing circuit. Causes of increased FICO$_2$ include an incompetent expiratory valve, exogenous source of $CO_2$, low fresh gas flows with a partial or nonrebreathing circuit, and expired $CO_2$ absorbent. The initial evaluation should include a rapid assessment of the integrity of the breathing circuit, the presence of bilateral breath sounds and absence of wheezing, and examination of the $CO_2$ absorbent.

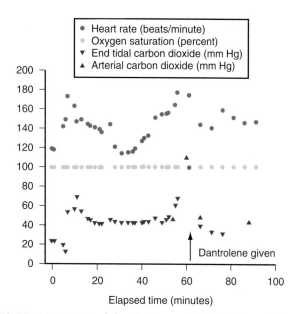

FIGURE 40-3 Response of physiologic parameters to dantrolene during an apparent intraoperative episode of malignant hyperthermia. Notice the rapid fall in arterial and end-tidal carbon dioxide pressures after dantrolene (2.5 mg/kg) administration (*arrow*). (Courtesy Steven C. Hall, MD.)

During airway obstruction and hypermetabolic states such as thyrotoxicosis and sepsis, an increased PETCO$_2$ can be readily corrected with mild to moderate hyperventilation. During MH reactions, however, it is very difficult to restore the PETCO$_2$ to the normal range, even with vigorous mechanical hyperventilation.[26] The $CO_2$ production is sometimes so great that the in-circuit $CO_2$ absorbent rapidly becomes exhausted in an exothermic reaction, and the absorbent container becomes hot to touch.

A child's response to surgery during light anesthesia often includes tachycardia and may sometimes include bronchoconstriction. However, a dramatic and unexpected increase in heart rate from 120 to 180 beats/min in a healthy, 7-year-old child (or an increase from 70 to 120 beats/min in an adult) strongly suggests a pathologic process, and a differential diagnosis beyond light anesthesia should be seriously considered. Before intervening, it is important to quickly scan all of the monitors to determine whether the aggregate indices point to a specific diagnosis. If tachycardia is associated with an increase in body temperature, a differential diagnosis of fever and tachycardia under anesthesia should be considered. Fever related to sepsis or viral infection usually has a slow onset, whereas fever from an MH reaction typically has a rapid onset. The differential diagnoses include iatrogenic external overheating and an MH reaction (see Table 40-4). A rapid increase in the inspired concentration of desflurane and isoflurane, but not sevoflurane, may cause a sympathetic-based tachycardia that in isolation should not suggest a diagnosis of MH because the PETCO$_2$ remains unchanged.[52,53] Of the inhalational anesthetics, halothane appears to be the most likely to trigger an MH reaction and the best discriminator for the CHCT. Enflurane provides the smallest trigger, sevoflurane and isoflurane are intermediate, and preliminary data suggest that xenon does not trigger MH reactions.[21,45,54-56] If none of these factors appears to be causative and a deeper level of anesthesia (achieved with propofol with or without an opioid) fails to abate the signs, simultaneous venous and arterial blood gases should be analyzed to determine whether the patient has or is developing a hypermetabolic state.

A moderate but gradual increase in body temperature may occur in children excessively draped, those with forced-air warming devices, those with bilateral limb tourniquets, and those covered with plastic occlusive wrap. However, the sudden onset of a high fever must be more thoroughly investigated because it may result from several potentially fatal causes (see Table 40-4).[57-60]

## Management, Susceptibility Screening, and Counseling

### TREATMENT

If the anesthesiologist suspects that a child is experiencing an MH episode, the inhalational anesthetic should be immediately discontinued, 100% oxygen administered at a large fresh gas flow rate (≥10 L/min), and the surgeon informed; if surgery cannot be aborted, it must be completed expeditiously. Charcoal filters should be inserted into both limbs of the breathing circuit until a clean breathing circuit is available (E-Fig. 40-2). They prevent the child from being contaminated by residual anesthetic in the AWS and to prevent the AWS from being contaminated by anesthetic in the patient.[50] The MH cart and additional personnel to assist in dissolving the dantrolene should be brought to the operating room immediately (Table 40-8). Minute ventilation should be increased to control the PaCO$_2$ and PETCO$_2$.

**40**

| TABLE 40-8 | Contents of a Pediatric Malignant Hyperthermia Emergency Cart | | | |
|---|---|---|---|---|

**Fluids**

2000 mL of $D_5$ 0.2 NaCl, 500-mL IV bottles

3000 mL of 0.9 NaCl, 500-mL IV bottles

1 regular insulin, 100 units/mL, 10-mL vial

4 ice packs

| Drug Number | Drug | Dose | Vessel |
|---|---|---|---|
| 10 | Dantrolene IV* | 20 mg (dilute with 60 mL of sterile water) | |
| 10 | 100 mL of sterile injectable water *for dantrolene use only* (red label) | | |
| 10 | 18- and 20-gauge needles | | |
| 4 | Sodium bicarbonate | 1 mEq/mL | 50-mL vial |
| 1 | Sodium bicarbonate | 1 mEq/mL | 50-mL syringe |
| 1 | 50% dextrose | 500 mg/mL | 50-mL vial |
| 10 | Sterile injection NaCl | | 10-mL vial |
| 4 | Mannitol 25% | 12.5 g/50 mL | 50-mL vial |
| 10 | Furosemide (Lasix) | 10 mg/mL | 4-mL ampule |
| 10 | 20- and 22-gauge IV catheters | | |
| 8 | Syringes, TB: 6, 12, 20, and 60 mL | | |

*To rapidly mix dantrolene, use 18-gauge needles on 60-mL syringes to transfer sterile water to dantrolene vials. Have a colleague vigorously shake the vial while diluting the next dantrolene vial to ensure adequate dissolution and reduce the time of preparation. Final concentration is 0.33 mg/mL. Administer 2.5 mg/kg. For larger patients, several individuals may be needed to vigorously shake multiple dantrolene vials.
*IV,* Intravenous; *TB,* tuberculin.

The anesthesia should be converted to total intravenous anesthesia, and if charcoal filters are not available, hyperventilation should be continued using an external self-inflating or anesthesia-type bag with an exogenous source of oxygen that is uncontaminated by inhalational anesthetics. If the airway was not intubated, tracheal intubation should be performed and ventilation controlled mechanically to achieve a normal $P_{ETCO_2}$.

Because native dantrolene is quite insoluble in water, several strategies have been developed to speed its solubility. The current formulation is packaged as a lyophilized yellow powder in 20-mg vials that contain 3 g of mannitol and enough base to maintain a pH of about 9.5 (E-Fig. 40-3). The lyophilized formulation, mannitol, and the alkaline pH all speed the dissolution of dantrolene in water. Sixty milliliters of sterile water should be added to each vial to dissolve the dantrolene, with a resultant dantrolene concentration of 0.33 mg/mL. Warming the sterile water speeds dissolution.[61] Most of the dantrolene in a vial dissolves within 60 seconds of adding the water. When the vial is vigorously shaken, any residual crystals dissolve, and the solution turns clear orange. The solution should be withdrawn immediately and administered intravenously as rapidly as possible. Occasionally, 1 or 2 additional minutes may be required to dissolve the last few crystals of dantrolene. Given the extreme alkaline pH of the

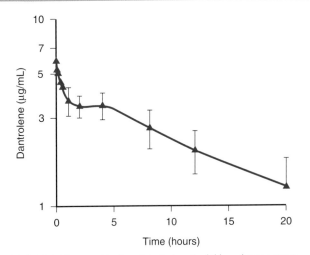

**FIGURE 40-4** Pharmacokinetics of dantrolene in children. (From Lerman J, McLeod ME, Strong HA. Pharmacokinetics of intravenous dantrolene in children. Anesthesiology 1989;70:625-9.)

dantrolene solution, it should be rapidly infused into a large vein to reduce the risk of phlebitis. Extravasation of dantrolene or prolonged continuous infusions of dantrolene may cause thrombophlebitis or thrombosis of large and small veins.[62-64] Some have recommended continuous infusions of dantrolene in adults after the initial bolus, although the risk/benefit ratio of this practice is unproved in adults and untested in children.[65] A new formulation of nanocrystalline dantrolene that rapidly dissolves and is available in a much greater concentration than the current formulation is undergoing federal review.[66]

The pharmacokinetics of intravenous dantrolene have been studied in MH-susceptible children 2 to 7 years of age.[67] A loading dose of 2.5 mg/kg produced predictable blood concentrations (≥3 µg/mL) for about 6 hours after the loading dose (Fig. 40-4).[67] Based on these pharmacokinetic data, if half of the loading dose of dantrolene were repeated at 6 hours after the loading dose, therapeutic blood concentrations of dantrolene would be maintained for a total of 15 hours and possibly prevent a recrudescence.[67]

An initial bolus dose of 2.5 mg/kg can control most MH reactions if the dantrolene is administered as soon after the onset of the reaction as possible (see Fig. 40-3).[68] Delay in instituting dantrolene therapy increases the probability of failed therapy and death.[36] For a 70-kg patient, this corresponds to 8 vials of dantrolene. The response to dantrolene should be evident within minutes, with a marked reduction in $P_{ETCO_2}$, heart rate, and respiratory rate (see Fig. 40-3). If there is no response within 3 to 5 minutes, the initial dose should be repeated until signs that the physiologic variables are abating. The clinical end points include resolution of the hypercapnia, tachypnea, and tachycardia; resolution of muscle rigidity; restoration of clear urine output; return of normal consciousness when sedation is discontinued; self-correction of blood gas abnormalities; and resolution of electrolyte disturbances. If these do not occur or are incomplete, additional doses of dantrolene should be administered until all signs and symptoms of the MH reaction have abated or the diagnosis reevaluated.[68] There is no upper limit to the amount of dantrolene that can or should be given acutely to stop an MH reaction. In rare instances of persistent MH or recrudescence, a cumulative dose of up to 40 mg/kg has been required.[69]

Dantrolene is a fairly potent muscle relaxant, and a child with an unintubated airway (particularly one with respiratory disorders) may become weak and require controlled respirations.

Although dantrolene is effective in terminating acute MH reactions, this effect may wane as the blood concentration of dantrolene decreases. In this case, the MH reaction may recrudesce. The prevalence of recrudescence has been reported to be as great as 20% and associated with several predictive factors, including muscular body type and a greater time interval between induction of anesthesia and the development of the initial reaction.[70] However, the first episode of recrudescence may occur any time after the initial reaction was successfully treated, up to and as late as 36 hours.[71] The possibility of recrudescence must always be considered during the first 2 to 3 days after an MH reaction has occurred. Because recrudescence cannot be predicted, all children who experience an MH reaction must be admitted to the pediatric intensive care unit or a monitored bed until the reaction resolves and the child's metabolic indices return to and remain normal for 2 to 3 days. MHAUS recommends that 1 mg/kg of dantrolene be administered intravenously every 6 hours for 24 to 48 hours after an MH reaction to prevent recrudescence. This recommendation remains empirical because there are no data to support the effectiveness of dantrolene in preventing recrudescence, although these dosages are consistent with pharmacokinetic data in children.[67] We recommend continued vigilance, frequent physical examinations for muscle tightness, and repeated laboratory tests (e.g., blood gas analyses), and monitoring of vital signs, particularly heart rate and expired $CO_2$ tension for evidence of a recrudescence during the first 48 hours after an MH episode. If recrudescence does occur, additional intravenous dantrolene should be administered until the reaction again abates.

Acute administration of dantrolene causes skeletal muscle weakness that can lead to respiratory embarrassment. Not surprisingly, neostigmine is ineffective in reversing the effects of dantrolene because the latter acts intracellularly, not at the neuromuscular junction (see the section on molecular mechanisms of dantrolene). It may be advisable to maintain control of the airway (combined with intravenous sedation) until there is no further need for dantrolene. Preoperative, orally administered dantrolene, initially recommended in MH-susceptible children 2 decades ago, caused skeletal muscle weakness, dysarthria, sialorrhea, and diplopia and was ineffective in preventing MH.[72] As a result, this practice has been discontinued.[72] There have been no reports of acute dantrolene toxicity, although reported adverse effects after intravenous administration include muscle weakness (about 22%), phlebitis (9%), gastrointestinal upset (about 4%), and respiratory failure (3.8%).[63] Long-term use in the treatment of chronic skeletal muscle spasticity has been reported to cause liver dysfunction and fatal hepatitis in about 1% and 0.1% of patients, respectively.[73] Given the risks of an MH reaction, there seems little downside to treating a child with dantrolene before the diagnosis is certain, provided all the necessary blood work and laboratory tests have been collected, because early treatment reduces mortality and morbidity (see Fig. 40-1).[36] The probability of developing a complication from an MH reaction increases almost threefold for every 2° C increase in body temperature and 1.6-fold for every 30-minute delay in administering intravenous dantrolene during a reaction.[36] Cardiac arrest and death during an MH reaction correlate with a muscular physique and greater time intervals between induction of anesthesia and the maximal value of $P_{ET}CO_2$.[24] Other possible diagnoses should continue to be considered while the treatment for the suspected MH reaction

is organized (see Table 40-4). A positive response to dantrolene is not pathognomonic of an MH reaction, because other conditions may respond with resolution of their signs.

Moderate external cooling measures may be instituted to control a rapidly increasing temperature, although ice should never be applied directly to the skin because it may cause tissue injury and intense cutaneous vasoconstriction. The latter may decrease heat loss further by accelerating acidosis and pyrexia. It is important to avoid overshooting with cooling measures (i.e., stop aggressive cooling at a temperature of about 38.5° C), because hypothermia may ensue, particularly if dantrolene has been administered. A urinary catheter should always be inserted during an MH reaction to identify myoglobinuria and to facilitate bladder emptying because 0.375 g of mannitol/kg body weight is given as part of the initial (2.5 mg/kg) loading dose of dantrolene.

Initial laboratory assessments should be obtained before the initial bolus dose of dantrolene, and in addition to arterial and venous blood gases, determinations should include electrolyte, glucose, blood urea nitrogen, and creatinine levels; a complete blood cell count with platelets; prothrombin and partial thromboplastin times; creatine kinase concentrations; and serum and urine myoglobin levels. Because creatine kinase concentrations peak 12 to 24 hours after the onset of an MH reaction, it is prudent to obtain a baseline blood sample as soon as an MH reaction is suspected. The provider should be especially aware of the potential for hyperkalemia due to muscle breakdown and for acute renal failure as a late complication. An arterial catheter should be inserted to continuously monitor blood pressure and for serial determinations of arterial blood gas and serum levels of electrolytes and creatine kinase.

The potential for life-threatening acidosis—a pure respiratory acidosis early in the syndrome, followed later by a mixed metabolic/respiratory acidosis—always exists. Metabolic acidosis should be treated with sodium bicarbonate (1 to 2 mEq/kg IV initially), as would be done for any acutely acidotic child, and continue treatment guided by pH and base deficit, although if hypercapnia persists despite aggressive hyperventilation, administration of sodium bicarbonate should be reconsidered because the severity of the respiratory acidosis may increase. Because an acute MH episode is associated with catecholamine stress, hemodynamic instability, particularly due to dysrhythmias, may develop and should be treated according to advanced cardiac life support protocols. Calcium channel blockers should be avoided when treating MH reactions because they may cause cardiovascular collapse or acute hyperkalemia in the presence of dantrolene.[74-76] Acute hyperkalemia is common in patients with MH complicated by rhabdomyolysis and acidosis. Glucose and insulin should be immediately available and combined with the judicious use of exogenous calcium for treatment. There is no evidence that the use of calcium in this setting exacerbates an MH reaction.

After the acute crisis has been treated, late complications, particularly severe rhabdomyolysis, are possible. It is important to follow serial concentrations of creatine kinase; if they are greater than 10,000 IU or urinary myoglobin concentrations increase, the urine should be alkalinized, and forced diuresis (>2 mL/kg/hr) with mannitol should be induced to prevent myoglobin from precipitating in the renal tubules, causing acute myoglobinuric renal failure. The enormous fluid requirements and edema associated with rhabdomyolysis may produce a compartment syndrome, which requires immediate surgical treatment.

Other organ systems may be affected after an acute episode of MH. It is common for markers of liver function to increase 12 to 36 hours after the crisis; some liver enzymes, including lactate dehydrogenase, aspartate aminotransferase, and alanine aminotransferase, can also originate from muscle. A concomitant increase in creatine kinase to more than 10,000 IU strongly suggests a severe and acute muscle disorder. Accompanying increases in γ-glutamyltransferase and bilirubin suggest liver involvement. Disseminated intravascular coagulation as part of multisystem organ failure is a common and ominous late complication.[77] Coagulation profiles should be followed frequently to guide treatment appropriate to the case.

When necessary, the MH treatment algorithm should be accessed, available on the MHAUS web site (http://www.mhaus.org/). We think that an updated MH treatment algorithm should be attached to every MH cart and anesthesia machine and that operating room personnel should hold practice drills for the treatment of an MH crisis (see "Emergency Therapy for Malignant Hyperthermia" on the inside back cover of this text and at ExpertConsult.com). If the patient experiences what is thought to be an MH reaction, the care provider should call the MH emergency response line (1-800-644-9737 or 001-1-315-464-7079 if calling from outside the United States) for consultation with experienced anesthesiologists who are available 24 hours every day. We strongly encourage completion of an adverse metabolic reaction to anesthesia (AMRA) report by members of the team who provided anesthesia and postoperative care to the child. These forms can be downloaded (www.mhreg.org), sent by the hotline consultant, or obtained from the MHAUS office through regular mail. The data contained in the completed AMRA forms allow the North American Malignant Hyperthermia Registry (NAMHR) and MHAUS to produce better data regarding the variability of MH crises and the effectiveness of treatment. Because anesthesiologists should take a leading role in managing these patients, the families should be strongly encouraged to register the proband before leaving the hospital for MedicAlert identification (www.medicalert.org) that provides critical health information, such as "malignant hyperthermia susceptible, avoid inhaled anesthetics and succinylcholine."

## STRESS-TRIGGERED MALIGNANT HYPERTHERMIA

In 1974, Wingard described an MH-susceptible family with a history of exercise- and emotion-induced fevers and sudden death not associated with anesthesia or surgery; he considered the possibility that MH was part of a spectrum of human stress syndromes.[78] Likewise, the porcine model of MH, also known as porcine stress syndrome, was first described as an awake, stress-induced syndrome brought about by tightly packing pigs in a train, car, or truck for shipment.[79] Dantrolene-responsive cases of awake and heat stroke–induced MH have been reported.[80,81] Heat stress–induced MH also seems to be characteristic of susceptible animal models.[82-84] A fatal case of exercise-induced MH in a 12-year-old boy who had previously survived a suspected episode of MH during general anesthesia to set a fractured humerus has been reported.[85] Eight months after surgery, while playing a game of football, the child became hyperthermic, collapsed, and died. Postmortem DNA testing revealed an MH-associated *RYR1* mutation in the child and his surviving father.[85] More cases of stress-induced MH have been reported, substantiated by genetic testing and in vitro contracture testing (IVCT).[86,87]

Screening for MH susceptibility in heat stroke patients and those suffering postexercise cramps or rhabdomyolysis using the in vitro CHCT has led to the laboratory diagnosis of MH susceptibility in some patients.[88-92] Although there is laboratory evidence of similarities in skeletal muscle metabolism in exertional heat stroke and MH,[93] and one of the mouse MH knock-in models exhibits environmental heat triggering,[51] there is as yet little evidence that these are anything more than clinically similar presentations.[92] For this reason, dantrolene has rarely been an effective treatment for heat stroke.[94] Nonetheless, it seems reasonable to suggest that subsets of MH susceptible patients may be more sensitive to heat stroke. Therefore it may be helpful to test children with exertional heat illness for MH susceptibility.[95]

MH reactions have been reported infrequently in susceptible patients who received a nontriggering anesthetic.[96-98] Of 2214 patients who presented for muscle biopsy for MH susceptibility, 5 (0.46%) of 1082 who had MH-positive biopsy results developed MH reactions in the recovery room. None of the patients with negative biopsy results developed MH reactions. There is a small incidence of MH reactions among susceptible individuals that may occur despite a safe anesthetic regimen. Whether this is caused by stress or trace anesthetic concentrations that were inhaled is unclear. Massive rhabdomyolysis has been reported on rewarming from cardiopulmonary bypass despite the patient having received a nontriggering anesthetic.[96,97] The mechanism of these responses may be stress, but evidence is lacking.

## POSTEPISODE COUNSELING

Ideally, after treating a child for MH, the anesthesiologist should arrange for referral of the child and first-degree relatives to an MH diagnostic biopsy center. It is only at such centers that the CHCT can be performed in adults. The CHCT is the only test that can produce a true negative diagnosis (i.e., not MH susceptible),[99] but the sensitivity and specificity of this test are less than 100%. False-negative test results may occur, albeit rarely.[100] When the anesthetic management of a small number of MH biopsy-negative patients was reviewed, more than one half were given inhalational anesthetics, although the biopsy results for the remainder may not have been known at the time of anesthesia because they were given trigger-free anesthetics.[101]

Because there are no control muscle biopsy data for prepubescent children, contracture testing is not performed in this age group. Instead, children are more often fitted with MedicAlert bracelets, and the parents are counseled regarding their own need for biopsies. The children may be reconsidered for muscle biopsy upon reaching puberty.

Many persons suspected of having MH have normal muscle responses on the CHCT. In the event that an adult who experienced an MH reaction has a normal CHCT result, he or she should be referred to a neurologist with an interest in muscle diseases to determine whether an occult myopathy is responsible for the clinical events. Alternatively, the diagnosis may be incorrect, and other diagnoses should be considered (see Table 40-4). Individuals suspected of being MH susceptible should undergo CHCT; the family should also be evaluated and counseled.

Patients with strongly positive CHCT results should undergo screening for the ryanodine receptor 1 gene *(RYR1)*, because mutations in this gene have been found in about 60% of family members who had an MH episode. If an MH-associated mutation (discussed later) is found in *RYR1*, first-degree relatives have a 50% probability of having a similar defect. Diagnostic testing for *RYR1* is performed on DNA obtained from a blood specimen, obviating the need to travel to an MH diagnostic biopsy center or undergo muscle biopsy for the genetic test. Genetic testing of relatives can be undertaken through the office of the primary care physician or by the anesthesiologist, a process that will simplify evaluation of the family. Failure to identify an MH-causative *RYR1* mutation (E-Fig. 40-4) does not confirm a negative diagnosis (i.e., not MH susceptible) because more than one gene is associated with MH susceptibility, and not all are known.

Genetic testing and counseling can be arranged by the anesthesiologist or primary care physician by scheduling an appointment; one such center is located at the Center for Medical Genetics at the University of Pittsburgh. The genetic counselors have extensive experience in counseling patients on the utility of the ryanodine receptor gene test for evaluation of MH susceptibility. The center currently screens 12 exons of genomic *RYR1* that commonly contain MH mutations (exons 6, 9, 11, 14, 17, 39, 40, 44, 45, 46, 101, 102). A private commercial laboratory that also offers *RYR1* testing is Prevention Genetics (www.preventiongenetics.com), which screens for MH mutations. It has adopted a two-tiered approach: Tier 1 involves bidirectional sequencing of exons 2, 6, 8, 9, 11, 12, 14, 15, 17, 39, 40-41, 44-47, 95, and 100-104. These 22 exons contain most of the conclusively documented MH and central core disease causative mutations in the *RYR1* gene (http://www.emhg.org/genetics/). If the first tier is uninformative, their second-tier screen covers the remaining 84 exons of the 106 making up the human *RYR1* gene. The Prevention Genetics company corresponds only with physicians and does not provide patient or family counseling.

As DNA sequencing has become more automated and the cost has drastically declined, many private companies have arisen that purport to diagnose the entire panoply of human genetic diseases and resultant predispositions, including MH. We have no information about the reliability of their screening or the recommendations based on their findings. If no causative *RYR1* mutations are found, nothing more can be determined from genetic testing about susceptibility, because more than one mutated gene is linked to MH.

## Genetics

MH in humans follows an autosomal dominant inheritance pattern with incomplete penetrance and variable expressivity.[27,102,103] In the context of MH, incomplete penetrance means that there are fewer patients with MH susceptibility than would be predicted by simple autosomal dominant inheritance. Variable expressivity means that the presence of a genetic mutation defining susceptibility is documented, but it does not mean that a patient will have an MH reaction when first exposed to triggering agents. One patient in the NAMHR received 30 anesthetics before an MH reaction was triggered.[36] Another was discovered to be MH susceptible by IVCT during screening of a proband's family and later was inadvertently anesthetized with succinylcholine and isoflurane, but they did not trigger a reaction.[104] However, it seems that once an MH reaction has been triggered, the reaction will always be triggered when the patient is exposed to the offending agents.

The molecular and cellular bases of these phenomena remain unknown. Naturally occurring susceptibility to MH seems to follow autosomal dominant inheritance patterns in dogs[105] and horses[106] but follows a recessive inheritance pattern in pigs.[107] This suggests that other genetic and epigenetic factors may play a role in determining the degree and timing of MH susceptibility.

The first breakthrough in finding a gene that predisposed to MH was the serendipitous finding of a similar syndrome in pigs.[108,109] When anesthetized with halothane and succinylcholine or with halothane alone, the pigs developed full-blown MH reactions (E-Fig. 40-5). The pig model has been a primary pathophysiologic, genetic, and pharmacologic model for the study of MH over the past 5 decades. A second, serendipitous event introduced a South African anesthesiologist, GG Harrison, to dantrolene, and he successfully tested it in his pig model of MH.[110,111] This observation was quickly followed by the successful treatment of a patient with dantrolene.[112] An interview about Harrison's discovery of dantrolene is available from the Wood Library-Museum of the American Society of Anesthesiologists (http://www.woodlibrarymuseum.org/library/media).

One of the most surprising findings was that six separate breeds of pigs at different locations worldwide shared this MH susceptibility to inhalational anesthetics and succinylcholine. All reactions were treated successfully with dantrolene, and all were determined to have an autosomal recessive inheritance pattern. It was established that MH was associated with an uncontrolled increase in intramyoplasmic $Ca^{2+}$, presumably the result of an exaggerated release of $Ca^{2+}$ from the sarcoplasmic reticulum (SR).[113,114] Much effort has been expended in understanding the physiologic basis of excitation–$Ca^{2+}$-release coupling (ECRC) as part of the general mechanism of skeletal muscle excitation-contraction coupling.

By the mid-1980s, a large channel in the SR membrane, now known as the ryanodine receptor (RyR1), was identified by its ability to bind a plant toxin, ryanodine. It was discovered to have properties consistent with being a $Ca^{2+}$ channel.[115-117] In 1988, this presumed primary $Ca^{2+}$-release channel of the SR was found to have gap junction–like channel properties.[118] It was hypothesized that the ryanodine receptor might be the site of mutations that caused MH. Within a year, the cDNA for the skeletal muscle ryanodine receptor was cloned.[119] Two years after the initial cloning of RyR1 the identical single amino acid mutation (Arg-615Cys) was discovered in this channel in all six breeds of MH susceptible pigs.[120] *RYR1* was immediately acknowledged as a potential target gene in MH susceptibility studies.

Detailed genetic evaluations have linked MH susceptibility to chromosome 19q12-13.2, the location of the human *RYR1* gene (19q13.1), in most MH-susceptible families. This is the locus for malignant hyperthermia susceptibility type 1, symbolized by *RYR1* (formerly designated MHS1) (Table 40-9).[102,121,122] More than 300 variants have been identified in *RYR1*,[123] only about 30 of which have been documented as causing MH (www.emhg.org

### TABLE 40-9  Malignant Hyperthermia Loci

| Designation | Chromosome Locus | Gene |
| --- | --- | --- |
| Ryanodine receptor 1 (skeletal) (formerly malignant hyperthermia susceptibility 1 [MHS1]) | 19q13.1 | *RYR1* |
| Malignant hyperthermia susceptibility 2 | 17q11.2-q24 | *MHS2* |
| Malignant hyperthermia susceptibility 4 | 3q13.2 | *MHS4* |
| Calcium channel, voltage-dependent, L type, alpha 1S subunit (formerly malignant hyperthermia susceptibility 5 [MHS5]) | 1q32 | *CACNA1S* |
| Malignant hyperthermia susceptibility 6 | 5p | *MHS6* |

provides a comprehensive list of known causative mutations in *RYR1*). Not all MH-susceptible families have disorders linked to this chromosome (see Table 40-9), indicating that this syndrome is genetically heterogeneous.

The next gene identified, *MHS2*, was found on chromosome 17q11.2-q24 in North Americans. The previously designated MHS3 locus, a voltage-dependent calcium channel *(CACNA2D1)*, is no longer thought to be linked to MH susceptibility.[123] Although the data identify single genes that seem to affect individuals with MH susceptibility, there is discordance between a genetic marker and the likelihood of being MH susceptible.[124-126] Linkage analyses of six loci for MH susceptibility and other candidate loci suggest that multiple interacting genes may modify the primary genetic defect and subsequent clinical susceptibility to developing MH.[127,128]

Complicating the potential of genetic testing for MH even further is the phenomenon of gene silencing. This phenomenon mimics a recessive mutation in heterozygous individuals by allowing expression of only the affected allele while silencing the other, normal, allele.[129] Because MH is an autosomal dominant susceptibility, it is conceivable that a mechanism underlying the variability in MH triggering seen in patients with identical, monoallelic *RYR1* mutations results from skeletal muscle–specific silencing of the affected gene. It follows that inhalational anesthetics or succinylcholine, after multiple exposures, may release a gene from the silenced state, allowing triggering to occur. This may be an explanation for discordance between genetics, linkage analysis, and trait expressivity.

Although the inheritance of human MH is described as autosomal dominant, there are a few individuals who are allelically homozygous for an *RYR1* mutation,[130,131] intraallelically heterozygous for two different *RYR1* mutations, or compound heterozygotes containing one mutation in *RYR1* and a second mutation at another locus for MH susceptibity.[132] Surprisingly, no overt myopathies have been reported in these affected individuals.

# Physiology

## NORMAL SKELETAL MUSCLE: EXCITATION-CONTRACTION COUPLING

The neurochemical signal that triggers excitation-contraction coupling begins with the release of acetylcholine from the motor nerve terminal at the skeletal muscle nicotinic synapse, resulting in depolarization of the surface membrane, the sarcolemma. Sarcolemmal membrane depolarization is transmitted into the interior of the muscle cell by specialized invaginations of the surface membrane known as transverse tubules (TTs), which occur at regular intervals along the muscle cell (Fig. 40-5). The TT membrane is studded with the skeletal muscle isoform of the voltage-dependent $Ca^{2+}$ channel known as the dihydropyridine receptor (DHPR). In skeletal muscle, this channel does not transmit $Ca^{2+}$ in response to sarcolemmal depolarization. Rather, it functions as a sarcolemmal voltage sensor.

In response to depolarization, intrachannel charge movement across the TT membrane results in a conformational change of the DHPR. The TT is surrounded by specialized portions of the cellular organelle (i.e., SR) that are responsible for maintaining the cellular $Ca^{2+}$ store, and the SR contains a high-capacity $Ca^{2+}$ storage protein called calsequestrin, which regulates the ability of the RyR1 channel to open.[133] The face of the SR junctional membrane apposing the TT contains a packed, regular array of RyR1 proteins in close apposition to the DHPR. Physically, the

DHPR and RyR1 receptor proteins overlie each other in a unique arrangement of four DHPRs (tetrad) per one RyR1, with every other RyR1 lacking a tetrad (Fig. 40-6).[134] Physical interaction of the DHPR with RyR1 after depolarization causes the RyR1 channel to open, and SR-stored $Ca^{2+}$ is released into the myoplasm. Orthograde and anterograde communication between the DHPR and RyR1 results in reciprocal regulation of both entities.[135,136]

In the myoplasm, the troponin C subunit of the troponin complex is bound to tropomyosin, which in the resting state inhibits myosin interaction with actin and maintains a relaxed muscle. $Ca^{2+}$ binding to troponin C causes a conformational change in troponin and allows the complex to move away from tropomyosin, which rotates along the actin filament in a way that permits myosin head interaction with this fibrous protein. Fiber shortening and muscle contraction then occur in a myosin-ATPase–driven ratcheting reaction. The muscle relaxes when the SR membrane–bound $Ca^{2+}$-ATPase transports free myoplasmic $Ca^{2+}$ back into the SR against its concentration gradient in an energy-dependent reaction, thereby driving myoplasmic $Ca^{2+}$ concentrations down to resting levels. Troponin I, with its bound $Ca^{2+}$ removed, moves back to block the myosin interaction with actin, thereby preventing muscle contraction and inducing its relaxation. Although a detailed description of the complexity of this process is beyond the scope of this chapter, reviews of excitation-contraction coupling are available.[137,138]

## PATHOPHYSIOLOGY OF MALIGNANT HYPERTHERMIA

Advances in the pathophysiology of MH have been reviewed in great detail elsewhere.[139-142] In brief, at the cellular level, MH is characterized by an inhalational anesthetic–induced, uncontrolled increase in intramyoplasmic $Ca^{2+}$ levels,[143,144] which precedes the metabolic and clinical signs of this syndrome[145] (see Fig. 40-6). Increased intramyoplasmic $Ca^{2+}$ has been demonstrated by directly measuring intracellular $Ca^{2+}$ in anesthetic-triggered pigs[143] and by substantiating the sensitivity of stored $Ca^{2+}$ release by isolated SR from MH-susceptible pigs.[113,114,146,147] There is also a significant loss in the ability of magnesium ($Mg^{2+}$), the natural inhibitory divalent cation that competes with $Ca^{2+}$ for binding sites on RyR1, to inhibit $Ca^{2+}$ release in MH-susceptible skeletal muscle.[148-150] RyR1 isolated from MH-susceptible pigs demonstrate greater open probabilities, greater sensitivity to $Ca^{2+}$ activation, less sensitivity to $Ca^{2+}$ inactivation, and reduced inhibition by $Mg^{2+}$. As a result, the affected RyR1 channels spend more time in the open state and less time in the closed state than normal channels.[151-155] Although not formally confirmed, this mechanism presumably underlies the sensitivity of RyR1 channels to volatile anesthetics and to the increase in intramyoplasmic $Ca^{2+}$ seen in MH-susceptible skeletal muscle.

Similar single-channel studies of the $Ca^{2+}$ responsiveness of human MH-susceptible RyR1 channels have yielded more equivocal results,[156] presumably because of the genetic heterogeneity of the human MH-susceptible population. Even within a single individual, heterozygosity for an MH mutation permits a given RyR1 channel that is supposed to be made up of four identical subunits to contain any combination of zero to four MH susceptibility subunits in combination with wild-type, normal RyR1 subunits. When examining single channels from a population of channels isolated from a heterozygous, MH-susceptible patient, the clinician can expect a wider range of channel responses than in the homozygous, inbred, porcine population used for MH models.

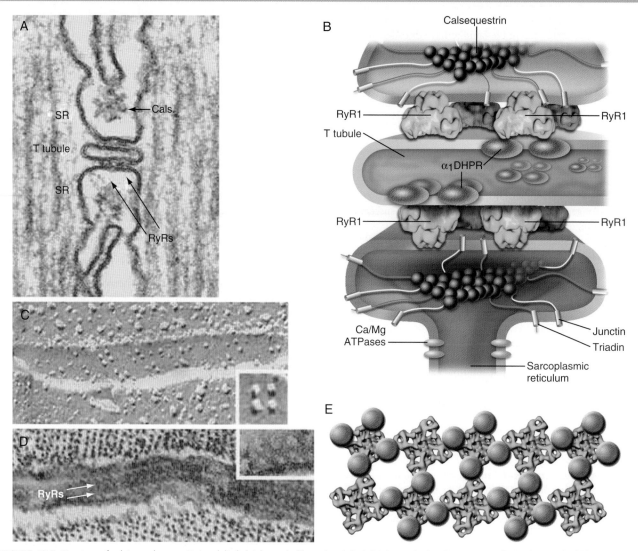

**FIGURE 40-5** Structure of calcium release units in adult skeletal muscle fibers. In adult skeletal muscle, junctions are mostly triads: two sarcoplasmic reticulum (*SR*) elements coupled to a central transverse tubule (*T tubule*). **A,** A triad from the toadfish swimbladder muscle in thin-section electron microscopy shows the cytoplasmic domains of the SR $Ca^{2+}$ release channel (*RyR1*), or feet, and calsequestrin (*Cals.*), the SR $Ca^{2+}$ storage protein. **B,** A tridimensional reconstruction of a skeletal muscle triad shows the ultrastructural localization of ryanodine receptors (RyRs), dihydropyridine receptors (DHPRs), calsequestrin, triadin, junctin, and $Ca^{2+}/Mg^{2+}$-ATPases. Notice the localization of DHPRs in the T-tubule membrane; DHPRs are intramembrane proteins that are not visible in thin-section electron microscopy but can be visualized by freeze-fracture replicas of T tubules (in **C**). **C,** DHPRs in skeletal muscle form tetrads, a group of four receptors (*inset*), that are linked to subunit of alternate RyRs (in **B** and **E**). **D,** In sections parallel to the junctional plane, RyR feet arrays are clearly visible in toadfish swimbladder muscle; the feet touch each other close to the corner of the molecule (*inset*). **E,** The model summarizes the findings of **C** and **D**: RyRs (*green*) form two (rarely three) rows, and DHPRs (*orange*) form tetrads that are associated with alternate RyRs. The T tubule is shown in *blue* in **B,** and sandwiched between two portions of the SR in **A.** (**A,** Courtesy Clara Franzini-Armstrong; **B,** courtesy T. Wagenknecht; from Protasi F. Structural interaction between RYRs and DHPRs in calcium release units of cardiac and skeletal muscle cells. Front Biosci 2002;7:d650-8.)

Several laboratories have reported the creation of knock-in mice containing one of two known MH-related RyR1 mutations: Tyr522Ser and Arg163Cys.[83,84] In contradistinction to the pig model, and like their MH-susceptible human counterparts, the knock-in MH mice are heterozygous. Their homozygous littermates die in utero on day 17. These heterozygous mice become rigid, hyperthermic, and hypermetabolic; die after exposure to inhalational anesthetics or heat stress; and respond therapeutically to dantrolene. They display exaggerated responses to the RyR1 agonists caffeine and 4-chloro-*m*-cresol and to potassium depolarization. As with MH-susceptible humans and pigs, their

muscle is less sensitive to inhibitory $Mg^{2+}$ and possesses higher resting $Ca^{2+}$ concentrations than wild-type animals. These experimental animals display a physiologic MH phenotype remarkably similar, if not identical, to the human syndrome and should prove extraordinarily useful in working out the details of MH pathophysiology.

Development of MH seems to require some form of neural input to muscle, because epidural anesthesia in the porcine MH model completely inhibits expression of MH.[157] However, complete inhibition of neural input into skeletal muscle in this model by the use of competitive, nondepolarizing, nicotinic cholinergic

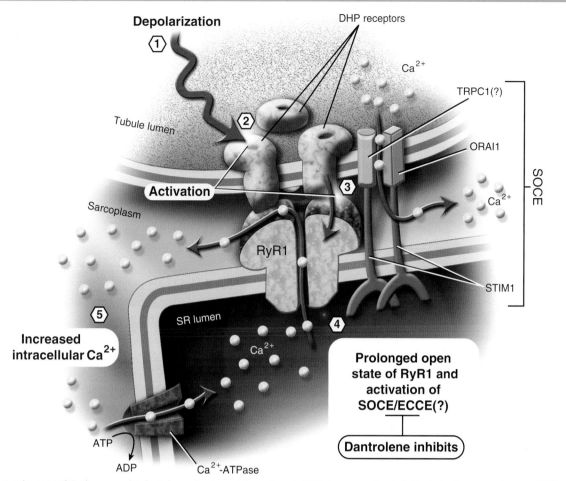

**FIGURE 40-6** Schematic of the known pathophysiology of malignant hyperthermia (MH). Exposure of an individual who has a genetic susceptibility because of a ryanodine receptor (*RyR1*) or dihydropyridine (*DHP*) receptor mutation to an anesthetic triggering agent may result in MH. Normally, muscle cell depolarization (*1*) is sensed by the DHP receptor (*2*), which signals RyR1 opening by a direct physical connection (*3*). The conventional view of the genesis of MH is that RyR1 opening is easier and more sustained in the presence of volatile anesthetics (*4*), allowing a sustained rise in the $Ca^{2+}$ concentration in the myoplasm (*5*) that surpasses the sarcoplasmic reticulum $Ca^{2+}$ reuptake activity of the $Ca^{2+}/Mg^{2+}$-ATPase. This results in unrelenting muscle contraction and uncontrolled anaerobic and aerobic metabolism, which translate into the clinical manifestations of respiratory and metabolic acidosis, muscle rigidity, and hyperthermia. If the process continues unabated, adenosine triphosphate (*ATP*) depletion eventually causes widespread muscle fiber hypoxia with resultant cell death and rhabdomyolysis. Rhabdomyolysis manifests clinically as hyperkalemia and myoglobinuria and an increase in the serum creatine kinase level. Dantrolene sodium binds to RyR1, presumably causing it to favor the closed state and stemming the uninhibited flow of calcium into the myoplasm. The contributions of store-operated $Ca^{2+}$ entry (*SOCE*) to myoplasmic $Ca^{2+}$ fluxes and its inhibition by dantrolene suggest that MH may have a significant component from SOCE or excitation-coupled $Ca^{2+}$ entry (*ECCE*), or both, and dantrolene may inhibit the RyR1-dependent activation of SOCE or ECCE. TRPC1, ORAI1, and STIM1 are proteins involved in calcium transport. *SR*, Sarcoplasmic reticulum. (Modified from Litman RS, Rosenberg H. Malignant hyperthermia: update on susceptibility testing. JAMA 2005;293:2918-24.)

receptor antagonists such as D-tubocurarine, pancuronium, and vecuronium before a halothane challenge does not inhibit development of MH.[158,159] Together, these results suggest that a neurologically significant contribution to MH arises from the central nervous system by means of sympathetic outflow or the neuroendocrine axis, rather than direct skeletal muscle stimulation. This theory is consistent with the awake or stress-related episodes of MH described earlier.

## MOLECULAR MECHANISMS AND PHYSIOLOGIC EFFECTS OF DANTROLENE

Dantrolene (Fig. 40-7) is a hydantoin derivative originally synthesized as part of an effort to examine the muscle relaxant properties of a series of substituted furan derivatives.[160] Thinking that they might have an NMBD, scientists investigated its mechanism of action but found that it was different from the known skeletal muscle relaxants. It affected the intrinsic properties of skeletal muscle without affecting the central nervous system, neuromuscular transmission, electrical properties of the sarcolemma or the T tubule, electromyogram, or train-of-four method for testing neuromuscular blockade. Its action was intracellular (Fig. 40-8).[161] Indirect evidence pointed to dantrolene affecting the $Ca^{2+}$ fluxes that were intrinsic to skeletal muscle contraction.[162-164] Direct observations[165,166] demonstrated that dantrolene suppressed the rate and amount of $Ca^{2+}$ released from the SR without completely abolishing it. Subsequently, it was

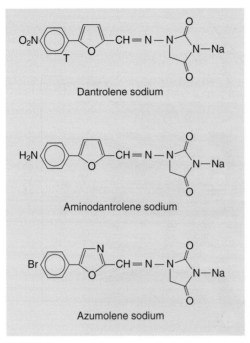

**FIGURE 40-7** Dantrolene and its congeners. Dantrolene and azumolene are equipotent drugs, but azumolene is far more water soluble. Only dantrolene is approved by the U.S. Food and Drug Administration for treatment of malignant hyperthermia. Aminodantrolene is a poorly active congener, demonstrating how small changes in drug structure can result in large changes in activity. (Modified from Parness J, Palnitkar SS. Identification of dantrolene binding sites in porcine skeletal muscle sarcoplasmic reticulum. J Biol Chem 1995;270:18465-72.)

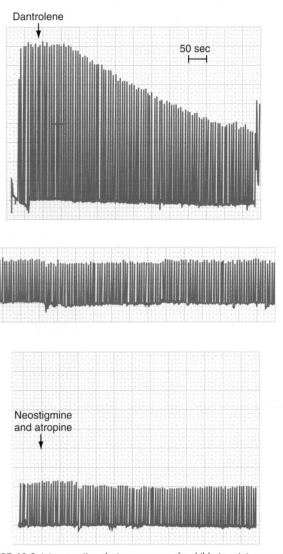

**FIGURE 40-8** Intraoperative electromyogram of a child given intravenous dantrolene (2.4 mg/kg). The twitch tension decreased about 75% after dantrolene but was not reversed by administration of neostigmine, demonstrating the lack of involvement of the neuromuscular junction in the action of dantrolene.

demonstrated that dantrolene inhibited halothane-induced $Ca^{2+}$ release from the isolated SR of MH-susceptible pigs,[146,167,168] while the drug had no effect on calcium reuptake into the SR.[169,170]

After SR $Ca^{2+}$ release was identified as the likely target of dantrolene activity, several unsuccessful attempts were made at identifying a dantrolene binding partner in the SR, mainly because of the difficulties of doing detailed pharmacologic receptor analyses with a drug as hydrophobic as dantrolene.[171,172] In 1995, an assay for radioactively labeled dantrolene helped to elucidate specific binding sites in porcine skeletal muscle SR.[173] Dantrolene inhibits RyR1-dependent cellular $Ca^{2+}$ fluxes in skeletal muscle, albeit incompletely, but it does not seem to affect RyR1 channel activity or its ability to transport $Ca^{2+}$.[174] With what does dantrolene interact, and how does this interaction relate to reduced $Ca^{2+}$ fluxes in skeletal muscle and MH?

A second physiologic process, called store-operated $Ca^{2+}$ entry (SOCE), contributes to the increase in intracellular $Ca^{2+}$ as a result of the RyR1 channel opening in skeletal muscle.[175-177] SOCE is a process by which the SR store of $Ca^{2+}$ is replenished from the extracellular milieu after significant loss of $Ca^{2+}$ from the SR.[178] Experiments with azumolene, a more water-soluble congener of dantrolene, have demonstrated inhibition of skeletal muscle RyR1-dependent SOCE, not SR $Ca^{2+}$ release.[179] These results raise profound questions. Do the induced $Ca^{2+}$ fluxes during excitation-contraction coupling, experimental manipulation, and MH that result in an increase in intracellular $Ca^{2+}$ all result from RyR1-dependent $Ca^{2+}$ release or RyR1-dependent $Ca^{2+}$ entry, or both?

Evidence of a dantrolene-sensitive, excitation-coupled $Ca^{2+}$ entry mechanism of skeletal muscle (ECCE) that is more easily activated in MH skeletal muscle has been described, as well.[180-183] ECCE is different from SOCE in that it does not require depletion of the SR $Ca^{2+}$ store and is activated by high-frequency electrical stimulation of the skeletal muscle membrane. ECCE and SOCE present new physiologic targets of investigation in to the pathophysiology of MH that involve $Ca^{2+}$ entry rather than $Ca^{2+}$ release (see Fig. 40-6).

Elucidation of the pathophysiology of MH and the mechanism of action of dantrolene has radically transformed our understanding of muscle physiology and pathophysiology. As our understanding continues to evolve, the future for advances in therapy and testing capabilities hold great promise.

## Laboratory Diagnosis

### CONTRACTURE TESTING

The standard for testing susceptibility to MH in the human population is an in vitro contracture test that assesses live human

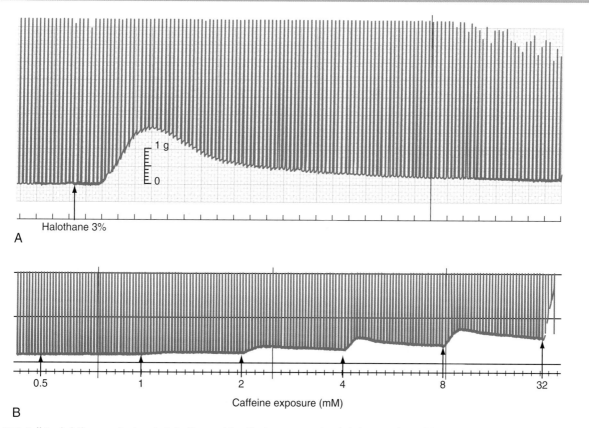

**FIGURE 40-9** Caffeine-halothane contracture test. **A,** Abnormal (positive) response to 3% halothane. Each small box represents 0.1 g of tension. The contracture response in this case is 1.6 g. A normal response to 3% halothane is a contracture up to 0.7 g. After exposure to halothane, 32 mmol/L of caffeine is added to the bath to determine maximal response. **B,** Abnormal (positive) response to caffeine. Caffeine exposure is increased to 0.5, 1.0, 2.0, 4.0, 8.0, and 32 mmol/L for 4 minutes. A contracture of greater than 0.3 g to 2 mmol/L of caffeine or less indicates susceptibility. (Modified from Rosenberg H, Antognini JF, Muldoon S. Testing for malignant hyperthermia. Anesthesiology 2002;96:232-7.)

muscle fibers from the vastus lateralis in a physiologic bath. With one end of the muscle tissue attached to a strain gauge, the degree of tension developed at baseline and on electrical stimulation is measured as a function of the concentrations of halothane or caffeine. The test is based on the observation that fresh muscle isolated from MH-susceptible patients behaved abnormally when exposed to halothane or caffeine in vitro (Fig. 40-9).[184-187] Two variations of this test have been developed and adopted: the CHCT by the North American Malignant Hyperthermia Group (NAMHG) and the IVCT by the European Malignant Hyperthermia Group (EMHG). The NAMHG test measures the response in separate muscle fascicles to a bolus of 3% halothane or incremental increases in the caffeine concentration,[22,188,189] and it requires a positive response to one of the challenges for a diagnosis of MH susceptibility. Those not responding are considered normal. The EMHG test measures the response to graded increases in the halothane concentration up to 2% and incremental increases in the caffeine concentration in different fascicles. The diagnosis of MH susceptibility by the IVCT requires a positive response to both challenges, whereas a positive response to one of the challenging agents results in equivocal diagnostic categorization (i.e., malignant hyperthermia equivocal [MHE]).[190-192]

Even though the EMHG protocol may prevent excess false-positive and false-negative results compared to the NAMHG protocol, overall results are comparable.[193] The EMHG reports that the sensitivity and specificity of its protocol are 99% and

94%, respectively,[191] whereas the NAMHG reports that its sensitivity and specificity are 97% and 78%, respectively.[194] Because the North American protocol is less specific and tends to overdiagnose MH susceptibility, it has a very small likelihood of failing to diagnose an MH-susceptible individual. The fact that there are some false-positive findings in the contracture testing demonstrates that other myopathic conditions that are not necessarily concordant with MH have muscle tissue that is also capable of giving an abnormal response to halothane and caffeine exposures. Discordance between the results of an IVCT and the presence of MH mutations in *RYR1* can occur in MH families such that 3.1% to 19.4% of family members who do not carry an MH mutation respond positively to an IVCT challenge.[75,191] This presumably indicates that there are other factors (e.g., a second MH susceptibility mutation in *RYR1*, another MH sensitivity locus, a sensitivity to caffeine and halothane that does not reflect MH susceptibility) in these individuals that give a positive IVCT result, but it does not necessarily mean that they are MH susceptible.

## GENETIC TESTING

Limited examination of the *RYR1* gene is available for the purpose of diagnosing MH susceptibility at two Clinical Laboratory Improvement Amendments (CLIA)–approved laboratories in North America as discussed earlier. Any physician can write a prescription for the ryanodine receptor gene test for MH susceptibility or fill out the requisition form and send blood for genetic testing. However, the probability of a positive outcome with genetic testing depends in part on the results of the in vitro CHCT because the clinical signs of MH are nonspecific. Current genetic testing indicates that about 60% of those who are positive with the CHCT also have positive genetic test results, whereas only 20% of those without a positive CHCT result yield positive genetic results.[75]

# Other Disorders and Malignant Hyperthermia

## MYOPATHIC SYNDROMES

An incriminatory association between various myopathies and malignant hyperthermia susceptibility, now known to be far more restricted than originally thought, was described in the 1970s and 1980s with much debate over the biochemical and pathophysiologic character of the clinical episodes that resulted from exposure to MH-triggering agents.[195,196] Did the clinical episodes represent true MH, did the episodes relate to the instability of myopathic muscle membrane with attendant destruction of muscle cells and release of intracellular proteins, and was there sometimes an associated hyperthermic reaction with these exposures? Although both types of episodes may result in increased creatine kinase levels, hyperkalemia, myoglobinemia, and myoglobinuria, one results from exaggerated ramping of cellular energy and heat production, and the other results from cellular destruction that does not involve abnormal cellular metabolism as a primary cause. Of the congenital myopathies, central core disease, the related multi-minicore disease, and the myopathy of King-Denborough syndrome are the only myopathies known to have a definite relationship with true MH (see Chapter 22).[197]

## MALIGNANT HYPERTHERMIA MIMICS

### Malignant Hyperthermia–like Syndrome in Pediatric Diabetes Mellitus

Diabetes mellitus has two well-characterized, life-threatening childhood presentations: diabetic ketoacidosis (DKA) and hyperglycemic hyperosmotic nonketotic syndrome (HHNS).[198-201] DKA, which is associated with type 1 diabetes, usually manifests as nausea, vomiting, dehydration, and weakness, but shock and coma are uncommon (1% to 2%) in the absence of cerebral edema. Fever is rarely a symptom and usually spurs a search for an underlying infection. HHNS is usually associated with type 2 diabetes and classically manifests with symptoms of increasing polyuria, polydipsia, and lethargy that develop over a few days. The estimated mortality rate is between 12% and 46%, somewhat more dramatic than that seen for DKA (2% to 10%), presumably because most cases of HHNS occur in adults with many other medical problems. The greatest rates of mortality with HHNS occur in adults older than 75 years of age or those with osmolarity values greater than 350 mOsm/L. The incidence of HHNS among U.S. children has been increasing rapidly and appears to be associated with the increase in childhood obesity. Despite this increase, pediatric HHNS is rare, and the presence of fever, as in DKA, usually prompts the search for an underlying infection.

A novel malignant hyperthermia–like syndrome (MHLS) against the background of pediatric diabetes mellitus was described in six adolescent boys between 14 and 18 years of age; the cases were culled from three tertiary care facilities in the United States.[202] The features of the syndrome included HHNS

with coma, fever, rhabdomyolysis, and severe cardiovascular instability. Among the six adolescents with MHLS, five were obese, five had acanthosis nigricans, four were African American, and four died. Two more cases were later described; one patient died 14 hours after admission due to too rapid a correction of serum osmolarity and resultant cerebral edema and cardiovascular collapse, and a second patient was treated with dantrolene and completely recovered despite developing compartment syndrome in her left upper extremity due to rhabdomyolysis.[203] The survivor was tested for metabolic abnormalities, and a deficiency in short-chain acyl-coenzyme A (acyl-CoA) dehydrogenase was found.

Investigators recommend that anyone presenting with symptoms of HHNS and MHLS should be treated with dantrolene as soon as the syndrome is recognized and that fluid and insulin therapy be used for an appropriate rate of correction of serum osmolarity. A search of the literature reveals a similar case described 10 years earlier as fulminant MH associated with DKA in a patient who survived with the addition of dantrolene to his treatment regimen.[204] Although it is difficult to ascertain the efficacy of dantrolene in abrogating the deleterious effects on skeletal muscle and in saving critically ill patients with MHLS during HHNS with such a small number of successfully treated patients, it seems prudent to initiate immediate treatment with dantrolene in these cases until the data can inform us about the true efficacy of this drug in MHLS.

### Disorders of Fatty Acid Metabolism

Growing numbers of reports have documented cases of rhabdomyolysis in patients with disorders of fatty acid metabolism that in some ways mimic awake MH. These disorders arise from mutations in the enzymes responsible for the metabolism of various fatty acids and for ensuring adequate energy substrate for the mitochondria during periods of reduced glucose availability, such as during stress. Although these disorders have profound effects on energy metabolism, they should not be confused with mitochondrial myopathies, which result from completely different molecular defects and have mutations in the proteins of the mitochondrial respiratory chain (see Chapter 22). In neither case has a real association with MH been established, but there have been case reports of rhabdomyolysis and cardiac arrest in patients with carnitine palmitoyltransferase II deficiency.[205-207]

Various forms of acyl-CoA dehydrogenase deficiencies (i.e., very-long-chain, long-chain, medium-chain, and short-chain forms) lead to different types of myopathy that can have severe clinical consequences, including hypoglycemia and rhabdomyolysis with attendant multiple-organ dysfunction, which in some deficiencies are brought about by stress, particularly heat and severe exercise.[208,209] These diseases can manifest early in childhood or late in adolescence or young adulthood, and they can be a particular problem for individuals in the military or those who participate in intense sports.[209] Patients with the very-long-chain acyl-CoA dehydrogenase deficiency can present with acute hypercapnic respiratory failure.[210] Dantrolene has been used successfully to treat one case of recurrent rhabdomyolysis in a patient with very-long-chain acyl-CoA dehydrogenase deficiency,[211] and it may be useful to treat acute intraoperative rhabdomyolysis in these patients, although there is a dearth of evidence in this regard.

Children may present for surgery without a diagnosis of an inborn error of fatty acid metabolism and develop intraoperative rhabdomyolysis, mimicking aspects of a fulminant MH reaction.

This may be the first manifestation of the child's fatty acid metabolism disorder. Preoperative increases in serum creatine kinase and uric acid levels, presumably due to subclinical rhabdomyolysis, suggest an inborn error of metabolism or myopathy,[212] but these tests are not part of the usual preoperative panel of blood tests in normal pediatric anesthesia practice. Perioperative stress that may result from fasting, fear, disease states, and other causes can induce metabolic decompensation and hypoglycemia. As a consequence, an intravenous glucose-electrolyte solution is recommended for affected children.[213] Because of a few reports of rhabdomyolysis when these children are anesthetized with inhalational anesthetics, there has been some reluctance to use inhalational anesthetics in them.[213,214] It is, however, likely that the number of patients with inborn errors of fatty acid metabolism who undergo surgery is far greater than the paucity of reports of adverse outcomes with inhalational anesthetics. Because these patients vary considerably in their responses to stress, it is not surprising that most do well with any well-managed anesthetic. The available evidence suggests that the perioperative risk is no greater with any particular anesthetic in these children.

If the clinician elects to avoid inhalational anesthetics, two alternatives remain: regional anesthesia and total intravenous anesthesia (TIVA). In children, peripheral limb surgery often allows for the use of intravenous sedation and regional anesthesia that may be suitable depending on the age of the child,[191] but most children do not tolerate this technique. However, TIVA often is used in children, most commonly with propofol.[215]

Propofol infusion syndrome, a rare, usually lethal complication of prolonged infusions of propofol, is diagnosed by cardiovascular collapse associated with lipemic plasma, enlarged fatty liver, severe metabolic acidosis, and rhabdomyolysis or myoglobinuria.[216-218] In this syndrome, a large increase in particular fatty acids (i.e., malonylcarnitine and C5-acylcarnitine) that points to impaired entry of long-chain fatty acids into mitochondria and to resultant failure of mitochondrial respiration at complex II has been identified.[219] Others suggest that propofol infusion syndrome may uncover medium-chain acyl-CoA dehydrogenase deficiencies, although this remains unproved.[216] The notion that propofol can impair fatty acid uptake and subsequent oxidation raises the possibility that the acute administration of propofol to a patient with a defect in fatty acid metabolism can precipitate a metabolic crisis, although this has never been reported. It has also been suggested that the lipid load from a propofol infusion in the absence of adequate carbohydrate intake can expose a carnitine deficiency as a model for propofol infusion syndrome.[220] Moreover, propofol itself has been shown to inhibit mitochondrial respiration, possibly compounding the effects of fatty acid oxidation deficiencies.[216] In these children, the use of propofol may be associated with an unclear risk of inducing a metabolic crisis. If their metabolic abnormalities are subclinical, there is no easy, inexpensive preoperative screening tool to establish a diagnosis for a rare abnormality. Even if the child is diagnosed with one of the subsets of fatty acid oxidation deficiencies, it is impossible to predict preoperatively which children will be sensitive to propofol and, if they are, how sensitive they are.

Other TIVA regimens that may be considered include ketamine, dexmedetomidine, benzodiazepines, and opioids. In these instances, the preoperative discussion with the parents, children, and surgeons must address the perioperative risks, including the lack of evidence that any particular anesthetic is more likely to precipitate rhabdomyolysis and a MH-like reaction than another.

### Neuroleptic Malignant Syndrome

Neuroleptic malignant syndrome (NMS) is a rare, potentially lethal reaction to neuroleptics (0.1% to 2.5% of patients), which is characterized clinically by the slow onset of fever, muscle rigidity, altered consciousness, and autonomic instability over a protracted period of time.[221] Laboratory findings include increased creatine kinase levels, leukocytosis, increased liver enzyme values, and reduced serum iron or potassium concentrations.[221] NMS is similar to MH, and the distinction between the two is often difficult to make, except by medication history; neuroleptics are associated with NMS, and inhalational anesthetics and succinylcholine are associated with MH.

NMS has developed in children taking neuroleptics that block all dopamine $D_2$ receptors (i.e., high-potency neuroleptics, such as haloperidol; atypical neuroleptics, such as thiothixene; low-potency $D_2$-receptor antagonists, such as metoclopramide; and tricyclic antidepressants) and in those with the withdrawal of antiparkinsonian medications. It is suggested that the syndrome results from a deficiency of central dopamine, but other pathophysiologic mechanisms have been proposed to explain the many clinical findings that cannot be explained by lack of dopamine.

Successful therapy for NMS requires early recognition, cessation of offending medications, and intensive medical and nursing care geared toward hydration and restoration of electrolyte balance.[221] Specific pharmacologic therapy with dopamine agonists such as bromocriptine or with dantrolene has been advocated, although use of dantrolene is controversial. Despite the fact that textbooks of psychiatry list dantrolene as the first-line pharmacologic treatment for NMS, there are no good data that it has a therapeutic effect in NMS, except for the occasional case report declaring that dantrolene is effective.[221-223]

Children with psychiatric diagnoses requiring treatment with neuroleptics make up a significant percentage of these pediatric patients. NMS in this pediatric population continues to be a problem, even with the newest of drugs. The perioperative period for the pediatric patient on neuroleptics is one fraught with potential diagnostic dilemmas. For example, one report described postoperative NMS in a child with severe cerebral palsy and seizure disorder who was not taking any neuroleptics and who was successfully treated three times with dantrolene.[224] Was this NMS or a mild form of MH? The answer is unclear.

## Summary

Many clinical scenarios in pediatric anesthesia can mimic MH and challenge our diagnostic acumen and our ability to deliver anesthesia safely. Not all metabolic syndromes that reveal themselves under inhalational anesthesia are MH, and not all metabolic syndromes that respond to dantrolene are MH. The examples given here underscore the need for expert advice during a case of suspected MH, and providers are urged to make use of the Malignant Hyperthermia Hotline when the need arises.

## ANNOTATED REFERENCES

Hirshey Dirksen SJ, Larach MG, Rosenberg H, et al. Special article: Future directions in malignant hyperthermia research and patient care. Anesth Analg 2011;113:1108-19.

*This article is a summary of a meeting held by MHAUS in 2010, outlining what we know and what we need to know about MH.*

Hopkins PM. Malignant hyperthermia: pharmacology of triggering. Br J Anaesth 2011;107:48-56.

*Excellent, most up-to-date review of the ability of all drugs used in the anesthetic pharmacopaeia and their capacity to trigger MH.*

Kolb ME, Horne ML, Martz R. Dantrolene in human malignant hyperthermia. Anesthesiology 1982;56:254-62.

*This is a classic report of dantrolene efficacy in treating malignant hyperthermia.*

Krause T, Gerbershagen MU, Fiege M, et al. Dantrolene—a review of its pharmacology, therapeutic use and new developments. Anaesthesia 2004;59:364-73.

*Different aspects of dantrolene pharmacology are well reviewed.*

Larach MG, Localio AR, Allen GC, et al. A clinical grading scale to predict malignant hyperthermia susceptibility. Anesthesiology 1994; 80:771-9.

*A retrospective clinical grading scale is used to predict a malignant hyperthermia episode.*

Lerman J, McLeod ME, Strong HA. Pharmacokinetics of intravenous dantrolene in children. Anesthesiology 1989;70:625-9.

*The paper describes the first and only treatment of malignant hyperthermia.*

Litman RS, Rosenberg H. Malignant hyperthermia: update on susceptibility testing. JAMA 2005;15:2918-24.

*The authors offer an excellent, simple review of the clinical pathophysiology and testing strategies for malignant hyperthermia.*

Robinson R, Carpenter D, Shaw MA, Halsall J, Hopkins P. Mutations in RyR1 in malignant hyperthermia and central core disease. Hum Mutat 2006;27:977-89.

*This comprehensive clinical and genetic review of malignant hyperthermia (MH) and central core disease (CCD) offers an up-to-date annotation of all published RyR1 mutations, comparing data from the United States and the United Kingdom and showing that hot spots of mutations in RyR1 may be population specific. Combined data show that there are many mutations outside of the hot-spot regions. Some mutations are concordant for both MH and CCD, and some are not.*

Rosenberg H, Sambuughin N, Dirksen R. Malignant hyperthermia susceptibility. In: Pagon RA, Bird TD, Dolan CR, Stephens K, Adam MP, editors. GeneReviews [Internet]. Seattle: University of Washington; 1993-Dec. 19, 2003 [updated Jan. 19, 2010].

*The most comprehensive review available in the literature to date.*

Rossi AE, Dirksen RT. Sarcoplasmic reticulum: the dynamic calcium governor of muscle. Muscle Nerve 2006;33:715-31.

*The article reviews the current state of knowledge of the molecular pathophysiology of malignant hyperthermia and central core disease from experts.*

## REFERENCES

Please see www.expertconsult.com

# Regional Anesthesia

## 41

SANTHANAM SURESH, DAVID M. POLANER, AND CHARLES J. COTÉ

THE USE OF REGIONAL anesthesia techniques in children has increased dramatically in the past two decades.[1-9] Regional anesthesia is most commonly used in conjunction with general anesthesia, although in certain circumstances regional anesthesia may be the sole technique. In addition to central neuraxial blocks, peripheral nerve blocks are now employed with increasing frequency, in part because of the introduction of high-resolution portable ultrasound imaging. Ultrasound-guided visualization of anatomic structures permits both greater precision of needle or catheter placement and confirmation that the drug has been deposited at the site of choice (see Chapter 42). The advent of ultrasound guidance has also facilitated the performance of several blocks, including truncal blocks, which could not be otherwise performed safely using landmark techniques, especially in children. Evidence from recent large-scale collaborative studies of regional blockade in children supports the contention that peripheral nerve blockade is assuming greater prominence in pediatric anesthesia, and data from the Pediatric Regional Anesthesia Network (PRAN) suggests that increased use of ultrasound guidance may be, at least in part, driving this trend.[10] Supplementing a general anesthetic with a nerve block can result in a pain-free awakening and postoperative analgesia without the potentially deleterious side effects associated with parenteral opioids (see Chapter 43).[11] This benefit may be of particular importance to neonates, former preterm infants, and in children with cystic fibrosis and other conditions.[4] There is also evidence that suggests that regional anesthesia may improve pulmonary function in children who have undergone thoracic or upper abdominal surgery.[12-15] Lastly, the greatly increased number of "same day surgery" cases in recent years has made the advantages of regional anesthesia, such as the rapid awakening, enhanced postoperative analgesia

with no sedation or altered sensorium, and lack of opioid-induced nausea or vomiting, even more apparent. The safe and effective use of these techniques in children, however, requires an understanding of both the developmental anatomy of the region in which the block is placed and the developmental pharmacology of local anesthetics. This chapter will focus on landmark-guided techniques for those who do not have the advantage of ultrasound imaging; ultrasound techniques are described in Chapter 42.

## Pharmacology and Pharmacokinetics of Local Anesthetics

There are two classes of clinically useful local anesthetics, the amino amides (amides) and the amino esters (esters) (Table 41-1). The amides are degraded in the liver by cytochrome P450 enzymes, whereas the esters are hydrolyzed primarily by plasma cholinesterases.[16-20] These degradation pathways account for some of the differences in distribution and metabolism of local anesthetics, particularly in neonates when compared with adults.

### AMIDES
Amide local anesthetics commonly used in children include lidocaine, bupivacaine (and its isomer levobupivacaine), and ropivacaine. The choice of agent most often depends on the desired speed of onset and duration of action of the block, but in small infants and children issues related to potential toxicity are also important. Compared with an adult, the neonatal liver has limited enzymatic activity to metabolize and biotransform drugs (E-Fig. 41-1; see also Chapter 6). The ability to oxidize and to

**TABLE 41-1** Commonly Used Local Anesthetics

| Esters | Amides |
| --- | --- |
| Procaine | Lidocaine |
| Tetracaine | Mepivacaine |
| 2-Chloroprocaine | Bupivacaine |
| | Levobupivacaine |
| | Ropivacaine |
| | Etidocaine |

reduce drugs, in particular, is immature.[19-25] Clearance is immature in preterm neonates and matures rapidly through infancy. Neonates do not metabolize mepivacaine, with most of it excreted unchanged in the urine.[26-32] Conjugation reactions are limited at birth and do not reach adult rates until approximately 3 to 6 months of age.[21-24,28]

Older children also differ from adults with respect to the pharmacokinetics of local anesthetics. Children achieve peak plasma concentrations of amide local anesthetics more rapidly than adults after intercostal nerve blocks, but at similar times (approximately 30 minutes with lidocaine and bupivacaine) after caudal epidural administration.[33-35] Ilioinguinal nerve blocks in children weighing less than 15 kg may produce plasma concentrations of bupivacaine in the toxic range if more than 1.25 mg/kg is administered.[36]

The nature of the epidural space in infants differs from that in the adult with increased vascularity, less fat, and a smaller absorptive surface for local anesthetics. Anatomical studies have shown that the epidural fat is spongy and gelatinous in appearance, with distinct spaces between individual fat globules.[37] With increasing age, fat becomes more tightly packed and fibrous. The absorption half-time of epidural levobupivacaine decreases from 0.36 hours at 1 month postnatal age (PNA) to 0.14 hours at 6 months PNA. This, combined with reduced clearance (by the cytochrome P450, CYP3A4), causes a time to maximum plasma concentration (Tmax) to decrease from 2.2 hours at 1 month PNA to reach 80% of the mature value (0.75 hours) by 6 months PNA.[38] The steady-state volume of distribution (Vdss) for amides in children is greater than that in adults, whereas their clearances (Cl) are similar.[35,39,40] Because the elimination half-life (t$_{1/2}$) is related to the volume of distribution and clearance,

$$t_{1/2} = (0.693 \times Vdss)/Cl,$$

a larger steady-state volume of distribution directly prolongs the elimination half-life. However it is clearance that determines steady-state concentrations with continuous amide infusion; reduced clearance in neonates implies that repeated doses and continuous infusions will cause an accumulation of local anesthetic (see E-Fig. 41-1).[41-43] Thus infusion rates and local anesthetic concentrations must be reduced in this vulnerable age group when prolonged administration of amides are employed for postoperative analgesia.

### Bupivacaine

Bupivacaine may still be the most commonly used amide local anesthetic agent for regional blockade in infants and children, although ropivacaine (and in Canada and Europe, levobupivacaine) is being increasingly used. After a single administration, analgesia may be expected for up to 4 hours, although its duration of action is somewhat less in small infants. The

concentration used depends on the site of injection, the desired density of blockade, consideration of the toxic threshold of the drug, and the dosage limitations imposed by the concomitant administration of other local anesthetics, such as local infiltration by the surgeon or intravenous (IV) or topical laryngotracheal administration of lidocaine. The most commonly used concentration for peripheral nerve blocks is 0.25%, with reduced concentrations of 0.0625% to 0.1% used for continuous epidural administration. The 0.5% concentration is less commonly used in children, although it may be employed for peripheral nerve blocks where subsequent doses and drug accumulation are not of concern and where the volume of administered drug is sufficiently low to permit that concentration to be used without toxicity. Greater concentrations also increase the density of the motor block, an effect that may be desirable depending on the clinical situation.

Bupivacaine is highly bound to plasma proteins, particularly to α1-acid glycoprotein. It is a racemic mixture of the levorotary and dextrorotary enantiomers; the *l*-isoform is the bioactive one with regard to clinical effect, and the *d*-isoform contributes more to toxicity. Levobupivacaine, the *l*-enantiomer of bupivacaine, retains similar efficacy and duration of blockade as the racemic formulation (demonstrated in both an ovine model and in adult volunteers), yet carries up to a 30% reduced risk of cardiac and central nervous system (CNS) toxicities.[44,45] Although levobupivacaine's beneficial toxicity profile has resulted in its widespread use, it is currently unavailable in the United States.[46]

Several new experimental preparations of bupivacaine (for example, the recently approved liposome extended-release formulation) have the prospect to dramatically prolong analgesia with a reduced potential for toxicity.[47-49] Bioerodible encapsulated microspheres of bupivacaine administered for peripheral neural blockade[50] release local anesthetic over many hours to several days, depending on the formulation of the microsphere, thus producing very prolonged analgesia.[51] The addition of dexamethasone to the microspheres prolongs the block up to 13-fold, and plasma bupivacaine concentrations in animal studies were far below the toxic threshhold.[52] No adverse local reactions were noted. Several different preparations have been developed and studied, including synthetic bioerodible microspheres, protein-lipid-sugar spheres, or liposomes.[53-55] The first such preparation (Exparel, Pacira Pharmaceutical, Inc., Parsippany, N.J.) has recently been approved for use in patients 18 years of age or older by the FDA for surgical incision pain; toxicology studies suggest a low risk because of the slow rate of drug release.[47,56-58] If this and other formulations become available for use in children, they may be particularly useful for those who cannot have an indwelling catheter for a regional anesthetic, but still require prolonged neural blockade for analgesia. Potential applications include intercostal blockade for children with rib fractures, postoperative analgesia for ambulatory surgery, and children in whom an indwelling epidural catheter poses an excessive risk of infection.[59]

### Ropivacaine

Like levobupivacaine, ropivacaine is an *l*-enantiomer that has reduced risks of cardiac and neurologic toxicities compared with bupivacaine.[60] The lethal dose in 50% of animals (LD$_{50}$) appears to be greater than that of bupivacaine. Rats of different maturity exhibit a threefold greater tolerance to equipotent doses of ropivacaine than of bupivacaine, when administered for a femoral nerve block.[61] Ropivacaine is also reputed to produce a less dense motor block at equianalgesic potency to other local anesthetics, although the data are conflicting in this regard. Some studies report a greater sparing of motor function compared with bupivacaine, whereas others have report no difference in motor and sensory block. Ropivacaine produces a denser blockade of the Aδ and C fibers than bupivacaine when low concentrations are used, lending mechanistic credence to the idea of differential blockade.[62] Much of the infant animal data, however, do not support the existence of a greater sensorimotor differential block than that after bupivacaine. The few clinical studies in infants and children currently available do not report a detectable motor-sensory differential, in contrast to the data in adults.[61,63] Several clinical studies in infants and children report a prolonged duration of analgesia with ropivacaine, despite using a solution of reduced potency.[63-65] Although there are still only limited data available in children, the decreased potential for toxicity makes ropivacaine an attractive agent in this age group. Most clinical studies have used a 0.2% solution (2 mg/mL) with a volume of drug that was similar to that of bupivacaine but that depended on the type of block and size of the child. We use concentrations of 0.1% for infusions with opioid for continuous postoperative analgesia.

### Lidocaine

Because lidocaine has a relatively short duration of action compared with bupivacaine and ropivacaine, it is not commonly used for single injection blocks in pediatric regional anesthesia, where a prolonged effect for postoperative analgesia is usually a priority. However, it can be used effectively in continuous blocks where the drug is continuously infused via a catheter, although here too, ropivacaine, levobupivacaine and bupivacaine are far more commonly employed. In vitro laboratory experiments have suggested that lidocaine might have greater potential for neurotoxicity in the developing nervous system than other local anesthetics, although the clinical implications of these findings remain unclear and unproved.[66]

### ESTERS

The pharmacokinetics of the ester local anesthetics are also affected by the quantitative and qualitative difference in plasma proteins. Plasma pseudocholinesterase activity in neonatal umbilical blood is decreased compared with adults.[67] The impact of this reduced activity on clearance is less certain. Other drugs that depend on plasma cholinesterase have mature clearance at birth (e.g., remifentanil). Limited data suggest that 2,3-chloroprocaine may be safe for neonatal regional techniques, and that potentially toxic accumulation does not occur after several hours of use with a 1.5% concentration.[68,69]

Another enzymatic system with decreased activity in neonates is methemoglobin reductase, which is responsible for maintaining hemoglobin in a reduced valence state where it is capable of binding and transporting oxygen. Hepatic metabolism of prilocaine yields o-toluidine, which can produce methemoglobinemia, thereby rendering red blood cells less capable of carrying oxygen.[70] The decreased activity of methemoglobin reductase and the increased susceptibility of fetal hemoglobin to oxidization make prilocaine an unsuitable local anesthetic for use in neonates. Although prilocaine is no longer available for use in the United States as an injected local anesthetic, it is one of the components of EMLA cream (Eutectic Mixture of Local Anesthetics, AstraZeneca, Wilmington, Del.), a commonly employed transdermal local anesthetic. The total dose and surface area for EMLA application is therefore limited in neonates because methemoglobinemia has been reported; however,

the dose must be carefully chosen even in infants and toddlers.[71] Other local anesthetics, particularly topical agents, such as benzocaine, are potentially dangerous in infants because of the risk of methemoglobinemia by this same mechanism.[72] EMLA should only be applied to normal intact skin in appropriate doses[73] (less than 5 kg, 1 g applied to a maximum of approximately 10 $cm^2$ surface area; 10 to 20 kg, 10 g applied to a maximum of approximately 100 $cm^2$ surface area; greater than 20 kg, 20 g applied to a maximum of approximately 200 $cm^2$ surface area. The dose must be reduced if EMLA is applied to mucosal surfaces (such as the glans of the penis) compared with intact skin. The duration of action is 1 to 2 hours after the cream is removed. Adverse reactions include skin blanching, erythema, itching, rash, and methemoglobinemia. EMLA should be used with caution and with strict attention to the amount of cream and surface area of application in children younger than 1 month of age. Infants receiving drugs that may induce methemoglobinemia, such as phenytoin, phenobarbital, and sulfonamides may be at increased risk, and caution is warranted. It is contraindicated in children with congenital or idiopathic methemoglobinemia. Topical amethocaine (Ametop) has a more rapid onset of analgesia and increased depth of penetration through the skin and produces minimal vasoconstriction of the skin compared with EMLA.[74] Iontophoresis of lidocaine can also produce excellent transdermal skin analgesia with much faster onset of action (10 minutes) and greater depth of skin penetration than EMLA.[74]

### TOXICITY OF LOCAL ANESTHETICS

With the exception of uncommon effects, such as producing methemoglobinemia, the major toxic effects of local anesthetics are on the cardiovascular system and the CNS. Local anesthetics readily cross the blood-brain barrier to cause alterations in CNS function. A consistent sequence of symptoms can be observed as plasma local-anesthetic concentrations progressively increase, although this may not be readily apparent in infants and small children. Because of the smaller threshold for cardiac toxicity with bupivacaine, cardiac and CNS toxicity may occur virtually simultaneously in infants and children, or cardiac toxicity may even precede CNS toxicity. During the intraoperative use of bupivacaine, the risk of cardiac toxicity may be increased by the concomitant use of inhalational anesthetics and the CNS effects of the general anesthetic may obscure the signs of CNS toxicity until devastating cardiovascular effects are apparent.[75]

In awake adults, the earliest symptom of local-anesthetic toxicity is circumoral paresthesia, which is because of the high tissue concentrations of local anesthetic rather than CNS effects. The development of circumoral paresthesia is followed by the prodromal CNS symptoms of lightheadedness and dizziness, which progress to both visual and auditory disturbances, such as difficulty in focusing and tinnitus. Objective signs of CNS toxicity during this time are shivering, slurred speech, and muscle twitching. As the plasma concentration of local anesthetic continues to increase, CNS excitation occurs, resulting in generalized seizures. Further increases in the local anesthetic concentration depresses the CNS, with respiratory depression leading to a respiratory arrest. In adults, cardiovascular toxicity usually follows CNS toxicity. In this case, the systemic blood pressure decreases because the peripheral vasculature dilates, and because of direct myocardial depression, leading to a progressive bradycardia. These effects culminate in a cardiac arrest. In large doses, bupivacaine produces ventricular dysrhythmias, including ventricular tachycardia, peaked T waves, and ST segment changes

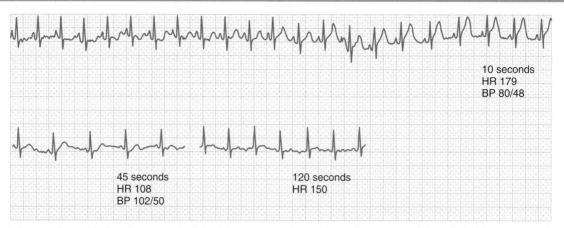

**FIGURE 41-1** Electrocardiographic changes associated with the intravenous injection of bupivacaine and epinephrine 1:200,000. Note the marked increase in the height of the T waves at 10 seconds. *BP*, Blood pressure; *HR*, heart rate. (From Freid EB, Bailey AG, Valley RD. Electrocardiographic and hemodynamic changes associated with unintentional intravascular injection of bupivacaine with epinephrine in children. Anesthesiology 1993;79:394-8.)

suggestive of myocardial ischemia, especially when epinephrine-containing solutions are used. Bupivacaine has a particularly strong affinity for the fast sodium channels, as well as the calcium and slow potassium channels in the myocardium. These effects explain why it is so difficult to resuscitate children from a toxic dose of bupivacaine.[76-78] Stereoselectivity of the sodium channel in the open state, however, has not been demonstrated. There is also evidence that the slow or "flicker" potassium channels may play a significant role in bupivacaine toxicity.[79]

With an intravascular injection of bupivacaine with epineph-rine, characteristic changes on the electrocardiogram (ECG) may be seen without any observable symptoms of CNS toxicity. Figure 41-1 shows an ECG tracing obtained during an IV injection of bupivacaine with and without epinephrine. Even a small IV dose of 1 to 2 µg/kg of epinephrine in a 1:200,000 solution with 0.25% bupivacaine produces peaked T waves with elevated ST segments, particularly in the lateral chest leads.[80-82] As opposed to the serious risk of ischemia and dysrhythmias with larger unintended doses of bupivacaine with epinephrine, small test doses result in only brief, transient changes in the ECG and may therefore be useful in the detection of an intravascular catheter or needle placement. Tachycardia is not a reliable indicator of an intravascular injection of bupivacaine, occurring in only 73% of intravascular injections during general anesthesia. When the ECG effects of bupivacaine, with and without epinephrine, and epinephrine alone were compared in children, the most reliable ECG changes (peaked T waves at 1 minute), and an increase in arterial pressure and heart rate, required the presence of epineph-rine.[83] It should be noted, however, that these changes in the T waves depended on age, diminishing in responsiveness beyond 8 years of age. These data suggest that careful observation of the ECG during test-dose administration may be a sensitive indicator of unintended intravascular injection of bupivacaine in the child anesthetized with an inhalational anesthetic.[84]

Plasma protein binding is the most important pharmacologic factor that determines the toxicity of local anesthetics, particularly for amides, because it is the free (unbound) fraction of the drug that produces toxicity. Reduced plasma protein concentrations cause more drug to remain in the unbound active form with greater potential for toxicity (see Chapter 6). Plasma concentrations of α1-acid glycoprotein are less in neonates than in older children, and adults, producing a clinically crucial greater free fraction of amide local anesthetics.[41,85-89] Current data suggest that the plasma concentration of free drug may be 30% greater in infants younger than 6 months of age and even greater in preterm infants than in adolescents[90] as a result of reduced clearance and reduced α1-acid glycoprotein concentrations. α1-Acid glycoprotein is an acute phase reactant whose concentration increases after surgery. Concentrations of α1-acid glycoprotein in infants are less in those undergoing elective rather than emergency surgery.[91] This increased concentration of α1-acid glyco-protein increases the total plasma concentrations for low to intermediate extraction drugs, such as bupivacaine. The unbound concentration, however, will not change because the clearance of the unbound drug is affected only by the intrinsic metabolizing capacity of the liver (i.e., clearance).[92,93]

Plasma concentrations of lidocaine that depress the cardiovascular and respiratory systems in human neonates are about half those that cause similar toxicity in adults.[94] In contrast, 2-day-old guinea pigs were less susceptible to the toxic effects of bupivacaine than 2-week or 2-month-old guinea pigs, even though the blood concentrations in the 2-day-olds were greater.[75] Data regarding toxicity in infant versus adolescent versus adult rats for both bupivacaine and ropivacaine are similar.[61] Young dogs, however, have a decreased threshold to both seizure and cardiac toxicity caused by excessive doses of bupivacaine.[95] Because the responses to toxic concentrations of local anesthetics vary among species, it is difficult to know which animal model and thus which study results are most applicable to human neonates.[96] No data exist in humans regarding age-dependent differences in the toxic threshold of bupivacaine at a given blood concentration. Seizures and cardiovascular collapse have been reported in human infants at the same blood concentrations of bupivacaine as in adults. Whereas data from some animal studies suggest that the greater volume of distribution of amides in younger children may protect against bupivacaine toxicity, retrospective analyses of large databases of infants who have received epidural infusions indicate that these findings may not be applicable to the human infant, particularly during continuous infusions or with repeated dosing. Current data on the pharmacokinetic and pharmacodynamic differences associated with early infancy suggest that caution should be exercised when using local anesthetics in infants. Several reports document that infants and children may develop systemic toxicity, including dysrhythmias, seizures, and cardiovascular depression from the accumulation of bupivacaine administered via epidural infusions.[41,97-100] Meticulous attention must be paid to the total dose of local anesthetic administered, the rate of administration, the site of injection, and the use of vasoconstrictors to diminish the rate of uptake of the local anesthetic. This is particularly important when a continuous regional anesthetic technique is used postoperatively or when repeated doses of local anesthetic are administered during prolonged surgery.

We recommend that both the bolus and infusion doses of bupivacaine and lidocaine be reduced by approximately 30% for infants younger than 6 months of age to decrease the risk for toxicity. This would mean that the maximum rate of bupivacaine administration should not exceed 0.2 to 0.3 mg/kg/hr.[42] Whereas these recommendations are particularly applicable to continuous infusions of bupivacaine for postoperative analgesia, the same caveats apply to large single injections, repeated injections, and continuous infusions of local anesthetics during prolonged surgeries.

The *l*-stereoisomer (or enantiomer) of racemic mixtures of local anesthetics is associated with less cardiac and CNS toxicity compared with the *d*-enantiomer in the mixture.[78] Both ropivacaine and levobupivacaine, which are *l*-enantiomers, the latter the *l*-enantiomer of bupivacaine, induce less cardiac toxicity than the racemic mixture of bupivacaine in adults and experimental animals.[79] This may be due in part, to the reduced affinity of the *l*-enantiomers for cardiac and CNS binding sites.[60] The inclusion of levobupivacaine and ropivacaine into the clinical armamentarium may decrease the toxicity of local anesthetics.

## PREVENTION OF TOXICITY

There are few data that correlate the anesthetic block, blood concentration of local anesthetic, and dose in infants and children. Most dosing guidelines have been extrapolated from studies in adults. Table 41-2 lists the maximum recommended doses of local anesthetics, as well as their approximate durations of action. To avoid overdose and the possibility of toxic effects, it is prudent to remain within these guidelines until studies in children clarify the pharmacokinetics and pharmacodynamics of local anesthetics for specific nerve blocks. As discussed earlier, all of these doses should be reduced by approximately 30% in infants younger than 6 months of age.

**TABLE 41-2** Maximum Recommended Doses and Duration of Action of Commonly Used Local Anesthetics

| Local Anesthetic | Maximum Dose (mg/kg)* | Duration of Action (minutes)† |
|---|---|---|
| Procaine | 10 | 60-90 |
| 2-Chloroprocaine | 20 | 30-60 |
| Tetracaine | 1.5 | 180-600 |
| Lidocaine | 7 | 90-200 |
| Mepivacaine | 7 | 120-240 |
| Bupivacaine | 2.5 | 180-600 |
| Ropivacaine | 3 | 120-240 |

*These are maximum doses of local anesthetics. Doses of amides should be decreased by 30% in infants younger than 6 months of age. When lidocaine is being administered intravascularly (e.g., during intravenous regional anesthesia), the dose should be decreased to 3 to 5 mg/kg; there is no need to administer long-acting local anesthetic agents for intravenous regional anesthesia, and such a practice is potentially dangerous.
†Duration of action is dependent on concentration, total dose, site of administration, and the child's age.

Toxic reactions from local anesthetics are a function of (1) the total dose administered, (2) the site of administration, (3) the rate of uptake, (4) pharmacologic alterations in toxic threshold, (5) the technique of administration, (6) the rate of degradation, metabolism, and excretion of local anesthetic, and (7) the acid-base status of the child.[101-106] Thus recommendations (including those of the authors) of a specific dose limit for a given drug are both overly simplistic and potentially misleading.[107] Because of the multiplicity of factors that drive the final concentration of unbound local anesthetic, and in the absence of definitive and comprehensive data, conservative dosing remains the most prudent course.

### Total Drug Dose

The dose of local anesthetic should be determined by a child's age, physical status, the area to be anesthetized, and *weight according to lean body mass*. A severely ill child who is in congestive heart failure, for example, has a reduced capacity to metabolize amide local anesthetics because of a reduced cardiac output and hepatic blood flow. Similarly, a markedly obese child must not be given a larger dose simply on the basis of increased weight. If a large volume of local anesthetic is required for a particular procedure, a dilute concentration should be used to avoid exceeding maximal safe dosage recommendations. Doses are calculated based on the lean body weight of the child (e.g., a 20-kg child could receive up to 50 mg of bupivacaine). An easy approximation for bupivacaine is 1 mL/kg of 0.25% bupivacaine, reduced by approximately one-third for infants younger than 6 months of age.

### Site of Injection

Injection of local anesthetics into very vascular areas leads to greater blood concentrations than the same dose injected into less vascular areas. The order of uptake (i.e., maximum blood concentration) of local anesthetics (in order from greatest to least) with regional blocks in adults is (1) intercostal nerve blocks, (2) caudal blocks, (3) epidural blocks, and (4) brachial plexus and femoral-sciatic nerve blocks.[108] An easy way to remember this is by the mnemonic ICE Block:

I = intercostal
C = caudal
E = epidural
Block = peripheral nerve blocks

Studies are required to determine whether this order holds true for children. Blood concentrations of bupivacaine twice those measured in older children have been reported in children weighing less than 15 kg after ilioinguinal nerve block for herniorrhaphy using only 1.25 mg/kg of 0.5% bupivacaine without epinephrine, which is half the usual recommended maximal dose.[36] However, the fascia iliaca block in older children produced blood concentrations of bupivacaine that were within the acceptable safe range.[109] Local infiltration of the wound in herniorrhaphy has not been associated with increased blood concentrations of local anesthetics,[110] but scalp infiltration during neurosurgery may produce relatively greater blood concentrations.[111] As would be expected, spinal anesthesia results in very small blood concentrations, even in neonates.[89]

### Rate of Uptake

The rate of uptake of a local anesthetic depends on the vascularity of the site of injection. Increased perfusion increases uptake, whereas decreased perfusion decreases uptake.[112] The rate of uptake in children is usually more rapid than in adults. In general, the addition of a vasoconstrictor to the local anesthetic reduces the rate of uptake and prolongs the duration of the block. In adults, the dose of epinephrine is usually limited when used in conjunction with potent anesthetic agents because of the risk of inducing cardiac arrhythmias. If epinephrine is combined with the ester anesthetics, there is no increased risk of arrhythmias. For example, in adults anesthetized with halothane, the maximum recommended dose of epinephrine is 1.0 to 1.5 µg/kg. In children, however, larger doses of epinephrine may be safe.[113-115] We have used as much as 10 µg/kg of epinephrine in children, with a maximum dose of 250 µg, during halothane anesthesia without evidence of ventricular irritability, and these doses are likely to be even more safe with currently used inhalational anesthetics, which do not sensitize the myocardium to the arrhythmogenic effects of epinephrine. An epinephrine concentration of 1 : 100,000 should not be exceeded, and 1 : 200,000 or less is generally used. A quick reference for converting local anesthetic concentrations and the amount of epinephrine in various dilutions is presented in Tables 41-3 and 41-4. *Epinephrine is contraindicated in blocks in which vasoconstriction of an end-artery could lead to tissue necrosis, such as for digital and penile blocks, although this historical practice has recently been challenged, setting the stage for prospective studies.*[116-118]

### Alteration in Toxic Threshold

Medications, such as diazepam or midazolam, that increase the seizure threshold (i.e., the threshold for CNS toxicity) can be valuable adjuncts to regional anesthesia. Premedication with diazepam (0.15 to 0.3 mg/kg) decreases a child's anxiety but also offers some protection from the toxic CNS effects of a local anesthetic overdose.[119] Although diazepam is no longer in common clinical use in children in the perioperative period, evidence in animal models and considerable clinical experience in humans suggests that midazolam is also effective in terminating seizure activity.[120] Animal data, however, suggest that the concomitant use of diazepam and bupivacaine decreases the elimination of bupivacaine from serum and cardiac tissue in mice.[121] This effect is not a result of changes in protein binding.[122] It is not known if this is true for all benzodiazepines or if this is also the case in humans. Although premedication with a benzodiazepine prevents manifestations

of CNS toxicity, the threshold for cardiovascular toxicity is unchanged.[123] Thus after premedication with a benzodiazepine, cardiovascular collapse can occur without warning because the symptoms of CNS toxicity may be blunted. Because most regional anesthesia administrations that are performed in children are placed after induction of general anesthesia (with the exception of some blocks in former preterm infants), this may be a moot point in most circumstances.

### Technique of Administration

Whenever regional anesthesia is performed, the operator must be prepared for an adverse reaction and resuscitation supplies, including drugs, suction, and airway equipment, must be immediately available. The needle or catheter must always be inspected for blood as soon as it is positioned, but before injecting the local anesthetic, to determine if the tip is within an artery or vein. It is preferable to observe the needle or catheter for passive blood flow rather than to actively aspirate for blood because the blood vessels, such as the epidural venous plexus, are thin walled and collapse readily when negative pressure is applied. As a result, the inability to aspirate blood is not absolute proof that the needle or catheter is not in a blood vessel. For this reason, a small volume of local anesthetic with a marker for intravascular injection, such as epinephrine in a concentration of 1 : 200,000, is administered first, while the ECG is observed for 30 to 60 seconds. Data from awake adults indicate that the heart rate will increase within 1 minute of intravascular administration.[124] When the drugs are administered during general anesthesia, however, the efficacy of the test dose to detect an intravascular injection may be greatly reduced. Heart rate increases in only 73% of children after an IV injection of 0.5 µg/kg of epinephrine during halothane anesthesia, suggesting that this marker of an intravascular injection is not completely reliable.[125] Administration of atropine several minutes before the test dose increased the rate of positive responders to 92%, suggesting that vagal tone and the anesthetic's blunting of the sympathetic reflexes are responsible for the reduced sensitivity to the test dose. Test doses during isoflurane anesthesia appear to have the same limitations.[126] With sevoflurane, positive results were obtained in 100% of children, if the threshold for a positive response was an increase in heart rate of 10 beats per minute and a dose in excess of 0.5 µg/kg of epinephrine was used; positive results were obtained in 85% if 0.25 µg/kg of epinephrine was used.[127] In all children, a change in the T-wave amplitude was a reliable indicator of intravascular injection with both doses of epinephrine (see Fig. 41-1). All children in that study were pretreated with atropine. It is not known if increasing the dose of epinephrine to 1.0 µg/kg or increasing the concentration of epinephrine in the test dose solution to 1 : 100,000 during general anesthesia would increase the sensitivity of the heart rate response test without atropine. Systolic blood pressure increased by more than 10% within 60 seconds of the test dose injection, suggesting that an increase in blood pressure may be a more sensitive indicator of intravascular injection than heart rate during inhalation anesthesia. ST-segment and T-wave changes also appear to be sensitive indicators of intravascular injection of local anesthetic. Observation of the ECG yields a highly sensitive indicator of an intravascular injection of bupivacaine with epinephrine. These ECG changes were present in 97% of infants and children who received an IV dose of bupivacaine and epinephrine.[81] These investigators did not confirm the efficacy of pretreatment with atropine on the heart rate. Isoproterenol (added to the local anesthetic rather than

**TABLE 41-3**   Epinephrine Dilution and Conversion to µg/mL

| Epinephrine Dilution | µg/mL |
| --- | --- |
| 1 : 100,000 | 10 |
| 1 : 200,000 | 5 |
| 1 : 400,000 | 2.5 |
| 1 : 800,000 | 1.25 |

**TABLE 41-4**   Local Anesthetic Concentration and Its Conversion to mg/mL

| Concentration (percent) | mg/mL |
| --- | --- |
| 3 | 30 |
| 2.5 | 25 |
| 2 | 20 |
| 1 | 10 |
| 0.5 | 5 |
| 0.25 | 2.5 |
| 0.125 | 1.25 |

epinephrine), 0.075 to 0.1 µg/kg, increases the heart rate in 90% to 100% of children during halothane anesthesia.[128,129] It also increases the heart rate in adults during isoflurane and sevoflurane anesthesia, but this has not been extensively studied in children.[130-132] During total intravenous anesthesia (TIVA) with propofol and remifentanil, however, quite different results have been reported. A prospective study of children who received an IV injection of bupivacaine with epinephrine as a simulated positive test dose during TIVA, found that T-wave alterations were inconsistent and could not be relied on as an indicator of intravascular injection.[107] Only blood pressure (particularly diastolic) was a consistent and reliable marker of intravascular injection, increasing more than 10% in all subjects during TIVA.

Even though no test dose regimen is completely infallible, it appears most prudent to use an epinephrine-containing test dose before administering the therapeutic dose of local anesthetic, particularly if the block is administered in an anatomic location near a blood vessel.[127] The test dose should be repeated before subsequent bolus injections through a catheter. If the drug injection is visualized in real time using ultrasound, test dosing may be less critical, as the actual drug deposition can be visualized during the injection, although this, too, may not be infallible. If the child is receiving a general inhalation anesthetic, blood pressure and the ST-segment configuration, in addition to the heart rate, should be carefully and frequently observed after injection of the test dose.[84] Pretreatment with atropine may increase the rate of detecting an unintended intravascular injection. In addition, the rate of injection may also be a factor in the development of toxicity. If injection is partially or completely intravascular, a slow injection may not exceed the toxic threshold, whereas a rapid injection could. Thus slow, incremental injection of the therapeutic blocking dose of local anesthetic (over several minutes), even though repeated injections within a brief period might also result in toxic reactions, may further increase the safety of regional blockade.

## TREATMENT OF TOXIC REACTIONS

Treatment of toxic reactions to local anesthetic overdose requires knowledge of the signs and symptoms previously described. The signs of local-anesthetic toxicity, with the exception of the catastrophic cardiovascular events, are all masked by general anesthesia. Indeed, inhaled anesthetics may actually raise the threshold for seizures and thereby delay the detection of toxicity until cardiovascular collapse occurs. Even in the nonanesthetized child, the progression from prodromal signs to cardiovascular collapse may be very rapid and the initial resuscitative therapy in some cases may need to be directed at reestablishing circulation and normal cardiac rhythm, including the timely institution of chest compressions, while definitive treatments are being readied. As always, initial management should consist of establishing and maintaining a patent airway and providing supplemental oxygen. The timely administration of a CNS depressant that alters the seizure threshold may prevent seizures. Midazolam (0.05 to 0.2 mg/kg IV), thiopental (2 to 3 mg/kg IV), or propofol (1 to 3 mg/kg IV) effectively prevent or terminate seizure activity, however the latter two agents are also potent myocardial depressants and should be used with caution. If seizure activity is present and the airway is not secured, the use of succinylcholine or other relaxant may facilitate tracheal intubation but does not prevent seizure activity. It should be remembered, however, that the acute morbidity from seizures is the result of airway complications (hypoxia and aspiration) and that securing the airway

takes precedence over the actual control of the electrical activity of the seizure. CNS excitability is exacerbated in the presence of hypercarbia; it is, therefore, important to mildly hyperventilate children who have seizures. None of these interventions should in any way supplant or delay the administration of lipid emulsion to directly treat the toxic levels of local anesthetic, and help should be sought to carry out these treatments simultaneously. Indeed, two case reports suggest that lipid emulsion may reverse the CNS symptoms of local-anesthetic toxicity in the absence of cardiovascular collapse, and might be a preferable first line therapy.[133,134]

Advances in the treatment of local-anesthetic toxicity have dramatically altered the therapeutic interventions that should be initiated in the event of cardiovascular collapse after a large intravascular injection of an amide local anesthetic. IV lipid emulsion has been shown to be effective for resuscitation of cardiac arrest caused by both bupivacaine and ropivacaine toxicity. In dogs, successful resuscitation after cardiac arrest and 10 minutes of external cardiac massage was demonstrated after lipid administration.[135] Although 100% of the dogs that received an infusion of 20% lipid emulsion were successfully resuscitated, none of the controls that received a saline infusion survived. A clear relationship between the tissue concentration and the response has also been established.[136] These animal studies have been corroborated by several anecdotal reports of rescue from cardiac arrest in humans that followed intravascular injections of all of the amide local anesthetics in common use.[137-140] The mechanism of action of lipid emulsions in bupivacaine toxicity is not entirely understood, but studies in isolated rat heart preparations concluded that lipid treatment promotes the elution of bupivacaine from the myocardium and accelerates the recovery from bupivacaine-induced asystole.[141] This "lipid sink" hypothesis suggests a novel mechanism of action as compared with more conventional antidysrhythmic drugs, and the treatment appears to be more effective as well. An inverse relationship between the concentration of lipid emulsion and the myocardial bupivacaine concentration (greater lipid concentrations were more effective at decreasing the bupivacaine concentration in the myocardium) suggests that this lipid sink hypothesis is correct.[136] In support of this theory, in vitro evidence indicates that the lipid solubility of the local anesthetic determines, in part, its responsiveness to lipid resuscitation.[142] Although long-chain lipids are recommended for resuscitation after the pH is normalized, recent evidence suggests that a lipid formulation that contains a mixture of medium- and long-chain lipids is superior to long-chain lipid to extract local anesthetic, and that the binding efficiency of the former is independent of blood pH.[143]

In a rat study of cardiac arrest, excessive epinephrine during the initial arrest phase may actually impair resuscitation with lipid emulsion and prevent a sustained response to treatment, and whereas the initial return to cardiac function may be quicker after epinephrine, sustained recovery was better after the lipid emulsion when compared with the high-dose (greater than 10 µg/kg) epinephrine group. This contrasts with a pig model of severe bupivacaine toxicity (50% reduction in arterial pressure) in which initial treatment with epinephrine more rapidly restored vital signs than did Intralipid (lipid emulsion) administration.[144] The same investigators also demonstrated that during bupivacaine-induced cardiac arrest in a pig model, survival after epinephrine alone or the combination of epinephrine and Intralipid was greater than after Intralipid alone or in combination with vasopressin.[144]

The anecdotal human reports and experimental literature suggests that 1.5 mL/kg of 20% lipid emulsion should be administered over 1 minute and repeated every 3 to 5 minutes, up to a maximum of 3 mL/kg, followed by a maintenance infusion rate of 0.25 mL/kg/min until the circulation is restored.[145] Several pediatric events report success with this intervention, with a range of doses similar to those reported in adults.[138,146,147] Therefore, although the dose of lipids in children remains speculative and has not been subject to controlled investigation, the adult guidelines appear to be effective in children. There is a growing consensus that 20% lipid emulsions should be immediately available in any location where regional anesthesia is performed, to permit rapid treatment of cardiac toxicity. Although propofol is compounded in a lipid emulsion, it is *not* recommended as a substitute for Intralipid for resuscitation from local-anesthetic toxicity.

Because the initial stage of cardiovascular toxicity consists of peripheral vasodilation, supportive treatment should include IV fluid loading (10 to 20 mL/kg of isotonic crystalloid) and, if necessary, titration of a peripheral vasoconstrictor, such as phenylephrine (initial rate of 0.1 µg/kg/min), to maintain vascular tone and systemic blood pressure at acceptable limits. As toxicity progresses to cardiovascular collapse, profound decreases in myocardial contractility occur, followed by dysrhythmias. In dogs, echocardiography showed that decreased systolic function always preceded the development of dysrhythmias. Before lipid emulsion treatment was described, norepinephrine was shown to be more effective than epinephrine, dopamine, isoproterenol, or amrinone to treat bupivacaine cardiac toxicity in rats.[148,149] In infants, a report suggested that phenytoin (5 mg/kg administered by a slow IV infusion) treated bupivacaine cardiac toxicity.[150] Many toxic reactions are self-limited because the local anesthetic redistributes throughout the body and plasma concentrations rapidly decrease. Excretion of local anesthetic is hastened by hydration and alkalization of the urine by IV administration of sodium bicarbonate.[151,152] Cardiopulmonary bypass has also been used to successfully resuscitate an adult with bupivacaine-induced cardiac toxicity.[153] All current data, however, strongly suggest that, in addition to the standard CPR algorithm, lipid infusion is the most successful treatment, and immediate administration of this agent should be the next first line of therapy.

### HYPERSENSITIVITY TO LOCAL ANESTHETICS

Hypersensitivity reactions to local anesthetics are rare.[154-156] Ester local anesthetics are metabolized to *p*-aminobenzoic acid, which is usually responsible for allergic reactions in this group. However, these agents may cause allergic phenomena in children who are sensitive to sulfonamides, sulfites, or thiazide diuretics.[157,158] Among the amide local anesthetics, only one case of a true allergic reaction has been documented. These drugs may contain the preservative, methylparaben, which can produce allergic reactions in those sensitive to *p*-aminobenzoic acid.[158,159] When in doubt, local anesthetic allergy must be ruled out. Detailed protocols are described elsewhere.[160]

## Equipment

### USE OF ULTRASOUND

Recently there has been great interest in the use of ultrasound-guided peripheral nerve blocks in children.[161] The availability of high-resolution portable ultrasound machines has become increasingly commonplace and ultrasound-guided treatment will likely soon become the new standard of care for many peripheral nerve blocks. Although this requires sophisticated expensive equipment and the acquisition of new skills, it is likely to have a larger role in pediatric regional blockade because most blocks are performed while the child is anesthetized. Several manufacturers make ultrasound machines that are about the size of a laptop computer and have been designed for ease of use by the anesthesiologist. The cost-effectiveness of acquiring these devices is justified because they serve a dual purpose for placing invasive central lines. Direct visualization of the nerve may facilitate correct placement of the local anesthetic and may also help reduce the total dose of local anesthetic needed for successful blockade. It is imperative to use an ultrasound machine that is capable of scanning superficially because most of the nerves in children are usually less than a few millimeters from the skin. A more in-depth discussion of ultrasound guidance for peripheral nerve blocks can be found in Chapter 42. Because ultrasound might still not be available to every practitioner, a complete discussion of landmark and nerve-stimulator guided peripheral blockade is included in this chapter.

### USE OF A NERVE STIMULATOR

The use of a peripheral nerve stimulator is an alternative safe and effective method to locate the nerve to be blocked. Despite the increasing use of ultrasound guidance for placement of peripheral nerve blocks, some anesthesiologists still use nerve stimulation to verify the position of the tip of the needle when ultrasound is not available, or in combination with ultrasound, particularly when imaging is suboptimal. A nerve stimulator is not a substitute for anatomic knowledge, but is a useful adjunct that allows the performance of the block in an unconscious or uncooperative heavily sedated child. It avoids the need to seek sensory paresthesias or to rely purely on anatomic landmarks. The tiny amount of current flowing from the uninsulated needle tip stimulates the nerve and produces a motor response when the needle is in close proximity to the nerve. The nerve stimulator is attached to the child as shown in E-Figure 41-2. The cathode (negative pole) cable is attached to the low output terminal of the nerve stimulator at one end and to the proximal (uninsulated) shaft of a Teflon-insulated needle via a sterile alligator clip, or to the plug-in lead of a specially designed block needle at the other end (the child). The anode (positive lead) cable is attached to the high-output terminal of the stimulator at the one end and to the child, distant to the block site, via an ECG electrode at the other end.[162,163] The needle is advanced in the appropriate anatomic direction, and when it appears to be in the correct position, the nerve stimulator is adjusted to approximately 0.5 mA with repetitive single pulse output at 1-second intervals. Local muscle contraction should be minimal at this setting, although direct muscle stimulation can occur and must be distinguished from neural stimulation. The area innervated by the nerves to be blocked is observed for the appropriate muscle contractions. As the uninsulated needle tip approaches the nerve, the muscle contractions will increase in intensity and become less strong as the needle tip moves away from the nerve. One should be able to decrease the current to approximately 0.2 mA with continued elicitation of easily perceptible muscle contraction to be sure that the needle tip is correctly positioned. It should be noted that the injection of even a very small volume of local anesthetic will ablate or dramatically attenuate responses produced by the low current of the nerve stimulator, so the needle position should be

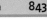

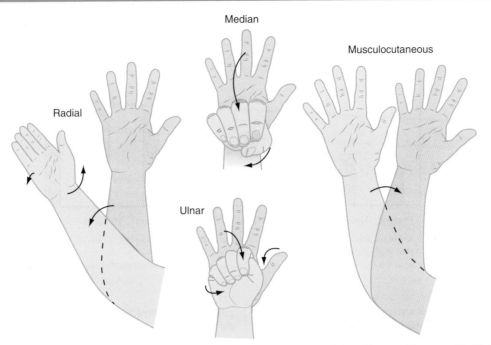

**FIGURE 41-2** Characteristic movements of the fingers, wrist, and elbow in response to nerve stimulation of four specific nerves. (Modified from Cousins MJ, Bridenbaugh PO, editors. Neural blockade in clinical anesthesia and management of pain. 2nd ed. Philadelphia: JB Lippincott; 1988, p. 406.)

optimized before injection (Video: Popliteal Fossa Block of Sciatic Nerve with Nerve Stimulator). The responses to stimulation of the radial, median, ulnar, and musculocutaneous nerves are shown in Figure 41-2.

Nerve stimulation has been used to verify the dermatomal level to which the tip of an insulated epidural catheter has been threaded. A low-dose current applied to a fine wire within the lumen of the epidural catheter stimulates motor paresthesias in the muscles of the abdomen and thorax and the most cephalad responses represent the dermatomal level corresponding to the tip of the catheter.[164,165]

## Specific Procedures

### CENTRAL NEURAXIAL BLOCKADE

#### Anatomic and Physiologic Considerations

Several anatomic and physiologic differences between adults and children affect the performance of regional anesthetic techniques. The conus medullaris (the terminus of the spinal cord) in neonates and infants is located at the L3 vertebral level, which is more caudal than in adults. It does not reach the adult level at L1 until approximately 1 year of age (E-Fig. 41-3) owing to the difference in the rates of growth between the spinal cord and the bony vertebral column. Thus lumbar puncture for subarachnoid block in neonates and infants should be performed at the L4-5 or L5-S1 interspace to avoid needle injury to the spinal cord. The vertebral laminae are poorly calcified at this age, so a midline approach is preferable to a paramedian one in which the needle is "walked off" the laminae. Another anatomic difference is noted in the sacrum. In neonates, the sacrum is narrower and flatter than in adults (see E-Fig. 41-3). The approach to the subarachnoid space from the caudal canal is much more direct in neonates than in adults, making dural puncture more likely, so the needle must not be advanced deeply in neonates.[166] The presence of a deep sacral dimple may be associated with spina bifida

occulta, greatly increasing the probability of dural puncture. Thus a caudal block may be contraindicated in these children.

The distance from the skin to the subarachnoid space, which is very small in neonates (approximately 1.4 cm) and increases progressively with age (Fig. 41-3).[167] The ligamenta flava are much thinner and less dense in infants and children than in adults, which makes the engagement of the epidural needle more difficult to detect and unintended dural puncture during epidural catheter placement a greater risk for the infrequent operator. Cerebrospinal fluid (CSF) volume as a percentage of body weight is greater in infants and young children than in adults (E-Fig. 41-4), although these studies are limited.[168-172] This finding may account in part for the comparatively larger doses of local anesthetics required for surgical anesthesia with subarachnoid block in infants and young children. The CSF turnover rate is also greater in infants and children, accounting in part for the much briefer duration of subarachnoid block with any given agent compared with adults. These anatomic differences necessitate meticulous attention to detail to achieve successful and uncomplicated spinal or epidural anesthesia.

In contrast to older children and adults, subarachnoid and epidural blockade in infants and small children is characterized by hemodynamic stability, even when the level of the block reaches the upper thoracic dermatomes.[173,174] Although heart rate variability, as determined by spectral analysis, is less, the heart rate is preserved, because the parasympathetic activity modulating heart rate appears to be attenuated in infants who receive spinal anesthesia.[175] This attenuated vagal tone allows the heart rate to compensate for any changes in peripheral vascular tone, an effect that may be the most important factor in preserving hemodynamic stability compared with any other factor, such as the relatively small venous capacitance in the lower extremities in infants, and the relative lack of resting sympathetic peripheral vascular tone.[176] Very high levels of spinal anesthesia can cause significant bradycardia that may require an anticholinergic.[177]

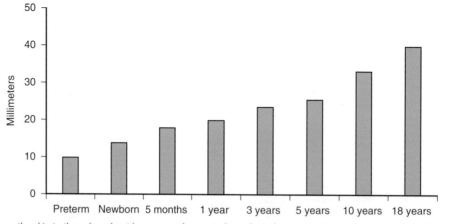

**FIGURE 41-3** Distance from the skin to the subarachnoid space as a function of age. (Data from Bonadio WA, Smith DS, Metrou M, et al. Estimating lumbar puncture depth in children. N Engl J Med 1988;319:952-3; Kosaka Y, Sato K, Kawaguchi R. [Distance from the skin to the epidural space in children.] Masui 1974;23:874-5; Lau HP. [The distance from the skin to the epidural space in a Chinese patient population.] Ma Tsui Hsueh Tsa Chi 1989;27:261-4.)

Nonetheless, data suggest that alterations in vascular resistance and blood flow to some vascular beds may occur, at least under certain conditions, in infants. In former preterm infants who received isobaric bupivacaine for subarachnoid block, cerebral blood flow decreased concomitant with changes in systemic blood pressure, although the conditions under which the baseline pressures were measured were not clear.[178] In a study in which changes in regional temperature were used as a surrogate sign of sympathetic activity, extremity but not truncal temperature increased during subarachnoid block, together with small insignificant changes in blood pressure.[179] In our clinical experience, and that of others, including the University of Vermont neonatal spinal anesthesia database, clinically significant systemic blood pressure changes do not occur in young infants after a subarachnoid block.[177]

Central neuraxial blockade can affect the respiratory mechanics of the chest wall and diaphragm by diminution in intercostal muscle activity. This may be particularly relevant in infants and young children, whose chest walls are very compliant because of limited ossification of the ribs.[180] Infants rely on the diaphragm for the maintenance of tidal volume to a greater extent than older children and adults. One may also observe some chest wall paradox, that is, inward displacement of the rostral edge of the rib cage in infants during deep sleep, even in the absence of airway obstruction. Studies of infants during sleep have demonstrated that during rapid eye movement (REM) and deep sleep, paradoxical chest wall motion occurs commonly and increases as the force of diaphragmatic excursion increases.[181] In a similar fashion, suppression of intercostal muscle activity, leading to decreased rib cage contribution to ventilation, has also been measured during spontaneous breathing in infants undergoing halothane anesthesia.[182] When respiratory inductance plethysmography was used to study rib cage and diaphragmatic contributions to breathing in seven former preterm infants who underwent spinal anesthesia for herniorrhaphy,[180] high thoracic (T2-4) levels of motor blockade were achieved, outward motion of the lower rib cage decreased, and paradoxical motion of the lower rib cage was noted in more than half of the infants. The diaphragmatic contribution to respiration, as estimated by abdominal displacement, was increased in all infants. This suggests a shift of respiratory workload from rib cage to diaphragm in compensation for the loss of the intercostal muscle

contribution to breathing. Other factors, such as the alteration of the conformation of the diaphragm relative to the chest wall, with concomitant changes in the size of the zone of apposition (the portion of the anterior diaphragm that lies against the lower rib cage), may also contribute. These measurements were compared with each infant's measurements before administration of the spinal anesthetic, but it is not known if these findings would be different if measured in unanesthetized infants during deep sleep. It is likely that these effects are well tolerated and that the ability of the diaphragm to compensate for loss of the contribution of the rib cage to breathing is adequate in the vast majority of infants.

Upper abdominal and thoracic surgery causes changes in respiration in the postoperative period by neurally inhibiting diaphragmatic function.[183-185] The afferent pathways that induce this inhibition are presumed to arise from the chest and abdominal walls and perhaps the diaphragm itself, although they have not been conclusively identified.[186] Contrary to popular belief, pain itself is not a major contributor to postoperative respiratory dysfunction. Numerous studies have demonstrated that opioids administered either parenterally or in the central neuraxis exert little effect on postoperative respiratory function.[187-189] Regional blockade, on the other hand, has been shown to improve several measures of postoperative respiratory function.[15,184,190] These data suggest that regional anesthesia has an important role to play in the attenuation of postoperative diaphragmatic dysfunction. Although the mechanism for this improvement has been attributed to blockade of the putative inhibitory neural pathways, other data suggest that alterations in respiratory mechanics, in particular an increase in the resting length of the diaphragm to its control value and the shift of the workload from rib cage to diaphragm, may play a greater role.[14] These data also suggest that the beneficial effects of regional anesthesia on postoperative respiratory function may, in part, be related to the degree of motor blockade. It is not known if the preoperative administration of regional blockade enhances respiratory function compared with postoperative application of the blockade, as has been postulated in "preemptive analgesia."

## Spinal Anesthesia

Spinal anesthesia has been successfully performed in children since the first published reports in 1900 to 1910.[191-194] The observation of postanesthetic apnea in former preterm infants led to a resurgence in the use of spinal anesthesia in infants, particularly for herniorrhaphy in the latter 20th century.[195,196] Spinal anesthesia has even been administered for myelomeningocele repair[197] by direct injection of tetracaine into the sac and supplemented as needed by direct application of tetracaine by the surgeon. It has also been used with success for a variety of other surgical procedures performed on infants.[197-200] It has been recognized since the early 1980s that preterm and former preterm infants are at significant risk for developing perioperative apnea after undergoing general anesthesia.[201-203] The reason for these postanesthetic apneas is not well understood. Spinal anesthesia has been proposed as an alternative to general anesthesia to reduce the incidence of perioperative apnea. However, when the spinal anesthetic was supplemented with ketamine, the incidence of postoperative apnea was even greater than with general anesthesia.[204] Both retrospective and prospective studies of infants undergoing spinal anesthesia demonstrated fewer or no episodes of postanesthetic apnea compared with those undergoing general anesthesia.[196,204] Although most of these studies were confounded by the absence of preoperative and postoperative pneumograms to control for baseline apnea and bradycardia, a prospective investigation confirmed that neonates who received a subarachnoid block exhibited no changes in heart rate and oxygen saturation when preoperative and postoperative pneumograms were compared.[205] The infants in the general anesthesia group, however, exhibited both reduced oxygen saturation and slower heart rates in the postoperative period and these episodes were more severe than those seen preoperatively. However, these events were not consistently associated with central apnea, which was defined as a cessation of respirations lasting more than 10 seconds with no demonstrable chest wall movement. These data suggest that the several case reports of apnea after subarachnoid block may have occurred even in the absence of the anesthesia and surgery; however, one cannot entirely discount that they may have indeed been caused by the anesthetic or, perhaps, by the stress of surgery itself. Although the data from this study are persuasive, we remain cautious and have not modified the use of routine postoperative monitoring in these infants. Until studies with greater numbers of infants can distinguish which criteria would define a group with low apnea risk, all former preterm infants less than approximately 60 weeks postconceptional age should be treated similarly, regardless of the anesthetic technique.[206-208] However, the best data available at this time suggest that for surgeries amenable to neuraxial blocks, spinal anesthesia (or caudal epidural analgesia) is preferable to general anesthesia for former preterm infants. It should be noted that the use of epidural anesthesia has also been reported for lower extremity and abdominal surgery in former preterm infants. Continuous spinal and epidural anesthesia for surgical procedures that outlast the duration of a "single shot" subarachnoid block have also been reported and are alternative strategies that can achieve the same goals as single injection subarachnoid block. The risk of local-anesthetic toxicity with a continuous caudal epidural blockade must be recognized; some have suggested that 2,3-chloroprocaine may be the prudent choice for local anesthetic in this situation.[209] For cardiac surgery, high spinal anesthesia with tetracaine (2.4 mg/kg) has been used for ligation of the patent ductus arteriosus. Total spinal anesthesia has been used in conjunction with isoflurane general anesthesia for cardiac surgery in infants and children.[210,211] Those infants whose tracheas were not intubated before surgery were successfully extubated

immediately after the operation. Hemodynamic stability was maintained without the use of inotropic agents in most children. A series of infants with gastroschisis closures, as well as open pyloromyotomies, have been reported using subarachnoid block.[200,211] Because spinal anesthesia in infants is associated with hemodynamic stability, it has been advocated as an ideal anesthetic for cardiac catheterization in infants with congenital heart defects and has been used, in conjunction with a light general anesthetic, for cardiac surgery.[212-214]

Recent concerns regarding the potential for adverse neurodevelopmental sequelae of general anesthetics administered to infants has led to additional interest in spinal anesthesia even in term infants. Although animal and retrospective human data are worrisome, a recent neonatal rat study demonstrated that memory was not impaired after sevoflurane anesthesia if the rats were exercised after the anesthetic.[215] There are no prospective data yet from which to make definitive conclusions, and several longitudinal prospective studies that will evaluate long-term neurocognitive development are in progress, including one in which infants undergoing herniorrhaphy are randomized to receive general or spinal anesthesia (see Chapter 23).[216-219]

When a solid block[37,208,220-223] is achieved, the majority of neonates fall asleep. This has been attributed to *deafferentation*, that is, a reduced level of consciousness because of diminished sensory input to the reticular activating system from the periphery, a mechanism confirmed in an animal model using spectral edge frequency analysis.[224] Sedation levels have been measured using bispectral index and spectral edge frequency analysis in infants undergoing spinal anesthesia without the use of adjunctive agents.[225] The investigators found a significant decrease in bispectral index, from 97 to 66.5 after 30 minutes, and in spectral edge frequency, from 26.1 to 9.9. These data indicate that sedation with dense regional blockade is a real physiologic phenomenon and can be used to the anesthesiologist's advantage during spinal anesthesia in infants. They also suggest that if sedation is administered to these infants, smaller doses than usual should be considered to avoid oversedation.

### Technique

After routine monitors (ECG, blood pressure cuff, pulse oximeter, and precordial stethoscope) are affixed, the child is placed in a sitting or lateral decubitus position. For neonates and infants, care must be taken to avoid excessive flexion of the neck (as in adults) because this position may obstruct the airway (Fig. 41-4, *A*).[226,227] The sitting position may aid in recognizing successful dural puncture by the increased CSF hydrostatic pressure and greater flow through the spinal needle. The skin is infiltrated with a minute quantity of 1% lidocaine (less than 0.25 mL should be sufficient; the authors use a 30-gauge needle on an insulin syringe), or a small amount of EMLA or other transcutaneous local anesthetic cream is applied to the infant's lumbar area at least 1 hour before spinal placement. The lumbar puncture is performed using a midline approach with a 22-gauge or smaller, 1.5-inch styletted spinal needle (see Fig. 41-4, *B* and *C*). We do not routinely use a 25-gauge spinal needle because of the time delay between entering the subarachnoid space and the appearance of CSF in the needle hub. This delay may make it difficult to recognize that the subarachnoid space has been entered. Whitaker, Sprotte, Marx, and other "pencil point" needles are available in pediatric sizes.[228,229] Lumbar puncture is performed only at the L4-5 or L5-S1 interspaces, for reasons previously described. The subarachnoid space in infants less than 60

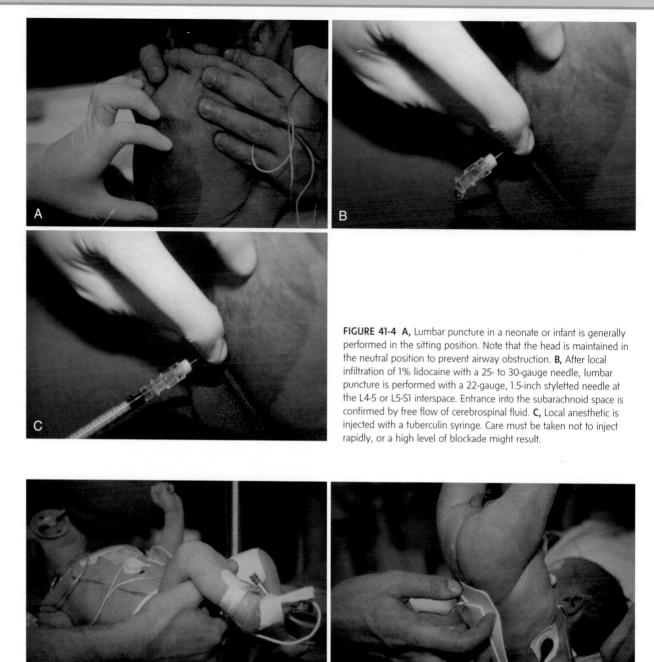

**FIGURE 41-4 A,** Lumbar puncture in a neonate or infant is generally performed in the sitting position. Note that the head is maintained in the neutral position to prevent airway obstruction. **B,** After local infiltration of 1% lidocaine with a 25- to 30-gauge needle, lumbar puncture is performed with a 22-gauge, 1.5-inch styletted needle at the L4-5 or L5-S1 interspace. Entrance into the subarachnoid space is confirmed by free flow of cerebrospinal fluid. **C,** Local anesthetic is injected with a tuberculin syringe. Care must be taken not to inject rapidly, or a high level of blockade might result.

**FIGURE 41-5 A,** The proper method of applying an electrocautery pad; the infant's entire body is elevated while maintaining the horizontal position or the infant is log-rolled along its long axis to avoid excessively high spread of subarachnoid blockade. **B,** Improper method of applying an electrocautery pad in a neonate after subarachnoid administration of local anesthetic; the legs should never be elevated as this may lead to a total spinal.

weeks postconceptional age is approximately 1.5 cm from the skin (see Fig. 41-3); care must be taken not to pass the needle too deeply, passing beyond the subarachnoid space.[167] When the subarachnoid space is located, the local anesthetic is slowly administered and the child is immediately placed in the supine position. After subarachnoid administration of local anesthetic, the child's body should remain completely horizontal to preclude cephalad spread of the local anesthetic. If the legs are raised, a "total" spinal anesthetic results (Fig. 41-5, *A* and *B*).[230] The grounding pad can be safely placed by lifting the entire infant, while maintaining the body in the horizontal plane or log-rolling

the infant, or the pad can be affixed to the anterior thigh if sufficient space and muscle mass are available. *The legs should never be raised above the torso as this may produce a high spinal block.*

Spinal anesthesia maintains remarkable hemodynamic stability in infants, even when a high spinal block occurs. Some pediatric anesthesiologists advocate starting the IV line after the onset of the block to avoid pain associated with inserting an IV, although if the airway had to be instrumented or resuscitation drugs administered, not having IV access would be very problematic. In addition, should IV access prove difficult, valuable operating time and spinal block time would be lost while searching for a suitable vein. We apply the pulse oximeter to a toe of one leg and the blood pressure cuff to the thigh of the other which avoid disturbing the neonate during the surgical procedure (e.g., inguinal herniorrhaphy) (E-Fig. 41-5).

Because the addition of sedatives has been associated with postanesthetic apnea with an incidence at least as great as that of general anesthesia, we try to avoid all sedatives, especially ketamine.[204] Most neonates will fall asleep once the block has set. A pacifier dipped in 50% dextrose will also help the infant to remain quiet and still. Gentle restraint is necessary in many cases, particularly during the most stimulating phase of the operation, when there is traction on the hernia sac, and thus on the peritoneum. It is particularly important for the infant to be still and not bear down when the hernia sac is dissected to avoid both tearing of the sac and of the extrusion of abdominal contents through the open hernia.

### Selection of Drug

NEONATES AND INFANTS. The proportional dose of local anesthetic required for subarachnoid block in neonates is much greater than that required for adults. When calculated on a per kilogram basis, there is a 5- to 10-fold greater drug requirement in neonates as for adults to reach a similar dermatomal distribution. In addition, the duration of the relatively larger dose lasts only about one-third to one-half as long as in the adult. As discussed previously, this appears to be due in part to the greater volume of CSF per kilogram and to the more rapid turnover of CSF in this age group. The drugs that have commonly been used for spinal anesthesia in neonates and infants include tetracaine, bupivacaine, and lidocaine.[168,231-235] Reported doses of tetracaine range from 0.22 to 1.0 mg/kg, with larger doses used more commonly to achieve an adequate height and duration of blockade. We use hyperbaric tetracaine (0.75 to 1.0 mg/kg [equal volumes of tetracaine 1.0% and 10% dextrose]) with 0.01 mL/kg of epinephrine (1 : 100,000) or hyperbaric bupivacaine (0.75 mg/kg of 0.75% bupivacaine in 8.25% dextrose). Epinephrine prolongs the duration of tetracaine blockade by more than 30%.[236] We draw a 1 : 1,000 epinephrine solution into a tuberculin or glass syringe and expel the contents in the manner of heparinizing a blood gas syringe. This leaves only a residual amount of epinephrine "wash" in the hub of the needle. The tetracaine dose and dextrose, if they are packaged separately, are combined. This dose usually provides adequate analgesia for inguinal hernia repair with a duration of motor block of 90 to 120 minutes and a dermatome height in the mid to upper thoracic region. For surgeries of limited duration that involve a lower extremity, smaller doses (0.5 to 0.6 mg/kg) may be used. The duration of bupivacaine is similar. Both isobaric and hyperbaric bupivacaine (0.5 to 1.0 mg/kg of a 0.5% solution) have been used in neonates and infants, with a reported duration similar to that of tetracaine, although the duration of action of the isobaric solution is slightly greater than for the hyperbaric solution.[234,235,237] A dose-ranging study reported that the addition of clonidine (1 μg/kg) prolonged the duration of blockade from a mean of 67 minutes (plain bupivacaine) to 111 minutes.[238] The use of larger doses of clonidine (2 μg/kg), however, caused transient hypotension and apnea, which required treatment with caffeine. Although lidocaine (2 mg/kg) is useful for a block of brief duration, such as for a muscle biopsy of the lower extremity, the duration of useful block is only approximately 30 minutes. In light of concerns regarding lidocaine in the subarachnoid space, we no longer recommend it in infants.[239-241] A summary of doses for commonly

**TABLE 41-5** Local Anesthetics for Spinal Anesthesia in Neonates and Infants

| Anesthetic Drug | Usual Dose (mg/kg) | Range (mg/kg) |
| --- | --- | --- |
| 1% Tetracaine in 5% dextrose | 0.75 | 0.6-1 |
| 0.5% Bupivacaine (isobaric) | 0.8 | 0.5-1 |
| 0.75% Bupivacaine in 8.25% dextrose | 0.75 | 0.5-1 |

used local anesthetics for subarachnoid block in neonates and infants is provided in Table 41-5.

CHILDREN. There is little information on the doses of local anesthetics for spinal anesthesia in children, as subarachnoid block is much less commonly used beyond infancy. When a regional technique is desirable in children, an epidural or caudal block together with a "light" general anesthetic is often preferable. For spinal anesthesia, 0.3 to 0.5 mg/kg of bupivacaine (5 mg/mL concentration) may be used in children 2 months to 12 years of age.[229] Doses of 0.3 to 0.4 mg/kg hyperbaric tetracaine have been used for subarachnoid block in children between 12 weeks and 2 years of age, and 0.2 to 0.3 mg/kg in children older than 2 years of age.[242-244] Based on these limited data, the dose requirement for spinal anesthesia decreases with increasing age. Because there are few data available on drug doses and the height of anesthetic block produced in this age-group, it is prudent to use these values as an appropriate reference point and to revise the dose as determined by clinical experience.

### Complications

Complications after spinal anesthesia include total spinal anesthesia, post–dural puncture headache, backache, neurologic sequelae, and the risk of lumbar epidermoid tumors if nonstyletted needles are used for subarachnoid puncture.[228-230,245-251]

Total spinal anesthesia has been reported in neonates. It is most commonly manifested by apnea with no change in systemic blood pressure or heart rate, although should pronounced bradycardia occur, a reduction in cardiac output is likely and should be treated aggressively.[177,230,252] It can occur after a dose of as little as 0.6 mg/kg of tetracaine.[230] Alteration in position, particularly by raising the lower body above the level of the head or thorax, may be the most common cause of a high spinal block. Although the rate of administration of the local anesthetic does not appear to affect the level of spinal anesthesia in adults, similar studies have not been conducted in neonates or infants.[253] It is possible that factors, such as the use of a relatively large-bore needle (22 gauge) and a tuberculin syringe providing the means for injecting with high pressure, along with the small distance between vertebrae, combine to make the rate of injection an important consideration in neonates and infants by producing unintended barbotage. We have also observed this complication with rapid drug administration. Management consists of assisted or controlled ventilation until the return of spontaneous respiratory function.

The incidence of post–dural puncture headache appears to be infrequent in infants and children, although the incidence in preverbal children is unknown. An early study reported an incidence of spinal headache of approximately 2% using 20- to 22-gauge needles in children 2 to 17 years of age.[244] However, no details were provided about the distribution of headache with respect to age. Other studies reported a 5% incidence of headaches in children ranging from 2 months to nearly 10 years of age, but, again, no age distribution was cited.[228,229] A prospective study of pediatric oncology patients undergoing diagnostic or therapeutic lumbar puncture with a 20-gauge needle reported that post–dural puncture headache was relatively rare in children younger than 13 years of age.[246] In most instances, the headaches were mild and resolved spontaneously. It is not entirely clear why young children should have a very low incidence of post–dural puncture headache. Several possible reasons include reduced CSF pressure,[247] the increased rate of CSF production, and hormonal changes with age.[246] As more pediatric regional anesthesia equipment becomes readily available, we expect that the use of "pencil point" (e.g., Whitaker, Marx, or Sprotte) needles will become more commonplace and will further reduce this already low incidence of headache.

Backache is a frequent postoperative complaint after both general and regional anesthesia in adults. It is thought to occur because of flattening of the normal lordotic lumbar curve secondary to muscle and ligament relaxation that occurs with spinal anesthesia. The incidence in children is unknown. Neurologic sequelae after spinal anesthesia are exceedingly rare. There are no reports in the literature of permanent neurologic injury caused by subarachnoid block, but good data in children are lacking. There have been no cases detected in over 1700 consecutive spinal anesthesias at the University of Vermont Medical Center, in another large series from Schneider Children's Medical Center (Petah Tiqva, Israel), or in the PRAN database.[10,177,252]

### Epidural Anesthesia

Epidural anesthesia administered by the caudal, lumbar, or thoracic route can be used for the same types of surgical procedures and indications as spinal anesthesia. Our most common indication, however, is for augmentation of general anesthesia and for postoperative pain management.

#### Caudal Epidural Anesthesia

Caudal epidural anesthesia is the regional technique that is used with the greatest frequency in children, although this may decline as familiarity with lumbar and thoracic epidural techniques and peripheral nerve blocks grows. Although its use was first described in 1933,[254] it was not until the early 1960s that caudal anesthesia gained any degree of popularity.[255-270] Improvements in catheter material and the availability of pediatric-sized needles and catheters, and the growing recognition of the benefits of regional analgesia in general, have increased the interest in this technique for children.

TECHNIQUE. The child is placed either in the lateral decubitus or prone position with a small roll beneath the anterior iliac crests. The cornua of the sacral hiatus are most easily palpated as two bony ridges, about 0.5 to 1.0 cm apart, when the examiner moves his or her finger in a medial to lateral direction (Fig. 41-6, *A*). When the sacral cornua are not prominent or easily appreciated, it may prove easier to locate the space by palpating the L4-5 intervertebral space in the midline and then palpate in a caudal direction until the sacral hiatus is reached. Because the space between the sacrum and coccyx may be mistaken for the sacral hiatus, the latter technique may make identification of the landmarks easier. The proper location is often, but not always, located just at the beginning of the crease of the buttocks. A short-bevel styletted needle, 22-gauge, should

be used because a long-bevel needle may increase the risk of intravascular injection.[271] Some practitioners think that a styletted needle avoids the possibility of introducing a dermal plug into the caudal space whereas others think that if the skin and subcutaneous tissues are punctured with an 18-gauge needle, an IV catheter can be inserted without entraining a dermal plug and transferring it to the subarachnoid space. Still others suggest that if using an IV catheter, it should be inserted with the bevel facing down because once in place, easy advancement of the IV catheter off the needle suggests that the caudal canal has been entered and may reduce the risk of intravascular placement. Although smooth and easy advancement of the cannula off the stylet is not a completely reliable sign that placement is correct, difficulty in doing so is virtually always a sign that the needle has penetrated bone or another extra-spinal structure. The needle is initially directed cephalad at a 45- to 75-degree angle to the skin until it "pops" through the sacrococcygeal ligament (see Fig. 41-6, *B*) into the caudal canal, which is contiguous with the epidural space. If bone is encountered before the sacrococcygeal ligament, the needle should be withdrawn 1 to 2 mm, the angle with the skin decreased to approximately 30 degrees, and the needle again should be advanced in a cephalad direction until the sacrococcygeal ligament is pierced (see Fig. 41-6, *C*). As the needle is advanced slightly farther, bone (the anterior table of the sacrum) is encountered, and the needle should be leveled in orientation before further advancement, so that it is nearly parallel to the child's back. Once the caudal-epidural space has been entered, the needle should be advanced only a few millimeters. If an IV catheter was used, the catheter should be advanced off the needle several millimeters in distance, while transfixing the latter. Advancing the needle any further should not be attempted because the dural sac lies relatively caudad in infants and may be entered a very short distance from the ligament (Video: Single Shot Caudal Epidural).[166,272]

Assessing whether the tip of the needle is outside the caudal epidural space may be difficult. Some clinicians aspirate the needle with a syringe, concluding that the absence of blood rules out an intravascular injection. Unfortunately, most unsupported veins collapse when negative pressure is applied (not yielding blood), and bone marrow does not yield much marrow through such small diameter needles. Another approach to rule out a vascular cannulation is to simply observe the needle and/or catheter for a passive return of blood. An effective means to identify an intraosseous cannulation is that attempts to slide the catheter off the needle are met with resistance; the catheter actually accordions or buckles. A subarachnoid puncture will yield a "gush" of CSF (without the need for negative pressure aspiration) immediately through the needle once the space has been breached.

After the caudal epidural location has been confirmed, a test dose of local anesthetic is administered. If neither ECG changes during inhalational anesthesia nor blood pressure changes during TIVA are evident after the test dose, the remainder of the dose of local anesthetic should be slowly injected in an incremental fashion over at least 1 to 2 minutes. Some view the entire volume of local anesthetic as simply an aggregate of multiple (1 to 2 mL) test doses and administer the entire in increments while observing the ECG for peaked T waves and changes in heart rate and/or blood pressure. Data from the PRAN showed that positive test doses occurred in 20 of 5,958 single injection neuraxial blocks, a rate of 0.34%, when there was no aspiration of blood [unpublished data, PRAN].[273] We strongly recommend the use of a test dose, even with "single shot" caudal anesthesia.

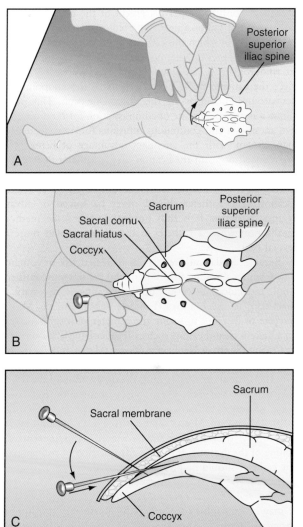

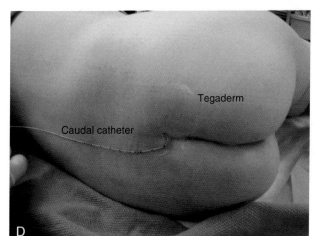

**FIGURE 41-6** Performing a caudal block. The child is placed in a lateral decubitus position (**A**). The posterior superior iliac spines are located and the sacral cornu is palpated; either an intravenous needle, an intravenous catheter, or a Crawford needle of appropriate size is advanced at an angle of approximately 45 degrees until a distinct "pop" is felt as the needle pierces the sacrococcygeal ligament (**B**). The angle of the needle with the skin is reduced parallel to the sacrum, and the needle or intravenous catheter is advanced into the caudal canal (**C**). If a continuous technique is used, the caudal catheter is advanced to the mid level of the surgical incision (it usually readily passes in children younger than 5 years of age), and the introducing needle or catheter is withdrawn. The catheter is secured with benzoin and an occlusive dressing (**D**).

Intraosseous injection of drugs results in very rapid uptake, similar to direct IV injection. The authors are aware of at least one case of circulatory collapse that occurred from this complication when a test dose was not employed.

The block may be placed before the onset of surgery without a significant decrement in duration of postoperative analgesia for short surgical procedures.[274] This has the advantage of reducing the amount of general anesthesia needed, resulting in a more rapid recovery. In addition, there is adequate time for the block to "set up," improving the chances of a pain-free awakening.

Inserting a catheter for a continuous caudal block follows a similar procedure (Video: Caudal Catheter Placement). First, one should determine the length of catheter that should be inserted into the caudal space by measuring the distance from the sacral hiatus to the desired site where the catheter tip will be positioned. Instead of a small-gauge needle or catheter, an 18-gauge IV catheter[275] or an 18-gauge Crawford needle is used to enter the epidural space (see Fig. 41-6, *D*). Because the internal diameters of

different IV cannulae vary, it is advisable to test that the epidural catheter easily passes through the IV cannula before puncturing the sacrococcygeal membrane. Once the epidural space has been accessed, the IV catheter and needle are advanced several millimeters. The catheter is then advanced off the needle several millimeters. Localization of the IV catheter tip in the epidural space is confirmed by lack of resistance to the injection of a small volume of saline and the absence of CSF or blood. If the needle had perforated the sacrum, the cannula will not easily advance off the needle. During injection, the area of the back overlying the IV catheter tip should be palpated; swelling or a fullness on injection of local anesthetic indicates a subcutaneous (SC) rather than an epidural catheter placement. The epidural catheter is advanced through the IV catheter and the IV catheter is withdrawn. After confirming the presence of neither blood nor CSF, a test dose of local anesthetic containing 1:200,000 epinephrine may be administered (see earlier). Test doses should be repeated each time a catheter is reinjected with a bolus dose of local anesthetic.

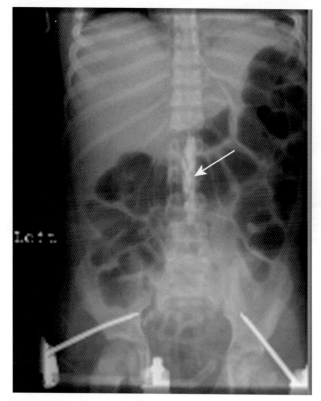

**FIGURE 41-7** Epidurogram, performed with 0.5 to 2 mL (max) of iopamidol nonionic contrast agent, demonstrating the "bubbly" appearance of contrast in the epidural space (*arrow*). Note the central localization of contrast within the borders bounded by the vertebral bodies. On occasion, contrast may be seen only on one side of the epidural space, with a sharp line of demarcation in the midline. This usually results in unilateral blockade, and is theorized to result from septation or some other impediment to bilateral spread of anesthetic within the epidural space.

For those younger than 5 years of age, the catheter can often be advanced to any level desired without exiting a dural sleeve or becoming tangled or knotted, although one study found a surprisingly high rate of catheter misplacements as detected using epidurograms, that were not suspected clinically.[37,276] Epidurograms are easily performed in the operating room when the catheter is placed. A small (0.5 to 2 mL max) volume of iopamidol is injected and imaged using fluoroscopy. A characteristic "bubbly" pattern in the midline is diagnostic of proper placement (Fig. 41-7). In addition to confirming placement in the epidural space and the location of the catheter tip, spread of the contrast may give a sense of how much volume is needed to cover the desired dermatomes. Besides epidurography, there are two other useful localizing techniques. The Tsui stimulating catheter, described earlier, produces motor twitches in the myotome at the catheter's tip. One can mark the catheter's advance by watching the motor paresthesias move up the legs, abdomen and thorax. Ultrasound has also been used to visualize the catheter in the epidural space, although this technique becomes more difficult with increasing age because of ossification of the posterior spinal column, and is frequently not possible in children older than 6 months of age.[277,278] For infants less than 5 kg, successful catheter advancement may be less reliable than in older children, and an epidurogram, ultrasound, or use of a stimulating catheter may be

needed to confirm proper placement of the catheter tip if the catheter is not radiopaque.[279] An epidurogram can be useful in any situation in which the catheter is threaded or when there is concern for proper catheter position, although the routine use of an epidurogram is not standard practice. We usually strive to place the catheter tip at a level near or at the midpoint of the dermatomes encompassing the surgical incision. This position allows a more specific site of administration for both intraoperative anesthesia and continuous infusions for postoperative pain management, with the attendant advantage of being able to use reduced doses of medication. If the catheter does not pass easily to the desired level, it should be withdrawn several millimeters and a localizing technique employed to ascertain its location. The catheter should never be forced or advanced against resistance. It is thus prudent to use some method of localization when a catheter is threaded cephalad more than several centimeters.

Because caudal catheters are at increased risk of contamination from fecal soiling in children who are not yet continent of stool, meticulous attention to the dressing is necessary. Our practice is to use Mastisol (Ferndale Labs, Ferndale, Mich.) or tincture of benzoin to secure the catheter with several layers of an adherent clear dressing, such as Tegaderm (3M, St Paul, Minn.) or OpSite (Smith & Nephew, Andover, Mass.), to affix the dressing in the crease of the buttocks (Video: Tegaderm Application). This transparent dressing permits the observation of the insertion site, which is the most likely source of infection (see later). A piece of single adhesive-edged plastic drape (e.g., Steri-Drape 1010; 3M, St Paul, Minn.) can be affixed just caudad to the lower edge of the dressing in a similar manner; this prevents direct soiling of the dressing. If there is any question of contamination, the catheter should be promptly removed.

### Lumbar and Thoracic Epidural Anesthesia

It may be preferable to place epidural catheters at a lumbar or thoracic interspace when the area of operation is innervated by higher dermatomes. Advantages include less risk of contamination by stool and urine, closer proximity to the desired tip location and smaller volume of drug required for a more cephalad dermatomal level (if the caudal catheter is not threaded cephalad). Both lumbar and thoracic epidural catheters may be safely placed in anesthetized infants and children by experienced anesthesiologists.[280] Although the adult literature has raised concerns about the risks of neural injury in the unconscious patient, no longitudinal studies have shown this to be the case in practice. An expert panel has recommended that, although caution must be used in all cases, there are few contraindications to the performance of regional blocks in anesthetized or heavily sedated children, and little evidence to support the notion that blocks placed while the patients are awake have fewer complications.[281,282] All large-scale prospective studies of regional anesthetics in children have found that the risk of permanent neural injury related to regional anesthetics in children, the vast majority of which are performed under general anesthesia, is exceedingly small when performed by experienced pediatric anesthesiologists.[11,66,283,284] Indeed, many of the arguments against regional anesthesia in the unconscious child are speculative, especially when one considers as the alternative a moving and uncooperative child.[280]

The technique for both lumbar and thoracic epidural catheter placement is similar to that in adults, with certain important exceptions (see Chapter 42 for ultrasound techniques). The midline approach is most commonly used, for the same reasons cited earlier regarding subarachnoid block. The ligamenta flava are considerably thinner and less dense in infants than in older children and adults. This makes recognition of engagement in a ligament more difficult and requires both extra care and slower, more deliberate passage of the needle to avoid subarachnoid puncture. It takes experience to perceive the more subtle differences in "feel" that are characteristic of the tissue planes in small children. The angle of approach to the epidural space is slightly more perpendicular to the plane of the back than in older children and adults, owing to the orientation of the spinous processes in infants and small children. The loss of resistance technique should be used with saline, not air. There are several reports of venous air embolism in infants and children when air was used to test for loss of resistance.[285-287] Another method used to identify the epidural space is to attach an IV infusion chamber with a mini-drip or other free-flowing fluid delivery device to the epidural needle. When the epidural space is entered, the IV set begins to drip (Video: Hanging Drop Technique).[288-290] We use a short (5 cm) 18-gauge Tuohy needle and a 20- or 21-gauge catheter in infants and children. The shorter length offers much better control than an adult-length (9 to 10 cm) needle. These catheters have fewer problems than the 24-gauge catheters, which in our experience are prone to kinking under the skin and have very high resistance to flow. Epidural kits specifically for infants and children are available, but aside from the substitution of a shorter needle they are identical to the adult sets.

SELECTION OF DRUG. The drug dose required to place an epidural block at a given dermatomal level depends on the volume (not concentration) of the local anesthetic and the volume and capacitance of the epidural space, which changes with age. There is a general impression that it takes greater volume on a per kilogram basis to achieve equal block heights in smaller children as compared with their older counterparts, but this has not been confirmed. Numerous studies have discussed the doses of local anesthetic drugs used for caudal anesthesia in children.[255,257-259,261,262,264-270] The volumes of local anesthetic that block from a T4 to a T10 dermatome level span a fivefold range. In our experience, the formula of Takasaki and colleagues[262] has best approximated good clinical results: Volume (mL) = 0.05 mL/kg/dermatome to be blocked.

Thus, in a 10-kg child in whom we wish to produce a T10 dermatome level, we would use a volume of (0.05 mL/kg/dermatome) × (10 kg) × (12 dermatomes) = 6 mL.

Another simple method is to administer 1 mL/kg (up to 20 mL) of local anesthetic (usually 0.125% bupivacaine with 1:200,000 epinephrine). This generally provides a sensory block with minimal motor block up to the T4-6 level; this volume limits the potential for toxicity for children over 6 months of age and is on the border for younger infants. If repeated doses are anticipated, or in infants less than 6 months of age, it is prudent to reduce the concentration or volume to avoid the risk of accumulation.

A third simple regimen for a caudal block used in UK and Australasia is that of Armitage[269]: 0.5 mL/kg for lumbosacral, 1 mL/kg thoracolumbar, and 1.25 mL/kg mid thoracic. If the total volume is less than 20 mL then use bupivacaine 0.25%. If the volume exceeds 20 mL then use bupivacaine 0.19%.

Because the level of the block depends on the volume of drug administered, the concentration of the local anesthetic should be based on the desired density of the block (less dense for postoperative analgesia, more dense for intraoperative anesthesia) and on the risk of toxicity.

### Continuous Epidural Infusions

Although intermittent doses of local anesthetic are often used to maintain epidural anesthesia during a prolonged surgical procedure, it is also common practice to initiate continuous infusions of local anesthetics during surgery. Continuous infusions maintain the block at a constant level, assuming that the infusion rate is appropriate. This obviates the need for repetitive test dosing. Theoretically, fewer entries into the epidural catheter may reduce the risk of infection and the risk of accidental administration of the wrong drug. Strict attention to the total drug administered per hour (i.e., the drug concentration and infusion rate) is required to preclude potentially toxic drug doses. We recommend that the same dosing guidelines for postoperative infusion rates be followed intraoperatively: *a maximum of 0.4 mg/kg/hr of bupivacaine after the initial block is established, with this dose reduced by approximately 30% for infants younger than 6 months of age.*[42] The concentration of local anesthetic solution depends on the age of the child, the surgical procedure, and the extent of area that needs to be blocked. When a more dense block is required in a small infant, it may be beneficial to use 2,3-chloroprocaine because its action is terminated by ester hydrolysis and has a minimal risk of accumulation compared with amide local anesthetics. A denser block with a more concentrated solution may then be achieved. The amides ropivacaine and levobupivacaine, because they are levorotary enantiomers and carry reduced risks of toxicity, may also successfully address these issues and allow the administration of more concentrated agents to produce denser blockade with less potential for adverse effects (see Chapters 42 and 43). In a study of children 1 to 9 years of age, infusion rates of up to 0.4 mg/kg/hr of ropivacaine that followed a 2 mg/kg bolus were found to result in stable levels of unbound ropivacaine in plasma, all well below the toxic threshold; clearance did not differ with age.[291]

### Epidural Opioids

Epidural opioids can be safely used to augment intraoperative anesthesia in children, as well as to provide postoperative analgesia. Their use is discussed in detail in Chapter 43. If extubation of the trachea is expected at the end of the surgical procedure, one must take into account both the systemic and the central neuraxial opioid doses to avoid excessive respiratory depression.

### Adjunctive Drugs

Numerous agents have been injected into the epidural space in attempts to prolong analgesia, to improve the quality of analgesia while reducing the dose of opioid and local anesthetic, or to replace the local anesthetic or opioid with a drug thought to possibly have fewer side effects. It is concerning, however, that several of these agents have not undergone exhaustive neurotoxicity testing and are not prepared or labeled for neuraxial use.[292] In the United States, the only adjunctive drug accepted for epidural administration is clonidine, an $\alpha_2$-adrenoceptor agonist. There is some controversy in the literature regarding the beneficial effect of clonidine on the duration of epidural analgesia. Several studies, including a meta-analysis, found a significant prolongation of analgesia (2 hours), as measured by the time to first supplemental analgesic requirement.[292-296] Other investigators found no significant increase in the duration of analgesia, including one double blind, randomized trial.[297,298] In neonates, neuraxial clonidine, particularly at doses of 2 μg/kg or greater, has been associated with apnea. Increased sedation is often reported in older infants and children at those doses as well.

## Complications

Complications after epidural anesthesia or analgesia include cardiac arrest from an intravascular or intraosseous injection, hematoma, neural injury, and infection. E-Figure 41-6 illustrates sites of unintended needle placement during the performance of a caudal epidural block. Injection of local anesthetic into an epidural blood vessel or intraosseous injection into the marrow cavity may result in a rapid increase in the blood concentration of the local anesthetic and a toxic reaction as discussed previously. It is also possible to pass the needle through the sacrum and perforate bowel or the pelvic organs, particularly in infants in whom ossification of the sacrum is incomplete.

There are now several large-scale prospective audits that have examined both the incidence and the nature of complications in regional anesthetics in children. The prospective audit from the UK and Ireland is the largest and most carefully described study on complications of epidural anesthesia in pediatrics to date. 10,633 cases were accrued over a period of 5 years, and all complications were reviewed and categorized by severity and type. Only five complications were graded as serious, and of these only one, the result of a drug error, had lasting sequelae. The French-Language Society of Pediatric Anesthesiologists (ADARPEF) published a follow-up prospective study on regional anesthetics in children in which they reported on 10,098 epidural blocks.[66] There were no permanent sequelae seen in any child. The PRAN consortium in the United States, reported data from their first prospective cohort in which 9087 epidural and caudal blocks were accrued, 6210 single injection (mostly caudal) and 2946 continuous caudal or epidural anesthesias.[10] In this study there were no complications of any kind lasting more than 3 months. The most common complication was catheter displacement or malfunction in the postoperative period in continuous blocks.

*Infection* is of grave concern when it occurs in either the subarachnoid or the epidural space.[299] A study of 1620 children over a 6-year period found no incidence of epidural abscess.[300] Catheters remained in situ for a mean of 2 days (maximum 8 days). The adult literature also suggests that infection is an uncommon complication.[301,302] However, both superficial and deep abscesses may rarely occur, particularly in those children with immunodeficiency syndromes and cancer who are receiving long-term infusions.[303] Epidural abscess and meningitis are the most potentially serious complications.[299,304] The development of an epidural abscess is a surgical emergency, because failure to treat it can lead to a permanent neurologic injury. The signs and symptoms (Table 41-6) are the same as for epidural hematomas, although fever, increased erythrocyte sedimentation rate, and increased leukocyte count with a leftward shift are also often present. Surgical drainage may be necessary. In the British audit, three serious infections (two epidural abscesses and one case of meningitis) were noted. These infections were all related to insertion site infections. All cultures grew *Staphylococcus aureus.* Twenty-five local infections were reported, mostly *S. aureus,* and 80% were associated with catheters left in place more than 48 hours. Of note is that some localized infections that developed at the catheter insertion site only became apparent several days after the catheter had been removed (see Fig. 43-11). Similar findings were reported in the PRAN data. In the British study one case progressed to an epidural abscess. Whether these infections developed while the catheter was in place leaving bacteria to track through the open site in the skin after the catheter was removed, or by hematologic spread is unknown, although the former etiology is most frequently cited. Infants and toddlers who are in

diapers require meticulous management of these catheters and their insertion site. A mild erythema occasionally occurs at the site of catheter insertion when children have indwelling catheters in place for several days, and this must be distinguished from a cellulitis (see Fig. 43-11). In most cases these superficial infections resolve with removal of the catheter and local care. On occasion these superficial infections may require treatment with a systemic antibiotic. If there is any question that the site is infected, the catheter should be removed. Although no serious systemic infection occurred in a prospective study of 210 children with 170 caudal catheters (age 3 ± 1 years) and 40 lumbar epidural catheters (age 11 ± 3 years) that were in place for 3 ± 1 days, 35% were colonized with bacteria.[305] This rate of colonization was similar with both caudal (25%) and lumbar epidural (23%) approaches. These results suggest that colonization is not synonymous with infection and that caudal catheters are not necessarily associated with greater infectious risk than lumbar epidural catheters. The factors that transform colonization into infection remain unknown.

It is common to have epidural fluid leak from the insertion site in caudal epidural catheters, especially in the presence of presacral edema. If an indwelling caudal epidural catheter is in place when a child develops a fever of unknown origin, the catheter should be removed because it may be causing the infection or become seeded by the infection (see Chapter 43).

*Epidural hematoma* is also a rare complication after epidural blockade. Optimal outcome depends on rapid diagnosis and prompt treatment and decompression. Signs and symptoms are presented in Table 41-6. The presence of clinically important coagulopathy or thrombocytopenia is an unacceptable risk for developing an epidural hematoma and is a contraindication to central neuraxial blockade. Guidelines for the conduct of neural blockade in the anticoagulated patient have been published by the American Society for Regional Anesthesia.[306] Of particular note is that there is a difference in the management of the patient who is receiving conventional (unfractionated) heparin and low molecular weight heparins, such as enoxaparin. Guidelines for the management of patients who are anticoagulated are shown

| TABLE 41-6 Signs and Symptoms of Epidural Hematoma and Abscess | |
| --- | --- |
| **Abscess** | **Hematoma** |
| Fever | Afebrile |
| ± Increased WBC | WBC normal |
| ± Increased sedimentation rate | Sedimentation rate normal or slightly increased |
| ± Left WBC shift | |
| Localized back pain | Localized back pain |
| Radicular pain | Radicular pain |
| Paraplegia | Paraplegia |
| Sensory loss | Sensory loss |
| Urinary and fecal retention | Urinary and fecal retention |
| Incontinence | Incontinence |
| Local tenderness | Local tenderness |
| Defect on myelography | Defect on myelography |
| Localized lesion on magnetic resonance imaging | Localized lesion on magnetic resonance imaging |

*WBC,* White blood cell count.

**TABLE 41-7** Guidelines for the Use of Regional Anesthesia in the Anticoagulated Patient

| Drug (Generic) | Common Trade Names | Interval for Catheter Placement after Last Dose | Interval for Catheter Removal after Most Recent Dose | Time Interval to Restart Med after Catheter is Removed |
|---|---|---|---|---|
| Enoxaparin* (therapeutic) | Lovenox (>60 mg daily or 1 mg/kg bid or 1.5 mg/kg daily) | 24 hours | Catheter should be removed before first dose. If med given, wait >24 hours | 2-4 hours after catheter removed |
| Enoxaparin* (prophylactic) | Lovenox (≤60 mg per day) | 12 hours | 12 hours | 2-4 hours |
| Heparin SC bid | Heparin | No significant risk at dose of 5000 units bid | | |
| Heparin SC tid | Heparin | Unknown risk at 5000 units tid: suggest check PTT. 10,000 units tid: check PTT | | |
| Heparin IV | Heparin | 2-4 hours, PTT < 35 | 2-4 hours, PTT < 35 | 2 hours |
| NSAID, ASA | Celebrex, Motrin, Naprosyn, etc. | No significant risk | | |
| Streptokinase | Streptase | 10 days | 10 days | Uncertain; at least 24 hours |
| Warfarin | Coumadin | 3-5 days, INR ≤ 1.5 | If >24 hours, check INR ≤ 1.5 | Same day |

Modified from the guidelines of the Massachusetts General Hospital Department of Anesthesia, Critical Care and Pain Medicine, 2011.
*ASA*, Acetylsalicylic acid; *INR*, international normalized ratio; *IV*, intravenous; *NSAID*, nonsteroidal antiinflammatory drug; *PTT*, partial thromboplastin time; *SC*, subcutaneous.
*Note for *low molecular weight heparin*: Prophylactic dosing may be started 6 to 8 hours postoperatively. Therapeutic dosing or bid dosing should be started at least 24 hours postoperatively. Epidural catheters should be removed before initiation of therapy.

in Table 41-7; however, each case must be decided on an individual basis.[306] Postoperatively, *urinary retention* has been associated with the presence of both epidural and spinal anesthesia. In this regard, it is important to distinguish between the effects of local anesthetics and central neuraxial opioids in the blocks. There is no evidence to support the notion that regional anesthesia with local anesthesia causes urinary retention, and, indeed, there are data to the contrary. In a prospective study of infants and children undergoing inguinal herniorrhaphy or orchiopexy, caudal blockade, ilioinguinal-iliohypogastric nerve block by the surgeon, or a control consisting of caudal injection of 1 : 200,000 epinephrine (no local anesthetic) yielded similar times to voiding postoperatively.[307] In a retrospective study of 326 children undergoing inguinal herniorrhaphy and urologic surgery, 237 received a caudal block and 66 received local anesthesia by the surgeon. The incidence of urinary retention was similar for the two groups, with the type of surgery being the primary determinant of urinary retention.[308]

The epidural and subarachnoid use of opioids, however, is associated with an increased incidence of urinary retention. Epidural morphine in a dose of 70 μg/kg (a dose that would now be considered excessive) was associated with a 50% incidence of urinary retention[309]; 70% of those with urinary retention required treatment. Another study reported an incidence of urinary retention of 27% after caudally administered morphine, 33 to 100 μg/kg, although most of the children had urinary catheters.[310] Finally, 50 μg/kg diacetylmorphine was associated with an 11% incidence of urinary retention.[311] A dose of 33 μg/kg epidural morphine is the most common recommended in current practice.

Data from the large prospective databases indicate that the incidence of *neural injury* after epidural blockade is very small and that long-term neurologic sequelae of neuraxial blockade is rare. One must slightly temper these conclusions, however, based on the limited follow up of children in these studies who did not have problems reported within the immediate time frame of the block. A prospective study of more than 2,500 infants and children who received epidural blocks demonstrated no evidence of neurologic complications, although a retrospective review of the first ADARPEF data determined that 1 in 5000 infants younger than

3 months of age had neurologic complications with MRI evidence of spinal cord ischemia.[99,312] In four of the five cases reported in that study the epidural space was located using loss of resistance to air (in the fifth the technique was not specified) and the authors thought that air embolus was the etiology of the neurologic injury. Based on these data, the use of air for loss of resistance in infants and children has been strongly discouraged, and saline should be used instead. In the follow up ADARPEF study there were no cases of neurologic injury.[66] The British epidural audit found six cases of neural injury in 10,633 children in this prospective study. Of particular note was the delay in recognition of the injury, as no cases were discovered before 2 days had elapsed from the time the block was placed, and some diagnoses were not made for 10 days after the block. All children had complete resolution of their symptoms within 1 year. Two children were referred to a chronic pain service and treated with gabapentin, and one child developed a common peroneal nerve injury that was attributed to malpositioning of the leg during surgery. We have had one child who developed symptoms of complex regional pain syndrome after common peroneal nerve injury from positioning in the postoperative period. This child had persistent motor block, which emphasizes (1) the importance of early recognition of motor blockade as a potential for injury after surgery and (2) the critical importance of positioning and nursing care in preventing pressure injuries. There were no cases of persistent neurologic injury in the initial PRAN data cohort. An in vivo study in young rabbits, using colored microspheres to assess spinal cord and organ blood flow, found that a decrease in blood pressure, when accompanied by epidural anesthesia with lidocaine, decreased spinal cord blood flow.[313] The addition of epinephrine to the local anesthetic solution did not increase the incidence of ischemia. These studies suggest that it may be particularly important to maintain adequate systemic blood flow during "combined technique" anesthesia in infants and children, and to treat hypotension promptly. Because blood pressure changes caused by neuraxial blockade are uncommon in infants and small children, hypotension in these patients is likely to be due to other causes and should prompt an assessment of intravascular filling pressures, inotropic state, and the depth of general anesthesia.

## PERIPHERAL NERVE BLOCKS

Peripheral nerve blocks are useful adjuvants to general anesthesia. These blocks are also useful as a means for providing postoperative pain relief. Peripheral nerve blocks differ from central neuraxial blocks in several respects:

- A targeted area is anesthetized.
- Side effects, such as weakness of extremities, are minimal.
- The dose of local anesthetic is reduced.
- There is no risk of an unintended spinal anesthetic.
- There is no risk of urinary retention.
- They can be used in areas where a central neuraxial block is not possible (e.g., face and scalp).

There are many peripheral nerve blocks that can be used in the practice of pediatric anesthesia and each is described below (Table 41-8; see also Chapter 42).

### Selection of a Local Anesthetic

Local anesthetics commonly used for peripheral blocks in children include lidocaine, mepivacaine, bupivacaine, and, more recently, levobupivacaine and ropivacaine.[63,65,314] Longer-acting agents have a greater role in peripheral blocks than shorter-acting agents because of the increased duration of postoperative analgesia. Lidocaine can be combined with bupivacaine to provide both a rapid onset and a long duration of action, a practice that we advocate if the child is having the procedure performed with a local block under sedation. If this is done, one must be careful to calculate the doses of the two drugs properly to avoid toxicity. Alternatively, the addition of sodium bicarbonate (1 mEq of bicarbonate/10 mL of local anesthetic [lidocaine]) can speed the onset and reduce the pain of injection of the block by increasing the pH of the solution.[315-318] This alters the $pK_a$ of the solution,

increasing the active cationic form of the local anesthetic in the solution.[319] Bicarbonate should be added to the local anesthetic solution immediately before administration because precipitation of the local anesthetic and therefore loss of bioavailability increases over time (it should be administered within 10 minutes after alkalinization).[320,321] This is particularly a problem with mepivacaine, bupivacaine, and ropivacaine in which the addition of 0.1 mL of 8.4% bicarbonate results in precipitation within 10 minutes.[319,320] The total drug dose administered should not exceed the maximum milligram per kilogram dose permitted for the local anesthetic (see Table 41-2). The addition of epinephrine (1 : 200,000) may decrease both the vascular absorption and the potential for toxicity; for some local anesthetics the addition of epinephrine will also extend the duration of the block. The exact dose of local anesthetic in terms of volume or concentration needed for most peripheral blocks in children has not been adequately studied. Most blocks performed in children are based on adult experience. Suggested dosing for common peripheral blocks based on volume per kilogram and our experience is presented in Table 41-9.

### Head and Neck Blocks

Peripheral nerve blocks for postoperative pain relief for the head and neck can be performed with the child under general anesthesia.[322] These blocks can also be used for the provision of pain relief in children with chronic painful problems, such as headaches. Anatomically, two major nerves, the ophthalmic division ($V_1$) of the trigeminal nerve and the branches of the cervical root C2, supply the sensory innervations of the face and scalp (Fig. 41-8).

#### Supraorbital and Supratrochlear Nerve Block

ANATOMY. The supraorbital and supratrochlear are the end branches of the ophthalmic division ($V_1$) of the trigeminal nerve. The supraorbital nerve, the terminal branch of $V_1$, exits the supraorbital foramen to supply the scalp anterior to the coronal suture. The supratrochlear nerve leaves the orbit between the trochlea and the supraorbital foramen and innervates the lower part of the forehead (Fig. 41-9, *A*). We use this combined block to provide pain relief in children undergoing frontal craniotomies and in children undergoing frontal ventriculoperitoneal shunt revisions. The technique can be used as the sole anesthetic in very sick neonates,[323] and also to control postoperative pain in children undergoing excision of scalp lesions.[324] The major advantage is the avoidance of opioids, thereby facilitating an early hospital discharge.

TECHNIQUE. With the child supine and the head in the neutral position, the supraorbital notch is palpated by running

---

### TABLE 41-8 Peripheral Nerve Blocks

**Head and Neck**

Supraorbital and supratrochlear
Infraorbital nerve
Greater occipital nerve
Great auricular nerve

**Chest Wall**

Intercostal nerve

**Upper Extremity**

Brachial plexus
Elbow blocks (ulnar, radial, and median nerves)
Wrist blocks (ulnar, radial, and median nerves)
Digital

**Abdomen and Genitalia**

Ilioinguinal nerve
Penile
Rectus sheath

**Lower Extremity**

Femoral nerve
Lateral femoral cutaneous
Fascia iliaca
Sciatic nerve
    Classic approach
    Lateral approach (popliteal fossa)
Ankle
Digital

---

### TABLE 41-9 Suggested Dosing for Local Anesthetic Volumes for Common Peripheral Nerve Blocks

| Technique | Dose (mL/kg) | Usual Volume (mL) |
|---|---|---|
| Head and neck blocks | 0.05 | 3 |
| Brachial plexus blocks | 0.2-0.3 | 10 |
| Ilioinguinal nerve block | 0.075 | 4 |
| Rectus sheath block | 0.1 | 4 |
| Femoral nerve block | 0.2-0.3 | 10 |
| Sciatic nerve | 0.2-0.3 | 15 |
| Digital nerves | 0.05 | 2 |

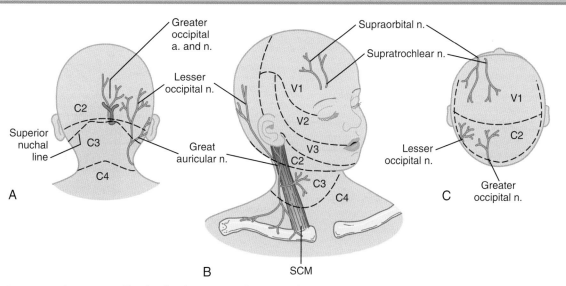

**FIGURE 41-8** Dermatomal innervation of head and neck. Sensory and dermatomal innervation of greater and lesser occipital nerves and the innervation of the anterior head by the first division of the trigeminal nerve. Note the sensory innervation anterior to the coronal suture is from the first division of the trigeminal nerve (supraorbital and supratrochlear nerves) and posterior to the coronal suture is from branches of C2 (greater and lesser occipital nerves). These nerves can be blocked individually and in combination to provide postoperative analgesia for a wide variety of procedures; see text for details. **A,** Posterior view. **B,** Anterolateral view. **C,** Axial view. *a,* Artery; *C2, C3, C4,* cervical sensory branches of the nerve roots; *n,* nerve; *SCM,* sternocleidomastoid muscle; *V1, V2, V3,* branches of the trigeminal nerve. (Modified from Brown DL, Wong GY. Occipital nerve block. In: Waldman S, Winnie AP, editors. Interventional pain management. Philadelphia: WB Saunders; 1996, p. 227.)

a finger from the midline laterally along the eyebrow (the supraorbital notch is usually located in line with the pupil with the eye in midline position). The skin is prepared with povidone-iodine or chlorhexidine and care is taken to avoid spilling the solution into the eye. A 27-gauge needle is inserted in the proximity of the supraorbital notch; 0.5 to 1.0 mL of bupivacaine (0.25% with epinephrine 1:200,000) is injected into the space after careful aspiration to prevent intravascular placement (see Fig. 41-9, *B*). To block the supratrochlear nerve, the needle is withdrawn to the skin level and then directed and advanced several millimeters medially toward the apex of the nose; 0.5 to 1.0 mL of bupivacaine (0.25% with epinephrine 1:200,000) is injected (Video: Supraorbital Nerve Block).

COMPLICATIONS. Because of the loose adventitious tissue of the eyelid, gentle pressure should be applied to the supraorbital area; this prevents the dissection of the local anesthetic into the eyelid and supraorbital tissue, and may reduce the potential for ecchymosis and/or hematoma.

### Greater Occipital Nerve Block
The greater occipital nerve block is used to diagnose and treat occipital pain. If this technique is used for the diagnosis of occipital neuralgia, a careful history and physical examination is performed to rule out other pathologic causes of headaches, including posterior fossa tumors and Arnold-Chiari malformation.[325] It can also be used to treat postoperative pain in the posterior fossa after posterior fossa surgery, and in children undergoing posterior ventriculoperitoneal shunt revisions.[326]

ANATOMY. The cervical spinal nerves innervate the posterior head and neck. The dorsal rami of C2 end in the greater occipital nerve, which provides the cutaneous innervation to the major portion of the posterior scalp (Fig. 41-10, *A*). The nerve becomes subcutaneous slightly inferior to the superior nuchal line by passing above the aponeurotic sling; here it is in close proximity and medial to the occipital artery.

TECHNIQUE. With the child supine and the head laterally rotated or with the child prone, the occipital artery is palpated at the level of the superior nuchal line. The occipital artery is usually located at approximately one-third of the distance from the external occipital protuberance to the mastoid process on the superior nuchal line (see Fig. 41-10, *B*). A total volume of 2 mL of bupivacaine (0.25% with 1:200,000 epinephrine) is injected SC (Video: Greater Occipital Nerve Block). A recent technique using ultrasound guidance has been used in children for performing occipital nerve blocks.[327]

COMPLICATIONS. It is rare to see complications with this block because of the superficial location of the nerve. One has to bear in mind the close proximity to the spinal canal, particularly in children who have had surgery in the area. Thus the needle must remain just beneath the skin during injection of local anesthetic. It is more difficult to perform this block at the C2 nerve root without the aid of either ultrasonography or fluoroscopy and hence it cannot cover the entire distribution of the greater occipital nerve. Intravascular injection may be avoided with incremental injection and frequent aspiration.

### Infraorbital Nerve Block
ANATOMY. The infraorbital nerve is the termination of the second division of the trigeminal nerve, the maxillary nerve (Fig. 41-11, *A*). This nerve is entirely sensory in function. It leaves the skull through the foramen rotundum and enters into the pterygopalatine fossa. It then enters the infraorbital groove and passes through the infraorbital canal. The nerve emerges in front of the maxilla through the infraorbital foramen and then divides into four branches: the inferior palpebral, the external nasal, the internal nasal, and the superior labial. The anatomic location of the infraorbital foramen has been studied using CT scans: the average distance from the midline (in millimeters) is $21.3 + 0.5 \times$ age (years).[328,329] The branches of the infraorbital nerve innervate the lower eyelid, the lateral inferior portion of the nose and

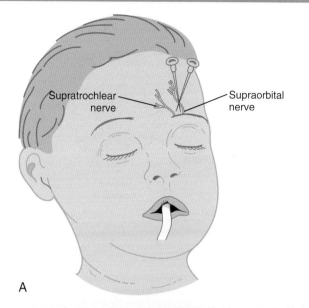

A

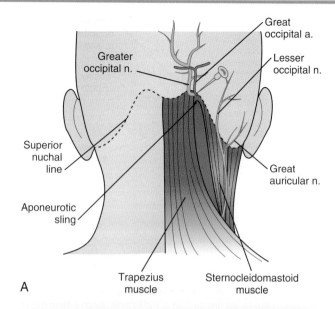

A

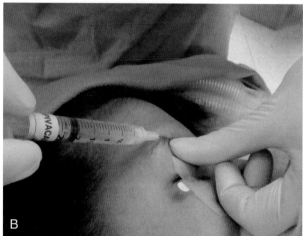

B

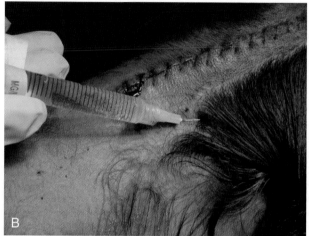

B

**FIGURE 41-9 A,** Supraorbital and supratrochlear nerve block. The supraorbital notch is palpated by running a finger from the midline laterally along the eyebrow. A 27-gauge needle is inserted into the supraorbital notch perpendicularly; bupivacaine (1 mL, 0.25% with 1:200,000 epinephrine) is injected into the space after careful aspiration (**B**). To block the supratrochlear nerve, the needle is withdrawn to skin level and then directed medially several millimeters toward the apex of the nose; bupivacaine (1 mL, 0.25% with 1:200,000 epinephrine) is injected. This block provides postoperative pain relief for children undergoing frontal craniotomies or frontal ventriculoperitoneal shunt insertion.

**FIGURE 41-10 A,** Greater occipital nerve block. With the patient supine and with the head turned to one side or with the patient prone, the occipital artery is palpated at the level of the superior nuchal line. The occipital artery is located about one-third of the distance from the external occipital protuberance (*dashed line*) to the mastoid process on the superior nuchal line. A total volume of 2 mL of bupivacaine (0.25% with 1:200,000 epinephrine) is injected subcutaneously to form a skin wheal (**B**). Frequent aspiration and incremental injection may avoid intravascular injection. This block is used to diagnose occipital neuralgia and as a means for providing postoperative pain relief for children undergoing posterior fossa tumor resection or posterior ventriculoperitoneal shunt insertion. *a*, Artery; *n*, nerve. (Modified from Brown DL, Wong GY. Occipital nerve block. In: Waldman S, Winnie AP, editors. Interventional pain management. Philadelphia: WB Saunders; 1996, p. 228.)

its vestibule, the upper lip, the mucosa along the upper lip, and the vermilion. This block is effective for surgery of the upper lip and the vermilion after a cleft lip repair,[330] for reconstructive procedures on the nose (including septal reconstruction and rhinoplasty),[331] and for endoscopic sinus surgery.[332] There are two approaches to the infraorbital nerve: intraoral and extraoral.

INTRAORAL APPROACH. This is our preferred method for this block. The infraorbital foramen is located by palpation of the infraorbital notch. After folding back the upper lip, a 27-gauge needle is inserted through the buccal mucosa approximately parallel to the maxillary second molar and passed SC with the tip of the needle directed toward the infraorbital foramen. It is important to place a finger over the infraorbital foramen so as to palpate the progress of the needle beneath the skin and prevent unintended passage of the needle into the orbit. With the tip of

the needle at the level of the infraorbital foramen and after careful aspiration, 0.5 to 1.0 mL of local anesthetic is injected (see Fig. 41-11, *B*, and Video: Infraorbital Nerve Block). Bupivacaine (0.25% with epinephrine 1:200,000) provides prolonged postoperative analgesia with this block.

EXTRAORAL APPROACH. The infraorbital ridge of the maxillary bone should be identified and the infraorbital foramen palpated. A 27-gauge needle is advanced toward the foramen at a 45-degree angle to the maxilla (see Fig. 41-11, *C*). After careful aspiration, 0.5 to 1.0 mL of bupivacaine (0.25% with epinephrine 1:200,000) is injected.

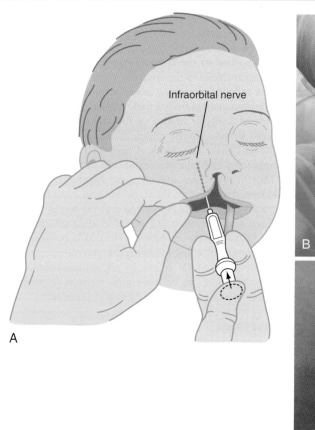

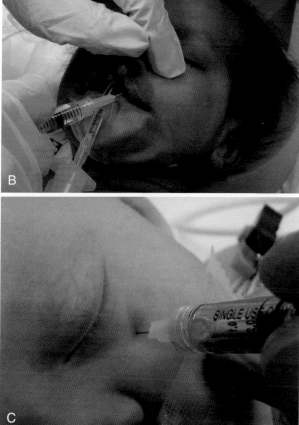

**FIGURE 41-11 A,** Infraorbital block (intraoral approach): The infraorbital foramen is located by palpation of the infraorbital notch (right-sided block). **B,** The lip is folded back and a 27-gauge needle is inserted through the buccal mucosa approximately parallel to the maxillary second molar. The tip of the needle is directed toward the infraorbital foramen. A finger is placed over the infraorbital foramen to avoid accidental placement of the needle into the orbit. After careful aspiration to avoid intravascular injection, 0.5 to 1.0 mL of bupivacaine (0.25% with 1:200,000 epinephrine) is injected (left-sided block). **C,** For the extraoral approach (left-sided block) the infraorbital ridge of the maxillary bone should be identified and the infraorbital foramen is palpated. A 27-gauge needle is advanced toward the foramen at a 45-degree angle to the maxilla (midpupillary point). After careful aspiration, 0.5 to 1.0 mL of bupivacaine (0.25% with epinephrine 1:200,000) is injected. This block is used to provide postoperative pain relief for children undergoing upper lip or cleft lip repair, reconstructive procedures of the nose (e.g., rhinoplasty), and endoscopic sinus surgery.

COMPLICATIONS. Because of the loose adventitious tissue, children can develop ecchymosis and swelling. Pressure should be applied to the infraorbital area to retain the solution within the infraorbital foramen, prevent dissection of the local anesthetic into the periorbital area, and reduce the potential for the formation of a hematoma or ecchymosis. Care should be taken to avoid direct injection into the orbit or eye. Intravascular injection may be avoided with incremental injection and frequent aspiration. This block can be achieved with low volumes in infants and toddlers and hence every attempt should be made to decrease the volume of the local anesthetic solution. Using other additives, including clonidine, may be helpful, although there are no randomized controlled trials to demonstrate the improved efficacy of this block using additives.

### Great Auricular Nerve Block

The great auricular nerve supplies the sensory innervation to the mastoid area and the external ear. It is a branch of the superficial cervical plexus. Cervical plexus blocks were first performed by

Halstead in 1884. This block has been used to provide postoperative analgesia in children undergoing otoplasty repair,[333] as well as in tympanomastoid surgery.[334] We found that the great auricular nerve block decreases the incidence of nausea and vomiting, which is a major morbidity associated with tympanomastoid surgery.[334] It provides surface analgesia but not muscle relaxation and hence can be used for intraoperative analgesia despite the need for facial nerve monitoring in children undergoing tympanomastoid procedures.

ANATOMY. The cervical plexus is formed by the anterior primary division of the anterior and posterior roots of cervical nerves C2-4. The great auricular nerve is derived from C3, which was described by McKinney. The anatomic location of the nerve for blockade has been described as the McKinney point.[335] The great auricular nerve wraps around the belly of the sternocleidomastoid muscle at the level of the cricoid cartilage and emerges to supply the area of the mastoid and external ear (Fig. 41-12, *A*).

TECHNIQUE. With the child under general anesthesia, the cricoid cartilage is identified. A line is drawn from the superior

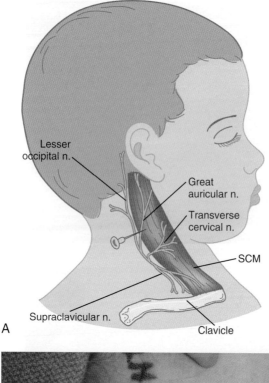

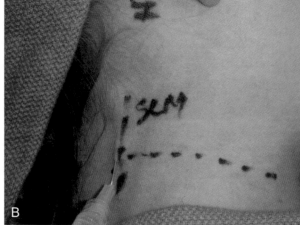

**FIGURE 41-12 A,** Great auricular nerve block. The cricoid cartilage is identified. A broken line drawn from the superior border of the cricoid cartilage laterally to the posterior border of the sternocleidomastoid (*SCM*) (McKinney point) is identified; bupivacaine (2.0 to 3.0 mL, 0.25% with 1:200,000 epinephrine) is injected subcutaneously at this point (**B**). Gentle massage after the injection allows spread of the local anesthetic in the injected site. This block is used to provide postoperative analgesia for children undergoing tympanomastoid surgery or otoplasty. *n,* Nerve. (Modified from Brown DL, editor. Atlas of regional anesthesia. Philadelphia: WB Saunders; 1999, p. 185.)

margin of the cricoid cartilage laterally to the posterior border of the sternocleidomastoid muscle (McKinney point). Bupivacaine (2 to 3 mL, 0.25% with epinephrine 1:200,000) is injected superficially at this point (see Fig. 41-12, *B,* and Video: Great Auricular Nerve Block).

COMPLICATIONS. Deep rather than superficial injection can result in a deep cervical plexus block and the risk of Horner syndrome, phrenic nerve block, or unintended central neuraxial blockade. A small erythematous area may be seen at the site of the needle injection. Intravascular injection may be avoided by incremental injection of the solution and frequent aspiration.

### Nerve of Arnold (Auricular Branch of Vagus)

The auricular branch of the vagus supplies the sensory nerve that supplies the innervation to the auditory canal, as well as the inferior portion of the tympanic membrane. This is useful for providing analgesia to the tympanic membrane following myringotomy and tube placement, as well as for tympanoplasty surgery. In a randomized controlled trial, intranasal fentanyl and blockade of the auricular branch of the vagus provided equivalent analgesia without adverse effects.[336]

INDICATIONS. This block is used to provide analgesia for myringotomy and tube placement, and for tympanoplasty.

TECHNIQUE. After induction of anesthesia, and with the child turned to one side, the tragus is cleaned and reflected laterally, a 30-gauge needle is inserted into the tragus to pierce the cartilage, after aspiration, 0.2 mL of local anesthetic solution is injected (Video: Nerve of Arnold Block). Mild pressure is applied to prevent any bleeding following the procedure.

COMPLICATIONS. It is rare to see complications, although occasionally there can be some brisk bleeding from the needle entry site, which can be offset by applying pressure.

### Truncal Blocks

Truncal blocks are performed in children for a variety of different surgical procedures. The most common blocks include intercostal blocks,[33] ilioinguinal blocks, penile blocks, rectus sheath blocks, and paravertebral blocks.

### Intercostal Nerve Block

Intercostal blocks after thoracotomy are useful in reducing opioid requirements, optimizing respiratory mechanics, and encouraging early ambulation.[33,337,338] Their major disadvantage is the limited duration of analgesia. Currently, we more commonly employ epidural blockade for this purpose. The development of degradable bupivacaine microspheres and the recent approval of liposomal encapsulated bupivacaine, which produce analgesia of dramatically greater duration, may change this practice in the future.[47,56-59,61] There are, however, still situations in which intercostal blocks are useful, particularly in children who cannot have a neuraxial catheter placed.

The uptake of local anesthetic after intercostal blocks is the most rapid of all sites of regional anesthesia, yielding the greatest plasma concentrations of local anesthetics following any other regional block. Furthermore, plasma concentrations in children increase more rapidly than after identical blocks in adults.[339] For this reason, epinephrine (1:200,000) should be added to reduce the absorption of local anesthetic. We commonly use 0.25% bupivacaine with epinephrine in a dose of 1 to 5 mL for each nerve being blocked, depending on the size of the child and the number of ribs to be blocked. A maximum of 2 mg/kg of bupivacaine is used, although this amount should be reduced by about 30% for infants younger than 6 months of age. The concentration of bupivacaine should be decreased to provide adequate volume for the desired number of intercostal blocks while avoiding the risk of systemic toxicity.

ANATOMY. The intercostal nerves are derived from the ventral rami of the first through twelfth thoracic nerves. There are four branches: the first is the gray rami communicans, which goes to the sympathetic ganglion; the second branch arises as the posterior cutaneous branch, which supplies the skin in the paravertebral area; the third branch, the lateral cutaneous branch, arises anterior to the midaxillary line and sends subcutaneous branches both anteriorly and posteriorly; and the final branch

41

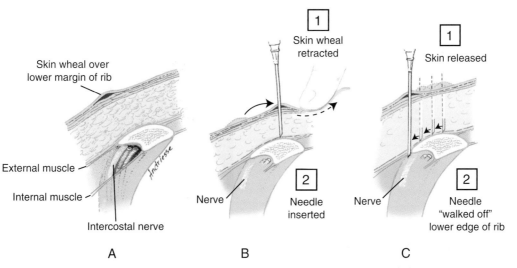

**FIGURE 41-13** Intercostal block. A skin wheal is inserted on the lower rib margin (**A**). The skin wheal is retracted over the body of the rib, and a needle is inserted until contact is made with the rib (**B**). The skin is released, and the needle is carefully "walked" off the edge of the rib margin (**C**). After negative aspiration for blood, the appropriate volume of drug is injected. This block is used for postoperative analgesia for thoracotomy or chest tube insertion (see also E-Fig 41-7).

provides cutaneous innervation to the midline of the chest and abdomen. The dura mater and the arachnoid membrane fuse with the epineurium as they exit the vertebral foramen. This could lead to subarachnoid block if the posterior paravertebral approach is used.

TECHNIQUE. The site of injection may be either paravertebral or in the midaxillary line. The lower rib margin is located, and the skin is retracted cephalad (Fig. 41-13, *A*). The needle is inserted perpendicular to the skin over the rib and advanced until the rib is encountered (see Fig. 41-13, *B*). The skin through which the needle is passed is allowed to retract caudally, and the needle is then walked off the lower edge of the rib a distance of 2 to 3 mm (see Fig. 41-13, *C*). This method may reduce the potential for pneumothorax, because the needle strikes the rib and is not advanced more than half of the thickness of the rib. A distinct pop may be felt as the needle enters the neurovascular sheath. After negative aspiration for blood, an appropriate volume of anesthetic is injected. Recently, with the use of ultrasound guidance, we can visualize the pleura, thereby avoiding puncturing the pleura because it can be adequately visualized while performing the block (E-Fig. 41-7; see also Fig. 42-11).

COMPLICATIONS. Pneumothorax has been reported after intercostal blockade, with an incidence of approximately 0.07% in adults.[340] However, the majority of the blocks in that study were performed by residents in training. If a small pneumothorax occurs, reabsorption is facilitated with the use of oxygen. Placement of a chest tube is only indicated if respirations are compromised. A more significant complication is the toxic effect of absorbed local anesthetic drugs. Using smaller volumes of more dilute local anesthetic may reduce the risk of achieving toxic plasma concentrations. The risk of intravascular injection may be reduced with incremental injection and frequent aspiration. A third complication is a high subarachnoid block, usually associated with the posterior paravertebral approach.

### Inguinal Block (Ilioinguinal and Iliohypogastric Nerves)
Inguinal block, supplemented by wound infiltration, is sometimes used in adult patients undergoing inguinal hernia repair. However, in children, it is used almost exclusively as an adjunct to general anesthesia and for postoperative pain management. This block is as effective as caudal anesthesia for inguinal repairs.[341,342] Blockade of the ilioinguinal and iliohypogastric nerves is very successful for this purpose and has few associated complications, although injection into the femoral vessels and potential femoral nerve block is a possibility.[343,344] The risks of toxicity from excessive drug doses may be greater than previously recognized, as discussed earlier, but ultrasound guidance has demonstrated adequate analgesia with reduced doses of local anesthetic solution because of the optimal drug placement.[345] This block may be (and commonly is) performed in conjunction with infiltration of the wound. The use of ultrasound may also avoid the risk of bowel perforation (see also Chapter 42, and Figs. 42-35 and 42-36).[346]

ANATOMY. The inguinal area is innervated by the subcostal nerve (T12), iliohypogastric and ilioinguinal nerves (derived from L1). These nerves lie in close proximity to each other medial and superior to the anterior superior iliac spine (Fig. 41-14, *A*). After piercing the internal oblique 2 to 3 cm medial to the anterior superior iliac spine, the nerve then lies between the internal oblique and the external oblique aponeurosis. Here it accompanies the spermatic cord (in males) to the genital area.

TECHNIQUE. The block may be performed either at the beginning of surgery or before the end of general anesthesia. If bupivacaine is used, a minimum of 15 minutes is usually required from the completion of the block until maximal analgesia is obtained. Thus blocks placed at the beginning of the surgical procedure (our preference) are usually more effective than those performed at the end of surgery. Blocks performed before skin incision may also provide "preemptive analgesia," although the evidence for this is still under debate and somewhat confusing.[347-350] The duration of postoperative analgesia is unaffected by the timing of placing the block: at the beginning of the procedure, assuming that the surgical procedure is not of more than 1.5 hours in duration or at the end. A short-bevel 27-gauge needle is inserted at a 45-degree angle at a point one-fourth of the way toward the midline along a line drawn from the anterior superior iliac spine to the umbilicus (1.0 to 1.5 cm cephalad and toward

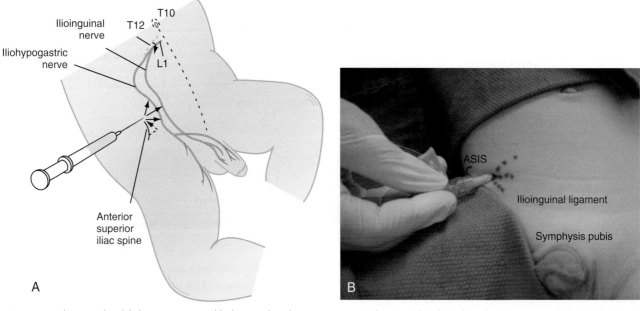

**FIGURE 41-14** Ilioinguinal and iliohypogastric nerve blocks. **A** and **B,** The anterior superior iliac spine *(ASIS)* is palpated, and a point 1.0 to 1.5 cm cephalad and toward the midline is located (*dashed line*). A 22-gauge needle is passed through the external and internal oblique muscles, and 1.0 to 5.0 mL of local anesthetic is deposited in a fan-like fashion cephalad toward the umbilicus, medially, and caudad toward the groin (*solid arrows*). Just before removal from the skin, another 0.5 to 1.0 mL of local anesthetic is injected subcutaneously to block the iliohypogastric nerve. Blockade of these nerves provide postoperative analgesia for inguinal hernia and orchiopexy procedures (see also E-Fig. 41-8).

the midline from the anterior superior iliac spine in a 10- to 15-kg child). As the needle is advanced through the external and internal oblique muscles (see Fig. 41-14, *B*), two pops are elicited and provide useful guides of proper needle placement. Negative aspiration should be confirmed several times during the incremental injection of local anesthetic. A volume of 0.3 mL/kg of local anesthetic solution is injected in a fan-like fashion, cephalad toward the umbilicus, caudad toward the groin, and medially. Before removal of the needle from the skin, an additional 0.5 to 1.0 mL of local anesthetic is injected SC to block the iliohypogastric nerve (Video: Ilioinguinal Nerve Block with Ultrasound). Care must be taken to avoid entering the peritoneum, which has been reported after the blind injection approach.[346] For inguinal herniorrhaphy, orchiopexy, or other inguinal procedures, local anesthetic deposited directly into the wound before it is closed has also proved effective for postoperative analgesia.[342] The volume of drug used by this approach, like the volume of drug used for wound infiltration, must be accounted for when calculating the maximal dose of local anesthetic that can be used. It is important to note that this block will not provide pain relief for scrotal procedures because this is supplied by the genitofemoral nerve and hence it is important to have the surgeon infiltrate the scrotum for complete pain relief following orchiopexy or any other scrotal procedures. As mentioned earlier, an ultrasound-guided technique may be easier and leads to fewer complications while performing the block (E-Fig. 41-8).[345]

COMPLICATIONS. Complications are rare. Care should be taken not to enter the peritoneal cavity. Intravascular injection may be avoided by incremental injection with frequent aspiration.

### Penile Block

A penile block is used for anesthesia and postoperative analgesia for circumcision, urethral dilatation, and hypospadias repair.

Caudal anesthesia is superior for proximal shaft or penoscrotal hypospadias repair because a penile block provides analgesia only for the distal two-thirds of the penis.[266,351,352] The block is easily performed and has a high success rate. Bupivacaine, levobupivacaine, and ropivacaine are the most useful agents because of their prolonged duration of action. *Epinephrine must never be used for this block because the dorsal artery of the penis is an end artery and vasospasm caused by epinephrine could cause necrosis.*

ANATOMY. The nerve supply of the penis is from the pudendal nerve and the pelvic plexus (Fig. 41-15, *A*). Along the dorsal artery to the penis are two dorsal nerves that separate at the level of the symphysis pubis; they supply the sensory innervation to the penis.

TECHNIQUE. There are two commonly used techniques for penile block: (1) a ring block and (2) blockade of the dorsal nerve. One investigation compared the efficacy of these techniques and concluded that the ring block provided analgesia of prolonged duration, although both techniques provided analgesia superior to EMLA cream.[353] The ring block is performed by inserting a 27-gauge needle at the base of the penis and, after negative aspiration, injecting the local anesthetic without epinephrine in a ring-shaped pattern around the base of the penile shaft. The needle may be inserted once in the midline and then redirected to each side (see Fig. 41-15, *B*). The alternate dorsal nerve block is performed with a 27-gauge needle inserted 1 cm above the symphysis pubis, in the midline, at a 30-degree angle and directed caudally (see Fig. 41-15, *C*). The needle is advanced 1 cm after it pierces the penile fascia. After negative aspiration for blood, 1 to 4 mL of local anesthetic *without epinephrine* is injected slowly. There is a small risk of injury to the adjacent neurovascular structures.

COMPLICATIONS. The major complication is compromise of organ blood flow. *Vasoconstrictors, such as epinephrine, must never be used for this block.* Applying pressure after the injection may

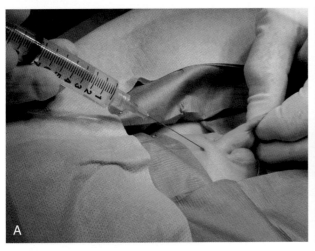

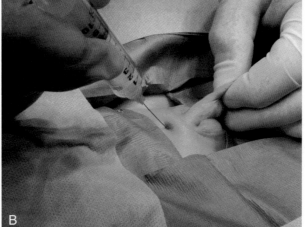

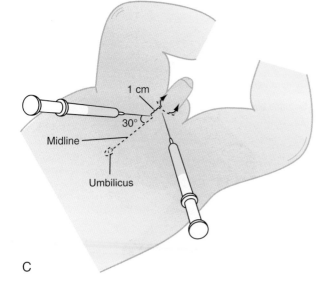

C

FIGURE 41-15 Penile block. **A,** Dorsal nerve block: a 27- or 25-gauge needle is inserted in the midline, 1 cm above the symphysis pubis at an angle of 30 degrees from the plane of the abdominal wall and directed caudad. **B,** After piercing the penile fascia (0.5 to 1.0 cm) and negative aspiration for blood, 1.0 to 4.0 mL of local anesthetic without epinephrine is injected. **C,** Ring block: a 25-gauge needle is inserted at the base of the penis at a 45-degree angle, and a ring of local anesthetic is deposited (*curved arrows*). This may be done through a single needle placement by redirecting the needle. This block may be used in children in whom a caudal block is contraindicated.

minimize hematoma formation. Intravascular injection may be avoided with incremental injection and frequent aspiration.

### Rectus Sheath Block

Although reported almost 20 years ago,[354] this block has recently become popular for children undergoing repair of an umbilical hernia.[355-357] The rectus sheath contains the thoracic intercostal nerves (T-10) that can be blocked at the paraumbilical area using a small volume of local anesthetic solution.

TECHNIQUE. On either side of the umbilicus, about 1 cm from midline a needle is inserted into the rectus sheath (Fig. 41-16, *A*). A pop can be felt as the needle advances beyond the anterior rectus sheath, through the rectus abdominis muscle and then just anterior to the posterior rectus sheath. After aspiration, a volume of 0.1 mL/kg of local anesthetic solution is injected (Video: Rectus Sheath Block with Ultrasound). This provides excellent analgesia for most umbilical area surgery, including laparoscopic surgery. Use of ultrasound may facilitate performing this block[358] (see Fig. 41-16, *A* and *B*; see also Chapter 42, and E-Figs. 42-2 and 42-3).

### Paravertebral Block

This block is also gaining some popularity for use in children. The main advantage is that deposition of local anesthetics in the paravertebral space will lead to strict unilateral anesthesia of one or more adjacent dermatomes (Fig. 41-17); the main indications for a paravertebral nerve block are unilateral thoracic or abdominal surgical procedures.

ANATOMY. The paravertebral space is a triangular wedge-shaped area situated in the angle between the lateral border of the vertebral body and the anterior surface of the transverse process (Fig. 41-18). The paravertebral space exists only between T1 and T12. Below T12 the space is sealed off by the origin of the psoas muscle from the vertebral body and the transverse process.[359] Cranially the space appears to communicate with fascial planes in the neck, because an upper thoracic paravertebral block may cause Horner syndrome. The communication of different thoracic levels of the paravertebral space is the foundation for spread of local anesthetic to multiple segments (see Fig. 41-17). The medial boundary of the paravertebral space is the lateral part of the vertebral body and disc, the dorsal limitation is the transverse process and costotransverse ligament, and the anterolateral boundary is the parietal pleura. Structures that pass through the paravertebral space include the spinal nerve root–intercostal nerve, the sympathetic chain, and the intercostal vessels. The paravertebral space is not like the epidural space, because the pleura are very adhesive to the other structures but should instead be viewed as a "potential space." This accounts

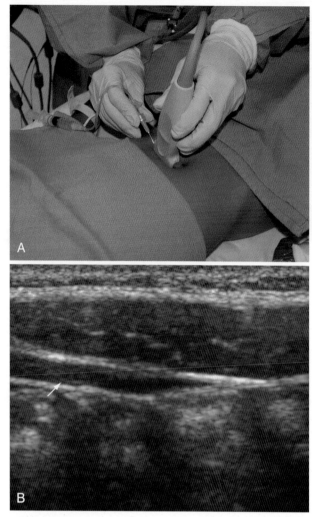

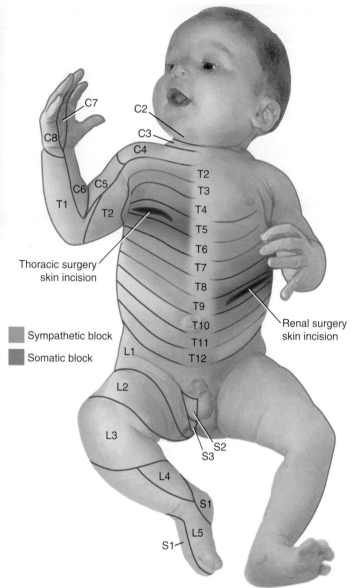

**FIGURE 41-16** Rectus sheath block. The rectus sheath is encompassed between the rectus abdominis muscle anteriorly and the posterior rectus sheath. **A,** A linear ultrasound probe is placed lateral to the umbilicus, and the anterior rectus sheath, the rectus abdominis muscle, and the posterior rectus sheath are identified. **B,** With the use of an in-plane approach, a 27-gauge needle is inserted through the rectus abdominis muscle anterior to the posterior rectus sheath and 0.1 mL/kg of local anesthetic solution is injected (*arrow*).

**FIGURE 41-17** Distribution of somatic and sympathetic blockade after thoracic paravertebral blocks. *Blue shading* indicates the approximate spread of somatic blockade and *pink shading* indicates the approximate extent of sympathetic blockade. (See text for details.) (From Lönnqvist PA, Richardson J. Use of paravertebral blockade in children. Tech Region Anesth Pain Manage 1999;3:184-8.)

**FIGURE 41-18** Anatomic relationship of the paravertebral block and correct position of Tuohy needle and catheter. (From Lönnqvist PA, Richardson J. Use of paravertebral blockade in children. Tech Region Anesth Pain Manage 1999;3:184-8.)

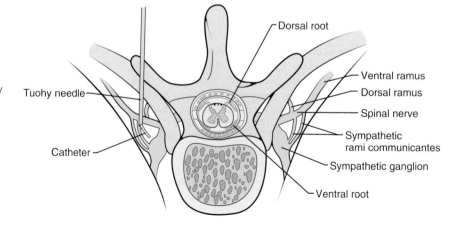

for the slight difficulty in introducing a percutaneous catheter into the paravertebral space. In the lumbar region a paravertebral block is still possible but each individual space must be blocked separately because there are no communications between adjacent lumbar levels.

TECHNIQUE. Three approaches to perform a paravertebral block in children have been described:

*Loss-of-Resistance Technique*[359]: The skin is punctured laterally to the spinous process and the needle is advanced in a perpendicular manner until contact is made with the transverse process. A Tuohy needle (19 to 20 gauge if younger than 1 year of age, 18 gauge if older than 1 year of age) is then "walked" below (underneath) the transverse process and by means of a loss-of-resistance technique the costotransverse ligament is pierced and the paravertebral space located. Alternatively the needle can be "walked" above (over the top of) the transverse process, but by using this approach there is the risk of striking the neck of the rib before entering the paravertebral space. Occasionally this will redirect the needle, making it virtually impossible to obtain access to the paravertebral space. The approach from below the transverse process is clearly advantageous.

Once in the paravertebral space, the bolus dose of local anesthetic can be injected after careful aspiration to exclude the presence of blood or air. If a continuous technique is preferred, a catheter can be introduced 1 to 2 cm into the paravertebral space through the Tuohy needle. The insertion of the catheter frequently needs manipulation of the Tuohy needle to be successful, and occasionally one will have to make the injection of the bolus dose to "open up" or "create" a space to allow catheter insertion. One should not insert more than 1 to 2 cm of the catheter into the paravertebral space because further advancement may cause the catheter to migrate into the spinal canal through the intervertebral foramen (causing an epidural distribution of the block) or to go laterally, following the path of the intercostal nerve (giving a dense block of only one dermatome).

An estimate of the distance from the spinous process to the skin puncture site (spinous process to paravertebral space distance) and the distance from the skin to the paravertebral space can be approximated by the following equations[360,361]:

$$\text{Spinous process to paravertebral space distance (mm)} = 0.12 \times \text{kg} + 10.2$$

$$\text{Skin to paravertebral space distance (mm)} = 0.53 \times \text{kg} + 21.2.$$

The level of the puncture depends on the surgical intervention, but for a thoracotomy the puncture is best performed at T5-6 and for renal surgery at T9-10.

*Nerve-Stimulator–Guided Technique.*[362] The intervertebral lines corresponding to the specific dermatomes are determined by manual palpation. The site of injection is marked 1 to 2 cm laterally from the midline on the intervertebral line according to the child's weight. A 21-gauge insulated needle of appropriate length, attached to a nerve stimulator (initial stimulating current: 2.5 to 5 mA, 1 Hz), is introduced perpendicularly to the skin in all planes. A contraction of the paraspinal muscles is initially observed, and the needle is advanced until the costotransverse ligament is reached. At this point the contraction of the paraspinal muscles will disappear. After piercing the costotransverse ligament, muscle contractions of the corresponding level are sought and the needle tip is manipulated into a position allowing continued muscular contractions while reducing the stimulating

current to 0.4 to 0.6 mA; the desired local anesthetic dose and volume is injected. Manipulation of the needle tip within the paravertebral space is not an "in and out" movement but is rather an angular manipulation and circumferential rotation around the axis of the needle to reach an optimal position of the needle tip with regard to the nerve within the paravertebral space.

*Ultrasound-Aided Approach.* With the aid of ultrasound the position of the transverse processes and the depth to the paravertebral space can be determined; ultrasound is very helpful regardless of whether a loss-of-resistance or nerve-stimulator–guided technique is used.

SELECTION OF DRUG. After a negative aspiration test and administration of a test dose, 0.5 mL/kg of the local anesthetic (levobupivacaine 0.25% with epinephrine 1:200,000, bupivacaine 0.25% with epinephrine 1:200,000, or lidocaine 1% with epinephrine 1:200,000) is injected in toddlers and older children. This dose will usually spread to cover at least five dermatomes. A typical distribution of the block will be unilateral analgesia of the trunk ranging from T4 to T12 (see Fig. 41-17). In neonates and infants, slightly modified dosage regimens are recommended[363-365]; these dosages have been found to be both effective and associated with acceptable plasma concentrations of bupivacaine.[363]

COMPLICATIONS. The use of a percutaneous loss-of-resistance technique in a mixed adult and pediatric population was found to be associated with an overall failure rate of approximately 10% and the complications experienced were hypotension (5%; only adults), vascular puncture (4%), pleural puncture (1%), and pneumothorax (0.5%).[366] The risk for block failure is reduced to less than 5% when a nerve-stimulator–guided technique is used, and this technique also appears to be associated with a reduced risk for complications.[362,367] Use of ultrasound may further improve success while reducing complications.

### Upper Extremity Blocks
#### Brachial Plexus Block
Of the four techniques used to block the brachial plexus (axillary, infraclavicular, supraclavicular, and interscalene), the axillary approach is most commonly used in children when using nerve stimulation or landmark technques.[368] Advantages include ease of insertion, a high rate of success in experienced hands, and low morbidity. The block is also well suited for orthopedic or plastic surgical repairs on the hand or forearm in a child with a full stomach.[369,370] In this situation, deeper levels of sedation, intravascular injection, or drug overdose places the child at risk for aspiration of gastric contents. Because it is unnecessary to elicit a sensory paresthesia, the block can also be performed in an anesthetized child for postoperative pain management. Toxicity is avoided if the dose of bupivacaine is less than 2.5 mg/kg.

Infraclavicular, supraclavicular, and interscalene blocks are not as frequently used as the axillary block in children. The infraclavicular block is our preferred technique for the placement of a continuous catheter in the postoperative period. Unintentional block of the phrenic and recurrent laryngeal nerves is much more common in young children because these nerves are close to the site of injection, especially with an interscalene block. Data suggest that some degree of phrenic nerve blockade is present in all children receiving interscalene blocks.[371,372] Phrenic nerve blockade may cause respiratory failure in very young children whose breathing is almost totally dependent on the diaphragm, whereas block of the recurrent laryngeal nerve may cause increased airway resistance because of vocal cord paralysis. The risk of pneumothorax is greater because the apex of the lung is situated more rostral in infants and small children. Total spinal anesthesia is also more likely with the interscalene approach to axillary plexus blockade.[373]

ANATOMY.  The brachial plexus arises in the neck from spinal nerves C5, C6, C7, C8, and T1, passes between the clavicle and first rib, and extends into the axilla. At that point, the axillary artery is surrounded by a narrow fascial sheath that contains the median nerve anteriorly, the ulnar nerve posteriorly, and the radial nerve on the posterolateral aspect (Fig. 41-19, *A*). In children, the axillary artery and, at times, the axillary sheath itself may be palpable.

TECHNIQUE.  Several techniques can be used to establish that the needle is within the axillary sheath. The first is by eliciting a sensory paresthesia with the needle, but this has little application

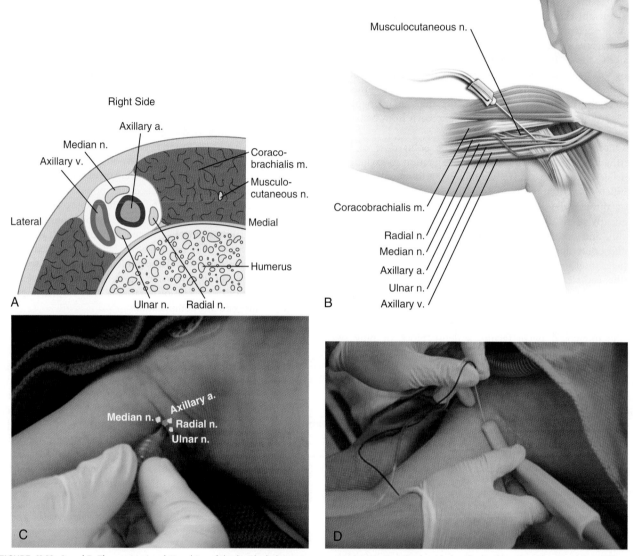

FIGURE 41-19  **A** and **B,** The anatomic relationships of the brachial plexus are presented. Note that the fascial sheath envelops the nerves and the axillary artery and vein; the musculocutaneous nerve lies within the body of the coracobrachialis muscle. Local anesthetic injected within the sheath (on either side of the axillary artery) produces a satisfactory block. There may be septation within the sheath in some individuals (not pictured). **C,** The axillary artery is palpated with the arm in abduction in the axilla. A needle is introduced superior to the pulsation to block the median nerve. If a nerve stimulator is used, opposition of the thumb can be elicited as the median nerve is stimulated. The needle is then gently positioned below the artery; the ulnar nerve can be blocked in this position. If a nerve stimulator is used, flexion of the fifth finger is elicited. For blocking the radial nerve that is situated posterior to the artery, it may be necessary to pass the needle posterior to the artery while constantly aspirating to avoid intravascular placement. If the needle does encounter the axillary artery, continue to advance the needle so that the aspirate is negative while the needle is situated posterior to the artery. If a nerve stimulator is used, biceps flexion may be observed. A total volume of 0.1 to 0.15 mL/kg in divided doses between all three nerves will provide an adequate blockade of the nerves. If the axillary artery is encountered while accessing the radial nerve, it is imperative to apply pressure after the block is placed to avoid hematoma formation. **D,** An ultrasound is particularly useful for successful placement of an axillary block. A linear ultrasound probe or a hockey stick probe is placed on the axilla. With the use of an in-plane approach, the median nerve (located anterior to the artery), then the radial nerve (located posterior to the axillary artery), and then the ulnar nerve (located below the artery) are blocked individually. Careful aspiration before injection may prevent intravascular injection. *a,* Artery; *m,* muscle; *n,* nerve; *v,* vein.

in pediatric practice, particularly in young children and in those who are anesthetized. The use of a nerve stimulator allows precise placement of the needle in the neurovascular sheath without either the cooperation of the child or the need for painful sensory paresthesias (see Fig. 41-2). In thin children, the sheath can often be palpated as a cord-like structure inferior to the coracobrachialis muscle, allowing the placement of the needle in the sheath by "feel." A transarterial approach can also be used.[374] With all techniques, it is useful to attach a short piece of extension tubing between the needle and syringe to facilitate precise handling during needle placement, aspiration, and drug injection.

The use of a nerve stimulator for the axillary approach to the brachial plexus is best accomplished by abducting the arm to 90 degrees (see E-Fig. 41-2). Care should be taken not to hyperabduct the arm, obscuring the axillary pulse. The artery is palpated in the axilla, and a short beveled needle is advanced toward it (see Fig. 41-19, *B*). When using a nerve stimulator, a distal motor response is elicited in the distribution of the radial, ulnar, or median nerves at a threshold of less than 0.2 mA (see E-Fig. 41-2). If one is not using a nerve stimulator, the needle is advanced until a distinct pop is felt as the needle pierces the axillary sheath. The axillary sheath may be divided into fascial compartments for each nerve, and these may limit the spread of local anesthetic within the axillary sheath. Although distinct paresthesias to the distribution of all three nerves may be elicited with the nerve stimulator, and divided doses of anesthetic may be administered to each of those locations, in practice it becomes extremely difficult to find the second and third motor paresthesia after the administration of even a very small amount of local anesthetic with the first injection (Video: Axillary Block with Ultrasound Guidance). Alternatively, the transarterial technique, which involves direct puncture of the axillary artery, allows deposition of local anesthetic in two sites within the sheath. The needle is aimed directly toward the axillary pulse. As soon as blood is aspirated, the needle is advanced through the posterior wall of the artery. When blood can no longer be aspirated, half of the dose of local anesthetic is deposited posterior to the artery. The needle is withdrawn through the anterior wall of the artery, and the remainder of the dose is deposited anterior to the artery after reconfirming a negative aspiration for blood. Regardless of technique, the local anesthetic is administered in incremental quantities with intermittent aspiration to confirm that the needle is still outside the blood vessel. Some practitioners advocate applying a tourniquet distal to the site where the block is to be performed. It is sometimes difficult to block the musculocutaneous nerve, which carries sensory fibers to the radial aspect of the forearm, because it exits the brachial plexus proximal in the axillary fossa. Applying a tourniquet may promote proximal spread of local anesthetic and enhance the chances of a successful block of this nerve. Alternatively, the musculocutaneous nerve may be blocked by infiltrating 1 to 3 mL (proportional to the size of the child) of local anesthetic into the body of the coracobrachialis muscle. Regardless of the technique chosen, an additional 1 to 3 mL of local anesthetic is deposited as a subcutaneous cuff to block the intercostobrachial nerve and its communications with the musculocutaneous nerve. These additional quantities of local anesthetic must be accounted for when calculating the total drug dose. An ultrasound may also be used in conjunction with a nerve stimulator to further improve the localization of each nerve bundle (see Figs. 42-16 and 42-21).[370]

SELECTION OF DRUG. Local anesthetics commonly used in our practice include lidocaine and bupivacaine (see Table 41-2).

As with other regional techniques that involve larger volumes of local anesthetic, the addition of both levobupivacaine and ropivacaine to the armamentarium is likely to prove beneficial in reducing the risk of toxicity from local anesthetics. Because it is desirable to have a prolonged duration of postoperative analgesia, longer-acting agents are usually used in place of lidocaine. To help ensure block of the musculocutaneous nerve, we use large volumes (0.5 mL/kg), diluting the concentration of local anesthetic with normal saline as needed to avoid toxicity. Care must always be taken not to exceed the maximal allowable doses of bupivacaine on a milligram per kilogram basis (2.5 mg/kg).[375] Adding epinephrine (1:200,000) may decrease vascular absorption and the potential for toxicity. Sodium bicarbonate (1 mEq/10 mL of local anesthetic) added to the local anesthetic will speed the onset of blockade by increasing the pH of the solution; this is particularly the case with the premixed anesthetic-epinephrine formulations that have a reduced pH.

COMPLICATIONS. All of the nerves of the brachial plexus occupy a neurovascular bundle and hence are prone to unintended injection into a blood vessel. A hematoma may form at the site of injection. If it is large enough, the hematoma may compress the neurovascular bundle, rendering the limb ischemic. Hence it is important to know the child's coagulation status before attempting the block. Intravascular injection may be avoided with incremental injection and frequent aspiration. Intraneural injection may be minimized by use of a nerve stimulator. Surgeons may feel the importance to check the viability of the radial, median, and ulnar nerves before injecting local anesthetic solution. This block can be carried out in the recovery room after the function of the nerves are determined. A simple rule of thumb is to check the radial nerve (extension of the thumb), median nerve (flexion of the proximal interphalangeal joint of the thumb), and ulnar nerve (scissoring of the fingers) (Video: Finger Examination). This can functionally check the nerves before injection of local anesthetic solution.[376]

INFRACLAVICULAR APPROACH. This approach to the brachial plexus is very helpful, particularly in children who may have fractures making it painful to abduct the arm. A vertical approach to the infraclavicular brachial plexus is performed using the coracoid process as a landmark to access the nerve.[377] We routinely use this technique in children who require continuous infusions of local anesthetic solution in the postoperative period.

TECHNIQUE. With the arm in abduction or adduction, the acromial process is palpated. A line drawn 2 cm below and medial to the coracoid process is usually where the needle is introduced (Fig. 41-20, *A*). At this level, the pleura is not usually affected. A sheathed needle with a nerve stimulator is introduced, and the nerve is stimulated at about 1 mA. Any stimulation other than forearm flexion is taken as a positive stimulation of the brachial plexus. Forearm flexion denotes stimulation of the musculocutaneous nerve. The needle should then be directed medial to provide a blockade of the cords of the brachial plexus (see Fig. 41-20, *B*). An ultrasound-guided technique may also be used (see also Chapter 42 and Figs. 42-17 to 42-19).

COMPLICATIONS. There is the potential for intrapleural injection and pneumothorax, especially if the needle is directed medially. Because of the proximity of the plexus to the subclavian vein and artery, it is imperative that the procedure not be attempted on children who have coagulation abnormalities.

SUPRACLAVICULAR APPROACH. This is an easy approach to the brachial plexus in children and can be readily performed, particularly with the aid of ultrasound guidance. The risk with

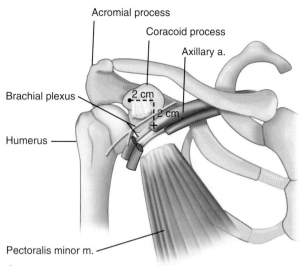

Acromial process

Coracoid process

Axillary a.

Brachial plexus

2 cm

2 cm

Humerus

Pectoralis minor m.

**A**

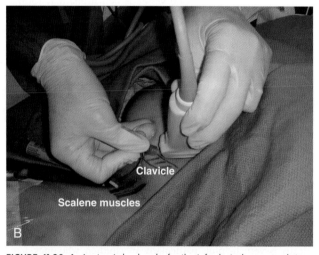

Clavicle

Scalene muscles

**B**

**FIGURE 41-20  A,** Anatomic landmarks for the infraclavicular approach to the brachial plexus. Note that the arm is in an abducted position, which may be quite useful for children with fractures. **B,** The coracoid process is palpated. With the arm abducted, a needle is inserted 2 cm medial and inferior to the coracoid process. A nerve stimulator is used and stimulation is initiated at 1 mA and then decreased to 0.4 mA as the nerve is accessed. Elicitation of hand flexion or extension is used as an indicator of being close to the nerve. After aspiration, 0.2 mL/kg of local anesthetic solution is injected. Use of ultrasound may also improve the success of this block. *a,* Artery; *m,* muscle. (Modified from Wilson JL, Brown DL, Wong GY, et al. Infraclavicular brachial plexus block: parasagittal anatomy important to the coracoid technique. Anesth Analg 1998;87:870-3.)

performing this procedure without ultrasound guidance is the potential for injection into the vertebral artery. It can be used for most procedures performed on the upper arm and forearm. The cervical pleura is also located close to the supraclavicular plexus; thus caution should be exercised while performing this block. The entire brachial plexus, including the musculocutaneous and the axillary nerves, is located lateral to the artery. Occasionally, the suprascapular nerve may leave the upper trunk more cranially.

INDICATIONS. This block is used for analgesia or anesthesia for upper arm surgery and can be performed with either a single injection or catheter technique.

TECHNIQUE. The supraclavicular plexus is located above the clavicle and is located superficially approximately at the middle

of the sternocleidomastoid. A stimulating needle (1 mA) is passed above the clavicle lateral to the arterial pulsation and close to the inferior margin of the anterior scalene. The plexus is located superficially and can be easily stimulated as soon as the skin is pierced. Any movement of the child's fingers or arm is accepted as an adequate stimulation to the plexus. The energy is reduced to 0.4 mA and, if continued response to the stimulation is observed, 0.15 to 0.2 mL/kg of local anesthetic solution is injected in graduated doses after careful aspiration.

*The ultrasound-guided technique* is now our preferred method for blocking the supraclavicular plexus. We use a linear probe or a hockey stick probe and, using the in-plane technique, pass the needle close to the plexus. If a stimulating needle is used, the needle is advanced until we see movement of the hand. We have been able to decrease the dose of local anesthetic solution to 0.15 to 0.2 mL/kg (Fig. 41-21 and Video: Ultrasound-Guided Supraclavicular Block; see also Fig. 42-16).

COMPLICATIONS. Pleural puncture and intravascular injection can occur from misplacement of the needle.

INTERSCALENE APPROACH. This approach is not commonly used in children. The main indication for this technique is for children undergoing shoulder surgery; this approach is generally reserved for the older teenager or young adult.

ANATOMY. The interscalene groove is formed by the anterior and middle scalene muscles and is located in most children at the lateral border of the sternocleidomastoid muscle (see Fig. 41-21, *A*). The upper three nerve roots are superficial, whereas the lower two roots are in a deeper position. In children the lower nerve roots are close to the pleura, which may increase the potential for a pneumothorax. The phrenic nerve is also close to the nerve roots and may often be unintentionally blocked on the side of the intended nerve block. Therefore this block is clearly avoided in children who may have a compromised pulmonary system. The vertebral artery is located in close proximity to the lower nerve roots (C7) and hence it is important to aspirate and ensure that the needle is not in a vessel.

INDICATIONS. Shoulder and upper arm surgery and ensuing postoperative analgesia can be provided with this block.

*Conventional Techniques.* Dalens and associates reported a technique of parascalene brachial plexus blockade for pediatric shoulder surgery using an extended head position and placing the puncture between the lower and middle thirds of the line extending from the center of the clavicle to the C6 transverse process (Chassaignac; see Fig. 41-21, *A*).[378] The rationale for selecting this puncture site was to avoid the vertebral artery and pleura. With the use of a perpendicular needle orientation, the lower roots (C8 and T1) are not blocked at all or require very large amounts of local anesthetic to be successfully blocked. Ultrasound guidance is greatly advantageous in this situation because it paves the way for safe blockade of both roots (C8 and T1). With the use of a nerve stimulator, diaphragmatic stimulation may be observed as a result of ventromedial needle position (the phrenic nerve runs ventral to the body of the anterior scalene muscle).

*Ultrasound-Guided Technique* (see Chapter 42). To visualize the anatomic structures of a child's neck, a high-frequency linear ultrasound probe is used. The process is facilitated by slightly turning the child's head to the contralateral side. The probe should be oriented from the medial to the lateral aspect. Medially, the thyroid gland and the major vessels in the neck area (carotid artery and internal jugular vein) are easily identified. Then the probe is moved along the sternocleidomastoid muscle

41

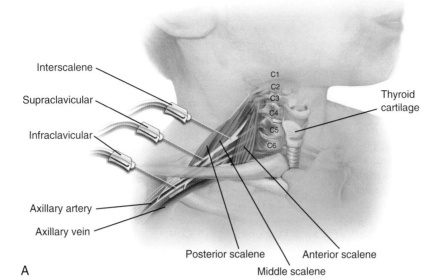

Interscalene

Supraclavicular

Infraclavicular

Axillary artery

Axillary vein

C1
C2
C3
C4
C5
C6

Thyroid cartilage

Posterior scalene

Middle scalene

Anterior scalene

**A**

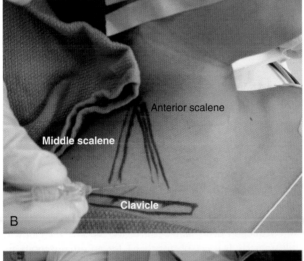

Anterior scalene

Middle scalene

Clavicle

**B**

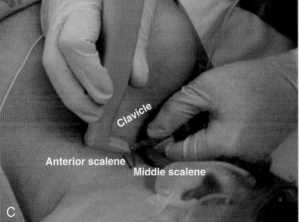

Clavicle

Anterior scalene

Middle scalene

**C**

**FIGURE 41-21** A right-sided supraclavicular block (landmark technique): The supraclavicular block is used frequently in children for most procedures on the hand and elbow. **A,** The divisions and cords are located around the carotid artery cephalad to the clavicle at the inferior margins of the scalene muscles. **B,** A stimulating needle, using 0.5 mA of energy, is introduced at the inferior border of the anterior scalene muscle. Any movement of the patient's fingers (including flexion or extension) suggests adequate positioning of the needle. After aspiration to avoid intravascular injection, 0.15 mL/kg of local anesthetic solution is injected. **C,** Supraclavicular block with ultrasound guidance. A linear ultrasound probe or a hockey stick probe is placed lateral to the suprasternal notch and above the clavicle. The carotid artery is identified. The supraclavicular plexus is located around the carotid artery at this location like a "bunch of grapes." A needle is placed in an in-plane approach (along the axis of the probe), and the plexus is penetrated. Injection of local anesthetic solution will be seen as a hypoechoic spread around the plexus.

until its lateral border is reached. At the same time, the transducer is moved in a caudal direction such that the posterior scalene gap and the upper anterior roots (C5-7) of the brachial plexus become visible between the anterior and medial scalene muscles. In very small children, all roots of the brachial plexus (C5-T1) can be simultaneously visualized. The puncture is performed in a tangential direction relative to the neck above the transducer. The C5 nerve root will be encountered superficially, within a few millimeters. As a rule, the needle should be oriented lateral to the C7 root, which will ensure that the neck vessels remain at an adequate distance from the needle insertion site. As soon as the local anesthetic has been injected, it will spread toward the C5 root, which can be visualized in the ultrasound image. Depending on the blockade required, the needle can be advanced to a deeper level for injection after the deep roots (C8 and T1) have been visualized. If the local anesthetic fails to spread adequately in a medial direction, the needle is retracted toward the subcutaneous level and is then repositioned on the medial side of the posterior scalene gap in the area of the C7 root. In the majority of cases, however, the local anesthetic will spread in an adequate manner even when the needle is in a lateral position. The injected volume of local anesthetic should not exceed the amount necessary to fully cover the root surfaces. It is, therefore, inappropriate to recommend a specific volume. In general, however, complete blockade via the interscalene route can be expected with local anesthetic volumes of 0.15 to 0.25 mL/kg.

COMPLICATIONS. Pneumothorax, intravascular injection, and temporary phrenic nerve injury are risks of this block.

### Intravenous Regional Anesthesia

IV regional anesthesia was first described in 1908 by August Bier and is frequently referred to as the Bier block.[379] This technique has been advocated for upper extremity procedures lasting 30 to 60 minutes in children because of its rapid onset of anesthesia and its ease of performance.[380-382] *Only dilute lidocaine (0.25% or 0.5%) can be used because of the risk of local-anesthetic toxicity.* This can be a useful block for upper extremity fracture reduction or suture of a large laceration in children with a full stomach. It is also helpful for chronic painful conditions, including complex regional pain syndrome type 1, in children and adolescents.[383] The exsanguination and manipulation of the limb before administering the local anesthetic may prove to be unduly painful for children with a fracture, and many children may not tolerate the discomfort of the tourniquet without significant sedation. Another disadvantage is the possibility of toxic reactions in the event of tourniquet failure. Strict attention to detail—elevation or exsanguination of the extremity to be blocked, proper application of a double pneumatic cuff, careful attention to anesthetic dose, and care not to deflate the tourniquet until 30 minutes after injection of the local anesthetic—is important to avoid serious complications and provide a successful block. This block is unsuitable for children younger than 1 year of age because of the risk of toxic reactions in infants. This technique may also be contraindicated for children in whom the prolonged use of a tourniquet is inadvisable.

TECHNIQUE. A small-gauge IV cannula is inserted in a vein on the dorsum of the hand. Exsanguination of the arm may be accomplished either by wrapping the limb with an Esmarch bandage, or by elevation of the limb if wrapping is too painful. The proximal compartment of a double tourniquet is inflated to a pressure of 200 to 250 mm Hg, although some have

recommended that it be inflated to 150 mm Hg above the child's systolic blood pressure. If tourniquet pain develops during the course of the procedure, the distal cuff may be inflated, followed by deflation of the proximal cuff. The tourniquet must remain inflated for a minimum of 30 minutes to prevent a rapid IV infusion of lidocaine. It is best to deflate the tourniquet incrementally. Because no residual blockade persists after the tourniquet is released, supplementary analgesia must be considered (e.g., IV opioids, local infiltration with a long-acting local anesthetic).

SELECTION OF DRUG. Only *preservative-free* 0.25 to 0.5% lidocaine without epinephrine (1 mL/kg) should be used for this block because the duration of the block is limited by tourniquet time and because of the potential for cardiac toxicity with longer-acting agents. A very low dose of a nondepolarizing neuromuscular blocking agent, such as rocuronium (0.03 mg/kg), may improve the quality of the motor blockade.[384-386]

COMPLICATIONS. Unintended deflation of the tourniquet results in release of drug into the intravascular compartment; hence, only a short-acting local anesthetic, such as lidocaine, should be used. *Bupivacaine should never be used for this block because of the risk of cardiotoxicity.*

### Peripheral Blocks at the Elbow

There is usually no great advantage to blocking the peripheral nerves at the elbow compared with blocking them at the wrist for analgesia or anesthesia of the hand because the forearm is supplied by cutaneous branches that originate in the upper arm. However, on some occasions (e.g., to avoid injections into surgical fields or areas of infection), anesthesia of the hand may be achieved by blocking the appropriate nerves at the elbow because the cutaneous nerve supply to the hand arises at the elbow.

### Radial Nerve

ANATOMY. The radial nerve supplies the radial side of the dorsum of the hand and the proximal parts of the radial three-and-a-half digits. Block at the elbow is useful for the provision of anesthesia for an arteriovenous fistula. It is also useful to supplement an inadequate brachial plexus block at the axillary level. The radial nerve passes over the anterior aspect of the lateral epicondyle (Fig. 41-22, *A*).

TECHNIQUE. The intercondylar line is marked. After identification of the biceps tendon, a 27-gauge needle is inserted directly toward the bone of the lateral epicondyle toward the lateral margin; 2.0 to 5.0 mL (depending on the child's weight) of bupivacaine (0.25% with epinephrine 1 : 200,000) is injected into the area (see Fig. 41-22, *B*). Ultrasound guidance can help with determination of exact location of the nerve in the forearm (see Chapter 42 and Fig. 42-25).

COMPLICATIONS. Intravascular injection and intraneural injections are potential complications. The use of a nerve stimulator or ultrasound can reduce unintended intraneural injection. Intravascular injection may be avoided with incremental injection and frequent aspiration.

### Median Nerve

ANATOMY. This nerve supplies the radial side of the palm and the three-and-a-half digits of the palmar aspect (see Fig. 41-22, *A*). It accompanies the brachial artery in its course down the arm. It is initially lateral and then crosses the ventral side of the artery and eventually lies medial to the artery at the bend of the elbow.

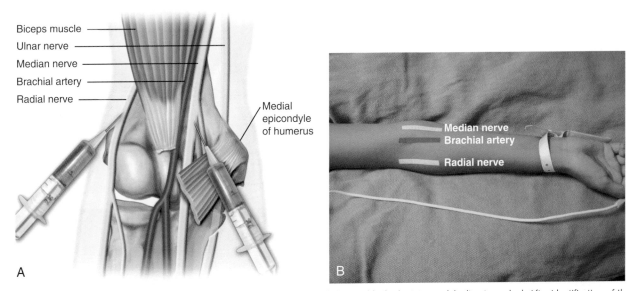

Biceps muscle
Ulnar nerve
Median nerve
Brachial artery
Radial nerve

Medial
epicondyle
of humerus

A

B

Median nerve
Brachial artery
Radial nerve

**FIGURE 41-22  A,** Anatomic relationship of the nerves around the elbow. **B,** Radial nerve block: the intercondylar line is marked. After identification of the biceps tendon, a 27-gauge needle is inserted directly toward the bone of the lateral epicondyle toward the lateral margin; 2.0 to 5.0 mL (depending on the patient's weight) of bupivacaine (0.25% with epinephrine 1:200,000) is injected into the area. To block the median nerve, the brachial artery is palpated at the elbow crease. The median nerve is located immediately medial to the brachial artery. A nerve stimulator is used, and flexion of the patient's fingers denotes adequate localization of the nerve.

It is deep to the bicipital fascia and superficial to the brachialis muscle.

TECHNIQUE.  The arm is abducted and the forearm supinated. After marking the intercondylar line between the medial and the lateral epicondyle of the humerus, the brachial artery is palpated (see Fig. 41-22, *A*). A 27-gauge needle is inserted just medial to the artery and directed perpendicular to the skin; 2.0 to 5.0 mL (depending on the child's weight) of bupivacaine (0.25% with epinephrine 1:200,000) is injected to the site. Caution must be exercised to avoid the artery because it is in close proximity to the nerve. Surface mapping employing a nerve stimulator probe generating 5 mA or greater can be used to locate the nerve in the forearm if there is difficulty in palpating the artery (see Fig. 41-22, *A*).[387] An ultrasound-guided technique may also be used for this block (see Chapter 42 and Fig. 42-23).

COMPLICATIONS.  Intravascular injection and intraneural injections are potential complications. The use of a nerve stimulator can prevent the unintended intraneural injection. Intravascular injection may be avoided with incremental injection and frequent aspiration.

### Ulnar Nerve

ANATOMY.  The ulnar nerve is the superficial nerve to the arm and the ulnar side of the forearm and the hand. It is the terminal continuation of the medial cord of the brachial plexus. At the elbow, it pierces the medial intermuscular septum and follows along the medial head of the triceps to the groove between the olecranon and the medial epicondyle of the humerus. It is covered only by skin and fascia and can be easily palpated and blocked at this level (see Figs. 41-22, *A*, and 41-23; see also Fig. 42-24).

TECHNIQUE.  With the child supine, the elbow is flexed. The medial epicondyle and the ulnar groove are palpated (see Fig. 41-23). A 27-gauge needle is advanced perpendicular to the skin along the line of the nerve; 2.0 to 3.0 mL (depending on

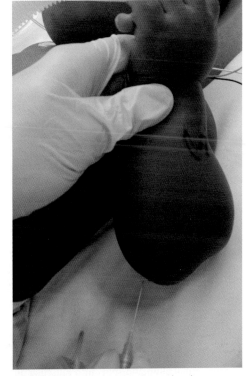

**FIGURE 41-23** Ulnar nerve block at the elbow. The olecranon process is palpated. The ulnar nerve is located in the olecranon groove; after aspiration, 1 to 3 mL of local anesthetic solution is injected. It is important not to deposit the local anesthetic deep into the olecranon groove because the nerve is superficial and can be easily blocked by a subcutaneous injection.

the child's weight) of bupivacaine (0.25% with epinephrine 1:200,000) is injected in the area. An ultrasound-guided technique may also be used for this block (see Chapter 42 and Fig. 42-24).

COMPLICATIONS. Intravascular injection and intraneural injections are potential complications. Because this is a very superficial nerve, injection just after the skin is pierced in the area of the ulnar nerve usually produces a good block. Intravascular injection may be avoided with incremental injection and frequent aspiration.

### Wrist Blocks
Blocking the median, radial, and ulnar nerves at the wrist can be easily achieved. These blocks provide very good analgesia and, because they are easy to perform, they generally have a predictable successful outcome.

### Radial Nerve
The cutaneous branches of the radial nerve supply the radial side of the dorsum of the hand and the proximal parts of the radial three-and-a-half digits.

ANATOMY. The superficial branch of the radial nerve runs along the lateral border of the forearm under the brachioradialis muscle. In the distal third of the forearm it angles dorsally under the tendon of the brachioradialis toward the dorsum of the wrist. It pierces the deep fascia and divides into two branches: (1) the lateral branch supplies the radial side and the tip of the thumb and (2) the medial branch communicates with the dorsal branch of the ulnar nerve. This then divides into the four digital nerves that supply the ulnar side of the thumb, the radial side of the index finger, and the space between the index finger and thumb. A communicating branch with the ulnar nerve supplies the adjacent sides of the middle and ring finger (Fig. 41-24, *A*).

TECHNIQUE. This is essentially a field block of the superficial terminal branches. An attempt to make the "anatomic snuffbox" prominent by extension of the thumb before anesthesia is desirable. The extensor pollicis and brevis tendons are marked. A 27-gauge needle is inserted close to the dorsal radial tubercle over the extensor longus tendon, and 2.0 mL of bupivacaine (0.25% with epinephrine 1:200,000) is injected SC. An attempt to fan the local anesthetic in the anatomic snuffbox helps to distribute the local anesthetic over the radial nerve (see Fig. 41-24, *B*).

COMPLICATIONS. Intravascular injection may be avoided with incremental injection and frequent aspiration. Post–nerve block dysesthesia may be occasionally experienced with a radial nerve block and is usually self-limited.

### Median Nerve
ANATOMY. In the palm of the hand, the median nerve is very superficial and is covered only by skin and the palmar aponeurosis and rests on the tendons of the flexor muscles. It emerges from under the retinaculum and splits into muscular and digital branches. The muscular division of the median nerve supplies the muscles of the thenar eminence. The palmar digital nerve supplies the thumb, index finger, middle finger, and ring finger. These nerves also supply the lumbricals (Fig. 41-25, *A*).

TECHNIQUE. The palmaris tendon is identified. This may be done before general anesthesia by asking the child to flex the wrist against resistance. The radial border of the tendon is identified. Cutaneous landmarks include both distal wrist skin creases. A 27-gauge needle is inserted at the level of the second skin crease

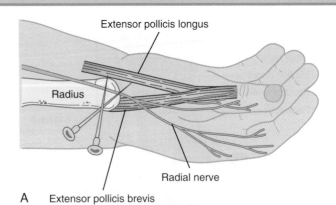

A

FIGURE 41-24 Wrist block: radial nerve. **A,** This is a superficial block of the terminal branches of the radial nerve. An attempt to make the "anatomic snuffbox" prominent by extension of the thumb before anesthesia is desirable. The extensor pollicis and brevis tendons are marked. **B,** A 27-gauge needle is inserted close to the dorsal radial tubercle over the extensor longus tendon; bupivacaine (2 mL, 0.25% with 1:200,000 epinephrine) is injected subcutaneously. Fanning the local anesthetic in the anatomic snuffbox helps to distribute the local anesthetic over the radial nerve. (Modified from Raj P, Pai U. Techniques of nerve blocking. In: Raj P, editor. Handbook of regional anesthesia. New York: Churchill Livingstone; 1985, p. 185.)

(1 to 1.5 cm proximal to the distal crease in teenagers) perpendicular to the skin. The nerve is at a depth of less than 1 cm in the teenager and less in younger children; 1.0 to 2.0 mL of bupivacaine (0.25% with epinephrine 1:200,000) is injected in the area (see Fig. 41-25, *B*). If the child is awake, it is better to elicit paresthesias because the needle may be anterior to the neurovascular bundle and the nerve could be missed altogether.

COMPLICATIONS. Intravascular placement should be avoided by repeated aspiration before injection.

### Ulnar Nerve
ANATOMY. The palmar cutaneous branch of the ulnar nerve arises near the middle of the forearm and accompanies the ulnar artery into the hand (see Fig. 41-25, *A*). It then perforates the flexor retinaculum and ends in the skin of the palm

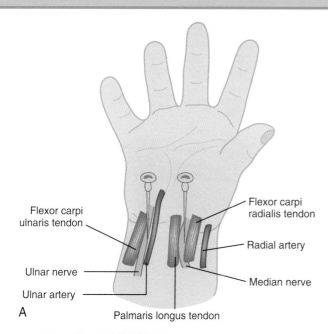

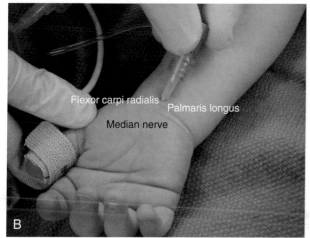

**FIGURE 41-25** Wrist block: median and ulnar nerves. **A,** Median nerve: identify the palmaris tendon by asking the child to flex the wrist against resistance. Distal skin creases are identified. **B,** A 27-gauge needle is inserted at the level of the distal skin crease perpendicular to the skin. The nerve is at a depth of less than 1 cm in teenagers and less than that in younger children; 1.0 to 2.0 mL of bupivacaine (0.25% with 1:200.000 epinephrine) is injected in the area. If the child is awake, it is better to elicit paresthesias because the needle may be anterior to the neurovascular bundle, which can be missed altogether. Ulnar nerve: identify the flexor carpi ulnaris tendon, which lies proximal to the pisiform bone. A 27-gauge needle is inserted just proximal to the pisiform bone and directed radially a distance of approximately 0.5 cm. Bupivacaine (2 mL, 0.25% with epinephrine 1:200,000) is injected. (Modified from Raj P, Pai U. Techniques of nerve blocking. In: Raj P, editor. Handbook of regional anesthesia. New York: Churchill Livingstone; 1985, p. 185.)

communicating with the palmar branch of the median nerve. There are two dorsal digital nerves and a metacarpal communicating branch. The more medial digital nerve supplies the ulnar side of the little finger and the digital branch supplies the adjacent sides of the little and ring finger. The palmar or the terminal portion of the ulnar nerve crosses the ulnar border of the wrist in company with the ulnar artery.

TECHNIQUE. Blocking the ulnar nerve at the wrist is easier than at the elbow. The nerve is blocked at the wrist where it lies under cover of the flexor carpi ulnaris tendon just proximal to the pisiform bone. The best way to access the nerve is to approach it from the ulnar side of the tendon. A 27-gauge needle is inserted just proximal to the pisiform bone and directed radially a distance of approximately 0.5 cm; 2.0 to 3.0 mL of bupivacaine (0.25% with epinephrine 1:200,000) is injected (see Fig. 41-25, *A*).

COMPLICATIONS. The ulnar artery runs in close proximity to the ulnar nerve; every possible effort should be made to avoid intravascular placement. Intravascular injection may be avoided with incremental injection with frequent aspiration.

### Digital Nerve Blocks: Hand

Digital nerve blocks are useful for providing pain relief to children who are undergoing procedures to individual fingers. These are useful for postoperative analgesia in procedures, such as trigger finger release, and also for the provision of pain relief in children undergoing laser therapy for warts on their fingers.[388]

ANATOMY. The common digital nerves are derived from the median and ulnar nerves and divide in the palm to volar digital nerves that supply the fingers. All digital nerves are usually accompanied by digital vessels. There are three digital nerves derived from the median nerve: the first divides into three palmar digital nerves that supply the sides of the thumb; the second common digital nerve supplies the web between the index and middle finger; and the third common palmar digital nerve communicates with a branch of the ulnar nerve and supplies the web space between the middle and ring fingers. These common digital nerves then become the proper digital nerves (digital collaterals) that supply the skin of the palmar surface and the dorsal side of the terminal phalanx of their respective digits. All digital nerves ultimately terminate in two branches: one ramifies in the skin of the fingertips and the other ends in the pulp under the nail. Smaller digital nerves are derived from the radial and ulnar nerves and supply the back of the fingers. These tend to lie on the dorsolateral aspect of the finger. There are four dorsal digital nerves: (1) ulnar side of the thumb; (2) radial side of the index finger; (3) adjacent sides of index and middle fingers; and (4) communication to the adjacent sides of middle and ring finger.

TECHNIQUE. There are two techniques for blockade of the digital nerves.

For blockade at the base of the thumb (Fig. 41-26, *A* and *B*), with the thumb extended, on the palmar surface of the hand, a 27-gauge needle is inserted into the web space between the index finger and thumb. The needle is advanced to the junction of the web space and the palmar skin of the hand, a distance of about 1 cm; 0.5 mL of bupivacaine *without epinephrine* is injected. A second needle is inserted into the thenar eminence on the radial aspect of the thumb; 1.0 mL of bupivacaine *without epinephrine* is injected. Caution has to be exercised if the child has collagen vascular disease, because this may precipitate acute vascular spasm that may not be relieved.

Blockade of the other fingers is accomplished at the bifurcation between the metacarpal heads (see Fig. 41-26, *B* and *C*). With the fingers extended, a 27-gauge needle is inserted into the web about 3 mm proximal to the junction between the web and the palmar skin; 1.0 to 2.0 mL of bupivacaine *without epinephrine* is injected. This can be performed either from a dorsal approach or a volar approach.

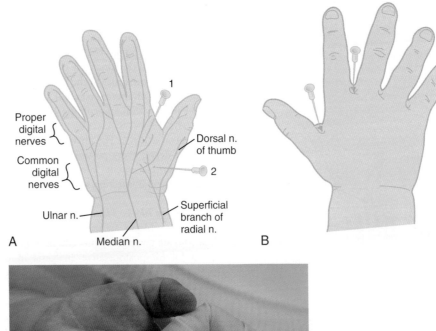

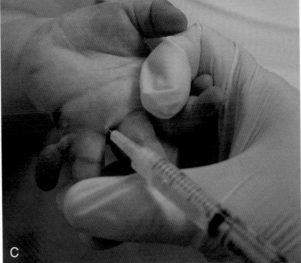

**FIGURE 41-26** Digital nerve blocks. **A,** Blockade of the thumb: with the thumb extended, on the palmar surface of the hand, a 27-gauge needle is inserted into the web space between the index finger and thumb (*1*). The needle is advanced to the junction of the web space and the palmar skin of the hand a distance of about 1 cm; bupivacaine (0.5 mL, *without epinephrine*) is injected. A second needle is inserted into the thenar eminence on the radial aspect of the thumb, and 1.0 mL of bupivacaine *without epinephrine* is injected (*2*). Caution has to be exercised if the patient has collagen vascular disease because this may precipitate acute vascular spasm that may not be relieved. **B,** Blockade of other digits: blockade of the other fingers is accomplished at the bifurcation between the metacarpal heads. With the fingers widely extended, a 27-gauge needle is inserted into the web about 3 mm proximal to the junction between the web and the palmar skin; bupivacaine (1.0 to 2.0 mL, *without epinephrine*) is injected. **C,** This can be performed either from a dorsal approach or a volar approach. The web on either side will have to be blocked to provide analgesia for each finger to be anesthetized. *n,* Nerve.

*Caution:* Vasoconstrictors are avoided when blocking digital nerves because these are end vessels and acute vasospasm caused by epinephrine can lead to permanent damage or necrosis of the digits.

COMPLICATIONS. Large volumes of local anesthetic are contraindicated because of the possibility of pressure and vascular compromise. Vasoconstrictors should be avoided because they may cause necrosis of the digit. Intravascular injection may be avoided with incremental injection and frequent aspiration.

### Lower Extremity Blocks
The major use of nerve blocks of the lower extremity in children is for managing postoperative pain and as an adjunct to general anesthesia. When considering the sensory and cutaneous innervation of the lower extremity (Fig. 41-27), it is not surprising that

few surgical procedures can be accomplished under single nerve blocks. However, combinations of sciatic, femoral, and lateral femoral cutaneous blockade can provide both excellent postoperative analgesia and surgical anesthesia for selected operations; the fascia iliaca block produces anesthesia of multiple nerves with a single injection.

### Sciatic Nerve Block
ANATOMY. The sciatic nerve arises from the L4 through S3 roots of the sacral plexus, passes through the pelvis, and becomes superficial at the lower margin of the gluteus maximus muscle. It then descends into the lower extremity in the posterior aspect of the thigh, supplying sensory innervation to the posterior thigh, as well as to the entire leg and foot below the level of the knee, except for the medial aspect, which is supplied by the femoral

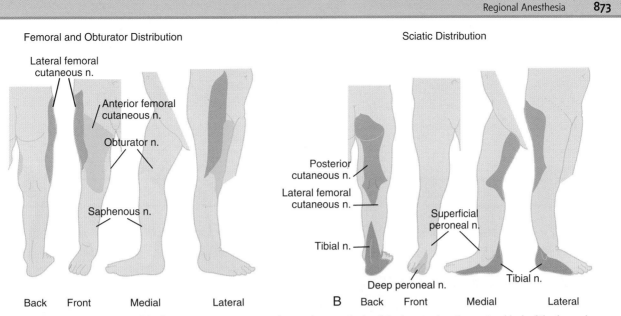

Femoral and Obturator Distribution

Lateral femoral
cutaneous n.

Anterior femoral
cutaneous n.

Obturator n.

Saphenous n.

**A**    Back    Front    Medial    Lateral

Sciatic Distribution

Posterior
cutaneous n.

Lateral femoral
cutaneous n.

Superficial
peroneal n.

Tibial n.

Deep peroneal n.

Tibial n.

**B**    Back    Front    Medial    Lateral

**FIGURE 41-27** The sensory innervation of the lower extremity is presented. Note that anesthesia of the lower extremity requires block of the femoral nerve (**A**) (and its branches), as well as the sciatic nerve (**B**). *n*, Nerve.

nerve (see Fig. 41-27, *A*). Although a sciatic nerve block alone is useful for few surgical procedures, it can be combined with a femoral nerve block (see Fig. 41-32; cited early) for operations below the knee and for postoperative pain relief. There are multiple approaches to the sciatic nerve.[389] All blocks are performed with the aid of a nerve stimulator to elicit a motor paresthesia in the foot, and, if the block is performed in a lightly sedated trauma victim, the approach that places the child in a greater position of comfort should be chosen. Ultrasound guidance improves the performance of the nerve block (see Chapter 42). A newer approach to the sciatic nerve using a lateral approach to the popliteal fossa has been described. This offers the additional advantage of being able to provide the block in the supine position. An infragluteal-parabiceps approach is another easy method of providing a sciatic nerve block in children.[390]

APPROACH OF LABAT (POSTERIOR APPROACH). The child is placed in the lateral decubitus position lying on the nonoperative leg. The leg to be blocked is flexed and the lower leg is extended (Fig. 41-28, *A*). A line is drawn from the posterior superior iliac spine to the greater trochanter of the femur. Another line is drawn from the greater trochanter to the coccyx. The first line is bisected, and a perpendicular line is drawn from that point to the second line; the point at which it intersects the second line is the site of needle insertion (see Fig. 41-28, *B*). A 22-gauge insulated needle is advanced in the perpendicular plane until it strikes bone. It is possible for the needle to pass through the sciatic notch without either encountering bone or causing a paresthesia. In that case, the needle is redirected in a cephalad direction until bone is encountered. A motor paresthesia is then sought using an organized grid-like approach, fanning medially to laterally.

ANTERIOR APPROACH. As the sciatic nerve emerges from the lower border of the gluteus maximus to extend down the thigh, it passes medial and deep to the lesser trochanter of the femur (Fig. 41-29, *A*; see also Figs. 42-31 and 42-32).

With the child in the supine position, a line is drawn from the anterior superior iliac spine to the pubic tuberosity. The greater trochanter is then located, and another line is drawn

parallel to the first line (see Fig. 41-29, *B*); at the medial one-third of the first line, a perpendicular is dropped to the second line. The point of intersection with the line originating at the greater trochanter marks the point of needle entry. The needle is inserted in a perpendicular plane until bone is encountered. It is then partially withdrawn and redirected medially. When the needle is posterior to the medial margin of the femur, ease of injection is determined after negative aspiration for blood. This approach carries a greater risk of unintended puncture of the femoral vessels, and repeated negative aspirations must precede incremental injection. If the needle is in muscle or a fascial bundle, resistance to injection will be felt. In this case, the needle is advanced until minimal resistance to injection is felt. Motor paresthesia is a helpful indicator.

For the previous two techniques, a dose of 0.2 mL/kg of bupivacaine (0.25% with epinephrine 1:200,000) is the dose usually administered for children older than 6 months of age. If the sciatic nerve block is used in conjunction with a femoral nerve block, consideration should be given to diluting the local anesthetic concentration further to limit the injected dose to 2.5 mg/kg of bupivacaine.[391]

### Lateral Popliteal Sciatic Nerve Block

This approach to the sciatic nerve can be performed with the child in the supine position.[392] This block provides postoperative analgesia in children undergoing surgery to the foot and knee, such as clubfoot repair or triple arthrodesis, and in children having knee surgery, particularly when combined with a femoral nerve block.[393] It has the advantage of preserving hamstring function and allows early ambulation with crutches.

ANATOMY. The popliteal fossa is a diamond-shaped area located behind the knee. It is bordered by the biceps femoris laterally, medially by the tendons of the semitendinosus and semimembranosus muscles, and inferiorly by the heads of the gastrocnemius muscle. The sciatic nerve, after its formation from L4 through S5, innervates all areas of the leg and foot below the knee except the anteromedial cutaneous areas of the leg and foot, which are supplied by the femoral nerve. The sciatic nerve divides

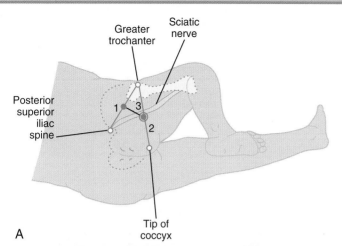

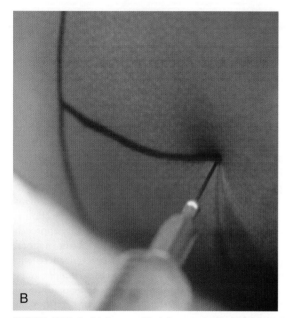

**FIGURE 41-28 A,** Sciatic nerve block (approach of Labat). The patient is placed in a lateral position with the lower leg extended and the upper leg, the one to be blocked, flexed; a line is drawn from the greater trochanter of the femur to the posterior superior iliac spine (*line 1*). A second line is drawn from the greater trochanter to the coccyx (*line 2*). Line 1 is bisected, and a perpendicular line is drawn from that point to line 2 (*black line 3*); the point at which the perpendicular broken line intersects line 2 (*circle with dot*) is the point of needle insertion. **B,** A 22-gauge needle is advanced perpendicular to the skin until it strikes bone or, if the child is awake, a paresthesia is elicited. Use of a nerve stimulator will produce either plantar flexion or dorsiflexion of the foot.

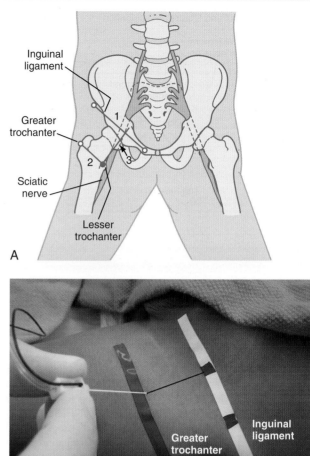

**FIGURE 41-29 A,** Sciatic nerve block (anterior approach). With the patient supine, a line is drawn from the anterior iliac spine to the pubic tuberosity (*line 1*). The greater trochanter is located, and another line is drawn parallel to the first (*line 2*). A perpendicular line is drawn from line 1 at a point one third the distance laterally from the pubic tuberosity to the anterior iliac spine (*solid line 3*). **B,** Left sciatic nerve block. A needle is inserted at the intersection of line 2 and the perpendicular line (in **A,** *solid dot*) until bone is encountered. The needle is redirected off the edge of the femur to the approximate posterior margin of the femur and, after negative aspiration for blood, ease of injection is ascertained. Resistance to injection indicates that the needle is within muscle or fascial bundle; the needle should be advanced until there is minimal resistance to injection or until a paresthesia is elicited.

into two branches, the larger tibial nerve located medially and the common peroneal nerve located laterally. The nerves are together at the apex of the popliteal fossa where they are in close proximity to each other and are enclosed in a connective tissue sheath for a few more centimeters before dividing into the component nerves (Fig. 41-30, *A*).

TECHNIQUE.  After induction of general anesthesia, the lower leg is elevated on a pillow. The biceps femoris tendon is palpated. The tendon is then traced upward for 3 to 5 cm. A 22-gauge insulated needle is inserted anterior to the tendon in a horizontal plane with a cephalad angulation (see Fig. 41-30, *B*). A nerve stimulator is attached to the sheathed needle and with low voltage stimulation (0.2 to 0.5 mV), the foot is observed for

plantar flexion or dorsiflexion. On injection of a test dose of 1 mL bupivacaine (0.25% with epinephrine 1:200,000), the twitching is abolished. This confirms the correct placement of the needle (see Fig. 41-30, *C*); 5 to 10 mL of additional local anesthetic is then injected (Video: Ultrasound-Guided Popliteal Nerve Block). In adult studies, it has been shown that the sciatic nerve block is longer lasting than an ankle block or subcutaneous infiltration, and it provides excellent postoperative analgesia.[392] Continuous catheter techniques can be used to provide effective analgesia in children in the postoperative period.[394] An ultrasound-guided technique may also be used (see Chapter 42 and Figs. 42-33 and 42-34).

COMPLICATIONS.  Intraneural injection must be avoided. Using a low-voltage nerve stimulator ensures the proper placement of the needle. It is rare to see intravascular placement of

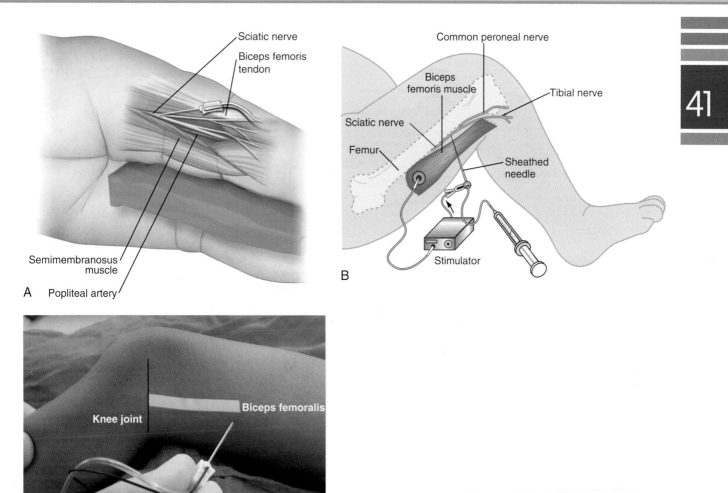

**FIGURE 41-30** Lateral popliteal sciatic nerve block. **A,** Anatomy for lateral popliteal approach to the sciatic nerve. The lower leg is elevated on a pillow and the biceps femoris tendon is palpated. The tendon is traced proximally for 3 to 5 cm. **B,** A 22-gauge insulated needle is inserted anterior to the tendon in a horizontal plane with a cephalad angulation. A nerve stimulator is attached to the needle and with low voltage stimulation (0.2 to 0.5 mV), the foot is observed for plantar flexion or dorsiflexion. With injection of the test dose of 1.0 mL of bupivacaine (0.25% with 1:200,000 epinephrine), the twitching is abolished. This confirms the correct placement of the needle. **C,** Then 5 to 10 mL of additional local anesthetic is injected.

the needle with this approach. Intravascular injection may be avoided with incremental injection and frequent aspiration.

### Infragluteal-Parabiceps Approach

This approach is a simple way to access the sciatic nerve.[390] It offers an advantage over the popliteal fossa technique because the posterior cutaneous nerve supplying the posterior portion of the thigh can be blocked with this approach.

TECHNIQUE. The child is placed in the supine position or a lateral position to perform this block. The biceps femoris tendon is palpated and traced cephalad to the distal crease of the buttocks (Fig. 41-31, *A*). A stimulating needle is then inserted perpendicular to the femoral shaft, along the biceps femoris tendon (parabiceps) until a twitch is obtained (see Fig. 41-31, *B*). Either inversion or eversion of the foot is a reasonable response for localization of the nerve. Next, 0.2 mL/kg of local anesthetic solution is injected into the area (Video: Subgluteal Sciatic Ultrasound Nerve Block). An ultrasound-guided

approach may facilitate this block (see also Chapter 42 and Figs. 42-31 to 42-33).[395]

COMPLICATIONS. Profound motor block can be seen in most children after a subgluteal (infragluteal) parabiceps sciatic nerve block. If the child is discharged home, caution should be exercised because of the motor weakness produced. More recently, we have used continuous catheters in hospitalized children having major lower extremity surgical procedures, with very good results.[396]

### Femoral Nerve Block

A femoral nerve block is particularly useful in children with a fractured femoral shaft so that transport, radiographic, and other manipulations are not painful.[397-399] This block provides analgesia and relieves muscle spasms around the fracture site.

ANATOMY. The femoral nerve is located immediately lateral to the femoral artery and deep to both the fascia lata and fascia iliaca (Fig. 41-32, *A*).

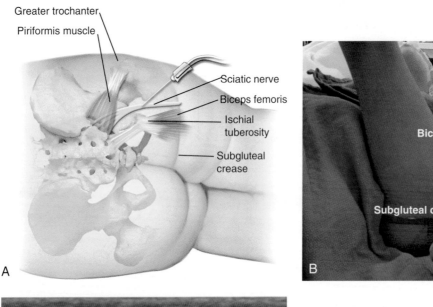

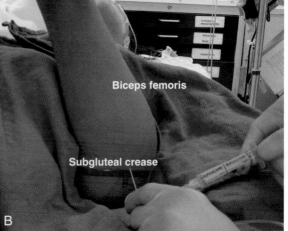

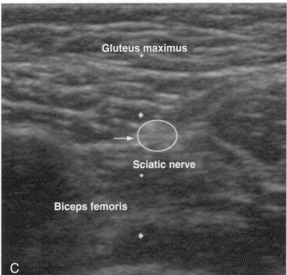

**FIGURE 41-31  A,** Artist's rendering of infragluteal-parabiceps block. **B,** The gluteal crease is identified (left leg) in the prone or supine position. The biceps femoris muscle is identified (distal portion not illustrated) and followed cephalad to the gluteal crease. A stimulating needle is inserted at the level of the gluteal crease along the medial border of the biceps femoris muscle; with stimulation at 0.5 mA, plantar flexion or extension or inversion or eversion denotes adequate positioning of the needle. After aspiration to rule out intravascular injection, 0.2 mL/kg of local anesthetic solution is injected to provide an adequate blockade of the sciatic nerve. **C,** An ultrasound technique may also be used. A linear ultrasound probe is placed along the inferior border of the gluteus maximus along the gluteal crease. The biceps femoris muscle and the semitendinosus muscle are identified. The sciatic nerve is seen as a hyperechoic shadow. In this location, the nerve may be isoechoic. This may require mild rotation or movement of the ultrasound probe to recognize the nerve completely. With the use of an in-plane approach, the needle is advanced close to the sciatic nerve. After aspiration, 0.2 mL/kg of local anesthetic solution is injected. A "donut sign" is seen as the nerve is surrounded by the local anesthetic solution.

TECHNIQUE.  A 22-gauge blunt B-bevel needle is advanced lateral to the pulsation of the femoral artery. Two fascial planes can be located by the distinct pop that is felt as the needle traverses these fascial tissues. The nerve is blocked by depositing an appropriate volume (5 to 10 mL) of local anesthetic lateral to the femoral pulse and deep to the fascia iliaca. The needle is advanced in a perpendicular plane (see Fig. 41-32, *B,* and Video: Femoral Nerve Block). It is not necessary to elicit a motor paresthesia, provided that the two fascial planes are penetrated. Performance of this block may, on occasion, produce a fascia iliaca block. Repeated aspiration and incremental injection should be used to avoid injection into the femoral artery. With ultrasound guidance,

the femoral nerve can be easily visualized and can be blocked (see also Chapter 42 and Fig. 42-29).[395] A catheter can be placed to provide continuous analgesia in the postoperative period.[397]

COMPLICATIONS.  It may be preferable to avoid this technique in children who are on anticoagulants or who may have blood dyscrasias, owing to the close proximity of the nerve to the femoral artery. Intravascular injection may be avoided with incremental injection and frequent aspiration.

### Lateral Femoral Cutaneous Nerve
ANATOMY.  The lateral femoral cutaneous nerve arises from the L2 and L3 roots of the lumbar plexus. It emerges from the lateral

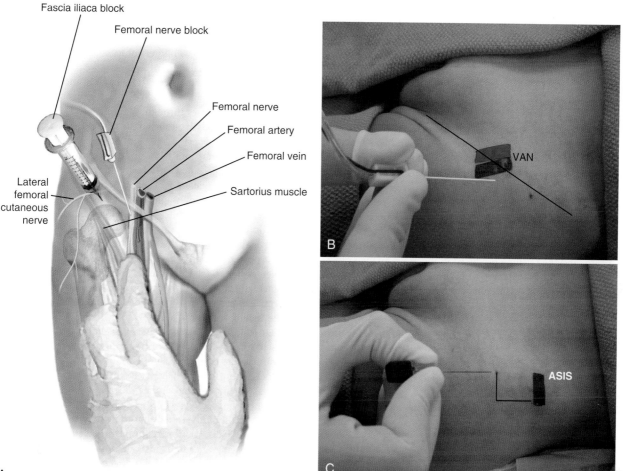

A

**FIGURE 41-32  A,** Right femoral nerve block and fascia iliaca compartment block. Note that the femoral nerve lies lateral to the femoral artery. The appropriate dose of local anesthetic is administered while maintaining pressure on the nerve sheath distal to the site of injection just below the inguinal ligament; local anesthetic is thus forced proximally. **B,** For a left femoral nerve block, the point of injection is lateral to the pulse, over the site of the nerve (*V,* vein; *A,* femoral artery; *N,* femoral nerve). **C,** The left lateral femoral cutaneous nerve is blocked by injecting 1.0 to 2.0 mL of local anesthetic 1 to 2 cm medial to the anterior superior iliac crest (*ASIS*). A caudal needle is used so as to better feel the "pop" through tissue planes. For the fascia iliaca block, the point of injection is just lateral to the site depicted for the femoral nerve block, 1 cm inferior to the lateral and middle thirds of the inguinal ligament. An injection at this location will bathe all three nerves in the compartment, resulting in blockade with a single injection.

border of the psoas muscle and passes obliquely under the fascia iliaca to enter the thigh 1 to 2 cm medial to the anterior superior iliac crest (Fig. 41-32, *A*). The nerve innervates the lateral aspect of the thigh. One of its anterior branches forms part of the patellar plexus; thus it must be blocked for regional anesthesia of the knee. Blockade is also indicated for supplementation of femoral and sciatic nerve blocks to provide relief of tourniquet pain. It is also suitable for anesthetizing the lateral aspect of the thigh as a donor site for small skin grafts, fascia iliaca grafts, or muscle biopsy for muscular disorders.[400,401] This block can also be used for both diagnostic and therapeutic purposes in treating meralgia paresthetica, a condition that leads to chronic pain along the lateral aspect of the thigh.[402,403] In most cases, a fascia iliaca block will block this nerve along with the femoral and obturator nerves, thus obviating the need for performing an isolated lateral femoral cutaneous block.

TECHNIQUE. A point approximately 2 cm caudal and 2 cm medial to the anterior superior iliac spine is located (see Fig. 41-32, *C*). A blunt needle is then advanced through the skin and then through the fascia lata. A distinct pop is felt at this point. The fascia lata and fascia iliaca compartments are entered as two

distinct pops can be felt as the needle advances into the fascia iliaca compartment. Two to 10 mL of local anesthetic, depending on the size of the child, is deposited in a fan-like fashion (Video: Lateral Femoral Cutaneous Nerve Block with Ultrasound). Recently we have used an ultrasound-guided technique that allows us to visualize the fascia iliaca compartment as it fills up with the local anesthetic solution on injection.

COMPLICATIONS. It is rare to see any complications associated with a lateral femoral cutaneous nerve block. However, care must be taken to avoid an intraneural placement of the local anesthetic solution. Intravascular injection may be avoided with incremental injection and frequent aspiration.

### Fascia Iliaca Block

This block is particularly useful in children to provide unilateral anesthesia or analgesia of the lower extremity. The block has been reported to be less reliable in adults than in children.[404] It produces blockade of the femoral, lateral femoral cutaneous, and obturator nerves with a single injection of local anesthetic.

ANATOMY. The compartment is bounded superficially by the fascia iliaca and iliacus muscle, superiorly by the iliac crest, and deeply by the psoas muscle (see Fig. 41-32, *A*). It has the advantage of producing blockade without requiring the needle to be in the close proximity to any major nerves or blood vessels. One study reported a greater than 90% success rate and found it far superior in children to the "3 in 1" block described by Winnie.[404]

TECHNIQUE. The injection is made approximately 1 cm inferior to the junction of the outer and middle thirds of the inguinal ligament (see Fig. 41-32, *A*). As the needle is inserted at a perpendicular angle of about 75 degrees to the skin, two characteristic pops are felt as the needle pierces the fascia lata and then the fascia iliaca. Slight pressure on a fluid-filled syringe attached to the needle may aid in placement of the block by producing a subtle loss of resistance when the fascia iliaca compartment is entered. The angle of needle insertion is decreased and directed cephalad, and the local anesthetic is incrementally injected. One should feel little resistance to injection. Digital pressure is exerted distally to the site during the injection and for a short time afterward, and the swelling produced in the groin by the volume of local anesthetic is massaged to promote proximal flow of the drug. A long-acting local anesthetic, such as bupivacaine, ropivacaine, or levobupivacaine, is usually chosen so that postoperative blockade can provide prolonged analgesia. A volume of 0.3 to 0.5 mL/kg is sufficient in most cases. An ultrasound-guided technique similar to that for the lateral femoral cutaneous block may also be used for this block.

COMPLICATIONS. Because of the larger volume that is required to provide an adequate block, care has to be taken to not exceed the maximum dosage of the local anesthetic. Intravascular injection may be avoided with incremental injection and frequent aspiration.

### Ankle Block

Block of the nerves of the foot at the ankle is a technique that is valuable to produce both surgical anesthesia and postoperative analgesia for procedures on the foot.

ANATOMY. Three nerves can be blocked from the dorsal aspect of the foot. The deep peroneal nerve (L4, L5, S1, and S2) innervates the web space between the great and second toes. This nerve extends down the anterior aspect of the leg medial to the extensor hallucis longus and lateral to both the anterior tibial

muscle and the anterior tibial artery. It is blocked at the level of the ankle crease in the lower part of the leg by inserting a 25-gauge needle through the skin until it contacts the tibia (Fig. 41-33, *A*). Several milliliters of local anesthetic are injected, and then an additional amount as the needle is being withdrawn. The superficial peroneal nerve (L4, L5, S1, and S2) innervates the medial and lateral aspects of the dorsum of the foot. Its anatomic course passes through the crural fascia on the anterior aspect of the distal two-thirds of the leg and subcutaneously along the lateral aspect of the foot. It is blocked immediately above the talocrural joint. It can be blocked by subcutaneous infiltration of local anesthetic from the anterior border of the tibia to the lateral malleolus. The last nerve that lies on the dorsal aspect of the foot is the saphenous nerve, which innervates the skin over the medial malleolus. It is blocked by subcutaneous infiltration around the great saphenous vein at the level of the medial malleolus. The tibial and the sural nerves are blocked using a posterior approach. The tibial nerve (L4, L5, S1, S2, and S3) lies posterior to the posterior tibial artery and divides into the medial and lateral plantar branches, which innervate their respective aspects of the sole of the foot. It is blocked at the level of the medial malleolus.

TECHNIQUE. It is not necessary to elicit paresthesias, and an ankle block can be satisfactorily performed in sedated children without the use of a nerve stimulator. Five principal nerves must be blocked to provide analgesia to the entire foot: (1) the deep peroneal, (2) superficial peroneal, (3) saphenous, (4) tibial, and (5) sural nerves (see Fig. 41-33). The technique is the same as in the adult. It should be noted that there might be some variation in the precise distribution of distal innervation from child to child. A 25-gauge needle is inserted at a 90-degree angle to the posterior aspect of the tibia and is directed lateral to the posterior tibial artery until the tibia is contacted. Several milliliters of local anesthetic are deposited at this level and several more are injected as the needle is withdrawn. The sural nerve innervates the heel. It is blocked by subcutaneous infiltration of local anesthetic from the Achilles tendon to the lateral malleolus (see Fig. 41-33, *B*). The deep peroneal nerve is located next to the extensor hallucis longus tendon. Usually it can be located by palpating the dorsalis pedis artery. The needle is inserted lateral to the extensor hallucis

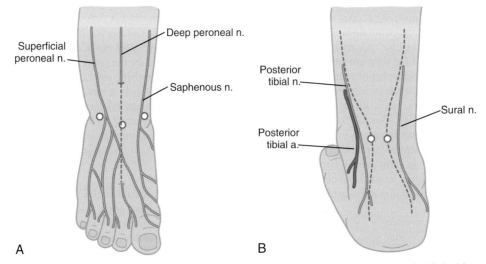

**FIGURE 41-33** Ankle block. Block of the ankle generally requires five separate nerves to be blocked. Three nerves can be blocked from the dorsal aspect of the foot (**A**) and two on either side of the Achilles tendon (**B**). Sites of injection are indicated by the *circles. a*, Artery; *n*, nerve.

longus tendon and is advanced until it meets the periosteum of the metatarsal. It is then withdrawn a few millimeters. After careful aspiration, a volume of 2 to 3 mL of local anesthetic is injected. The superficial peroneal nerve is located under the dorsum of the foot. A superficial injection from the lateral malleolus to the extensor hallucis longus tendon area blocks all the branches of the superficial peroneal nerve.

COMPLICATIONS. It is very rare to see complications from an ankle block. However, the use of vasoconstrictors can cause necrosis of the toes. Care should be taken to avoid the use of an ankle block in children who may have compromised blood flow to the lower extremity.[405]

### Digital Nerve Blocks: Foot

This is an easy block to perform and is useful for surgeries that include trauma to the nails and toes, ingrown toenail surgery, and laser treatment of warts.[388]

ANATOMY. The digital nerves of the foot are derived from the plantar cutaneous branches of the tibial nerve. The proper digital nerve of the great toe pierces the plantar aponeurosis posterior to the tarsal-medial joint and supplies the medial side of the great toe. The three common digital nerves pass between the divisions of the plantar aponeurosis and split into two proper digital nerves each. The first supplies the adjacent areas of the great and second toes; the second supplies the adjacent sides of the second and third toes; the third supplies the adjacent sides of the third and fourth toes. Each proper digital nerve gives off cutaneous and articular filaments that terminate in the tip of the toe. The superficial peroneal nerve gives off branches that supply the dorsum of the foot. They are derived from two nerves: (1) the dorsal cutaneous divides into two branches, a medial one that supplies the great toe and a lateral one that supplies the adjacent sides of the second and third toes; and (2) the intermediate dorsal cutaneous nerve, which passes along the lateral part of the foot supplying the lateral part of the dorsum of the foot and communicating with the sural nerve. This latter nerve terminates by dividing into two dorsal digital branches, one of which supplies the adjacent sides of the third and fourth toes and another one that supplies the adjacent sides of the fourth and little toes.

TECHNIQUE. Digital blocks of the foot can be difficult owing to the thickness of the overlying skin. We prefer using an approach in which we access the nerve from the web space or at the dorsolateral aspect of the toe. Bupivacaine *without epinephrine* is injected (1 to 2 mL) after aspiration to rule out intravascular placement. These blocks should be avoided in children with already compromised blood flow to the toes.

COMPLICATIONS. Large volumes of local anesthetic are contraindicated because this may cause pressure and vascular compromise. *Vasoconstrictors should be avoided because this may cause necrosis of the digit.* Intravascular injection may be avoided with incremental injection with frequent aspiration.

## Summary

Most regional techniques that are suitable for adults can be used in children. Although in most children sedation or general anesthesia is necessary in addition to the regional anesthetic, in certain neonates, regional anesthesia is often used as the sole technique and may reduce the incidence of postanesthetic apnea in former preterm infants. In addition to the intraoperative benefits, regional anesthesia may improve postoperative analgesia and may offer some improvement to postoperative respiratory function in selected children. Regional anesthesia is particularly useful in outpatient surgery, providing postoperative analgesia with rapid emergence and a low incidence of side effects. It is important to realize, however, that anatomic, physiologic, and pharmacologic factors that are unique to children can affect the performance and safety of regional anesthetic techniques. The advent of ultrasound guidance for placement of peripheral, as well as central, neuraxial blockade may increase the use of these blocks. Continuous catheter techniques can also increase the postoperative pain control in these children, with fewer adverse effects related to opioid use.[406] Once these differences are understood, regional anesthesia can be safely and efficaciously used, either as the sole anesthetic or as a supplement to general anesthesia, to provide a smooth intraoperative course and pain-free awakening.

### ACKNOWLEDGMENT

The authors wish to thank Per-Arne Lönnqvist, MD, DEAA, FRCA, PhD, for his generous contribution to the paravertebral block section of this chapter.

## REFERENCES

Please see www.expertconsult.com.

# Ultrasound-Guided Regional Anesthesia

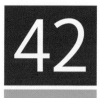

## MANOJ K. KARMAKAR AND WING H. KWOK

PERIPHERAL NERVE BLOCKS ARE frequently performed in children to provide anesthesia or analgesia during the perioperative period.[1-3] Success depends on the ability to accurately place the needle and thereby the local anesthetic close to the target nerve without causing injury to the nerve or adjacent structures. Peripheral nerve blocks are not without risk and can pose a serious challenge even to the experienced anesthesiologist because they are usually performed after the child is anesthetized. In the past, clinicians relied on anatomic landmarks,[1-3] fascial clicks,[4] loss of resistance,[5] or nerve stimulation[6] to position the needle in the vicinity of the nerve (see Chapter 41). Anatomic landmarks provide valuable clues to the position of the nerve, but they are surrogate markers, lack precision,[7] vary among children of different ages, and may be difficult to locate in obese children. Even nerve stimulation, which has been recommended as the gold standard for nerve localization, may not always elicit a motor response[8] and its use does not guarantee success or preclude complications.[9] Moreover, the accuracy of needle placement cannot be predicted with any of these methods,[8] which may lead to multiple attempts to place the needle that may result in pain and possibly an incomplete or failed nerve block.

Various imaging modalities, such as fluoroscopy,[10] computed tomography (CT),[11] and magnetic resonance imaging (MRI),[7] improve the accuracy of block placement in adults. However, these adjuncts are rarely used in children[1-3] and are not practical in the operating room. Recently, increased interest has been shown in the use of ultrasound (US) to guide peripheral and central neuraxial blocks in both adults and children.[12-21] In this chapter, the basic principles of US imaging and US-guided regional anesthesia (USGRA) in children are described. It is assumed that the reader has a basic understanding of common landmark-based nerve block techniques in children.

The use of US for regional anesthesia dates to 1978, when La Grange and associates[22] used a Doppler flow detector to locate the subclavian artery and guide supraclavicular brachial plexus blocks. In 1994, Kapral and colleagues[23] published the first report on direct sonographic visualization in regional anesthesia. They used US to directly visualize the brachial plexus and observe the spread of the local anesthetic in real time during supraclavicular brachial plexus block. Today, US is used to guide peripheral nerve blocks and central neuraxial blocks in both adults and children.[12-21] This has become possible owing to improvements in US technology and the availability of portable US machines with high-resolution imaging capabilities. The ability to directly visualize the peripheral nerves and central neuraxial structures in children is truly exciting and can be compared to removing a blindfold from the anesthesiologist performing regional anesthesia. Currently, outcome data that prove US increases the safety and efficacy of regional anesthesia in children are rapidly accumulating. For example, when compared with nerve stimulation, US speeds the onset time of infraclavicular block.[20] A greater success rate of pediatric truncal blocks is seen when US guidance is used.[21]

# Principles of Ultrasound

Sound is a form of mechanical energy that propagates through a medium as a wave of alternating pressure, causing local regions of compression and rarefaction (Fig. 42-1). The frequency (f) of sound is the number of cycles of oscillation per second made by the sound source and the particles in the medium through which it moves. It is expressed in hertz (Hz, cycles per second). Sound waves propagate symmetrically away from the source at a constant velocity (v), which is the speed of sound in the medium. Distance between the wavefronts is the wavelength ($\lambda$) of the sound. The speed of sound through a medium can thus be represented as:

$$v = f \times \lambda$$

Amplitude is the strength of a sound wave, and the unit used to describe it is decibels (dB). The velocity of transmission of sound through a medium depends on its acoustic impedance and is determined by factors such as the stiffness, elasticity, and density of the medium. This accounts for the varying velocity of sound transmission through different tissues in the human body (Table 42-1). The average velocity of sound transmission through biologic tissue is 1540 m/sec. If the time taken by the US signal to return to the transducer is known, the distance of the target from the transducer (depth) can be computed.

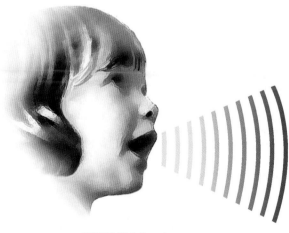

**FIGURE 42-1** Sound wave.

**TABLE 42-1** Propagation Velocity of Sound in Body Tissues

| Tissue | Propagation Velocity of Sound (m/sec)* |
|---|---|
| Bone | 4080 |
| Muscle | 1580 |
| Blood | 1570 |
| Kidney | 1560 |
| Liver | 1550 |
| Soft tissue (average) | 1540 |
| Water | 1480 |
| Fat | 1450 |
| Lung | 600 |
| Air | 330 |

*m/sec*, Meters per second.
*Medical ultrasound device measurements are based on an assumed average propagation velocity of 1540 m/sec.

The human ear can detect sound between 20 and 20,000 Hz. US is sound with a frequency beyond 20,000 Hz (20 KHz). For medical imaging, US typically uses a frequency between 1 million and 15 million Hz (megahertz [MHz]) and is produced by a piezoelectric crystal (element) within the transducer. Artificial ferroelectric materials, such as lead zirconate titanate or lead zirconium titanate (PZT), are commonly used as elements in transducers, and their thickness determines the resonant frequency. When an electrical field is applied to the surface of an element in a transducer, it undergoes dimensional changes that cause it to vibrate and produce sound. The element is typically driven by a pulsed alternating voltage. This results in the generation of short pulses of US that are emitted into body tissues. Between successive short pulses of US generation, the transducer does not transmit but rather functions as a receiver of the reflected US energy (i.e., the echoes). The percentage of time that a transducer is transmitting is termed the *duty factor* and is typically less than 1%. The US transducer thus has a dual function—it functions as both a transmitter and a receiver.

The emitted US signal travels through the tissue medium, and when it encounters a tissue interface it is reflected back. The degree of reflection of US from tissues is related to the changes in acoustic impedance (Z) between two tissue interfaces. The reflected echoes are detected by the transducer and converted into electrical energy; they are then processed by the US machine according to their strength and displayed as dots on the monitor. The brightness of each dot corresponds to the strength of the echo signal. Strong echoes produce bright white dots, weak echoes produce gray dots, and anatomic structures that do not reflect US appear as black dots. The position of the dot on the monitor represents the depth from which the echo is received. When all of these dots are combined, they produce a complete image of the area scanned.[24-26]

## MODES OF ULTRASOUND
### A-Mode (Amplitude)
In amplitude, or A-mode, the echoes from tissue interfaces are represented on the monitor as a spike, and the spike height represents the amplitude of the echo.[27] The distance of the interface from the transducer is calculated from the time taken for the signal to be sent and received, the "round-trip time." A-mode US imaging is rarely used and is considered obsolete.

### B-Mode (Brightness or Two-Dimension Mode)
Brightness, or B-mode, is the most commonly used US mode. In this mode, the spike is converted to a dot and the brightness of the dot represents the amplitude of the returning signal.[24-26] The position of the dot on the display represents the depth from which the signal is returning and depends on the round-trip time of the US signal. Multiple scan lines across a plane are combined to produce a single two-dimensional (2D) image. A series of frames are then displayed in rapid succession to give the impression of constant motion, the quality of which depends on the number of images displayed per second, that is, the frame rate.

### M-Mode (Motion)
Motion, or M-mode, US is directed along a single scan line (sample line), and reflected signals along this scan line are converted to a brightness scale and displayed against a time axis. Because M-mode is produced from US signals along a single scan line, the 2D anatomy of the underlying body tissues should be studied first using the 2D mode (see later). M-mode is of

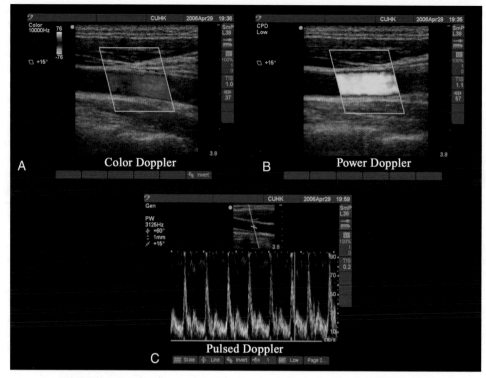

**FIGURE 42-2** Doppler ultrasound. **A,** Color Doppler. **B,** Power Doppler. **C,** Pulsed Doppler.

particular interest when time resolution is necessary, such as when examining a target with rapid movement (e.g., the mitral valve during echocardiography).[28]

### Doppler Ultrasound

Doppler US (based on the Doppler principle) detects a shift in frequency between the emitted US waves and their echoes.[29-32] It is used to detect and measure blood flow, and the major reflector for this purpose is red blood cells. Several modes are available:

- *Color Doppler* measures and color codes the direction and magnitude of the mean Doppler frequency shifts that occur in moving red blood cell and superimposes a color depiction of these data on the gray-scale image (Fig. 42-2, *A*).
- *Power color Doppler* depicts the amplitude, or power, of the Doppler signals (see Fig. 42-2, *B*). This allows better sensitivity for visualization of small vessels, but at the expense of directional information.
- *Pulsed Doppler* allows a sampling volume (or gate) to be positioned in a vessel visualized on the gray-scale image and displays a spectrum of the full range of blood velocities within the gate plotted as a function of time (see Fig. 42-2, *C*).

### THE ULTRASOUND MACHINE

US machines are either cart-based or portable systems. Irrespective of their shape or size, US machines are made up of the following components: a *monitor* (where the clinical images are displayed), the *US unit* (where the signals are processed), the *control panel* (with the knobs and controls), one or more *transducers*, and a *data storage device.*[33-35] For an anesthesiologist, the first encounter with an US machine can be quite intimidating. The wide array of knobs and controls that are available may be

confusing. However, several controls are common in most US machines, and a clear understanding of their function ("knobology") is essential for optimal imaging.

### Presets

Most US machines have a number of presets, which are factory set, to allow optimal US imaging of a specific area of the body or type of examination. Some of the categories of presets that are available include small part, vascular, breast, nerve, musculoskeletal, abdominal, and so on. For example, if a small part preset is chosen, the US machine assumes that the operator is scanning for small, relatively superficial structures and automatically adjusts the depth, power, focus, gain, and time-gain compensation (TGC) (see later) to allow optimal imaging of superficial structures. Some US machines also allow the operator to customize presets according to clinical requirements. Power output is the amount of energy transmitted from the US transducer. In most machines, the power cannot be adjusted by the operator but is automatically set when a particular preset is chosen.

### Frequency

This control is used to select the desired frequency, within certain limits, of a broadband transducer, that is, a transducer that serves a range of frequencies. In some US systems (M-Turbo, SonoSite Inc, Bothell, Wash.), this is available as an image optimization control. In the "Res" (resolution) setting the highest frequency of the broadband transducer is selected; in the "Pen" (penetration) setting the lowest frequency is selected; and in the "Gen" (general) setting an intermediate frequency is selected.

### Gain

The gain control adjusts the amplification of the returning acoustic signals and is used to optimize the US image (Fig. 42-3). Reduced gain produces a dark image (see Fig. 42-3, *A*) and detail

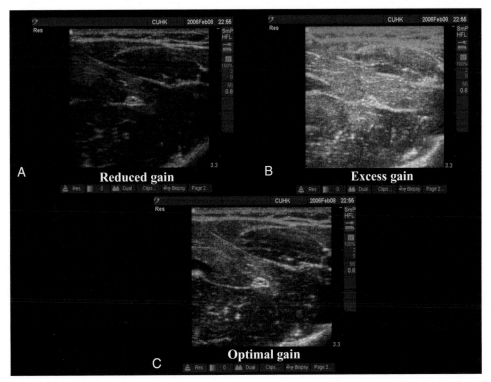

**FIGURE 42-3** Transverse sonogram of the forearm demonstrating reduced gain (**A**), excess gain (**B**), and optimal gain (**C**).

is masked. In contrast, too much gain produces a white image and detail is saturated (see Fig. 42-3, *B*). In some US machines there are separate controls for overall gain and gain for the near and far fields. "Auto-gain," by which the US machine automatically adjusts the gain, is also available in some machines.

### Time-Gain Compensation

US energy is progressively attenuated as it travels through tissue. Therefore signals returning from reflectors at a depth are weaker in strength. By selectively amplifying the echoes from greater depths, using the TGC method or depth-gain compensation (DGC), equal reflectors at unequal depths are displayed as structures of equal brightness on the monitor. TGC is preset to a large degree, and the operator can make fine adjustments if necessary. The TGC control is presented as a series of sliders arranged in a vertical fashion on the control panel. Each of the sliders adjusts the amplification of the returning US signals at a specific image depth.

### Depth

Adjustment in the displayed depth may be necessary depending on the location of the target, the patient's body size, or other anatomic factors. A depth greater than necessary should not be chosen because this reduces the frame rate and resolution of the image.

### Focus (Focal Zone)

The focus of the US signal occurs at a point at which the beam is at its narrowest width. It is also the region where lateral resolution is the best. The focus point should therefore be positioned at the depth at which the pertinent anatomic structures are located. In some US machines, the operator can select multiple focal zones, but this markedly reduces the frame rate and thus should not be routinely used.

### Freeze and Unfreeze

The "freeze" function allows the operator to lock a static image on the monitor. A number of frames (usually 20 or more) are also simultaneously stored in a memory bank. A trackball or an "arrow" key is then used to scroll back and forth through these frames. The selected still image can then be used for annotation, documentation, storage, review, or teaching. Pressing the freeze button once again will unfreeze the image.

### Ultrasound Transducers

The transducer functions both as a transmitter and a receiver of the ultrasound signal.[33-35] Three types of transducers are currently used (Fig. 42-4): (1) in a linear-array transducer, the piezoelectric crystals are arranged in a linear fashion and sequentially fired to produce parallel beams of ultrasound in sequence, creating a field of view that is rectangular and as wide as the footprint of the transducer (see Fig. 42-4, *A*); (2) a curved linear-array transducer has a curved surface, creating a field of view that is wider than the footprint of the probe (see Fig. 42-4, *B*), but at the cost of reduced lateral resolution in the far field as the scan lines diverge; (3) a phased-array transducer has a small footprint, but the ultrasound beam is steered electronically to produce a sufficiently wide far field of view. The ultrasound beam diverges from virtually the same point in the transducer (see Fig. 42-4, *C*). Phased-array transducers are routinely used for transthoracic echocardiography.[34] The footprints of these transducers are small enough to fit between the ribs and still produce a wide far field of view to image the heart. US transducers serve either a single frequency or a range of frequencies (broadband). For example, a transducer with the notation HFL38/13-6 indicates that it is a high-frequency broadband (13-6 MHz) linear transducer with a 38-mm footprint. Note that the nomenclature used for transducers varies among manufacturers of US devices.

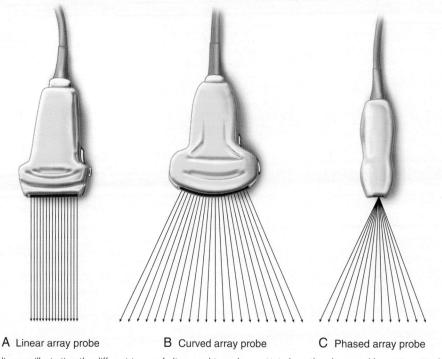

A Linear array probe    B Curved array probe    C Phased array probe

**FIGURE 42-4** Schematic diagram illustrating the different types of ultrasound transducers. Note how the ultrasound beam is emitted from each of these transducers.

## Ultrasound Transducer Selection

*Resolution* is the ability to distinguish two objects that are close together. Axial resolution is the ability to distinguish two objects that are along the axis of the US beam, and lateral resolution is the ability to distinguish two objects that are side by side. High-frequency US (13-6 MHz) has a higher axial and lateral resolution compared with low-frequency US but cannot penetrate as deeply into body tissue. Therefore high-frequency US is used to image superficial structures such as the brachial plexus in the interscalene groove or supraclavicular fossa. A lower-frequency US transducer (10-5 MHz) is suited for slightly deeper structures, such as the brachial plexus in the infraclavicular fossa, whereas a low-frequency US transducer (5-2 MHz) is used to image deep structures, such as the lumbar plexus or the sciatic nerve. Broadband transducers allow a single transducer to be used for scanning over a wide range of depths. Because regional blocks are performed at relatively shallow depths in neonates, infants, and young children, high-frequency linear transducers are perfectly adequate for most procedures in these age groups. High-frequency linear transducers with a small footprint (13-6 MHz, hockey stick, 25 to 26 mm) are particularly suited for young children.

## Essentials of Musculoskeletal Ultrasound Imaging

### AXIS OF SCAN

In diagnostic ultrasonography, scans are performed in the transverse, longitudinal (sagittal), oblique, or coronal axis. During a transverse (axial) scan the transducer is oriented at right angles to the target, producing a cross-sectional display of the structures (Fig. 42-5, *A*). During a longitudinal scan, the transducer is oriented parallel to and along the long axis of the target (e.g., a

blood vessel or nerve) (see Fig. 42-5, *B*). During USGRA procedures, US scans are most commonly performed in the transverse axis. In this axis, the nerves, the adjoining structures, and the circumferential spread of the local anesthetic are easily visualized.

### PROBE AND IMAGE ORIENTATION

The US image must be properly oriented to accurately identify the anatomic relations of the various structures on the monitor. To facilitate this, all US probes have an orientation marker, which is usually represented by a groove or a ridge on one side of the transducer and corresponds to a green dot (or a logo) on the monitor. By convention, the orientation marker on the transducer is directed cephalad when performing a longitudinal scan and directed toward the right side of the patient when performing a transverse scan. This way the orientation marker on the left upper corner of the monitor always represents the cephalad end during a longitudinal scan or the right side of the patient during a transverse scan. The top of the display monitor therefore represents superficial structures and the bottom of the monitor the deep structures.

### ECHOGENICITY

Certain terms are frequently used to describe the sonographic appearance of musculoskeletal structures (Fig. 42-6):

*Echogenic:* A bright white structure against a dark background
*Reflective:* Synonymous with an echogenic structure
*Isoechoic:* A shade of gray that is of the same brightness or echogenicity as the surrounding tissues
*Hyperechoic:* A shade of gray that is bright white or brighter than the surrounding tissues
*Hypoechoic:* A shade of gray that is dark or less bright than the surrounding tissues
*Anechoic:* An absence of echoes, hence blackness

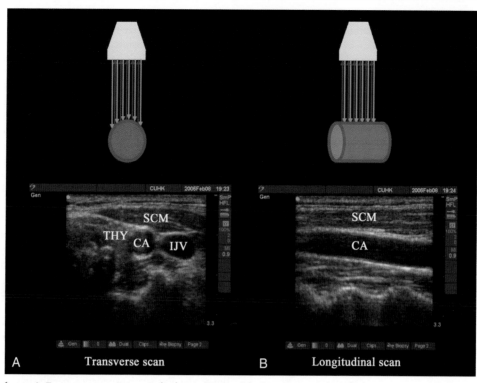

**FIGURE 42-5** Axis of scan. **A,** Transverse scan. **B,** Longitudinal scan. *CA,* Carotid artery; *IJV,* internal jugular vein; *SCM,* sternocleidomastoid muscle; *THY,* thyroid.

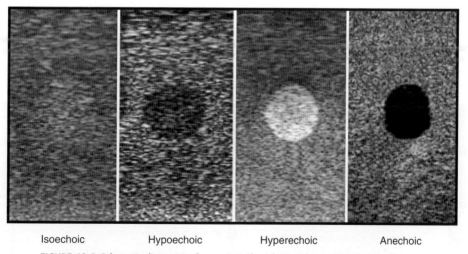

FIGURE 42-6 Schematic diagram to demonstrate the relative echogenicity of various tissues.

## AXIS OF INTERVENTION

The plane of US imaging is only 1 mm thick (Fig. 42-7); for a needle to be visible during US imaging it must lie within this narrow plane of imaging. During USGRA procedures, the block needle is inserted either outside of the plane (out-of-plane approach) (Fig. 42-8, *A*) or within the plane of the US beam (in-plane approach) (see Fig. 42-8, *B*). In the out-of-plane approach, the needle is inserted in the short axis and is initially outside the plane of imaging and therefore not visible. It becomes visible only when the needle crosses the plane of imaging and is seen as an echogenic dot on the monitor (see Fig. 42-8, *A*). It is important to note that this echogenic dot may be just the cross-sectional image of the shaft of the needle as it passes through the plane of the US beam and thus may not represent the tip of the needle. In the in-plane approach, the needle is inserted along the long axis of the transducer in the plane of imaging and therefore both the shaft and tip of the needle are visible on the monitor.

Both approaches are commonly used, and no data have shown that one is better than the other. Proponents of the out-of-plane approach[13,14,36] have had great success with this method and claim that it causes less needle-related trauma and pain because the needle is advanced through a shorter distance to the target. However, critics of the short-axis approach express concerns that the inability to reliably visualize the needle and to use tissue movement as a surrogate marker to locate the needle tip during a procedure can lead to complications. The needle is better visualized in the in-plane approach,[37,38] but this requires good hand and eye coordination and reverberation artifacts from the shaft of the needle can be problematic. Moreover, there are claims that the in-plane approach also causes more discomfort in awake patients because longer needle insertion paths are required.[13,14,36]

## NEEDLE VISIBILITY

The ability to visualize the needle during a US-guided procedure is critical for precision, safety, and success. However, this is often limited by the dispersion of the reflected US signals away from the transducer. Several factors have been identified that can influence needle visibility. The shaft of the needle is better visualized in the long axis than in the short axis, and its visibility decreases linearly with steep angles of insertion and smaller needle diameters. The needle tip is better visualized when it is inserted in the long axis for shallow angle of insertion (less than 30 degrees) and in the short axis when the angle of insertion is steep (greater than 60 degrees). This is also true when the needle is inserted with its bevel facing the US transducer. To overcome the effect of angle on needle visibility, some high-end US machines allow the operator to steer the US beam toward the needle during steep needle insertions. However, this requires experience and decreases in needle visibility can still occur. Needle visibility is also enhanced in the presence of a medium-sized guidewire. Priming a needle with saline or air, insulating it, or inserting a stylet before insertion does not improve visibility.[39-41]

We think that the anesthesiologist's skill in aligning the needle along the plane of imaging is by far the most important variable influencing needle visibility because minor deviations of even a few millimeters from this plane will result in inability to visualize the needle. Even with experience, needle tip visibility is a problem when performing blocks at a depth in areas that are rich in fatty tissue. Under such circumstances, gently jiggling (rapid in-and-out movement) the needle and observing tissue movement or performing a test injection of saline or 5% dextrose (1 to 2 mL) and observing tissue distention can help locate the position of the needle tip. Five percent dextrose is preferred for the latter when nerve stimulation is used because it does not increase the electric current required to elicit a motor response.[42]

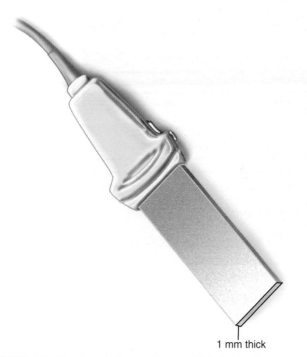

1 mm thick

**FIGURE 42-7** The plane of ultrasound imaging. Note that the ultrasound beam is only 1 mm thick and for a needle to be visible during an ultrasound-guided intervention it must lie within this plane of imaging.

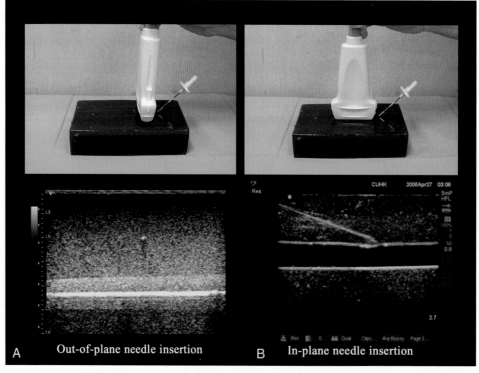

A  Out-of-plane needle insertion     B  In-plane needle insertion

**FIGURE 42-8** Axis of intervention. Out-of-plane (**A**) and in-plane (**B**) techniques.

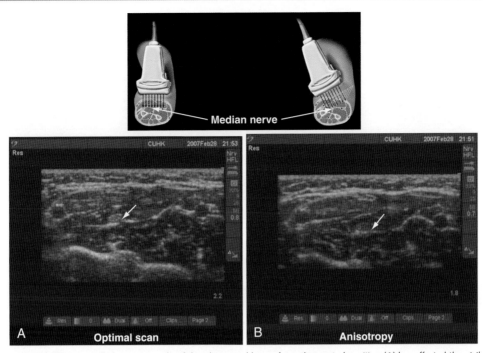

**FIGURE 42-9** Anisotropy. Note how a small change in angle of the ultrasound beam from the neutral position (**A**) has affected the visibility of the median nerve (*white arrow,* **B**) in the forearm.

## ANISOTROPY

*Anisotropy,* or angular dependence, is a term used to describe the change in echogenicity of a structure with a change in the angle of insonation of the incident US beam (Fig. 42-9).[43] It is frequently observed during scanning of nerves, muscles, and tendons. This occurs because the amplitude of the echoes returning to the transducer varies with the angle of insonation. Nerves are best visualized when the incident beam is at right angles (see Fig. 42-9, *A*); small changes in the angle away from the perpendicular can significantly reduce their echogenicity (see Fig. 42-9, *B*). Therefore, during USGRA procedures, the transducer should be tilted, from side to side, to minimize anisotropy and optimize visualization of the nerve.[44] Although poorly understood, different nerves also exhibit differences in anisotropy, which may be related to the internal architecture of the nerve.

## Identification of Nerves, Tendons, Muscle, Fat, Bone, Fascia, Blood Vessels, and Pleura

### NERVES

On a transverse scan, nerves appear round, oval, triangular, lip shaped, or even flat.[45,46] Nerves also assume different shapes along their course depending on the surrounding structures. The echogenicity of nerves also varies and depends on the nerve and area scanned. They are generally hyperechoic and stand out in the background of the hypoechoic muscles (Fig. 42-10, *A*), but they can also appear hypoechoic with a hyperechoic rim (see Fig. 42-10, *B*). They also have been described to have a fascicular or honeycomb appearance (i.e., echogenic structures with internal punctate, echo-poor spaces) (see Fig. 42-10, *C*). On longitudinal scan, the appearance of peripheral nerves has been likened to a "tram track"; that is, parallel hyperechoic lines are seen against a background of echo-poor space (see Fig. 42-10, *D*). Nerve motion also can be demonstrated on dynamic US imaging.

### TENDONS

Tendons appear to have numerous fine parallel hyperechoic lines separated by fine hypoechoic lines (*fibrillar* pattern) on long-axis scans.[46] Compared with nerves, tendons have more hyperechoic lines and move more than adjacent nerves when the corresponding muscle is contracted or passively stretched.

### MUSCLE

Muscle fibers are hypoechoic, but the connective tissue structure enveloping the entire muscle *(epimysium)* is hyperechoic.[47,48] The *perimysium* that envelops individual muscle fascicles is also hyperechoic. Muscle fibers converge to become tendons or aponeurosis.

### FAT

Fat lobules appear as round to oval hypoechoic nodules that are separated by fine hyperechoic septa. Fat tends to be superficially distributed (subcutaneous fat), slightly compressible, and similar on transverse and longitudinal scans.

### BONE

Bone reflects most of the US energy. Therefore it appears bright and has a hyperechoic edge on US imaging, with a large anechoic shadow (acoustic shadow) distal to it (Fig. 42-11).

### FASCIA

Fascia, peritoneum, and aponeurosis appear as thin hyperechoic layers on US imaging.

### BLOOD VESSELS

Arteries are identified by their intrinsic pulsatility, are not compressible, and have anechoic lumens. Veins are not pulsatile, are

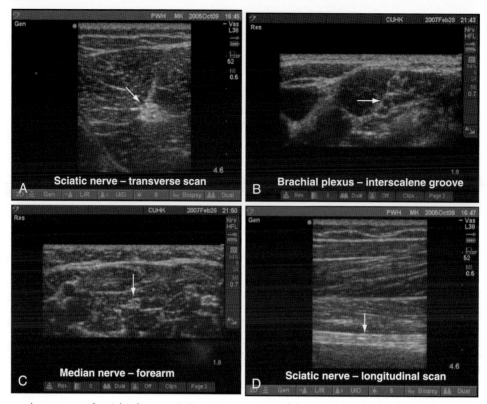

FIGURE 42-10 Ultrasound appearance of peripheral nerves. **A,** Transverse sonogram of the sciatic nerve in the thigh. **B,** Transverse sonogram of the brachial plexus in the interscalene groove. **C,** Transverse sonogram of the median nerve in the forearm. **D,** Longitudinal sonogram of the sciatic nerve in the thigh.

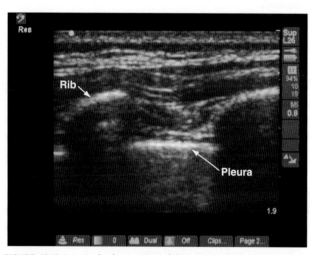

FIGURE 42-11 Longitudinal sonogram of the intercostal space demonstrating the ultrasound appearances of bone and pleura.

compressible, and have anechoic lumens. Color Doppler or power Doppler modes can also be used to demonstrate blood flow and differentiate arteries from veins (see Fig. 42-2).

### PLEURA

The pleura appear as a hyperechoic line on US imaging (see Fig. 42-11).[49-51] During scanning of the intercostal space, the pleural line is located slightly below the hyperechoic ribs. "Comet-tail" artifacts may be present as a series of vertical lines arising from the pleura. On real-time imaging, lung sliding movement between

the parietal and visceral pleura can be discerned from movement of the comet-tail artifacts ("lung sliding sign").

## Special Techniques

### TISSUE HARMONIC IMAGING

The term *harmonic* refers to frequencies that are integral multiples of the frequency of the transmitted pulse (which is also called the fundamental frequency or first harmonic). The second harmonic has a frequency of twice the fundamental frequency. Harmonics are generated in the tissues by the nonlinear propagation of sound. Tissue harmonic imaging (THI) is a technique in which the harmonic signals reflected from tissue interfaces are selectively displayed.[52-54] This results in reduced image artifacts, haze, and clutter and improved contrast resolution (Fig. 42-12).

### COMPOUND IMAGING

US imaging depends on the reflection of the US from tissue interfaces. Not all tissues are good reflectors, and certain structures also cause scattering of the US signals. Unlike reflected signals, scattered signals radiate in all directions. As a result, only a small amount of energy is reflected back to the transducer. The scattering of the US signal results in speckle artifacts, also described as noise, which reduces image resolution and makes the US image appear grainy. Compound imaging is a technique used to improve resolution by reducing the contrast-to-noise ratio (speckle).[55] The US beam from the transducer is electronically steered, and the same structure is imaged from several different angles. The returning echoes are then processed with simultaneous filtering of the artifacts in real time, producing a

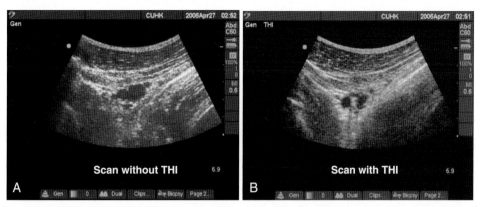

**FIGURE 42-12** Tissue harmonic imaging (*THI*). Sagittal sonogram of the infraclavicular fossa. **A,** Conventional scan. **B,** Conventional scan with THI.

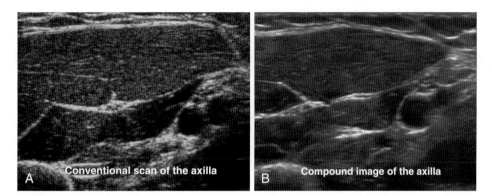

**FIGURE 42-13** Compound imaging. Transverse sonogram of the axilla. **A,** Conventional scan. **B,** Conventional scan with compound imaging.

composite image that has reduced noise or speckle and improved definition (Fig. 42-13).

## PANORAMIC IMAGING

B-mode (2D) ultrasonography has a limited field of view and allows visualization of only a small portion of any large structure. Panoramic imaging, as the name implies, is a technique used to extend the field of view so that larger structures and their surrounding tissues can be visualized together.[56] During a panoramic scan, the operator slowly slides the US transducer across an area of interest. During this motion, multiple images are acquired from many different transducer positions across the area of interest. The registered image data are accumulated in a large buffer and then combined to form the composite panoramic image (Fig. 42-14). Although useful for annotation, documentation, teaching, and research, it is rarely used in children during USGRA procedures.

## ARTIFACTS

US artifacts are structures that are visible in the US image that do not correlate with any anatomic structure.[57] The US machine makes the following assumptions when generating an image:

1. The US beam is considered to travel only in a straight line, with a constant rate of attenuation.
2. The average speed of sound through body tissue is considered to be 1540 m/sec.
3. The US beam is assumed to be infinitely thin, with all echoes originating from its central axis.
4. The depth of a reflector is calculated by determining the round-trip time of the US signal.

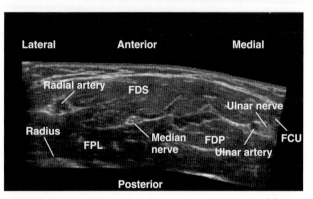

**FIGURE 42-14** Panoramic imaging. Transverse panoramic scan of the forearm. *FCU,* Flexor carpi ulnaris; *FDP,* flexor digitorum profundus; *FDS,* flexor digitorum superficialis; *FPL,* flexor pollicis longus.

When a deviation from any of these assumptions occurs, the US machine is unable to determine it. This results in the display of an echo that has no relation with the interface that actually produced the echo; that is, an artifact is produced. Some artifacts are undesirable and interfere with interpretation, whereas others help identify certain structures. It is essential to recognize them to avoid misinterpretation. Therefore, when a structure appears abnormal on ultrasonography, it must be examined in two planes to avoid making a wrong interpretation. Real anatomic structures are visible in both planes of imaging, whereas artifacts are visible in only one plane.

## Contact Artifact

The contact artifact is the most common artifact produced when loss of acoustic coupling occurs between the skin and the transducer. This could occur because the transducer is not touching the skin, but more frequently it is due to air bubbles that are trapped between the skin and the transducer. Therefore it is prudent to apply liberal amounts of gel to exclude air from the skin and transducer interface.

## Reverberation Artifact

Reverberation artifacts, also known as repetitive echoes, occur when repeated reflection of US occurs between two highly reflective surfaces.[58] Some of the US signals returning to the transducer are reflected back, then strike the original interface, and are reflected back toward the transducer a second time. As a result, the first reverberation artifact is twice as far from the skin surface as the original interface. A second or third reverberation artifact also may be seen. Because of attenuation, the intensity of the artifacts decreases with increasing distance from the transducer. Reverberation artifacts are frequently seen during US-guided axillary brachial plexus block, particularly when the needle is inserted in the long axis.

## Mirror Image Artifact

Mirror image artifact is a type of reverberation artifact that occurs at highly reflective interfaces.[59] The first image is displayed in the correct position, and a false image is produced on the other side of the reflector because of its mirrorlike effect.

## Propagation Speed Artifact

Propagation speed artifacts occur when the medium through which the US beam passes does not propagate at 1540 m/sec, resulting in echoes that appear at incorrect depths on the monitor. An example of propagation speed artifact is the "bayonet artifact,"[60] which has been reported during an US-guided axillary brachial plexus block. The shaft of the needle appeared bent when it accidentally traversed the axillary artery. This happens because of the difference in the velocity of sound between whole blood (1580 m/sec) and soft tissue (1540 m/sec).

## Acoustic Shadowing

Acoustic shadow is an echo-free area behind surfaces that are highly reflective or attenuating, such as bone (see Fig. 42-11) or metallic implants. The implication for regional anesthesia is that tissues in the area of the shadow cannot be imaged.

## SCANNING ROUTINE

Being able to consistently produce high-quality images of the area scanned is vital for safety and success during any USGRA procedure. Without optimal images, it is not possible to accurately identify musculoskeletal structures or perform interventions with precision. We have found that following a "scanning routine" or a set of simple steps, which is repeatable, is essential for optimal imaging; the routine that we follow is outlined in Table 42-2. Although the suggested routine may appear complicated at first, with repetition these steps are gradually internalized. Attaching a card with the scanning routine to the US machine facilitates easy recall.

## Scout Scan

The aim of the scout scan, or the preintervention scan, as the name implies, is to examine the area of interest before the

**TABLE 42-2** Scanning Routine

1. Turn on the ultrasound machine.
2. Select a scanning mode.
3. Select an appropriate transducer.
4. Dim the lights in the room.
5. Assume a comfortable position.
6. Apply liberal amount of ultrasound gel.
7. Perform a scout scan.
8. Orient the transducer and image.
9. Select the appropriate ultrasound settings (preset, frequency—for broadband transducers, depth, gain, and focus point).
10. Mark the position of the transducer on the patient's skin once an optimal image is obtained before the intervention.

intervention. This has also been referred to as a "mapping scan." During the scout scan, steps 8 and 9 described in Table 42-2 are performed, the sonoanatomy of the area is visualized, and the image is optimized. Once an optimal view with the target structure is obtained and the best possible site for needle insertion is determined, it is advisable to mark the position[44] of the transducer on the patient's skin so the transducer can be returned to the same position after sterile preparations have been completed. It is common to diagnose anatomic variations during the scout scan. The operator can then decide whether to continue with the block in the same location or to choose an alternative approach or technique that may be safer. This assessment of anatomic variation is one of the major benefits of using US for regional anesthesia.

## GENERAL CONSIDERATIONS IN CHILDREN

Preparations for an ultrasound-guided nerve block should begin during the preoperative visit by adequately explaining the technique, its benefits and risks, and, more importantly, the possibility of a failed block to the parents. In the event of failure, a contingency plan to quickly convert to general anesthesia or another form of postoperative analgesia must always be in place. In children, most regional anesthetic procedures are performed while the child is anesthetized. However, in a cooperative child or under special circumstances, such as in a child with difficult airway or a child predisposed to malignant hyperthermia, it is possible to perform the block after light sedation. We find that it is easy to explain the procedure to children who are older than 8 years of age. Some of them may even express a wish to stay awake and observe the US images during the block. Eutectic mixture of local anesthetic (EMLA) cream applied an hour before the procedure to the skin over the area where the block needle and the intravenous catheter are to be inserted helps reduce needle-related pain. Parental presence during the nerve block may also be helpful. In older children, allowing the child to listen to favorite music through a personal stereo or watch a video are useful distraction techniques that make the whole experience a more pleasant one for the child. We have connected a DVD player to our US machine, and this is used to play movies or cartoons through the monitor during the surgical procedure (E-Fig 42-1).

Before any USGRA procedure, intravenous access is established, standard monitoring is applied, and equipment and drugs appropriate for the child are prepared. Aseptic precautions are maintained, and the skin over the needle puncture site is prepared with antiseptic solution in the usual fashion. The US probe is prepared by covering the footprint with a sterile transparent dressing. It is important to avoid trapping any air between the transparent dressing and the footprint. This is done by gently stretching the transparent dressing before applying it on the footprint. The transducer and cable are then covered using a sterile plastic cover. We use the same plastic cover that our surgeons use to cover their laparoscopic camera.

## TIPS AND TRICKS FOR SUCCESS

Certain steps are common to all US-guided procedures, and, if followed, they may increase success. The lights in the room must be dimmed to avoid any glare or reflection from the US monitor. The operator must assume a comfortable position (Fig. 42-15). For upper extremity blocks, the operator sits at the ipsilateral head end of the child and the US machine is placed directly in front. For lower extremity blocks, such as femoral nerve block, the operator stands on the ipsilateral side of the child and the US machine is placed on the opposite side. For lower extremity or central neuraxial blocks in the lateral position, the operator sits behind the child and the US machine is placed in front, with the monitor in the line of view of the operator. Because of the small muscle bulk in young children the nerves are relatively superficial and can most frequently be easily visualized using high-frequency linear transducers. The exact choice of transducer depends on the area scanned, but a high-frequency linear transducer with a small footprint (13-6 MHz, 25-mm footprint) is particularly suited for young children. The 15-6–MHz broadband linear-array transducer, which has recently become available, is also useful for most blocks in young children. In older children, a 10-7–MHz broadband linear-array transducer, which allows greater flexibility with the depth of scan, is adequate for most procedures. Low-frequency (5-2 MHz) curved-array transducers are rarely used in children but are useful for imaging deeper structures such as the lumbar plexus and sciatic nerve in older children.

To improve dexterity, hold the transducer with the nondominant hand and perform interventions with the dominant hand.

Holding the transducer steady for even short periods can be quite testing. We have found that gently resting the hand that is holding the transducer on the child during a procedure helps to keep the transducer steady (see Fig. 42-15). It is important to maintain light contact between the transducer and the skin because excessive pressure in a child will cause the veins to collapse or distort the anatomy of the area of interest. Always apply liberal amounts of US gel to maintain adequate acoustic coupling between the skin and the transducer because even small amounts of air trapped between the two can result in artifacts. We use sterile US gel from single-use sachets for all US-guided peripheral nerve blocks. At any given time during an US-guided intervention either the transducer or the needle must be moved. It is impossible to maintain the needle within the plane of imaging if both are moving, a common error by novices. This results in an inability to visualize the needle. If the needle is not visible in the US image, a good strategy is to keep the needle steady and manipulate the transducer (slide, tilt, or rotate) until the needle becomes visible on the monitor. Thereafter the transducer should be held steady and the needle should be gently advanced to the target nerve, maintaining it in the imaging plane. When the angle of insertion of the needle is steep (greater than 60 degrees), it is preferable to introduce the needle in the short axis using the out-of-plane technique. However, if the in-plane approach is used for all US-guided interventions, as in our case, inserting the needle a few centimeters away from the edge of the transducer may improve needle visibility by decreasing the angle between the needle and the imaging plane.

Injecting air into the area of the intervention must be avoided at all cost because air bubbles in the field of imaging will degrade the US image. We routinely introduce the needle into the subcutaneous tissue and then purge it with saline or the local anesthetic to remove any air from the shaft of the needle, extension, and syringe system before proceeding with the block. An assistant aids with the injection. When the needle tip is close to the target nerve, the assistant gently aspirates to exclude unintended intravascular placement. The assistant must avoid generating excessive negative pressure because small blood vessels are prone to

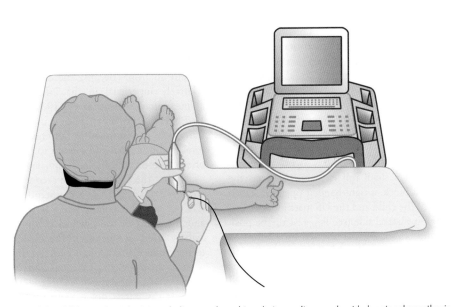

**FIGURE 42-15** Position of the child, anesthesiologist, and ultrasound machine during a ultrasound-guided regional anesthesia procedure.

collapse. A short length of extension tubing attached between the needle and the local anesthetic syringe allows the operator to hold the needle steady while the assistant performs the injection.[61] We routinely perform a test injection with 1 to 2 mL of saline or 5% dextrose (when nerve stimulation is also used) and visualize the distribution of the injectate in real time before injecting the local anesthetic. Failure to visualize the injectate in the US image indicates that the needle is not in the plane of imaging or it is intravascular until proven otherwise. No further injection should be made until the needle is repositioned and the distribution of the injectate is confirmed.

## ANCILLARY EQUIPMENT

Other than the US machine, equipment required for US-guided nerve block procedures in children is relatively simple. We are not aware of any needle that has been specifically designed for US-guided interventions in children but do believe that such equipment will be available in the future. In our experience, most single-shot peripheral nerve blocks can be performed with a standard short-bevel needle designed for regional anesthesia. In older children, we have found the 22-gauge Tuohy needle (B. Braun Medical Inc., Bethlehem, Pa.) to be a very useful alternative. The tip of the needle is relatively blunt, and its design (when introduced with the bevel facing upward) also allows it to be easily identified on US imaging. Moreover, graduations on the shaft of the needle provide useful cues about the depth to which the needle has been inserted. Insulated needles used for peripheral nerve stimulation (Stimuplex A, 50 or 100 mm, B. Braun Melsungen AG, Melsungen, Germany) are also suited for US-guided peripheral nerve blocks in children. Indwelling catheters also can be placed under US guidance; however, compared with single-shot techniques, experience with US-guided catheter placement for continuous peripheral nerve blocks in children is still limited. A standard epidural kit or an insulated continuous peripheral nerve block kit of an appropriate size can be used for catheter placement.

# Specific Ultrasound-Guided Nerve Blocks

## UPPER EXTREMITY BLOCKS

### Supraclavicular Brachial Plexus Block

Supraclavicular brachial plexus block has been described in children, although it is rarely used because of fear of pleural puncture and pneumothorax.[62] US-guided supraclavicular brachial plexus block has recently been successfully performed in a series of 17 children aged younger than 6 years for orthopedic upper limb surgeries.[63] Even though the brachial plexus and cervical pleura are clearly delineated using US in the supraclavicular fossa, this technique should be performed only by experienced operators because of the close proximity between the cervical pleura and the brachial plexus.

The child's head rests on a head ring and is slightly turned to the contralateral side, and a small roll is placed between the scapula. For a right-sided block, a right-handed operator stands or sits at the head end of the child and the US machine is placed directly in front on the ipsilateral side (see Fig. 42-15). The position of the operator and US machine is reversed for a left-sided block. In the supraclavicular fossa, the subclavian artery lies on top of the first rib. The trunks and divisions of the brachial plexus are superficial and lateral to the subclavian artery and sandwiched between the scalenus anterior and scalenus medius muscle (Fig. 42-16). A linear-array transducer (13-10 MHz) is used to perform

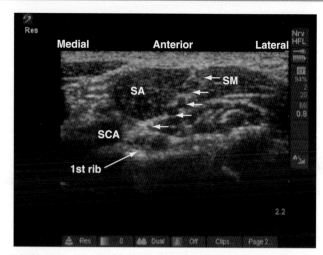

**FIGURE 42-16** Sonographic appearance of the brachial plexus (*white arrows*) in the supraclavicular fossa. *SA,* Scalenus anterior; *SCA,* subclavian artery; *SM,* scalenus medius.

the block; the hockey stick probe or a linear-array transducer with a small footprint (25 mm) is particularly suited for this block.

During the scout scan the transducer is positioned parallel to and against the clavicle and the subclavian artery is identified. The trunks and divisions of the brachial plexus often look like a bunch of grapes on the superficial and lateral aspect of the subclavian artery (see Fig. 42-16). The cervical pleura and lung are deep to the first rib. The operator should bear in mind that the acoustic shadow of the first rib can obscure the view of the pleura and lung (see also Fig. 41-21 and Chapter 41 for the landmark-guided techniques). The block needle is inserted in the long axis (in-plane) of the transducer in a lateral to medial direction, keeping the pleura in view. A test injection with saline is performed to ensure optimal needle position, after which the calculated dose of local anesthetic is injected in aliquots.

## INFRACLAVICULAR BRACHIAL PLEXUS BLOCK

US-guided infraclavicular brachial plexus block is performed with the child in the supine position. The block can be performed with the arms by the side, but it is preferable to abduct the arm (to 90 degrees) whenever possible because it elevates the lateral part of the clavicle, which makes more space available below the clavicle for transducer placement. The operator sits at the ipsilateral head end of the child, and the US machine is positioned directly in front. Because the cords of the brachial plexus are relatively superficial in the infraclavicular fossa in children, a linear-array transducer (13-10 MHz in young children and 10-7 MHz in the older child) is used to perform the block. The transducer is positioned in the sagittal plane over the deltopectoral region, medial and inferior to the coracoid process, with its orientation marker directed cephalad.

During the scout scan the second part of the axillary artery and the axillary vein are identified deep to the pectoral muscles (Fig. 42-17). The axillary artery is located superior to the vein, and the cords of the brachial plexus are closely related to the axillary artery at this level. The medial cord is situated caudal to the axillary artery, often between the axillary artery and vein, whereas the posterior and lateral cords are posterior and cephalad to the artery, respectively (see Fig. 42-17). Despite this relation, in most cases it is not easy to identify all three cords of the brachial plexus in a single plane of imaging. If the transducer is

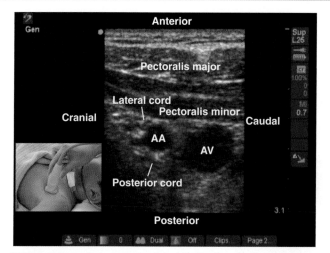

**FIGURE 42-17** Sagittal sonogram of the left infraclavicular fossa. *AA*, Axillary artery; *AV*, axillary vein.

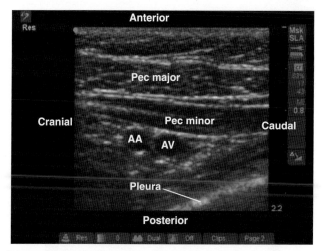

**FIGURE 42-18** Sagittal sonogram of the infraclavicular fossa with the transducer positioned medially. Note the hyperechoic pleura in the lower right corner of the image. *AA*, Axillary artery; *AV*, axillary vein; *Pec*, pectoralis.

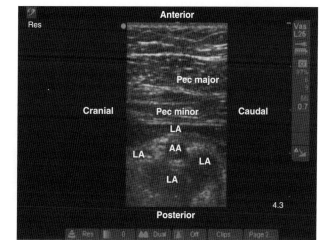

**FIGURE 42-19** Infraclavicular brachial plexus block. Sagittal sonogram of the infraclavicular fossa after local anesthetic injection demonstrating the circumferential spread of local anesthetic around the axillary artery—the "doughnut sign." *AA*, Axillary artery; *LA*, local anesthetic; *Pec*, pectoralis.

moved medially, the pleura usually comes into view (Fig. 42-18). In infants and young children, the margin of safety between the cords of the brachial plexus and the pleura is relatively small and pleural puncture is a risk if the block is performed in this medial position. Therefore we recommend that the infraclavicular brachial plexus block be performed laterally where the pleura is not visible in the US image.

We prefer to perform multiple injections targeting the areas where the three cords of the brachial plexus are located. The aim is to produce a circumferential spread of the local anesthetic around the axillary artery, the "doughnut sign" (Fig. 42-19), which correlates well with successful brachial plexus anesthesia.[64-71] This perivascular injection technique is best visualized by imagining the transverse image of the axillary artery as a clock face with its 12-o'clock position in its anterior aspect and the 6-o'clock position in the posterior aspect of the artery (Fig. 42-20). The block needle is inserted using in-plane technique from a cranial to caudal direction (see Fig. 42-20), and one third of the total dose of local anesthetic is injected close to each of the posterior (6-o'clock position), lateral (9-o'clock position), and medial (3-o'clock position) cords.[38] Because the angle of needle insertion

is fairly steep with this approach, the needle is rarely seen on the US image and the operator has to gently jiggle the needle to locate the needle tip. A subtle pop may be felt as the needle tip traverses the epimysium of the pectoralis minor muscle. A test injection with 1 to 2 mL of saline should be performed before the local anesthetic injection to ensure optimal needle position and distribution of the injectate (see also Fig. 41-20 and Chapter 41 for landmark-guided techniques).

## AXILLARY BRACHIAL PLEXUS BLOCK

US-guided axillary brachial plexus block is typically performed with the child in the supine position.[72-74] The arm is abducted (to 90 degrees) and externally rotated so that the palm of the hand is facing the ceiling. The operator sits at the ipsilateral head end of the child, and the US machine is positioned directly in front (see Fig. 42-15). Because the nerves of the brachial plexus are relatively superficial in the axilla a high-frequency linear-array transducer (13-6 MHz) is used. During the scout scan, the transducer is positioned just below the lateral border of the pectoralis major muscle, with its orientation marker directed laterally (Fig. 42-21). The resultant image in the monitor is a transverse scan of the axillary structures. The pulsatile vessel in the image is the axillary artery. The axillary vein is located medial to the artery. It is common to see more than one vein in the scan (see Fig. 42-21).

At this level, the three major nerves of the brachial plexus (the median, ulnar, and radial nerves) lie very close to the axillary artery. In adults, when the arm is abducted and externally rotated, the median nerve is located on the anterior or anterolateral side of the axillary artery (97.9%), the ulnar nerve is located on the anteromedial side of the artery (91.3%), and the radial nerve is located posterior to the axillary artery (89.9%) (Fig. 42-22).[75] No comparable data exist in children, but we find that the location of the median, ulnar, and radial nerves in children closely reflect those in adults. To accurately identify these three nerves it may be necessary to trace the nerve distally along its course. The musculocutaneous nerve is frequently seen between the coracobrachialis and the biceps muscle or within the substance of the coracobrachialis muscle (see Fig. 42-21).[76,77] Occasionally, the musculocutaneous nerve also may be located very close to the median nerve, and local anesthetic injected close to the median

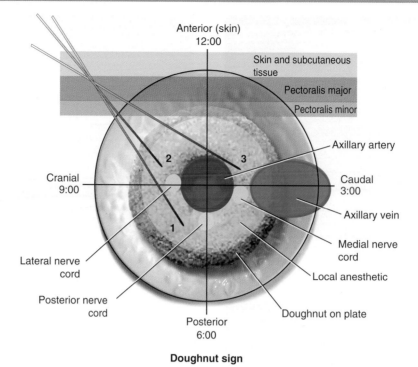

**Doughnut sign**

**FIGURE 42-20** Infraclavicular brachial plexus block. Schematic diagram showing the positions of the cords of the brachial plexus and the sites at which the local anesthetic is injected: (*1*) posterior cord, (*2*) lateral cord, and (*3*) medial cord.

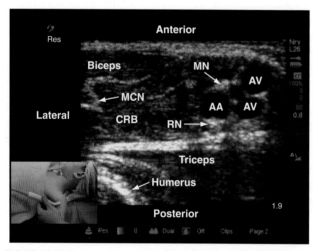

**FIGURE 42-21** Transverse sonogram of the left axilla. *AA,* Axillary artery; *AV,* axillary vein; *CRB,* coracobrachialis muscle; *MCN,* musculocutaneous nerve; *MN,* median nerve; *Res,* resolution; *RN,* radial nerve.

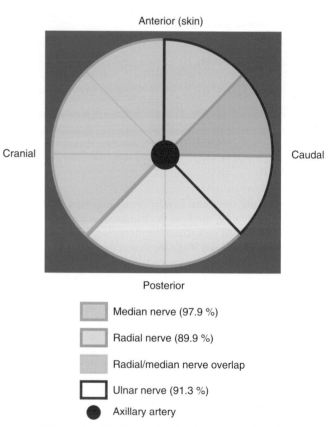

Median nerve (97.9 %)

Radial nerve (89.9 %)

Radial/median nerve overlap

Ulnar nerve (91.3 %)

Axillary artery

**FIGURE 42-22** Schematic diagram showing the positions of the three main nerves (median, radial, and ulnar) of the brachial plexus in relation to the axillary artery, as identified on transverse ultrasonography, at the axilla.

nerve may affect the musculocutaneous nerve. The shape of the musculocutaneous nerve varies along its course, and it may appear oval, round, elliptical, or even triangular.

We prefer the in-plane approach for needle insertion during axillary brachial plexus block in both sedated and anesthetized children. The block needle is inserted from the lateral to the medial side of the arm, keeping it within the plane of the US imaging. A subtle pop is often felt when the tip of the needle traverses the epimysium of the biceps muscle and enters the fascial plane containing the neurovascular bundle. Multiple injections are required to block the median, radial, and ulnar nerves. The objective is to produce a circumferential spread of local anesthetic around the artery (i.e., "the doughnut sign" in the US image). To achieve this, local anesthetic is injected close to the anterior (12-o'clock position), posterior (6-o'clock position), and lateral (9-o'clock position) aspects of the axillary artery. The musculocutaneous nerve is then identified and selectively blocked using a few milliliters of local anesthetic.[77] We have found this approach to be technically simple, safe, and effective in producing brachial plexus blockade in children (see also Fig. 41-19 and Chapter 41 for landmark-guided techniques).

## SELECTIVE PERIPHERAL NERVE BLOCKS OF THE UPPER EXTREMITY

Selective blockade of the nerves of the upper extremity is very rarely performed in children. It can be used to rescue incomplete or partial axillary brachial plexus block or provide analgesia or anesthesia over a specific dermatome.[78] We have also found it to be useful for US-guided differential nerve blockade in adults undergoing ambulatory hand surgery, and the same also may be applicable in children. In this technique an axillay brachial plexus block is performed using a short-acting local anesthetic agent such as lidocaine and combined with a peripheral nerve block (e.g., a median or ulnar nerve block, depending on the dermatomes involved) in the forearm using a long-acting drug (bupivacaine or ropivacaine). Because of the shorter duration of action of lidocaine compared with bupivacaine or ropivacaine, the child

regains protective motor function of the elbow fairly quickly after surgery (2 to 4 hours) while still enjoying prolonged postoperative analgesia from distal nerve blockade. All of the major nerves of the upper extremity (median, ulnar, and radial) can be identified using high-frequency linear-array transducers (13-10 MHz), and it is possible to selectively block these nerves at various sites along their course with only 1 to 2 mL of local anesthetic. We prefer the in-plane needle insertion technique and use a short-beveled block needle for this purpose.

### Median Nerve

The median nerve is closely related to the brachial artery throughout its course in the arm. In the upper part, it is lateral to the artery; in the middle of the arm it crosses the artery from the lateral to medial side and continues on the medial side all the way up to the elbow. In the antecubital fossa, the median nerve lies medial to the brachial artery, behind the bicipital aponeurosis, and in front of the brachialis muscle (Fig. 42-23). In the forearm, the median nerve is deep to the flexor digitorum superficialis and on the surface of the flexor digitorum profundus (Fig. 42-24) and accompanied by the median artery that is a branch of the anterior interosseous artery. Pulsations of the latter can occasionally be observed on the US image. A few centimeters proximal to the wrist, the median nerve becomes superficial and lies between the tendon of the flexor carpi radialis (laterally) and the

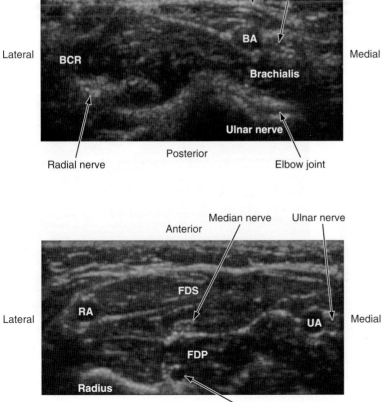

**FIGURE 42-23** Transverse sonogram of the cubital fossa. *BA,* Brachial artery; *BCR,* brachioradialis.

**FIGURE 42-24** Transverse sonogram of the forearm. *FDP,* Flexor digitorum profundus; *FDS,* flexor digitorum superficialis; *RA,* radial artery; *UA,* ulnar artery.

flexor digitorum superficialis (medially) and may also be over-lapped by the tendon of the palmaris longus. Because the nerve is superficial at this level and it can be difficult to differentiate the nerve from the tendons, we prefer to perform median nerve block at the midforearm, where it is clearly delineated (see also Fig. 41-22 and Chapter 41 for landmark-guided techniques).

### Ulnar Nerve

In the arm, the ulnar nerve runs on the medial side of the brachial artery up to about the midhumeral level or the insertion of the coracobrachialis muscle, where it pierces the medial intermuscular septum and enters the posterior compartment of the arm. At the elbow, it passes behind the medial epicondyle to enter the ulnar nerve sulcus. Although the nerve is palpable and superficial at the sulcus, it is often difficult to visualize using US because of bony and contact artifacts. The ulnar nerve then enters the proximal forearm and runs between the flexor digitorum profundus (posterior) and the flexor digitorum superficialis (laterally) muscles, and in the distal forearm it is accompanied by the ulnar artery (lateral) (see Fig. 42-24). Close to the wrist, the ulnar nerve is lateral to the flexor carpi ulnaris muscle. The ulnar artery may be used as a reference to locate the ulnar nerve. Once the artery is located, the nerve is traced backward and the local anesthetic injection is performed away from the artery (see Chapter 41 for landmark-guided techniques).[79]

### Radial Nerve

In the arm the radial nerve is posterior to the brachial artery. It then leaves the artery to enter the radial (spiral) groove on the back of the arm, where it is accompanied by the profunda brachii artery. In the distal arm the radial nerve pierces the lateral intermuscular septum and enters the anterior compartment. In the antecubital fossa it is lateral to the biceps tendon and lies in an intermuscular gap between the brachialis (medially), the brachioradialis, and the extensor carpi radialis longus (laterally) (Fig. 42-25). At the level of the lateral epicondyle the radial nerve gives off the posterior interosseous nerve (deep branch of the radial nerve), which leaves the fossa by piercing the supinator muscle. In the forearm, the radial nerve (superficial branch of the radial nerve) continues as a pure cutaneous nerve and supplies the radial half of the dorsum of the hand and the proximal parts of the dorsal surfaces of the thumb and index finger. The radial nerve is best blocked before its division in the antecubital fossa (see also Figs. 41-2, 41-23, and Chapter 41 for landmark-guided techniques).[78]

## LOWER EXTREMITY BLOCKS

### Lumbar Plexus Block

The lumbar plexus results from the union of the ventral rami of the first four lumbar spinal nerves within the substance of the psoas major muscle[80] The plexus may also receive contributions from the 12th thoracic nerve or the 5th lumbar nerve. In adults, the plexus is located between the fleshy anterior part of the psoas major muscle, which arises from the anterolateral part of the vertebral bodies and the intervertebral disc, and the accessory posterior part of the muscle that originates from the anterior surface of the transverse process.[81] Local anesthetic injected into this intramuscular plane, also referred to as the *psoas compartment*, produces ipsilateral lumbar plexus block.

An US scan for the lumbar plexus block can be performed in the transverse or sagittal axis at the L3-4 vertebral level. The child is positioned in the lateral position with the side to be blocked uppermost with the hip and knees flexed. A linear-array transducer (10-5 MHz) is adequate for imaging in young children, whereas in the older child (older than 6 to 8 years) a curved-array transducer (8-5 or 5-2 MHz) is required.

For a transverse scan,[82] the US transducer is positioned approximately 2 to 3 cm lateral to the lumbar spine at the L3-4 vertebral level, with its orientation marker directed laterally. We also prefer to align the transducer slightly medially so as to produce a paramedian oblique transverse scan (PMOTS) of the lumbar paravertebral region. Also during a PMOTS of the lumbar paravertebral region, the US beam can be insonated either at the level of the transverse process (PMOTS-TP, Fig. 42-26) or through the gap between the two adjacent transverse process (i.e., the intertransverse space [ITS]) producing a PMOTS-ITS scan (Fig. 42-27). In a typical PMOTS-ITS sonogram of the lumbar paravertebral region, the erector spinae muscle, the vertebral body, the psoas major muscle, quadratus lumborum muscle, and the

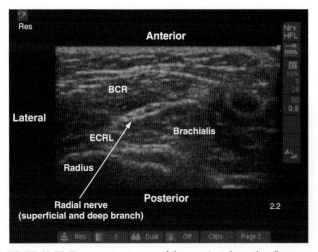

**FIGURE 42-25** Transverse sonogram of the arm, just above the elbow, showing the radial nerve. *BCR*, Brachioradialis; *ECRL*, extensor carpi radialis longus.

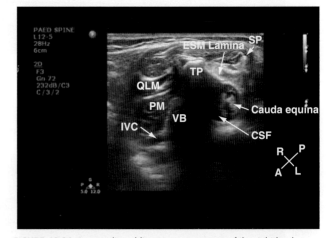

**FIGURE 42-26** Paramedian oblique transverse scan of the right lumbar paravertebral region at the level of the transverse process (PMOTS-TP) in a 11-month old infant. Note how the acoustic shadow of the transverse process (*TP*) obscures the posterior part of the psoas muscle (*PM*) and how parts of the spinal canal and neuraxial structures (dura, intrathecal space, and cauda equina) are seen through the interlaminar space. *CSF*, Cerebrospinal fluid; *ESM*, erector spinae muscle; *IVC*, inferior vena cava; *QLM*, quadratus lumborum muscle; *SP*, spinous process; *VB*, vertebral body.

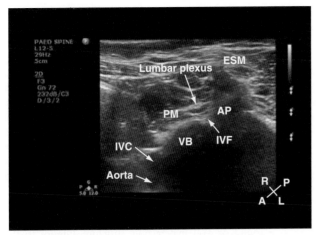

**FIGURE 42-27** Paramedian oblique transverse scan of the right paravertebral region through the gap between two adjacent transverse processes (PMOTS-ITS) in a 14-month old child. Note the intervertebral foramen (*IVF*), articular process (*AP*), and the lumbar plexus in the posterior part of the psoas muscle (*PM*). *ESM,* Erector spinae muscle; *IVC,* inferior vena cava; *PM,* psoas muscle.

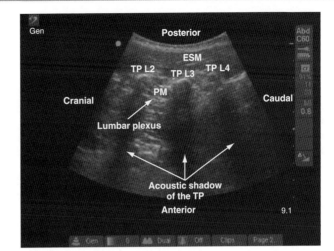

**FIGURE 42-28** Longitudinal sonogram of the lumbar paravertebral region showing the lumbar plexus. *ESM,* Erector spinae muscle; *PM,* psoas muscle; *TP,* transverse process ("trident sign").

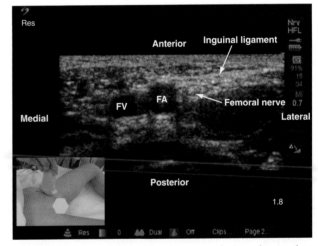

**FIGURE 42-29** Transverse sonogram of the inguinal region showing the femoral nerve and its relations. *FA,* Femoral artery; *FV,* femoral vein.

anterolateral surface of the vertebral body are clearly visualized (see Fig. 42-27). The inferior vena cava (on the right side) and the aorta (on the left side) are also identified anterior to the vertebral body. The lower pole of the kidney is closely related to the anterior surfaces of the quadratus lumborum and psoas muscle and is seen as an oval structure that moves with respiration in the retroperitoneal space. The lumbar plexus is not sonographically visualized in all patients, but when it is visualized, it appears as an oval hyperechoic structure in the posterior part of the psoas muscle (see Fig. 42-27) and close to the intervertebral foramen. In contrast, because the acoustic shadow of the transverse process obscures the posterior part of the psoas muscle and the area close to the intervertebral foramen during a PMOTS-TP, the lumbar plexus is rarely visualized in this US scan window (see Fig. 42-26). Therefore, if a transverse scan is performed during an ultrasound-guided lumbar plexus block, it is our recommendation to use the PMOTS-ITS.

For a sagittal scan of the lumbar paravertebral region, the US transducer is positioned approximately 2 to 3 cm lateral and parallel to the lumbar spine,[83] with its orientation marker directed cranially. In a typical sagittal sonogram of the lumbar paravertebral region, the L2, L3, and L4 transverse processes with their acoustic shadow produce what we refer to as the "trident sign" (Fig. 42-28) because of its similarity to the trident (*Limia tridens* or *tridentis*) that is often associated with Poseidon (the god of the sea in Greek mythology) and the trishula of the Hindu god Shiva. The hypoechoic psoas muscle is seen between the transverse processes, and the lumbar plexus is identified as hyperechoic longitudinal striations within the posterior aspect of the muscle. A laterally positioned transducer will produce a suboptimal scan without the trident, and the lower pole of the kidney, which can reach the L4-5 level in young children, will come into view.

Once an optimal image of lumber paravertebral region is obtained, the insulated block needle is inserted in the plane of the US beam. The needle is inserted from the medial side of transducer when a PMOTS-ITS is used or from the caudal end of the transducer when a sagittal scan is used. The needle is slowly advanced under ultrasound guidance to the posterior part of the psoas muscle, and the correct position of the needle tip close to

the lumbar plexus is confirmed by observing ipsilateral quadriceps muscle contraction. After negative aspiration, an appropriate dose of local anesthetic is injected in aliquots over 2 to 3 minutes and the patient is closely monitored.

### Femoral Nerve Block

The femoral nerve is the largest branch of the lumbar plexus and is the major nerve of the anterior (extensor) compartment of the thigh. It is formed by the dorsal division of the anterior primary rami of spinal nerves L2, L3, and L4. It exits the pelvis and enters the femoral triangle in the thigh by passing under the inguinal ligament just lateral to the femoral artery. In the thigh it lies in the groove between the iliacus and the psoas major muscle, outside the femoral sheath, and lateral to the artery. A high-frequency (13-10 MHz) linear-array transducer is used to scan the femoral nerve.[36,84] On a transverse sonogram the femoral nerve is seen as an oval or triangular hyperechoic structure lateral to the femoral artery (Fig. 42-29). The femoral nerve exhibits marked anisotropy, and it may be necessary to tilt or rotate the transducer during the scan before it can be visualized. In young children one must avoid exerting too much pressure during the scan because it is easy to collapse the femoral vein.

A femoral nerve block is used to provide postoperative analgesia after femoral fractures. It is performed with the child in the supine position. The ipsilateral lower limb is slightly abducted and externally rotated, and the knee is also slightly flexed. A right-handed operator stands on the right side of the child, and the US machine is positioned directly in front on the contralateral side. The sides of the operator and the US machine are reversed for a left-handed operator. The scout scan is performed with the transducer positioned parallel and just below the inguinal ligament. This ensures that the femoral nerve is scanned before its division. Once an optimal view of the femoral nerve is obtained, the block needle is inserted in the long axis (in-plane) of the US transducer from the lateral to medial side and directed to the lateral aspect of the femoral nerve. A test injection with saline (1 to 2 mL) is performed before the local anesthetic is injected to confirm that the needle is deep to the fascia iliaca and to observe the distribution of the injectate in relation to the femoral nerve (see also Fig. 41-32 and Chapter 41 for landmark-guided techniques).

### Subsartorial Saphenous Nerve Block

The saphenous nerve is a branch of the anterior division of the femoral nerve and supplies the skin on the medial aspect of the leg and foot up to the ball of the big toe. In the thigh, the saphenous nerve is located in the subsartorial canal and local anesthetic injected into this intramuscular space produces a saphenous nerve block.[85-87] The subsartorial canal is also referred to as the adductor canal or Hunter's canal and is situated on the medial side of the middle one third of the thigh and extends from the apex of the femoral triangle, above, to the tendinous opening in the adductor magnus muscle, below. The canal is triangular in cross section, and its anterior wall is formed by the vastus medialis muscle, the posterior wall or floor is formed by the adductor longus, and the medial wall or roof is formed by a strong fibrous membrane that is overlapped by the sartorius muscle (Fig. 42-30). The subsartorial canal contains the following structures: femoral artery and vein, saphenous nerve, nerve to vastus medialis, and the two divisions of the obturator nerve. The femoral vein lies posterior to the artery in the upper part and

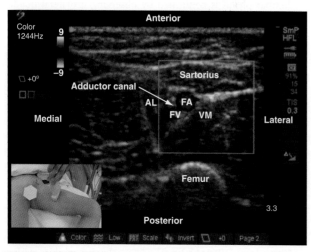

**FIGURE 42-30** Transverse sonogram of the thigh showing the adductor canal. *AL,* Adductor longus; *FA,* femoral artery; *FV,* femoral vein; *VM,* vastus medialis.

lateral to the artery in the lower part of the canal. The saphenous nerve crosses the femoral artery anteriorly from the lateral to the medial side in the canal.

A high-frequency (13-6 MHz) linear-array probe is used to scan the saphenous nerve in the subsartorial canal with the child the supine position. The ipsilateral lower limb is slightly abducted and externally rotated, and the knee is also slightly flexed. For a right-sided block, a right-handed operator stands on the right side of the patient and the US machine is positioned directly in front on the contralateral side. The transducer is positioned in the transverse axis over the middle one third of the thigh. The triangular subsartorial canal can be identified between the epimysium of the vastus medialis (closely related to the femur), the adductor longus, and the sartorius muscles. The pulsatile femoral artery lies anterior to the vein in the canal, and the saphenous nerve is seen as a round or oval hyperechoic structure anterior to the artery (12-o'clock position). Because the saphenous nerve is a small nerve, it may not always be visible on US imaging in children. However, owing to the close relation of the saphenous nerve to the femoral artery in the subsartorial canal, a perivascular (arterial) injection in the canal will produce saphenous nerve block. The block needle is inserted in the long-axis (in-plane) of the US transducer from the medial to lateral side and is directed to the anterior aspect of the femoral artery. A test injection of saline (1 to 2 mL) is performed to confirm that the tip of the needle is in the canal, after which the local anesthetic is injected.

### Sciatic Nerve Block

The sciatic nerve is the largest mixed nerve in the body and arises from the lumbosacral plexus (L4, L5, S1-3). It innervates the posterior aspect of the thigh and the entire lower limb below the knee except for a small patch of skin on the medial aspect of the leg and ankle, which is innervated by the saphenous nerve. Sciatic nerve block is frequently used to provide analgesia for foot (clubfoot) and leg surgery in children. Several different approaches to the sciatic nerve have been described in the literature. Most approaches described to date rely on surface anatomic landmarks (anterior, transgluteal, infragluteal, lateral, posterior subgluteal, proximal thigh, or at the popliteal fossa). Recently, US-guided sciatic nerve block also has been described.[88,89] A proximal approach to the sciatic nerve is selected when surgery involves the hip (rare in children) or block of the posterior cutaneous nerve of the thigh is warranted. Because sciatic nerve block is most frequently used for foot (clubfoot) surgery in children, a distal approach to the sciatic nerve at the popliteal fossa is usually preferred (see also Fig. 41-31 and Chapter 41 for landmark-guided techniques).

### Sciatic Nerve Block at the Subgluteal Space

The sciatic nerve exits the pelvis through the greater sciatic foramen, between the piriformis and the superior gemelli muscles, and enters the subgluteal space below the piriformis muscle. It then descends over the dorsum of the ischium, lying on the dorsal surface of the gemellus superior muscle, tendon of obturator internus, gemellus inferior muscle, and quadratus femoris muscle (in a cranial to caudal relation) before it enters the hollow between the greater trochanter and the ischial tuberosity and then goes on to the posterior compartment of the thigh. The anterior surface of the gluteus maximus covers the upper part of the sciatic nerve; and immediately distal to its lower border (infragluteal position), the sciatic nerve is fairly superficial. In between the greater trochanter and the ischial tuberosity, the sciatic nerve lies

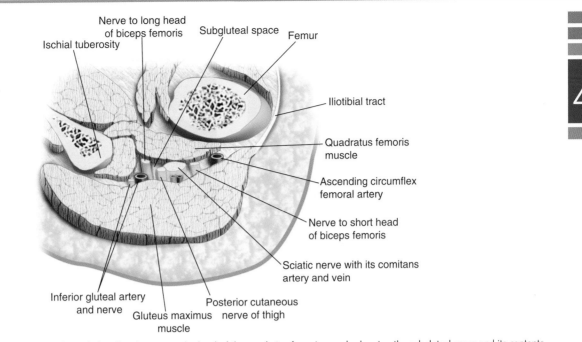

**FIGURE 42-31** Transverse section through the gluteal region at the level of the quadratus femoris muscle showing the subgluteal space and its contents.

in the subgluteal space, which is a well-defined anatomic space between the anterior surface of the gluteus maximus and the posterior surface of the quadratus femoris muscle (Fig. 42-31).[88,89] Other structures that are present in the subgluteal space include the posterior cutaneous nerve of the thigh, inferior gluteal vessels and nerve, nerve to the short and long head of the biceps femoris, the comitans artery and vein of the sciatic nerve, and the ascending branch of the medial circumflex artery (see Fig. 42-31). Local anesthetic injected into the subgluteal space blocks not only the sciatic nerve but also the posterior cutaneous nerve of the thigh. The latter is useful when anesthesia over the posterior aspect of the thigh is needed.

US-guided sciatic nerve block at the subgluteal space is performed with the child in the lateral position. The side to be anesthetized is placed uppermost, and the hip and knees are flexed (Fig. 42-32). The operator sits or stands behind the child, and the US machine is positioned directly in front. In young children, a linear-array transducer (10-5 MHz) is adequate for imaging the sciatic nerve. In children older than 6 to 8 years, the sciatic nerve can also be imaged using a linear-array transducer (10-5 MHz). However, the increased depth of scan required (as a result of increased muscle bulk) limits the field of vision because as the depth of scan increases the field of vision becomes narrower when a linear transducer is used. Therefore a curved-array transducer (8-5 or 5-2 MHz) with a wide field of vision is preferable in older children.

The greater trochanter and the ischial tuberosity are identified, and a line is drawn between these two landmarks. The US transducer is placed parallel to this line, with its orientation marker directed toward the greater trochanter to obtain a transverse scan of the sciatic nerve and the subgluteal space. It may be necessary to slide the transducer slightly cephalad or caudad before an optimal image of the sciatic nerve in the subgluteal space can be obtained. On a sonogram, the subgluteal space is seen as a hypoechoic area between the hyperechoic epimysium of the gluteus maximus and quadratus femoris muscle (see Fig. 42-32) extending from the greater trochanter laterally to the ischial

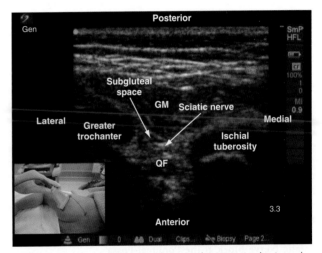

**FIGURE 42-32** Transverse sonogram between the greater trochanter and the ischial tuberosity showing the hypoechoic subgluteal space between the hyperechoic perimysium of the gluteus maximus and the quadratus femoris muscle. The sciatic nerve is seen as a hyperechoic structure in the medial aspect of the subgluteal space. *GM*, Gluteus maximus; *QF*, quadratus femoris.

tuberosity medially.[88,89] The subgluteal space is not so well delineated in young children and is better visualized in older children. The sciatic nerve is seen as an oval or triangular hyperechoic structure within the subgluteal space (see Fig. 42-32). The medial limit of the space is obscured by the attachments of the semimembranosus, semitendinosus, and biceps femoris muscles to the ischial tuberosity. Pulsationf of the inferior gluteal artery often can be detected medial to the sciatic nerve on the sonogram.

The block needle is inserted using in-plane technique from the ischial tuberosity side and advanced slowly toward the sciatic nerve. Once the block needle is deemed to be in the subgluteal space, the position is confirmed by injecting 1 to 3 mL of saline through the needle and observing a distention of the subgluteal space (i.e., separation of the epimysium of the gluteus maximus

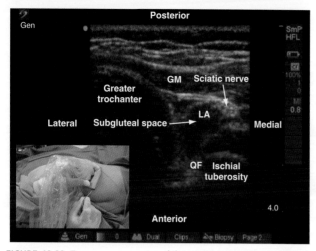

**FIGURE 42-33** Transverse sonogram of the sciatic nerve at the subgluteal space after local anesthetic injection. Note the distention of the subgluteal space caused by the local anesthetic and the distribution of local anesthetic around the sciatic nerve. *GM,* Gluteus maximus; *LA,* local anesthetic; *QF,* quadratus femoris.

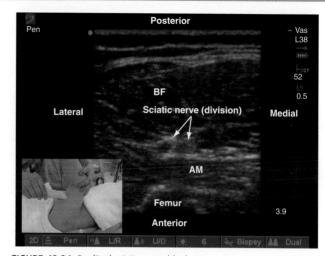

**FIGURE 42-34** Popliteal sciatic nerve block. Transverse sonogram of the sciatic nerve at the apex of the popliteal fossa. *AM,* Adductor magnus; *BF,* biceps femoris.

and quadratus femoris muscle) on the US image (Fig. 42-33). However, if the test injection of saline is seen to spread posterior to the epimysium of the gluteus maximus muscle, it indicates that the tip of the needle is not in the subgluteal space. The needle should be reoriented and advanced a little farther until the typical distention of the subgluteal space to the saline test injection is seen. Occasionally, a subtle pop is felt when the needle tip traverses the epimysium of the gluteus maximus muscle and enters the subgluteal space. Local anesthetic is then injected in aliquots over 2 to 3 minutes while observing for the distention of the subgluteal space and the spread of local anesthetic in relation to the sciatic nerve. It is also easy to pass a catheter into the subgluteal space when a continuous sciatic nerve block is planned. Because the catheter is inserted into an anatomic space, the catheter is also more likely to stay in situ (see also Figs. 41-28, 41-29, and 41-31, and Chapter 41 for landmark-based techniques).

### Sciatic Nerve Block at the Popliteal Fossa

The sciatic nerve block at the popliteal fossa is also referred to as the *popliteal fossa block* and is the preferred approach for sciatic nerve block in children undergoing foot surgery. The popliteal fossa is a diamond-shaped space lying behind the knee joint, the lower part of the femur, and the upper part of the tibia. It is bound superolaterally by the tendon of biceps femoris, superomedially by the tendon of semitendinosus and the semimembranosus, inferolaterally by the lateral head of gastrocnemius, and inferomedially by the medial head of gastrocnemius. The sciatic nerve enters the posterior aspect of the thigh at the lower border of the gluteus maximus and runs vertically downward to the apex of the superior triangle of the popliteal fossa, where it terminates by dividing into the tibial and the common peroneal nerve, usually 3 to 7 cm above the popliteal crease.[90,91] The division of the sciatic nerve into its terminal branches may, however, take place anywhere above this level. This accounts for the occasional sparing of either division of the sciatic nerve after distal sciatic nerve block techniques using nerve stimulation.

Although the classic teaching is to perform popliteal sciatic nerve block with the patient in the prone position, it is very

commonly performed in children with the child in the supine position with the leg elevated by an assistant (Fig. 42-34). During US-guided popliteal sciatic nerve block the operator sits on the ipsilateral side facing the head of the patient and the US machine is positioned directly in front. In young children, a linear-array transducer (10-5 MHz) is adequate for imaging the sciatic nerve in the popliteal fossa. In the adolescent child or children with muscular thighs, a curved-array transducer (8-5 MHz) may be preferable. The transducer is positioned just above the apex of the upper triangle of the popliteal fossa in the transverse axis (see Fig. 42-34). It may be necessary to first scan for the sciatic nerve in the middle of the thigh and then trace it distally to the popliteal fossa, where the sciatic nerve is seen as a round, hyperechoic structure. Division of the sciatic nerve into the tibial and common peroneal nerve can also be visualized in children; location of this division varies widely among children. In the popliteal fossa and proximal to the popliteal crease, the tibial and common peroneal nerve are seen as hyperechoic structures superficial and lateral to the popliteal artery.

The block needle is inserted using in-plane technique from the lateral aspect of the thigh with its point of entry being anterior to the tendon of the biceps femoris (if it is palpable). This places the needle in the same orientation as for the lateral approach to the sciatic nerve at the popliteal fossa. The exact point of needle entry will depend on where the sciatic nerve is best visualized. The needle is gradually advanced under US guidance, and the tip is positioned just posterior to the sciatic nerve. This is confirmed by injecting 1 to 3 mL of saline through the needle, after which half of the calculated dose of local anesthetic is injected. The same process is repeated by repositioning the tip of the needle anterior to the sciatic nerve. This ensures that the local anesthetic spreads optimally around the sciatic nerve (see also Fig. 41-30 and Chapter 41 for landmark-guided techniques).

### TRUNCAL BLOCKS

### Rectus Sheath Block

Rectus sheath block is the technique of injecting local anesthetic into the potential space between the rectus muscle and the posterior rectus sheath. This produces anesthesia of the ventral rami of the intercostal nerves as they traverse the rectus muscle to supply the skin of the anterior abdominal wall on either side of the midline. Because the seventh and eight intercostal nerves also provide motor innervation to the rectus abdominis muscle, a rectus sheath block at this level should also produce relaxation of the muscle. Bilateral rectus sheath blocks are frequently used in children to provide perioperative analgesia during umbilical and paraumbilical hernia.[92] We have also found it to be useful for analgesia after laparoscopic procedures in children in whom the port insertion sites are close to the midline.

The rectus abdominis muscle arises as two tendinous heads from the lateral part of the pubic crest and the anterior pubic ligament. The fibers run vertically upward and are inserted to the front of the chest wall through the xiphoid process and the 5th, 6th, and 7th costal cartilages. The muscle is enclosed in a fibrous aponeurotic sheath, the rectus sheath, which is formed by the aponeurosis of the external oblique, internal oblique, and transversus abdominis muscles. The anterior rectus sheath is complete and covers the muscle from end to end. However, the posterior rectus sheath is incomplete, being deficient above the costal cartilage and below the arcuate line (or the fold of Douglas), which is located midway between the umbilicus and the pubic symphysis. The rectus sheath on both sides is held together in the midline by a raphe, the linea alba, which is formed by the fusion of the fibers of the three aponeuroses that form the rectus sheath. The ventral rami of the 7th to 12th intercostal nerves pass anteriorly and downward from the intercostal spaces and pierce the posterolateral aspect of the rectus sheath before passing anteriorly through the muscle to supply the skin of the anterior abdominal wall. Three transverse fibrous bands (tendinous insertions), one at the level of the umbilicus, one at the level of the xiphoid process, and one midway between the two, divide the rectus muscle into three smaller parts. These fibrous bands are adherent to the anterior rectus sheath and traverse only the anterior half of the rectus muscle. Therefore a potential space exists between the rectus muscle and the posterior rectus sheath that communicates from the xiphisternum to the pubic crest. Local anesthetic injected into this space can spread up and down the sheath and is the basis of a rectus sheath tumor.

A linear-array transducer (13-10 MHz) with a small footprint (25 mm) is used for imaging in children (E-Fig. 42-2). The operator stands or sits on one side of the anesthetized child, and the US machine is positioned directly opposite on the contralateral side. The transducer is positioned in the longitudinal axis midway between the umbilicus and the xiphisternum. The rectus muscle is seen as a hypoechoic structure between the hyperechoic anterior and posterior rectus sheath (see E-Fig. 42-2). Deep to the posterior rectus sheath the hyperechoic peritoneum can be recognized by its typical peritoneal sliding movement and the "comet-tail" artifacts produced. The fibrous bands (tendinous insertions) in the rectus sheath can also be recognized in the longitudinal sonogram as hyperechoic areas on the anterior surface of the hypoechoic muscle that do not traverse the whole muscle belly.[93,94] The linea alba can be recognized on a transverse sonogram, and the posterior deficiency of the rectus sheath is also readily recognized below the level of the arcuate line.

The block needle is inserted using in-plane technique in a caudal to cranial direction (E-Fig. 42-3). When the tip of the needle is visualized in the potential space between the rectus muscle and the posterior rectus sheath, a test injection of saline (1 to 3 mL) is performed to confirm the longitudinal spread of the injectate between the muscle and the rectus sheath and the widening of the space (see E-Fig. 42-3, *C* and *D*). Injection into the muscle will offer resistance to injection and is readily

recognized in the sonogram. The needle should be repositioned, and the typical spread of the test injection under the rectus muscle should be confirmed before a calculated dose of the local anesthetic is injected. For umbilical hernia surgery, bilateral rectus sheath blocks are performed just above the umbilicus on either side (see also Fig. 41-16 and Chapter 41 for landmark-guided techniques).

## Ilioinguinal and Iliohypogastric Nerve Blocks

Ilioinguinal and iliohypogastric nerve blocks are used to provide analgesia after inguinal hernia repair, orchidopexy, or hydrocele surgery. The analgesia is comparable to caudal epidural analgesia, and it offers the advantage of not affecting micturition after surgery,[95] making it ideal for analgesia in children undergoing an outpatient procedure. Currently, anatomic landmarks and tactile sensations are relied on to perform the block,[95] which unfortunately can result in failure in up to 20% to 30% of cases. Moreover, it can also lead to complications such as femoral nerve palsy,[96,97] pelvic hematoma,[98] and bowel perforation.[99] A US-guided ilioinguinal iliohypogastric nerve block has been described in children.[21,100] Compared with the traditional landmark-based method, US-guided ilioinguinal iliohypogastric nerve block is accomplished more accurately, using smaller volumes of local anesthetic, and has a greater success rate.

The ilioinguinal and iliohypogastric nerves are branches of the primary ventral ramus of L1, which arises from the lumbar plexus. It also receives contributions from the T12 spinal nerve. Superomedial to the anterior superior iliac spine (ASIS), the two nerves pierce the transversus abdominis muscle to lie between it and the internal oblique muscle. The iliohypogastric nerve is situated superior to the ilioinguinal nerve and continues inferomedially for a short distance, after which their ventral rami transverse the internal oblique muscle to lie between the internal and external oblique muscles before giving off branches that pierce the external oblique muscle to provide cutaneous sensation. The iliohypogastric nerve supplies sensory innervation to the skin over the inguinal region. The ilioinguinal nerve continues anteroinferiorly with the spermatic cord or the round ligament of the uterus in the inguinal canal and becomes superficial by emerging through the superficial inguinal ring to innervate the skin of the upper medial aspect of the thigh and either the skin of the upper part of the scrotum and the root of the penis or the skin covering the labia majora and mons pubis.

A linear-array transducer (13-10 MHz) is used for the imaging and the ilioinguinal and iliohypogastric nerves, which are best visualized close to the ASIS. The operator stands on the ipsilateral side to be blocked, and the US machine is positioned directly opposite on the contralateral side. The transducer is positioned close to the ASIS and parallel to a line joining the ASIS and the umbilicus (Fig. 42-35). The ilioinguinal and iliohypogastric nerves are identified as two small, rounded structures lying side by side between the internal oblique and transversus abdominis muscle (see Fig. 42-35). The external oblique is frequently identified only as a hyperechoic aponeurotic layer at the point of needle insertion. Deep to the transversus abdominis muscle the peritoneum and the bowel are also visualized (see Fig. 42-35).

The block needle is inserted in the long axis (in-plane) of the US beam in a medial to lateral direction (Fig. 42-36). We prefer this orientation because it facilitates visualization of the needle (in-plane) and, in the event that the needle is inadvertently inserted too deep, further passage is obstructed by the iliac bone,

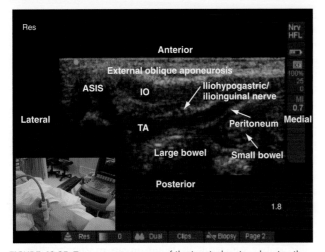

**FIGURE 42-35** Transverse sonogram of the inguinal region showing the ilioinguinal and iliohypogastric nerves and its relation to the abdominal musculature. *ASIS,* Anterior superior iliac spine; *IO,* internal oblique; *TA,* transverse abdominis.

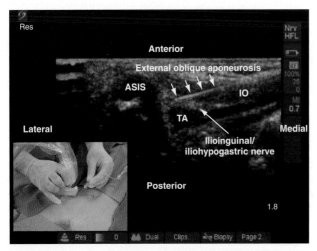

**FIGURE 42-36** Ilioinguinal iliohypogastric nerve block. The in-plane needle insertion technique. *ASIS,* Anterior superior iliac spine; *IO,* internal oblique; *TA,* transverse abdominis.

thus reducing the potential for a major complication such as bowel perforation. When the tip of the needle is close to the two nerves, a test injection is performed with 0.5 to 1 mL of normal saline. Correct position of the needle tip is confirmed by observing the widening of the tissue plane between the internal oblique and the transversus abdominis muscle. A calculated dose of a long-acting local anesthetic (0.2 mL/kg) is then injected through the needle, and the spread of the local anesthetic to both nerves is visualized (see also Fig. 41-14 and Chapter 41 for landmark-guided techniques).

### Transversus Abdominis Plane (TAP) Block

The sensory supply of the abdominal wall is provided by the anterior rami of the T7 to L1 thoracolumbar nerves. T7 to T9 innervate the skin above the umbilicus, T10 innervates the skin around the umbilicus, and T11, T12 (cutaneous branches of the subcostal nerve), and L1 (iliohypogastric and ilioinguinal nerves) innervate the skin below the umbilicus. These nerves pass infero-anteriorly in a plane between the internal oblique and transversus

abdominis muscles, also known as the transversus abdominis plane (TAP). The lateral cutaneous branch is given off at the midaxillary line and innervates the abdominal wall up to the lateral edge of the rectus abdominis muscle. The segmental nerve then courses anteriorly and medially toward the midline in the TAP to penetrate the lateral margin of the rectus sheath and emerge anteriorly though the rectus muscle as the anterior cutaneous branch. The lateral and anterior cutaneous branches of the thoracolumbar nerves supply the skin form the midline to the anterior axillary line. The thoracolumbar nerves, as they course through the TAP, also supply muscular branches to the abdominal musculature.

Local anesthetic injected into the TAP plane produce sensorimotor blockade (segmental) of the abdominal wall, and two techniques, the posterior TAP block and subcostal TAP block, have been described.[101,102] In the posterior TAP block the local anesthetic is injected in the TAP plane between the iliac crest and the costal margin, and during a subcostal TAP block the local anesthetic is injected into the TAP plane just below the costal margin at the midclavicular line. Anesthesia and analgesia produced by a TAP block is unilateral; thus it is useful for surgical procedures (e.g., orchidopexy, herniotomy, appendicectomy) in which the incision does not cross the midline. Bilateral TAP blocks are indicated for abdominal surgical procedures in which the surgical incision is in the midline or across the midline. It is also the authors' practice to perform bilateral TAP blocks for laparoscopic procedures. Because TAP blocks do not produce visceral analgesia, they should be used as part of a multimodal analgesic regimen for perioperative analgesia. Currently, published data on the use of TAP blocks for perioperative analgesia in children are limited[101,103] but may be useful as an alternative when central neuraxial blocks are contraindicated (e.g., in children with underlying coagulopathy or spinal dysraphism).

For a posterior TAP block, a high-frequency linear array transducer (15-7 MHz) is placed midway between the iliac crest and the costal margin along the midaxillary line (Fig. 42-37, *A*). For infants and young children, a linear transducer with a small footprint (25 mm) is preferred. The operator stands or sits on one side of the anesthetized child, and the US machine is positioned directly opposite on the contralateral side. The various layers of the abdominal wall are identified on the sonogram (see Fig. 42-37, *B*). From superficial to deep, they include a layer of subcutaneous tissue and fat and the three abdominal muscles with their fascial layers (i.e., the external oblique, internal oblique, and the transversus abdominis muscles, respectively). Deep to the transversus abdominis muscle the hypoechoic peritoneum is also visualized (see Fig. 42-37, *B*). The block needle (50 mm) is inserted 1 to 2 cm medial to the medial edge of the ultrasound transducer (Fig. 42-37, *C*), depending on the depth at which the TAP is located (can be determined using the electronic caliper in the US system), and in the plane of the US beam. Because the abdominal wall in infants and young children is relatively thin, and to avoid inadvertent deep needle insertion and visceral puncture it is the authors' practice to initially insert the block needle directed toward the US transducer rather than in an anteroposterior direction. Once the needle tip penetrates the skin and enters the abdominal muscle, it is redirected and slowly advanced under direct vision and penetration of the tip through the external oblique and internal oblique muscles, and finally the TAP is identified between the internal oblique and transversus abdominis muscles. A test injection (1 mL) of saline is performed to confirm correct needle placement in the TAP, which is indicated

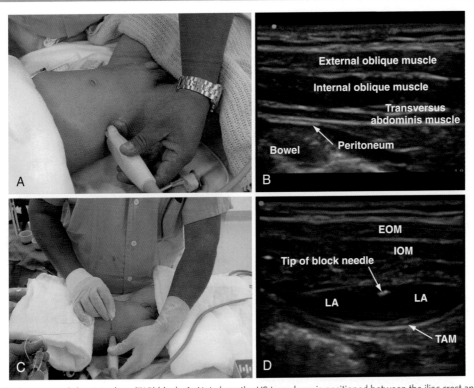

**FIGURE 42-37** Posterior transverse abdominis plane (TAP) block. **A,** Note how the US transducer is positioned between the iliac crest and the costal margin along the mid-axillary line. **B,** The three layers of the abdominal musculature. **C,** In-pane needle insertion during a posterior TAP block. **D,** Distention of the TAP by the injected local anesthetic (*LA*). *EOM,* External oblique muscle; *IOM,* internal oblique muscle; *TAM,* transversus abdomen muscle.

by distention of the TAP by the hypoechoic fluid. A calculated dose of a long-acting local anesthetic (0.2 mL/kg) is then injected through the needle, while distention of the TAP is visualized in realtime (see Fig. 42-37, *D*).

For a subcostal TAP block, a high-frequency linear array transducer (15-6 MHz) is placed immediately below the costal margin along the midclavicular line and the block needle (50 to 80 mm) is inserted in the plane of the US beam and from a medial to lateral direction until the tip is identified to be in the TAP. As described earlier, saline 1 to 2 mL is injected to confirm correct needle placement in the TAP. A calculated dose of local anesthetic (0.2 mL/kg) is then injected, and as the local anesthetic hydro-dissects the TAP plane, the block needle is advanced posteriorly in the TAP to improve spread of the local anesthetic. Bilateral subcostal TAP blocks are indicated for midline upper abdominal incision. Currently, no published data exist on the use of subcostal TAP blocks in children and its role in children is still not defined.

### Thoracic Paravertebral Block

Thoracic paravertebral block is the technique of injecting local anesthetic alongside the thoracic vertebra close to the intervertebral foramen.[104] This produces ipsilateral, segmental, somatic, and sympathetic nerve blockade that is effective for relieving postoperative pain of unilateral origin from the chest[105] and abdomen.[106] Traditionally, thoracic paravertebral block is performed using surface anatomic landmarks[106] or a catheter is placed in the paravertebral space under direct vision during thoracic surgery (see Chapter 41).[105] Currently, no published data exist on US-guided thoracic paravertebral block in children, although there are several reports in adults.[107,108] The following section describes how the authors perform real-time, in-plane

US-guided single-shot thoracic paravertebral block and paravertebral catheter placement in young infants.

US-guided thoracic paravertebral block is performed with the child in the lateral position and with the side to be blocked uppermost. The operator sits or stands behind the child, and the US machine is positioned directly in front on the opposite side of the operating table. In most children a 15-6–MHz linear array transducer is adequate for imaging the paravertebral anatomy. However, a high-frequency linear array transducer with a small footprint (25 mm) is ideal for US-guided thoracic paravertebral block in neonates and young infants. For a US-guided thoracic paravertebral block for thoracotomy, the US transducer is placed at the midthoracic region and a transverse scan of the thoracic paravertebral region is performed with the orientation marker directed laterally. On a transverse sonogram of the thoracic paravertebral region and with the US beam being insonated between two adjacent ribs, the paraspinal muscles are identified as hypoechoic structures on either side of the midline and posterior to the spinal osseous elements (Fig. 42-38). The spinous process and lamina are identified as hyperechoic structures. Because the posterior spinal elements are cartilaginous in neonates and young infants, the acoustic window for imaging is relatively large and it is possible to visualize the neuraxial elements in the same transverse sonogram (see Fig. 42-38). Anterior to the lamina and transverse process the pleura can be visualized as a hyperechoic structure that moves synchronously with respiration or ventilation (see Fig. 42-38). A hypoechoic triangular space may also be visualized lateral to the paravertebral region and posterior to the pleura, which represents the apex of the thoracic paravertebral space (see Fig. 42-38).

For a US-guided thoracic paravertebral block, the block needle (50 mm) is inserted lateral to the US transducer and advanced

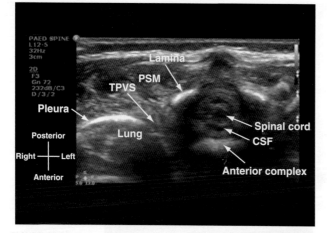

**FIGURE 42-38** Transverse sonogram demonstrating the sonoanatomy of the right thoracic paravertebral region in a neonate. Note the hyperechoic pleura anteriorly and the hypoechoic apical part of the thoracic paravertebral space (*TPVS*) posterior to the pleura. Also note the large acoustic window resulting from incomplete ossification of the posterior spinal elements that allows visualization of the neuraxial structures within the spinal canal. *CSF*, Cerebrospinal fluid; *PSM*, paraspinal muscles.

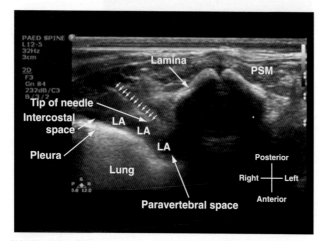

**FIGURE 42-39** Transverse sonogram of the right thoracic paravertebral region in a neonate after an ultrasound-guided thoracic paravertebral block. Note the direction of needle insertion and distention of the right thoracic paravertebral and intercostal spaces, adjacent to the level of injection, with the local anesthetic (*LA*). *PSM*, Paraspinal muscle.

toward the apical part of the paravertebral space in the plane of the US beam. The advancing needle is visualized in real time, and entry into the apex of the thoracic paravertebral space is confirmed using a test bolus injection (1 mL) of saline. Correct placement of the needle in the paravertebral space is indicated by anterior displacement of the parietal pleura, distention of the paravertebral space, and increased echogenicity of the parietal pleura (Fig. 42-39). A calculated dose of local anesthetic (0.2 mL/kg) is then injected with the needle in situ before a catheter is inserted through the needle, leaving approximately 2 cm of catheter in situ if a continuous thoracic paravertebral block is planned (see also Figs. 41-17, 41-18, and Chapter 41 for landmark-guided techniques).

### Spinal Sonography and Central Neuraxial Blocks

Since the early 1980s, spinal ultrasonography has been used as a diagnostic screening tool in neonates and infants suspected of

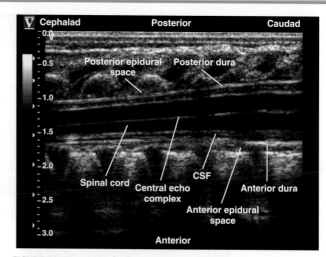

**FIGURE 42-40** Longitudinal paramedian sonogram of the thoracic spine in a neonate. *CSF*, Cerebrospinal fluid.

spinal dysraphism and for detecting spinal tumors, vascular malformations, and trauma.[109,110] Today it is considered the first-line screening test for spinal dysraphism, with a diagnostic sensitivity comparable to that of MRI. Spinal ultrasonography is possible in neonates and infants because the incomplete ossification of the predominantly cartilaginous posterior spinal elements creates an acoustic window that allows the transmission of the US beam. The overall visibility of neuraxial structures decreases with age.[109] Neuraxial structures are best visualized in neonates and infants younger than 3 months of age; progressive ossification of the posterior spinal elements makes detailed sonographic evaluation of the spine difficult beyond 6 months of age unless the child has a persistent posterior spinal defect.[111] Some reports have demonstrated that neuraxial structures can be visualized in older children, although their details are limited. The overall visibility of neuraxial structures also decreases as one progresses up the spine, with the best visibility in the sacral level followed by the lumbar and then at the thoracic level.

In diagnostic radiology, spinal US is most frequently performed with the child in the prone position, whereas in an anesthetized child it is generally performed with the child in the lateral position. Because the neuraxial structures are relatively superficial in children, they are best visualized using high-frequency (10-5 MHz) transducers, which also produce better images than sector transducers. Scans are obtained in both the transverse (axial) and longitudinal (sagittal) axes, and they are performed either through the midline or parallel and lateral (paramedian) to the spinous processes. The paramedian scan is preferable in older children because it avoids the ossified spinous processes that can interfere with US transmission. In neonates and young infants, the spinal canal can be scanned with the transducer placed directly over the spinous processes (i.e., a median longitudinal scan). Beyond this age group a paramedian longitudinal scan provides the best overall view of neuraxial structures.[112-114]

On a longitudinal sonogram, the neonatal spinal cord is seen as a hypoechoic tubular structure with hyperechoic anterior and posterior walls (Fig. 42-40). A thin strip of variable intense echo, "the central echo complex" (see Fig. 42-40), extends longitudinally through the center of the spinal cord and represents the area between the myelinated ventral white commissure and the

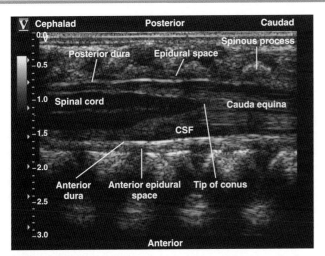

FIGURE 42-41 Longitudinal paramedian sonogram of the thoracolumbar spine in a neonate showing the termination of the spinal cord. *CSF*, Cerebrospinal fluid.

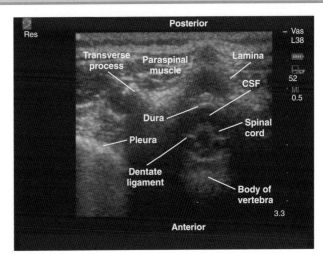

FIGURE 42-42 Transverse sonogram of the thoracic spine in a neonate. *CSF*, Cerebrospinal fluid.

42

central portion of the anterior median fissure. This produces the "triplet echoes" that are characteristic of the spinal cord at all levels (see Fig. 42-40). The diameter of the spinal cord varies, being largest in the cervical and lumbar regions and smallest at the thoracic region. Anterior and posterior to the spinal cord are two well-defined linear and hyperechoic echoes that represent the arachnoid-dural layer (see Fig. 42-40). The ligamentum flavum, which is relevant for epidural access, is also readily visualized in young children and appears less echoic than the dura (E-Fig. 42-4). The dural layers taper distally to close the thecal sac at the S2 level. The epidural space is the hypoechoic area between the dura and the ligamentum flavum (see E-Fig. 42-4), and arterial pulsations also may be visible on US between these two layers. The cerebrospinal fluid (CSF) surrounds the spinal cord as an anechoic layer between the dura and spinal cord (E-Fig. 42-5). The vertebral bodies are seen as echogenic structures anterior to the spinal cord. The spinal cord tapers distally to form the conus medullaris (Fig. 42-41) at the level of first and second lumbar vertebral bodies. The conus medullaris is continuous with the filum terminale, which extends into the sacral canal as a hyperechoic structure. It is surrounded by the roots of the cauda equina, which appear as multiple parallel echogenic lines surrounding the filum terminale (E-Fig. 42-6). Differentiation of the filum terminale from the roots of the cauda equina can sometimes be difficult. The cauda equina typically lies in the anterior half of the spinal canal when the child is in the prone position, but it moves freely within the CSF with change in position and with crying. Slight anteroposterior movement of the spinal cord, superimposed on the arterial pulsations, is commonly seen during real-time imaging.

On a transverse (axial) sonogram, the spinal cord is seen as a round or oval hypoechoic structure, with its bright central echo complex (Fig. 42-42). The spinal cord is fixed laterally by the dentate ligament (see Fig. 42-42), which represents the transversely oriented, echogenic arachnoid duplications that are seen in parts of the thoracic spinal canal. Paired (ventral and dorsal) echogenic nerve roots are seen below the L2 level. Farther caudally in the lumbar region, a transverse scan shows the filum terminale surrounded by the nerve roots of the cauda equina (E-Fig. 42-7). The arachnoid–dura mater complex is hyperechoic and forms the anterior and posterior border of the subarachnoid

space with the anechoic CSF and the spinal cord in the thoracic region (see Fig. 42-42) and the cauda equina in the lumbar region (see E-Fig. 42-7). The vertebral bodies are the hyperechoic structures anterior to the spinal canal. The vertebral arches are also echogenic and cast an acoustic shadow anteriorly (see E-Fig. 42-7). The paraspinal muscles appear hypoechoic on US.

## CAUDAL EPIDURAL ANESTHESIA

Single-shot caudal epidural injection is the most frequently used regional anesthetic technique in children and almost always is used in combination with general anesthesia for surgery involving the lower thoracic, lumbar, and sacral dermatomes.[115] Several methods are used to perform a caudal epidural injection.

Detecting the characteristic pop or give as the needle traverses the sacrococcygeal ligament to enter the caudal epidural space is by far the most commonly used method in children.[115,116] However, even in experienced hands it can result in failure, and the overall failure rate varies between 2.8% and 11%.[117] US has been used to guide caudal epidural injection in children.[118,119] The correct position of a needle or catheter in the caudal epidural space is confirmed by real-time US visualization of the needle in the sacral canal or by observing dural displacement after a saline test bolus (0.2 to 0.3 mL/kg to a maximum of 10 mL) injection.

The anesthetized child is positioned in the lateral position with the knee and hips flexed. The operator sits or stands behind the child, and the US machine is positioned directly in front. A linear-array transducer (13-10 MHz) is used to image the sacrum. A transducer with a wide footprint is preferable because it allows a greater length of the spine to be examined in a single view. The transducer is initially positioned directly over the sacral cornua in the transverse axis (Fig. 42-43). On a transverse sonogram at the level of the sacral hiatus, the sacral cornua are seen as two hyperechoic reverse U-shaped structures, one on either side of the midline. Connecting the two sacral cornua and deep to the skin and subcutaneous tissue is a hyperechoic band, the sacrococcygeal ligament (see Fig. 42-43). Anterior to the sacrococcygeal ligament is another linear hyperechoic structure, which represents the posterior surface of the sacrum. The hypoechoic area between the sacrococcygeal ligament and the bony posterior surface of the sacrum is the sacral hiatus (see Fig. 42-43). The two sacral cornua and the posterior surface of the sacrum produce a US

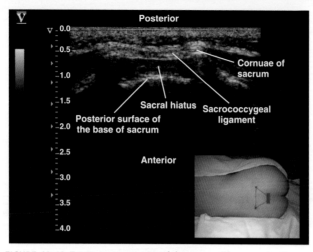

**FIGURE 42-43** Transverse sonogram of the sacrum ("frog eye sign").

image that we refer to as the "frog-eye sign" because of its resemblance to the eyes of a frog (see Fig. 42-43). On a longitudinal sonogram of the sacrum, the sacrococcygeal ligament, the base of the sacrum, and the sacral hiatus can be clearly seen (E-Fig. 42-8). In neonates and young infants the tapered end of the thecal sac with CSF, the anterior and posterior epidural space filled with fat, and the cauda equina may be visualized in the sacral canal (see E-Fig. 42-8).

For US-guided caudal epidural injection, either in-plane or out-of-plane technique can be used. We prefer the in-plane approach, and the needle is advanced under real-time guidance into the sacral canal through the sacrococcygeal ligament. During insertion, the needle is maintained at an angle (approximately 20 degrees) so that it is parallel to the posterior surface of the sacrum. Correct position of the needle in the caudal epidural space is confirmed objectively by performing a test bolus injection of saline and observing in real time the displacement of the dura (E-Fig. 42-9).[119,120] Anterior displacement of the posterior dura is more frequently seen than posterior displacement of the anterior dura. If dural displacement is not seen in the US image, it implies that the needle or catheter is not in the correct position, the needle or catheter is not in the plane of US imaging, or the needle is intravascular. The needle should be withdrawn and the procedure repeated until the typical dural displacement is visualized. The calculated dose of local anesthetic is then injected in aliquots. The cephalad spread of the local anesthetic within the epidural space also can be visualized in real time. Depending on the volume of local anesthetic injected, progressive widening of the epidural space and a resultant compression of the thecal sac occur (see E-Fig. 42-9). These changes are visualized in the sacral canal and at the lumbar and thoracic levels. In some cases the thecal sac is almost completely obliterated in the sacral and lumbar region (see E-Fig. 42-9). Because the compression and obliteration of the thecal sac occurs in a caudal to cranial direction, it indicates that there is a net cranial displacement of CSF.

US guidance during a caudal epidural injection in children offers several advantages. It is safe, noninvasive, radiation free, simple, and quick to perform; it provides real-time images that are easy to interpret; and, unlike the nerve stimulation technique, is not affected by the use of neuromuscular blocking drugs or epidural local anesthetics. Moreover, US can demonstrate the underlying caudal anatomy, which is useful in children with

cutaneous markers of dysraphism when it can be used to screen the underlying spinal anatomy. Thus many children who may have otherwise been excluded from a caudal block can benefit from its effects. It is also a useful tool for teaching and learning of caudal anesthesia (see also Fig. 41-6 and Chapter 41 for landmark-guided techniques).

## Epidural Catheterization

Continuous epidural analgesia via an indwelling epidural catheter is a well-established method of providing perioperative analgesia in children.[121] The loss-of-resistance technique[5,122] is the most frequently used method of identifying the epidural space. Although popular, this technique relies on the operator's tactile sensation and can rarely result in dural puncture and serious neurologic complication, such as spinal cord injury. Alternative methods for identifying the epidural space in children have been described[123] but have not gained widespread acceptance. Epidural catheters have been successfully placed in young children under US guidance.[122,124] Compared with the traditional loss-of-resistance method, when epidural catheterization is performed using the loss-of-resistance method in conjunction with US guidance, fewer bony contacts occur during the procedure and the time required for catheter placement is reduced. The spread of local anesthetic in the epidural space can also be visualized in real time. In addition, the underlying anatomy and the depth from the skin to the ligamentum flavum, dura, and epidural space can be assessed before needle insertion. However, epidural catheterization under US guidance requires two anesthesiologists who are familiar with epidural anesthesia and spinal sonography in children. The first anesthesiologist performs the scan in the longitudinal paramedian axis and maintains a steady image while the second anesthesiologist performs the needle insertion through the midline. Entry of the needle into the epidural space is confirmed by the loss of resistance to saline and observing the local sonographic changes resulting from the saline injection (i.e., anterior displacement of the posterior dura, widening of the epidural space, and compression of the thecal sac). US-guided epidural catheterization in young children is a very demanding procedure and requires a great deal of skill and dexterity. It should be undertaken only by pediatric anesthesiologists who have acquired adequate training and skill in US-guided regional anesthesia (see Chapter 41 for landmark-guided techniques).

### Assessment of Indwelling Epidural Catheters

For optimal epidural anesthesia or analgesia, the epidural catheter tip must be located in the correct dermatomal level. This is often achieved by directly placing the catheter in the desired level via the lumbar or thoracic route. Even with this approach, and in particular when loss of resistance is used to locate the epidural space, it is not possible to determine with any certainty the exact location of the catheter tip. Epidurography can locate the catheter tip,[125] but this exposes the child to radiation and the risk of anaphylaxis from the contrast medium (see Figure 41-7). An epidural catheter inserted via the caudal route can be advanced to the lumbar or thoracic epidural space. However, this is technically difficult in children older than 1 year of age,[126] and even in children younger than 6 months of age, the catheter can be misplaced in the sacral, lumbar, and even the cervical region.[127,128] Whether styleted epidural catheters are easier to advance from the caudal to the thoracic epidural space than nonstyleted ones is not known, although better success has been reported with styleted catheters.[129] Even if a catheter is successfully advanced

42

to the thoracic epidural space, radiographic confirmation is still required to confirm the position of the catheter tip.[127] Electric nerve stimulation through an indwelling styleted epidural catheter and observation of myotomal contractions have been used to locate the position of the catheter tip.[130] In experienced hands this technique has a success rate of 89%. However, this test cannot be performed if neuromuscular blocking drugs or local anesthetics have been administered. Epidural electrocardiography also can be used to locate the position of a thoracic epidural catheter[131] and is not affected by the use of neuromuscular blocking drugs or local anesthetics in the epidural space. This method relies on matching the evolving electrocardiogram (ECG) recorded from the tip of a specially adapted epidural catheter, as it is advanced, to the surface ECG recorded at the target vertebral level. However, this method is not specific because even a subcutaneous electrocardiographic electrode at the same position relative to the heart will produce a similar electrocardiographic pattern.

US has been used to directly visualize the position of epidural catheters in children (E-Fig. 42-10).[132,133] US localization is noninvasive, does not involve exposure to radiation or contrast medium, and is not affected by the use of neuromuscular blocking drugs or epidural local anesthetics. It also provides real-time images of the catheter during catheter insertion. However, not all epidural catheters or their tips can be identified using US, and it may be limited by the acoustic window available for scanning in children of different ages. Gently jiggling the catheter and observing tissue movement within the epidural space also has been used to facilitate epidural catheter localization.[133] Injecting saline with air bubbles may improve catheter localization using US, but the use of air in the injectate can lead to inadvertent air embolism or a patchy block.[134] Therefore it is suggested that observing surrogate markers such as the widening of the epidural space, dural displacement, and compression of the thecal sac, subsequent to a saline test injection, may be more accurate in locating the position of an epidural catheter in children.

### ADVANTAGES OF ULTRASOUND IMAGING

US-guided regional anesthetic blocks appear to offer several advantages. US imaging is noninvasive and simple to use and does not involve exposure to radiation. It allows the target nerves and the surrounding structures to be directly visualized during block placement, which is particularly advantageous in children with difficult or variant anatomy, obesity, or amputated limbs in whom the evoked motor responses cannot be visualized. US is also useful in young children because the majority of regional anesthetic procedures in this age group are performed under general anesthesia when the use of a muscle relaxant makes nerve stimulation impractical. US guidance also helps determine the best possible site and maximum safe depth for needle insertion, allows real-time guidance of the needle and needle tip to the target site, avoids unintended vascular or pleural puncture, and allows visualization of the spread of the injected local anesthetic in real time. Together, these should lead to fewer needle insertions, improved comfort during block placement in awake and sedated children, reduced complications, improved quality of block, and greater success rates. However, limited studies exist comparing US with conventional methods of performing regional nerve blocks in children. Cumulative evidence (from adults and children) suggests that US speeds the execution of peripheral nerve and central neuraxial blocks, reduces the discomfort experienced during block placement, reduces the amount of local anesthetic required, speeds the onset of sensory blockade, improves the quality of sensorimotor blockade, and prolongs the duration of sensory block. Additional studies are required to determine whether US guidance reduces complications related to regional anesthesia in children.

## Education and Training

Learning US-guided nerve block techniques takes time and patience. The state of the art of regional anesthesia demands a high degree of manual dexterity and hand–eye coordination and an ability to conceptualize 2D information into a 3D image. In addition, to produce good-quality US images, the anesthesiologist must also possess a sound knowledge of anatomy, the physical principles of US, and musculoskeletal imaging. Therefore individuals who intend to perform US-guided regional anesthesia should start by learning the basics of US and US-guided interventions by attending a course or workshop and by working with individuals who already possess these skills. Initial experience of musculoskeletal scanning can also be acquired in volunteer situations, and US-guided interventions can be practiced using a US phantom.[135-139] Once the basic skills are acquired, it is best to start by performing superficial peripheral nerve block procedures (e.g., axillary brachial plexus block, femoral and sciatic nerve block) under supervision before attempting deeper blocks (e.g., lumbar plexus block), which can be technically demanding even for an experienced operator. Whenever possible, it is advisable to use a peripheral nerve stimulator in conjunction with US during the learning phase of US-guided nerve blocks. With proficiency, it is possible to perform most techniques without nerve stimulation. Fortunately, the learning curve is steep[140] and most anesthesiologists are able to acquire the required skills very quickly, probably owing to their inherent good hand–eye coordination and ability to think in three dimensions. It is preferable to perfect these techniques in adults or older children before performing them in young children. US-guided epidural techniques, other than single-shot caudal epidural injections, demand a high degree of skill and dexterity and should be performed only by anesthesiologists experienced in US-guided regional anesthesia.

## Summary

US-guided RA is a promising alternative to anatomic landmark-guided techniques, and almost all regional anesthetic techniques that are commonly performed in children can be performed using US guidance. US imaging is noninvasive, is easy to use, does not involve exposure to radiation, and is not affected by the type of anesthesia administered. US allows the anesthesiologist to visualize the target nerves and surrounding structures in real time during block placement, which is particularly advantageous in children because the majority of regional anesthetic procedures in this age-group are performed under general anesthesia. Currently, the use of US for regional anesthesia in children is still in its infancy and the evidence to support its use is sparse. USGRA is facing the same challenges for widespread acceptance that laparoscopic surgery faced during the 1980s. Today, laparoscopy is the standard of surgical care. We envision that as more anesthesiologists who care for children acquire the skills necessary to perform USGRA and embrace this technology, US guidance will be the standard of care in pediatric regional anesthesia in the future.

**ACKNOWLEDGMENT**

Figures, sonograms, and videos in this chapter were reproduced with permission from www.aic.cuhk.edu.hk/usgraweb.

## ANNOTATED REFERENCES

Kapral S, Krafft P, Eibenberger K, et al. Ultrasound-guided supraclavicular approach for regional anesthesia of the brachial plexus. Anesth Analg 1994;78:507-13.

*In 1994, Kapral and colleagues, from Vienna, Austria, published the first randomized control study on direct sonographic visualization in regional anesthesia. They used ultrasound to directly visualize the brachial plexus and observe the spread of the local anesthetic in real time during supraclavicular brachial plexus block.*

La Grange P, Foster PA, Pretorius LK. Application of the Doppler ultrasound bloodflow detector in supraclavicular brachial plexus block. Br J Anaesth 1978;50:965-7.

*In 1978, La Grange and associates were the first to describe the use of a Doppler flow detector to locate the subclavian artery and guide supraclavicular brachial plexus block.*

Marhofer P, Frickey N. Ultrasonographic guidance in pediatric regional anesthesia. I. Theoretical background. Paediatr Anaesth 2006;16: 1008-18.

*In this review article, Marhofer and Frickey, from Vienna, Austria, discuss the basic principles of ultrasound that are a prerequisite for the safe application of ultrasound for regional anesthesia in children.*

Roberts S. Ultrasonographic guidance in pediatric regional anesthesia. II. Techniques. Paediatr Anaesth 2006;16:1112-24.

*In this review article, Roberts, from Liverpool, England, describes the practice of ultrasound-guided peripheral and central neuraxial blocks in children.*

## REFERENCES

Please see www.expertconsult.com.

# Acute Pain

SHOBHA MALVIYA, DAVID M. POLANER, AND CHARLES B. BERDE

THE PRACTICE OF PAIN MANAGEMENT in children continues to advance. Since the early 1980s, clinicians have come to recognize that neonates and infants experience pain and process those learning experiences. Research has demonstrated the adverse long-term consequences of unrelieved pain, including harmful neuroendocrine responses, disrupted eating and sleep cycles, and increased pain perception during subsequent painful experiences.[1-3] Disparities in pain treatment led organizations, such as the Agency for Healthcare Research and Quality (AHRQ) and the American Pain Society (APS), to provide guidelines and the Joint Commission (formerly the Joint Commission on Accreditation of Healthcare Organizations [JCAHO]) to issue mandates that further enhanced the practice of pediatric pain management.[4-6] The availability of reliable and valid pain assessment tools for children and governmental incentives encouraged the inclusion of children in analgesic drug trials. Sufficient research data regarding children's pain became available, making it possible to develop pediatric evidence-based pain management guidelines. Many children's hospitals now have dedicated specialized multidisciplinary pain teams that manage acute and chronic pain. The increasing use of regional analgesia techniques led to the development of the Pediatric Regional Anesthesia Network (PRAN), a registry of practice patterns and complications of regional anesthetics in children. An enormous expansion of the breadth of techniques for acute pain management in children, the establishment of pediatric pain services, and the investigation and introduction of innovative modalities of therapy all attest to the importance accorded to this aspect of perioperative care.

## Developmental Neurobiology of Pain

Nociceptive pathways in the periphery, spinal cord, and brain develop in a series of stages through the second and third trimester in humans. By 26 weeks postconception, there is sufficient maturation of peripheral and spinal afferent transmission for the late-gestation fetus or preterm neonate to respond to tissue injury or inflammation with withdrawal reflexes, autonomic arousal, and hormonal metabolic stress responses. There are also changes in responsiveness after injury or repetitive stimulation indicative of central sensitization. In general, preterm neonates have reduced thresholds for withdrawal to noxious thermal and mechanical stimuli compared with older infants and children. One mechanism that may contribute to these low-threshold responses involves projections of low-threshold peripheral afferents to superficial as well as deep laminae in the spinal dorsal horn; later in development these afferents project only to deeper dorsal horn laminae.

Investigators have examined indices suggestive of cortical activation, including near-infrared spectroscopy[7] and electroencephalography,[8] in response to noxious events. Using near-infrared spectroscopy, a unilateral heelstick (performed for clinical purposes) produces signal changes suggestive of contralateral cortical activation.[7-9]

Despite these lines of evidence, the nature of pain in neonates, viewed as conscious suffering, remains unknown. Other investigators have looked for long-term consequences of painful events (with or without treatment) in humans and in animal models. Despite attempts by these investigators to correct for confounding factors, in our view, the interpretation of these studies, especially in humans, should be quite cautious. Neonates who undergo painful procedures are commonly those who are more medically ill. It appears difficult to distinguish consequences of pain per se from the consequences of other factors, such as prematurity, critical illness (including episodes of hypoxia or ischemia), deprivation of tactile and social contact, and nutritional deprivation. Many clinicians and investigators have adopted the view that, in the absence of better information about either the nature of suffering experienced by neonates or the potential adverse consequences of pain in terms of long-term development, caregivers should err on the side of providing, rather than withholding, analgesia. Although this is a compelling perspective, it is important to highlight three concerns: (1) in general, available studies have had difficulty showing effects of routine administration of analgesia (e.g., morphine infusions) on immediate behavioral indices of distress in neonates undergoing intensive care; (2) repeated or prolonged administration of anesthetics and sedatives in animal models have been shown to have deleterious effects on brain development, (the human implications of these animal studies remain unclear at this time [see also Chapters 6 and 23]);[10-16] and (3) as will be detailed later, younger organisms develop tolerance to opioids and benzodiazepines more rapidly than older organisms, so that the management of tolerance and withdrawal has now become a nearly universal consequence of prolonged administration of these medications to critically ill neonates, infants, and children.

## Pain Assessment

The International Association for the Study of Pain (IASP) has defined *pain* as an unpleasant sensory and emotional experience associated with actual or potential tissue damage, or *described* in terms of such damage. The IASP and others have acknowledged that the inability to communicate verbally, as in the preverbal, nonverbal, or the cognitively impaired, does not preclude the possibility that an individual is experiencing pain and is in need of appropriate pain management.[17,18] Physicians and nurses have been very creative in developing tools to evaluate pain in children of all ages; most of these tools are discussed below. Table 43-1 summarizes various pain assessment tools in terms of appropriate age, target population, ease of use, and practicality.

## SELF-REPORT MEASURES

Because pain is a subjective experience, self-report measures, in which a patient is asked to quantify the severity of the pain between 0 (no pain) and 10 (maximum pain), are considered to most accurately reflect acute pain. Because many children lack the cognitive skills to use such scales, pain assessment measures that include developmentally appropriate self-report tools, behavioral-observational tools, and physiologic-biologic measures have been developed. Given the multidimensional nature of the individual pain experience, and the complexity and inherent biases associated with self-report, use of unidimensional numeric scales alone to reflect pain is overly simplistic.[19-22] Therefore, regardless of the measure used, it must be emphasized that a complete pain assessment is more than just a number attempting to quantify the severity of pain. Estimating the impact of pain on the suffering and the quality of the individual's life, targeting appropriate therapeutic measures, and evaluating the effectiveness of such measures are additional key components of a global and ongoing pain assessment and treatment strategy.

For children to use numeric scales, they must understand the concepts of magnitude and ordinal position, that is, they must be able to identify which of different-sized objects is bigger and place them in order from smallest to largest. They must also be able to arrange geometric figures or numbers in a series *(seriation)*.

**TABLE 43-1** Appropriate Pain Assessment Measures by Age-Group: Self Report, Observational/Behavior, and for the Cognitively Impaired

| Self-Report Tools | Appropriate Age-Groups | Comments |
|---|---|---|
| Faces Pain Scale | 3-18 years | Simple and quick to use; extensively validated in healthy schoolchildren with postoperative and cancer pain |
| Oucher | 3-18 years | Photographic for ≥3-year-olds, numeric 0-10 scale for ≥6-year-olds; less clinical utility and feasibility compared to other faces scales |
| Manchester Pain Scale | 3-18 years | Panda bear faces eliminate gender and ethnic bias; tested in emergency department setting |
| Computer Face Scale | 4-18 years | Offers option for continuous rather than categorical format; good construct validity; preferred by children over the Wong Baker Faces Scale; further testing needed |
| Sydney Animated Facial Expression Scale (SAFE) | 4-18 years | Animated version of Faces Pain Scale; rated by children as easiest to use; no psychometric advantage compared to other scales |
| Visual Analog Scale (VAS) | 6-18 years | Simple and quick to use; requires the concepts of order, magnitude, and seriation (the ability to place or visualize in series); widely used across settings; preferred to other self-report tools by children ≥8 years old and adolescents |
| Numeric Rating Scale (NRS) | 7-18 years | Simplest and most commonly used in clinical as well as research settings |
| **Observational/Behavioral Measures** | | |
| Comfort Scale | 0-18 years | Developed for use in intensive care settings; useful in mechanically ventilated children and in the postoperative setting |
| Face, Legs, Activity, Cry, Consolability (FLACC) | 2 months to 7 years | Excellent pragmatic and psychometric qualities; widely adopted in clinical and research settings; has been translated into several languages other than English |
| Children's Hospital of Eastern Ontario Pain Scale (CHEOPS) | 1-7 years | Good psychometric properties; lengthy with inconsistent scoring among categories; cumbersome; extensively used both in clinical and research settings |
| **Cognitively Impaired Children** | | |
| Revised FLACC | All ages | Allows for scoring individualized pain behaviors; good psychometric properties; highest clinical utility compared to the Non-Communicating Children's Pain Checklist—Postoperative Version (NCCPC-PV) and Nurses' Assessment of Pain Intensity (NAPI) |
| Non-Communicating Children's Pain Checklist (NCCPC) | All ages | Requires 5-minute observation period; comprehensive but cumbersome; used in clinical and research setting |
| University of Wisconsin Pain Scale | All ages | Inconsistent scoring style compared to other clinical scoring systems; scoring style may permit flexibility but limits precision |
| The Pain Indicator for Communicatively Impaired Children | All ages | Useful for pain assessment in cognitively impaired children in the home setting. |

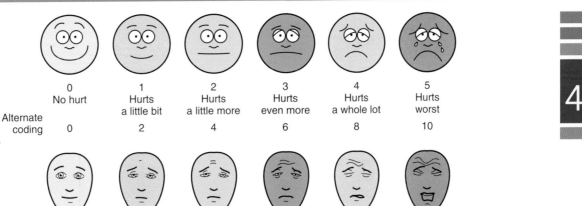

FIGURE 43-1 **A,** The Wong-Baker Faces Pain Scale. **B,** The Bieri Faces Pain Scale. (**B** modified from Bieri D, Reeve RA, Champion GD, et al. The Faces Pain Scale for the self-assessment of the severity of pain experienced by children: development, initial validation, and preliminary investigation for ratio scale properties. Pain 1990;41:139-50.)

These skills are typically not present until 7 years of age; thus several pain assessment tools that most commonly use graphic facial displays representing different degrees of pain expression are used to facilitate self-report of pain in young children.

### Faces Pain Scales

Faces pain scales comprise a series of line diagrams of faces with expressions of increasing distress.[23-28] Some versions have a smiling face whereas others have a neutral face to represent the "no pain" end of the scale (Fig. 43-1). Unlike the numeric scales, the faces scales do not require the concept of magnitude or seriation and can therefore be used by preschool aged children. The Wong Baker Faces Pain Scale has been extensively studied and its reliability and validity confirmed in children 3 to 18 years of age. Strong correlations have been reported between the Wong Baker Scale scores and other faces scales, the Visual Analog Scale (VAS), as well as nurses' ratings based on behavior.[29-32] Recent data suggest that versions with the smiling face at the no-pain end of the spectrum, such as the Wong Baker Scale, may overestimate pain because children without pain, but with distress from other sources, may be reluctant to choose the smiling face.[28] The Wong-Baker scale was preferred by children to the numeric rating scale, the graphic rating scale, and the Color Analog Scale.[23,25,30,33] Overall, the Faces Pain Scale–Revised is the faces scale with the largest support for its validity.[34]

### Oucher

The Oucher combines a photographic faces scale with a 0 to 10 vertical numeric scale. Different versions of the Oucher incorporate photographs of Caucasian, African American, Asian, and Hispanic children to minimize biases related to ethnicity (Fig. 43-2 and E-Fig. 43-1, *A* to *C*).[35,36] Strong correlations have been demonstrated between Oucher scores and those obtained using the Pieces of Hurt tool, faces pain scales, and VAS.[37-39] The Oucher also demonstrates responsivity, that is, the ability to detect change in pain intensity before and after surgery and after administration of an analgesic.[37] The numerical rating component of the Oucher requires that the child be able to count to 10 and has been used successfully in children older than 6 years.

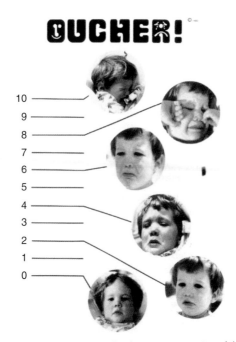

FIGURE 43-2 The Oucher Pain Scale. The Caucasian version of the Oucher Pain Scale.

### The Manchester Pain Scale

The Manchester Pain Scale (Fig. 43-3), which was designed to overcome the gender and ethnic biases of the Oucher, is composed of a pain ruler on which panda facial images are superimposed.[40] It includes verbal descriptors of the extent of pain and how pain possibly interferes with normal functions. A study of children presenting to an emergency department found a very good correlation between scores assigned using the Manchester Scale and the Oucher.[40]

### Novel Self-Report Tools

These self-report tools use a categorical format and the static faces do not allow for "fine tuning" of the ratings before a final

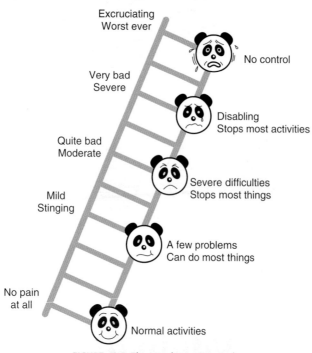

**FIGURE 43-3** The Manchester Pain Scale.

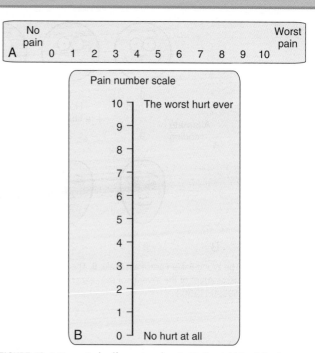

**FIGURE 43-4** Numerical self-report scales. **A,** Horizontal Visual Analog Scale. **B,** Vertical Visual Analog Scale.

assessment regarding the severity of pain is reached.[41] In recent years, there has been interest in developing computer-based self-report assessment tools that use a continuous rather than categorical format.[42]

The Computer Face Scale allows the child to adjust the shape of the mouth of a cartoon face from smiling to frowning and simultaneously to adjust the eyes from completely open to completely closed.[41,43] The suggested benefits of this scale include increased sensitivity (given the ability to select from a wide range of faces) and computerized storage of the results, with ready access and data display. Preliminary work with this scale has demonstrated its construct validity and it was preferred by children over the Wong Baker Faces Scale.[41]

The Sydney Animated Facial Expression Scale (SAFE) is an animated version of the Faces Pain Scale[44] and comprises of a series of 101 faces (Video 43-1). To administer this scale, the child pushes the left or right arrow key on a computer causing the expression of the single face to change until it corresponds with the child's pain intensity (www.usask.ca/childpain/research/safe). At this point, a keystroke records a score between 0 and 100. The SAFE scale was rated to be easiest to use by children aged 4 to 16 years compared with other scales, including the Faces Pain Scale, the Color Analog Scale, and Pieces of Hurt,[45] although it offered no psychometric advantage over the other scales. At this time, further research with this tool is needed before its role can be clearly defined.

### Numeric Scales
#### Visual Analog Scale
Several versions of the VAS are available, including horizontal and vertical lines, word anchors representing extremes of pain, and lines with divisions and numeric values (Fig. 43-4). When using the vertical versions of this scale, the severity of the pain increases as one ascends the ladder. Although moderate to strong correlations have been reported between the VAS, faces pain

scales, and the Oucher,[37,46] the effect of user age on VAS ratings are conflicting.

#### Numeric Rating Scale
The Numeric Rating Scale (NRS) is the simplest and most commonly used numeric scale in which the child rates the pain from 0 (no pain) to 10 (worst pain). Its validity has been established with good correlations between NRS and Faces Pain Scale-Revised scores in children 7 to 17 years of age and NRS and VAS scores in children 9 to 17 years of age.[47] An important caveat when using numeric scales is to be sure of the denominator that the child is using. For example a pain score of 9 on a 0 to 100 scale would reflect mild pain and may not require treatment whereas a score of 9 on a 0 to 10 scale would reflect severe pain that warrants aggressive treatment.

### Selection Criteria
Selection of a self-report tool for a child requires careful consideration of the age and cognitive and developmental level. Figure 43-5 depicts the percentages of children of different ages who are able to self-report their pain and the tools most appropriate for various age ranges. Children who are unable to use a self-report tool may be able to report their pain intensity using simple words, such as "small," "medium," and "big." However, self-reports of pain are subject to the modulating influences of a number of factors, including the child's previous pain experience and response to treatment, psychosocial factors, and parental preferences and influences. In many cases, therefore, it may be necessary to complement self-reported pain scores with behavioral observations, particularly in preschool-aged children. Regardless of the tool selected, assessment of postoperative pain is greatly facilitated by the introduction of the concept of rating pain and of the tool itself during the preoperative preparation of the child.

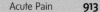

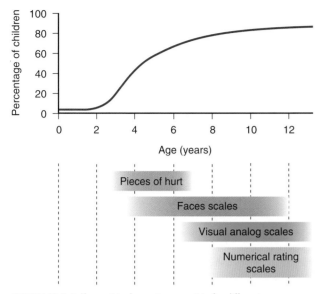

FIGURE 43-5 Self-report tools most appropriate for different age ranges.

**TABLE 43-2** Content Validity of Behavioral Pain Tools: Categories of Behavior in Pain Assessment Tools

| FLACC | CHEOPS | OPS | TPPPS | Büttner/Finke |
|---|---|---|---|---|
| Face | Facial expression | | Facial pain expression | Facial expression |
| Legs | Leg movement | Movement | | Leg position |
| Activity | Torso movement | Agitation | Bodily pain expression | Position of torso |
| | | | | Motor restlessness |
| Cry | Cry | Cry | Vocal pain expression | Cry |
| Consolability | Touching of the wound | Blood pressure | | Consolability |
| | Verbal report of pain | Verbal complaint and body language | | |

*CHEOPS,* Children's Hospital of Eastern Ontario Pain Scale; *FLAAC,* Face, Legs, Activity, Cry, Consolability scale; *OPS,* Objective Pain Scale; *TPPPS,* Toddler Preschool Preoperative Pain Scale.

## OBSERVATIONAL-BEHAVIORAL MEASURES

Despite several age-appropriate methods for self-reporting, assessing pain in children who are unable or unwilling to self-report depends on observations of their behaviors. Five behaviors that have been shown to be reliable, specific, and sensitive when predicting analgesic requirements are facial expression, vocalization or cry, leg posture, body posture, and motor restlessness.[48] Variations in these behaviors have been used in several observational pain tools. Table 43-2 describes the content validity of some of the observational tools that are commonly used in clinical practice. Behavior checklists provide a list of pain behaviors that are marked as present or absent and the extent of pain is estimated on the basis of the number of behaviors present at the time of the assessment.[49,50] Behavior rating scales also incorporate a rating of the intensity or frequency and duration of each behavior.[51] Global rating scales provide a rating of the observer's global impression of the child's pain.

### Children's Hospital of Eastern Ontario Pain Scale

The Children's Hospital of Eastern Ontario Pain Scale (CHEOPS), one of the earliest behavioral rating scales (Table 43-3),[52] incorporates six categories of behavior scored individually from 0 to 2 or 1 to 3 and then sums them to provide a pain score ranging from 4 to 13. Scores of 6 or less indicate no pain. Its validity and reliability for brief painful events and for postoperative pain has been well established, with good to excellent correlations with faces pain scales and the VAS.[46,53] However, the time required to complete the evaluation and inconsistent scoring among categories of the CHEOPS makes it cumbersome and impractical to use in a busy clinical setting.

### Face, Legs, Activity, Cry, Consolability Scale

The Face, Legs, Activity, Cry, Consolability (FLACC) scale was developed in an effort to improve on the pragmatic qualities of the existing behavioral pain tools by providing a simple framework for quantifying pain behaviors in children.[51] This tool includes five categories of behaviors previously found to reliably correlate with pain in young children, including: facial expression, leg movement, activity, cry, and consolability (Table 43-4).[48] The acronym FLACC facilitates recall of these categories, each of which is scored from 0 to 2 to provide a total pain score ranging from 0 to 10. The FLACC tool has been extensively tested and determined to have good inter-rater reliability and excellent validity based on changes in pain scores from before to after analgesic administration and excellent correlation with the Objective Pain Scale (OPS), the CHEOPS, the Toddler Preschool Preoperative Pain Scale (TPPPS), and good correlation with self-reported pain scores using faces pain scales.[51,53-55] The FLACC scale has been translated into several languages, including Chinese, Swedish, French, Italian, Portuguese, Norwegian, and Thai.

### Comfort Scale

The Comfort scale (Table 43-5), developed for use in an intensive care setting, consists of six behavioral and two physiologic measures, each of which has five response categories, thereby allowing detection of subtle changes in the child's distress.[56] Initial evaluation of the Comfort scale found acceptable inter-rater reliability and good correlations with VAS scores in 37 mechanically ventilated infants.[56] Another study evaluated the reliability and validity of the Comfort scale as a postoperative pain instrument in children after thoracic or abdominal surgery.[57] This study found good to excellent inter-rater agreement for all categories except respiratory response, for which there was moderate agreement. Additionally, strong correlations between Comfort and VAS pain scores support the use of the Comfort scale as a postoperative pain measurement instrument in children.

After a systematic review of observational pain measures, the FLACC and the CHEOPS[52] scales were recommended for assessment of pain associated with medical procedures, the FLACC for postoperative pain, and the Comfort Scale for pain in children in critical care.[19] Despite the extensive science supporting the use of behavioral tools, it may be difficult to separate behaviors caused by pain from those caused by other sources of distress in some children.[58] Accurate pain assessment in children,

**TABLE 43-3** Children's Hospital of Eastern Ontario Pain Scale (CHEOPS)*

| Item | Behavioral | Score | Definition |
|------|-----------|-------|------------|
| Cry | No cry | 1 | Child is not crying. |
| | Moaning | 2 | Child is moaning or quietly vocalizing silent cry. |
| | Crying | 2 | Child is crying, but the cry is gentle or whimpering. |
| | Scream | 3 | Child is in a full-lunged cry; sobbing; may be scored with complaint or without complaint. |
| Facial | Composed | 1 | Child has neutral facial expression. |
| | Grimace | 2 | Score only if definite negative facial expression. |
| | Smiling | 0 | Score only if definite positive facial expression. |
| Child Verbal | None | 1 | Child is not talking. |
| | Other complaints | 1 | Child complains, but not about pain, e.g., "I want to see mommy" or "I am thirsty." |
| | Pain complaints | 2 | Child complains about pain. |
| | Both complaints | 2 | Child complains about pain and about other things, e.g., "It hurts; I want my mommy." |
| | Positive | 0 | Child makes any positive statement or talks about others things without complaint. |
| Torso | Neutral | 1 | Body (not limbs) is at rest; torso is inactive. |
| | Shifting | 2 | Body is in motion in a shifting or serpentine fashion. |
| | Tense | 2 | Body is arched or rigid. |
| | Shivering | 2 | Body is shuddering or shaking involuntarily. |
| | Upright | 2 | Child is in a vertical or in upright position. |
| | Restrained | 2 | Body is restrained. |
| Touch | Not touching | 1 | Child is not touching or grabbing at wound. |
| | Reach | 2 | Child is reaching for but not touching wound. |
| | Touch | 2 | Child is gently touching wound or wound area. |
| | Grab | 2 | Child is grabbing vigorously at wound. |
| | Restrained | 2 | Child's arms are restrained. |
| Legs | Neutral | 1 | Legs may be in any position but are relaxed; includes gentle swimming or discrete movements. |
| | Squirming/kicking | 2 | Definitive uneasy or restless movements in the legs and/or striking out with foot or feet. |
| | Drawn up/tensed | 2 | Legs tensed and/or pulled up tightly to body and kept there. |
| | Standing | 2 | Standing, crouching, or kneeling. |
| | Restrained | 2 | Child's legs are being held down. |

*Recommended for children 1 to 7 years old; a score greater than 6 indicates pain.

**TABLE 43-4** The FLACC Behavioral Pain Scale

| Categories | SCORING | | |
| | 0 | 1 | 2 |
|-----------|---|---|---|
| Face | No particular expression or smile | Occasional grimace or frown, withdrawn, disinterested | Frequent to constant frown, clenched jaw, quivering chin |
| Legs | Normal position or relaxed | Uneasy, restless, tense | Kicking, or legs drawn up |
| Activity | Lying quietly, normal position, moves easily | Squirming, shifting back and forth, tense | Arched, rigid, or jerking |
| Cry | No cry (awake or asleep) | Moans or whimpers, occasional complaint | Crying steadily, screams or sobs, frequent complaints |
| Consolability | Content, relaxed | Reassured by occasional touching, hugging, or being talked to, distractible | Difficult to console or comfort |

Each of the five categories, (F) Face; (L) Legs; (A) Activity; (C) Cry; (C) Consolability, is scored from 0 to 2, which results in a total score between 0 and 10. ©2002, The Regents of the University of Michigan. All Rights Reserved.

therefore, requires careful consideration of the context of the behaviors. Input from the parents or caregivers may be valuable as proxy measures, although some parents may lose objectivity in such a situation. Similarly, a regular caregiver may best assess older children with significant developmental delay. When in doubt regarding the source of distress, a trial of analgesics is appropriate and may be both diagnostic and therapeutic.

## LIMITATIONS OF PAIN ASSESSMENT

It remains unclear whether integration of routine pain assessment into clinical practice significantly improves patient outcomes. A critical review of the studies that addressed this question determined that in 2 of 6 studies, children experienced a reduction in pain intensity when a standardized pain assessment tool was used, in 2 studies there was no change in pain intensity, and in

**TABLE 43-5** Comfort Scale

| | 1 | 2 | 3 | 4 | 5 |
|---|---|---|---|---|---|
| Alertness | Deeply asleep | Lightly asleep | Drowsy | Fully awake and alert | Hyper-alert |
| Calmness or Agitation | Calm | Slightly anxious | Anxious | Very anxious | Panicky |
| Respiratory Response | No coughing and no spontaneous respirations | Spontaneous respiration with little or no response to ventilation | Occasional cough or resistance to ventilator | Actively breathes against ventilator or coughs regularly | Fights ventilator; coughing or choking |
| Physical Movement | No movement | Occasional, slight movement | Frequent slight movement | Vigorous movement limited to extremities | Vigorous movement including torso and head |
| Blood Pressure | Less than baseline | Consistently at baseline | Infrequent increases of 15% or more (1 to 3 episodes during observation period) | Frequent increases of 15% or more (>3 episodes) | Sustained increase >15% |
| Muscle Tone | Muscles totally relaxed; no muscle tone | Reduced muscle tone | Normal muscle tone | Increased muscle tone and flexion of fingers and toes | Extreme muscle rigidity and flexion of fingers and toes |
| Facial Tension | Facial muscles totally relaxed | Facial muscle tone normal; no facial muscle tension evident | Tension evident in some facial muscles | Tension evident throughout facial muscles | Facial muscles contorted and grimacing |

43

2 studies pain intensity decreased when pain assessment was combined with pain management interventions.[59] Studies that examined sustainability of the benefits over time reported conflicting results, and most studies were identified to have major methodologic problems.[60,61] Additional investigation is required to determine whether routine pain assessment has any effect on pain outcomes.

Despite the large body of evidence supporting the psychometric properties of numerous structured pain assessment tools described previously and elsewhere, there remains considerable variability in the interpretation of the clinical relevance of pain scores.[22] Attempts have been made to define what range of pain scores is associated with a perceived need for medicine or what magnitude of change in pain score is associated with a perception of better or worse pain.[62-64] A survey of 6- to 16-year-old hospitalized children found that a median pain score of 3 on a 0-to-6 Faces Pain Scale was associated with the child's perceived need for medicine.[62] Others have reported that a 10-mm change in a 0-to-100-mm VAS score was the minimum difference whereby children in the emergency department perceived their pain to be slightly better or slightly worse.[63] In the postoperative period, children with a median pain score of 6 on a 0-to-10 NRS scale perceived the need for an analgesic whereas those with a score of 3 felt there was "no need" for treatment.[64] In addition, children felt "a little better" or "worse" if the NRS scale changed by at least 1. Despite these findings, there was large variability and overlap in scores associated with these outcomes.

It has been suggested that the widespread adoption of a pain score as the fifth vital sign may contribute to the overprescribing of analgesics and sedatives.[65] A review of trauma center site surveys reported a fivefold increase in deaths from excessive pain medicines during two time periods (1994 through 1998 and 2000 through 2004). Evaluations of the effectiveness of pain treatment algorithms based on numerical pain scores have yielded conflicting results. One study reported increased prescription for opioid and nonopioid analgesics, an increased administration of non-opioids, and reduced pain scores in children who received postoperative pain treatment based on a pain score–based algorithm.[66] Children whose pain management was algorithm-based

experienced more nausea, but no other adverse effects. In contrast, hospitalized adults whose pain management was based on a numerical pain treatment algorithm, experienced a twofold increase in episodes of oversedation and a 49% increase in opioid-related adverse drug events.[67] This latter study highlights the potential for harm when numeric pain scores alone are used guide decisions regarding pain treatment. A comprehensive approach to pain assessment that includes consideration of the child's self-reporting (when available), combined with behavioral observation and the overall clinical context, is required to direct treatment decisions.[68]

## SPECIAL CONSIDERATIONS FOR THE COGNITIVELY IMPAIRED CHILD

Children who are cognitively impaired experience pain more frequently than cognitively intact children because of a number of inherent conditions, such as spasticity, muscle spasms, the need for assistive devices for positioning and mobility, and the need for invasive surgical procedures. Indeed, as many as 60% of children with cerebral palsy undergo orthopedic surgery by 8 years of age, and many of them require repeated procedures.[69] Yet both children and adults who are cognitively impaired receive fewer analgesics than those who are cognitively intact with similar painful conditions.[70,71] Barriers to effective pain management in the cognitively impaired include the complexity of pain assessment in those who cannot verbalize their pain, outdated beliefs that these children have altered or blunted pain perception, limited evidence for the safety and efficacy of analgesic regimens, and an exaggerated concern regarding opioid adverse effects, particularly respiratory depression. Difficulties with pain assessment have led to the virtual exclusion of these children from clinical drug trials, leading to deficits in our knowledge of how to effectively manage their pain. A survey of clinicians who treat children who are cognitively impaired identified inadequate pain assessment tools and inadequate training and knowledge of providers as significant barriers to effective pain management, despite respondents beliefs that children who are cognitively impaired perceive pain to a similar extent as cognitively intact children.[72]

### The University of Wisconsin Pain Scale for Preverbal and Nonverbal Children

This scale is composed of five behavior categories with four descriptors for each (E-Table 43-1).[73] The overall rating using this tool is not a sum of scores of individual behaviors but a score assigned on a 0- to 5-scale based on the clinician's judgment relative to assessment of individual categories. The scoring style of this tool does allow for flexibility, but limits its precision. This scale has been tested in 59 preverbal children and 15 children who were nonverbal because of cognitive impairment. Although these investigators reported good validity and reliability in their overall sample, the reliability and validity of this tool for the subset of children with cognitive impairment was not reported.

### The Non-Communicating Children's Pain Checklist—Postoperative Version

This tool comprises a checklist of 27 pain behaviors across six categories.[74] Each of these behaviors (E-Table 43-2) is scored on a 0- to 3-point scale based on the frequency of observation of that behavior over a 10-minute observation period. The scores of all items are summed to provide a total pain score. This tool has been evaluated in 25 children who were cognitively impaired,[74] with good inter-rater reliability in four of the six behavior categories and good correlations between the Non-Communicating Children's Pain Checklist—Postoperative Version (NCCPC-PV) scores and VAS scores. Although this checklist provides a comprehensive pain assessment method for children with cognitive impairment undergoing surgery, it may be cumbersome for frequent and repeated pain assessments in the clinical setting.

### The Pain Indicator for Communicatively Impaired Children

One group of investigators interviewed parents and/or caregivers of 30 communicatively impaired children regarding cues they used to identify pain in their child.[75] Six core pain cues were reported by 90% of the caregivers as signs of definite or severe pain in their child (E-Table 43-3). Each of these cues is scored on a 4-point Likert scale (not at all, a little, often, all the time), based on the frequency of occurrence of the behavior over the observation period. Caregivers of children with severe cognitive impairment, who evaluated this scale at home over a 7-day period, reported no significant relationship between crying and the presence of pain. Yet, they found that a "screwed up or distressed looking face" had the strongest relationship with the presence of pain. In fact, they found that facial expression alone correctly identified 71% of children in pain and 93% of those not in pain, with an overall correct classification rate of 87%. This tool provides a simple method of assessing pain in children with cognitive impairment in the home setting. Further testing of this tool is required in the hospital setting, and using shorter observation periods, to determine its feasibility of use by clinicians.

### Face, Legs, Activity, Cry, Consolability Observational Tool

Initial evaluation of the FLACC tool in children with cognitive impairment found a good correlation between scores assigned independently by different observers and by parent global ratings of pain.[76] Although measures of exact agreement between observers were acceptable for the face, cry, and consolability categories, measure of agreement for the legs and activity categories were less acceptable, likely because of coexisting motor impairments such as spasticity. The FLACC tool was therefore revised to incorporate additional descriptors of behaviors most consistently associated with pain in children with cognitive impairment (Table 43-6).[77] Inter-rater reliability for the total FLACC scores, as well as for each of the categories, improved when the evaluation included the revised FLACC (r-FLACC) in 52 cognitively impaired children. Also, good correlation between FLACC, parent, and child scores supported its criterion validity. FLACC scores were noted to decrease after an opioid was administered, supporting the construct validity of the tool. The pragmatic attributes of the r-FLACC were compared with those of the Nurses' Assessment of Pain Intensity (NAPI) and the NCCPC-PV.[78] Clinicians using these tools to score pain rated the complexity as less and the relative advantage and overall clinical utility of the FLACC and the NAPI to be greater compared with the NCCPC-PV, suggesting that these tools may be more readily adopted into clinical practice.

## Strategies for Pain Management

Pain is a complex phenomenon that occurs because of the transmission of nociceptive stimuli from the peripheral nervous system through the spinal cord to the cerebral cortex. Pain perception is further influenced by emotions, behavior, and previous pain experiences via multiple synapses in the limbic system,

| **TABLE 43-6** Revised FLACC for Pain Assessment in the Cognitively Impaired* | | | |
|---|---|---|---|
| | 0 | 1 | 2 |
| Face | No particular expression or smile | Occasional grimace/frown; withdrawn or disinterested [Appears sad or worried] | Consistent grimace or frown; frequent/constant quivering chin, clenched jaw [Distressed-looking face; expression of fright or panic] |
| Legs | Normal position or relaxed | Uneasy, restless, tense [Occasional tremors] | Kicking, or legs drawn up [Marked increase in spasticity, constant tremors or jerking] |
| Activity | Lying quietly, normal position, moves easily | Squirming, shifting back and forth, tense [Mildly agitated (e.g., head back and forth, aggression); shallow, splinting respirations, intermittent sighs] | Arched, rigid, or jerking [Severe agitation head banging; shivering (not rigors); breath holding, gasping or sharp intake of breath; severe splinting] |
| Cry | No cry (awake or asleep) | Moans or whimpers, occasional complaint [Occasional verbal outburst or grunt] | Crying steadily, screams, or sobs; frequent complaints [Repeated outbursts, constant grunting] |
| Consolability | Content, relaxed | Reassured by occasional touching, hugging, or "talking to"; distractible | Difficult to console or comfort [Pushing away caregiver, resisting care or comfort measures] |

*Revised descriptors for children with disabilities shown in *brackets*.

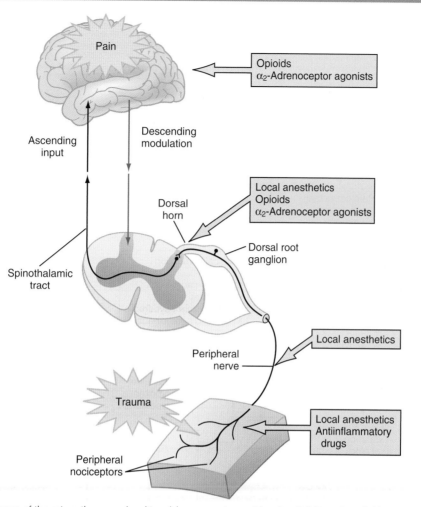

**FIGURE 43-6** Schematic diagram of the pain pathways and multimodal measures to provide pain relief. (From http://old.cvm.msu.edu/courses/VM545/ Evans/Pain%20Management%20PDA.htm.)

frontal cortex, and thalamus. Given the complexity of the pain mechanism, effective treatment of pain requires the use of multimodal therapies that target multiple sites along the pain pathways, as illustrated in Figure 43-6. Analgesics with additive or synergistic activity and different adverse effect profiles should be selected so that adequate analgesia can be provided with fewer adverse consequences. Thus pain can be treated at the peripheral level using local anesthetics, peripheral nerve blockade, nonsteroidal antiinflammatory drugs (NSAIDs), antihistamines, or opioids. At the spinal cord level, pain can be treated with local anesthetics, neuraxial opioids, $\alpha_2$-adrenoceptor agonists, and N-methyl-D-aspartate (NMDA) receptor antagonists. Finally, at the cortical level systemic opioids, $\alpha_2$-agonists, and voltage-gated calcium channel $\alpha_2\delta$ proteins (targets for anticonvulsants) can be used.[79] Most cases of moderate to severe pain are best treated with a combination of analgesic techniques.

The strategy for postoperative pain management is an integral part of the preanesthetic plan, so that informed consent for procedures, such as placement of peripheral or regional blocks, can be obtained (see Chapters 41 and 42). Additionally, appropriate teaching for techniques, such as patient-controlled analgesia (PCA), should begin in the preoperative period. An honest discussion with the child that, although some discomfort is inevitable, every effort will be made to minimize pain after surgery, decreases the anxiety related to the perioperative experience. This, together with the use of nonpharmacologic techniques, may even reduce the need for opioids and other analgesics. Selection of an analgesic regimen requires careful consideration of a number of factors, including scope and requirements of the surgical procedure, age and cognitive abilities of the child, the child's previous pain experience and response to treatment, underlying medical conditions that might alter the response to pain medications, and child and family preferences. The goal should be for the child to emerge from anesthesia in reasonable comfort, because it is generally easier to maintain analgesia in a pain-free child than to achieve analgesia in a child with severe pain. Figure 43-7 presents a flowchart describing strategies for assessment and management of acute postoperative pain in a child.

## SURGICAL CONSIDERATIONS

The scope and requirements of the surgical procedure, as well as specific postoperative issues, should be discussed with the surgical team before choosing an analgesic regimen, particularly if a regional technique is planned. For example, the site of placement of an epidural catheter and choice of epidural solution will differ in a child with a vertical midline incision from a child with a transverse suprapubic incision. With certain procedures,

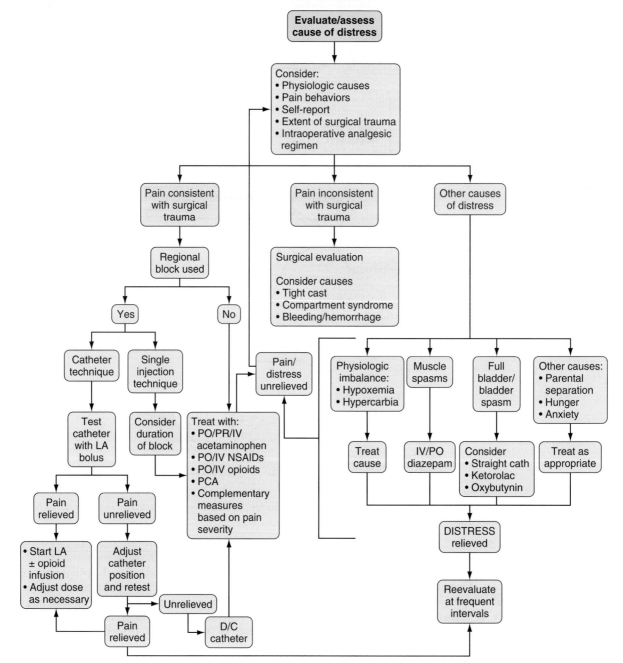

**FIGURE 43-7** Flowchart for assessment and management of acute postoperative pain in a child. *D/C*, Discontinue; *IV*, intravenous; *LA*, local anesthetic; *NSAIDs*, nonsteroidal antiinflammatory drugs; *PCA*, patient-controlled analgesia; *PO*, orally; *PR*, per rectum.

an epidural catheter may intrude into the surgical field or access to the catheter site in the postoperative period may be obscured by a cast or dressing. In such cases, the catheter may be tunneled subcutaneously away from the surgical field. Alternatively, one or more epidural catheters may be placed under direct vision by the surgeon at the end of the procedure (e.g., spinal fusion or selective dorsal rhizotomy).[80-83] Postoperative pain is managed by the pain service, using infusion of local anesthetic and/or opioid solutions through the catheter.[80] Painful muscle spasms after certain procedures are often well managed with continuous epidural analgesia.[80,84,85] Refractory spasms of the bladder, which can be quite problematic after some surgeries (e.g., ureteral reimplantation), can also be effectively treated with NSAIDs (e.g., ketorolac) or anticholinergics.[86] Intravesical bupivacaine has

also been used to manage bladder spasm.[87,88] Muscle spasms after orthopedic surgery may be prevented by dense levels of regional blockade, but may also require supplementation with oral or parenteral benzodiazepines if epidural analgesia alone is ineffective. Epidural blockade may favorably alter diaphragmatic mechanics after thoracotomy and upper abdominal surgery. This effect is likely a result of the motor blockade of the intercostal muscles and alteration in the resting length of the diaphragm, and not solely a result of reversal of diaphragmatic inhibition.[89-92] However, it remains uncertain whether analgesia alone, achieved by systemic opioids or central neuraxial blockade, is of value in diminishing postoperative diaphragmatic inhibition or significantly improving postoperative pulmonary function.[93,94] Effective analgesia, however, does improve child compliance with measures such as deep breathing and early mobilization, thereby reducing the incidence of postoperative complications.[95]

### Child-Related Considerations

#### Age and Cognitive Abilities

Analgesic techniques, such as infiltration of the wound with local anesthetics, peripheral nerve blocks, or regional blockade that minimize the use of opioids and central respiratory depressants, may be ideal for preterm or very young infants with impaired central respiratory drive.[96,97] Acetaminophen can be a useful adjunct, because when used within its recommended dose range it has a large therapeutic window with few untoward effects. Although the judicious use of opioids is not contraindicated, preterm or term infants younger than 1 month of age who receive these medications require careful observation and monitoring to detect respiratory depression.[98] The use of local anesthetics in infants also requires more careful attention to dose, to avoid accumulation and toxicity.

Although analgesia for the preterm infant was often neglected in the past, we now understand that these infants have reduced thresholds to painful or noxious stimuli when compared with older children.[99] Most of the neural pathways that conduct nociception from the periphery through the central nervous system (CNS) are present and functional at 24 weeks gestational age, although the central connections, particularly in the thalamocortical pathways that are involved in the integration and perception of conscious pain, are not as well developed.[100-102] Controversy remains as to the meaning and implications of this neural immaturity. Opioid receptors and responses are present in the spinal cord at the time of birth, although spinal glial inflammatory mechanisms are immature. Because these mechanisms are central to the cyclooxygenase (COX-1 and COX-2) responses, this may imply that there is limited or no analgesic response to NSAIDs and COX inhibitors in preterm infants or neonates, whereas opioid responses are active. GABAergic pathways, which play an important role in the effects of analgesics and anesthetics, can be either excitatory or inhibitory, depending on the stage of development.[103] The neuroplasticity that is characteristic of these infants may be a double-edged sword. Animal models and some clinical evidence suggest that repeated noxious stimuli may result in heightened sensitivity to nociceptive input and adverse behavioral sequelae.[2,10,104-107] On the other hand, nerve injury in infant animals may result in less pain than it does in older animals.[106,107] In humans, the neural injury to the brachial plexus after shoulder dystocia during delivery rarely results in chronic pain.[108] It may be that there are both vulnerable periods and periods of greater resiliency during development, so that the consequences of pain in our youngest children may not be easily predictable.

Older infants and toddlers who are expected to experience moderate to severe pain may be adequately treated with oral opioids when oral intake resumes. Alternatively, low-dose continuous opioid infusions, nurse-controlled analgesia,[109] or regional blockade may be required in those undergoing extensive surgery. Nonpharmacologic techniques, such as child life therapy and the presence of a comforting parent, can do much to supplement analgesic therapy.

Preschool and school-aged children have greater fears and better understanding of the postoperative experience than do their younger counterparts. Most cognitively intact children 7 years of age or more are able to understand the concept of patient-controlled analgesia (PCA), which may be helpful in giving a sense of control back to the child during a period in which all other aspects of control are removed.[110] Such issues of control and dependency assume even greater importance in adolescents; allowing them to participate in decision-making will contribute to the success of any analgesic technique.[110] Regional techniques are excellent for providing analgesia in all age groups and are associated with a reduced incidence of adverse effects compared with systemic opioids (e.g., nausea, vomiting, excessive sedation, dysphoria and respiratory depression). Children with significant developmental delay require special consideration of their physical disability, as well as cognitive abilities, although in most cases the pharmacologic actions of the drugs are not altered.

#### Previous Pain Experience

A detailed history regarding the child's previous pain experience, analgesic history, response to treatment, and adverse effects from previous analgesic regimens should be carefully considered when selecting a pain management technique. An opioid-naive child undergoing surgery for the first time requires smaller doses of opioids for a smaller duration compared with a child with chronic pain who has developed opioid tolerance as a result of long-term or repeated opioid use. Analgesic selection should also be modified based on the effectiveness of analgesics for that particular child in the past. For example, a child with a history of not responding to codeine may be deficient in the cytochrome P-450 2D6 isoenzyme (see also Chapter 6). These children cannot metabolize codeine (methylmorphine) to morphine (its active moiety) and experience reduced analgesia after codeine. Ineffective conversion of codeine to morphine may be present in up to 7% to 10% of Caucasian children, whereas the incidence of fast metabolizers is 5% in North America. These incidences differ with ethnicity, with a significantly greater incidence of polymorphisms in North African descendants.[111-115] On the other hand, another polymorphism, present in about 0.5% of children, results in rapid demethylation of codeine to morphine, producing exaggerated sedation and respiratory depression when codeine is administered.[116,117] Overall, we strongly discourage routine use of codeine as a first-line opioid for children. Oxycodone, hydrocodone, hydromorphone, or morphine are superior alternatives to codeine. Alternatively, if pain is of moderate or smaller intensity, another class of analgesics (e.g., NSAIDs) can be substituted.

## Pharmacologic Treatment of Pain

### NONOPIOID ANALGESICS

Nonopioid analgesics may be used as sole agents for the treatment for mild pain and as important adjuncts for the multimodal treatment of moderate to severe pain. Although most nonopioid analgesics produce dose-dependent responses, they are limited by a ceiling effect in the analgesia achieved, that is, larger doses of the medication provide no additional analgesia. Hence, more severe pain is resistant to therapy from these medications alone.[118] Therefore they are frequently prescribed in combination with opioids to reduce both the opioid requirements and the adverse effects (Table 43-7).

### Acetaminophen

Acetaminophen is the most common antipyretic and nonopioid analgesic used in children. It exerts its analgesic effects by blocking central and peripheral prostaglandin synthesis, reducing substance P–induced hyperalgesia, and modulating the production

**TABLE 43-7**  Oral Dosing Guidelines for Commonly Used Nonopioid Analgesics

| Medication | Individual Dose for Children <60 kg (mg/kg) | Individual Dose for Children ≥60 kg (mg) | Dosing Interval (hours) | Maximum Daily Dose for Children <60 kg (mg/kg) | Maximum Daily Dose for Children ≥60 kg (mg) |
|---|---|---|---|---|---|
| Acetaminophen | 10-15 | 650 | 4 | 75[†] | 3000 |
| Ibuprofen | 6-10 | 400-600 | 6 | 40 | 2400 |
| Naproxen | 5-6 | 250-375 | 12 | 10 | 1000 |
| Diclofenac | 1 | 50 | 8 | 3 | 150 |
| Ketorolac* | 0.5 | 30 | 6-8 | 2 | 120 |
| Tramadol | 1-2 | 50 | 6 | 8 | 400 |

Modified from Berde CB, Sethna NF. Analgesics for the treatment of pain in children. N Engl J Med 2002;347:1094-103.
*Ketorolac should be administered for a maximum of 5 days or 20 doses up to 15 mg per dose for children <50 kg or 30 mg per dose for children >50 kg.
†See text for new age-related dosing.

of hyperalgesic nitric oxide in the spinal cord.[119-121] In addition, it has been suggested that acetaminophen produces analgesia via activation of descending serotonergic pathways.[122-124] However, it is likely that its primary site of action may be inhibition of prostaglandin $H_2$ synthetase at the peroxidase site.[123] Effective analgesic and antipyretic effects have been described with plasma concentrations of 5 to 20 μg/mL[125-129]; a target effect-site concentration of 10 μg/mL reduces pain after tonsillectomy by 3.6/10 pain units.[130] The total daily dose of acetaminophen via any route is age- and weight-based but should not exceed 75 mg/kg for children; term and preterm infants require further downward dosing adjustment (60 mg/kg and 45 mg/kg, respectively).

The recommended dose for oral administration is 10 to 15 mg/kg every 4 hours. Acetaminophen has a wide margin of safety when administered in the recommended therapeutic dose range. However, hepatotoxicity has been reported with doses only slightly above the recommended 10- to 15-mg/kg/dose orally for a total of five doses or 75 mg/kg/day, suggesting that acetaminophen may have a narrow therapeutic index in some children.[131,132] Because of these reports and on the advice of a U.S. Food and Drug Administration panel, the manufacturers have reduced the maximum single dose of oral acetaminophen in adults to 650 mg and the maximum daily dose to 3 grams. Acetaminophen is available in a wide variety of formulations, alone or in combination with decongestants, for oral use in a variety of cold remedies, and with opioids for the treatment of moderate to severe pain. There are currently more than 600 over-the-counter acetaminophen-containing products, increasing the risk of an overdose because children may take more than one formulation that contains the drug. Frequent review of medications and parental education is needed to minimize the risk of overdose. In the past, pediatric liquid formulations of acetaminophen as in infant drops were commonly supplied in larger concentrations than that in elixirs, resulting in dosing errors. The current recommendation is to standardize liquid formulations to a single concentration of 32 mg/mL. Acetaminophen can be given orally before surgery; both gastric fluid volume and pH are unchanged after acetaminophen was administered orally 90 minutes before induction of anesthesia.[133]

Slow and unpredictable absorption of acetaminophen after rectal administration results in variable blood concentrations, with peak concentrations reached between 60 and 180 minutes after administration.[128,134,135] There is a dose-response relationship for rectal acetaminophen. The morphine-sparing effects of 40 mg/kg and 60 mg/kg of rectal acetaminophen were greater than those of 20 mg/kg and placebo in children undergoing ambulatory surgery.[136] In children undergoing orthopedic surgery, a loading dose of 40 mg/kg rectal acetaminophen followed by 20 mg/kg every 6 hours yielded serum concentrations of 10 to 20 μg/mL, with no evidence of accumulation over a 24-hour period.[134] This dosing scheme is now the one most commonly recommended when the rectal route is employed.

Intravenous (IV) formulations of paracetamol (acetaminophen) and its prodrug propacetamol have been used in Europe and Australia for several years and are now available in the United States. IV acetaminophen is available as a 10 mg/mL solution and should be infused over at least 15 minutes in a dose of 10 mg/kg, with a total daily dose not to exceed 75 mg/kg. The maximum dose, regardless of weight, is 750 mg every 6 hours (3 grams per day).

After IV administration of acetaminophen, analgesic onset occurs in 15 minutes and that of antipyresis in 30 minutes.[137,138] IV paracetamol rapidly penetrates the blood-brain barrier in children, yielding detectable concentrations in the cerebrospinal fluid (CSF) within 5 minutes of administration, and peak CSF concentrations within 57 minutes after injection (compared with 2 to 3 hours after rectal or oral administration), thus explaining the fast onset of its analgesic and antipyretic effects.[139] A large multicenter trial reported that 1 gram of IV paracetamol and 2 grams of IV propacetamol (equivalent to 1 gram acetaminophen) provided superior analgesia with a reduced need for morphine compared with placebo in adults after lower extremity joint replacement.[140] The propacetamol group experienced a greater incidence of local skin reactions and pain on injection compared with the IV paracetamol group. A controlled randomized trial reported that both rectal acetaminophen, 40 mg/kg, and IV acetaminophen, 15 mg/kg, administered after induction of anesthesia in children undergoing adenotonsillectomy, provided good analgesia for the first 6 hours after surgery.[141] However, children who received acetaminophen rectally had a greater duration of analgesia and did not require rescue analgesia as early as those in the IV group.[141] This is attributable to the slow absorption of rectal acetaminophen causing sustained effective concentrations. A prospective randomized trial comparing rectal acetaminophen to IV propacetamol in infants after craniofacial surgery reported that the IV formulation provided superior analgesia,[142] in part because of reduced bioavailability of acetaminophen by the rectal route.

Another controlled randomized study compared the analgesic efficacy and side effects of fentanyl-placebo versus fentanyl-acetaminophen administered via PCA in 6- to 24-month-old children undergoing ureteroneocystostomy.[143] Children in the acetaminophen group required significantly less fentanyl and demonstrated a reduced incidence of vomiting and excessive sedation compared with those in the placebo group. Lastly, a large retrospective study reported no differences in alanine transaminase and γ-glutamyl transferase concentrations, and a progressive decrease in aspartate aminotransferase levels, in term and preterm neonates before, during and after IV acetaminophen injection.[144]

## Nonsteroidal Antiinflammatory Drugs

NSAIDs provide excellent analgesia for mild to moderate pain resulting from surgery, injury, and disease. Their principle mechanism of action is via inhibition of the enzyme prostaglandin $H_2$ synthetase at the COX site, causing a reduction in the production of prostaglandins at the site of tissue injury, and attenuation of the inflammatory cascade. In addition to their peripheral effects, the NSAIDs have also been shown to exert a direct spinal action by blocking the hyperalgesic response induced by activation of spinal glutamate and substance P receptors.[145] Decreased production of leukotrienes, activation of serotonin pathways, and inhibition of excitatory amino acids, NMDA-mediated hyperalgesia, and central inhibition of prostaglandin biosynthesis have been proposed as additional mechanisms of action.[146,147] The COX-1 enzyme is present in the brain, gastrointestinal tract, kidneys, and platelets and is expressed constitutively. It preserves gastric mucosal integrity and function, platelet aggregation, and renal perfusion. COX-2 expression is induced by inflammation or tissue injury. Selective COX-2 inhibitors reduce inflammation but have less effect on gastric mucosal function and have fewer effects on platelet aggregation, thereby resulting in fewer adverse effects. Their deleterious effects on renal perfusion, however, are no different than the nonselective COX drugs, because COX-2 is constitutively expressed in renal tissues and may be involved in prostaglandin-dependent renal homeostatic processes.[148] The risks of renal toxicity increase in the presence of hypovolemia, cardiac failure, preexisting renal dysfunction, or with the concurrent use of other nephrotoxic drugs. Reports of thrombotic cardiovascular and CNS events after both long-term and short-term use in adults led to withdrawal of two of the COX-2 inhibitors, rofecoxib and valdecoxib from the market.[149,150] Similar data are unavailable to date in children; consequently, the risk of these agents causing thrombotic complications in children remains unknown. Most pediatric studies have evaluated the use of nonselective COX medications. In adult studies, COX-2 inhibitors have generally, but not always, produced analgesia roughly equivalent to that of traditional NSAIDs. Ibuprofen, one of the oldest orally administered NSAIDs, has been used extensively for treatment of fever and pain related to surgery, trauma, arthritis, menstrual cramps, and sickle cell disease. A large, controlled, randomized, double-blind study reported a greater decrease in VAS pain scores with ibuprofen than with acetaminophen or codeine in children presenting to the emergency department with acute pain after musculoskeletal trauma.[151] Additionally, more children who received ibuprofen had VAS scores less than 30 on a 0-to-100-mm VAS scale than in the other two groups. The recommended dose of ibuprofen is 6 to 10 mg/kg every 6 hours. Like acetaminophen, ibuprofen is available in a variety of formulations and concentrations, placing children at risk for an overdose. For pediatric use, ibuprofen is available as:

- Concentrated drops containing 50 mg ibuprofen in 1.25 mL
- Oral suspension containing 100 mg of ibuprofen in 5 mL
- Junior-strength chewable tablets or caplets containing 100 mg of ibuprofen in each

Diclofenac provides effective analgesia after minor surgical procedures in children. It is available only as an oral tablet in the United States, but it is available as a suppository and in the injectable form in several countries. The pediatric dose of diclofenac is 1 mg/kg every 8 hours orally, 0.5 mg/kg rectally, and 0.3 mg/kg IV.[152] The oral and rectal doses reflect bioavailabilities of 0.36, 0.35, and 0.6 for suspension, dispersible tablets, and suppository, respectively. When diclofenac was administered rectally, the relative bioavailability was greater and the peak concentration was reached earlier than after enteric coated tablets administered orally.[153] Children who received diclofenac experienced comparable analgesia to those who received caudal bupivacaine or IV ketorolac for inguinal hernia repair.[154-156] In children undergoing tonsillectomy and/or adenoidectomy, diclofenac yielded superior analgesia with less supplemental opioid dosing, less nausea and vomiting, and earlier resumption of oral intake compared with acetaminophen.[157,158] Although there are occasional reports of increased bleeding and restlessness in the recovery room in children who received diclofenac compared with those who had received papaveretum during tonsillectomy,[159] a Cochrane review established that NSAIDs did not cause any increase in bleeding that required a return to the operating room (OR) for children. There was significantly less nausea and vomiting with NSAIDs compared with alternative analgesics, suggesting their benefits outweigh their negative aspects.[160]

Ketorolac, indomethacin and ibuprofen are the only injectable NSAIDs available in the United States. Indomethacin is the only NSAID used for closure of patent ductus arteriosus in preterm neonates. The IV formulation of ibuprofen is only labeled for adults in the United States. Clinical trials are currently under way in children. Ketoprofen and diclofenac are other injectable NSAIDs that are available outside the United States. A large multicenter study compared the risks of serious adverse events from IV ketorolac, ketoprofen, and diclofenac in more than 11,000 adults undergoing major surgery.[161] The results indicated that 1.4% of adults experienced a serious adverse outcome, including surgical site bleeding (1%), death (0.17%), severe allergic reactions (0.12%), renal failure (0.09%), and gastrointestinal bleeding (0.04%), with no differences in outcomes among the groups; similar large-scale studies are not available for children.

Ketorolac has been shown to provide postoperative analgesia similar to opioids, in children of all ages.[162-165] Its benefits include lack of opioid adverse effects (respiratory depression, sedation, nausea, and pruritus) making it an attractive choice for the treatment of postoperative pain. However, in common with all NSAIDs, it carries risks of platelet dysfunction, gastrointestinal bleeding, and renal dysfunction. Ketorolac (1 mg/kg) given to 18 preterm and term neonates undergoing painful procedures in the OR or the neonatal intensive care unit,[163] revealed reduced pain scores (Neonatal Infant Pain Scale) with no incidents of systemic or local bleeding and no hematologic, hepatic, or renal complications (note that this dose is twice the usually recommended dose of 0.5 mg/kg). Similarly, no adverse effects on surgical drain output, renal or hepatic function tests, or oxygen saturation after major surgery were noted in 37 infants and toddlers between 6 and 18 months of age.[166] Children in that study received continuous morphine infusions postoperatively, confounding the evaluation of the analgesic efficacy of ketorolac. Finally, ketorolac has been used to supplement opioid analgesia, with no increase in renal or bleeding complications in infants and children after open heart surgery.[167-169] Nevertheless, because ketorolac can reduce renal blood flow, many recommend that its course be limited to 48 to 72 hours, and that renal function be checked if a course of administration greater than 72 hours is required. In single dose studies, the pharmacokinetics (PK) of ketorolac in infants less than 12 months of age appear to be homogeneous, although there was a trend toward reduced clearance in the infants less than 6 months of age.[170]

In an effort to avoid the respiratory depressant effects of opioids after airway surgery, several studies investigated the safety and benefits of ketorolac in children undergoing tonsillectomy.[171-175] These early reports of ketorolac adversely skewed analyses of the adverse effects of NSAIDs after tonsillectomy. All but one of these studies[171] found a two- to fivefold increase in bleeding complications, including measured blood loss, ease of achieving hemostasis, and bleeding episodes in the postanesthesia care unit (PACU), necessitating reexploration and hospital admission in some cases. Two of these studies were terminated prematurely, when preliminary data showed an unacceptably greater risk of bleeding in children who had received ketorolac.[172,175] In one of these two studies, ketorolac was given at the end of surgery after hemostasis had been achieved.[172] The benefits of ketorolac, including adequacy of analgesia, resumption of oral intake, and reduction in nausea, vomiting, and sedation were modest. This issue is further confounded by conflicting results yielded by two meta-analyses that evaluated the related literature. In one of these, the use of aspirin, but not of NSAIDs (diclofenac or ibuprofen), significantly increased the risk of posttonsillectomy hemorrhage compared with either acetaminophen with codeine or tramadol for postoperative analgesia.[176] The other reported no increase in intraoperative blood loss, postoperative bleeding, or admission because of bleeding, but did show a statistically significant increase in the rate of reoperation for bleeding in children who received an NSAID in the postoperative period compared to those who did not.[177] Taken together, these data suggest that the use of NSAIDs during or after tonsillectomy is best avoided, and alternative analgesics, such as acetaminophen and tramadol, be considered to reduce opioid requirements. A large multicenter study in adults found that the risk of gastrointestinal and operative site bleeding associated with ketorolac was larger and clinically important when ketorolac was used in larger doses, in older subjects, and for more than 5 days.[178]

Another contentious issue regarding NSAIDs relates to their effects on bone healing and their use in children undergoing spinal fusion. Prostaglandins play an integral role in bone metabolism and significantly influence bone resorption and formation; however, their effects on bone formation predominate. NSAIDs inhibit the formation of prostaglandins, thereby raising the concern that they could promote nonunion after spinal fusion. Studies in rabbits and some studies in adults have reported a greater incidence of nonunion or pseudarthrosis, particularly with the use of large doses of ketorolac.[179,180] However, no differences in curve progression, hardware failure, pseudarthrosis, or need for reoperation have been found in children and adolescents who received ketorolac in the immediate postoperative period compared with those who did not.[181-183] Of note, the majority of the pediatric data are from otherwise healthy children with idiopathic scoliosis, making it problematic to extrapolate these data to children with comorbidities or those with neuromuscular scoliosis. There is no unique advantage of the IV route with NSAIDs. There is also no evidence that IV ketorolac is a more potent analgesic than comparable (i.e., equipotent) doses of a number of other NSAIDs, administered by oral or rectal routes.[184]

A recent meta-analysis of the use of NSAIDs for postoperative pain included 27 studies and compared 567 children who received NSAIDs to 418 children who did not.[185] This study found that coadministration of NSAIDs and opioids during the perioperative period decreased opioid requirement in the PACU and the first 24 hours after surgery, decreased pain intensity in the PACU, and postoperative nausea and vomiting (PONV) during the first 24 hours postoperatively. Additionally, coadministration of acetaminophen with NSAIDS and opioids reduced pain intensity for the first 24 hours postoperatively. Other investigators demonstrated up to a 30% opioid-sparing effect in children who receive acetaminophen and diclofenac in addition to PCA. Therefore, in the absence of contraindications, it has been recommended that NSAIDs be used as part of a multimodal regimen to manage postoperative pain and to decrease opioid consumption in children.[185]

### Tramadol

Tramadol is a synthetic analogue of codeine that exerts its analgesic properties by two complementary mechanisms. One of its metabolites has a weak affinity for the μ opioid receptor with no affinity for the δ or the κ receptors. In addition to its mild opioid effects, it also inhibits serotonin and norepinephrine uptake. Its main advantages over opioids include reduced incidences of respiratory depression, sedation, nausea, and vomiting. Additionally, because it does not inhibit prostaglandin synthesis, it does not cause the adverse effects commonly reported with NSAIDs, including peptic ulceration and renal and platelet dysfunction. Adverse effects associated with its use include nausea and vomiting (9% to 10% of cases), pruritus (7%), and rash (4%).[186] It is known to cause dizziness and its use has been associated with seizures. Tramadol is available only in tablet form alone or in combination with acetaminophen in the United States. However, it is available in a liquid formulation (and as oral drops for infants), as a suppository, and as an injectable solution in other countries, allowing for greater flexibility of dosing. Therefore, it has been used to provide analgesia by a number of routes, including oral, rectal, IV (including PCA devices), into the caudal epidural space, and by local infiltration.

Tramadol is used for postoperative pain treatment in children undergoing ambulatory surgery and has also been used when transitioning from IV opioids to oral analgesics. Two doses of tramadol (1 mg/kg and 2 mg/kg orally) were compared in children who were being transitioned from morphine PCA. Children who received 2 mg/kg required fewer supplemental analgesics with no difference in adverse effects compared with those who had received 1 mg/kg.[186] Tramadol, 2 mg/kg IV, produced similar analgesia and sedation, with fewer episodes of oxygen desaturation compared with morphine 0.1 mg/kg IV, in children with obstructive sleep apnea undergoing adenotonsillectomy.[187] Tramadol has also been found to produce a similar analgesic effect as that of ilioinguinal and iliohypogastric nerve blocks in children undergoing herniorraphy.[188] The tramadol group, however, experienced a greater incidence of nausea and vomiting. Tramadol PCA has also been found to provide adequate analgesia with less sedation, earlier awakening, and earlier extubation in children undergoing atrial or ventricular septal defect repair compared with those who received morphine via PCA.[189]

Tramadol has also been effective when administered via the neuraxial space. Caudal tramadol (2 mg/kg) produced reliable postoperative analgesia comparable to that produced by caudal morphine (30 μg/kg) in children undergoing inguinal hernia repair.[190] No additional pain medications were required in the first 24 hours in more than 90% of children in each group. Rigorous drug-specific neurotoxicity studies, however, are lacking. Another study compared the analgesic efficacy of 2 mg/kg tramadol administered IV or by peritonsillar infiltration in children undergoing adenotonsillectomy.[191] Both groups experienced excellent analgesia in the first hour. However, the local infiltration group experienced more prolonged analgesia and required fewer rescue doses of acetaminophen compared with the IV group. Overall, tramadol appears to be an analgesic of medium potency with a low incidence of adverse effects that may be used alone for mild to moderate pain and for its opioid-sparing effect in children with severe pain.

### Ketamine

There has been increasing interest in the use of ketamine, an NMDA-receptor antagonist, in the treatment of both chronic and acute pain. Its professed benefits include an opioid-sparing effect, avoidance of opioid tolerance, prevention of central sensitization and wind-up, mitigation of opioid-induced hyperalgesia, and provision of synergistic analgesia in multimodal regimens by virtue of its own antinociceptive properties. Case series in children with intractable pain resulting from advanced stages of cancer have reported reduction in opioid requirement, decreased opioid adverse effects, improvement in pain control and function, and increased ability to interact with their families.[192-194]

Studies evaluating the use of ketamine alone or in combination with opioids for acute postoperative pain in children have yielded equivocal results. In one study, children undergoing tonsillectomy who received IV ketamine 0.5 mg/kg after induction or at the end of surgery experienced reduced pain scores and required fewer rescue analgesics compared with those who received placebo.[195] All children in this study received a standardized analgesic regimen, including rectal diclofenac before the start of surgery and oral acetaminophen at scheduled intervals postoperatively. Another study reported reduced pain scores and reduced requirement for rescue analgesics in children who received ketamine as a bolus dose and by infusion that began before the start of a tonsillectomy, compared with those who received a single bolus dose of ketamine at the end of surgery.[196] Intramuscular (IM) ketamine 0.5 mg/kg has also produced equivalent analgesia in terms of similar pain scores and need for rescue analgesics compared with IM morphine 0.1 mg/kg as sole analgesics for tonsillectomy.[197] Other studies have found no such benefits when ketamine was compared with placebo for tonsillectomy, urologic, and orthopedic surgery.[198-201]

A meta-analysis of 35 randomized controlled trials compared 567 children who received ketamine as an adjuvant analgesic by a variety of routes for a variety of surgical procedures with 418 who did not receive ketamine.[202] This study found that, although the use of ketamine was associated with reduced pain intensity in the PACU and a reduced need for nonopioids, it did not demonstrate an opioid-sparing effect. A systematic review of 37 studies included 4 studies in children, two of which demonstrated beneficial effects of ketamine administered as an adjuvant analgesic and two found no benefits.[203] The investigators could draw no conclusions regarding the use of ketamine as an adjuvant analgesic. The use of ketamine in all the above studies was associated with only a few mild and self-limiting adverse effects. Further investigation is needed to evaluate the benefits of low-dose ketamine for acute postoperative pain before its routine use can be recommended.

## OPIOID ANALGESICS

Opioids are indicated for moderate to severe pain after surgery or trauma, for acute painful crisis in children with sickle cell disease, as well as for chronic painful conditions such as cancer. Opioids mimic the effects of endogenous ligands known as endorphins, exerting their effects by binding to specific opioid receptors located at presynaptic and postsynaptic sites in the brain, spinal cord, and peripheral nerve cells. Opioid receptors in the CNS are classified as μ, κ, δ, and σ.[204-206] Activation of these receptors causes neuronal inhibition by decreasing the release of excitatory neurotransmitters from presynaptic terminals. The μ receptors are further subdivided into $μ_1$ receptors, responsible for supraspinal analgesia and physical dependence, and $μ_2$ receptors, responsible for respiratory depression, bradycardia, physical dependence, and gastrointestinal dysmotility.[207] Activation of the κ receptors causes analgesia without significant respiratory depression, whereas activation of the σ receptors causes dysphoria, tachycardia, tachypnea, hypertonia, and mydriasis. The δ receptors modulate the activity of the μ receptors.

Drugs that exert their effects on opioid receptors are classified as agonists, antagonists, partial agonists, and mixed agonist-antagonists. Agonists are neurotransmitters that bind to a receptor and exert their pharmacologic effects. Antagonists, on the other hand, bind to the receptor but do not initiate any effects; yet by occupying the receptor they block the effects of agonists. Partial agonists have reduced intrinsic activity and produce less than a maximal response. They act as antagonists as well because they block the agonists from access to the receptor. The mixed agonist-antagonist drugs act as agonists at certain opioid receptors and antagonists at others. E-Table 43-4 depicts the various opioid receptors, their effects, as well as the drugs that exert activity on each of them. The opioids that are used most commonly in the management of pain are μ-receptor agonists, including morphine, hydromorphone, the fentanyls, methadone, hydrocodone, and oxycodone. Of these, morphine is the opioid that is most commonly used as first-line therapy for moderate to severe pain in children and, consequently, is the agent with which clinicians have the greatest experience. Table 43-8 lists the relative potencies and suggested initial doses of the opioids in common clinical use. Developmental pharmacology, PK, and side effects of opioids are discussed in depth in Chapter 6.

### Delivery Techniques

The blood concentration of opioids must be maintained within a therapeutic range to provide effective analgesia and avoid undesirable adverse effects, such as excessive sedation and respiratory depression. Both the dose and the route by which the opioid is delivered determine how well one is able to maintain the blood concentration within this therapeutic window and minimize adverse effects.

#### Oral Administration

Oral administration of opioids at regular intervals can lead to reasonably constant blood concentrations if dosed appropriately. Oral opioids are well-tolerated and suitable for children with mild to moderate pain, for those who undergo outpatient surgery, or as adjuncts to regional anesthetics. For those with regional

**TABLE 43-8** Opioid Analgesics: Relative Potency and Initial Dosing Guidelines*

| Drug | Potency Relative to Morphine | Oral Dose | Intravenous Dose | PO:IV Dose Ratio |
|---|---|---|---|---|
| Morphine | 1 | 0.3 mg/kg every 3-4 hours<br>Sustained release:<br>20-35 kg: 10-15 mg every 8-12 hours<br>35-50 kg: 15-30 mg every 8-12 hours | Bolus: 0.1 mg/kg every 2-4 hours<br>Infusion: 0.03 mg/kg/hr | 1:3<br>1:6 for opioid-naive child |
| Hydromorphone | 5-7 | 0.04-0.08 mg/kg every 3-4 hours | Bolus: 0.02 mg/kg every 2-4 hours<br>Infusion: 0.006 mg/kg/hr | 1:4 |
| Fentanyl | 80-100 | NA | Bolus: 0.5-1 μg/kg every 30 minutes to 2 hours<br>Infusion: 0.5-2 μg/kg/hr | NA |
| Codeine | 0.1 | 0.5-1 mg/kg every 4-6 hours | NR | NA |
| Oxycodone | 1-1.5 | 0.1-0.2 mg/kg every 4-6 hours | NA | NA |
| Hydrocodone | 1-1.5 | 0.1-0.2 mg/kg every 4-6 hours | NA | NA |
| Methadone† | 1 | 0.1-0.2 mg/kg every 6-12 hours | 0.1 mg/kg every 6-12 hours | 1:2 |
| Nalbuphine | 0.8-1 | NA | 50-100 μg/kg every 3-6 hours | 4-5:1 |

Modified from Berde CB, Sethna NF. Analgesics for the treatment of pain in children. N Engl J Med 2002;347:1094-103.

*IV*, Intravenous; *NA*, not applicable; *NR*, not recommended; *PO*, oral.

*Recommended doses are for infants >6 months of age. For younger infants, reduce initial doses to 25% of these doses and increase as needed.

†Methadone has a long half-life and can accumulate, causing delayed sedation or respiratory depression. If sedation or respiratory depression occurs, doses should be withheld until sedation resolves. Then the drug is restarted at a smaller dose and extended dosing interval.

anesthetics, oral administration of an opioid before the block dissipates may provide a virtually pain-free recovery period. In most cases, oral opioids are better tolerated after resumption of oral intake.

Hydrocodone and oxycodone are two of the most commonly prescribed oral opioids. Both are available in a variety of formulations either alone or in combination with acetaminophen. Oxycodone causes significantly less nausea and vomiting than codeine and is usually better tolerated postoperatively when oral intake has resumed. Both hydrocodone and oxycodone are available in liquid form, making them easy to prescribe for infants and young children. Oxycodone is available in 1 mg/mL and 20 mg/mL strengths. The 1 mg/mL strength is easy to dose and administer to infants, whereas the 20 mg/mL strength is reserved for older children with chronic pain and should rarely be used to treat acute postoperative pain. Although the different formulations allow flexibility in dosing, extreme caution is required in prescribing and dispensing the correct concentration to avoid a potentially lethal overdose. Another important caveat when prescribing combination formulations of oral opioids and nonopioid adjuvants (such as acetaminophen) is to ensure that the recommended daily dose of the adjuvant is not exceeded. For children who require large doses of the opioid component to treat their pain, it may be necessary to prescribe the medications separately.

Although codeine has been widely used as an oral opioid analgesic, our strong preference is to avoid prescribing it in almost all situations, for several reasons. First, in recommended doses, it is a weak analgesic. Second, because it is a prodrug that requires conversion via demethylation to morphine (as detailed in Chapter 6), there is marked developmental and pharmacogenetic variation in this conversion that may result in ineffective conversion and thus reduced analgesia in some cases, or an overdose in others. Third, when the dosing is escalated, the frequencies of adverse effects, such as nausea, vomiting,

constipation, and dysphoria increase. It is important to note that with active metabolites of codeine excreted in breast milk, there has been a report of an opioid overdose in a neonate who was breastfed by a mother who was an extensive metabolizer.[208]

Methadone is a synthetic opioid with a very prolonged elimination half-life (mean of 19 hours) in children between 1 and 18 years of age, and a large bioavailability (approximately 80%) after oral administration. Oral or IV methadone has been considered a good alternative to the use of continuous opioid infusions because repeated dosing at intervals of every 4 to 8 hours can achieve relatively stable plasma drug concentrations.[209] Although it is used most frequently to facilitate weaning of opioid-tolerant children, it has also been recommended for postoperative analgesia and for transitioning children from parenteral to oral opioid therapy.[210-212] Methadone is especially useful for children with cancer, burns, or other serious illnesses who require a long-acting oral opioid, because it is available in an elixir formulation. Unlike some sustained-release formulations of other opioids, oral methadone is also relatively inexpensive. Note that crushing tablets of most sustained-release formulations of other opioids renders them into immediate-release, relatively short-acting medications. Methadone should be thought of as virtually a combination analgesic. It is supplied as a racemic mixture. The *l*-isomer acts as a μ opioid, whereas the *d*-isomer acts as an antagonist at the NMDA subclass of excitatory amino acid receptors. Action at NMDA receptors makes methadone uniquely effective in the treatment of neuropathic pain. This NMDA-blocking action, and a differential activation of receptor-mediated endocytosis versus protein kinase activation,[213,214] may lead to a relatively slower rate of development of tolerance for methadone compared with some other opioids. Despite these advantages of methadone, it requires careful titration and repeated reassessment to avoid delayed oversedation. This challenge in methadone dosing is due, in part, to its slow and widely variable clearance, as well as to its effects on NMDA antagonism, generating incomplete cross tolerance on conversion to methadone from other opioids. In opioid-naive subjects, a single dose of IV morphine is roughly equipotent to a single dose of methadone. Although morphine has active metabolites, the slower clearance of methadone compared with morphine translates in opioid-naive subjects, into daily IV methadone requirements that are roughly one-third those of morphine. *However, in the setting of marked opioid tolerance, such as in the case of children with advanced cancer or in the setting of intensive care, the equipotent daily dose of IV methadone may be as small as one-tenth the preceding daily dose of IV morphine.*[129,209,215-217] A convenient web-based calculation tool (www.globalrph.com/narcoticonv.htm) has synthesized the information from these and other studies to aid in opioid conversions in both opioid-naive and opioid-tolerant subjects. In our practice, this calculation tool appears quite useful, although it must be noted that it has not received independent assessment for use in children. Smartphone applications for multiple platforms are also available.

### Intravenous Administration

Intermittent IV injections with opioids of short or moderate duration administered on an as-needed basis (pro re nata, or PRN) do not achieve stable blood concentrations and predispose to periods of excessive sedation alternating with periods of inadequate analgesia. Yet this technique remains the most common method of treating postoperative pain in many centers. A partial solution to this problem is to prescribe the opioid at closer intervals (such as 2 hourly) and then use a "reverse-PRN" schedule, in which the medication is offered at the prescribed interval but the child can choose to take it or refuse it. Children should be assessed frequently, with the goal of administering the next dose before moderate to severe pain recurs. The use of a long-acting opioid, such as methadone, has been recommended to provide more prolonged and even periods of analgesia than could be achieved with shorter-acting opioids, approaching the efficacy of continuous infusions.[218] However, careful titration of dosing and frequent assessment of the child are required because of methadone's slow and variable clearance. Alternatively, administration of shorter-acting opioids via continuous infusion or a PCA device should be considered.

Continuous IV opioid infusions are an excellent means of providing analgesia to children with moderate to severe pain who are unable to use PCA, such as infants, young children, and those who are cognitively impaired or physically disabled.[219] Once a therapeutic blood concentration of the opioid is achieved by administering an initial loading dose, an infusion rate can be selected to maintain that concentration without excessive fluctuations. Additionally, rescue doses of IV opioids may be required for breakthrough pain. Opioids, however, cause a dose-dependent respiratory depression by shifting the $CO_2$ response curve, reducing its slope, and decreasing the hypoxic ventilatory response. Residual and synergistic effects of sedatives and hypnotics in the early postoperative period further increase the risk of opioid-induced respiratory depression. This is particularly true in preterm and term infants because of age-related differences in elimination and clearance of opioids and other sedating medications (see also Chapter 6). This is of particular concern with the use of continuous opioid infusions because inappropriate dosing or prolonged elimination may lead to drug accumulation, placing children at risk for side effects. In a recent prospective audit of 10,726 opioid infusions in the UK and Ireland, the overall risk of permanent harm was found to be 1 in 10,000 cases, and serious events without permanent harm 1 in 383, with half of

the serious events being respiratory depression.[220] Therefore, the rate of the infusion should be carefully selected, based on the child's age, comorbidities, and clinical condition. Additionally, children who receive opioid infusions should be monitored and assessed frequently for depth of sedation and respiratory rate. The onset of sedation is an important clinical index of incipient respiratory depression and should alert the nursing staff and physicians to decrease the infusion rate and observe the child more closely. Use of continuous pulse oximetry is widely recommended during continuous opioid infusions, especially in opioid-naive children and other children at increased risk for respiratory depression. Another method of IV opioid delivery is via PCA, which is discussed below. With any infusion technique, scrupulous attention must be paid to protocols for checking pump settings to avoid errors. Pump programming errors, none of which caused serious harm, but which had the potential to do so, occurred in 17 instances in the UK audit, all from a single center, highlighting the critical importance of system safeguards to prevent patient harm.[220]

### Intramuscular and Subcutaneous Routes

Intermittent IM and subcutaneous injections of opioids are obsolete because they are frightening and unpleasant for children and are often perceived as worse than the pain for which they are administered.[221] Additionally, they have the PK disadvantage of unpredictable and erratic uptake if regional blood flow is impaired, and they produce pronounced wide swings in blood concentrations. The goal of maintaining an even level of analgesia is thus nearly impossible to achieve with these routes of administration. An important exception is the use of indwelling subcutaneous catheters for continuous infusions and PCA as in palliative care.

### Selection of Opioids for Parenteral Use

Morphine is the opioid most commonly used for postoperative analgesia and has been extensively studied in all pediatric age groups. After major abdominal, thoracic, and orthopedic surgery, children who received continuous morphine infusions had reduced pain scores compared with those who received intermittent IM or IV injections.[222-224] However, other investigators were only able to demonstrate reduced pain scores with continuous morphine infusions compared with intermittent IV injections of morphine in children between 1 and 3 years of age, and not in infants in the first year of life.[225,226] Similarly, evidence of the beneficial effects of opioid analgesia in ameliorating the postoperative response to surgical stress are conflicting. A significant reduction in serum β-endorphin concentrations has been reported in neonates after the initiation of a continuous infusion of morphine in the postoperative period.[227] In neonates whose lungs were mechanically ventilated, both epinephrine and norepinephrine concentrations decreased significantly after the initiation of morphine or fentanyl infusions.[228] However, β-endorphin concentrations decreased only in the children who received fentanyl. When the effects of continuous infusions of morphine were compared with those of intermittent IV injections of morphine on the stress response in children between 1 and 3 years of age, reduced glucose concentrations in the continuous infusion group suggested only a modest ablation of the stress response in this age group.[225]

Several studies have described the PK of morphine administered as a continuous infusion and evaluated the pharmacodynamic effects of morphine on respiratory indices in neonates, infants, and children after various surgical procedures. In children 14 months to 17 years of age who underwent cardiac surgery,[229] morphine infusions were adjusted between 10 and 50 μg/kg/hr to minimize discomfort and avoid excessive sedation. Supplemental boluses of 100 μg/kg morphine were administered for breakthrough pain. Steady-state morphine concentrations were achieved in 4 hours. Those children who could self-report their pain reported good analgesia with morphine concentrations in excess of 12 ng/mL. Morphine infusions of 10 to 30 μg/kg/hr yielded mean serum concentrations between 10 and 22 ng/mL with less than 2% experiencing evidence of respiratory depression ($PaCO_2$ greater than 50 mm Hg). Furthermore, children who received morphine infusions of 10 to 30 μg/kg/hr breathed spontaneously after extubation of the trachea, and those who were weaned from assisted to spontaneous ventilation maintained a normal $PaCO_2$. On the other hand, 60% (3 of 5 children) who received a greater infusion rate of morphine, 40 to 50 μg/kg/hr, experienced hypercarbia ($PaCO_2$ 48 to 66 mm Hg). A subsequent study by the same investigators evaluated the severity of respiratory depression in infants and children aged 2 days to 18 months treated with morphine. Of those whose morphine concentrations exceeded 20 ng/mL, approximately 70% experienced respiratory depression ($PaCO_2$ greater than 55 mm Hg and/or a depressed slope of the $CO_2$ response curve) compared with 15% to 28% of those whose concentrations were less than 20 ng/mL.[230] The investigators suggested a steady-state morphine concentration of 20 ng/mL as a threshold concentration for respiratory depression in this age group.

Previous studies determined that the clearance of morphine is impaired in preterm infants and that clearance increases with postconception age.[231] Additionally, morphine clearance is impaired in full-term infants up to 1 to 2 months of age, at which time it is comparable with that in older children and adults.[98,232] Preterm and full-term neonates, therefore, have a narrower therapeutic window for morphine analgesia compared with older children. Indeed, these groups have reduced morphine requirements postoperatively, requiring fewer rescue doses of morphine when receiving continuous infusions or intermittent bolus doses.[233] Therefore, opioids should be carefully titrated in infants in a monitored environment with significantly reduced continuous infusion rates. Based on PK modeling and morphine clearance predictions, a target morphine concentration of 10 ng/mL can be achieved with morphine infusions ranging from 5 μg/kg/hr in term neonates to 16 μg/kg/hr in 1- to 3-year-old children (see Chapter 6).[234]

Pharmacodynamic differences between infants and children have been postulated as the mechanism responsible for the greater sensitivity of infants (compared with older children) to the respiratory depressant effects of opioids. However, this may not be the case. Although rodent data suggest that the brain concentrations of opioids in neonates are greater than those in older children at similar serum concentrations,[235] these findings may not be applicable to humans. Neonatal rats have a relatively immature brain and a far more permeable blood-brain barrier than that in human infants. Consequently, the rodent may not be an appropriate model to depict the human condition.[236] It appears that the "increased sensitivity" is related, at least in part, to PK variables, perhaps in some measure as a result of a neonate's decreased conjugating ability.

Regardless of the mechanism, respiratory depression remains the most feared adverse effect of opioids administered by any route. Neonates and infants younger than 6 months of age are at greater risk for opioid-induced respiratory depression because the ventilatory responses to airway obstruction, hypoxemia, and hypercapnia are immature at birth and mature over the first several months of life in preterm as well as full-term infants (see also Figs. 4-8 and 4-9). Indeed, there was a 4.5% incidence of failure to wean from the ventilator and a 13.5% incidence of apnea (30 seconds or more that required intervention) or severe respiratory depression in spontaneously breathing neonates who received opioids for postoperative pain.[237] Another report of a 3-year surveillance period for adverse drug reactions described 15 children aged 2 days to 17 years who experienced opioid-induced respiratory depression.[238] Respiratory depression in the latter study was defined as apnea, hypoxemia, cyanosis, a marked decrease in respiratory rate, or a need for naloxone. Although this study was unable to define the incidence of respiratory depression because the denominator was unknown, it did identify several predisposing factors, including age younger than 1 year (7 of 15 children), drug errors (including prescription and administration errors; 6 of 15 children), concurrent medical problems (diminished respiratory reserve, hepatic, and/or renal impairment), and concurrent sedative drugs. The prospective UK audit found 14 cases of respiratory depression (out of 10,726 total infusions, or 0.13%), 10 with nurse-controlled anesthesia (NCA), 2 with continuous infusions, and 2 with PCA.[220] Potentially contributing risk factors in half of the cases included very young age and neurodevelopmental, respiratory, or cardiac disease. In contrast to the above studies, no case of respiratory depression was reported in 110 children older than 3 months of age who received opioid infusions postoperatively.[239] Interpretation of this literature is confounded by different monitoring techniques and different definitions of respiratory depression. For instance, in the latter study, a 4.5% incidence of clinically significant hypoxemia was reported but was not included in their definition of respiratory depression. Additionally, children in that study were monitored with hourly documentation of respiratory rate, but oxygen saturation was not monitored after discharge from PACU, thereby reducing their ability to detect the more subtle episodes of respiratory depression. In summary, the results of these studies suggest that children who receive opioids require careful monitoring for respiratory depression, with appropriate age-based reduction of dosage, particularly for neonates and infants younger than 6 months of age.

The most common adverse effect of opioid therapy is nausea and vomiting. One study reported nausea and vomiting in 34 of 80 children (42.5%) who received postoperative morphine infusions. These were well managed with antiemetic therapy in all but 2 children who required discontinuation of the opioids.[239] In the same study, the incidence of pruritus and urinary retention were both 13% and that of dysphoria was 7%. Seizures have been reported in two neonates who had received bolus doses of morphine followed by infusions of 32 and 40 μg/kg/hr and whose serum morphine concentrations were 61 and 90 ng/mL, respectively.[240] Irregular jerking movements, as well as one case of a generalized seizure, have been reported in children 1 to 15 years of age receiving postoperative morphine infusions.[222] Metoclopramide, 0.10 to 0.15 mg/kg (100 to 150 μg/kg) given IV, is an effective antiemetic but may also cause sedation and dystonia. The serotonin-receptor antagonist antiemetics, such as ondansetron and dolasetron, have the advantage of virtually eliminating the risk of dystonic or oculogyric reactions that occur with phenothiazines, butyrophenones, and metoclopramide. However, headaches occur in a small number of those who receive serotonin-receptor antagonists. A "micro-dose" naloxone infusion (0.25 to 1.0 µg/kg/hr) reverses the incidence of both nausea and pruritus after opioids without affecting the analgesia or opioid consumption.[241,242] A more recent dose-escalation study demonstrated that doses of 1 to 1.65 µg/kg/hr resulted in greater efficacy in reducing side effects, particularly pruritus, without degrading analgesia.[242] It is likely that these results may be generalized to other routes of opioid administration.

Opioid-induced bowel dysfunction reported in more than 90% of patients on opioid therapy, occurs by blocking propulsive peristalsis, inhibiting secretion and increasing reabsorption of intestinal fluids, and decreasing the activity of excitatory and inhibitory neurons in the myenteric plexus. Bowel dysfunction manifests as abdominal distension and bloating, delayed gastric emptying, and constipation. Aggressive prophylactic measures, including osmotic, lubricant, or stimulant laxatives, should be prescribed early in the course of treatment. A newer selective gastrointestinal peripheral µ-opioid receptor antagonist, methylnaltrexone, was approved for use in adults in 2008. Although adult studies have shown promising results with the use of this agent,[243,244] its pediatric use has been described in only one case report.[245] A neonate who experienced a severe ileus during fentanyl administration after major abdominal surgery was noted to have resolution of the signs within 15 minutes of IV methylnaltrexone (0.15 mg/kg). She received 5 daily doses of methylnaltrexone without reversal of analgesia or occurrence of withdrawal.[245]

Fentanyl may be a useful substitute for morphine in children with hemodynamic instability, in whom a decrease in peripheral vascular tone is undesirable, and in whom histamine release caused by morphine is not well-tolerated. Additionally, its rapid onset of analgesia makes it ideal for children with severe escalating pain who require urgent pain relief. Fentanyl is metabolized by the liver into an inactive metabolite, norfentanyl, which is excreted via the kidneys. It is 80 to 100 times more potent than morphine. Although its elimination half-life is significantly less than that for morphine, its context-sensitive half-life during chronic infusion increases exponentially as a result of growing tissue storage (see Chapter 6). Like morphine, the elimination half-life of fentanyl in neonates is nearly twice that in adults, predisposing them to a greater risk for accumulation compared with older infants.[246,247] As with morphine, a reduction in hepatic blood flow in very young infants further decreases fentanyl conjugation. For a given bolus of fentanyl, plasma concentrations in infants between 3 months and 1 year of age are less than those in older children and adults.[248] This finding is consistent with the almost twofold greater clearance of fentanyl in children compared with neonates. In children 18 days to 14 years of age who were mechanically ventilated, the clearance of fentanyl was age related yet quite variable, with the slowest clearance occurring in infants younger than 6 months of age and the most rapid in those between 6 months and 6 years of age.[249] The clearance of fentanyl is slow in preterm infants, with the clearance correlating with the postnatal age.[250]

Fentanyl is known to cause all of the adverse effects reported with opioids, including pruritus, nausea, vomiting, constipation, and sedation. Respiratory depression and chest wall and glottic rigidity, however, are its most feared adverse effects. One study compared the incidence of respiratory depression in full-term and former preterm infants and young infants receiving 2 µg/kg bolus doses of fentanyl every 2 hours or a continuous infusion of 1 µg/kg/hr after abdominal or thoracic surgery.[251] Randomization was terminated prematurely because of a sixfold greater incidence of apnea that required intervention in the bolus dose group compared with the continuous infusion group (89% vs. 14%). The continuous infusion arm was continued for another 20 children, resulting in a 25% incidence of apnea in this group. In contrast, the incidence of respiratory depression (based on transcutaneous $PaCO_2$ measurements and the incidence of apnea) for a given plasma fentanyl concentration in infants 1 to 12 months of age and children 1 to 5 years of age was less than that in adults undergoing hernia repair or other peripheral surgery.[252] Differences in surgical procedures and the inclusion of preterm infants in the former study may account for the significant difference in the incidence of apnea found in these two studies.

Although chest wall rigidity usually occurs after the rapid bolus administration of high-dose fentanyl, it has also been reported in an infant after a low-dose continuous infusion of fentanyl. Chest wall rigidity was reported in 9% of preterm and full-term neonates who received an average of 4.9 µg/kg over a 2 to 3 minute period for a procedure or for perioperative analgesia.[253] In every case, naloxone reversed the chest wall rigidity. Additionally, a case of chest wall rigidity has been reported in a preterm neonate after high-dose fentanyl was administered to the parturient before a cesarean section.[254] Although administration of naloxone has been used successfully to treat cases of chest wall rigidity, severe cases associated with rapid oxygen desaturation may require the use of neuromuscular blocking drugs and mechanical ventilation.

The use of continuous fentanyl infusions in infants and children has been associated with a rapid development of tolerance, as indicated by a steady increase in infusion rate to maintain the desired effect[255,256] and a large incidence of opioid withdrawal syndrome after termination of the infusion.[256,257] The incidence of opioid withdrawal is directly related to the total dose administered and the duration of infusion.[256,257] Neonatal abstinence syndrome has been reported in 21 of 37 neonates (57%) after continuous fentanyl infusions during extracorporeal membrane oxygenation.[256] Both a total fentanyl dose in excess of 1.6 mg/kg and extracorporeal membrane oxygenation that lasted more than 5 days were predictors of opioid withdrawal. A similar incidence has been reported in 23 children 1 week to 22 months of age who received continuous fentanyl infusions during mechanical ventilation.[257] This study also found that a total dose of 1.5 mg/kg of fentanyl over 5 days was associated with a greater than 50% incidence of withdrawal symptoms. Furthermore, a total dose of 2.5 mg/kg as a continuous infusion over 9 days was 100% predictive of the occurrence of withdrawal. Finally, movement disorder and irritability have been reported after withdrawal of fentanyl infusion in five infants who were mechanically ventilated.[258] None of the infants who developed the movement disorder had received another opioid after withdrawal of fentanyl, whereas five of eight controls who did not develop withdrawal during the same period had received a substitute opioid. These data suggest that opioid withdrawal occurs earlier and with greater frequency after fentanyl infusions compared with other opioids. Therefore it seems prudent to use fentanyl infusions for pain relief during periods of hemodynamic instability, such as in the early postoperative period, and to transition to another opioid, such as morphine, as soon as the child is stabilized. Children who require fentanyl infusions for 5 days or more should undergo a slow taper (e.g., 10% decrease every 12 hours) or be transitioned to another parenteral or oral opioid regimen.

Hydromorphone has a spectrum of action similar to that of morphine. Adult opioid equipotency data suggest that it is 3.5 to 7 times as potent as morphine.[259-261] The only pediatric study that was performed in children with mucositis pain after bone marrow transplant reported that a 7:1 conversion ratio of morphine to hydromorphone, underestimated hydromorphone requirements by 27%.[262] These data suggest that a 5:1 conversion ratio may be more appropriate, particularly in children with chronic pain. Despite its widespread use, there are very few studies that evaluated the use of hydromorphone in children. A Cochrane review of studies related to the use of hydromorphone for acute and chronic pain in adults and children found little difference between the analgesic efficacy and adverse effect profile of morphine and hydromorphone.[263] However, several of the studies in this review included small numbers of patients, some were of low quality and only four of them included children. It remains common practice to prescribe a trial of hydromorphone in children who experience unacceptable side effects with morphine.

Meperidine is an opioid that has been used clinically for many years.[264,265] Its potency is approximately one-tenth that of morphine. Accumulation of its active metabolite, normeperidine (which has CNS stimulant properties), after repeated doses of meperidine, places children at risk for seizures.[266] Therefore, its use has been restricted to the treatment of postoperative shivering[267,268] or rigors after amphotericin. A single dose of dexmedetomidine (0.5 µg/kg) has been used successfully for the treatment of postoperative shivering and may replace meperidine for this indication.[269] Although its short-term use continues by some clinicians for procedural sedation and analgesia, it is preferable to use other analgesics for this purpose. Meperidine is not recommended for PCA or as a continuous infusion in children.

## Patient-Controlled Analgesia

PCA was first studied in adults in 1965. The initial interest with this technique was as a research tool for the study of pain. By the early 1970s, it was identified as an excellent strategy for treating pain in the clinical setting, with studies demonstrating that pain relief was achieved by PCA with relatively smaller doses of opioids and with greater patient satisfaction than with conventional methods.[270] However, it was not until the late 1980s that PCA was studied in children.[271] Since that time, it has become the preferred method for opioid delivery in children older than 5 to 6 years of age for acute pain, as well as chronic pain associated with cancer or sickle cell disease.[262,271-274] The primary benefit of PCA is that it allows children to titrate the analgesic to the extent of their pain. The goal is for the child to self-regulate a blood opioid concentration within the therapeutic range. Most children strike a balance between adequate pain relief on the one hand and adverse effects of the drug on the other. This approach, which grants the child some degree of autonomy, is the rationale given for the fact that pain is an entirely subjective and individual experience and that opioid metabolism and pain perception are quite variable among individuals. It also reduces the apprehension that older children and adolescents have about pain relief because they can control it and they can tailor the opioid delivery to the extent of pain they have at a given time, for example, before physical therapy, removal of tubes or drains, dressing changes, or getting out of bed. Additionally, the use of PCA avoids delays in administration of analgesics associated with standard "as needed" orders of IV opioids and allows smaller doses of opioids to be delivered more frequently without increasing nursing workload. Therefore, PCA is thought to provide more consistent pain relief with less total opioid dosing, resulting in fewer side effects, such as sedation, nausea, and vomiting. Purportedly, children using PCA report better analgesia and reduced pain scores compared with children who have to rely on the nursing staff to administer analgesics when they are in pain. These and other benefits of PCA have been extensively touted in the medical literature,[274-276] as well as in the lay press.[277] Recently, however, risks associated with PCA use have also been highlighted and are discussed later.[278-280] Recognition of these risks has led to recommendations for careful dosing and monitoring of all children who are receiving opioids, particularly those receiving continuous infusions and those with specific risk factors.[281]

Child training is a necessary part of PCA, because successful use of PCA requires that both the child and family understand how it works.[282] The instructions should be clear that the pump should be activated whenever the child feels pain, that children cannot give themselves "too much medication" because of the computer lockout interval, that the child should not wait for severe pain to activate the pump, and that a dose can also be given in anticipation of painful stimuli, such as ambulation or chest physiotherapy. Most importantly, PCA does not mean *parent*-controlled analgesia, and parents should never activate the pump unless specifically authorized to do so by the primary care or pain service physician (see Nurse/Caregiver-Controlled Analgesia, later).[281]

### PCA Equipment

PCA devices are microprocessor-driven pumps that are connected to the child's IV line via Y tubing. For safety reasons, the IV tubing should incorporate a one-way valve to prevent backflow of the PCA drug up the tubing and an unintended delivery of a large bolus of opioid. Alternatively, PCA may be delivered through a separate IV line. These pumps allow programming of the individual dose to be administered, the minimal interval between doses (lockout interval), and the maximal cumulative allowable dose over a 4-hour period. Some pumps allow programming of a maximum number of doses per hour. Most pumps allow delivery of a continuous basal infusion (CBI) in addition to the demand dose. All PCA pumps should have a locking mechanism, so that neither the settings nor the medication cartridge can be changed without using a key, making the device virtually tamper proof. The child is able to self-administer the preprogrammed doses by pushing a button. A liquid crystal display on the pump displays the programmed settings, the cumulative dosage, the number of doses administered, and the number of times that the button was pushed but no dose was given because either it was during the lockout interval or the 4-hour limit had been reached. This information allows clinicians to track opioid usage and make appropriate changes to the PCA prescription based on the usage pattern. Most children 5 to 6 years of age and older are able to push the button themselves. In general, a child who is able to play video games has the cognitive skills required to push a button to achieve a desired response and can, therefore, use PCA quite effectively.

### Choice of Drug and Drug Dosages

Morphine remains the most common opioid administered via PCA, with hydromorphone and fentanyl being second-line drugs usually reserved for children who are intolerant to morphine. Suggested initial dosages for opioids via PCA for opioid-naïve

**TABLE 43-9** Patient-Controlled Analgesia Dosing Guidelines

| Drug | Demand Dose (µg/kg) | Lockout Interval (minutes) | Continuous Basal Infusion (µg/kg/hr) | 4-Hour Limit (µg/kg) |
|------|---------------------|----------------------------|--------------------------------------|----------------------|
| Morphine | 10-20 | 8-15 | 0-20 | 250-400 |
| Hydromorphone | 2-4 | 8-15 | 0-4 | 50-80 |
| Fentanyl | 0.5 | 5-10 | 0-0.5 | 7-10 |

children are presented in Table 43-9. Children with opioid tolerance will require adjustments to these settings, taking into account the previous opioid history and the opioid doses that the child was receiving before the acute painful stimulus. Indeed, one study reported that children with sickle cell disease self-administered more than double the dose of morphine via PCA, required more nonopioid adjuvant analgesics, reported greater pain scores, and stayed in the hospital for twice the duration compared with non–sickle cell disease–affected children after laparoscopic cholecystectomy.[283]

Fentanyl PCA has been used with success as a first-line and a secondary drug in children with cancer pain, as well as acute postoperative pain.[276,284] Most of the adverse effects, including nausea and pruritus, were mild and easily managed. However, some reported an overall incidence of apnea and hypoxemia of 3.5% in 212 children receiving PCA, of whom 144 had received fentanyl.[276] Finally, children who received tramadol PCA after heart surgery were extubated earlier and had less sedation, comparable pain scores, and a similar incidence of emesis as those who received morphine PCA.[189] The IV formulation of tramadol is not yet available in the United States, but some studies from Europe and China support its use in the postoperative period.[189,285] The benefits that hydromorphone PCA offers over morphine PCA in the chronic and acute pain settings require further investigation.

### Pump Settings

Most PCA pumps have five settings to adjust:

- A *loading dose* of opioid ranging from 0.025 to 0.1 mg/kg morphine divided into incremental doses is usually given to establish adequate analgesia before therapy is turned over to the child, because self-administered doses with this technique are generally small. A sufficient interval between incremental doses must be allowed, so that the morphine achieves its peak effect before the next dose, thereby avoiding an overdose. If PCA is started in the PACU, opioid doses administered during surgery must be considered before prescribing a loading dose. Additionally, it may be desirable to administer the loading dose via the PCA pump so that it is included in the initial 4-hour or hourly limit of the PCA. That is because children who receive IV-PRN doses of opioids in the PACU, followed by initiation of PCA, may be at risk for oversedation and respiratory depression resulting from opioid stacking. Children who have received opioids toward the end of surgery, those who awaken in comfort, or those who receive nerve blocks may not need a loading dose and may start to use the demand doses as needed on awakening.
- A *patient bolus dose*, that is, the dose that will be administered with each child's activation of the pump, must be prescribed. These small boluses are usually in the range of 0.01 to 0.02 mg/kg of morphine in opioid-naive subjects.
- A *lockout interval* of usually 5 to 15 minutes prevents a child from activating the pump until the full effect from the

previous bolus is achieved, and it should correspond to the time from IV injection to the peak effect of the drug.

- A *continuous basal infusion* ranging from 0.00 to 0.02 mg/kg/hr of morphine (or more, in opioid-tolerant subjects) may be used in selective cases (see later).
- A *maximum hourly dose or a 4-hour limit* may be chosen to limit the cumulative amount of drug a child can administer. Once this limit is reached, the child cannot activate the pump until the 4-hour limit has passed. Four-hour limits allow for increased flexibility in dosing over greater periods of time and pain intensity. Typically, the maximum hourly dose ranges from 0.05 to 0.1 mg/kg and 4-hour limits from 0.25 to 0.4 mg/kg of morphine in opioid-naive subjects. This amount may be chosen based on the average hourly use of morphine during the past 24 hours or, in children started on PCA immediately after surgery, at the reduced range of the dosage scale. Figure 43-8 presents sample PCA orders, including choice of drugs, dosing, and suggested monitoring.

### Continuous Basal Infusions (CBI)

The use of a CBI of the opioid to supplement child-administered doses remains a subject of controversy. The rationale for the use of CBI is to maintain near-therapeutic plasma opioid concentrations, particularly during periods of sleep when there may be no self-administered doses, as illustrated in Figure 43-9, *A*. On the other hand, as depicted in Figure 43-9, *B*, a child who receives only PCA bolus dosing with no CBI is likely to awaken with unrelieved pain that may require multiple doses to again achieve adequate pain relief. Decreased nocturnal awakenings secondary to pain, improved restfulness or sleep patterns, reduced total opioid consumption, fewer adverse effects, and improved analgesic effectiveness have all been proposed as potential reasons in favor of using CBI. However, the use of CBI commits the child to receiving a fixed dose of opioid regardless of the level of sedation, and has the theoretical potential for overriding one of the inherent safety features of PCA, that is, an excessively sedated or somnolent child is unlikely to push the button and therefore receives no additional opioid but, with a fixed infusion, drug may accumulate (Fig. 43-9, *C*), with the potential for hypoventilation.[286] Furthermore, it has also been argued that programming errors with CBI can lead to more serious adverse events because the opioid medication is delivered regardless of the child's level of sedation.[285,287]

Some adult studies have suggested that the use of CBI has limited benefit in terms of efficacy and is associated with a greater incidence of opioid adverse effects, including respiratory depression.[288-290] Studies in children, however, have yielded conflicting results.[273,274,291-295] Children 7 to 19 years of age who received PCA with CBI after orthopedic surgery reported significantly reduced pain scores compared with those who received PCA boluses alone or IM morphine.[274] There were no differences in morphine consumption or in opioid adverse effects among the three groups, with no incidents of respiratory depression.

| | | | BIRTHDATE |
|---|---|---|---|

**Pediatric Acute Pain Service (APS)**

NAME

**Patient Controlled Analgesia (PCA) Initial Orders**

Reg. No.

Date: _____ Time: _____

Clerk's Initials: _____ Unit: _____

No other OPIOIDS or SEDATIVES to be administered while on PCA unless Pain Service has ordered them or been notified.
Please page Pain Service before discontinuing PCA at pager xxxx.

AGE: _____ mo/yr    WEIGHT: _____ kg

MODE: ☐ PCA ONLY
   ☐ PCA & Continuous
   ☐ Nurse Controlled
   ☐ Continuous
   ☐ Other: _____

| Select drug to be used | ☐ Morphine | | ☐ Hydromorphone<br>Anesthesia faculty/fellow approval needed.<br>Must start at 100 µg/mL concentration. | | ☐ Fentanyl<br>_____ |
|---|---|---|---|---|---|
| **Drug Concentration** | ☐ 1 mg/mL | ☐ 100 µg/mL<br>(3000 µg/30 mL<br>use for pts ≤10 kg) | ☐ 0.5 mg/mL (use only for pts requiring excessive dosing) | ☐ 100 µg/mL<br>(3000 µg/30 mL) | 20 µg/mL |
| **PCA Dose** | _____ mg<br>0.02-0.03 mg/kg | _____ µg<br>20-30 µg/kg | _____ mg<br>0.002-0.004 mg/kg | _____ µg<br>2-4 µg/kg | _____ µg<br>0.20-0.5 µg |
| **Lockout Interval** | _____ minute<br>8-15 minutes | _____ minute<br>8-15 minutes | _____ minute<br>8-15 minutes | _____ minute<br>8-15 minutes | _____ minute<br>8-15 minutes |
| **Continuous Infusion Rate** | _____ mg/hr<br>0.01-0.02 mg/kg/hr | _____ µg/hr<br>10-20 µg/kg/hr | _____ mg/hr<br>0.002-0.004 mg/kg/hr | _____ µg/hr<br>2-4 µg/kg/hr | _____ /hr<br>0.1-0.5 µg/kg/hr |
| **4-Hour Limit** | _____ mg<br>0.25-0.4 mg/kg | _____ µg<br>250-400 µg/kg | _____ mg<br>0.05-0.08 mg/kg | _____ µg<br>50-80 µg/kg | _____<br>7-10 µg/kg |
| **Double Check** | Double check pump settings against the order. Document double check on the PCA/Epidural Flowsheet. | | | | |
| ***Emergency Measures*** | **For sedation score >2 or respiratory rate < _____ :**<br> Hold PCA and page Pain Service<br><br>**For sedation score = 4 or respiratory rate < _____ :**<br> Hold PCA, give Naloxone and STAT page Primary Service **FIRST**, then Pain Service<br>  **Naloxone Dose:**<br>  Under 10 kg _____ mg IV STAT (0.01 mg/kg/dose, maximum of 0.1 mg), may repeat every 2 minutes × 2<br>  Over 10 kg 0.1 mg IV STAT, may repeat every 2 minutes × 2<br><br> For O₂ Saturation < _____ : (Consider baseline saturation) Stimulate patient and encourage deep breathing<br>  Administer O₂ by face mask or nasal cannula and page the Primary Service and Pain Service | | | | |
| **Antipruritic** | ☐ Naloxone (Narcan) 0.25 µg/kg/hr. Add 0.25 mg to 100 mL normal saline (0.1 mL/hr = 0.25 µg/kg/hr) to be infused at 0.1 mL/hr × weight (kg) = _____ mL/hr or Nalbuphine 0.05 mg/kg = _____ mg IV every 4 hours | | | | |
| **Antiemetic** | ☐ Ondansetron (Zofran) _____ mg IV every 6 hours PRN (0.1 mg/kg/dose up to 4 mg) MAX single dose: 4 mg<br>☐ Per Primary Service<br>☐ Other: _____ | | | | |
| **Other** | ☐ Other: _____ | | | | |

1. Monitoring:

 Continuous pulse oximetry while on PCA except while patient is out of bed. Record pulse oximetry readings at same frequency as respiratory rate. Respiratory rate and sedation level:

  Initiation of therapy: every 30 minutes × 1 hour and then every 2 hours for the first 24 hours and then every 4 hours
  Transfer to a new unit: every 30 minutes × 1 hour then either every 2 or 4 hours (depends upon start of PCA therapy)
  With loading dose and increases in doses, infusions, limits: every 30 minutes × 2 then every 2 or 4 hours (depends upon start of PCA therapy)
  Regularly scheduled Day/Night changes: every 4 hours if therapy has been initiated longer than 24 hours.

 *Pain Scores:*
  every 2 hours × 8 hours, then every 4 hours. If pain not controlled after 1 hour, page xxxx or xxxx

2. The Acute Pain Service (APS) nurse may change PCA orders by increasing or decreasing pump settings by 20% and stop the continuous infusion.
3. Any order changes in #2 must be documented on a subsequent PCA order form.

| Verbal ☐ | | | | |
|---|---|---|---|---|
| Telephone ☐ Print name/title of person giving order | Signature/title of person taking order | | Date | Time |
|     Physician Signature | Dr. # | | Date | Time |

**FIGURE 43-8** Sample patient-controlled analgesia orders. (Modified from the University of Michigan Hospitals & Health Centers.)

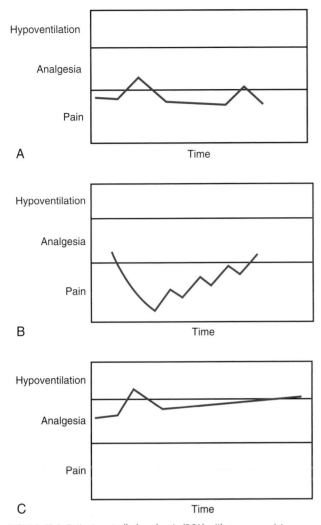

**FIGURE 43-9** Patient-controlled analgesia (PCA) with an appropriate dose of continuous basal infusion. **A,** Use of an appropriate dose of continuous basal infusion (CBI) maintains near-therapeutic plasma opioid concentrations during sleep with rapid increase to analgesic concentrations as soon as the child awakens and activates the PCA button. **B,** Chart depicts plasma opioid concentrations in a child who is receiving PCA bolus doses only, with no CBI. Plasma concentrations decrease significantly when the child is asleep, necessitating multiple doses to achieve analgesic concentrations. **C,** An excessive dose of CBI results in opioid accumulation with delayed hypoventilation even when the PCA button is not activated. (Reproduced with permission from Berde CB, Solodiuk J. Multidisciplinary programs for management of acute and chronic pain in children. In: Schecter NL, Berde CB, Yaster M, editors. Pain in infants, children and adolescents. 2nd ed. Philadelphia: Lippincott Williams and Wilkins; 2003, p. 476.)

Notably, child satisfaction was greatest in the PCA with CBI group. Similar pain scores with improved sleeping patterns have also been reported with the use of PCA with CBI, compared with those who received PCA alone, on the first two postoperative nights in children after abdominal surgery. No incidents of respiratory depression or excessive sedation were reported in either group.[273] Children who received CBI with PCA or NCA in one study reported slightly reduced pain scores without differences in morphine use or adverse effects after spine fusion surgery compared with those who received PCA or NCA alone.[295] In contrast, others have reported greater morphine use and a greater

incidence of hypoxemia with similar pain scores in children who received PCA plus CBI after surgery compared with those who received PCA alone.[293,294] A subsequent study found that children who received PCA with a CBI of morphine (4 μg/kg/hr) experienced fewer adverse effects and less hypoxemia than children who received PCA with 20 μg/kg/hr CBI or those who received PCA bolus doses alone, noting similar pain scores in all three groups.[292] Both of the PCA with CBI groups reported better sleep at night than did the PCA alone group. Differences in opioid doses, age groups, and surgical procedures may account, in part, for these apparent conflicting observations in the pediatric studies. Based on these studies and our own experience, we hold the view that the use of CBI may be beneficial in some children, although it requires careful selection of dose, based on the surgical severity and the child's comorbid conditions and vigilant monitoring to ensure safety. CBI should be used as a routine for most children with pain resulting from cancer, for most children with mucositis resulting from cancer treatment or bone marrow transplantation, and for a significant percentage of children with sickle cell vasoocclusive episodes. At our institutions, the standard practice is to use CBI, unless limited by somnolence or hypoventilation, for the first night for a majority of children undergoing selected major painful surgeries, such as scoliosis surgery, pelvic osteotomies, and thoracotomies.

### Nurse/Caregiver-Controlled Analgesia

Activation of the PCA pump by the bedside nurse, a parent, or a caregiver (such as a grandparent) has been used with success in children who are unable to push the button because of young age or because of physical or cognitive impairments.[275,276,295-297] In much of the literature, and in some policy statements by the Joint Commission and other organizations, there is, in our view, too little distinction between activation of PCA pumps by nurses and activation by nonclinician surrogates. The term *caregiver* is used variably in this literature; here it is used to mean nonclinician surrogates. In pediatrics, this means primarily parents and other family members. A small study of 12 children who received NCA after spine fusion surgery reported adequate analgesia, parent and nurse satisfaction, and no complications.[295] Children who received NCA received smaller total morphine doses compared with those who were able to use the PCA device themselves, likely because of the tendency for nurses to underestimate their patients' pain. A larger observational study of 212 children who received parent- or nurse-controlled analgesia with morphine, fentanyl, or hydromorphone reported effective analgesia (pain scores 3/10 or 2/5 or below) in more than 80% of children.[276] Pruritus occurred in 8% and vomiting in 15% of the children on the first day of treatment. Nine children (4.2%) required naloxone for the following: apnea (N = 4), hypoxemia (N = 1), excessive sedation (N = 3), or to facilitate extubation (N = 1). Six of these children had significant comorbid conditions, and 5 received additional sedatives. These investigators emphasized the importance of close monitoring to minimize risk and permit early intervention when using nurse/caregiver-controlled analgesia (NCA/CCA). Another study found that the incidence of overall adverse events in opioid-naive children who received NCA was similar to that in children who received PCA after surgery (22% and 24%, respectively).[297] However, children who were able to self-administer PCA required only minor interventions (stimulation, reduction in opioid dosage, or supplemental oxygen), whereas those who received NCA were more likely to require more aggressive interventions, such as opioid reversal, airway management, or escalation of care. This study found that cognitive impairment and opioid dose on the first postoperative day were independent predictors of adverse events. Although the mean time to the occurrence of adverse events was 16 to 27 hours, some events occurred during the third postoperative day, suggesting that monitoring, including continuous pulse oximetry, should be continued as long as the PCA is used. In a study of children with cancer, five respiratory and/or neurologic serious adverse effects were reported, with 1 child requiring naloxone during the 576 days of treatment with NCA/CCA.[296] In that study, pulse oximetry was used only at the discretion of the provider, perhaps reducing the investigator's ability to recognize hypoxemia in some children. Furthermore, the reduced incidence of adverse events may be explained by the fact that most children in that study were not opioid naive and may have developed some degree of opioid tolerance. A study of 10,000 pediatric patients receiving NCA further confirms the safety and tolerability of this delivery method.[109]

For safety reasons, however, it is important to distinguish between authorized and unauthorized use of the PCA button by an individual other than the child. Several reports describe serious adverse events, including excessive sedation, severe respiratory depression, respiratory arrest, and death, attributed to unauthorized activation of the PCA device by parents, spouses, other family members, and health care providers.[297-301] The practice of PCA by proxy has therefore come under scrutiny and its safety questioned by the Joint Commission and the Institute for Safe Medication Practices (ISMP).[302-304] In 2004, the Joint Commission issued a sentinel event alert based on PCA errors reported to the U.S. Pharmacopeia. Of 460 errors that resulted in death or some level of harm to the patient, 15 resulted from PCA by proxy, including 12 attributed to family members, 2 to a nurse, and 1 to a pharmacist.[302] In interpreting this report and some other reports, it should be emphasized that many do not cite denominator data (total numbers of patients receiving PCA vs. NCA/CCA), so that it is difficult to assign numbers for relative or absolute risks of these techniques. Recognition of these risks has led the Joint Commission and ISMP to strongly recommend that specific policies and procedures be developed and implemented related to the use of PCA by individuals other than the child. Such policies must address the following issues:

- Appropriate selection of children. Many pediatric centers restrict parent-controlled analgesia to children with chronic pain, those who require palliative care, and in special circumstances for children who undergo repeated and extensive surgery. In pediatric centers worldwide, NCA is increasingly being used, with appropriate observation, for both opioid-naive and opioid-tolerant children.
- The specific process of identifying suitable caregivers who will be allowed to activate the PCA button.
- Communication among clinicians, including the primary service physician, the pain service team, and the primary bedside nurse, regarding the suitability of CCA.
- An educational plan for health care providers involved in the decision-making.
- Education of caregivers, including pain assessment, recognition of opioid adverse effects, and scenarios when not to activate the PCA button (e.g., when the child is asleep or somnolent). The caregiver should be encouraged to call the nursing staff when in doubt.
- Monitoring protocols, including assessment of sedation depth, respiratory status, and pain assessment at regular intervals. It

must be emphasized that the primary responsibility for monitoring the safety and effectiveness of analgesia remains with the nursing staff. Electronic monitoring, including pulse oximetry, is widely used in this setting.

With carefully defined policies and procedures, adequate education of clinicians and caregivers, prevention of unauthorized dosing, and vigilant monitoring, it may be possible to reduce the frequency of adverse events from PCA, NCA, and, especially, CCA. However, large outcomes studies are needed after implementation of such policies to confirm the safety and efficacy of practice based on these recommendations. Our view is that NCA is a well-established practice and should be encouraged as a generally safe and effective means for delivering opioids to children who are unable to self-administer.

### Risks and Adverse Events with PCA

Despite its numerous benefits, the use of PCA has been associated with a wide range of adverse effects, adverse events, and unfavorable outcomes in adults.[278,279,299,305-308] Although some adverse effects from PCA therapy may be attributed to the opioid drugs themselves or to patient comorbidities, a significant number of harmful effects occur as a result of human error, with incorrect prescribing, dispensing, administration, or equipment failure. E-Table 43-5 describes the causes of PCA medication errors as identified by the ISMP.[303-305,309] Increasing awareness of preventable adverse events from PCA has led to improved pump technology directed at minimizing the likelihood of programming errors, including the development of smart PCA pumps that use bar-coded syringes and an integral bar-code reader to prevent incorrect programming of drug concentration. Potential PCA pump errors have been reduced with these "smart pumps."[310] Children are at greater risk for medication-related adverse events resulting from calculation errors in drug doses (because all doses are based on body weight or body surface area) and to developmental differences in PK. However, data for PCA-related adverse events in children are limited.[280,311-313] The reported incidence of respiratory depression in children receiving PCA ranges from 0% to 25%.[297,311,312,314,315] Risk factors for respiratory depression identified by these studies include cumulative opioid dose, use of basal infusions, concomitant administration of sedatives, and comorbid conditions, including renal failure and cognitive impairment. Recognition of the risks from PCA[316,317] has led organizations, such as the ISMP, to emphasize the importance of monitoring children who use PCA and of detailed child and staff education regarding its use.[318]

### Monitoring the Child Using PCA

Despite the recommendation from the ISMP that practitioners should identify children at risk for opioid-related respiratory depression and define the appropriate level of monitoring, there remains no consensus regarding the risk-to-benefit ratio and effectiveness of any specific forms of monitoring for children receiving PCA, NCA, or CCA. The Anesthesia Patient Safety Foundation (APSF) recommended the use of continuous respiratory monitoring (minimally pulse oximetry and a continuous measure of respiratory rate) for children receiving PCA, neuraxial, or serial doses of parenteral opioids.[319] Additionally, the APSF recommended that reliable alerting methods, such as audible alarms, central stations, or pagers, be implemented to ensure timely and appropriate clinician response to deteriorating respiratory status of those receiving opioid therapy. Recently a nurse notification system was implemented at one of the authors' institutions, where pulse oximetry alarms generated automated nurse call-light notification after 15 seconds, a page to the bedside nurse and charge nurse after 1 minute, and an emergency group page after 3 minutes of sustained oxygen desaturation.[297] The impact of implementing such technology on the incidence of PCA-related adverse events requires investigation. It must be emphasized that pulse oximetry can detect hypoventilation only if the child is breathing room air. Oximetry is *not* a measure of ventilation but rather of oxygenation. The use of supplemental oxygen interferes with the ability of pulse oximetry to detect respiratory depression by delaying the onset of desaturation.[320,321]

Side stream sampling of end-tidal $CO_2$ via a nasal cannula or noninvasive capnography detects respiratory depression earlier and more frequently than does pulse oximetry or periodic checks of respiratory rate in adults who are receiving opioids via PCA, or for procedural sedation/analgesia.[322,323] Although similar data for children receiving PCA therapy are not available, studies in children undergoing procedural sedation in the emergency department and intensive care unit have reported that capnography detected respiratory events that would have been unrecognized by pulse oximetry, periodic respiratory rate monitoring, and/or clinical examination.[324-327] Additionally, these studies identified instances of respiratory depression that were recognized by abnormal capnography before oxygen desaturation was detected. Thus capnography may provide the earliest warning of impending respiratory compromise and may alert clinicians to carefully evaluate the children under their care and adjust opioid doses accordingly. Conversely, in real-world practice, capnography cannulas can be difficult to maintain in proper position in children on a busy postoperative ward, readings can be influenced by mouth breathing, and this technology also has the potential for false-positive and false-negative conclusions. Newer technology incorporates a fully integrated PCA system with modules for continuous monitoring of oxygen saturation and end-tidal $CO_2$.[328] Some of these pumps also have a feature that shuts off PCA delivery if preset threshold parameters for oxygen saturation and end-tidal $CO_2$ are reached. Studies evaluating the benefits of such technology in reducing PCA-related adverse events in children are needed. Although electronic monitoring has an important role in patient safety, all available methods are imperfect. Moreover, they generate frequent false alarms that annoy children and families, disturb the restorative sleep of both children and parents, and contribute to desensitization of nurses' vigilance. Despite these limitations of electronic monitoring, it has been reported that the use of computerized physician order entry and involvement of dedicated pediatric pain teams improved compliance with routine monitoring and increased the likelihood of early identification of adverse events.[329]

## REGIONAL BLOCKADE AND ANALGESIA

The use of local anesthetics, both with and without the addition of central neuraxial opioids and other adjuncts, offers many advantages in the postoperative setting. Blockade with long-acting local anesthetics, or continuous peripheral nerve blockade with infusion of local anesthetics via catheters and elastomeric infusion pumps can provide postoperative analgesia for outpatient surgery so that a child can be discharged home in comfort. Reducing or eliminating the need for systemic analgesics diminishes the potential for adverse effects associated with their use (see Chapters 41 and 42). Regional blockade affords the ability to provide excellent analgesia to children who might otherwise

not tolerate larger doses of opioids. This group includes some neonates, especially preterm and former preterm infants who are at risk for apnea; children with problems of central ventilatory control, respiratory disease, precarious airways; or those who risk obstruction with sedation (e.g., children with obstructive sleep apnea).

There are few absolute contraindications to regional blockade. Anatomic anomalies, such as myelodysplasia, sacral dysgenesis, and other abnormalities, either disrupting the epidural space or making access to it impossible, may prevent the performance of a caudal or epidural block. A report of epidural analgesia in children with myelodysplasia, however, suggests that catheters may be used safely in these children when placed at a level above the anatomic neural abnormality.[330] In cases involving these types of anatomic anomalies, we encourage consultation with experts in pediatric regional anesthesia, prior review of imaging studies, and consideration of fluoroscopic guidance. A needle and block should never be placed through infected tissue or in close proximity to it. Children with burn injuries may be candidates for continuous regional techniques, provided the burned area is distant from the catheter insertion site (see Chapter 34). We do not believe that the benefits of regional analgesia outweigh the potential risks inherent in inserting catheters through burned tissue or close to it.

Sepsis presents a similar problem. In general, it is not advisable to place caudal or epidural catheters in children who are septic, for fear of seeding the epidural space during a period of bacteremia. Peripheral nerve, plexus, or intrapleural catheters may pose less of a problem in this regard, but there are no data to provide guidance regarding this issue. Coagulopathy and thrombocytopenia are relative contraindications to regional anesthesia, with mild abnormalities in hemostasis not necessarily precluding a regional block. In unusual cases, and with proper consideration of risk-benefit issues, fresh frozen plasma or platelets can be infused at the time of a regional procedure to provide temporary correction of coagulopathy. The considerations regarding regional anesthesia, coagulopathy, and anticoagulation are complex and have been reviewed extensively for adults by consensus groups from the American and European Societies of Regional Anesthesia, and suggested guidelines regarding regional blockade in the anticoagulated patient can be found in Table 41-7.[331] In the absence of additional pediatric data, we recommend that clinicians review these adult publications as provisional guides for pediatric regional anesthesia as well. When placing a catheter for continuous blockade, consideration of the state of coagulation must include the time of catheter withdrawal as well as placement. If a child is to receive postoperative anticoagulation, for example, a continuous block should not be considered unless anticoagulation therapy can be stopped for 2 hours before the catheter is removed.

When a nerve repair or revision is planned for an extremity, some surgeons may wish to assess motor or sensory function postoperatively. In these cases, consultation with the surgeon should precede a plan for postoperative regional analgesia. If the surgery involves the legs, a caudal or lumbar epidural catheter can be used with opioids or adjunctive drugs such as clonidine without local anesthetics. Very dilute concentrations of local anesthetics (e.g., 0.05%-0.075% bupivacaine or ropivacaine) often can provide some additive analgesia if needed without significantly impairing motor function.

There is no consensus on the timing of a regional block (at the beginning or end of the surgical procedure). Placing a single-injection caudal block before incision confers a similar duration of postoperative analgesia, after a brief surgical procedure of 1 hour or less, as placing it at the end of surgery. For example, the times from recovery until the first request for analgesics after caudal blocks placed before incision or after surgery for inguinal herniorrhaphy were similar.[332] For more prolonged procedures, the block may be renewed with a second caudal injection before emergence or a catheter placed and redosed at appropriate intervals (usually approximately 1.5 hours). A volume of half of the original dose is usually sufficient if less than 2 hours have elapsed. A reduced concentration of local anesthetic is usually effective for postoperative analgesia. Adjunctive additives, such as clonidine, have also been shown in some studies to prolong the action of "single shot" central neuraxis and some peripheral blocks (see later discussion) permitting a single-injection block placed before the incision to augment both intraoperative and postoperative analgesia for longer operations. In cases of major surgery on the extremities and shoulders, there is a growing trend toward placement of indwelling plexus or peripheral nerve catheters for local anesthetic infusions for several days, both for adults and children, as detailed subsequently in the section on catheter techniques.[333,334]

Evidence suggests that placing a block at the beginning of surgery offers several potential advantages.[335] Although preemptive or preventive analgesia is a reproducible phenomenon in laboratory studies, the results in humans have been conflicting. For example, initial studies in adults demonstrated a dramatic decrease in the incidence of phantom limb pain when an epidural block was administered before an amputation, although subsequent studies did not consistently reaffirm the initial observations.[336-338] Similarly, children who receive intraoperative neural blockade may experience less postoperative pain than those managed with general anesthesia alone, with the duration of analgesia in some cases lasting beyond the pharmacologic action of the block. On the other hand, a blinded study of caudal anesthesia administered either before or after inguinal surgery failed to show a difference in postoperative analgesia.[339]

It is theorized that interruption of nociceptive impulses at the spinal cord level attenuates imprinting of painful stimuli on the sensory cortex or forestalls the development of spinal cord hyperexcitability and "wind up," thereby reducing the neural input and persistent postoperative pain.[338,340-343] It has also become increasingly evident however, that if preemptive or preventative analgesia is to have a beneficial effect, other conditions must be met: the block must be of sufficient duration in relation to the nociceptive stimulus, it must extend into the postoperative period, and it must be effective at preventing central transmission of the nociceptive signals.[335] This third requirement suggests that a multimodal analgesic approach may offer the greatest benefit. The presence of poorly controlled preoperative pain may sensitize the CNS, rendering pain difficult to control via intraoperative or postoperative interventions.[344] Additionally, epidural opioids have been shown to reduce the inflammatory response after surgery in adults, as indicated by interleukin-2 concentrations, suggesting that attenuating the stress response to surgery may improve postoperative analgesia.[345]

Further evidence suggests that local anesthetic infiltration of the incision site, especially when performed in conjunction with a regional anesthetic technique, may be an effective means of providing prolonged analgesia after surgery.[346,347] This simple and effective approach can be used before or at the end of virtually any surgical procedure. A major limitation of wound infiltration

with currently available local anesthetics is that the duration of analgesia is usually only 4 to 6 hours. Because postoperative pain commonly persists for several days, it would be more useful to administer local anesthetics for 2 to 4 days. To achieve this, the surgeon must place a multi-orifice catheter in the tissue planes of the wound during closure, through which local anesthetics can be infused.[334,348-352] Several commercially available kits using these "soaker hoses" have been shown to be effective. A disposable elastomeric pump, filled with local anesthetic that infuses local anesthetic continuously into the surgical tissues, can be placed at the end of surgery and the child sent home with it infusing for several days. Although this is an effective supplemental strategy to achieve postoperative analgesia, practitioners should be aware of complications that have been reported in adults.[353] *A note of caution: the concentration of local anesthetics, such as bupivacaine, and the infusion rate must be carefully prepared to avoid a local anesthetic overdose if such an approach is planned, particularly after chest surgery and in neonates and small infants.* A novel method of providing prolonged analgesia that is currently under investigation involves injection of a suspension of biodegradable polymer microspheres or lipospheres that contain bupivacaine. Dexamethasone can further prolong the duration of this method of block. After injection, these microspheres release bupivacaine in a controlled manner to provide blockade of peripheral nerves for periods of 2 to 6 days, depending on dose, formulation, and site of injection.[354-357] An alternative experimental approach to providing prolonged analgesia is the use of modified neurotoxins. Site 1 sodium channel blockers, such as tetrodotoxin and neosaxitoxin, have very strong affinity for sodium channels in vitro. Tetrodotoxin and neosaxitoxin are nonneurotoxic, and do not significantly block sodium channels in the myocardium.[358]

In animals, the combination of these toxins with bupivacaine, epinephrine, or clonidine markedly prolongs the nerve block and reduces systemic toxicity. Neosaxitoxin shows no cardiotoxicity in animals,[359] and has shown promise in a recent Phase 2 clinical trial for abdominal surgery in adults.[360]

Peripheral nerve and plexus blocks tend to provide blocks of greater duration than do central neuraxial blocks, the former lasting 8 to 12 hours, and on occasion exceeding 24 hours. Depending on the nature of the surgery, this may permit the child to transition to nonopioid analgesics at the time the block wears off, thereby eliminating or reducing the use of opioids and their potential untoward effects. Children undergoing outpatient surgery may be discharged after a single-injection regional block, but follow-up the next day with the family is necessary to ensure that the block has receded and no complications have developed. This is especially the case after peripheral nerve blocks. Parents must further be cautioned that there may be some degree of motor blockade present, and that the blocked limb must be protected from injury. If a lower extremity is blocked, assistance with ambulation is mandatory. Techniques for regional anesthesia and analgesia are discussed in detail in Chapters 41 and 42.

### Choice of Local Anesthetics, Additives, and Dosing

Dilute long-acting local anesthetics, such as bupivacaine 0.125% to 0.25% or ropivacaine 0.1% to 0.2%, are the most commonly used local anesthetics for regional blockade. In Europe and Canada, levobupivacaine is available and has the advantage of smaller risk of toxicity than bupivacaine (see Chapter 41). Ropivacaine and levobupivacaine have the dual advantages when compared with bupivacaine of a relatively prolonged duration of action and decreased motor blockade. Epinephrine (1:200,000)

is often added to bupivacaine to decrease systemic absorption and increase duration of action but *should be omitted when a digital or penile block is performed, because of the risk of inducing ischemia by direct vasoconstriction.* (Note that the avoidance of epinephrine for digital blocks is based on limited and historical evidence, and current proponents of the practice have not found adverse complications to occur).[361-363]

Initial studies concluded that the optimal concentration of bupivacaine that provides maximum sensory blockade without motor blockade for caudal analgesia was 0.125%,[364] although subsequent studies demonstrated that the optimal concentration was actually 0.175% (7 mL of 0.25% bupivacaine combined with 3 mL of saline).[365] More concentrated solutions of bupivacaine (0.2% to 0.25%) may be used for blocks that do not significantly affect motor function, such as for an ilioinguinal-iliohypogastric nerve block after herniorrhaphy. Bupivacaine 0.5% offers no advantage in most settings, and limits the volume that can be administered because of the risk of toxicity. The maximum allowable dose of bupivacaine is 2.5 mg/kg. Furthermore, the use of solutions with many different concentrations may increase the risk of calculation errors and potential overdoses. For this reason, it is prudent to restrict the choice of the concentrations of local anesthetics to a manageable number. Our clinical impression is that thoracic epidural analgesia after Nuss bar placement may be enhanced with a denser blockade. For these blocks, motor block is of less significance because most lung expansion is produced by the diaphragm.[92] For thoracic epidural blocks, we use ropivacaine 0.2% with an opioid and clonidine.

Ropivacaine, an *l*-enantiomer amide local anesthetic, is widely used in children, particularly in neonates and infants.[366-369] In both pediatric and adult studies, the duration of analgesia after ropivacaine is similar to that after bupivacaine. Although data in adults suggest that there is a more selective sensory than motor blockade, this has not been demonstrated in studies of immature animals or children.[366-368,370-376] Ropivacaine, is less cardiotoxic than bupivacaine. In terms of developing terminal apnea, infant rats tolerate 1.5 times the dose of ropivacaine as compared with bupivacaine. The doses for the onset of respiratory distress and seizures are similarly increased with ropivacaine.[368] These differences are more pronounced in infant rats than in adult rats. Animal data suggest that the toxic thresholds for both CNS and cardiovascular toxicity are increased 20% to 30% with this agent in both adults and infants, although seizures can still occur with ropivacaine if the dose exceeds the toxic threshold. The authors recommend using a levorotatory enantiomer (levo-enantiomer), such as ropivacaine, in preference to bupivacaine in infants younger than 6 months of age, because of the potential increased margin of safety.[369,377] Another local anesthetic with a similar decreased toxicity is levobupivacaine (the levorotatory isomer of bupivacaine). This drug possesses properties similar to bupivacaine with a moderate reduction in the toxicity risks inherent with bupivacaine.[378-380] Levobupivacaine has become difficult to obtain in the United States, although it is commonly used in place of bupivacaine elsewhere.[381]

Opioids have been injected in the epidural and intrathecal space for analgesia in children, both with and without local anesthetics. Central neuraxial opioids have been used for more than two decades to produce effective analgesia in children. However, opioids administered into the central neuraxis have the potential to cause delayed respiratory depression, and are generally avoided in the outpatient setting to ensure the safety of children after discharge.[382] Their use is described in detail later.

Adjuvant drugs have been added to the local anesthetic administered for caudal blockade to prolong the duration of the sensory block, an obviously desirable attribute for a single-injection block. However, their use is not without controversy. Many drugs have been injected into the epidural space with only limited laboratory evidence for safety and lack of neurotoxicity, and some caution is necessary.[383] Clonidine, 0.5 to 2 µg/kg, has been shown to lack evidence of neurotoxicity. It increases the duration of analgesia after bupivacaine in caudal blocks by approximately 3 hours, with insignificant hemodynamic effects, mild sedation, and no delay in recovery times.[384-390] Despite these reported beneficial effects of clonidine, one double-blind investigation found no difference between IV and caudally administered clonidine in a dose of 2 µg/kg as an adjunct to caudal blocks using bupivacaine, and another found no difference in duration or quality of analgesia when compared with caudal bupivacaine alone.[391,392] Conversely, when clonidine was used in conjunction with levobupivacaine, children who received clonidine in the caudal space demonstrated a significant delay in the need for rescue analgesia and reduced pain scores compared with those who received IV clonidine, suggesting that the prolonged analgesia occurs at a spinal cord site of action.[389,390,393] Caudal clonidine produces less nausea, itching, ileus, and urinary retention than opioid additives, although it may increase postoperative somnolence or respiratory depression at doses in excess of 1 µg/kg, particularly in the neonate.[392,394-396] The clearance of clonidine in infants is approximately one-third that of older children.[397] The preponderance of evidence supports the use of clonidine to prolong the analgesic effect of central neuraxial blocks, but we caution against the use of more than 1 µg/kg for outpatient procedures, especially in younger infants, because of an increased risk of respiratory depression.

*Preservative-free* ketamine has also been used for caudal analgesia, both alone and in combination with bupivacaine. Doses of 0.5 mg/kg appear to provide adequate analgesia, without untoward behavioral effects, such as those reported with IV or oral administration of ketamine.[398] When combined with bupivacaine, the duration of analgesia approached 24 hours.[203,399,400] In a comparison with IV ketamine, caudal (*S*)-(+)-ketamine significantly prolonged the duration of analgesia, despite similar plasma concentrations.[400] One clinical study suggested a specific spinal site of action. *Only preservative-free ketamine should be used because preservatives have been associated with neurotoxicity.*[401,402] In the United States, preservative-free ketamine is currently unavailable.[386,403]

When performing a regional block, the total safe dose of local anesthetic should be calculated first and the volume and concentration of the solution adjusted if necessary, to avoid administering a toxic dose. Because most infants and children will have a regional block placed in combination with general anesthesia, surgical concentrations of local anesthetics are not necessary and dilute medications can still provide excellent postoperative analgesia. This is particularly important when performing blocks in infants. For example, a 7-kg infant has a maximal allowable dose of 17.5 mg of bupivacaine (or 2.5 mg/kg). If a 0.25% solution (2.5 mg/mL) were administered, the total volume would be limited to 7 mL. The maximum dose should probably be slightly more restrictive in infants less than 6 months of age. At this age, a cautious approach is to further reduce the allowable dose by 25% to 30%. For example, a 4-kg 2-month-old infant would be permitted to receive 2.7 mL (6.6 mg) of the same solution.

## Choice of Block and Techniques

### Single-Injection Techniques

There are many circumstances in which the simplicity and duration of action of a single-injection block is desirable. Both neuraxial blocks and peripheral plexus and nerve blocks can be effective as single-injection techniques. The caudal block remains the most commonly used technique in pediatric regional anesthesia. It provides analgesia of the lower extremity and lower abdomen, and is easily and quickly performed in most infants and children (see Chapter 41). When an operation is performed on both legs it is often preferable to bilateral lower extremity blocks.

The use of ultrasound makes the identification of plexuses and peripheral nerves much easier in an anesthetized child. Peripheral nerve stimulation using Teflon-coated needles remains an effective technique, but is becoming less frequently used as familiarity with ultrasound and its benefits increases. It is plausible, but unproven, that ultrasound reduces the risk of injury to nerves and adjacent structures (see Chapters 41 and 42).[404] To precisely position the needle in the target area and avoid piercing adjacent structures, one must develop skill in coordinating its trajectory with the ultrasound image so that the needle tip does not pass out of the plane of view. Although it remains unknown whether ultrasound and more precise needle placement will reduce nerve injury, there is evidence that it reduces the volume of local anesthetic needed to produce an effective block.[405,406] Ultrasound visualization of the local anesthetic surrounding a nerve or plexus provides reliable confirmation that a block will be successful. Nerve blocks of the lower extremity can, in some circumstances, be used instead of caudal blockade (see Chapters 41 and 42). They provide a field of analgesia limited to the operative site, have a prolonged duration of analgesia (usually at least twice that of caudal block), and eliminate some of the potential undesirable effects of central neuraxis blockade, such as urinary retention, motor blockade (wobbly legs), and, occasionally, numbness. The fascia iliaca block, which produces analgesia in the distribution of the femoral, obturator, and lateral femoral cutaneous nerves, has been described in children as an excellent alternative for postoperative analgesia of a lower extremity.[407] Blockade of the femoral nerve, the sciatic nerve, and the nerves of the ankle is easily performed in children by using similar techniques to those in adults (see Chapters 41 and 42). Regional blockade of the upper extremity may involve an axillary block, interscalene, supraclavicular, or infraclavicular block, or less commonly, blockade of the individual nerves at the level of the arm or wrist. Intercostal nerve blocks may be used after thoracic or upper abdominal surgery. This block may be considered for procedures of limited scope, such as open-lung biopsy or thoracostomy for drainage, but the duration of blockade is limited to several hours. In our view, for most thoracic procedures, the duration of single-injection percutaneous intercostal blockade is generally too short to warrant the risk of pneumothorax. For open-chest procedures, intercostal blocks by the surgeon pose a low risk and may be indicated, although again, their effectiveness is limited by their short duration. Epinephrine is commonly included in the local anesthetic for these blocks to limit the rate of uptake. More extensive surgery anticipated to cause postoperative pain of longer duration may be best managed with a catheter (continuous infusion) technique.

Ilioinguinal-iliohypogastric nerve block provides excellent postoperative analgesia for inguinal herniorrhaphy, a common outpatient procedure in children (see Chapters 41 and 42). It appears similar in efficacy to a caudal block, with a duration of analgesia of at least 4 hours when bupivacaine with epinephrine is used. For orchiopexy, ilioinguinal nerve block has been found to be as effective as caudal blockade to the T10 level in a randomized and blinded investigation.[408] In our experience, however, postoperative analgesia for procedures that involve considerable manipulation and traction on the spermatic cord and testis may be better managed with caudal blockade. Penile block is effective for both circumcision and distal, simple hypospadias repair. More extensive procedures on the penis, especially repair of penile-scrotal hypospadias, require a caudal, rather than a penile block, to produce effective analgesia.[409] The use of single-injection neuraxial opioids is an additional technique that can provide longer-lasting analgesia, but must be used in inpatients only, because of the need for respiratory monitoring. Intrathecal morphine has been administered to infants and children for several decades and provides long-acting analgesia (up to 24 hours) after a single injection.[410,411] It is absolutely essential that only preservative-free preparations of the drug be used because preservative-containing solutions may result in injury to the central neuraxis. Doses ranging from 5 to 10 μg/kg are usually chosen. Because of the hydrophilicity of this agent, respiratory monitoring is mandated. Respiratory depression, as well as pruritus, nausea, and urinary retention, are reported after intrathecal morphine. We most commonly employ this modality for analgesia after posterior spinal fusion. The drug is often administered by the surgeon under direct vision of the dura, but if administered at the beginning of the case, it has been reported to reduce intraoperative blood loss.[412,413] This route of administration has also been employed before cardiac surgery.[414] The effective intrathecal dose of opioid is roughly one-fifth to one-tenth that of the epidural dose, and the duration of action, especially with morphine, is significantly prolonged. Therefore, observation in a monitored setting must be continued for 24 hours or until no further evidence of respiratory compromise exists (without the use of naloxone). A novel extended-release preparation of morphine uses a liposomal foam suspension of the drug (DepoDur, EKR Therapeutics, Bedminster, N.J.) that is injected in the lumbar epidural space (note that it should not be used intrathecally) and provides 48 hours of analgesia, with no increase in untoward effects compared with conventional neuraxial morphine.[415-418] To date there are no pediatric data, but clinical trials in children are currently in progress.

### Catheter Techniques

A catheter placed in the epidural space or adjacent to a nerve or plexus can be used to provide continuous uninterrupted analgesia for prolonged periods after surgery. These catheters are commonly used for about 3 days but may be used for more prolonged periods in selected situations. With proper care, catheters tunneled under the skin may be left in situ for more than 7 days.[419,420] Catheters can also be placed in intrapleural or extrapleural and/or retropleural locations to provide analgesia after thoracic surgery.[421] In our experience, intrapleural analgesia reduces but does not eliminate the need for systemic opioids, especially if thoracostomy drains are present. We rarely use this technique because toxic concentrations of local anesthetic and seizures have been reported.[422] Continuous extrapleural, intercostal, and paravertebral catheters can be placed either through the operative field or percutaneously. In adult studies, and in a smaller series of pediatric studies, these techniques appear to provide excellent analgesia at rest, but with movement they provide only partial

opioid sparing. Some clinicians regard these techniques as pro-viding many of the advantages of thoracic epidural analgesia, with the potential for reducing the risks and adverse effects of thoracic epidural analgesia.

Continuous regional blockade is remarkably effective and safe, although as with any technique, monitoring for untoward effects is necessary to prevent complications. New technology for the delivery of drugs to peripheral nerves and plexuses have made it possible for children to receive the benefits of continuous neural blockade after discharge from the hospital or day surgery unit.[333] Catheters may deliver local anesthetics and other medica-tions via controlled infusion devices that use a pressurized elastomer-bulb reservoir that controls the infusion rate with a flow limiter (ON-Q pump, I-Flow LLC, Lake Forest, Calif.; Infusor, Baxter, Deerfield, Ill.; Accufusor, Moog Medical Devices, Salt Lake City; Easypump, B Braun Melsungen AG, Melsungen, Germany; and others) (E-Fig. 43-2). These devices can be used at home after discharge, for infusion of medication into a tissue plane to provide a continuous field blockade or a continuous peripheral nerve block. Infusion of local anesthetics in the sub-cutaneous tissues at the incision site or into the surgical plane using these devices provides prolonged analgesia in both adults and children. Several types of these infusion systems are avail-able, including ones that have options for fixed, variable, or continuous infusion rates with a bolus option. The latter two must be used with caution in smaller children in whom local anesthetic toxicity from excessive dosage may be a risk; we gener-ally use the fixed-rate devices. When continuous peripheral nerve or plexus blocks are used for outpatients, a carefully designed system must be in place to follow these children, to avoid com-plications and achieve early detection of potentially adverse events. Daily follow-up, either by visiting nurses or by phone, is mandatory. We are aware of a small number of anecdotal cases of possible excessive doses of local anesthetic from a continuous infusion pump used at home that resulted in adverse effects, although no catastrophic events have been reported.

CAUDAL AND EPIDURAL CATHETERS. With experience and proper equipment, the lumbar route is feasible at any age, but specific expertise is required for infants and toddlers. Practitio-ners who have less experience with lumbar epidural catheteriza-tion in children should consider placing the catheter via the caudal route for children less than 6 years of age. In infants and children up to about 6 years of age, catheters may be advanced freely from the caudal canal cephalad to lower thoracic levels with excellent success.[423] This is possible in part because young children have a less developed vascular plexus and more compact and globular fat than do older children and adults.[423,424] However, other authors describe less reliability with caudal-to-thoracic advancement of catheters in children larger than 10 kg.[425] This has been attributed to the more mature composition of the contents of the epidural space and the lumbar lordosis that occurs with walking. With age, the epidural fat appears to lose the spongy gelatinous character noted in infants and the spaces between the fat globules become less distinct.[423,424] Catheters made of nylon or polyamide may be less likely to kink beneath the skin and seem to thread more easily than those made of Teflon or other materials. The catheter should never be advanced if resistance is felt. Similar difficulties in advancing catheters that resulted in catheters looping backwards, or kinking, or punc-turing the dura have been reported in neonates weighing less than 3.5 kg.[426] In one series of 20 preterm infants, epidurography revealed misplaced catheters in 3 infants or 15%. New data

suggest that misplacement of threaded catheters in all ages may be more common than is generally recognized.[427] In this series of 724 epidurograms, unexpected misplacement was detected in 11 or 1.5%, including 3 intravascular catheters, despite negative test doses, 2 intrathecal without cerebrospinal fluid aspiration, 4 that were intraperitoneal, and 1 each in the rectum and psoas compartment. These authors recommended epidurography in all cases, although this is not the current standard of practice. If specific dermatomal placement of a catheter is sought, one should consider obtaining an imaging study to confirm the dermatomal level of the tip of the catheter, and the aforemen-tioned data suggest that imaging might be advisable whenever a catheter is advanced to a level substantially more rostral than its insertion level.

As an alternative to epidurography, a nerve-stimulating cath-eter may be used, which allows real-time monitoring of the loca-tion of the tip of the catheter as it is advanced cephalad (with the stylet in place, using one system available in Canada), or at least confirmation of tip location on removal of the stylet (using a convenient modification of equipment readily available in the United States).[428,429] The technique requires the use of saline loss-of-resistance and avoiding air bubbles in the epidural space or in the catheter-connector-injection system, because air impedes electrical conduction. In addition, neuromuscular blockade must be avoided because it abolishes the motor response. Used in conjunction with a nerve stimulator set to very low milliamper-age (approximately 6 mA), the muscles supplied by a nerve root will twitch as the catheter approaches the segments that supply that dermatome, thereby confirming the catheter tip's location. Specifically, twitches in the feet and ankles occur with catheter tips around L5 to S1, hip flexion occurs with catheter tips around T12 to S1, abdominal muscle twitches without hip flexion imply thoracic positioning above T12, intercostal muscle twitches imply midthoracic tip positioning. Finger twitches would imply advancement to around T1. This technique can also be used to detect catheter malpositioning. Bilateral twitching at a current less than 0.6 mA generally implies subarachnoid positioning. Unilateral twitches in a narrow motor distribution at a current less than 1 mA may suggest advancement out a root foramen. Unilateral twitches at a current less than 1 mA in a very broad motor distribution may indicate subdural positioning. Absence of twitches as the current is increased to about 15 mA (in the absence of air bubbles or neuromuscular blockade) generally indicates that the epidural catheter is not in the epidural space. Our experience is that the use of one of these confirmatory techniques can help avoid problems with failed or incomplete blocks in the postoperative period.

Choice of drugs for epidural infusions depends on a number of factors, including site of surgery, site of the epidural catheter tip, and child risk factors. Local anesthetics, lipophilic opioids, and, to some extent, clonidine all have more restricted cephalad distribution of action during infusions, compared with hydro-philic opioids, such as hydromorphone or morphine. Conse-quently, optimal positioning of the catheter tip during insertion can improve the analgesic action postoperatively. Experience in adults suggests that when local anesthetics are used, analgesia is optimized when the tip of the epidural catheter is positioned at or slightly above the dermatomal levels involved in the surgery. This effect may be more pronounced when children are moving than when they are at rest. Positioning at levels slightly above the dermatomal levels involved in surgery is more relevant for surgery in lumbosacral dermatomes compared with upper

thoracic dermatomes because of the greater distance between root level and dorsal horn level in these two circumstances.[430]

Placement of catheters at thoracic levels requires consideration of risk-benefit trade-offs. Therefore, if a catheter tip is at the lumbar or caudal level and the surgery is in thoracic and upper abdominal dermatomes, continuous infusions containing local anesthetics alone or with lipophilic opioids, such as fentanyl or sufentanil, are likely to be ineffective. Increasing the infusion volume is limited by maximum allowable systemic local anesthetic concentrations. In this circumstance, a reasonable alternative is to administer hydrophilic opioids (e.g., morphine or hydromorphone) through lumbar or caudal catheters. The hydrophilic properties of these opioids permit a greater rostral spread, such that a wider range of dermatomes can be covered after caudal or lumbar catheter placement, with only small increases in dose for surgical sites remote from the catheter tip. This same characteristic, unfortunately, also appears to increase the risk for adverse effects, including respiratory depression, as a result of rostral spread of morphine to the central respiratory center in the brainstem. Hydromorphone may offer some advantages because its rostral spread is intermediate compared with fentanyl and morphine and it causes slightly less pruritus compared with morphine.[431,432] Lumbar administration of hydromorphone spreads sufficiently to provide thoracic analgesia.[433] It should be noted that the potency of hydromorphone relative to morphine in the epidural space, is less than when it is administered systemically (2-3 : 1 epidural vs. 5 : 1 systemic).[434] Such a technique, however, precludes the optimal use of local anesthetics, and the considerable benefit that may accrue from a multimodal approach to regional analgesia.

A thoracic epidural catheter can be placed in an awake, sedated, or anesthetized child. Some clinicians are hesitant to perform thoracic epidural puncture in anesthetized children because of the inability to use child reports (e.g., paresthesia or lancinating pain) as an indicator of improper catheter or needle placement. However, there are few, if any, data to suggest that the risk of inserting a thoracic epidural catheter in an anesthetized child by an experienced clinician is actually greater than attempting such placement in an awake child who may not be able to remain still, nor is it clear that a well-sedated child can accurately report sensations of paresthesia or differentiate the discomfort of needle passage from more ominous pain.[435] The prospective data from the British National Epidural Audit do not support the contention that there is increased risk with this practice, and those data are corroborated by the PRAN study, which found no neural injury regardless of patient state during epidural placement.[436-438] We believe that data and experience support the safety of placement of thoracic epidural catheters in anesthetized children by anesthesiologists trained and experienced in this procedure, although the tolerances for error are smaller than in adults and older children.[439-441]

It is extremely important to secure caudal catheters to the skin with a clear occlusive dressing, to avoid contamination or dislodgment and to allow daily inspection of the site. In addition, tincture of benzoin or other adhesive solution reduces the incidence of catheter and dressing displacement. For a caudal catheter, the use of an adhesive-edged plastic drape, covering the area from the gluteal crease over the dressing, also helps prevent fecal soiling of the dressing by children who are in diapers. Despite these precautions, if a dressing becomes detached and the insertion site is contaminated it is prudent to remove the catheter. The use of lumbar catheters removes the insertion site from the diaper area and thereby further reduces the potential for contamination of the catheter and the insertion site.

Successful management of children with an epidural catheter requires carefully coordinated monitoring protocols, nursing management, and medical management of drug selection and dosing. As with PCA or continuous-infusion opioids, the orders should be standardized and written in consultation with the nursing staff, so that misinterpretations are less likely to occur (Fig. 43-10). Because the single most sensitive monitor of children receiving epidural opioids is the nurse, rather than a mechanical or electronic device, education of the nursing staff is of paramount importance to ensure safety. Nursing staff can also assess the adequacy of analgesia and thereby help to titrate the drug dose. Catheter insertion sites should be inspected at least once daily by the pain service, both for the integrity of the dressing and for any evidence of erythema or skin infection (Fig. 43-11). *When continuous infusions are used, the tubing connecting the infusion pump to the catheter should not have any injection ports and it should be clearly labeled as an epidural catheter to preclude unintended epidural administration of drugs intended for IV use.* We use color-coded tubing and a color-coded drug cassette for the continuous administration of regional agents. Although the same pumps are used for IV PCA administration, it is immediately obvious what route the drug is intended for simply by recognizing the tubing and cassette color.

A variation of traditional epidural analgesia and PCA is the technique of patient-controlled epidural analgesia (PCEA).[442] With this variation of traditional PCA, children are generally maintained with an infusion of epidural analgesics (frequently opioid alone or an opioid–local anesthetic mixture) and have the capability of self-administering supplemental doses when needed. When using this technique, the background infusion is used to provide the majority of the analgesia and the child can add to this when needed. It must be emphasized that the time needed for a bolus dose to effect a change with epidural administration is more prolonged than it is with IV agents. Therefore, with PCEA, lockout intervals are greater (often 15 to 30 minutes) than with PCA.[443,444] The considerations one would employ for choosing this technique include the same child-monitoring factors for IV PCA and epidural analgesia, and maximum local anesthetic doses must be carefully calculated to cover the contingency of the greatest possible activation of the PCEA demand doses. "Smart pump" technology has been demonstrated to improve safety of this technique.[445]

SELECTION OF DRUGS AND DOSES. Local anesthetics, opioids, and adjuvant agents were discussed previously; this section addresses the specifics of drug choices for continuous infusion through indwelling catheters. Many drugs and combinations have been administered via continuous infusion to the epidural space to provide postoperative analgesia.[390] The most common choices involve mixtures of local anesthetics and opioids, such as bupivacaine and fentanyl, although, increasingly, clonidine is being added (Table 43-10). Continuous infusions for peripheral nerve and plexus blocks are generally limited to local anesthetics, as evidence for the efficacy of other agents in these blocks is equivocal at best.

The choice of drug is based on several factors: the age and size of the child, the operation, and the underlying medical conditions that may decrease the margin of safety of one of the agents. The volume of solution required to fill the epidural space on a milliliter-per-kilogram basis appears to decrease with age; therefore, older children and adolescents may require less volume

43

Child's weight: _____ kg
Allergies: _____

**Continuous regional analgesia via (check appropriate modality)**
☐ Caudal epidural    ☐ Lumbar epidural    ☐ Thoracic epidural    ☐ Plexus or peripheral nerve catheter (specify)

_____

The catheter is _____ cm at the skin.    Loss of resistance (for lumbar and thoracic epidurals) was at _____ cm.

**Infusion:**
(Choose one only) ☐ Bupivacaine    ☐ Ropivacaine    ☐ Chloroprocaine
(Concentration) ☐ 0.075%    ☐ 0.1%    ☐ 0.2%    ☐ 1% (chloroprocaine only)

**Additives (caudal and epidural only):**
Opioid (choose one only) ☐ Fentanyl    ☐ Hydromorphone    ☐ Morphine
Concentration (µg/mL):    ☐ 1    ☐ 2    ☐ 3    ☐ 5 (hydromorphone and morphine only)    ☐ 7 (morphine only)
                                       ☐ 10 (morphine only)
☐ Clonidine    Concentration (µg/mL):    ☐ 0.5    ☐ 1

**Infusion rate:**  Start at _____ mL/hr. Range: _____ to _____ mL/hr. This is a maximum of _____ mg/kg/hr of local
anesthetic and _____ µg/kg/hr of opioid.

**Dosing guidelines for regional anesthesia/analgesia solution**

| | Local anesthetics | | | Opioids | | | |
|---|---|---|---|---|---|---|---|
| | Bupivacaine or ropivacaine | Chloroprocaine | Fentanyl | Hydromorphone | Morphine | Clonidine |
| Concentration | 0.05%-0.1% (0.5-1 mg/mL) May use up to 0.2% for ropivacaine | 1%-1.5% (10-15 mg/mL) | 1-3 µg/mL | 3-7 µg/mL | 5-10 µg/mL | 0.5-1 µg/mL |
| Suggested dose | Less than 6 months of age: 0.2-0.3 mg/kg/hr; Maximum dose: 0.3 mg/kg/hr 6 months of age or older: 0.2-0.4 mg/kg/hr Maximum dose: 0.4 mg/kg/hr | 0.2-0.8 mL/kg/hr (neonates)* | 0.3-1 µg/kg/hr | 1-2.5 µg/kg/hr | 1-5 µg/kg/hr | 0.1-0.5 µg/kg/hr |

*Note that the concentration of additives must be proportionally reduced with chloroprocaine if higher infusion rates are administered
to avoid overdose.

**Treatment of side effects:**
*Respiratory depression:*   For RR < ____ BPM, immediately stop epidural infusion and call acute pain service STAT. Administer $O_2$,
ensure clear airway, and assist ventilation if necessary.
                          ☐ Naloxone (Narcan) 1 µg/kg IV = _____ µg, repeat q1min as needed

*Nausea and vomiting:* ☐ Ondansetron 0.1 mg/kg (4 mg maximum) = _____ mg IV q6hr
                          ☐ Metoclopramide 0.1 mg/kg (10 mg maximum) = _____ mg IV q6hr

*Pruritus:*          ☐ Nalbuphine 0.05 mg/kg = _____ mg IV q4hr

☐ *For any of above,* begin naloxone infusion at 0.25 µg/kg/hr = _____ µg/hr
Adjunctive medications: ☐ Acetaminophen 10 mg/kg PO q4hr for 24 hours then q4hr prn
Inadequate analgesia:  ☐ Morphine 0.05-0.1 mg/kg IV = _____ mg q3-4hr prn for pain
                          ☐ Ketorolac 0.5 mg/kg IV = _____ mg q6hr prn for pain (up to 15 mg ≤ 50 kg; up to 30 mg > 50 kg)
Muscle spasms:        ☐ Diazepam 0.05-0.1 mg/kg IV = _____ mg q6hr prn

**Monitoring and equipment:** *must choose for patients receiving epidural opioids*
           ☐ Continuous pulse oximetry and respiratory monitoring
           ☐ $O_2$ and bag/mask delivery system, suction at the bedside

**Nursing orders:**
VS:     ☐ q4hr: temp, HR, RR, BP, pain score
           ☐ Dermatome level for caudal and epidural
           ☐ $SpO_2$ and sedation score (required if opioids are used). Call acute pain service for RR < _____bpm.
           ☐ Record Bromage score q8hr; call acute pain service if 4 or less (choose for children receiving local anesthetics).

Call acute pain service for any questions or problems: inadequate analgesia despite intervention, loose or contaminated
dressing, catheter disconnect, sedation score >3, increased somnolence, confusion, agitation, dizziness, tinnitus, hypotension,
bradycardia, fever >38.2° C; inflammation, tenderness or swelling at catheter site; Bromage score >0.

Maintain IV access.

For epidural or peripheral nerve block of lower extremity: Ambulate with assistance only with order from primary service and Bromage
score of 0. Pad blocked extremities and elevate heels off of bed.

**FIGURE 43-10** Sample epidural orders. (Modified from the University of Michigan Hospitals & Health Centers.)

**TABLE 43-10** Commonly Used Medications for Epidural Administration

| | Dose Range | Untoward Effects | Comments |
|---|---|---|---|
| **Local Anesthetics** | | Motor block | Reduce dose by 30% in infants younger than 6 months of age |
| Bupivacaine | 0.2-0.4 mg/kg/hr | | |
| Ropivacaine | 0.2-0.5 mg/kg/hr | | Levo-enantiomer; may have 20%-30% less toxicity than |
| Levobupivacaine | 0.2-0.5 mg/kg/hr | | racemic amino amides |
| Chloroprocaine | 1%-1.5%; 0.2-0.8 mL/kg/hr (neonates) | | |
| **Opioids** | | Respiratory depression, sedation, pruritus, urinary retention | |
| Fentanyl | 0.3-1 µg/kg/hr | | Lipophilic; use when catheter tip is positioned near surgical dermatomes and wide spread is not needed |
| Hydromorphone | 1-2.5 µg/kg/hr | Most rostral spread of opioids | Hydrophilic; use when surgery is more extensive and/or |
| Morphine | 1-5 µg/kg/hr | | catheter tip is positioned farther from surgical dermatomes |
| **Adjuncts** | | | |
| Clonidine | 0.1-0.5 µg/kg/hr | Sedation, respiratory depression at greater doses, hypotension (possibly postural) at high doses | Increased risk of apnea with high doses in neonates |

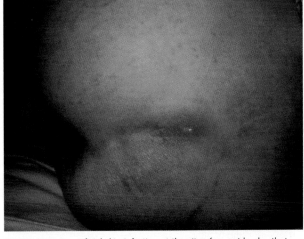

**FIGURE 43-11** Superficial skin infection at the site of an epidural catheter insertion. The catheter was withdrawn, and the problem resolved with local skin care only.

than infants and young children, based on weight. In children over 1 year of age, continuous infusions of ropivacaine up to 0.4 mg/kg/hr for up to 72 hours produced stable blood concentrations of unbound ropivacaine without evidence of accumulation or toxicity.[446,447] In very young or preterm infants, however, the risk of accumulation of the amino-amide local anesthetics, and thus the potential for toxicity, is particularly problematic.[448,449] Neonates are at increased risk for potential local anesthetic toxicity because of decreased protein binding (resulting in increased unbound drug) and possibly immature drug metabolism. The manifestations of local anesthetic toxicity in infants and neonates may be more difficult to recognize than in adults. Hence, we recommend a conservative maximum infusion dose for bupivacaine of 0.2 mg/kg/hr for no more than 48 hours in neonates.[450-452] Because safe infusion rates of bupivacaine in the neonate frequently provide insufficient analgesia when wide dermatomal coverage is needed, the amino-ester local anesthetic chloroprocaine may be used in an epidural infusion instead.[453]

Although the amino-amide local anesthetics are slowly cleared in neonates and young infants, the amino-ester chloroprocaine is cleared extremely rapidly, even in preterm infants, via ester hydrolysis, with an elimination half-life of several minutes.[453] This permits large doses and infusion rates with a reduced risk for systemic toxicity. Previous concerns regarding neurotoxicity after chloroprocaine involved a succession of formulations with preservatives, including metabisulfite, methylparaben, and ethylenediaminetetraacetic acid, although the current formulation is preservative-free. An epidural solution of 1% to 1.5% chloroprocaine can be infused at rates of 0.2 to 0.8 mL/kg/hr. If chloroprocaine is not available, the levorotatory enantiomers ropivacaine or levobupivacaine may be preferable to bupivacaine in this age group, because of their better toxicity profile.

When a block is not previously established in the OR, it is useful to dose catheters with local anesthetic (without opioids) at a volume of 0.05 mL/kg per spinal segment or between 0.5 and 1 mL/kg of local anesthetic, not to exceed 5 mg/kg of lidocaine, or 2.5 mg/kg of bupivacaine or ropivacaine. Some clinicians administer a loading dose of opioid as well, such as 1 µg/kg of fentanyl or 1 to 3 µg/kg of hydromorphone. Bupivacaine infusion rates should not exceed 0.4 mg/kg/hr (e.g., 0.4 mL/kg/hr for 0.1% bupivacaine) for children, because toxicity may result.[454] Similarly, starting epidural fentanyl infusion rates should not exceed 1 µg/kg/hr. The upper limits of the epidural fentanyl dose should be determined by clinical effect. If epidural local anesthetic infusions are begun without either opioids or clonidine (e.g., 0.0625% to 0.125% bupivacaine) and inadequate analgesia occurs at infusion rates of 0.3 to 0.4 mL/kg/hr (a maximum dosage of 0.4 mg/kg/hr), further increases in local anesthetic infusion rate or concentration should be avoided. Instead, correct placement of the catheter should be confirmed (e.g., with an epidurogram or chloroprocaine/lidocaine test dose) if dermatomal levels cannot be unequivocally determined. If the catheter is properly located, an epidural opioid or clonidine can be added to the local anesthetic infusion. It is imperative to confirm that an epidural catheter is properly functioning immediately after an infant or child arrives in the PACU, or if there is any question of its proper location later. If an amino-amide local anesthetic has been given during or after surgery as an initial bolus followed by a continuous infusion, then use of a repeat bolus dose of these amino amides may result in a "stair casing" of plasma concentrations, with a risk for systemic toxicity. Although administration of epidural or systemic opioids may provide analgesia, they may not clarify the site of the epidural catheter. For this reason, confirmation of the catheter location is imperative whenever the clinical picture is not clear. Several means of accomplishing this are described later.

Local anesthetic and opioid combinations (e.g., 0.1% bupivacaine or ropivacaine with fentanyl 2 to 3 μg/mL or hydromorphone 3 to 5 μg/mL at infusion rates of 0.2 to 0.4 mL/kg/hr), via lumbar epidural catheters or caudal catheters advanced to a lumbar position, provide adequate analgesia in the majority of children undergoing lower abdominal or lower extremity surgery. Fentanyl alone (0.3 μg/kg/hr) has been shown to provide 90% effective postoperative analgesia after a levobupivacaine block was established during surgery.[455] Epidural opioids should be used with great caution, or at considerably reduced doses, in children at risk for apnea or hypoventilation (e.g., former preterm infants, children with chronic respiratory failure or disorders of central control of ventilation, or those with obstructive sleep apnea). In very young infants, epidural infusions of both local anesthetics and opioids and other adjuvants can be used safely, but require increased surveillance and reduced initial infusion rates. This is because (1) drug clearance may be reduced; (2) protein binding, which is decreased, may increase the free serum drug concentrations; and (3) titration to clinical end points (e.g., pain scoring) is less precise. A double-blind randomized study demonstrated that the combination of 0.1% bupivacaine with 1 μg/mL of fentanyl provided superior analgesia compared with local anesthetic alone, with no increase in adverse effects, when infused through thoracic catheters in infants under 6 months of age after thoracotomy.[456] In contrast, another study found no incremental benefits in children after abdominal surgery from the addition of fentanyl to epidural catheters with greater local anesthetic concentrations (e.g., 0.125% bupivacaine at 0.3 mL/kg/hr).[455,457] The use of fentanyl as an adjunct may increase PONV.[457] In some centers, application of epidural infusions, especially with opioids, for children younger than 3 to 6 months of age is restricted to intensive care areas. Acetaminophen or NSAIDs can also be administered if adjunctive analgesia is needed.

If the catheter tip is positioned at the thoracic dermatomes, bupivacaine-fentanyl[85,95,458-461] or ropivacaine-fentanyl solutions may be used for thoracic and upper abdominal surgery.[462] Infusion rates may need to be decreased for thoracic catheters compared with lumbar catheters because the capacitance or volume of the epidural space appears to be less than in lumbar regions. The authors have noted that some older children and adolescents require greater than expected infusion rates to achieve adequate dermatome levels for analgesia. Using hydromorphone in place of fentanyl may be of benefit in these instances, as its greater hydrophilicity results in wider spread. If thoracic placement is not possible, other agents may be administered through lumbar or caudal catheters. For example, epidural bolus doses of morphine 0.03 mg/kg (30 μg/kg) may be administered every 6 to 12 hours as needed.[463] Because the time to onset of analgesia is between 30 and 90 minutes, the doses must be administered at the earliest sign of return of pain. Alternatively, an epidural morphine infusion may be administered at a rate of 0.005 mg/kg/hr (5 μg/kg/hr; doses usually range from 4 to 8 μg/kg/hr) after a small initial bolus. We now rarely use epidural morphine and prefer a continuous epidural infusion of hydromorphone when greater spread is desired, as its adverse effect profile appears to be preferable. Studies in adults suggest an epidural potency ratio of between 2 and 3:1, compared with 5:1 for systemic morphine.[433] For thoracic or upper abdominal epidural infusions, hydromorphone is commonly administered at infusion rates of 0.001 to 0.003 mg/kg/hr (1 to 3 μg/kg/hr). When mixed with a local anesthetic for lumbar epidural infusion, concentrations of 3 to 5 μg/mL of hydromorphone yield a solution that results in an appropriate infusion rate of both drugs.

Hydrophilic opioids, especially when administered by infusion, require prolonged careful observation (see later discussion). If somnolence, shallow breathing, or hypopnea occurs, the infusion must be stopped, not simply decreased, until these effects subside, and appropriate therapy instituted (Table 43-11). Rather than administering a large dose of naloxone, it is preferable to titrate it at 1 μg/kg every 1 to 2 minutes until the respiratory

**TABLE 43-11** Treatment of Untoward Effects of Epidural Opioids

| Adverse Effect | Treatment | Infusion Rate |
|---|---|---|
| Pruritus | Naloxone, 0.5-1 μg/kg IV or infusion at 0.25-1 μg/kg/hr<br>Nalbuphine, 0.025 mg/kg IV every 6 hours | No change, or decrease opioid concentration, or decrease by 10%-20% (if dermatome level permits) |
| Nausea and vomiting | NPO for 24 hours<br>Naloxone, 0.5 μg/kg IV or infusion at 0.25-1 μg/kg/hr<br>Ondansetron 0.1 mg/kg (maximum 4 mg) IV every 6 hours<br>Metoclopramide, 0.1-0.15 mg/kg IV every 6-8 hours | Decrease opioid concentration or decrease by 10%-20% (if dermatome level permits) |
| Urinary retention | Bladder catheterization (one time; some institutions keep urinary catheters in these children routinely)<br>Naloxone, 0.5 μg/kg IV or infusion at 0.25-1 μg/kg/hr<br>Indwelling urinary catheter | Decrease opioid concentration |
| Respiratory depression;* child unarousable, hypoxemic, hypercarbic, or apneic | Oxygen by mask; assisted ventilation if needed<br>Naloxone, 5-10 μg/kg IV<br>Transfer child to monitored setting until episode is fully resolved.<br>Consider naloxone infusion (0.25-1 μg/kg/hr) | Discontinue infusion; consider possibility of intrathecal catheter migration (check by aspirating) |

*IV*, Intravenous; *NPO*, nothing by mouth.
*Stop infusion until the child is alert, if using morphine or hydromorphone.

drive improves, assuming that the airway can be adequately supported. In this manner, analgesia can be preserved. The duration of action of naloxone is considerably less than the respiratory depressant effect of the neuraxial opioids, thus continued respiratory monitoring is required and usually an infusion of naloxone (0.25-1 μg/kg/hr) until resolution of the respiratory depression. Common epidural infusions and alternative modalities for pain management of sample cases are provided in Appendix 43-1.

The sympathetic blockade that may occur in older children as a result of epidural or plexus blocks with local anesthetics may also be used advantageously to provide postoperative vasodilation in children undergoing replantation or vascularized flaps of the extremities.

Adjuvant agents, particularly clonidine, can be administered continuously via epidural catheter, most commonly in combination with or in place of local anesthetics and opioids. The primary analgesic effect appears to be via an α-adrenergic mechanism. Although epidural clonidine has been found to be less potent in terms of analgesic efficacy compared with epidural opioids, such as fentanyl, it has occasionally been substituted for neuraxial opioids because it is associated with a smaller incidence of untoward effects, such as respiratory depression, nausea, and pruritus.[464-467] This also suggests that the combination of all three agents, each at smaller concentrations than required individually, might be beneficial at reducing the incidence of adverse effects while optimizing analgesia, but carefully controlled studies have yet to be performed.

### Risks and Untoward Effects

Adverse effects associated with regional analgesia can be grouped according to those caused by the technique (e.g., the catheter) and those related to the medications (e.g., local anesthetics, opioids, other adjuvants). Three recent large prospective studies have confirmed the safety of regional anesthetics in children, detecting very small complication rates.[436-438,468]

*Local anesthetics* in the dilute concentrations used for postoperative analgesia have a very small incidence of untoward effects. Motor blockade occurs less frequently with dilute concentrations, but can be observed even with small concentrations of bupivacaine, such as 0.1%. As discussed earlier, children with neuromuscular disorders causing motor weakness should be observed carefully for exacerbation of their motor weakness. Motor weakness and blockade can result in several problems. Inability or difficulty in ambulation may impede recovery. The inability of a child to move a limb can result in skin breakdown or peripheral nerve compression injuries, especially if meticulous attention to frequent repositioning does not occur. We are aware of a case of complex regional pain syndrome in the distribution of the peroneal nerve that arose in this manner. Motor blockade should be avoided, if at all possible, and frequent examinations may quantify motor function using the Bromage score, if possible (Table 43-12). At our institutions, motor function is assessed every 8 hours along with the other vital signs pertinent to regional blockade (see Fig. 43-10). If motor blockade occurs, the clinician should (1) reduce the concentration of local anesthetic, (2) pay strict attention to padding and to frequent repositioning of the extremity involved, and (3) consider stopping the infusion until motor function returns. *Rapid onset of more profound motor block during epidural infusion should raise immediate concern about erosion of the catheter into the subarachnoid space.* Motor blockade may occur more frequently with peripheral nerve or plexus analgesia than with epidural blocks, and is subject to the same precautions.

| TABLE 43-12 Bromage Score* for Assessment of Motor Function of the Legs | |
|---|---|
| Full motor function: can flex hip, knee, and ankle | 0 |
| Can't flex hip (unable to perform straight-leg lift) | 1 |
| Can't flex hip or knee | 2 |
| Can't flex hip, knee, or ankle | 3 |

*Note that alternative scoring schemes for the Bromage scale exist that range from 1-4 (sometimes denoted I-IV) that directly correspond to the 0-3 scale depicted here.

When children are discharged home with a peripheral nerve catheter, it is particularly important to teach the parents how to deal with motor blockade.

The PK of bupivacaine have been studied in infants and children after both single-injection doses[469] and continuous infusions. Data suggest that in children younger than 6 months of age, reduced protein binding increases the free fraction of circulating bupivacaine, which increases the risk of bupivacaine toxicity.[470] Neonates and infants with impaired hepatic blood flow may be at particular risk for bupivacaine accumulation. Seizures and cardiac arrest have been reported when large doses of bupivacaine have been administered, usually after excessive infusion rates or unintended intravascular injection. Limited information is available regarding extended administration over days, although low concentration solutions (and therefore low total doses) reduce the risk for toxicity. *l*-Enantiomers of amino amides (ropivacaine and levobupivacaine) have toxic thresholds that are greater than that of bupivacaine by as much as 30%, and such drugs should be considered in smaller children and for blocks that require greater infusion rates and for greater durations. A particular "hidden" risk occurs when a block is functioning less than optimally and bolus doses are administered in an attempt to broaden the dermatome level. Even though the infusion rate is kept within the recommended range, the bolus doses can raise the blood concentration above the toxic threshold. *Whenever a local anesthetic is administered by continuous infusion, nursing and medical staff must be aware of the signs and symptoms of local-anesthetic toxicity, be vigilant in monitoring for the early detection of those signs, and be familiar with the use of lipid rescue protocols to treat toxicity if it occurs.* The use of lipid emulsion for treating local anesthetic toxicity is discussed in detail in Chapter 41. Tachyphylaxis during prolonged administration of local anesthetics is a theoretic consideration, although no systematic studies have addressed this phenomenon in children. In animal models, tachyphylaxis is accelerated by hyperalgesia and prevented by agents that prevent hyperalgesia at spinal sites. One rationale for coadministration of opioids or clonidine in epidural infusions may be to reduce the incidence or severity of tachyphylaxis. As discussed in Chapter 41, hemodynamic stability is maintained in children younger than 6 years of age during spinal or epidural blockade, even with extensive sympathetic blockade. As children approach school age, however, rapid position changes may produce hemodynamic responses after extensive sympathetic blockade, and this must be considered in children who receive continuous epidural blockade. Orthostatic changes may be exacerbated when epidural clonidine is infused, and extra caution should be taken.

*Neuraxial opioids* confer several potential adverse effects, including respiratory depression, nausea, urinary retention, and pruritus. Indeed, despite their proven analgesic efficacy, not all authorities are proponents of their use because of these effects, preferring other adjuvants instead.[471] The most effective means of treating or preventing the adverse effects is the use of opioid antagonists or mixed agonist-antagonists. This approach directly targets the etiology of the signs rather than simply treating their manifestations. Low-dose naloxone infusions, which have been shown to be effective in children receiving parenteral opioids, are also effective for treating the adverse effects of neuraxial opioids, although pediatric data are lacking.[472-476] We have used similar rates to those shown effective in the PCA studies, beginning at 0.25 μg/kg/hr.[241] This infusion rate can be titrated upwards as needed to 1 μg/kg/hr without adversely affecting analgesic efficacy.[242]

The most worrisome and dangerous complication is respiratory depression. The lipophilic agents (fentanyl and sufentanil) have the widest therapeutic indices. This results from greater receptor binding in the substantia gelatinosa of the spinal cord adjacent to the area of drug administration, thus limiting the rostral spread of the drug. Despite the fact that the hydrophilic opioids, hydromorphone and morphine, pose a greater risk for respiratory depression, the incidence remains low. Nevertheless, reports in the pediatric literature of respiratory depression after epidural administration of morphine demonstrate that vigilance in monitoring is mandatory.[382,477,478] The incidence of complications with caudal morphine is reduced if a dose of 0.033 mg/kg (33 μg/kg) or less is used in children older than 1 year of age.[463] The adequacy of analgesia at this dose was virtually unchanged from 0.1 mg/kg (100 μg/kg), with the exception of a prolongation of action with the greater dose. *The hallmark of impending overdose of central neuraxial opioids is increasing sedation and decreasing DEPTH AND RATE of respirations. It is important to recognize that the depth of respiration must be assessed, not just the rate, because children frequently develop decreased tidal volume before the respiratory rate decreases, leading to alveolar hypoventilation and the potential for hypercarbia and hypoxemia.*[479]

In addition to clinical assessment, quantitative capnography and pulse oximetry can be valuable monitors for these children and provide more useful information than impedance-type respirometers, which count only respiratory rate. Impedance-based respiratory monitors may continue to register breathing efforts when significant airway obstruction exists, as long as the chest wall is still moving, thereby potentially delaying the recognition of respiratory depression. Because electronic monitors that alarm only in the child's room can be ignored, it is important that these monitors are configured to either alarm at the nurses' station and in the hallways, or notify the nurse directly using portable communication devices. Such advanced communication systems are now commercially available and may help to provide early warning of impending complications, although the risk of false alarms, and the complacency caused by their frequent activation, must also be considered. Again, it is emphasized that no monitor can replace vigilance and frequent clinical assessment.

Oversedation, diminished respiratory depth, and slowing of the respiratory rate are treated by decreasing the rate of opioid administration and, if necessary, administering small incremental doses of naloxone (0.5 to 1 μg/kg) every few minutes until the adverse effects are reversed (see earlier discussion). A continuous low-dose infusion of naloxone, as described earlier (0.25 to 1 μg/kg/hr) may need to be started. More profound respiratory depression, including inability to arouse the child and apnea, must be treated more aggressively. In this circumstance, the infusion should be discontinued, positive-pressure ventilation with oxygen instituted if respirations are very slow, shallow, or absent, and up

to 5 to 10 μg/kg of naloxone administered IV. As long as respirations are adequately supported, there is no need to administer very large doses of naloxone. *The new development of respiratory depression in a child receiving what appears to be an appropriate opioid dose, should always raise the question of catheter migration into the subarachnoid space. Whenever central neuraxial opioids are administered, facilities must be immediately available at the child's bedside for resuscitation, in the unlikely event of respiratory depression.* It is recommended that emergency equipment, including a bag-valve device, appropriate sizes of masks and airways, and suction, be at the child's bedside or in a "code cart" that is accessible within seconds, should the need arise. Naloxone should similarly be immediately available, without the need to obtain the drug from the pharmacy. All children receiving continuous regional analgesia should also have an IV line (a heparin lock is adequate in those children not requiring IV fluids).

Pruritus is a common adverse effect associated with epidural or intrathecal opioid use, occurring in as many as 30% to 70% of children. Antihistamines are less effective antipruritics in this situation, because the primary mechanism is a central opioid, not a histamine, effect. Thus opioid antagonists, used in small doses, are most effective. Again, low-dose infusions of naloxone can be employed with good results.[242,472,473,475,476] Some practitioners have found low-dose nalbuphine to be effective to antagonize pruritus (25 to 50 μg/kg every 6 hours, PRN).[473,474] Although we have found this treatment to be effective, others have found it to be no more effective than placebo in reducing pruritus in children.[480]

Nausea and vomiting can also occur in association with opioids (both systemic and neuraxial) and may be more common with morphine than with fentanyl. Children who are fasted during the first 24 hours after surgery do not vomit excessively, even when given caudal morphine.[481] As with all other opioid adverse effects, nausea and vomiting respond to the previously mentioned doses of naloxone or mixed agonist-antagonists, such as nalbuphine. Some antiemetics, such as antihistamines and butyrophenones (e.g., droperidol), may cause sedation and should be used with caution. Serotonin receptor antagonists, such as ondansetron (0.1 to 0.15 mg/kg, maximum 4 mg) or dolasetron (0.35 mg/kg, maximum 12.5 mg), may be effective and not cause sedation.[482] Metoclopramide in doses of 0.1 to 0.15 mg/kg (100 to 150 μg/kg) IV every 6 to 8 hours may provide adequate relief, with less sedation than other drugs of its class. It is sometimes prudent to decrease the infusion rate of the epidural (if the block level permits) or the opioid concentration in the infusate when untoward effects require treatment. If additional analgesia is required, acetaminophen, oral NSAIDs, or ketorolac may be administered. Untoward effects of epidural opioids and their treatment are summarized in Table 43-11.

Urinary retention is a relatively common complication of neuraxial opioids. Studies of single-injection caudal blocks have found that this complication does not occur when epidural local anesthetics are used, only when neuraxial opioids are added.[372] Neuraxial opioids depress detrusor contractility in a dose-dependent manner, and this effect may actually outlast the analgesic effect of the drug by hours.[483,484] Different approaches have been used for this problem, including indwelling urinary catheterization and the use of opioid antagonists.[485]

Concerns have been raised that regional analgesia could mask or delay the detection of compartment syndrome of an extremity because of the intensity or quality of analgesia produced by neural blockade.[486] Despite the theoretical worries, this has not been demonstrated in numerous studies, and indeed, the opposite has been observed, that the onset of pain in a patient with previously adequate analgesia from an epidural or nerve block is an early warning sign that may herald the onset of compartment syndrome.[487,488] The concentration of local anesthetics used for postoperative analgesia appears to be inadequate to mask the intensity of pain caused by compartment syndrome. In addition, epidural blockade is not effective in controlling the discomfort from intense pressure (as demonstrated by the parturient's ability to perceive pressure during labor contractions despite being pain-free). The loss of effective analgesia in a child at risk of compartment syndrome should raise suspicion and prompt investigation before any changes are made to the analgesic regimen (see also Chapter 30).

### Catheter-Related Complications

Inadequate analgesia must prompt an examination of the child and a review of the operative procedure and the analgesic technique. The dermatome level should be determined using differentiation between cold and warm sensation in children who are cognitively and developmentally able to cooperate. Presence of a dermatome level suggests a successful block of inadequate height. No demonstrable blockade suggests a primary malfunction, although low concentrations of local anesthetic may make differentiation of the level difficult in some children. If there were difficulties during catheter placement coupled with a lack of effective analgesia when the child emerges from general anesthesia, the catheter is likely malpositioned. We often use epidurography in this situation to determine whether the catheter is in the epidural space. Misplacement in various locations has been reported, including the subdural space, paravertebral space, tissue planes adjacent to the spine, and even in an epidural blood vessel after a negative test dose.[427,489-491] The catheter's location can be easily visualized on a plain radiograph (or with fluoroscopy in the OR) after the injection of a small volume of nonionic contrast agent. Contrast agent in the epidural space has a characteristic "bubbly" appearance, with the contrast agent centrally located over the spinal column (Fig. 43-12). The existence of a median raphe in the epidural space has been postulated and may be the cause of unilateral multi-dermatome blockade.[492] This has been demonstrated on epidurography when unilateral blockade has occurred (Fig. 43-13). A single unilateral dermatomal band of analgesia or temperature-sensation change may indicate that the catheter has passed through a spinal foramen. In some cases, simply withdrawing the catheter 1 or 2 cm may allow proper repositioning within the epidural space. A functional, rather than anatomic, method of confirming epidural placement is the "chloroprocaine test," which has the advantage of both providing rapid analgesia (with a properly located catheter) and confirming the site of placement. A chloroprocaine test is presented in Figure 43-14.

On occasion, a collection of fluid may be found at the skin insertion site and pooling under the dressing. Experience suggests that in most cases this is not, as one may fear, cerebrospinal fluid, but rather edema fluid, or occasionally local anesthetic solution, tracking along the catheter's course and leaking through a hole in the skin from the subcutaneous tissues. Local anesthetic solutions would test negative for glucose and protein, whereas cerebrospinal fluid and edema fluid would test positive for glucose and protein. It usually requires no special treatment except reinforcing the dressing. It subsides as the edema and third space fluids are mobilized in the first days after surgery. If troublesome

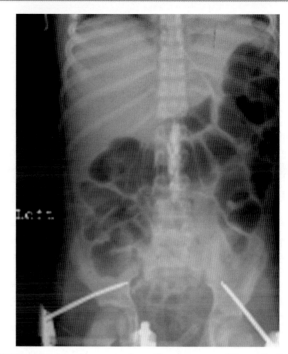

**FIGURE 43-12** An epidurogram shows the appearance of the contrast agent centered in the spinal column and also the bubbly appearance of the contrast agent, presumably produced by the epidural fat and plexus.

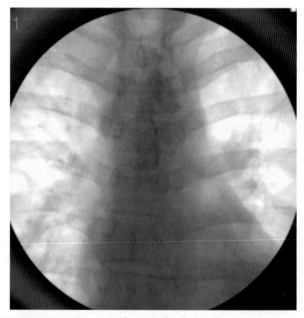

**FIGURE 43-13** Epidurogram taken with fluoroscopy demonstrating unilateral spread of contrast agent. The contrast agent appears to have a very sharp edge precisely in the center of the spinal column, demarcating one side of the epidural space from the other.

and persistent leakage occurs, a drop of collodion or Dermabond (Ethicon, Inc. Cornelia, Ga.) over the skin site may be effective in sealing the hole.

The catheter site should be inspected daily to ensure that the dressing is intact and to assess for the presence of infection. Infections are exceedingly rare, perhaps in part because of the bactericidal properties of the local anesthetics themselves.[493]

## PROCEDURE FOR THE CHLOROPROCAINE TEST

An anesthesiologist is present for the procedure with use of standard monitors and supplies for providing respiratory or hemodynamic support.

1. A loading dose of chloroprocaine 3% is divided in five equal increments, each given at 1- to 2-minute intervals (over 5-10 minutes total) according to weight approximately as follows: (doses may be adjusted according to clinical circumstances)

| Weight Group | Increment Volume | Total Volume |
|---|---|---|
| 0-10 kg | 0.125 mL/kg | 0.6 mL/kg |
| 10-20 kg | 0.1 mL/kg | 0.5 mL/kg |
| 20-35 kg | 2.5 mL (fixed volume) | 12.5 mL (fixed volume) |
| 35-60 kg | 3 mL (fixed volume) | 15 mL (fixed volume) |
| ≥60 kg | 3.5 mL (fixed volume) | 17.5 mL (fixed volume) |

2. Incremental dosing is stopped before giving the full dose if there are clear signs of bilateral lower extremity sensory or motor block, or a very definite reduction in heart rate (e.g., 30 beats per minute) and blood pressure (e.g., 25 mm Hg drop in systolic pressure). In most cases, because you are performing this test because of signs of pain, there is some tachycardia and hypertension relative to baseline values at the start of the test. Transient cessation of crying in an infant or toddler is not a sufficiently specific positive response to warrant interruption of the test.

3. A catheter positioned in the **thoracic** epidural space will generally not show lower extremity sensory or motor block with the chloroprocaine test, but should give a very clear drop in heart rate and blood pressure, as well as a clear and persistent reduction in pain reports or pain behaviors.

4. If the chloroprocaine test is positive (i.e., confirms epidural placement), this implies that a stronger or different epidural solution is needed for steady-state pain relief. Because hydromorphone is sufficiently hydrophilic to spread from lumbar to thoracic spinal levels, **switching the solution from bupivacaine-fentanyl to bupivacaine-hydromorphone will provide good steady-state pain relief in >90% of these cases**. A typical loading dose of hydromorphone of 2 μg/kg (0.002 mg/kg) will provide analgesia within 30 minutes in most cases.

If the chloroprocaine test fails to confirm epidural placement, the catheter is repositioned, removed, or replaced according to clinical circumstances.

**FIGURE 43-14** Chloroprocaine test to determine regional catheter function as performed at Children's Hospital, Boston. (Personal communication, C. Berde.)

Although colonization of catheters, usually with *Staphylococcus epidermidis* and other gram-positive organisms, appears common, adult and pediatric studies have shown that this is not associated with neuraxial infection.[494,495] In the UK epidural audit, there were three cases of deep tissue infection and 25 local infections reported out of 10,660 epidural catheters.[436] Tunneling a catheter subcutaneously may reduce the risk of bacteriologic contamination and permit the use of a catheter for a greater period of time.[420] A study of the microbiology of the infusion fluids and delivery systems has demonstrated that catheter-related infections of the deep tissues, including epidural abscess, appear to have their origin in local skin infections that track along the catheter's path or via a bacteremia.[496] *Any sign of local infection is cause for immediate catheter removal.* Epidural abscess is a catastrophic complication that can be generally avoided if the catheter is removed early, when only a localized cutaneous infection is present.[497] Clinical signs include fever, malaise, and back pain. Specific neurologic signs, paresthesias, and motor symptoms (e.g., flaccid paralysis as cord compression develops, eventually progressing to spasticity) may occur late in the course, if early warning signs are not heeded, but may progress rapidly once established. Children who develop fever or sepsis need to be evaluated on an individual basis. If a clear source for the fever is found, it is acceptable to leave the catheter in place with regular and frequent observation and reassessment, although we remove it if a child is overtly septic or if the situation is unclear.

### Intrapleural Catheters

Continuous intrapleural analgesia has been used in children after thoracic, upper abdominal, and retroperitoneal surgery, although this technique has fallen out of favor in recent years as familiarity with paravertebral and thoracic epidural blockade has increased.[498-500] A standard epidural catheter can be introduced to the intrapleural space in the same fashion as for a thoracentesis, that is, over the *upper* margin of the rib to avoid the neurovascular structures. The catheter is threaded several centimeters, anchored at the skin site with a suture to prevent its migration, and affixed with a clear occlusive dressing. Infusing 0.25% bupivacaine with epinephrine (1:200,000) at 0.5 mL/kg/hr has provided effective analgesia.[498] Because the local anesthetic solution flows with gravity, the position of the child is important in determining the efficacy of analgesia. The risks associated with this technique include rapid uptake of drug into the circulation from the large and efficient absorptive surface of the pleura. Although none of the children in the initial reports of this technique had signs of clinical toxicity, total blood concentrations of bupivacaine (bound and unbound) reached the toxic range of 4 μg/mL after 24 hours of therapy in some children. Anecdotally, seizures have been reported with intrapleural analgesia in children. Given these concerns, *hourly bupivacaine infusion rates should generally not exceed 0.5 mg/kg/hr.*[452] Ropivacaine or levobupivacaine may be safer alternatives than bupivacaine because of their reduced risk of cardiotoxicity. The potential also exists for paresis of the phrenic, recurrent laryngeal, and vagus nerves, and the thoracic sympathetic chain, as well as for direct effects on the diaphragm. Pneumothorax remains a risk with percutaneous placement through a closed chest. In our experience, epidural analgesia is more effective and has a wider margin of safety than intrapleural analgesia for major thoracoabdominal surgery. Thoracic paravertebral block has also been described in children, and is another preferable alternative with less risk of local anesthetic toxicity (see Chapter 41). With the widespread use of ultrasound guidance, thoracic paravertebral catheters are being used much more commonly in major pediatric centers.[501-503]

### Plexus Catheters

Catheters may be placed adjacent to the brachial plexus via an axillary, infraclavicular, or supraclavicular approach with the latter two affording improved stability and security of the catheter.[352,504,505] Ultrasound guidance is rapidly becoming the standard of practice for regional anesthesia in children (see Chapter 42). The prolonged duration of analgesia after a single-injection brachial plexus block reduces the need for an indwelling catheter in many instances, although it may be useful in some operative circumstances, and for postoperative management of reimplantation of an arm or hand, because sustained vasodilation from the block may improve revascularization.[506] Specialized kits for peripheral nerve and plexus cannulation are commercially available. These catheters are inserted using the same landmarks and techniques as for placing a single-injection block. After initial dosing, 0.125% bupivacaine or 0.2% ropivacaine at 0.1 to 0.2 mL/kg/hr may be infused. Potential complications of continuous brachial plexus blockade include infection and nerve injury, although these are quite rare and none have been reported to PRAN to date).[438] In a retrospective study of complications from axillary catheters in adults, the rate of localized infection was less than 3 per 1000 and of new neurologic symptoms was 5 per 1000.[507]

### Peripheral Nerve Catheters

Catheter techniques have been used with increasing frequency for peripheral nerve blocks in outpatients and inpatients, in part because of the increased use of ultrasound guidance to confirm placement. Infusions can be delivered with conventional infusion pumps or disposable elastomeric controlled infusion devices described earlier. We usually use conventional infusion pumps for inpatients owing to reduced cost and to the increased safety that may be inherent in the familiarity of the inpatient nurses with such systems. The disposable devices permit the child to be discharged home and still receive long-lasting analgesia with a regional anesthetic. This technique can be used for many of the nerve blocks mentioned in Chapters 41 and 42 and is most commonly used for femoral or fascia iliaca, sciatic, and brachial plexus blocks. Most commonly, 0.2% ropivacaine is used at rates of 0.1 to 0.2 mL/kg/hr.[352] An organized system of daily follow-up by telephone or visiting nurses is essential for safety and efficacy of such a service, but both limited published and anecdotal experience suggests that ambulatory analgesia with peripheral neural blockade can be an effective modality in pediatric outpatients.[333,508]

### Fascial Plane and Wound Catheters

Catheters with multiple side holes can be placed in a fascial plane or wound bed by the surgeon at the time of closure and local anesthetics infused over several days for postoperative analgesia.

There are very limited data in children, but such techniques have been reported to be effective.[508,509] There are no studies to date comparing infusion rates; volumes of 2 to 5 mL/hr of 0.2% ropivacaine have most commonly been used, infused via the elastomeric pumps previously described.

### Removal of Catheters and Transition to Oral Analgesics

The transition from continuous regional blockade to oral analgesics should ideally be achieved without a significant decrement in the quality of pain relief for the child and should permit the clinician to revert to more aggressive modalities, should the decision prove to be premature. The duration of continuous blockade is, of course, in large part dependent on the type of operation and the underlying medical and/or surgical problems of the child. Some children do well with transition to oral analgesics on the morning after surgery. This is often the case for the child who has undergone an uncomplicated ureteral reimplantation. For more painful procedures, such as Nuss bar placement for pectus excavatum in an adolescent, strong analgesics will be required for a greater duration. The norm in this situation is 3 days. We find it most effective to begin the transition from regional analgesia to oral therapy early in the morning. As soon as the regional infusion is discontinued, a dose of oral analgesic, usually an oral opioid, such as oxycodone, in combination with acetaminophen, is administered. This ensures that the oral agents have provided their full effect before the block recedes. The catheter is not removed until the child has demonstrated that the oral agents provide adequate comfort without any residual analgesia from the block, so that blockade can be reestablished if transition fails. The oral agents are best administered on a schedule, rather than as needed, for the first 12 to 24 hours after transition.

Children who are anticoagulated require special consideration before removing epidural catheters. Although there are no specific pediatric data, the recommendations of the consensus panel of the American Society for Regional Anesthesia are generally accepted.[331] The report notes *"the initiation of systemic therapeutic heparin therapy for medical or surgical indications in the presence of a neuraxial catheter potentially increases the risk of hematoma formation during catheter removal"* and that systemic heparinization is recommended to be discontinued for 2 to 4 hours before catheter removal. At least 1 hour should elapse before heparin therapy is restarted, and careful neurologic assessment should be performed for at least 12 hours after removal of the catheter. Fractionated or low molecular weight heparins pose a risk as well, compounded by several different regimens in common clinical use (once-a-day vs. twice-a-day dosing) and the inability to assess the degree of anticoagulation with commonly available tests of coagulation (prothrombin time and partial thromboplastin time). The consensus panel recommends that catheters should be removed no sooner than 10 to 12 hours after the last dose of low molecular weight heparin, and dosing should resume no sooner than 2 hours after the catheter's removal.

# Pain Management in the Cognitively Impaired Child

The goals of pain management in the child with cognitive impairment are to minimize discomfort, maximize function, and improve the quality of life. With these goals in mind, the child's pain management plans should include multimodal pharmacologic and nonpharmacologic strategies tailored to the severity and etiology of pain. The World Health Organization's analgesic ladder provides a framework for decision-making related to analgesic use based on severity and persistence of pain.

## OPIOID ANALGESICS

The use of opioids in children with cognitive impairment has been limited by concerns regarding potential adverse effects and a perceived reduced margin of safety because of diminished cardiorespiratory reserve and neurologic impairment. Indeed, a recent study identified cognitive impairment to be an independent predictor of adverse events from PCA/NCA.[297] It is, therefore, necessary to carefully balance the goals of providing adequate analgesia while minimizing adverse events related to analgesic treatments. For moderate to severe pain, the judicious use of opioids in small doses titrated to effect are a suitable option. Children with cognitive impairment may lack the cognitive and motor skills to use PCA devices successfully. In these children, NCA or CCA will permit titration of small amounts of opioids to effect, without significantly increasing nursing workload.[510] A study of children whose postoperative pain was managed by parent- or nurse-controlled analgesia, reported low pain scores and modest opioid requirements with the use of basal infusions in addition to bolus dosing, in the majority of children.[511] Adverse effects included nausea and vomiting, and pruritus requiring treatment, in 14% and 32% of children, respectively. Supplemental oxygen was required in 79% of the children, and respiratory depression requiring naloxone was noted in 2.8%. The management of two children was remarkable, in that one had received an average morphine dose of 0.045 mg/kg/hr and four concomitant sedatives, including diphenhydramine, diazepam, droperidol, and chloral hydrate, and the second had only received a small dose of morphine and no other sedatives, but the basal infusion of morphine was implicated as the cause of respiratory depression. Both recovered without sequelae. The above studies highlight the importance of frequent and careful assessment of pain, depth of sedation, and respiratory status (using continuous pulse oximetry and/or noninvasive capnography) to ensure the safety and the comfort of children with cognitive impairment receiving opioid therapy

## NONOPIOID ANALGESICS

Nonopioid adjuvants, such as acetaminophen, nonsteroidal anti-inflammatory drugs, or tramadol, should be added to provide synergistic analgesia and to reduce opioid requirements. They may be administered orally or via gastrostomy tubes. IV ketorolac provides excellent analgesia in children who have not initiated oral intake after surgery, although the risks of platelet dysfunction must be considered if ongoing bleeding is an issue. The $\alpha_2$-agonist clonidine has also been used for its synergistic analgesic effects. However, it has the potential to cause sedation and hypotension.

Muscle spasms and clonus are an ongoing source of pain in children with cognitive impairment, and may be exacerbated after surgical procedures, particularly orthopedic and neurosurgical procedures. Diazepam and baclofen have been effective for treating acute painful muscle spasms after surgery in children with spasticity. Because benzodiazepines have a synergistic respiratory depressant effect when used in conjunction with opioids, they must be used judiciously.

## EPIDURAL AND REGIONAL ANALGESIA

Epidural analgesia has been used with success in children with cognitive impairment who are undergoing lower extremity orthopedic procedures, selective dorsal rhizotomy, and Nissen fundoplication.[80,512] Epidural catheters may be technically difficult to place in some children with cognitive impairment because of contractures and spine deformities. However, when feasible, this technique provides excellent analgesia, reduces muscle spasms, and promotes overall child comfort, with a small incidence of sedation and respiratory depression. Some children will still experience muscle spasms and will require intermittent doses of midazolam or oral diazepam. Intermittent bolus epidural morphine or continuous fentanyl and bupivacaine provided excellent analgesia in 91 of 92 children with cerebral palsy undergoing subumbilical procedures.[512] The children who received epidural morphine experienced a 6.5% incidence of excessive sedation and hypopnea and a 7.6% incidence of oxygen desaturation to less than 90%. Other adverse effects included emesis (52%), pruritus (29%), and urinary retention (70%). These authors recommended the use of fentanyl and bupivacaine in an effort to avoid the excessive sedation and hypopnea observed in the children who received epidural morphine. Urinary catheters are also routinely placed, given the frequency of urinary retention, particularly when neuraxial opioids are used. Epidural morphine infusions have been compared with morphine PCA in children with cerebral palsy undergoing selective dorsal rhizotomy.[80] Epidural catheters were placed under direct visualization by the neurosurgeon at the end of surgery. Children in the epidural group experienced reduced pain scores and fewer muscle spasms and tolerated activity better in the early postoperative period than did the PCA group. Respiratory depression did not occur in any of the groups, and the incidence of vomiting and pruritus was similar between groups. In summary, these studies support the attributes and safety of epidural analgesia in children with cognitive impairment.

Children with cerebral palsy who received continuous infusion of local anesthetics via catheters tunneled into the incision site following orthopedic surgery experienced significantly lower pain scores and required less oral analgesics on the first two postoperative days, compared to controls who received oral analgesics alone.[508] Although data related to peripheral and plexus blocks in cognitively impaired children are limited, our experience suggests that these, too, are safe and effective in this population, and can contribute to reducing the reliance on systemic analgesics and, thereby, their adverse effects.

Emerging data must be used to guide treatment plans and protocols that incorporate frequent evaluation and careful monitoring of children with cognitive impairment. Involvement of a multidisciplinary pain team that includes the primary care provider, pain specialist, psychologist, nurse, physical therapist, and occupational therapist is required to provide the level of expertise required to care for these children with special needs.

## Summary

Postoperative analgesia is an integral and essential component of any pediatric anesthetic plan. Contemporary knowledge of anatomy, physiology, PK, and pharmacodynamics in infancy and childhood permits the anesthesiologist to apply advanced anesthetic and analgesic techniques with excellent efficacy and safety to all children. Clinical examples of postoperative management strategies are presented in Appendix 43-1. The optimal use of these modalities requires an understanding of the techniques outlined in this chapter, as well as the integration of multiple medical and nursing disciplines in the assessment and care of these children. A well-organized pediatric pain service and an educated nursing staff are the keys to the successful management of acute pain, which, in turn, can be expected to result in improved care for infants and children.[513]

## ANNOTATED REFERENCES

Berde CB, Sethna NF. Analgesics for the treatment of pain in children. N Engl J Med 2002;347:1094-103.

*This authoritative reference provides a succinct yet complete review of the pharmacology of effective analgesic regimens in children.*

Llewellyn N, Moriarty A. The national pediatric epidural audit. Paediatr Anaesth 2007;17:520-33.

*The largest prospective study on epidural anesthesia to date followed patients into the postoperative period and highlights the incidence and nature of complications and adverse events, which were rare. This should be read in conjunction with the French study.[468]*

Lynn AM, Nespeca MK, Opheim KE, Slattery JT. Respiratory effects of intravenous morphine infusions in neonates, infants, and children after cardiac surgery. Anesth Analg 1993;77:695-701.

*This important study identified the threshold serum morphine concentration for respiratory depression in neonates, infants, and children receiving continuous morphine concentrations following heart surgery to be 20 ng/mL, and, as such, provides a framework to guide appropriate dosing of morphine in these populations. The authors recommended careful observation of all children receiving morphine because of the wide variability in the $CO_2$ response slope seen in their subjects.*

Malviya S, Voepel-Lewis T, Burke C, et al. The revised FLACC observational pain tool: improved reliability and validity for pain assessment in children with cognitive impairment. Paediatr Anaesth 2006;16: 258-65.

*The FLACC tool was revised to incorporate behavioral descriptors consistently associated with pain in cognitively impaired children. This paper describes the development of the revised FLACC and demonstrates its reliability and validity in assessing pain in this vulnerable population.*

Maxwell LG, Kaufmann SC, Bitzer S, et al. The effects of a small-dose naloxone infusion on opioid-induced side effects and analgesia in children and adolescents treated with intravenous patient-controlled analgesia: a double-blind, prospective, randomized, controlled study. Anesth Analg 2005;100:953-8.

*This study demonstrated that a low-dose naloxone infusion significantly reduced the incidence and severity of opioid-induced adverse effects, including pruritus and nausea, without affecting opioid-induced analgesia. These data address the important clinical problem of opioid-induced adverse effects that frequently limits the utility of opioids in the treatment of pain.*

Michelet D, Andreu-Gallien, Bensalah T, et al. A meta-analysis of the use of nonsteroidal anti-inflammatory drugs for pediatric postoperative pain. Anesth Analg 2012;114:393-406.

*This meta-analysis shows that perioperative NSAID administration reduces opioid consumption and PONV during the postoperative period in children. In 27 randomized controlled trials, perioperative administration of NSAIDs reduced opioid requirement in the PACU and for the first 24 hours after surgery, decreased pain intensity in the PACU and PONV during the first 24 hours postoperatively. Results from this study suggest that multimodal analgesia should be used in an effort to reduce opioid consumption and adverse effects in children undergoing surgery.*

Morton NS, Errera A. APA national audit of pediatric opioid infusions. Pediatr Anesth 2010;20:119-25.

*This very large prospective audit of opioid infusions of all types (continuous, PCA, NCA) confirmed the safety of these techniques, but highlights the potential complications and pitfalls that are always present. Respiratory depression and pump programming errors each occurred in about 1 of 766 cases and 1 of 631 cases respectively, and there was one permanent injury (1 of 10,000 cases).*

Polaner DM, Taenzer AH, Walker BJ, et al. Pediatric Regional Anesthesia Network: a multi-institutional study of the use and incidence of complications of pediatric regional anesthesia. Anesth Analg 2012 Jun 13 [Epub ahead of print].

*This is the first report from this network in the United States that prospectively examined the incidence of adverse events and complications in nearly 15,000 regional blocks in children. There were no permanent complications detected. PRAN now has over 37,000 cases accrued. These data are similar to those reported in the French study.[468]*

Voepel-Lewis T, Burke CN, Jeffreys N, et al. Do 0-10 numeric rating scores translate into clinically meaningful pain measures for children? Anesth Analg 2011;112:415-21.

*This study provides important information regarding the clinical interpretation of NRS pain scores in children. )-10 NRS scores were found to be reliably associated with the child's perceived need for medicine, perceived pain relief, and satisfaction with pain treatment. However, a significant overlap in scores associated with the above outcomes suggests that the use of specific cutoff scores to guide treatment decisions would be inappropriate in children.*

von Baeyer CL, Spagrud LJ. Systematic review of observational (behavioral) measures of pain for children and adolescents aged 3 to 18 years. Pain 2007;127:140-50.

*This is a comprehensive review of the numerous behavioral observational measures of pain for children and identifies the most appropriate tools for assessing pain in various settings, including the postoperative period and in critical care.*

## REFERENCES

Please see www.expertconsult.com.

# Appendix 43-1    Clinical Examples of Postoperative Analgesic Management Strategy

**43**

## Case 1

A 2-year-old child, ASA 1 (American Society of Anesthesiologists physical status classification system, category 1), presented for inguinal hernia repair, weight 15 kg.

### CONSIDERATIONS

- Mildly painful surgery
- Outpatient setting–avoidance of nausea and oversedation is helpful

### ALTERNATIVES

1. Ilioinguinal nerve block: bupivacaine 0.25% with epinephrine 1 : 200,000, 0.5 mL/kg × 15 kg = 7.5 mL (3.75 mL on each side)
2. Wound infiltration with bupivacaine 0.25% with epinephrine 1 : 200,000, 0.5 mL/kg × 15 kg = 7.5 mL (3.75 mL on each side)
3. Caudal block using bupivacaine 0.125% to 0.25% with epinephrine 1 : 200,000, 0.5 to 0.75 mL/kg × 15 kg = 7 to 11 mL
4. Add acetaminophen, 10 to 15 mg/kg every 4 to 6 hours (oral), or ibuprofen, 6 to 10 mg/kg every 6 hours, as needed at home.

## Case 2

A 6-month-old, 6-kg child, ASA 1, presented for ureteral reimplantation.

### CONSIDERATIONS

- Moderately painful surgery, bladder spasms
- Urinary retention is not an issue
- Pain assessment using behavioral tools such as FLACC

### ALTERNATIVES

1. Epidural analgesia
   - Need to cover approximately 10 dermatomes (5 sacral, 5 lumbar); initial bolus, 10 × 0.05 mL/kg/dermatome × 6 kg = 3.0 mL.
   - Bupivacaine 0.1% with fentanyl, 2 µg/mL, starting at 0.2 mL/kg/hr × 6 kg = 1.2 mL/hr
   - Apnea monitoring, pulse oximetry, and frequent observation
   - Add acetaminophen as needed, 10 to 15 mg/kg every 4 hours (oral) or 10 mg/kg every 6 hours (IV), or 35 to 40 mg/kg initial dose (rectal) followed by 20 mg/kg every 6 hours (rectal) not to exceed 100 mg/kg/day (rectal).
   - Add ketorolac 0.5 mg/kg every 6 hours for 48 hours for bladder spasms as needed.
2. Continuous intravenous morphine infusion
   - Loading dose of up to 0.075 to 0.1 mg/kg × 6 kg = 0.45 to 0.6 mg in incremental doses if needed
   - Infusion starting at 0.02 mg/kg/hr (20 µg/kg/hr) × 6 kg = 0.12 mg/hr
   - Apnea monitoring, continuous pulse oximetry, and frequent observation
   - Add acetaminophen as needed.

3. Nurse-controlled analgesia with morphine
   - Loading dose 0.05 to 0.1 mg/kg × 6 kg = 0.3 to 0.6 mg administered via PCA pump in PACU
   - Continuous basal infusion of 0.01 to 0.02 mg/kg/hr
   - Bolus dose of 0.02 to 0.03 mg/kg
   - Lockout interval: 8 to 15 minutes
   - Four-hour limit of 0.25 to 0.3 mg/kg
   - Apnea monitoring, continuous pulse oximetry, and frequent observation
   - Add acetaminophen as needed.

## Case 3

A 6-week-old, 3-kg child, ASA 3, presented for thoracoabdominal incision for excision of a Wilms tumor.

### CONSIDERATIONS

- Painful surgery
- Pain assessment using behavioral tools such as FLACC
- Impairment of respiration
- Many dermatomes involved
- Bladder catheter warranted

### ALTERNATIVES

1. A continuous epidural infusion (catheter inserted through the caudal approach and threaded to the mid-portion of the surgical incision)
   - Need to cover approximately 16 dermatomes (5 sacral, 5 lumbar, 6 thoracic): Initial bolus 16 × 0.05 mL/kg/dermatome × 3 kg = 2.4 mL loading dose. The infusion could be chloroprocaine 1.5% with fentanyl 0.4 µg/mL *or* chloroprocaine 1.5% with clonidine 0.2 µg/mL
   - To be infused at a starting rate of 0.3 mL/kg/hr up to 1.2 mL/kg/hr
   - Apnea monitoring, continuous pulse oximetry, and frequent observation
   - *Note that the concentration of clonidine and fentanyl per mL of local anesthetic solution is reduced compared with that which would be used with older children because of the more rapid epidural infusion rate used to take maximal advantage of the local anesthetic.*
2. Nurse-controlled analgesia with morphine
   - Loading dose of 0.05 to 0.1 mg/kg × 6 kg = 0.3 to 0.6 mg administered via PCA pump in PACU
   - Continuous basal infusion of 0.01 to 0.02 mg/kg/hr
   - Bolus dose of 0.02 to 0.03 mg/kg
   - Lockout interval: 8 to 15 minutes
   - Four-hour limit of 0.25 to 0.3 mg/kg
   - Apnea monitoring, continuous pulse oximetry, and frequent observation
   - Add acetaminophen as needed 10 to 15 mg/kg every 4 hours (oral) or 35 to 40 mg/kg initial dose (rectal) followed by 20 mg/kg every 6 hours (rectal) not to exceed 100 mg/kg/day. IV acetaminophen 10 mg/kg every 6 hours may also be added.

# Case 4

An 8-year-old, 18-kg girl with cerebral palsy, severe cognitive impairment, ASA 3, presented for femoral osteotomy.

## CONSIDERATIONS

- Painful surgery
- Altered/individual pain behaviors: use specific tools for pain assessment such as r-FLACC
- Potential for altered pain perception
- Increased risk of opioid-induced respiratory depression
- May need benzodiazepines for muscle spasms

## ALTERNATIVES

1.  Continuous epidural analgesia
    - Need to cover approximately 10 dermatomes (5 sacral, 5 lumbar); initial bolus, 10 × 0.05 mL/kg/dermatome × 18 kg = 9 mL.
    - Bupivacaine 0.1% with fentanyl, 2 μg/mL, starting at 0.2 mL/kg/hr × 18 kg = 3.6 mL/hr
    - Apnea monitoring, pulse oximetry, and frequent observation
    - Add acetaminophen as needed, 10 to 15 mg/kg every 4 hours (oral) or 35 to 40 mg/kg initial dose (rectal) followed by 20 mg/kg every 6 hours (rectal) not to exceed 100 mg/kg/day (rectal). IV acetaminophen 10 mg/kg every 6 hours may also be added.
2.  Femoral nerve, fascia iliaca, or lumbar plexus block
    - There is the need to block the distribution of the femoral nerve and possibly (depending on the location of the incision) the lateral femoral cutaneous and obturator nerves.
    - Single-injection block of the peripheral nerves will provide analgesia for 8 to 16 hours; a continuous catheter technique will provide greater duration of analgesia.
    - Blockade of just the upper leg is provided without risks of urinary retention or motor block of the contralateral leg
    - 0.2% ropivacaine or 0.125% to 0.25% bupivacaine; initial dose of 0.3 mL/kg = 5.4 mL, followed by infusion of 0.2 mL/kg/hr = 3.6 mL/hr
    - Add acetaminophen and diazepam as needed.
3.  Continuous intravenous morphine infusion
    - Loading dose of up to 0.05 to 0.1 mg/kg × 18 kg = 0.9 to 1.8 mg in incremental doses if needed
    - Infusion starting at 0.02 mg/kg/hr (20 μg/kg/hr) × 18 kg = 0.36 mg/hr
    - Apnea monitoring, continuous pulse oximetry, and frequent observation
    - Add acetaminophen as needed.
    - Consider IV/PO diazepam, 0.05 mg/kg, for muscle spasms.
4.  Nurse-controlled analgesia with morphine
    - Loading dose 0.05 to 0.1 mg/kg × 18 kg = 0.9 to 1.8 mg administered via PCA pump in PACU
    - Continuous basal infusion of 0.01 to 0.02 mg/kg/hr
    - Bolus dose of 0.02 to 0.03 mg/kg
    - Lockout interval: 8 to 15 minutes
    - Four-hour limit of 0.25 to 0.3 mg/kg
    - Apnea monitoring, continuous pulse oximetry, and frequent observation
    - Add acetaminophen as needed.
    - Consider IV/PO diazepam, 0.05 mg/kg, for muscle spasms.

# Chronic Pain

ALEXANDRA SZABOVA AND KENNETH GOLDSCHNEIDER

THE PRACTICING PEDIATRIC ANESTHESIOLOGIST sees chronic pain in one of three main venues: a child coming to the operating room for a procedure, after a request for a consultation from a colleague of another specialty, or when making acute pain management rounds. In this chapter, we focus on the essential approaches to children with chronic pain and provide guidelines to help the children and colleagues who request your assistance.

## Chronic Pain in Children

Chronic pain affects a large number of children.[1] Back pain has been reported in up to 50% of children by the mid-teens,[2] and abdominal pain occurs weekly in up to 17%.[3] Other conditions such as headaches, complex regional pain syndrome (CRPS), fibromyalgia, limb pain, chest pain, and joint pain are common and affect quality of life.[4-7]

Several chronic medical conditions are strongly associated with pain and blur the boundaries between acute and chronic pain treatment, including sickle cell disease, cystic fibrosis,[8] epidermolysis bullosa,[9] and cancer. These children require frequent hospitalizations, and their pain can be severe. Because the children present with pain in the hospital, treatment often follows the model for acute pain management based on medication use. However, psychosocial factors heavily influence the child's ability to cope and can improve or worsen the child's suffering, depending on personal and family factors.[10,11] It is appropriate to seek psychology, child life, and physical therapy consultations as part of the therapeutic plan. The ultimate goal for each of these medical conditions is to stabilize the child's condition and return her or him home. For many, the painful disease and dysfunction continue, and having a long-term plan that is integrated with acute management is vital.

## Multidisciplinary Approach

The model of care that appears to work optimally for children with chronic pain is one in which multiple disciplines are involved in developing a coordinated care plan.[4,12] In the outpatient setting, there is a pain physician, a psychologist, nurses, and a physical therapist. Sometimes, a neurologist or physiatrist may be involved. Anesthesiologists managing children with chronic pain should make use of these disciplines when recommending a plan of care. Advocating for the involvement of other therapeutic specialties can advance the patient's care beyond suggesting a regional block or medication.

### THE PAIN PHYSICIAN

The consulting anesthesiologist in an inpatient setting may be called on to provide care for one of three reasons. First, the patient may need a regional nerve block, such as an epidural steroid injection for magnetic resonance imaging–confirmed discogenic pain or epidural catheter placement to assist physical therapy. This consultation is fairly straightforward and is an extension of basic regional anesthesia principles. Second, a child who has been prescribed opioids chronically or other medications that have implications for anesthesia or postoperative pain management may present for consultation. The anesthesiologist must investigate possible drug interactions and determine which chronic medications have been prescribed; this approach is an extension of basic perioperative anesthesia skills. Third, a consultation may be requested to assess and diagnose the source of pain. This scenario is the most complex and requires taking a detailed history and performing a thorough physical examination. These children often require multidisciplinary care beginning with the initial evaluation and extending through treatment.

## THE PSYCHOLOGIST

Pain is more than just a physical phenomenon. It can cause and be worsened by stress, suffering, family dysfunction, social tension, anxiety, and depression.[5,13] Pain can disrupt almost any aspect of the life of the child or family. Family and school problems can worsen a painful condition and dramatically reduce a child's level of function. The family is always involved in the child's suffering and should therefore be included in the pain evaluation process.

Families often are wary about seeing a psychologist and are afraid of being stigmatized. It is important to emphasize that pain is what the child says it is, regardless of whether an obvious organic cause is identified. The child is being treated as a person, not just as the painful body part, and this approach should be emphasized for the child's family.

Psychology-based therapy includes relaxation training, biofeedback, hypnotherapy, coping skills training, and psychotherapy. Biofeedback is a modality that trains the child to become more aware of his or her body, enhancing the sense of control over it. Therapies aimed at parental and familial aspects of the child's pain include teaching strategies for behavioral interventions (e.g., distraction), activity pacing, consistent discipline, coaching skills training, stress management, and occasionally, family therapy.

## THE PHYSICAL THERAPIST

Physical therapy is a crucial component of evaluating and treating chronic pain. The painful condition can cause loss of muscle strength and range of motion. Alterations in the use of a limb affect the biomechanics and daily function of the body. Children can become deconditioned and require a conditioning program to regain lost strength and stamina. These changes affect the original pain site and generate secondary pain problems that need to be addressed.

Physical therapy can benefit many painful conditions (e.g., myofascial pain improves with stretching and range-of-motion exercises) and is the cornerstone of treatment for others (e.g., chronic regional pain syndromes [CRPS]).[14] Emphasizing self-reliance and responsibility for their own care is an important aspect of caring for adolescents. However, young children and older ones in pain cannot be expected to work aggressively at home without beginning with a structured program. Parental involvement is especially important for younger children, but the caretakers must be taught to be encouraging and supportive while not making them the child's taskmasters.

Therapies provided by physical therapy include stretching, strengthening, and reconditioning programs. Range-of-motion exercises and endurance training are also important. Aquatic therapy is very useful for children who cannot bear weight on lower limbs or have limited range of motion or strength. Massage, heat, and cold therapies are helpful adjuncts to increase functioning and enhance other physical therapy modalities.

Transcutaneous electrical nerve stimulation (TENS) is an effective,[15] low-risk, analgesic therapy that is usually provided under the guidance of a physical therapist. TENS is excellent for localized pain. The fact that it is portable, can be used discreetly, and has few side effects makes it attractive for use at school. Because tolerance to TENS can develop with prolonged use, children need to limit use to no longer than 2 hours at a time. They can take a break for an amount of time equal to the TENS use and then restart it.

## THE NURSE

Pain nurses play a major role in hospital-wide education of floor nurses regarding assessment and treatment of pain, including the use of epidural and patient-controlled analgesia (PCA) pumps. When starting to see chronic pain patients, the first personnel recruitment should be an advanced practice nurse who can be trained to triage, perform the initial evaluation and intake assessment, and assist with all subsequent pain-related issues that do not require the direct input of a physician.

## THE CONSULTANT

Anesthesiologists should be cognizant of their limitations and judiciously use of consultants to help make or confirm diagnoses and fashion the best treatment plan. Neurologists typically are well versed in headache management and in the use of many of the medications used for neuropathic pain. Physical medicine and rehabilitation specialists can assist in structuring a treatment plan for a variety of musculoskeletal pains and are accomplished in the treatment of spasticity.

# General Approach to Management

Most children with chronic, noncancer pain are adolescents who require special considerations in terms of their history and physical examination. Because they are between childhood and adulthood, their behavior can fluctuate broadly and often. It is important to address them directly but also involve the parents to the extent needed to obtain the relevant and complete history. The clinician should not try to be "cool" with the adolescent patient, because teenagers tend to find that approach condescending and will respond negatively. The examiner should instead find a point of common interest and use it to establish greater rapport.

Adolescents tend to be very image conscious. They may or may not want to discuss body functions such as defecation or menstruation, even when these functions are directly relevant to the problem. If patients seem uneasy with the questions, the physician should proceed in a straightforward manner, acknowledge their feelings, and reassure them that the information is needed to help them. When discussing these pediatric patients with parents, clinicians should use a phrase such as "children and young adults" rather than just "children" because even 12 and 13-year-olds like to think they are no longer children.

## HISTORY

The basic history focuses on the pain: location, duration, quality, intensity, aggravating and alleviating factors, associated symptoms, therapies that have been tried, and which tests have been performed and by whom. Pain intensity is often assessed by a 0 to 10 numeric rating scale for children older than approximately 8 years of age. The child must be asked about the current pain level and about the best and worst pain levels to obtain an idea of the pattern of pain and when it peaks. Quality descriptors include *burning, sharp, aching, throbbing, tingling, numb, weird,* and others; each may give a clue about the type of pain the child is experiencing. Odd descriptors, burning, and tingling suggest neuropathic pain; sharp, tight, and aching may indicate bony or muscular causes; throbbing suggests a vascular component; cramping or pain that comes in waves often suggests spasms of a muscle or hollow viscus.

A vital part of the chronic pain evaluation process is to look for *red flags*, which are signs or symptoms that may indicate a serious illness. Some of the red flag signs and symptoms for major pain types can be found in Tables 44-1, 44-2, and 44-3. For example, a child with back pain who also has weak legs and incontinence may have a tethered spinal cord. Headache that is worse in the morning and associated with vomiting suggests increased intracranial pressure. Back pain with loss of ankle jerk suggests compression of the S1 nerve root.

A complete pain evaluation comprises further history regarding medications, allergies, family history, and a thorough review of systems. Certain painful conditions, such as migraine headaches,[16] fibromyalgia,[17] irritable bowel syndrome,[18] and sickle cell disease, have a genetic basis. Knowing the family history can assist in making the diagnosis. The child sometimes may model his or her behavior after a family member. For example, if a parent has a "bad back" and is functionally compromised, the child also may complain of back pain. This does not mean the child is faking the complaints but simply patterning the behavioral response to pain after a model that he or she understands. Treatment can include reassurance, cognitive behavioral therapy, and gentle physical therapy to restore the child's functional ability and help him or her with any underlying issues. Family and social histories can be useful in fashioning a treatment plan in conjunction with the general history, physical examination, and relevant testing.

## PHYSICAL EXAMINATION

The physical examination should focus on the area of interest, but a brief general examination is also important. A full screening examination, including a neurologic examination, takes only a few minutes and can be combined with the social history. A systemic illness may manifest as a localized complaint; for example, diabetes can manifest as abdominal pain or leukemia as focal bone pain

When examining a child of the opposite sex, the physician should have a nonfamily observer of the same gender as the child present. Some children are very conscious of their bodies and may consider routine examination maneuvers as invasions of their privacy. The occasional child has a history of being abused and can be further traumatized by even a standard examination. Physicians can demonstrate examination techniques that may make the child uneasy. For example, a pinprick examination requires a needle or sharp object; the examiner should touch his or her own skin with a pin first to demonstrate that blood is not being drawn. Children are often fascinated by the deep tendon reflexes and usually have fun with that examination. Children with chronic pain often have had many examinations, and doing something a little different or fun can help them accept the current evaluation and enhance rapport.

## ANCILLARY DATA

By the time chronic pain patients have reached a pain clinic, they usually have undergone several investigative tests, and those data should be reviewed. After it becomes clear that there is no life-threatening illness, the focus should shift away from further testing. This is often a hard transition for families and children to accept, especially if no concrete diagnosis has been made to explain the pain. It is a challenge for them to embrace the thought that the pain itself is the disease rather than something that is still undiagnosed. Any study that may help to explain the pain or make a diagnosis that had not been entertained should be recommended. However, pursuing tests and imaging in an unfocused manner wastes resources and causes families to postpone treatment while waiting for a diagnosis. Until the patient wholeheartedly endorses the treatment plan and becomes active in it, the child or adolescent's pain will continue unabated.

# Chronic Pain Conditions

Any part of the body can hurt, but in practical terms, several diagnostic clusters represent most pediatric pain conditions. The frequency and intensity of the pain can be striking. One study on the 3-month prevalence, characteristics, consequences, and provoking factors of chronic pain described the experience of 749 children and adolescents in one elementary and two secondary schools[19]: 83% experienced pain during the preceding 3 months. The leading sources of pain were headaches (60.5%,

| TABLE 44-1 Red Flag Signs and Symptoms for Abdominal Pain |
|---|
| Persistent right upper or right lower quadrant pain |
| Dysphagia |
| Persistent or cyclic vomiting |
| Gastrointestinal blood loss |
| Family history of inflammatory bowel disease, celiac disease, or peptic ulcer disease |
| Pain that wakes the child from sleep |
| Arthritis |
| Nocturnal diarrhea |
| Involuntary weight loss |
| Deceleration of linear growth |
| Delayed puberty |
| Unexplained fever |
| Hepatosplenomegaly, masses, or perianal lesions |
| Bilious emesis |
| Costovertebral angle tenderness |

| TABLE 44-2 Red Flag Signs and Symptoms for Secondary Headache |
|---|
| Persistent vomiting |
| Focal neurologic signs |
| Meningeal signs |
| Unexplained fever |
| Increased intracranial pressure |
| Changes in behavior or mental status |
| Sudden onset of severe headache |
| Morning headaches |
| Headaches awakening the child from sleep |

| TABLE 44-3 Red Flag Signs and Symptoms for Back Pain |
|---|
| Unexplained fever |
| Night sweats |
| Weight loss |
| Night pain |
| Constant pain |
| Bowel function changes |
| Urinary retention |
| Neurologic changes in legs: trouble walking, footdrop, weakness, loss of reflexes, sensory changes |

also perceived as most bothersome), abdominal pain (43.3%), extremity pain (33.6%), and back pain (30.2%). Many subjects reported associated sleep problems, restriction in hobbies, and eating problems. School absenteeism reached 48.8% in the population with pain. The use of health care resources by children and adolescents with pain was extensive: 50.9% visited the physician's office, and 51.5% reported use of pain medication.

## ABDOMINAL PAIN

Abdominal pain is a major source of distress in children that causes anxiety and invites a large amount of testing. This painful condition, formerly referred to as *recurrent abdominal pain*, is now described as *functional gastrointestinal disorders* (FGIDs).[20] Specific criteria exist for the major categories so that FGIDs are no longer considered diagnoses of exclusion. The pain is thought to be caused by abnormal interactions between the enteric nervous system and central nervous system.[21] Research suggests that peripheral sensitization and abnormal central processing of afferent signals at the level of the central nervous system play roles in the pathophysiology of visceral hyperalgesia—a decreased threshold for pain in response to changes in intraluminal pressure.[22] The history and physical examination focus on excluding warning signs and symptoms of underlying disease (see Table 44-1).[20,23] The role for testing, endoscopy, and radiographic evaluation is limited.

Multidisciplinary treatment of FGIDs includes medication, psychological interventions, and education, which often need to be ongoing. The most important aspect of the treatment plan is to establish realistic goals, which frequently means return of function rather than complete elimination of pain. Although the literature for treatment is sparse, tricyclic antidepressants such as amitriptyline, nortriptyline, or doxepin have been used effectively for FGID-related pain. Anticonvulsants also are useful because they modify nerve conductivity and transmission. Antacids, antispasmodic agents, smooth muscle relaxants, laxatives, and antidiarrheal agents can be added to address symptoms. Data support the use of peppermint oil capsules in managing irritable bowel syndrome, although gastroesophageal reflux can be a limiting adverse effect.[24] Children with functional bowel disorders can have abnormal bowel reactions to physiologic stimuli, noxious stressful stimuli, or psychological stimuli (e.g., parental separation, anxiety). Children benefit from cognitive-behavioral therapy, coping skill development, biofeedback, hypnosis, and relaxation techniques (Table 44-4).[25,26]

## HEADACHE

Headaches can be categorized as primary or secondary. Primary headaches include migraine, tension, cluster, and trigeminal neuralgia headaches. Secondary headaches are those attributable to head and neck traumas; muscle spasms; vascular disorders; nonvascular intracranial disorders; infection; eye, ear, cranium, nose, sinus, and teeth or mouth diseases; homeostatic disturbances; and psychiatric disorders. Headaches represent one of the more poorly tolerated types of chronic pain, with greater medication use than for other types. Of 77 children with long-term headaches who were followed up to 20 years after the initial diagnosis, 27% were headache free, and 66% had improved.[27]

Migraines (especially migraine without aura) and tension-type headaches are the most common types of pediatric headaches. The prevalence of migraine ranges from 2.7% to 10%. It occurs more frequently in boys than girls between 4 and 7 years of age, and then the prevalence equalizes between 7 and 11 years of age.

**TABLE 44-4** Care Pathway for Abdominal Pain

**Evaluation**

Medical examination

Behavioral medicine assessment

Review of records, treatments, history, and physical findings

Consultations with pediatrics, surgery, and gastroenterology specialists as indicated by presence of red flags; assessment may include laboratory testing, ultrasound, computed tomography or magnetic resonance imaging, endoscopy, lactose testing

**Treatment of Functional Gastrointestinal Disorders**

*Medications:* tricyclic antidepressants; consider selective serotonin reuptake inhibitors or serotonin-norepinephrine reuptake inhibitors; peppermint oil

*Behavioral medicine:* important and effective to de-medicalize therapy; de-emphasize testing and search for organic diagnoses; redirect focus to treatment and improved function

*Physical therapy:* not usually involved; trial of transcutaneous electrical nerve stimulation (TENS) if abdominal wall origin found

*Other therapy:*
Blocks are rare, except in palliative situation; celiac plexus with local anesthetic and steroid; epidural
Trigger point injections if abdominal wall trigger points found
Acupuncture
Hypnosis
Meditation
Dietary management

After 11 years of age, three times more girls than boys have migraines.[28,29] Studies are not routinely recommended in the absence of focal neurologic findings. However, the practitioner must be alert to red flag signs and symptoms that warrant imaging and laboratory studies to rule out an underlying condition as a cause of the headaches (see Table 44-2).

There is a genetic component to migraine and chronic tension headaches; 50% to 77% of children with migraines have a positive family history for migraine headaches, especially on the maternal side. The clearest genetic link has been established for familial hemiplegic migraine.[16]

Children with frequent headaches often suffer from medication overuse headaches due to chronic or repeated use of over-the-counter analgesics. If possible, children should be weaned off analgesics gradually.

Treatments for migraine and tension-type headaches overlap greatly. Pharmacologic interventions can be divided in two types. In the first, abortive treatment focuses on stopping the acute headache. In the second, prophylactic therapy is indicated for patients with more than two headaches per month, for children with severe attacks, and for those with frequent headaches unresponsive to medication (Table 44-5).[30]

Older medications that have been used successfully to prevent headaches in adolescents include amitriptyline and trazodone. These medications tend to make children drowsy and are prescribed 30 to 60 minutes before bedtime each night. Younger children appear to respond well to the antihistamine cyproheptadine. Overall, few evidence-based recommendations can be made; the lack of randomized, controlled pediatric trials precludes an evidence-based recommendation.[31] However, the anticonvulsant topiramate is a promising medication for the prevention of migraine headaches.[32-34]

**TABLE 44-5** Care Pathway for Headaches

**Evaluation**

Medical examination

Behavioral medicine assessment

Physical therapy if neck or upper back tightness occurs

Review of records, treatments, history, and physical findings

Magnetic resonance imaging and neurology consultations as indicated by red flag signs and symptoms

**Treatment**

*Medications:* tricyclic antidepressants, topiramate, trazodone, cyproheptadine

*Behavioral medicine:* biofeedback, relaxation, coping and pacing skills

*Physical therapy:* transcutaneous electrical nerve stimulation (TENS) unit on shoulders, posterior neck; stretching

*Other therapy:*
  Yoga
  Acupuncture
  Meditation
  Occasional neck trigger point injection or occipital nerve block

**TABLE 44-6** Care Pathway for Complex Regional Pain Syndromes

**Evaluation**

Medical examination

Behavioral medicine assessment

Physical therapy assessment

Review of records, treatments, history, physical findings, and radiographic studies

**Treatment**

*Medications:* tricyclic antidepressants, gabapentin, oxcarbazepine

*Behavioral medicine:* very important, especially in refractory cases

*Physical therapy:* activate, range of motion, desensitization, strength training. Structured home program extremely important; may use transcutaneous electrical nerve stimulation (TENS) unit

*Other therapy:*
  Consider intravenous regional block for hand or foot
  Consider lumbar sympathetic block catheter and admission for structured program for lower extremity complex regional pain syndrome (CRPS) that is refractory despite best efforts of patient and family
  Consider high thoracic epidural or continuous brachial plexus catheter for upper extremity CRPS

## COMPLEX REGIONAL PAIN SYNDROME

Type I and type II CRPS are different only in the presence of a documented nerve injury in type II (formerly called *causalgia*). Pain is an obligatory feature, often occurring alongside allodynia or hyperalgesia. There must be evidence at some time (not necessarily at the time of diagnosis) of edema, changes in skin blood flow, or abnormal sudomotor activity in the region of pain. There are often features of a motor disorder such as tremor, dystonia, and weakness that sometimes lead to a loss of joint mobility. Nail and hair growth can also be affected. In the past, three distinct stages were described. However, it may be that there are phenotypic subtypes instead of stages.[35]

From a clinical standpoint, the typical pediatric CRPS patient is older than 10 years of age, Caucasian, female, and very active or a high achiever from an active family, and the child or adolescent presents with lower extremity pain.[36] A genetic predisposition is suggested by the clinical observation that CRPS is rare in the African American population. The rarity of CRPS in preadolescent children suggests a developmental aspect to its origin.

It is important to obtain a detailed history of the mechanism of trauma and the signs and symptoms. The examiner should specifically look for pain, allodynia, hyperalgesia, and hyperpathia. Edema and color changes do not have to be present at the time of diagnosis, but there should be a history of such changes in the recent past (Fig. 44-1). A complete neurologic examination includes testing muscle strength, reflexes, sensory responses (e.g., cold, touch, pinprick), capillary refill, temperature, and color differences. The physician should also look for deep tissue hyperalgesia. Occasionally, noninvasive or invasive testing may be helpful, but it is not sensitive or specific. These evaluations may include an electromyogram with nerve conduction velocity (EMG/NCV), quantitative sensory testing (QST), and quantitative sudomotor axon reflex testing (QSART) to detect small fiber dysfunction; thermography; and bone scans. Sympathetic ganglion blocks are not considered necessary for diagnosis, but they can be part of the therapeutic approach.

The therapeutic goal for CRPS is restoration of function. It may seem simple, but in daily practice, this may represent the

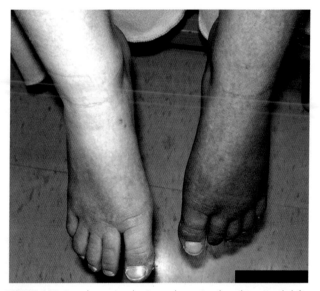

**FIGURE 44-1** Complex regional pain syndrome involves the patient's left foot and ankle. Notice the cyanosis and mottling. The affected foot was cool, and allodynia was prominent. Left foot toenails had not been trimmed in 3 months.

biggest challenge for the physician and the child. The therapeutic approach to the child with CRPS is multidisciplinary, with a focus on the psychosocial and physical aspects of the disease (Table 44-6). Education is important, and the information available on the Internet is ubiquitous, although it is often discouraging and not applicable to children with CRPS. No isolated treatment technique has been helpful for this condition. Children and physicians should follow an algorithm and adjust the therapeutic strategy every 4 weeks if the child does not respond satisfactorily to chosen measures.

The mainstay of CRPS treatment is physical therapy. However, the pain can be severe and disabling enough to prevent active participation by the child in the physical therapy program. Pharmacologic therapy is often initiated to facilitate physical therapy. Medications for neuropathic pain (described later) take time to titrate to effect. It is reasonable to use nonsteroidal antiinflammatory drugs (NSAIDs) and opioids for a short time until the primary medications take effect. The psychology team must play an active role in the overall treatment program. Psychosocial issues must be aggressively addressed. With physical therapy, psychology, and medications, most children achieve good results and disease resolution. In unusual refractory cases, for which interdisciplinary outpatient programs are insufficient, inpatient pain rehabilitation programs are recommended.

The role of interventional therapy in the treatment of CRPS is to alleviate the pain and provide the child with the opportunity to tolerate and advance in physical therapy. Sympathetic nerve blocks are widely used in adults although a systematic review revealed a lack of randomized, controlled trials to confirm the effectiveness of this approach in short-term and long-term pain relief.[37] Interventional therapies can be a double-edged sword, representing an easy solution that can demotivate the child from taking an active role in his or her physical therapy. However, pain may be too severe to allow physical therapy and thereby accelerate loss of function.

Several techniques enjoy popularity among pediatric pain specialists. For isolated limb CRPS, intravenous regional blockade with local anesthetic and adjuncts such as clonidine, ketamine, or ketorolac is performed. General anesthesia or deep sedation is frequently required because placement of intravenous catheters in the affected limb and inflation of the tourniquet are poorly tolerated. More invasive alternatives include placement of a lumbar sympathetic plexus catheter (Fig. 44-2) and a tunneled epidural catheter in the upper thoracic or lumbar area. The duration of infusion ranges from 3 to 5 days to as long as 4 to 6 weeks, and the procedure requires extensive logistical support. An alternative approach is to place a peripheral nerve catheter for a continuous block.[38] Spinal cord stimulation and intrathecal drug delivery are rarely used for pediatric CRPS due to the overall good prognosis with more conservative treatment and the continued growth of the skeleton, which can change the area of paresthesias in the case of spinal cord stimulators.

## MUSCULOSKELETAL AND RHEUMATOLOGIC PAIN

Musculoskeletal pain is a recognized problem in children and adolescents, and back pain commonly affects adolescents.[39,40-42] Although many factors are blamed for musculoskeletal pain (e.g., heavy backpacks, participation in sports, sedentary lifestyle, scoliosis, increased body mass index), only a few have been proved to contribute to musculoskeletal pain. According to one study, in more than half of cases the cause could not be identified, and only a minority of children had an underlying disease process (e.g., spondylolysis, infection, tumor, disk problem). Radiologic findings correlated poorly with the pain and failed to distinguish between individuals with pain and those without pain.[42] Selected red flags for back pain are provided in Table 44-3. A care pathway for the evaluation and treatment of back pain in children and adolescents is presented in Table 44-7.

A special group of children with musculoskeletal pain are those with rheumatologic diseases. Most children referred to the rheumatologist's office complain of musculoskeletal pain. Only some of them are diagnosed with a true rheumatologic disease; juvenile idiopathic arthritis is the most common form. Besides pain, the diseases often manifest as morning stiffness, fatigue, and sleep problems. The process may progress and cause joint deformities and destruction due to osteoporosis, with resulting growth abnormalities and functional disability. Management combines pharmacologic and nonpharmacologic interventions. The mainstay of therapy is the use of NSAIDs, acetaminophen, and rarely, opioids for severe breakthrough pain. The rheumatologist may prescribe agents such as methotrexate, cyclophosphamide, or systemic corticosteroids for severe flare-ups. Splints, physical therapy, and psychological interventions such as cognitive-behavioral therapy are often used.[43] Children with Ehlers-Danlos syndrome or other connective tissue disorders suffer from unstable joints that become very painful from repeated dislocations and mechanical stress.

Some young women present with fatigue, poor sleep, and pain or unusual tenderness in multiple sites. Fibromyalgia is more common in adolescents than expected, and it can be a significant problem. Therapy includes education, medications, and general restorative therapy, with a focus on aerobic reconditioning. Traditionally, tricyclic antidepressants and cyclobenzaprine have

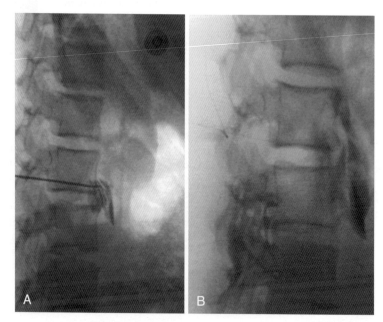

**FIGURE 44-2** Lumbar sympathetic block. **A,** In the lateral view, the Tuohy needle is in the proper position. Notice the prepsoas spread of contrast agent. **B,** The dye spreads and clears due to injection of local anesthetic through the catheter. The catheter is tunneled and can be left in place for a week.

## TABLE 44-7 Care Pathway for Back Pain

### Evaluation

Medical examination

Behavioral medicine assessment

Physical therapy assessment

Review of records, treatments, history, and physical findings

Consultation with specialists in orthopedics; magnetic resonance imaging or computed tomography, as indicated by history and examination findings

### Treatment

*Medications:*

Tricyclic antidepressants

Muscle relaxants (e.g., baclofen, cyclobenzaprine)

Anticonvulsant (if radicular component)

Nonsteroidal antiinflammatory drug of choice

Cyclooxygenase-2 inhibitor for gastrointestinal or bleeding issues

If disk disease with radicular pain is documented, up to three epidural steroid injections may be helpful

*Behavioral medicine:* biofeedback, coping skills, and relaxation techniques

*Physical therapy:*

Stretching, postural rehabilitation, general reconditioning, and lifting techniques

Limit bed rest; reactivate

Transcutaneous electrical nerve stimulation (TENS)

Exercise program

*Other therapy:*

Acupuncture

Yoga

Chiropractic (older patients, lumbar only)

Massage

Trigger-point injections

Additional modalities for specific indications include back bracing, surgery, bisphosphonate therapy

## TABLE 44-8 Care Pathway for Nonverbal Patients

### Evaluation

Medical examination

Often tricky; go slowly

May need more than one visit to complete the examination

Try to isolate body part during examination, to avoid generalized effect

Watch facial or vocal and parent reaction to each examination maneuver

Behavioral medicine assessment: often not possible

Physical therapy assessment: often already engaged in therapy

Review of records, treatments, history, and physical findings

Video documentation: parent may be able to capture pain behaviors for examiner to view

### Treatment

*Medications:* often on multiple agents at baseline and coordination with other practitioners is important; apply general principles in choosing medications; long-acting opioid is sometimes beneficial for refractory musculoskeletal pain; watch for worsening of constipation.

*Behavioral medicine:* often not possible if patient's cognitive ability is too low, but the family sometimes can benefit because they carry a large burden when caring for children with multiple medical problems

*Physical therapy:* often already engaged; if not, engage for musculoskeletal pain or help therapist focus efforts of a particular region of the body

*Other therapy:*

Nerve blocks can be used to identify painful areas, if more than one seems active

Rarely, a patient must be brought to the operating suite for an infusion of remifentanil to differentiate opioid responsiveness from potentially centralized or behavioral pain phenomena; the latter may respond to anticonvulsant therapy

Intrathecal baclofen (and occasionally morphine)

Surgical therapy for selected conditions

### Cautions

Site of pain is often unclear.

Do not forget to look in the ears.

If patient is spastic, strongly consider hip pathology (e.g., subluxation, bursitis, infection).

Constipation, gallbladder pain, and gastroesophageal reflux are possible.

These patients often require more testing than verbal patients.

Be careful with use of nonsteroidal antiinflammatory drugs because gastroesophageal reflux can be a problem and reporting abdominal pain as a signal of gastrointestinal side effects may not be possible.

been used, and duloxetine and milnacipran are helpful in adults.[44,45] As with many chronic pain conditions, cognitive-behavioral approaches are valuable components of treatment.[46]

Musculoskeletal pain is a particularly difficult problem in children with cerebral palsy.[47] Spasticity itself can be painful, and the daily stretching exercises are reported to be painful by many children. Some children with cerebral palsy are nonverbal, making assessment even more difficult. The parents or guardians can provide information about how the child expresses pain and how the pain manifests during daily life. If diaper changes seem to hurt, the practitioner should suspect hip or perineal pain. Pain after eating or a history of hard stools may point to constipation-based abdominal pain. A careful and sometimes staged examination is required. A thoughtful, empirical approach to therapy and judicious use of radiologic and laboratory evaluations can often lead to the diagnosis (Table 44-8).

## PAIN IN SICKLE CELL DISEASE, TRAIT, AND VARIANTS

Sickle cell disease is a hereditary disorder characterized by abnormal hemoglobin S (see Chapter 9). About 8% of African Americans carry the sickle gene. The homozygous form (sickle cell disease [HbSS]) manifests as a hemolytic anemia with unique vaso-occlusive features. The heterozygous form (sickle cell trait [HbAS]) is milder and manifests as a borderline anemia and rarely with vaso-occlusive features. Sickle cell/hemoglobin C disease (HbSC) has a clinical presentation similar to that of HbSS, but its vaso-occlusive episodes are fewer and usually less intense.

From a pain management perspective, the homozygous HbSS genotype manifests as acute pain attacks (e.g., pain crisis, vaso-occlusive episodes, acute chest syndrome) or as underlying chronic pain with acute exacerbations (e.g., avascular necrosis, vertebral collapse, joint involvement). Treatment frequently requires a multidisciplinary approach with close cooperation between the hematologist, psychologist, and pain physician.[48] Most of the episodes can be managed at home with NSAIDs or acetaminophen, supplemented with opioids such as codeine or oxycodone or with tramadol. In severe cases, children often are hospitalized and treated with intravenous opioids, although they should be gradually weaned off the opioids as the primary process improves. For episodes of localized, hard-to-control pain or if acute chest syndrome develops, epidural analgesia can provide

**TABLE 44-9** Care Pathway for Sickle Cell Disease

**Evaluation**

Medical examination

Behavioral medicine assessment: may be limited to social support in acute setting

Review of records, treatments (need opioid exposure history for dosing), and history

Hematology almost always directly involved, with focused evaluation

**Treatment of Vaso-occlusive Episodes**

*Medications:* opioid (often requires basal infusion for the first days); nonsteroidal antiinflammatory drug; consider neuropathic medication for hyperalgesia

*Behavioral medicine:* can be helpful, although learning techniques in the acute setting may be difficult; introducing this modality early in life may be more helpful

*Physical therapy:* transcutaneous electrical nerve stimulation (TENS) for localized pain

*Other therapy:*
Regional anesthesia may be helpful.
Strongly consider thoracic epidural for acute chest crisis.

**Treatment of Chronic Problems**

*Medications:* may involve chronic opioids; otherwise follows treatment of particular pain condition

*Behavioral medicine:* per particular pain condition; early involvement may reduce need for hospitalizations

*Physical therapy:* per particular pain condition; may have joint, bone, and deconditioning issues from recurrent vaso-occlusive episodes

excellent relief.[49] Rarely, children require opioid maintenance with long-acting preparations of morphine or oxycodone (Table 44-9). Hyperalgesia over the affected area suggests peripheral or central sensitization, although the role for neuropathic medications is undefined.

# Pain Pharmacotherapy

Pain treatment has received less study in children than adults, as it is true for much pediatric pharmacologic therapy. In the absence of U.S. Food and Drug Administration (FDA)–approved indications and experimental data, off-label use of many medications used to treat chronic pain is common. In this situation, the decision to use a particular medication is most often based on extrapolation from adult literature, expert consensus, applied theory, and clinical judgment (see Chapter 6). Three categories of medications are available for consideration: nonopioid analgesics (i.e., NSAIDs and acetaminophen), opioid analgesics, and a broad spectrum of adjuvant analgesics, including anticonvulsants, antidepressants, muscle relaxants, local anesthetics, *N*-methyl-D-aspartate (NMDA) receptor antagonists, $\alpha_2$-agonists, and corticosteroids.

## NONSTEROIDAL ANTIINFLAMMATORY DRUGS AND CYCLOOXYGENASE-2 INHIBITORS

NSAIDs come from various chemical groups (e.g., salicylates, propionic acid, oxicams, naphthylalkalones, fenamates). The mechanism of action is inhibition of cyclooxygenases (COXs) at the prostaglandin $H_2$ synthetase enzyme. COX-1 is constitutive and always present, and COX-2 is inducible and produced in the body under proper conditions. NSAIDs have different selectivities for COX-1 or COX-2; selective COX-2 inhibitors have predominant action on inducible COX-2. The benefit of selective blockade is decreased risk of gastrointestinal bleeding. Celecoxib is the only selective COX-2 inhibitor available in the United States.

The analgesic and antiinflammatory actions of NSAIDs exhibit a dose-dependent response until they reach maximum effect; beyond which there is no further benefit of dose increase (i.e., ceiling effect). Unlike opioids, there is no development of physical dependence or tolerance with NSAIDs.

The choice of NSAID is empirical and based on clinical judgment. If the child provides a history of good response to a particular NSAID, we tend to continue the same medication or adjust the dose. If the response is inadequate, we select a different medication until we find an effective one. In children with a history of gastrointestinal adverse effects, we prescribe combination preparations with protective agents (e.g., misoprostol) or a histamine$_2$ ($H_2$) receptor or proton pump inhibitor, or we switch to a selective COX-2 inhibitor. Preexisting renal disease and disorders that reduce actual or effective intravascular volume vastly increase the risk for renal toxicity, and NSAIDs must be used cautiously in these situations.

## OPIOIDS

The use of opioids for treating chronic nonmalignant pain has been associated with many myths and controversies. Their use in the past was reserved for children with acute and cancer-related pain. In selected cases, with appropriate monitoring, opioids can improve quality of life and functional capacity without significant risk of addiction, tolerance, and toxicity. However, a history of substance abuse (mainly in adolescent and young adult populations) and a family member with substance abuse and a dysfunctional social situation are red flags for opioid prescribing.

Opioid agonists are used almost exclusively; agonist-antagonists have less popularity because of their ceiling effect and the potential to precipitate withdrawal when administered alongside a pure agonist. We typically use opioids in two scenarios. The first features opioids as a bridge while titrating other classes of medications to effect or while awaiting physical therapy or an intervention to exert its effect. In the second scenario, we use opioids as maintenance analgesics in carefully selected children (e.g., chronic musculoskeletal pain in a child with cerebral palsy, children with juvenile rheumatoid arthritis or Ehlers-Danlos syndrome). Medication is titrated in increments toward the main goals of optimal (although rarely complete) pain relief, improved function, and minimal adverse effects. Escalations are seen usually with exacerbations of the primary disease process. Common opioid adverse effects that occur with long-term use can be found in Table 44-10.

A special medication in this group is methadone. Besides being an opioid agonist, methadone is also reasonably effective in controlling neuropathic components of pain. There are a few exceedingly important caveats for its use. It has a long half-life and presents a risk of accumulation leading to sedation and respiratory depression. The usual 1:1 methadone to morphine equianalgesia ratio does not work for dose conversion. The greater the dose of opioid being converted, the more skewed the conversion ratio; the methadone to morphine ratio ranged from 1:2.5 to 1:14.3 in one study.[50] Because of the long half-life, dose adjustments should be made no more frequently than every 5 days. A unique adverse effect of methadone among opioids is its potential to prolong the QT interval and modestly increase

**TABLE 44-10** Opioid Side Effects Associated with Chronic Use

**With Development of Tolerance**

Cognitive impairment
Itching
Miosis
Nausea
Prolonged reaction time
Respiratory depression
Sedation
Urinary retention

**Without Development of Tolerance**

Constipation

**Side Effects with Long-Term Use**

Hypogonadism
Immunosuppression

the dispersion of repolarization on the electrocardiogram.[51] Because the dispersion of repolarization is less than 100 msec, it remains unlikely that methadone can trigger torsades de pointes.

When a child who is taking long-term opioids presents in the operating room, a thorough medication history is essential for developing a perioperative plan. If the child has not taken a morning dose of opioid, that dose should be replaced by the intravenous route to avoid withdrawal. It is essential to convert the home medication into morphine equivalents, and the daily dose of home opioids should be provided as a baseline, with all further dosing being in addition to the baseline, to avoid pain at the time of emergence. Because of tolerance to long-term opioids, larger doses than usual may be required, and it is advisable (as in all children) to titrate to comfort in the immediate postoperative period and use the amount required to achieve optimal analgesia. Opioid consumption during the perioperative period may be more than three times that observed in patients not taking chronic opioids. Sparing use of opioids in the perioperative period results in poor pain management and withdrawal phenomena.[52,53]

## ADJUVANT DRUGS

### Anticonvulsants

Anticonvulsant medications have been widely used in the pharmacologic treatment of chronic pain since the 1960s. Often referred to as membrane stabilizers, anticonvulsants work on neural receptors, ion channels, and nerve conductivity. They modify the level of excitatory and inhibitory neurotransmitters and activation of nerve cells. They are most effective in controlling neuropathic pain. First-generation agents (e.g., carbamazepine) have been used less often due to significant adverse effects, and they have been replaced by second-generation agents that have a better adverse effect profile.

Therapeutic effect is achieved with all membrane stabilizers by gradual titration. The purposes of this approach are to avoid development of adverse effects by allowing enough time for the child to develop tolerance (mainly to sedation) and to find the lowest effective dose for the child. The treatment course usually lasts 3 to 6 months. At the end, the child is gradually weaned off the medication in reverse order of its titration. Although weaning is not necessary to prevent seizures, rapid discontinuation may result in pain and in sleep or mood disturbances. Gradual weaning allows rapid re-escalation in case the pain begins to return in children for whom the pain has been controlled but

not completely eliminated. In that case, we would determine the child's minimal effective dose. If pain recurs, we continue medication for 3 to 6 months longer.

Although use of anticonvulsants for pain in children represents an off-label use and studies are lacking (even for adults), this class of medications is a mainstay of therapy for selected pain conditions in children. The choice of drug is based on thoughtful consideration and expert consensus, as with all therapies for which randomized, controlled trials are lacking.

### Gabapentin and Pregabalin

Gabapentin is an anticonvulsant with a complex mechanism of action. Its name is deceiving; gabapentin does not interact with the γ-aminobutyric (GABA)-ergic system. It binds to the $\alpha_2$-delta subunit of the voltage-dependent calcium channel[54] and reduces the release of glutamate in the dorsal horn of the spinal cord. This leads to decreased production of substance P, less activation of α-amino-3-hydroxy-5-methylisoxazole-4-propionate (AMPA) receptors on noradrenergic synapses, decreased transmitter release, and decreased neuronal activity.[55] This mechanism is shared by gabapentin and pregabalin.

Gabapentin is usually a drug of first choice due to good tolerability, minimal adverse effects, and positive clinical experiences. Besides sedation, patients can retain sodium and water, develop peripheral edema, and gain weight. In teenagers, gabapentin can cause mood swings, irritability, and suicidality. Despite these concerns, we use gabapentin frequently after a detailed explanation and discussion with the patient and parents. We use two titration schedules. For younger children, the target dose is 10 to 15 mg/kg/dose three times per day. In older children weighing more than 60 kg, we use adult-type titration to effect. Gabapentin does not have to be adjusted in liver failure patients because it is not metabolized by the liver; however, the dosage needs to be adjusted in children with compromised renal function. Pregabalin is chemically related to gabapentin but has fewer adverse effects and a significantly faster titration schedule. It is approved for postherpetic neuralgia, diabetic neuropathy, and fibromyalgia in adults; experience in children is growing.

### Topiramate

Best studied for the treatment of migraine headaches, topiramate can be applied to the full spectrum of neuropathic pain states.[33] Because a unique adverse effect is appetite suppression, we may choose it for a patient with neuropathic pain who is concerned about weight gain. Topiramate has carbonic anhydrase–inhibiting properties and can result in metabolic acidosis and lead to renal stones in some cases.

### Oxcarbazepine

Oxcarbazepine is the second-generation relative of carbamazepine and has potential for the treatment of neuropathic pain states. Although rare, Stevens-Johnson syndrome can occur with oxcarbazepine and with several other anticonvulsants. Hyponatremia also may occur in addition to adverse effects common to anticonvulsants, such as sedation, difficulty concentrating, ataxia, and mood instability.

### Carbamazepine, Valproic Acid, and Phenytoin

The effectiveness of carbamazepine, valproic acid, and phenytoin has been discussed elsewhere.[56] Carbamazepine has proved effective in the treatment of trigeminal neuralgia, spasticity in multiple sclerosis, and spinal cord injury (compared with tizanidine).

Phenytoin has been used alone or in combination with buprenorphine for cancer pain, and it has provided good pain relief in more than 60% of patients.

Despite their effectiveness, the use of these medications is limited because of the possibility of serious adverse effects. For carbamazepine and phenytoin, adverse effects include liver and renal toxicity (regular laboratory tests are necessary), aplastic anemia, Steven-Johnson syndrome, and a syndrome of inappropriate secretion of antidiuretic hormone (SIADH)-like picture. Valproate lacks renal side effects but can cause pancreatitis.

### Antidepressants

Two major groups of antidepressants are used in the treatment of chronic pain: tricyclic antidepressants (TCAs) (e.g., amitriptyline, nortriptyline, desipramine, doxepin, imipramine) and the newer selective serotonin reuptake inhibitors (SSRIs) (e.g., fluoxetine, paroxetine) and serotonin-norepinephrine reuptake inhibitors (SNRIs) (e.g., venlafaxine, duloxetine, milnacipran).[57] The efficacy of TCAs in the treatment of neuropathic pain has been confirmed in meta-analyses.[58,59] The doses required to control chronic pain are usually less than those used in the treatment of depression. The effectiveness of antidepressants has been demonstrated in neuropathic and nonneuropathic pain such as fibromyalgia and low back pain.

When prescribing antidepressants, we recommend vigilance about the potential increase in suicidal ideation and attempts in adolescents and young adults. We inform patients and families in detail to ensure that they will communicate with us about such ideation. We refer patients at greater risk for psychiatric comorbidity to a psychologist for evaluation before prescribing this class of medications.

#### Tricyclic Antidepressants

The major limiting factor in prescribing TCAs is their adverse effects. Onset of adverse effects can be reduced by slow dose escalation, as is done with anticonvulsants. The most frequent side effect is sedation, which is often beneficial in chronic pain patients who have difficulties sleeping. We prescribe the drug to be taken at bedtime. It is important to monitor the child in the mornings for carryover sedation. In such cases, it is reasonable to decrease the dose or encourage the child to take the medication earlier in the evening. Because of the anticholinergic effects of TCAs, children often notice a dry mouth and may experience constipation, urinary retention, or weight gain.

TCAs prolong the cardiac QT interval, which can cause a lethal arrhythmia. We obtain a careful history of cardiac symptoms and conduction abnormalities in the child and family members. It is reasonable to order a baseline electrocardiogram to rule out congenital prolonged QT interval before initiation of therapy. Because concomitant use of SSRIs, SNRIs, or tramadol can decrease the seizure threshold in children with a seizure disorder, their simultaneous use is discouraged. Amitriptyline and nortriptyline are the most commonly used medications of this group. The usual starting dose for both medications is 5 to 10 mg orally at night, which is increased to 20 or 25 mg at night 1 week later. Analgesic effects can be seen in 1 to 3 weeks, as with antidepressants effects. Nortriptyline is a metabolite of amitriptyline, with similar utility for pain but less sedation. If top-range dosing is required, periodic electrocardiographic monitoring for QTc changes is suggested.

#### Selective Serotonin and Norepinephrine Reuptake Inhibitors

Venlafaxines starting dose is 37.5 mg/day in adults, which can be increased by 37.5 mg every week up to 300 mg/day. Adverse effects include headaches, nausea, sweating, sedation, hypertension, and seizures. If the dose is less than 150 mg/day, the effects are mostly serotoninergic. If it exceeds 150 mg/day, the effects are mixed serotoninergic and noradrenergic. Duloxetine has antidepressant effects and analgesic effects for neuropathic pain, fibromyalgia, and back pain.[45,57,60] It is usually started at 20 to 60 mg daily to a maximum dose of 120 mg/day. The major adverse effects are nausea, dry mouth, constipation, dizziness, and insomnia. Use of both medications in younger children is best left to those who prescribe the medications frequently because dosing has not been well established in the pediatric age group.

### Muscle Relaxants

Muscle relaxants are frequently used as an adjunct to other medications (mostly NSAIDs) in patients with myofascial pain.

#### Cyclobenzaprine

Cyclobenzaprine is a centrally acting muscle relaxant. Its major adverse effects are somnolence, dizziness, and asthenia. The usual starting dose is 5 mg at night, which can be increased to 10 mg after 5 to 7 days unless the child has difficulties awakening in the morning. The dose can be escalated up to 10 mg three times per day.[61]

#### Baclofen

Baclofen is one of the most powerful centrally acting muscle relaxants. It interacts with the GABA$_B$ receptor subtype. It is usually indicated in patients with spasticity such as children with cerebral palsy or multiple sclerosis. In children 2 to 7 years old, the daily dose is 10 to 15 mg, divided into two or three doses. The dose can be escalated every 3 days by 5 mg to a maximum dose of 40 mg/day. In children older than 8 years of age, the maximum dose is 60 mg/day. Baclofen is one of a few medications approved for intrathecal administration by implanted pumps and is usually administered to children with spasticity (e.g., cerebral palsy, spinal cord injury).

#### Tramadol

Tramadol is a unique analgesic. It is a very weak μ-receptor opioid agonist. It also blocks monoamine reuptake in the central nervous system (similar to antidepressants). For the latter reason, tramadol is a popular analgesic for neuropathic pain, especially for controlling paresthesias, allodynia, and touch-evoked pain. The likelihood of tolerance or development of dependence is small, although it has been reported. Despite its weak opioid properties, sudden discontinuation of tramadol can cause withdrawal symptoms.

The doses used for chronic pain vary from 25 mg up to 100 mg four times per day (400 mg/day maximum).[62] The dose should be limited in renally impaired children with creatinine clearance less than 30 mL/min up to a maximum of 200 mg/day and in those with impaired liver function up to 100 mg/day.

Common adverse effects include nausea, vomiting, sedation, constipation, diarrhea, dizziness, headache, seizures, and hallucinations. Rare side effects include orthostatic hypotension, syncope, and tachyarrhythmia.

### Local Anesthetics, α$_2$-Adrenergic Receptor Agonists, Topical Agents, and N-Methyl-d-Aspartate Receptor Antagonists

Many drugs are used in the treatment of chronic pain, and they have a wide array of mechanisms of action. Oral medications with local anesthetic properties such as mexiletine have been used in the treatment of neuropathic pain in patients with CRPS. The $\alpha_2$-adrenergic receptor agonist clonidine finds its application in the same arena. It is used orally, as a transdermal patch, or added to local anesthetic solutions in intravenous regional techniques. The major limiting factor in the use of these drugs is their adverse effect profile, which includes hypotension, sedation, bradycardia, and nausea (especially with mexiletine). $\alpha_2$-Adrenergic agonist blocking properties are also part of the mechanism of action of the muscle relaxant tizanidine.

The topical agent capsaicin, derived from hot chili peppers, is also helpful in managing neuropathic pain, but its application can cause a burning sensation where applied, which is often poorly tolerated. The topical lidocaine patch has been effective in the controlling symptoms of postherpetic neuralgia and has been used for localized myofascial pain, hyperpathia, and allodynia in other neuropathic conditions.[63] Pharmacokinetic studies in adults have found minimal lidocaine blood concentrations, suggesting a large margin of safety,[64] although similar studies have not been carried out in children.

NMDA receptor antagonists such as ketamine, amantadine, or dextromethorphan have anecdotal evidence supporting their utility in the treatment of neuropathic pain. It is also thought that NMDA receptor antagonists exert an opioid-sparing effect. An important limiting factor of the broader use of ketamine in the treatment of chronic pain symptoms is the potential for psychotropic side effects.

## Complementary Therapies

Alternative therapies have appealed to patients for a long time. Because traditional medical therapies have a high failure rate, patients continue to search for better treatments. Many types of therapies are useful in treating chronic pain. As a consultant, the anesthesiologist should consider suggesting some of these therapies when they seem appropriate. TENS and biofeedback have been discussed earlier.

Acupuncture and its derivative, acupressure, originated in China and constitute an important part of traditional Chinese medicine (Fig. 44-3). In acupuncture, the body energy or qi (pronounced *chi*) circulates in body meridians and collaterals. Meridians and collaterals are pathways that represent body organ systems called the Zang-Fu organs. In Chinese medicine, pain is caused by obstruction in the circulation of qi in these channels due to multiple causes. Acupuncture has been used in acute and chronic pain conditions such as neck and back pain, dental pain, musculoskeletal and arthritic pain, CRPS, migraine, facial pain, and fibromyalgia. The data from randomized, controlled trials is controversial or insufficient to support or deny efficacy of acupuncture.[65]

## Summary

The pediatric anesthesiologist may be called on to assist with the care of a child or adolescent with chronic pain. The basic tenets of care apply, and a careful history and focused physical examination remain key components of the evaluation. Determining that the child is not being physically harmed by the painful condition (i.e., ensuring safety) is the first step, followed by focused diagnostic evaluation and therapy. Treatment for all but the simplest painful conditions employs multiple disciplines in a coordinated attack on the pain. The input of psychologists is a prominent part of chronic pain management, and psychological treatment is not a sign of psychiatric disease or malingering but a tool that can be powerful and effective. Physical therapy and judicious use of medications round out the approach to most chronic pain problems in children. The occasional use of interventional modalities and opioids is warranted, but success is limited if the problem is viewed in a unidimensional manner. Many patients benefit from alternative approaches to therapy, and these disciplines can be used in a prudent fashion to expand the range of therapies that can be recommend.

## ANNOTATED REFERENCES

Perquin CW, Hazebroek-Kampschreur AA, Hunfeld JA, et al. Pain in children and adolescents: a common experience. Pain 2000;87:51-8.
*This survey article describes the prevalence of chronic pain in children, which is a much more common problem than previously recorded in the general population.*

Ripamonti C, Groff L, Brunelli C, et al. Switching from morphine to oral methadone in treating cancer pain: what is the equianalgesic dose ratio? J Clin Oncol 1998;16:3216-21.
*This is an intriguing discussion about the conversion ratio between morphine and methadone. It explodes the commonly held belief (seen in so many opioid conversion tables) that the two opioids are equianalgesic.*

Stanton-Hicks M, Baron R, Boas R, et al. Complex regional pain syndromes: guidelines for therapy. Clin J Pain 1998;14:155-66.
*The article outlines the multidisciplinary approach to complex regional pain syndromes (CRPS). Multidisciplinary treatment is not just for children with CRPS.*

Turk DC. Clinical effectiveness and cost-effectiveness of treatments for patients with chronic pain. Clin J Pain 2002;18:355-65.
*The author takes a look at the big picture. Blocks make us money; comprehensive treatment makes patients better.*

Wilder RT, Berde CB, Wolohan M, et al. Reflex dystrophy in children: clinical characteristics and follow-up of seventy patients. Am J Bone Joint Surg 1992;74:910-9.
*The classic paper describes complex regional pain syndrome in children, its treatment, and patient outcomes. Its observations hold up today.*

## REFERENCES

Please see www.expertconsult.com.

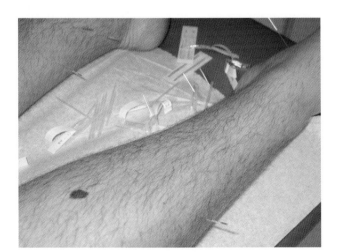

**FIGURE 44-3** Acupuncture needles in situ.

# SPECIAL TOPICS

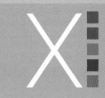

# Anesthesia Outside the Operating Room

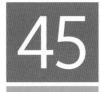

**45**

JOSEPH P. CRAVERO

THE APPROACH TO PROVIDING ANESTHESIA outside the operating room (OR) for children (also known as non–operating room anesthesia [NORA] or off-site anesthesia) varies greatly among organizations and even from one anesthesia provider to another. NORA practice is not as standardized as anesthesia delivered within the OR setting. As such, it is a difficult topic to cover using an evidence-based approach. Although most anesthesiologists would agree (generally) on the optimal methodology for delivering anesthesia to a 2-year-old child for inguinal hernia repair, much more variability (in terms of drugs used, airway management techniques, and general organization) exists in providing anesthesia for a magnetic resonance imaging (MRI) scan. This issue is made even more confusing by the fact that procedures that are performed with sedation in one institution may be accomplished with general anesthesia in another. Furthermore, a procedure that is performed under sedation with an *anesthesia* provider in one institution may have sedation provided by a specialist *other* than an anesthesiologist at a different institution.[1]

The discussion of anesthesia services outside the operating room must also include the recognition that the level of sedation or anesthesia for a given child at any moment during a procedure is often a matter of some conjecture. Almost any procedure that involves pain, or the requirement for absolute movement control in a child, necessitates deep sedation or general anesthesia. The distinction between these two states–defined by the presence or absence of movement in reaction to painful stimuli–is often difficult to determine.[2] For anesthesiologists, the difference

between these two states is more of semantic interest than practical importance. Anesthesia services are often requested outside the OR when sedation is actually what is required. Finally, anesthesia is often provided outside of the OR for patients with significant comorbidities undergoing routine procedures. Many of these children would be managed with sedation by other specialists were it not for the complexity of the coincident condition(s). Comorbid conditions that require referral to an anesthesiologist vary with institutions but common (generally accepted) examples include:

1. Extremely young age, including well children younger than 1 month of age
2. History of significant prematurity (younger than 32 weeks at birth) and post–conceptional age younger than 60 weeks.
3. History of ongoing apnea and bradycardia episodes
4. Craniofacial anomalies or any known difficult functional or anatomic airway problem
5. Cyanotic congenital heart disease or cardiomyopathy
6. Any serious coexisting disease such as sickle cell disease or muscular dystrophy that would qualify a patient as American Society of Anesthesiologists (ASA) III-IV.
7. Procedures that require elective airway control (intubation) or respiratory control such as breath holding

With these considerations in mind, this chapter focuses on issues specifically related to the delivery of anesthesia and deep sedation outside of the OR *provided by anesthesiologists*. Issues concerning minimal, moderate, and deep sedation, as well as issues involving care by providers other than anesthesiologists, are covered Chapter 47.

## Standards and Guidelines

Anesthesia outside of the OR must meet the same standards as anesthesia given in the OR. Specifically, Medicare's *Conditions for Participation* for hospitals are enforced by The Joint Commission (TJC) regardless of location of care. The *Conditions for Participation* are principles that are articulated to surveyors as instructions in the Interpretive Guidelines published in January, 2011, and available at http://www.cms.gov/SurveyCertificationgeninfo/dounloads/SCLetter11_10.pdf. These guidelines describe appropriate training, credentialing, and oversight of sedation and anesthesia providers and some of the specific requirements for care documentation. The ASA has developed templates for the required policies that help institutions meet the standards of the new Interpretive Guidelines. These resources can be downloaded from the ASA website at http://www.asahq.org. With particular reference to NORA, there are several notable templates, as follows:

1. Preanesthesia Evaluation Policy, Form and Note (template) Within 48 hours immediately before the delivery of the first dose of medication for the purpose of inducing anesthesia, a qualified practitioner must perform a preanesthesia evaluation of the patient that includes, at a minimum: a) a review of the medical history, including anesthesia, drug and allergy history, and b) an interview, if possible, given the patient's condition, and examination of the patient. In addition, the following must be reviewed and updated within 48 hours prior to anesthesia:

   a) Notation of the anesthesia risk. b) Identification of potential anesthesia problems. c) Additional preanesthesia data or information, if applicable and as required in accordance with standard practice prior to administration of anesthesia (i.e., stress tests). d) Development of the plan for the patient's anesthesia care, including the type of medications for induction, maintenance and postoperative care and discussion with the patient (parents) of the risks and benefits of the delivery of anesthesia.

2. Intraoperative record policy. Standard data elements and timing must be included in the intraoperative record–just as in the OR.

3. Postanesthesia Evaluation Policy, Note and Form (template) A postanesthesia note must be completed within 48 hours after surgery. The person completing the evaluation does not have to be the person who delivered the anesthetic. The elements of the postanesthesia note include assessment of the following: a) respiratory function, b) cardiovascular function, c) mental status, d) temperature, e) pain, f) nausea and vomiting, and g) postoperative hydration.

NORA Services must be organized in such a way as to meet the *Conditions for Participation* (and thus TJC) standards mentioned earlier, just as they are met in the OR environment. Depending on how NORA is organized in a particular institution, this can be challenging. The departments that require anesthesia services must appreciate the need to meet these standards and allow for the infrastructure to meet or exceed them, particularly in the preanesthesia and postanesthesia timeframes.

## Off-Site Anesthesia: Structure

Anesthesia services outside of the OR can be organized in various ways. In some institutions these services are organized through an off-site anesthesia unit or sedation unit. These units have the advantage of providing all anesthesia-related care through one location that contains all of the personnel and equipment required for anesthesia. Ideally, these units provide for preanesthesia assessment, induction, procedure location, and a recovery area. Children may be transported to remote locations when equipment (such as MRI) cannot be brought to the sedation unit. The advantages of this organizational scheme are clear. The uniform environment leads to maximum consistency in the equipment and personnel that interact with children and their families and thus adds to safety, efficiency, parent satisfaction, and effectiveness of care. Many experts (along with TJC) advise the formation of specialty teams or microsystems for provision of anesthesia out of the OR. Microsystems are coordinated groups of professionals who deliver a specific service, to achieve the best outcomes by developing reliable, efficient, and responsive systems that have the capability of meeting the individual needs of one child, continually improving care for the next child, and creating a great place to work for all staff. The sedation microsystem should be made up of pediatric anesthesiologists and nursing, technical, and administrative personnel who are familiar with the service and dedicated to this care.[3] The microsystem can provide structure and expertise for this care. As members gain expertise and comfort with the off-site environment, their care is consistent and reproducible, leading to less confusion with other services. Such systems of care lead to improved effectiveness (decreasing failed anesthesia and sedation cases) and improve patient and family and staff satisfaction.[4-6]

Another option for anesthesia organization outside the OR is the use of standard same-day unit admission and assessment services and postanesthesia care unit recovery capability while providing induction and procedural anesthesia at the site of the procedure (e.g., endoscopy suite or hematology and oncology unit). This organizational paradigm makes use of existing anesthesia ancillary services but often requires patient transport before and after anesthesia.

Finally, anesthesia services outside of the OR may be primarily organized at the site of procedural care. Most typically these services are organized in radiology departments or gastrointestinal procedure suits, where a majority of pediatric sedation and anesthesia takes place outside of the OR. For this organizational setup, the procedure unit itself may be outfitted for admission and preanesthesia assessment. An anesthetizing location can be provided and recovery of children can be accomplished in a space contiguous within the immediate location of the procedural equipment. This kind of organization is most common in children's hospitals, where high volumes of procedures are performed in a given location such as the MRI scanner.[7] In locations such as this, where anesthesia services are required on a daily basis for a multitude of children, the investment in the infrastructure for anesthesia support services makes economic sense in addition to optimizing patient care.

### PERSONNEL REQUIREMENTS

The environment and the demands of providing anesthesia outside of the OR are unique regardless of the specific organization that has been chosen for NORA. To create the kind of functioning sedation microsystem discussed earlier, several common themes lead to optimal safety and effectiveness of off-site anesthesia care:

1. Anesthesia providers should rotate on this service and have a frequency of experience with the environment and ancillary personnel that allow familiarity among the anesthesiologists, nurse anesthetists, respiratory therapists, registered nurses, patient care technicians, biomedical engineers, and child life specialists. This familiarity should be based on a common understanding of the routines and protocols for standard procedures and a common agreement on the goals of the service.

2. Effective and efficient communication among personnel is critical to optimize outcomes. Logically, help from all members of the care team, including the supervising anesthesiologist, should be available within time frames that would allow optimal outcomes for children with critical events—specifically within 3 to 4 minutes. The use of cell phones, Internet phones, or other devices to optimize communication in NORA locations is often helpful.

3. The ancillary personnel in each location must be familiar with the needs and processes of providing anesthesia to children.

4. Equipment and monitoring standards should mimic that of the OR environment (see later discussion). Anesthesia carts and machine preparation and setup should mirror the OR environment as much as possible to maximize the similarity to the most common workspace. It is critical to have a system that allows appropriate restocking and security of anesthesia carts in all of the off-site locations. All off-site carts should include a full range of drugs, intravenous equipment, fluids, and airway equipment such as tracheal tubes, laryngeal mask airways (LMAs), laryngoscopes, oral and nasal airways, masks, and suction equipment in sizes that would fit all possible pediatric age groups.

5. Scheduling off-site anesthesia resources is complex and personally demanding. Timing for some procedures is inexact. In addition, anesthesia time requirements can vary with the child and the associated pathology. Success is enhanced by focusing the task of scheduling NORA procedures with one individual (or a small group) (similar to scheduling cases for the OR) who intimately understands the process involved in anesthesia. This type of organization allows the NORA service to have one focal point for communication between the individuals who perform procedures and the anesthesia service, thus maximizing communication among services and minimizing incorrect assumptions of staffing or timing for procedures.

## SPECIFIC ENVIRONMENTAL REQUIREMENTS

Equipment (see earlier discussion) and monitoring standards (see later discussion) must meet those of the main OR environment. Regardless of whether the anesthetizing location is inside or outside the OR, the ASA has established minimum standards for equipment, monitors, and conditions of anesthesia delivery. These guidelines may, of course, be exceeded at any time based on the judgment of the involved anesthesia personnel. The ASA specifically requires that remote locations must have two sources of oxygen ($O_2$) (preferably a central source of piped $O_2$ and a backup E cylinder), suction, an anesthesia machine if administering inhalational anesthetics, a scavenging system for waste anesthetic gases, a self-inflating hand resuscitator bag able to deliver 90% $O_2$ and positive-pressure ventilation, standard of care monitors and equipment,[7,8] and sufficient electrical outlets,

illumination, and space. The ASA Standards for Basic Anesthetic Monitoring include the following:

- Pulse oximetry with audible pulse tone and low-threshold alarm
- Adequate illumination and exposure of the patient to assess color
- Anesthesia machine with $O_2$ analyzer
- Continuous end-tidal carbon dioxide ($ETCO_2$) analysis with an audible alarm
- Continuous electrocardiogram (ECG)
- Arterial blood pressure and heart rate every 5 minutes or more frequently as indicated
- Temperature, if there is potential for clinically significant changes in body temperature

In addition, it is important to make further adaptations in the non-OR setting. Duplicates of critical equipment, such as laryngoscope handles and blades, should be immediately available. In the MRI unit, it is essential to have MRI-compatible laryngoscope blades and handles, as well as compatible monitoring devices. Each site should be carefully evaluated for important items, such as presence or absence of wall-delivered gases ($O_2$, nitrous oxide [$N_2O$], and air), location of suction equipment, and Ambu bag. Every site must have backup gas supplies. If pipeline $O_2$ is not available, $O_2$ should be drawn from H cylinders (6600 L) rather than the smaller E tanks (659 L).

Many off-site areas do not have wall suction, especially in the MRI environment. MRI-compatible wall suction is not widely available. An alternative method for providing suction in the MRI suite is to mount a suction canister with 30 feet of suction tubing outside the scanner room.[9] The suction tubing can then be threaded through a hole in the console wall to access for use in the MRI unit.

Scavenging systems should be carefully evaluated in out of OR locations. When passive scavenging is not possible, active scavenging may be developed by using the wall-source vacuum or wall suction canisters. Ideally, a scavenging system dedicated solely to waste gases should be present.

Electrical circuitry in off-site locations must be upgraded to meet OR standards. Specifically, although the outlets tend to be grounded and hospital grade, plug and outlet incompatibility may be a problem. Adapters and conversion plugs must be available. Although off-site locations tend not to have as great a risk of electrical shock or electrocution to the child as in the OR, it is important to remember that these sites do not have line-isolation monitors. In the event of excessive leakage of current, the anesthesiologist would not be warned. Although the National Electrical Code no longer requires line-isolation monitors in nonflammable anesthetizing locations, it is strongly recommended in areas with multiple power sources. To ensure child and health care personnel safety, biomedical engineers must be attentive to the safe maintenance of all electrical equipment.

It is in the nature of off-site anesthesia that the physical environment and practice patterns are typically that of another medical specialty. It should also be noted that these other specialties practice under standards developed by their own professional organizations that apply to the procedures within their locations reflecting the different procedure goals. The varying specialties involved include (but are not limited to) gastroenterology, dentistry, cardiology, oncology, intensive care, emergency medicine, and radiology.[10] Anesthesia providers who work in these environments are well served by familiarizing themselves with the standards for the given specialty area they are working in, as published on the individual websites for the various professional organizations.

## Quality Assurance of Anesthesia Services and Outcome in the Off-Site Areas

This chapter reviews issues related to care delivered by members of anesthesiology departments outside of the OR. In this case the quality improvement (QI) and assurance (QA) activities center in the anesthesiology department. Issues relating to sedation services provided by other services are discussed in Chapter 47. Just as is the case in the OR, it is important to have a consistent tracking tool to follow all clinically important complications. Each department can set its own thresholds for review; however, certain incidents logically require inquiry, as follows[11]:

- Aspiration events
- Unscheduled admissions to the hospital as a direct result of the sedation (i.e., because of protracted emesis, prolonged sedation, respiratory or cardiac complication)
- Failed procedures resulting from inadequate or problematic anesthesia or sedation
- Cardiovascular compromise that requires assistance from an outside rescue team
- Cardiac arrest

Many institutions choose to follow other outcomes such as prolonged nausea and vomiting after anesthesia or $O_2$ desaturation events. Regardless of the data that the QI committee chooses to review, the process should include anesthesiologists, nurses, and other technical personnel who are routinely involved in anesthesia care and support. It is particularly important to note that in the case of off-site anesthesia, it is critical to include members of the departments that are served by the service in the quality improvement process. The timing of QI meetings depends on the number and acuity of the non-OR anesthesia provided at a given institution. Review committee meetings should be considered not just an opportunity to evaluate complications but also a forum for exchange of ideas, expertise, and information that can lead to improvements in patient care.

## Anesthesia versus Sedation for Non–Operating Room Procedures and Tests in Children

Anesthesiologists can deliver either deep sedation or anesthesia for procedures outside of the OR. The choice of whether to deliver general anesthesia with a secured airway (tracheal tube or LMA) using potent inhalational anesthetics versus deep sedation with facemask $O_2$ and propofol infusion depends on many factors, including the child's comorbid conditions, the procedure, and the experience and comfort level of the anesthesia provider. Several reviews are available on this topic. For MRI scans, propofol sedation has been suggested as an (overall) safe and effective option in children with airway pathologic conditions or who are premature or very young.[12] Similarly, multiple reports have recommended both propofol sedation and general anesthesia with tracheal intubation (GETA) techniques for endoscopies.[13,14]

No clear evidence exists on which to conclude that one technique is specifically better than another for procedures in which both techniques are effective and safe, such as MRI or endoscopy procedures. Recognizing this fact, it is still important for anesthesiologists to avoid providing GETA in every case (ignoring the possible advantages that deep or moderate sedation could provide in terms of rapidity of emergence and lack of side effects). It is appropriate to carefully evaluate the nature of the sedation/anesthesia provided in the non-OR setting and consider all of the possible implications of a given technique. For instance, how efficient and effective is the care that is provided? How well does the care provided meet the requirements of the procedure in terms of pain and movement control? What are the nature and rapidity of the emergence from sedation or anesthesia and the time that children should remain in the hospital or ambulatory unit between emergence and discharge after a specific procedure with a given technique? Only after careful analysis can guidelines be established for the optimal technique for a given procedure.[15]

When delivering general anesthesia to children out of the OR, the risk benefit of instrumenting the airway must be carefully evaluated. The LMA is perhaps most useful in the MRI or computed tomography (CT) setting because it maintains spontaneous ventilation, enables the anesthesiologist to monitor $ETCO_2$ continuously and provides a clear airway in a child who may otherwise have obstruction with a natural airway. With the LMA in place, the child can be maintained with a relatively low level of anesthesia, allowed to breathe spontaneously, and then rapidly awakened at the conclusion of the scan. After the LMA is placed, anesthesia can be provided with either a continuous infusion of propofol or with a low-dose inhalation agent (sevoflurane 1.5% in 50% $N_2O/O_2$). In some circumstances, the LMA may provide a suitable airway in children with bronchopulmonary dysplasia, cystic fibrosis, severe asthma, or active respiratory issues. In children with upper respiratory tract infections, the incidence of mild bronchospasm, laryngospasm, breath holding, and major $O_2$ desaturation (less than 90%) in those whose airway was managed with an LMA was reduced compared with those whose airway was managed with a tracheal tube.[16] Similarly, the use of LMAs in ex-preterm infants with bronchopulmonary dysplasia resulted in less coughing and wheezing and greater hemodynamic stability than in those managed with tracheal tubes. In children who underwent a vitrectomy for retinopathy of prematurity, the time to discharge after an LMA was less than that after a tracheal tube.[17] LMAs provide more hemodynamic stability during their removal than during tracheal extubation and thus the former may be useful in children with hemodynamic instability.[18]

Others think any instrumentation of the airway theoretically increases the risk of triggering airway reflexes or regurgitation compared with no airway instrumentation. In healthy children, some clinicians prefer a deep sedation technique, for example, for brain MRI that includes a propofol infusion, an optimally positioned upper airway (with a roll under the cervical spine and the neck extended) and noninvasive monitoring (nasal capnometry supplemented with oximetry, an electrocardiogram, and noninvasive blood pressure).[19] Some note that the majority of children do not require an airway during deep sedation for medical procedures. However, in some (e.g., those with excess secretions or upper airway obstruction during the sedation), the following algorithm of airway intervention may be followed to relieve the obstruction: reposition the head and shoulders, insert an oral airway, insert a nasal airway, place an LMA, and finally, if the LMA fails to clear the airway, place a tracheal tube.

# Logistics of Managing Acute Emergencies and Cardiopulmonary Arrest Outside the Operating Room

Although the actual management of a cardiopulmonary arrest should not vary between the OR setting and the non-OR setting, the logistics of performing a resuscitation may be challenged by unanticipated factors, such as personnel who may not be familiar with code situations, an environment that makes performing a resuscitation difficult, or equipment that may be unsafe if used in the particular location (e.g., the MRI environment). It is important that all personnel in the off-site location be familiar with the location and operation of the code cart. The anesthesia cart and the code cart in the off-site location should be stocked in the same precise configuration as all others throughout the hospital and ORs. Standardizing the code carts throughout the hospital ensures that all ancillary personnel can be helpful in locating critical items. If the code cart is kept locked, the key or access code must be readily accessible and in a location that is known to all essential personnel. A hard board on which chest compressions may be performed should also be readily available. Each off-site location should have an identified and rehearsed routine for announcing a code situation and summoning aid. The use of human patient simulation can be very helpful in testing the team response to critical events. Simulators can be used in place in off-site locations to replicate critical events and evaluate the ability of the care team and backup systems to resuscitate a patient. Blike and colleagues used exactly this methodology to document significant variation in the ability of rescuers to resuscitate children from sedation or anesthesia critical events in locations outside the OR.[20]

Of all the non-OR environments in which anesthesiologists are asked to provide care, the MRI scanner poses a unique challenge for cardiopulmonary resuscitation. The MRI environment is divided up into four zones that correlate with the intensity of the magnetic field and the risk to children and health care providers. These zones are delineated in Table 45-1.

In 2009 the ASA published a report titled Practice Advisory on Anesthetic Care for Magnetic Resonance Imaging: A Report by the American Society of Anesthesiologists Task Force on Anesthetic Care for Magnetic Resonance Imaging.[21] This document advises that in the case of a medical emergency in a patient within the scanner, the anesthesia providers should (1) initiate cardiopulmonary resuscitation while immediately removing the patient from zone IV, (2) call for help, and (3) transport the patient to a previously designated safe location in proximity to the MRI suite. This designated location should contain a defibrillator, vital signs monitors, and a code cart with all resuscitation drugs, airway equipment, $O_2$, and suction. Other acute emergencies that are unique to the MRI environment include a "quench" or a fire in the scanner. Quenching occurs when the liquid that cools the magnet boils off rapidly and results in helium escaping from the cryogen bath. The magnetic field of the magnet is rapidly decreased because the coils in the magnet cease to be superconducting and become resistive. In addition to performing the institution's protocol in reaction to either of these events, the ASA consultants involved in writing the advisory agree that in the event of a quench, (1) the child should be removed from zone IV immediately and (2) $O_2$ should be administered immediately; (3) because of the powerful magnetic field that can exist after a quench or a fire, emergency response personnel should be restricted from entering zone IV.

# Difficult Airway Management in the Non–Operating Room (Off-Site) Environment

Two potential difficult airway scenarios may occur in non-OR locations: the child with a known difficult airway and the child with an unrecognized difficult airway. Extensive literature addresses these scenarios, but logic would dictate that children who were preidentified as having potentially difficult airways should have their airways secured in the controlled environment of the OR. Regardless of an anesthesiologist's comfort level and familiarity with the intended off-site environment, the critical backup personnel and the full array of airway equipment are not always available in remote locations. It is important to note that a fiberoptic bronchoscope and light source are not MRI compatible. It is easier to perform a fiberoptic intubation or to have the fiberoptic equipment readily available in an OR. In this environment, both the nursing and anesthesia support staff (technicians, other anesthesiologists, and otolaryngologists) are readily available and prepared to provide assistance. After intubation, the child may be safely transported to the off-site location for subsequent care.

The more difficult scenario is that of the unrecognized difficult airway[22]; this scenario may best be handled by establishing a local management protocol that can be activated when the situation arises. Each institution has peculiar equipment, space, and personnel resources. NORA leaders should establish a local protocol for management of the unanticipated difficult airway in an off-site location. In some cases this might involve bringing advanced airway management equipment to the location in a rapid, organized manner. In other cases the best option would include "temporizing" management with alternative airway devices and transporting the child to a location where a definitive airway can be placed in a controlled manner. For this reason, it is important to have alternative airway devices such as LMAs stocked in all anesthesia carts that are designated for off-site locations. In the event that the lungs cannot be ventilated or the trachea intubated, the LMA can provide a lifesaving temporary airway until more definitive action can be taken.[23,24]

**TABLE 45-1** Descriptions of the American College of Radiology's Four Zones in the Magnetic Resonance Imaging Suite

| ACR Zones | Occupants | Hazards |
|-----------|-----------|---------|
| Zone I | General public | Negligible |
| Zone II | Unscreened MRI patients | Immediately outside area of hazard |
| Zone III | Screened MRI patients and personnel | Potential biostimulation interference, access to magnet room |
| Zone IV | Screened MRI patients under constant direct supervision of trained MRI personnel | Biostimulation interference, radiofrequency heating, missile effect, cryogens |

From the Joint Commission International Center for Patient Safety. Available at: http://www.acr.org/~/media/ACR/Documents/PDF/QualitySafety/MR%20Safety/SafeMR07.pdf.
*ACR*, American College of Radiology; *MRI*, magnetic resonance imaging.

45

# Specific Locations for Non–Operating Room Anesthesia

### COMPUTED TOMOGRAPHY

CT involves ionizing radiation and can provide a good modality for differentiating between high-density (calcium, iron, bone, contrast-enhanced vascular and cerebrospinal fluid [CSF] spaces) and low-density ($O_2$, nitrogen, carbon in air, fat, CSF, muscle, white matter, gray matter, and water-containing lesions) structures. Because the scan time for current devices is brief, with actual imaging time ranging from 5 to 50 seconds per sequence, many children are able to tolerate CT without sedation or anesthesia. In cases in which anesthesia is required, it is often for those who have a fragile or unstable respiratory or cardiovascular status. Anesthesia or sedation is often required for children who are unable to cooperate (cognitively impaired children and those younger than 2 to 3 years of age) or require CT emergently. Emergent indications for CT include head trauma, unstable respiratory status in need of a pulmonary diagnosis, unexplained changes in mental status, or neoplasm workup in severely debilitated children. Anesthesia management is also necessary with a potentially unstable airway (peritonsillar abscess, anterior mediastinal mass, craniofacial anomaly, tracheoesophageal fistula, uncontrolled vomiting, or gastroesophageal reflux), or the need for breath holding during acquisition of images (three-dimensional dynamic airway studies) (Figs. 45-1 and 45-2). Some CT units are particularly concerned about children moving when contrast is injected (because of dose restrictions the contrast injection cannot be repeated) and therefore request anesthesia services for any child they cannot confidently predict will stay motionless for the study.

Children with Down syndrome present a particular area of interest for the anesthesiologist working with the CT scanner. These children pose a unique risk for atlantoaxial instability and may require a head or neck CT to evaluate cervical and temporomandibular anatomy, recurrent sinusitis, or choanal atresia. The incidence of atlantoaxial instability varies from 12% to 32%.[25] Many children with Down syndrome require cervical spine radiographs before entering grade school or participating in the Special Olympics. Usually, the parents know the outcome of these tests and can relay the results of cervical spine radiographs. These studies alone do *not* indicate to the practitioner whether the child is at risk of dislocation.[23] Rather, it is the presence of neurologic signs or symptoms that would herald a spine that is "at risk": abnormal wide-based gait, incontinence, increased clumsiness,

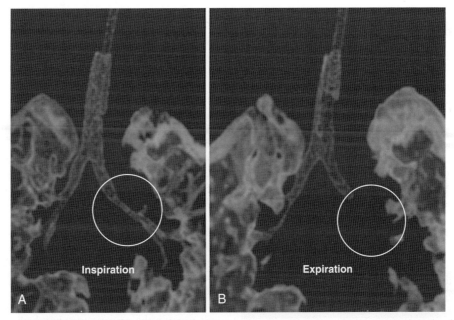

**FIGURE 45-1** Three-dimensional dynamic computed tomography scan demonstrating change in caliber of left main-stem bronchus (*circle*) in an intubated child at end-inspiration (pressure held at 15 to 18 mm Hg) (**A**) versus end-expiration (**B**).

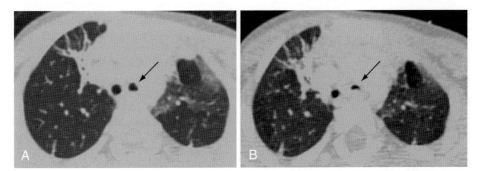

**FIGURE 45-2** Three-dimensional CT scan demonstrating change in caliber of left main-stem bronchus (*arrows*) on inspiration (**A**) versus expiration (**B**).

fatigue with ambulation, complaints of numbness, tingling in an extremity, weakness of an extremity, or a new preference for sitting games. In infants, these clinical signs may be difficult to assess. In younger children, developmental milestones (e.g., crawling, sitting up, reaching for objects) should be evaluated. Physical signs may include clonus, hyperreflexia, quadriparesis, neurogenic bladder, hemiparesis, ataxia, and sensory loss. Children with atlantoaxial instability on a radiograph are at less risk for dislocation if they do not exhibit any signs or symptoms of instability. Children who are capable of following commands are asked to perform full neck flexion and extension maneuvers to determine whether pain, sensory, or motor manifestations of cord compression develop.

Perhaps the most controversial issue facing anesthesiologists with regard to CT scans is the issue of oral contrast for CT. Because children lack abundant retroperitoneal fat, they do not have the natural contrast needed to elucidate abdominal images. For this reason, children may be required to ingest (orally or via nasogastric tube) diatrizoic acid (Gastrografin) to opacify the stomach and bowel. Oral contrast is useful in the identification of an intraabdominal abscess, mass, fluid collection, bowel injury, pancreatic injury, or other traumatic injury. The oral contrast comes as Gastrografin 3% and may be diluted to a 1.5% to 2.5% strength concentration. Gastrografin 3% is the full-strength concentration; in this undiluted form, Gastrografin is hypertonic (2200 mOsm/L). At this concentration, it can cause pulmonary edema, pneumonitis, osmotic effusions, and death if aspirated. Fortunately, when Gastrografin is administered to children for CT it is diluted to 1.5% to 2.5% strength, which is thought to be much less dangerous if aspirated. The volume of oral contrast that is administered can be quite large. Neonates typically receive 60 to 90 mL. Infants between 1 month and 1 year of age may receive up to 240 mL. Children between the ages of 1 and 5 years receive between 240 to 360 mL of contrast medium. Risk is introduced when these children require anesthesia within an optimal window after ingestion (usually 30 minutes to 1 hour after receiving the contrast agent) to enhance visualization. By most fasting guidelines (nil per os [NPO]), Gastrografin consumption within 1 to 2 hours of an anesthetic or sedation does not fall within the usual NPO guidelines. Yet, the scan must be completed while the Gastrografin is present in the gastrointestinal tract. Despite the large volume of Gastrografin that may be ingested, there does not appear to be a significant aspiration risk in this population, and many anesthesiologists do not secure the airway with a tracheal tube (Fig. 45-3). A review of the pediatric and adult literature confirms that over the last 35 years only a few case reports have been published of aspiration syndrome attributed to Gastrografin, all in extremely high-risk patients.[24-26] Several investigators have evaluated this issue from different perspectives. In one study, a cohort of 50 patients who received oral contrast after blunt abdominal trauma were evaluated for radiologic evidence of aspiration pneumonia or clinical complications of aspiration.[27] Some of the patients received general anesthesia, and some were neurologically impaired (including several with increased intracranial pressure). In this very high-risk group, only one patient had a question of aspiration on a chest radiograph after the CT scan, and that patient did not develop pulmonary symptoms. Another study evaluated the volume of gastric contents of 365 patients undergoing deep sedation or general anesthesia for abdominal CT scans.[25] Gastric contents exceeded 0.4 mL/kg in 49% of those who received gastric contrast. Two cases of vomiting were recorded. None of the patients in the

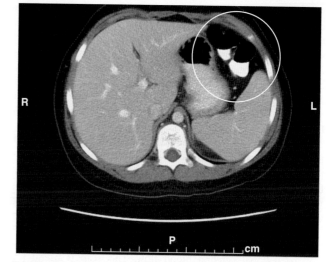

**FIGURE 45-3** Four hours after ingestion of Gastrografin, oral contrast is still present in the stomach and small intestine. Although dilute Gastrografin is still frequently present in the stomach at the time of computed tomography, there are as yet no case reports validating an increase in risk of pulmonary aspiration.

study developed clinical evidence of aspiration. When dilute Gastrografin is used, the risks associated with pulmonary aspiration appear to be small, even in children who are moderately to deeply sedated.[28] In spite of this evidence, no large cohort studies have been conducted that have the power to determine the actual incidence of aspiration in this setting. Therefore no accepted standard of care for the airway management of these children has been determined. Some anesthesiologists induce anesthesia with an intravenous or inhalational technique and maintain the anesthetic without securing the airway with a tracheal tube. Others perform rapid-sequence induction and tracheal intubation. The lack of consensus among anesthesiologists and the absence of evidence preclude a clear and consistent recommendation for managing the airway in these children.

## NUCLEAR MEDICINE

Nuclear medicine is one of the oldest functional imaging disciplines. Because of the advances in instrumentation and radiopharmaceuticals, nuclear scanning is becoming an increasingly popular imaging modality. Nuclear imaging can be used to evaluate an incredible range of pathologic conditions. These scans are useful for identification of the extent of disease for a large number of neoplasms.[29] They can also be used to detect epileptic foci in refractory epilepsy, evaluate cerebrovascular disease (e.g., moyamoya disease) and cognitive and behavior disorders, and detect and delineate renal function and disease, including detection of reflux and acute pyelonephritis.[23] Improvements in the hardware for nuclear imaging has greatly decreased the scan time, although even with the advent of two-level emission and transmission scans and combined CT imaging, a child must remain motionless for 20 to 60 minutes. The nuclear medicine environment is quiet, and the scan is pain-free. Accordingly, the indications for anesthesia or sedation include only those children who could not be reasonably expected to hold still for the 20 to 60 minutes, such as those with cognitive or behavioral impairment, young age, or severe pain or who are claustrophobic.[29] Sedation providers should be aware that the equipment in nuclear medicine imaging emits no ionizing radiation, but rather the radiation is contained

within the child and is of very low energy levels. Depending on the nature of the study, the children require intravenous access for administration of the nuclear tracer well in advance of the scan and therefore usually have intravenous access for the anesthesia or sedation. Many nuclear scans also require an empty bladder to avoid interference from concentrated tracer in an enlarged bladder. Accordingly, the bladder is often catheterized after anesthesia is induced and the radioactive urine that is collected is disposed of in a radioactive-safe manner.

Two relatively new nuclear scans that involve anesthesia and present particular challenges are single-photon emission computed tomography (SPECT) and positron emission tomography (PET) scans. SPECT scans use single-photon gamma-emitting radioisotopes and rotating gamma cameras to produce three-dimensional brain images. SPECT scans involve the use of radio-labeled technetium-99m (half-life of 6 hours), which has a high rate of first-pass extraction and intracellular trapping in proportion to regional cerebral blood flow. This scan is useful for localizing seizure foci. It appears to be as accurate as invasive direct cortical mapping in this regard.[30] Injection of the radio-nuclide during a seizure will tag areas of increased cerebral blood flow and localize the seizure foci. The child should be scanned within 1 to 6 hours of the seizure and injection of the tracer. Logistically this can pose a problem because there is no way to predict exactly when a seizure will occur. Therefore the neurology service needs to communicate to the anesthesiology service the importance of being flexible in providing anesthetic services within the window of time allowed to complete the test whenever the next seizure occurs.

PET scans use radionuclide tracers of metabolic activity such as $O_2$ usage and glucose metabolism. Radionuclide tracers of glucose may be useful when seeking seizure foci or tumor recurrence.[29,31,32] Unlike SPECT scans, PET scans should be performed during the seizure itself. Because of the short half-life of the glucose tracer (110 minutes), the scan is best completed during the seizure or within 1 hour thereafter. The logistical problem in providing this service is even more difficult than that of SPECT scans. In addition to the need to have a team available to provide anesthesia on very short notice, there is a risk of hypovolemia, especially in infants, who remain on NPO status and without intravenous hydration while anticipating a seizure. It is therefore important to work with the neurology and neurosurgery services to plan these scans in advance, to ensure intravenous access to avoid hypovolemia, and to arrange anesthesia coverage when needed.

## STEREOTACTIC RADIOSURGERY

Stereotactic radiosurgery (gamma knife) is a major advance in the treatment of selected malignant tumors (ependymoma, glioblastomas), vascular malformations, acoustic neuromas, and pituitary adenomas in children.[33,34] Radiosurgery is indicated, especially for those children with a tumor located deep in the brain or in an area that could put the child at significant surgical risk (e.g., speech, motor, cerebellum, brainstem areas) or for the recurrent brain tumor that has failed prior treatment. Radiosurgery involves the use of a single large fraction of radiation that is directed at a specific target with minimal radiation exposure to the surrounding normal tissues. Optimal results are achieved with small tumor volumes (14 cm$^3$ or less).[35]

Stereotactic radiosurgery requires the coordination of the departments of radiology, radiation therapy, and anesthesiology. The procedure averages 9 hours but can take up to 15 hours. The stereotactic portion of the procedure begins in the morning in a CT scanner. A stereotactic head frame is applied after induction of general anesthesia and tracheal intubation. Some older children can tolerate the application of the head frame with local anesthesia alone but then develop anxiety because the pressure sensation produced by the head frame that can lead to anxiety, nausea, or vomiting. The vast majority of children require general anesthesia for application of the frame and subsequent imaging and surgery. When the head frame is in place, the key to unlock and remove it should be taped to the frame itself, in the event of a situation necessitating its emergent removal (e.g., vomiting, airway obstruction, or accidental tracheal extubation). For smaller children, nasal intubation may be considered to provide better stability during transport from the radiology suite to the OR. After the head frame is in place and the imaging study is completed, the child is transported (trachea intubated, sedated, and appropriately monitored) to the postanesthesia care unit while the radiologists and neurosurgeons review the images and plan radiosurgery. The postanesthesia care unit stay can range from 3 to 5 hours, during which time these children require continuous physiologic monitoring.

After the images are reviewed and the radiosurgery planning is complete, the child is transported to the stereotactic radiosurgery linear accelerator for treatment. In the treatment room full anesthesia monitoring and an anesthesia machine are present. To minimize radiation exposure to health care personnel, only the child remains in the scanner during treatment, observed at a distance with video cameras focused on both the child and monitors. The actual treatment lasts approximately 1 hour.

After radiosurgery is completed, the child is returned to postanesthesia care unit, where the trachea is extubated under controlled conditions. Risks are inherent with this prolonged anesthesia, which requires multiple transports between sites. One study examined 68 radiosurgery procedures in 65 children and reported four potentially serious anesthesia-related events.[36] In those children who received general anesthesia, serious complications included obstruction of the tracheal tube while in the head frame and lobar collapse requiring prolonged mechanical ventilation.

## RADIATION THERAPY

Radiation therapy for children uses ionizing photons to destroy lymphomas, acute leukemias, Wilms tumor, retinoblastomas, and tumors of the central nervous system. Improved three-dimensional imaging and enhanced computing power have allowed radiation oncologists to conform radiation dose to the shape of the tumor and minimize radiation to the surrounding tissues.[37] The energy absorbed by the tissues is measured in *grays* (Gy), which has replaced the term *rad*. One Gy is equivalent to 100 rad. Although most children receive standard x-ray therapy, specific lesions may respond better to bombardment with electron, proton, or neutron beam therapy. The anesthetic considerations are identical regardless of the type of therapy in this respect.[38] A planning session in a simulator is typically scheduled before the initiation of radiation therapy to map the fields that require irradiation while the child is in a fixed position. For proton beam treatments, a planning session is carried out in a CT scanner. A fiberglass immobilization cast of the head is made while the child is anesthetized with propofol and with a natural airway (Fig. 45-4). This cast allows secure positioning to ensure that the child does not move during treatment, but considerable care is required to configure the mask for optimal airway patency

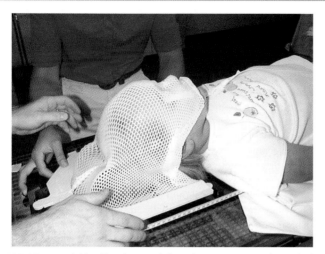

**FIGURE 45-4** Child in fiberglass mask for radiation treatment of a cerebral neoplasm.

45

while ensuring proper windows for treatments because the mask may interfere with airway access.

Radiation therapy involves "fractionated" exposure. Repeat sessions are typical. The child must be motionlessness during therapy to precisely target malignant cells. Radiation therapy is typically administered by dividing the total radiation therapy course among daily or twice-daily sessions. In general, most treatment sessions last between 15 and 30 minutes and the planning simulation session may take as long as 2 hours, depending on the nature and location of the target lesion or area for therapy. For children who require neuraxial treatments for spinal metastases, as many as four fields may be irradiated and in both the supine and prone position. Dividing the total radiation therapy course into discrete daily sessions allows normal tissue repair between sessions while the tumor burden is lessened or destroyed. These children are optimally managed via central venous access that obviates the need for repeated venipunctures. Unless there is a specific airway anomaly, daily anesthetic management typically consists of general anesthesia using a propofol infusion (with or without midazolam pretreatment),[39] blow-by oxygen via nasal cannula or face mask, and spontaneous ventilation monitored with $ETCO_2$. Tachyphylaxis does not appear to be an issue even with multiple, frequent, treatments.[40] One retrospective review of 177 patients undergoing 3833 radiation treatments documented a 1.3% complication rate.[41] This rate compares favorably with the rate of complications for children undergoing propofol-based anesthesia without cancer.[42]

Dexmedetomidine sedation has been used for radiation therapy, but its use has not become widespread, most likely because of the need for a 10-minute loading dose and relatively frequent need for repeated boluses at the doses that have so far been studied.[43] Single-dose IV ketamine 0.5 to 0.8 mg/kg provides effective sedation, albeit with a greater half-life and more adverse effects (e.g., vomiting) than propofol.[44]

One exception to the technique of moderate or deep sedation for radiation therapy is the treatment of retinoblastoma. In this case, the eye must be completely immobile during the treatment. General anesthesia or very deep propofol sedation is indicated in these cases to ensure appropriate irradiating conditions; ketamine, with its side effect of lateral nystagmus, is not appropriate in these cases.[44]

The logistics of radiation therapy anesthesia or sedation are complex, even though the treatments themselves are not challenging. First and foremost, because of the large dose of radiation involved, only the child remains in the room during treatment. All monitoring must be performed via video observation. All radiation therapy units are equipped with video monitoring, but it must be adjusted to allow viewing of the physiologic monitors used for anesthesia. Children are often moved during treatment to allow different angles of access for the radiation treatment, and this must be taken into consideration when placing the monitors and the data or power cords associated with them. As with any anesthetic, positioning of the child must be considered. Many cases of spinal irradiation require the patient to be prone for treatment with the head at a specific angle with respect to the back. In addition, because of the need for the children to be in the close fitting mask during treatments, it is impossible to place an oral airway, LMA, or tracheal tube, thus the importance of monitoring expired carbon dioxide.

Most children undergoing radiation therapy are also receiving adjuvant and simultaneous chemotherapy. As the treatment progresses, nausea, vomiting, and respiratory illness stemming from local radiation effects and chemotherapy can challenge the anesthesiologist. It is important to work with the child's oncologist to manage symptoms and complete the treatment series as close to the planned treatment regimen as possible, because this is critical to the child's survival and maximizing quality of life.

## MAGNETIC RESONANCE IMAGING

MRI, magnetic resonance spectroscopy (MRS), magnetic resonance angiography (MRA), and magnetic resonance venography (MRV) are employed for the evaluation of neoplasms, nonhemorrhagic trauma, vascular lesions, cardiac lesions, orthopedic lesions (including joint disorders, osteomyelitis), central nervous system and spinal cord lesions, craniofacial disorders, detecting the origin of developmental delay, behavioral disorders, seizures, failure to thrive, apnea, cyanosis, hypotonia, and in the workup of mitochondrial and metabolic diseases.[45-48] MRA and MRV are especially helpful in evaluating vascular flow and often can replace invasive angiography in follow-up evaluations of vascular malformations, interventional therapy, or radiotherapy.[49,50] All of these imaging modalities are essentially equivalent in terms of the requirements for the provision of anesthesia or sedation and thus can be considered the same as for MRI in the following discussion.

Most MRI systems are superconducting magnets set up in a horizontal configuration within the bore so that the magnetic field is directed lengthwise to the child. The magnet is cooled by liquid nitrogen to a temperature of 39.2° F (4° C). The strength of the magnetic field in these scanners is described in tesla (T) units and range from 0.5 to 3.0 T. To put this into perspective, a 1.5-T magnet is the equivalent of 30,000 times the earth's magnetic field.

A variety of safety issues with respect to MRI are important, as mentioned in the earlier discussion of management of acute emergencies during anesthesia outside the OR. A useful review of these issues has been published by the American College of Radiology entitled "ACR Guidance Document for Safe MR Practices: 2007."[51] All individuals who work in the MR environment should be familiar with the primary recommendations in this paper.

First and foremost is the risk of injury from ferromagnetic objects that can become attracted to the magnetic core of

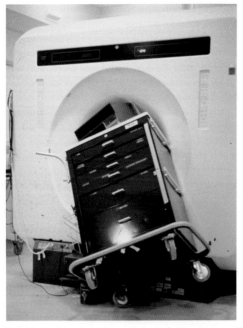

**FIGURE 45-5** Magnetic resonance imaging cart that is not compatible inadvertently brought into scanner room.

the MRI scanner and cause significant morbidity and mortality (Fig. 45-5). In the presence of an external magnetic field, a ferromagnetic object can develop its own intrinsic magnetic field. The attractive forces created between the intrinsic and extrinsic magnetic fields can propel the ferromagnetic object toward the MRI scanner. Numerous injuries have been reported from this mechanism. Objects that have been reported as accidentally attracted to the MRI magnet include a metal fan, pulse oximeter, shrapnel, wheelchair, cigarette lighter, stethoscope, pager, hearing aid, vacuum cleaner, calculator, hair pin, $O_2$ tank, prosthetic limb, pencil, insulin infusion pump, keys, watches, clipboards, and steel-toe or heeled shoes.[52,53] Mortality can result from projectile disasters, as in the case of a death in 2001 in which a ferrous $O_2$ tank was inadvertently brought into the MRI scanner after the wall $O_2$ source failed. The $O_2$ tank was "pulled" from the hands of the respiratory therapist and crushed the skull of the child being scanned (*New York Times,* July 31, 2001:B1, B5). It is absolutely essential that all portable $O_2$ tanks are MRI compatible and that anesthesia carts are not brought into the MRI. Many MRI scanner units now have screening protocols that include a small handheld magnet to test whether objects are ferromagnetic and thus at risk of being pulled into the magnet.

The other major potential morbidity related to MRI scanning results from implanted devices (i.e., cardiac pacemakers, spinal cord stimulators, programmable ventriculoperitoneal shunts) that may malfunction in the powerful magnetic field of the MRI scanner and can cause injury. These injuries are most often caused by inappropriate patient screening or unfamiliarity with a particular implant's MRI compatibility. Recently the U.S. Food and Drug Administration (FDA) changed the terminology for designating MRI safe objects from MRI-compatible and MRI-incompatible to MRI-safe, MRI-unsafe, and MRI-conditional (www.fda.gov/MedicalDevices/DeviceRegulationandGuidance/GuidanceDocuments/ucm107705.htm). This terminology will not be applied retrospectively to objects previously designated as MRI-non-compatible. *MRI-safe* is defined as not posing any known hazard in any MR environment. *MRI-conditional* refers

to objects that may or may not be safe, depending on the specific conditions that are present. Examples include a laryngoscope, cardiac occluder device (e.g., for closure of an atrial septal defect), halo vest, or cervical fixation device. *MRI-unsafe* means the object should never be brought into the MRI environment because it poses a potential or realistic risk or hazard.

All implanted objects should be carefully evaluated before a patient or health care provider enters the MRI suite. The website http://www.MRIsafety.com is a useful resource for identifying MRI-safe objects. Note that stainless steel or surgical stainless objects may interact with the external magnetic field, potentially resulting in translational (attractive) and rotational (torque) forces. Special attention should be paid to intracranial aneurysm clips (may move and potentially dislodge), vascular stents, cochlear and stapedial implants, shrapnel, intraorbital metallic bodies, and prosthetic limbs. In fact, some eye make-up and tattoos may contain metallic dyes and are at risk of causing skin, ocular, periorbital, and cutaneous irritation and burning.[54-56] Bivona (Smiths Medical, Dublin, Ohio) tracheostomy tubes pose a risk in the MRI environment because of the ferrous material within the tracheostomy tube. Bivona tracheostomy tubes are not FDA approved as MRI-compatible or MRI-safe. These tubes may produce rotational and translational motion on the tracheostomy tube itself, may create artifact on MRI images of the head or neck, and may create a thermal hazard from the heating of the ferrous elements in the magnetic environment. All Bivona tracheostomy tubes should be replaced with an MRI-safe tracheostomy tube or a tracheal tube until the FDA confirms otherwise.[57-58]

Cardiac pacemaker compatibility is a matter of some debate.[59] Historically, the presence of a pacemaker has been considered a contraindication for the MRI environment. Most pacemakers have a reed relay switch that can be activated when exposed to a strong magnetic field and convert the pacemaker to the asynchronous mode. In at least two known cases, patients with pacemakers died from cardiac arrest while in the MRI scanner.[57] Adverse events associated with pacemakers in the MRI scanner include ventricular fibrillation, rapid atrial pacing, asynchronous pacing, inhibition of pacing output, and movement of the device.[58,60]

Since 1996, however, changes in pacemaker electronics have included decreased ferromagnetic content and increased sophistication of the computer capabilities. In 2004, one study reported no changes in pacemaker capabilities or adverse outcomes after 56 patients with pacemakers underwent 62 MRI procedures.[61] Similar results were reported in 68 patients whose pacemakers were reprogrammed to asynchronous or demand mode before undergoing scans in a 1.5-T MRI scanner. Unfortunately, there is a paucity of data on children with pacemakers or implanted defibrillators who underwent MRI scans, particularly with respect to scanners with 3-T field strength. Extreme caution and consultation with local experts is advisable before administering sedation or anesthesia in children with pacemakers in these environments.

Auditory considerations exist with respect to MRI. Specifically, a loud banging sound and vibrations are produced as the forces generated within the gradient coils of the MRI scanner cause the gradient coils to vibrate. The noises generated range from 65 to 95 dB in a 1.5-T magnet. Cases have been reported of temporary hearing loss after an MRI scan.[62] This report suggests that earplugs may prevent the temporary hearing loss associated with MRI. Given these data, earplugs or MRI-compatible headphones are routinely used in children undergoing MRI scans.

Temperature regulation for children during sedation or analgesia for MRI has been the source of significant discussion and speculation. Cool temperatures and humidity are required for proper magnet function. These conditions are a setup for radiant and convective heat loss. Anesthesia limits intrinsic thermoregulation. On the other hand, the MRI generates radiofrequency radiation (RFR) that is absorbed by the child and may offset heat lost to the environment. The specific absorption rate (SAR) is measured in watts per kilogram and is used to follow the effects of RF heating. The FDA allows a SAR of 0.4 watts/kg averaged over the whole body.[63] Data suggest that children can increase their core body temperature by 0.5° C during MRI of less than 1 hour duration in a 1.5-T environment.[64,65] The temperature of infants who underwent MRI scans of the brain increased 0.2° C with a 1.5-T scanner and 0.5° C with a 3-T scanner, with minimal efforts to prevent passive heat loss.[66] Accordingly, it seems appropriate to minimize efforts to avoid passive heat loss in the MRI scanner and to monitor temperature in the 3-T environment particularly for long scans.

Focal heating remains a concern with respect to monitoring equipment in the MRI scanner. For example, the ECG leads should not have frays or exposed wires; *any coils or loops in a conductor such as ECG wires or a pulse oximeter probe can cause tissue burns* (Fig. 45-6). Cases of first-, second-, and third-degree burns after MRI have been reported.[67] To avoid patient injury, the following precautions should be taken: (1) Avoid creating a conductive loop between the child and a conductor (ECG monitoring or gating leads, plethysmographic gating wire, and fingertip attachment), (2) do not leave any unconnected imaging coils in the magnet during imaging, and (3) prevent all exposed wires or conductors from touching the child's skin during the scan.

Many MRI scans require contrast administration. Gadolinium (gadopentetate dimeglumine) is an FDA-approved contrast agent that is intravascularly administered for MRI enhancement. Approved for use in 1998, gadolinium provides greater contrast between normal and abnormal tissue throughout the body. Gadolinium forms a complex with chelating agents that facilitates biodistribution to the extracellular compartment and excretion via the kidneys. Unlike iodinated contrast agents, gadolinium complexes do not present a significant osmotic load. Gadolinium agents are considered to be safer than iodine agents with respect to adverse reactions. It is reportedly easily removed with dialysis.[68] On the other hand, recent warnings from the FDA suggest that gadolinium-containing contrast agents may be associated with the development of nephrogenic systemic fibrosis (NSF) or nephrogenic fibrosing dermopathy (NFD) in patients with moderate to end-stage kidney disease. The FDA suggests that gadolinium be administered only if necessary in children with advanced kidney failure and that, in those children, prompt dialysis be considered after gadolinium administration for MRA studies (http://www.fda.gov/Drugs/DrugSafety/DrugSafetyNewsletter/ucm142889.htm). The incidence of severe anaphylactic reactions to gadolinium is less than that of iodine-based contrast media. The incidence of severe anaphylactic or anaphylactoid reactions is 0.01% to 0.0003%.[69] Care must be taken to ensure the proper dose by weight and creatinine if renal function is compromised. Dosing estimates may be obtained from the following website based on the glomerular filtration rate: https://www.radiologyprotocols.com (free trials available for 1 month).

MRI-compatible equipment continues to be developed and improved. Multiple MRI-compatible anesthesia machines (with ventilators), monitors (including wireless models), and infusion pumps are now available. Unfortunately the cost for this equipment is substantial. An MRI-compatible anesthesia machine costs approximately $60,000, MRI-compatible monitors range up to $140,000, and compatible infusion pumps are $12,000 to $18,000. This cost may be overwhelming, especially in facilities with limited financial resources or limited need for MRI anesthetics. However, it is highly advisable for institutions to make the investment. If patient volume is not high enough or financial backing to support such an investment is lacking, then special planning may be instituted to deliver anesthesia without a full complement of MRI-compatible equipment. Specifically, a non–MRI-compatible anesthesia machine could be used in the following manner: the machine must be positioned outside the MRI suite, and 30 feet of parallel ventilator circuit (Bain Mapleson D) or circle system extension may be threaded through the appropriate-sized hole in the console wall to the child within. Alternatively, intravenous sedation or anesthesia can be delivered using MRI-compatible infusion pumps and $O_2$ can be delivered using a facemask or nasal cannula. If an MRI-compatible $ETCO_2$ monitor is not available, a conventional carbon dioxide ($CO_2$) monitor may be situated outside the MRI room and the 30-foot-long tubing threaded through the console wall in a similar fashion to attach to the child within.[66] If GETA is required without an MRI-compatible anesthesia machine, it is safer to anesthetize the child outside the scanner (anesthesia circuit threaded through the console wall and then back out the entrance door to an induction area), secure the airway, and then move the child into the scanner. Similarly, if propofol sedation is intended, the propofol infusion pump can also be situated outside the scanner and equipped with 30 feet of intravenous infusion tubing. It is important to determine whether the pump is able to infuse accurately through the resistance of the long tubing and that the caliber of the tubing is sufficiently large that the length of tubing required does not trigger the pump's high-pressure alarm. An Ambu bag or Mapleson circuit must always be situated in the MRI suite and connected directly to an $O_2$ source within the scanner. This is critical, especially when the anesthesia machine is far from the child.

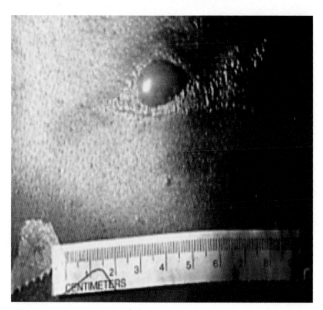

**FIGURE 45-6** Burn at site of electrocardiogram pad from a frayed lead.

MRI-safe stethoscopes, stylets, laryngoscope, and flashlights should be available. If they are not available, standard equipment can be used with some modification and testing. The only component of the laryngoscope that is usually *not* MRI-safe is the battery. Replacing the standard battery with a lithium battery may be a simple, safe, and less expensive alternative to purchasing a marketed MRI-compatible and safe laryngoscope. Before introducing any equipment into the MRI environment, a rudimentary safety check should be performed by first passing a handheld magnet over the object to confirm that there is no ferrous material within. As a final safety check, an MRI safety expert should carefully introduce the object into the scanner (before bringing in a child) to confirm safety.

Anesthetic management of children in the MRI suite depends to a large extent on the availability of support personnel and equipment, the anesthesiologist's personal anesthetic practice, and the child's medical history. In clinical practice, the choice of anesthetic varies greatly among anesthesiologists. Airway management may include an LMA, a tracheal tube, or a natural airway (with a roll placed under the shoulders). With an LMA or tracheal tube, either inhalational or intravenous anesthesia may be used to establish a motionless child. With a natural airway, only intravenous sedation or anesthesia with propofol or dexmedetomidine is commonly used.[7,70-75] ETCO$_2$ should be monitored; in the case of nasal prongs, a septate design that delivers O$_2$ (2 to 4 L/min) through one nostril while aspirating gas for CO$_2$ (capnometry) through the other allows for continuous assessment of respirations during spontaneous ventilation. If respiratory problems occur, immediate access to the airway is not possible while the child is in the bore of the scanner; for this reason, some anesthesiologists may prefer to insert an LMA or tracheal tube in all children. Most LMAs are MRI-compatible, although the pilot balloon should be taped to the circuit tubing when imaging the head or neck because it may create imaging artifacts (Figs. 45-7 and 45-8).

Few studies have directly compared general anesthesia with a controlled airway to intravenous sedation or anesthesia techniques during MRI. One randomized study of 200 children demonstrated no difference in airway complications between the two groups. However, more pauses occurred during scans (for movement, etc.) with propofol sedation, but much less agitation was experienced on emergence after the scan.[76] To ensure MRI scans without interruption in the majority of children, many begin with infusion rates of propofol 200 to 250 μg/kg/min in children and either maintain that infusion rate throughout or taper the infusion rate as described previously.[77] For younger children (infants) and children with severe cognitive dysfunction, infusion rates 20% to 50% greater than 250 mg/kg/min may be required to prevent movement during MRI scans. Other studies documented agitation[78] and prolonged nausea and vomiting[79] after MRI scans performed under general anesthesia with inhalation agents. Some MRI scans (cardiac, thoracic, or abdominal) require breath holding to obtain adequate images. In such cases, it is necessary to control the airway with an LMA or endotracheal tube and deliver general anesthesia. After reviewing the literature, insufficient evidence exists to recommend a particular anesthetic technique for MRI scans. Anesthesiologists still must consider their own practice environment and expertise, the demands of the scan itself, and the comorbidities of the particular child when selecting an anesthetic technique, particularly for children undergoing a cardiac MRI.

## INTERVENTIONAL RADIOLOGY AND INVASIVE ANGIOGRAPHY

Interventional radiology has evolved greatly in the last decade; many procedures that previously required operative treatment now can be accomplished with minimal intervention. In spite of the relatively little painful stimulation involved in most of these procedures, general anesthesia is often required particularly in children. Control of movement is often critical, and even the simplest procedures such as angiography often require a general anesthetic to ensure motionless conditions in children. In addition, many procedures require intermittent breath holding to acquire clear images. Furthermore, when the radiologist encounters vasospasm or needs to vasodilate arteries to enhance the images, the anesthesiologist may be requested to induce hypercarbia.

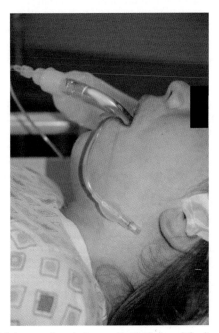

**FIGURE 45-7** Laryngeal mask airway with pilot balloon left adjacent to face.

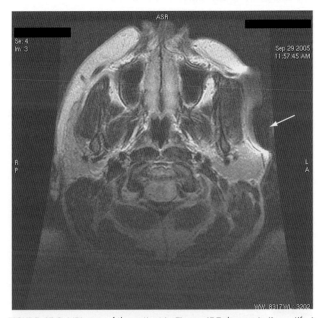

**FIGURE 45-8** MRI scan of the patient in Figure 45-7 demonstrating artifact (*arrow*) created by ferrous material in pilot balloon.

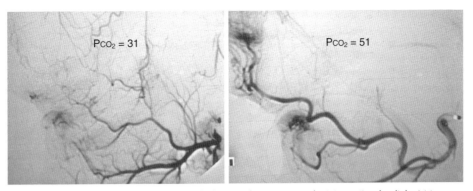

**FIGURE 45-9** Effect of hypercarbia on caliber of cerebral blood vessels; hypercarbia may assist the interventional radiologist to pass a catheter into small vessels (*right*).

Interventions involving the abdomen and pelvis have unique considerations; $N_2O$ can diffuse into the bowel, causing distention and, in some cases, distort or mask the vasculature of interest; it should be used with caution. In addition, when angiographic imaging of the abdomen is required, the interventional radiologist may request that the anesthesiologist administer intravenous glucagon, usually in 0.25-mg increments. Glucagon reduces peristalsis and, as a consequence, reduces motion artifact during image acquisition.[80] Glucagon has been reported to have side effects, including nausea, vomiting, hyperglycemia, depression of clotting factors, and electrolyte disturbances[70]; close monitoring is warranted, particularly in neonates and small infants.

Cerebral angiograms and interventions can be complex and carry significant risk. Cerebral studies may be indicated in the workup or postoperative follow-up of vascular malformation or tumor resections, stroke, hemorrhagic events, vascular disease, and unexplained mental status changes. These interventions typically require GETA to provide hypercarbia and breath holding. Hypercarbia to $ETCO_2$ values of 50 mm Hg or greater promote vasodilation to allow better access and visualization of cerebral vasculature (Fig. 45-9). During these cases, orogastric and nasogastric tubes, esophageal stethoscopes, and esophageal temperature probes should be used with caution because they may cause artifacts on the angiographic images.

Any child who requires a study for the potential or confirmed diagnosis of moyamoya disease should be treated with utmost precaution. These children should have an anesthetic that minimizes the risk of transient ischemic attacks and stroke during the procedure.[71] Anesthetic care should begin with the preinduction administration of 10 mL/kg of intravenous fluid to minimize the risk of hypotension (and potential cerebral ischemia) on induction of anesthesia. Hypocarbia should be avoided throughout and mild hypercarbia promoted. In the event of vasospasm or difficult access of small, tortuous vessels, locally administered (through the catheter) nitroglycerin in small doses (25 to 50 µg) may facilitate visualization and access. Although often effective for discretely vasodilating specific areas, nitroglycerin will generally not have a clinically important systemic effect on blood pressure. Consequently, intraarterial blood pressure monitoring usually is not required. Specific protocols have been suggested for minimizing perioperative strokes in these children.[72] Sedating the child before starting the intravenous line decreases crying and hyperventilation that can lead to cerebral ischemia. Close attention to postoperative pain control can similarly improve outcomes (see Chapter 24).

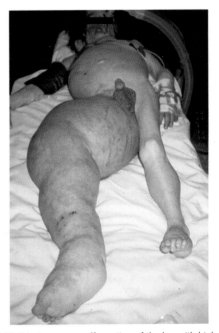

**FIGURE 45-10** Arteriovenous malformation of the leg with high output cardiac failure.

The anesthetic management of children with vascular malformations who present for embolization or sclerotherapy can be challenging. These lesions, although present at birth, are often discrete and not clearly visible. As the child grows, the vascular malformation may expand rapidly, growing with the child. In one review, only 18% of lesions presented before 15 years of age.[73] This rapid proliferative phase may occur in response to hormonal changes (pregnancy, puberty), trauma, or other stimuli. Vascular malformations may be classified as high-flow or low-flow lesions, depending on which vessels are involved. High-flow lesions may include arteriovenous fistulas, some large hemangiomas, and arteriovenous malformations. Symptoms of high-output cardiac failure predominate in the neonate, and symptoms of stroke, seizures, or hydrocephalus are more common in infants and older children.[73] The potential for pulmonary edema should be anticipated and assessed in the physical examination and past medical history (Fig. 45-10). Low-flow lesions consist of venous, intramuscular venous, and lymphatic malformations. Surgical resection of symptomatic vascular malformations may be hazardous, as well as unsuccessful—any vascular element that is not resected may enlarge and cause further problems. It is for this reason that invasive angiography and embolization is a popular alternative to surgical resection.

When embolizing vascular malformations, radiologists often strive to cut off the feeding vessels with agents such as ethanol, stainless steel coils, absorbable gelatin pledgets and powder, polyvinyl alcohol foam, glues, thread, and ethanol. The choice of agent depends on the clinical situation and the size of the blood vessel. Absolute ethanol (99.9% alcohol) is a powerful sclerosing agent that thromboses vessels even at the level of the capillary bed. It is particularly useful in the embolization of symptomatic vascular malformations. Ethanol causes thrombosis by injuring the vascular endothelium. Ethanol also denatures blood proteins. When permanent occlusion is the goal, polyvinyl alcohol foam and ethanol are often employed because they both occlude at the level of the arterioles and capillaries. Medium to small arteries may be occluded with coils, which are the equivalent of surgical ligation. In trauma situations, when only temporary (days) occlusion is the goal, absorbable gelatin pledgets or powder are employed.[74]

The embolization and sclerotherapy of vascular malformations usually requires a general anesthetic to ensure motionless conditions, especially during high-risk procedures that involve injection of a contrast agent and potentially painful sclerosants. These procedures require careful planning and discussion between the interventional radiologist and the anesthesiologist for safe airway management, intraprocedural and postprocedural care, and disposition. The anesthesiologist must have a basic understanding of the procedure and the risks involved. Some of the risks are inherent to the procedure and the agents used for embolization or sclerotherapy. Pulmonary emboli have been reported after these procedures as a result of the inadvertent migration of embolization material to the lungs. The incidence of pulmonary embolization after cerebral interventions has been reported to be as great as 35% in children after embolization or coiling.[75] Before each procedure, the anesthesiologist and radiologist should discuss the radiologist's specific requirements and concerns and decide on an anesthetic plan. Some procedures, especially embolizations of the head and neck, carry an increased risk of neurologic or cardiovascular complications.[81] It is important that the anesthesiologist anticipate these potential complications and modify the anesthetic technique to permit neurologic assessment soon after extubation.

The anesthesiologist should be familiar with the mechanism of action and potential risks associated with the various agents and devices used for embolization and sclerotherapy. All sclerosants produce local hemolysis when administered into the vascular bed. Large amounts of sclerosant, particularly sodium tetradecyl and ethanol, can cause hemoglobinuria, which can result in renal injury if the child is not adequately hydrated during and after the procedure.[82] Most children have a urine catheter placed to monitor the urine output, facilitate generous hydration, and monitor for hematuria. The anesthesiologist should generously hydrate the child with intravenous saline. On average, it has been our practice to administer as much as 50 mL/kg intravenous fluids over the course of the procedure. When hemoglobinuria is noted during the procedure, the anesthesiologist should notify the radiologist coincident with increasing the rate of fluid administration (Fig. 45-11). Hemoglobinuria may not occur until the end of the procedure, sometimes after a cumulative large dose of sclerosant has been administered or the tourniquet (if used) has been released. During procedures that

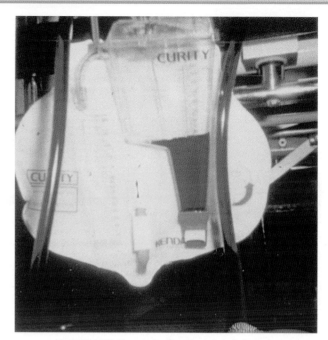

**FIGURE 45-11** Hematuria after ethanol embolization.

involve lower extremity lesions and tourniquets, hemoglobinuria can develop soon after the tourniquet is released. Promoting diuresis with furosemide 0.5 to 1 mg/kg helps resolve gross hematuria. Occasionally, hemoglobinuria develops 1 to 2 hours after the procedure, usually while in the postanesthesia care unit. It is important to carefully balance fluid administered with urine output. In the event of persistent hemoglobinuria, sodium bicarbonate 75 mEq/L in $D_5W$ may be administered at two times maintenance rate to alkalinize the urine and minimize precipitation of hemoglobin in the renal tubules.[8]

Administering ethanol to sclerose a vascular malformation has the potential for severe complications.[83] The most infrequent but serious risk is cardiovascular collapse, which is generally preceded by hypoxemia and bradycardia. Most reported cases of cardiovascular collapse involved lower extremity malformations.[84] The cause of the cardiovascular collapse associated with ethanol is unclear, although it is reported to occur uniquely when there is direct release of ethanol into the systemic veins. Collapse can occur after release of tourniquets in extremities that have been injected with ethanol. It is critical that the radiologist communicate with the anesthesiologist whenever ethanol is being injected, as well as before the deflation of the tourniquet. It has been recommended that any child at significant risk of systemic ethanol egress should have a pulmonary artery catheter placed before the procedure to identify changes in pulmonary artery pressure that might herald electromechanical dissociation. Significant increases in pulmonary artery pressure resulting from pulmonary vasoconstriction necessitate interrupting the administration of ethanol until the pressure normalizes. Significant fluctuations in vital signs include an increase in pulmonary artery pressure, a decrease in systemic blood pressure, decrease in $ETCO_2$, or $O_2$ saturation, cardiac arrhythmias, or full cardiac arrest.

Ethanol can produce a state of intoxication. The ethanol used for embolization and sclerotherapy is 95% to 98% pure. Children who receive greater than 0.75 mL/kg can become clinically intoxicated. Blood levels correlate with the volume of ethanol administered, regardless of the location or type of vascular malformation

(Fig. 45-12). On extubation, these children display either significant agitation or excessive sedation and analgesia; opioids should be administered with caution because they have a synergistic effect with ethanol and potentially cause unwanted respiratory depression. It is generally advisable to administer minimal or no opioids until the child is extubated and confirms the presence of pain. Ketorolac may be administered intravenously after soliciting the agreement of the radiologist, removing the invasive catheters, and ensuring hemostasis has been achieved.

Children with vascular malformations, especially venous malformations, can have preexisting coagulation disturbances that resemble disseminated intravascular coagulation.[85] Children with laboratory indices consistent with preexisting consumptive coagulopathy should have a hematology consultation and, if possible, receive heparin for 2 weeks before the procedure to replenish their fibrinogen levels. The anesthesiologist may be asked to

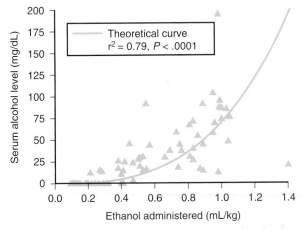

Serum Alcohol Levels

FIGURE 45-12 Positive relationship between serum ethanol level and amount of ethanol administered. (From Mason KP, Michna E, Zurakowski D, Koka BV, Burrows PE. Serum ethanol levels in children and adults after ethanol embolization or sclerotherapy for vascular anomalies. Radiology 2000;217:127-32.)

administer cryoprecipitate or platelets during the procedure to promote clotting and successful sclerosis. The use of ethanol for sclerosis or embolization can also elicit a coagulation disturbance that resembles disseminated intravascular coagulation. There is a statistical relationship between the amount of ethanol administered and the degree of coagulation disturbance elicited.[86] Additional cryoprecipitate or fresh frozen plasma transfusions are given only in severe cases, because the coagulopathy is generally not symptomatic and resolves within 5 days. However, major surgery should be deferred until the coagulation parameters have normalized.

It is important to be aware of the potential morbidity associated with embolization procedures. Type and crossmatch should be performed for all children scheduled for embolization in anticipation of possible major hemorrhage. Embolization therapy has been associated with multiple potentially devastating outcomes, including stroke, cerebral abscess, bleeding, cyanosis, and pulmonary embolism.[87] Postprocedural mortality is reported to be 5% to 6%.[88] It is important to document full return of neurologic status after the child recovers and the trachea is extubated. Vascular malformations involving the airway are particularly challenging (Fig. 45-13). The anesthesiologist and radiologist should review the imaging studies (usually MRI) before the procedure. The scans should be evaluated for patency of the nares, nasopharynx, hypopharynx, and oropharynx, as well as for an uncompromised trachea, carina, and bronchi. MRI will also confirm that there is no malformation in the nares or nasopharynx, which could be damaged or bleed during intubation. Most interventional radiology suites are not situated in the OR. If there is any potential for airway compromise, difficulty in attaining a mask airway, or failure to intubate, the airway should be secured in the OR before transport to the radiology suite. In general, an otolaryngologist or another specialist skilled in bronchoscopy and tracheotomy should be present in the OR prepared to perform bronchoscopy (fiberoptic or rigid) or tracheostomy should the airway be lost.

If postsclerotherapy edema and vascular congestion involving the airway structures are anticipated, the child's trachea should be intubated nasally and remain intubated for 48 hours or

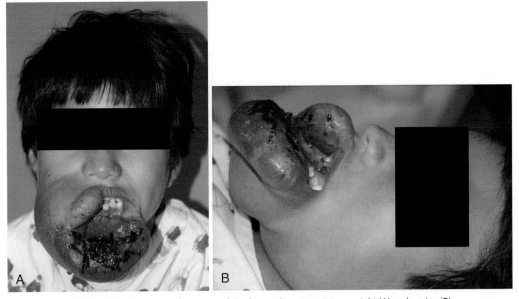

FIGURE 45-13 Venous malformation of the face with patient sitting upright (**A**) and supine (**B**).

until the swelling subsides. Nasal intubation is preferred to minimize the risk of dislodging the tracheal tube or premature extubation. The decision to have the child remain intubated postoperatively is usually made before the start of the procedure, after the anesthesiologist and radiologist review the MR images together. If the trachea remains intubated postoperatively, the trachea is extubated in the intensive care unit after the presence of an air leak around the tracheal tube is confirmed or a flexible nasal fiberoptic view of the airway can be performed at the bedside. If there is any doubt about the patency or self-sufficiency of the airway, these children should be transferred to the OR for tracheal extubation in a controlled setting with an otolaryngologist present.

Venous malformations involving the head, neck, or airway structures typically swell with dependency or Valsalva maneuver (e.g., crying). Before extubating the trachea, these children should be positioned head-up to promote venous drainage and reduce swelling. Efforts should be made to minimize coughing before tracheal extubation. In the event of respiratory compromise, venous malformations can enlarge when the child coughs, increases intrathoracic pressure, or uses accessory muscles. Attempts at reintubation, cricoid pressure, head extension, and mask ventilation can further enlarge the malformation. Mask ventilation can be challenging, sometimes impossible, if the malformation is swollen and firm. Achieving an occlusive mask seal is particularly difficult when there is swelling of the cheek, tongue, lip, chin, or nares. Venous malformations of the lips and tongue, because of their blue color, can make it difficult to assess the child for hypoxemia in the event of respiratory distress. Reintubation can become impossible in these situations because all of the maneuvers to achieve a mask seal increase venous pressure and swelling. When attempting to reintubate the trachea of a child with intraoral or pharyngeal malformations, special care should be taken to avoid damaging the malformation: even a small nick can create significant bleeding. In the event of oropharyngeal bleeding and inability to mask ventilate and/or intubate, it is critical to have alternative airway devices immediately available. LMAs in particular can be lifesaving. Proper insertion and inflation of the LMA can secure an airway and, more importantly, tamponade bleeding. However, because the LMA rests above the vocal cords, it does not protect the airway from pulmonary aspiration.

## INTRAVASCULAR CONTRAST MEDIA

The use of intravascular contrast media is ubiquitous in interventional radiology and cardiac catheterization. It is important that the anesthesiologist be aware of the risks and potential side effects of these agents. Almost all life-threatening reactions occur immediately or within 20 minutes of contrast agent administration. Low-osmolality ionic and nonionic contrast media are associated with a reduced incidence of adverse events, especially non–life-threatening events compared with high-osmolality contrast media. Serious contrast reactions are estimated at 1 to 2 per 1000 studies using high-osmolality contrast media versus 1 to 2 per 10,000 studies with low osmolality contrast media.[89,90] Adverse reactions include nausea, vomiting, hypotension, urticaria, bronchospasm, anxiety, chills, fever, facial flushing, seizures, pulmonary edema, and cardiovascular collapse. Anaphylactic shock is the most worrisome of all contrast reactions and may occur as early as 1 minute and as late as several hours after administration of the contrast material. Although adverse reactions to intravascular contrast media are unpredictable, some risk factors are identifiable. These include children who suffer from allergies or an atopic disease, children with asthma, significant cardiovascular disease, and paraproteinemia, and children with prior contrast reactions have an increased incidence of adverse reactions.[91] Children who have been identified as being at increased risk of a contrast reaction should be premedicated with corticosteroids and antihistamines. The American College of Radiology suggests that corticosteroid premedication, along with low osmolality contrast media, should be used for those at risk.[91,92]

Because the contrast agent is hypertonic relative to plasma, attention needs to be paid to the risk of a triphasic response: initial but transient (30 to 60 seconds) hypotension, followed by hypertension as the contrast material draws fluid intravascularly, followed by a hyperosmotic diuresis with the potential for hypotension. Equilibration with the extracellular fluid compartment occurs within 10 minutes, heralded by the onset of diuresis. For this reason, special attention should be paid when administering iodine contrast to any child with a history of congestive heart failure. The initial increase in blood volume may precipitate cardiovascular compromise. Renal failure from contrast media can occur with high- and low-osmolality contrast media. Although the cause of the acute renal failure is not known, risk factors include preexisting renal insufficiency (serum creatine 1.5 mg/dL or greater), diabetes mellitus, dehydration, cardiovascular disease, hypertension, and hyperuricemia. For these at-risk children, good hydration must be maintained, along with careful follow-up of renal function.[93] It should be noted that those with paraproteinemias (multiple myeloma, Waldenström macroglobulinemia) are predisposed to irreversible renal failure from protein precipitation in renal tubules, which is preventable with proper hydration.[94]

## ENDOSCOPIC PROCEDURES

Gastrointestinal endoscopy is a common procedure for pediatric gastroenterologists. Both upper and lower endoscopies involve significant stimulation, which requires deep sedation or general anesthesia in infants and children. A range of sedation and anesthesia options may be used for both simple[95,96] and more complex procedures such as foreign body removal, endoscopic retrograde cholangiopancreatography (ERCP), and percutaneous endoscopic gastrostomy (PEG) placement.[97] The choice of deep sedation versus general anesthesia (with or without a tracheal tube) depends on the medical condition of the child, the risks associated with the specific procedure, and the anticipated duration. Upper esophagogastroduodenoscopy (EGD) in infants (less than 10 kg) generally requires tracheal intubation to avoid airway compression caused by the endoscope pressing the trachealis muscle into the trachea. However, few definitive data exist on this issue (few studies include infants less than 1 year of age). At Dartmouth Hitchcock Medical Center, we have found that if the endoscopist is willing to use the smallest available pediatric scopes, successful sedation or anesthesia without a tracheal tube is possible for infants as small as 6 to 7 kg. In some cases an LMA may be used to secure the airway and the cuff deflated to allow passage of the endoscope and then reinflated once the scope has entered the esophagus. It is advised to hold on to either a tracheal tube or an LMA during the procedure to reduce the risk of the endoscopist dislodging it during their manipulations.

Many techniques may be employed successfully to maintain adequate conditions for upper and lower gastrointestinal endoscopy. Although all anesthesia-delivery areas must meet ASA standards, scavenging and ventilation in endoscopy suites may not always be effective in allowing the safe use of inhalational anesthetics. In these cases, total intravenous anesthesia can substitute for potent inhalation agents.[98-100] Over the last several years, various combinations of intravenous agents have been described for the delivery of sedation and anesthesia in the endoscopy suite for children. As a general rule, propofol is used either alone,[101] in combination with an opioid (fentanyl or remifentanil),[102,103] or with ketamine.[104] Outcomes after deep sedation or anesthesia with propofol and inhalational anesthesia were similar.[99] However, the time to awakening was more rapid after the inhalational anesthetic, the incidence of agitation on emergence was less, and the time to hospital discharge earlier after propofol.

Access to the airway is obviously limited once a transoral endoscope is in place. The two most stimulating portions of the esophagogastroduodenoscopy are transoral and transpyloric passage of the endoscope. After endoscope insertion, the sedation or anesthesia can often be reduced without adverse effect on the procedure conditions. Smooth insertion of the endoscope can be aided by topical spray of local anesthesia to the oropharynx to reduce the discomfort of passing the endoscope and to prevent coughing and gagging. For older children, topicalization of the oropharynx can be accomplished before sedation and the child can position himself or herself for the gastroenterologist (lateral position). Sedation can be subsequently accomplished with the child prepositioned. For cases performed without tracheal intubation, a $CO_2$ sampling nasal cannula can be placed and used over the nose or near the mouth (for those who do not breath through the nose) to supplement $O_2$ and allow a monitor of respiration.

Upper endoscopies have the inherent risk of apnea, laryngospasm, bronchospasm, and airway obstruction. Most problems resolve after withdrawal of the endoscope and positive-pressure ventilation with a face mask.[105] In rare situations, tracheal intubation may be required to complete the procedure or resolve an airway issue. In young infants, abdominal distention secondary to air introduced into the stomach may impair diaphragmatic excursion, leading to hypoventilation. Little published evidence exists on which to base age-related practice in endoscopy sedation and analgesia, experience led several groups to select all infants up to 6 months of age as the age interval for which general anesthesia with tracheal intubation is required, because of a greater frequency of respiratory complications.[95,96] When extubating the tracheas in these infants, be wary that residual air in the stomach can impair effective ventilation and contribute to desaturation or $O_2$ dependence in the recovery room. Thus it is important to remind the endoscopist to suction any residual air from the stomach before removing the endoscope.

Few large studies have reported outcomes after pediatric gastrointestinal endoscopy. The Clinical Outcomes Research Initiative (CORI) is a national registry of endoscopic procedures that was started in 1995. The PEDS-CORI is the pediatric component that was started in 1999. A 2007 report collected the complications from pediatric upper endoscopy involving 10,236 encounters from 13 different institutions over 4 years.[106] Overall, there was a 2.3% incidence of complications (of any kind). Of these, 79.9% were cardiopulmonary, 18% were gastrointestinal complications, and 5.9% were other complications, including prolonged sedation, drug reactions, or rash. Not surprisingly, children who developed complications were younger and had a greater ASA physical status. General anesthesia was associated with a reduced overall complication rate (1.2%) compared with that in the IV

sedation group (3.7%). Although these data were not controlled or randomized, it does shed some insight into the complication rates associated with pediatric sedation outside the OR.

## Summary

As the need for anesthesia services for children outside the OR continues to expand, anesthesiologists will be more frequently called on to provide anesthesia services for this venue. It is in our patients' interests and our own professional interest to accept this responsibility and provide the most effective, efficient, and safe anesthesia and sedation and anesthesia outside of the OR. Each site and procedure may pose particular anesthetic implications and challenges. It remains important that a core group of anesthesiologists become familiar with these challenges and that they communicate amongst each other and with the proceduralists with whom they work. The anesthetic configuration and equipment demands may be unique at each center. Emergency situations should be role-played in advance so that all personnel are familiar with the location of code equipment and emergency airway equipment. All morbid conditions and untoward events should be reviewed regularly to make improvements and implement any changes in practice. Working in the areas outside the OR can be rewarding and challenging and should be approached with a commitment to ensure that children will receive a standard of care that is equal to the care provided in the OR.

**ACKNOWLEDGMENT**
We wish to thank Leira P. Mason and Babu V. Koka for their prior contributions to this chapter.

## ANNOTATED REFERENCES

Coté CJ, Wilson S. Guidelines for monitoring and management of pediatric patients during and after sedation for diagnostic and therapeutic procedures: an update. Pediatrics 2006;118:2587-602.

*The most recent American Academy of Pediatrics sedation guideline, this is a landmark paper because it was jointly published by the American Academy of Pediatric Dentistry. Many new recommendations have been added to improve the safety net of medical supervision during and after procedural sedation.*

Cravero JP, Beach ML, Blike GT, et al. The incidence and nature of adverse events during pediatric sedation/anesthesia with propofol for procedures outside the operating room: a report from the Pediatric Sedation Research Consortium. Anesth Analg 2009;108:795-804.

*This is the largest study to date that examines the side effects and adverse events associated with the use of propofol for sedation of children during procedures outside the operating room.*

Kanal E, Borgstede JP, Barkovich AJ, et al. American College of Radiology White Paper on MR Safety: 2004 update and revisions. AJR Am J Roentgenol 2004;182:1111-4.

*Updated paper details the standards and recommendations for providing safe patient care in the MR environment.*

Shellock FG, Crues JV. MR procedures: biologic effects, safety, and patient care. Radiology 2004;232:635-52.

*This detailed article reviews the biologic effects and important safety issues in delivering safe patient care in the MR environment.*

## REFERENCES

Please see www.expertconsult.com.

**45**

# The Postanesthesia Care Unit and Beyond

# 46

ANDREAS H. TAENZER AND JEANA E. HAVIDICH

CHILDREN'S RECOVERY FROM ANESTHESIA is substantively different from that of adults. Although both age groups share the key elements of regaining consciousness, controlling pain, and maintaining a patent airway, the nature and timing of these elements are different. In young children, emergence from inhalational agents can be quite rapid because of the increased minute ventilation, increased blood flow to the vessel-rich group (see Chapter 6), and decreased total body muscle and fat stores, whereas emergence from intravenous agents in infants may be delayed because of decreased clearance as a result of reduced liver blood flow and enzyme activity. The quality of the emergence is different in children and adults because agitation (i.e., emergence delirium) after sevoflurane and desflurane is more common in young children than in adults. The criteria used to evaluate emergence from anesthesia or sedation must be consistent with the developmental level of the child. The nature and rapidity of complications that can occur during emergence require careful planning and anticipation of problems. Parents should be considered partners and active participants in effective postoperative management.

The environment in the pediatric postanesthesia care unit (PACU) is unique and challenging. The staff and facility of any institution in which children recover after surgery must understand these challenges and be prepared to manage children through the difficult process of emerging from the anesthetized state to the new reality of postoperative consciousness. Early admission of parents to PACU and use of rocking chairs to permit parents to comfort their children is a common means of facilitating recovery.

## Perioperative Environment

The ideal perioperative environment is one that combines aspects of safety, ergonomics, and comfort for the child, family, and caregivers. The environment should be child specific and staffed by experts in child care. This should start with the admission process and conclude with the discharge to home or the hospital ward. Ideally, a child should be under the care of the same team throughout his or her hospital stay. For example, the child can be admitted by the nurse who will later take care of the child and the family in the PACU. In some hospitals, this is achieved by creating an integrated perioperative environment, in which children are admitted, prepared, and allowed to recover in the same space, with the same nurses and child life specialist. Familiarity with personnel and surroundings is a great stress reliever for children and families; it also fosters trust and comfort.

Privacy and shelter from noise is an important aspect of the setup. The ability to spend time with the child without being disturbed is something that many families appreciate, and this helps the child to deal with the stress of a strange environment. Most modern PACUs have moved to individual patient rooms or cubicles for preoperative and postoperative care, similar to a typical pediatric intensive care unit (PICU).

Equipment (Table 46-1) and available medications (Tables 46-2 and 46-3) should be standardized throughout the unit and be compatible with transport monitors and other devices used in corresponding high care facilities (e.g., PICU). An important safety precaution is the use of preprinted weight-based emergency drug doses for each child; these rapid reference sheets can be attached to each child's bed or chart on admission so that a quick dose recommendation is readily available. Alternatively, the electronic record should have precalculated emergency drug doses for each child. This practice may also reduce the risk of drug errors in an emergency situation.

Nurses, residents, fellows, attending physicians, and other personnel working in the perioperative area should be competent in the provision of neonatal and pediatric advanced life support.

Opioids are indicated during the immediate postoperative period for any procedure in which moderate or severe pain is not being managed by other means. Morphine, fentanyl, and hydromorphone have a long history of safe use for infants and children in the PACU. Repeated doses of meperidine are not recommended for children because of the potential for seizures from epileptogenic metabolites (e.g., normeperidine).[99] Opioid dosing should be initiated according to body weight, physiologic development, underlying medical or surgical conditions, coadministered medications, and severity of pain. The goal should be effective and rapid pain relief. Subsequent dosing of the medications should be titrated based on response to the initial dose. Administration of multiple, small, ineffective doses results in prolongation of pain, stress, and anxiety without improving the safety of care provided. With this caveat in mind, patient-controlled analgesia and patient-controlled epidural analgesia (see Chapters 41 and 43) may be used in the PACU environment, but either intervention should be started only after acute pain has been adequately treated. The small doses administered by patient-controlled analgesia typically are not adequate to completely treat acute postoperative pain and may add to a sense that the method is not working for a given child.[100]

Regional analgesia is a common mode of intraoperative pain control in the child that extends into the PACU (see Chapters 41 to 43). The PACU personnel need to know how well it is working, and this assessment can be approached in a systematic manner.

The regional block should be placed in a manner that provides analgesia for the surgical incision site and visceral pain. Evidence that the regional block is effective should first be detected during surgery. If the regional block is effective, the anesthetic requirements are usually reduced. For instance, a caudal block is not effective for a midabdominal incision unless the catheter has been threaded to the region of the incision or relatively large volumes of local anesthetic have been administered. The addition of hydrophilic opioids or clonidine may extend the level of analgesia to some extent over the course of several hours; however, a block that is many dermatome segments away from the site of the surgical incision is unlikely to remain adequate for long. The addition of opioids to an epidural or spinal block increases the risk of pruritus, urinary retention, and emesis. Similarly, visceral pain such as bladder spasms (which have thoracic innervation) or the sore throat after intubation are not attenuated by a lumbar epidural catheter and must be managed by other measures.[101]

The anesthesiologist must verify that the catheter is in the epidural space. Older children can be questioned about their sensation level using ice or other cold sensation to determine the level of sympathectomy. Preverbal or developmentally disabled patients require some other objective form of confirmation. Previous reports have focused on electrical stimulation through the epidural catheter at the time of catheter placement to determine the level of insertion.[102] Ultrasound methods for detecting epidural catheter placement have been described.[103] Perhaps most practical in the PACU may be radiographic confirmation of the dermatome level of the tip of the catheter, often with the use of an appropriate contrast material (i.e., epidurogram) to ensure appropriate placement in the epidural space.[104,105] A small amount (<1 mL) of contrast (e.g., Omnipaque 180 or 240) can be infused into the catheter while one radiograph is taken to confirm placement (see Fig. 41-7).[105]

## TEMPERATURE MANAGEMENT

Intraoperative normothermia is key to maintaining a normal temperature postoperatively. Hypothermia is associated with discomfort, bleeding, infections, altered metabolism of drugs, delayed return of cognitive functions, and prolonged recovery.[106-110] Because about 90% of heat loss occurs through the skin, only heat exchange through the skin provides an adequate way of warming children. This method of warming is enhanced by the vasodilation properties of most anesthetic agents. Forced-air warming blankets are the most effective way of maintaining body temperature in children.[111] Given the vasoconstriction that occurs after anesthesia, attempts at warming are less effective postoperatively than intraoperatively, and most of the detrimental physiologic changes have already taken place. A growing body of literature documents the detrimental effects of hypothermia and shows that it is best when children arrive in the PACU with a normal body temperature.

Infants and children may suffer burns from overly aggressive rewarming measures. This is particularly true for nonverbal children, children who are somnolent, and children who have decreased sensation due to disease or use of regional anesthesia techniques. Recommendations from manufacturers and recent literature should be carefully reviewed before instituting routine use of warming devices.

## DISCHARGE CRITERIA

The recovery process and discharge criteria vary from institution to institution. Various criteria are used to determine readiness for discharge from the PACU. Some institutions require an assessment by a physician before discharge for all patients, but others require an evaluation only if routine discharge criteria are not met. The modified Aldrete scale is the most common system used to assess discharge readiness, but specific criteria depend on the particular situation or environment to which the child will be discharged. For example, a child with a slight degree of postextubation croup or stridor may be discharged for monitoring on a pediatric floor or ICU, but the same child is not discharged to parental care and a 2-hour drive home. The criteria for discharge of children to a general inpatient setting are summarized in Table 46-6. For outpatients, these criteria hold, and the additional criteria outlined in Table 46-7 usually must be met before discharge.

Traditionally, pediatric patients have been allowed to recover in a first-stage recovery unit until the airway was considered stable, consciousness is regained, baseline motor activity is

---

**TABLE 46-6** Discharge Criteria for Inpatients

1. Recovery of airway and respiratory reflexes adequate to support gas exchange and to protect against aspiration of secretions, vomitus, or blood
2. Stability of circulation and control of any surgical bleeding
3. Absence of anticipated instability in criteria 1 and 2
4. Reasonable control of pain and vomiting
5. Appropriate duration of observation after opioid or naloxone flumazenil administration (minimum of 60 minutes after intravenous naloxone and up to 2 hours after flumazenil)
6. Return to baseline level of consciousness unless transfer is to an intensive care unit environment

received a single dose of dexamethasone (0.15 to 1 mg/kg) were two times less likely to vomit after tonsillectomy and adenoidectomy than those who did not receive dexamethasone.[77,78] In a randomized, prospective dose-finding study of dexamethasone administered to children undergoing tonsillectomy, there was no difference in the incidence of vomiting after prophylactic doses of dexamethasone between 0.0625 and 1.0 mg/kg (see Fig. 31-5)[79]; a similar trial has not been conducted in the PACU for children who are already vomiting. Before the black box warning was added for droperidol, it was also recommended for prophylaxis of PONV in the United States,[80] but for medicolegal reasons alone, it is no longer a first-tier antiemetic. Droperidol is commonly used in low doses, which limit extrapyramidal and sedation side effects.

Adequate fluid resuscitation plays in important role in PONV prevention. Children given 10 mL/kg of lactated Ringer's solution during strabismus correction had more PONV than those given 30 mL/kg (54% versus 22%).[81]

The most effective prophylaxis strategy in children at moderate or high risk for PONV is to use combination therapy that includes hydration, a 5-HT$_3$ receptor antagonist, and a second drug such dexamethasone. Antiemetic rescue therapy should be administered to children who vomit after surgery. An emetic episode more than 6 hours postoperatively can be treated with any of the drugs used for prophylaxis except dexamethasone and transdermal scopolamine.[82]

### Rescue Therapy

The consensus panel recommends that children who did not receive intraoperative prophylaxis or those who fail prophylaxis should receive a 5-HT$_3$ receptor antagonist at the first signs of PONV.[69] The recommended dose should be one fourth of that used for prophylaxis. For all other therapies, the data on efficacy for rescue are sparse, and doses are unknown. In adults, promethazine and droperidol have been as effective as ondansetron in the general surgical population, but comparable studies have not been conducted in children. The sedative properties of promethazine may last for many hours and may be a problem for patients with OSA.

### Alternative Treatments

Alternative methods for nausea and vomiting prophylaxis deserve consideration. Isopropyl alcohol reduces PONV, although the effect is transient.[83] In a meta-analysis of alternative antinausea and vomiting techniques, acupuncture, electroacupuncture, transcutaneous electrical nerve stimulation, acupoint stimulation, and acupressure each exert antiemetic effects compared with placebo in adults, but not in children.[84]

## Postoperative Care and Discharge

### PAIN MANAGEMENT IN THE POSTANESTHESIA CARE UNIT

Acute postoperative pain management strategies are discussed in detail in Chapter 43. A child's level of pain (or the perception of pain) changes more rapidly in the PACU than in any other unit of the hospital. Frequent and consistent use of pain scores for children of all ages, including those with developmental disabilities, is essential. Many pain scales have been validated for use in children. More important than the specific scale employed, the scale should be used consistently and follow simple principles. For instance, children who are verbal and developmentally appropriate should be encouraged to describe their pain using a self-report scale (e.g., Oucher scale). Young children or those without verbal skills should be assessed using an objective pain behavior scale (e.g., Face, Legs, Activity, Cry, Consolability [FLACC] scale).[85,86] Just as important is the consistent application of protocols to treat pain; treatment of a given pain level should not vary from shift to shift or from one nurse to another.[87]

As with other areas of pediatric pain control, a multimodal approach to postoperative pain is recommended. A plan for pain management should be discussed among the family, surgical team, and anesthesia team before surgery.[88] Depending on the surgery, the plan may include any or all of the following: acetaminophen, nonsteroidal agents, local anesthesia, nerve blocks, regional anesthesia, clonidine, opioids, patient-controlled analgesia, and patient-controlled epidural analgesia.

Acetaminophen and nonsteroidal drugs act through inhibition of prostaglandins and their metabolites. Most of these drugs are given orally and should be given preoperatively or intraoperatively to be effective in the PACU. Occasionally, they may be indicated in the PACU if they were not administered before arrival. Oral acetaminophen (15 mg/kg) or ibuprofen (10 mg/kg) has been shown to decrease opioid requirements by 20% to 30% after a variety of surgical procedures. Intravenous acetaminophen has become available in the United States for children 2 years of age or older, and it is likely to become a popular analgesic for mild to moderate pain in the PACU and as an opioid-sparing drug.[89,90] The U.S. Food and Drug Administration (FDA) has approved the use of intravenous acetaminophen for children 2 years or older for the treatment of mild to moderate pain or fever. The intravenous dose of 15 mg/kg every 6 hours is recommended for patients weighing less than 50 kg and should be administered over 15 minutes.[91] Studies on intravenous formulations of propacetamol and paracetamol have mostly been conducted in the European Union since drug approval in 2002. Several randomized, controlled studies and meta-analyses have demonstrated efficacy of intravenous administration in adults and children for the treatment of mild to moderate pain or fever.[92,93] It is effective as an adjuvant to other analgesic modalities for moderate to severe pain.[94]

Acetaminophen can also be given rectally in doses of 35 to 45 mg/kg; however, because absorption varies and is delayed (i.e., peak concentration at 60 to 180 minutes after rectal administration), this route is not recommended for use in the PACU.[95] Because of the pharmacokinetics of the rectal route, a greater interval (6 hours) between doses is recommended, and subsequent doses are reduced (20 mg/kg) so that the total dose per 24 hours does not exceed 100 mg/kg.[96] There are no data to provide guidance for rectal acetaminophen beyond 24 hours. If a child has received rectal acetaminophen, the first oral dose should be delayed until 6 hours after the rectal dose.

The nonsteroidal antiinflammatory drug ketorolac can decrease opioid requirements by approximately 30%. The recommended dosage is 0.2 to 0.5 mg/kg, which is given intravenously every 6 hours.[97] Caution is warranted in postoperative children with significant bleeding or a history of renal insufficiency. The manufacturer recommends limiting the total doses to 15 mg for children weighing less than 50 kg and to 30 mg for children weighing more than 50 kg.[98]

vary with the duration of anesthesia and the coadministered medications. Differences in the times to discharge from the PACU and the hospital between inhalational agents are even more difficult to detect when specific comparisons are made because so many other factors, such as pain management, agitation, availability of hospital beds, and family circumstances, affect discharge readiness.

The age of the child exerts a minimal influence on the washout of inhalational anesthetic agents and has little impact on the rapidity of emergence, although age may be a factor for infants younger than 1 year of age.[4] However, the overall clinical implications of age-related differences in emergence are exceedingly difficult to detect.[5] The speed of emergence correlates more closely with the duration of anesthesia. The greater the duration of anesthesia, the more the tissue compartments become filled with these anesthetics and the more time it takes to eliminate these anesthetics and for the child to recover. For example, emergence from 30 minutes of sevoflurane anesthesia is significantly faster than emergence from 2 hours of anesthesia, which is more rapid than from 8 hours of anesthesia.[6] This relationship between emergence time and the duration of anesthesia has less relevance as inhalational anesthetics have become less soluble (e.g., desflurane).

Emergence from intravenous agents can vary significantly from that of inhalational agents. Several studies have evaluated the quality and rapidity of emergence after intravenous anesthetic agents compared with that after inhalational agents. For outpatient surgery, emergence after propofol anesthesia is as rapid as that after sevoflurane but with far less agitation and pain behaviors.[7,8] The recovery characteristics of propofol with remifentanil total intravenous anesthesia have been compared with those after desflurane inhalational anesthesia. Recovery is as rapid as that after desflurane with nitrous oxide, with a similar incidence of nausea and vomiting but with much less agitation.[9]

Midazolam is rarely used for maintenance of anesthesia but is often used as an oral or intravenous premedication for anxiolysis and amnesia in the preinduction period. There is evidence that the addition of midazolam in the preinduction period to an inhalational or propofol anesthetic may delay early emergence after brief anesthesia. However, this effect of midazolam is attenuated after anesthesia of greater duration, or when considering late emergence, this effect is minimal.[10] Midazolam does not affect the incidence of postoperative agitation.[11,12]

## EMERGENCE AGITATION OR DELIRIUM

Emergence agitation (i.e., emergence delirium [Videos 46-1 and 46-2]) was first described in a large cohort of postsurgical patients

almost 40 years ago.[13] From a clinical perspective, it is often impossible to differentiate pure agitation from delirium. Delirium implies a specific set of thought disorders and hallucinations based on the American Psychiatric Association's *Diagnostic and Statistical Manual of Mental Disorders,* 4th edition (DSM-IV). Despite numerous investigations, differentiating emergence delirium from postoperative pain has also proved difficult. Emergence delirium usually manifests as thrashing, disorientation, crying, and screaming. The child is unable to recognize parents, familiar objects, or surroundings; is inconsolable; and talks irrationally during early emergence from anesthesia. Emergence delirium occurs more often in children (rate of 10% to 20%) than in adults, particularly in those younger than 6 years of age.[14,15] It may in part reflect differences in clearance of insoluble inhalational agents from the central nervous system.

An emergence delirium scale has been developed and validated that may provide clinicians and investigators with a tool to differentiate emergence delirium from pain.[16] Tables 46-4 and 46-5 show two scoring systems used to evaluate emergence behaviors in children. In evaluating emergence delirium with the Pediatric Anesthesia Emergence Delirium (PAED) scale after anesthesia, preliminary evidence suggested that values greater than 10 were consistent with emergence delirium in 37% of patients,[17] although that cutoff value has not been useful for others.[18] Later evidence suggested that values greater than 12 provided greater sensitivity and specificity.[17] In the PICU, evidence suggests that a PAED score greater than 8 predicts emergence delirium.[19]

Our understanding of emergence delirium or agitation continues to evolve, but it is clear that it occurs after surgical procedures and after procedures that are free from pain, such as magnetic resonance imaging.[14,20,21] Emergence delirium appears to occur more frequently after use of less-soluble inhalational anesthetics such as sevoflurane and desflurane than after more-soluble inhalational anesthetics such as halothane and isoflurane,[22,23] even though some data suggest otherwise.[24] There may be a greater incidence of emergence delirium after painful procedures; emphasizing the difficulty separating agitation due to pain from agitation due to the direct effects of the inhalational agents on the sensorium.[25] Emergence delirium occurs more commonly in children younger than 6 years of age than in older children, usually lasts 5 to 15 minutes, and resolves spontaneously if the children are left undisturbed or they are held by their parents.[14]

Several strategies have been used to decrease the duration and intensity of emergence delirium. Effective regional analgesia, opioids, ketamine, $\alpha_2$-agonists, and propofol can prevent or treat

---

**TABLE 46-4** Pediatric Anesthesia Emergence Delirium Scale

| Scored Factor | SCORING | | | | |
| --- | --- | --- | --- | --- | --- |
| | 0 | 1 | 2 | 3 | 4 |
| Child makes eye contact with caregiver | Extremely | Very much | Quite a bit | Just a little | Not at all |
| Child's actions are purposeful | Extremely | Very much | Quite a bit | Just a little | Not at all |
| Child is aware of surroundings | Extremely | Very much | Quite a bit | Just a little | Not at all |
| Child is restless | Not at all | Just a little | Quite a bit | Very much | Extremely |
| Child is inconsolable | Not at all | Just a little | Quite a bit | Very much | Extremely |
| *Total score** | | | | | |

Modified from Sikich N, Lerman J. Development and psychometric evaluation of the pediatric anesthesia emergence delirium scale. Anesthesiology 2004;100:1138-45.
*Preliminary evidence suggested that a total pediatric anesthesia emergence delirium (PAED) score greater than 10 defined emergence delirium, but later evidence suggested that a total score greater than 12 might be more specific.

**TABLE 46-5** Postanesthesia Behavior Assessment Scale

Perceptual disturbances (maximal score 3)*
0   None evident
1   Feelings of depersonalization (says that situation is not real, comments on "out of body" feelings)
2   Visual illusions or misperceptions (misidentifies objects, such as urinates in trash can)
3   Markedly confused about external reality (misidentifies self or surroundings, such as being at school)

Hallucination type (maximal score 6)*
0   None evident
1   Auditory hallucinations only (responds to questions not asked)
2   Visual hallucinations or misperceptions (responds to things only the child can see)
3   Tactile, olfactory (responds to sensations not obvious to others, such as a bug crawling on the leg)

Psychomotor behavior (maximal score 3)*
0   No significant agitation
1   Mild restlessness, tremulousness, or anxiety
2   Moderate agitation with pulling at intravenous lines
3   Severe agitation, needs to be restrained, combative

From Przybylo HJ, Martini DR, Mazurek AJ, et al. Assessing behavior in children emerging form anaesthesia: can we apply psychiatric diagnostic techniques? Pediatr Anesth 2003;13:609-16.
*A higher postanesthesia behavior assessment (PABA) score is associated with a greater degree of postanesthetic distress.

emergence delirium. Low-dose fentanyl (2 μg/kg intranasally or 1 to 2 μg/kg intravenously) decreases the duration and intensity of emergence delirium,[26] even in the absence of significant painful stimuli.[20] Other adjunctive agents used to treat this phenomenon include ketorolac and acetaminophen (for myringotomy with ventilation tube placement) and midazolam; the effectiveness of midazolam, however, has been mixed.[27,28] Dexmedetomidine can decrease the incidence of emergence delirium,[29,30] but the cost-effectiveness of this treatment compared with others requires evaluation. Administration of propofol by continuous infusion or by bolus at the end of surgery appears to be preventative,[31,32] although these findings have not been consistent.[18] The induction dose of propofol administered at the start of the case does not appear to prevent postoperative emergence delirium.[33] Regional analgesia in the form of caudal blocks can reduce the incidence of emergence delirium, although this effect is probably related to improved pain control, which eliminates pain as a source of agitation.[34,35]

Although there is no evidence of long-term consequences, in the current era of fast-tracking anesthesia, emergence delirium can represent a significant time expenditure for nurses in the PACU. Discharge from the PACU may be delayed while waiting for the delirium to wane or for the effects of the interventional drugs to dissipate. Injury to the child who is extremely agitated is a concern. Parental satisfaction decreases when severe emergence delirium occurs. Although the impact of extreme delirium is not fully known, evidence suggests that the incidence of postoperative maladaptive behaviors increases among children who experience marked emergence delirium.[36]

## Respiratory System

### CRITERIA FOR EXTUBATION

In most cases, extubation may be safely performed in the operating room. However, a child's condition may necessitate delayed extubation at a more appropriate time in the PACU or PICU. There is widespread agreement that children who have been anesthetized with a full stomach, children at risk for airway obstruction, those with difficult airways, premature infants, and other infants predisposed to apnea should be awake before extubation of the trachea is attempted. Beyond this, the timing of extubation is a matter of individual judgment. For example, the practice at some institutions is to extubate the trachea when a child is awake and demonstrating eye opening and other purposeful movements; the practice at others is to extubate while the child is under a deep plane of inhalational anesthesia. Clinicians report only rare problems with either approach. Most clinicians agree that either approach is preferable to extubating the trachea during a very light plane of anesthesia, when laryngospasm is more likely and vomiting may occur while protective reflexes are impaired.

### EXTUBATION IN THE OPERATING ROOM OR POSTANESTHESIA CARE UNIT

Immediately after extubation, oxygen should be administered, and the child should be observed for adequate ventilation, satisfactory oxygen saturation, color of the mucous membranes, and laryngospasm or vomiting. Transport of children should not be undertaken until the patency of the airway and the adequacy of oxygenation and ventilation have been confirmed in the form of stable and satisfactory oxygen saturation and adequate respiratory effort. Our criterion for transporting the child from the operating room to the PACU without oxygen is a stable oxygen saturation of 95% or greater while breathing room air. If the child cannot sustain this level of oxygen saturation, more time for recovery in the operating room is taken, or the child is transported with supplemental oxygen and a means for providing positive-pressure ventilation.

For children who are extubated in the PACU, respiratory insufficiency is the most worrisome and most frequent complication. It comprises approximately two thirds of critical perioperative events when it is associated with emergence from anesthesia.[37] Respiratory insufficiency may manifest in the form of difficulty breathing, or it may be more subtle as anxiety, unresponsiveness, tachycardia, bradycardia, hypertension, arrhythmia, or seizures. Cardiac arrest is a late manifestation. When any of these conditions are present, respiratory insufficiency must be considered as the root cause. Hypoxemia, hypoventilation, and upper airway obstruction are the three most common adverse respiratory events that occur in children in the PACU, and this is particularly true for children after tonsillectomy complicated by obesity and possible obstructive sleep apnea and for those who have undergone diagnostic bronchoscopy.

### HYPOXEMIA

Hypoxemia may result from hypoventilation, diffusion hypoxia, upper airway obstruction, bronchospasm, aspiration, pulmonary edema, pneumothorax, atelectasis, or rarely from postobstructive pulmonary edema or pulmonary embolism. Hypoxia occurs more rapidly and may be more profound during emergence from general anesthesia because general anesthesia inhibits the hypoxic and hypercapnic ventilatory drive, reduces functional residual capacity, and alters hypoxic pulmonary vasoconstriction. Shivering may further increase oxygen consumption by a factor of two to five[38,39] and exacerbate hemoglobin desaturation.

Postoperative hemoglobin desaturation is more common in children with or recovering from an active upper respiratory tract

infection due to increased airway reactivity, atelectasis, and increased secretions than in children without a history of upper respiratory tract infection.[40,41] In neonates, hypoxia *increases* ventilation for approximately 1 minute but then *depresses* the respiratory drive (i.e., respiratory rate and tidal volume).[42] The ventilatory response to hypoxia in formerly preterm infants with severe bronchopulmonary dysplasia who sustained an hypoxic injury is delayed for several months, placing them at particular risk for desaturation in the perioperative period.[43]

## HYPOVENTILATION

Minute ventilation is the product of tidal volume and respiratory rate. It decreases when tidal volume, respiratory rate, or both values decrease. Hypoventilation leads to hypercarbia and promotes alveolar collapse, known as *atelectasis*. Severe hypoventilation causes respiratory acidosis, hypoxemia, carbon dioxide narcosis, and apnea. The ventilatory response to carbon dioxide depends on the child's age. For example, during halothane anesthesia and spontaneous ventilation, 3.7% inspired carbon dioxide triggers no ventilatory response in infants younger than 6 months of age, but it triggers a 34% increase in minute ventilation in infants and children older than 6 months of age.[44,45]

Hypoventilation results from a decrease in ventilatory drive, insufficiency of the muscular system, or mechanical effects. Inhalational anesthetics, opioids, benzodiazepines, and other sedating medications decrease the ventilatory drive in children in a dose-dependent manner. At particular risk for postoperative hypoventilation are children with underlying disturbances in respiration, such as infants with apnea of prematurity (formerly preterm infants of less than 60 weeks postconceptual age [PCA]); those with central nervous system injury such as head injury, strokes, and intracranial surgery; and obese children, especially those with obstructive sleep apnea (OSA). Some of these children require prolonged observation in a setting with continuous monitoring capabilities.

Muscular weakness may contribute to respiratory insufficiency. Preexistent muscular disease (e.g., muscular dystrophy) and inadequate reversal of neuromuscular blockade, electrolyte abnormalities, neurologic disorders, drugs, infection, and endocrine disease may impair the respiratory effort sufficiently to cause hypoventilation and respiratory insufficiency.

Respiratory insufficiency may result from upper airway obstruction. Airway obstruction is a feature in children with known airway problems due to congenital anomalies of the face (particularly those with midfacial hypoplasia as in trisomy 21, achondroplasia, and Crouzon disease) and obese children with a history of OSA. Inadequate analgesia can lead to splinting and hypoventilation, which may depress oxygen saturation.

## AIRWAY OBSTRUCTION

Among the most common and serious problems in the PACU is an extrathoracic airway obstruction. Clinical hallmarks of airway obstruction include hemoglobin desaturation with inspiratory stridor, inspiratory retraction, and paradoxical chest wall motion. Common interventions include stimulating the child, repositioning, suctioning, performing a jaw thrust, insertion of an oral or nasal airway, and application of positive end-expiratory pressure (PEEP) (see Fig. 12-10). If these measures fail, patency of the upper and lower airways should be considered because gas exchange may be compromised by

laryngospasm, subglottic narrowing as the result of edema, bronchospasm, atelectasis, or tracheal secretions. Incomplete recovery from general anesthesia or neuromuscular blockade, wound hematoma, and vocal cord paralysis may also lead to upper airway obstruction.

If the airway is not cleared by any of the previously described maneuvers, placement of a tracheal tube preceded by administration of oxygen by mask with continuous positive airway pressure and indicated medications may be necessary. Postobstructive pulmonary edema is a complication of acute upper airway obstruction and the relief of chronic airway obstruction after tonsillectomy. The mechanism appears to be generation of extreme negative intrathoracic pressure against a closed glottis or obstructed airway and its sudden release, resulting in a dramatic increase in pulmonary blood flow and causing noncardiogenic or neurogenic pulmonary edema. This complication should be suspected when significant hypoxia, persistent tachypnea, or tachycardia follows a prolonged episode of laryngospasm, airway obstruction, or tonsillectomy and the child has pink, frothy secretions. Treatment of noncardiogenic pulmonary edema includes tracheal intubation, positive-pressure ventilation with PEEP, 100% oxygen to maintain an adequate oxygen tension, furosemide, and morphine. Furosemide (1 to 2 mg/kg) should be given immediately intravenously because it is thought to act instantaneously by decreasing venous return to the heart by direct venodilatation.[46-48]

Postintubation croup or subglottic edema has been associated with factors such as traumatic intubation, tight-fitting tracheal tubes, multiple intubation attempts, coughing with an in situ tracheal tube, a change in the child's position during surgery, prolonged duration of intubation, surgery of the head and neck, and a history of croup.[49] Treatment should be initiated with the inhalation of cool mist. If the symptoms do not abate, nebulized epinephrine should be administered, although its effects are temporary and its repeated use may be followed by rebound edema. The use of nebulized epinephrine indicates the need for a prolonged period of observation. Outpatients may have to be admitted to the hospital overnight or observed for an extended period.

## RESPIRATORY EFFORT

If the airway is patent, attention turns to the adequacy of ventilatory effort. Residual neuromuscular blockade can be diagnosed by observation (i.e., the patient's ability to lift extremities against gravity or perform a sustained head lift) and quantitatively by assessment with a peripheral nerve stimulator. Depending on the severity and the clinical situation, this condition may be treated with supplemental doses of reversal agents or ventilatory assistance. If the respiratory rate is slow, suggesting opioid-induced respiratory depression, titrated incremental doses of naloxone (0.01 to 0.1 µg/kg) reverses the respiratory depression without precipitating acute anxiety, pain, or pulmonary edema. If naloxone is effective, continuous monitoring of respiratory status is advised because naloxone has a short half-life of 20 minutes. The same effective total dose should be given intramuscularly to prevent recrudescence of the opioid-induced respiratory depression. Residual sedation after benzodiazepines may be antagonized with flumazenil.

Children who have an adequate airway and adequate muscular strength may experience difficulty breathing because of pain, restriction from bandages or casts, abdominal distention,

pneumothorax, atelectasis, aspiration pneumonitis, or cardiogenic or postobstructive pulmonary edema. In most cases, the history and physical examination focus the differential diagnosis, and when necessary, investigations that include a chest radiograph, blood gas analysis, and possibly invasive hemodynamic monitoring can identify the underlying cause and determine an effective treatment.

### DISCHARGE OF PRETERM INFANTS FROM THE POSTANESTHESIA CARE UNIT

Preterm infants (<37 weeks gestation at birth) are at risk for apnea after sedation and general anesthesia.[50,51] As the PCA (i.e., age since conception) increases, the risk for apnea decreases.[52] Guidelines are lacking because there are inadequate randomized, controlled trials and underpowered institutional studies, and apnea has been reported even after more modern anesthetic agents (i.e., desflurane and sevoflurane). However, it is recommended that formerly preterm infants who are 55 to 60 weeks PCA who are not anemic and not experiencing apnea be observed for an extended period and, if stable, later discharged. Infants younger than 55 weeks PCA, those who are anemic (hematocrit <30%), and those with ongoing apnea should be admitted for monitoring.[53-59] Prophylactic administration of caffeine (10 mg/kg intravenously) may reduce the risk of apnea after general anesthesia for infants at high risk,[60,61] although it should not supplant postoperative admission and monitoring. Administration should be discussed with neonatologists, because it does not change management (i.e., infants are monitored in the hospital), and the administration of caffeine resets the number of apnea or bradycardia-free days (i.e., used as a discharge criterion for preterm infants) to zero. Preterm infants younger than 55 weeks PCA, particularly those with anemia or those with major cardiorespiratory or neurologic disorders, should be admitted and monitored for at least 12 apnea-free hours after general or regional anesthesia or sedation (see Chapter 4).[54,62]

Although preterm infants who undergo surgery under spinal anesthesia have fewer respiratory and cardiovascular complications compared with those undergoing general anesthesia,[54,55,58,61] the infants remain at risk for apnea. It is unknown whether the risk is greater after a spinal anesthetic without supplemental sedation (with no other medication given) than the preoperative baseline risk. Similarly, caudal anesthesia has been reported as an effective alternative to spinal anesthesia in preterm infants undergoing herniotomy.[62,63] Infants who have received a spinal anesthetic supplemented with ketamine or midazolam are at greater risk for apnea than those who received no supplemental sedation. Despite evidence of a reduced risk of apnea after regional anesthesia[61,64] and no postdischarge complications on the day of surgery in some institutions,[61,65] there is insufficient evidence to make general recommendations regarding this practice. Our recommendation is to admit and monitor these infants.

Full-term neonates typically have a reduced risk of apnea and bradycardia after general anesthesia compared with preterm infants. Opinions vary on the minimum PCA for ambulatory surgery in infants 44 to 50 weeks PCA; many children's hospitals admit all full-term neonates (<28 days of age) for overnight monitoring after general anesthesia, although this is not evidence-based practice. All full-term infants with a history of apnea and bradycardia or those who have siblings with sudden infant death syndrome should be observed for an extended period or admitted for overnight monitoring after general anesthesia.

# Cardiovascular System

## BRADYCARDIA

Bradycardia is the most common dysrhythmia in children and requires immediate attention because of its association with decreased cardiac output. *Until proved otherwise, the most common cause of bradycardia in infants and children is hypoxemia.* Other possible causes for the bradycardia include vagal responses (e.g., passage of a nasogastric tube), medications (e.g., neostigmine, β-adrenergic blockade, high spinal blockade, opioids such as fentanyl), increased intracranial pressure, and high neuraxial anesthetic block. The definition of bradycardia depends on the age of the child; the incidence decreases with increasing age (see Chapter 2).

Treatment is directed at correcting the underlying cause, including the administration of oxygen and ensuring a patent airway. Bradycardia should be immediately treated with oxygen and, if necessary, with ventilation. If intervention with oxygen does not immediately restore the heart rate, atropine (0.02 mg/kg) should be administered; and if no response is observed within 30 seconds, administration of epinephrine (2 to 10 μg/kg) is indicated. For symptomatic bradycardia (e.g., hypotension, decreased level of consciousness), immediate administration of epinephrine is indicated. If there is no response to epinephrine, chest compressions should be instituted and standard cardiopulmonary resuscitation algorithms followed (see Chapter 39).

## TACHYCARDIA

Tachycardia is an important postoperative sign that is a marker for one of several disorders, such as inadequate cardiac output or oxygen delivery, or it may be a response to pain or a direct drug effect (e.g., epinephrine, atropine). Tachycardia may occur in response to hypoxemia, hypercarbia, hypovolemia, hypervolemia, emergence delirium, anxiety, sepsis, fever, a full bladder, a previously unrecognized cardiac conduction abnormality (see Chapters 14 and 16), or heart failure. The threshold for diagnosing tachycardia varies with the age of the child, and the threshold decreases with age.

Treatment is directed at correcting the underlying cause. Occasionally, children present with a sustained tachycardia unrelated to the previously described conditions that is refractory to the usual therapy. A cardiac consultation is required to investigate and identify less common causes, such as an aberrant conduction system or ectopic foci as a source of supraventricular tachycardia (SVT). SVT, which is defined as more than 220 beats/min in infants and more than 180 beats/min in children, may be treated with adenosine when there are no other symptoms. However, SVT with accompanied hypotension or decreased level of consciousness may require cardioversion. Children who have had prior cardiac surgery are particularly at risk.

## OTHER ARRHYTHMIAS

With the exception of bradycardia and tachycardia, postoperative arrhythmias are rare in children. Isolated premature ventricular or atrial beats may be observed in the PACU and, unless they progress, are not important. Multifocal premature ventricular beats are uncommon in children. They may occur as a result of inadequately treated pain, cardiac conduction defects, or in rare instances, may be a harbinger of malignant hyperthermia (see Chapters 14, 16, and 40), acute rhabdomyolysis with hyperkalemia, inadequately treated pain, a congenital conduction defect, or a structural cardiac defect. Electrolyte and arterial

blood gas status should be checked. Children with known congenital heart disease should have continuous ECG monitoring in the PACU (see Chapters 14 and 16); all arrhythmias should be recorded and a cardiologist consulted because this may be the first manifestation of a developing ectopic focus.

## BLOOD PRESSURE CONTROL

### Hypotension

The anesthesiologist should be familiar with the normal blood pressure ranges of infants and children (see Chapter 2). The measurement should be obtained with an appropriately sized blood pressure cuff; the width of the cuff should be two thirds of the length of the upper arm. An improperly sized cuff produces spurious readings. Small cuffs may yield a false high reading, whereas large cuffs may yield a false low reading. Proper placement of the cuff is essential to avoid errors in interpretation.

*The most common cause of hypotension in children is hypovolemia* from inadequate replacement of blood and fluids lost during the surgical procedure or ongoing blood loss. Clinical hallmarks of hypovolemia are tachycardia, urine output of less than 0.5 to 1 mL/kg/hr, slow capillary refill (>3 seconds), and narrowing of the pulse pressure. If the hematocrit is adequate, hypovolemia may be treated with an initial bolus of 10 to 20 mL/kg of isotonic crystalloid solution or albumin. This may be repeated until the blood pressure is normalized. If the hematocrit is inadequate, packed red blood cells (PRBCs) or whole blood should be administered. In this case, a rough guide for the volume of blood required is 4 mL/kg of packed cells or 6 mL/kg of whole blood to raise the hemoglobin 1 g/dL in children and adults (see Chapter 10). To achieve a desired hematocrit more precisely, the volume of PRBCs may be estimated as follows:

$$\frac{(\text{Desired hematocrit} - \text{present hematocrit}) \times \text{estimated blood volume}}{\text{The hematocrit in the PRBCs}}$$

If the child does not respond to volume expansion, other causes for the hypotension need to be considered, such as occult blood loss (e.g., intraabdominal, retroperitoneal, intrathoracic [blocked chest tube], cardiac tamponade), sepsis, or other disorders. Any factor that interferes with venous return can cause hypotension, including positive-pressure ventilation, auto-PEEP, tension pneumothorax, pericardial tamponade, and compression of the inferior vena cava.

Large end-tidal concentrations of inhalational anesthetics, local anesthetics, or opioids and interactions between benzodiazepines and opioids may produce hypotension through vasodilation (i.e., relative hypovolemia) and direct myocardial depression. However, these factors are rarely important in the PACU. Uncommon causes include anaphylaxis (e.g., latex allergy, antibiotics), transfusion reaction, adrenal insufficiency, systemic inflammation, infection, severe liver failure, and administration of antihypertensive, antidysrhythmic, and anticonvulsant medications. Increased body temperature may cause vasodilation and a relative hypovolemia. The increased metabolic demands of fever may compromise an already stressed myocardium. If a child arrives in the PACU requiring vasopressors and subsequently develops hypotension, consider a disconnect or kink in the vasopressor infusion, disruption of the intravenous access, a disconnect from the pump, or pump failure.

Vasodilation caused by sympathetic blockade associated with regional anesthesia occasionally causes hypotension, especially with a high-level blockade and restricted fluid intake. This typically is a problem only in children older than 6 years of age. Because of the developmental changes in the sympathetic nervous system, most children younger than 6 years of age are normally peripherally vasodilated and therefore have little response to further vasodilation with a regional block.

Decreased inotropy, dysrhythmia, cardiomyopathy, calcium channel blockers, sepsis, hypothyroidism, negative inotropic agents, and congestive heart failure are uncommon causes of hypotension in children. Treatment is directed at the underlying cause, such as correcting hypovolemia with volume loading, treating the allergic reaction, or treating the sepsis. Decreased cardiac contractility may be treated by diuresis and the administration of inotropic agents that also decrease the afterload (i.e., inodilators).

### Hypertension

Postoperative hypertension in children is less common than hypotension and most often reflects incorrect measurement or pain. A blood pressure cuff that is too small may yield a spuriously high blood pressure reading and should be one of the first considerations in the differential diagnosis, especially if the child has no other symptoms consistent with pain. Causative factors besides pain include hypervolemia, preexisting hypertension (e.g., renal disease with inadequate continuity of antihypertensive medications), distended bladder, hypercarbia, hypoxemia, agitation and delirium, increased intracranial pressure, and exogenous vasoactive drugs (e.g., epinephrine).

## Renal System

Complications related to the renal system are rare in the postoperative period. The most likely cause of low urine output (<0.5 to 1 mL/kg/hr) is hypovolemia as discussed previously (e.g., postoperative hypotension). Mechanical obstruction downstream from the kidneys may result from direct surgical interference or a misplaced or dysfunctional urinary catheter (i.e., blood clot or kink). If the child has regional (spinal or epidural) anesthesia that includes an opioid and there is no urinary catheter in place, placement of a Foley or straight catheter may be indicated. Renal failure is a rare possibility in children who have had major operations or have systemic inflammatory disease. If screening tests such as blood urea nitrogen, serum creatinine, and urine analysis suggest renal insufficiency, a pediatric nephrologist should be consulted (see also Chapter 26).

## Gastrointestinal System

### INCIDENCE OF POSTOPERATIVE NAUSEA AND VOMITING

Postoperative nausea and vomiting (PONV) is one of the most bothersome adverse effects of anesthesia and surgery. Unlike adults, most children are unfamiliar with and have never experienced nausea. It is unlikely that they will warn the PACU personnel that they are nauseated. In children, vomiting and complaining about a "sore tummy" are likely the first and only manifestations of gastrointestinal upset. Among children, PONV is inversely related to age.[66] The incidence of PONV is small in very young children, increases throughout childhood, and reaches a zenith in adolescents, for whom the incidence exceeds that for adults.[66]

The type of surgery influences the incidence of PONV. The incidence of PONV in children is greatest after tonsillectomy, strabismus repair, hernia repair, orchiopexy, microtia, and middle ear procedures.[67] Before puberty, there are no gender-related differences in PONV; after puberty, girls experience much more PONV than boys. The medical complications of PONV include pulmonary aspiration, dehydration, electrolyte imbalance, fatigue, wound disruption, and esophageal tears. PONV can produce psychological effects that may produce anxiety in the children and parents and lead them to avoid further surgery. The cost implications of PONV can be major because of delayed recovery and discharge, increased medical care, and reoperation. Although these problems are seldom life-threatening, the cumulative costs in terms of prolonged PACU stays, unplanned admissions, and patient dissatisfaction are serious.[68]

## EVIDENCE-BASED CONSENSUS MANAGEMENT

Management of PONV is complex, and many treatment strategies have been formulated (Fig. 46-1). Most have been shown to be effective in one study or another. However, the superiority of some treatments over others has not been established, in part because of study design flaws such as inadequate dosing, small sample sizes, or various periods of observations and data collection; some studies monitored PONV only during the first few hours after surgery, whereas others monitored the children for 24 to 48 hours after surgery. To make sense of the conflicting data that exist, a consensus-based management strategy for the prevention and management of PONV has been devised.[69] These guidelines advise first identifying the children at significant risk for PONV as outlined earlier; prophylaxis for PONV is recommended for children in high-risk categories. Studies frequently focus on postoperative vomiting as the primary outcome because nausea may be difficult to identify in children.

The consensus guidelines recognize that the choice of anesthetic can influence the incidence of PONV in children. Propofol-based anesthesia during operations associated with a large incidence of PONV dramatically reduces the incidence of PONV compared with isoflurane-based anesthesia, even when both groups are given prophylactic 5-hydroxytryptamine type 3 (5-HT$_3$) receptor inhibitors.[70] Similarly, multimodal therapy that is a combination of PONV treatment strategies is more effective than a single-treatment strategy.[71] For instance, the combination of propofol anesthesia plus ondansetron has been shown to significantly reduce the incidence of PONV compared with the use of propofol alone (7% versus 22%).[72] The combination of dexamethasone and ondansetron is more effective than either intervention in isolation and permits the dose of ondansetron to be reduced by 50%.[73] A slightly more contentious effect has been the elimination of nitrous oxide, which decreases the incidence of PONV among those undergoing highly emetogenic surgery, with a number needed to treat of only five patients.[74] However, that meta-analysis also revealed a 2% incidence of awareness under anesthesia if nitrous oxide was omitted.[74]

Other strategies recommended to decrease the rate of PONV include the use of the smallest dose of opioids that still provides adequate pain control and the use of regional anesthesia if possible. The use of nonopioids such as acetaminophen, ketamine, and ketorolac should be considered. Adequate parenteral hydration and avoidance of early postoperative fluid ingestion can reduce the incidence of PONV (see Chapter 4).

## PROPHYLACTIC THERAPY

Ondansetron has been studied extensively and shown to decrease early and late PONV at doses of 50 to 100 μg/kg.[75] Because the 5-HT$_3$ receptor antagonists as a group have greater efficacy in the prevention of vomiting than nausea, they are the drugs of first choice for prophylaxis in children. Dexamethasone also is effective in decreasing PONV.[76] Administration of dexamethasone alone or in combination with other antiemetics can extend the period of effective treatment up to 24 hours. In a systematic review, Steward and associates demonstrated that children who

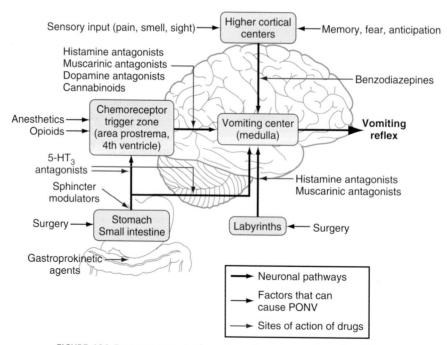

**FIGURE 46-1** Treatment strategies for postoperative nausea and vomiting (*PONV*).

intravenous lines, the arterial line, chest tubes, drains, and the urinary catheter should be checked before transport. Children should be in presentable condition (e.g., removal of blood and secretions) before and kept normothermic during transport to the PACU or PICU.

Unless children are awake, with protective airway reflexes intact, or unless there is a specific contraindication, it is sensible to transport extubated children in the lateral position (i.e., tonsillectomy recovery position) so that the tongue lies away from the larynx, and secretions and vomitus leave the mouth rather than enter the larynx, causing aspiration or airway obstruction. To assess ventilation and maintain a patent airway with the child in the decubitus position, we recommend applying the thumb to the forehead to extend the neck and holding the fingers (the finger tips are the most sensitive part of the hand) over the mouth (or nose) to feel for exhalation. A precordial stethoscope may also be used to auscultate respirations. If the child is breathing room air, a pulse oximeter can indicate oxygenation and serve as a crude measure of ventilation because desaturation will occur quickly if hypopnea develops. However, if oxygen is provided to the child, the oximeter can no longer serve as a guide to ventilation, because desaturation will not occur until a sustained apnea occurs. For sleepy children, the precordial stethoscope and portable oxygen saturation monitor can trend ventilation, oxygenation, and the heart rate within the previously described provisos. We recommend that children in a potentially unstable condition be transported with a pulse oximeter, capnogram, an electrocardiographic (ECG) monitor, and a blood pressure cuff or a transduced arterial line. The monitoring lines, intravenous drips, infusion pumps, and other equipment should be clearly labeled and simplified before transport. For sick children, those with intubated tracheas, and children with potentially difficult airways, an appropriate resuscitation bag, facemask, oral airway, oxygen tanks (oxygen levels should be checked), functioning laryngoscopes, tracheal tube, and medications (including atropine and succinylcholine) should be carried en route to the PACU or PICU. A tackle box containing all of this equipment is helpful, especially when children are transported to the PICU in an elevator. Children receiving vasoactive drugs require infusion pumps so that these agents can be continuously administered at precise titrated rates.

Transport to the PACU or PICU is a time of potential danger. Distance and duration of travel should be minimized. When designing pediatric perioperative areas or reallocating space, strong emphasis should be placed on ergonomics.

A child often appears awake after the stimulation of tracheal extubation and transfer to the stretcher but may subsequently become obtunded and obstruct the airway during transit to the PACU or PICU. Just as frequently, children may become restless during transit. Although restless behavior has many causes, hypoxia should never be overlooked. The guard rails on the stretcher should always be raised when the child is in it. Most importantly, the anesthesiologist must remain vigilant throughout the transfer.

### ARRIVAL IN THE CARE UNIT

On arrival in the PACU, attention should first be directed to the airway, ensuring it is patent and not obstructed; to the color of the lips and mucous membranes; to the oxygen saturation; and to the adequacy of ventilation, perfusion, and central nervous system function. Admission heart rate, blood pressure, oxygen saturation, respiratory rate, and temperature should be recorded on arrival. The nurse-to-patient ratio should be 1 to 1 for sick children and 1 to 2 or 1 to 3 for routine cases. Supplemental oxygen is administered as indicated, recognizing the limitations of the monitors to detect ventilation in such cases. Many children object to having an oxygen mask fixed to their faces; a funnel-type mask or open hose with large flow rates may be less objectionable (although less optimal). Thereafter, report should be given to the nurses and physicians in attendance. Ideally, the nurses taking care of the child postoperatively are already familiar with the child and family from the preoperative setting.

The standardized transfer of care report should include, at a minimum, the child's name, institutional identification code, age and gender, preoperative vital signs, and specific circumstances, such as a language barrier or developmental delay. The size and location of catheters, a description of the child's current problem, medical history, medications, allergies, operative procedure, and pertinent surgical problems should be outlined. The anesthetic should be summarized and include the premedication and anesthetic agents used at induction and for maintenance, techniques used, reversal of neuromuscular blockade (i.e., adequacy of the train-of-four response), estimated blood loss, fluid replacement (including amount and type of solution), urine output, and vasoactive drugs, bronchodilators, and intraoperative medications (e.g., antibiotics) used. Regional anesthesia issues, such as epidural use and location, drug choice and concentration, use of adjuvants, effective level of analgesia, and drug infusion rate should be clearly communicated. Administration of analgesics (time and dose), local blocks and wound infiltration with local anesthetics, problems with surgery or anesthesia (e.g., difficult intravenous access, difficult intubation, intraoperative hemodynamic instability, cardiac changes), and potential problems in the PACU should be listed.

The anesthesia team must remain with the child until he or she has stable vital signs and the PACU team is comfortable and ready to assume responsibility for the child. Physicians who will be in charge of taking care of the child in the PACU after the anesthesia team leaves must be clearly identified by name, and ways to reach them (e.g., pager number) must be given to surgeons, anesthesiologists, and regional block and pain services.

All children should be monitored continuously in the PACU. At the very least, this should include continuous pulse oximetry and intermittent noninvasive blood pressure and temperature monitoring. Most PACUs also monitor the electrocardiogram continuously, although some limit this to children with cardiac disease or complex multiple-organ disease. During emergence, many children are so active that it is impossible to maintain the monitoring devices in place. If the child is not hypoxic and is sufficiently awake to remove the monitors, he or she probably does not require the monitors any longer. If the child falls back to sleep, then a pulse oximeter probe should be reapplied, particularly for at-risk children such as those with obstructive sleep apnea. For a child who is physically or mentally challenged, it may be necessary to apply light restraints until he or she is oriented and awake.

## Central Nervous System

### PHARMACODYNAMICS OF EMERGENCE

Emergence from anesthesia is faster after a relatively insoluble inhalational anesthetic agent such as sevoflurane or desflurane than it is after a more soluble agent such as halothane.[3] However, the clinical importance of these differences may be minimal and

**TABLE 46-1** Suggested Essential Bedside Equipment

Oxygen supply with regulated flows

Oxygen facemasks and face tents for spontaneous ventilation (various sizes)

Stethoscope

Resuscitation bags, self-inflating (Ambu)

Anesthesia facemasks for positive-pressure ventilation (pediatric sizes: 0, 1, 2, 3; adult sizes: small, medium, large)

Oral airways (sizes 00, 0, 1 to 5)

Nasal airways (sizes 12F to 36F)

Suction and appropriate suction catheters (sizes 6.5F to 14F); tonsil-type (Yankauer) attachment

Needles, syringes, alcohol wipes, Betadine solution, gauze pads

Arterial blood gas kit

Gloves (preferably nonlatex)

Pulse oximeter and sensors (size appropriate, stick-on type preferred to clip-on type)

Electrocardiograph, monitor and pads

Manual and automated blood pressure device

All sizes of blood pressure cuffs

**TABLE 46-2** Suggested Emergency Supplies for a Crash Cart or Central Location

Laryngoscopes with blades: Miller 0, 1, 2, 3; Macintosh 2, 3, 4; extra laryngoscope bulbs and batteries

Endotracheal tubes, sizes 2.0-mm internal diameter (ID) through 8-mm ID; cuffed and uncuffed tubes for all sizes when available

Laryngeal mask airways, sizes 1, 1.5, 2, 2.5, 3, 4, 5

ProSeal laryngeal mask airway, sizes 1.5, 2, 2.5, 3, 3.5, 4, 5

Fast-track intubating laryngeal mask airway

Stylet appropriate for each endotracheal tube size

Syringe for endotracheal cuff inflation

Tape and liquid adhesive for endotracheal tube fixation

Intravenous catheter (14 gauge) with 3-mm ID endotracheal tube adapter for emergency cricothyroidotomy (see Fig. 12-25)

Cricothyrotomy kits appropriate for age (see Figs. 12-25 and 12-26; see also E-Figs. 12-5 through 12-10)

Backup resuscitation bags and masks and oral airways for each bedside

Nasogastric tubes

Intravenous infusion solutions, tubing, drip chambers

Supplies for intravenous cannulation, catheter sizes 24 to 14 gauge

Cutdown tray, tracheostomy, and suture sets

Central venous catheter insertion sets (3F to 7F single and multiple lumen)

Tube thoracotomy set and system for suction and underwater seal

Defibrillator (adult, child paddles)

Electrocardiograph

Pressure transducer system and oscilloscope monitor

Sterile gowns, gloves, masks, towels, drapes

Urinary catheters of appropriate pediatric size

Bed board for cardiopulmonary resuscitation

**TABLE 46-3** Suggested Recovery Room Medications

**Suggested Emergency Medications on Crash Cart***

Amiodarone

Atropine

Calcium chloride or gluconate

Dextrose

Diphenhydramine

Dopamine

Epinephrine

Etomidate

Flumazenil

Furosemide

Heparin

Hydrocortisone, dexamethasone, methylprednisolone

Lidocaine (intravenous and topical)

Mannitol

Naloxone

Neostigmine

Norepinephrine

Phenytoin or fosphenytoin

Physostigmine

Propranolol, atenolol, esmolol, labetalol

Sodium bicarbonate

Sodium nitroprusside

Succinylcholine and rocuronium

Thiopental and propofol

Verapamil

For inhalation: racemic epinephrine (2.2% at 0.05 mL/kg, common in the United States) or epinephrine 1:1000 (0.1%), 0.5 mL/kg, maximum of 5 mL

**Medications to Be Kept under Lock***

Diazepam

Fentanyl

Ketamine

Meperidine

Midazolam (intravenous and oral)

Morphine

Phenobarbital

Potassium chloride

**Other Medications for Central Location***

Acetaminophen (oral, rectal, and intravenous)

Antibiotics

Antiemetics (e.g., 5-HT$_3$ antagonist, promethazine, metoclopramide)

Dantrolene

Digoxin

Insulin

Pancuronium, rocuronium, vecuronium

Potassium chloride

Protamine

*Alternative or additional medications may be needed.

The team should participate in mock codes and simulations to train for an emergency. Patient sign outs should be standardized, include checklists, and follow an institution-specific protocol.[1] All personnel should be familiar with resuscitative equipment and be able to use it instantaneously. We recommend instituting equipment and policies according to the guidelines for the pediatric perioperative anesthesia environment published by the American Academy of Pediatrics.[2]

## TRANSPORT TO THE CARE UNIT

Transport from the operating room to the PACU should be carried out under the direct supervision of a trained expert. The security and patency of the airway, intravenous and arterial lines, drains, and urinary catheters should be checked before transport. The security and patency of the tracheal tube (if the airway remains intubated) or laryngeal mask airway, all

**TABLE 47-5** The Dartmouth Operative Conditions Scale (DOCS)

| Patient State | Observed Behaviors | | | |
|---|---|---|---|---|
| Pain/stress | (0) Eyes closed or calm expression | (1) Grimace or frown | (2) Crying, sobbing, screaming | |
| Movement | (0) Still | (1) Random little movement | (2) Major purposeful movement | (3) Thrashing, kicking, biting |
| Consciousness | (0) Eyes open | (−1) Ptosis, uncoordinated, "drowsy" | (−2) Eyes closed | |
| Sedation side effects | (−1) SpO₂ < 92% | (−1) Noise with respiration | (−1) Respiratory pauses >10 seconds | (−1) BP decrease of > 50% from baseline |

The Dartmouth Operative Conditions Score (DOCS). Patients are scored in four state categories at any one time during sedation for a procedure. The sum of the scores in all four categories is used to determine the DOCS score for any discrete point during a sedation encounter.
$SpO_2$, Oxygen saturation as measured by pulse oximetry.

which a child developed apnea. Given that the expected incidence of a sedation-induced crisis should be on the order of one in tens of thousands, it is not surprising that the majority of similar studies are underpowered to report a critical event.[87]

Another approach to assessing safety is to carefully observe relatively small groups of children and track minute-to-minute changes in their level of sedation. This has been accomplished by the creation of the Dartmouth Operative Conditions Scale (DOCS) (Table 47-5).[88] This scale was derived from observing 110 videos of pediatric sedation outside the OR. The DOCS quantifies the child's "state" based on observable behavior. Continuously applying this scale allows for careful tracking of level of sedation, effectiveness of sedation, uncontrolled adverse effects, and the timing of induction of sedation and recovery without poking or prodding the child to determine their depth of sedation. These data can help to quantify the quality of sedation and best practices.

Simulations have been used to carefully examine rare adverse effects in pediatric sedation and ability to rescue.[89,90] In a simulated scenario of a sedation complication, a standard reproducible event was introduced in which physiologic variables degraded with inappropriate interventions and improved when effective treatment was introduced. The simulation was distributed throughout the hospital and used with different sedation provider teams (e.g., postanesthesia care unit, emergency department [ED], radiology, and sedation unit). The event was videotaped and scored based on deviations from best practice; it quantifies episodes of hypoventilation, apnea, hypoxia, and cardiovascular collapse. Hypoxia and hypotension lasted 90 seconds in the pediatric sedation unit and 360 seconds in the ED and radiology setting.[91] Such studies demonstrate that prospective and retrospective analysis of simulated but rare adverse events can identify areas within the hospital that are in need of improving their clinical skills, and have a positive impact on patient safety.

There has been a recent effort to capture information from the large numbers of pediatric sedation procedures necessary to understand the nature and frequency of adverse reactions to sedation. The Pediatric Sedation Research Consortium (PSRC) comprises a group of over 30 institutions in North America who share prospective data on pediatric sedation.[14] Analysis of the first 30,000 records identified demographics, procedures, sedation techniques, outcomes, and adverse events: (1) there were no deaths and only one cardiac arrest reported; (2) unanticipated admission occurred infrequently, 1 per 1500 sedations; (3) vomiting occurred 1 per 200 sedations, including one aspiration;

(4) stridor, laryngospasm, wheezing, and apnea occurred in 1 of 400 procedures; and (5) airway or ventilatory manipulations occurred in 1 time per 200 sedations.[91] Risk factors included age younger than 3 months, ASA physical status 3 or greater, and multiple drug combinations for sedation. The PSRC has also reviewed the incidence of adverse events in 49,386 propofol sedation and/or anesthesia encounters for procedures outside of the OR.[15] Propofol was delivered by multiple providers (anesthesiologists, intensivists, emergency medicine, pediatricians, and radiologists). No deaths were recorded. CPR was required in 2 children (anesthesiologists were not involved in their care) and aspiration occurred in 4 children. Desaturation of less than 90% for more than 30 seconds occurred 154 times per 10,000 sedations/anesthesias; central apnea or obstruction occurred 575 times per 10,000. Stridor, laryngospasm, excessive secretions, and vomiting occurred 50, 96, 341, and 49 times per 10,000, respectively. The most prominent type of complication was related to the airway and occurred 1 out of 65 sedations; 1 in 70 children required airway rescue. Unexpected admissions occurred 7.1 times per 10,000 sedations. When all possible adverse events are considered, anesthesiologists report fewer events than nonanesthesiologists, with an odds ratio of 1.38 (95% confidence interval [CI] of 1.21 to 1.57, $P < 0.001$).[15] No difference, however, was noted when outcomes were limited only to major pulmonary complications. The authors concluded that propofol sedation and/or anesthesia when given under these strict organized conditions, i.e., following the AAP sedation guideline, with very well-trained providers, can result in effective sedation with a minimal incidence of severe adverse events. The safety of this practice is contingent on the ability to quickly and safely manage less serious events. In a prospective cohort study of 131,751 procedural sedations[92] in radiology (62%), hematology–oncology (11%), and minor medical or surgical procedures (16%), in which sedation included primarily propofol (60%), midazolam (25%), and others provided by anesthesiologists, emergency physicians, intensivists, pediatricians, and "other" (pediatric residents, radiologists, dentists, surgeons, and nurses), the rate of major complications per 10,000 sedations (and 95% CIs) were: anesthesiologist 7.6 (4.6 to 12.8), emergency physician 7.8 (5.5 to 11.2), intensivist 9.6 (7.3 to 12.6), pediatrician 12.4 (6.9 to 20.4) and "other" 10.2 (5.1 to 18.3). There were no statistical differences between any providers before or after potential confounding variables (age, ASA status, fasting status, propofol use). A significant limitation of the study was the selection bias that was introduced because not all sedation areas within each hospital

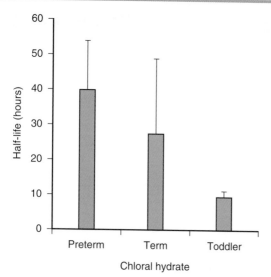

FIGURE 47-3 β-Elimination half-life of the active metabolite of chloral hydrate, trichloroethanol, in preterm infants, term infants, and toddlers. Note the extremely prolonged half-lives and the large standard deviations in all age groups. Although often thought of as a short-acting sedative, chloral hydrate can have profoundly long sedative effects, with a real possibility of re-sedation after a procedure when the child is left undisturbed. It is for this reason that we recommend a longer period of observation in a step-down area before discharge.

well. A second individual must monitor the child, administer drugs, and record vital signs.

- Minimize physical discomfort and pain.
- Control anxiety, minimize psychological trauma, and maximize the potential for amnesia.
- Control behavior and/or movement, to allow the safe completion of the procedure.
- Rapidly return of the child to a state in which he or she is safe for discharge from medical supervision, as determined by recognized criteria.
- Create an optimal and efficient system that is not a burden to the health care providers

## Risks and Complications Associated with Sedation

The foremost goal is to optimize patient safety and thereby decrease the risk and associated complications. The assessment of risk for pediatric sedation must include age, type of procedure, underlying medical conditions and how these might influence the response to sedating medications, intended level of sedation, pharmacology (pharmacokinetics [PK] and pharmacodynamics [PD]) of the medications used, guidelines (i.e., training, equipment, personnel, monitoring), appropriate-for-age fasting, and strict discharge criteria.

A recent area of concern that was not previously recognized in providing safe sedation or anesthesia to small children is whether drugs used for sedation or anesthesia are neurotoxic to children[64-71]; this topic is covered in detail in Chapter 23. More important than the theoretical concern regarding potential neurotoxicity of sedating medications is the more practical risk assessment regarding both inadequate and excessive sedation. Sedation centers in the United States are less likely to offer sedation for painful procedures than similar centers in Europe. Thirty percent

of U.S. respondents to a mail survey reported performing bone marrow biopsies in children without significant sedation more than 50% of the time, as compared with 0% of European centers![72] When 1140 children (mean age 2.96 ± 3.7 years) were sedated by nonanesthesiologists who followed AAP guidelines for procedures,[73] approximately 13% received inadequate sedation.

The psychological consequences of inadequate sedation have not been specifically studied but can be inferred from children's responses to other stressful situations. Inadequate preoperative sedation is clearly linked to increased anxiety in children and their families. Of children undergoing a stressful anesthesia induction, 54% have postoperative maladaptive behaviors for up to 2 weeks after the experience.[74] The incidence of these behaviors decreases with the use of appropriate preoperative sedation. Similar sequelae have been reported after repeated invasive procedures in pediatric intensive care units (ICUs).[75] Although the number of children who developed posttraumatic stress syndrome because of no sedation or less than optimal sedation during diagnostic and therapeutic procedures is unknown, one can assume that it would be similar to that found in the study situations.

There have been many approaches to assess the risk involved in oversedation of children. One approach is to review sedation-related deaths and critical incidents to find common causes. In 2000, a now classic retrospective review was undertaken of 95 cases of sedation-related deaths and critical incidents derived from the U.S. Food and Drug Administration's (FDA) adverse drug event reporting system, the U.S. Pharmacopeia, and a survey of pediatric specialists.[54] Although a number of the incidents cited in this study occurred over 20 years ago, the findings remain applicable today. The analysis revealed that, rather than being related to a specific medication, the overwhelming majority of critical events were preventable and caused by operator error or lack of robust rescue systems. Drug interactions were the most common factor, followed by drug overdose, inadequate monitoring, inadequate cardiopulmonary resuscitation skills, inadequate evaluation before sedation, and premature discharge from medical supervision. The report emphasizes that most sedation complications are related to adverse respiratory events (80%); a majority progressed to cardiac arrest, indicating a lack of rescue skills of the practitioners. A disproportionately large number of severe complications and deaths occurred when sedation was performed in offices outside of hospitals, pointing to a lack of trained personnel available for rescue. There was no relationship with class of drug or route of administration, although there was a positive correlation when three or more sedating medications were administered.[55] Indeed, the combination of a sedative, hypnotic, and an opioid is well recognized as a precursor to significant respiratory depression.

There are many underpowered reports with relatively few patients (n <200) receiving a variety of sedative medications in a variety of settings declaring successful completion of the procedures and no fatalities.[76-86] Most studies describe adequate conditions and successful completion with no severe outcomes, but with varying frequencies of transient airway obstruction or desaturation. Conclusions often state that the particular technique and sedation providers are safe and effective. An example is a study that prospectively followed 1140 children (mean age 2.96 ± 3.7 years) sedated for procedures by nonanesthesiologists following AAP guidelines and using a quality-assurance tool.[73] Neither death nor sedation-induced crises occurred, although they reported a 5.3% incidence of respiratory events, including one in

**47**

## TABLE 46-7 Discharge Criteria for Outpatients

**All criteria in Table 46-6, plus the following:**

1. Cardiovascular function and airway patency are satisfactory and stable.
2. The child is easily arousable, and protective reflexes are intact.
3. The child can talk (if age appropriate).
4. The child can sit up unaided (if age appropriate).
5. For a very young or handicapped child, incapable of the usually expected responses, the preanesthetic level of responsiveness or a level as close as possible to the normal level for that child should be achieved unless the child is to be transferred to another monitored location.
6. The state of hydration is adequate.
7. It may be permissible for parents to carry their children without full recovery of gait (parents must be advised that the child is at risk of injury if improperly supervised).
8. Control of pain should be achieved to permit adequate analgesia by the oral route thereafter.
9. Control of nausea and vomiting should be achieved to allow for oral hydration (see "Discharge Criteria" in text).

## TABLE 46-8 Discharge Criteria for Fast-Tracking

| Criteria | Score |
| --- | --- |
| **Level of Consciousness** | |
| Aware and oriented | 2 |
| Arousable with minimal stimulation | 1 |
| Responsive only to tactile stimulation | 0 |
| **Physical Activity** | |
| Able to move all extremities on command | 2 |
| Some weakness in movement of extremities | 1 |
| Unable to voluntarily move extremities | 0 |
| **Hemodynamic Stability** | |
| Blood pressure <15% of baseline MAP value | 2 |
| Blood pressure 15% to 30% of baseline MAP value | 1 |
| Blood pressure >30% of baseline MAP value | 0 |
| **Respiratory Stability** | |
| Able to breathe deeply | 2 |
| Tachypneic with good cough | 1 |
| Dyspneic with weak cough | 0 |
| **Oxygen Saturation Status** | |
| Maintains value >95% on room air | 2 |
| Requires supplemental oxygen (nasal prongs) | 1 |
| Saturation <90% with supplemental oxygen | 0 |
| **Postoperative Pain Assessment** | |
| None or mild discomfort | 2 |
| Moderate to severe pain controlled with intravenous analgesics | 1 |
| Persistent, severe pain | 0 |
| **Postoperative Emetic Symptoms** | |
| None or mild nausea with no active vomiting | 2 |
| Transient vomiting or retching | 1 |
| Persistent, moderate to severe nausea and vomiting | 0 |
| *Total** | 14 |

From White PF, Song D. New criteria for fast-tracking after outpatient anesthesia: a comparison with the modified Aldrete's scoring system. Anesth Analg 1998;88:1069-72.
*MAP*, Mean arterial pressure; *PACU*, postanesthesia care unit.
*Pediatric patients must score 14 to bypass the phase 1 (PACU) recovery unit to be admitted directly to the step-down care unit.

confirmed, vital signs are stable, and oxygen saturation values are stable in room air (or at baseline) without respiratory support (unless needed at baseline). Pain should be well controlled. Children then can be transferred to a second-stage recovery unit, where more complete recovery takes place with a reduced nurse-to-child ratio, until children have met criteria for adequate hydration, minimal emesis, appropriate wound status, good vital signs, and appropriate ambulation and mental status.

The requirements for children to eat, drink, and void before leaving the secondary recovery area significantly delay discharge. Efforts should be made to reinstate volume homeostasis during surgery, negating any physiologic imperative for oral intake in the immediate postoperative period. Postoperative maintenance fluids should consist of isotonic rather than hypotonic solutions for those expected to remain as inpatients to reduce the risk of hyponatremia (see also Chapter 8).[112] Other than children who are at high risk for urinary retention (e.g., history of urinary retention, urethral surgery), there is little evidence that discharge before voiding results in readmission for voiding problems, and this requirement is therefore no longer part of standard discharge criteria.[113] Children who have received a caudal block for surgery are likewise at low risk for urinary retention as long as opioids have not been added to the caudal medication.[114]

Although there are few data on the current status of recovery processes across the country, there appears to be a trend toward one-stage (fast-track) recovery for pediatric outpatients.[115,116] This process allows selected children to bypass the first-stage recovery and go directly to the second-stage unit based on appropriate level of consciousness, physical activity, vital signs, respiratory status, and pain control (Table 46-8). This approach has proved successful and quite safe, although appropriate attention to issues such as pain control must be addressed when initiating such a program.

## ACKNOWLEDGMENT

The authors wish to thank A.J. de Armendi, MD, I.D. Todres, MD, and J.P. Cravero, MD, for their prior contributions to this chapter.

## ANNOTATED REFERENCES

Anderson BJ, Woolard GA, Holford NH. Pharmacokinetics of rectal paracetamol after major surgery in children. Paediatr Anaesth 1995;5:237-42.

*The authors conducted a pharmacokinetic study in 20 children from 12 months to 17 years of age and demonstrated that paracetamol reached therapeutic plasma concentrations 1 to 2 hours after administration at a dose of 40 mg/kg. Anderson's research group subsequently defined the use paracetamol in various forms of administration (e.g., oral, rectal, intravenous) in children of all ages.*

Choong K, Arora S, Cheng J, et al. Hypotonic versus isotonic maintenance fluids after surgery for children: a randomized controlled trial. Pediatrics 2011;128:857-66.

*This important paper addresses the issue of postoperative hyponatremia in children. The authors randomized 258 children to two groups receiving isotonic or hypotonic maintenance solutions. Children in the isotonic group had hyponatremia at a rate of 22.7% (versus 40.8%), with no increased risk for hypernatremia.*

Cravero JP, Beach M, Thyr B, Whalen K. The effect of small dose fentanyl on the emergence characteristics of pediatric patients after sevoflurane anesthesia without surgery. Anesth Analg 2003;97:364-7.

*The authors performed a prospective, randomized, blinded trial in which they studied patients undergoing magnetic resonance imaging with general inhaled sevoflurane anesthesia through a laryngeal mask airway. They concluded that small doses of opioids decrease emergence agitation without increasing unwanted side effects.*

Gan TJ, Meyer T, Apfel CC, et al. Consensus guidelines for managing postoperative nausea and vomiting. Anesth Analg 2003;97:62-71.

*The authors review the available literature concerning postoperative nausea and vomiting. They use strength of evidence criteria when possible and expert opinion when data are lacking.*

Hackel A, Badgwell JM, Binding RR, et al. Guidelines for the pediatric perioperative anesthesia environment. American Academy of Pediatrics. Section on Anesthesiology. Pediatrics 1999;103:512-5.

*The American Academy of Pediatrics guideline for the pediatric perioperative anesthesia environment addresses the facility- and personnel-based components of the postoperative care setting for children.*

Kain ZN, Caldwell-Andrews AA, Maranets I, et al. Preoperative anxiety and emergence delirium and postoperative maladaptive behaviors. Anesth Analg 2004;99:1648-54.

*This study is extremely unusual in its ability to correlate perioperative anxiety with the incidence of emergence agitation. Preoperative anxiety is significantly related to the incidence of emergence agitation, and the incidence of agitation is related to the rate of postoperative maladaptive behaviors. This study argues strongly for identifying children at risk for emergence agitation and gives some evidence for why it is worth the effort to prevent or ameliorate this phenomenon.*

McNicol ED, Tzortzopoulou A, Cepeda MS, et al. Single-dose intravenous paracetamol or propacetamol for prevention or treatment of postoperative pain: a systemic review and meta-analysis. Br J Anaesth 2011;106:764-75.

*The authors performed a meta-analysis of 36 randomized, controlled trials and 3896 patients to look at the effect of a single, intravenous dose of acetaminophen. They found that 37% of patients with acute postoperative pain had pain relief for about 4 hours.*

## REFERENCES

Please see www.expertconsult.com.

# Sedation for Diagnostic and Therapeutic Procedures Outside the Operating Room

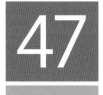

RICHARD F. KAPLAN, JOSEPH P. CRAVERO, MYRON YASTER, AND CHARLES J. COTÉ

THE USE OF SEDATION and analgesia for diagnostic and therapeutic procedures performed by anesthesiologists and nonanesthesiologists outside the operating room (OR) continues to dramatically increase. Millions of such procedures are performed each year throughout the world. Great progress has been made in understanding the need for and the risks associated with sedation and analgesia outside the OR; the mere restraint of a child for a frightening and/or painful procedure is difficult to justify.[1-4] Indeed, the time-honored techniques of immobilization by physical restraint or sedation with archaic medications, such as the "lytic cocktail" (meperidine, promethazine, and chlorpromazine), are unacceptable and were made possible only because children were easily overpowered, not routinely asked if they were in pain, and were unable to withdraw consent. Furthermore, many of these techniques were inefficient and failed to provide the conditions necessary to complete required procedures. Sedation/analgesia for painful procedures performed outside the OR (e.g., bone marrow aspiration, lumbar puncture, repair of minor surgical wounds, insertion of arterial or venous catheters, burn dressing changes, fracture reduction, bronchoscopy, and endoscopy) requires the same attention to detail as for procedures performed in the OR, because sedation levels needed often achieve the state of deep sedation or general anesthesia, particularly in children 6 years of age and younger. Nonpainful procedures often require sedation, immobility, and sometimes breath-holding. Children undergoing diagnostic studies (e.g., computed tomography [CT], magnetic resonance imaging [MRI], positron emission tomography, electroencephalography [EEG], electromyography), or who require high doses of ionizing radiation, also require deep levels of sedation or general anesthesia because they must remain absolutely motionless.[5] Given these requirements, a team approach is required to provide appropriate care for the child and to provide optimal conditions for the procedure.

Young and developmentally delayed children, are often unable to remain motionless for even short periods of time. Even some older children and adults may be unable to enter the confined space and often frightening environment of a diagnostic imaging scanner. The fear and anxiety associated with procedures are difficult to control and may be exacerbated by parental anxiety, separation from parents, and the pain (or anticipation of pain) from the procedure. Although distraction, guided imagery, and the use of videos and music have clear and documented benefit, they are often not enough to efficiently and successfully complete procedures.[6-10]

The pharmacologic armamentarium for sedation for diagnostic and therapeutic procedures has greatly expanded to include drugs classified as sedatives, as well as those classified as general anesthetics. Who uses these drugs and what qualifications are needed by those who provide such sedation is controversial.[11] The demand for safe efficient sedation and analgesia outside the OR comes from many sources, including hospital administrators, insurance companies, and medical specialists. Failed sedations for diagnostic or therapeutic procedures are no longer acceptable, as this increases costs and frustrates parents[12]; however, this manpower need has far outstripped the available supply of anesthesiologists. This led to the demand to create sedation services for diagnostic or therapeutic procedures by nonanesthesiologists (i.e., nurse practitioners, pediatricians, emergency medicine physicians, intensivists, and dentists) who often use sedative agents, including general anesthetics. The development of pediatric sedation services has taken many directions. In a 2005 survey of pediatric sedation practice in 116 children's hospitals in the United States and Canada,[13] only 50% of the hospitals had a formal pediatric sedation service. Anesthesiologists were the sole sedation providers in only 26% of institutions. A consortium of pediatric hospitals heavily involved in sedation noted that anesthesiologists were involved in 19% of sedation procedures.[14] Even when looking at the use of drugs such as propofol, which is considered a "general anesthetic," this group noted anesthesiologists involvement only 10% of the time.[15] This chapter will focus on the current definitions of sedation for diagnostic and therapeutic procedures and the goals, risks, and guidelines for creation of safe conditions for children who require sedation for procedures outside the OR.

As anesthesiologists we need to ask—why should we care? We believe that we provide the best, most efficient, and safest conditions for procedures, whether they are painful or not and whether they are in the OR or not. However, there simply aren't enough anesthesia care providers to meet the ever-increasing demand. Further, after years of training and the ability to provide anesthesia for "big" cases (e.g., liver transplants, craniofacial reconstruction, trauma, etc.), we need to ask ourselves whether we are "overtrained" to care for children who require sedation or anesthesia for procedures outside of the OR, or whether it can be safely done by others with less training. Federal regulatory agencies, hospital administrations, and professional societies have recognized the expertise of anesthesiologists to provide sedation and have required us to lead, teach, and be responsible for oversight and credentialing of all sedation providers. We must "grab this tiger by its tail."[12,16]

## Definition of Levels of Sedation

Several organizations have created guidelines and definitions of sedation for diagnostic and therapeutic procedures in children.[17-20] The definitions of the American Academy of Pediatrics (AAP), the American Society of Anesthesiologists (ASA), The Joint Commission (previously called the Joint Commission on Accreditation of Healthcare Organizations), and the American Academy of Pediatric Dentistry (AAPD) are the most frequently cited and agreed-upon position statements.[18,19,21-23] These organizations defined sedation and analgesia for procedures as a continuum of consciousness to unconsciousness, ranging from minimal sedation (anxiolysis) to moderate sedation (previously, "conscious sedation") to deep sedation and general anesthesia (Fig. 47-1). Note that a child's depth of sedation may easily pass from a light level all the way to general anesthesia.[24]

A clear understanding of the definition of sedation is mandatory to recognize when the child has progressed to a deeper level of sedation than anticipated (i.e., from moderate sedation to deep sedation or from deep sedation to general anesthesia). Recognition of this transition allows escalation of monitoring and care to avoid complications. The AAP, ASA, and The Joint Commission formalized and defined the concepts of minimal sedation, moderate sedation, deep sedation, and general anesthesia. The definitions that follow are taken from The Joint Commission (2010)[25,26] and are in agreement with AAP, AAPD, and ASA definitions[18,19,21]:

- *Minimal sedation (anxiolysis):* A drug-induced state during which patients respond normally to verbal commands. Although cognitive function and coordination may be impaired, ventilatory and cardiovascular functions are unaffected (Video 47-1).
- *Moderate sedation* (previously called "conscious sedation" or sedation/analgesia): A drug-induced depression of consciousness during which patients respond purposefully to verbal commands, either alone or accompanied by light tactile stimulation. No interventions are required to maintain a patent airway, and spontaneous ventilation is adequate. Cardiovascular function is usually maintained (Video 47-2).
- *Deep sedation:* A drug-induced depression of consciousness during which patients cannot be easily aroused but respond purposefully after repeated or painful stimuli (*note:* reflex withdrawal from a painful stimulus is not considered a purposeful response). The ability to independently maintain ventilatory function may be impaired. Patients may require assistance in maintaining a patent airway and spontaneous ventilation may be inadequate. Cardiovascular function is usually maintained (Video 47-3).
- *General anesthesia:* A drug-induced loss of consciousness during which patients are not arousable, even to painful stimuli. The ability to independently maintain ventilatory function is often impaired. Patients often require assistance in maintaining a patent airway, and positive-pressure ventilation may be required because of depressed spontaneous ventilation or drug-induced depression of neuromuscular function. Cardiovascular function may be impaired (Video 47-4).

Painful procedures or nonpainful procedures requiring complete immobility (e.g., diagnostic imaging or radiation therapy) cannot be performed in a child who is moderately ("consciously") sedated. Most pediatric procedures require deep sedation. The myth that a state of moderate sedation in which children are conscious and simultaneously responsive to voice command while immobile in the face of pain is just that, a myth.[27]

Assessing the depth of sedation based on the child's responses to stimulation is illustrated in Figure 47-2. This is a difficult challenge in children and depends on their verbal abilities, age, level of maturity, and underlying condition. A common problem with classifying a child as either moderately or deeply sedated is to misinterpret any movement in response to touch as "purposeful" and therefore a sign of "moderate sedation." A child who is moderately sedated should respond to touch or firm rubbing by an appropriate response, such as saying "ouch," pushing your hand away, and pulling up the covers. *An inappropriate response, such as nonpurposeful movement, is a sign that the child has progressed to a deeper sedation level, which should lead to an escalation of care because respiratory depression may occur.*[28-31] Similarly, children who are deeply sedated should respond purposefully to painful stimuli. *Reflex withdrawal, a nonpurposeful response or no response to painful stimuli, is a sign that the child has progressed to a level of*

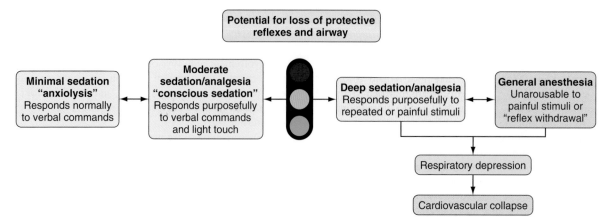

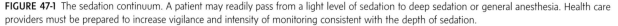

**FIGURE 47-1** The sedation continuum. A patient may readily pass from a light level of sedation to deep sedation or general anesthesia. Health care providers must be prepared to increase vigilance and intensity of monitoring consistent with the depth of sedation.

reported data and the providers were not randomized. The study did not track whether high-risk patients were referred to practitioners outside of their sedation practice (i.e., the anesthesia service). Only major complications and not minor but dangerous complications (i.e., desaturation, hypoventilation, and need for airway support) were monitored. The participants in these hospitals are highly motivated, and application of these data outside of the consortium requires rigorous evaluation of safeguards and training. The ASA thinks that anesthesiologist participation in all deep sedation is the best means to achieve the safest care. The ASA acknowledges that nonanesthesiologists administer or supervise the administration of deep sedation and has created guidelines to help anesthesiologists provide leadership in this area.[93,94]

## Guidelines

The first sedation guidelines were published in 1985 from the Committee on Drugs, Section on Anesthesiology, American Academy of Pediatrics.[95] These guidelines provided the first framework to improve safety for children requiring sedation for a procedure. The guidelines emphasized systems issues, such as the need for informed consent, appropriate fasting before sedation, frequent measurement and charting of vital signs, the availability of age- and size-appropriate equipment, the use of continuous physiologic monitoring, the need for basic life support skills, as well as proper recovery and discharge procedures. The guidelines stated that an independent observer whose only responsibility was to monitor the child was required for deep sedation. Advanced airway and resuscitation skills were encouraged but not required. In 1992, the guidelines were revised[96] emphasizing that a child could readily progress from one level of sedation to another and that the practitioner should be prepared to increase vigilance and monitoring as indicated. In 2002, the same Committee on Drugs of the AAP updated and amended the guidelines.[97] It eliminated the use of the confusing term *conscious sedation* and replaced it with the term *moderate sedation*. It also emphasized the application of these guidelines outside the hospital, in recognition of the relatively high complication rate in non–hospital-based settings. The ASA guidelines in use today were updated in 2002 and, in many respects, modeled after the AAP guideline.[98] These guidelines were systematically developed by a task force of 10 members. The task force reviewed the strength of evidence and made recommendations that include the following:

- *Patient Evaluation:* Clinicians should be familiar with the sedation-related aspects of the patient's medical history. These include (1) abnormalities of major organ systems, (2) previous adverse effects with sedation and general anesthesia, (3) drug allergies, current medications, and drug interactions, (4) time and nature of oral intake, and (5) history of tobacco, alcohol, or substance abuse. A focused physical examination, including vital signs, auscultation of the heart and lungs, and evaluation of the airway, is recommended.
- *Preprocedural Preparation:* Patients should be informed of and agree to sedation, including its risks, benefits, limitations, and alternatives. Sufficient time should elapse before a procedure to allow gastric emptying in elective patients. Minimum fasting periods of 2 hours (clear liquids), 4 hours (breast milk), and 6 hours (infant formula, nonhuman milk, and light meal), are recommended for healthy patients. If urgent, emergent, or other situations impair gastric emptying,

the potential for pulmonary aspiration of gastric contents must be considered in determining the target level of sedation, delay, or intubation.

- *Monitoring Level of Consciousness:* Monitoring of verbal commands should be routine during moderate sedation, with the exception of young children and mentally impaired, uncooperative patients, or when the response would be detrimental. During deep sedation the response to a more profound stimulus should be sought to be sure the patient has not drifted into general anesthesia.
- *Physiologic Monitoring:* All patients undergoing sedation/analgesia should be monitored by pulse oximetry with appropriate alarms. In addition, ventilatory function should be continually monitored by observation or auscultation. Monitoring of end-tidal carbon dioxide ($ETCO_2$) should be considered for all patients receiving deep sedation and for patients whose ventilation cannot be directly observed during moderate sedation. Multiple studies have confirmed the usefulness in $ETCO_2$ monitoring especially during deep sedation. Although not currently required, adverse events can be anticipated and corrected by using $ETCO_2$ monitoring.[99] It should be noted that ASA standards for basic monitoring have been amended to include $ETCO_2$ monitoring for all sedated patients beginning in 2012.[99,100] When possible, blood pressure (BP) should be determined before sedation/analgesia is initiated. Once sedation/analgesia is established, BP should be measured at regular intervals during the procedure, unless such monitoring interferes with the procedure (e.g., pediatric MRI, in which stimulation from the BP cuff could arouse an appropriately sedated child). Electrocardiographic (ECG) monitoring should be used in all children during deep sedation, and during moderate sedation in those with significant cardiovascular disease or those who are undergoing procedures in which dysrhythmias are anticipated.
- *Recording of Monitored Parameters:* For both moderate and deep sedation, the child's level of consciousness, ventilatory and oxygenation status, and hemodynamic variables should be assessed and recorded at a frequency that depends on the type and amount of medication administered, the length of the procedure, and the general condition of the patient. At a minimum, this should be (1) before the beginning of the procedure; (2) after administration of sedative/analgesic agents; (3) at regular intervals during the procedure; (4) during initial recovery; and (5) just before discharge. If recording is performed automatically, device alarms should be set to alert the care team to critical changes in patient status. (Children's National Medical Center [CNMC] hospital policy requires recording of vital signs every 15 minutes and every 5 minutes for moderate and deep sedation, respectively.)
- *Availability of an Individual Responsible for Patient Monitoring:* A designated individual, other than the practitioner performing the procedure should be present to monitor the child throughout procedures performed with sedation/analgesia. During deep sedation, this individual should have no other responsibilities. However, during moderate sedation, this individual may assist with minor, interruptible tasks once the patient's level of sedation/analgesia and vital signs have stabilized, provided that adequate monitoring for the child's level of sedation is maintained.
- *Training of Personnel:* Individuals responsible for children who receive sedation/analgesia should understand the pharmacology of the medications that are administered, as well as the

**47**

role of pharmacologic antagonists for opioids and benzodiazepines. Individuals who monitor children who receive sedation/analgesia should be able to recognize the associated complications. At least one individual capable of establishing a patent airway and positive-pressure ventilation, as well as a means for summoning additional assistance, should be present whenever sedation/analgesia is administered. It is recommended (although not specifically stated) that an individual with advanced life support skills be immediately available (within 5 minutes) for moderate sedation; such an individual must be within the procedure room for deep sedation.

■ *Availability of Emergency Equipment:* Pharmacologic antagonists, as well as appropriately sized equipment for establishing a patent airway and providing positive-pressure ventilation with supplemental oxygen, should be present whenever sedation/analgesia is administered. Suction, advanced airway equipment, and resuscitation medications should be immediately available and in good working order. A functional defibrillator should be immediately available whenever deep sedation is administered and when moderate sedation is administered to those with mild or severe cardiovascular disease.

■ *Use of Supplemental Oxygen:* Equipment to administer supplemental oxygen should be present when sedation/analgesia is administered. Supplemental oxygen should be considered for moderate sedation and should be administered during deep sedation unless specifically contraindicated for a particular child or procedure. If hypoxemia is anticipated or develops during sedation/analgesia, supplemental oxygen should be administered.

■ *Combinations of Sedative/Analgesic Agents:* Combinations of sedative and analgesic agents may be administered as indicated for the procedure being performed and the condition of the child. Ideally, each component should be administered individually to achieve the desired effect (e.g., additional analgesic medication to relieve pain; additional sedative medication to decrease awareness or anxiety). The propensity for combinations of sedative and analgesic agents to cause respiratory depression and airway obstruction emphasizes the need to appropriately reduce the dose of each component, as well as the need to continually monitor respiratory function (Fig. 47-4).

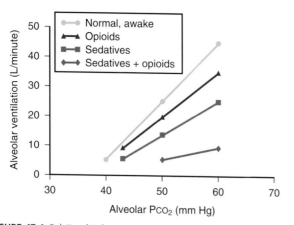

**FIGURE 47-4** Relationship between ventilation and carbon dioxide is represented by a family of curves. Each curve has two parameters, an x-intercept and a slope. Sedatives and opioids increase the intercept and decrease the slope. The combination of sedatives and opioids produce the most profound effect. (From Yaster M, Nichols DG, Deshpande JK, Wetzel RC. Midazolam-fentanyl intravenous sedation in children: case report of respiratory arrest. Pediatrics 1990;86:463-7.)

■ *Titration of Intravenous Sedative/Analgesic Medications:* Intravenous (IV) sedative/analgesic drugs should be given in small, incremental doses that are titrated to the desired end points of analgesia and sedation. Sufficient time must elapse between doses to allow the effect of each dose to be assessed before subsequent drug administration. When drugs are administered by non-IV routes (e.g., oral, rectal, intramuscular [IM], transmucosal), allowance should be made for the time required for drug absorption before supplementation is considered. Because absorption may be unpredictable, administration of repeat doses of oral medications to supplement sedation/analgesia is not recommended.

■ *General Anesthetic Induction Agents Used for Sedation/Analgesia (Propofol, Methohexital, Ketamine):* Even if moderate sedation is intended, children who are sedated with either propofol or methohexital by any route should receive care consistent with that required for deep sedation. Accordingly, practitioners who administer these drugs should be qualified to rescue the children from any level of sedation, including general anesthesia. Children who are sedated with ketamine should be cared for in a manner consistent with the level of sedation that is achieved.

■ *Recovery Care:* After sedation for diagnostic and therapeutic procedures, the children should be observed in an appropriately staffed and equipped area until they are near their baseline level of consciousness and are no longer at increased risk for cardiorespiratory depression. Oxygenation should be monitored periodically until they are no longer at risk for hypoxemia. Ventilation and circulation should be monitored at regular intervals until the children are suitable for discharge. Discharge criteria should be designed to minimize the risk of central nervous system (CNS) or cardiorespiratory depression after discharge from observation by trained personnel.

■ *Consultation and Availability of an Anesthesiologist:* Whenever possible, appropriate medical specialists should be consulted before sedating children with significant underlying conditions. The choice of specialists depends on the nature of the underlying condition and the urgency of the situation. For severely compromised or medically unstable children (e.g., anticipated difficult airway, severe obstructive pulmonary disease, or congestive heart failure), or if it is likely that sedation to the point of unresponsiveness will be necessary to obtain adequate conditions, practitioners who are not trained in the administration of general anesthesia should consult an anesthesiologist (Table 47-6).

The above ASA guideline pertains to all age-groups. The AAP's most recent guideline update was published in 2006.[18] In general, their updated guideline reinforces the ASA guideline. The AAP updated revision retains the same definitions of the continuum of sedation that are identical to the ASA and Joint Commission definitions. The AAP guidelines emphasize a systematic approach to sedation that includes:

■ No administration of sedative medications without the safety net of medical supervision (i.e., no sedative medications given at home)

■ Careful presedation evaluation to include review of pertinent medical and surgical conditions

■ Careful history for ingestion of nutraceuticals and other medications that may alter drug metabolism and prolong sedation

■ A "time out" should be performed before sedation

■ Appropriate fasting guidelines for elective and urgent procedures. There should be a balance between the depth of

**TABLE 47-6** Guidelines for the Consultation of an Anesthesiologist

1. Medical Problems
   - ASA Physical Status III or IV
   - Pulmonary: airway obstruction (tonsils/adenoids)—loud snoring, obstructive sleep apnea. Poorly controlled asthma, congenital or acquired anomalies of the airway or face (Trisomy 21, Pierre Robin syndrome, Treacher Collins syndrome, Crouzon disease, tracheomalacia)
   - Morbid obesity ($\geq$2 times ideal body weight, BMI > 30 kg/m$^2$)
   - Cardiovascular: cyanosis, repaired or unrepaired congenital heart disease with significant symptoms of cyanosis or congestive heart failure
   - Prematurity: less than 60 weeks postconceptional age at time of sedation
   - Residual pulmonary, cardiovascular, gastrointestinal, neurologic problems
   - Neurologic: developmental disabilities, poorly controlled seizures, central apnea
   - Gastrointestinal: uncontrolled gastroesophageal reflux
   - Severe liver of renal disease

2. Procedures requiring deep sedation in patients with a full stomach
   - Emergency Procedures

3. Management problems
   - Severe developmental delay
   - Patients who are difficult to control
   - Severe attention deficit disorder (paradoxically, the child may develop increased agitation during or after the procedure)

4. History of failed sedation
   - Oversedation (loss of airway reflexes)
   - Inability to adequately sedate
   - Hyperactive (paradoxical) response to sedatives

*ASA*, American Society of Anesthesiologists; *BMI*, body mass index.

sedation and the risk for those who are unable to fast because of the urgent nature of the procedure
- Focused airway examination with particular attention to anatomic airway abnormalities and enlarged tonsils
- Understanding of the pharmacologic and PD effects of sedation medications and drug interactions
- Appropriate training and skills in airway management to allow for rescue. Deep sedation requires training in pediatric advanced life support
- Immediate availability of size- and age-appropriate airway, monitoring, and resuscitation equipment
- Appropriate medications and reversal agents
- Sufficient numbers of sedation providers to carry out the procedure and monitor the child
- Appropriate physiologic monitoring during and after the procedure; use of capnography is encouraged
- Appropriate recovery personnel, monitoring, and discharge criteria with return to baseline condition before discharge
- Prolonged observation in a step-down unit of children who have been sedated with drugs known to have a long half-life (e.g., chloral hydrate, "lytic cocktail" [see later discussion])
- Continuous quality improvement to track common markers of potential safety issues, such as desaturation events, airway obstructions, laryngospasm, unplanned hospital admission, unsatisfactory sedation, and medication errors
- Use of simulators to practice how to manage rare adverse events

- Assume all children younger than 6 years of age to be deeply sedated from the beginning of the sedation process

Other organizations, including the American College of Emergency Physicians (ACEP), published their own sedation guidelines.[101-105] The latter guidelines are distinguishable from the AAP and ASA guidelines in several respects, including the definition of the continuum of sedation. The ACEP guideline does not use the terms "moderate" or "deep" sedation but rather the term "procedural sedation." It is defined "as a technique of administering sedatives, analgesics, dissociative agents, alone or in combination to induce a state that allows the child to tolerate unpleasant procedures while maintaining cardiopulmonary function." It is intended to result in a depressed level of consciousness but one that allows the child to "independently and continuously" control their own airway. Unfortunately, the lack of uniform agreement on definitions and overlap of "procedural sedation" into "deep sedation" and "anesthesia" has led to considerable confusion and debate among practitioners. In 2006 the ASA asserted that "privileges to administer deep sedation should be granted only to practitioners who are qualified to administer general anesthesia."[93,94] Intensivists and emergency room physicians took umbrage with the ASA "usurping" control over their sedation practice.[11] They pointed out that their specialties have been using drugs, such as propofol and ketamine, for procedural sedation with minimal complications at levels that are considered deep sedation or anesthesia for many years,[106,107] and that they resent an outside organization imposing guidelines on their practices. In 2010 the ASA acknowledged that Medicare regulations permit some non–anesthesia practitioners to administer deep sedation and created guidelines to help hospital directors of anesthesia services grant privileges to such individuals.[93] The guidelines include: formal training in administration of deep sedation during residency training (within 2 years) or an Accreditation Council for Graduate Medical Education accredited training program; experience and competency in managing sedated patients; clinical experience with more than 35 patients; knowledge of ASA guidelines; advanced cardiac life support training; and quality assurance tracking. Separate privileging is required for the care of children. The exact nature of these requirements are not specified, but are over and above baseline competencies and dependent on the hospital's director of anesthesia services.

It is mandatory that sedation policies used in hospitals conform to Joint Commission standards that have been derived from the Department of Health & Human Services (DHHS) Centers for Medicare & Medicaid Services (CMS). In the 1990s, the Joint Commission recognized that there is considerable variation in the level of care provided to sedated children, depending on where the sedation is administered, even within one institution. They mandated that the standard of care for all sedated patients be uniform throughout any one institution Thus institutionally standardized documentation (e.g., medical history, physical status, and record-keeping during the procedure and the recovery from the procedure), fasting guidelines, and informed consent procedures are mandatory for all patients undergoing sedation, regardless of the nature, duration, patient's history, and location of the procedure. Similarly, the sedation personnel, monitoring equipment, and recovery facilities must be standardized or uniform within an institution. All of this must be part of an active quality improvement process. Hospitals risk losing federal funding if they fail to comply. In 2004, 18% of hospitals were found noncompliant in planning the administration of

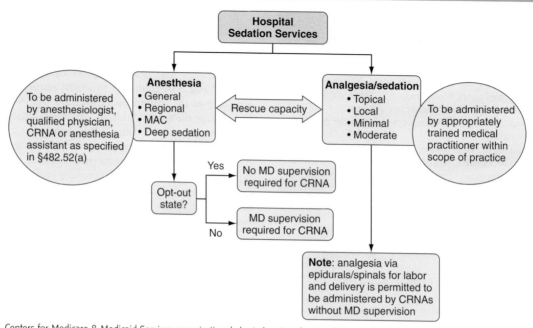

**FIGURE 47-5** Centers for Medicare & Medicaid Services organizational chart showing deep sedation under the category of "Anesthesia" and supervised by "Hospital Sedation Services." *CRNA*, Certified registered nurse anesthetist; *MAC*, monitored anesthesia care; *MD*, physician.

moderate or deep sedation.[108] In the most recent Joint Commission regulations, 2010,[25] the leadership and responsibilities for the delivery of deep sedation fall on the shoulders of the anesthesia department (Fig. 47-5).

*Deep sedation* is placed under Anesthesia and *subject to the anesthesia administration requirements at 42 CFR 482.52(a):* whereas *minimal and moderate sedation* are placed under analgesia/sedation and therefore not subject to anesthesia administration requirements. CMS states that one anesthesia service has authority and responsibility of all anesthesia services throughout the institution. Anesthesia must be administered by a (1) qualified anesthesiologist; (2) CRNA (certified registered nurse anesthetist) or AA (anesthesiologist assistant) with appropriate supervision; (3) doctor of medicine or osteopathy (other than an anesthesiologist); and (4) dentist, oral surgeon, or podiatrist who is qualified to administer anesthesia under state regulations. Credentialing and privileging must be done per hospital policy and is the responsibility of the hospital's director of anesthesia services. The appropriateness and quality of anesthesia, including sedation, must be reviewed and approved by the director of anesthesia services.

Specific standards for sedation are mentioned in Provision of Care, Treatment and Services (PC.03.01.01, .03, .05 .07), Improving Organization Performance (PI.01.01.01), and records (RC.02.01.03).[23] These standards address moderate and deep sedation, as well as anesthesia services. The standards require that each hospital develop specific appropriate protocols for patients receiving sedation. These protocols must be consistent with professional standards and address the following:

1. Qualified individuals in sufficient numbers to perform and monitor patients during and after the procedure. A registered nurse must supervise perioperative nursing care.
2. Competency-based education, training, and experience in evaluating patients. These must include the following:
   a. Evaluating patients before the sedation
   b. Performing moderate and deep sedation, including rescuing patients who slip into a deeper than desired level of sedation. These include the following:
      i. Moderate sedation—are qualified to rescue patients from deep sedation and are competent to manage a compromised airway and to provide adequate oxygenation and ventilation
      ii. Deep sedation—are qualified to rescue patients from general anesthesia and are competent to manage an unstable cardiovascular system, as well as a compromised airway and inadequate oxygenation and ventilation
3. Appropriate equipment for care and resuscitation
4. The following must occur before moderate or deep sedation:
   a. Appropriate needs of the patient are assessed
   b. Preprocedural education is provided to the patient according to a plan of care
   c. A "time out" is conducted immediately before starting, as described in universal protocol
   d. A licensed independent practitioner plans or concurs with the planned procedure
5. Appropriate monitoring of vital signs during and after the procedure, including, but not limited to, heart rate and oxygenation using pulse oximetry, respiratory frequency and adequacy of pulmonary ventilation, monitoring of BP at regular levels, and cardiac monitoring (by ECG or use of a continuous cardiac monitoring device) in patients with significant cardiovascular disease or when dysrhythmias are anticipated or detected
6. Documentation of care before, during, and after the procedure
7. Monitoring of outcomes. In particular, analysis of data is performed on adverse events or patterns of adverse events during moderate or deep sedation.

## IMPLEMENTATION OF SEDATION GUIDELINES

Institutions and health care organizations (e.g., offices or freestanding centers) may choose to provide a range of sedation services to meet their particular needs. Large institutions, in which sedation is performed in multiple areas within the hospital at all hours, may choose to decentralize the approach, where individual departments have practitioners who perform sedation under strict guidelines and oversight. Other institutions may designate one area where most children who require sedation are prepared and a small team of sedation providers care for them. The latter is the organization model at Dartmouth Medical Center in New Hampshire. Other institutions may have teams of sedation nurses or hospitalists who go where sedation is required. CNMC has expanded sedation services to include non–operating room anesthesia locations on burn, hematology-oncology, and MRI units, where anesthesiologists provide deep sedation or anesthesia to these children; in all cases, institutional and anesthesia oversight is required.

The implementation of a successful institution-wide policy involves organization, education, record keeping, enforcement, and continuing quality improvement.[109] A sedation committee must be carefully organized and involves many departments, practitioners, and geographic areas within the institution. The goal of the committee is to create a sedation policy that can facilitate patient care without placing undue burden on practitioners. Ideally, the committee should be composed of representatives from at least one and preferably two to three sedation practitioner services (e.g., an endoscopist, intensivist, dentist, surgeon, or emergency medicine physician) and departments: anesthesiology, nursing, pharmacy, hospital administration, and—very importantly—risk management. The responsibilities of the sedation committee include the creation of hospital- or institution-wide sedation policies, determination of hospital- or institution-wide personnel and equipment needs, creation of educational programs, monitoring of sedation problems, modification of policies as needed, and granting sedation privileges.

The department of anesthesiology (chairperson or their designee) must play a central role in formulating policy, educating nonanesthesiology sedation practitioners, acting as consultants for potentially complex cases, particularly those patients with a difficult airway, and determining when sedation by a nonanesthesiologist is or is not appropriate. The department of anesthesiology should approve sedation flow sheets and records, and be involved, along with the committee and the institution's risk management department, in periodic review of the records and compliance with documentation and institutional policies and procedures. A member of the department of anesthesiology is responsible for the process of continuous quality improvement. Continuous quality improvement is needed to review complications, incident reports, and sedation flow sheets to ensure compliance with policy and recommend changes to the sedation committee. Finally, sedation and analgesia require a treatment plan. The department of anesthesiology must play a leading role in determining which sedatives, hypnotics, general anesthetics, and analgesics can be safely used alone and in combination in each institution. Several drugs in particular can easily produce deep sedation or general anesthesia, airway obstruction, an unprotected airway, and cardiorespiratory collapse, namely, methohexital, thiopental, nitrous oxide (when combined with other sedating medications), ketamine, propofol, and remifentanil. Which drugs can be used and by whom should be made on an institution-by-institution basis. Education is vital to maintain safety. An institution-wide ongoing educational program on sedation, emphasizing physician (and dentist) responsibility, nursing responsibility, guidelines, and the pharmacology of drugs, should

be given frequently enough to train the staff and to accommodate staff turnover (usually one to two times a year). Teaching modules, videos, handouts, simulations, and hands-on supervision have been used to supplement such programs.[87] One institution (CNMC) uses a computerized teaching module that includes a review of hospital policy, equipment, personnel, pharmacology of drugs used, and rescue from deeper levels of sedation (see Children's Exchange [CHEX] course module). A quiz must be successfully completed at the end of the computerized teaching module. The module is part of the orientation and hospital privileging procedure for each physician and nurse, and must be successfully completed before they can administer sedation; the module must be reviewed and successfully completed every 2 years. Staff privileges also require training for Basic Life Support or equivalent for those providing moderate sedation and Pediatric Advanced Life Support or equivalent for those administering deep sedation. Each division chief or section supervisor must attest to the practitioner's competency to provide the desired level of sedation.

Specialty organizations are also becoming involved in training of sedation providers. The Society for Pediatric Sedation provides an extensive "primer" on pediatric sedation on its web site at www.pedsedation.org. This organization also provides a credentialing course for pediatric sedation that uses a test of knowledge based on its written materials (see previous) and the completion of a full day "Sedation Provider Course," which includes lectures, interactive sessions, and human patient simulation sessions (developed from data relating to pediatric sedation adverse events) to teach and test core competencies.

Education should also emphasize the limits of sedation and appropriate referral to an anesthesiologist. Of particular concern is upper airway obstruction that would likely become worse with the administration of sedatives (Table 47-6).[54] Tonsil and adenoid hypertrophy is common in children aged 2 to 12 years, and is associated with loud snoring or obstructive sleep apnea. Obstructive sleep apnea occurs in 1% to 3% of all children, in up to 12% of adolescents, is threefold more frequent in African American children and fivefold more frequent in obese children.[110] Parents will frequently report that their child snores loudly and then "stops breathing." These children are at increased risk for airway obstruction and should be referred to an airway specialist (anesthesiologist, pediatric intensivist, pediatric emergency medicine specialist) if sedation will be required for their procedures. They may also require postsedation overnight admission and monitoring (see also Chapters 4 and 31).[98,111-113] Children with developmental disabilities should raise concern for sedation because they have a high incidence of airway obstruction during sedation and anesthesia.[114] Problems for which consultation with an anesthesiologist or other expert is suggested are listed in Table 47-6.

The importance of nursing in the provision of safe and effective sedation for children cannot be overemphasized. Nurses are the "front line" in sedation safety and frequently the part of the sedation team that identifies variation in policy compliance. Their support and education is mandatory. In addition, state nursing restrictions on nurses administering certain drugs (such as propofol and ketamine) must be taken into consideration.

The performance improvement administrative part of sedation implementation is the final piece of the puzzle. Compliance can be monitored by the medical and dental staff office, the department of nursing, as well as a committee charged with the responsibility of continuing quality improvement. *This committee should fall under the purview of risk management.* Nursing and medical staff offices should monitor compliance with educational certification for appropriate credentialing. The medical staff office should report to the department chairman and nursing office a list of individuals who need to be recertified in sedation. It is the responsibility of the department chairman and nursing supervisors to secure individual staff compliance. Finally, variance reports should be generated when sedation policy is not followed or when a critical incident occurs. The appropriate institutional committee reviews the incident and informs the sedation committee. Educational and corrective action should take place as quickly as possible. This committee should not be viewed as "sedation police," but rather as a resource to objectively and unemotionally review critical sedation-related events. The committee can then determine where the "system" broke down, to define what went wrong and why (e.g., inadequate history taking combined with sedation, inadequate monitoring combined with delay in problem recognition, or inadequate recovery procedures combined with re-sedation at home). Tracking common problems, such as desaturation events, the need for bag-mask ventilation, apnea, unplanned hospital admissions, unsatisfactory sedation, and so on, can provide direction for developing changes in policy that will prevent more severe but much less frequent events from occurring (Fig. 47-6). This type of critical incident analysis allows recommendations to be made for future prevention.[115-117] An example of a successful hospital sedation policy is that of the CNMC (see Appendix 47-1).

## DOCUMENTATION

Although differing departmental procedures, practice requirements, patient needs, and location limitations produce unique problems, a unified systematic approach to sedation creates a safety net that will protect children while providing sedation/analgesia for procedures. A single sedation flow sheet that is used wherever sedation is given within the institution will allow for uniformity of care and compliance with sedation policy. The universal sedation flow sheet allows for nurses to rotate to different areas and feel familiar with sedation requirements in different locations. The sedation flow sheet should be organized such that the practitioners have a practical guide to the sedation policy. Following and completing the sedation flow sheet will ensure compliance with hospital policy (E-Fig 47-1). CNMC is in the process of converting to electronic records. As such we have an opportunity to move to an electronic paperless sedation document, which can "pull in" data from other databases and automatically add vital signs (Video 47-5). Our first draft will be available through this book. We still use the paper form when we are in areas that are remote or that do not have electronic record keeping (e.g., MRI, offsite locations) (see E-Fig 47-1). The flow sheet (both paper and electronic) is organized into Presedation, During Sedation, and Postsedation responsibilities of the registered nurse and licensed independent practitioner (physician or dentist) providing sedation. The electronic version has various dropdown menus which allows the practitioner to access rating scale information and automatically enter vital signs (see Video 47-5).

- *Presedation responsibilities:* During this time, the responsibilities of the registered nurse include evaluation of the child to include learning assessment, NPO (nothing by mouth) status, allergies, current medications, and review of medical problems. The licensed independent practitioner verifies this information with emphasis on airway assessment. A sedation plan is identified and informed consent is obtained. The licensed independent practitioner assigns an ASA physical status and reassesses the child immediately before the procedure.
- *Presedation pause:* A "time out" is performed immediately before sedation medications are given. The "time out" includes a process of verbal confirmation of the patient and procedure identification, verification of informed consent, as well as ASA physical status and confirmation of the procedure and site of the procedure. No medications will be administered without completion of the "time out." One advantage of the electronic form is that it forces the licensed independent practitioner to verify "time out" before it allows further access to the rest of the sedation flow sheet.
- *During sedation:* The time-based flow sheet identifies the type of stimulation needed to elicit a response, as well as what monitors and how frequently vital signs should be recorded for both moderate and deep sedation. A summary of monitoring, documentation, personnel, and equipment during sedation is given in Table 47-7.
- *Postsedation:* The criteria for discharge from the sedation area, pain score, and disposition of the child, as well as discharge teaching are specified. This includes documentation and signature by the licensed independent practitioner and nurse. Space is given for additional documentation and medications given.

Most importantly, both the paper and electronic form have critical parts of the sedation policy for immediate bedside review. This includes pain assessment scales, NPO guideline variations, reassessment by the licensed independent practitioner before sedation, and the opioid medication order verification. A table that defines the levels of sedation, required monitors, and

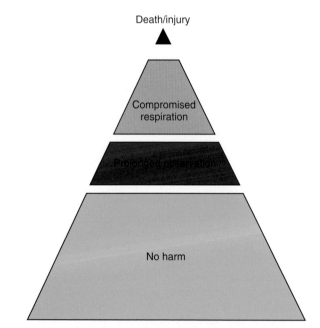

**FIGURE 47-6** The sedation accident pyramid. The majority of adverse sedation events result in no harm. A smaller number result in no harm but require prolonged observation. An even smaller number result in the need for some intervention, usually related to respirations (repositioning the head, a jaw thrust, bag or mask respirations or intubation). A very small number result in injury or death because the sentinel event was missed or inadequately treated. The latter cases are the types that occasionally are reported in newspapers, but in general go unreported. The reported cases likely represent just the tip of the pyramid in terms of events that could have indicated a developing problem.

**TABLE 47-7** Recommended Intensity of Monitoring, Documentation, Personnel, and Equipment for Different Levels of Sedation

| | Moderate Sedation | Deep Sedation |
|---|---|---|
| Monitoring | Pulse oximetry continuous<br>Heart rate continuous<br>Respiratory rate every 15 minutes<br>Level of consciousness every 15 minutes (if possible) | Pulse oximetry continuous<br>Heart rate continuous<br>Respiratory rate every 5 minutes<br>Level of consciousness every 5 minutes (if possible) |
| Documentation | Pulse oximetry every 15 minutes<br>Heart rate every 15 minutes<br>Respiratory rate every 15 minutes<br>Level of consciousness every 15 minutes, if possible | Pulse oximetry every 5 minutes<br>Heart rate every 5 minutes<br>Respiratory rate every 5 minutes<br>Level of consciousness every 5 minutes, if possible<br>ETCO$_2$ monitoring |
| Personnel | The same individual may observe the child and assist with procedure. | Dedicated independent observer—may not assist with procedure |
| Equipment | Pulse oximeter, blood pressure device, stethoscope<br>Resuscitation equipment immediately available | Pulse oximeter, blood pressure device, stethoscope, ECG monitor<br>Resuscitation equipment immediately available |
| Airway equipment | Age and size appropriate | Age and size appropriate (including a defibrillator) |

ECG, Electrocardiography; ETCO$_2$, end-tidal carbon dioxide.

**47**

frequency of monitoring is also present. This, in addition to the online availability of the hospital policy, ensures that sedation practitioners have all information available to be in compliance, to safely and successfully sedate children.

Individual departments may have special needs or situations that require addenda to the hospital sedation flow sheet. In addition, individual departments may find it helpful to create information sheets on presedation assessment, telephone interviews, and postsedation follow-up. The radiology–nursing database that consists of presedation telephone information, presedation instructions, NPO guidelines, health history, and postexamination telephone call information is shown in E-Figures 47-2 and 47-3. Samples of presedation and postsedation instruction sheets for pediatric dentistry are shown in E-Figures 47-4 and 47-5, respectively. These forms are available in Spanish and are explained via interpreters if necessary.

## Specific Sedation Techniques

A *sedation treatment plan* analyzing the requirements for analgesics, anxiolytics, or both is necessary for each child and will vary depending on the procedure and the anxiety of the child and family. Psychological techniques to allay anxiety (cuddling, parental support, warm blankets, a gentle reassuring voice, and hypnosis) are extraordinarily useful adjuncts to the sedation plan.[6-10]

Although the FDA is responsible for approval of the use of drugs, for a variety of reasons many of the drugs used for sedation and analgesia in children are not approved by the FDA for use in young children (e.g., fentanyl less than 2 years; morphine less than 12 years, bupivacaine less than 12 years, propofol less than 2 months, and dexmedetomidine less than 18 years of age). Although midazolam is approved even in preterm infants, the reversal agent flumazenil is not approved in children younger than 1 year of age! The lack of "approval" by the FDA does not imply that a drug should not be used; rather, it only means that the manufacturer never carried out the appropriate studies to gain FDA approval.[28,118-121] A number of legislative changes are intended to improve drug research in children and improve drug labeling; however, some of the drugs are no longer under patent

protection and there is no motivation for drug companies to study their use in children.[122-124] It is hoped that the continuing legislative efforts will improve drug labeling for children; see Chapter 6 for a more complete discussion of this issue.

It is important to review the child's presedation medications. Particular note of the use of protease inhibitors (used by many patients with human immunodeficiency virus infection) must be sought. These protease inhibitors (e.g., nelfinavir, ritonavir, saquinavir) are potent inhibitors of the cytochrome P-450 CYP3A metabolic pathway. This pathway is responsible the metabolism of many sedatives, including midazolam, and may markedly prolong duration of action and may lead to life-threatening respiratory depression. Erythromycin and some calcium channel blockers may also inhibit the cytochrome system and delay metabolism of midazolam.[125-127] Dexmedetomidine should not be combined with digoxin in infants because severe bradycardia has been reported.[128] Another concern for the practitioner is the widespread use of herbal medicines that can enhance or shorten sedative medication activity.[129-133] Herbal medicines (e.g., St. John's wort or echinacea) may alter drug PK through inhibition of the cytochrome P450 system, resulting in prolonged drug effect and altered (increased or decreased) blood drug concentrations. Kava may increase the effects of sedatives, and valerian may itself produce sedation (see also E-Table 4-4).[134]

The main classes of drugs used for sedation and analgesia for diagnostic and therapeutic procedures in children are:

- Local anesthetics
- Anxiolytics and sedatives
- Barbiturates
- Opioid analgesics
- General anesthetics

### LOCAL ANESTHETICS

*Local anesthetics* play a critical role in analgesia for painful procedures and greatly reduce requirements for systemic opioids. Unlike most drugs used in medicine, local anesthetics must be physically deposited at their site of action to produce their effect. Cessation of action often depends on the rapidity of removal of drug from this site. Systemic toxicity is related to how much and how rapidly local anesthetics are absorbed into the blood. Thus

**TABLE 47-8** Maximum Recommended Doses and Duration of Local Anesthetics

| Local Anesthetic | Maximum Dose (mg/kg) without Epinephrine | Maximum Dose (mg/kg) with Epinephrine | Approximate Duration (minutes) |
|---|---|---|---|
| Procaine | 7 | 10 | 60-90 |
| 2-chloroprocaine | 15 | 20 | 30-60 |
| Tetracaine | 1 | 1.5 | 180-600 |
| Lidocaine | 5 | 7 | 90-200 |
| Mepivacaine | 5 | 7 | 120-240 |
| Bupivacaine | 2 | 3 | 180-600 |
| Levobupivacaine | 2 | 3 | 180-600 |
| Ropivacaine | 2 | 3 | 180-600 |
| Articaine (dental procedures) | | 7 | 60-230 |

Modified from American Academy of Pediatrics; American Academy of Pediatric Dentistry; Coté CJ, Wilson S. Work Group on Sedation. Guidelines for monitoring and management of pediatric patients during and after sedation for diagnostic and therapeutic procedures: an update. Pediatrics 2006;118:2587-602.

small amounts of local anesthetics can be toxic if injected intra-arterially or IV. On the other hand very large amounts of local anesthetics can be safely administered in vascular-poor structures like fat. For most blocks and local skin infiltration, epinephrine (1:200,000 [5 µg/mL]) is used as a vasoconstrictor to lengthen the duration of blockade, decrease bleeding, and reduce systemic toxicity by decreasing vascular uptake. Local anesthetics should only be prepared in labeled syringes immediately before use. They should never be prepared before a procedure starts because of the possibility of inadvertent and catastrophic injection of the local anesthetic into an IV catheter or infusion. Finally, no more than the maximum allowable dose (mg/kg) should be prepared in the syringe to minimize the risk of an accidental overdose (Table 47-8). *Epinephrine-containing local anesthetics can cause tissue ischemia and are contraindicated in end-arterial areas (digits, ear, and penis), as well as in Bier blocks.* Local anesthetics can obtund airway reflexes when sprayed in the mouth for bronchoscopy or gastrointestinal endoscopy.

Specific blocks used in the sedated child include subcutaneous (SC) infiltration, field blocks, and IV regional anesthesia. A discussion of these topics and treatment of local anesthetic toxicity is found in Chapters 41 and 42. Topical administration of local anesthetics is useful in the sedated patient. EMLA cream is a eutectic mixture of local anesthetics (lidocaine 2.5% and prilocaine 2.5%) (AstraZeneca Pharmaceutical LP, Wilmington, Del.). When placed on the skin for 60 minutes,[135,136] it is useful for reducing the pain of skin incision, IV cannula insertions, lumbar punctures, and circumcision.[137-139] Absorption of large amounts of prilocaine can cause methemoglobinemia. It should be applied only to normal intact skin in appropriate doses[31] (i.e., for children weighing less than 10 kg, apply to a maximum of approximately 100 cm² surface area; for those 10 to 20 kg, apply to a maximum of approximately 600 cm² surface area; and for those more than 20 kg, apply to a maximum of approximately 2000 cm² surface area). The duration of action is 1 to 2 hours after the cream is removed. Adverse reactions include erythema, itching, rash, and methemoglobinemia. It also causes blanching of the skin, which can make IV access difficult. It is contraindicated in children younger than 1 month of age, in children with congenital

or idiopathic methemoglobinemia, or in infants receiving methemoglobinemia-inducing drugs (e.g., phenytoin, phenobarbital, acetaminophen, and sulfonamides).

ELA-Max and LMX4 (Ferndale Healthcare, Ferndale, Mich.) are topical 4% liposomal lidocaine solutions whose effects occur in 30 minutes.[140] The S-Caine patch (ZARS, Inc., Salt Lake City) is a eutectic mixture of 70 mg of lidocaine and 70 mg tetracaine in a bioadhesive layer that contains a heating element. The 20-minute application is effective in lessening pain from venipuncture procedures.[141]

## ANXIOLYTICS AND SEDATIVES

The most commonly used anxiolytics or sedatives in pediatric sedation are chloral hydrate, diazepam, and midazolam.

*Chloral hydrate* is one of the most widely used sedatives in neonates and children younger than 3 years of age (Table 47-9).[142-145] It is used as a sedative to facilitate nonpainful diagnostic procedures, such as EEG, CT, or MRI.[144] It is rapidly and completely absorbed when given orally. Rectal administration is erratically absorbed and therefore not recommended. The onset of sedation is 30 to 60 minutes, and the usual clinical duration is 1 hour. Although it has a long safety record, it can cause respiratory depression as a result of airway obstruction. Deaths have been associated with its use alone and when combined with other sedating medications.[54,113,146-149] One large series showed a 0.6% incidence of respiratory depression, especially at larger doses (75 to 100 mg/kg).[150] Its effect is primarily mediated by the active metabolite trichloroethanol, which is formed by the liver and erythrocytes.[151] Trichloroethanol has a half-life of 10 hours in toddlers, 18 hours in term infants, and 40 hours in preterm infants (see Fig. 47-3).[152] The prolonged effects of chloral hydrate warrant a longer period of postsedation observation; chloral hydrate can also cause adverse effects after discharge, which include motor imbalance (31%), gastrointestinal effects (23%), agitation (19%), and restlessness (14%). Agitation and restlessness lasted more than 6 hours in more than one-third of children who experienced these effects, 5% of whom did not return to baseline activity for 2 days after the procedure![44,153] The unpredictable onset and active metabolites dictate that this drug (as well as all sedatives for sedation) is given only in facilities capable of resuscitation (AAP guidelines) and that discharge occurs when sedation is clearly lessening and the child meets discharge criteria. Airway obstruction and death occurred after chloral hydrate sedation in a child who was in a child's car seat in the back of a car.[54] Despite being restricted in some countries as a result of potential carcinogenicity, in the United States the AAP states that there is insufficient evidence to avoid single doses of chloral hydrate.[154]

The *benzodiazepines* are commonly used in pediatric sedation. They are anxiolytic, amnestic, sedative hypnotics with anticonvulsant activities but without analgesic properties. Their high lipid solubility at physiologic pH accounts for the rapid CNS effects. As opposed to diazepam, midazolam is delivered in a water-soluble form (pH 3.5), which markedly decreases the incidence of pain on injection and thrombophlebitis.[151] However, the resulting decrease in fat solubility markedly delays transport into the CNS (peak EEG effect 4.8 minutes for midazolam vs. 1.6 minutes for diazepam; Fig. 47-7).[155,156] Benzodiazepines exert their effects by occupying the benzodiazepine receptor that modulates γ-aminobutyric acid (GABA), the major inhibitory neurotransmitter in the brain. The clearance of benzodiazepines is decreased in neonates and also by liver enzyme inhibition that

**TABLE 47-9** Sedation Regimens for Children

| Drug Regimen | Dose/Route | Onset (minutes) | Duration (minutes) | Comments |
|---|---|---|---|---|
| Pentobarbital | 4-6 mg/kg IV or PO | IV: 2-5<br>PO: 20-60 | IV: 15-45<br>PO: 60-240 | Long history of safety. Slow onset. Prolonged emergence. May have paradoxical excitement. Half-life increased by valproic acid and MAO inhibitors. Contraindicated in porphyria. |
| Midazolam | 0.25-0.75 mg/kg PO<br>0.025-0.05 mg/kg IV<br>0.2 mg/kg intranasal<br>0.1-0.15 mg/kg IM | 15-30<br>1-3<br>10-15<br>10-15 | 60-90<br>45-60<br>60-90 | Paradoxical response not infrequent. Intranasal route very irritating and should be avoided. Increased respiratory depression when used with opioids; reduce midazolam dose by 25%. Prolonged duration with protease inhibitors. Antagonist: flumazenil. |
| Chloral hydrate | 50-100 mg/kg PO (maximum not to exceed 2 grams) | 30-60 | 60-120 | Very popular for nonpainful radiologic procedures in small children when IV not available. Effects unreliable over 1-2 years of age. Prolonged sedation and paradoxical responses noted. Respiratory depression and obstruction reported with tonsil hypertrophy and anatomic abnormalities. Moderate sedation guidelines required. Markedly prolonged half-life in neonates. Contraindicated in porphyria. |
| Etomidate | 0.1-0.4 mg/kg IV | <1 | 5-15 | No analgesic effect. Greater doses cause general anesthesia, respiratory depression, and loss of airway. Stable cardiovascular profile. Little data in children. Must be credentialed for deep sedation/anesthesia. No reversal drug. Causes adrenal suppression ~12 hours. |
| Methohexital | 0.25-0.50 mg/kg IV<br>20-25 mg/kg rectal<br>10 mg/kg IM | <1<br>10-15<br>10-15 | 10-20<br>30-60<br>30-60 | Avoid if temporal lobe epilepsy or porphyria. IV doses quickly lead to general anesthesia. Rectal doses cause high frequency of apnea and should be avoided. Deep sedation/anesthesia credentialing. Contraindicated in children younger than 3 months of age, psychosis, stimulation of oropharynx, increased intracranial pressure, head injury, glaucoma. |
| Dexmedetomidine | IV: 1-3 μg/kg bolus (over 10 minutes)<br>Infusion: 0.5-3.0 μg/kg/**hr** | 10 | Clinical 30 minutes to 1 hour; half-life 1.5-3 hours | Mimics natural sleep. Rapid bolus may cause hypertension. Minimal respiratory depression. Dose-dependent hypotension and bradycardia. Use with caution with digitalis medications. Glycopyrrolate treatment of bradycardia may induce sustained hypertension of unknown mechanism. |
| Fentanyl with propofol | Fentanyl 1-2 μg/kg IV with propofol 50-150 mg/kg/min infusion IV | 1-2 | 30-60 | Child may rapidly become anesthetized with loss of airway. Advanced airway management skills required, with appropriate credentialing. |
| Midazolam with fentanyl | Midazolam 0.02 mg/kg IV with fentanyl 1-2 μg/kg IV | 2-3 | 45-60 | Commonly used for painful procedures. Careful titration needed to avoid deep sedation/anesthesia with apnea and hypoxia. Reduce dose of fentanyl when combined with benzodiazepine. Reduce dose with protease inhibitors. |
| Ketamine | 3-4 mg/kg IM<br>1-2 mg/kg IV<br>4-6 mg/kg PO | 5<br>1<br>10-20 | 30-60<br>30-60<br>30-90 | Nausea and vomiting common after procedure. Laryngospasm, apnea, agitation, hallucinations reported but uncommon. Midazolam may not help emergence delirium. Anticholinergic to control secretions. Larger doses can produce state of general anesthesia. Usually causes tachycardia, hypertension, and bronchodilatation. Paradoxical hypotension in critically ill patients. No antagonist available. Advanced airway management skills required, with appropriate credentialing. |
| Propofol | Bolus 1-2 mg/kg<br>Infusion 50-250 μg/kg/min | 30 seconds | 5-15 minutes after discontinuation | Profound, dose-related respiratory depressant. Assume deep sedation/anesthesia when using in children. Infusions > 5 hours may cause propofol infusion syndrome. Caution when used in mitochondrial myopathies. Pain on injection mitigated by IV lidocaine. Advanced airway management skills required, with appropriate credentialing. |

*Continued*

**TABLE 47-9** Sedation Regimens for Children—cont'd

| Drug Regimen | Dose/Route | Onset (minutes) | Duration (minutes) | Comments |
|---|---|---|---|---|
| Remifentanil | 0.1-0.25 μg/kg/min | 1 | 10-15 | Difficulty in titration frequently leads to apnea and general anesthesia. Few studies in children. Exclusively used by anesthesiologists. |
| Nitrous oxide | 50% in 50% oxygen for "minimal sedation"; up to 70% used by some for moderate sedation | <5 | On discontinuing | Requires specialized equipment for delivery, monitoring, and scavenging. When used alone or with local anesthesia is considered "minimal sedation." Greater doses or addition of other sedatives/analgesics requires a minimum of "moderate sedation" guidelines. Contraindications include respiratory failure, altered mental status, otitis media, bowel obstruction, and pneumothorax. No antagonist available. |
| Opioid antagonist: naloxone | 0.01-0.1 mg/kg IV or IM Max 2 mg/dose May repeat every 2 minutes | 1-2 | IV: 20-40 IM: 60-90 | Specifically antagonizes opioid effects. Should not be used for routine reversal of opioid effect. Adverse reactions: nausea, vomiting, tachycardia, hypertension, delirium, pulmonary edema. Reversal after long-term opioid use may lead to acute withdrawal. Children may renarcotize 1 hour after IV dosing. |
| Benzodiazepine antagonist: flumazenil | IV 0.01-0.02 mg/kg May repeat every 1 minute to 1 mg | 1-2 | 30-60 | Specific benzodiazepine antagonist. Does not antagonize opioids or other sedatives. Re-sedation may occur in 1 hour. Prolonged observation (2 hours) required. Not for routine sedation reversal. Children using benzodiazepine to control seizures or drug dependency may have exacerbations with flumazenil. |

Data modified from Cravero JP, Burke GT. A review of pediatric sedation. Anesth Analg 2004;99:1355-64; Krauss B, Green SM. Procedural sedation and analgesia in children. Lancet 2006;367:766-80; and Coté CJ, Stafford MA. The principle of pediatric sedation. Boston: Tufts University School of Medicine; 1998.
*IM*, Intramuscularly; *IV*, intravenously; *MAO*, monoamine oxidase; *PO*, by mouth.

occurs during concomitant use of erythromycin, cimetidine, or protease inhibitors.[126]

The sedated child usually becomes compliant but does not lose consciousness. Children frequently move, and another agent, such as an opioid, may be necessary if the child must not move to successfully accomplish the procedure. Although many children initially act disinhibited and "drunk" after small doses of benzodiazepines, some have a true paradoxical response.[157] Paradoxical responses, such as combativeness, disorientation, hyperexcitability, and agitation may appear in 1% to 15% of treated children.[158] It is prudent to switch to a different sedative drug in these children, because increasing the dose of benzodiazepines may lead to severe agitation followed by unconsciousness and respiratory compromise. The benzodiazepines have the advantage of antegrade amnesia in a significant number of children.[159,160] The markedly prolonged and variable elimination half-life and active metabolite of diazepam (desmethyldiazepam) make midazolam a superior sedative drug in children, particularly infants.[161-166] The time to peak effect after IV administration of midazolam is 2 to 4 minutes, and its duration is 45 to 60 minutes. Midazolam can be given IV, intranasally, sublingually, orally, or rectally (see Table 47-9). It is the only drug in this class approved for neonates. A manufactured oral cherry-flavored form is available. The oral route has become very popular and is well tolerated. The oral route can lead to variable effects, dependent on gastric emptying and first-pass hepatic metabolism. Nasal administration causes nasopharyngeal burning and should be avoided.[167,168] Rectal administration is usually well tolerated in children who have not been toilet trained (younger than approximately 1 year of age), but absorption may be irregular owing to many factors, including superior versus inferior hemorrhoidal vein absorption within the rectum. Benzodiazepines produce mild respiratory depression and upper airway obstruction.[169-171] Even small doses of oral midazolam (0.3 mg/kg) that cause minimal sedation were associated with a 6.5% decrease in functional residual capacity and a 7.4% increase in respiratory resistance.[172,172]

Respiratory depression may become severe in compromised children or in children with tonsil hypertrophy. Benzodiazepines must be given according to appropriate guidelines.[18,56,74] The combination of benzodiazepines and opioids is particularly troubling because they can produce a "super additive effect" on respiratory depression where the total depressant effect from the combination of drugs is much greater than the sum of their anticipated individual effects.[173,174]

*Flumazenil* is a specific benzodiazepine-receptor antagonist and will rapidly reverse the sedative and respiratory effects of benzodiazepines.[175-179] It is the first specific reversal agent for benzodiazepines and rapidly reverses CNS-induced unconsciousness, respiratory depression, sedation, amnesia, and psychomotor dysfunction. Children who take benzodiazepines for seizures or drug dependency may have those symptoms rapidly recur if flumazenil is given.[180] It should also be used with caution in children with benzodiazepine dependence, increased intracranial pressure, and in those taking drugs that decrease the seizure threshold (e.g., cyclosporine, theophylline, and lithium). The recommended dose of flumazenil is 10 μg/kg up to 0.2 mg every minute to a maximum cumulative dose of 1 mg IV. Antagonism begins within 1 to 2 minutes and lasts approximately 1 hour. Because re-sedation after 1 hour may occur, any child who receives flumazenil must be carefully monitored for at least 2 hours. Repeat flumazenil may be necessary. It should be noted that flumazenil will not antagonize respiratory depression caused

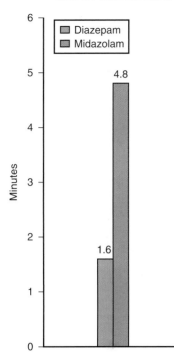

FIGURE 47-7 Time to peak electroencephalographic (*EEG*) effect of diazepam vs. midazolam in adults. Note that it takes nearly three times longer to achieve a peak EEG effect after intravenous (IV) midazolam than after IV diazepam. This is likely caused by the difference in fat solubility; because midazolam is less fat-soluble than diazepam, midazolam does not cross biologic membranes as easily. The clinical importance of this observation is the need to wait 3 to 5 minutes between IV doses of midazolam to avoid stacking of doses and excessive drug effect. (Data from Buhrer M, Maitre PO, Crevoisier C, Stanski DR. Electroencephalographic effects of benzodiazepines: II. Pharmacodynamic modeling of the electroencephalographic effects of midazolam and diazepam. Clin Pharmacol Ther 1990;48:555-67.)

by opioids.[181] Flumazenil should not be administered for the routine reversal of the sedative effects of benzodiazepines, but reserved for reversal of respiratory depression.

## BARBITURATES

*Pentobarbital* is the most commonly used intermediate-acting barbiturate for sedation. It has no analgesic effect and produces sedation, hypnosis, and amnesia. It has a long history of use during radiologic procedures. Sedation starts in 3 to 5 minutes and peaks in 10 minutes. Studies have shown a low incidence of respiratory obstruction and transient desaturation, as well as hypotension.[182,183] The barbiturates tend to make children more sensitive to pain and should be combined with analgesics when used during painful procedures. Pentobarbital's relatively long duration of action (1 to 2 hours or greater) and slow recovery sometimes leaves children in a prolonged disinhibited state that necessitates prolonged recovery and restraint[143]; pentobarbital "rage" occasionally occurs. The alkaline pH of barbiturates can lead to local erythema and thrombophlebitis if subcutaneous infiltration occurs. Newer, shorter-acting, faster recovery drugs are quickly replacing pentobarbital (see Table 47-9).

## OPIOIDS

*Opioid analgesics* are rarely used alone for diagnostic and therapeutic procedures in children. These potent analgesics are important during painful diagnostic and therapeutic procedures. They bind with four primary opioid receptor types ($\mu$, $\kappa$, $\delta$, and $\sigma$) that are located in the brain, spinal cord, and periphery. Once opioids bind to the receptor, they trigger the production of signaling proteins (such as G proteins) whose end effects are modulation of pain neurotransmission.[184] The $\mu_1$ subgroup is responsible for supraspinal analgesia and the development of dependence. The $\mu_2$ and $\kappa$ receptors are responsible for sedation. Although the opioids provide some sedation, the sedation produced is usually inadequate, therefore requiring combination with a sedative. The "super-additive" respiratory depressant effects of the combination of opioids and sedatives must be reemphasized (see Fig. 47-1).[173,185] This is especially true in infants and children with upper airway obstruction (e.g., tonsil and/or adenoid hypertrophy, trisomy 21, mucopolysaccharidosis). In addition, infants younger than 3 months of age and children who were born preterm have very large patient-to-patient drug metabolism variability.[186] Other serious effects of opioids include bradycardia, hypotension, seizures, and opioid-induced glottic and/or chest wall rigidity.

*Morphine* may be considered for painful procedures (lasting more than 1 hour) or when the child will also be in pain after the procedure. The duration of action is 3 to 5 hours after IV administration.[186] Morphine may be given orally (0.2 to 0.5 mg/kg), IV (0.05 to 0.1 mg/kg [maximum 0.3 mg/kg]), or IM (0.1 to 0.2 mg/kg). Rectal administration may cause delayed respiratory depression from erratic absorption and should be abandoned.[187] Time to peak effect for oral, IV, or IM administration is 60 minutes, 3 to 5 minutes, and 10 to 30 minutes, respectively. Its slow onset and prolonged duration have caused it to be replaced by shorter-acting opioids when used for sedation and analgesia for procedures.

*Meperidine* (Demerol) was also once used for sedation for procedures. Its clinical duration of action is 2 to 4 hours.[31] In addition to respiratory depression, the active metabolite of meperidine (normeperidine) may cause seizures, particularly after repeated doses of meperidine. Other adverse reactions include delirium, nausea, vomiting, urinary retention, pruritus, smooth muscle spasm, and hypotension (histamine induced). Special considerations include avoiding its use in children taking monoamine oxidase inhibitors (effects can include serotonin-induced hyperpyrexia and cardiovascular instability). CNS toxicity may occur in children taking tricyclic antidepressants and phenothiazines. Children taking phenytoin (Dilantin) may have a reduced analgesic effect. Reversal of meperidine-induced respiratory depression by antagonists may precipitate seizures caused by normeperidine. Because of these undesirable effects and prolonged duration, meperidine is not recommended for use as an analgesic or sedative in children.

*DPT "lytic cocktail"* is meperidine (Demerol [25 mg/mL]), promethazine (Phenergan [6.25 mg/mL]), and chlorpromazine (Thorazine [6.25 mg/mL]). Its long sedation duration (7 to 19 hours), hypotension, seizures, extrapyramidal reactions, and severe, prolonged, life-threatening respiratory depression[143,188-191] have caused its use to be abandoned.[189-195]

*Fentanyl* has replaced morphine and meperidine as the opioid of choice for sedation/analgesia for procedures in children. Fentanyl is available in parenteral form, in a transdermal patch delivery form (Duragesic), and in an oral transmucosal fentanyl citrate (OTFC; Actiq) form. *Duragesic is not to be used for sedation/analgesia during procedures.* Similarly, OTFC is only approved for breakthrough cancer pain in children 16 years of age or older, and has a box warning that it should be used only in opioid-tolerant children.

IV fentanyl is a potent, pure opioid (i.e., approximately 50 to 100 times more potent than morphine) with no amnesic properties. Its high lipid solubility allows for onset within 30 seconds and a peak effect at 2 to 3 minutes. It has a brief clinical duration of 20 to 40 minutes when given in small doses, owing to its rapid redistribution to skeletal muscle, fat, and other inactive sites. Unlike morphine, it has no active metabolites. The clearance of fentanyl is decreased and its half-life increased in preterm and term infants compared with older infants.[196] It is fully antagonized by naloxone. Fentanyl is frequently used with a short-acting anxiolytic (midazolam). IV doses usually start at 0.5 to 1 µg/kg and are titrated every 5 minutes to effect but not to exceed 5 µg/kg.[197] Doses must be given in small aliquots and carefully titrated to avoid chest wall and glottic rigidity. When carefully titrated and appropriately monitored, fentanyl has few adverse effects. Chest wall rigidity is a centrally mediated idiosyncratic reaction that can interfere with respiratory function. The mechanism of action is partially modulated by GABA pathways at the spinal level. Chest wall rigidity can be reversed with either naloxone or muscle relaxants. The rigidity is quite rare and not described after these small doses were given in boluses for sedation in neonates.[198-200] Other adverse reactions from fentanyl include bradycardia, dysphoria, delirium, nausea, vomiting, pruritus, urinary retention, hypotension, and smooth muscle spasm. Close postprocedural observation is required because respiratory depression can outlast analgesia (see Table 47-9).

*Remifentanil* an ultrashort-acting, rapid-acting, extremely potent, lipophilic opioid that is metabolized by plasma cholinesterase and must be administered as a continuous infusion. It has a context-sensitive half-life of 3 to 6 minutes that is independent of the duration of infusion. Remifentanil, when used as a sole agent in adults in the ED, caused a 17% incidence of respiratory complications that required bag mask ventilation or the placement of an laryngeal mask airway.[201] This suggests a need to clearly understand the PK and PD when used outside of the OR.[201]

Remifentanil has been used for intraoperative and procedural sedation by anesthesiologists and in intubated children in the ICU.[202-207] It has been suggested that children may develop opioid tolerance to this drug after several hours of infusion.[208] Remifentanil is associated with a substantial incidence of apnea, hypoxemia, chest wall and glottic rigidity, and should not be used as a sole agent for pediatric sedation (see Table 47-9).[204,206,209]

*Opioid antagonists* specifically reverse the respiratory and analgesic effects of opioids, and should be readily available when opioids are used (see Table 47-9). Naloxone (Narcan) is the most commonly used antagonist.[210] Opioid antagonists should not be used to routinely reverse the sedative effects of opioids, but reserved for reversal of respiratory depression or respiratory arrest. Naloxone may be given IV, IM, or SC.[211] The initial dose for respiratory depression is 0.01 mg/kg titrated to effect every 2 to 3 minutes. A dose of 10 to 100 µg/kg up to 2 mg may be required for respiratory arrest. Adverse reactions from reversal of analgesia include nausea, vomiting, tachycardia, hypertension, delirium, and pulmonary edema.[212-214] Children on long-term opioid therapy should be given opioid reversal agents in low doses and with extreme caution, because withdrawal seizures and delirium may occur. Children given naloxone may have recurrence of opioid effects after 1 hour. *If naloxone is used, the child should be observed for a minimum of 2 hours.* Repeat naloxone may be necessary. To avoid recrudescence of respiratory depression, some clinicians administer the same dose that was effective IV as an IM injection. Nalmefene (Revex) has a greater half-life (approximately 10 hours) than naloxone.[215] Although experience in children is limited, it has been shown to accelerate recovery from sedation.[216] Because of its relatively long half-life, it outlasts the effects of fentanyl and negates the treatment of pain with opioids for several hours.

## α₂-ADRENOCEPTOR AGONIST: DEXMEDETOMIDINE

*Dexmedetomidine* is the most recent addition to the list of sedative drugs used in pediatrics. Unlike other sedatives, it is an imidazole $\alpha_2$ agonist that is similar to clonidine but with an even greater $\alpha_2$- to $\alpha_1$-adrenoceptor specificity ratio of 1600 to 1. Clearance is predominantly by glucuronide conjugation, as well as by CYP2A6 action in the liver. The drug is highly lipid soluble and quickly crosses the blood-brain barrier. Its CNS effect is to stimulate receptors in the medullary vasomotor center, which decreases sympathetic tone. It also stimulates central parasympathetic outflow and decreases sympathetic outflow from the locus ceruleus of the brainstem. The decreased outflow from the locus ceruleus allows for increased activity of the inhibitory GABA neurons, which cause sedation and analgesia.[217] Dexmedetomidine is approved for sedation of ventilated adult patients in the ICU, and for procedural sedation, but as of 2012, it is not approved for use in children younger than 18 years of age. In addition to IV use, it has been administered via the buccal and IM routes in adults.[218] When administered in clinical doses, it causes limited effects on ventilation in adults and may mimic natural rapid-eye-movement sleep.[219-221] Because rapid IV boluses can cause transient systemic hypertension, the initial loading dose must be given over 10 minutes, followed by an infusion. When given in the recommended fashion, it decreases BP and heart rate in a dose-dependent manner. It should be used with caution in children with preexisting bradycardia, atrioventricular conduction defects, hypotension, and decreased cardiac output.[222,223] It has been associated with severe bradycardia in infants receiving digitalis.[128] The minimal effects on ventilation have led to a surge in its use in children.[224-227]

Sedation after IV administration has a relatively rapid onset of 10 min and a half-life of 1.5 to 3 hours. It is unique among sedatives in that it mimics natural sleep. Its minimal effect on respiration has led to its use alone in nonpainful procedures (e.g., EEG, CT, and MRI), in children with Down syndrome, and children with obstructive sleep apnea. It has also been used in combination with ketamine and propofol for painful procedures and syndromes (e.g., cardiac catheterizations and complex regional pain syndrome)[228,229]; however, caution is advised in children with known congenital heart disease, as it depresses sinus and atrioventricular node function and may pose an increased risk for children prone to bradycardia.[228-232] It has also been used as a novel approach to control the adverse effects of opioid and sedative withdrawal in children in the ICU.[233-235] The minimal respiratory effects of dexmedetomidine has been demonstrated both anatomically and physiologically in healthy children. Analyzed by MRI, the dose-response effects of dexmedetomidine (1 to 3 µg/kg/min) on upper airway morphology in children without obstructive sleep apnea[236,237] demonstrated minimal changes in upper airway dimensions in several planes, with no clinical evidence of airway obstruction. Infants and children 5 months to 16 years of age who were sedated with dexmedetomidine for nonpainful procedures (e.g., MRI, MRI plus EEGs, and nuclear medicine procedures) showed minimal effects on respiration.[57] Boluses of 0.5 to 1.0 µg/kg dexmedetomidine were infused over 5 to 10 minutes, followed by an infusion of 0.5 to 1.0 µg/kg/hr. Heart rate, BP, and respiratory rate decreased but remained within normal limits for age. The ETCO$_2$ exceeded 50 mm Hg in only 7 of 404 measurements. Maximum ETCO$_2$ was 52 mm Hg; mean recovery time was 84 minutes. The minimal effect of dexmedetomidine on respirations has also been verified in children with obstructive sleep apnea.[236,237]

Initial studies demonstrated that standard doses of dexmedetomidine could not consistently provide optimal conditions for sedation for these procedures. Some clinicians increased the initial loading dose and maintenance infusion dose of dexmedetomidine, whereas others supplemented the original dosing regimen with midazolam 0.1 mg/kg, in search of a successful regimen for sedation for radiologic investigations. In the case of sedation for MRI,[238] a loading dose of 3 µg/kg administered over 10 minutes IV followed by an infusion of 2 µg/kg/hr minimized the need for rescue with pentobarbital (2.4%). Mean arterial pressure was maintained in all children and oxygen saturation remained greater than 95% in all children. However, most importantly, in 30 of the 747 (4%) children, the heart rate decreased to less than the 20th percentile for age. Heart rates in the 1- to 3-year-old and 3- to 6-year-old age-groups were as low as the 30 to 40 beats per minute, although no adverse effects were noted, nor were any treatments required. *Although not apparently harmful in this cohort, we do not recommend use of such large doses of dexmedetomidine, because heart rates of 30 to 40 beats per minute are well below the acceptable range of normal heart rates in children!* Caution should also be used when administering glycopyrrolate to treat the bradycardia from dexmedetomidine in children, because severe and sustained hypertension after traditional doses of 5 µg/kg have occurred (e.g., BP 161/113 in a 3-year-old); the mechanism of this unusual response remains elusive.[239] An alternative approach[240] included a loading dose of 1 µg/kg dexmedetomidine over 10 minutes followed by an infusion of 0.5 µg/kg/min plus a 0.1 mg/kg bolus of midazolam after a sevoflurane inhalational induction for IV placement. With this regimen, all MRI scans were completed successfully, with only small changes in ETCO$_2$ (maximum 57 mm Hg). Hemodynamically, systemic BP and heart rate were maintained, with the lowest systolic BP being 70 mm Hg and the lowest heart rate 64 beats per minute in 3 children. This regimen was compared with propofol at 300 µg/kg/min for 10 minutes and a dose of 250 µg/kg/min thereafter, with equivalent hemodynamic responses and no complications.

## GENERAL ANESTHETICS

General anesthetics traditionally have been used in the OR by anesthesiologists. With appropriate monitoring and skilled personnel, these agents are safely used outside the OR for diagnostic and therapeutic procedures. In the following discussion we will emphasize the use of IV drugs for sedation outside the OR when an anesthesiologist may not be directly involved.

*Ketamine* has been available since the 1960s. It is one of the few sedatives that produce both amnesia and analgesia. It is structurally similar to phencyclidine and exerts its dissociative properties by interacting with the limbic and thalamic systems. Additional mechanisms postulated are antagonism of

*N*-methyl-D-aspartate (NMDA) receptors and agonism of opioid subgroups.[151] The clinical appearance is that of a child who has open eyes (usually with horizontal nystagmus) but does not respond to pain, the so called "dissociative" state. Ketamine preserves cardiovascular function and exerts limited effects on respiratory mechanics, allowing spontaneous respirations in most children.[241] Although it is certainly not a new drug, ketamine has recently experienced a resurgence in popularity, particularly in the ED for procedural sedation. Some emergency medicine physicians suggest that ketamine not be considered an anesthetic, but rather a "dissociative sedation" drug with unique properties that warrant their own separate monitoring guidelines.[242] New clinical practice guidelines for EDs have been written which emphasize this position[107]; however, given the fact that airway obstruction, apnea, and laryngospasm occur with some regularity (approximately 1% to 2%), we strongly disagree with attempts to reclassify the drug as a means of side-stepping the AAP sedation guidelines.[107,243-245]

IM and IV ketamine (with and without midazolam) are frequently used for closed fracture reductions and other painful minor procedures in the ED (see Table 47-9).[245-247] In a review of 1022 children sedated with ketamine in the ED, there were no instances of aspiration, and airway reflexes were preserved, although complications included the need for airway management (0.7%), laryngospasm (0.4%), and apnea or respiratory depression (0.3%). Unpleasant reactions were rare and were not improved by prophylactic benzodiazepines.[104] In a more recent review of 4252 children, respiratory complications occurred in 2.4%, with serious airway events occurring more frequently: of this 2.4%, laryngospasm occurred in 28%, hypoxia in 79%, and apnea in 10%.[99,248] The risks in children younger than 2 years during ketamine with midazolam (62% of children) and morphine with midazolam (16% of children) showed a 6% incidence of complications in which all but one incident were related to ketamine with midazolam. Most were considered minor in severity, although one child required tracheal intubation.[249] Ketamine (1 to 3 mg/kg) has also been studied in children undergoing gastroendoscopy procedures, with transient laryngospasm occurring in 8.2%, emesis in 4.1%, emergence agitation in 2.4%, partial airway obstruction in 1.3%, apnea and respiratory depression in 0.5%, and excessive salivation in 0.3%.[83] The analgesic effects of ketamine make it very appealing for use during burn dressing changes. In one study, 4.9% of the sedations resulted in adverse outcomes, of which 2.9% required an intervention. Eight events were related to the airway.[250] Ketamine sedation/analgesia has a very long history of safety, perhaps having advantage over other sedation regimens, although these studies indicate that potentially life-threatening events can and do occur during ketamine sedation. Ketamine is also associated with nonpurposeful motion, which limits its usefulness when immobility is necessary (e.g., use during CT).

Ketamine is contraindicated in a number of clinical scenarios. It may increase cerebral blood flow and is contraindicated in children with increased intracranial pressure, particularly without controlled respirations. Similarly, it is contraindicated in those with head injury, open globe injury, hypertension, and psychosis. Ketamine decreases the ventilator response to hypercarbia, as well, it may cause laryngospasm, coughing, and apnea. No antagonist is available.

Typical starting doses[251] of ketamine are 1 to 2 mg/kg IM, 0.25 to 1.0 mg/kg IV, and 4 to 6 mg/kg orally.[252-254] The onset after IM injection is 2 to 5 minutes, with a peak at ~20 minutes;

duration can be 30 to 120 minutes. Onset after IV administration occurs in less than 1 minute, with a peak effect in several minutes and duration of action of approximately 15 minutes. Oral doses of 4 to 6 mg/kg are usually combined with atropine and have an effect in 30 minutes and last up to 120 minutes.[31] Larger doses or supplementation with other sedatives or opioids may produce deep sedation or general anesthesia. We advise that ketamine be administered with an antisialagogue (atropine, 0.02 mg/kg, or glycopyrrolate, 0.01 mg/kg) because copious secretions from ketamine alone may induce laryngospasm.[255]

*Etomidate* is a carboxylated imidazole that is primarily used as an induction agent for anesthesia. Its mechanism is thought to be potentiation of GABA inhibitory neurotransmission via alteration of chloride conductance. Loss of consciousness occurs in 15 to 20 seconds, and recovery results from redistribution and occurs in 5 to 10 minutes. It is hydrolyzed in the liver to inactive metabolites and excreted (90%) in the urine.[151] Etomidate produces sedation and anesthesia, anxiolysis, and amnesia similar to the barbiturates and propofol. Its major advantage is its lack of adverse cardiovascular effects. Etomidate has been used in adults and children for procedural sedation, although the end point of sedation is not well described and often is a state of general anesthesia.[79] Using data from the Pediatric Sedation Research Consortium, etomidate has been compared with pentobarbital for CT sedation. Adverse events were more common with pentobarbital (4.5%) than etomidate (0.9%); one child who received etomidate experienced apnea.[256] Etomidate with fentanyl has been compared to ketamine with midazolam for reduction of limb fractures in children in the ED. Etomidate with fentanyl had a quicker recovery time but was less effective in reducing observed patient distress.[257] Transient adrenal suppression can occur after multiple doses and has been described after single-dose administration in septic patients.[258-262]

*Propofol* is an anesthetic that is widely used for pediatric sedation and anesthesia. It is an isopropyl phenol derivative whose mechanism of action appears to be activation of the sodium channel of the $\beta_1$ subunit of GABA receptors, thereby enhancing inhibitory transmission.[263] Its onset is within 30 seconds. It is highly lipid soluble and is provided in a lipid solution that is the same as the lipid component in total parenteral solutions. The lipid solubility makes the drug effect diminish extremely quickly (5 to 15 minutes).[264] It has no analgesic properties, but it does have antiemetic and antipruritic properties. Although small doses of propofol (25 to 50 µg/kg/min) can provide moderate sedation in adults, deep sedation and airway obstruction quickly occurs in some children at greater rates of administration. Dosing in adults for sedation is recommended at 25 to 200 µg/kg/min, whereas children, particularly infants and those with cognitive impairment, require larger doses (150 to 250 µg/kg/min). Propofol is also a profound respiratory depressant and can cause apnea. Respiratory complications have been reported in 8% to 30% of children.[265] It is generally best administered by titration with an infusion pump. Other adverse reactions include increased salivary and tracheobronchial secretions, myoclonic movements, anaphylactic reactions, and bacterial contamination. Pain on injection can be lessened by several strategies, although the two most effective strategies are pretreatment with nitrous oxide by inhalation, or a mini–Bier block with 1 mg/kg lidocaine applied for 1 minute.[266,267] Hypotension is mild and usually not clinically significant. Cases of fatal metabolic acidosis, myocardial failure, and lipemic serum have been reported in children who received propofol infusions for more than 48 hours at doses exceeding

5 mg/kg/hr (83 µg/kg/min), with sporadic cases, which may have been exacerbated by an underlying mitochondrial disorder, of the syndrome appearing after only 5 to 6 hours in some cases.[268-273] Propofol should only be administered by practitioners with advanced sedation training and airway skills, because the propofol-sedated child will always be deeply sedated.

The use of all sedatives drugs in children continues to grow. All providers must be aware of the potency and risks of sedative drugs. There are many anecdotes and reviews with small numbers of incidents that attest to the risks of propofol. This is especially true when sedatives with general anesthetic potential are used by health care providers who are not specifically trained to use them in children. Propofol sedation frequently causes anesthesia with an inability to maintain and protect the airway. In a study of propofol sedation (2.5 to 3 mg/kg IV loading dose with an infusion up to 200 µg/kg/min) in 105 painful procedures in the pediatric ICU, 21% of the children required airway repositioning, 17% had apnea, 5% had hypotension, and 45% had events that required intervention.[86] In the ED, propofol was administered to 113 children in a dose (4.5 mg/kg in addition to fentanyl 1 to 2 µg/kg)[274] sufficient to ensure the children were motionless during the reduction of fractures. The net effect was an incidence of desaturation of 21%, laryngospasm in 1%, and a supplemental oxygen requirement in 25%. A study of sedation by nonanesthesiologists for bone marrow procedures, lumbar punctures, and esophagoscopies titrated propofol to a target of "not arousable"; 21 children 27 weeks to 18 years of age were studied. Only after a BIS score of 45 or less was 100% adequate sedation accomplished. Propofol total doses were 520 µg/kg/min for these short procedures.[275] These responses to stimulation, effects on the airway, doses of propofol, and BIS levels are beyond the range of deep sedation, and more in keeping with the definition of general anesthesia, with the inherent risk of loss of the airway. More recent studies that reviewed the use of propofol by ED physicians specifically trained in sedation and performed in highly monitored environments, show that propofol can be used with much less severe adverse outcomes (and much smaller doses) than previously reported.[15,92,106,276] The debate about who is best to provide sedation with all drugs and especially propofol will continue. The key to safety is training and environment.

The risks associated with propofol were brought into the international spotlight with the death of Michael Jackson in 2009. Michael Jackson's physician who administered the propofol was tried for homicide and found guilty of involuntary manslaughter. This was not the first reported case of homicide using propofol.[277]

Sedatives also pose risks to providers. Propofol and all sedative drugs have severe abuse potential. The *New York Times* reported in August 2009 that 18% of anesthesia training programs reported propofol abuse. There is an effort to classify propofol as a "Class IV" drug by the U.S. Drug Enforcement Agency. This is the same category as benzodiazepines and this categorization will likely lead to tighter control of this drug.

*Fospropofol* (Lusedra) is a water-soluble prodrug of propofol. Fospropofol is hydrolyzed by plasma alkaline phosphatase to propofol, formaldehyde, and phosphate.[278,279] As fospropofol must first undergo dephosphorylation to propofol, time to onset of action is delayed (4 to 8 minutes).[280,281] Because of its slower onset, it was proposed as a safe alternative to propofol with fewer restrictions on its administration. In December 2008, the FDA qualified fospropofol to be administered only by persons trained in the administration of general anesthesia (i.e., the same wording as propofol). Currently, there are no data on fospropofol use in children. The slow onset, adverse effect of perineal burning, and formaldehyde and formate byproducts may make this drug less appealing for sedation and only useful during general anesthesia.[278,282] One possible advantage for this preparation may be for long-term sedation because it is free of any fatty acids and thus may avoid possible propofol infusion syndrome. Further studies are needed, particularly because preliminary PK data were flawed.[283]

There has been increasing use of a combination of ketamine (10 mg/mL) with propofol (10 mg/mL), so called "ketofol," for painful procedures in the ED and for oncology patients.[284-289] This combination is administered in incremental doses of 0.5 mg/kg of each drug at approximately 1-minute intervals. The limited number of prospective studies at this point preclude assessment of safety and efficacy. A literature review found insufficient evidence to recommend routine use of this combinaiton.[288] A prospective study of adults found one patient in each group to require positive pressure ventilation.[285]

*Methohexital* is a short-acting oxybarbiturate that is rapidly metabolized and redistributed, and has a rapid recovery (see Table 47-9).[290] Induction of anesthesia occurs with IV doses of 1 to 2 mg/kg. Apnea, hiccups, and methohexital-induced seizures in children with temporal lobe epilepsy have been reported.[291] Methohexital has been used IM in doses of 8 to 10 mg/kg but has a slow onset[292] and is not generally recommended. Rectal methohexital (20 to 25 mg/kg [from a 100 mg/mL solution]) can induce deep sedation in 7 to 11 minutes[293] with a duration of action of about 30 to 45 minutes.[294] Absorption through the rectal route is erratic.[295] Children given methohexital (1 mg/kg) completed their head CT more quickly and needed less total sedation monitoring than those given pentobarbital (2 mg/kg).[296] The variability of absorption, tendency to deep sedation, and airway problems have decreased the use of methohexital in favor of newer drugs. This medication is rarely used and should be used only by individuals with advanced airway skills, because upper airway obstruction and apnea may readily occur.[297]

*Nitrous oxide* ($N_2O$) is a potent inhalation analgesic with a peak effect in 3 to 5 minutes and very rapid return to baseline when discontinued (see Table 47-9). A premixed tank of no more than 50% $N_2O$ is available (Entonox). Administration of $N_2O$ can be used for "minimal sedation" under the following AAP guidelines: (1) only ASA physical status I or II patients; (2) only 50% nitrous oxide or less is used; (3) inhalation equipment must have the capacity to deliver 100% oxygen and never less than 25% oxygen; and (4) a calibrated oxygen analyzer must be used. The child is able to maintain verbal communication throughout the procedure. Although $N_2O$ in 50% concentration with oxygen usually produces "minimal" sedation, the addition of any sedatives or hypnotic may rapidly produce a deeper level of sedation and require increased monitoring and vigilance.[148,169] Nitrous oxide is frequently used by dentists for sedation. A recent questionnaire showed that all respondents performed dental treatment as a trainee, to patients who were under sedation, and the majority used nitrous oxide inhalation sedation.[298,299] Extensive guidelines, following the ASA and AAP definitions and guidelines, have been written by the American Academy of Pediatric Dentistry that detail the accepted use of nitrous oxide.[299] Adverse reactions, drug interactions, and special concerns are listed in Table 47-9.

## ANNOTATED REFERENCES

Coté CJ, Notterman DA, Karl HW, Weinberg JA, McCloskey C. Adverse sedation events in pediatrics: a critical incident analysis of contributory factors. Pediatrics 2000;105:805-14.

*Landmark study that collated severe adverse outcomes from multiple sources and allowed the identification of sedation practices that led to injury and death. In particular, it highlighted the need for appropriate personnel, monitors, and rescue capability to ensure safety.*

Cravero JP, Beach M, Gallagher SM, Hertzog JH. The incidence and nature of adverse events during pediatric sedation/anesthesia for procedures with propofol outside the operating room: report from the Pediatric Sedation Research Consortium. Anesthesia Analgesia 2009;108:795-804.

*A review of nearly 50,000 sedation encounters using propofol by a variety of sedation providers. The participating providers were highly trained members of organized sedation services with advanced airway education and ongoing quality improvement efforts. Adverse events and requirements for airway interventions are analyzed. The information is useful in understanding the critical competencies necessary for the safe use of this drug.*

Cravero JP, Blike GT, Beach M, et al. Incidence and nature of adverse events during pediatric sedation/anesthesia for procedures outside the operating room: report from the Pediatric Sedation Research Consortium. Pediatrics 2006;118:1087.

*A review of more than 30,000 sedation cases from the Pediatric Sedation Research Consortium. This study is useful as it supplements anecdotal information on sedation complications and aids in understanding the nature and frequency of adverse events in a large group of patients cared for by a variety of sedation providers.*

## REFERENCES

Please see www.expertconsult.com.

# Procedures for Vascular Access

## 48

### SAMUEL H. WALD AND CHARLES J. COTÉ

| Venous Cannulation | Arterial Cannulation |
|---|---|
| Peripheral Intravenous Cannulation | Umbilical Artery |
| Central Venous Pressure Measurement | Radial Artery |
| Central Venous Catheterization | Temporal Artery |
| Intraosseous Infusion | Femoral Artery |
| Umbilical Vein Catheterization | Dorsalis Pedis and Posterior Tibial Artery |

VASCULAR CANNULATION is an important procedure in the anesthetic and perioperative management of children. Its routine use was introduced in the 1950s.[1] The indications are to provide routes for fluid, drug, and blood product administration, monitoring of cardiopulmonary function, and provision of access for blood sampling. Although the technique of insertion may be extremely difficult, especially in the very young or small child, no child should be denied an indicated procedure because of an operator's inexperience; appropriate consultation should be sought, if necessary. Regardless of the procedure, gloves should be worn to maintain clean or sterile technique and to protect health care professionals from exposure to blood.[2-6] An update from the Pediatric Perioperative Cardiac Arrest Registry suggests that lack of good vascular access may contribute to the underestimation of fluid or blood loss and inadequate replacement of fluid or blood in anesthetized children, emphasizing the importance of appropriate and adequate vascular access and monitoring.[7,8]

## Venous Cannulation

### PERIPHERAL INTRAVENOUS CANNULATION

#### Indications

Percutaneous intravenous cannulation should be used in almost all anesthetized children for the following purposes[9,10]:

- Provision of a route for postoperative pain relief
- Administration of drugs, fluids and electrolytes, glucose, and blood products, including resuscitation medications
- Indirect central venous pressure measurement; the accuracy of this method for central venous pressure measurement does not appear to vary by location of the catheter[11] but does depend on ensuring direct continuity between the central and peripheral circulation.[12,13] This can be assessed by providing a large, sustained inspiration or occluding the venous return of the extremity, which both cause an increase in the peripheral pressure.[14-16] Hypothermia may impair the accuracy of such measurement.[17]

#### Equipment

- Alcohol pads or chlorhexidine swabs
- Gloves
- Tourniquet
- Gauze
- Clear plastic dressing (Tegaderm, 3M Medical-Surgical Division, St. Paul, Minn., or OpSite, Smith + Nephew, Inc., Largo, Fla.)
- Tape
- Armboard

Consider the possible need for latex-free equipment. In cases of difficult access, the availability of a transillumination light source (Karl Storz, 485 B Type, Tutlingen, Germany) may improve the success rate of catheter placement.[18] Ultrasonography also may be used for obtaining peripheral venous access at the basilic, cephalic, or brachial veins.[19,20] Finally, new near-infrared and infrared technology is available to aid in the identification of peripheral veins (AccuVein, Accuvein, Huntington, N.Y.; Vein-Viewer, Christie Digital Systems, Cypress, Calif.).[21]

#### Practical Suggestions

1. Awake intravenous line placement can be facilitated by any combination of good patient rapport, EMLA cream (lidocaine 2.5% and prilocaine 2.5%), lidocaine and tetracaine patch, lidocaine by iontophoresis, lidocaine by topical cream, topical tetracaine (Ametop), ethyl chloride spray, and/or pre-medication.[22-31]
2. Prefilling the cannula with saline may reduce menisci tension and allow a more rapid blood flash back.
3. A butterfly needle can be inserted for induction, followed by an appropriate-size catheter after anesthesia.
4. A T-connector (Abbott Hospitals, Inc., Chicago) may be used to minimize the fluids necessary to flush drugs administered through the intravenous line; this is particularly important for infants.[32]
5. A calibrated burette should be used to limit the total infusion and provide a means to titrate fluids accurately in infants and young children.
6. A flow-limiting infusion pump may be used for preterm and full-term neonates.
7. Flow rates may be significantly changed by catheter brand, tubing type, and addition of extensions and stopcocks.[33]
8. One-way valves in the intravenous tubing are useful in preventing back-flow of drugs or infusions.
9. Air filters also may be useful for children at risk for paradoxical gas embolization.

**TABLE 48-1** Comparison of Intravenous Safety Mechanisms

| Safety Mechanism | Operator Activation Required | Syringe Attachment | Rapid Flash | Bulky | Advantages | Disadvantages | Devices (Manufacturers) |
|---|---|---|---|---|---|---|---|
| Retractable needle | Yes | No | Yes | Yes | Unobstructed and rapid blood flash Similarity in use to nonsafety devices | Bulky Requires operator activation No syringe attachment | Angiocath Autoguard (BD Medical, Franklin Lakes, N.J.), Secure IV (Span America Medical Systems, Inc., Greenville, S.C.) |
| Blunted needle | No | Yes | No | No | Passive action requiring no operator activation Syringe attachment possible | Slow blood flash if needle has been partially withdrawn | Introcan Safety IV (B. Braun, Bethlehem, Pa.), Protectiv Acuvance (Smiths Medical, U.K.) |

## Complications

Hematoma from a failed vascular cannulation is usually of no serious consequence. Infection or thrombosis may be limited by aseptic technique.[34-36] One study of 642 Teflon catheters in 525 patients showed that the risk of catheter complications in children was extremely small and would not be reduced significantly by routine replacement of the catheters.[37] Catheter life span has been found to be unrelated to insertion site, cannula size, or brand in infants younger than 12 months of age.[38,39]

Skin sloughing is usually caused by subcutaneous infiltration of calcium, potassium, or hypertonic solutions; it may be avoided by frequent inspection of the intravenous line before injecting medications.[40] The risk of subcutaneous infiltration increases with the administration of medications versus no medications and with parenteral nutrition solutions compared with 5% or 10% dextrose solutions, but the risk of infiltration is no different with solutions that contain potassium ($\leq$20 mEq/L vs. >20 mEq/L). In addition, there is no difference between gravity-controlled versus infusion delivery devices.[41]

There are insufficient data to support the routine use of heparin to prolong the patency of peripheral intravenous catheters in neonates and children.[42]

## CENTRAL VENOUS PRESSURE MEASUREMENT

Some studies in children and adults describe a reasonable correlation between peripheral intravenous catheters and central venous catheters, even in critically ill children. Hypothermia (peripheral vasoconstriction) decreases the accuracy of such measurements, but it is useful to understand that transducing the pressure of a peripheral vein may provide valuable information regarding right-sided cardiac filling pressures.[9,10,43-46]

### Establishing a Large Intravenous Catheter in Small Patients
#### Indications
The following procedure is used for any child in whom there is the potential for massive, rapid hemorrhage:
1. Prepare and drape the appropriate area using standard sterile techniques.
2. Perform a standard intravenous cannulation of an antecubital, saphenous, or external jugular vein with a small (22-gauge) intravenous catheter.
3. Pass a small, flexible guidewire (0.018 inch) through the intravenous catheter, remove the catheter, and with a number 11 blade make a small incision at the entry point of the wire at the skin.

4. Pass the next larger size intravenous catheter over the wire to dilate the vein and leave in place; stiff intravenous catheters are more effective. An alternative is to use a small dilator from a pulmonary artery catheter introducer and leave the sheath in place. The wire is removed, and the next larger size wire is inserted (0.025 inch). The catheter (or sheath) is removed, leaving this larger wire within the vein. This process may be repeated with larger catheters and wires until the desired size cannula or sheath is reached. An alternative is to leave progressively larger pulmonary artery introducer sheaths in the vein; both techniques provide a reasonably rapid method of establishing a large-bore intravenous infusion site.

### Rapid Infusion Catheters and Introducer Sheaths
Special rapid volume catheters (6F and larger, Arrow International, Reading, Pa.) allow venipuncture with a needle or small intravenous catheter, passage of a guidewire, and then introduction of a dilator and sheath, with fewer steps required (see E-Fig. 10-1).

### Intravenous Cutdown
#### Indications
- Percutaneous cannulation is unsuccessful.
- Percutaneous cannulation is tenuous.
- The catheter in place is inadequate for the planned surgical procedure.

The most common sites for insertion are the saphenous vein at the medial malleolus and the brachiocephalic vein at the antecubital fossa. This procedure may require considerable time to perform and has limited utility for emergent access.[47]

#### Complications
Intravenous cutdown has a high incidence of infection and therefore should be used only on a short-term basis.

### Saphenous Vein Cannulation
The saphenous vein is often a reliable point for intravenous access in infants and children that may be directly visualized or cannulated with a "blind" technique (Fig. 48-1). It is consistently found lateral to the medial malleolus of the ankle one-half to one finger breadth over the anterior quadrant.
1. Cleanse the area in the standard fashion after a tourniquet is applied to the lower extremity below the knee.

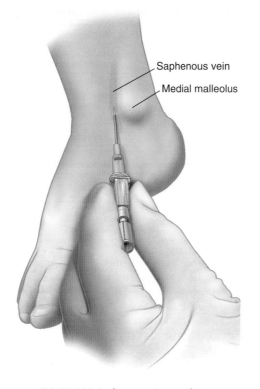

Saphenous vein

Medial malleolus

**FIGURE 48-1** Saphenous vein cannulation.

2. The saphenous vein may or may not be palpated, and visualization may not be possible.

3. Enter the skin at a 30-degree angle at the expected site of the saphenous vein at the level of the medial malleolus, with the tip of the needle directed toward the upper two thirds of the calf. If no evidence of venipuncture is seen on insertion, slowly withdraw the needle because the flash of blood may occur while exiting the vein.

4. If unsuccessful on the first attempt, fan medially and then laterally from the same insertion point, slowly advancing and withdrawing the catheter until blood return is obtained.

5. Once a flashback is seen, gently advance the entire unit 2 to 3 mm into the lumen before advancing the catheter off the needle.

### Safety Intravenous Catheters

In the United States, federal law requires that retractable or sheathed needles designed to reduce the potential for needlestick injury are available for use by health care personnel (see Table 48-1).[48] A study that compared traditional intravenous catheters to safety devices found that a larger proportion of children younger than 3 years of age required more than one catheter to successfully gain intravenous access. The retractable intravenous catheter was associated with a nearly fourfold greater incidence of splattering and spilling of blood compared with traditional catheters.[49] Retractable needles require activation of a button to trigger the safety device; therefore sheathed catheters are regarded as inherently safer because they require no action on the part of the operator to protect the needle tip. Note that the U.S. federal legislation requires that these devices be available but the ultimate decision to use them rests with the physician. *Therefore the*

*type of catheter should not be dictated by the hospital but rather by the individuals who place the catheters.*

## CENTRAL VENOUS CATHETERIZATION

### Indications

- Provision of a secure means for administration of fluid and blood when major shifts in intravascular volume are anticipated (e.g., multiple trauma, intestinal obstruction, burns)
- Monitoring of cardiac filling pressures
- Infusion of drugs and fluids that are sclerosing to peripheral veins (e.g., antibiotics, vasopressors, and hyperalimentation fluids)
- Need for blood sampling
- Measurement of mixed venous acid-base balance, estimation of cardiac output (Fick principle) or measurement of cardiac output (dye dilution)
- Route for aspiration of air emboli

The common sites for central venous cannulation are the external and internal jugular veins, the subclavian and brachiocephalic veins, the femoral vein in infants and children, and the umbilical vein in neonates. Approaches such as the internal jugular and subclavian veins should be used with extreme caution in the presence of a bleeding diathesis as stopping bleeding may be difficult. The percutaneous approach to central venous cannulation is often successful using a modified Seldinger technique (Fig. 48-2).[50,51] The advantages of this technique are that it avoids the need for a cutdown, only one venipuncture is made with a thin-walled small-gauge needle, a guidewire directs the catheter within the blood vessel, introducing a large catheter through the small venipuncture site minimizes the chances of significant hematoma formation even after systemic heparinization, and the procedure often can be accomplished when access is required emergently. Whenever a central line is inserted into the heart from above, care must be taken to ensure that the catheter tip is positioned at the junction of the superior vena cava and the right atrium, because positions within the heart have been associated with perforation of large vessels and the myocardium (Fig. 48-3) with triggering of ventricular arrhythmias.[52]

Ultrasound guidance, pressure waveform analysis, or electrocardiographic guidance may help prevent complications related to central catheter placement.[53,54] Ultrasound-guided access assists successful cannulation of the internal jugular vein,[53] the infraclavicular axillary vein,[54] and the subclavian vein.[55,56] A meta-analysis of 18 trials with 1646 participants, including infants, children, and adults, showed a benefit from the use of two-dimensional ultrasound guidance compared with the landmark method. The greatest benefit was for internal jugular vein cannulation rather than subclavian or femoral veins.[57] See Chapter 42 and Video 48-1 for ultrasound-guided techniques.

### Complications

Pneumothorax, arrhythmia, hematoma, bleeding, infection, thrombosis, inadvertent arterial puncture, cardiac tamponade, air embolus, thoracic duct injury, and malposition are all possible complications associated with central venous cannulation. Data in adults suggest that the smallest catheter and placement from the left subclavian approach may have the least complication rate; similar studies have not been conducted in children.[58] The infection rate reported after 1056 central venous catheters were inserted into 289 children with burn injury varied from 2.0% to 7.3% for catheters in place for 11 or fewer days, but that the rate

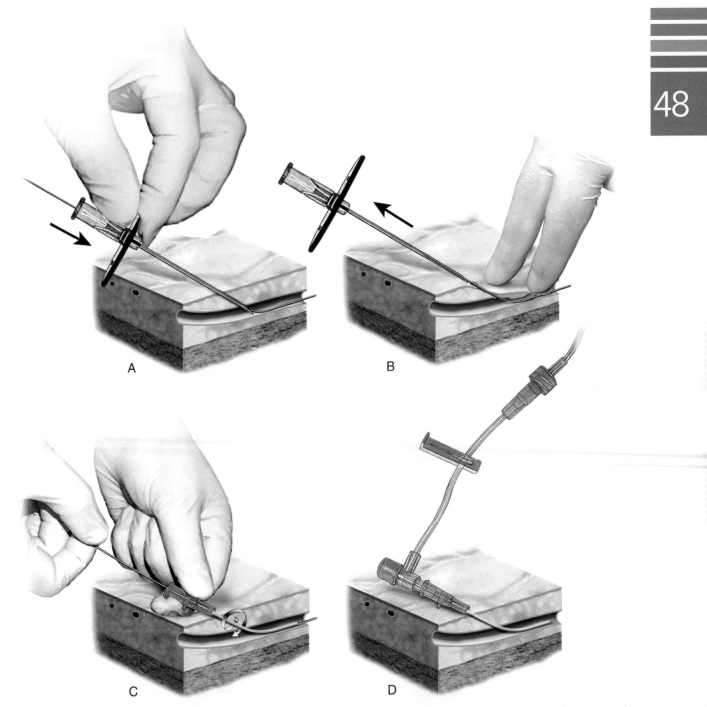

A

B

C

D

**FIGURE 48-2 A,** Seldinger technique for catheter placement. The needle is inserted into the target vessel, and the flexible end of the guidewire is passed freely into the vessel. **B,** The needle is then removed, leaving the guidewire in place. **C,** The catheter is advanced with a twisting motion into the vessel. **D,** The wire is removed, and the catheter is connected to an appropriate infusion or monitoring device. (Redrawn with permission from Schwartz AJ, Coté CJ, Jobes DR, et al. Central venous catheterization in pediatrics. Scientific exhibit, American Society of Anesthesiologists, New Orleans, 1977.)

increased dramatically to 15.8% to 37.5% for catheters left in place for 12 to 14 days.[59]

### *Aseptic Technique*

Contamination of catheters during insertion may result in catheter colonization or bacterial infection. Evidence suggests that the use of maximum barrier precautions during placement, including the use of sterile gloves, long-sleeved gowns, full-size drape, and a nonsterile mask and cap, decrease the risk of

catheter-related infection.[34,36,60,61] The efficacy of chlorhexidine versus povidone-iodine for preventing bacteremia remains unclear, and the safety of chlorhexidine in infants and children has not been fully established.[62] For older infants and children, chlorhexidine may be safe and effective, but it can cause severe local contact dermatitis in low-birth-weight infants.[63,64] In a case-controlled, prospective, active surveillance study in a pediatric intensive care unit (ICU), independent risk factors for central line-associated bloodstream infection were the duration of central

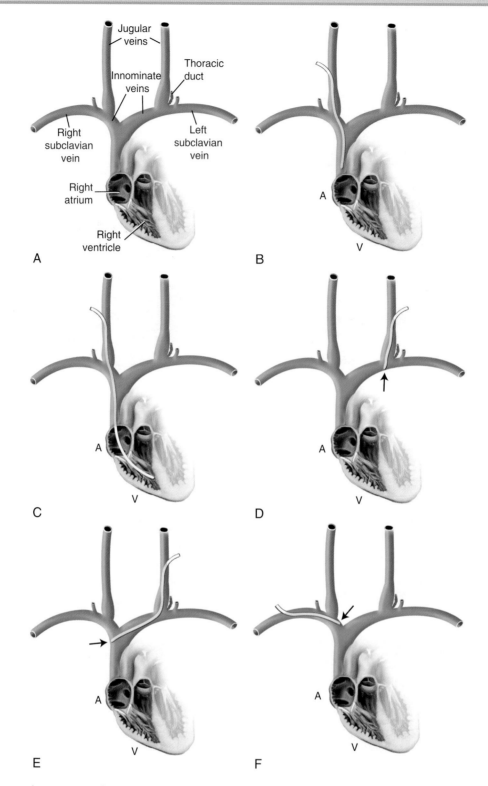

**FIGURE 48-3** Proper and improper central venous pressure catheter placement. **A,** Normal vascular anatomy. **B,** Proper location for right internal jugular catheter (i.e., high right atrium or superior vena cava). **C,** Ventricular location of any catheter is dangerous and contraindicated. **D,** A short left-sided internal jugular catheter may erode through the innominate vein (*arrow*). **E,** A left-sided internal jugular catheter striking the lateral wall of the superior vena cava (*arrow*) may erode through it and must be partially withdrawn or advanced. **F,** A short right subclavian catheter may strike the lateral wall of the innominate vein (*arrow*) and erode through it; this catheter should be advanced or withdrawn.

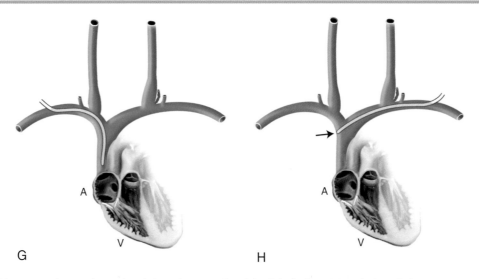

G          H

FIGURE 48-3, cont'd **G,** Proper location for a right subclavian line. **H,** A short left subclavian line may erode through the superior vena cava (*arrow*); this catheter should be advanced or withdrawn. *A,* Atrium; *V,* ventricle.

venous catheterization in the ICU, nonoperative cardiovascular disease, gastrostomy tube, parenteral nutrition, central line placement in the ICU, and red blood cell transfusion.[65]

### External Jugular Vein Catheterization

1. Place the child in the Trendelenburg position with the head turned 45 degrees away from the side of cannulation.
2. Place a pillow or rolled sheet under the shoulders to extend the head and allow complete access to the neck.
3. Under aseptic conditions, venipuncture and catheter insertion are completed according to the techniques shown in Figure 48-2. A J-wire is usually more useful to circumvent the plexus of veins at the clavicle.[66,67]
4. Suture or tape appropriately and cover with an occlusive dressing. Many catheters will not pass beyond the clavicle or will pass into the axillary vein; success is generally more often attained on the right side.[68,69] If a shorter catheter is used, infusion and pressure monitoring are very dependent on the position of the head.[70] Continuous free-flowing infusion is best maintained when the head is turned away from the side of catheter insertion. This vein is particularly valuable in children with difficult peripheral venous access and in an emergent situation that suddenly develops intraoperatively that requires establishment of additional intravenous access.

### Internal Jugular Vein Catheterization

Numerous approaches and techniques are used for internal jugular vein cannulation.[71-74] A high approach using the apex of a triangle formed by the two bellies of the sternocleidomastoid muscle and the clavicle may be used as a landmark for insertion (Fig. 48-4). With the use of the Seldinger technique, the success rate, even in neonates, approaches 75% on the first attempt and 90% to 95% on the second attempt.[50] Cannulation of the right side virtually ensures a central location because the internal jugular vein, the superior vena cava, and the right atrium are in a straight line (see Fig. 48-4). Left-sided cannulation risks injury to the thoracic duct and possible pneumothorax because the apex of the lung is more cephalad on the left. In addition, if the catheter inserted on the left is too short, it is not unusual for the tip to rest against the wall of the superior vena cava, be position dependent, and possibly erode through the wall of the vessel.

Figure 48-3 illustrates less desirable sites for catheter tips that may result in perforation. The principal advantage of the high approach is that the most common complication (arterial puncture, approximately 10%) is easily recognized and usually treated uneventfully. In one study, the effect individually and in combination of the simulated Valsalva maneuver (positive inspiratory pressure of 25 mm Hg for 10 seconds), liver compression, and Trendelenburg position to increase the cross-sectional area of the right internal jugular vein was investigated.[75] A maximal mean increase in cross-sectional area of the right internal jugular vein was $17.4 \pm 16.1\%$ from baseline when all three maneuvers were combined. This effect was most pronounced in children 1 to 6 years of age and was clinically negligible in infants younger than 12 months of age. The effect on ease of catheter placement was not investigated.[75] For neonates, a study using skin traction in infants less than 5 kg showed that a technique using tape for skin traction combined with ultrasound guidance increased internal jugular cross-sectional area and decreased the time for catheter placement.[76-78]

### Technique

1. Position the child as for external jugular vein cannulation but with a rolled towel under the center of the back to allow the head to be slightly extended (see Fig. 48-3 and Video 48-1 for positioning and the use of ultrasound to guide insertion). The head is turned slightly away from the side of insertion; *turning the head too far to the side may result in compression of the vein and moving the vein in closer proximity to the carotid artery.*
2. Locate the apex of a triangle formed by the two bellies of the sternocleidomastoid muscle. This point is usually where the external jugular vein crosses the sternocleidomastoid muscle or the midpoint between the mastoid process and the sternal notch.
3. Palpate the carotid artery. Introduce the needle just lateral to this artery at an angle of 30 degrees to the skin surface. If the internal jugular vein is superficial, a less acute angle may be indicated. While continuously aspirating, advance the needle toward the ipsilateral nipple a distance of no more than 2.5 cm. If no blood is freely obtained, slowly withdraw the needle while maintaining aspiration. The

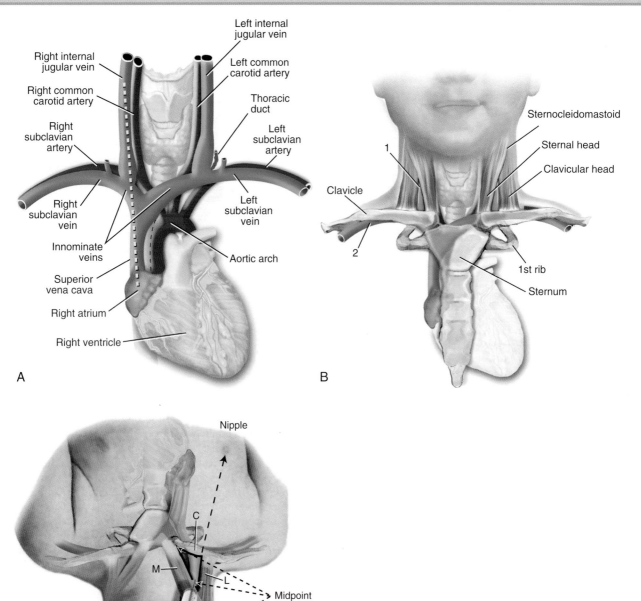

**FIGURE 48-4 A,** The anatomic relationships of major chest and neck structures. Note how the internal jugular vein is in close proximity to the carotid artery. Also note that a nearly straight line is formed by the internal jugular vein, innominate vein, superior vena cava, and right atrium (*yellow hatched line*); thus it is rare for a right internal jugular catheter to migrate anywhere but to the right atrium. **B,** The relationship of external anatomic landmarks to the anatomy illustrated in **A.** Note the triangle formed by the two bellies of the sternocleidomastoid muscle and the clavicle. *1,* The preferred point of needle insertion at the apex of this triangle for internal jugular vein puncture. *2,* The point of needle insertion for subclavian vein puncture. **C,** The anatomic landmarks as they would appear to an anesthesiologist. The needle is introduced at the apex of the triangle outlined in **C** and is directed at an angle of 30 degrees to the skin toward the ipsilateral nipple. This point of entry is generally half the distance between the mastoid process and the sternal notch. *C,* Clavicle; *M* and *L,* medial and lateral bellies of the sternocleidomastoid muscle (*SCM*).

needle can compress the vessel on entry, and it straightens during withdrawal, allowing free aspiration of blood.

4. Once venipuncture is accomplished, carefully remove the syringe and occlude the end of the needle (to prevent entraining air if the child is breathing spontaneously) until a flexible guidewire is inserted (see Fig. 48-2).[51] The wire should advance easily. However, if the wire cannot be advanced, the needle has passed out of the vessel lumen or its tip rests against the vessel wall. In this situation, the wire and needle should be withdrawn simultaneously to avoid shearing the wire. If the wire passes without difficulty, then cannulation proceeds as demonstrated in Figures 48-2 and 48-4. Catheter tip location should be confirmed with a radiologic study and repositioned as necessary (see Fig. 48-3).

5. Suture the catheter in place, and protect the area with an occlusive dressing.

### *Contraindications*

- A bleeding diathesis (relative contraindication); in life-threatening emergencies, the benefit may outweigh the risk.
- Contralateral pneumothorax
- Raised intracranial pressure (Trendelenburg position and venous occlusion by the catheter may increase intracranial pressure); this is a relative contraindication and ultrasound-guided insertion may provide a great advantage because Trendelenburg position may not be required.
- Aberrant vessels (e.g., cervical aortic arch)

### Subclavian Vein Catheterization

The subclavian vein is a site frequently used for central vein cannulation.[79,80] Success rates of over 80% have been reported even in infants younger than 4 weeks of age.[81-83] The advantages include fixed landmarks, ease of securing the line to children for long-term management, and patient comfort. Disadvantages include pneumothorax and hemothorax.[84,85] If this site is chosen, we suggest obtaining a chest radiograph after the catheter is inserted and before surgery begins to preclude an unrecognized intraoperative tension pneumothorax. The use of the Seldinger technique (our preference) may reduce the incidence of damage to intrathoracic structures compared with other techniques. As with left-sided internal jugular vein cannulation, if a left subclavian catheter tip rests against the wall of the superior vena cava, it can erode through, resulting in hemothorax or hydrothorax (see Fig. 48-3, *H*). In a comparison of neutral versus lowered shoulder position in 361 adult patients, neutral position significantly reduced the incidence of misplacement of the catheter tip (ipsilateral internal jugular or brachiocephalic vein) with no difference in the rate of arterial puncture or pneumothorax.[86] This maneuver remains to be tested in children.

### *Technique*

1. Prepare and position the child as previously described for external jugular vein puncture.
2. Insert a needle immediately inferior to the clavicle at a point one-half to two-thirds its length from the sternoclavicular junction; while "hugging" the undersurface of the clavicle, the needle is directed toward the suprasternal notch while continuously aspirating.
3. As soon as free blood flow is obtained, proceed as in Figure 48-2. If the Seldinger technique is not used, then first

locating the subclavian vein with a small-gauge finder needle is recommended.

4. Suture the catheter in place, and apply an occlusive dressing.

If the child's ventilation is controlled, the risk of pneumothorax may be decreased by momentarily ceasing ventilation so that the apex of the lung is away from the needle tip. While probing for the subclavian vein, once successful venipuncture has been achieved, maintaining positive end-expiratory pressure reduces the possibility of air embolism. Optimal depths for right subclavian catheterization have been studied in infants 2 to 5 kg using transesophageal echocardiography and found to be 40 to 55 mm for catheter tip placement at the junction of the superior vena cava and the right atrium.[87] Contraindications are the same as for internal jugular vein catheterization (see Video 48-1 for illustration of technique).

### Brachiocephalic Vein Catheterization

The brachiocephalic vein offers the advantage of being far removed from the intrathoracic structures.[88] The main disadvantage is that a significant number of catheters introduced at this site do not pass centrally, that is, they are caught in the axilla or pass up the jugular vein (internal or external).[89-91] Other disadvantages include significant catheter migration with movement of the arm and possibly an increased incidence of infection. This approach is commonly used by radiologists and pediatric nurses for placement of peripherally inserted central catheters (PICCs), which can be used on a long-term basis.[92-94] These catheters often markedly improve patient care and the quality of life for the child because of the reduced need for peripheral venous access and the reduced number of venipunctures for blood testing. The routine use of heparin to prevent catheter thrombosis and occlusion is not supported by published studies, but the data are inadequate to reach a conclusion one way or the other.[95]

### *Technique*

1. Prepare and drape the arm with aseptic technique.
2. Cannulate the brachiocephalic vein either by using the modified Seldinger technique (special long catheters and wires for this purpose) or by passing a catheter through a needle (Intra Cath, New Delhi, India). If the catheter cannot be threaded once the vein is entered, initiating rapid intravenous fluid administration, cephalad positioning of the arm, and anterior displacement of the shoulder may assist advancement. If percutaneous techniques are not possible, direct venous cutdown may be performed.

### Femoral Vein Catheterization

The femoral vein may also be used for access to the central circulation.[96] The catheter must pass into the thorax to provide accurate cardiac filling pressure measurements, although there seems to be a reasonable correlation with central filling pressures even when the catheter tip is within the abdomen.[97] One advantage of this route is that the vein is large and presents easy access distant from the vital intrathoracic structures (Fig. 48-5). Disadvantages include difficulty in securing the catheter to the child, kinking of the catheter with leg flexion, and problems in maintaining insertion site sterility. Short-term catheterization can provide large-bore venous access for the duration of a procedure with expected large and rapid blood loss if other veins are not accessible. Surprisingly, this site is not associated with a greater

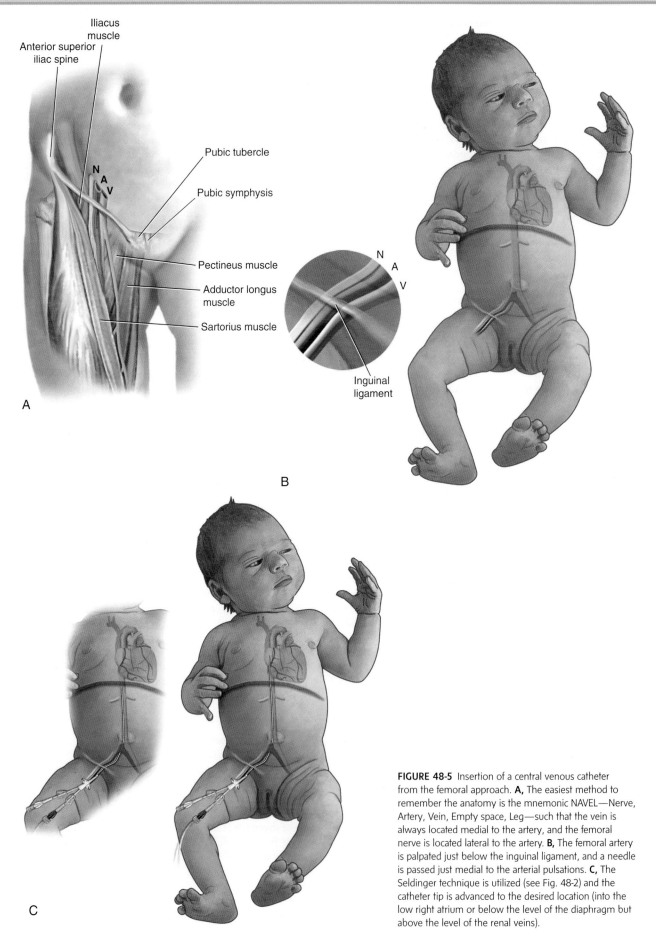

**FIGURE 48-5** Insertion of a central venous catheter from the femoral approach. **A,** The easiest method to remember the anatomy is the mnemonic NAVEL—Nerve, Artery, Vein, Empty space, Leg—such that the vein is always located medial to the artery, and the femoral nerve is located lateral to the artery. **B,** The femoral artery is palpated just below the inguinal ligament, and a needle is passed just medial to the arterial pulsations. **C,** The Seldinger technique is utilized (see Fig. 48-2) and the catheter tip is advanced to the desired location (into the low right atrium or below the level of the diaphragm but above the level of the renal veins).

incidence of catheter-related sepsis compared with other insertion sites.[59,98] This site is not appropriate if disruption of inferior vena cava blood flow is possible (e.g., Wilms tumor resection with invasion of the inferior vena cava, abdominal trauma). The tip of the catheter should be located either low in the atrium or inferior to the level of the diaphragm but superior to the level of the renal veins to reduce the potential for renal vein thrombosis. Use of this technique also has been reported to be safe in infants weighing less than 1000 g with the caution of careful catheter advancement to avoid cardiac perforation.[99]

### Technique

1. Prepare and drape the groin using an aseptic technique with the legs at 90-degree angles ("frog-leg position") (see Fig. 48-5, *B*) A roll under the hips also may provide optimal conditions by slightly elevating the hips.
2. Palpate the femoral artery at a point midway between the pubic tubercle and the anterior superior iliac spine (see Fig. 48-5, *A*).
3. Using the Seldinger technique, enter the vein at a point just medial to the femoral artery and 1 to 2 cm below the inguinal ligament. A catheter is inserted as in Figure 48-2. As for the brachiocephalic vein, special long catheters and wires are needed to achieve a central location (see Video 48-1). As with many vascular access methods, ultrasound guidance can be quite useful.[100-102]
4. Protect the catheter insertion site as previously described (see discussion of internal jugular vein catheterization). If an alternative technique is used (e.g., catheter through the needle), maintain compression of the cannulation site until hemostasis is ensured. The saphenous vein may be cannulated by direct venous cutdown at its junction with the femoral vein if percutaneous techniques are unsuccessful.

## INTRAOSSEOUS INFUSION

The administration of intravenous fluid into the medullary cavity of long bones is a proven method for volume resuscitation in a hypovolemic child and even in teenagers.[103-109] This method can effectively deliver drugs to the central circulation as quickly as using peripheral intravenous infusion sites.[110] It is a particularly valuable emergency route of drug administration, even in the hands of emergency medical technicians[111-113] and as part of emergency department resuscitation of pediatric trauma patients.[107] Complications such as cellulitis, abscess, fractures, and osteomyelitis have been reported in less than 1% of cases, and this technique does not appear to affect later growth of the tibia with proper insertion technique.[114-116] These complications relate in part to duration of infusion, underlying medical conditions, and aseptic technique. The major difficulties with this technique are due to failure to adhere to proper landmarks[117] and bending and clotting of the needle. This technique is used in an emergency situation if several attempts at peripheral or central venous cannulation have failed (suggested "if you cannot achieve reliable access quickly," which generally means after three attempts or 90 seconds).[118,119] Sites for insertion include the upper medial tibia just below the tibial tuberosity, the lower medial tibia just superior to the medial malleolus (to avoid growth plates), the lower femur and the anterior iliac crest. Intraosseous infusions are discontinued once an alternative intravenous infusion site has been secured. This technique has been successfully used for

resuscitation of burn victims.[120,121] Intraosseous devices should not be used in a fractured leg. For the most recent, complete information, please refer to a review directed to the anesthesiologist caring for pediatric patients.[122]

### Technique

1. Palpate the tibial tuberosity.
2. Locate a point on the medial surface of the tibia at least 1 to 2 cm below and medial to the tibial tuberosity for the site of needle puncture, because the mantle of the tibia is thin at this location (Fig. 48-6, *A*).
3. Use a special short needle with a stylet to puncture the mantle of the tibia at a 75-degree angle directed toward the feet to avoid the epiphyseal plate (see Fig. 48-6, *B* and *C*). A styleted spinal needle also may be used.
4. The appropriate position is readily achieved with the loss of resistance; take care to avoid advancing the needle too far (i.e., out the opposite side or against the opposite mantle of the tibia). The needle is usually quite stable if properly positioned.
5. Attach standard intravenous infusion equipment. Fluid should flow freely without extravasation (see Fig. 48-6, *D*). A new device for intraosseous access is the EZ-IO (VidaCare, San Antonio, Tex.), which is a handheld battery-powered device that works much like an electric drill (E-Fig. 48-1). This device should be immediately available in all operating rooms and prenatal intensive care units because this is the simplest and easiest means for establishing emergent intraosseous access even in out of hospital venues.[123-127]

## UMBILICAL VEIN CATHETERIZATION

### Indications

The umbilical vein provides convenient access to the central circulation of a neonate for restoration of blood volume and for administration of glucose and drugs. This procedure is often carried out blindly with later radiographic confirmation of correct position. A large fraction of catheters are initially malpositioned, which if unrecognized, can lead to life-threatening complications.[128-132] A change in the configuration of the electrocardiogram (ECG) suggests that a small QRS complex reflects catheter position below the diaphragm; a normal-sized QRS complex with a small P wave was associated with location within the inferior vena cava at the thoracic level; and the appearance of a tall P wave indicated positioning within the right atrium.[128] Umbilical vein catheterization also provides a route for the procedure of exchange transfusion and for measuring central venous pressure.

### Equipment

- Umbilical artery catheter sizes 3.5 and 5F
- Scalpel and blade
- Fine-curved forceps
- Mosquito hemostats
- Umbilical tape
- Scissors
- Sutures with needle (3-0 silk)
- Antiseptic solutions (povidone-iodine and alcohol)
- Three-way stopcocks
- 10-mL syringe
- Sterile drapes

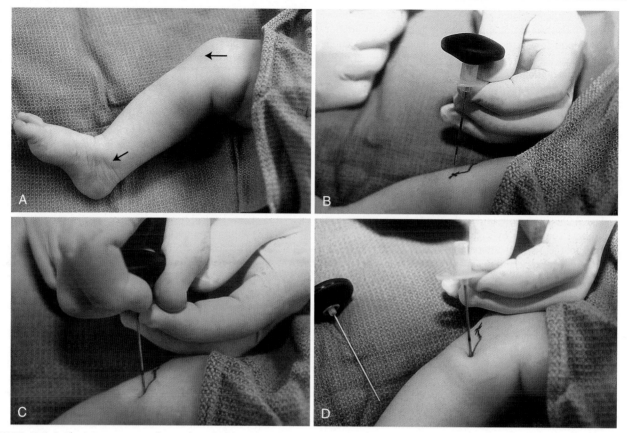

**FIGURE 48-6 A,** The intraosseous needle may be inserted in either of two locations: at a point 1 to 2 cm below and medial to the tibial tuberosity or at the medial malleolus (*arrows*). **B** and **C,** The leg is prepared, and the intraosseous needle punctures the skin (note the *X mark* connecting the tibial tuberosity with the point of needle insertion); the needle is advanced with a twisting motion in a caudal direction. **D,** The stylet is removed, and the selected solution is infused.

- Infusion solution of 10% dextrose in water, with 1 to 2 units of heparin per milliliter at 1 mL/hour
- Calibrated transducer/monitoring system if used for central venous pressure measurement

*Technique*

1. Prepare and drape the umbilicus with sterile technique; cut the cord approximately 1 cm above the umbilicus. The umbilical vein orifice is more patulous and thin walled than the two umbilical arteries (Fig. 48-7).

2. Holding the catheter filled with heparinized solution 2 cm from the tip, gently introduce it into the vein. In some situations, forceps can aid in directing the catheter. Traction of the umbilical stump *caudad* may facilitate the catheter's advancement (see Fig. 48-7). The catheter is passed a distance that approximates the length between the umbilical stump and the right atrium. Blood should freely aspirate into a syringe. Inability to withdraw blood may occur if the tip of the catheter is resting against a vessel wall or if a clot is present within the catheter lumen. *It is important that the tip of the catheter be placed in the proper position, that is, at the junction of the inferior vena cava and right atrium.* A radiograph confirms proper catheter position. Monitoring changes in the configuration of the ECG during insertion may allow for a more accurate placement within the right atrium but is limited to neonates with a

normal tracing.[128] At times, the catheter may fail to traverse the ductus venosus and become wedged in the liver. This position is potentially dangerous because portal necrosis and subsequent cirrhosis may result should hyperosmolar or sclerosing solutions be injected (calcium, sodium bicarbonate, 25% to 50% glucose).[132,133] A low position might be acceptable for short-term use if it is not possible to pass the catheter centrally, but the distance of insertion should be no more than 3 to 4 cm or just until blood is freely aspirated.

3. Suture the catheter in place, cover the insertion site with antibiotic ointment, and tape it to the abdominal wall. The catheter is then connected to a constant-infusion system and should be removed as soon as the indications for its insertion have passed. Complications appear to relate in part to the duration of insertion.[130,132,134]

*Complications*

- Thrombosis of portal or mesenteric veins[132,135]
- Infection (septicemia)[130]
- Endocarditis
- Pulmonary infarction (misplacement of the catheter into the pulmonary vein through a patent foramen ovale)
- Portal cirrhosis and esophageal varices later in life[136-139]
- Cardiac tamponade[140]
- Liver abscess and subcapsular hematoma[129,133]

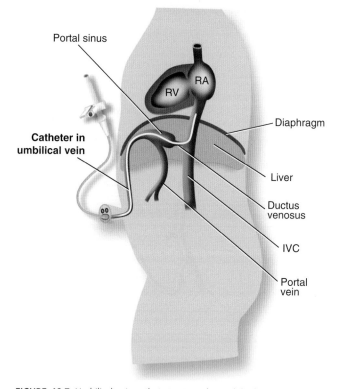

Portal sinus

RV | RA

Diaphragm

**Catheter in umbilical vein**

Liver

Ductus venosus

IVC

Portal vein

**FIGURE 48-7** Umbilical vein catheterization. The umbilical vein is thin walled and patulous, whereas umbilical arteries are thicker walled and of smaller diameter. *Caudal* traction on the umbilical stump may facilitate catheter advancement. The catheter should be advanced through the liver into the central circulation within the low right atrium (*RA*) before administration of any medications. *IVC*, Inferior vena cava; *RV*, right ventricle.

## Arterial Cannulation

### UMBILICAL ARTERY

The umbilical artery in a neonate is a convenient site for monitoring arterial blood pressure, blood gases, and pH. It provides emergency access to an infant's circulation for restoration of blood volume and administration of glucose and drugs.[141-144] Continuous monitoring of arterial $O_2$ saturation is also possible.[145]

#### Equipment

The materials used for cannulation are identical to those described for umbilical venous catheterization. Equipment is required for continuous monitoring of blood pressure. *End-hole rather than side-hole catheters may have a lower incidence of thrombosis or associated ischemic events.*[146]

#### Technique

1. Prepare and drape the area with sterile technique; cut the umbilical cord approximately 1 cm above the umbilicus. The two umbilical arteries are identified (Fig. 48-8). The cut vessel ends have thicker walls, are smaller than the vein, and are usually in spasm. The artery is entered in the manner described for umbilical vein catheterization, except that *cephalad* traction is applied to the umbilical stump (see Fig. 48-6, *A*) to encourage *caudal* direction

of the catheter. The catheter should course through the umbilical artery into the iliohypogastric artery and then into the descending aorta. Proper positioning of the catheter tip is crucial. If the catheter is advanced too far up the aorta, it may pass through the ductus arteriosus and into the pulmonary artery. If this situation is not recognized, blood pressure and blood gas measurements may be misleading. Care should be taken to ensure the placement of the catheter tip in the descending aorta (at T7 to T9). Early reports suggested that a cephalad position, at or above the level of the diaphragm, is easier to maintain but predisposes infants to increased risk of embolization to renal or mesenteric vessels (see Fig. 48-8, *B*).[147-150] However, positioning just above the bifurcation of the descending aorta, that is, at L3 to L5 (see Fig. 48-8, *A*) (below the origin of the renal arteries and visceral branches of the aorta) has not been supported by a Cochrane review; a cephalad position is recommended.[151] The caudad position is difficult to maintain, and the catheter tip may slip into one of the iliac arteries, resulting in tissue ischemia (see Fig. 48-8, *C*).

2. Confirm the position radiographically. Once the catheter is properly positioned, the system is connected to a constant-infusion pump and heparinized fluids (10% dextrose in water or normal saline) are infused. Suture and tape the catheter and apply antibiotic ointment as for umbilical vein catheters. A Cochrane review of the use of heparin suggested that low-dose heparinization of the infusate (0.25 unit/mL) has been shown to reduce the likelihood of catheter occlusion compared with intermittent flushing with heparinized solutions.[152]

#### Complications

Using the umbilical artery as a source for blood pressure monitoring and blood gas analysis only and reserving alternative sites for glucose and drug administration may minimize complications. Changes in cerebral blood flow are associated with intraventricular hemorrhage and have been documented to occur with umbilical artery blood sampling; fewer changes in cerebral blood flow occur with low-positioned catheters.[153] The incidence of documented intraventricular hemorrhage appears to have a stronger relation with age than with catheter position and is not associated with the use of low-dose heparin.[152,154] Other complications are as follows:

- Accidental disconnection of stopcocks and catheters can lead to potentially dangerous exsanguination.
- Blood clots may embolize retrograde or, more likely, distally, leading to ischemia or infarction of the infant's gut, kidneys, or lower limbs (see Fig. 48-8, *C*).[155]
- Vascular spasm is usually transitory and may be resolved by withdrawal of the catheter. Several cases of flaccid paraplegia have been reported resulting from spasm or embolic phenomena.[156]
- The infant is always at risk for sepsis; therefore clear indications for the insertion of this catheter are mandatory. The catheter should be removed at the earliest possible time. A Cochrane review failed to establish a role for prophylactic antibiotics in reducing catheter-related infections.[157]
- Hypertension as a result of renal artery emboli may cause ischemia and infarction of the kidney.[150,158]
- Aortic thrombosis may occur.

48

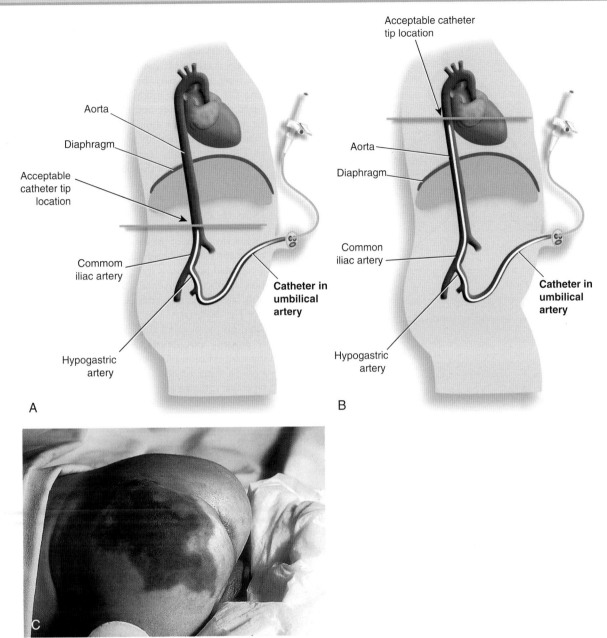

**FIGURE 48-8** Umbilical artery catheterization. *Cephalad* traction on the umbilical stump may facilitate catheter advancement. **A,** The catheter tip at L3-4 just above the aortic bifurcation and below the renal arteries is one acceptable location (*arrow to yellow line*). **B,** An alternative acceptable location is in the descending aorta between T7 to T9 (*arrow to yellow line*). **C,** An area of necrosis in the left buttock that resulted from a catheter migrating into the internal iliac vessel, occluding one of its branches.

## RADIAL ARTERY

Radial artery cannulation is a reasonable alternative to umbilical artery cannulation in a neonate and is the primary site of arterial cannulation in infants and children in most pediatric institutions. Percutaneous radial artery cannulation is widely practiced, with minimal morbidity.[130,159-164] Failure to cannulate the artery percutaneously may be followed successfully by direct arterial cutdown. Of children with Down syndrome (trisomy 21), 16% to 19% have abnormal radial vessels (both size and location), which can make arterial cannulation particularly difficult; some children with Down syndrome have a single median artery.[166,167] The ulnar artery also has been used as an alternative site for arterial catheterization when attempts at insertion in other locations have been unsuccessful; to ensure adequate perfusion of the hand, this site should not be used if previous attempts at cannulation of the ipsilateral radial artery had been attempted.[165]

### Indications

Indications for radial artery cannulation include monitoring of arterial blood pressure, arterial blood gases, and pH. The right radial artery is preferred in neonates because it is representative of preductal blood flow.

### Technique

1. Confirm the adequacy of ulnar artery collateral flow by the modified Allen test (Fig. 48-9, *A*). The color of the hand is noted. The hand is passively clenched, and the radial and ulnar arteries are simultaneously compressed at

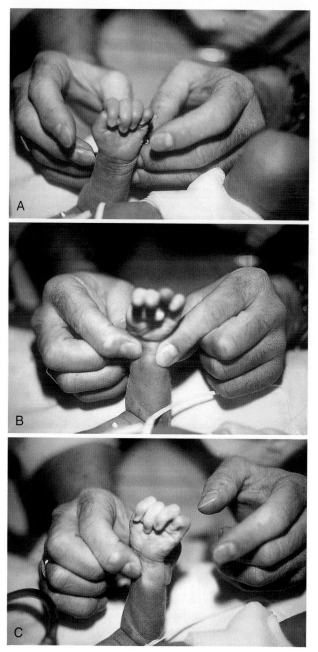

**FIGURE 48-9** Modified Allen test. **A,** Color and perfusion of the hand are noted. **B,** The hand is first passively clenched, and then both radial and ulnar vessels are occluded. **C,** The ulnar artery is released while the radial artery remains occluded. If flow through the ulnar artery and collateral arch in the hand is adequate, the color and perfusion should rapidly return.

3. Observe the course of the radial artery in a neonate with the aid of a fiberoptic light source directed toward the lateral side or dorsal aspect of the wrist. Use of a Doppler device may also be of great value.[169,170]

4. Use a 20-gauge needle to make a small skin puncture over the maximal pulsation of the radial artery, usually at the second proximal wrist crease. This step eases passage of the cannula by reducing resistance offered by the skin and prevents a burr from forming on the catheter tip as it passes through the dermis. A method to avoid accidental puncture of the artery is to pull the overlying skin laterally to make the skin nick.

5. Perform cannulation with a 24- or 22-gauge catheter either on direct entry of the artery at an angle of 15 to 20 degrees or on withdrawing the cannula after transfixion of the artery (Fig. 48-10, *A* to *C*). A wire (0.018 inch) may be used as an aid to advance 22-gauge and nontapered 24-gauge catheters.

6. Attach the catheter firmly to a T-connector to permit continuous infusion of isotonic saline (1 unit/mL) at the rate of 1 to 2 mL/hr via a constant-infusion pump (see Fig. 48-10, *D*). The catheter is securely taped in place. A pressure transducer is connected to allow continuous arterial pressure monitoring. To ensure accurate blood pressure measurement, it is essential that the transducer be calibrated to the neonate's or child's heart level, that all air bubbles be removed from the system, and that no more than 3 feet of tubing be used between the neonate or child and the transducer to minimize artifacts caused by the monitoring tubing.[171]

7. Obtain blood samples by clamping off the distal end of the T-connector, cleaning the injection port of the T-connector with povidone-iodine, introducing a 22-gauge needle, and withdrawing 1 mL of blood. A sample of blood is obtained by heparinized syringe, with minimal blood loss and minimal manipulation of the system.[159,172] An alternative is the use of a 3-mL syringe on a three-way stopcock: aspirate 2 to 3 mL, clamp the system, and then take the sample of blood from the T-connector as just described. After sampling, the clamp is released, the aspirated blood is readministered, and continuous infusion is resumed or flush is run into the 3-mL syringe and then the system is gently manually flushed intermittently with the syringe but the flush syringe is changed just once per 24 hours. This method of sampling maintains a closed system with reduced potential for sources of infection. Bolus flushes are avoided, which is an important consideration because bolus flushing has been associated with retrograde blood flow to the brain. Disastrous results may occur if an air bubble or blood clot should accompany a bolus flush.[173-177] *All arterial lines must be clearly identified (red tape) to avoid accidental infusion of hypertonic solutions and sclerosing medications.*

***Complications***

■ Infection at the site of the catheter insertion, with possible septicemia.

■ Arterial thrombus formation. This depends on the size of catheter inserted, the material of which it is constructed, the technique of insertion, and the duration of cannulation.

■ Emboli. A blood clot or air may embolize to the digits, resulting in arteriolar spasm or more serious ischemic necrosis.

the wrist (see Fig. 48-9, *B*). The ulnar artery is then released, and flushing (reperfusion) of the blanched hand is noted (see Fig. 48-9, *C*). If the entire hand is well perfused while the radial artery remains occluded, indicating adequate collateral flow, catheterization of the radial artery is performed. Note that the sensitivity of the Allen test is approximately 73%, with a specificity of 97%.[168]

2. Secure the hand using an arm board with slight extension of the wrist to avoid excessive median nerve stretching. The fingertips should be left exposed when the hand is taped down so that any peripheral ischemic changes from spasm, clot, or air can be observed.

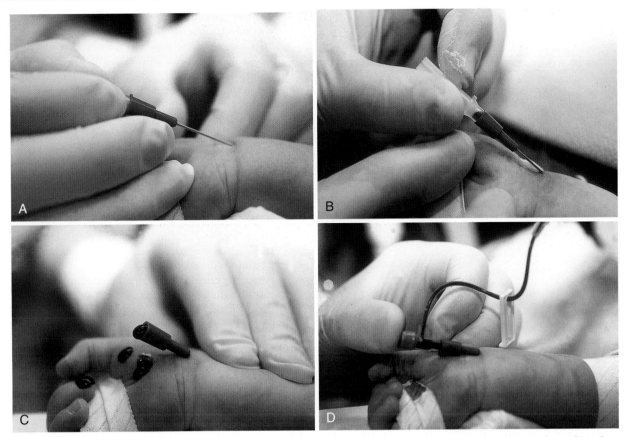

**FIGURE 48-10 A,** After adequate collateral circulation has been ensured, the radial artery is palpated and the appropriate catheter is advanced into the vessel. **B,** After blood return is noted, the catheter is threaded over the needle and into the artery. **C,** Pulsatile backbleeding confirms intraarterial position. **D,** A T-connector with appropriate flush solution is connected; the catheter is aspirated to clear air bubbles and then gently flushed. Antibiotic ointment and benzoin are applied. The injection port should be clearly marked as "arterial" so as to minimize accidental drug administration into the artery. A Luer-Lok connection is preferred to prevent accidental disconnection.

- Disconnection of the catheter from the infusion system. Blood loss may be life-threatening, especially in an infant.
- Ischemia. The radial artery cannula should be withdrawn if ischemic changes develop.
- Vasospasm. Usually transient but requires careful observation.

The method just described is the traditional percutaneous radial artery cannulation at the ventral aspect of the wrist. The radial artery on the dorsal aspect of the wrist within the anatomic snuff box may be used as an alternative site.[178] Once an attempt at cannulation of the radial artery is made, the ipsilateral ulnar artery should not be instrumented to ensure adequate perfusion of the entire hand. Strict indications for inserting radial artery catheters are necessary, and their removal must be considered at the earliest possible time.[147-150]

### TEMPORAL ARTERY

When the radial artery has been previously cannulated or is inaccessible, the temporal artery may be used.[179] Cerebral infarction has been described as a complication of this technique. It appears to be related to retrograde embolization of air or a blood clot.[180]

An advantage of this sampling site is that it provides preductal blood gas values. However, in our experience, the tortuous course of the artery and the resultant apposition of the distal tip of the catheter and the arterial wall have caused difficulties in freely drawing blood samples.

### FEMORAL ARTERY

Femoral catheterization in infants and children includes a greater risk of vascular injury or thrombosis resulting in ischemia[181] and is not recommended if other peripheral sites are available. In situations in which peripheral arterial cannulation is impossible (e.g., in burned patients or children with poor peripheral perfusion), the femoral artery should be used rather than not having any invasive arterial monitoring; the remote possibility of a complication must be balanced versus a greater likelihood of life-threatening complications owing to less than ideal monitoring.[182]

### Technique

1. Locate the femoral artery by palpation at the groin; this can be confirmed with ultrasonic guidance. Anatomically, it is situated midway between the anterior superior iliac spine and the pubic tubercle.
2. After sterile preparation of the skin, insert a catheter of appropriate size into the femoral artery using the Seldinger technique. The artery is entered at the point of maximal pulsation, approximately 1 cm below the line joining the anterior superior iliac spine and the pubic tubercle.
3. After cannulation, connect the catheter to a continuous-flow system and pressure transducer. The catheter is

sutured in place, the insertion site is covered, and an occlusive dressing is applied. The likelihood of fecal and urinary contamination makes this last step particularly important.

### Complications

- Infection
- Emboli of clot and air, leading to ischemic necrosis of the lower limb
- Poor arterial puncture technique, leading to osteoarthritis of the hip joint; severe trauma to the femoral artery has resulted in gangrene of the lower limb, retroperitoneal hemorrhage, and arteriovenous fistula formation.[183-185] A late complication can be partial arrest of bone growth likely as a result of thrombus formation.[186]
- Vasospasm. Usually transient but requires careful observation.

## DORSALIS PEDIS AND POSTERIOR TIBIAL ARTERY

The dorsalis pedis and posterior tibial arteries are additional sites for arterial cannulation in children when more desirable locations are inaccessible. Collateral circulation should always be checked. If cannulation is attempted or performed in one artery in the foot, the ipsilateral artery should not be instrumented, to ensure adequate collateral blood flow.

### Technique

The artery is cannulated in the same manner as for the radial artery at a point of maximal pulsation. An understanding of the anatomy of the dorsalis pedis and posterior tibial arteries before attempting this procedure is important. If percutaneous cannulation is impossible, the cutdown technique may be performed. The complications are similar to other arterial line sites of insertion.

## REFERENCES

Please see www.expertconsult.com.

**48**

# Infectious Disease Considerations for the Operating Room

ANDRE L. JAICHENCO

## 49

---

Causative Agent
Host
Methods of Transmission
Air Transmission
Contact Transmission
Accidents with Cutting or Piercing Devices
Strategy for Preventing Infection Transmission
in Health Care Institutions

Measures for Prevention of Infection
Transmission in the Operating Room
Prevention of Airborne
Pathogen Transmission
Standard Precautions
Antimicrobial Prophylaxis

---

THE TRANSMISSION OF INFECTION depends on the presence of three interconnected elements: a causative agent, a source, and a mode of transmission (Fig. 49-1). Understanding the characteristics of each element provides the practicing anesthesiologist with a methodologic aid to protect susceptible patients and health care workers and to avoid spreading infection.

There has always been concern about the transmission of infectious agents both to the patient from the anesthesiologist as well as from the anesthesiologist to the patient.[1] In addition, there are many sites within the hospital environment where moist or desiccated organic material with the ability to host potentially pathogenic microbes may survive for extended periods of time (Table 49-1)[2,3]; some may even resist the usual cleaning and disinfection techniques.[4] Their transmission from the source to the host may occur via indirect nonapparent mechanisms (e.g., most commonly through hand contact).

## Causative Agent

The infectious vector may be any microorganism capable of causing infection. The pathogenicity is the ability to induce disease, which is characterized by its *virulence* (infection severity, determined by the germ morbidity and mortality rates) and the level of *invasiveness* (capacity to invade tissues). No microorganism is completely avirulent. An organism may have a very low level of virulence, but if the host (i.e., patient or health care provider) is highly susceptible, infection by the organism may cause disease. The risk of infection increases with the *infecting dose* (the number of organisms available to induce disease), the *reservoir* (the site where the organisms reside and multiply), and the *infection source* (the site from where it is transmitted to a susceptible host either directly or indirectly through an intermediary object). The infection source may be a human (e.g., health care providers, children, visitors, housekeeping personnel) with a symptomatic or an asymptomatic infection during the incubation period. The source may also be temporarily or permanently colonized (the most frequently colonized tissues are the skin and digestive and respiratory tracts).

## Host

The presence of a susceptible host is an increasingly important element in the chain of infection that paradoxically results from advances in current medical therapies and technology (e.g., children undergoing organ transplantation, chemotherapy, or extremely premature neonates) and the presence of children with diseases that compromise their immune systems (e.g., acquired immunodeficiency syndrome [AIDS], tuberculosis, malnutrition, or burns). The organism may enter the host through the skin, mucous membranes, lungs, gastrointestinal tract, genitourinary tract, or the bloodstream via intravenous (IV) solutions, after laryngoscopy, or from surgical wounds. Organisms may also infect the individual as a result of work accidents with cutting or piercing devices. The development of infection is influenced by the host defense mechanisms that may be classified as either nonspecific or specific:

- *Nonspecific defense mechanisms* include the skin, mucous membranes, secretions, excretions, enzymes, inflammatory responses, genetic factors, hormonal responses, nutritional status, behavior patterns, and the presence of other diseases.
- *Specific defense mechanisms or immunity* may occur as a result of exposure to an infectious agent (antibody formation) or through placental transfer of antibodies; artificial defenses may be acquired through vaccines, toxoids, or exogenously administered immunoglobulins.

## Methods of Transmission

Microorganisms are transmitted in the hospital environment through a number of different routes; the same microorganism may also be transmitted via more than one route. In the operating room (OR), three main routes of transmission are possible: air, direct, and indirect contact.

### AIR TRANSMISSION

Airborne infections that may infect susceptible hosts are transmitted via two mechanisms: droplets and droplet nuclei.

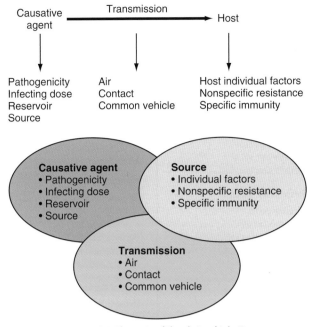

FIGURE 49-1 Elements of the chain of infection.

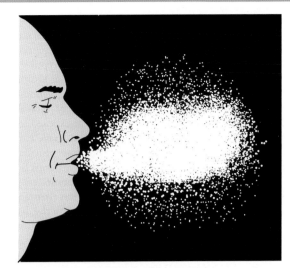

FIGURE 49-2 Droplets expelled during sneezing. (From www.vaccineinformation.org/flu/photos.asp.)

## Droplets

Droplet contamination is considered a direct transmission of organisms because there is a direct transfer of microorganisms from the colonized or infected person to the host. This generally occurs with particles whose diameters are greater than 5 μm that are expelled from an individual's mouth or nose, mainly during sneezing, coughing, talking or during procedures such as suction, laryngoscopy, and bronchoscopy (Fig. 49-2). Transmission occurs when the microorganism-containing droplets, expelled or shed by the infected person (source), are propelled a short distance (usually not exceeding 60 cm or about 2 feet through the air) and deposited on the host's conjunctivae or oral or nasal mucous membranes. When a person coughs, the exhaled air may reach a speed of up to 965 km/hr (600 mph).[5] However, because the droplets are relatively large, they tend to descend quickly and remain suspended in the air for a very brief period, thus obviating the need for special handling procedures for the OR air. Examples of droplet-borne diseases include influenza, respiratory syncytial virus, severe acute respiratory syndrome (SARS), and others commonly found in droplets from the respiratory tract.

## Droplet Nuclei

Droplet nuclei result from the evaporation of droplets while suspended in the air. Unlike droplets, the nuclei have an outer layer of desiccated organic material and a very small diameter (1 to 5 μm) and remain suspended in air indefinitely. The microorganisms contained within these nuclei may be spread by air drafts over great distances, depending on the environmental conditions (dry and cold atmosphere, with limited or no exposure to sunlight favoring the spread).[6] In contrast to droplets, which are deposited on mucous membranes, droplet nuclei may enter the susceptible host by inhalation; examples of droplet nuclei–borne diseases include tuberculosis, varicella, and measles.

## CONTACT TRANSMISSION

Direct and indirect contacts are the most significant and frequent methods of hospital infection transmission.

**TABLE 49-1** Nosocomial Pathogens and Environmental Contamination

| Pathogen | Types of Environmental Contamination | Organism Survival Time |
|---|---|---|
| Influenza virus | Aerosolization after cleaning; fomites | 24-48 hours on nonporous surfaces |
| Parainfluenza virus | Clothes and nonporous surfaces | 10 hours on nonporous surfaces; 6 hours on clothes |
| Norovirus | Extensive environmental contamination, possible aerosolization | ≤14 days on fecal specimens, ≤12 days on carpets |
| Hepatitis B virus | Environmental contamination with blood | 7 days |
| Coronavirus-SARS | Possible results from emergency department specimens; super-spreading events | 24-72 hours on fomites and fecal specimens |
| Candida | Fomite contamination | 3 days for Candida albicans and 14 days for Candida parapsilosis |
| Clostridium difficile | Extensive environmental contamination | 5 months on hospital floors |
| Pseudomonas aeruginosa | Drain sink contamination | 7 hours on glass slides |
| Acinetobacter baumannii | Extensive environmental contamination | 33 hours on laminated plastic surfaces |
| MRSA | Extensively contaminated burn units | ≤9 weeks after drying; 2 days on laminated plastic surfaces |
| VRE | Extensive environmental contamination | ≤58 days on working surfaces |

Modified from Hota B. Contamination, disinfection, and cross-colonization: are hospital surfaces reservoirs for nosocomial infection? Clin Infect Dis 2004;39: 1182-9.
MRSA, Methicillin-resistant *Staphylococcus aureus*; VRE, vancomycin-resistant enterococci.

## Direct Contact

This type of disease transmission involves direct physical contact between two individuals. The physical transfer of microorganisms from an infected or colonized person to a susceptible host may occur from child to health care provider or from health care provider to child during professional practice (e.g., venous cannulation, laryngoscopy, burn care, or suction of secretions). Health care providers working in the OR may be exposed to skin contamination by body fluids. This is an issue of grave concern because of the potential exposure of health care providers to patients with unrecognized infections, especially hepatitis B virus (HBV), hepatitis C virus (HCV), and human immunodeficiency virus (HIV). Hepatitis B is a highly infectious virus that requires a small amount of blood ($10^{-7}$ to $10^{-9}$ mL) to transmit the disease. The incidence of skin contamination of anesthesiologists and related personnel by blood and saliva is substantial. One study examined 270 anesthetic procedures during 7 consecutive days. The blood of 35 patients (14%) contaminated the skin of 65 anesthesiologists in 46 incidents. Of these contamination events, 28 (61%) occurred during venous cannulation. Of anesthesiologists who had been contaminated by blood, 5 of 65 (8%) had cuts in the skin of their hands.[7] The importance of this observation is that seroconversion of health care providers has been reported after skin contamination by infected blood from HIV carriers[8] and HBV infection after blood splashing into health care workers' eyes.[9] Scabies, pediculosis, and herpes simplex are among the diseases most frequently transmitted by direct contact.[10-17] These studies explain why meticulous hand washing and routine use of barriers such as gloves and eye protection are such an important part of protecting ourselves even during routine procedures such as starting an IV line or performing laryngoscopy.[18]

## Indirect Contact

Indirect contact involves the transmission of microorganisms from a source (animate or inanimate) to a susceptible host by means of a vehicle (e.g., an intermediary object) contaminated by body fluids. Tables 49-2 and 49-3 provide examples of diseases associated with bodily fluids to which health care workers may be exposed. The vehicle for transmission may be the hands of a health care provider who is not wearing gloves or a provider who fails to wash his or her hands after providing care to a child.[19-22]

**TABLE 49-2** Body Fluids and Diseases They May Transmit

| Body Fluid | Disease Transmitted |
|---|---|
| Blood | HBV, HIV, HCV, CMV, EBV, NANBH |
| Seminal fluid | HIV, HBV, CMV |
| Vaginal discharge | HIV, HBV, CMV |
| Saliva and sputum | HSV, TB, CMV, respiratory diseases |
| Cerebrospinal fluid | Encephalopathic organisms (see Table 49-5), HIV |
| Breast milk | HIV, HBV, CMV |
| Urine | CMV, EBV, HBV |
| Feces and intestinal fluid | HAV, gastrointestinal diseases (see Table 49-5) |

Modified with permission from Browne RA, Chenesky MA. Infectious diseases and the anaesthetist. Can J Anesth 1988;35:655-65.
*CMV,* Cytomegalovirus; *EBV,* Epstein-Barr virus; *HAV,* hepatitis A virus; *HBV,* hepatitis B virus; *HCV,* hepatitis C virus; *HIV,* human immunodeficiency virus; *HSV,* herpes simplex types I and II; *NANBH,* non-A, non-B hepatitis; *TB,* tuberculosis.

**TABLE 49-3** Infectious Agents That May Be Found in the Operating Room

| Viral Hepatitis | Viruses |
|---|---|
| Hepatitis A virus | Rhinovirus |
| Hepatitis B virus | Influenza |
| Hepatitis C virus | Parainfluenza |
| Delta hepatitis virus | Adenovirus |
| Non-A, non-B hepatitis | Respiratory syncytial virus |
| Human immunodeficiency virus | Measles |
| Cytomegalovirus | Rubella |
| Epstein-Barr virus | Cytomegalovirus* |
| Herpes simplex virus | |
| | **Gastrointestinal** |
| **Respiratory Bacteria** | Viruses: hepatitis A virus, |
| Streptococcus | rotavirus, adenovirus, |
| Pneumococcus | enterovirus |
| Meningococcus | Bacteria: *Giardia,** |
| Diphtheria | *Cryptosporidium, Isospora** |
| Mycobacterium* | Fungi: *Candida** |
| Legionella* | |
| | **Central Nervous System** |
| **Fungi** | Viruses: Human |
| Candida* | immunodeficiency virus,* |
| Nocardia* | herpes simplex virus,* |
| Cryptococcus* | Epstein-Barr virus* |
| | Parasites: *Toxoplasma** |
| **Parasites** | Fungi: *Cryptococcus* |
| Pneumocystis* | |

Modified with permission from Browne RA, Chenesky MA. Infectious diseases and the anaesthetist. Can J Anesth 1988;35:655-65.
*Opportunistic infections in immunocompromised patients, especially those with acquired immunodeficiency.

This type of contact can also come from health care providers who touch (with or without gloves) contaminated monitoring or other patient care devices (e.g., blood pressure cuffs, stethoscopes, electrocardiographic cables, or ventilation systems [respirators, corrugated tubes, Y pieces, valves]), which are used with several children without proper cleaning or disinfection between each use.[23-25]

There are also reports of equipment, fomites, and drugs (mainly propofol) that have resulted in hospital-acquired infections.[14,26-44] However, many of the following situations could potentially cause an infection:

- Up to 40% of the anesthetic equipment in the OR that was in direct or indirect contact with the child (blood pressure cuffs, cables, oximeters, laryngoscopes, monitors, respirator settings, and horizontal and vertical surfaces) may be contaminated with blood because of inadequate cleansing procedures between uses.[2,3,23,45,46]
- In some institutions, up to 8% of the Bain circuits that were reused without previous sterilization were contaminated.[47]
- Contamination of syringe contents has occurred with glass particles during ampule opening, which in turn may compromise the sterility of the contents, presumably because of the passage of bacteria contained on glass particles into the solution.[48-50]
- IV tubing has a significant blood contamination rate as well as contamination by blood from syringes used to inject medications. This can occur with the absence of visible blood reflux in the tubing or syringe. Simply replacing the needle on a syringe that will be reused is ineffective in preventing

cross-infection. The only certain strategy to prevent infection is to not use the same syringe in multiple patients.[51]

■ Refilling both glass and plastic syringes several times has been shown to result in contamination of the contents; single use is therefore recommended.[51,52]

■ Some drug formulations, especially propofol, can sustain bacterial growth under certain conditions. Thus great care should be given to aseptic technique when transferring drugs from the vial to a syringe and to use the contents of the syringe within 4 hours.[53-57]

■ Needles that had been used for spinal or epidural anesthesia were found to be contaminated with coagulase-negative staphylococci (15.7%), yeasts (1.5%), enterococci (0.8%), pneumococci (0.8%), and micrococci (0.8%), suggesting that despite standard skin preparation and cleansing there may be a significant rate of needle contamination.[58] It is unclear whether these skin organisms can be transmitted and cause an infection during administration of a neuraxial block.

■ Blood and saliva frequently contaminate the skin of anesthetic personnel during routine anesthetic practice.[7]

■ Violations of contemporary guidelines for preventing infections (e.g., hand-washing, wearing gloves, surgical masks, ocular protection, scrubs, or syringe reuse) by anesthesiologists are frequent.[18] Anesthesia staff are aware that they work in a potentially infectious environment, but whether they adopt the protective measures to prevent infections in both themselves and their patients is quite variable (11% to 99%).[23,59-61]

## ACCIDENTS WITH CUTTING OR PIERCING DEVICES

Percutaneous contamination as a result of a cutting or piercing accident is the most effective means to transmit bloodborne pathogens. Evidence suggests that this is the main route of HIV, HBV, and HCV infection,[62-64] especially if the injury is caused by hollow-bore needles that were used to draw blood or establish IV access.[65,66] Over 20 other bloodborne pathogens have been transmitted by this means, including those causing herpes, malaria, and tuberculosis.[67] The infectious risk after a percutaneous exposure to blood or body fluids from an HIV positive person is approximately 0.3%. Among health care providers lacking protective antibodies, the risk of HBV infection after an injury with a cutting or piercing device contaminated with hepatitis B antigen is approximately 37%; in the case of HCV it is approximately 1.8% (range 0% to 7%). Anesthesia staff lacking HBV protective antibodies are at great risk for acquiring the disease.[68,69] These infection rates underscore the need for the use of "safe" needles and the need to advocate the use of "needleless" systems even though they are significantly more expensive. This also emphasizes the need for meticulous handling and disposal of needles and other sharp instruments as well as the use of special "sharps boxes" designed to minimize accidental needle sticks (e.g., "mail box" type boxes that do not allow the hand to enter the disposal area).[70-85] The U.S. Centers for Disease Control and Prevention (CDC) has estimated that in the United States there are approximately 385,000 cutting and piercing accidents annually among health care providers in hospitals; 25% of these occur in the OR.[67] However, the actual prevalence is thought to be much greater, because many of these events are unreported. The distribution of these accidents among anesthesiologists is shown in Figure 49-3, *A*; the distribution of the items most frequently associated with cutting and piercing injuries in health care providers is shown in Figure 49-3, *B*. Should such an accident occur

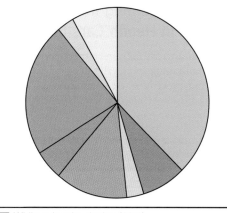

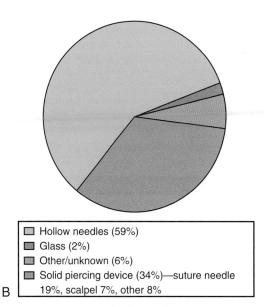

☐ While using the device (38%)
☐ Between steps or during complex procedures (8%)
☐ While removing the needle from the rubber stopper or other resistant material (3%)
☐ While capping a used needle (13%)
☐ While setting components apart (5%)
☐ After use, before disposal (23%)
☐ While dumping the device in the waste container (3%)
☐ Other (8%)

A

☐ Hollow needles (59%)
☐ Glass (2%)
☐ Other/unknown (6%)
☐ Solid piercing device (34%)—suture needle
B    19%, scalpel 7%, other 8%

**FIGURE 49-3 A,** Percentage distribution of percutaneous injury to anesthesiologists caused by contaminated cutting or piercing devices. **B,** Percentage distribution of items associated with percutaneous injuries in health care work.

(e.g., needle puncture, exposure to nonintact skin, or mucous membrane exposure) there are now specific recommendations regarding immediate assessment of risk, assessment of the exposure source (chart review, inform the patient that an accident has occurred and ask permission to determine HBV, HCV, and HIV serologic status) and initiation of appropriate treatment of the health care worker. It is advised to obtain as much information regarding the patient as possible, if the patient is known, to obtain a sample of blood from the patient for determination of potential carrier state (Table 49-4), and to report to the health service for immediate institution of prophylaxis and follow-up (Table 49-5), especially for HIV exposure (Tables 49-6 and 49-7).

## Strategy for Preventing Infection Transmission in Health Care Institutions

Institutional administrative measures aimed at developing, implementing, and monitoring specifically designed accident prevention policies and procedures are key factors in reducing and preventing transmission of infectious agents in health care centers. To this end, the center must take the following actions[67,86,87]:

■ Include infection control as a major goal in the organizational mission statement and implement safety programs, both for patients and health care workers.
■ Provide sufficient administrative and financial support to carry out this mission.

### TABLE 49-4 Recommendations for the Contents of the Occupational Exposure Report

- Date and time of exposure
- Details of the procedure being performed, including where and how the exposure occurred; if related to a sharp device, the type and brand of device; and how and when in the course of handling the device the exposure occurred
- Details of the exposure, including the type and amount of fluid or material and the severity of the exposure; for example, for a percutaneous exposure, depth of injury and whether fluid was injected and for a skin or mucous membrane exposure, the estimated volume of material and the condition of the skin (e.g., chapped, abraded, intact)
- Details about the exposure source (e.g., whether the source material contained hepatitis B virus, hepatitis C virus, or human immunodeficiency virus; if the source is infected with human immunodeficiency virus, the stage of disease, history of antiretroviral therapy, viral load, and antiretroviral resistance information, if known)
- Details about the exposed person (e.g., hepatitis B vaccination and vaccine-response status)
- Details about counseling, postexposure management, and follow-up

Modified with permission from Updated U.S. Public Health Service guidelines for the management of occupational exposures to HBV, HCV, and HIV and recommendations for postexposure prophylaxis. MMWR Recomm Rep 2001;50:1-52. Available at www.cdc.gov/mmwr/PDF/rr/rr5011.pdf

### TABLE 49-5 Factors to Consider in Assessing the Need for Follow-up of Occupational Exposures

**Type of Exposure**

Percutaneous injury
Mucous membrane exposure
Nonintact skin exposure
Bites resulting in blood exposure to either person involved

**Type and Amount of Fluid/Tissue**

Blood
Fluids containing blood
Potentially infectious fluid or tissue (semen; vaginal secretions; and cerebrospinal, synovial, pleural, peritoneal, pericardial, and amniotic fluids)
Direct contact with concentrated virus

**Infectious Status of Source**

Presence of HBsAg
Presence of HCV antibody
Presence of HIV antibody

**Susceptibility of Exposed Person**

Hepatitis B vaccine and vaccine response status
HBV, HCV, and HIV immune status

From Updated U.S. Public Health Service guidelines for the management of occupational exposures to HBV, HCV, and HIV and recommendations for postexposure prophylaxis. MMWR Recomm Rep 2001;50:1-52. Available at www.cdc.gov/mmwr/PDF/rr/rr5011.pdf
HBsAg, Hepatitis B virus surface antigen; HBV, hepatitis B virus; HCV, hepatitis C virus; HIV, human immunodeficiency virus.

### TABLE 49-6 Recommended HIV Postexposure Prophylaxis for Percutaneous Injuries

| Exposure Type | INFECTION STATUS OF SOURCE | | | | |
|---|---|---|---|---|---|
| | HIV-Positive Class 1* | HIV-Positive Class 2* | Source of Unknown HIV Status† | Unknown Source‡ | HIV-Negative |
| Less severe§ | Recommend basic 2-drug PEP | Recommend expanded ≥3-drug PEP | In general, no PEP warranted; however, consider basic 2-drug PEP‖ for source with HIV risk factors¶ | In general, no PEP warranted; however, consider basic 2-drug PEP‖ in settings in which exposure to HIV-infected persons is likely | No PEP warranted |
| More severe** | Recommend expanded 3-drug PEP | Recommend expanded ≥3-drug PEP | In general, no PEP warranted; however, consider basic 2-drug PEP‖ for source with HIV risk factors¶ | In general, no PEP warranted; however, consider basic 2-drug PEP‖ in settings in which exposure to HIV-infected persons is likely | No PEP warranted |

Updated U.S. Public Health Service guidelines for the management of occupational exposures to HBV, HCV, and HIV and recommendations for postexposure prophylaxis. MMWR Recomm Rep 2001;50:1-52. Available at www.cdc.gov/mmwr/PDF/rr/rr5011.pdf
HIV, Human immunodeficiency virus; PEP, postexposure prophylaxis.
*HIV-positive class 1: asymptomatic HIV infection or known low viral load (e.g., <1500 ribonucleic acid copies/mL). HIV-positive class 2: symptomatic HIV infection, acquired immunodeficiency syndrome, acute seroconversion, or known high viral load. If drug resistance is a concern, obtain expert consultation. Initiation of PEP should be delayed pending expert consultation, and because expert consultation alone cannot substitute for face-to-face counseling, resources should be available to provide immediate evaluation and follow-up care for all exposures.
†For example, deceased source person with no samples available for HIV testing.
‡For example, a needle from a sharps disposal container.
§For example, solid needle or superficial injury.
‖The recommendation "consider PEP" indicates that PEP is optional; a decision to initiate PEP should be based on a discussion between the exposed person and the treating clinician regarding the risks versus benefits of PEP.
¶If PEP is offered and administered and the source is later determined to be HIV-negative, PEP should be discontinued.
**For example, large-bore hollow needle, deep puncture, visible blood on device, or needle used in patient's artery or vein.

**TABLE 49-7** Recommended HIV Postexposure Prophylaxis for Mucous Membrane Exposures and Nonintact Skin* Exposures

| | INFECTION STATUS OF SOURCE | | | | |
|---|---|---|---|---|---|
| Exposure Type | HIV-Positive Class 1[†] | HIV-Positive Class 2[‡] | Source of Unknown HIV Status[‡] | Unknown Source[§] | HIV-Negative |
| Small volume[‖] | Consider basic 2-drug PEP[¶] | Recommend basic 2-drug PEP | In general, no PEP warranted** | In general, no PEP warranted | No PEP warranted |
| Large volume[††] | Recommend basic 2-drug PEP | Recommend expanded ≥3-drug PEP | In general, no PEP warranted; however, consider basic 2-drug PEP[¶] for source with HIV risk factors** | In general, no PEP warranted; however, consider basic 2-drug PEP[¶] in settings in which exposure to HIV-infected persons is likely | No PEP warranted |

Updated U.S. Public Health Service guidelines for the management of occupational exposures to HBV, HCV, and HIV and recommendations for postexposure prophylaxis. MMWR Recomm Rep 2001;50:1-52. Available at www.cdc.gov/mmwr/PDF/rr/rr5011.pdf

*PEP*, Postexposure prophylaxis.

*For skin exposures, follow-up is indicated only if evidence exists of compromised skin integrity (e.g., dermatitis, abrasion, or open wound).

[†]HIV-positive class 1: asymptomatic HIV infection or known low viral load (e.g., <1500 ribonucleic acid copies/mL). HIV-positive class 2: symptomatic HIV infection, acquired immunodeficiency syndrome, acute seroconversion, or known high viral load. If drug resistance is a concern, obtain expert consultation. Initiation of PEP should be delayed pending expert consultation, and because expert consultation alone cannot substitute for face-to-face counseling, resources should be available to provide immediate evaluation and follow-up care for all exposures.

[‡]For example, deceased source person with no samples available for HIV testing.

[§]For example, splash from inappropriately disposed blood.

[‖]For example, a few drops.

[¶]The recommendation "consider PEP" indicates that PEP is optional; a decision to initiate PEP should be based on a discussion between the exposed person and the treating clinician regarding the risks versus benefits of PEP.

**If PEP is offered and administered and the source is later determined to be HIV-negative, PEP should be discontinued.

[††]For example, a major blood splash.

■ Provide sufficient administrative and financial support for the microbiology laboratory and implement an infection surveillance plan, especially for postsurgical infections.

■ Establish a multi-discipline cross-functional team (e.g., a team manager, an epidemiologist, a representative from industrial health, and a person trained in quality control) to identify health and safety issues within the institution, analyze trends, assess outcomes, implement interventions, and make recommendations to other members of the organization.

■ Provide sufficient administrative and financial support to develop and implement education programs for health care providers, patients, and their families. One positive example of such education is that anesthesiologists who have read the CDC's Universal Precaution Guidelines for the Prevention of Occupational Transmission of HIV and HBV develop better hygienic practices.[59]

■ Provide health care workers with hepatitis B vaccine and document that an appropriate immunologic response was achieved. Provide hepatitis B immune globulin (HBIG) for those exposed who do not have established immunity.[4]

■ Provide a health care service for employees for counseling and postexposure prophylaxis should an exposure to HIV occur.[88]

■ Provide regular surveillance of health care workers to determine established immunity to infectious diseases such as tuberculosis, measles, mumps, rubella, and chickenpox. Lack of immunity may require immunization; several studies have demonstrated the cost-effectiveness of immunization (for prevention of disease) versus the cost of replacement of health care workers who have become infected.[63,89-94]

## Measures for Prevention of Infection Transmission in the Operating Room

### PREVENTION OF AIRBORNE PATHOGEN TRANSMISSION

Airborne pathogens may be transmitted through the OR heating, ventilation, and air conditioning systems. Thus it is vital to have

**TABLE 49-8** Ventilation System Specifications for the Operating Room

- Minimize the circulation of people during surgeries. It has been proved that the level of microbes in the operating room air is directly proportional to the number of people moving inside the room.
- Maintain humidity under 68% and temperature control to prevent environmental conditions that favor the development of germs.
- Maintain positive pressure compared with corridors and surrounding areas to prevent microorganisms from entering the operating room.
- Provide at least 15 air changes per hour in the operating room, 20% of which should be fresh air. Air should be recirculated through a high-efficiency particulate air (HEPA) filter.
- Air should be introduced at ceiling level and disposed of at ground level.

From Guidelines for environmental infection control in healthcare facilities: recommendations of CDC and the Healthcare Infection Control Practices Advisory Committee (HICPAC). 2003. http://www.cdc.gov/mmwr/preview/mmwrhtml/rr5210a1.htm

in place proper systems to (1) remove contaminated air, (2) facilitate air management requirements to protect susceptible health care providers and children against hospital-related airborne pathogens, and (3) minimize the risk of airborne pathogens being transmitted by children. Table 49-8 shows the 2003 HICPAC's (Healthcare Infection Control Practices Advisory Committee) and CDC's general recommendations for ventilation system specifications for the OR.[95] Children with tuberculosis require special consideration because of the high risk of occupational transmission of *Mycobacterium tuberculosis*,[96,97] especially after the emergence of multidrug-resistant strains (Table 49-9). An easy preventive measure is to screen all children before coming to the OR to determine recent exposure to infectious disease such as measles, mumps, rubella, and chickenpox because these infections can pose a significant risk to health care providers and patients, especially those who are immunocompromised.[63,93] Another potential source for airborne spread of pathogens is through the anesthesia circuit; this may be reduced

**TABLE 49-9** Summary of Recommended Tuberculosis Control Guidelines

Early diagnosis
Availability and access to diagnostic tests
Improved tests and reporting of results
Source controls
Containment of infectious nuclei from coughs and sneezes
Patient isolation
Personal respirators
Engineering controls
Negative-pressure patient environments*
Minimum of 6 air changes per hour
Ultraviolet light sources
High-efficiency particulate air (HEPA) filters
Decontamination
Sterilization and disinfection of equipment
Screening and treatment
Annual tuberculin testing
Availability and compliance with chemoprophylaxis
Bacille Calmette-Guérin (BCG) vaccination

From Tait A. Occupational transmission of tuberculosis: implications for anesthesiologists. Anesth Analg 1997; 85:444-51.
*Negative-pressure rooms are to prevent the escape of contaminated air to the outside.

**TABLE 49-10** Indications for Hand Washing and Antisepsis

*Hand washing* is defined as a process for removal of soil and transient microorganisms from the hands. Hands should be washed with soap and water or disinfected.

1. When hands are visibly dirty or contaminated with proteinaceous material or are visibly soiled with blood or other body fluids, wash hands with either a non-antimicrobial soap and water or with an antimicrobial soap and water.
2. If hands are not visibly soiled, use an alcohol-based hand rub for routinely decontaminating hands in all other clinical situations described in items 3 to 10. Alternatively, wash hands with an antimicrobial soap and water in all clinical situations described in items 3 to 10.
3. Decontaminate hands before having direct contact with patients.
4. Decontaminate hands before donning sterile gloves when inserting a central intravascular catheter.
5. Decontaminate hands before inserting indwelling urinary catheters, peripheral vascular catheters, or other invasive devices that do not require a surgical procedure.
6. Decontaminate hands after contact with a patient's intact skin (e.g., when taking a pulse or blood pressure and lifting a patient).
7. Decontaminate hands after contact with body fluids or excretions, mucous membranes, nonintact skin, and wound dressings if hands are not visibly soiled.
8. Decontaminate hands if moving from a contaminated body site to a clean body site during patient care. Decontaminate hands after contact with inanimate objects (including medical equipment) in the immediate vicinity of the patient.
9. Decontaminate hands after removing gloves.
10. Before eating and after using a rest room, wash hands with a non-antimicrobial soap and water or with an antimicrobial soap and water.
11. Antimicrobial agent–impregnated wipes (i.e., towelettes) may be considered as an alternative to washing hands with non-antimicrobial soap and water. Because they are not as effective as alcohol-based hand rubs or washing hands with an antimicrobial soap and water for reducing bacterial counts on the hands of health care workers, they are not a substitute for using an alcohol-based hand rub or antimicrobial soap.
12. Wash hands with non-antimicrobial soap and water or with antimicrobial soap and water if exposure to *Bacillus anthracis* is suspected or proven. The physical action of washing and rinsing hands under such circumstances is recommended because alcohols, chlorhexidine, iodophors, and other antiseptic agents have poor activity against spores.

Modified from Boyce JM, Pittet D. Guideline for hand hygiene in health-care settings. Recommendations of the Healthcare Infection Control Practices Advisory Committee and the HIPAC/SHEA/APIC/IDSA Hand Hygiene Task Force. Am J Infect Control 2002;30:S1-46.

by the use of circuit filters. However, at present there are no regulatory requirements to use such devices, and performance characteristics vary widely.[24,25,98-102]

## STANDARD PRECAUTIONS

*Standard precautions*[103] assume that any person or patient is potentially infected or colonized by microorganisms that could be transmitted and cause an infectious process. Standard precautions must be implemented with all patients and include:

- *Universal precautions–blood and body fluid precautions*, developed to reduce bloodborne pathogen transmission
- *Body substance isolation*, designed to reduce the risk of pathogen transmission by moist body substances

Standard precautions are used to reduce the transmission of all infectious agents from one person to another, thus protecting health care providers and children against exposure to the most common microorganisms. Standard precautions are implemented for any contact with blood and body fluids, secretions, and excretions (except sweat), whether or not they contain visible blood, as well as for any contact with nonintact skin, mucous membranes, and intact skin that is visibly soiled with blood and/or body fluids. Summaries of standard precautions, droplet precautions, airborne precautions, and contact precautions are available on line.[87,104-107]

### Hand Washing

Hand washing is considered the most important and cost-effective individual intervention in the prevention of hospital-acquired infections in children and health care providers.[108] Its significance in medical practice had not been universally accepted, despite the pioneering work by Oliver Wendell Holmes[109] (1843) and Ignaz Semmelweis[110] (1846), who separately recognized that the contaminated hands of physicians performing autopsies were the vectors responsible for the spread of puerperal fever caused by streptococci, and how by washing their hands before delivering a baby, they could reduce the risk of infectious transmission and maternal mortality, the latter by 90%! Unfortunately, the

scientific basis for hand washing was not established until the introduction of the germ theory of disease by Louis Pasteur[111] and the discovery of the microorganism that caused anthrax *(Bacillus anthracis)* by Robert Koch[112] in the late 19th century. More than one-and-a-half centuries later, and with strong evidence that health care providers are a leading source of hospital acquired infections,[19,20,113] health care providers' compliance with hand hygiene protocols in the hospital environment is generally poor (5%-48%) and difficult to change,[114-120] especially in intensive care areas, ORs, and postanesthesia care units. The risk of pathogen transmission via the hands is proportional to the power of the number of times a child is touched.[121] Table 49-10 presents a summary of the indications for hand washing and antisepsis. Compared with soap and water, alcohol-based hand rubs are more effective in reducing microbial colonization of hands.[122,123] The use of alcohol-based hand rubs prompted some authors to change the term *hand washing* to *hand hygiene*. An important addition to the 2002 CDC Hand Washing Guide[120] is to use alcohol-based hand rubs, because they work more rapidly (10 to 20 seconds compared with 90 to 120 seconds for hand washing) and can be used while ambulating. These advantages preclude the usual objections of health care workers to hand washing that include a lack of time, absence of sinks, and skin damage.[18,124] Furthermore, the scarcity of water in developing countries no longer needs to be a constraint against hand hygiene.

After hand washing, it is very important to dry the hands properly with appropriate paper towels, hot air flow, or both, because the level of pathogen transmission from a health care worker's hands to a patient is greatly increased if the hands are wet.[125] Transmission may also occur from patients' wet sites, such as groins or armpits, or when a health care worker gets his or her hands wet when opening parenteral solutions. It is critical for health institutions to establish written procedures and protocols to support adherence to the recommended hand hygiene practices.

## Gloves

Wearing clean or sterile gloves while caring for children is an effective means of reducing hospital-acquired infections. Gloves remain a supplementary barrier to infection that should not replace proper hand hygiene. Gloves protect patients by reducing health care provider hand contamination and the subsequent transmission of pathogens to other children, provided the gloves are changed after providing care to each child. Additionally, when the use of gloves is combined with CDC standard precautions, they protect the health care provider against exposure to bloodborne infections or infections transmitted by any other body fluids, such as excretions, secretions (except sweat), mucous membranes, and nonintact skin.

Recommendations for the use of gloves include[126-128]:

- Wear gloves in case of contact with blood or any other potentially infecting body fluid such as excretions, secretions (except sweat), mucous membranes, and nonintact skin.
- Remove the gloves immediately after providing care to a child. Staff should not wear the same pair of gloves to take care of more than one child, nor should they touch the surfaces of any equipment, monitoring devices, or even light switches. Contaminated gloves can pass blood or other body fluids to working surfaces and are vectors for hepatitis transmission.[62]
- Change gloves when taking care of a child if you must move from a contaminated to a clean body site.
- Apply hand hygiene measures immediately after removing the gloves because, despite the use of gloves, hands may get contaminated through small (microscopic) holes in the gloves.[113,129,130] Microbial contamination of hands and possible infection transmission have been reported even with the use of gloves.[131]
- Remove the gloves by using an appropriate technique (so as not to contaminate your hands with the contaminated surface of the gloves).
- Alcohol-based hand rub dispensers and clean glove boxes (at least two sizes) should be in place near every patient care site (e.g., on top of every anesthesia cart, medication cart, or in the nursing station).

- Disposable gloves should not be washed, re-sterilized, or disinfected. If gloves are reused, appropriate reprocessing methods should be in place to ensure the physical integrity of the gloves and their full decontamination.
- Sterile gloves are much more expensive than clean, disposable gloves and should be used only for certain procedures, such as when hands are in contact with normally sterile body areas or when inserting intravascular or urinary catheters. Clean gloves should be used during any other procedure, including wound dressing.
- Latex-free gloves should be worn when caring for children at risk for latex allergy.

## ANTIMICROBIAL PROPHYLAXIS

Surgical antimicrobial prophylaxis is an essential tool to reduce the risk of postoperative infections, and the anesthesia team plays a central role in ensuring the proper timing of drug administration.[132,133] The aim of the perioperative administration of antibiotics is to obtain plasma and tissue drug concentrations exceeding the minimal inhibitory concentration of those organisms most likely to cause an infection. This will reduce the microbial load of the intraoperative contamination to a level not exceeding the host defenses; it is not the intent to cover all possible pathogens, because this can lead to the selection of drug-resistant bacteria.

### Selection of the Antimicrobial Agent

Several antimicrobial prophylaxis guidelines have been published (Table 49-11). For most surgical procedures that do not involve chronically colonized organs, the most common pathogens are the skin flora, *Streptococcus* and *Staphylococcus*. A first-generation cephalosporin (i.e., cefazolin) can provide cost-effective coverage for these organisms. Surgical procedures that involve contamination from the bowel require antibiotic treatment against gram-negative and anaerobic pathogens. For these procedures, cefoxitin, cefotetan, or a second-generation cephalosporin is appropriate.[134] The selection of antibiotics requires consideration of resistance patterns as determined by local microbiology or health center infectious disease departments. The newer-generation broad-spectrum antibiotics should not be used for routine antibiotic prophylaxis but should be reserved for the treatment of resistant organisms. Moreover, the dose of antibiotic selected should be based on the child's weight or body mass index; administration should be repeated intraoperatively if surgery exceeds more than two half-lives after the first antibiotic administration (see Table 49-11), if the duration of surgery exceeds 4 to 8 hours, if blood loss is extreme, or if the drug has a particularly short half-life (e.g., penicillin or cefoxitin) to ensure appropriate tissue concentrations of antibiotic until wound closure.[135]

### The Timing of Antibiotic Prophylaxis

A key element in the prevention of surgical site infection is the timely administration of prophylactic antibiotics. For most surgical procedures, a single prophylactic dose of antibiotics should be administered 30 to 60 minutes before the skin incision. This should provide appropriate plasma concentrations of the antibiotic.[136,137] However, in the case of children, IV access is often established after induction of anesthesia. With a brief time interval between establishing IV access and skin incision, it is important to administer the antibiotics as soon as possible after IV access is established and before surgical incision. If vancomycin must be used for prophylaxis, it should be infused slowly over 60 minutes (to minimize the risk of severe hypotension, ["red

**TABLE 49-11** Suggested Initial Dose and Time to Redosing for Antimicrobials Commonly Used for Surgical Prophylaxis

| Antimicrobial | Half-Life Normal Renal Function (hours) | Half-Life End-Stage Renal Disease (hours) | Recommended Infusion Time (minutes) | Standard Intravenous Dose (g) | Weight-Based Dose Recommendation* (mg) | Recommended Dosing Interval[†] (hours) |
|---|---|---|---|---|---|---|
| Aztreonam | 1.5-2 | 6 | 3-5[‡] | 1-2 | Max 2 g (adults) | 3-5 |
| Ciprofloxacin | 3.5-5 | 5-9 | 60 | 400 mg | 400 mg | 4-10 |
| Cefazolin | 1.2-2.5 | 40-70 | 3-5[‡] 15-60[§] | 1-2 | 20-30 mg/kg 1 g < 80 kg 2 g ≥ 80 kg | 2-5 |
| Cefuroxime | 1-2 | 15-22 | 3-5[‡] 15-60[§] | 1.5 | 50 mg/kg | 3-4 |
| Cefamandole | 0.5-2.1 | 12.3-18[ǁ] | 3-5[‡] 15-60[§] | 1 | | 3-4 |
| Cefoxitin | 0.5-1.1 | 6.5-23 | 3-5[‡] 15-60[§] | 1-2 | 20-40 mg/kg | 2-3 |
| Cefotetan | 2.8-4.6 | 13-25 | 3-5[‡] 20-60[§] | 1-2 | 20-40 mg/kg | 3-6 |
| Clindamycin | 2-5.1 | 3.5-5.0[¶] | 10-60 (do not exceed 30 mg/min) | 600-900 mg | <10 kg: at least 37.5 mg ≥10 kg: 3-6 mg/kg | 3-6 |
| Erythromycin base | 0.8-3 | 5-6 | NA | 1 g orally at 19, 18, and 9 hours before surgery | 9-13 mg/kg | NA |
| Gentamicin** | 2-3 | 50-70 | | 1.5 mg/kg[#] | [#] | 3-6 |
| Neomycin | 2-3 hours (3% absorbed under normal GI conditions) | 12-≥24 | NA | 1 g orally at 19, 18, and 9 hours before surgery | 20 mg/kg | NA |
| Metronidazole | 6-14 | 7-21 no change | 30-60 | 0.5-1 | 15 mg/kg (adult) 7.5 mg/kg on subsequent doses | 6-8 |
| Vancomycin | 4-6 | 44.1-406.4 (CLcr <10 mL/min) | 1 g: ≥60 minutes (use extended infusion times if dose <1 g) | 1.0 | 10-15 mg/kg (adult) | 6-12 |

*CLcr*, Creatinine clearance; *NA*, not applicable.
*Weight-based doses are primarily from published pediatric recommendations.
[†]For procedures of long duration, antimicrobials should be redosed at intervals of 1 to 2 times the half-life of the drug. The intervals in the table were calculated for patients with normal renal function.
[‡]Dose injected directly into vein or running intravenous fluids.
[§]Intermittent intravenous infusion.
[ǁ]In patients with a serum creatinine value of 5 to 9 mg/dL.
[¶]The half-life of clindamycin is the same or slightly increased in patients with end-stage renal disease compared with patients with normal renal function.
[#]If the patient's weight is 30% above the ideal body weight, dosing weight can be determined as follows: Dosing weight = ideal body weight + 0.4 (total body weight − ideal body weight).
**Gentamicin may also be given as a single daily dose 5 to 8 mg/kg. Dose is dependent on postmenstrual age, renal function, and subsequent therapeutic drug monitoring.

man" syndrome]) beginning within 2 hours of skin incision. If a tourniquet is required, the full antibiotic dose should be administered before the tourniquet is pressurized.[138] Postsurgical prophylactic antibiotics are not necessary for most procedures and should generally be stopped within 24 hours after the surgical procedure.[138]

### Allergy to β-Lactams

Several studies have shown that the true incidence of allergy to antibiotics is less than that reflected in medical charts.[139] For surgical procedures where cephalosporins are the prophylaxis of choice, alternative antibiotics should be administered to those children at risk of anaphylaxis to β-lactams, based on their history or diagnostic tests (e.g., skin testing). However, the incidence of severe allergic reactions to first-generation cephalosporins in children with reported allergy to penicillin is rare (but not zero)[140,141]; furthermore, skin testing does not reliably predict the likelihood of adverse reactions to cephalosporins in those with reported

allergy to penicillin.[142-144] There is no evidence of any risk of cross-reactivity between penicillin and second- and third-generation cephalosporins. For the most part, "allergies" to oral antibiotics that appear on children's charts (rash, vomiting, gastrointestinal disturbances) are most likely reactions to the additives in the antibiotic formulation, including food dyes, fillers, and other compounds, or a manifestation of the underlying infection. IV administration of small test doses of the pure antibiotics in a fully monitored (and anesthetized) child with a so-called allergy will determine whether the child is at risk for an allergic reaction to the antibiotic. In the case of surgical procedures where antibiotic prophylaxis is mainly directed at gram-positive cocci, children who are truly allergic to β-lactams (cephalosporins) should receive either vancomycin or clindamycin.[134]

### Indications for Prophylactic Antibiotics

Surgical wounds are classified in four categories (Table 49-12). The use of antibiotic prophylaxis for postoperative infections is

| TABLE 49-12 Wound Classification System | |
|---|---|
| **Wound Category** | **Description** |
| Class I/clean | Uninfected wound with no inflammation and the respiratory, alimentary, genital, or uninfected urinary tract is not entered. Clean wounds primarily are closed and drained, when necessary, with closed drainage. Operative wounds after blunt trauma may be included in this category if they meet criteria. |
| Class II/clean contaminated | Operative wound in which the respiratory, alimentary, genital, or urinary tract is entered under controlled conditions and without unusual contamination. Specifically, operations involving the biliary tract, appendix, vagina, and oropharynx are included in the category, provided no evidence of infection or major break in technique is encountered. |
| Class III/ contaminated | Open, fresh, accidental wounds; operations with major breaks in sterile technique (e.g., open cardiac massage) or gross spillage from the gastrointestinal tract; and incisions in which acute, nonpurulent inflammation is encountered |
| Class IV/dirty-infected | Old traumatic wounds with retained devitalized tissue and those that involve existing clinical infection or perforated viscera, suggesting that the organisms causing postoperative infection were present in the operative field before operation. |

From Neville HL, Lally KP. Pediatric surgical wound infections. Semin Pediatr Infect Dis 2001;12:124-9.

administration of antibiotics is a therapeutic, not a prophylactic, measure. The use of antibiotics in children has implications not only for the response to the current treatment, but also to future treatments. Thus all medical professionals are jointly responsible for the rational use of antibiotics.

Protocols, although effective, require continuous feedback on their acceptance and surgical-site infection results.[147] No surgical protocol can replace the judgment of the medical professional; clinical reasoning must be tailored to the individual circumstances. Finally, children with congenital heart disease and a subgroup of those with repaired congenital heart disease may require bacterial endocarditis prophylaxis (see also Tables 14-2 and 14-3).[148]

## ANNOTATED REFERENCES

Hota B. Contamination, disinfection, and cross-colonization: are hospital surfaces reservoirs for nosocomial infection? Clin Infect Dis 2004;39:1182-9.

*Although much about the spread of nosocomial infection remains unknown, several facts have been established by existing data: (1) inanimate environmental surfaces can become durably contaminated after exposure to colonized patients; (2) although an organism may be endemic within an institution, specific isolates may predominate in the inanimate environment (e.g., vancomycin-resistant enterococci); and (3) contaminated rooms may be a risk factor for the acquisition of nosocomial pathogens by unaffected patients. This author elaborates on the need for improved infection control measures for preventing nosocomial infections.*

Rizzo M. Striving to eliminate catheter-related bloodstream infections: a literature review of evidence-based strategies. Semin Anesth Perioper Med Pain 2005;24:214-25.

*This paper reviews and emphasizes the need for preventive measures that could help to avoid or reduce most nosocomial catheter-related infections. The use of evidence-based standardized protocols will result in "best practices" and markedly reduce such infections.*

Sagoe-Moses CH, Pearson R, Perry J, Jagger J. Risks to health care workers in developing countries. N Engl J Med 2001;345:538-41.

*Protecting health care workers in developing countries from exposure to bloodborne pathogens will involve some cost. Health care workers are a crucial resource in the health care systems of developing nations. In many countries, including those in sub-Saharan Africa, workers are at high risk for preventable, life-threatening occupational infections. This paper expands on the need for improved support of health care workers throughout the world with appropriate supplies of gloves, barriers, sharps disposal, and the need for accident education programs.*

well established for clean-contaminated procedures. Within the clean category, prophylaxis has been traditionally reserved for surgical procedures involving a foreign body implantation or for any surgical procedure where a surgical site infection would be catastrophic (e.g., cardiac surgery or neurosurgical procedures). However, there is evidence that postoperative infections resulting from procedures not involving prosthetic elements are underreported; estimates show that over 50% of all complications occur after the patient is discharged and are thus unrecognized by the surgical team. Therefore, antibiotic prophylaxis is also recommended for certain procedures, such as herniorrhaphy.[145,146] The direct and indirect costs of these complications may not affect the hospital budget; however, they represent a substantial cost for the community at large. In the case of contaminated or dirty procedures, bacterial contamination or infection is established before the procedure begins. Accordingly, the perioperative

## REFERENCES

Please see www.expertconsult.com.

# Pediatric Anesthesia in Developing Countries

## 50

ADRIAN T. BÖSENBERG

THE POPULATION IN THE DEVELOPING WORLD CONTINUES TO GROW while world demographics trend toward an aging population in an urbanized, developed world. Children, many orphaned by the ravages of war, human immunodeficiency virus (HIV) infection,[1] and famine, constitute more than one half of the population in many of these countries.[2] Eighty-five percent of them will require surgery before their 15th birthday.[3] The burden of surgical disease requires safe anesthesia,[4,5] but provision of safe pediatric anesthesia[6] and intensive care[7-9] in the developing world presents serious challenges.[10-12] Poverty, poor educational standards, and limited health resources characterize the developing world.[5,6,13] Debt repayment, housing, education, social service, and health care provision are near-impossible tasks for most governments of these countries. Of the world's poorest countries, 70% are in sub-Saharan Africa, and they are ravaged by HIV, malaria, and tuberculosis and are desperately short of health care providers.[4,5]

Pediatric anesthesia in these low-income countries has not kept pace with the advances made in the developed countries.[4] International standards for the safe practice of anesthesia, adopted by the World Federation of Societies of Anaesthesiologists (WFSA) in 1992, are seldom met in developing countries.[14-16] In one survey, only 13% of anesthesiologists were able to provide safe anesthesia for children.[3] Consequently, perioperative mortality and morbidity rates in these countries are high by developed world standards[5,17-21] although local expectations are commensurate with the facilities and quality of the available care.

This chapter outlines some of the many challenges that anesthesiologists face when providing anesthesia for children in a developing country. Different countries have different problems requiring different solutions. The problems faced in many tropical countries,[8,13] for example, are completely different from those on a tropical island in the South Pacific[22] or West Indies,[23,24] at altitude in Nepal[25] and Afghanistan,[26] or in the humidity of sub-Saharan Africa.[2,3,19,21,27-30] These diverse situations necessitate that generalizations be made. The main differences among the sites, however, are related to the personnel, the spectrum and nature of the pathology, the facilities and equipment available, and a tenuous supply of cheap, generic, and perhaps outmoded drugs.[10,31]

## The Child

Children of the developing world are for the most part victims of circumstance; natural disasters, war, social unrest,[32] and economic crises. For many, medical care or timely access to care is a remote or nonexistent possibility.[10,25,30,33,34] Fear, poor understanding, and poor education often result in delayed presentation. Frequently, prior visits to well-meaning traditional healers expose the child to additional risks caused by potions that may be hepatic-renal toxic or enemas that may perforate the bowel.[35] Further delays occur when patients have to undertake long journeys to the hospital, and if the initial diagnosis is wrong, tertiary referral is made only when complications arise (Fig. 50-1).[10,30,36,37]

A typical example is acute appendicitis, a relatively uncommon condition in the developing world, where many other causes for a change in bowel habit are initially suspected.[37,38] Most patients present for surgery with generalized peritonitis, and perforation is common. In the developing world, the prospect of providing anesthesia for a toxic, acidotic, and dehydrated child is daunting.

Another example is infantile hypertrophic pyloric stenosis, also uncommon in developing countries, where symptoms other than the classic triad of bile-free vomiting, visible peristalsis, and a palpable tumor are more likely. The unsuspecting anesthesiologist, who may have no access to a laboratory[2,13-15] and is limited in the choice of fluid for resuscitation, would be challenged to manage the extreme metabolic derangements in these infants.

Superstition plays a role in compounding the anesthesia risk. For example, rural Vietnamese believe that it is not good to die with an empty stomach. Parents consider surgery to be an enormous risk so they feed their children beforehand. In these circumstances, passage of a nasogastric tube before induction is routine, although it is quite likely that the stomach cannot be completely emptied of solids despite the tube.[24]

Perinatal mortality in some parts of the developing world is ten times greater than those in developed countries.[5,39-41] The common denominators are early childbearing, poor maternal health, and lack of appropriate and quality medical services. Although lifesaving practices for most infants have been known

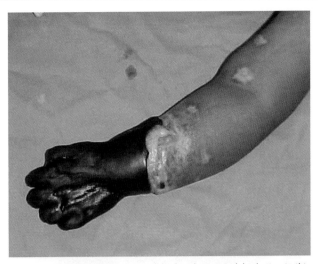

FIGURE 50-1 Peripheral gangrene of the hand. Severe dehydration in this infant was caused by severe gastroenteritis. Dehydration associated with delayed presentation, hypernatremia, herbal medications, and pneumonia are common contributors to this disastrous outcome.

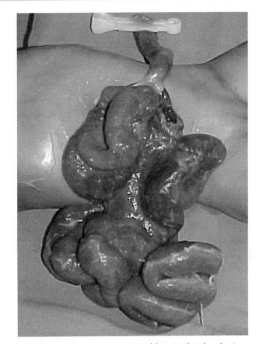

FIGURE 50-2 Gastroschisis is a major problem in the developing world. The outcome is poor because of a paucity of facilities for neonates. This defect was not diagnosed antenatally, and the patient presented late for closure, which proved difficult. Ventilatory support was not available, and a silo was fashioned. Unfortunately, the child died of overwhelming sepsis a week later.

for decades, one third of pregnant women still have no access to medical services during pregnancy, and almost 50% do not have access to medical services for childbirth.[30,34,41] Most parturients give birth at home or in rural health centers,[34] where basic neonatal resuscitation equipment is deficient or nonexistent.[30] Those who require surgery may need to be transferred, but specialized transport teams rarely exist.

In some hospitals, neonates are not candidates for surgery because "they always die,"[42] whereas in others, they undergo surgery without anesthesia[23] because "it's safer" and because some still believe that neonates do not feel pain. When surgery is performed on neonates, there are additional challenges, particularly in emergency situations.[23] Appropriately sized equipment is lacking,[36] and it may be extremely difficult to maintain normothermia even in relatively warm climates without improvisation. Regional anesthesia can play a significant role in neonatal anesthesia[30,36,43] and in some centers may be the only choice for anesthesia.[34,44] Apart from providing analgesia without respiratory depression, the need for postoperative ventilatory support for conditions such as esophageal atresia,[45] congenital diaphragmatic hernia,[46] and abdominal wall defects is reduced by continuous epidural analgesia (Fig. 50-2).

Regrettably, even neonates who have skillful anesthesia and surgery may die because of inadequate postoperative care.[44] Overwhelming infection, sepsis, respiratory insufficiency, and surgical complications are the main causes of morbidity and mortality.[30,34] The development of highly specialized neonatal anesthesia and surgical services,[7,40-42] essential for a good outcome after neonatal surgery,[30,34,36] is a low priority.

Although the burden of disease is dominated by infections and malnutrition,[4,5] pediatric trauma has a low level of advocacy and is given scant attention.[30,36,47] Socioeconomic advances in some countries have introduced a new danger in the form of faster, more powerful vehicles without the necessary maintenance culture or road discipline. Road traffic accidents are inevitable, and effective systems to handle the polytrauma victims that result are hard to find.[36]

Road traffic accidents are common. Even simple bone fractures have disastrous outcomes. Inappropriate management by traditional bonesetters frequently results in compartment syndromes or gangrene.[47] Trauma prevention strategies are given low priority despite the acknowledged impact trauma has on the economy of any country. Many developing countries are at war, and this has led to massive trauma and injuries to children who are participants in the fighting or innocent bystanders.

## CHILDREN AND WAR

Children may be victims of all aspects of violence. They face an intense struggle for survival as a consequence of displacement, separation from or loss of parents, poverty, hunger, and disease. They are vulnerable to the abuse of abandonment, abduction, rape, and forced soldiering. An estimated 300,000 children are used as child soldiers in more than 30 countries.[48] Many sustain physical injuries and permanent disabilities, and a large number acquire sexually transmitted disease, including HIV infection and acquired immunodeficiency syndrome (AIDS). These HIV-positive child soldiers then become vectors in communities where they are deployed.[49]

For many of these children, acts of violence become their form of normality, and the former victims become the perpetrators.[32] Survivors are subjected to the total collapse of economic, health, social, and educational infrastructures. Lost and abandoned children sleep on the streets and are forced to beg for food while trying to find their families. Many become child laborers or turn to crime or prostitution for survival.[50]

Children in war-torn areas sustain bullet, machete, or shrapnel wounds, and others are burned. They often sustain mutilating injuries (Figs. 50-3 and 50-4) that are not commonly seen in civilians.[51] Land mines are responsible for killing or maiming an estimated 12,000 civilians per annum. In Angola, a country with

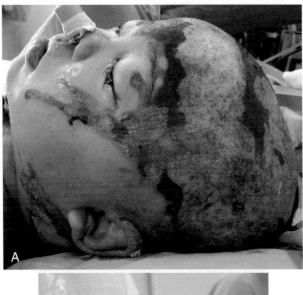

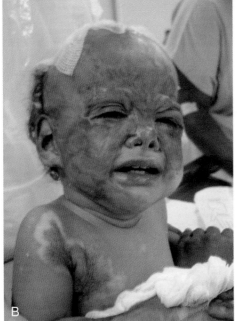

FIGURE 50-3 Facial burn injuries are common in the developing world, and these children may require multiple episodes of anesthesia. **A,** Flame burns of the face are invariably associated with inhalation injuries that may necessitate ventilatory support in intensive care facilities, which are not readily available. **B,** Pain management and pain assessment are challenging. The pained expression on this child's face is one of fear (and possible indignation about having the photograph taken) rather than actual pain.

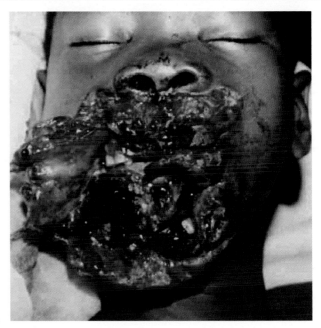

FIGURE 50-4 Children fare poorly in war. This 8-year-boy bit a detonator he found while playing. Endotracheal intubation proved a major challenge without a fiberoptic laryngoscope, which is a luxury in the developing world.

The terrible psychological effects of war persist even though the armed conflict may be over. Mental and psychiatric disorders with all the ramifications of posttraumatic stress disorder are common among child survivors.

## PAIN

Pain management modalities for children in a First World environment are vastly different from those available to practitioners working with limited resources.[52] Attempting to apply similar standards is fraught with difficulty. Illiteracy, malnutrition, poor cognitive development, different coping strategies, altitude (e.g., chronic hypoxia),[53] and pharmacogenetic, cultural, and language differences all contribute to the complexity of the problem.[54]

Children of the developing world learn to cope with vastly different problems. They may be victims of poverty, malnutrition, violence (e.g., war, trauma, abuse), and their attitudes about pain and pain tolerance are diverse. Children from an impoverished background seem more stoic and indifferent to even severe pain. After cardiac surgery, for example, some appear to need very little pain relief and are easily soothed by lollipops (A. Davis, personal communication) or play therapy.[33] Many walk from the intensive care unit to the general ward on the first postoperative day (A. Davis and R. Ing, personal communication).

Pain assessment of children from an impoverished background is difficult[55] (see Fig. 50-3, *B*). Many children in acute pain do not show facial expressions. Is this stoicism or simply a reflection of malnutrition, lack of social stimulation, severity of illness, or even cultural attitude? Language difficulties, cultural barriers, willingness to share information, emotional expressiveness, and outdated attitudes of the caregiver may endorse this quandary. Some societies convey pain readily, but others teach that expression of pain is inappropriate. Although many pain assessment instruments are available, few have been validated in the developing world.[55-57]

the highest rate of amputees in the world, there were an estimated 5.5 land mines for every child. Continuing land mine explosions remain a legacy of this conflict.[51] These blast injuries leave children without feet or lower limbs and with genital injuries, blindness, and deafness—a pattern of injury that has become a post–civil war syndrome encountered by surgeons worldwide.[51] Although the war in Angola is essentially over, the cost of mine removal is beyond the means of local governments. Ironically, artificial limb manufacture has become a developing industry.[51] Tragedies such as these are likely to be repeated in the ongoing conflicts in Afghanistan, Iraq, and Somalia.

There is an urgent need to develop pain treatment strategies that can be applied to the children of the developing world. Local conditions dictate their use and applicability. Simple pain management strategies may produce the most benefit with the least risk, whereas more complex techniques, which offer the most benefit, require a minimum standard of monitoring and regular reassessment to allow individualized titration of analgesia. These devices and personnel are seldom available to children of the developing world. The final choice of analgesia is therefore dictated by economic pressures or by the facilities available rather than what would be considered best for the child.

## Human Resources

Anesthesia does not enjoy a high profile and lacks the voice to demand access to resources in developing countries. The critical shortage of manpower is a barrier to progress.[5,8] Anesthesia is frequently delivered by nonphysicians,[3,6,58] a reality that has remained constant over many decades. Most anesthetics are administered by nurses or unqualified personnel who have little medical background and are "trained on the job."[3,36] In many African[5,59] and Asian countries,[5,60] the ratio of doctors to patients often is so small that the ideal of employing a physician specifically to provide routine anesthesia is out of the question.[5,61,62] Salaries are insufficient to attract suitably trained and qualified practitioners for more than short periods. Emigration of scarce trained personnel to developed countries in search of better salaries and improved lifestyles exacerbates these human resource difficulties.[3,5,10,58,61-64]

Anesthesia is not perceived as an attractive career for many undergraduates,[63] who receive little or no exposure to the specialty.[64] In some countries, surgery is performed without the "luxury" of anesthesia.[65] Few developing countries can afford specialist anesthesiologists, except possibly in the principal hospitals. Supervision of "nonphysician anesthesiologists" is invariably inadequate,[66] and access to textbooks, journals, or other medical literature is limited. Internet access depends on a reliable electrical supply, telecommunications network, and a computer, luxuries that are considered the norm in the developed world.[67,68]

Despite these problems, many individuals provide high-quality anesthesia for a limited range of surgical procedures, but few receive formal training in pediatric or neonatal anesthesia. Inadequately trained anesthesiologists tend to shy away from children, particularly neonates and infants, because of the perceived difficulty and fear. This is understandable in view of the lack of supervision, the severity of the child's condition, and the equipment that is more suited for adults. Invariably, the "pediatric anesthesiologist" is someone who may have a special interest in or affinity for children or who has been allocated to pediatric anesthesia for the day because there is no one else. A genuine pediatric anesthesiologist is a luxury.

On a more positive note, the World Health Organization (WHO) has recognized that surgery is a public health issue and has launched the Safe Surgery Saves Lives program.[5,16,17,62,69] The WHO has emphasized that safe surgery does not exist without safe anesthesia.[10,11,16,17] Training anesthesiologists in the skills required for pediatric anesthesia is a slow process. It is hoped that the WFSA program[69-78] will snowball so that children undergoing surgery in developing countries will reap the benefit.

## Pathology

Many pathologic conditions that are seldom seen in industrialized countries are more prevalent in developing countries because of poor health education, malnutrition, proximity of livestock to humans, earth-floored homes, poor sanitation, and contaminated water supplies (Fig. 50-5). Some conditions that are prevalent worldwide and relevant to the anesthesiologist are considered in the following sections.

### HUMAN IMMUNODEFICIENCY VIRUS INFECTION AND ACQUIRED IMMUNODEFICIENCY SYNDROME

An estimated 33.4 million people are living with HIV. Most cases occur in the developing world (90%), with sub-Saharan Africa (22.4 million) and Southeast Asia (3.8 million) making up two thirds of the global total; approximately 6% are children (see Fig. 50-5, *A*).[79] More than 25 million have died of HIV-related diseases since 1981, and as a consequence, there are an estimated 14 million orphans in sub-Saharan Africa alone.[79] Worldwide, more than 1000 children are newly infected with HIV each day; most of these children are in sub-Saharan Africa.[80] The prevalence of HIV seropositivity varies from one country to another. In this environment, it is prudent for the anesthesiologist and surgeon[81] to assume a positive status for every patient until proved otherwise.[36]

Although some success has been achieved in slowing the transmission of HIV in developed countries,[81-87] there are numerous barriers to the treatment of HIV-infected children in the developing world. Only 4 million people in low- to middle-income countries have access to treatment.[79] Treatment of children has lagged behind that of adults, in part because of the expense and the lack of pediatric antiretroviral drug formulations[84] but mainly due to poor human resources and infrastructure for administration of treatment.[88] Only an estimated 38% children infected with HIV receive treatment.[79]

Children can be infected by vertical transmission from the mother (>90%) or when sexually abused (≈2%) by an infected adult.[89] Transmission through blood products remains a risk, but with the global trend toward volunteer donors and more sophisticated testing of blood, this risk is expected to diminish. Vertical transmission can occur in utero, during labor and delivery, or postnatally. Risk factors include maternal plasma viral load and breastfeeding.[80,86] Data indicate that mixed feeding (i.e., breast-feeding with other oral foods and liquids) is associated with the greatest risk of transmission.[90] Perinatal transmission rates have been dramatically reduced by universal HIV testing of pregnant women, provision of antiretroviral therapy (when needed for maternal health) or prophylaxis, elective cesarean delivery, and avoidance of breastfeeding.[80,86] Highly active antiretroviral therapy (HAART), the triple antiretroviral therapy, has changed HIV from a fatal illness to a chronic disease with decreased mortality rates and improved quality of life[86]; however, these strategies require resources.

In practical terms, it is difficult to differentiate infants who are infected by vertical transmission from those who are not infected because differentiating between actively or passively acquired antibodies is virtually impossible in low-income countries. All children born to HIV-positive mothers have acquired HIV antibodies for the first 6 to 18 months. Only 30% to 40% of the infants who are infected may go on to develop AIDS. The presence of HIV antibody is therefore not a reliable indicator of infection. More sophisticated and expensive tests have been

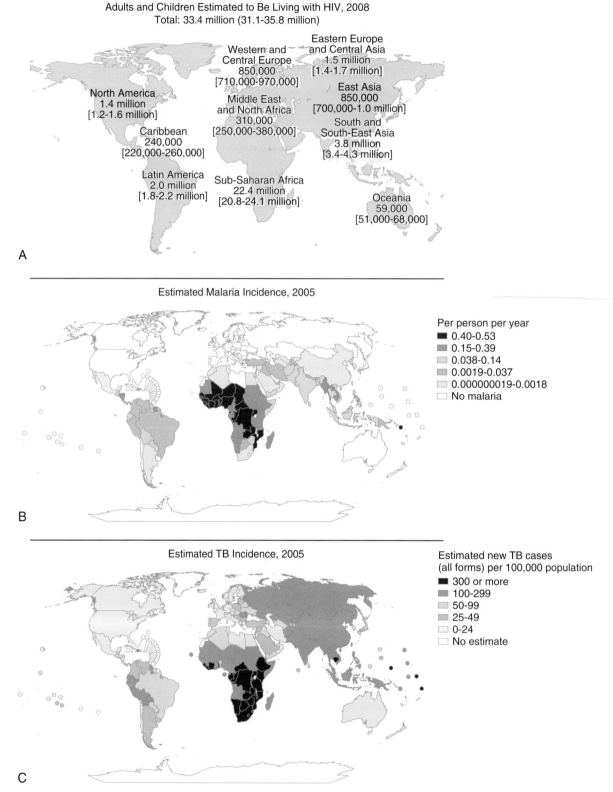

**FIGURE 50-5  A,** Global distribution of human immunodeficiency virus infection and acquired immunodeficiency syndrome (HIV/AIDS). Developing countries, particularly sub-Saharan Africa, carry the greatest health burden with the poor resources. **B,** The global distribution of malaria is remarkably similar to that of HIV/AIDS. Blood products in these regions carry an enormous risk, even if family members act as donors. **C,** Global distribution of tuberculosis (*TB*) in 2005. (**A,** From AIDS Epidemic Update, p. 66. Available at http://data.unaids.org/pub/EpiReport/2006/2006_EpiUpdate_en.pdf, page 66 [accessed July 2012]; **B,** from World Malaria Report. Available at http://www.rbm.who.int/wmr2005/html/map3.htm [accessed July 2012]; **C,** from World Health Report, 2006. Available at http://www.who.int/whr/2006/en/ [accessed July 2012].)

developed but are not widely available. All children born to HIV-positive mothers should be considered infected; if antibody persists beyond 15 months, infection should be assumed.

Progression of the disease depends on the mode of transmission; vertically acquired infection is more aggressive than other forms. Between 20% and 30% of untreated HIV-infected children will develop profound immunodeficiency and AIDS-defining illnesses within a year, whereas two thirds will have a slowly progressive disease. The course of the disease depends on a variety of factors, including timing of infection in utero, the viral load, the mother's stage of the disease, and whether the mother is receiving antiretroviral therapy. Treatment of children depends on clinical category, CD4 T-cell cell count, viral load, and age at the time of diagnosis. According to the current state of knowledge, after HAART is started, it must be carried on lifelong. This implies great challenges in adherence to avoid development of resistance and to evade long-term adverse effects of HIV therapy. Emerging drug resistance in children in low- and middle-income countries has necessitated new treatment strategies.[84,87]

The clinical manifestation of HIV in infants and children depends on whether they have been managed with antiretrovirals.[81,84,87] Most have asymptomatic infections, and the presentation may be subtle, such as failure to thrive, lymphadenopathy, hepatosplenomegaly, interstitial pneumonia, chronic diarrhea, or persistent oral thrush. Some present for the first time with life-threatening disease. Chronic diarrhea, wasting, and severe malnutrition predominate in Africa, whereas systemic and pulmonary pathologies are more common in the United States and Europe. Recurrent bacterial infections, chronic parotid swelling, lymphocytic interstitial pneumonitis (LIP), and early onset of progressive neurologic deterioration are characteristic of children with AIDS.

Pulmonary disease remains the leading cause of morbidity and mortality.[91-93] Bacterial pneumonia, viral pneumonia, and pulmonary tuberculosis are common in children throughout the developing world. The course of these infections is more fulminant when associated with HIV infection.[94] Acute opportunistic infections occur when the CD4 T-cell count falls; they include *Pneumocystis (carinii) jiroveci* pneumonia (PCP or PJP), cytomegalovirus infection, and the more typical *Haemophilus influenzae, Streptococcus pneumoniae,* and respiratory syncytial virus infections.[91,92,94] The classic presentation of PCP is fever, tachypnea, dyspnea, and marked hypoxemia, but in some children, the presentation is more indolent, with hypoxemia preceding clinical or radiologic changes.[95]

LIP is a slowly progressive, chronic form of lung disease seen in older children. It can lead to an insidious onset of dyspnea, cough, and chronic hypoxia with normal auscultatory findings and can cause pulmonary lymphoid hyperplasia in AIDS patients. In contrast to adults, LIP in children may cause acute respiratory failure, which is treated with steroids and bronchodilators. The clinical manifestations affecting otolaryngologists[96] and dental surgeons[97] have been outlined. Management of the upper airway may be difficult in the presence of stomatitis and gingival disease. Intubation may be difficult in the presence of acute (i.e., candidal infection) or chronic epiglottitis (i.e., lymphoid hyperplasia), necrotizing laryngotracheitis, Kaposi sarcoma (Fig. 50-6), or laryngeal papillomas (Fig. 50-7). These comorbid respiratory disorders can challenge even the most experienced pediatric anesthesiologist (Fig. 50-8).

Cardiac disease is being recognized with increasing frequency in HIV-infected children. The pathogenesis of cardiomyopathy is multifactorial and includes pulmonary insufficiency, anemia,

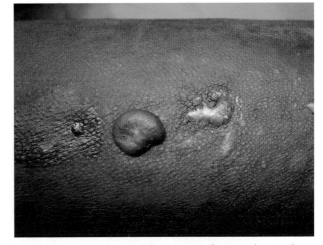

**FIGURE 50-6** Human immunodeficiency virus infection and acquired immunodeficiency syndrome (HIV/AIDS) are an increasing problem is developing countries, particularly in sub-Saharan Africa. The skin manifestations in this 8-year-old boy indicate Kaposi sarcoma, an AIDS-defining tumor.

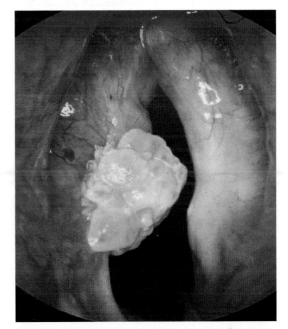

**FIGURE 50-7** Laryngeal papilloma. Papillomas, caused by the human papillomavirus, are prevalent in low socioeconomic groups and have the highest incidence in the 2- to 5-year-old age-group. This age distribution is changing in the human immunodeficiency virus–exposed population. Even in well-equipped institutions, anesthesia for these patients can be challenging.

nutritional deficiencies, specific viral infections, and drug therapy. Left and right ventricular dysfunction, arrhythmias, and pericardial effusions occur, but pulmonary hypertension is rare.[98] HIV may directly infect the myocardium, leading to early electrocardiographic (ECG) changes and abnormal echocardiograms showing hyperdynamic left ventricular dysfunction or evidence of diminished contractility (e.g., dilated cardiomyopathy, myocarditis).

The gastrointestinal tract is commonly involved,[99] particularly in those living in tropical countries, and affected children show evidence of malabsorption (i.e., slim), chronic recurrent diarrhea,

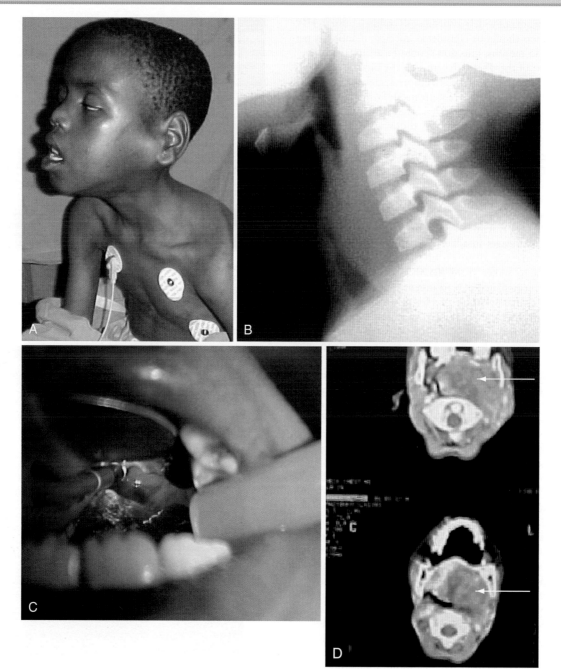

**FIGURE 50-8** Kaposi sarcoma is a marker for acquired immunodeficiency syndrome (AIDS). **A,** AIDS was previously considered to be rare in children, but it may affect the airway at different levels, as shown in this 12-year-old girl. She is clearly fatigued from the respiratory distress caused by Kaposi sarcoma at three levels: base of the tongue, tonsil, and trachea. She also has an underlying pneumonia. Significant supraclavicular recession suggests upper airway obstruction. **B,** The Kaposi sarcoma of the base of the tongue, tonsil, and trachea is shown on a poor-quality, lateral neck radiograph, which illustrates one of the many difficulties faced in remote areas, high quality imaging. **C,** Laryngoscopic view of the Kaposi sarcoma at the base of the tongue and the tonsil. **D,** Computed tomography shows a large retropharyngeal Kaposi sarcoma *(arrows)* obstructing the upper airway. The poor quality of the scan reflects inexperienced radiographers using the poor-quality equipment commonly found in developing countries.

dysphagia, failure to thrive, or enteric infection. They may require endoscopy for diagnostic studies. From the point of view of the anesthesiologist, there is an increased risk of reflux due to esophagitis, which may be caused by infection (e.g., *Candida*, cytomegalovirus) or drugs (e.g., zidovudine). Pseudobulbar palsy, a manifestation of central neurologic involvement, or esophageal strictures may occur.

Nausea and vomiting may have a neurologic, infectious, or drug-related cause. Pancreatitis, lymphomas, or smooth muscle tumors may delay gastric emptying. Hepatomegaly is invariably present, but severe hepatocellular dysfunction is seldom a major problem unless the patient has chronic hepatitis (e.g., hepatitis B or C, cytomegalovirus). Cholestasis and fluctuating transaminase levels may be caused by HIV infection, poor nutrition, or drugs. In theory, hepatic enzyme dysfunction caused by antiretroviral therapy should affect the metabolism and pharmacokinetics of some anesthetic agents, but little research has been done on this subject.

Medications used to manage HIV are involved in drug interactions on several levels.[100] The reverse transcriptase inhibitors

(e.g., zidovudine) are excreted by the kidney, and drugs affecting renal clearance reduce excretion. Reverse transcriptase inhibitors may induce CYP3A4 (e.g., nevirapine) or inhibit CYP3A4 (e.g., delavirdine) and affect other drugs (e.g., midazolam, levobupivacaine, ketamine, methadone) cleared by this enzyme. Protease inhibitors are inhibitors of CYP3A enzyme systems and are substrates and inhibitors of P-glycoprotein transporters. Coagulation status with the concomitant use of warfarin (which is metabolized by CYP2C9) may be altered by enzyme induction (e.g., ritonavir) or competition for clearance pathways (e.g., efavirenz, nelfinavir).[101]

Protease inhibitors also can inhibit specific uridine 5-diphosphoglucuronosyltransferase (UGT) pathways. This accounts for the increase in bilirubin concentration (i.e., UGT1A1 glucuronidates bilirubin) observed in some patients. UGT1A6 (i.e., acetaminophen glucuronidation) and UGT2B7 (i.e., morphine glucuronidation) are unaffected.[102] Gastric motility changes due to opioids (e.g., methadone) reduces absorption of some reverse transcriptase inhibitors.

HIV, a neurotrophic virus, can have a devastating effect on the immature brain, which is further compounded by the opportunistic infections and neoplasms that occur as a consequence of the associated immunosuppression.[103] Neurologic impairment is seen in most symptomatic HIV-infected children, commonly as a progressive encephalopathy with developmental delay, progressive motor dysfunction, and behavioral changes. Craniofacial dysmorphic features have been described. Hematologic abnormalities can reflect depression of all cell lines. Anemia may be caused by primary marrow failure, malnutrition, or drugs, whereas thrombocytopenia may reflect an autoimmune disorder.

Universal precautions should be strictly applied for all anesthesia procedures. Extra care should be taken when anesthetizing an HIV-infected child. Precautions should also be taken to prevent contamination of the anesthetic circuits. Disposable equipment, bacterial filters, and disposable circuits are recommended. The prohibitive cost for most institutions in developing countries limits the use of disposables. Reusable equipment should be cleaned, sterilized, and decontaminated according to the manufacturer's instructions. Fortunately, HIV is sensitive to a wide range of disinfectants.[104]

## TUBERCULOSIS

Tuberculosis remains an important cause of morbidity and mortality.[36,105-110] The epidemiology of pediatric tuberculosis is shaped by risk factors such as age, race, immigration, poverty, overcrowding, and prevalence of HIV/AIDS (see Fig. 50-5, C).[109,110] HIV and tuberculosis form a dangerous synergy that is difficult to manage in view of drug interactions between the antituberculosis and antiretroviral agents.[79,106] Even bacillus Calmette–Guérin (BCG) vaccinations can cause significant complications in immunocompromised HIV patients.[106] The emergence of drug-resistant tuberculosis adds to the burden and is a constant danger to health care workers in general and anesthesiologists in particular.

Primary tuberculosis infection usually does not produce clinical illness in well-nourished, immunized children, whereas reactivated pulmonary tuberculosis is a chronic or subacute disease that may present a variety of challenges for the anesthesiologist, including preventing transmission by contamination of the anesthetic circuits and the risks associated with pleural effusions, pulmonary cavitation, or bronchiectasis.[93,95] Mediastinal and hilar lymphadenopathy may severely compromise the airway.

Primary tuberculosis and its complications are more common in children than in adults. After young children are infected, they are at increased risk for progression to extrapulmonary disease.[109,110] *Mycobacterium tuberculosis* infection can cause symptomatic disease in any organ of the body and is usually a reactivation of a latent site of infection. The most common sites of reactivation are lymph nodes, bones, joints, and the genitourinary tract. Less frequently, the disease may involve the gastrointestinal tract, peritoneum, pericardium, or skin. Tuberculosis meningitis and miliary tuberculosis, both more common in children, carry a high mortality rate.[109] In view of the high prevalence of HIV infection among tuberculous children, HIV testing should be performed on all children with tuberculosis; conversely, tuberculosis should be sought in all HIV-positive children. Tuberculosis is, however, difficult to diagnose in young children, and the search for more sensitive tests continues.[105]

## MALARIA

Malaria (see Fig. 50-5, *B*) is a febrile, flulike illness caused by one of four species of malaria parasites: *Plasmodium falciparum, P. vivax, P. ovale, and P. malariae.* Effective and safe prophylaxis against malaria has become increasingly difficult because the species that causes the most severe illness, *P. falciparum*, has become widely resistant to chloroquine and to other antimalarial drugs in some areas.[110] Severe malaria, even when optimally treated, carries a mortality rate of 10% to 25%.[110-112]

Prompt diagnosis and early treatment is an important determinant of outcome. Uncomplicated malaria usually manifests as fever, headache, dizziness, and arthralgia. Gastrointestinal symptoms may predominate and include anorexia, nausea, vomiting, and abdominal discomfort or pain that may mimic appendicitis. In children, malaria can manifest with an acute, life-threatening disease or run a chronic course with acute exacerbations. The acute manifestations include three overlapping syndromes: respiratory distress due to a severe underlying metabolic acidosis (pH <7.3), usually a lactic acidemia; severe anemia (hemoglobin <5 g/dL) with hypovolemia[113] and thrombocytopenia; or neurologic impairment as a manifestation of cerebral malaria.[111-114] Seizures are an important presenting feature in 60% to 80% of cases. Prolonged seizures refractory to treatment and those that occur on antimalarial treatment are ominous signs and are usually associated with neurologic sequelae or death.[113] Cerebral malaria can also manifest as a prolonged postictal state, status epilepticus, severe metabolic derangement (i.e., hypoglycemia and metabolic acidosis), or a primary neurologic syndrome, ranging from diffuse cortical involvement to brainstem abnormalities.

Children with chronic malaria adjust physiologically to low hemoglobin levels but may decompensate rapidly when challenged with a febrile illness or surgery. The characteristic physical findings in children with severe anemia are respiratory distress and a hyperdynamic circulation. Blood transfusion may be administered rapidly in children with metabolic acidosis because most have a depleted intravascular volume.

Although controversial, exchange transfusion has been advocated for severe malaria, particularly for those with cardiorespiratory compromise, hyperparasitemia, or cerebral malaria. The rationale is to remove harmful metabolites, toxins, and cytokines; decrease the parasite load; remove deformed red cells; and restore normal red cell mass, platelets, and other clotting factors.[113] Unfortunately, many malaria-endemic areas also have a high prevalence of HIV, adding significantly to the risk of blood transfusions.

Chronic recurrent malarial infections may manifest with splenic enlargement. This may cause delayed gastric emptying

and pose an aspiration risk on induction of anesthesia. The spleen may enlarge acutely or rupture spontaneously during coughing, vomiting, or defecation. Rupture during external cardiac massage has also been described. Malaria may cause bloody diarrhea with massive fluid loss of fluid resembling dysentery in children.

### CARDIAC DISEASE

Pediatric cardiac services typically are too expensive for most developing countries, and the increasing economic divide threatens those services that do exist.[115,116] In North America, each cardiac center serves 120,000 people; by contrast, one center serves 16 million people in Asia and 33 million in Africa.[61] Despite the need, few third world units can treat the required volume of cases. Unless families have the financial means to travel to a developed country, the options for diagnostic or therapeutic cardiac procedures are poor.[33,115-117] Medical missions may provide immediate help, but their impact on a developing country is short term and potentially disruptive. These visiting teams ultimately have little effect on the complex socioeconomic and sociopolitical problems that exist.[116]

Rheumatic heart disease is more common than congenital heart disease in many developing countries,[115-117] reflecting the socioeconomic problems of poverty, overcrowding, malnutrition, and lack of antibiotics. Children often present late with life-threatening symptoms due to repeated infections and superimposed endocarditis. The acute deterioration precipitated by endocarditis may be the factor that prompts the search for medical attention. Valve replacement can be lifesaving, but long-term follow-up of anticoagulant therapy is often not feasible.

Congenital heart disease is an additional challenge, and it is common to see congenital heart defects in adults in developing countries. Those who have survived without the benefit of palliative or corrective surgery may present with pulmonary hypertension or endocarditis. Total correction of these defects usually is not feasible, and palliative surgery may be the more effective alternative. Excellent palliation with reasonable quality of life can be achieved relatively cheaply.[116]

### TETANUS

Tetanus is a disease characterized by painful tonic muscle spasms, hyperreflexia, and autonomic instability.[118] It is caused by the exotoxin of *Clostridium tetani*, an organism that is ever present in the soil and contaminated wounds. Although rarely seen in developed countries, tetanus is prevalent in countries where children are not routinely immunized. Tetanus neonatorum carries a high mortality rate and is still encountered in areas where it is customary to apply feces to the umbilical cord to stop bleeding.

The clinical manifestations of the disease are not the result of invasive tissue injury but are caused by production of a potent neurotoxin, tetanospasmin, at the site of the injury. The injury may be trivial and may not even be detectable at the time of presentation. The incubation period is inversely proportional to the distance between the site of the injury and the central nervous system. This usually occurs within 14 days of the injury in children.

Trismus is the presenting sign in most cases, and sustained trismus produces a characteristic sardonic smile (i.e., risus sardonicus). Persistent contractions of the chest and back muscles result in opisthotonos. Restlessness and irritability may be followed by tetanic seizures, which are often precipitated by trivial stimuli (e.g., touch, noise). Glottic or laryngeal spasm can cause sudden death. Late deaths may be caused by nosocomial infection, renal failure, sudden cardiac arrest, or cerebral hemorrhage as result of the autonomic instability.[118]

Treatment consists of surgical débridement of the wound, administration of human tetanus immunoglobulin, antibiotic therapy, and intensive supportive medical care. Ventilatory support is invariably necessary because the frequent spasms impair ventilation already compromised by sedative therapy. Benzodiazepines and opioids are the mainstay of treatment, but numerous protocols have been studied.[118] Magnesium sulfate has been successfully used to reduce spasms and has been shown to reduce circulating catecholamines,[119] whereas clonidine does not.[120] Pain management should also be considered, and I have been encouraged by the use of continuous epidural analgesia for these children. Further advantages of epidural analgesia include good control of autonomic instability, earlier weaning from ventilatory support, and possible reduction in the complication rate.[118] From the anesthesiologist's point of view, trismus is overcome by muscle relaxants and does not pose a significant intubation problem.

## Drugs

The supply of anesthetic gases and drugs for rural medical facilities is erratic and unreliable.[3,8] The cost of many drugs, particularly the modern anesthetics, has increased alarmingly beyond the reach of most health care budgets. Anesthesiologists in developing countries therefore must be resigned to using less expensive anesthetics or generic medications.

Ether and halothane remain the only inhalational anesthetics available in many countries and are the mainstay of anesthesia in many institutions.[2,3,10,31,121] Ether is cheaper and probably safer than halothane, although its use is limited by its flammability. This extreme flammability limits its transportability and therefore its availability in remote areas.

Ether and halothane have virtually disappeared from the operating rooms in the developed world and have been replaced by isoflurane, sevoflurane, and desflurane. As demand for the less-expensive agents has waned, some manufacturers claim a lack of profitability for them and have threatened their withdrawal. Although this may make commercial business sense, these agents sustain the anesthesia services for millions of patients in the developing world,[2] and their loss would be tragic.

Ketamine is probably the most commonly used intravenous anesthetic.[3,65,121] Ketamine is simple to use, effective, and relatively safe when used as a sole agent for short procedures, used in combination with muscle relaxants, or used to supplement general anesthesia for major surgery. It should be used with midazolam to reduce the hallucinatory side effects and nightmares after ketamine use. Benzodiazepines, however, are not always available. Morphine and other opioids may not be permitted in some cultures or even available in some institutions. It is sobering to realize that only 6% of the morphine consumption worldwide is used in the low- and middle-income countries that are home to 80% of the world's population.[52]

The choice of neuromuscular blocking drugs is limited. Suxamethonium, gallamine, curare, alcuronium, or pancuronium are the usual options, and the choice is dictated by their availability or the availability of reversal agents. For this reason, neuromuscular blocking drugs are not commonly used.

The cost of nitrous oxide is prohibitive in terms of storage, erratic delivery, and budgetary constraints.[122,123] Closed or semi-closed anesthetic systems are considered dangerous in an environment where the oxygen supply is erratic,[123] agent monitors are seldom available,[25] and the supply of soda lime and compressed gas cylinders is erratic. Consequently, the potential benefits and cost savings of low-flow anesthesia are lost.[123,124]

Regional anesthesia has many benefits in terms of safety, cost savings, and immediate postoperative analgesia.* Children in developing countries usually are very accepting of this form of analgesia. However there seems to be a general reluctance to perform regional anesthesia in children,[29,36] even in some institutions in the developed world. Possible reasons include lack of training or expertise, fear of failure, and the unavailability of drugs, disposables, and other ancillary equipment such as ultrasound.

Improvisation may be the key. In the absence of appropriate equipment, access to the epidural space can be achieved by using a technique first described before the introduction of pediatric epidural needles into clinical practice. A catheter can be threaded through an intravenous cannula into the epidural space through the sacral hiatus in neonates and small infants.[127] Cheap, uninsulated needles can be used for peripheral nerve blocks when more expensive, insulated needles are not available.[128]

## Blood Safety

An estimated 70% of all blood transfusions in Africa are given to children with severe anemia caused by malaria. Blood transfusion services, when they exist, aim to provide a lifesaving service by ensuring an adequate supply of safe blood.[129-131] Patients, particularly children, in developing countries face the greatest risks from unsafe blood and blood products.[130-133]

Less than 30% of developing countries have a nationally coordinated blood transfusion service. Many do not perform the most rudimentary tests for diseases such as HIV or hepatitis B and C because of economic constraints.[133] Even limited testing doubles the basic cost of a unit of blood. It is estimated that about 6 million tests that should be done globally to check for infections are not done annually.

Many countries still rely on paid donors or family members to donate blood before surgery.[133] In Argentina, for example, up to 92% of the blood supply is derived from family members. Although voluntary, unpaid blood donation has increased to 20% in the past 5 years in Pakistan, family donors comprised 70% and paid donors 10% of the blood donors in 2004.[131] Public education about the value of blood transfusion is vital to improve supply.[129,130] Through concerted efforts by the World Health Organization to improve blood safety worldwide over the past decade, the number of voluntary, unpaid donors has increased considerably. For example, voluntary blood donation in China increased from 45% of donations in 2000 to 90% in 2004. Similarly, the rate of voluntary, unpaid donations in Bolivia increased from 10% in 2002 to 50% in 2005. Malaysia, China, and India reached 100% screening of donated blood for HIV by the year 2000.[132]

There are risks in any system.[129,130] Family and paid donors may hide aspects of their health and lifestyle that could make the blood unsafe for different reasons. Family members may feel pressured to donate, whereas paid donors are driven by need and avoid important details about their health status that would

negate the transaction. The commercial plasma industry and blood trade can fuel the transmission of HIV. In 1999, 26 million liters of plasma were fractionated for global use,[133] and the major source was paid donors from developing countries. Voluntary, unpaid donors have a greater sense of responsibility to their community and keep themselves healthy to be able to keep giving safe blood. South Africa has had 100% voluntary, unpaid donations since it established a national blood service. With HIV prevalence approaching 30% among the adult population of Africa, only 0.02% of its regular blood donors in South Africa have contracted HIV.

Storage of blood is difficult considering the unreliable and unpredictable electricity supply in many developing countries. To obviate the risk of transmission of malaria, HIV, and other infectious diseases, blood should be transfused only when absolutely necessary. In sophisticated blood transfusion units, the use of predonated autologous blood is an option.[134-135] In poorer countries, this is not practical because malnutrition and chronic anemia are common. There is often a lack of appropriate equipment, and cost is prohibitive. Similarly, intraoperative blood salvage and cell savers appropriate for use in children are not available. Recombinant factor VII, which is being used increasingly to reduce blood use by those who can afford it,[134] is beyond the scope (and cost) of practice in many countries.[135]

## Equipment

Electricity is unreliable in many hospitals in the developing world. In some, particularly in rural areas, neither power-line electricity nor a reliable functional generator is available.[3,4] General facilities for infection control, such as running water, disinfectants, or gloves, are also unreliable, even though recycling disposable equipment such as endotracheal tubes is considered normal practice in many countries.[2]

Essential equipment to provide safe anesthesia for children and particularly for neonates is lacking.[3,25,30,36] Neonatal or pediatric ventilators are virtually nonexistent outside the main centers.[30] Small intravenous cannulae are a precious commodity, and butterfly needles are still used and sometimes reused. Syringe pumps and other control devices are impractical in environments that have an erratic electricity supply. Metal and plastic laryngoscopes usually are available but not well maintained. Batteries may be in short supply and light bulbs unreliable. A full range pediatric tracheal tubes is considered a luxury. Laryngeal mask airways in pediatric sizes are usually unavailable. Intravenous fluids are very expensive if not manufactured locally, and many developing countries do not have local production facilities.[10] The choice of intravenous fluid is therefore limited and in short supply.

Monitoring is very basic: a precordial stethoscope and a finger on the pulse.[2,11] ECG monitoring is used when available, but it depends on a continuous electricity supply and proper maintenance. Appropriately sized blood pressure cuffs are scarce. Pulse oximetry has been the most useful monitor and should be available in all centers where pediatric surgery is performed.[2,25] Unfortunately, this ideal is far from reality, but it is hoped that the global pulse oximetry project will be rewarded with universal quality improvement.[17]

Anesthetic machines in developing countries fall into two categories: modern, sophisticated machines and simple, low-maintenance equipment. The electronic machines provided by well-meaning donors have a poor track record in austere

*References 2, 23, 30, 34, 36, 43, 125-127

environments. Sophisticated equipment needs to be understood, but operating manuals printed in foreign languages are not helpful. Sophisticated machines require ongoing maintenance, but individuals trained to repair such equipment are seldom available. Service contracts are not considered viable. Unfortunately, these machines are invariably discarded when the first fault occurs, because guarantees are unlikely to be honored and faults are considered too expensive to repair. Poorly maintained equipment becomes hazardous and even life-threatening in untrained hands.

Simplicity and safety has long been the key to anesthetic equipment in developing countries.[2-4,136] Ideally, a suitable anesthetic machine should be inexpensive, versatile, robust, and able to withstand extreme climatic conditions; able to function even if the supply of cylinders or electricity is interrupted; easy to understand and operate by those with limited training, economical to use; and easily maintained by locally available skills.[136-138] The cheapest, most practical, and most widely used method is inhalational anesthesia administered through an Epstein

Macintosh Oxford drawover vaporizer (EMO, Penlon Ltd., Oxford, United Kingdom) or Oxford Miniature Vaporizer (OMV, Penlon Ltd.). Oxygen concentrators supplement oxygen delivery and eliminate the need for expensive oxygen cylinders, whose reducing valves are often faulty or destroyed in these situations. The most appropriate ventilator is the Manley Multivent Ventilator, which essentially functions like a mechanical version of the Oxford Inflating Bellows (OIB) and can be used with a drawover system.[138]

A general scheme for inhalational anesthesia, which was first proposed by Ezi Ashi and colleagues in 1983,[124] for use in developing countries is shown in Figure 50-9.[136] Applying this scheme, four different modes can be used and modified according to the available supplies and services. The basic mode A is used when there is no electricity and no supply of compressed gases. The apparatus consists of a low-resistance vaporizer linked by valves to the child to act as a drawover system with room air as the carrier gas. The self-inflating bag or hand bellows makes it possible to provide artificial ventilation while the

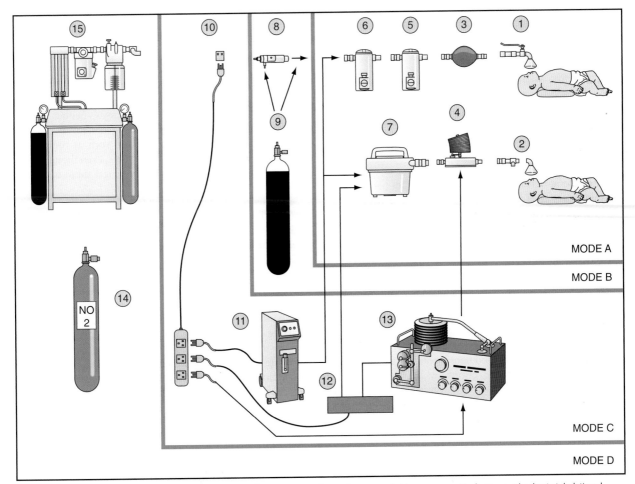

**FIGURE 50-9** The schematic diagram shows the use of anesthetic systems, depending on available resources. **Mode A** provides basic inhalational anesthesia with air, spontaneous ventilation, or self-inflating bags. Drawover vaporizers are required. **Mode B** provides oxygen enrichment but requires the availability of oxygen cylinders. Plenum vaporizers can be used. **Mode C** requires electricity to power the oxygen concentrator, air compressor, and ventilator. A mechanical ventilator (e.g., Manley) does not require electrical power. **Mode D** requires a Boyles machine and nitrous oxide cylinders. *1*, T-piece with reservoir tube and facemask; *2*, Ambu Pedi valve; *3*, self-inflating bag (Ambu); *4*, Oxford Inflating Bellows (OIB); *5*, Oxford Miniature Vaporizer (OMV) with halothane; *6*, OMV with trichloroethylene; *7*, Epstein, Macintosh, Oxford (EMO) vaporizer with ether. These circuits and manual ventilators are interchangeable, and ether, halothane, and trichloroethylene can be used on their own or in series. Farman entrainer (*8*) with an oxygen cylinder (*9*) can be used to supplement oxygen, or an electrical power source (*10*) with an oxygen concentrator (*11*), air compressor (*12*), or Manley ventilator (*13*). Nitrous oxide (*14*) and Boyles apparatus (*15*) allow anesthesia practice equivalent to that of developed countries.

vaporizer remains as a drawover device. The addition of low-flow oxygen to the inspired gas in mode B depends on the availability of an oxygen cylinder. The addition of a length of reservoir tubing to the circuit enables oxygen to be stored on expiration and to be used on the next inspiration, substantially improving its economy.

When electricity is available (mode C), operation of the anesthetic apparatus can be extended by permitting the use of an air compressor to provide continuous gas flow (allowing use of a Boyles apparatus and plenum vaporizer), an oxygen concentrator, and ventilators. When nitrous oxide is available (mode D), all types of inhalational anesthesia available in developed countries can be practiced. When services and supplies are interrupted even briefly, it is possible to change from one mode to another without requiring other anesthetic apparatuses.

These techniques may be of little interest to the anesthesiologist working comfortably in the well-maintained, sophisticated environment of developed nations. Their roles, however, are essential in field situations (e.g., war, natural disasters), and all anesthesiologists should be acquainted with their functioning in this unpredictable world (Videos 50-1 and 50-2).

## DRAWOVER ANESTHESIA

Drawover anesthesia enables inhalational anesthesia to be administered using atmospheric air as the carrier gas. The essential features of this system consist of a calibrated vaporizer with sufficiently low resistance (i.e., EMO and OMV) to allow the negative pressure created by the child's inspiratory effort to draw room air through the vaporizer during spontaneous ventilation. Positive-pressure ventilation can be provided by means of a self-inflating bag or bellows (OIB), using a valve to prevent the gas mixture from reentering the vaporizer and a unidirectional valve at the child's airway to direct expired gases to the atmosphere, preventing rebreathing (see mode A, Fig. 50-9). In this way, an anesthetic can be administered in the absence of compressed gases. The vaporizer has an inlet for supplementary oxygen that can be attached to the oxygen output tube of an oxygen concentrator or oxygen cylinder when available (see modes B and C, Fig. 50-9).

The EMO and OMV are the more commonly used low-resistance vaporizers. The EMO is calibrated only for ether, but its performance is linear for other agents. The OMV is calibrated for a variety of agents;[42,137-139] despite the lack of temperature compensation, its performance is stable under most conditions. Both vaporizers have been used successfully in pediatric anesthetic practice,[33] but it is recommended that they be converted to form a T-piece for greater safety.

The OMV has been evaluated as a simple drawover system for pediatric anesthesia. Wilson and Bem[42] showed that when a self-inflation bag is used in a drawover mode, more efficient vaporization occurs despite vaporizer cooling. However, the respiratory efforts of neonates or weak infants are insufficient to operate the valve mechanisms of the self-inflating bag (e.g., Ambu bag), necessitating continuous assisted ventilation even in the presence of ether, which stimulates ventilation.

## OXYGEN CONCENTRATORS

Improved oxygen availability, independent of compressed gas and electrical power supply, can be provided by linking oxygen concentrators[140,141] to a drawover anesthetic apparatus as first described by Fenton.[121] Maintenance requirements are low, and servicing is recommended only after approximately 10,000 hours

of usage. The benefits are enormous, but a reliable electricity supply is critical.

The concentrator functions by using a compressor to pump ambient air alternately through one of two canisters containing a molecular sieve of zeolite granules that reversibly absorbs nitrogen from compressed air.[121,136,140] The controls are simple and comprise an on/off switch for the compressor and a flow-control knob to deliver 0 to 5 L/min. Flow of oxygen continues uninterrupted as the canisters are alternated automatically so that oxygen from one canister is available while the other regenerates. A warning light on a built-in oxygen analyzer illuminates if the oxygen concentration is less than 85%, and the concentrator switches off automatically when the oxygen concentration is less than 70%. This action is heralded by visual and audible alarms. Air is then delivered as the effluent gas. Modern machines are relatively silent.

The oxygen output of the concentrator depends on the size of the unit, the inflow of oxygen, the minute volume, and pattern of ventilation. The addition of dead space (or oxygen economizer tube) at the outlet improves the performance, and predictable concentrations of more than 90% oxygen can be obtained with flows between 1 and 5 L/min, independent of the pattern of ventilation. Much lower concentrations and less predictability were observed when the dead space tubing was omitted.[142]

The possible hazards of oxygen concentrators are few if they are positioned in the operating room so that the in-draw area is free from pollutants. Failure of the power supply or failure of the zeolite canisters results in the delivery of ambient air. A bacterial filter at the outlet combined with the use of dust-free zeolite should prevent contamination of the delivered gas. Dirty internal air filters may produce lower oxygen concentrations and must be checked. An oxygen storage tank and booster pumps afford protection against the vagaries in electrical supply.

## The Visitor

Personality traits compatible with survival have been suggested as a prerequisite for working in the developing world. These traits include an almost pathologic desire for work, a willingness to merge or at least sympathize with different cultures, patience in relating to and teaching people sometimes far removed educationally, the ability to withstand prolonged periods of cultural isolation, and mostly a never-failing ability to improvise and make the best of a bad situation.[143-147] There is no place for risk-taking "cowboy anesthesiologists."[139,147]

International travel, particularly visits to many parts of the developing world, needs careful preparation and planning, whether the anesthesiologist is part of a volunteer organization[33,145-148] or traveling as an individual.[146] Detailed advice[144-149] is beyond the scope of this chapter, but some generalizations are made based on personal experience and that of colleagues. Changing political climates and international health guidelines dictate visa and vaccination requirements. Expert advice should be sought to tailor the traveler's needs according to the individual's medical and immunization history, the duration of stay, and proposed itinerary.

Physical acclimatization to jet lag, altitude sickness, and heat or sun exposure is necessary, as is adjustment to the local culture and cuisine. Social graces acceptable in a Western culture may be deemed offensive in some other cultures. An interpreter is an important ally. However, the inability to understand a language or the local dialect places a visiting anesthesiologist at a serious disadvantage, particularly when dealing with children. Children often use subtle ways to describe their feelings that even a skilled interpreter may fail to convey.

The hospital environment may be disconcerting for some. In contrast to the familiar comforts of a clean, child-friendly hospital, the visitor may be struck by the relatively shabby, bland appearance of many hospitals in developing countries. The buildings may not have received a coat of paint since they were built, and broken windowpanes provide the only air conditioning. Children are usually cared for in adult wards.

In the operating room, the visitor may be faced with anesthetic equipment barely recognizable from its original manufacture or in a state of disrepair with nonstandard improvisations in attempts to make it functional. The choice of drugs may be limited, and the names of locally manufactured generic drugs and the presentation of intravenous solutions may add to the perplexity. Surgical safety may be the next issue. Informed consent as we know it is unlikely, and identification of the child in the absence of parents may not be obvious to the newcomer. A local or itinerant surgeon may suggest an extensive procedure on a malnourished child without consideration for monitoring, blood transfusion, or availability of intensive care or postoperative analgesia in an unmonitored environment. The anesthesiologist is obligated to consider the risks and benefits carefully in such circumstances.

# Conclusions

The practice of anesthesia in a developing country will always be challenging, particularly for those who provide anesthesia for children. The challenges vary, and it is wise to expect the unexpected and have the flexibility to improvise in the face of an ever-changing world racked by famine, violence, natural disasters, and political unrest.

Attracting trained anesthesiologists to work in the developing world is difficult.[5,62,70-74,146-150] Temporary sojourns with volunteer medical groups are for the most part stimulating, but volunteers are unlikely to return for longer periods, let alone permanently.

Can anything be done to improve the lot of children who undergo anesthesia in the developing world? The Pediatric Anesthesia Fellowship Program established through the WFSA is commendable, but it produces only a small number of trainees each year.[70,73,74] Audits of morbidity and mortality are the first steps toward improvement if action is taken to address the problems uncovered. Publications reflecting outcomes in developing countries have increased over the past decade.[19-21] Purchasing equipment without ensuring subsequent maintenance is wasteful. Disposables are short-lived items even if they are recycled. Human resources are needed.

Different standards may emerge from different parts of the world. These standards need not necessarily be considered inferior but may open the way for the assimilation of new ideas.[149] The nuances of practice in different communities inevitably vary and may challenge some fondly held beliefs in pediatric anesthesia. A safe anesthetic is not necessarily the most expensive one. It is usually not the agents that we use but the skill with which we use them that determines outcome. It should never be necessary to depart from the dictum *primum non nocere*. Simplicity may be the key, but there is no place for double standards. Guidelines that have evolved over time in the United Kingdom, United States, and Australasia may be untenable in many parts of the world,[147] but every attempt should be made to exercise the same standard of care as expected in developed countries. Our children deserve no less.

## ANNOTATED REFERENCES

Hodges SC, Mijumbi C, Okello M, et al. Anaesthesia services in developing countries: defining the problems. Anaesthesia 2007;62:4-11.
*This paper identifies the difficulties of providing anesthesia in Uganda. The disturbing result was that only 23% of anesthesiologists have the facilities to provide safe anesthesia to adults, 13% for a child, and only 6% for caesarean section.*

Walker IA, Merry AF, Wilson IH, et al. Global oximetry: an international anaesthesia quality improvement project. Anaesthesia 2009;64:1051-60.
*This paper describes the initial quality assurance program for pulse oximetry in four pilot studies of pulse oximetry in Uganda, Vietnam, India, and the Philippines. The studies determined that formal training in pulse oximetry needed to be a central part of the WHO Safe Surgery Saves Lives project.*

Walker IA, Newton M, Bosenberg AT. Improving surgical safety globally: pulse oximetry and the WHO Guidelines for Safe Surgery. Paediatr Anaesth 2011;21:825-8.
*This paper describes the fact that approximately 78,000 operating rooms lack pulse oximetry. It discusses the WHO Safe Surgery Saves Lives Program as well as the Global Pulse Oximetry Program.*

Zoumenou E, Gbenou S, Assouto P, et al. Pediatric anesthesia in developing countries: experience in the two main university hospitals of Benin in West Africa. Paediatr Anaesth 2010;20:741-7.
*This article describes anesthesia in Benin. Cardiac arrests occurred at a rate of 156 per 10,000 cases with a mortality rate of approximately 60%, even in two University Hospitals. The authors are to be congratulated for studying this issue to gain more financial support from their government for better equipment and monitoring.*

## REFERENCES

Please see www.expertconsult.com.

# Pediatric Equipment

RICHARD H. BLUM AND CHARLES J. COTÉ

## Heating and Cooling Systems

The operating room (OR), which is comparable to a large infant incubator, provides the physical environment for the conduct of anesthesia. Readily controlled heating and cooling systems are crucial for thermal stability of the child, that is, control of the external environment. Neonates and small infants require a warmer room temperature than adults; they should be considered poikilothermic, particularly if they are preterm, critically ill, or stressed. With approximately 40% of heat loss by radiation and 35% by convection, heating the OR temperature warms the walls, which decreases radiation heat loss and warms the air, which decreases convection heat loss (see Chapters 35 and 36). Exposure to a cool room temperature during induction of anesthesia and surgical preparation may cause significant thermal stress, particularly in the neonate and young infant. Mild to moderate hypothermia may cause acidosis and apnea in infants, alter the pharmacokinetics of medications, cause difficulty in antagonizing the neuromuscular blockade, and increase oxygen ($O_2$) consumption with shivering.[1] Once the child is prepared and draped, the OR temperature may be reduced to a more comfortable level.

## Warming Devices

### RADIANT WARMERS

Overhead radiant heating units with servomechanism temperature control were useful to maintain the temperature of small neonates and infants in the past, but these have been replaced with other strategies. Given the risk of skin burn, the servomechanism control sensor must be applied to the warmed skin and should not measure body core temperature.[1] A maximum skin temperature of 98.6° F (37° C) should preclude surface burns, although the risk persists in poorly perfused skin. The radiant warmer may be used during induction and surgical preparation; it may be used again as the drapes are removed. If infrared light bulbs are used, care must be taken to ensure that the heat lamp is an appropriate distance from the child to avoid thermal injury[2]; note that the red cast from the light may make evaluation of a child's color difficult.

## WARMING BLANKETS

Circulating water mattresses help maintain normothermia in children with body surface areas of 0.5 m² or less (approximately 10 kg).[3] For most children, conductive heat loss accounts for less than 5% of total body heat loss; therefore these devices have limited usefulness in maintaining thermal homeostasis and virtually no benefit for children weighing more than 10 kg. To avoid surface burns, the fluid temperature should never exceed 102.2° F (39° C) and must be monitored[4]; several layers of material should be interposed between the child and the warming blanket to avoid direct contact. In many institutions these have been replaced by forced air warming mattresses.

## FORCED WARM AIR DEVICES

The most useful device for maintaining thermal homeostasis is the warm air mattress that can be wrapped around the head and upper or lower torso.[5-9] These devices rely on the combination of convection with warm air and plastic wrap that also serves to reduce evaporative heat losses. They are the single most effective means for warming children, even when only a portion of the body is covered.[5,10] One report suggests that simple delivery of warm air beneath bed sheets without the use of a plastic blanket can be effective,[10] but significant thermal injuries have been reported without the use of a licensed blanket or when used in children with poor skin perfusion.[6] Therefore unlicensed use of these devices is *not* recommended. In extreme cases of hypothermia (cardiac surgery or liver transplant), a blanket can be placed both beneath and on top of the child to speed the warming process. Two concerns have been raised regarding these devices. First, concern has been expressed that these devices may incubate infections and distribute them into the OR. The standard design and design changes in the hardware may, unbeknownst to the operator, increase the infectious risk from some warmers.[7-9] Concern also exists that under laminar airflow conditions for joint replacement, these devices increase the infectious risk.[11] Also, the cost of these disposable air mattresses may be a considerable expense.

## PASSIVE HEAT AND MOISTURIZER EXCHANGERS, "ARTIFICIAL NOSE"

Heat moisture exchangers are effective in preserving body heat, but ineffective to raise the child's body temperature.[12-14] In infants and children, these devices add humidity to the circuit[15] and may also function as filters for infectious pathogens and reduce the transmission of infectious agents between children.[16,17] These devices may increase the resistance to breathing during spontaneous ventilation and completely obstruct the circuit with prolonged use.[18-20]

## FLUID AND BLOOD WARMERS

The effectiveness of standard fluid warmers depends on the time that the intravenous fluids or blood products are in contact with the warmer. Excessive heating may cause hemolysis of red blood cells.[21] With slow intravenous fluid therapy, the fluid warmer does not contribute significant heat transfer because heat is lost along the intravenous tubing between the warmer and the child, before the fluid enters the child's body. Warming intravenous fluid during maintenance therapy is virtually useless for temperature regulation.

Blood warmers vary from simple coiled tubing in a warming bath to the more sophisticated rapid transfusion devices. Rapid transfusion systems are vitally important in any institution that manages trauma patients or performs major surgical procedures. The new generation of warming devices is far superior to water-bath warmers. They use countercurrent heat exchange or microwave technology as a means of rapidly warming fluid along the length of the column of fluid. The choice of device depends on the size of the child, the anticipated rate of blood loss, and cost. The length of the intravenous tubing and the diameter of the intravenous catheter also limit the rate of rapid infusion. An example of these devices with the lowest capacity is the Hot Line (Smiths Medical ASD, Rockland, Mass.), which is extremely effective at rates up to 75 mL/min.[22] The manufacturer's data suggest that approximately 90 mL/min of refrigerated blood products can be warmed to 95° F (35° C) with this device. Another device that has a low volume (6 mL priming volume) and is inserted within the intravenous system just before the intravenous catheter is the Belmont Buddy fluid warmer (Belmont Instrument Corp., Billerica, Mass.). The manufacturer claims a warming capacity of cold fluids to 100.4° F (38° C) at flow rates as low as "keep vein open" (KVO) and as great as 100 mL/min.[23] This device should be inserted close to the intravenous catheter because it may help maintain the child's temperature by minimizing heat loss along the length of the intravenous tubing. A more complex and larger capacity system is the Level 1 System 1000 (Smiths Medical ASD, Rockland, Mass.), which uses countercurrent warming technology combined with the capacity to infuse fluid, blood, or plasma in bags under pressure. *Because this device infuses bags of fluid under pressure, it is important to eliminate all air from the bags to avoid the possibility of air embolization.* This system is capable of warming fluids at rates up to approximately 500 mL/min.[24] The Level 1 device is capable of warming blood starting at 41° F (5° C) to 42.8° F (6° C) to at least 91.4° F (33° C) at rates as high as 250 mL/min.[25] The manufacturer's data suggest that up to 600 mL/min of red cells diluted to a hematocrit of 60% can be delivered through a 14-gauge intravenous catheter and 750 mL/min through an 8.5F introducer sheath. The addition of an air detection device with automatic flow interruption has improved safety.[26] Another high-capacity system is the Belmont FMS warmer (Belmont Instrument Corp, Billerica, Mass.) uses microwave warming and is capable of fluid delivery at rates of 10 to 750 mL/min; this device has two air detectors and an in-line pressure detector. One study compared the flow rates and warming capabilities of the Level 1 system with the Rapid Infusion System (no longer manufactured but equivalent to two Belmont FMS systems); both devices were comparable when used with 18- or 20-gauge intravenous catheters in terms of warming and flow rates. However, for any catheter larger than 18 gauge, the Rapid Infusion System was superior for both flow and fluid warming, particularly for flows greater than 200 mL/min (Figs. 51-1 and 51-2).[27,28] A similar comparison has been made with the Level 1 and the Belmont FMS systems, with a similar difference in terms of better warming capacity during high flows.[29]

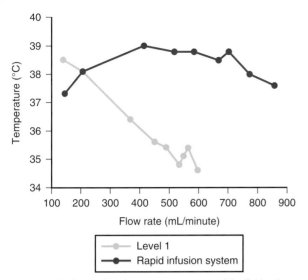

**FIGURE 51-1** This figure plots the mean temperature of the fluid at the end of two 2-liter infusions of crystalloid for the Level 1 versus the Rapid Infusion System. Note that both devices have equivalent warming capacities with flow rates 200 mL or less per minute but that there is markedly less warming capacity with the Level 1 system at higher flow rates. (From Barcelona SL, Vilich F, Coté CJ. A comparison of flow rates and warming capabilities of the Level 1 and Rapid Infusion System with various-size intravenous catheters. Anesth Analg 2003;97:358-63.)

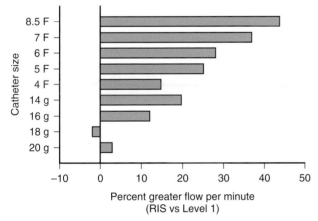

**FIGURE 51-2** Percent differences in flow rates for the Rapid Infusion System versus the Level 1 for various catheter sizes. Note that the Rapid Infusion System produced greater incremental changes in flow with progressively larger catheters (16 gauge or larger). The Belmont FMS system should have performance characteristics similar to those of the Rapid Infusion System. (From Barcelona SL, Vilich F, Coté CJ. A comparison of flow rates and warming capabilities of the Level 1 and Rapid Infusion System with various-size intravenous catheters. Anesth Analg 2003;97:358-63.)

In general, the Level 1 Hotline (Smiths Medical) or the Belmont Buddy appear most suited for low-volume, relatively slow blood loss. The Level 1 system seems most appropriate for children weighing 40 kg or less with expected rapid blood loss and the Belmont FMS for larger children with expected massive and rapid blood loss. The advantages and disadvantages of these warming devices are compared in Table 51-1.[30]

### HEATED HUMIDIFIERS

Airstream warming and humidification devices are useful for maintaining body temperature.[31-33] If a humidifier is used, the anesthesiologist should be familiar with the potential hazards: overheating, leaks, "rain out," changes in compression volume, and obstruction if connected in reverse. Humidifiers with servomechanism-controlled temperature regulation may prevent overheating and overhydration of infants. Anesthesia breathing circuits with internal heating elements may further reduce the rainout problem and minimize the risk of overheating; these advantages must be weighed against the additional expense. However, with the advent of warm air mattresses and more common use of circle systems in children of all sizes, there appears to be less of a need for in-line humidification as a means of warming children. The main indication for in-line humidification is to prevent secretions from drying when nonrebreathing circuits are used.

### WRAPPING

Any form of wrapping can reduce radiant and convective heat losses; plastic wrap used for food is particularly effective and inexpensive. Covering an infant's head is of greatest value because the head represents such a large proportion of the body surface area. As with any warming device, there are hazards; the plastic drapes reduce conductive losses but also eliminate sweating as a mechanism of thermal regulation, so that hyperthermia may result.[34] "Space" blankets with reflective aluminized Mylar layers have been very effective in preventing heat loss in the past.[35] With effective room temperature control and forced air heating mattresses, the importance of wrapping the child has diminished.

## Intravenous Therapy

It is necessary to have the appropriate range of intravenous equipment for the patient population being anesthetized. In general, it is safest to establish intravenous access in all anesthetized children. The only exception to this practice may be a brief, noninvasive procedure such as myringotomy and tube insertion or suture removal; in this situation, an infusion set is primed and ready for use should it be needed.

The volume of the infusion fluid container should not exceed the child's estimated fluid deficit unless a volume-limiting device is interposed between the intravenous container and the child. Generally, an intravenous set with a microdrop outlet (60 drops/mL) is most practical for children weighing less than 50 kg. Infusion sets that include a one-way valve to prevent retrograde flow in the intravenous administration set are most useful. The infusion setup should include easily accessible injection ports; intravenous extension tubing may be required if the access is in the lower extremities. A three-way stopcock within the system is also helpful should an "adult" intravenous line be needed to give a rapid bolus of intravenous fluid. Recent practice has shifted from needle injection ports to needleless. Both the needleless ports and stopcocks are reservoirs for small volumes of air that may be injected into the intravenous tubing if the air is not cleared during the initial setup or aspirated into the medication syringe before delivering the syringe contents. It is best to purge infusion sets of all air bubbles, especially at each injection port, before use with infants and children.[36] In children with known cardiac defects with shunts or arteriovenous malformations, and in infants with patent foramen ovale, the potential for paradoxical air emboli is always present (up to 27% of adults).[37] In these circumstances, intravenous air traps may reduce this risk, but caution is advised because blood cannot pass through such

**TABLE 51-1** Comparison of Three Blood and Fluid Warming Devices

| | WARMING DEVICE | | |
| --- | --- | --- | --- |
| | Level-1 | FMS2000 | Buddy |
| Manufacturer | Level-1 Technologies, Rockland, Mass. | Belmont Instrument Corp., Billerica, Mass. | Belmont Instrument Corp., Billerica, Mass. |
| Cost* | Without air detector, ~$5500<br>With air detector, ~$8950 | ~$20,000 | ~$1600 |
| Footprint | Medium | Medium | Small |
| Setup | Stand-alone system mounted on its own IV pole | Mounted on IV pole | Power module mounted on IV pole, warming unit mounted on IV tubing |
| Weight (kg) | ~32 with IV pole | ~12 | ~4.4 (unit on IV tubing only 105 g) |
| Air detection | Single detector (optional) | Two detectors | Pressure-regulating valve and venting membrane |
| Ease of fluid loading | Requires venting of air from IV bags to prevent air embolization | No air venting required | No air venting required but not designed to deliver fluid under pressure |
| Ease of setup | Easy | Relatively easy | Very easy |
| Other | No reservoir for blood mixing | Does not heat at flows <10 mL/min | Unclear effectiveness with rapid blood transfusion |

Modified from Barcelona SL, Thompson AA, Coté CJ. Intraoperative pediatric blood transfusion therapy: a review of common issues: I. Hematologic and physiologic differences from adults; metabolic and infectious risks. Paediatr Anaesth 2005;15:716-26.
*IV*, Intravenous.
*In U.S. dollars; cost may vary from country to country and with multiple purchases.

devices.[38] In the smallest patients, a T-connector placed at the hub of the intravenous catheter allows direct injection of drugs with minimal fluid dead space. It should also be noted that stopcocks and injection ports may act as a reservoir for administered drugs; it is thus important to always flush through any medications administered with these systems. With standard injection ports, long needles will bypass the injection port and deliver drug into the main body of the intravenous tubing (see later).

When carefully metered transfusion of colloid or blood is necessary, a multiple-stopcock manifold, preferably with Luer-Loks to avoid disconnections, added to the infusion line allows the main line to continue infusing maintenance fluid except during the actual administration of either blood or colloid. This arrangement provides an outlet for blood administration, another for colloid administration, and a third for a metering syringe. Careful titration of intravenous fluid and medication infusion rates may be facilitated by the use of electronic pumps or intravenous rate controllers. The infusion pump chosen for a child must suit the circumstances. In most situations, a device with precise volume limits and air bubble and pressure alarms is the safest. Multiple stop-cock manifolds allow the administration of several medications (e.g., vasopressors) simultaneously; special narrow-bore tubing also reduces the dead space of such a setup, thus minimizing delays in response to changes in the vasopressors because of the reduced dead space of the system (see later).

The flow of crystalloid is not a simple linear function of perfusion pressure; the relationship deviates substantially from linearity. Additionally, elements of the intravenous system have isolated effects on one factor or another. For example, a 5-$\mu$m filter increases resistance and reduces flow at all pressures. A check valve significantly increases resistance but reduces flow primarily at high flow rates.[39] A similar nonlinear function describes the pressure and flow relationship of intravenous cannulas.[40] Studies of crystalloid solutions demonstrate steep increases in resistance with increasing pressure in a nonlinear manner with smaller-gauge cannulas (E-Fig. 51-1). The effects of the tubing set add to the effects of the cannula; connecting large-diameter tubing to a smaller-diameter catheter limits flow according to the diameter of the catheter. In situations in which massive and rapid blood loss is anticipated, insertion of extra-large peripheral intravenous catheters such as 5, 6, 7 or 8F pulmonary artery flow catheter introducers or specially designed rapid infusion catheters will provide the most efficient method for rapid volume administration. Special placement kits are available that allow the dilation of small veins by the placement of a guidewire through either a small needle (Seldinger technique) or a small-gauge intravenous line followed by dilation of the vein and placement of a larger-diameter cannula (see Chapter 48).

Accelerating flow through an intravenous line is a concern in emergency situations. Rapid transfusion devices are the best method for increasing flow rates (see earlier).[22,24,25] For bags of crystalloid, colloid, or blood components a pressure infusion cuff is a relatively fast, readily available, and the least expensive method for rapidly administering large volumes.[41] *It is important to remove air from these bags so as to avoid air embolization because an air detector is not used with this technique.* Next in order of efficacy are in-line blood pumps or a stopcock and syringe arrangement; gravity is the slowest method of infusion. The syringe technique is often used in infants and children (primarily for accurate measurement in infants); it is similar in efficiency to the in-line blood pump. Intravenous tubing designed for administering blood has better flow characteristics than standard intravenous tubing.[42] Large-bore "resuscitation" tubing provides the best flow characteristics; however, the final common pathway, the lumen of the intravenous catheter itself, is the major limitation of flow capacity.[25,39-44] Larger-diameter, short catheters allow greater flow than long narrow-diameter catheters.[44] This factor is particularly important when rapid volume administration is required but the only intravenous access is through a central venous catheter. This problem is greatly magnified when multilumen catheters are used.[44-45] *If rapid volume resuscitation is a significant potential problem, then one single-lumen, large-bore peripheral intravenous line is of much greater value than a multilumen central venous catheter. Peripherally inserted central catheters (PICC) lines are a potential problem as well because of their very large resistance they cannot be relied on for rapid volume administration* (see further discussion of laminar and turbulent flow).

The choice of fluid and its temperature also have effects on the rate of infusion, primarily because of differences in viscosity. Crystalloid passes most readily, followed by colloid, whole blood, and packed red blood cells. Dilution of packed red blood cells with normal saline markedly improves the flow rate and decreases hemolysis during rapid infusion.[46] Hemolysis and associated hyperkalemia of packed red blood cells transfused through short or long catheters under high pressure appears to not be clinically important when the rate of transfusion is moderate. However, rapid transfusion may be associated with hyperkalemia, particularly in infants.[47-51]

One further concern that has very important clinical implications is the interaction among intravenous tubing design, infusion pumps, and carrier flow rates regarding timing of actual drug delivery to the child. This is an even greater issue in infants and neonates in whom the volumes of drugs and the carrier infusion rates are small. Several studies of adult equipment have examined the interactions of dead space volumes and carrier rates on the time lag to initial drug delivery, time to steady-state drug delivery, and then offset once the infusion is stopped. These interactions also vary whenever a change in carrier flow rate occurs (e.g., when a slow carrier infusion is suddenly increased, this will result in a bolus of drug). Conversely, when a rapid carrier rate is suddenly reduced, this will result in a marked reduction in drug delivery. The importance of these interactions increases the further upstream in the system that a drug is administered; for example, the administration of a drug directly into the T-connector will be the least susceptible to these variables than a drug administered into a side port of an intravenous line 10 to 30 cm away from the intravenous catheter. Thus, when life-support medications are being administered, it is vital to avoid fluctuations or interruptions in carrier rate and to reduce as much as possible the dead space in the system between the child's bloodstream and the point of drug entering the intravenous system. This is true for the OR, during transit to the intensive care unit (ICU), and at the time of transfer of care. This is particularly an issue when OR pumps and intravenous equipment are switched over to new tubing and pumps in the ICU. Figure 51-3 illustrates the time delay in drug delivery comparing the dead space of an injection port with and without a needle that bypasses the dead space of the injection port and how this time delay can be minimized by "priming" the dead space of the injection port.[52,53] Figure 51-4 illustrates several multidrug administration manifolds that allow administration of many medications simultaneously, each with differing dead space characteristics that could cause considerable delay in drug delivery if the dead space within each is inadequately primed. The best way to avoid this problem is to flush each drug through the system from entry to exit point, shut off the infusion, flush the carrier through the system to remove any medications from the carrier portion of the manifold, then attach the system to the patient, so that all infusions will immediately be discharged into the carrier intravenous fluid when turned on, rather than having a delay while the dead space at the connection is filled.

## Airway Apparatus

### MASKS

The importance of elimination of mechanical dead space increases with decreasing size of the child. Rendell-Baker/Soucek masks,

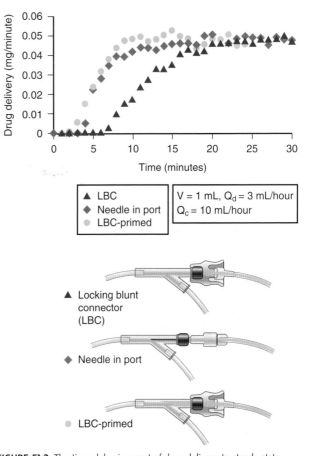

**FIGURE 51-3** The time delay in onset of drug delivery to steady-state drug delivery as affected by a needle in an injection port, a blunt locking connector or "priming" of the dead space of the injection port are illustrated. Note that the time to initiate drug delivery is delayed by several minutes and the time to achieve a steady-state rate of drug administration may be delayed by 10 minutes or longer when the dead space is not primed or a needle is not used to bypass the dead space of the injection port (in this example, the parameters were: carrier rate [$Qc$] 10 mL/hr, drug flow rate [$Qd$] 3 mL/hr, dead space volume [$V$] 1 mL). This concept has important implications regarding drug delivery to all patients, but this is particularly important in infants and neonates in whom small volumes of drug may be administered into a relatively large dead space that must be filled before any drug enters the flow of the intravenous fluid and the hourly rate of the carrier is low. (From Lovich MA, Doles J, Peterfreund RA. The impact of carrier flow rate and infusion set dead-volume on the dynamics of intravenous drug delivery. Anesth Analg 2005;100:1048-55.)

developed from molds of the facial contours of Caucasian children, were designed to minimize mechanical dead space without the inflatable cuff or high dome of adult masks. Transparent disposable plastic models are preferable to the classic black conductive rubber because they allow observation of a child's color and condensate from exhaled humidity with respirations. Plastic disposable masks with soft inflatable cuffs around the periphery of the mask are particularly well suited for children with anatomic or mechanical problems that interfere with normal mask application. An especially useful mask has a built-in port, which allows passage of an endotracheal tube over a fiberoptic scope, thus providing excellent fiberoptic intubation conditions while maintaining spontaneous respiration, oxygenation, and depth of anesthesia (see E-Fig. 12-13).[54]

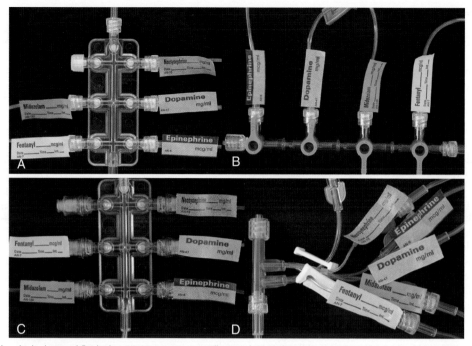

**FIGURE 51-4** Several multiple-drug and fluid administration systems are illustrated. Note the wide variation in dead space volume among the screw-in connectors (**A**), simple stopcocks (**B**), screw-in connectors with one-way valves (**C**), and multiple short tubing connections (**D**). To avoid variations in rate of drug delivery, it is advised to use a dedicated carrier on a pump. To ensure that the initiation of drug delivery is timely, the following steps are necessary: (1) each dead space port must be flushed and primed with the desired infusion as it is attached to the delivery manifolds; (2) after priming, the stopcock is turned to the off position or the tubing clamped; (3) the carrier portion of the system is then run through or flushed with the carrier intravenous fluid; and (4) the system is attached to the patient with just the carrier ensuring a constant flow to the patient. When the drug infusion is initiated, the stopcock is turned to the on position or the tubing unclamped and each drug infusion pump turned on at the desired rate. This ensures that no drug is accidentally administered and reduces the time to initial drug delivery by priming the dead space of the system for each drug infusion. It should be borne in mind that this system should be connected as closely as possible to the intravenous catheter to avoid further delay in drug delivery because of the need to fill the dead space between the multiple drug manifolds and the entry into a vein. The use of a pump for the carrier solution also prevents retrograde drug infusion.

## ORAL AIRWAYS

A complete selection of oral airways must be readily available. Infants have a relatively large tongue, which easily obstructs the airway once they lose consciousness. If too large an airway is inserted, damage to laryngeal structures (traumatic epiglottitis, uvular swelling) may result in postoperative airway obstruction (see Fig. 12-13).[55] Improperly inserted airways, by obstructing venous and lymphatic drainage, also may result in airway obstruction secondary to swelling of the tongue.[56,57] A tongue blade is useful to help insert the airway without kinking the tongue or catching the tongue or lips between the airway and the teeth.

## NASOPHARYNGEAL AIRWAYS

Nasopharyngeal airways are not as frequently used in children because the internal diameter is often small, resulting in increased work of breathing and increased chance of blockage by sections or blood. In addition, adenoid hypertrophy makes a child susceptible to bleeding after nasopharyngeal airway insertion. Despite its limitations, it can help provide a patent airway in spontaneously breathing infants and children (particularly after pharyngoplasty or cleft palate repair) and is better tolerated in awake children. Nasopharyngeal airways range in sizes to accommodate neonates through to adolescents and may have a movable ring to set the length or a flange on the end to prevent loss in the nasal cavity. If a stiffer airway is necessary, a well-lubricated tracheal tube, cut to the appropriate length (to reach the nasopharynx only), may be used; however, it must be safely secured because it may accidentally pass into the nasopharynx.

## LARYNGEAL MASK AIRWAY

The laryngeal mask airway (LMA) has proved to be a great addition to the airway management of children. Minimal practice is required to develop the skills for insertion. In some circumstances the LMA can be lifesaving (see Chapter 12).[58-64] This device generally provides a clear airway for maintaining spontaneous respirations; however, it cannot be relied on if controlled ventilation is required. Controlled ventilation has been described but holds the risk of gastric dilation.[65] We think that this device should be used primarily for spontaneous ventilation and with great caution with controlled ventilation in infants and children. Modern anesthesia ventilators provide the alternative and likely safer pressure-assisted mode of ventilation.[66] The LMA is particularly useful in children with anatomic airway abnormalities, because it provides a clear airway while other measures are planned for successful tracheal intubation or a tracheotomy.[64,67] Fiberoptic intubation through the LMA is possible in children with midfacial hypoplasia syndromes and in those with redundant airway tissue such as mucopolysaccharidoses (see also E-Fig. 12-22, *A* through *C*). Fiberoptic intubation is easier through the LMA because the child can be well oxygenated while using the fiberoptic scope to find the laryngeal inlet. Emergency placement of this device can also be lifesaving in children who are difficult to ventilate with bag and mask with or without a nasal or oral airway.[68]

Variations to the classic LMA include disposable LMAs of all sizes, intubating LMAs in larger sizes, LMAs with reinforced tubing, and the ProSeal LMA (LMA, La Jolla, Calif.) with a distal opening that provides the ability to pass an orogastric tube (see

Fig. 12-18, *A* and *B*). This variation to the classic LMA produces a better laryngeal seal and provides the ability to ventilate the lungs without a significant leak at greater peak inflation pressures.[69] This variation would seem to offer the greatest advantage in the child with a known difficult airway or in the emergency management of the child with a difficult airway who also has a full stomach. Many other LMA variants are available, each with claimed advantages. Each practitioner should assess which device is most effective in the practice environment[70] (see also Chapter 12 for a more in-depth discussion).

## TRACHEAL TUBES

A variety of tracheal tubes must be available with appropriate sizes of stylets. There may be considerable variations from one manufacturer to another in wall thickness, external diameter, kink resistance, and direction and angle of bevel, as well as differences in tracheal tube cuff length and thickness of cuffed tracheal tubes.[71] All tracheal tubes should be implantation tested and manufactured in accordance with the Z79 international agreement for safe products. Tracheal tubes are sized by the internal diameter (ID) in millimeters. Despite differences in endotracheal tube wall thickness among manufacturers, a first approximation for the correct tracheal tube size for an average child older than 2 years of age is[72]:

$$4 + \frac{\text{age in years}}{4}$$

Preterm infants weighing less than 1500 g generally require a 2.5-mm ID tracheal tube, whereas preterm infants of more than 1500 g require a 3.0-mm ID tube, full-term neonates require a 3.0- to 3.5-mm ID tube, a 1-year-old requires a 4.0-mm ID, and a 2-year-old requires a 4.5- to 5.0-mm ID. Although it has been suggested that the correct diameter of the tracheal tube may be determined by examining the diameter of the distal phalanx of the child's first or fifth digit, evidence suggests that this is unreliable.[69] Tracheal tubes at least one half-size larger and smaller than estimated should be immediately available to accommodate airway size variability. The only true test for appropriate size selection is that the tube passes through the subglottis easily and has an appropriate leak (e.g., between 10 and 40 cm $H_2O$ peak inflation pressure). The leak may be easily assessed by closing the circuit pop-off valve and slowly increasing the pressure by gently squeezing the anesthesia bag while listening over the larynx with a stethoscope. This technique has been demonstrated to be a sensitive and accurate measure of fit between the tracheal lumen and the endotracheal tube.[73] It should be borne in mind that a leak is dependent in part, upon the child's head position and degree of paralysis.[74] For example, if the neck is flexed or the head is turned from side to side, a leak may become worse or decrease. If the trachea was intubated without the use of muscle relaxants, the child must be well anesthetized to assess the leak properly. If a child is coughing, it is difficult to make this assessment. Conversely, if the child has laryngospasm around the tube, then it will appear to be too large because a leak may not be present. On the other hand, too large a leak may prevent adequate ventilation should positive-pressure ventilation be required, pollute the OR excessively, and dilute the inspired gases during spontaneous respirations. In this circumstance, the tracheal tube should be replaced with the next larger size and the leak reassessed. The relationship of age, tracheal tube sizes and inhalaton pressure leak is commonly used to estimate laryngeal size (see Fig. 31-13).

The past decade has seen a transition from the routine use of uncuffed tubes in children during general anesthesia to the routine use of cuffed tubes. Uncuffed tubes are available for use from 2.0-mm ID to 6-mm ID and have been used as a standard in children up to 8 years of age. Indeed, traditional teaching suggests that the use of uncuffed tubes is the most appropriate practice[75]; however, this is not evidence-based. The use of cuffed tracheal tubes has been demonstrated to reduce costs of inhalation agents use because of the ability to use lower fresh gas flows.[76] With the introduction of the MICROCUFF (Kimberly-Clark Health Care, Roswell, Ga.) tube and publication of several clinical studies, practice has shifted from the routine use of uncuffed to cuffed tracheal tubes. The external diameter of cuffed tracheal tubes is approximately 0.5 mm larger than uncuffed because of the cuff, so one must use a smaller-ID tube for a given tracheal size. Cuffed tracheal tubes as small as 3.0 mm ID are available for use in elective and emergency surgery in infants and children. Some have proposed that the advantages of a cuffed tracheal tube for children include reduced number of reintubations, decreased leak around the tracheal tube leading to less contamination of the operating room, greater ease and consistency of ventilation, reduced cost if low-flow anesthesia is used, and a theoretical attenuated incidence of aspiration.[76-82] If a cuffed endotracheal tube is used, the cuff is generally inflated just enough to provide a leak between 20 and 30 cm $H_2O$ peak inflation pressure or cuff pressure can be monitored using a device that continually monitors cuff pressure.[83] It must recognized that the endotracheal tube cuff pressure will increase during a nitrous oxide ($N_2O$)-supplemented anesthetic because of diffusion of $N_2O$ into the cuff,[84] unless saline is used to fill the cuff.[85] However, because the MICROCUFF tube seals the airway at a reduced pressure compared with polyurethane cuffed tubes, the time until the pressure within the cuff becomes excessive with the MICROCUFF tube is greater than with traditional tracheal tubes.[86] Excessive cuff pressures may present a special additional hazard to children, in whom swelling of the pseudostratified columnar epithelium that lines the inside of the cricoid ring may critically reduce the diameter of the upper airway. To date, studies have not investigated long-term complications such as subglottic stenosis that might occur in the intensive care unit. Tracheal tubes used in the OR remain in the trachea for only a brief time; thus it is unlikely that such use could result in long-term complications. An important advantage of the MICROCUFF tube is that the cuff is located closer to the tip of the tube (thereby reducing the potential for cuff pressure on the vocal cords or the cricoid cartilage, but eliminating the Murphy eye), lower cuff sealing pressure (again potentially reducing injury to the mucosa of the trachea), and less leakage around the cuff (less microaspiration) (see Fig. 12-15).[87-92] However, the marked nearly fivefold difference in cost will likely prohibit the routine use of this tracheal tube for short term intubation. Additionally, reports of easy kinking in the smaller size tubes resulted in a product recall.[93] The authors' practice has increased the use of the Mallinckrodt Lo-Pro Endotracheal Tubes (Nellcor, Pleasanton, Calif.), which is not a new product but anecdotally provides a low-pressure cuff that has a lower contour, aiding the view during tracheal intubation, and has a smaller effect on the size of the outer diameter of the tracheal tube. No specific studies have demonstrated any differences in complications when comparing different low-pressure endotracheal tubes. The original Khine formula (4 + age [years]/4)[79] has been critically evaluated, and a new formula with greater tracheal tube size accuracy has been proposed (3.5 + age [years]/4).[79,94] However, these studies did not adequately examine the infants in the lowest age range, nor did they examine these specific brands of tracheal tubes. The argument could be made that long-term follow-up data for complications has not been adequately investigated.[95] *Currently, we do not recommend the routine use of 3.0-mm ID cuffed tracheal tubes in neonates because the potential for laryngeal/tracheal damage far outweighs the advantage of avoiding an extra laryngoscopy and intubation.*

Molded preformed tracheal tubes are especially useful for head and neck surgery because they remove the anesthesia circuit connections from the surgical field.[96] When excessive external pressure may be applied to the tracheal tube or when extreme flexion of the neck is likely to kink a standard endotracheal tube, a tracheal tube with Tovell spiral wire reinforcement may be used. Its kink resistance is well-known, but the additional wall thickness limits its applicability in younger children. The spiral springlike construction has caused the tube to pop out of the airway; in addition, repeated improper sterilization of nondisposable models may lead to bubble formation within the rubber, leading to airway obstruction when used with $N_2O$.[97]

The carbon dioxide ($CO_2$) laser for treatment of laryngeal polyposis and other airway lesions has introduced the problem of ignition of the tracheal tube or other material in the airway. Avoiding high levels of $O_2$ and $N_2O$, which both support combustion, diminishes the risk of fire. Special stainless steel and metal implanted tracheal tubes are available but are quite expensive. Protecting the tube surface with aluminum or copper foil or wet sponges and red rubber tracheal tubes, which have a much reduced ignition potential, may offer the greatest protection (see Chapter 31).[98-102] Electrocautery can ignite standard tracheal tubes, esophageal stethoscopes, oral airways, feeding tubes, tissue, and packs if the correct circumstances combine.[103-105] Rubber tracheal tubes may soon no longer be manufactured because they are made of latex rubber but are still being advocated by some practitioners for laser surgery.

The tracheal tube itself creates significant resistance to airflow, and this phenomenon is described in the physics of resistance to flow for all gases and fluids. Flow of gases and fluids through airways and blood vessels and at branching points may be described as either laminar or turbulent. Reynolds number, a dimensionless value, is calculated as the ratio of inertial to viscous forces in the following equation:

$$NRe = DV\rho/\mu$$

where *NRe* is the Reynolds number, *D* is the diameter of the airway or blood vessel, and *V* is the velocity, $\rho$ is the density, and $\mu$ is the viscosity of the gas or fluid. An NRe less than 2100 denotes flow that is laminar, whereas an NRE of 3000 or greater denotes turbulent flow. Flows that have NRe between 2100 and 3000 may be either laminar or turbulent. Conceptually, laminar flow is organized flow in which each plate of fluid, air, or gas moves in parallel at the same speed, with zero velocity at the interface between the wall of the airway or blood vessel and the gas or fluid. Laminar flow occurs in blood beyond the aortic arch and in airways beyond the fifth bronchial division. In contrast, turbulent flow is chaotic, unpredictable flow in which the fluid, air, or gas does not flow in parallel plates but rather develop eddies and lateral as well as forward flow, thus dissipating large amounts of energy. Turbulent flow occurs in the aortic arch and in the large airways of the tracheobronchial tree down to the fifth bronchial division.

Laminar flow is characterized by the Hagen-Poiseuille equation:

$$\Delta P = 8Q\eta l/\pi r^4$$

Where $\Delta P$ is the pressure drop, $Q$ is the flow rate, $\eta$ is the viscosity of the fluid (air or gas), $l$ is the length of the airway or blood vessel, and $r$ is the radius of the airway or blood vessel. Thus pressure drop is proportional to the flow rate and viscosity of the fluid and inversely proportional to the radius to the *fourth power*.

Turbulent flow is not easily characterized by an equation. Unpredictable losses such as friction are difficult to quantify. Hence, no single equation exists or turbulent flow as in the case of laminar flow. However, for large NRe, we know that:

$$\Delta P \alpha Q^2 \rho/r^5$$

Where $\Delta P$ is the pressure drop, $Q$ is the flow rate, $\rho$ is the density and $r$ is the radius of the airway or blood vessel. Note that in contrast to laminar flow, pressure drop is proportional to the square of the flow rate and inversely related to the *fifth power* of the radius.

Therefore the resistance to gas or fluid flow is greater in relation to the longer and narrower tracheal tube (or intravenous catheter) used; anything that increases turbulence may proportionally increase the resistance to gas or fluid flow. In practical terms, this means that with a tracheal tube, when the respiratory rate is increased, turbulent flow results (meaning that resistance changes with radius to the fifth power, not the fourth power), decreasing the size of the delivered tidal volume.[106] In addition, flow may vary from laminar to turbulent at different portions of the respiratory cycle. Studies with in vivo models have shown that this effect is less pronounced with progressively larger tracheal tubes; however, larger tubes may result in reductions in delivered tidal volume when the respiratory rate is increased in children who require a smaller than normal endotracheal tube; that is, an increase in respiratory rate from 10 to 20/min does not double the delivered minute ventilation.[106-108] Data suggest that in children with poorly compliant lungs, lung compliance seems to be the most important factor, even with very small tracheal tubes.[106] The implications of these observations are that accurate measurement of end-expired $CO_2$ or arterial blood gases are the only way to be certain of the effectiveness of ventilation. In patients with severe pulmonary disease with ventilation-perfusion mismatch, only arterial blood gases or transcutaneous $CO_2$ monitoring will provide the needed information.

## Intubation Equipment

### ROUTINE EQUIPMENT

Intubation equipment must suit pediatric children of all sizes. Laryngoscopes are available with lightweight small handles and a full range of blades (see Chapter 12). An Oxyscope (Foregger, Inc. Langhorne, Pa.), which incorporates a small-bore $O_2$ delivery tube, reduces the incidence of cyanosis and bradycardia in spontaneously breathing neonates should laryngoscopy be prolonged (see E-Fig. 12-12, *A* and *B*).[109] Magill forceps are available in several sizes for children of different ages.

### SPECIAL AIRWAY EQUIPMENT

Difficult airways require special intubation equipment; flexible and rigid fiberoptic laryngoscopes and bronchoscopes are available for infants and children. Flexible fiberoptic laryngoscopes are available as small as 1.8 mm external diameter; these are suitable for passage of 2.5-mm ID endotracheal tube.[110] The small scope is limited because it does not provide suction. Fiberoptic endoscopic skills should be developed during routine elective cases and in training exercises using airway or full manikin simulators to acquire these skills before encountering emergency cases or children with abnormal airway anatomy (see Chapter 12).[110] Fiberoptic intubation through the LMA in infants and neonates with midfacial hypoplasia allows the maintenance of a clear airway, delivery of $O_2$ with or without inhalation anesthetic and provides optimal conditions for successful placement of the tracheal tube.[61,62,111-114]

Lighted stylets provide an alternative technique for management of a difficult airway.[115-118] Other airway devices such as the Bonfils fiberscope (Karl Storz, Tuttlingen, Germany), the Airtraq disposable optical laryngoscope (Prodol Meditec, Vizcaya, Spain), the GlideScope video laryngoscope (Verathon, Bothell Wash.), the Storz DCI video laryngoscope (Karl Storz, Tuttlingen, Germany), and the Trueview PCD Infant (Truphatek, Netanya, Israel) can optimize the management of difficult pediatric airways[119-125] (see Chapter 12 for a more in-depth discussion).

## Suction Apparatus

A functioning suction apparatus must be available before beginning any anesthetic administration. The device should be capable of regulated pressures; suctioning the oropharynx requires a greater vacuum level than suctioning the tracheal tube. Special circumstances (e.g., a full stomach and arterial bleeding in the oropharynx) may require a second suction device. A separate vacuum system is needed to scavenge waste anesthetic gases. Several sizes of suction catheters are helpful, depending on the indication—tracheal, gastric, or oropharyngeal suction. A 6 or 8F suction catheter with a thumb-controlled side port is useful for suctioning through small tracheal tubes, whereas 10, 12, and 14F catheters are useful for larger tracheal tubes. Routine suction of stomach contents after induction of anesthesia may reduce the potential for gastric fluid regurgitation and serious pulmonary aspiration of gastric contents. In larger patients, vented catheters (e.g., Salem Sump; Sherwood Medical, St. Louis) may be more efficacious than unvented catheters. Suctioning the stomach with the child in the supine position and in left and right lateral decubitus positions has been shown to be most efficient in evacuation of stomach contents.[126]

Yankauer suction devices are commonly used for oropharyngeal suctioning. When purchasing Yankauer suction devices, it is best to choose a plastic model rather than metal to minimize the risk of damage to the teeth. These suction devices are more efficient at removing large fluid volumes (e.g., during regurgitation) than suction catheters.

## The Anesthesia Machine and Its Appendages

### ANESTHESIA MACHINE

All children can be anesthetized with standard adult machinery as long as the anesthesiologist is aware of the pitfalls and limitations. No anesthesia machines are currently marketed solely for pediatric use; however, anesthesia machines that have the ability to be customized for pediatric use may be of value, but not necessary. If one wishes to use special circuits, a Mapleson D system may be permanently mounted, allowing the choice of either a circle or open system. Modifying the anesthesia machine has inherent danger, especially for inexperienced users; the circuit or other components could be assembled incorrectly and potentially be unsafe. In addition, air should be available from a central

pipeline or a cylinder with an appropriate yoke and flow meter. This is particularly advantageous in circumstances in which $N_2O$ or a high inspired $O_2$ concentration is contraindicated (avoiding hyperoxia in a premature infant, $N_2O$ in a patient with bowel distention, or laser airway surgery).[127-129] Even though machines are designed not to allow the delivery of a hypoxic gas mixture, an in-line $O_2$ analyzer and pulse oximetry are indicated to use an air–oxygen blend safely. The anesthesia machine should also be equipped with an alternative means of providing $O_2$ and positive-pressure ventilation (self-inflating bag) in case of a machine failure or malfunction.

### SCAVENGER

The scavenging of anesthetic waste gases to limit exposure of anesthetic gases to health care providers is important. However, during pediatric anesthesia, exposure to anesthetic gases occurs during inhalational inductions by mask where high fresh gas flows are used and a poor mask seal exists because of patient anxiety or movement. The use of uncuffed tracheal tubes with large leaks also increases exposure. Modern scavenging systems are designed to avoid applying either negative or positive pressure to a patient circuit by using an *open system,* in which a reservoir is used to collect the waste gases and active (suction) or passive pressures are used to remove waste gases from the OR.[130] In a *closed scavenging system,* positive or negative relief values are used in the reservoir or waste gas exhaust hose to ensure that positive pressure does not build up in the system or if the system is blocked so negative pressure is not applied to the patient circuit.[131,132] In addition to scavenging systems, exposure to anesthetic gases is also related to adequate ventilation of the OR.[133]

### CIRCUITS

A full spectrum of anesthetic circuits have been used in infants and children.[134] Adolescents and older children may be anesthetized with a standard adult semiclosed circle absorber system, perhaps with the substitution of a smaller rebreathing bag. Younger children may be anesthetized with the circuit modified by replacing the hoses with small-diameter pediatric tubing and by substituting a smaller reservoir bag. In the past, most infants and neonates (10 kg or less) were anesthetized with nonrebreathing open systems, such as the Mapleson D or F variety. These circuits are used infrequently today and may soon be of historical interest only because the increasing pressure for cost containment and the expense of the newer anesthetic agents has forced most children's hospitals to convert to circle systems. In our institutions, we use only circle systems; this has simplified teaching and markedly reduced anesthetic agent costs. However, because Mapleson D systems are still being used, the advantages and disadvantages of open and closed systems for infants and neonates are reviewed in the following discussion.

Mapleson D systems do not have directional valves or a $CO_2$ absorber, thus eliminating the resistance intrinsic to the opening pressure of circuit valves and to turbulent flow through soda lime.[135] This may be an advantage in spontaneously breathing neonates during induction before intubation. The main disadvantage of open systems is the need for relatively high fresh gas flows and waste of expensive anesthetic agents, as well as unnecessary pollution of the environment. The work of breathing may be important for spontaneously breathing infants, so most pediatric circuits and masks are designed to eliminate both dead space and resistance. The classic example of this type of system is the Ayre T-piece; this circuit includes no valves or

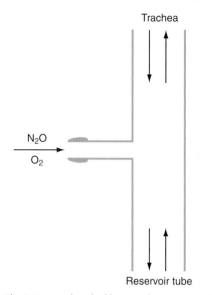

Trachea

N₂O

O₂

Reservoir tube

**FIGURE 51-5** The T piece as described by Ayre. (From Ayre P. The T-piece technique. Br J Anaesth 1956;28:520-3.)

reservoir bags (Fig. 51-5).[136] Later modifications included changes to the T-piece and expiratory limb.[137] The Jackson-Rees modification involves the addition of a reservoir bag to the expiratory limb (Mapleson F).[138]

The Magill circuit and its various modifications, Mapleson A to E (Fig. 51-6) remain popular.[139] These systems consist of a source of fresh gas flow into the circuit, a reservoir bag, a pressure-relief (pop-off) valve, tubing of various lengths connecting all of these parts, and an adapter for the mask or tracheal tube. Each of these has advantages and disadvantages, which are well reviewed elsewhere.[130,134,140,141] The Mapleson D variety is the most commonly used because of its safety and versatility with both controlled and spontaneous ventilation.[141] The pop-off valve is at the end of the expiratory limb, just before the reservoir bag; thus, fresh gas washes alveolar gas out of the expiratory limb during expiration. The efficiency of this washout (to prevent rebreathing) depends on the volume of the expiratory limb, the fresh gas flow, and the size of the tidal volume.[130] Larger children (heavier than 15 kg) require greater fresh gas flow rates to prevent rebreathing during spontaneous ventilation.[141,142] Fresh gas flow rates as low as 1 times minute ventilation may be used with controlled ventilation without an increase in expired $CO_2$ values.[143] Rebreathing (an increase in inspired $CO_2$) can occur in children with controlled ventilation when the respiratory rate increases above 20 breaths per minute; this apparent rebreathing can be diminished by using greater fresh gas flows (E-Fig. 51-2). The reason for this phenomenon may relate to inadequate washout of expired alveolar gas before the onset of the next breath. The advantages of minimal dead space and low resistance to flow with nonrebreathing circuits are counterbalanced by the disadvantages of heat and humidity lost to the anesthetic gases and significant waste of anesthetic agents because of the high flows required.[134,141] A clinically important factor is that whenever a change in anesthetic gas concentration is made at the vaporizer, this change is immediately reflected at the airway. This allows a more rapid induction of anesthesia, which may be an advantage but also means a greater risk of producing an anesthetic overdose when compared with a circle system. The most common and efficacious use of the Mapleson D circuit is for the safe transport

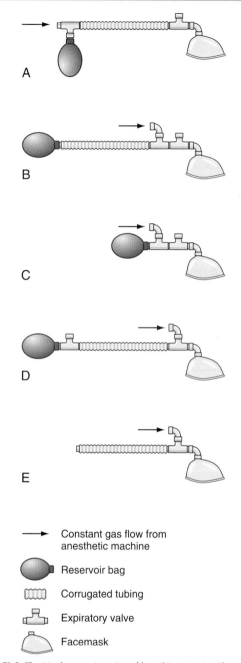

A

B

C

D

E

⟶  Constant gas flow from anesthetic machine

⬤  Reservoir bag

▭  Corrugated tubing

⬚  Expiratory valve

◺  Facemask

**FIGURE 51-6** The Mapleson categories of breathing circuits. The most commonly used circuit for infants is the Mapleson D configuration. (From Mapleson WW. The elimination of rebreathing in various semi-closed anaesthetic systems. Br J Anaesth 1954;26:323-32.)

of a child to and from the OR and for intrahospital transport. In this situation the light weight of the system, the ability to easily adjust peak inflation pressure and provide positive end expiratory pressure, and the ability to use relatively low $O_2$ flows make this system far superior to self-inflating (Ambu type) devices.

The circle system offers the advantage of using reduced fresh gas flows that decreases cost and decreases pollution of the atmosphere with waste anesthetic gases.[144,145] The use of the circle system in neonates and small infants generally requires assisted or controlled ventilation. Newer anesthesia machines use valves that require reduced pressure to open and close and the $CO_2$ absorbers are now wider and shorter, thus reducing the resistance. The main resistance to spontaneous ventilation in infants and

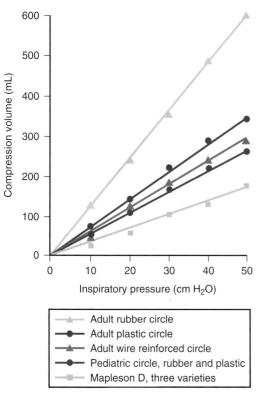

**FIGURE 51-7** The differences in compression volumes among five anesthetic circuits. The Mapleson D systems are the most efficient with the lowest compression volume, whereas the adult rubber circle system has the highest compression volume and is the least efficient circuit. (From Coté CJ, Petkau AJ, Ryan JF, Welch JP: Wasted ventilation measured in vitro with eight anesthetic circuits with and without in-line humidification. Anesthesiology 1983;59:442-446.)

neonates is the inner diameter and length of the tracheal tube. It is particularly important for practitioners using older systems with ventilators that do not compensate for circuit compliance or fresh gas flow to be aware of the different pressure and volume characteristics of circle systems compared with nonrebreathing systems (Fig. 51-7). Because most pediatric anesthesiologists recommend controlled ventilation in this age group, there no longer seems to be a great need for special circuits. The most important pitfall is that a tidal volume is selected based solely on weight rather than examining chest wall excursion, listening to breath sounds, observing the peak inflation pressure, and measuring end-tidal carbon dioxide (ETCO$_2$) tension. Our in vitro studies have found that the main determinants of delivered tidal volume are peak inflation pressure, inspired to expired ratio, and respiratory rate.[106-108] As long as careful attention is paid to these important variables, even tiny infants can be successfully ventilated with adult circuits and adult bellows with pressure-limited ventilation (see further). No difference exists between adult circle systems and a Bain (Mapleson D) type system if pressure-limited ventilation is used and the same peak inflation pressure is generated.[108] The most important factor is that tidal volume per kilogram will be very large with an adult circle system compared with nonrebreathing systems, especially in infants. Many of these issues of delivering accurate small tidal volumes relative to the compliance of the circuit are simplified with the newer generation ventilators that compensate for the compliance of the system and the fresh gas flow (see later). In the final analysis,

however, the practitioner must be cognizant of the fact that the only physiologic measure of the adequacy of ventilation is the CO$_2$ tension—ETCO$_2$ or arterial CO$_2$.

**Carbon Dioxide Absorption**

When using a closed or semiclosed circle system, removal of CO$_2$ from the circuit is required. This is accomplished by inserting a CO$_2$ absorption canister into the anesthetic circuit. The canister is usually placed between the anesthesia bag or ventilator and the fresh gas inlet. In some anesthesia machines, the canister contains two levels of a CO$_2$ absorbent in series. The replacement of the absorbent can create leaks in the circuit if the seal is not reapplied tightly,[146] complete obstruction if the plastic packaging is not removed from the prepackaged absorbent before insertion, or intermittent obstruction if part of the packaging is left in place.[147] The size of the absorbent is designed to maximize CO$_2$ reabsorption while minimally increasing the resistance in the circuit. Many different commercially manufactured absorbents are available whose chemistry involves the use of materials such as calcium hydroxide, sodium hydroxide, potassium hydroxide, and barium hydroxide, so that CO$_2$ is converted into calcium carbonate, water and heat. CO$_2$ absorption, cost and chemistry are reviewed in detail elsewhere.[148] The most common absorbents are soda lime and Baralyme (Allied Healthcare Products, Inc., St. Louis). Soda lime contains 95% calcium hydroxide, either sodium or potassium hydroxide and the balance as water. Baralyme has been voluntarily withdrawn from the market (see later). It contains 80% calcium hydroxide, 20% barium hydroxide, and the balance as water. Newer agents exist, such as Amsorb (Armstrong Medical Limited, Coleraine, Northern Ireland), which contains 70% calcium hydroxide, 0.7% calcium chloride, 0.7% calcium sulfate, 0.7% polyvinyl pyrrolidine, and the balance as water. Potassium hydroxide and sodium hydroxide have been incriminated in the degradation of halogenated anesthetic agents in CO$_2$ absorbers; thus the absence of these compounds in Amsorb prevents the degradation of inhaled anesthetics to carbon monoxide (CO) and compound A (see later). Most absorbents contain a dye such as ethyl violet that turns color as the pH of the absorbent decreases because carbonic acid is formed as CO$_2$ reacts with water. The change in the color in the absorbent indicates it is time to replace the absorbent.

Significant concern exists regarding the interaction of anesthetic agents with CO$_2$ absorbents because this interaction is an exothermic reaction that produces potentially toxic degradation products and a large amount of heat. Sevoflurane is degraded in the presence of CO$_2$ absorbent to produce five compounds, the most common of which is an olefin compound known as compound A.[149] Although compound A has been shown to cause renal corticomedullary necrosis in rats, extensive studies in humans have not yielded any substantive consequences or similar renal damage.[150-155] Factors that increase production of compound A include use of low-flow anesthesia, use of large sevoflurane concentrations, increased minute ventilation, anesthetics of prolonged duration, increased absorbent temperature, and fresh absorbent (Baralyme > soda lime >> Amsorb).[156-159] The safety of low-flow (less than 2 L/min fresh gas flow) sevoflurane is still a question because of the limited number of studies in children, although no anecdotal or animal evidence exists to suggest that children may be at greater risk with compound A.[160] Other toxic degradation products, including CO, formaldehyde, and methanol are produced when inhaled anesthetic agents interact with desiccated carbon dioxide absorbents (see Chapter 6). Carbon

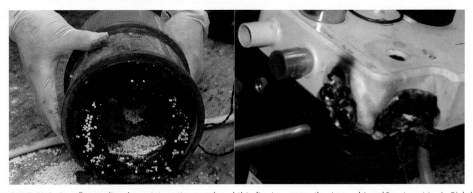

**FIGURE 51-8** Sevoflurane/Baralyme interaction produced this fire in an anesthesia machine. (Courtesy Mr. A. Rich.)

monoxide poisoning has been reported in patients with carboxy-hemoglobin levels reaching 30% or more.[161-163] These case reports were often after several days of anesthesia machine inactivity, in particular, on a Monday morning (i.e., after a weekend with a large fresh gas left flowing through the machine all weekend while it was not in clinical use and usually without a reservoir bag attached).[160,161,164] In some anesthetic machines in which the fresh gas enters at or near the $CO_2$ canister rather than downstream of the inspiratory valve, fresh gas can dry the $CO_2$ absorbent by flowing retrograde through the absorber and exiting where the reservoir bag would usually be connected, because of lower resistance to retrograde flow when a reservoir bag is not in the circle system. In vitro studies demonstrated that CO production from the currently used inhaled agents occurs only when the $CO_2$ absorbent has been desiccated. The order of CO production from greatest to least is desflurane > isoflurane >> halothane and sevoflurane.[165,166] Other factors that increase the production of CO include the degree of desiccation and type of $CO_2$ absorbent (Baralyme > soda lime), increased temperature, increased anesthetic concentration, and low fresh gas flow rates.[160,167-170] Newer $CO_2$ absorbents with little or no potassium or sodium hydroxide produce significantly less or no CO and compound A when they become dehydrated.[158,171,172] The Anesthesia Patient Safety Foundation developed a consensus statement in 2005 to address the problem of desiccation of $CO_2$ absorbents: *"The APSF recommends use of carbon dioxide absorbents whose composition is such that exposure to volatile anesthetics does not result in significant degradation of the volatile anesthetic."*[173] The report discusses the difficulty and impracticality of monitoring $CO_2$ absorbent for desiccation and makes specific recommendations (if absorbents are used that degrade anesthetic agents), including turning off all fresh gas flow when the machine is not in use, changing the $CO_2$ absorbent frequently (e.g., every Monday morning), and changing the absorbent when there is concern about the state of hydration of the absorbent, such as when the machine is found with high fresh gas flows for an uncertain period.[173] New multiwavelength pulse oximeters are now available (e.g., Masimo Rainbow SET Pulse CO-Oximetry; Masimo Corporation, Irvine, Calif.) that have the ability to measure carboxyhemoglobin and methemoglobin levels noninvasively (see later discussion of multiple wavelength pulse oximetry); however, the costs of this technology make its routine use prohibitive.

A very important interaction of the modern halogenated anesthetics and desiccated $CO_2$ absorbent is a poorly defined exothermic reaction that has resulted in fires and explosions, specifically with sevoflurane and Baralyme. There have been several reports of extremely high heat in the $CO_2$ canister and

inspiratory circuit in conjunction with fires, explosions, and various detrimental effects to patients, including burns, acute respiratory distress syndrome, and carbon monoxide poisoning (Fig. 51-8).[174-176] These cases often reported a very slow increase in sevoflurane concentration in the inspiratory circuit with a large gradient between the vaporizer setting and the measured inspiratory sevoflurane concentration along with a rapid color change of the $CO_2$ absorbent presumably from rapid degradation of sevoflurane and possibly a rapid change in pH or other substances causing the indicator color change. In 2003, Abbott Laboratories (North Chicago, Ill.), in conjunction with the U.S. Food and Drug Administration (FDA), released a practice alert and revised the product information about this phenomenon. This highly exothermic reaction occurs with other inhalation agents and other absorbents such as soda lime, but the highest temperatures of 392° F (200° C) and fires were associated with sevoflurane and desiccated Baralyme; Baralyme was voluntarily withdrawn from the market in 2004.[177-179]

### HUMIDIFIERS

The benefits of heating and humidifying inspired gases include maintenance of body temperature, improved mucociliary function, and prevention of drying secretions, particularly with non-rebreathing circuits.[180,181] A heated humidifier also helps maintain body temperature.[31-33] When using a circle system partial heat and humidification occur as part of the exothermic reaction used in the $CO_2$ absorber that adds heat and humidity to the circuit. Low fresh gas flows do increase the rebreathing of humidified and warmed gases, and when combined with passive humidification "artificial nose," provides warm, humidified gases.[15] However, small fresh gas flows add little heat and humidity in infants ventilated through a circle circuit.[182] Humidification can be further increased by active humidification systems.[15] Active humidification systems may create problems such as additional connections that may leak or become disconnected, "rain out" from humidified gas (resulting in water collection within the circuit or the tracheal tube and blockage of the capnograph), added resistance to gas flow, and bubbling noises that distract from the ability to auscultate heart tones and breath sounds. Inhalation of excessively heated inspiratory gases may result in "hot pot tracheitis."[183] Whenever a heated humidifier is added, the extra gas-containing volume of the tubing and humidifier increases the total volume of the anesthetic circuit,[184] in turn increasing compression volume. The degree to which anesthetic circuit efficiency is affected depends on the gas-containing volume of the humidifier and the distensibility of the tubing used.[184] Because of significant complexity and potential for complications, these devices are no longer commonly used and likely soon to be of historic interest only.

## VENTILATORS

### First-Generation Anesthesia Ventilators

Nearly any adult-volume ventilator may be used with children by making appropriate adjustments to the respiratory rate, fresh gas flow, tidal volume, and inspiratory-to-expiratory time ratio. The use of first-generation adult ventilators in children, particularly neonates, requires meticulous attention to the settings before initiation of controlled respiration, to avoid barotrauma. In old anesthesia machines, most volume ventilators could be converted to pressure ventilators by adjusting the pop-off valve to the desired peak inflation pressure. When this modification is made, special attention must be paid to the peak inflation pressure because a fractional turn of the pop-off valve in either direction could result in either excessively high or inadequate peak inflation pressures.

The next generation of anesthesia machines, which have a switch at the $CO_2$ canister to change from manual to mechanical ventilation, do not allow adjustment of peak inflation pressure at the pop-off valve because in the mechanical ventilation mode the pop-off valve is out of the circuit. When such a configuration is used, *the pop-off valve of the ventilator must be used to limit the peak inflation pressure.* The excursion of the ventilator bellows may also be adjusted to limit the size of each tidal volume. Additionally, limiting the inflow of gas to the bellows will limit the bellows inflation. Any of three techniques for adjusting the excursion of the adult bellows provides equal tidal volume as long as the anesthesiologist pays careful attention to peak inflation pressure.[106-108] Using the adult ventilator in pressure pop-off mode allows safe use even in neonates with a very small tidal volume. The following is a suggested means for setting up an older adult ventilator for use with children in the pressure-controlled mode:

1. Set pop-off limit on ventilator to 20 cm $H_2O$.
2. Set rate to appropriate age.
3. Set inspiratory to expiratory ratio to 1:2.
4. Set gas flow to the middle range.
5. Set tidal volume to a minimum of 10 mL/kg or minute ventilation (VE) to a minimum of 200 mL/kg/min.
6. Turn lever to ventilator mode (new systems) or attach ventilator hose to replace bag (old system).
7. Observe peak inflation pressure to be certain that it is 20 cm $H_2O$ or less. If the peak inflation pressure is less than 20 cm $H_2O$, recheck pressure pop-off limit to make sure it is set at 20 cm $H_2O$, and, if correctly set, slowly increase the size of the tidal volume until 20 cm $H_2O$ is achieved.
8. Auscultate both lungs and observe chest excursion and $ETCO_2$.
9. Make certain fresh gas flow is adequate to maintain bellows at full capacity.
10. Reassess the entire process based on Step 8.
11. For noncompliant lungs or with a small-diameter tracheal tube (e.g., 2.5 mm ID), greater peak inflation pressures may be required.[106-108]

It is our bias that manual bag ventilation provides immediate feedback about a child's lung compliance or problems with the circuit (e.g., kinked tube, disconnections, or bronchospasm). However, the literature is unclear regarding this issue. Some experienced anesthesiologists have been able to detect an occluded endotracheal tube, whereas others have not.[185,186] This

may in part depend on fresh gas flow, the size of the child, and the configuration of the circuit. The use of a ventilator provides valuable assistance by freeing the anesthesiologist's hands for other use when the immediate hand-bag feedback is given up for the convenience of a mechanical ventilator. A disconnect, apnea, or peak inflation pressure alarm system is helpful to aid vigilance for these types of adverse events, although these alarms are not perfect.[187] A $CO_2$ detector with the alarm enabled is optimal; the American Society of Anesthesiologists' (ASA) Standards for Basic Anesthetic Monitoring require "continual monitoring for the presence of expired $CO_2$" and the "alarm shall be audible to the anesthesiologist or the anesthesia care team personnel."[188]

With many first-generation ventilators, fresh gas flow may have considerable impact on tidal volume during volume-controlled ventilation[189]; fresh gas flow into the circuit is added to the ventilator output during the inspiratory time. This augmentation effect may result in serious errors in calculating delivered VE during volume-controlled ventilation. The following examples illustrate this situation in volume-controlled ventilation:

1. An adult has a VE of 7 L/min, I:E ratio of 1:2, and fresh gas flow of 6 L/min. If there were no compliance or compression volume losses, the patient would receive 7 L/min + ($\frac{1}{3}$ × 6 L/min) = 9 L/min. If the fresh gas flow were reduced to 3 L/min, the patient would receive 7 L/min + ($\frac{1}{3}$ × 3 L/min) = 8 L/min. This is a change of about 11%.
2. A child has a VE of 2 L/min, I:E ratio of 1:2, and fresh gas flow of 6 L/min. Again, assuming no compression or compliance volume losses, the child would receive 2 L/min + ($\frac{1}{3}$ × 6 L/min) = 4 L/min. If the fresh gas flow were now reduced to 3 L/min, the child would receive 2 L/min + ($\frac{1}{3}$ × 3 L/min) = 3 L/min. This is a 25% decrease in delivered minute ventilation (E-Fig. 51-3). Compared with the earlier example in adults, the impact on the minute ventilation in a child is magnified 2.5-fold.

Thus when using first-generation anesthesia ventilators, increases and decreases in fresh gas flow during volume-controlled ventilation result in changes in delivered VE. The potential for clinically important effects on ventilation is greatest in infants (e.g., several study patients were found to have a 40% difference in VE when fresh gas flow was changed from 1.5 L/min to 6.0 L/min without any change in the ventilator settings.[190] When using volume-controlled ventilation, if a change is made in fresh gas flow for any circuit used in children, the adequacy of chest expansion, breath sounds, peak inspiratory pressure, and $ETCO_2$ must be reevaluated, particularly when using older ventilators that do not automatically compensate for such changes (see later discussion of new ventilators).[191] This effect does not occur during pressure-controlled ventilation because excess flow is simply diverted out of the pop-off valve. However, if fresh gas flows were reduced such that the tidal volume was less than the peak pressure setting, the tidal volume delivered to the child could be reduced.

### Intensive Care Ventilators in the Operating Room

It has been suggested that ventilators used in the ICU may be of greater value compared with standard OR ventilators in children with very poor lung compliance.[144] One study failed to demonstrate any clinically important differences among several commonly used ICU ventilators compared with standard operating room ventilators using pressure-controlled ventilation in an infant lung model with low compliance.[192] However, other modes of ventilation such as volume-limited or pressure-assisted ventilation have not been systematically examined. It would appear that there may not be an advantage to using ICU ventilators in pressure-limited ventilation and there may even be a disadvantage because the anesthesiologist may not be as familiar with these ICU devices, thus leading to the potential for errors in ventilator adjustments. Additionally, this requires the use of total intravenous anesthesia because these devices do not interface with the anesthesia machine.

### Current Anesthesia Ventilators

Newer anesthesia ventilators with ICU performance capabilities are now incorporated into modern anesthesia machines. The most common systems in North American are the Datex-Ohmeda systems (GE Medical, Madison, Wis.) and the Dräger systems (Dräger Medical, Telford, Pa). These ventilators have been designed to accurately volume ventilate the small lungs of neonates and infants and deliver other modes of ventilation, such as pressure-controlled ventilation, synchronized intermittent mandatory ventilation (SIMV) and pressure support ventilation, either alone or in combination with volume- or pressure-controlled ventilation. Significant advances that aid in accurate volume ventilation include fresh gas flow decoupling and compliance compensation. Unlike the older anesthesia ventilators, fresh gas flow decoupling allows the tidal volume to remain constant regardless of changes to the fresh gas flow. Compliance compensation provides measurement of breathing system compliance and accurately delivers a constant tidal volume in spite of changes in lung compliance (while compensating for the compliance of the circuit, e.g., low-volume pediatric or high-volume adult circuit). Fresh gas flow decoupling and compliance compensation can prevent unsafe changes in tidal volume that could lead to hypoventilation or hyperventilation. The Datex-Ohmeda system uses a pneumatically driven ventilation system; the Dräger uses an electronic piston-driven ventilation system.

Delivered and set tidal volume and pressure, as well as flow volume loops, can be monitored with these new machines. These machines also can detect lost volume resulting from system leaks (e.g., tracheal tube leak). Other safety features include electronic machine checkout procedures that may detect problems not detected by the anesthesiologist and more electronic control and monitoring of ventilator settings, including positive end expiratory pressure (PEEP); in older ventilators this was mechanically set or added separately.

The newer modes of ventilation may offer advantages in certain patient populations under specific conditions, but further research is required to demonstrate whether they improve patient care or patient outcomes in the OR. Examples of potential uses of the alternative modes of ventilation include SIMV for children who have not received a neuromuscular blocking drug and situations in which the anesthesiologist is attempting to establish spontaneous ventilation; the child triggers a breath by creating negative pressure or positive-flow gas flow in the circuit. Pressure support ventilation may help overcome increased resistance and improve ventilation when patients are breathing spontaneously through an endotracheal tube or LMA[193]; pressure support ventilation can be used in combination with SIMV to ensure adequate ventilation if a child becomes apneic.

In limited comparison study of earlier versions of the modern anesthesia ventilation systems compared with ICU ventilation systems, the anesthesia systems performed reliably under a wide range of infant conditions, including high respiratory rates, poor compliance, and small tidal volumes.[192]

## Equipment Cart

It is advantageous to use mobile multidrawer carts to stock the wide range and sizes of items necessary to care for the full spectrum of infants and children. The drawers should be organized for ease of use: airway equipment, drugs, intravenous supplies, monitoring equipment, circuits, and suction catheters, separated into appropriately labeled drawers. To facilitate efficient and safe delivery of anesthesia, it is prudent to design and stock each cart identically. Because pediatric anesthesia is often administered outside of the OR suite, these mobile carts simplify the safe practice of anesthesia for children and guarantee the availability of all necessary equipment in these remote locations (Table 51-2).

## Defibrillator and External Pacemakers

Every operating room facility should be equipped with a direct-current defibrillator. It is not necessary to have a unit specifically for use with children, as long as the energy range may be adjusted to the appropriate levels (2 joules/kg) and pediatric paddles are kept with the device. Ideally, the design should incorporate all controls in the paddles, facilitating use without leaving the child's side. A desirable feature is a sensing circuit, providing the capacity for synchronous defibrillation should it be needed. External defibrillators with disposable pads applied to the front and back or right chest and left lateral chest of the child have improved the rapidity of response in some circumstances. These can be placed on high-risk children (e.g., cardiac surgery, cardiomyopathy, conduction defects) before induction of anesthesia.[194-197] Similar devices that allow for external cardiac pacing represent a major new advance for high-risk infants and children.[198-200]

## Ultrasound for Regional Anesthesia and Vascular Cannulation

Ultrasound technology has advanced greatly in the last 10 years and now is routinely used in children for regional and neuraxial anesthesia and central venous cannulation (see Chapters 41, 42, and 48).[201-209] The advent of portable, less expensive ultrasound machines has made this more practical for most pediatric institutions. Visualization of nerves and vascular structures in children requires small probes that can provide high-frequencies (10 to 14 MHz); high-frequency is necessary for visualization of shallow tissue structures.[201] Most regional blocks described in children use a small high-frequency probe shaped like a hockey stick and use small needles (21 or 22 gauge) for single injection blocks or continuous infusion techniques and a Tuohy type of needle or an intravenous catheter (18 or 20 gauge) for threading an indwelling catheter.[201,210-212] Ultrasound-guided techniques provide real-time visualization of nerves, blood vessels, and other structures that may improve the success rate of regional nerve blocks and central venous cannulation while decreasing the complication rate[210] (see Chapter 41 for a more detailed description). This is particularly true in children, in whom the risk is greater than in adults because of the small size of the structures involved and the potential need to perform these procedures after induction of general anesthesia.[201,202] An additional potential advantage is the greater ability to perform these procedures in awake-sedated children compared with the use of nerve stimulation or blind percutaneous cannulation, which can be painful. Other potential advantages are decreased adverse effects such as

**TABLE 51-2** Suggested Pediatric Equipment Cart Inventory

| Drawer 1 | Laryngoscope handles (functioning) (2)<br>Laryngoscope blades (functioning) |
|---|---|

|  | Miller | Macintosh | Wis-Hipple |
|---|---|---|---|
|  | 0 (2) | 1 (2) | 1½ (2) |
|  | 1 (2) | 2 (2) |  |
|  | 2 (2) | 3 (2) |  |
|  | 3 (2) |  |  |

| | Magill forceps: 1 pediatric, 1 adult; 1-inch tape (4); ½-inch waterproof tape (4); 4 each ¾-inch and ¼-inch (tourniquets of nonlatex material); scissors; flashlight; extra batteries for laryngoscope handle |
|---|---|
| Drawer 2 | Masks: neonate (3), infant (3), toddler (3), child (3), medium adult (3), large adult (3)<br>Airways: 3.5 cm (5), 5.0 cm (5), 6.0 cm (5), 7.0 cm (5), 8.0 cm (5), 9.0 cm (5) |
| Drawer 3 | Gauze sponges (sterile and nonsterile), double-stick disks, rubber bands, adhesive bandages, alcohol swabs, antibiotic ointment, water-soluble surgical lubricant, lidocaine ointment 5%, bulldog clips, safety pins, corneal lubricant, pediatric blood tubes (blue, red, purple, and green), eye patches |
| Drawer 4 | Adult sodium bicarbonate (2), pediatric sodium bicarbonate 8.4% (2), infant sodium bicarbonate 4.2% (2), cardiac lidocaine 100 mg (2), dextrose 50% (1), mannitol 25% (1), diphenhydramine 50 mg (2), calcium chloride 10% (4), calcium gluconate 10% (4), sterile water, lidocaine 1% (5), phenylephrine (5), neostigmine 1:2000 (10), ephedrine (5), atropine (10), isoproterenol (1), furosemide (3), epinephrine 1:1000 (10), succinylcholine (1), rocuronium (1), dexamethasone 4 mg/mL (2), dopamine (2), ondansetron (10), propofol (10) |
| Drawer 5 | Pediatric uncuffed endotracheal tubes: 2.5 (6), 3.0 (6), 3.5 (6), 4.0 (6), 4.5 (6), 5.0 (6), 6.0 (6); pediatric cuffed endotracheal tubes: 5.0 (3), 5.5 (3); adult cuffed endotracheal tubes: 2 each of 6.0, 6.5, 7.0; stylets in various appropriate sizes |
| Drawer 6 | Pediatric and adult esophageal stethoscopes (6), adult electrocardiography pads (10), pediatric electrocardiography pads (10), 6.5F suction catheters (6), 10 of each size 8F and 14F |
| Drawer 7 | Syringes: 60 mL (2), 20 mL (6), 12 mL (10), 6 mL (10), 3 mL 22 gauge (20), 3 mL 25 gauge (20), 1 mL 27 gauge (20) |
| Drawer 8 | Intravenous catheters: 24 gauge, 22 gauge, 20 gauge, 18 gauge, 16 gauge, 14 gauge; pediatric intravenous boards: 2 sizes (4), T-connector, three-way stopcocks |
| Drawer 9 | Pediatric intravenous sets (6); pediatric Buretrol (2); intravenous extension sets (2); lactated Ringer solution 250 mL 0.9 normal saline (5); air trap filters (6); head strap; blood pressure cuffs (2 each size), 1 adult size with stethoscope; oximeter sensors for infants and children |

*NOTE: These are only suggested equipment cart materials. Each hospital should alter the order of drawers and their contents to suit its particular needs and for convenience.*

intravascular and intraneuronal injection, reduced dosage of local anesthetic, faster onset, longer duration, and improved quality of blocks.[202,213,214] Studies of central venous and peripheral venous cannulation in infants and children demonstrate quicker times to cannulate the vessel, fewer attempts before success, and significantly fewer failures compared with landmark-based techniques.[215-220] Quality randomized, controlled trials are difficult to perform owing to the difficulty in defining the level of training and experience of the care providers and the relatively low rates of complications.[221,222] More studies are needed to better define the use of ultrasound techniques in infants and children; optimal outcomes require significant education, training, and hands-on experience.

# Monitoring Equipment

## THE ANESTHESIA RECORD AND BAR CODE DRUG ADMINISTRATION

In addition to its obvious role as a medicolegal document, the anesthetic record can be a very important monitor. Proper recording of a child's status on arrival in the OR encourages evaluation of the effects of any premedication, confirmation of nil per os (NPO) status, allergies, current medications, and assessment of weight and fluid balance. Careful recording of intraoperative fluid administration and losses allows assessment of a child's fluid replacement. Concurrent charting of vital signs and anesthetic drugs administered allow correlations to be made and encourages trend analysis. Many changes that are too subtle to interpret on a moment-to-moment basis become obvious when graphed out over time. In addition, a numbering system correlating events with time on the anesthesia record documents the sequence of anesthetic management and may prove very useful should a medicolegal issue arise.

Automated anesthesia records or automated anesthesia information management systems (AIMS) are increasingly used and will eventually replace hand-recorded records and likely improve the accuracy of data collection.[223-226] These systems can provide timely reminders for administration of antibiotics, documentation of start and stop times, compliance with regulatory requirements, reminders of blood pressure measurement gaps, and automatically provide cumulative totals in infusions of drugs, such as propofol or remifentanil.[227-230] Most importantly, the automated recording of physiologic data in real time provides improved accuracy, particularly at times when the anesthesiologist is multitasking or when an emergency occurs. In fact, such data may actually be protective from medical malpractice because the veracity of the data is far improved over retrospective data recording.[231,232] Conversely some data recorded are spurious and may in fact be nonreflective of an actual event; neither system is perfect.[233,234] Currently, the widespread introduction of automated record-keeping has been very slow for several reasons, including the large capital and contract expenses for implementation, difficulty integrating all hospital-wide digitized systems in real-time terms, and costs for 24-hour support staff.[225]

Medication errors are quite common, particularly in high acuity areas such as the OR and the ICU.[235] The next area of technology improvement may be the adoption of bar code confirmation of drug administration in the operating room.[236-242] Such systems are currently available to provide accurate labeling of syringes (date, time, concentration) and have had great success in reducing medication errors.[235,243-251] Several studies have demonstrated reduced medication errors in the OR when bar coding is used.[236,242,251] These systems will be incorporated into the automated anesthesia record in the future as well.

## PRECORDIAL AND ESOPHAGEAL STETHOSCOPE

In infants, neonates, and small children, an experienced ear can easily detect arrhythmias but also may be able to assess changes in cardiac output and blood pressure (soft heart tones compared with baseline).[252] The continuous use of a stethoscope is of particular value in situations in which more advanced noninvasive blood pressure monitoring (NIBP) is unavailable. The precordial stethoscope may be stabilized with a double adhesive disk. For specialized needs, such as bronchography, angiography, or magnetic resonance imaging, a plastic stethoscope that is not radiopaque or ferromagnetic may be used. The optimal site where both heart tones and breath sounds can be heard is usually at the apex of the heart, but occasionally the suprasternal notch provides better listening conditions. The latter position may be more advantageous during induction and emergence, because information regarding airway patency is more readily obtained. The stethoscope can provide early indications of developing airway obstruction or laryngospasm, allowing the practitioner to take corrective action (PEEP) before a full-blown episode of laryngospasm develops. However, the perception is growing among clinicians that current monitors have superseded the need for the precordial stethoscope.[253]

Whenever the trachea has been intubated, the precordial stethoscope may be exchanged for an esophageal stethoscope. The pediatric size esophageal stethoscope may be introduced atraumatically, even in neonates. The optimal position for the stethoscope within the esophagus can be ascertained by inserting the scope while listening for the position that provides the loudest heart and breath sounds. The less expensive adult variety is often usable in children age 6 years or older. Some disposable esophageal stethoscopes incorporate a thermistor, allowing the introduction of two monitors at once. One possible relative contraindication to using or inserting an esophageal stethoscope is during a tracheostomy. Misidentification of an esophageal stethoscope as an endotracheal tube has resulted in the surgeon opening the esophagus.[254] During a tracheostomy in a child, either the esophageal stethoscope should not be used or the surgeon should be informed that two stiff tubes pass through the neck structures, because this complication has occurred even in the hands of very experienced surgeons.[255]

The major drawback of a stethoscope as a monitor is that it provides information only when it is connected to the anesthesiologist. Custom-molded earpieces, which better exclude room noises, are much more effective and more comfortable to wear than the conventional binaural stethoscope. These earpieces have the added advantage of leaving one ear open for communication with the surgeon and ancillary personnel. Even with pulse oximetry and capnography the stethoscope can provide great reassurance that the patient has an adequate blood pressure and cardiac output. *If both the NIBP and the oximeter fail, but the child has strong heart tones, a technical problem likely exists. However, if the other monitors fail and the heart tones are very weak, then cardiac output may be compromised and attention should be immediately focused on resolving that problem rather than wasting time trying to search for a problem with the monitor.*

## BLOOD PRESSURE DEVICES

Blood pressure must be monitored in every child who requires our care. An appropriate-size blood pressure cuff should cover approximately two thirds of the length of the upper arm or thigh.[256,257] The cuff bladder should rest over the artery; in older children a stethoscope may be secured over the artery to listen for Korotkoff sounds. In smaller children, the flicker of the needle in an aneroid sphygmomanometer dial may be used as an indicator of systolic pressure.[258] If the flicker is not clearly visible, a distal pulse sensor may be used. Such a sensor can

be either a photoelectric plethysmograph on a digit that detects the return of the signal as the cuff deflates or a Doppler flow detector that is positioned over a distal artery.[259] Electronic oscillometer units (NIBP) are capable of repeated, frequent, and accurate measurements.[260-263]

If an automatic NIBP device is used, it is important that proper application, function, and adequate deflation time be ensured; venous stasis, petechiae, and nerve compression damage are possible, especially with early models.[264] Most automated NIBP machines have specific cuff sizes for infants, neonates, and preterm infants, as well as a requirement that the monitor settings be matched with the size of the patient (neonate, child, adult). For neonates and infants, special tubing is required to connect the cuff with the monitor. If cuffs are improperly matched with the tubing and monitor settings, the built-in algorithms will produce factitious data.[265] It appears that these devices offer reasonable accuracy for systolic blood pressure but may be less accurate for diastolic blood pressure.[266,267] NIBP monitors provide very useful information during induction of anesthesia, particularly important during that period before establishing intravenous access. The results of one study showed greater consistency and accuracy with these devices than with standard auscultatory methods.[263] One common practice is to place the cuff on the calf of infants as a substitute for upper extremity measurements. There is poor correlation between arm and calf blood pressures; because of this variability, one should not simply assume that one site is a substitute for the other.[268-271] Another study determined that the loss of the pulse oximeter waveform correlated with systolic arterial pressure in children weighing less than 15 kg.[272]

## ELECTROCARDIOGRAPH

Although many arrhythmias may be diagnosed by careful attention to the heart sounds conducted through the precordial or esophageal stethoscope, the electrocardiogram (ECG) remains a mandatory monitor for all instances of sedation, regional anesthesia and general anesthesia. In a healthy child, lead placement may differ from that selected for adults because the principal need is for diagnosis and resolution of arrhythmias rather than detection of ischemia. One report emphasized that children undergoing cardiac surgery or children with severe anemia may develop ST depression consistent with ischemia, although it occurs extremely rarely.[273] With the greater right heart predominance in the younger ages, a cross-chest lead generally provides the optimal combination of atrial and ventricular voltage signals. A QRS detector with a beeper is a useful accessory, particularly when vagal stresses occur. The ECG heart rate is used for comparison with the pulse oximeter heart rate to confirm appropriate application and function of the pulse oximeter. A built-in lead fault detector is also useful to check the cables and a patient's leads when a poor signal is obtained. Cleaning, gently abrading, and defatting the skin with alcohol can improve the contact. Tincture of benzoin may also help maintain secure adhesion in areas near the application of surgical preparation solutions. Care must be taken not to allow the leads to become wet with preparation solutions and to isolate the leads from the electrocautery dispersive electrode to avoid electrical burns.[274] Special ECG leads and monitors are required for use in the MRI scanner (see Chapter 45).

## OXYGEN MONITOR

Assessment of the inspired $O_2$ concentration is one aspect of the monitoring guidelines published by the ASA and Harvard

Medical School.[193,275] It is necessary in preterm infants and neonates to be alert to the possible relationship between high arterial $O_2$ tension ($PaO_2$) resulting from high inspired $O_2$ concentrations and ocular toxicity, although recent evidence suggests that this relationship is not a quid pro quo.[276] This monitor is also helpful in guiding inspired $O_2$ concentrations in certain types of congenital heart disease in which low inspired $O_2$ is key to optimizing pulmonary artery pressures and pulmonary blood flow. An $O_2$ monitor allows easy blending of air and $O_2$ to achieve the desired inspired $O_2$ concentration. In all children, $O_2$ monitoring can help prevent hypoxemia. The standard, so-called fail-safe device built into most anesthesia machines is generally keyed only to pressure in the $O_2$ line; should the $O_2$ flow be turned off, a child may receive a potentially hypoxic mixture (air plus a large concentration of inhalational anesthetic such as sevoflurane or desflurane) without warning from the fail-safe alarm. An $O_2$ monitor on the inspiratory limb would indicate a decrease in the inspired fraction of $O_2$ and provide an accurate alarm. With the more frequent use of closed-circuit anesthesia and air–$O_2$ blends, $O_2$ monitoring assumes even greater importance. *Anesthesia machines generally provide a mechanical or electronic coupling system that delivers minimal $O_2$ flow and prevents the delivery of hypoxic mixtures of $N_2O$ and $O_2$. However, some newer machines do not have a minimum $O_2$ flow and disable their electronic coupling system when air and $O_2$ are combined; thus it is possible to intentionally or unintentionally turn on the air without $O_2$ to deliver 21% $O_2$. The delivery of low inspired $O_2$ is sometimes desirable in certain conditions such as hypoplastic left heart syndrome or to decrease the risk of airway fire when laser or electrocautery are being used. When high concentrations of sevoflurane or desflurane are used with air it is possible to dilute the $O_2$ and deliver a potentially hypoxic mixture. Careful monitoring of inspired $O_2$ is vital to prevent this from occurring unintentionally.* A high inspired $O_2$ alarm device is also desirable; this may detect when an air tank is empty. The $O_2$ analyzer should be calibrated and alarm limits set before anesthetic induction; a narrow band of alarm limits allows early detection of changes in gas flow ratio.

## TEMPERATURE MONITORS

Although there is medicolegal pressure to monitor temperature in every child because of the potential danger of malignant hyperthermia, in reality temperature monitoring is mandated for other reasons. Hypothermia is much more common in the OR than hyperthermia and may be associated with acidosis, myocardial irritability, coagulopathy, respiratory depression, prolonged neuromuscular blockade, greater absorption of inhalation agents, and delayed emergence from anesthesia.[277-280]

## NONINVASIVE OXYGEN SATURATION MONITORS
### Pulse Oximetry
Nothing has changed anesthetic practice more in the past few decades than the introduction of mandatory pulse oximetry for all cases requiring sedation and general anesthesia. This monitor determines the $O_2$ saturation of hemoglobin by spectrophotoelectric oximetric techniques. Measuring the amount of light transmitted through tissue between a two-wavelength light source (930 and 660 nm) and a detector allows continuous calculation of arterial $O_2$ saturation.[281] The use of two frequencies helps eliminate interfering absorption by other molecules, although intravenous dyes (indocyanine green, methylene blue) and colored nail polish may interfere with normal sensor function and cause the oximeter into reading a factitiously low $O_2$ saturation value.[275,282,283] Additionally, dyshemoglobinopathies such as carboxyhemoglobinemia and methemoglobinemia may result in

significant artifact. Carboxyhemoglobinemia causes an overestimation of $O_2$ saturation because the photodetector incorrectly interprets carboxyhemoglobin as oxyhemoglobin; this artifactual change is roughly proportional to the concentration of carboxyhemoglobin.[284] Methemoglobinemia results in desaturation, but the saturation recorded tends to read greater than the actual saturation; at high levels of methemoglobin during episodes of desaturation, this disparity becomes greater.[285] Fetal hemoglobin, hyperbilirubinemia, and sickle cell disease have minimal effect on pulse oximetry.[286-290] This monitor is easy to use, noninvasive, and reasonably accurate, although not perfect.[291,292] Of greatest importance to the clinician is appreciating that the current oximeter technology underestimates the actual hemoglobin saturation as the saturation is decreasing; the more rapidly the saturation decreases, the more the saturation reading underestimates the true saturation.

The clinical efficacy of this monitor was demonstrated in a prospective single-blind study of pediatric patients; 50% of the cases were conducted with the saturation data and alarms made available to the anesthesia team, whereas in the remainder, the data were blinded and the alarms silenced. Several observations were reported[293,294]:

1. Twice as many "major" desaturation events (defined as saturation 85% or less for 30 seconds or longer) occurred in the blinded group.
2. The oximeter detected a greater number of desaturation events before clinical recognition by the anesthesiologist.
3. Major desaturation events were not accompanied by changes in vital signs in most cases (i.e., in only 4 of 19 such events was any change in blood pressure, heart rate, or respiratory rate noted).
4. The incidence of these events in ASA physical status 3 and 4 patients was greater than in ASA 1 and 2 patients.
5. Desaturation events occurred in children who were managed by both experienced and inexperienced anesthesia personnel.
6. Correlation between the observation of cyanosis and true desaturation was poor.
7. Desaturation events were as likely in brief as in procedures of extended duration.[293]

In a subsequent study, the efficacy of combined pulse oximetry and capnography was examined to determine if patient safety was improved with the addition of capnography.[294] In 400 children, 260 problems were observed (E-Fig. 51-4). The study confirmed that pulse oximetry was superior to the human eye in diagnosing hemoglobin desaturation. The incidence of major desaturation events when the oximeter data and alarms were blinded from the practitioners was threefold greater than when they were available. Capnography was not as helpful in diagnosing the majority of events leading to hemoglobin desaturation (E-Fig. 51-5). This is consistent with the Australia anesthesia incident study in which the authors reported that oximetry provides useful data in 85% of events.[295] In the pediatric study, 15 problems fulfilled the criteria of a major capnograph event. These were problems that posed a threat to life (e.g., kinked tracheal tube, circuit disconnect, esophageal intubation, accidental extubation) and would have been detected immediately by a capnograph, but 8 were diagnosed initially by pulse oximetry (E-Fig. 51-5). Capnography may have helped initially to diagnose the seven remaining events; however, pulse oximetry would have diagnosed these events as desaturation developed, 30 to 60 seconds later. This observation is also consistent with the Australia incident study.[296] This study also examined the incidence of "minor" capnograph events, defined as an abnormality of ventilation that was not a threat to a child's life (e.g., hypercarbia or hypocarbia). A significantly greater incidence of both hypercarbia and hypocarbia occurred in children whose anesthesiologist was blinded from the capnograph data and alarms.

Infants 6 months of age or younger are at greatest risk for experiencing at least one major desaturation event (E-Fig. 51-6) or a major capnograph event. The number of children with multiple problems in the group in which neither pulse oximetry nor capnography data were available to the anesthesia team was twice as great as in the group in which both were available. An interesting observation was the relatively high incidence of *clinically unrecognized endobronchial intubation that manifested as persistent, though minor, hemoglobin desaturation (93% to 95%).*[297]

These studies confirm that the pulse oximeter provides an early warning of developing desaturation well before a clinician is able to detect it clinically. This is easily explained by the fact that approximately 5 g of desaturated hemoglobin is required to detect cyanosis; if a child's hemoglobin level is 15 g/dL, the $O_2$ saturation would have to decrease to 66% (i.e., less than the normal venous hemoglobin desaturation before cyanosis would be clearly evident). Pulse oximetry detects evolving hemoglobin desaturation in advance of this value being achieved. There is some variability among manufacturers, and accuracy declines as the saturation values decrease (70% or lower).[284,298] The degree of inaccuracy of pulse oximeters is a function of many variables that should be carefully reviewed.[286,299,300] Pulse oximetry is a reliable monitor for the majority of children who are free of cyanotic congenital heart disease.

Quite apart from the hemoglobin $O_2$ saturation data, pulse oximetry provides additional information including data pertinent to the systemic blood pressure.[272] Pulsus paradoxus may be observed in hypovolemic children. Loss of the peripheral pulse when using pulse oximetry may accompany hypovolemia, vasoconstriction resulting from hypothermia, or inadequate cardiac output as a result of hypovolemia, allergic reaction, or anesthetic overdose.[301,302] Pulse oximetry is useful as a noninvasive trend monitor in individuals with anatomic or physiologic shunts, because the effects of anesthetic agents and positive-pressure ventilation are difficult to predict.[303-305] Pulse oximetry also can be an effective monitor for preventing hyperoxia in preterm infants by guiding the inspired $O_2$ concentration to values that correspond to hemoglobin saturations between 93% and 95%.[306] Preductal and postductal oximeters indicate opening and closing of a patent ductus arteriosus (PDA).

Various common OR events can affect the accuracy and reliability of pulse oximetry including electrocautery, flickering operating room lights, movement, blood pressure cuff inflation, bright light, vasoconstriction, stereotactic positioning systems,[307] and injected dyes (cardio green and methylene blue). Falsely high $O_2$ saturation measurements may occur despite severe hemoglobin desaturation in the presence of interference with the oximeter sensor. Darkly pigmented skin color may also affect accuracy with up to a 10% error in low saturation ranges.[308] Consequently, it is important to remember that this monitor is not foolproof.[309] One very important artifact, the penumbra effect, is caused when an adult clip-on sensor is placed on an infant's finger or toe.[310] *In this situation the oximeter senses the motion of the pulse but light is transmitted around the finger or toe, thus providing a falsely high hemoglobin saturation. Only appropriate-size oximeter probes should be used in infants and children.* In critically ill children and those with thermal injuries, problems with finding a suitable site to apply

the probe can be overcome by using a modified oximeter probe applied to the tongue (see E-Fig. 34-5, *A* to *D*).[311,312] The tongue provides a rich blood supply unaffected by vasoconstriction, and electrocautery interference is less. If the tongue moves, the sensor may dislodge or record a false heart rate. Thermal injury secondary to the interface of incompatible sensor probes and cables (i.e., equipment from more than one manufacturer) has been reported, as has pressure necrosis resulting from too tight an application.[313,314]

Recent advances in pulse oximetry technology have attempted to make several major improvements, including (1) software that provides motion artifact compensation; (2) software that allows uninterrupted readings even in low flow states; and (3) software that provides more accurate assessment of oxygenation in cyanotic patients.[315] Conventional pulse oximetry time-averages a signal over 5 to 10 seconds, depending on the default settings of the oximeter. This signal represents the ratio of transmitted red and infrared light, and the instrument uses this to determine the child's hemoglobin saturation. This averaging smoothes motion-induced artifacts but may ultimately lessen the sensitivity and response time of a conventional oximeter in situations of hypoxemia or even delay the recognition of asystole or severe bradycardia by several seconds. More recent models are designed to recognize motion artifact and discard signal aberrations secondary to motion using proprietary signal-filtering techniques. Some devices combine two different approaches to signal processing to arbitrate the correct saturation based on dual signal filtration techniques using both pattern matching and adaptive comb filtering. This technique is designed to detect motion and reject analysis of data generated during motion. Other oximeter manufacturers take a different approach, using spectrophotometer principles to generate a saturation signal. That saturation signal may contain several component saturations corresponding to different absorption artifacts of blood and other tissues, including venous blood. The signal is then processed using a discrete saturation transform (DST) algorithm that then extracts the highest and presumably the arterial component saturation and reports this value as the hemoglobin $O_2$ saturation.[316-319] Conventional pulse oximeters can overestimate or underestimate the degree of desaturation and therefore may have less accuracy and greater signal dropout rate (i.e., no reading or poor quality signal associated with an alarm, especially in children with hypoxemia). These deviations may be improved with the newer generation pulse oximeters, but this has yet to be definitively demonstrated.[320] The newer generation pulse oximeters perform better than conventional pulse oximetry in hypothermic low flow states during cardiopulmonary bypass.[321] Movement artifact is the main cause of false alarms in sedated or awake children who require oximetry monitoring. This artifact is significantly reduced with the current generation of pulse oximeters in both adult and pediatric patient populations.[322-326]

### Multiple Wavelength Pulse Oximetry

The latest advancement in pulse oximetry technology is multiple wavelength pulse oximetry, which was approved by the FDA in 2006 (Masimo Rainbow SET Pulse CO-Oximetry, Masimo Corporation, Irvine, Calif.). These systems use the principles of pulse oximetry and co-oximetry and at least seven wavelengths of light to calculate the standard measurements from new-generation pulse oximeters and continuous (1) hemoglobin, (2) carboxyhemoglobin, (3) methemoglobin, and (4) plethysmographic (Pleth) variability index. Several studies have examined the accuracy (bias and precision) of the measurements obtained via pulse co-oximetry, and data inconsistencies require further investigation. For the continuous measurement of hemoglobin it was estimated to be accurate within 1 g/dL in adult patients who had systematic hemodilution.[327] More studies are needed to determine whether this level of accuracy is reproducible.[328,329] The measurement of carboxyhemoglobin via pulse oximetry (SpCO) has been studied extensively because of its potential for screening large numbers of patients, especially in the emergency room setting. The accuracy data are not completely consistent, but in the authors' opinions are likely acceptable for patient screening. However, with the known degree of false positive and false negative results, SpCO should be used in conjunction with clinical data and blood co-oximetry to verify results when indicated.[315, 330-335] Initial studies of the accuracy of methemoglobin measurement by pulse co-oximetry (SpMet) demonstrated decreased accuracy with hypoxia[315,336] but the more recent studies using newer technology appear to be even more accurate than the measurement of SpCO and possibly as good or better than $SpO_2$ in the ranges measured in the studies—$O_2$ saturation 74% to 100% and methemoglobin 0 to 14%.[337-339]

All the measurements from pulse co-oximetry likely have a significant degree of decreased accuracy in the presence of abnormal hemoglobins; more studies need to be done to examine these complex interactions and the effect on the accuracy of the obtained measurements with the coexistence of different forms of hemoglobin. Pleth variability index is a measure of the degree of hypovolemia and potentially might provide guidance for decisions regarding volume administration. The measurement comes from respiratory variations in the plethysmographic waveform amplitude and uses an algorithm to determine the likelihood of improved blood pressure and cardiac index with fluid or colloid administration.[340] There are significant limitations in this technology and accurate assessment of volume status may require specific conditions, including general anesthesia, sinus rhythm, mechanical ventilation with a tidal volume of at least 8 mL/kg, PEEP less than 5 cm $H_2O$, location of sensor, and an invasive arterial line depending on the algorithm or commercial product used.[341,342] The use of invasive arterial blood pressure and plethysmographic variations in hemodynamic parameters during the respiratory cycle has potentially significant clinical utility but requires further investigation, including evaluation in the pediatric patient population.[342,343]

### Reflectance Oximetry

Reflectance pulse oximetry has been available for many years, but with recent technologic improvements, several devices have received FDA approval and are currently marketed. Reflectance oximetry technology was first created to improve $O_2$ saturation data in difficult clinical conditions, such as decreased perfusion, movement, and conditions in which optimal sites for standard transmission oximetry probes may not exist (e.g., burns). The technology behind reflectance oximetry involves the emission of multiple wavelengths of red and infrared light that are sensed in two or more photodetectors located a distance away from the diodes on the same probe sensor (Fig. 51-9). These devices measure reflected rather than transmitted light. The technology used to create these oximeter probes permit usage on the forehead, in the esophagus, and on the fetal scalp. The forehead devices have had the largest use among pediatric anesthesiologists. Studies of reflectance oximeters in general demonstrated that these devices are more susceptible to erratic measurements

when the probe is placed directly over an artery[344] and vein.[345] Some potential advantages to using reflectance oximetry on the forehead include better signals during conditions of poor perfusion, lack of motion, and faster response time than conventional peripheral oximeter probes.[346,347] However, possible disadvantages include a potentially high signal dropout rate (no measurable signal) and poor accuracy, often measuring lower than finger transmission oximetry, particularly in cases of venous congestion (e.g., Trendelenburg position or situations that impede venous return).[348] Several studies, including more recent studies, report good correlation between concurrent measurements of $O_2$ saturation comparing reflectance oximetry on the forehead,[349-351] the esophagus,[352] and around the chest of premature infants,[353] compared with extremity pulse oximetry and arterial co-oximetry measurements; these studies also report a clear dropout rate.

### Near-Infrared Spectroscopy

Near-infrared spectroscopy (NIRS) is a noninvasive, optical technology that bears similarities to pulse oximetry in that it uses the relative absorption of near-infrared light, 700 to 900 nm, through biologic tissues to determine tissue oxygenation (E-Fig. 51-7).[354] Oxyhemoglobin and deoxyhemoglobin absorb light at different frequencies, and the use of a probe that emits and detects different frequencies of near-infrared light can be used to estimate tissue oxygenation. This device has been most widely used to measure "regional" cerebral $O_2$ saturation ($rSO_2$),[355,356] but measurement of oxygenation in other areas, such as kidney, bowel, spinal cord, free tissue flaps, and other areas, is possible.[357-368] These recent developments provide an exciting new potential to detect ischemia to various tissues before it is evident clinically.[369-376] Pulse oximetry requires the measurement of the pulsatile (arterial) component of the total light transmitted by the biologic tissue. Because NIRS does not require the subtraction of the pulsatile component, the signal is more than 100 times stronger and unaffected by poor perfusion compared with pulse oximetry. However, it is susceptible to motion artifact and ambient light noise but software algorithms have significantly decreased these sources of error. A probe placed on the child's forehead measures the concentration of oxyhemoglobin and deoxyhemoglobin in the tissue underlying the probe. The device functionally measures the oxygenation of blood in the underlying tissues, including blood in the arterioles, capillaries, and venules. The majority (approximately 85%) of the signal originates from the venules; skin and bone and extracranial blood absorb only limited amounts of light, which is subtracted from the signal and does not have significant impact of the measurement in infants and children.[357,358] NIRS thus measures the $O_2$ saturation in venous and arterial blood and thus represents an average saturation across blood vessels and tissue. In cerebral oximetry, the $O_2$ saturation of the blood in the tissue (i.e., between the sending and emitting probe) depends on factors that affect $O_2$ transport, including cerebral blood flow, hemoglobin saturation, hemoglobin–$O_2$ binding affinity, and oxygenation saturation in the arterial blood. Therapies aimed at improving $O_2$ delivery or decreasing oxygenation consumption to the brain will potentially increase cerebral oxygenation ($rSO_2$).[359-361,376]

This technology is not new; however, only three devices are currently FDA approved for commercial use to measure cerebral oxygenation: the first, is the INVOS Cerebral Oximeter (Somanetics Corporation, Troy, Mich.). The absolute accuracy of the current Somanetics device is ±10% to 15%, making the

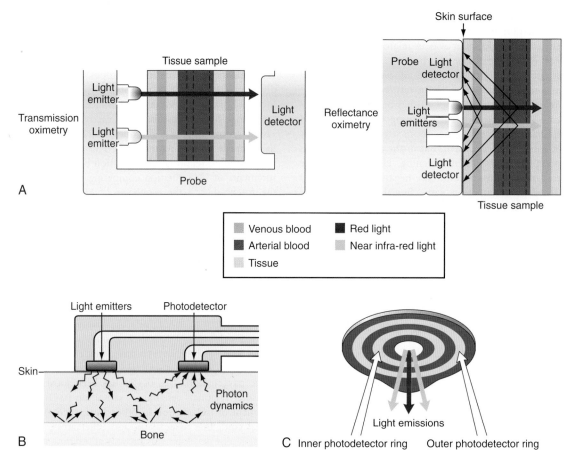

**FIGURE 51-9 A,** Comparison of conventional transmission pulse oximetry with reflectance oximetry. Note that with conventional oximetry the light detector is located directly opposite on the other side of a digit and detects light transmitted through the digit; with reflectance oximetry the light detector is located next the light emitters and detects the light reflected back through and from the tissues. **B,** The typical configuration of a reflectance oximeter. **C,** Another configuration, in which several light detectors are located at different distances from the light emitters. In addition, reflectance oximeters may emit light in more than just 2 wavelengths, which is typical of conventional transmission pulse oximeters. (Modified from Kugelman A, Wasserman Y, Mor F, et al. Reflectance pulse oximetry from core body in neonates and infants: comparison to arterial blood oxygen saturation and to transmission pulse oximetry. J Perinat 2004;24:366-71; and Keogh BF, Kopotic RJ. Recent findings in the use of reflectance oximetry: a critical review. Cur Opin Anesth 2005;18:649-54.)

measurement of absolute oxygenation unreliable. However, it is reasonably accurate for changes in oxygenation (±5%), making this device most useful for following trends in cerebral oxygenation.[362-365] This device is currently FDA approved for trend monitoring. The Somanetics Cerebral Oximeter has demonstrated that normal regional cerebral oxygen saturation ($rSO_2$) is 60% to 80%.[366,367] In controlled hypoxic-ischemic states in animals, electroencephalogram (EEG) slowing and increased tissue lactic acid levels occur at $rSO_2$ between 40% and 45%. The EEG becomes flat at $rSO_2$ between 30% and 35%, and if the cerebral ischemia is protracted, it may be associated with tissue infarction.[367]

The second device, the Fore-Sight Absolute Tissue Oximeter (CAS Medical systems, Branford, Conn.) has been approved for actual saturation estimation and not just trending. This device uses four wavelengths of light and multiple sensors incorporated into one sensor, which is usually placed over the forehead; three sensor sizes are available, and use is based on patient weight.

The most recent device to be approved by the FDA is the EQUANOX (Nonin Medical Inc., Minneapolis, Minn.), which uses light-emitting diode (LED) technology to transmit three wavelengths (EQUANOX Classic Sensor) and most recently four wavelengths (EQUANOX Advance Sensor, Model 8004CA).[368,377] The EQUANOX sensor differs from the others by having dual emitter and sensor sites. The company claims this technology decreases surface tissue variability and can obtain quicker measurements. The first sensor did not have sufficient accuracy for absolute measurements and would be best used in trend monitoring. The newest sensor claims to be very accurate (4.1%), but further study needs to confirm the accuracy of these new systems.

This technology has important limitations. The relationship between the amount of tissue damage and clinical outcome depends on the site of the tissue damage. Because these monitors only measure the saturation in tissue below the probes, they more accurately reflect on focal tissue oxygenation or damage. If the probe is placed on the forehead, it will reflect the state of the tissue in the frontal cortex and may not reflect other areas of the brain.

Although some studies suggest improved outcomes when cerebral oximetry is used including pediatric congenital heart surgery, in which neurologic complications are high (2% to 25%),[362,366,378,379] a fair degree of skepticism remains regarding the utility of cerebral oxygenation in clinical practice.[380,381] There is hope, however, that these devices may at some time in the future provide real-time guidance of regional tissue oxygenation and the effectiveness of interventions to improve the oxygenation. Additional research, further improvements in the technology, and reduced per-patient costs are needed to clarify the role of reflectance oximetry in pediatric patient management.[373]

## CARBON DIOXIDE ANALYZERS

The most commonly used gas monitor is the expired $CO_2$ analyzer. This monitor is particularly useful in teaching about ventilation, $CO_2$ elimination from alveoli, and airway management, provided the response time of the instrument is rapid enough to accurately reflect end-expired $CO_2$ tension.[382,383] Two configurations of infrared $CO_2$ monitors are in clinical use. They differ only in the location of the $CO_2$ analysis: (1) the side-stream analyzer, which involves the aspiration of expired gas from the anesthesia circuit and remote $CO_2$ analysis, or (2) a mainstream analyzer in which an optical sensor within a cuvette is inserted into the circuit just proximal to the elbow and where analysis of the $CO_2$ occurs based on a signal detected at the cuvette. Side-stream analyzers are less cumbersome than mainstream analyzers because the former requires no additional pieces to be inserted into the anesthetic circuit. Gas for side-stream analysis only requires a narrow-gauge flexible tube to transfer the expired gas unidirectionally from the elbow of the circuit to the analyzer. The gas sampling line and water trap can become obstructed with water or secretions, requiring replacement of the parts. Mainstream gas analyzers do not obstruct with secretions, but they are heavy, and if a tracheal tube of a small caliber is used, airway obstruction may occur as a result of kinking of the tracheal tube.[383] Furthermore, mainstream systems require a large inventory of cuvettes, which must be sterilized between patients. Most OR monitors today use side-stream sampling. The current generation of these monitors have improved precision that reduces the gas sampling rate to just 50 mL/min and excellent accuracy even with small rapid tidal volumes.[384-388]

Capnography is the gold standard to ensure that the tracheal tube has been inserted within the trachea.[188,389] If no expired $CO_2$ is detected after a presumed tracheal intubation, one must assume that the endotracheal tube is in the esophagus. However, if the stomach has been distended by manual ventilation or crying before tracheal intubation or if carbonated soft drinks were present in the stomach, $CO_2$ could be detected immediately after intubation, even after an esophageal intubation.[390] In such a case, the expired $CO_2$ will be very low or decrease rapidly in a stepwise manner after placing the tracheal tube. This artifact is very short lived. In addition, the presence of $CO_2$ during cardiopulmonary resuscitation is a very important sign of pulmonary blood flow.[391] Alternatively, its absence during resuscitation may indicate inadequate chest compressions and pulmonary blood flow (see Chapter 39).[392-395]

Measurement of expired $CO_2$ tension is also helpful in detecting other clinical problems. Clinically important air embolism causes a transient but marked reduction in $CO_2$ excretion because the lungs are ventilated but not perfused; hence dead space is suddenly increased (see Chapter 24). Quantitative measurement allows detection of change in circuit flows, disconnections, endotracheal tube kinking, or accidental extubations.[296,396-398] Capnography also signals the earliest clinical sign of a malignant hyperthermic reaction and the effectiveness of treatment[399] (see also Fig. 40-3). In critically ill neonates or children in a hypermetabolic state after thermal injuries, ventilatory requirements

may be as much as 4 times normal and capnography may be an effective noninvasive means of assessing the adequacy of ventilation in these children as well (see Chapter 34).[400]

A capnograph with a recorder or a display is most valuable because the $CO_2$ waveform may help in diagnosing other types of respiratory difficulties (Fig. 51-10). Bronchospasm and its response to treatment may be identified by changes in the $CO_2$ waveform; bronchospasm causes an increasing slope of the plateau during expiration, and resolution of the bronchospasm restores the plateau to the horizontal. Data also suggest that the shape of the $CO_2$ waveform changes with growth and development. The shape of the $CO_2$ waveform achieves the normal adult configuration by adolescence.[401] A slow-speed recorder also allows trending, which we have found particularly useful in diagnosing small circuit leaks, partially kinked endotracheal tubes, and rebreathing. In children free from pulmonary shunts, the arterial and alveolar $CO_2$ values ($PaCO_2$ and $PACO_2$ [as reflected by a true end-expired sample]) should be within 2 to 3 mm Hg. The severity of a shunt or the diagnosis of a shunt may be made if this difference is greater than 5 mm Hg and if the $CO_2$ sensor is properly calibrated. Children with a variety of pulmonary problems may have significant differences between arterial and expired $CO_2$ values. In such cases, expired $CO_2$ monitoring may be used only for trending and as a disconnect alarm.[402,403] This monitor is of great value in assessing the adequacy of ventilation in children whose trachea is intubated, but of possibly less value in children whose airway is managed by facemask when it is difficult to obtain an accurate end-expired sample.[294,396] The accuracy of $ETCO_2$ monitoring is slightly better with an LMA than with a facemask.[404]

No monitoring device is perfect, and it is possible to develop a false sense of security when monitoring the ECG, $O_2$ saturation, and expired $CO_2$ values. Anesthesiologists must not abandon stethoscopes and the powers of observation; the practitioner is still the ultimate monitor. It is our powers of observation and clinical judgment combined with our ability to synthesize and integrate the data that determine the appropriate course of action. The following case is an example:

> An 8-kg infant with a 45% scald burn was anesthetized, her trachea was intubated, and she was placed in the prone position. The child was monitored with an ECG, a temperature probe, an esophageal stethoscope, an expired $CO_2$ mainstream sampler, a pulse oximeter, and an arterial line. The arterial line malfunctioned, and it took approximately 45 minutes to replace it. An arterial blood gas sample was obtained, and at that time, the $O_2$ saturation was 100% and the expired $CO_2$ was 43 mm Hg (mainstream device, no wave form, and circle system); there had been no noticeable changes in vital signs. The blood gas results were pH 6.96, $PaO_2$ 214 mm Hg, and $PaCO_2$ 103 mm Hg. This child had a partially kinked endotracheal tube and a large shunt, both of which contributed to the false data from the capnograph.

Although this is an extreme example, it emphasizes that even in the presence of highly sophisticated, properly working, noninvasive monitors, they may fail to accurately depict physiologic derangements in some clinical scenarios. Recognizing the limitations of our monitors and their potential for errors and remembering to verify physiologic indices with blood gas analyses (either arterial or venous) in the critically ill can only improve the quality of care delivered to the smallest and most critically ill infants and children under our care.

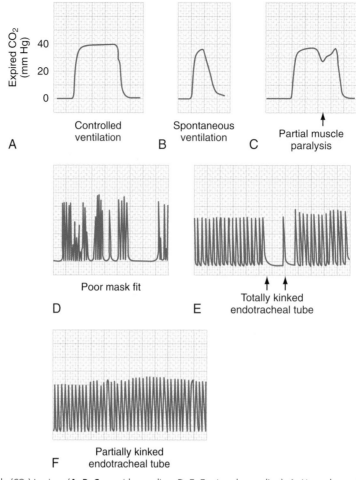

**FIGURE 51-10** Expired carbon dioxide ($CO_2$) tracings (**A, B, C** = rapid recording; **D, E, F** = trend recording). **A,** Normal waveform with a long alveolar plateau indicating good alveolar gas sampling during controlled ventilation. **B,** Spontaneous ventilation with rapid respiratory rate; minimal alveolar plateau. **C,** Patient with partial muscle paralysis; note change in $CO_2$ waveform (*arrow*) during inspiration, which took place during the ventilator expiration. **D,** Poor mask fit with many periods when no $CO_2$ was detected; this also results in many false alarms. **E,** A totally kinked endotracheal tube was detected by the absence of a $CO_2$ waveform (*between arrows*); a similar trace could result in a circuit disconnect, esophageal intubation, or a simple pause in respiration. **F,** A partially kinked endotracheal tube may result in a slow change in peak expired $CO_2$; a similar change could be noted with an unrecognized endobronchial intubation, change in pulmonary compliance, circuit leak, or increase in metabolic rate. The reverse would occur with air embolism, hypothermia (decreased metabolic rate), improved compliance, or, increased fresh gas flow without compensatory change in ventilator settings. (From Coté CJ, Liu LM, Szyfelbein SK, et al. Intraoperative events diagnosed by expired carbon dioxide monitoring in children. Can Anaesth Soc J 1986;33:315-20.)

### Transcutaneous Carbon Dioxide Measurement

Transcutaneous $CO_2$ monitoring has been available for many years, but this technology has been limited because of difficulties preparing and fixing the sensor, preparing the skin, having to rotate the sensor to prevent burns, and calibration time, as well as questions of its reliability. The most common use for transcutaneous monitoring has been in critically ill neonates.[405,406] Two monitors combine pulse oximetry with transcutaneous carbon dioxide ($PtcCO_2$) measurement through a probe designed for application to the ear lobe (TOSCA, Linde Medical Sensors AG, Basel, Switzerland; V-Sign Sensor, SenTec Digital Monitoring System; SenTec AG, Steinhausen, Switzerland). These products use a variant of the Severinghaus-type $CO_2$ electrodes in which the skin is warmed to 107.6° F (42° C) to increase blood flow to the capillary bed.[407,408] $CO_2$ is measured by change in pH of the electrode where pH is proportional to the logarithm of the change in $CO_2$. The $CO_2$ values are greater than the local arterial values because of the increased temperature and increased metabolic production locally. The system corrects for these

changes, is relatively easy to use because of self-calibration, and requires infrequent need for repositioning and changes of the electrolyte layer of the probe. Both systems are reliable and accurately reflect the $PaCO_2$ in a variety of settings in both pediatric[409,410] and adult patients.[411-413] Proponents of this type of $CO_2$ monitoring suggest that $ETCO_2$ monitoring is often inaccurate in some clinical conditions, including neonates with a large air leak around the tracheal tube, high respiratory rates, and sampling at the end of a tracheal tube such that a true end-tidal sample is not obtained, significant cardiopulmonary disease associated with increased dead space and/or right-to-left shunt, and conditions of frequent movement. A clear disadvantage is the lack of breath-to-breath monitoring capability for apnea and disordered breathing provided by end-tidal capnography.[414] Transcutaneous $CO_2$ monitoring may more closely approximate $PaCO_2$ in children who have large ventilation-perfusion mismatch.[415-417] Transcutaneous $CO_2$ monitoring may have a role in anesthetized children with severe pulmonary disease or other pathology that prevents accurate $ETCO_2$

measurement. More studies are needed to assess its role in the pediatric patient population in various settings such as the OR and ICU and for unintubated patients undergoing sedation.

## ANESTHETIC AGENT ANALYZERS

Most current anesthetic agent analyzers use ultraviolet or infrared monochromatic (only one agent detected) or polychromatic (more than one agent detected) absorption or mass spectroscopy and provide a rapid time response.[418,419] Polychromatic infrared analyzers are most useful because they can detect erroneously selected anesthetic agents.[420] Careful assessment of the end-expired vapor tensions may provide some indication of a child's anesthetic depth, but each child must be assessed on an individual basis. Vaporizer malfunctions and miss-fills may also be diagnosed. Mass spectroscopy may be particularly valuable in providing an early warning of air embolism (after a child has been denitrogenated), because the sudden appearance of expired nitrogen is abnormal (entrainment of room air into the circuit and release of nitrogen from extremities with a tourniquet also may provide a source of nitrogen).[421] The purported advantages of less waste of anesthetic gases and a more rapid awakening are effects that have not been proved. However, the ability to use low flows offers the potential for significant cost savings in the form of less waste of anesthetic agent and less pollution of the atmosphere.[422] The report of accumulation of methane with closed circuit anesthesia and the inaccuracy of agent analysis (methane additive to the agent used) is worrisome but can be obviated with simple periodic flushing of the system.[423,424]

## BLOOD LOSS MONITORS

Close observation of the surgical field is the best single monitor of blood loss. A small-volume trap on the suction line before the major evacuation trap is particularly useful for small children. Routinely weighing surgical sponges on a dietary scale, assuming that 1 g of weight is equivalent to 1 mL of blood, is also helpful. Greatest accuracy is obtained by immediate weighing as the sponges come off the surgical field, thus minimizing evaporative losses. Point-of-care testing devices such as the HemoCue (HemoCue AB, Ängelholm, Sweden) and the I-STAT (Abbott Point of Care Inc., Princeton, N.J.) provide a rapid means for assessment of hemoglobin values[425-431] but each may underestimate the hematocrit at lower values.[430,432-437] Noninvasive hemoglobin measurements using multiwavelength pulse oximetry in general may be useful for trend monitoring.[328,438] However, overall it tends to underestimate hemoglobin values and may not be sufficiently accurate at this time to use these data for clinical transfusion decisions because discrepancy of up to 1 g of hemoglobin have been reported.[327,329,436,437,439-442]

## NEUROMUSCULAR TRANSMISSION MONITORS

Measuring the indirectly elicited twitch response is indicated when neuromuscular blocking agents are used. Residual or incomplete reversal of neuromuscular blockade has been shown in adults to be a common cause for delay in leaving the OR, prolonged postanesthesia care unit (PACU) recovery time, and respiratory complications in the early postoperative period.[443-446] It has been clearly determined that even experienced anesthesiologists cannot determine decrement in the train-of-four (TOF) accurately. Clinical signs (e.g., sustained head lift) are often difficult to perform in older patients and can be done with a significant degree of residual blockade, thus leading to undetected residual neuromuscular blockade and presumably the

potential for respiratory complications.[444] In general, two types of neuromuscular monitoring devices are available, those using acceleromyography and those using mechanomyography. Mechanomyography models use constant current nerve stimulation. These devices self-calibrate and then deliver a constant stimulus (30 to 70 mA) to the skin regardless of other influences. Failure to deliver a supramaximal stimulus may result in overestimation of twitch suppression. The power should generally be left off between readings to avoid possible injury secondary to prolonged, repetitive exposure to electric current. Acceleromyography uses a piezoelectric sensor to quantitate the acceleration (proportional to force) of the thumb converting this to an electrical signal. There is considerable disagreement in the published literature as to which of these techniques is most accurate.[447-449] Monitors based on acceleromyography are becoming more commonly available; however, these are difficult to use in infants because of the small arc of the displaced thumb. Some consider this monitor to be more accurate than the standard mechanomyography based train-of-four monitors, but they are difficult to use in infants and are not user friendly.[445,446] Others think mechanomyography is more accurate because it is less influenced by external disturbances, that is, it does not go out of calibration.[450] Therefore at present for clinical purposes in infants and children, mechanomyography still seems to be the simplest and most helpful clinical monitor during the use of nondepolarizing competitive blockers. The TOF does not require recording capability or baseline measurement because it works strictly by comparing the fourth twitch with its own internal standard, the first twitch.[451,452] The unit may also be used with depolarizing relaxants, monitoring only the first twitch amplitude. A significant decrement (>50%) between the first and fourth twitch in this context suggests phase-two blockade (see E-Fig. 6-14).[453] Needle electrodes are hazardous because they may cause bleeding, infection, burns, or nerve injury; current density may be very high, owing to the limited contact surface and the resistance of surrounding skin. Needle electrodes should not be used. Self-adhesive electrodes designed specifically for twitch monitors are available, but they are unnecessary and expensive and tend to be too large for infants and small children. A reasonable alternative is a pair of infant-sized ECG electrodes. The choice of monitoring location depends on the nature of the surgery. Any site where a motor nerve is close to the body surface and its associated muscle group is available for observation may be chosen. The most common stimulation site is the ulnar nerve in the forearm, observing the thumb (adductor pollicis brevis); this is the standard site for most research reports. It should be noted that the majority of studies have been standardized to the ulnar nerve, thus quantitating the response of other motor nerves is less reliable. Using the facial nerve may result in false-positive responses because the muscles may be easily stimulated directly, potentially causing an overdosing of nondepolarizing neuromuscular blocking agents.

## PROCESSED ELECTROENCEPHALOGRAM MONITORS

Monitoring the processed EEG has become a common means for monitoring patients who are anesthetized or sedated, but its role has yet to be fully defined in the pediatric patient population.[454-457] Analysis of the EEG waveforms and EEG data from brain response to auditory input have been used to assess the depth of sedation and anesthesia and in turn to predict or avoid awareness under anesthesia in adults. Several excellent reviews are available regarding the technology and process of validation.[458,459]

Awareness under anesthesia has become a major source of litigation in the United States,[460] and public concern prompted The Joint Commission to issue a Sentinel Event Alert.[461] In response to this alert, the ASA instructed a taskforce to review the available literature and the existing monitors.[462] Their review included studies from several processed EEG monitors (Bispectral Index [BIS], Aspect Medical Systems, Natick Mass.; Entropy, General Electric Healthcare Technologies, Waukesha, Wis.; and Narcotrend, MonitorTechnik, Bad Bramstedt, Germany) and data for auditory evoked potentials (AEP Monitor/2 (Danmeter Aps, Odense, Denmark). This task force reached several important conclusions:

> *Intraoperative monitoring of depth of anesthesia, for the purpose of minimizing the occurrence of awareness, should rely on multiple modalities, including clinical techniques (e.g., checking for clinical signs such as purposeful or reflex movement) and conventional monitoring systems (e.g., electrocardiogram, blood pressure, heart rate, end-tidal anesthetic analyzer, capnography). The use of neuromuscular blocking drugs may mask purposeful or reflex movements and adds additional importance to the use of monitoring methods that assure the adequate delivery of anesthesia. . . . It is the consensus of the Task Force that brain function monitoring is not routinely indicated for patients undergoing general anesthesia, either to reduce the frequency of intraoperative awareness or to monitor depth of anesthesia.*

A few studies have suggested that the use of these monitors may decrease awareness in adults[463,464] but no definitive data exist in infants and children that these monitoring systems decrease the incidence of awareness under anesthesia.[465] The vast majority of studies have examined the Bispectral Index (BIS); therefore this section will primarily focus on this device with the understanding that other devices are available but have not been adequately evaluated in children.

Bispectral analysis generates a value (0 to 100) derived from processed electroencephalographic data that provide a measure of the depth of anesthesia.[458,466,467] There have been significant inconsistencies in data obtained from the BIS monitoring system in adults and even more inconsistencies in children. Some of the complexity and inconsistency of the BIS data will be reviewed to understand the possible uses and limitations of this and other EEG-based systems. Because of the nature of the data collection in the awake patient, artifacts may occur as a result of eye movement, blinking, and so forth at baseline if the device is applied before induction. Depth of anesthesia as measured by the bispectral analysis is more reliably assessed during propofol or inhalation-based anesthesia than during opioid-based anesthesia, although there is significant individual variation in the bispectral analysis reading.[468-470] $N_2O$ has a minimal effect on the bispectral analysis, whereas ketamine paradoxically increases the bispectral analysis.[458,471-473] Some well-controlled studies in adults examined the effects of a broad spectrum of medications on the bispectral analysis reading; this device monitored the effects of anesthetic drugs on awareness and patient responsiveness to painful and nonpainful stimuli.[463,464,468,469,474-479] Studies also have demonstrated decreased anesthetic requirement and improved recovery parameters in adults who were monitored with bispectral analysis.[480,481] However, although bispectral analysis technology appears to monitor the effects of hypnotics, it does not necessarily monitor the adequacy of anesthesia or analgesia.[462]

Bispectral analysis values in children anesthetized with sevoflurane were inversely proportional to end-tidal sevoflurane concentration in both infants and children, although the BIS values in anesthetized children had a much broader range than in adults.[482,483] In one study, the BIS values decreased with increasing end-tidal concentration of sevoflurane until 3%, after which the bispectral analysis value paradoxically increased with higher inspired concentrations.[482,483] At equi-minimal alveolar concentration (equi-MAC), bispectral analysis values are greater in children than in adults.[483-485] Additionally, the bispectral analysis values at equi-MAC concentrations of volatile anesthetics has been inconsistent; several studies have shown that the bispectral analysis values during halothane anesthesia are greater than those during isoflurane, sevoflurane, or desflurane in children.[486-488] *These data indicate that BIS values may be substantially greater with halothane than with the other inhalational anesthetics.*[489] In addition, several studies have demonstrated conflicting results in children compared with infants, suggesting greater bispectral analysis values for halothane in children but not in infants at equi-MAC.[482,485,488] All of these studies have suggested wide interindividual variability in the bispectral analysis values at comparable expired MAC concentrations of inhalational anesthetics. One disturbing study has found lower BIS values in intellectually impaired children compared with controls.[490] Other studies have found differences between the right and left side of the brain.[491] Limited data validate bispectral analysis readings in young children and infants. The algorithm was based on processed EEG readings from adults, and the EEG does change with age developmentally; therefore it seems reasonable that the algorithm will need to be adjusted for age if the bispectral analysis is to be used in infancy.

One study noted an incidence of awareness in children aged 5 to 12 years of approximately 0.8%.[492] This is fourfold to eightfold greater than the incidence of awareness reported in adults, although the clinical implications are not clear at this time. Indeed, unlike in adults, none of the children who had awareness reported distress as a result.[493,494] The use of $N_2O$ (when there is no contraindication) may be valuable in reducing the incidence of awareness without significantly adding to the duration of emergence.[495] No randomized, controlled trials in children have demonstrated a decrease in awareness using bispectral analysis or other commercially available processed EEG devices. A recently introduced device is the SEDLine (Masimo Corp., Irvine, Calif.). This device uses four EEG electrodes and therefore simultaneously measures both sides of the brain. Preliminary experience at one institution has found that $N_2O$ interferes with SEDLine monitoring (personal communication, CJC). At present, no validating studies in children have been reported; until further data are developed, we do not recommend adopting this technology.

The BIS has the longest track record, but again its value in children is still quite unsubstantiated. One study in children 3 to 18 years of age demonstrated a more rapid recovery when bispectral analysis monitoring was used. However, this did not hold true for children younger than 3 years of age.[496] Bispectral analysis monitoring is able to help predict voluntary patient movement during intraoperative wake-up tests during spinal fusions.[497] Bispectral analysis also has been used to assess the depth of sedation in children and to correlate bispectral analysis values with other measures of recovery, exclusive of ketamine-induced sedation.[498-500] Unfortunately, bispectral analysis values were unable to predictably separate moderate and deep sedation in children. In yet another study, a poor correlation was reported between the bispectral analysis values and a standardized Ramsay sedation score.[501] Bispectral analysis values do not appear to correlate with arousal from sevoflurane anesthesia.[502] Limitations on the usefulness of bispectral analysis monitoring in children include fear of probe placement while they are awake (thus in most cases the bispectral analysis monitor is applied after anesthetic induction). Because many procedures in children involve the head (e.g., strabismus, tonsillectomy, neurosurgical), the use of this monitor may be impractical in nearly half of the surgeries that involve children.

At this point, bispectral analysis and other depth of anesthesia monitoring systems appear to have some potentially useful applications in older children, whose EEG pattern is likely to be similar to that of adults, such as in trauma and during certain surgeries in which anesthetic drug use may be extremely limited (i.e., motor evoked potential monitoring for scoliosis surgery). However, the variability of response in any given child, the issues relating to the effects of specific drugs, and other technical factors such as probe placement in awake children, create significant limitations to its use in infants and toddlers. It is hoped that further, controlled studies will better define the possible role of depth of anesthesia monitoring in infants and children during sedation and general anesthesia.

## INTRACRANIAL PRESSURE MONITORS

In children with increased intracranial pressure (ICP), direct monitoring of ICP may be helpful. Measurement may be accomplished by transduced pressures through either a ventricular cannula placed through a burr hole or by a subarachnoid bolt or equivalent. Measurement also can be performed noninvasively in infants with an open anterior fontanelle (see Chapter 24).

## DISCONNECT AND APNEA ALARMS

When a ventilator is used, the tactile feedback from palpating the breathing bag is lost. A disconnect alarm is useful in this circumstance, particularly in the absence of capnography. Most anesthesia ventilators incorporate a disconnect alarm, but it may also be purchased as a separate add-on for older designs. These alarms generally sense time cycling of pressure events. Most of these alarms can detect complete ventilator disconnects but may not be sensitive enough to detect extubations with small endotracheal tubes or partial circuit disconnects because of the continued presence of flow resistance. Other types of alarms, such as heat-sensing devices or capnographs, provide a more reliable means of detecting inadequate ventilation, accidental extubation, or disconnect. Besides the sensing of pressure cycles, many newer monitors include high-pressure, continuous positive-pressure, and negative-pressure alarms. Some products include an automatic switch-on when shifting from hand to machine ventilation, thereby avoiding failure to monitor.

## APNEA MONITORS

Apnea monitors, whether based on transthoracic impedance, motion, or other patient parameters, are helpful in the perioperative and recovery room phases for former preterm infants younger than 60 weeks postconceptual age.[503] Infants with a history of apnea spells and children with ongoing apnea spells are much more likely to develop apnea in the postoperative period. Even if a child has had a period of some months with a normal respiratory pattern at home, the anesthetic state may bring about a temporary return of apnea spells, and such a monitor should be used according to current guidelines (see Chapters 2, 4, 35, and 36).

## VOLUME METER AND SPIROMETER

In some instances, monitoring a child's respiratory gas flow may be desirable. A Wright turbine respirometer, Dräger positive displacement spirometer, and newer designs based on the pneumotachograph operating principle, vortex detectors, or thermistor flow meters are available. Some devices allow measurement of flow–volume loops, which can be very useful in both diagnosing and correcting ventilatory issues related to bronchospasm, airway compression, or single-lung ventilation.[504-509] These monitors are not widely used in the clinical anesthesia care of children.

## INSPIRATORY PRESSURE GAUGE

In children who require ventilatory assistance, a pressure gauge applied at the airway allows the delivery of precise airway pressures and thus helps minimize barotrauma. When infants are treated with PEEP and continuous positive-airway pressure, airway pressures are best measured as close to the airway as possible. Such a device is useful in accurately determining leaks around an endotracheal tube when used to determine the size of the larynx (see Chapter 31).[510]

## URINARY CATHETER

Aseptically inserted, a catheter in the bladder connected to a closed drainage system is of little risk to most children. Urine output is a useful indicator of volume and perfusion status; the presence of hematuria or hemoglobinuria can aid in the diagnosis of surgical trauma to the urinary system, a bleeding dyscrasia, or a transfusion reaction. Indications for a urinary catheter include massive fluid shifts, prolonged radiologic procedures with large doses of contrast material, prolonged surgery, neurosurgery and cardiac surgery with osmotic diuretic therapy, and urinary reconstructive procedures. In infants, standard urinary catheters might be difficult to insert and therefore a feeding tube provides an excellent substitute. Because the urine output in infants may be scant, connecting a feeding tube to a syringe barrel may provide an adequate and accurate measurement system. Care must be taken to avoid using latex catheters, particularly in children who are latex sensitive.

## INVASIVE BLOOD PRESSURE MONITORS

When clinically indicated, arterial, central venous, or very rarely pulmonary artery pressure should be monitored. Percutaneous arterial cannulation is performed with a 22- to 24-gauge catheter-over-needle device in infants and neonates, respectively, and a 20-gauge device in older children (see Chapter 48 and Fig. 48-10, *A* to *D*).[511,512] Central venous and pulmonary artery cannulation are usually achieved using the Seldinger technique (see also Fig. 48-2, *A* to *D*).[513,514] The proper reference location for all pressure transducers is usually the level of the child's right atrium. If ICP monitoring is used or if the child is in the head-up or sitting position, a reference zero position at a reproducible cranial site (e.g., the external ear canal) is vitally important to accurately assess cerebral perfusion pressure. Placement of any of these invasive monitors provides additional benefits other than direct hemodynamic monitoring. Serial pH and arterial blood gas tension measurements from an arterial line or from determination of serial chemistries, ionized calcium, glucose concentrations, hematocrit, coagulation profiles, and osmolality allows continual assessment of a complex case. In operations performed in the sitting position, a right atrial catheter provides an approach to therapy for air embolism (see Chapter 24).

To withdraw a valid blood sample, an adequate volume of blood must be aspirated; 2 to 3 times the dead space (the point of aspiration to the tip of the catheter) usually accomplishes this.[515] In infants, these systems must be flushed with small volumes at slow rates. In infant arterial lines, this amount is 0.5 mL/5 sec, to avoid dangerous fluctuations in blood pressure and retrograde flow with the risk of stroke.[516]

## ECHOCARDIOGRAPHY

Some reports have examined the usefulness of transesophageal echocardiography as a means of continuously monitoring cardiac output and the cardiac response to surgery and anesthetic agents. This equipment is very expensive and requires a great deal of skill and experience to take full advantage of its capacity. The practicality of this device in children appears to be primarily limited to those undergoing corrective cardiac surgery (see Chapters 14 to 16).[517-524] However, this device is clearly of benefit in defining the source of an adverse cardiovascular event such as an air, clot, tumor embolism, or other source of right-sided outflow tract obstruction.[525-529]

## CONTINUOUS INVASIVE AND NONINVASIVE CARDIAC OUTPUT MONITORS

Traditionally, cardiac output has been estimated with thermodilution, Fick $O_2$ consumption, or echocardiography. Continuous invasive techniques such as continuous analysis of central venous $O_2$ saturation is feasible and accurate even in neonates but generally not applicable in the operating room.[530,531] Arterial pulse contour analysis is another invasive method that requires arterial and central venous catheters; data regarding the accuracy and reliability for children are still preliminary.[532-534] Other noninvasive techniques such as measurement of expired $CO_2$ have been attempted but with variable success.[535-542] The NICO device (Philips Respironics, Amsterdam, the Netherlands) estimates cardiac output as reflected by changes in expired $CO_2$ using a Fick partial rebreathing calculation.[541,542] This device requires that the child is intubated, and its accuracy in children is yet unproved.[536,539,541,543] A new device, Cardiotronic EC (Cardiotronic, Inc., La Jolla, Calif.), has been approved by the FDA for use in children of all ages, including neonates.[544-549] Electrical cardiometry continuously estimates stroke volume and left ventricular outflow to calculate cardiac output, cardiac index, and a variety of other parameters through quantitation of changes in impedance associated with changes in the orientation of red blood cells (Fig. 51-11). During diastole red cells are organized chaotically, but during systole they assume a position parallel to the direction of blood flow. Thus thoracic electrical bioimpedance relates to changes in thoracic aortic blood flow, and through the use of refined algorithms, noninvasive measurement of cardiac output is achieved.

The height (cm), gender, weight (kg), and age of the patient are entered into the handheld device. Four electrodes are applied to the neck and left chest at specified locations—in infants, one lead is placed on the cheek or forehead and the fourth lead placed on a thigh (see Fig. 51-11). The device records the heart rate and averages cardiac output every 10 to 60 heartbeats depending on how the device is configured. Studies in neonates, children, and adults suggest that this is a reasonable trend monitor to estimate cardiac output in a noninvasive manner. It certainly is not a

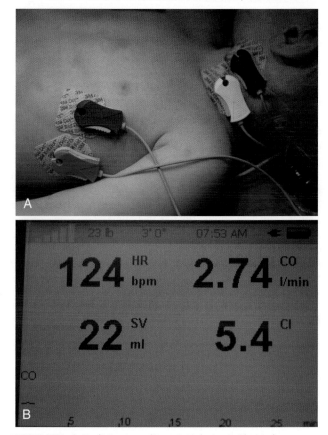

**FIGURE 51-11 A,** Cardiotronic cardiac output device. **B,** Electrical cardiometry continuously estimates stroke volume and left ventricular outflow to calculate cardiac output, cardiac index, and a variety of other parameters through quantitation of changes in impedance associated with changes in the orientation of red blood cells. During diastole red cells are organized chaotically, but during systole they assume a position parallel to the direction of blood flow. Thus thoracic electrical bioimpedance relates to changes in thoracic aortic blood flow and through the use of refined algorithms noninvasive measurement of cardiac output with four electrocardiography pads is achieved.

monitor that will replace the gold standard of echocardiography or thermodilution cardiac output, but the $r^2$ value of 0.86 and Bland-Altman plot suggest reasonable efficacy for monitoring and trending purposes in adults.[550] Preliminary experience (CJC) with this device is favorable as an early warning device of a developing adverse cardiovascular event and as an indicator of successful intervention of such events.

## ELECTROCAUTERY

Although anesthesiologists are not directly responsible for electrocautery devices, they should have a basic knowledge of how they function and the necessary precautions to prevent burn injury or a fire. The most important means of preventing injury is to ensure that an appropriate-size grounding pad has been applied and that no blood, urine, or preparation solutions have been allowed to pool around or under the grounding pad. Additionally, the electrocautery can ignite any flammable implements, drapes, and an $O_2$-rich environment. Severe injuries and deaths have occurred when high concentrations of $O_2$ have been allowed to build up beneath drapes (supplemental $O_2$ in awake or sedated patients) and have been ignited by the spark of the electrocautery on the other side of the surgical drape.[551-556]

# Operating Table

The operating table is a vital piece of anesthesia equipment. The table should provide the full range of positioning, including Trendelenburg controls in case of either regurgitation or the need to increase venous return. It must have appropriate padding to prevent patient contact with metal structures. The ability to remove the head support and to lower the foot section provides a smaller table appropriate for infants. For extremely long procedures, an alternating-pressure air mattress or silicone gel padding placed between the patient and the operating table guards against decubitus injuries.[557] Periodically changing the patient's head position may prevent bald spots as a result of prolonged contact pressure in one location.[558] The use of a silicone gel ring helps stabilize the head and reduces contact pressure at one point. The Jackson spinal table (Orthopedic Systems Inc., Union City, Calif.), along with other new tables with interchangeable modular components to maximize exposure of the surgical field and protect the patient from potentially harmful positions, have become popular for spine surgery in the past decade. This table may present unique challenges for the anesthesiologist, with access to the head of the table limited because of an immobile and obstructive block. If tracheal intubation must be performed in a smaller child who requires this table, provisions should be made to ensure that adequate access to the head can be obtained to facilitate laryngoscopy and intubation in advance of induction of anesthesia. An additional concern is to ensure that the operating table can handle the unfortunate increasing weight of the pediatric patient population; many centers are now performing bariatric surgery in teenagers.

# Transport Apparatus

Because transport environments (particularly outside the hospital in ambulances, helicopters, and fixed-wing aircraft) are exceedingly noisy, we depend on electronic monitoring for the heart rate more than we would in an operating theater (where we could use a stethoscope). The monitor must have battery-mode capability and, if possible, aircraft and ambulance power (direct current), as well as routine hospital power (alternating current). If the monitor incorporates a QRS beeper, it should be capable of high volume to compete with the noisy transport environment. The use of headphones connected directly to monitors may be useful in this circumstance. The oscilloscopic display must have bright phosphors to allow arterial, ECG, pulse oximetry, and expired $CO_2$ waveforms to be observed in minimal and bright light conditions.

# Purchasing Anesthesia Equipment

With the increasing sophistication of monitoring and life support equipment, purchasing decisions are no longer intuitive. A complete grounding in the underlying engineering concepts would probably require an advanced degree in engineering, but a reasonable working knowledge of the operating principles, advantages, and special hazards of the various types of apparatus is relatively easy to obtain. Most hospitals now have a full-time biomedical professional staff, which often have considerable engineering and practical experience to assist in the purchasing, maintenance, and safety of all of the equipment and systems used in the hospital setting. The biomedical professionals should be closely integrated into the purchasing, maintenance and ongoing safety monitoring of all devices. Although vendors are pleased to promote a product, the manufacturer's information literature should be obtained from an unbiased source such as the equipment periodical *Health Devices,* published by ECRI (formerly Emergency Care Research Institute, Plymouth Meeting, Pa.). The biomedical or hospital safety office of each hospital usually subscribes to this periodical.

Another useful source of information is the specialty pediatric hospital. Whether through inquiry at medical meetings or by direct solicitation, practitioners at these unique resource institutions are often willing to share their special expertise.

The following are useful principles for any equipment purchase:

1. New purchases should interface with equipment that is already present. Considerable cost savings can occur if the same or compatible equipment is used in all the perioperative areas, including the OR, PACU, and ICU. Another issue to consider is how the equipment will interface with automated record-keeping systems and other hospital information systems if they are present. If an automated recording device is a possible plan for the future, the equipment should be evaluated for how well it will interface with systems that will possibly be purchased. Another compatibility issue to carefully review is the software that is required to use the equipment. Review the product information carefully to identify the need for software upgrades and compatibility, which can be important for safety and cost-effectiveness.

2. Recognize that the salesperson is inherently biased.

3. Always test proposed equipment in the environment in which it will be used, with the personnel who will be using it. What appears attractive in a display as presented by a salesperson may not function well in practice. It is also important to test the device in unusual circumstances to see how well it performs. The use of simulation is becoming an important modality to test devices under normal and unusual circumstances. Human factors must be considered, such as how easy it is to use the equipment clinically (i.e., the user interface), and equally important, the safety of the equipment or product. Evaluate systems issues that could lead to error or misuse. Software-driven products are harder to test for how they may potentially fail when connected to existing systems and products in your workstations; always test new equipment in the environment where it will be used.

4. Do not use equipment for any purpose other than that for which it has been designed.

5. Have your hospital biomedical staff be intimately involved with the safety issues of your systems, as described earlier, and periodically check for electrical leakage and other safety issues.

6. Decide explicitly how the product will be maintained; are the biomedical professionals going to perform the necessary calibration, testing, and repair of the equipment, or is a member of your department going to take on this role? Spend the necessary resources to properly maintain the product; this is typically on the order of 10% of the cost of the device per year. Consider a maintenance contract, if available. Ask that the company ensure the future availability of parts and the compatibility of subsequent modifications or design evolutions with your equipment.

7. Consider the cost and quality of disposable components of the equipment. This can also have an impact on the safety and cost of the product.

8. If two products are comparable but one has local service facilities, that one may be the better choice.

9. If areas of special needs have been recognized, be as detailed as possible with specifications. For example, if a monitor is to be used strictly in the OR, it may be reasonable to operate it from wall power. Conversely, if the monitor is to serve in the OR, and also for transport between the operating theater and the recovery room or ICU, it must have internal battery backup.

The more precisely needs can be defined, the more accurate the comparisons will be between the bids of rival vendors. Note that any given piece of equipment will occasionally be out of service, whether for regular preventive maintenance or for some unanticipated repair, although it is often difficult in this era of cost containment to convince the hospital administration, this fact dictates a need for additional spare units.

## ANNOTATED REFERENCES

American Society of Anesthesiologists Task Force on Intraoperative Awareness. Practice advisory for intraoperative awareness and brain function monitoring. Anesthesiology 2006;104:847-64.
*Addresses the important issue of awareness and anesthesia and discusses recommendations including the possible use of depth of anesthesia monitors but making it clear that the data certainly do not support uniform use in children.*

Coté CJ, Liu LM, Szyfelbein SK, et al. Intraoperative events diagnosed by expired carbon dioxide monitoring in children. Can Anaesth Soc J 1986;33:315-20.
*This important article examines intraoperative events in children in which the diagnosis was aided by capnography.*

Coté CJ, Rolf N, Liu LM, et al. A single-blind study of combined pulse oximetry and capnography in children. Anesthesiology 1991;74:980-7.
*This sentinel article establishes adverse events in children undergoing anesthesia by the use of pulse oximetry and capnography.*

Eichhorn JH, Cooper JB, Cullen DJ, et al. Standards for patient monitoring during anesthesia at Harvard Medical School. JAMA 1986;256:1017-20.
*This is the key article developing uniform standards for anesthesia monitoring, which were adopted by the ASA.*

Lopez-Gil M, Brimacombe J, Alvarez M. Safety and efficacy of the laryngeal mask airway: a prospective survey of 1400 children. Anaesthesia 1996;51:969-72.
*This large-scale study demonstrates the safety and efficacy of LMA use in children that significantly changed anesthesia practice for infants and children.*

Morray JP, Geiduschek JM, Caplan RA, et al. A comparison of pediatric and adult anesthesia closed malpractice claims. Anesthesiology 1993;78:461-7.
*This key study helped define a subset of major anesthetic complications that had an impact through the judicial system.*

Olympio MA. Carbon dioxide absorbent desiccation safety conference convened by APSF. Anesth Patient Safety Found Newslett 2005;20.
*This article presents a detailed review and consensus report on the issues of interactions of anesthetic agents and carbon dioxide absorbents. Issues covered include fire with sevoflurane, carbon monoxide poisoning, and compound A. It also gives recommendations for managing these issues.*

Van der Spek AF, Spargo PM, Norton ML. The physics of lasers and implications for their use during airway surgery. Br J Anaesth 1988;60:709-29.
*Excellent detailed review of the concepts and safety issues (including airway fire) surrounding the use of lasers in anesthesia and airway surgery.*

## REFERENCES

Please see www.expertconsult.com.

# Medicolegal Issues

FREDERIC A. BERRY AND REBECCA W. WEST

MEDICOLEGAL ISSUES ARE a continuing concern for the anesthesia care team.[1-10] Taken too seriously, they can alter practice so that legal concerns rather than medical principles are in control. Taken too lightly, these concerns can transform into an adverse outcome disaster. This chapter enumerates some of the medicolegal issues faced in clinical anesthesia and describes ways to balance a safe practice with avoidance of litigation.

The opinions in this chapter reflect issues of practice within the United States, but the same issues are encountered in other countries. Two problems that were taken too seriously are provided as examples. First, the U.S. Food and Drug Administration (FDA) assigned a black box warning to droperidol because of droperidol-induced QT prolongation. Although these transient findings were associated only with high-dose droperidol, most anesthesiologists have stopped using even low-dose droperidol for fear of litigation if an adverse event occurs. Many hospitals have removed it from their formulary. As a consequence, this warning has resulted in the loss of a low-cost and demonstrably effective antiemetic from use in the perioperative period. Second, guidelines of The Joint Commission (TJC, formerly called the Joint Commission on Accreditation of Healthcare Organizations [JCAHO]) required anesthesia carts to be locked. Although intended to protect against entry by nonanesthesia personnel, this guideline created the potential for delayed access to essential rescue medications and airway equipment in an emergency situation as the anesthesia caregiver struggled to open the cart in a high-pressure situation. It is difficult for practitioners to place these kinds of issues in perspective.

## Policies and Procedures

The foundation of continually upgrading medical practice is knowledge of the medical literature. The use of evidence-based or outcomes-based studies allows safe and effective adjustments in practice. Practice within a department or hospital is further guided by its policies and procedures, and the applicable standard of care is predicated on the standards developed by the

American Society of Anesthesiologists (ASA) that are incorporated in the institutional policies and procedures. Departmental policies and procedures can be used to defend a practice but can also be used against the anesthesia caregiver if his or her practice is inconsistent with the rules and guidelines. Departmental policies and procedures must be written and available to all team members.

## Practice Areas of Controversy

There are several key areas of controversy about medical practice in the United States.

### DISCLOSURE OF UNANTICIPATED EVENTS

In July 2002, TJC released The Joint Commission Patient Safety Standards, which states, "Patients and, when appropriate, their families are to be informed about the outcomes of care, including unanticipated events." There is no clear information from TJC or agreement among institutions about what is required to meet this standard. Controversy exists over the types of conditions and the severity of the outcomes that should trigger this requirement for disclosure to the patient or family. Some suggest that it should be managed as part of the sentinel event process required by TJC, encouraging the health care facility to conduct a root cause analysis. Many health care facilities have created policies that determine when disclosure is required based on *when the patient is substantially harmed*. However, what constitutes substantial harm remains an issue of debate. Harm may be viewed from a patient or family's subjective view, or it may require a more concrete approach, such as the need for additional medical care or diagnosis of a patient's injury.

This TJC standard has created much discussion and different views about what information must be shared with patients and their families. The debate is likely to continue and produce more regulations in the future. In Canada, the judiciary has declared that health care providers should disclose any and all substantive risks related to a procedure that any reasonable individual would wish to know to provide informed consent for surgery or anesthesia. Being honest about care is always good policy, but a policy mandating disclosure of unanticipated events can be fraught with legal peril. If an adverse event occurs, the practitioner should seek risk management or legal advice to determine what information should be disclosed and the mechanism by which the information should be conveyed to the family. In many cases, avoiding a misunderstanding is crucial and may determine whether a frivolous lawsuit results.

## MANAGING ADVERSE OUTCOMES

An *adverse event* is an event that occurs during patient care that can cause an undesirable or unanticipated outcome. *Adverse outcomes* include the following:

- Patient injury
- Escalation of care
- Operational inefficiency

Patient injuries are adverse outcomes. A patient's care plan that is changed and requires an unanticipated escalation of care also is an adverse outcome. These situations may result in two types of discontent for patients and their families: disappointment in the medical outcome and disappointment with the way health care providers discuss the issues.

Preliminary research suggests that families and patients are much more distressed and disappointed when the health care providers who do not present straightforward, honest information or are perceived to be hiding the truth and facts. This has been the message of the Sorry Works movement, which advocates a proactive approach to patients and their families or legal guardians to fully disclose and discuss adverse events such as an untoward incident, therapeutic misadventure, iatrogenic injury, or undesirable outcome.

Communication must start with the medical or surgical team as they try to evaluate the unanticipated outcome, its cause, and its subsequent treatment. The entire team must fully comprehend the facts and come to a mutual understanding of the sequence and timing of the occurrence. Disclosures should be made after information has been gathered and analyzed and practitioners are comfortable with their position. Health care providers and risk management personnel should be consistently involved in the investigation and communication with the patient and family. Patients and their families desire and deserve a discussion of what transpired, an apology (e.g., Sorry Works program) that the unanticipated outcome occurred, and assurances that there will be ongoing dialogue to clarify the events and the future for the patient and family. Families also want reassurance that the event will not happen to other patients and that something good may come out of this experience through system improvements.

However, communication is often very difficult after such an event. Guilt, speculation based on incomplete information, and the need to blame something or someone can interfere with the investigative process and with communication with the patient and family.

In some centers, there is direct communication with the patient and family concerning an apology and settlement if it is determined there was an error by the hospital or the medical team. There is considerable support for apologizing for the unanticipated event, regardless of whether an error precipitated it. This process does not imply guilt, and most states have passed legislation to protect apologies from being used in litigation. However, a statement of fact that posits the cause of harm is not protected from discovery in a legal action. Rather, most legislation is intended to protect statements of empathy, such as, "I'm sorry you have experienced this unanticipated outcome." Other types of statements, such as, "I'm sorry the nurse or doctor gave too much of the medication," are not protected from discovery in a lawsuit.

In some cases, the cause of the unanticipated event cannot be ascertained in a timely manner to a reasonable degree of certainty (i.e., the legal standard that an expert must meet). When this occurs, a candid discussion of the situation should take place with the family members, and they should be informed that further investigation is anticipated, the results of which will be communicated to them. Families often seek legal assistance because an event occurred that resulted in questions that they think were not adequately addressed by the hospital or members of the medical team (e.g., an event occurred but no one followed up with the family to explain in lay terms what had transpired).

# Problem Areas for the Anesthesia Caregiver in Dealing with Children

## WHO SHOULD ANESTHETIZE CHILDREN?

Occasionally, when a child who has a significant medical problem presents for elective surgery at a location that does not routinely provide care for a child with a complex medical problem, an adverse outcome may result. The resulting lawsuit may be difficult to defend. The nature of the anesthesia services that are appropriate to perform in a particular location and the qualifications of those who provide the services must be addressed in the policies and procedures of the facility to avoid such an event, although guidelines in this area typically are arbitrary. Children in certain age groups with certain medical conditions and in certain types of emergencies should be designated for referral to a center that is more appropriately equipped or staffed to deliver expert care.

## ISSUES OF CONSENT AND ASSENT

Consent is a process that provides patients and families with sufficient information to allow them to make an informed decision about whether to proceed. The anesthesiologist must provide sufficient information in terms that are understandable by adults with a grade 5 or equivalent education. In most instances, the patient must be an adult (18 years of age or older) to consent to a procedure. However, in some states, minors are allowed to make decisions independently, without the participation of a parent or guardian. In some circumstances, the court has the authority to override the parent's rights based on the best interests of the patient. An example is providing lifesaving blood transfusions for children of parents who are Jehovah's Witnesses. Knowledge of these special provisions for minor consent in the state's laws is important. Virginia addressed the issue of pediatric assent and adult neglect in 2007 (VA code §63.2-100 et seq.). Assent may be given when a 14-year-old with a life-threatening condition or elective surgical issue is sufficiently mature to agree to the proposed treatment (see later for a complete definition). Dissent is when the child refuses. A judge threatened to remove a 14-year-old boy from his parents because they refused chemotherapy for lymphoma and instead trusted in prayer and herbal remedies.[11] These discussions and decisions are influenced by the severity of the issues and whether the procedure is elective or necessary to treat a life-threatening problem.

A common difficulty that arises with consent for minors is identifying the adult who is legally responsible to provide consent. State law governs who makes health care decisions for minors, and these laws vary from state to state. As an example, when the parents of a child are divorced, the custodial parent is most often the health care decision maker. However, this designation may vary based on the parents' custody agreement and according to state law. Reviewing the custody agreement is not feasible, and most often, the arbiter must rely on what a parent says. If questions or concerns remain regarding the appropriate decision maker, a facility administrator, risk manager, or legal advisor should be consulted. Lack of consent from the appropriate decision maker is the same as no consent, which can lead to liability.

The issue of assent deserves special consideration. *Assent* is defined as agreeing to something after thoughtful consideration. Children may not be able to assent to a procedure because they are unqualified to have thoughtful consideration. At what age and under what circumstances the minor's wishes should be followed because they mature enough to engage in thoughtful consideration is unclear. Unless there is a specific state law that grants decision-making authority to a minor in the current circumstances, the issue of a minor's assent is an ethical one, rather than a legal matter. Knowing whether the issue is ethical or legal is important in minimizing liability risks. If an older minor patient does not want a surgical procedure, a discussion should be held with the legally responsible adult, and any differences should be resolved before surgery. Even if the parents or guardians wish to proceed and the child does not, it is usually best to delay surgery and have a focused discussion to ensure that the wishes and thoughts of the minor patient have been considered and respected. Knowledge of state law and a low threshold for seeking consultation with the hospital lawyer are indicated in this situation.[11]

## COMMUNICATION WITH PATIENTS AND FAMILIES

The preoperative visit is an opportunity to develop rapport with the child and the family. It is important to establish a shared relationship, because children and families who feel they have communicated well preoperatively with their health care provider usually do not sue if there is an adverse outcome. Unfortunately, the time for preoperative evaluation and discussion is greatly limited. The physician should review the record before interviewing the child to focus the discussion and be aware of any underlying issues so that they can be directly addressed during the interview session. One technique for developing rapid communication with the child and the family is to recognize that they have major concerns about the surgical procedure, such as pain management, severe anxiety, nausea and vomiting, and safety issues. The anesthesiologist should clarify how he or she will address these issues preemptively so that the child and family understand that they have an advocate who can ensure safety and comfort throughout surgery (see also Chapter 4). The next step is to determine whether the child and family have specific concerns or suggestions. If the child has had multiple operations, the anesthesiologist should inquire whether any anesthetic technique has proved superior to others and incorporate it when possible. If the lines of communication have been opened before an unanticipated outcome occurs, it will be easier to maintain rapport, which reduces the likelihood of a lawsuit being filed.

## UNANTICIPATED EVENT RESULTING IN PATIENT INJURY OR DEATH

When a medical error in providing anesthesia results in injury or death, an anesthesia caregiver's worst nightmare has come true. One example of an unanticipated event is a perioperative allergic reaction such as latex anaphylaxis.[12] This event may be avoided by a careful preoperative history, and anticipation and preparation for this possibility can aid treatment. Little has been done to develop an algorithm for management of an adverse outcome that results in injury or death. An algorithm published by the Anesthesia Patient Safety Foundation emphasizes the need for an incident manager, who is the person who takes charge of the administrative aspects of the situation while the anesthesia caregivers continue to manage the patient's problems.[13]

Step 1 in this algorithm is taking care of the patient. Step 2 is making plans for dealing with the family, which can be done with the help of the surgical team, the anesthesia team, and/or the risk management team. Most anesthesia caregivers have an enormous emotional jolt of depression and guilt over the bad outcome because the American system of teaching through negative reinforcement suggests that they must have done something wrong. This likely response needs to be recognized by the anesthesia caregiver, so that when the issues are discussed with the family, the caregiver can avoid his or her own emotions taking over and instead focus on known facts while offering appropriate empathy to the family. Full disclosure (previously discussed) remains a critical issue, along with complete and accurate charting and discussion of the child's care with other key providers to ensure that there is a mutual understanding of what transpired and that the documentation is consistent.[14] The family will understandably be very emotional and angry. A note should be entered into the child's chart providing a summary of these family discussions.

Involved physicians should notify their medical malpractice insurance carrier in the event of a medical error or when there is a significant adverse outcome without error, but the family is very angry and threatening. The insurance carrier will conduct its own investigation of the event. If the carrier thinks there is a significant likelihood of a claim being filed, it may assign an attorney to represent the physician before a lawsuit is filed. The attorney can discuss the matter with confidentiality and offer advice as the facility's quality review takes place. Regardless of whether legal action will occur, it behooves the physician to record the precise sequence of events that occurred and then to sign, date, and file the narrative with his or her risk management office and insurance carrier.

Emotional support should be available for the involved care providers. The facility may have a mechanism to provide for this, but at the very least, the anesthesia department should have a plan. Sometimes, the anesthesia caregiver may need to seek professional help from psychologists or psychiatrists to help him or her cope with the emotional impact of the event. Doing so is important for the individual's well-being and professional career. These issues are well recognized, and assistance should be readily accessible for health care providers.[15]

# Reducing Unanticipated Events and Adverse Outcomes

## ANESTHESIA RECORD AND CHARTING

Poor anesthesia records and charting often lead to verdicts in favor of the plaintiff in lawsuits. A key strategy to avoid lawsuits is to ensure that documentation is complete, understandable, timely, and legible.[16,17] The use of automated anesthesia records (i.e., automated information management systems) is helpful in most cases.[16] We think that many malpractice cases that resulted in plaintiff verdicts could have been defended if greater attention had been paid to accurate documentation in the medical records. In the middle of a difficult or complicated case, it often is impossible to ensure thorough documentation of the events. However, many modern anesthesia monitors retain recent data (until they are powered off), allowing the anesthesia caregiver to retrieve information that is missing from the medical record and to document the details in a timely manner. When completed, a note that includes the date and time and the reason that the documentation was completed after the fact should be added to the child's record. Completing a record can only help as long as the entries added are accurate and properly identified.

The second area of record keeping is the anesthesia note about the incident. After some preparation, it is written in the chart and can be compared with what the other health care professionals state in their notes. The anesthesia note should be brief, factual, and without unsubstantiated conjecture regarding what occurred. Before writing the note, the anesthesia care provider should discuss the event with the nurses and the surgeons to clarify the sequence of events and any other pertinent information to ensure that there is a consistent understanding of what transpired. Occasionally, there is a difference of opinion regarding the events that occurred. It is preferable to clarify any discrepancies immediately rather than after inconsistent documentation has been entered into the child's chart and discussed with the parents. It is important to review notes written by other caregivers at the time of the event; for example drugs administered by the anesthesia care team that are entered in the anesthesia record must also be listed on the arrest log.

The international trend toward using automated medical information systems to create an anesthesia record has been encouraged by the provision of generous financial incentives. Whatever method is used, having a full, accurate, and timely record is essential for a successful defense. Correcting errors or making additions to the record should follow the policies and procedures of the department and hospital; on paper, errors should be indicated by using a single line through the text followed by the initials of the signer and the date. Errors should never be removed with whiteout or by removing the page. Late entries should be so indicated and initialed.

## MONITORING

The ASA has set standards for basic anesthesia monitoring (Table 52-1). Specific monitors must be used with all patients who are undergoing general anesthesia, regional anesthesia, or monitored anesthesia care. The anesthesia caregiver may waive certain monitoring requirements under extenuating circumstances. However, when this is done, the reasons should be stated in the anesthesia record. The second standard for basic anesthesia monitoring states, "during all anesthesia, the patient's oxygenation, ventilation, circulation, and temperature shall be continually evaluated." The ASA standards further state, "When the pulse oximeter is used, the variable-pitch pulse tone and the low-threshold alarm shall be audible to the anesthesiologist or the anesthesia care team personnel." The section on temperature monitoring provides this standard: "Every patient receiving anesthesia shall have temperature monitored when clinically significant changes in body temperature are intended, anticipated, or suspected." This can be interpreted to mean that brief procedures and certain anesthesia locations may make temperature monitoring unnecessary or impractical or potentially dangerous because of burns. It

is essential to document when and why standard monitoring procedures are not followed. If this is not done, it increases the risk of a decision against the defendant in a malpractice claim. Physicians also must be aware of changes in these standards. For example, expired carbon dioxide monitoring becomes a requirement for the updated ASA standard in 2012 for all patients receiving moderate or deep sedation by an anesthesiologist.[17a]

Delay in the recognition of ventilatory or circulatory difficulties is frequently caused by the anesthesia caregiver not believing that the monitor accurately reflects the child's condition. An example of this is the pulse oximeter. Movement and mechanical problems frequently interfere with pulse oximetry readings, suggesting that an erroneous reading is not a patient-related but rather an equipment-related problem. A basic premise of monitoring is that when there are changes in the monitor, the patient must be evaluated first and the monitor evaluated second. If the accuracy of the pulse oximeter is in doubt, the other monitors should be scanned to determine whether they show consistent changes. The most useful monitor for cross-checking the pulse oximeter is the capnograph. A decrease in the child's perfusion (i.e., cardiac output) reduces oxygen saturation and end-tidal carbon dioxide ($ETCO_2$). Another useful method is checking that the heart rates displayed on the pulse oximeter and the electrocardiogram are identical. If there is any question about the accuracy of the pulse oximeter after the child and the monitor readings have been carefully checked, the pulse oximeter sensor should be applied to the anesthesia caregiver to verify its function. Changes in $ETCO_2$ usually are caused by hyperventilation, hypoventilation, or decreased cardiac output.

Tracheal intubation may be problematic. When the breathing circuit is connected to the tracheal tube, the absence of the carbon dioxide waveform should immediately raise concerns that the tracheal tube is not in the trachea. If the functionality of the capnogram is in question, the caregiver can breathe into the sampling line for the capnogram, providing the child's oxygen saturation remains within normal limits. If the capnogram is functioning properly, laryngoscopy should be performed to confirm that the tracheal tube has passed through the vocal cords.

Another potential problem with monitoring systems is that the default alarms are set for adults, not children. This has resulted in the alarms sounding despite normal readings for children, prompting some clinicians to inappropriately disable the alarms. As irritating as these alarms may be, they should not be disabled but should be reset for the appropriate values. Alarms should only be temporarily silenced when the anesthesia caregiver knows the reason for the alarm and is taking steps to correct it. The alarms are set for the anesthesia caregiver and for the whole surgical team. If the anesthesia caregiver is having difficulty with the child's vital signs, the other members of the surgical team should be informed so that they can assist in correcting the problem. If the alarms are disabled, other members of the care team may not be aware that a problem is developing. If monitor alarms are ignored or turned off, the risk of a finding in favor of a plaintiff in a medical malpractice case increases dramatically.

## RESUSCITATION

If a child develops bradycardia and hypotension, the classic interventional sequence of airway, breathing, and circulation as taught by the American Heart Association should be followed. A common finding is that repeated doses of atropine are

## TABLE 52-1 Standards for Basic Anesthesia Monitoring

These standards apply to all anesthesia care, although in emergency circumstances, appropriate life support measures take precedence. The standards may be exceeded at any time based on the judgment of the responsible anesthesiologist. They are intended to encourage quality patient care, but observing them cannot guarantee any specific patient outcome. They are subject to revision from time to time, as warranted by the evolution of technology and practice. They apply to all general anesthesia, regional anesthesia, and monitored anesthesia care. This set of standards addresses only the issue of basic anesthesia monitoring, which is one component of anesthesia care. In certain rare or unusual circumstances, (1) some of these methods of monitoring may be clinically impractical, and (2) appropriate use of the described monitoring methods may fail to detect untoward clinical developments. Brief interruptions of continual* monitoring may be unavoidable. These standards are not intended for application to the care of the obstetric patient in labor or in the conduct of pain management.

1. STANDARD I

   Qualified anesthesia personnel shall be present in the room throughout the conduct of all general anesthesia, regional anesthesia, and monitored anesthesia care.

   1.1. Objective

   Because of the rapid changes in patient status during anesthesia, qualified anesthesia personnel shall be continuously present to monitor the patient and provide anesthesia care. In the event there is a direct known hazard (e.g., radiation) to the anesthesia personnel which might require intermittent remote observation of the patient, some provision for monitoring the patient must be made. In the event that an emergency requires the temporary absence of the person primarily responsible for the anesthesia, the best judgment of the anesthesiologist will be exercised in comparing the emergency with the anesthetized patient's condition and in the selection of the person left responsible for the anesthesia during the temporary absence.

2. STANDARD II

   During all anesthesias, the patient's oxygenation, ventilation, circulation, and temperature shall be continually evaluated.

   2.1. Oxygenation

       2.1.1. Objective: To ensure adequate oxygen concentration in the inspired gas and the blood during anesthesia

   2.2. Methods

       2.2.1. Inspired gas: During every administration of general anesthesia using an anesthesia machine, the concentration of oxygen in the patient's breathing system shall be measured by an oxygen analyzer with a low oxygen concentration limit alarm in use.[†]

       2.2.2. Blood oxygenation: During all anesthesias, a quantitative method of assessing oxygenation such as pulse oximetry shall be employed.[†] When the pulse oximeter is used, the variable-pitch pulse tone and the low-threshold alarm shall be audible to the anesthesiologist or the anesthesia care team personnel.[†] Adequate illumination and exposure of the patient are necessary to assess color.[†]

3. VENTILATION

   3.1. Objective

   To ensure adequate ventilation of the patient during anesthesia

   3.2. Methods

       3.2.1. Every patient receiving general anesthesia shall have the adequacy of ventilation continually evaluated. Observation of qualitative clinical signs such as chest excursion, observation of the reservoir breathing bag, and auscultation of breath sounds are useful methods. Continual monitoring for the presence of expired carbon dioxide shall be performed unless invalidated by the nature of the patient, procedure, or equipment. Quantitative monitoring of the volume of expired gas is strongly encouraged.[†]

       3.2.2. When an endotracheal tube or laryngeal mask is inserted, its correct positioning must be verified by clinical assessment and by identification of carbon dioxide in the expired gas. Continual end-tidal carbon dioxide analysis, in use from the time of endotracheal tube or laryngeal mask placement until extubation or removal or until initiating transfer to a postoperative care location, shall be performed using a quantitative method such as capnography, capnometry, or mass spectroscopy.[†] When capnography or capnometry is utilized, the end-tidal carbon dioxide alarm shall be audible to the anesthesiologist or the anesthesia care team personnel.[†]

       3.2.3. When ventilation is controlled by a mechanical ventilator, there shall be in continuous use a device that is capable of detecting disconnection of components of the breathing system. The device must give an audible signal when its alarm threshold is exceeded.

       3.2.4. During regional anesthesia (with no sedation) or local anesthesia (with no sedation), the adequacy of ventilation shall be evaluated by continual observation of qualitative clinical signs. During moderate or deep sedation, the adequacy of ventilation shall be evaluated by continual observation of qualitative clinical signs and monitoring for the presence of exhaled carbon dioxide unless precluded or invalidated by the nature of the patient, procedure, or equipment.

4. CIRCULATION

   4.1. Objective

   To ensure the adequacy of the patient's circulatory function during anesthesia

   4.2. Methods

       4.2.1. Every patient receiving anesthesia shall have the electrocardiogram continuously displayed from the beginning of anesthesia until preparing to leave the anesthetizing location.[†]

       4.2.2. Every patient receiving anesthesia shall have arterial blood pressure and heart rate determined and evaluated at least every 5 minutes.[†]

       4.2.3. Every patient receiving general anesthesia shall have, in addition to the above, circulatory function continually evaluated by at least one of the following: palpation of a pulse, auscultation of heart sounds, monitoring of a tracing of intraarterial pressure, ultrasound peripheral pulse monitoring, or pulse plethysmography or oximetry.

5. BODY TEMPERATURE

   5.1. Objective

   To aid in the maintenance of appropriate body temperature during anesthesia

   5.2. Methods

   Every patient receiving anesthesia shall have temperature monitored when clinically significant changes in body temperature are intended, anticipated, or suspected.

---

Modified from Standards for Basic Anesthesia Monitoring, Committee of Origin. Standards and practice parameters. Approved by the ASA House of Delegates on October 21, 1986, and last amended on October 20, 2010, with an effective date of July 1, 2011. Available at http://www.asahq.org/~/media/For%20Members/documents/Standards%20Guidelines%20Stmts/Basic%20Anesthetic%20Monitoring%202011.ashx (accessed July 2012).

*Continual means repeated regularly and frequently in steady, rapid succession, whereas continuous means prolonged without interruption at any time.

[†]Under extenuating circumstances, the responsible anesthesiologist may waive the requirements marked with a dagger; it is recommended that when this is done, it should be so stated (including the reasons) in a note in the patient's medical record.

administered before epinephrine; the latter is the first drug of choice for symptomatic bradycardia (see Chapter 39). A nurse or other assistant should accurately record the timing and doses of medications administered during these events, the names of the health care providers who were present, the timing of the call for additional help, and the name of the person who directed the resuscitation. In facilities without automated anesthesia records, the anesthesia record can often be filled in after the event if the monitor stores recent vital signs that can be interrogated later, and a note should be made in the record that this is how the data were retrieved.

After this type of event, the anesthesia machine should be quarantined and the monitors left on so that the stored data can be retrieved at a later time or date to better reconstruct the sequence of the events. If there is a problem retrieving data, a technician should be called to download the information to a permanent record. This should then be handed over to risk management for preservation. Any time discrepancy between the monitors and the operating room clock used to record events should be noted.

## Anatomy of a Medical Malpractice Case

### SERVICE OF PROCESS
A defendant physician in a medical malpractice case usually is served by an official of the court (often a local sheriff) with a copy of a medical malpractice lawsuit. The heading on the lawsuit indicates the location of the court where the lawsuit has been filed and the name of the person (i.e., plaintiff) who is filing the litigation, along with the names of any other defendants.

Service of process may be accepted by anyone, but the person accepting service must sign the suit papers as accepting them on behalf of the defendant. Others at the office and those at home must immediately notify the defendant of having received a lawsuit. The defendant should then immediately notify his or her medical malpractice insurance carrier that a lawsuit has been served, and then fax a copy of the suit papers to the insurance company. If an attorney has not already been assigned, one will be soon. The insurer undertakes its own investigation and requests a copy of the medical record if it does not already have it. The hospital administration should also be informed because the hospital also may become a defendant.

### COURT PLEADINGS
Different states use different names for a civil claim filed in court (as is the case for most medical malpractice insurance claims). It may be called a complaint, motion for judgment, or another name. The attorney must file a responsive pleading within the time specified by state law, usually 21 days. If a defendant does not file a response in the required time frame, a default judgment may be entered. After a lawsuit is filed, all further interactions between plaintiffs and defendants must be through their respective attorneys. It is inappropriate for a defendant to call a plaintiff or vice versa.

### DISCOVERY
The next step in the legal process is called the discovery process. It can continue for years. Discovery provides an opportunity to investigate the plaintiff's claim and the defendant's responses. The initial step in discovery is to file interrogatories, which are written questions answered under oath. The attorney sends them to the defendant with a deadline for returning them. The

defendant's answers are reviewed by his or her attorney, who may discuss them further. The final answers must be signed by the defendant and notarized. If needed, the answers may be amended later. However, if they are not amended and the answers are different from those given in a deposition at a later date or at trial, the interrogatory responses may be used to attack the defendant's credibility. It is vitally important to answer the interrogatories as accurately as possible. The defense also is asked to identify all witnesses they will use, including experts and their expected opinions to be testified to at trial. The number and detail of questions vary from case to case and attorney to attorney. The attorney may instruct the defendant not to answer some questions based on a legal objection. The defense attorney also poses interrogatories to the plaintiff.

In addition to interrogatories, the attorneys may request the defendant to produce certain documents. The attorney works with the defendant to determine if there are objections to these documents and will make any needed objections.

Dispositions constitute the most important tool in the discovery process. All witnesses, whether experts or general witnesses, may be deposed, in addition to all parties to the lawsuit. In a deposition, questions usually come only from the attorney on the opposing side. The defendant's attorney does not want to reveal information or strategy for your defense, so his or her questions will be reserved for trial. Objections to questions are usually made but reserved for argument later if the matter goes to trial. These objections are a distraction to the defendant but are a part of the legal process. Occasionally, the issue is so important that the matter may be taken to the judge during or shortly after the deposition. However, during a deposition, the attorney makes his or her objection and then instructs the client to answer the question.

The importance of the deposition in developing a defense cannot be underestimated. The physician must know the chart, his or her entries, and the medical issues of the case. Several points should be remembered during a deposition. The defendant should give short, concise answers, not try to educate the lawyers or impress them with a superb record as a health care practitioner. Persons being deposed should be prepared to avoid traps. For example, the attorney may ask, "Do you have an independent recollection of the case?" The lawyer does not want to know if the person generally remembers the tragedy of the event but instead wants specific details of the case. Because depositions usually occur 2 to 5 years after the event, it is often difficult to remember the details of a case, and the person being deposed should rely primarily on the patient's chart. Offering a best guess is never a good idea, and if a certain detail cannot be recalled, the person should answer, "I do not recall."

An example of such a case was provided in the deposition of a nurse anesthetist defendant, who gave excellent answers. She said that she remembered the tragedy of the event but that she did not remember any details. She was asked many times about her independent recollection of the case. Her answer was always the same: "The record speaks for itself. The times may be off a little bit, but the sequence of events is [recorded] as they occurred." The total time of her deposition was 1.5 hours. The anesthesiologist defendant in the case said that he did have an independent recollection, and he tried to remember details of the events. By the end of his deposition, which took 5.5 hours, he had tied himself completely in knots. The nurse anesthetist's deposition also demonstrates the importance of having an accurate chart that is complete.

## 52

During depositions, the defendant may become angry or frustrated with the plaintiff's attorney and the legal process. When anger becomes part of the defendant's answers, the deposition often becomes protracted and confrontational. This can lead to answers that are not well thought out and consistent with records and sometimes result in angry outbursts by the defendant.

The discovery process may take place over several years. After it is complete, a case may proceed to trial. The purpose of discovery is to avoid any surprises at trial by revealing as much of the evidence as possible in advance of trial. This extensive discovery process leads to most medical malpractice cases being withdrawn or settled before trial.

## TRIAL

At trial, the plaintiff has the burden of proving his or her case by the preponderance of the evidence. The jury will decide if this burden is met, which means that the jury members must find that it is more than 50% likely that negligence occurred.

A trial begins with selection of the jury. In civil cases, there are seven jurors. The trial begins with the opening statement of the attorney for the plaintiff, followed by the opening statement of the lawyer for the defendant. These statements are not evidence but preview for the jury what evidence the attorneys expect to present.

The plaintiff's case is presented first, which often means that the defendant is called by the plaintiff as an adverse witness. If so, the defendant should give short, concise answers that respond only to the question asked to avoid being boxed into an opinion or unintended admission. All witnesses called by the plaintiff are first questioned by the plaintiff's counsel. Defense's counsel may then cross-examine a plaintiff's witness. After that, the plaintiff's attorney may have a redirect examination. On cross-examination, leading questions may be used, such as, "Isn't it true that...." At this time, the attorney can go back to the prior answers to interrogatories and deposition testimony to make the defendant appear that he is contradicting himself or changing his story, which is why it is vital to keep the answers to all questions precise and concise.

At the completion of the plaintiff's case, the defendant's lawyer may move (i.e., make a motion to strike) the court to dismiss the plaintiff's case if all the elements of the claim made have not been established. A motion to strike is rarely granted by a court. Trial usually proceeds to the defendant's evidence, which seeks to rebut the evidence introduced by the plaintiff. New evidence may also be introduced in an effort to provide an alternative theory of what occurred.

At the close of the defendant's evidence, the plaintiff has one last opportunity to put on evidence that rebuts the defendant's case. The testimony by these rebuttal witnesses must be confined to contradicting evidence of the defendant.

Before a case goes to a jury, the defendant's attorney has another opportunity to ask the court to dismiss the case on the basis of the plaintiff's failure to establish his or her case. The attorneys also submit jury instructions to the judge, who selects from those submitted as he or she deems appropriate. These instructions are read to the jury by the judge before they enter into deliberations.

The last information provided to the jury is the closing statement of attorneys. These statements are not evidence but rather summations of what the attorneys think their cases showed. Jury deliberations may last minutes, hours, or days. At this point, all the defendant can do is wait because the verdict rests with the jurors or judges, depending on the jurisdiction.

## APPEAL

The plaintiff or defendant may appeal a case, although appeals are rare. There must be a legal basis for the appeal rather than an appeal based on the merits of the case. Rarely, an appeal may be granted because there is reasonable question that the evidence did not support the jury's decision. Because the courts give extreme deference to the jury, overturning the decision solely on this basis is unlikely. Most often, appeal is based on a mistake of law by the trial judge.

If the appeal is granted, an appellate judge usually hears oral arguments by the attorneys. No witnesses are presented. The arguments are based on evidence and events in the trial court. The appellate court may decide that there is no basis for appeal, remand the case for retrial in the lower court with instructions on the applicable law, or dismiss the case altogether. How many levels of appeal there are depends on the particular state in which the case is being heard or whether it is heard in federal court.

# Response to Being Sued for Medical Malpractice

Defendants should do the following:
- Review the record
- Analyze the case
- Look for other relevant documents
- Review the literature
- Identify experts in the field who might be willing to help with the defense
- Make a list of fact witnesses
  Defendants should *not* do the following:
- Discuss the case with anyone (including codefendants) but legal counsel, a member of defense team (which may include a psychologist or psychiatrist), or a spouse
- Change the records
- Accept calls from other attorneys or the patient or their family members
- Talk to media

The attorney and anesthesia caregiver should act as a team. The anesthesia caregiver should become educated about the issues of the case so that he or she and the defense expert can educate the defense attorney; often, this can be in the form of teaching physiology and pharmacology and providing questions to counter opinions raised by the experts for the plaintiff. Open and frank communication is essential. The anesthesia caregiver should be kept advised of all developments through correspondence and periodic meetings. Tactical and strategic considerations should be frequently discussed and decisions jointly made. The attorney and anesthesia caregiver need to work together to ensure a strong and effective defense.

Litigation stress syndrome is a well-recognized effect of being involved in a lawsuit. The emotional toll a lawsuit takes on the defendant and his or her family should not be ignored. The defendant needs appropriate support systems in place throughout the litigation process.[18] This involves family, colleagues, and occasionally, a psychiatrist. The most difficult emotion to deal with in the course of a trial is anger when it becomes apparent that the focus is less on the truth and more on how the lawyers can persuade the jury to their line of reasoning. Emotional stress also is engendered by the qualifications or lack of qualifications of the plaintiff's experts, which sometimes surprise those present with distortions or exaggerations of fact.[19]

## Summary

The manner in which anesthesia caregivers interface with the law in their daily practice of medicine varies greatly. The need for a pediatric anesthesia caregiver to be informed of legal issues arising from his or her practice has become essential. Educational materials to keep current with pertinent legal issues are a necessary part of any practice. Other legal issues, such as billing regulations and regulations that govern the relationships between group practices and health care facilities, are beyond the scope of this chapter, but they are equally important to understand to prevent legal challenges.

## ANNOTATED REFERENCES

Davidson AJ, Smith KR, Blusse van Oud-Alblas HJ, et al. Awareness in children: a secondary analysis of five cohort studies. Anaesthesia 2011;66:446-54.

*This paper defines the incidence of awareness under anesthesia among children, which may be greater than among adults, but further study is needed.*

Eichhorn JH. Organized response to major anesthesia accident will help limit damage: update of "adverse event protocol" provides valuable plan. APSF Newslett 2006;Spring:11. Available at http://www.apsf.org/newsletters/pdf/spring2006.pdf (accessed July 2012).

*This selected article from an issue of the Anesthesia Patient Safety Foundation's newsletter discusses management of an adverse event, including the adverse event protocol.*

Feldman JM. Do anesthesia information systems increase malpractice exposure? Results of a Survey. Anesth Analg 2004;99:840-3.

*This paper demonstrates with a small cohort that an automated record can be more helpful in defending an anesthesiologist if an adverse event occurs, primarily because there is more precise recording of the event at the time of occurrence compared with a record being completed hours after the event has occurred.*

Gazoni FM, Durieux ME, Wells L. Life after death: The aftermath of perioperative catastrophes. Anesth Analg 2008;107:591-600.

*This paper reviews surveys that dealt with physicians' attitudes toward a perioperative death. Cases included medical students, residents, interns, and attending physicians. It shows that perioperative catastrophes have a major effect on health care providers and suggests ideas about how to handle the aftermath of these catastrophes.*

Stemland C. Parental consent by proxy and adolescent assent for pediatric cases: implications for the pediatric anesthesiologist. Society for Pediatric Anesthesia (SPA) News 2010;Fall:8-9.

*This short paper offers a timely discussion of the issues of assent for medical decisions about the care of the adolescent patient.*

## REFERENCES

Please see www.expertconsult.com.

# Simulation in Pediatric Anesthesia

## CHRISTINE L. MAI, DEMIAN SZYLD, AND JEFFREY B. COOPER

| | |
|---|---|
| Simulation-Based Training in Anesthesia | Sites for Simulation |
| What Is Simulation? | Applications of Simulation in Anesthesia |
| Technologies Used in Simulation | Comparing Traditional Learning |
| Partial Task Trainers | with Simulation-Based Learning |
| Human Patient Simulators | Aspects of a High-Fidelity Simulation |
| Standardized Patient | What is a Debriefing? |
| Hybrid Simulation | Using Simulation for Evaluation |
| Screen-Based Simulator: Virtual Patients and Immersive | Challenges in Using Simulation |
| Environments | Future of Simulation |

THE FIELD OF PEDIATRIC anesthesia has become increasingly subspecialized, with unique challenges that demand high-quality teaching and training. Pediatric anesthesia is a subspecialty that has become increasingly refined and technically advanced, with the advancement of complex surgical techniques and patients with a low tolerance for error.[1] Radiologic progress and interventions have revolutionized the field to include caring for children in remote sites outside of the operating theaters. In many countries, tertiary pediatric services are becoming increasingly centralized, whereas medical working hours have been reduced, leading to a situation where there is a decline in exposure to difficult pediatric cases and emergencies for those who are not pediatric specialists. There is an inverse correlation between the level of specialization and perioperative morbidity and mortality associated with pediatric anesthesia.[2] Furthermore, a significant proportion of pediatric surgical procedures will continue to be performed outside tertiary centers, at community hospitals or outpatient surgical centers where the volume-to-outcome relationship may not be favorable.[3] The growth and increased sophistication of pediatric anesthesia, as well as the regionalization of specialty care, has profound implications for the ability to train anesthesiologists in the safe and effective delivery of routine and emergency pediatric anesthesia. Early portions of a trainee's learning curve are inconsistent with the demands of safe and efficient patient care, thereby posing challenges for the medical education infrastructure. Advancements in simulation education techniques and technology have led to a new paradigm in training and assessment. These advances provide opportunities to improve diagnostic and decision-making skills for common as well as rare events.

Current medical training emphasizes basic science knowledge and leaves most of the clinical practice to an apprenticeship model. The focus has been on individual knowledge and skills rather than on performance or clinical team dynamics. Once a clinician has completed training, the required level of continued education declines, both in structure and formality. Within the past decade, there has been rapid progress in simulation in health care training for purposes of improving patient safety and quality of care. Interest in simulation in health care derived from the historical utility of simulation for training purposes in nonmedical industries, such as commercial aviation, nuclear power production, and the military.[4] Similar to health care, these industries are known to be associated with hazards and complexities that benefit from simulation training. Many of the concepts in health care simulators, including systematic training, rehearsal, performance assessment, situational awareness, and team interactions, have been adopted from aviation flight simulators. Given that crises in pediatric anesthesia are rare, difficult to predict, and that trainees are expected to be able to successfully manage these situations, simulation technology can fill important gaps in many curricula. In this chapter, we review how simulation is applied in pediatric anesthesiology by describing its use for learning and practicing basic and advanced skills, and by defining key types of technologies and teaching approaches with illustrative videos.

## Simulation-Based Training in Anesthesia

In 1987, Gaba and colleagues identified gaps in decision making and crisis management in anesthesia training. They noted that diagnostic decisions tended to be relatively static.[5-7] However, in the complex, rapidly changing, time-pressured environment of the operating room (OR), anesthesiologists are challenged beyond static decision making, especially when identifying and resolving crises and leading interdisciplinary teams. As a result, the term *anesthesia crisis resource management* (ACRM), modeled after the Crew Resource Management of commercial aviation,[5-7] was developed. These investigators established a framework and curriculum to teach individual and team leadership skills, along with effective communication styles. ACRM provided anesthesia trainees with tools that were similar to those that made the complex dynamic world of aviation safer in the areas of decision making and crisis resource management. These skills were not systematically taught during anesthesia residency training.

ACRM was an outgrowth of the patient safety movement that began in anesthesia in the early 1980s in America. In the late 1980s, research grant funding from the Anesthesia Patient Safety Foundation (APSF) supported the early development of several forms of human patient simulators (HPS). Further publicity and advocacy from APSF propelled anesthesiology to the forefront of specialties in the application and adoption of simulators, with strong patient safety implications through education (residents attempting new skills for the first time on a manikin), training (teamwork, critical event management, and situational awareness), and research (human performance).[8] Today, simulation in anesthesiology is global, with emphasis not only on medical knowledge and skills training, but also on ACRM, disaster training, debriefing, and patient safety. The American Board of Anesthesiology now requires at least one simulation-based course to satisfy its Maintenance of Certification in Anesthesia requirement.[9] In some institutions, such training is required as a condition of credentialing for practice and insurance coverage.

## What Is Simulation?

Simulation is a *technique* to replace or amplify real experiences with guided experiences that evoke or replicate aspects of the real world. Simulation is enabled by a diverse set of emergent *technologies*.[4] The application of simulation in the health care field is focused on education and training of clinicians. *Education* emphasizes knowledge, skills, and introduction to the actual work. *Training* emphasizes the actual tasks and work to be performed.[4] The term "simulator" is used in the health care field to refer to a device that represents a simulated patient, and interacts appropriately in response to the actions of the simulation participant. In aviation, pilots are seated in the cockpit of a flight simulator whereas in health care, clinicians are in a simulated OR, emergency ward, or patient floor in simulated clinical scenarios, caring for a simulated "patient" experiencing a critical or otherwise challenging event.

Participants in a simulation are "immersed" into a task or setting to the extent necessary to achieve the learning objectives. This may be conducted in a normal classroom or in an environment that extensively replicates the real world. In the latter case, participants are asked to "suspend disbelief" and to interact and speak as they would do in their everyday jobs.[4] Most importantly, it is incumbent on those who create and implement the simulation to create sufficient *realism* to enable the learner to feel the reality of the situation and respond accordingly. Thus the participant agrees to accept the "fiction contract" with their instructors.[10,11]

Participants in a simulation scenario experience *realism* in three distinct domains: *physical, conceptual, and emotional*.[10] Simulations that address all three domains are more likely to instill the intended learning objectives. A high degree of realism appropriate for the specific learning objectives is central to ensure that the learners become mentally and physically engaged. The *physical* properties of the simulator (the patient) and the clinical environment (the simulation room, center, or OR), such as weight, flexibility, tensile strength, and color, are important for developing kinesthetic awareness and muscle memory. For example, the weight of the head and force required to effectively perform laryngoscopy are important for teaching tracheal intubation, whereas the rubbery feel of the manikin skin is not. *Conceptual realism* refers to the causal relationships observed in the scenario, such as a decrease in oxygen saturation during a period of apnea or the resolution of hypotension after an appropriate intravenous fluid bolus. High conceptual reality enhances clinical reasoning and decision making. Finally, *emotional* and *experiential* fidelity is achieved when participants experience familiar and authentic feelings, such as "emotional activation," anxiety, stress, fear, or excitement. Ultimately, realism in simulation is perceived as "an exciting simulation that captures the imagination, triggering

physiological responses and execution of ingrained clinical algorithms."[10] Although realism is important, investigators emphasize that, "when learning is the focus, the flawless recreation of the real world is less important." It is necessary to find circumstances that help participants learn, rather than circumstances that exactly mimic a clinical situation.[11] The degree of realism desired for a successful simulation education program is an amount sufficient to achieve the intended learning outcomes.

## Technologies Used in Simulation

### PARTIAL TASK TRAINERS

Partial task trainers are manikins or models (e.g., suturing board, IV arm, airway head, etc.) designed to allow participants to practice clinical skills and tasks (Fig. 53-1). They should be reliable, robust, and medically meaningful. Usually they represent a portion of a person rather than the whole. Although many are simple devices designed for learning or practicing a specific procedure (e.g., suturing, IV insertion, laryngoscopy, or intraosseous access), some are coupled with computers, robotic interphases, and digital graphics to provide sophisticated partial task simulators designed for learning or practicing more involved procedures (e.g., bronchoscopy and endoscopy, endovascular catheterization, or laparoscopic skills). These models are particularly useful for teaching invasive, risky, and rare procedures (e.g., emergency cricothyrotomy, transvenous pacing, or pericardiocentesis), complex psychomotor skills requiring repetitive training (e.g., ultrasound guided central venous catheterization or awake fiberoptic intubation), or those that are safe, but create increased anxiety for either the learner or the patient and their family (e.g., urethral catheterization, IV insertion, or arterial puncture), where coaching and deliberate practice can be done in a simulated environment.[12] Curricula that use these types of training devices focus on skills training at varying levels of skill goals, rather than a particular situation. For example, cricothyrotomy training on a partial task simulator aims to teach the procedure, regardless of the indication (e.g., angioedema, burns, obstructing mass, or hemorrhage). Specific partial task trainers for simulating aspects of children include products to learn or practice lumbar puncture, peripheral IV insertion, intraosseous needle insertion, laryngoscopy and intubation, umbilical vein and artery catheterization, and cardiopulmonary resuscitation (Video 53-1).

### HUMAN PATIENT SIMULATORS

An HPS is a representation of the human body constructed on a manikin, typically made of plastic and metal, without a bony skeletal frame. Although popularized in the 1990s, the first manikin-based simulator (SimOne) was developed at University of Southern California in the 1960s and was intended to facilitate medical education and training.[13] Adult HPSs became commercially available in the early 1990s; the first high-fidelity pediatric simulator was introduced in 1999. The METI PediaSIM (Medical Education Technologies, Inc., Sarasota, Fla.) represented a child between 5 and 7 years of age. Two models of integrated infant HPS became available in 2005: the METI BabySIM and the Laerdal SimBaby (Laerdal Medical, Stavanger, Norway) (Fig. 53-2). Both models exhibited standard vital signs and variable airway features (e.g., tongue swelling and laryngospasm), breathing patterns and sounds (e.g., retractions to illustrate upper airway obstruction, breath sounds [wheezing], and pneumothorax), cardiovascular features (e.g., heart sounds and peripheral pulses

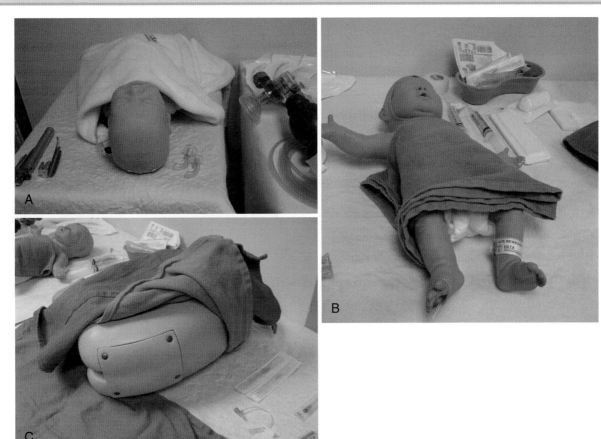

**FIGURE 53-1** Examples of partial task trainers to practice (**A**) intubation in neonates (Laerdal SimNewB [Laerdal Medical, Stavanger, Norway]), (**B**) peripheral intravenous placement (Nita Newborn Model #1800 Infant Venous Access Simulator [VATA, Canby, Ore.]), and (**C**) central neuraxial techniques (M43C Pediatric LP Simulator [Kyoto Kagaku, Kyoto, Japan]).

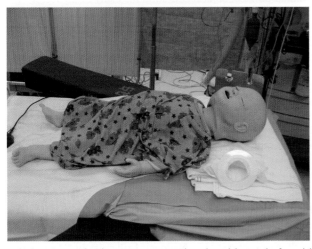

**FIGURE 53-2** An infant human patient simulator (Laerdal SimBaby [Laerdal Medical, Stavanger, Norway]) exhibits standard vital signs, variable airway features (tongue swelling, laryngospasm), breath sounds (retraction, wheezing), cardiovascular features (palpable pulses, heart sounds), and others (abdominal sounds, bulging fontanelle).

[diminished or absent]), and others (e.g., abdominal sounds and distension, and fontanelle bulging). Both infant simulators produce a variety of monitor signals and allow extensive treatment interventions (e.g., intubation, laryngeal mask and nasogastric tube insertion, intravenous and intraosseous cannulation, and thoracocentesis).[14] Incorporated into the clinical setting or

in a simulation room outfitted with biomedical equipment and teams of health care providers, the HPS can provide a high degree of clinical authenticity and realism to facilitate participants to fully engage in the care of the simulated patient. Typically, participants in simulation scenarios reflect on their performance during the simulation, for the purpose of sustaining and improving their practice with an instructor, in the process termed *debriefing*[15] (see Video 53-1).

## STANDARDIZED PATIENT

In some facilities, actors who are trained to represent a patient's condition (e.g., symptoms or social situation) and who are very reliable raters of clinicians' behaviors are used as standardized patients. It is common practice to use standardized patients when a simulation session focuses on interviewing, counseling, and examining a patient. Now a required part of the medical licensing exam in the United States (USMLE Step II Clinical Skills), Objective Structured Clinical Exams (OSCEs) are common in many undergraduate and graduate medical education programs. The OSCEs have been incorporated into the national board certification exams for anesthesiology in Israel.[16] In pediatrics, actors are more likely to play the role of a parent (e.g., a standardized parent) and team members (e.g., a standardized nurse), although child actors have also been reported, as well as the use of youthful appearing actors who role-play adolescents.[17] Going beyond standardized patients, actors can be employed as standardized nurses, surgeons, even residents for the purpose of teaching supervision skills (see Video 53-1).

## HYBRID SIMULATION

*Hybrid simulation* refers to a technique of combining any of the above simulators into a single activity. For instance, in the OR, the simulation scenario may take shape using a combination of three elements: an HPS, to provide the representation of the patient and clinical feedback in the form of the physiologic parameters that can be measured and monitored; a partial task simulator deployed to integrate a surgical skill that allows cutting and suturing of tissue; and an actor trained to represent the patient's parent and enact family presence during resuscitation.

*Hybrid learning* refers to the combination of web-based instruction incorporated with physical skills practice and validation for teaching and learning. As the field of simulation education has matured, it has become clearer that learning with simulation should not be isolated. Integration of simulation into course curricula has given way to hybrid learning techniques. For example, clinicians may complete precourse work to strengthen or activate prior knowledge in the days leading up to a simulation session. Subsequently, a simulation session can take place in the simulation-training environment, allowing for integration of new skills and attitudes. This model allows participants to obtain background knowledge to assist them with understanding the planned simulated procedural skills, which can save time and resources when conducting a training course for large numbers of clinicians (e.g., central line maintenance for nursing staff) (see Video 53-1).

## SCREEN-BASED SIMULATOR: VIRTUAL PATIENTS AND IMMERSIVE ENVIRONMENTS

Virtual patients are generally two-dimensional avatars on the computer screen that serve to help learners maneuver through clinical situations or perform a task, such as the proper technique for taking a patient's medical history. They can also be incorporated into OSCE training when standardized patients are not available. For example, the American Heart Association uses a screen-based simulation to teach and assess knowledge from advanced cardiac life support and pediatric advanced life support courses.[18]

Immersive environments, such as Second Life (Linden Lab, San Francisco), Advanced Disaster Management Simulator (Environmental Tectonics Corp., Orlando) and multi-user virtual environments, have been used to teach disaster management using interactive virtual simulation systems.[19-21] Other examples include Gas Man (Med Man Simulations, Inc., Boston) for teaching, simulating, and experimenting with the uptake and distribution of inhalational anesthetics,[22] and a virtual reality simulator for training in regional anesthesia.[23] Although virtual reality has been used in advanced cardiac life support and pediatric advanced life support education,[18] the use of virtual reality simulators in anesthesia is novel and not yet widely incorporated into curricula (see Video 53-1).

## Sites for Simulation

The growth of simulation education centers has been exponential from the mid-1990s through the first decade of this century. There is no exact count, but there are at least 1000 centers worldwide incorporated within medical schools and residency training programs in hospital settings, as well as nursing schools and allied health professions colleges.[24] Different settings of simulation education centers include: hospital-based or medical school-based simulation centers, freestanding simulation facilities, and in situ simulation located within the actual clinical work environment

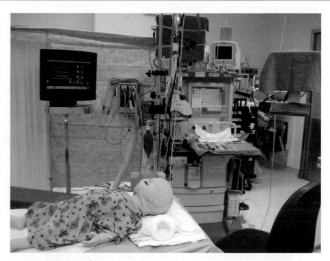

**FIGURE 53-3** Simulation in situ setup in an operating room at Massachusetts General Hospital. A human patient simulator (Laerdal SimBaby [Laerdal Medical, Stavanger, Norway]) is used in this setting.

(Fig. 53-3). Dedicated simulation facilities, either within an existing medical institution or a freestanding center, have been constructed throughout the industrialized world to house high-technology simulator equipment, such as manikins, laparoscopic surgical equipment, robotics, and audiovisual laboratories. For example, the Treadwell Library at Massachusetts General Hospital has a dedicated simulation learning lab that houses simulation equipment, high-fidelity manikins, partial task trainers, and simulators for students, residents, and faculty training. Although simulation education centers are expensive and require significant manpower to operate, they may serve to replace some traditional forms of clinical education for many of the reasons that simulation is generally becoming more accepted (e.g., patient safety, clinical production efficiency, and lack of standardized curricula in the apprenticeship mode). An in situ simulation location involves setting up the simulator equipment, trainers, and trainees within the actual work environment, such as the OR, emergency room, or intensive care unit. The benefits of an in situ simulation include imitation of the work environment with equipment, personnel and surroundings that are real and familiar to the trainee. Disadvantages of in situ simulation involve availability of the location, impromptu setup of equipment to operate in different locations, and increased manpower to help with set up and relocation (Table 53-1).

## Applications of Simulation in Anesthesia

Concern for patient safety has been growing since the Institute of Medicine of the U.S. National Academies of Sciences published a report, *To Err is Human*, which publicized medical errors in patient care.[25] Since then, numerous efforts and interventions have been implemented to mitigate medical hazards and improve patient safety.[26] The demand for pediatric simulation curricula is substantial, presumably driven by the perceived imbalance between the potential difficulties of incidents and emergencies, and the everyday clinical routine, particularly for anesthetizing infants and neonates. Simulator-based courses can effectively supplement bedside teaching in pediatric anesthesia for trainees, non–tertiary-center anesthetists, and pediatric anesthesiologists alike. Newer infant simulators can generate a wide range of

**TABLE 53-1** Features of Simulation-Based Education by Location

| | Distance | Features | Limitations | Operations |
|---|---|---|---|---|
| **Hospital Simulation Center** | *Pro*: Trainees available before during and after clinical duties. Other disciplines and professions available. *Con*: Interruptions may occur. Risk of simulation equipment or medication leakage back to clinical environment. | Multimodal education possible (human patient simulators, task trainer, standardized patients, hybrids). Hospital name, numbers, and infrastructure preserved. | Clinical environment may not be accurately represented (outdated equipment, medications not real). | Real estate might be at premium. Equipment and supplies must be ordered separately. |
| **Freestanding Simulation Center** | *Pro*: Greatest separation between working and learning environment. Psychological safety and confidentiality are easier to preserve *Con*: Environment and equipment may be significantly different from clinical practice. | Audio and video recording without compromising patient confidentiality. Ability to recreate different clinical environments. | Generic features required to represent multiple hospital systems may lead to environments that are significantly different from the clinical environment. | Must fund and staff independent organization. May need to pay for transportation. Equipment and supply chain not readily available. |
| **In Situ Simulation** | *Pro*: Shortest distance to travel. Participants present for work. *Con*: Interruptions are frequent. Family and other practitioners may be disturbed or bothered. Risk of simulation equipment or medication leakage back to clinical environment. | Ability to train in the intended environment enables evaluation of system-level safety features. Findings are readily applicable. | High acuity or census may lead to cancellation of sessions. Emergency equipment may go out of service (MH cart). Equipment may be used for clinical practice during the session (bronchoscope or Glidescope). Difficult to obtain video recording and guarantee patient confidentiality. | Low facility cost (If not charged). Training at work requires no overtime. Disposable material and restocking, including medications, time, and effort to transport equipment to location. |

*MH*, Malignant hyperthermia.

53

pediatric case scenarios and have the advantage of being mobile for in situ simulation in the OR, intensive care unit, or emergency department setting. Training and managing low-frequency, high-risk cases (e.g., malignant hyperthermia, difficult airway, venous air embolism, or neonatal resuscitation) can be effectively performed on these manikins.[27] In addition, evaluation of new procedures and technology or simulation of new hospital environments can be safely performed on these manikins before involving humans. For example, the anesthesia residents at Massachusetts General Hospital are taught basic pediatric anesthesia skills and airway management during a simulation orientation at the beginning of their dedicated pediatric month. This in situ simulation curriculum occurs monthly in the Massachusetts General Hospital ORs for residents new to the rotation, before they care for children. A combination of partial task trainers, standardized "parents," and high-fidelity HPS infant manikins are used to orient and teach residents about the typical flow of a pediatric anesthesia case.

## Comparing Traditional Learning with Simulation-Based Learning

The medical learner at each level of higher education (i.e., undergraduate, graduate, or postgraduate) is an adult learner. An adult learner is one who learns by several methods for different reasons at various stages in his or her education.[28] Adult learning theory teaches that active learning (with simulation) is an effective way to prepare for the dynamic clinical environment.[29] Five adult learning principles to help guide medical learners have been described[28-30] (Table 53-2).

**TABLE 53-2** Five Adult Learning Principles That Apply to the Medical Learner

1. Adult learners need to know why they are learning
2. Adult learners are motivated by the need to solve problems
3. The previous experiences of adult learners must be respected and built upon
4. The educational approach should match the diversity and background of adult learners
5. Adult learners need to be involved actively in the process

Modified from Okuda Y, Bryson E, Demaria S. The utility of simulation in medical education: what is the evidence? Mt Sinai J Med 2009;76:330-43, and Bryan R, Kreuter M, Brownson R. Integrating adult learning principles into training for public health practice. Health Promot Pract 2009;10:557-63.

Traditional medical education emphasizes learning and mastering cognitive skills based on textbook readings, lectures, and small group discussions. Evaluation of medical knowledge relies mainly on written or oral examinations. Training models are isolated and sometimes described as being within a "silo," in a static environment where nurses train with nurses, doctors with doctors, pharmacists with pharmacists, and so on. Retention and transfer is weak when passive learning models are employed. Simulation-based training allows for interdisciplinary, active learning, whereby participants are immersed into clinical scenarios and are able to experience how behavior and interactions and communication between disciplines affect patient care and, potentially, patient outcomes. The more realistic the case scenario, simulation environment, and actors are, the more those participating are able to become immersed in the task and engaged in the clinical scenario. This engagement with an authentic clinical problem and the need to resolve it as a team, serves as the foundation for the debriefing, which typically follows a simulation scenario.

## Aspects of a High-Fidelity Simulation

High-fidelity simulation requires considerable manpower and preparation. A typical team consists of the following: a team leader, actors, high-fidelity manikin, simulation room, audiovisual equipment, participants and learners, a facilitator, and a debriefer.[31] The team leader may be compared with a director of a film production. He or she is responsible for the smooth execution of the case scenario, from assigning and delegating roles to team members and directing the evolving scenario in the console room, to handling unexpected problems and situations that may arise during the simulation. This position may be the same or different from an "operator" who is responsible for operating the manikin behind the scenes in the console room. Actors, otherwise known as "confederate actors," are responsible for creating the realism of the case scenario by effectively performing impromptu in a case scenario. They may take roles, such as nurses, surgeons, technicians, or administrative staff, to help guide the participants in a way that is clinically familiar. The challenge for actors is to maintain their simulated character and to interact with participants to guide them, but without overt interference with the clinical decisions and management. Communication between confederate actors and control room personnel using wireless audio devices is helpful to maintain the smooth flow of the scenario.

The simulation room is ideally a flexible setting that can be converted into a range of patient care environments, such as the OR, emergency department, obstetric ward, a cafeteria or other public place—anywhere an anesthesia team might be called to respond. Elaborate scenery, anesthesia and surgical equipment used in everyday work, and moulage (e.g., fake blood and vomitus) may create very realistic scenarios. The rooms should be equipped with medical air, oxygen, and vacuum suction capabilities to run the high-fidelity manikins and to provide for their use in the scenario.[31] Audiovisual equipment, such as cameras and microphones, are strategically placed so as to not be obvious to the participants, whose actions are followed in the simulation for debriefing and feedback. The facilitator is responsible for observing the simulation scenario, and after the event to stimulate learning and discussion in a nonthreatening and organized way. The facilitator's role is to identify elements of the simulation that possess educational value pertinent to the learning objectives of the course, and to facilitate discussion of these learning nuggets (e.g., point out where communication broke down or where situational awareness was lost) (Video 53-2).

## What is a Debriefing?

A debriefing is a "conversation between two or more people to review a real or simulated event in which participants analyze their actions and interactions, and reflect on the roles of thought processes, psychomotor skills, and emotional states, to improve or sustain performance in the future."[32] It is generally thought that the debriefing is the most important component of simulation-based education, the time when learning is embedded. Many consider the scenario an excuse for the opportunity for debriefing. Facilitated by the debriefer, the debriefing usually follows the simulation. "Pause and discuss" style debriefing, where the faculty interjects during pauses in a scenario has been shown to be an effective teaching method.[33] Video review of portions of the scenario can be helpful during a debriefing, especially when used to observe key moments, clarify recall discrepancies among participants and faculty, and to offer a global view of the room to participants who might have been focused on a task or fixated on a portion of the action. This guided reflection of the scenario allows participants to bridge the gap between experiencing an event and making sense of it.

Debriefing can be approached in three phases: *reactions, understanding,* and *summary.*[15,32,34] The *reactions phase* asks participants to share how they felt, allowing the participants to vent and deactivate from the heightened emotional state that participating in a simulation provokes. The debriefer leads the group through a description of the facts of the case, to ensure that everyone understands the clinical scenario before tackling the learning objectives. The *understanding phase* is the richest and longest phase, and is intended to help participants analyze and apply what happened and explore deeper meaning of the interactions. Discussion and teachings are involved in this phase to help simulation participants gain new perspectives and insights into group dynamics and communication. Lessons learned during the simulation can be generalized and applied to the real world, preparing participants to transfer new knowledge into their clinical practice. In the *summary phase,* participants share lessons learned, including individual and group behaviors, skills, and thinking patterns that they wish to improve, as well as those that were productive and they wish to retain for future performance.[15,32,34] Becoming an effective debriefer requires training and practice to acquire new skills that are not taught in traditional health care educational programs. Instructors and facilitators are encouraged to learn about the principles of effective debriefing via the literature, formal courses, and mentoring. The Debriefing Assessment for Simulation in Healthcare (DASH) is an example of a testing instrument that was developed to assess and improve debriefing skills.[35]

## Using Simulation for Evaluation

Although patient simulators are well accepted as a core component of crisis resource management and other clinical training, their acceptance and validity as assessment tools for clinical performance has not yet been widely established or validated. In particular, a number of senior professionals are reluctant to be assessed in a simulator environment (e.g., in the process of their recertification). However, some scoring systems for simulator-based performance assessments have been developed, such as the Anaesthetists' Non-Technical Skills (ANTS) system.[14,36] Although validity is not yet rigorous (e.g., based on correlation of training with consistent transfer of skills into clinical use or improvement of patient care), there is increasing evidence that simulation-based assessment can be done with sufficient reliability to be used for testing (e.g., reproducible scenarios can be created and implemented, raters can be trained to assign reproducible scores of performance, and critical clinical skills can be simulated).[37] Multiscenario, simulation-based assessment has the potential to assess performance of pediatric anesthesia skills in anesthesia residents and pediatric anesthesia fellows; however, further measures of validity, including correlations with direct measures of clinical performance, are needed to establish the true utility and validity of these simulations as assessment tools.[27]

Simulation is widely thought to be effective in improving clinical skills in a way that is safer than the traditional apprentice model of training. Although there is not yet a large body of evidence regarding the effectiveness of simulation or the cost relative to its benefit, there is substantial literature that documents its utility. A meta-analysis has established the overall effectiveness of simulation-based training.[38] Furthermore, a study of simulation-based training showed improved outcomes, specifically in survival of children after cardiopulmonary resuscitation.[39]

## Challenges in Using Simulation

Although simulation centers are increasingly popular worldwide, there are many challenges in establishing and maintaining a simulation program. Trained educators in simulation are few and apprenticeship models require extensive time and effort. There are now several simulation programs that offer various types of courses for educators and instructors. Popular centers that consistently offer courses are the Center for Medical Simulation in Cambridge, Mass. (http://harvardmedsim.org/), the Multidisciplinary Simulation Center in Rochester, Minn. (http://www.mayo.edu/simulationcenter/), the Center for Immersive and Simulation-Based Learning in Palo Alto, Calif. (http://cisl.stanford.edu/), the Michael S. Gordon Center for Research in Medical Education in Miami (http://www.gcrme.miami.edu/), the Danish Institute for Medical Simulation in Herlev, Denmark (http://www.regionh.dk/dims-eng/menu/), and the Tübingen Center for Patient Safety and Simulation in Tübingen, Germany (http://www.tupass.de/). Fellowships in medical simulation are also becoming more widespread across the U.S., located within anesthesia, emergency medicine, and other departments, or at interdisciplinary centers, such as the Neil and Elise Wallace STRATUS Center for Medical Simulation in Boston (http://www.stratus.partners.org). However, availability of faculty members to develop curricula and routinely run simulation case scenarios has been a challenge due to operational costs and the high demands of clinical practice and patient care. Technical staff and support to help run a simulation center are also important factors that affect the overall cost of operating a center. Simulation equipment, computers, partial task trainers, and high-fidelity manikins are expensive, as is the maintenance of this equipment. In some institutions, funding may not be available to staff and operate a simulation center with a skills training laboratory. Other options may include implementing in situ simulations in existing hospital facilities, remodeling old facilities into a simulation room, or having mobile units that contain simulation equipment. Hence, operating and maintaining a simulation center poses monetary, time availability, and faculty availability concerns.

## Future of Simulation

Simulation-based education provides many opportunities for curriculum development in anesthesia residency training, with creative strategies to enhance clinical experiences, to practice caring for rare cases, and to improve mass-casualty training. This model will become of greater importance as residency work-hours are reduced. Although the apprenticeship model and patient care experience is unlikely to be replaced, incorporation of simulation-based training can help provide solutions to systems-based problems, improve interdisciplinary team training, ease relocation into facilities, and help adapt to new equipment and technology. Since 2004, the Society for Simulation in Healthcare has represented a growing community of educators and researchers who use simulation techniques for education, testing, and research in health care. This consistently growing international society (over 3000 members in 2012) is a broad-based, multidisciplinary, multispecialty network that ties together physicians, nurses, and allied-health professionals with educators and other social scientists, as well as with industry.[40] Other societies, including the Society for Simulation in Healthcare in America and the Society in Europe for Simulation Applied to Medicine, provide technical and political leadership for the simulation community.

The extent of the long-term impact of simulation on health care still remains to be determined; however, what is certain is that a large part of residency training and maintenance of skills will incorporate simulation-based education. The American Board of Anesthesiology now requires simulation-based crisis resource management training as part of its program for recertification. Other specialty medical boards are also considering using simulation as a requirement for certification and recertification. In Israel and the United Kingdom, simulation-based stations are included in the National Anesthesia Board exams and OSCEs in anesthesia, respectively.[16,41] Simulation-based education and research will become an integral part of health care. Future research must nonetheless focus on addressing questions of how best to use simulation to improve real-life quality of care, patient safety, and long-term care.

## REFERENCES

Please see www.expertconsult.com.

**53**

# INDEX